Brief Table of Contents

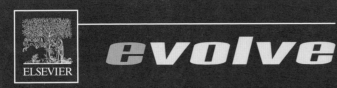

evolve

❖ *To access your Student Resources, visit:*

http://evolve.elsevier.com/Gutierrez/pharmacotherapeutics

Evolve® Student Resources for **Gutierrez:** *Pharmacotherapeutics: Clinical Reasoning in Primary Care,* **2nd Edition,** include the following features:

Student Resources

- **Bonus Content**
  Valuable reference tables provide additional information on food-drug interactions, effects of maternal drug ingestion, pharmacological resources, and more.

- **WebLinks**
  This dynamic resource lets you link to hundreds of websites carefully chosen to supplement the content of the textbook. The WebLinks are updated regularly, with new ones added as they develop.

- **Patient Teaching Handouts**
  A collection of Gold Standard® patient handouts, covering the drugs most commonly prescribed in primary care, are ready to print for use in clinical practice.

- **Elsevier ePharmacology Update Newsletter**
  An informative, full-color, quarterly newsletter, the ePharmacology Update provides current and well-documented information on new drugs, drug warnings, medication errors, and more.

- **Drugs@FDA—A Catalog of FDA Approved Drug Products**
  A link to this comprehensive and up-to-date database of FDA drug approvals and withdrawals is readily available for the very latest drug information.

Pharmacotherapeutics

Clinical Reasoning in Primary Care

Pharmacotherapeutics
Clinical Reasoning in Primary Care

2nd Edition

Kathleen Gutierrez, PhD, RN, ANP-BC, CNS-BC

Adult Nurse Practitioner in Private Practice,
Littleton, Colorado
and
Associate Professor of Nursing,
University of Colorado at Denver Health Sciences Center,
Denver, Colorado

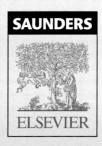

SAUNDERS

ELSEVIER

SAUNDERS
ELSEVIER

11830 Westline Industrial Drive
St. Louis, Missouri 63146

PHARMACOTHERAPEUTICS:
CLINICAL REASONING IN PRIMARY CARE   ISBN: 978-1-4160-3287-8

Notice

Knowledge and best practice in this field are constantly changing. As new research and experience broaden our knowledge, changes in practice, treatment and drug therapy may become necessary or appropriate. Readers are advised to check the most current information provided (i) on procedures featured or (ii) by the manufacturer of each product to be administered, to verify the recommended dose or formula, the method and duration of administration, and contraindications. It is the responsibility of the practitioner, relying on their own experience and knowledge of the patient, to make diagnoses, to determine dosages and the best treatment for each individual patient, and to take all appropriate safety precautions. To the fullest extent of the law, neither the Publisher nor the Editors/Authors assumes any liability for any injury and/or damage to persons or property arising out of or related to any use of the material contained in this book.

The Publisher

Library of Congress Control Number: 2007934781

Senior Editor: Lee Henderson
Senior Developmental Editor: Maureen Iannuzzi
Associate Developmental Editor: Jacqueline Twomey
Publishing Services Manager: Jeffrey Patterson
Project Manager: Amy Rickles
Cover Designer: Julia Dummitt
Text Designer: Julia Dummitt

Cover Art: The cover art is a photomicrograph of crystalline tibolone, a synthetic steroid that is included in a newer class of drugs known as selective estrogen receptor modulators (SERMs). It has been found to have antiresorptive properties in bone, and it is used outside of the United States in the treatment of the symptoms and osteoporosis associated with menopause.

Printed in Canada

Last digit is the print number: 9 8 7 6 5 4 3 2 1

Now that all is said and done once again, I dedicate this book to my family,
whose unwavering love, care, thoughtfulness, and guidance
supported me through another lengthy endeavor.

To my husband and soul mate Pat,
who stands beside me through thick and thin,
maintains our home, nourishes me, and helps me to keep my sanity;
I don't know what I would do without you.

To my daughter and friend Pam, and her husband Brad,
whose abilities to be forthright and honest keep my life in perspective,
particularly through life's challenges.

And to our son and brother Michael,
who remains the most honest, compassionate, devoted,
nonjudgmental individual I have ever known.

Preface

Most interactions between health care providers and their patients conclude with a prescription for drugs or orders for other therapies. Patients and their drug therapies are dynamic; pharmacotherapeutics is an interactive process involving competing or conflicting forces. In today's dynamic environment, health care providers and patients are confronted by drugs advertised and promoted in the media, by managed care systems with restricted formularies, and by time limitations that complicate decision-making processes in choosing one drug over another. Further, new over-the-counter and prescription drug information floods the market daily, requiring continual growth in knowledge.

Drug therapies often represent the best treatment for illness and disease, and the spectrum of useful drugs continues to grow at a remarkable pace. This tempo is likely to continue over the coming years, as our understanding of physiology, pathophysiology, diseases, and drugs expands, in turn fueling the discovery of new drugs and drug classes. For example, impressive advances in our understanding of the human genome and in technology ensure a new swell of targeted therapies and individualized treatment regimens. Nonetheless, most of our current drugs evolved from classical pharmacology and chemistry and stand on a foundation of imperfect knowledge of disease mechanisms. This may contribute in part to the tendency of many drugs to cause adverse drug effects or to exhibit limited efficacy. Nevertheless, these imperfect drugs will remain the cornerstone of therapeutics for years to come.

Throughout this edition, pharmacotherapeutics is discussed along with disorders for which the drugs are commonly used. Frequently, the indications for a drug change over time; either previous indications are made obsolete or new ones are added to the armamentarium. And, as evidenced-based practice dictates new and better treatment options, improved drug therapies will continually replace older treatment regimens. Yet there will always be areas in which a specific treatment engenders substantial debate, and this may cause a given drug regimen to seem inappropriate.

One of the goals for this second edition was to disseminate information that is clinically appropriate for both nurse practitioners and physician assistants. We began this effort by enlisting the aid of Patrick Auth, Director of the Physician Assistant Program at Drexel University. Dr. Auth was instrumental in helping to plan a text that incorporates the perspectives for professionals in both of these clinical roles. To further this goal, contributors to this volume included practicing nurses and physician assistants, academicians, and pharmacists. Experts were again drawn from all of these fields to extensively review the content. Their joint efforts have produced a resource that is in accordance with current clinical practice and standards of care across professional disciplines.

ORGANIZATION

Arranging the chapters by drug class or drug category proved effective in the previous edition. Wherever possible, that organizational structure has been retained in this edition. Coverage of generic and brand-name drugs, drug categories, and drug actions continues to be comprehensive and includes drugs available by prescription as well as selected over-the-counter drugs. New chapters on poisons, drugs used for migraines, and drugs used for bladder, prostate, and erectile dysfunction have been added. Each chapter has been thoroughly updated and revised to include current drugs and drug information. Additional information on investigational new drugs and orphan drugs can be found on the *Evolve* website (http://evolve.elsevier.com/Gutierrez/pharmacotherapeutics/).

Throughout the book, we persevere in our attempt to advance the safety and quality of patient care by doing the following:

- using clinical reasoning strategies that are grounded in sound pharmacotherapeutic principles
- stimulating the reader to accomplish higher levels of learning
- motivating novice health care providers to enhance the breadth, depth, and quality of care they provide to each of their patients
- challenging experienced health care providers to incorporate new concepts while helping to redefine their understanding of the basic doctrines of pathophysiology and pharmacotherapeutics
- informing health care communities about the standards of drug therapy and management toward which we all strive–standards that patients have come to expect and, yes, even demand

Unit I, Foundations of Professional Practice, focuses on the fundamentals of pharmacology and professional practice. This unit grounds the reader in the history of pharmacology and explains the concepts of pharmacotherapeutics, pharmacoeconomics, pharmaceutics and pharmacokinetics, pharmacodynamics, and clinical reasoning. Life-span variables are explored in chapters covering perinatal, pediatric, and geriatric pharmacotherapeutics and are highlighted throughout the clinical chapters.

Unit II, Community Pharmacotherapeutics, contains revised chapters on over-the-counter drugs, vitamins and minerals, complementary and alternative medicine, substance abuse, poisons, adherence to therapy, patient education, and community resources. The chapter on substance abuse discusses the use of both by-prescription and illicit drugs in a culture that sometimes promotes dependence.

Units III through XII are organized around the influence of drugs on various body systems, with chapters that employ a unique clinical reasoning format. The basic purpose for a clinical reasoning format is to focus on pharmacotherapeutics, thus ruling in some factors as germane to the drug decision and ruling out others because of their lesser importance to patient outcomes. The utility of the model comes from the systematic organization it provides for thinking, observing, and analyzing treatment regimens. In addition, it provides structure and rationale for specific activities and a mechanism for professional accountability. The model also provides criteria for knowing when a patient problem has been resolved.

Clinical reasoning begins with the assumption that competent health care providers usually know more than they put into words. They exhibit a kind of knowing in practice, most of which is tacit. Indeed, health care providers themselves often reveal a capacity to reflect on their intuition in the midst of action, and from time to time they use this capacity to cope with the unique, uncertain, and conflicted situations inherent in practice. Donald Schon ("Educating the Reflective Practitioner," Presentation to the 1987 meeting of the American Educational Research Association, Washington, DC) contends that a professional cannot be taught what he or she needs to know, but can be "coached." The clinical reasoning sections of each chapter provide not answers as such, but coaching.

INTEGRATED PHYSIOLOGY, PATHOPHYSIOLOGY, AND PHARMACOTHERAPEUTICS

The integration of physiology and pathophysiology with the study of pharmacotherapeutics provides readers with an understanding of the physical and cellular causes of specific diseases and the advantages of using specific drugs for therapy. Examples of physiologic and pathophysiologic processes discussed include pain and the use of opioid analgesics and nonsteroidal antiinflammatory drugs, multiple sclerosis and the role of skeletal muscle relaxants, the antimicrobial therapy used for tuberculosis, and the role of antiarrhythmic drugs in treating arrhythmias. Where possible, the generic name, brand names, and the Canadian equivalent drug names are included. Canadian drug names are identified with a maple leaf icon ❧.

FEATURES

CASE STUDIES

The second edition includes 48 *Case Studies* that present patient profiles and variables that influence the clinical reasoning process in pharmacotherapeutics. Each of these case studies, which feature a streamlined new format for this edition, explores how factors such as age, economic status, comorbidity, and drug characteristics affect drug selection.

EVIDENCE-BASED PHARMACOTHERAPEUTICS

Included throughout the book are 32 *Evidence-Based Pharmacotherapeutics* boxes. These boxes include background information for the research study cited, the purpose of the study, research design and methods, findings and conclusions, and implications for practice.

CLINICAL ALERTS

Clinical Alerts ⚠ appear throughout the chapters to highlight patient safety issues and to draw attention to important aspects of a drug or drug class.

CONTROVERSY BOXES

Controversy boxes, designed to increase awareness of the ethical, legal, and practical dilemmas associated with pharmacotherapeutics, appear throughout the text. The 39 Controversy boxes address such issues as why we question the use of generic drugs, the wisdom of administering opioids to chemically dependent patients, immunization policy issues, the use of the antidepressant fluoxetine for managing weight loss, and the wisdom of using directly-observed therapy in the management of tuberculosis, to name a few. Each Controversy presents divergent viewpoints on the issue, and posits questions for readers to consider so they can formulate their own opinions on the topic.

PHARMACOKINETICS TABLES

Pharmacokinetics describes what happens to a drug following administration—what the body does with the drug. *Pharmacokinetics* tables appear in each of the clinical chapters and provide an overview of the drugs' onset, peak, and duration of action, as well as their protein binding and half-life.

DRUG INTERACTIONS TABLES

Each of the clinical chapters contains at least one *Drug Interactions* table. Drug interactions are often the by-product of concurrent administration of two or more drugs or of a food-drug combination. Biologic effects as well as physical and chemical effects result. Although some drug interactions are intentional and often seen as beneficial, others may diminish a drug's therapeutic benefits or increase the risk of adverse effects. The number of potentially significant drug interactions increases as pharmacotherapy becomes more complex and drugs more potent.

DOSAGE REGIMEN TABLES

Dosage tables include the usual purposes and routes of drug administration, along with common adult and pediatric dosages.

ILLUSTRATIONS

The illustrations in this text begin with a timeline of drug development and progress through graphs, charts, algorithms, drug products, and human physiology at the systemic and cellular levels. All were carefully chosen and designed to maximize visual communication and enable readers to better understand drug action. Whether the illustrations show the pharmacokinetic phases, examine a toxic range, outline the nervous system, describe the drug actions of antidepressants or antibiotics, or follow the steps from an injured blood vessel to development of a fibrin-platelet plug, all are integral to the written text and are intended to enhance learning.

ADDITIONAL RESOURCES

The companion Evolve Resources can be found at http://evolve.elsevier.com/Gutierrez/pharmacotherapeutics/.

For Instructors

The teaching package includes a Test Bank, available in RTF format, an Image Collection including virtually all illustrations within the text, and 15 three-dimensional animations to enhance understanding of pharmacology.

For Students

The Evolve Resources offer Bonus Content for in-depth information on a variety of topics, "WebLinks" that are maintained throughout the life of this edition, and downloadable Patient Teaching Handouts for the most frequently prescribed drugs. Students may also sign up to receive the Elsevier *ePharmacology Update* newsletter and keep up to date on drug approvals, withdrawals, and changes in indications by subscribing to Drugs@FDA—A Catalog of FDA-Approved Drug Products.

As with the previous edition, every effort has been made to ensure that the text is accurate, well-organized, and user-friendly. We hope that it will provide both students and health care providers alike with a valuable frame of reference, as well as expand their understanding and enhance their practice of pharmacotherapeutics. We look forward to your comments and suggestions as you use this text and its companion resources.

Kathleen Gutierrez, PhD, RN, ANP-BC, CNS-BC

Acknowledgments

No author writes a book alone. A project of this size could not come to fruition without the collaboration of many people. First and foremost, my thanks and continued appreciation go to a friend and retired fellow educator, Janet Velazquez, RN, MS, who 40 years ago fostered my initial interest in pharmacology and facilitated my first opportunity to teach the subject. Over the years my students contributed valuable insight into sorting the information into categories referred to as *need-to-know, nice-to-know,* and *fluff.* Attempts have been made to avoid the last.

The limited efficacy and potential toxicities of many drugs used today, along with the rapid expansion of drugs for prevention and treatment of disease, creates enormous complexity in selecting optimal drug treatment for patients. Thus, the expertise of clinically educated pharmacists is increasingly important if we are to ensure that patients receive the most effective drugs in the dosages and combinations that are optimal for them. For this reason, our PharmD reviewers were invaluable in critically reviewing, analyzing, and making recommendations for content and format of the text.

I would like to thank Patrick Auth from Drexel University for his aid in planning a text to satisfy the needs of nurse practitioners and physician assistants. And of course thanks go to the many PAs and NPs who have reviewed the individual chapters and are listed on the following pages.

My thanks also go to the many educators and fellow health care providers who have collaborated over the years. Your patience and sharing of knowledge, skills, and expertise have permitted the development and revision of a text that will become a gold standard in pharmacotherapeutics education.

Thanks too to the contributors of the previous edition. You all helped me get my feet on solid ground.

And of course, last but not least, my thanks to the editors and staff at Elsevier:

- Senior Editor Lee Henderson, who was willing to take me under his wing again
- Senior Developmental Editor Maureen Iannuzzi, who continually provided sound advice and a realistic perspective, not to mention daily emails to keep me using the proper format
- Associate Developmental Editor Jacqueline Twomey, who coordinated reviewers with finesse
- Project Manager Amy Rickles, for keeping the text on schedule despite overwhelming odds
- Designer Julia Dummitt, whose creativity provided a lovely, functional design
- Copyeditor Judith Huober, for your patience and understanding as I once again waded through the copy editing process and for fielding the myriad changes, additions, and deletions with unwavering poise
- Graphic Artist Hans Neuhart of Electronic Illustrators Group in Fountain Hills, Arizona, who created the illustrations for the previous edition and who continued his fine work for this edition

To you all, my sincere thanks and appreciation for putting up with me once again; for the diligence, expertise, patience, and understanding few others would understand.

Kathleen Gutierrez, PhD, RN, ANP-BC, CNS-BC

Contributors

Reamer L. Bushardt, PharmD, PA-C
Director and Assistant Professor, Physician Assistant Program, Department of Clinical Services, College of Health Professions, Medical University of South Carolina, Charleston, South Carolina

Antineoplastic Drugs; Antiarrhythmic Drugs; Thrombolytic and Sclerosing Drugs

Sheryl J. Cator, RN, MSN, FNP, MAOM
Presbyterian Healthcare Services, Albuquerque, New Mexico; Instructor, University of St. Francis, Albuquerque, New Mexico

Opioid Analgesics and Related Drugs; NSAIDs, DMARDs, and Related Drugs; Biologic Response Modifiers

Gail Ladean Cross, MSN, RN-C, MSN, FNP
Private Practice, Saguaro Family Clinic, Castle Rock, Colorado

Antiasthmatic and Bronchodilator Drugs; Antihistamines and Related Drugs

Kathleen Gutierrez, PhD, RN, ANP-BC, CNS-BC
Private Practice, Littleton, Colorado; Associate Professor of Nursing, University of Colorado at Denver Health Sciences Center, Denver, Colorado

Introduction to Pharmacotherapeutics; Clinical Reasoning in Pharmacotherapeutics; Pharmacoeconomics; Pharmaceutics and Pharmacokinetics; Pharmacodynamics; Pharmacotherapeutics for Pregnant and Nursing Women; Pharmacotherapeutics for Older Adults; Vitamins and Minerals; Complementary and Alternative Medicine; Substance Abuse; Sympathetic Nervous System Drugs; Parasympathetic Nervous System Drugs; Anesthetics; Antianxiety and Sedative-Hypnotic Drugs; Antidepressant and Antimania Drugs; Antipsychotic Drugs; Skeletal Muscle Relaxants; Drugs Used for Migraines; Antiepileptic Drugs; Drugs for Parkinson's Disease and Myasthenia Gravis; Antibiotics; Antiviral and Antifungal Drugs; Antitubercular and Antileprotic Drugs; Anthelmintic, Antimalarial, and Antiprotozoal Drugs; Inotropic Drugs; Antianginal Drugs; Antihypertensive Drugs; Antilipidemic Drugs; Anticoagulant and Antiplatelet Drugs; Diuretics; Drugs Used for Bladder, Prostate, and Erectile Dysfunction; Drugs Used for Renal Dysfunction; Drugs for Hyperacidity, Gastroesophageal Reflux Disease, and Peptic Ulcer Disease; Cation-Exchange Resins and Ammonia-Detoxifying Drugs; Alkalinizing and Acidifying Drugs; Thyroid and Parathyroid Drugs and Drugs for Calcium Disorders; Pituitary Drugs; Adrenal Cortex Agonists and Inhibitors; Uterine Motility Drugs; Fertility Drugs; Dermatologic Drugs

Evolve: Effects of Selected Maternal Drug Ingestion on the Fetus or Neonate; Resources Supporting Orphan Drug Development; Dietary Considerations; Influence of Drugs on Laboratory Values; Selected Formulas Used in Pharmacotherapeutics

Christine C. Hansen, FNP
Private Practice, Sacramento, California

Hormonal Contraceptives and Related Drugs

Christina J. Hanson, MS, RN, FNP
Highlands Ranch, Colorado

Androgens and Anabolic Steroids

Elizabeth Wise Kissell, BSN, MSNE
La Casa–Quigg Newton Family Health Center; Denver Health and Hospital Authority, Denver, Colorado

Over-the-Counter Drugs; Poisonings; Sera, Vaccines, and Immunizing Drugs; Ophthalmic Drugs; Otic Drugs

Margaret Elaine McLeod, MSN, ADM-BC, APRN-BC, CDE
Tennessee Valley Healthcare System, Nashville, Tennessee

Drugs Used in the Treatment of Diabetes Mellitus

Sean M. Reed, RN, MS, CNS
Doctoral Student, University of Colorado at Denver and Health Sciences Center, Denver, Colorado

Central Nervous System Stimulants; Urinary Antimicrobials and Related Drugs

Martha A. Spangler, MSN, RN, ANP-BC
Castle Rock Family Physicians, Castle Rock, Colorado

Laxatives and Antidiarrheal Drugs; Antiemetics and Related Drugs; Decongestants, Expectorants, Antitussives, and Mucolytics

Arlys J. Williams, RN, MSN, APRN
Assistant Professor, Montana State University Northern, Havre, Montana

Pharmacotherapeutics for Children and Adolescents

Jonathan J. Wolfe, PhD, RPH
Associate Professor, University of Arkansas for Medical Sciences Department of Pharmacy Practice, Little Rock, Arkansas

Controversy boxes for Chapters 6, 8, 9, 10, 11, 12, 16, 17, 19, 20, 22, 23, 25, 27, 28, 29, 31, 32, 34, 36, 37, 38, 39, 45, 46, 51, 53, 57, 58, 59, and 60

Reviewers

Beth J. Alexander, PharmD, BCPS, RPh
Associate Professor
Department of Physician Assistant Studies
Augsburg College
Minneapolis, Minnesota

Frank Ambriz, Jr, MPAS, PA-C
Assistant Professor
University of Texas–Pan American
Edinburg, Texas

Patrick Auth, PhD, MS, PA-C
Director, Physician Assistant Program
Assistant Professor
College of Nursing and Health Professions
Drexel University
Philadelphia, Pennsylvania

Suleiman Bahouth, PhD, RPh
Associate Professor
Department of Pharmacology
The University of Tennessee Health Sciences Center
Memphis, Tennessee

Steven L. Bents, MPAS, PA-C
Physician Assistant Program
Rocky Mountain College
Billings, Montana

Mary Kay Betz, MS, RPA-C
Dent Neurologic Institute
Amherst, New York; and
D'Youville College
Buffalo, New York

Suzanne G. Bollmeier, PharmD, BCPS, AE-C
St. Louis College of Pharmacy
St. Louis, Missouri

Mary Jo Bondy, MHS, PA-C
Physician Assistant Program
Anne Arundel Community College
Arnold, Maryland

Reamer L. Bushardt, PharmD, PA-C
Assistant Professor
Department of Clinical Services
College of Health Professions
Medical University of South Carolina
Charleston, South Carolina

Eric W. Bussear, MPH, PA-C
Assistant Professor
Physician Assistant Program
Nova Southeastern University
Fort Lauderdale, Florida

Lisa B. Cohen, PharmD, CDE
Clinical Assistant Professor of Pharmacy
University of Rhode Island
Kingston, Rhode Island

Melissa Coughlin, MS, CRNA
State University of New York at Buffalo
Buffalo, New York

Gail Ladean Cross, MSN, RN-C, FNP
Private Practice, Saguaro Family Clinic
Castle Rock, Colorado

Sandra Cuellar, PharmD, BCOP
Clinical Assistant Professor
Clinical Oncology Professor
Director, Oncology Residence Program
University of Illinois at Chicago Medical Center
Chicago, Illinois

Paul T. Davis, MD
Physician Assistant Program
The University of Findlay
Findlay, Ohio

George DeMaagd, PharmD, BCPS
College of Pharmacy
Ferris State University
Kalamazoo, Michigan

Kathleen L. Ehrhardt, MMS, PA-C
Physician Assistant Program
DeSales University
Center Valley, Pennsylvania

Lea S. Eiland, PharmD, BCPS
Assistant Clinical Professor of Pharmacy Practice
Harrison School of Pharmacy
Auburn University
Auburn, Alabama

David Fahringer, MSPH, PA-C
Associate Professor
Physician Assistant Studies
College of Health Sciences
University of Kentucky
Lexington, Kentucky

James R. Fry, MS, PA-C
Physician Assistant Program
Marietta College
Marietta, Ohio

Catherine A. Gillespie, DHSc, MPAS, PA-C
Gannon University
Erie, Pennsylvania

Julie Golembiewski, PharmD
Clinical Associate Professor
College of Pharmacy
University of Illinois at Chicago
Chicago, Illinois

Gloria R. Grice, PharmD, BCPS
St. Louis College of Pharmacy
St. Louis, Missouri

Andy Grimone, PharmD, BCPS
Pharmacy Residence Director
Saint Vincent Health Center
Erie, Pennsylvania

Vicki Groo, PharmD, BS Pharmacy
Clinical Assistant Professor
College of Pharmacy
University of Illinois; and
Clinical Pharmacist
University of Illinois at Chicago Hospital
Section of Cardiology
Chicago, Illinois

Ahmad Hakemi, MD
Director, Physician Assistant Program
Central Michigan University
Mt. Pleasant, Michigan

Kristen Lehman Helms, PharmD
Harrison School of Pharmacy
Auburn University
Auburn, Alabama

James F. Hull, Jr, MPAS, PA-C
Assistant Professor
Seton Hill University
Greensburg, Pennsylvania

Federico Innocenti, MD, PhD
Assistant Professor of Medicine
University of Chicago
Chicago, Illinois

Rupali Jain, PharmD, BCPS
Clinical Assistant Professor
Pharmacotherapist, Infectious Diseases
Department of Pharmacy Practice
College of Pharmacy
University of Illinois at Chicago
Chicago, Illinois

Kathryn T. Janick, MSPAS, PA-C
Instructor, Hahnemann Physician Assistant Program
Drexel University
Philadelphia, Pennsylvania

Holly Jodon, MPAS, PA-C
Gannon University
Erie, Pennsylvania

Melissa M. Kagarise, MMS, PA-C
Assistant Professor
Director of MMS/MHS
Saint Francis University
Loretto, Pennsylvania

Darcie L. Keller, PharmD, BCPS
Assistant Professor
School of Medicine
University of Missouri–Kansas City
Kansas City, Missouri

Pat Kenney-Moore, MS, PA-C
Associate Professor
Division of Physician Assistant Education
Oregon Health and Science University
Portland, Oregon

Michael J. Koronkowski, PharmD
College of Pharmacy
University of Illinois at Chicago
Chicago, Illinois

Beverly Lassiter-Brown, MPH, PA-C
College of Science and Health
Charles R. Drew University
Los Angeles, California

Mary Ann Laxen, MAB, PA-C
Director, Associate Professor
Physician Assistant Program
School of Medicine and Health Science
University of North Dakota
Grand Forks, North Dakota

Jeffery J. Libra, MD
Medical Director, Associate Professor
Physician Assistant Studies
Grand Valley State University
Grand Rapids, Michigan

John E. Lopes, Jr, DHSc, PA-C
Physician Assistant Program
School of Rehabilitation and Medical Science
Central Michigan University
Mount Pleasant, Michigan

Celia P. MacDonnell, PharmD, BPharm, RPh
Clinical Assistant Professor
Director of Student Affairs
College of Pharmacy
University of Rhode Island
Kingston, Rhode Island

Jeanie McHugo, MS, PA-C
University of North Dakota
Grand Forks, North Dakota

Heidi B. Miller, PA-C, MPH
Director, Associate Professor
Physician Assistant Program
Rochester Institute of Technology
Rochester, New York

Lama H. Nazer, PharmD, BCPS
School of Pharmacy
Western University of Health Sciences
Pomona, California

Joshua J. Neumiller, PharmD
Geriatrics Resident/Clinical Research Associate
Department of Pharmacotherapy
College of Pharmacy
Washington State University
Spokane, Washington

Jeegisha R. Patel, PharmD
Assistant Professor
Department of Pharmacy Practice
University of the Sciences in Philadelphia
Philadelphia, Pennsylvania

Luis A. Ramos, MS, PA-C
Director, Physician Assistant Program
Anne Arundel Community College
Arnold, Maryland

Otilio Ramos, Jr, PA-C
Eastern Virginia Medical School
Norfolk, Virginia

Ellen Elizabeth Rhinard, PharmD, BCPS
Assistant Professor of Pharmacy Practice
St. Louis College of Pharmacy
St. Louis, Missouri

Mildred B. Roach, MS, PA-C
Associate Professor
Kettering College of Medical Arts
Kettering, Ohio

James Roch, MPAS, PA-C
Physician Assistant Program
University of North Texas Health Science Center
Fort Worth, Texas

Barbara L. Sauls, EdD, MS, PA-C
Associate Clinical Professor
Physician Assistant Program
King's College
Wilkes-Barre, Pennsylvania

Jaclyn Sauve, PharmD
University of Illinois at Chicago
Chicago, Illinois

Mark E. Schneiderhan, PharmD, BCPP
Department of Pharmacy Practice
College of Pharmacy
University of Illinois at Chicago
Chicago, Illinois

Stephen M. Setter, PharmD, CDE, CGP, DVM
Associate Professor of Pharmacotherapy
Elder Services/Visiting Nurses Association
Washington State University Spokane
Spokane, Washington

Nancy L. Shapiro, PharmD, BCPS
College of Pharmacy
University of Illinois at Chicago
Chicago, Illinois

Anita Siu, PharmD
Clinical Assistant Professor
Ernest Mario School of Pharmacy
Rutgers University Medical Center
Piscataway, New Jersey; and
Neonatal/Pediatric Pharmacotherapy Specialist
The K. Hovnanian Children's Hospital at Jersey
    Shore University Medical Center
Neptune, New Jersey

Dionne Marie Soares, MPAS, PA-C
Howard University
Washington, DC

Martha A. Spangler, MSN, RN, NPC
Certified Nurse Practitioner
Castle Rock Family Physicians
Castle Rock, Colorado

Curt C. Stilp, MS, PA-C
Rosalind Franklin University
North Chicago, Illinois

Debbie D. Sullivan, PhD, PA-C
Arizona College of Osteopathic Medicine
Glendale, Arizona

Eljim P. Tesoro, PharmD
Clinical Assistant Professor
Department of Pharmacy Practice
University of Illinois at Chicago
Chicago, Illinois

Hieu Trung Tran, PharmD
Dean, College of Pharmacy
Sullivan University
Louisville, Kentucky

Kurt A. Wargo, PharmD, BCPS
Harrison School of Pharmacy
Auburn University
Auburn, Alabama

Virginia A. Wilson, PharmD, BSN
University of Tennessee at Chattanooga
Chattanooga, Tennessee

James M. Wooten, PharmD
Associate Professor
Department of Medicine
Section of Clinical Pharmacology
University of Missouri–Kansas City
Kansas City, Missouri

Contents

CHAPTER 6
Pharmacotherapeutics for Pregnant and Nursing Women, 70
Kathleen Gutierrez

CHAPTER 7
Pharmacotherapeutics for Children and Adolescents, 82
Arlys Williams

CHAPTER 8
Pharmacotherapeutics for Older Adults, 91
Kathleen Gutierrez

Introduction to Pharmacotherapeutics

The history of pharmacology helps us understand the development and uses of drugs in religious, psychosocial, political, and economic frameworks. Because a drug is defined broadly as any chemical agent affecting living processes, the subject of pharmacotherapeutics is strikingly extensive. Although a drug's societal impact may be far reaching, we are concerned here in providing a clear understanding and appreciation for the principles of *pharmacodynamics* (what the drug does to the body) and *pharmacokinetics* (what the body does to the drug). Understanding these principles allows us to practice *pharmacotherapeutics* safely and effectively, because whether a drug is useful for therapy depends on its ability to produce desired effects with minimal adverse reactions.

HISTORICAL BACKGROUND

Four distinct stages evolved as humankind searched for substances to treat illness and cure disease. These stages chronicle the development of medicinal treatment by natural and derived substances.

MYSTICAL PERIOD

The mystical period persisted in primitive and prehistoric cultures before 3000 BC. These cultures used supernatural beliefs to explain disease and its cure. Illness was thought to be the result of malevolent external influences, such as evil spirits or hostile sorcerers. Treatments were magical and mystical, employing three primary modes of healing: prayer, crude surgeries, and potions. Each generation orally passed its knowledge on to the next. However, as knowledge about the effects of plant and animal compounds increased, their use moved from the supernatural to a more scientific base. This view implies a straight line of progress; in reality, however, history covers a broad spectrum of cultures moving forward at varying and overlapping rates across a lengthy period of development.

EMPIRICAL PERIOD

The empirical period began around 3000 BC and lasted until approximately 200 BC. During this period, treatment was based on observations of a substance's effectiveness even though the mechanism of its action remained unknown. The earliest records of this period were preserved in cuneiform script on a clay tablet by a Sumerian physician in the Euphrates River Valley, in what is now known as Iraq. The Sumerians are also credited with the first written prescriptions.

The empirical stage of pharmacotherapeutics was reached at different times in different cultures because it was dependent on the scientific and religious development of a particular region. In Europe, the empirical period lasted until the late Middle Ages, when the so-called period of specifics emerged and encouraged closer scrutiny of mysticism and superstitious practices.

MEDIEVAL PERIOD

The medieval period began in the 1200s AD and lasted through the 1800s. During these 600 years, many myths and superstitions about hygiene and health existed, just as they do in contemporary times. The body was viewed by the Greeks and Romans as part of the universe. Four balanced body fluids, or "humors," were seen as essential requirements for life: fire equaled yellow bile or choler, water equated to phlegm, the earth to black bile, and the air to blood. Natural functions, such as sneezing, were thought to be the best way to maintain health. When a build-up of any one humor created an imbalance, it could be disposed of through sweat, tears, feces, or urine. When these natural systems broke down, illness occurred.

It was also thought that sins of the soul resulted in disease. Many people sought relief from their disease through prayer and pilgrimages, meditation, and other nonmedical means. Bloodletting was a popular method for restoring a patient's health and humors.

After the fall of the Roman Empire, Muslims settled throughout Egypt, North Africa, Spain, and the Holy Land. They blended their culture's mathematical and scientific knowledge with that of the Greek, Roman, and Jewish peoples. The new formularies reflected the first drug standards and, along with the southern European compilations, served as models for the first *London Pharmacopoeia,* published in 1618. This book contained 1028 simple drugs and 932 preparations and compounds.

The best-known pharmaceutics authority of the late Middle Ages was Nicholas of Salerno, director of the University of Salerno Medical School. While at the university, Nicholas wrote a book entitled *The Antidotarium,* for centuries the standard for pharmaceutical preparations. According to laws drafted by Spanish Emperor Frederick II in 1240, ownership of an apothecary shop or any business relationship with an apothecary was limited to licensed pharmacists.

Pharmacy flourished during the Renaissance, with pharmaceutical advancements occurring on a regular basis. Paracelsus, the Swiss-born son of a German physician, advocated the use of simple preparations in the treatment of illness and disease. He introduced remedies such as sulfur and calomel (used today in powder form to treat ulcers and skin rashes), as well as other chemical compounds.

Two advances in the late 1700s were significant and remain so today. Digitalis, a cardiac glycoside derived from the foxglove plant, was introduced in 1785 by Englishman William Withering to treat heart disease. Edmund Jenner, also an Englishman, introduced smallpox immunization and began public inoculations in May 1796. The result was a dramatic reduction in the numbers of smallpox cases and confirmation that immunization could prevent disease.

CONTEMPORARY PERIOD

The early 1800s mark the advent of contemporary pharmacotherapeutics, which continues today. Pharmaceutical chemistry became a specialized science following the first significant discovery made by Frederick Serturner. He first isolated an active ingredient, opium, from the flowers of the poppy. The discovery led to further research and to the isolation of other active compounds in previously known drugs.

Problems related to drug efficacy were recognized during this period. Scientists examined dosage, time of drug action and time to drug effect; processes involved in the absorption, distribution, biotransformation, and elimination of drugs; sites of drug action; specific mechanisms of drug action; and relationships between chemical composition and biologic activity of substances.

Early in the 1900s, two significant advances were achieved: an improved understanding of the relationship between the pancreas and diabetes mellitus and the development of antimicrobial compounds. In 1899, Joseph von Mering and Oskar Minkowski conducted experiments that linked the pancreas to diabetes mellitus. Banting and Best formulated an early preparation of insulin in 1922. Four years later, John Abel became the first to crystallize insulin. His experiments revealed its molecular structure and hormonal action.

In 1907, German physician Paul Ehrlich introduced a specific drug against a specific microorganism. He experimented for years with chemical compounds while looking for a cure for syphilis. His six hundred and sixth experiment was a success, revealing arsphenamine as the chemical compound that could cure syphilis.

The discovery of penicillin by Alexander Fleming in 1928 dramatically changed the treatment of infectious diseases. He had observed that the *Penicillium notatum* mold secreted a substance that inhibited the growth of certain types of gram-positive organisms. The physicians Howard Florey, of Oxford University, and Ernest Chain went on in 1941 to demonstrate the value of penicillin in the treatment of infectious diseases, and penicillin became the best drug at that time for treating gonococcal infections and pneumococcal pneumonia.

Subsequent investigators developed other important therapeutic drugs including antihistamines, additional antimicrobials, glucocorticoids, oral contraceptives, and antihypertensives, as well as a parenteral poliomyelitis vaccine. Antiviral drugs and the oral form of polio vaccine were developed in the 1960s. During the 1970s, antineoplastic drugs such as doxorubicin and bleomycin and the histamine$_2$ antagonist cimetidine appeared. Calcium channel blockers were introduced in the 1980s for the treatment of arrhythmias, angina pectoris, and hypertension. Drugs effective in the prevention and treatment of conditions associated with the human immunodeficiency virus were developed throughout the 1990s. Today, virtually every body function can be enhanced, suppressed, or manipulated by pharmaceutical means.

NEW DRUG DEVELOPMENT

The term *pharmacognosy* refers to the study of natural drug sources. Plants were the earliest source of drugs, with their use dating back to the primitive-prehistoric period. Commonly used drugs derived from plant sources include digitalis (from the purple foxglove), vincristine (from the periwinkle plant), and morphine (from the opium poppy). Drugs derived from plant sources are organized by their physical and chemical characteristics. These include alkaloids (a group of nitrogen-containing compounds that are physiologically active as poisons or drugs), glycosides (compounds belonging to a group that reacts with water to form a sugar and a nonsugar), oils, gums, and resins. Drugs derived from animal sources include some insulins (from pork and beef pancreas) and pituitary hormones. A newer insulin product is derived from the saliva of a Gila monster found from extreme southwest Utah to Mexico's southern Sonora and northern Sinaloa, as well as from extreme southwest New Mexico to southern Nevada, and just into California.

The majority of drugs today are either inorganic or organic compounds. Synthetic drugs are far more easily standardized and less often associated with allergic reactions than those made of natural ingredients. In fact, many drugs in use today are directly related to the increasing sophistication of chemical synthesis. Recombinant DNA technology combines or incorporates one organism's DNA into another organism's DNA.

The process of new drug development, monitored by the Food and Drug Administration (FDA), begins with preclinical development (laboratory and animal studies), progresses through several phases of clinical testing, and ends with postmarketing surveillance studies (Fig. 1-1). The effectiveness and safety of a drug are based on the uniformity of its strength, the purity of the preparation, and the consistency of drug action. Biochemical assay testing is performed to determine identity and potency. Biologic assays measure the amount of drug required to produce a predetermined biologic effect. Clinical studies determine toxicity and dosing.

PRECLINICAL DEVELOPMENT

Promoters of new drugs or therapies often request a meeting with the FDA to discuss the results of preclinical findings and to review plans for development of the new drug. During this phase of new drug development, the primary goal is to establish (1) whether the product is reasonably safe for initial use in humans, and (2) if the compound is sufficiently effective against a disease (in chemical assay tests or in animal models) to justify the cost of development. When a product is identified as a viable compound, the drug's promoters focus on its effectiveness and on collecting dosing information and safety data. Obtaining this information is necessary to establish that the compound will not expose humans to unreasonable risk for harm when the compound is used in limited, early-stage clinical trials.

Stage		Subjects	Purpose	Outcome
Preclinical testing (~1-2 years)		Laboratory and animal studies	Attention to toxicity and reversal of toxic, carcinogenic, and teratotoxicity	5000 compounds evaluated
Clinical trials	Phase I (1 year)	20-100 healthy volunteers	Determine safety and dosage	5 drugs enter clinical trials
	Phase II (2 years)	100-300 patient volunteers	Evaluate effectiveness and adverse effects	
	Phase III (3 years)	1000-3000 patient volunteers	Verify effectiveness, monitor adverse effects from long-term use	
FDA Review (~2 years)			Approval of new drug application (NDA)	One drug approved

FIGURE 1-1 **New Drug Development.** (Adapted from Wierenga, D., and Eaton, C. (1993). *The drug development and approval process.* Office of Research and Development. Washington, DC: Pharmaceutical Manufacturers Association.)

During preclinical development, the FDA requires testing with both male and female animals of at least two different mammalian species. Special attention is given to toxicity and the reversal of toxic effects, carcinogenicity, and teratogenicity.

CLINICAL TRIALS

The clinical phase of product development extends from a sponsor's initial submission of the investigational new drug (IND) application to begin testing a new drug in humans (i.e., clinical studies), to submission of a complete new drug application (NDA) or biologic license application (BLA) to the FDA for marketing approval. The four phases of clinical trials are designed to provide information about a drug's purity, bioavailability, potency, efficacy, safety, and toxicity.

Phase 1 Clinical Trials
Phase 1 clinical trials involve the initial evaluation of a drug. A pharmacologist typically supervises studies involving 20 to 100 healthy persons. With a primary focus on safety, the goal of this phase is to determine the relationship between dosing and the patient's total drug exposure; the drug's most common adverse effects and whether they are related to dose; and how the drug is biotransformed and eliminated. The clinical data obtained determine the need for further testing.

Phase 2 Clinical Trials
Phase 2 studies commence if phase 1 studies do not uncover unacceptable toxicities associated with the compound. During this phase, emphasis is on effectiveness of the compound in people with specific diseases, and the relationship between dosage and effectiveness. The drug is tested on several hundred diseased or ill volunteers over a period lasting between 2 months and 2 years. In general, patients receiving the compound are compared with similar patients receiving another compound, usually a placebo or an entirely different drug. Also during this phase, safety evaluations continue and short-term adverse effects are studied.

Phase 3 Clinical Trials
Most of the risks associated with a new drug are determined during *phase 3* studies. Phase 3 studies start if and when preliminary evidence of effectiveness has been shown during phase 2. The goal is to gather information about the compound's safety and effectiveness, its effects on different populations, and the effects of different dosages. Data are also gathered on drug interactions. The therapeutic effectiveness of the drug is verified with larger numbers of individuals (1000 to 3000). To reduce bias from the study, double-blind research designs are used. In this process, neither the patient nor the health care provider knows who received the IND and who received an alternative therapy. The new drug is usually compared with a treatment known to be effective. There may be ethical problems with the use of placebo, particularly when an accepted effective therapy exists. A cross-over research design may be used in some clinical trials, in which the patients receive the drug for part of the time and an alternative for the remaining part of the study.

The compound's promoter and the FDA usually meet at the end of phase 2 clinical trials and again before an NDA or a BLA is submitted to the FDA for marketing review.

The marketing review team is made up of six different specialty groups: chemists, pharmacologists and toxicologists, physicians, clinical pharmacologists, statisticians, and microbiologists. *Chemists* direct their attention to how the compound is made and whether the manufacturing process and packaging are acceptable to ensure the identity, strength, quality, and purity of the product. *Pharmacologists* and *toxicologists* evaluate the effects of the compound in short- and long-term animal studies. *Physicians* evaluate the results of the clinical trials, including the compound's therapeutic and adverse effects, and whether the proposed labeling accurately reflects the effects of the compound. *Clinical pharmacologists* analyze the rate and the extent to which the compound's active ingredient is absorbed and distributed, biotransformed (also known as metabolized), and eliminated. *Statisticians* critique the controlled study designs and the analyses and conclusions regarding the compound's safety and effectiveness that are based on the study data. *Microbiologists* also participate in the review of antimicrobial drug products and of products formulated as solutions or as injectables. The microbiologist may also be a product specialist for new biologic products, focusing on how the agent is manufactured and packaged to ensure potency and purity.

The review team analyzes study results and looks for problems with the application, such as weaknesses in the study design or analyses, and missing information that may be critical in determining safety of the compound. Reviewers may agree with the sponsor's results and conclusions, or identify any additional information needed to make a decision about moving the compound forward in development.

The determination of whether the safety assessment is of adequate scope is based on consideration of observed adverse effects. Each reviewer prepares a written evaluation containing conclusions and recommendations about the application. Approval of the NDA means that the new drug has been accepted and can therefore be marketed exclusively by that company for a period of 7 years.

Postmarketing Surveillance

The FDA maintains a system for postmarketing surveillance and risk assessment to identify adverse effects that did not appear during the development and approval process of the compound (see Fig. 1-1). When a drug is suspected of producing a previously unknown adverse effect, that effect should be reported to the FDA, even if there is no unequivocal proof of the compound's involvement in the adverse effect. The postmarketing surveillance typically lasts 2 to 3 years. The purpose of the reporting system is to collect, sort, and scrutinize reports of clinically relevant adverse effects and to enable the following to take place: (1) evaluation of the likelihood that the event was drug related; (2) identification of patterns, which may help prevent further adverse effects; (3) investigation of product quality problems; (4) drug labeling updates; and (5) formulation of guidelines for managing reactions.

Health care providers may voluntarily report a serious adverse event, product quality problem, or product use error they suspect in connection with an FDA-regulated drug,

biologic, medical device, or dietary supplement. The FDA relies on the voluntary reporting of these events; it uses these data to maintain safety surveillance of all FDA-regulated products. The MedWatch form available from the FDA is used for reporting adverse events and product problems. It is available at the FDA website: www.fda.gov/opacom/background-ers/problem.html.

In the last few years a number of organizations have become more and more interested in safe drug practices. One such organization is the Institute for Safe Medication Practices (ISMP) (www.ismp.org). The ISMP is dedicated to learning about drug errors, understanding their system-based causes, and disseminating practical recommendations that help health care providers and consumers and the pharmaceutical industry prevent errors.

FINANCING NEW DRUG DEVELOPMENT

In 1992, Congress passed the Prescription Drug User Fee Act (PDUFA). This was reapproved by the Food and Drug Modernization Act of 1997, and again by the Public Health Security and Bioterrorism Preparedness and Response Act of 2002. The PDUFA authorizes the FDA to collect certain fees from companies that want the FDA to approve a new drug or biologic before marketing. In addition, companies pay annual fees for each manufacturing establishment and for each prescription drug marketed. The users' fees for fiscal year 2003 through 2007 have been established by the PDUFA (Table 1-1). Certain provisions of the PDUFA are intended to ensure that user fees supplement rather than replace Congressional appropriations intended to support the process of human drug review.

Fees are reestablished each year so that revenues from each category (see Table 1-1) approximate the revenue levels established in the statute (after adjustment for inflation and workload). In the past, taxpayers alone paid for product reviews through budgets provided by Congress. In newer programs, industry provides funding in exchange for an FDA agreement to meet drug-review performance goals, with an emphasis on timeliness.

Orphan Drugs

Orphan drugs are a special category found useful in the treatment of certain rare diseases. The Orphan Drug Act (ODA)

TABLE 1-1 Financing New Drug Review

Type of Fee Revenue*	FY 2003	FY 2004	FY 2005	FY 2006	FY 2007
APPLICATIONS AND SUPPLEMENTS	$74,300,000	$77,000,000	$84,000,000	$86,434,000	$86,434,000
Adjustment for inflation and workload	$533,400	$573,500	$672,000	$767,400	–
ESTABLISHMENT	$74,300,000	$77,000,000	$84,000,000	$86,433,000	$86,433,000
Adjustment for inflation and workload	$209,900	$226,800	$262,200	$264,000	–
PRODUCT	$74,300,000	$77,000,000	$84,000,000	$86,433,000	$86,433,000
Adjustment for inflation and workload	$209,900	$36,080	$41,710	$42,130	–
TOTAL FEE REVENUE	$222,900,000	$231,000,000	$252,000,000	$259,300,000	$259,300,000
TOTAL ADJUSTMENT FOR INFLATION AND WORKLOAD	$1,163,100	$836,380	$975,910	$1,073,530	–

*Any adjusted fee revenue amount must reflect the greater of the following: (1) The total percentage change that occurred in the Consumer Price Index (CPI) (all items; U.S. city average) during the 12-month period ending June 30 preceding the fiscal year for which fees are being set; or (2) the total percentage pay change for the previous fiscal year for Federal employees stationed in the Washington, DC, metropolitan area.

FY, Fiscal year.

See Federal Register Online via GPO Access [http://www.fda.gov/cber/pdufa/userfees07.htm] [DOCID:fr02au06–96] for more information, or the Federal Register of August 2, 2006 (Volume 71, Number 148).

provides special status for a product to treat a rare disease or condition (i.e., diseases or conditions affecting fewer than 200,000 people in the United States) upon request of a sponsor.

Because of patent laws or a limited market, these drugs often are not considered good financial investments for pharmaceutical companies who would rather spend money on drugs that will provide, with reasonable certainty, substantial returns on their research and development dollars. Congress therefore passed the Orphan Drug Act (Public Law 97–414) in 1983 to motivate companies to develop orphan drugs. The act, with its subsequent amendment in 1984, offers substantial tax incentives and longer patent protection to companies developing orphan drugs.

A drug with an orphan designation qualifies the sponsor of the product for the ODA tax credit and marketing incentives. A marketing application for a prescription drug designated as a drug for a rare disease or condition is not subject to a prescription drug user fee unless the application includes an indication for a disease or condition other than a rare one. Under the law, an application for designation as an orphan product can be made any time before the filing of a marketing application for the product.

For information on resources supporting orphan drug development, see the Evolve Resources Bonus Content at http://evolve.elsevier.com/Gutierrez/pharmacotherapeutics/.

NAMING NEW DRUGS

The name given a new drug is almost as important as the drug itself. A drug usually has three designations. The *chemical name* is based on the compound's precise chemical structure. Chemical names are complex and therefore not practical for everyday use.

A *generic name*, or common name, is generally an abbreviated or modified version of the chemical name and identifies or classifies the drug in scientific literature. The generic name is assigned to the compound by the United States Adopted Name (USAN) Council, with consultation with the company developing the drug. The USAN Council is jointly sponsored by the American Medical Association (AMA), the American Pharmaceutical Association (APA), and the United States Pharmacopeial Convention. As a general rule, the USAN Council accepts whatever name the company suggests. In clinical practice, using a drug's generic name facilitates communication and promotes safe, effective drug use.

TABLE 1-2 Comparison of Chemical, Generic, and Brand Names

Chemical Name	Generic Name	Brand Name
acetylsalicylic acid	aspirin	Bayer
N-acetyl-para-aminophenol	acetaminophen	Tylenol
ethyl 1-methyl-4-phenylisonipecotate hydrochloride	meperidine	Demerol
17,21-dihydroxypregna-1,4-diene-3,11,20-trione	prednisone	Deltasone
7-chloro-1,3-dihydro-1-methyl-5-phenyl-2H-1,4-benzodiazepin-2-one	diazepam	Valium

The *brand name, trade name,* or *proprietary name* identifies the drug as the product of a specific manufacturer (Table 1-2). Brand names are copyrighted, and they are important because they distinguish a company and its product from the competition. Patents issued before June 8, 1995, typically extend 17 years from the date the patent was issued. Patents granted after this date now have a 20-year patent life from the date of the first filing of the patent application. In effect, however, the patent term is frequently less than 20 years, because patents are often obtained before the drug is actually marketed. A patent can be extended for 5 years. However, the extension cannot postpone the patent's expiration to more than 14 years after the drug's approval date, or in other words, allow for more than 14 years of potential marketing time.

Pharmaceutical companies want names that are easily recognized by patients and health care providers. Unfortunately, multiple brand names for a single generic drug impair recognition of the drug and increase the possibility of errors. Sometimes similarities in drug names have been associated with errors that have caused harm to some patients. Most errors occur when the drug name is similar to that of a more frequently prescribed product: it could be misread, misheard, or miswritten (Table 1-3).

UNITED STATES DRUG LEGISLATION

Before 1906, there were no legal controls for the sale or use of any drug. Patented drugs and remedies were sold by traveling medicine men from the back of wagons, in drugstores, by mail order, and by real and self-professed physicians. In addition, drug manufacturers were not required to list ingredients on

TABLE 1-3 Drug Names Too Similar for Comfort

Instead of *(Prescribed Drug Name)*	for *(Patient's Condition)*	The Patient Received *(Mistaken Drug Name)*	for *(Other Condition)*
acetazolamide (Diamox)	Glaucoma	acetohexamide (Dymelor)	Diabetes
Anturane (sulfinpyrazone)	Gout	Antabuse (disulfiram)	Alcoholism
hydroxyzine (Vistaril)	Anxiety	hydralazine (Apresoline)	Hypertension
metolazone (Zaroxolyn)	Fluid retention	metaxalone (Skelaxin)	Muscle spasm
ritodrine (Yutopar)	Uterine contractions	Ritalin (methylphenidate)	Attention deficit hyperacidity disorder
Plavix (clopidogrel)	Anticoagulation	Paxil (paroxetine)	Depression
Foradil (formoterol)	Bronchodilation	Toradol (ketorolac)	Pain
Zyvox (linezolid)	Bacterial infection	Zovirax (acyclovir)	Viral infection
Avinza (extended-release morphine)	Pain	Evista (raloxifene)	Osteoporosis
Protonix (pantoprazole)	Gastric reflux	Protamine	Hemostasis
Cerebyx (fosphenytoin)	Seizure activity	Celebrex (celecoxib)	Arthritis

TABLE 1-4 Summary of U.S. Drug Legislation

Year	Title	Significance of Legislation
1906	Pure Food and Drug Act (The Wiley-Heyburn Act)	Restricted manufacture and sale of drugs; established the National Formulary and the U.S. Pharmacopeia as official standards Gave federal government authority to enforce standards.
1912	Sherley Amendment to FDA	Prohibited fraudulent therapeutic claims by drug manufacturers.
1914	Harrison Narcotic Act	Established word *narcotic* as legal term; regulated import, manufacture, sale, and use of habit-forming drugs.
1938	United States Federal Food, Drug, and Cosmetic Act	Mandated that drug manufacturers test all drugs for harmful effects before the drugs enter interstate commerce and that all drug labels must be accurate and complete. Made it mandatory to conduct toxicology tests on lab animals prior to seeking FDA approval to market any new drug by interstate commerce. Label must clearly identify if drug is habit forming. Required medical devices to be safe and effective, as well as cosmetics.
1938	FFDCA amendment to Sherley	Mandated drug manufacturers test all drugs for harmful effects before they enter interstate commerce. All drug labels must be accurate and complete.
1952	Durham-Humphrey Amendment	Distinguished between over-the-counter and prescription drugs and specified procedures for distribution of prescription drugs. Permits pharmacists to take a telephone order for noncontrolled drugs and for schedule III and IV drugs.
1962	Kefauver-Harris amendment to FFDCA	Tightened controls regarding safety and effectiveness of drugs; made statements about adverse reactions and contraindications; introduced drug-testing methods.
1970	Comprehensive Drug Abuse Prevention Act of 1970 (Controlled Substances Act)	Categorized controlled substances based on their abuse potential; established governmental programs to prevent and treat drug abuse; assigned drugs to schedules.
1978	Drug Regulation Reform Act	Established a more expedient process for release of new drugs to the public.
1983	Orphan Drug Act	Offers drug manufacturers incentives to develop drugs for rare disorders and those disorders with a limited market.

the container, permitting many products to contain alcohol, opium, or heroin. Illnesses and injuries occurred as a result of the tonic's ingredients, as well as the quantity of the ingredients.

The original drug legislation passed by Congress on June 30, 1906, and signed by President Theodore Roosevelt prohibits interstate commerce of misbranded and adulterated foods and drugs. According to the Center for Drug Evaluation and Research (CDER, 2006), the factors leading up to this drug legislation were disclosures of unsanitary conditions in meat-packing plants, the use of poisonous preservatives and dyes in foods, and cure-all claims for worthless and dangerous patent drugs.

Table 1-4 summarizes U.S. drug legislation.

FEDERAL FOOD, DRUG, AND COSMETIC ACT

The United States Federal Food, Drug, and Cosmetic Act (FFDCA) was passed by Congress in 1938 giving authority to the FDA to oversee the safety of food, drugs, and cosmetics. In 1968, the Electronic Product Radiation Control provisions were added to the FFDCA. In the same year, the FDA formed the Drug Efficacy Study Implementation (DESI), which incorporated into the regulations the recommendations made by a National Academy of Sciences investigation of the effectiveness of previously marketed drugs. The act was amended by the FDA Modernization Act of 1997. The original introduction of this act was influenced by the 1937 death of 107 children after sulfanilamide elixir was compounded using toxic diethylene glycol as the vehicle.

The Federal Trade Commission, under the Wheeler-Lea Act of 1938, was charged with oversight of advertising associated with products, including pharmaceuticals, otherwise regulated by FDA. The principle that certain drugs (nonnarcotic) should only be available by prescription evolved with the FDA policy of the same year that required a qualified expert to supervise the administration of sulfanilamide and selected other dangerous drugs.

During this same period, the Insulin Amendment was passed; it required the FDA to test and certify the purity and potency of this life-saving drug for diabetes. When nearly 300 deaths and injuries resulted from distribution of sulfathiazole tablets tainted with the sedative phenobarbital, the FDA turned its attention to what would later be called "good manufacturing practices" to drastically revise manufacturing and quality controls. The 1945 Penicillin Amendment requires FDA testing and certification of safety and effectiveness of all penicillin drugs. Later amendments would extend the requirement to all antibiotics. In 1983, such control was no longer considered necessary because of improved manufacturing methods and oversight and thus was abolished.

The act also designated the United States Pharmacopeia (USP) and the National Formulary (NF) as official drug references.*

SHERLEY AMENDMENT

The Supreme Court had ruled in 1911, in *United States v. Johnson*, that the 1906 Food and Drug Act did not prohibit false therapeutic claims, but only false and misleading statements about the ingredients or identity of a drug. In 1912, Congress went further and enacted the Sherley Amendment to prohibit drug labels containing false therapeutic claims intended to defraud the purchaser; CDER (2006) points out that this was a standard difficult to prove.

Although toxicity studies and an NDA were needed before a compound could be promoted and distributed, drug manufacturers were not required to establish drug efficacy (i.e., whether or not the drug is effective). Drugs went from the laboratory to the clinical arena without FDA approval. As a result, overstated claims of therapeutic uses were made. A 1938 amendment to the Sherley Amendment dealt

---

*The NF was established by the APA in 1888. In 1906, both the USP and the NF were established as official *standards* by the U.S. government. In 1974, the United States Pharmacopeial Convention purchased the NF from the APA, thereby merging the two resources.

primarily with truth in labeling and drug safety. According to the amendment, drug labels are to contain the following elements before products enter the marketplace:

- A statement describing package contents
- A reference to the presence, quantity, and proportion of certain drugs such as alcohol, atropine, digitalis, and bromides
- A statement that the product contains habit-forming substances and a listing of their effects, where appropriate
- The name of the manufacturer, the packager, and the distributor
- Directions for use, with recommendations for dosage and frequency
- A statement that the product has not yet been approved for interstate commerce, where appropriate
- The brand name and the generic name; no false or misleading statements are to appear

HARRISON NARCOTIC ACT

The Harrison Narcotic Act of 1914 followed the Sherley Amendment, aiming to set limits and controls on medicinal use of opium. The act put a limit on the amount of opium, opium-derived products, and cocaine allowed in products that were freely available to the public. Prescription drugs were still permitted to exceed the limit; however, physicians and pharmacists who dispensed opioids were subject to a stricter system of record-keeping. A separate law dealing with marijuana would be enacted in 1937 (CDER, 2006).

DURHAM-HUMPHREY AMENDMENT

The Durham-Humphrey Amendment of 1945 further altered the FFDCA, providing for direct supervision and inspection of drugs during their production and distribution. The FFDCA was amended again in 1952 to distinguish between over-the-counter (OTC) drugs and prescription drugs; it spelled out which drugs cannot be safely used without medical supervision and restricted their sale to prescription by a licensed health care provider.

KEFAUVER-HARRIS AMENDMENT

When thalidomide was found to cause birth defects in thousands of babies born in Western Europe, public support for stronger drug regulation helped lead to enactment of the Kefauver-Harris Amendment of 1962. For the first time, drug manufacturers were required to substantiate the effectiveness of their products to the FDA before marketing them. In addition, the FDA was given closer control over investigational drug studies, FDA inspectors were granted access to additional company records, and manufacturers were required to demonstrate the efficacy of products approved before 1962. The CDER (2006) credits this legislation for these milestone accomplishments.

CONTROLLED SUBSTANCES ACT

The most stringent drug-related regulation is the Controlled Substances Act (i.e., Title II of the Comprehensive Drug Abuse Prevention and Control Act). Passed by Congress in 1970, it was designed to contain the rapidly increasing problem of drug abuse. The act encouraged research into the prevention and treatment of drug abuse and dependency and promoted drug education programs. In addition, it provided for the establishment of treatment and rehabilitation centers. Drug enforcement was further strengthened by the creation of drug schedules based on the potential for abuse and dependency (Table 1-5).

Both the health care provider and the pharmacist are legally responsible for drugs covered by the Controlled Substances Act. In order to prescribe, dispense, or administer any controlled substance, the health care provider must be registered with the federal Drug Enforcement Administration (DEA). Once a provider's application is approved, the certificate is valid for 3 years. Separate registrations are required if the provider practices in more than one location. An outline of the Controlled Substances Act of 1970 may be obtained from the DEA (www.dea.gov). Many states require concurrent certification or registration with other agencies involved with the prescribing, dispensing, or administering of controlled substances.

Schedule I

Schedule I drugs have a high potential for abuse and no accepted medical use. They may be available for research use or for chemical analysis; an application and supporting protocols should be forwarded to the DEA. Under normal circumstances, health care providers cannot write, and pharmacists cannot fill, prescriptions for Schedule I drugs.

Schedule II

Schedule II drugs also have high abuse potential, but they have accepted medical uses as well. The inappropriate use of Schedule II drugs results in psychologic or physiologic dependence. A written prescription is required; however, federal law permits emergency telephone orders for Schedule II controlled drugs under the following circumstances:

- Immediate administration of the drug is necessary for proper treatment.
- There are no alternative treatments available.
- It is not possible to provide a written prescription for the drug at that time.

Under these circumstances, the quantity of drug prescribed is limited to that used to treat the patient during the emergency. A written, signed prescription must be provided to the pharmacy within 72 hours. In addition, the phrase "authorization for emergency dispensing" and the date of the verbal order must be written on the face of the prescription. The pharmacist is required to notify the DEA if the written prescription is not received within 72 hours.

Schedule III

Schedule III drugs have a lower potential for abuse than drugs in Schedules I and II. Abuse of these drugs may lead to low to moderate physical dependency or to high psychologic dependency. Schedule III drugs often contain a noncontrolled substance along with a controlled substance (e.g., acetaminophen [noncontrolled drug] with 30 mg of codeine [controlled drug]). Formulations with less than 1.8 grams of codeine per 100 mL, depressants such as butabarbital and glutethimide, and certain anabolic steroids fall into this schedule.

TABLE 1-5 U.S. Schedules for Controlled Substances

Schedule	Selected Examples	Schedule Characteristics	Restrictions Required
C$_I$	Cannabis, heroin, lysergic acid diethylamide (LSD), mescaline, methaqualone, peyote, psilocybin	All nonresearch, analysis, or instructional use prohibited High potential for abuse May lead to severe dependence	Approved research protocol only
C$_{II}$	Amphetamine, cocaine, codeine, hydromorphone, morphine, meperidine, methadone, methylphenidate, oxycodone, pentobarbital, secobarbital	May lead to severe dependence High abuse potential May lead to severe physical or psychologic dependence, or both	Written prescription necessary No telephone renewals May prescribe over the phone if an emergency Container must have warning label*
C$_{III}$	Drugs containing limited amounts or that are combined with one or more active noncontrolled ingredients: codeine, hydrocodone, morphine, and nonopioid drugs such as derivatives of barbituric acid except those listed in another schedule, chlorphentermine, paregoric, and others.	Accepted medical uses Potential for abuse lower than with drugs in Schedules I or II May lead to low to moderate physical dependence or high psychologic dependence	Written or verbal prescription required Prescription expires in 6 months No more than five refills permitted within 6 months Container must have warning label*
C$_{IV}$	Alprazolam, chlordiazepoxide, clorazepate, diazepam, dextropropoxyphene, flurazepam, lorazepam, oxazepam, pentazocine, and others	Accepted medical uses Potential for abuse lower than Schedule III drugs May lead to limited physical or psychologic dependence	Written or verbal prescription required Prescription expires in 6 months No more than five refills permitted within 6 months Container must have warning label*
C$_V$	OTC drugs used for relief of cough or diarrhea Contain limited amounts of select opioid ingredients	Accepted medical uses Potential for abuse lower than Schedule IV drugs May lead to limited physical or psychologic dependence	May require written prescription, or may be sold without a prescription Check state laws

*CAUTION: Federal law prohibits the transfer of this drug to any person other than the patient for whom it was prescribed.
OTC, Over-the-counter.
NOTE: Some states may impose their own schedules (e.g., pentazocine is a C$_{II}$ drug rather than a C$_{IV}$ in several states).

Prescriptions for Schedule III drugs may be presented in writing or given verbally to the pharmacist. If authorized on the prescription, the order may be refilled 5 times within 6 months of the date of issue. A new prescription is needed at the end of the 6-month period. Federal law permits verbal authorization for additional refills under the following circumstances:

- The total quantity does not exceed five refills or extend beyond 6 months from the date of the original prescription.
- The quantity of each additional refill is equal to or less than the quantity originally authorized.
- A new prescription must be provided for additional quantities beyond the five refills or 6-month limitation.

Schedule IV

Schedule IV drugs have a low abuse potential compared to Schedule III drugs and have medical use as accepted in the United States. The primary difference between Schedule III and Schedule IV drugs is the penalty for unlawful possession. Prescription requirements for drugs in Schedule IV are similar to those of Schedule III.

Schedule V

Drugs in this schedule are thought to have less abuse potential than those of Schedule IV. These drugs are generally used for their antitussive and antidiarrheal effects and contain moderate quantities of opioid. Schedule V drugs may be distributed without a prescription under the following conditions:

- The purchaser is at least 18 years of age and proper identification is obtained.
- Distribution is made only by a pharmacist.
- No more than 240 mL of any Schedule V substance containing opium, and not more than 120 mL or 24 solid-dosage units of any other controlled substance, can be sold to the same person in any 48-hour period without a valid prescription.
- Records are kept of the name and address of the person purchasing the drug, the name and quantity of the controlled substance, the date of sale, and the name or initials of the pharmacist.
- Other federal, state, and local laws do not require a prescription to obtain the drug.

CANADIAN DRUG LEGISLATION

CANADIAN FOOD AND DRUGS ACT

Canadian drug laws evolved in a manner analogous to those of the United States. The present Food and Drug Act was passed in 1953 and has been amended almost every year since. The legend CSD (Canadian Standard Drug) must appear on the inner and outer labels of drug packaging to indicate it meets standards contained in the following formularies and pharmacopeias:

- The British Pharmaceutical Codex
- Pharmacopeia Française

- Pharmacopoeia Internationalis
- The British Pharmacopoeia
- The Canadian Formulary
- The U.S. Pharmacopeia/National Formulary

The British Pharmacopoeia (BP) is similar in scope and purpose to the USP. The British Pharmaceutical Codex is published by the Pharmaceutical Society of Great Britain. It includes standards for new drugs that are prescribed in Canada but not included in the BP. The USP is used a great deal in Canada. Some drugs used in Canada conform to the USP instead of the BP because, although they are used in Canada, they are manufactured in the United States.*

The trade group, Canadian International Pharmacy Association (CIPA) has a checklist to help people with due diligence. All sites listed on the CIPA website have verified Canadian pharmacies filling prescriptions (www.ciparx.ca/art-steps-to-ensure-safety.html). Steps U.S. patients can take to ensure safety when obtaining prescription medications from Canada include the following:

- Look for the provincial pharmacy license number on the pharmacy website.
- Phone the Provincial Regulatory Authority to confirm the license (see www.napra.org or www.pharmacists.ca to view a list of the regulators).
- Look on the website for a physical address in Canada.
- Look for toll-free phone numbers to call from the United States.
- Call the toll-free number and speak to a customer service representative or pharmacist.
- Make sure the pharmacy requires a prescription from a licensed physician.
- Make sure the pharmacy requires a patient medical history, including allergies.
- Make sure the pharmacy requires the patient to sign a patient agreement to order.
- Look for the CIPA certification seal on the pharmacy website.
- Avoid following up on "spam" and pop-up ads that promise cheap prescription drugs or opioids.

The most important things a consumer should look for on the website are the name and address and license number of the Canadian pharmacy. By law, this information must be placed on the home page.

The Drugs Directorate of the Health Protection Branch (HPB) of the Department of National Health and Welfare is responsible for the administration and enforcement of the Foods and Drugs Act. The directorate is also responsible for the administration and enforcement of the Proprietary or Patent Medicine Act and the Narcotic Control Act. These acts are designed to control and continuously monitor the research, development, advertising, and product information for all drug products.

NARCOTIC CONTROL ACT

The most recent Canadian legislation is the Narcotic Control Act of 1996. The act is similar in scope to the U.S. Controlled Substances Act (1970). It designates drug classifications, with

drug schedules based on abuse potential (Table 1-6). Although the administration of the Narcotic Control Act is legally the responsibility of the Department of National Health and Welfare, the enforcement of the law falls primarily to the Royal Canadian Mounted Police. Health care providers are advised to check with appropriate government officials regarding drug controls and standards if they will be working within Canadian boundaries.

SOURCES OF DRUG INFORMATION

The need for objective, concise, well-organized, and accurate information about drugs is obvious. Unfortunately, there is no single source of drug information that covers all clinical situations. Resources include pharmacology and therapeutics textbooks, professional journals, drug compendia, continuing education seminars and meetings, advertising, drug information centers, and online computer databases.

OFFICIAL INFORMATION SOURCES

The only official book of drug standards in the United States is the United States Pharmacopeia-National Formulary (USP-NF), a privately issued compendium. The USP is revised every 5 years by a group of elected experts from a variety of fields including nursing, pharmacy, pharmacology, and chemistry, and by consumers. Drugs included in the reference meet high standards of quality, purity, and strength and are identified by the letters USP-NF following the official name.

NONOFFICIAL INFORMATION SOURCES

Numerous clinical reference books and guides are available. *Goodman and Gilman's The Pharmacological Basis of Therapeutics* is the classic reference on pharmacology. As the name implies, the primary focus is on the basic science information that underlies drug use and not on individual drugs. New editions are published approximately every 5 years.

Drug Facts and Comparisons is organized by drug classification and is updated monthly. It contains a comprehensive list of drugs with a cost index guide to the average wholesale price (AWP) for equivalent quantities of similar or identical drugs.

Two other valuable resources are the USP Dispensing Information (USPDI) and the *American Hospital Formulary Service* (AHFS) drug information book. These unbiased, relatively accessible sources of information provide data on the clinical uses of drugs. The USPDI is published annually, with regular updates issued during the year. It contains information for both the health care provider (volumes I and III) and the patient (volume II). The provider volumes offer information about approved drug products, drug indications, pharmacokinetics, dosing, warnings, adverse effects, and precautions. It does not require the user to obtain permission for its use from the publisher. Automatic permission is granted to health care providers who copy a limited quantity of monographs to distribute free of charge to their patients.

The AHFS is a collection of monographs published by the American Society of Health System Pharmacists (ASHP). The collection is kept current by annual republication. It frequently reviews newer or investigational uses for drugs.

*Canadian drugs within this book's drug lists are identified with a maple leaf icon (e.g., ampicillin [Omnipen; ◆ Apo-Ampi])

TABLE 1-6 Canadian Schedules for Controlled Substances

Sch	Selected Examples	Schedule Characteristics	Restrictions Required
RESTRICTED DRUGS			
H	N,N-diethyltryptamine (DET), N,N-dimethyltryptamine (DMT), 4-methyl-2,5-dimethoxyamphetamine, (STP, DOM), lysergic acid diethylamide (LSD), mescaline, peyote	No recognized medicinal use Sale is prohibited Possess dangerous physical and psychologic effects	Available for investigational use with authorization from Minister of National Health and Welfare
N	anileridine, cannabis, cocaine, codeine, morphine, opium, phencyclidine, and preparations containing controlled substances with noncontrolled substances (e.g., acetaminophen with codeine, diphenoxylate with atropine)	Stringently restricted High potential for abuse All parenteral narcotics containing less than two other nonnarcotic ingredients All narcotic compounds containing more than one narcotic drug	Letter *N* must appear on all labels and professional advertisements Refills not permitted Reorders require new written prescription Oral formulations require written or verbal order
CONTROLLED SUBSTANCES			
G	Amphetamines, anabolic steroids, barbiturates	Potential for abuse All combinations containing more than one controlled drug All combinations with one controlled drug and one or more ingredients in recognized therapeutic dosage	"c" symbol must appear on all labels and professional advertisements Refills not permitted if original order was verbal Refills authorized if identified on original prescription
F	Antipsychotics, benzodiazepines, oral antibiotics, oral contraceptives, steroids hormones	Some have relatively low abuse potential Can be sold and refilled only on prescription (Pr)	Orders may be written, verbal, or electronic Refills permitted at specified intervals but cannot exceed 6 months Drugs available only in pharmacy and used only on physician recommendation "Pr" symbol must appear on label
C & D	Anterior pituitary extracts, antibiotics, injectable liver extracts, low-dose codeine, insulin, muscle relaxants, nitroglycerin, radioactive isotopes, parenteral serums, vaccines not of bacterial origin	Nonprescription drug schedule Limited public access	Drugs available only in pharmacy and used only on physician recommendation

Objective journals not supported by drug manufacturers include the journals *Clinical Pharmacology and Therapeutics* and *Drugs*. The former is devoted to original articles that evaluate actions and effects of drugs on humans. The latter publishes timely reviews of individual drugs and drug classifications.

Three further publications provide objective information in an effective, easy-to-understand form. *The Medical Letter*, a biweekly newsletter-like publication of a nonprofit corporation, provides summaries of scientific reports and consultant evaluations as to the safety, efficacy, and rationale for using particular drugs. *Clin-Alert* consists chiefly of abstracts from the literature on drugs. *Rational Drug Therapy* provides a monthly review article on drug groups or on the management of specific conditions.

The *Nurse Practitioners' Prescribing Reference (NPPR)* and the *Physician Assistants' Prescribing Reference (PAPR)* are quarterly publications produced in New York. They provide the advanced practice nurse (APN) and physician's assistant (PA) with an up-to-date guide to commonly prescribed products available by prescription, as well as selected OTC drugs.

The *Physicians' Desk Reference (PDR)* is an unofficial source of information commonly used by health care providers. The information contained in the *PDR* is identical to that found in drug package inserts and is submitted and paid for by drug companies. The information is largely based on the results of phase III clinical trials. Its primary value is in identifying the clinical indications for an FDA-approved drug. It does not include the care implications of a particular drug.

Textbooks

Depending on their purpose and scope, pharmacology textbooks offer basic pharmacologic principles, critical appraisal of useful categories of therapeutic drugs, and descriptions of individual prototype drugs. Prototypes serve as standards of reference for assessing new drugs. Pharmacodynamics and pharmacokinetics are also covered in textbooks. Most include administration techniques, patient assessment and monitoring, and patient teaching.

Pocket reference books are another resource. These references provide specific information regarding administration, assessment and evaluation of patient responses, and patient education considerations.

Online Databases

A number of online computer databases have been developed that provide drug and treatment information to health care providers and the public alike. The most popular of these are accessed through the Internet. The Internet has its roots in the network designed to centralize military computing by the Department of Defense in the late 1960s. This network also linked researchers and defense contractors at colleges and universities across the country through a network of supercomputing centers accessible by personal computers for heavy-duty statistical analyses funded by the National Science Foundation (NSF). Today, the Internet is used by more than 70 million people.

Resources available through the Internet include medical subject directories; clinical resources; conditions and diseases;

consumer and patient information; dictionaries and glossaries; online medical journals; and news, statistics, and drug information. A working knowledge of computer databases and resources continues to be important to successful drug therapies as more information becomes available online.

For more information on internet-accessible information databases, see the Evolve Resources Bonus Content at http://evolve.elsevier.com/Gutierrez/pharmacotherapeutics/.

Pharmacists and Pharmacologists

Inevitably, clinical situations occur in which needed information is not contained in available resources. The health care provider is then wise to consult with a pharmacist. A pharmacist may provide a brochure or other reference material on the drug. As an expert in the field of drug therapy, the pharmacist is a valuable member of the health care team and should be actively involved in drug regimen decisions.

Each health care provider adopts sources found to be useful and convenient but should guard against undue reliance on any one reference or person for drug information. Periodic use of other resources helps minimize systematic bias in the selection of drugs and drug information data that influence clinical reasoning.

KEY POINTS

- Historical writings show that early pharmacotherapeutic efforts were for the most part mystical, based on magic, prayers, and incantations.
- The process of new drug development begins with preclinical studies, progresses through several phases of clinical testing, and ends with postmarketing surveillance studies.
- A drug usually has three designations: a chemical name, a generic name, and a brand name that identify the drug as the product of a specific manufacturer.
- The Harrison Narcotic Act of 1914 was the first significant legislation classifying certain drugs as habit-forming.

- The Controlled Substances Act of 1970 classified habit-forming drugs into five schedules and established drug education programs, treatment programs, and rehabilitation centers.
- The FDA monitors new drug development, often over a period of 6 to 12 years, before a drug reaches the marketplace.
- The only official books of drug standards in the United States are the United States Pharmacopeia/National Formulary (USP-NF) and the United States Pharmacopeia Dispensing Information (USPDI), whereas Canada uses the USP, the Canadian Formulary, and the British Pharmacopoeia.

Bibliography

AAPA. (2003). Physician assistant prescribing practices similar to medical doctors. Doctor's Guide. Available online: www.pslgroup.com/dg/2339CE.htm. Accessed June 13, 2007.

American Society of Health System Pharmacists. (2007). *American hospital formulary service (AHFS)*. Bethesda, MD: Author.

Center for Drug Evaluation and Research. Time Line: Chronology of drug regulation in the United States. Available online: www.fda.gov/cder/about/history/time1.htm. Accessed September 25, 2006.

The Food and Drugs Act, Part C, Drugs, Division 1 C.01.004 and C.01.003, Dec 30, 2002. p. 396. Available: www.hc-sc.gc.ca/fn-an/alt_formats/hpfb-dgpsa/pdf/legislation/e_e-drugs.pdf. Accessed October 3, 2006.

Code of Federal Regulations. (2006). Title 21, 1300. Washington, DC: Superintendent of Documents. Washington, DC: United States Government Printing Office.

Compendium of Pharmaceuticals and Specialties. (1990). (25th ed.). Ottawa, Ontario: Canadian Pharmaceutical Association.

Department of Justice. Canada. (1996). Controlled Drugs and Substances Act. Available online: http://laws.justice.gc.ca/en/C-38.8/37301.html. Accessed February 1, 2007.

Drug Enforcement Administration. (2006). *Physician's manual*. Washington, DC: Drug Enforcement Administration. Available online: www.deadiversion.usdoj.gov/pubs/manuals/index.html. Accessed February 1, 2006.

Facts & Comparisons. (2007). *Drug facts and comparisons*. Baltimore, MD: Lippincott, Williams, & Wilkins.

Farley, D. (1987–1988). How FDA approves new drugs. *FDA Consumer, 21*(10):6–13.

Food and Drug Administration. (2005). Center for Drug Evaluation and Research. *Approved Drug Products with Therapeutic Equivalence Evaluations*. (24th ed.). Available online: www.fda.gov/cder/ob/docs/preface/ectablec.htm. Accessed February 1, 2007.

Food and Drug Administration. (1981). *The story of the laws behind the labels*. Part I: 1906 Food and Drugs Act. *FDA Consumer*. June. Available online: vm.cfsan.fda.gov/~lrd/history1.html. Accessed February 1, 2007.

Food and Drug Administration. (1981). *The story of the laws behind the labels*. Part II: 1938–The Federal Food, Drug, and Cosmetic Act. *FDA Consumer*. June. Available online: vm.cfsan.fda.gov/~lrd/histor1a.html. Accessed February 1, 2007.

Food and Drug Administration. (1981). *The story of the laws behind the labels*. Part III: 1962 Drug amendments. *FDA Consumer*. June. Available online: vm.cfsan.fda.gov/~lrd/histor1a.html. Accessed February 1, 2007.

Goodman, L., Rall, T., Nies, A., Taylor, P. (2001). *Goodman and Gilman's the pharmacologic basis of therapeutics* (10th ed.). New York: Pergamon Press.

Leake, C. (1975). *An historical account of pharmacology to the twentieth century*. Springfield: Charles C Thomas.

National Association of Pharmacy Regulatory Authorities (Canada). *Controlled Drugs and Substances Act and Regulations*. Available online: www.napra.org/docs/0/93/143.asp. Accessed February 1, 2007.

Prescribing Reference. (2007). *Nurse practitioners' prescribing reference (NPPR)*. New York: Author.

Prescribing Reference. (2007). *Physician assistants' prescribing reference (PAPR)*. New York: Author.

Riley, D. (1998). *Drugs and drug policy in Canada: A brief review and commentary*. Available online: www.cfdp.ca/sen1841.htm. Accessed February 1, 2007.

Segal, M. (1993). *Rx to OTC: The switch is on*. Rockville, MD: Department of Health and Human Services, Public Health Service, Food and Drug Administration, Office of Public Affairs (Pub. No. 92–3195).

Stehlin, D. (1995). *Getting information from FDA.* Rockville, MD: Department of Health and Human Services, Public Health Service, Food and Drug Administration (Pub. No. 95–1167).

The Rx legend—an FDA manual for pharmacists. Rockville, MD: U.S. Food and Drug Administration.

Thomson Health Care. (2007). *Physicians desk reference.* Montvale, NJ. Author.

Thorwald, J. (1963). *Science and secrets of early medicine.* New York: Harcourt, Brace, and World.

United States Food and Drug Administration: Available online: www.fda.gov. Accessed February 1, 2007.

United States Pharmacopeial Convention. (1990). *The United States pharmacopeia* (22nd rev.). Easton, PA: Mack Printing.

United States Pharmacopeial Convention. (1990). *The national formulary* (17th ed.). Easton, PA: Mack Printing.

United States Pharmacopeia Dispensing Information (USPDI). (2006). *Approved drug products and legal requirements 2007.* (26th ed.). Volume III. Rockville, MD: Thomson PDR.

United States Pharmacopeia Dispensing Information (USPDI). (2005). *Drug information for the health care professional.* (26th ed.). Volume 1. Rockville, MD: Thomson PDR.

United States Pharmacopeia Dispensing Information (USPDI). (2002) *Advice for the patient: Drug information in lay language* (25th ed.). Volume II. Rockville, MD: Micromedex.

York, J. (1993). *FDA ensures equivalence of generic drugs.* Rockville, MD: Department of Health and Human Services, Public Health Service, Food and Drug Administration, Office of Public Affairs (Pub. No. 93–3206).

Ziporyn, T. (1985). The Food and Drug Administration: How those regulations came to be. *Journal of the American Medical Association, 254*(15), 2037–2039, 2043–2046.

Clinical Reasoning in Pharmacotherapeutics

2

PHARMACOTHERAPY AS ART AND SCIENCE

Health care providers make decisions all the time: what the problem is, what the diagnosis is, whether to do anything about it, and then what to do; which factors should be taken into account to come to a decision; and what processes should be used to decide on a course of action. The same holds true in pharmacotherapeutics. The information presented by a patient's history and physical exam findings, together with laboratory and imaging studies, guides the health care provider in selecting the correct drug for therapy, or choosing to institute lifestyle modifications or other non–drug therapies. However, numerous comparable drug therapies can exist for a specific condition, and differentiating one drug from another can be tedious and at times obscure. Because of these difficulties, simply accepting facts at face value may not be the shortest route to a plan for proper care and treatment of patients; optimal treatment may require deeper investigation into subtleties offered by the practice arena of pharmacotherapeutics.

There are different types of knowledge. *Operative knowledge* is collected during everyday practice, and experts' skills are reported and stored in the hospital information system. On the other hand, well-developed, *formalized knowledge* is reported in textbooks and clinical guidelines. We assert that all this assorted information should be secured and distributed, and made available to health care providers in the right form and at the right time, in order to support decision making. In reality, though, a decision support system cannot be conceived of as an independent tool, nor should it replace the human expert. Some clinical pathways, such as may be seen in some disease state management programs, make the assumption that all patients with a given problem will benefit from and will comply with standard medication regimens shown in large clinical studies to improve quality of life, alleviate symptoms, or reduce morbidity and mortality. However, patients with a comorbid condition may react very differently to drug therapy, thus the health care provider must combine evidence and experience to tailor an appropriate pharmacotherapeutic regimen to the individual. From the methodologic viewpoint, case-based clinical reasoning has proven to be a paradigm well suited to managing operative knowledge. On the other hand, *rule-based knowledge* is historically one of the most successful approaches to deal with formalized knowledge. To take advantage of all the available knowledge types, it is usually best to use a multimodal reasoning methodology that integrates and supports investigation into the clinical context, information retrieval, and decision support.

The concept of reflection is an epistemology (i.e., the branch of philosophy that studies the nature of knowledge, in particular its foundations, scope, and validity) for practice; such reflection enables health care providers to resolve problematic, everyday patient situations through conscious thought processes eventually leading to *practice-based knowledge*. In a general sense, how do we know what we know about drug therapies? Information may come from clinical study, anecdotal reports, clinical experience, or consensus from an expert panel. It is prudent to balance evidence and experience consistent with a provider's clinical exposure and to be cautious with following general expert opinion or clinical guidelines that have little support from empirical evidence. A hallmark of the health care provider who seeks to improve his or her ability to bestow quality care is ongoing study and quality improvement to ensure that his or her knowledge is current and balanced by experience and evidence.

COLLABORATION

Collaboration means to work together, to cooperate, or to unite, especially in a joint intellectual effort. The purpose of collaboration among health care providers is to enhance quality of care and improve patient outcomes. Although patient needs are the primary focus, collaboration is a synergistic link that optimizes the contributions of each professional participant. Historically, prescribing was exclusively a medical function and was not delegated to others. However, times have changed, and today there are a variety of health care providers involved in drug therapies.

Since there is much that remains to be learned about the actual mechanism of drug action as well as the effects of prolonged use, an awareness of each health care provider's role in pharmacotherapeutics and the ability and willingness to interact with each other are vital to safe and effective drug management.

MIDLEVEL PROVIDERS

Traditionally, physicians and dentists have been responsible for assessing the patient, building a diagnosis, and determining appropriate interventions. Increasingly, however, the responsibility for assessment, diagnosis, and treatment has expanded to include midlevel providers such as advanced practice nurses (APNs; i.e., nurse practitioners, clinical nurse specialists, nurse midwives, and nurse anesthetists) and physician assistants (PAs). When permitted by state law, they may write prescriptions for drugs to be dispensed by a pharmacist. The person prescribing a drug is responsible for monitoring patient response, treating adverse effects, and modifying the treatment regimen, if needed. In many cases, midlevel providers use protocols when prescribing, or they have some degree of legislated or delegated prescriptive authority. Protocols are written recommendations, rules, or standards to be followed for any situation in which rational procedures can be specified; they are essentially guidelines for practice. Table 2-1 provides an overview comparing the roles of APNs and PAs.

Advanced Practice Nurses

Prescriptive authority for APNs became important as education and expertise progressed to expanded nursing roles. Two early documents recognized the need for prescriptive authority: a 1970 report from the American Medical Association (AMA) and a 1971 report from the U.S. Department of Health, Education, and Welfare (HEW). Both documents clearly point out that prescribing may be a practice of medicine when carried out by a physician, and it may be a practice of nursing when carried out by the APN. As a result of the publication of these two documents, a number of states have

amended nurse practice acts (NPAs) to accommodate this perspective and the subsequent expansion of the nurse's role.

Because prescriptive authority is regulated by the state, the legislative process for obtaining prescriptive authority differs from state to state. In most states, APNs have the authority to prescribe by virtue of a nurse practice act, a pharmacy law, a medical practice act, or any combination of the three. Statutory authority indicates that an amendment to a practice act or a bill specifically addressing prescriptive authority has passed the state legislature with the governor's signature. In states without legislated prescriptive authority for APNs, many APNs are nonetheless actively prescribing for patients through one or more activities. For example, a physician writes the prescription for the patient, and the prescription is called into the pharmacy under the physician's name; or the APN cosigns the physician's prescription pad; or an APN carries out prescribing activities according to collaborative agreements.

Physician Assistants

The need for PA training programs became apparent in the 1960s as the result of a shortage of primary care physicians.

TABLE 2-1 Comparison of Advanced Practice Nurses and Physician Assistants

Characteristic	APNs	PAs
Definition	Registered nurses who perform independent nursing acts and delegated medical acts with physician collaboration	Health care professionals who perform medical care with physician supervision
Philosophy, practice model	*Medical and/or nursing model:* Biopsychosocial-oriented with emphasis on disease adaptation, health promotion, wellness, and prevention *Practice model:* Collaborative relationship with physicians	*Medical and/or physician model:* Disease-oriented; emphasis on biologic and pathologic aspects of health, assessment, diagnosis, and treatment *Practice model:* Team relationship with physicians
Education	*Prerequisite:* Bachelor of science in nursing *Affiliation:* Nursing schools and programs *Curriculum:* Advanced science–based. Approximately 500 hours didactic education; 500 to 700 clinical hours, depending on specialty area (in addition to 3 to 4 years of undergraduate clinical hours) APNs choose specialty track: Acute care, adult, family, pediatrics, women's health, nurse midwife, nurse anesthetist, gerontology. Emphasis on diagnosis, treatment, prevention, patient education. Master's degree awarded.	*Prerequisite:* Previous health care experience. Undergraduate degree in sciences preferred *Affiliation:* Medical schools, universities, liberal arts colleges, allied health science colleges *Curriculum:* Advanced science–based. Approximately 1500 hours didactic training; 3000 clinical hours Trained as generalists; a primary care model; some receive postgraduate specialty training Procedure- and skill-oriented with emphasis on diagnosis, treatment, surgical skills, and patient education To date, 79% of programs award master's degree.
Licensure Certification	Practice under state nurse practice act. Accreditation through credentialing organizations (ANPP and/or ANCC) MSN required for certification exam National certification voluntary; needed for specialty practice	Practice under state medical practice act Accreditation through national credentialing organization (e.g., NCCPA) Graduation from an accredited PA program and passage of the national certifying exam required for state licensure
Recertification	1500 direct patient care hours and 75 CEUs every 5 years for each certification held No exam required	100 CME hours every 2 years and an exam every 6 years (comparable to physician certification)
Scope of practice	Nursing care allowed as an independent function; collaborative agreement is required for prescriptive authority Does not require on-site supervision	Supervising physician has relatively broad discretion in delegating medical tasks within his or her scope of practice in accordance with state regulations Written guidelines are required for prescriptions May require on-site supervision a percentage of the time each week or month
Third-party coverage and reimbursement	Eligible for certification as Medicare and Medicaid providers; generally receive favorable reimbursement from commercial payors	Eligible for certification as Medicare and Medicaid providers; generally receive favorable reimbursement from commercial payors
References	www.ana.org www.aanp.org www.nonpf.org	www.aapa.org www.nccpa.org

AANP, American Academy of Nurse Practitioners; *AAPA,* American Association of Physician Assistants; *ANCC,* American Nurses Credential Council; *APN;* advanced practice nurse (can be nurse practitioner, nurse anesthetist, nurse midwife, clinical nurse specialist); *CEUs,* continuing education units; *CME(s),* continuing medical education (hours); *MSN,* master of science in nursing; *NCCPA,* National Commission on Certification of Physician Assistants; *NONPF,* National Organization Nurse Practitioner Faculties; *PA,* physician's assistant.

Dr. Eugene Stead began the first PA program at Duke University Medical Center in North Carolina. He chose Navy corpsmen who had provided medical care to soldiers during the Vietnam War to become the first PA students. Since that time, PA programs have grown across the United States.

The legal status of the PA varies from state to state, but in many areas, this person prescribes drugs following established protocols. PAs practice under the state medical practice act with certification through a credentialing organization (e.g., National Commission on Certification of Physician Assistants [NCCPA]). Graduation from an accredited PA program and passing a national certifying exam are required for state licensure.

PAs provide patient care with physician supervision, although their role can vary according to training, experience, and state law. In general, PAs see many of the same types of patients as the physician or an APN. Close consultation between the patient, the PA, and the physician is used for unusual or hard-to-manage cases. PAs are taught to "know their limits" and make appropriate referrals to physicians. Forty-nine states, the District of Columbia, and Guam have enacted laws permitting PAs to prescribe. In California, PA prescriptions are referred to as *written prescription transmittal orders*.

Pharmacologists and Pharmacists

A *pharmacologist* investigates how drugs and chemicals interact with biologic systems. Most pharmacologists have PhD degrees. Because pharmacology and medicine are closely related, some pharmacologists become physicians, and vice versa. Pharmacologists have knowledge of chemistry, biology, physiology, and mathematics.

A *pharmacist* has the legal authority to compound and dispense drugs upon written or verbal prescription from a licensed provider. Many practicing pharmacists hold baccalaureate degrees from a 5- or 6-year educational program. The profession of pharmacy includes the provision of drug and therapeutic information to other members of the health care team and the public. An important aspect of the pharmacist's role is to ensure the proper storage and security of drugs. The terms *pharmacologist* and *pharmacist* are often used interchangeably.

The *PharmD* is generally awarded after an additional 6 or 7 years of study and has become the terminal degree for most pharmacists graduating today. The education includes advanced, more comprehensive coursework in research, pathophysiology, pharmacokinetics, and pharmacotherapeutics. In recent years there has been a push in some states for pharmacists to be able to order drugs. The outcome is undecided at this time.

ASSOCIATE HEALTH CARE PROVIDERS

The role of the pharmacy technician is to provide technical and clerical support to pharmacists in hospitals or in retail pharmacies. Pharmacy technicians are trained to collect information about patient allergies, transcribe drug orders, prepare drug records or treatment sheets, and order drugs from the manufacturer or supplier. In some settings, they prepare simple prescriptions for dispensing; they may measure, mix, package, label and, in some cases, deliver drugs. In addition, they maintain computerized lists of drugs taken by patients to ensure that the correct drugs have been prescribed. Pharmacy technicians also look after home care products such as canes, vision aids, and hearing aids. Depending on their position, they may also manage third-party billing, answer telephones, receive written prescriptions, clean and prepare dispensing equipment, and so forth.

In some states, the institutionally employed pharmacy technician may be a licensed practical or vocational nurse (LPN, LVN) who is responsible for administering prescribed drugs. No formal license is required of pharmacy technicians in many instances. A licensed pharmacist remains responsible for delegated tasks. However, evaluation of therapeutic response still falls to the health care provider.

Registered respiratory therapists (RRTs) may administer drugs (other than anesthetics) that are given by inhalation, and they are well informed about machines that deliver drugs to the lungs. The educational background of an RRT varies from a 2-year associate degree to more advanced degrees. Students who successfully complete an accredited entry-level educational program take the certifying respiratory therapy (CRT) examination. After acquiring advanced education and additional clinical experience, CRTs take the registered respiratory therapist (RRT) examination.

Like many other health care providers, their scope of practice is dictated by health care agency policies and procedures, job descriptions, state licensure boards, and credentialing agencies. In tertiary-care institutions, professional nurses still monitor patient response.

CLINICAL REASONING

Schon (1993) maintains that professionals, helped by senior providers, learn by practicing decision making or performing a task in which they become adept. Schon contends that a professional cannot be taught what he or she needs to know, but can be "coached." A reflective educational environment is characterized by the following: people exchange information, there is an openness toward intellectual risk-taking, control is shared, there is a continuous flow of feedback (negative as well as positive), and the focus is on the ongoing process of learning.

Imagine yourself at the first day of a piano class. You have heard other people playing, and think this might be something you would like. So, why not give it a try? You register and meet the instructor. She plays a few songs, and after watching her, you wonder, "How does she do that so smoothly?" You begin to doubt if you will be able to complete the class, but still, you try. She explains all the notes, and counts out the music for you. It takes all of your energy just to watch, listen, and follow her directions. You try really hard to reproduce her moves exactly. You concentrate so much on which fingers to use, and which keys to play and in which sequence, that the activity lacks your own style. You are so focused on playing the correct notes that you are not even aware of what your classmates are really doing, even though they are just as intense in learning the same piece of music. You notice especially that you have problems when the tempo changes or the instructor leaves the room. "Wait a minute," you say to yourself, "How come that combination of notes doesn't sound the same when she changes the tempo of the music? How do I know when the music calls for this combination of notes at this rhythm and when it doesn't?"

Just as with music, a thought process guides our practice; for us, however, it is the thought process of clinical reasoning. When we first started playing the piano we focused on the actual combination of notes that made up the song (this is called *procedural reasoning*). These beginning steps are what seem most basic to us, and they are the easiest to follow. In a way, the combination of moves needed to play a song well can be compared to how well we use all of the knowledge that we've picked up in class and in our practice sessions. We have learned the steps of an assessment, the steps involved in formulating a diagnosis, and those in developing an intervention plan. Sure, in time we become okay at playing; but our moves are limited, even after graduation. We continue to have difficulty deciding which set of notes and rhythms go with which piece of music, and we struggle when the tempo or complexity of the music changes unexpectedly.

Suddenly, when we get into practice, the music changes, even more than ever happened in music class. We also have less time to think about what keys to play. We find that the tempo stays pretty much the same for two different songs, but the music sounds distinctly unique—like when we have two patients with identical diagnoses, but with whom our interactions and the intervention plans we develop are completely different.

With time and practice, we begin to recognize and accommodate for changes. We begin to feel more comfortable with the variety of decisions we make. As we concentrate less on the combination of notes, we suddenly become better able to interact with our classmates, not to mention our patients (this we call *interactive reasoning*). We actually begin to understand what "music" our patients enjoy and need, and what motivates him or her to be part of our music class. Or, perhaps, it is more appropriate to say that we become part of our patient's routine.

Expert health care providers are much like expert pianists. They are unaware of how many times they changed the notes, and may not realize that they were planning to play a piece in B-flat, and then at the last minute decided to play in the key of F. They are able to integrate available information and quickly know what to do. If any part of the program changes, they are able to quickly make accommodations. They may even think a lot of their moves are "common sense" and "logical," and may not even realize that they have moved on from novice player to "expert" pianist.

Clinical reasoning is also a way of perceiving. In simple terms, clinical reasoning is composed of the thinking and decision-making processes integral to clinical practice. However, clinical reasoning also results from a complex interplay of many factors including contextual and disciplinary parameters, emotions, knowledge, experience, cognitive skills, and personal frames of reference. Clinical reasoning is not separate from clinical practice; in fact, thought (i.e., the clinical reasoning) and action (i.e., clinical practice) are interdependent and intradependent. Moreover, clinical reasoning is not just about better meeting patient needs through quality care, but rather it refers to the clinical reasoning and actions required of health care providers to effectively provide care to our patients within a particular organizational and health care culture.

Another way to think about clinical reasoning is to compare it to "clinical jazz." Like jazz musicians who improvise melodies and the rhythms to make music, professionals must first take time to practice and study—and then go one step further. Pharmacology offers treatment options and skills, but how they are put together to make good music (i.e., good care) depends on the situation, what else is happening, patient preference, experience, and so on. Furthermore, like musical talent, some clinical reasoning ability is inborn, that is, talent for the practice of medicine.

Clinical reasoning requires more than technical skills or knowledge; it demands the ability to identify the assumptions underlying beliefs, values, and attitudes. It involves considerations about which action is appropriate in a particular situation, with one patient and at one point in time. So, by definition, clinical reasoning is a process of thinking, reflecting, and decision making that is grounded in patient interactions. Vital to talking about how health care providers think is understanding *how* they think; *what* they perceive when they view their patients; *what* they identify as the central problem and what information they choose to ignore; *how* they describe what is physiologically problematic; and even their view of *who* the patient is as a person.

The model used in this text provides a framework for clinical reasoning in pharmacotherapeutics (Fig. 2-1). The clinical chapters delineate the expected requisite drug information and then apply clinical reasoning analyses through a series of case studies. The model's basic purpose is to provide focus, factoring in some information as germane to the drug choice and ruling other information out as less important to patient outcomes.

The utility of the model comes from the systematic organization it provides for thinking, observing, and analyzing treatment regimens. In addition, it gives structure for and the rationale behind specific activities, as well as a mechanism for professional accountability. The model also offers general criteria for knowing when a patient's problem has been solved. It is important, however, to mention a few terms that are commonly misunderstood and misused, but that are relevant in considering drug regimens (Box 2-1).

Treatment Objectives

The first step of clinical reasoning is to develop treatment objectives based on all available patient and drug information. Treatment objectives are influenced by the severity, urgency, and prognosis of the disease. Prevention, cure, alleviation, and palliation therapies are interrelated and interdependent, in many instances. Drugs may be prescribed to accomplish any or all of these objectives, after a complete drug history is obtained (Table 2-2).

▮▮ Prevention

Primary preventive health behaviors are most commonly viewed as voluntary actions taken to decrease the threat of illness. Actions taken with this objective in mind are not curative or restorative because they occur before symptoms appear. Identification and correction of precipitating factors constitutes an important component of preventive regimens. Primary prevention measures such as proper diet, exercise, and immunizations help to avert a specific disease or illness.

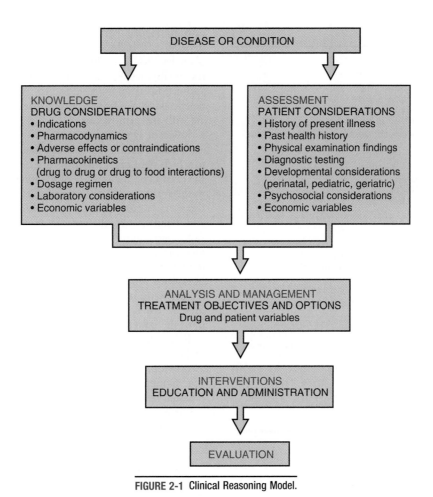

FIGURE 2-1 Clinical Reasoning Model.

BOX 2-1

Commonly Misused Word Pairs

Patient: The person cared for by the physician, nurse, or other health care provider	*versus*	**Case:** Not a patient but an episode or example of illness, injury, or asymptomatic disease
Effect: The result of an action; or to bring about or to cause to come into being	*versus*	**Affect:** The sum of feelings that accompany a mental state; the appearance of emotion or mood
Incidence: The number of cases developing in a specific unit of population in a specific time	*versus*	**Prevalence:** The number of cases existing in a specific unit of the population at a specific time
Sign: Any objective evidence of disease or dysfunction, an observable physical phenomenon frequently associated with a given condition	*versus*	**Symptom:** An indication of disease or illness perceived by the patient
Management: The process of controlling how something is done or used; a more active process	*versus*	**Planning:** Consciously setting forth a scheme to achieve a desired end or goal; applies to overall management of a disorder for which a drug is used and much less to the drug itself
Dosage: The amount of drug taken or given in a period; the total amount	*versus*	**Dose:** The amount of drug to be taken or given at one time; the sum of the doses may be dosage or total dose

---

Ensure that the patient has the knowledge necessary to make an informed decision. Explaining the consequences of the disease for which a patient is at risk and providing information about how to reduce vulnerability to the disease are vital components. Awareness of stigma, celebrity endorsement, and peer pressure have been used in some situations to promote preventive health behaviors.

Immunizations are a deliberate attempt to protect the individual against certain diseases. Antigenic stimulation is produced either by having the disease, or through inoculation with a vaccine. Active immunity is achieved by the person developing antibodies to a particular antigen of a disease. Passive immunity is acquired in utero from antibodies that pass from the mother through the placenta to the fetus, or that

---

TABLE 2-2 Drug History

PRESCRIPTION AND OTHER DRUG USE
- Prescription drugs used to treat illness or disease
- Self-prescribed drugs (over-the-counter drugs)
- Street drug use, borrowed prescriptions, home or folk remedies that include herbal preparations, use of obsolete prescriptions
- Caffeine use, smoking history
- Drugs prescribed by other providers that may be unknown to current care health care provider

RESPONSES TO DRUG USE
- Therapeutic responses to drugs used in the past
- Side effects, adverse drug reactions
- Idiosyncratic, paradoxic reactions
- Allergic reactions
- Tolerance and dependence

ATTITUDES TOWARD DRUG USE
- Attitudes toward drugs and reasons for use and chosen route
- Compliance with use or with any special monitoring required
- Placebo effects that may have occurred
- Knowledge of drug-drug and drug-food interactions
- Educational level (impact on current health status and future planned drug regimens)

CLINICAL REASONING
- Identify contraindications to drug use or factors warranting cautious use of a drug
- Determine the patient's risk for undesirable reactions
- Determine physiologic and psychologic response to previous drug use
- Use information in database to identify potential problems with planned regimen
- Identify factors affecting administration or adherence, or both

---

are acquired by the newborn through breastfeeding. Passive immunity may also be produced by injecting antibodies. Drugs used to cause active and passive immunity are discussed further in Chapter 31.

▥ Cure

Three sets of criteria are used in identifying a disease in the traditional biologic perspective of health and illness: (1) the patient's subjective experience of illness; (2) the finding (e.g., by laboratory tests) that the patient has some disorder of body system or function; and (3) symptoms are noted that form an identifiable pattern that meets diagnostic criteria. In other words, the person is said to be ill or diseased when patient complaints, signs and symptoms, or results of laboratory testing and physical exam fit a particular model or pattern of disease.

In one sense, illness is viewed as the body's attempt to adapt to internal and external stressors and noxious conditions. The signs and symptoms that result, when they are sufficiently disturbing or intense, tend to draw attention to bodily functions. There may be apprehension about minor alterations in body function that in health would go unnoticed. Unusual sensations act as stimuli to remind the patient of the illness or disease. Minor variations in temperature, pulse, digestion, or elimination take on particular importance. Relief of the alterations begins to take precedence over other needs.

However, for an individual to function in the sick role, those around him or her must perceive the illness. The classic components of the sick role (a social phenomenon that

disrupts regular patterns of living) were defined by Parsons in 1958 and include the right of the individual to be held blameless for the illness and to be released from routine responsibilities. Further, the patient has a duty to view illness and disease as undesirable and to try to get well, to seek competent assistance from a health care provider, and to cooperate with the plan of care.

Relief of signs and symptoms as well as curing the illness, are usually priority concerns for patients. However, the extent to which signs and symptoms can be relieved is dependent on the extent and the severity of the illness or disease. Drugs used in the treatment of disease and illness may be organized into three major groups: replacement therapy, supportive therapy, and maintenance therapy, or a combination of all three. *Replacement drug therapies* are appropriate when there is an identifiable deficiency and may be short- or long-term in nature. For example, a patient who has a deficiency of thyroid hormones requires lifelong supplemental thyroid hormone replacement. In contrast, ferrous sulfate is an iron preparation used in the short-term treatment of iron deficiency anemia until the patient's own iron reserves are replenished.

Relieving signs and symptoms of illness or disease also includes psychologic as well as physical interventions such as providing reassurance, limiting activity, or providing oxygen. Symptomatic illness management may require lifestyle redesign in some cases. For example, a patient with ulcerative colitis may elect to go only to events in locations where the restrooms are nearby.

▥ Alleviation

On the other hand, *supportive drug therapies* may be required when a certain illness threatens other body systems. Drugs may be used until the primary condition is alleviated or under control. For example, a patient hospitalized for treatment of an acute myocardial infarction may require a histamine$_2$ antagonist such as famotidine to minimize the potential for stress-related duodenal ulcers.

Supportive therapies may be used for patients who have chronic or long-term conditions. The objective of supportive therapy is to maintain a patient's level of wellness while halting further progression of the disease. For example, essential hypertension is not curable. However, it can be managed effectively with a variety of drugs and through lifestyle modification. A postmenopausal woman uses calcium supplements and hormones to prevent or minimize the debilitating effects of osteoporosis.

Drugs that are used for a specific disease or condition may be many and varied or limited. The most appropriate treatment regimen takes into account the specific characteristics of the drug and patient variables that relate to adherence, the benefits and risks of using a particular drug, serum drug levels desired, concerns related to toxicity, dosing frequency and, last but not least, the cost. At times, the identification and correction of precipitating factors may require drug therapy, surgery, or other interventions. For example, a patient with heart failure may require antiarrhythmic drugs to treat cardiac irregularities, surgery to correct a preexisting valvular dysfunction, or thrombolytic drugs to treat an ischemic problem. In this example, the drugs are used as a secondary intervention, because several other pathologic processes are present.

Palliation

The Latin *pallium* referred to a type of cloak worn in ancient Greece and Rome and, later, to a white woolen band with pendants in front and back worn by the pope or an archbishop as a symbol of full episcopal authority. Pallium was modified to form the English "palliate," an adjective meaning "cloaked" or "concealed," and a verb meaning "to cloak," "to clothe," or "to shelter." Today the term *palliation* or *palliative care* is defined as the following:

- Active total care of patients whose disease is not responsive to curative treatment. Control of pain, of other symptoms, and of psychologic, social, and spiritual problems, is paramount. The goal of palliative care is achievement of the best quality of life for patients and their families (World Health Organization).
- Active compassionate care of the chronically and terminally ill, primarily directed towards improving the quality of life at a time when the goal is not cure. The emphasis of palliative care is on the control of pain and symptoms, and meeting physical, emotional, spiritual, social, and cultural needs (Palliative Care Institute).

Treatment Options

Patient Variables

It is important to recognize that the locus of decision making includes both the patient and the family. Decision making about care should not be a unilateral process. Initial drug regimens are chosen from a variety of reasonable alternatives. Also note that reasonable alternatives and adjuncts include non–drug therapies. Specific interventions are directed at resolving or preventing problems identified in the analysis.

There are several considerations to take into account when considering a particular drug regimen. Acknowledge that there are risks inherent in every potentially beneficial therapy. Will possibly adverse effects compromise an already stressed cardiovascular, respiratory, renal, or hepatic system? Will the drug alter the patient's mental status to such an extent that it increases the possibility of injury or dependence on others? Do adverse effects of a drug include the possibility of bladder or bowel incontinence which, in turn, may cause a loss of dignity? Consider the patient's unique set of circumstances when weighing the benefits and risks of a particular drug regimen. Also, analyze the likelihood of patient adherence and, at times, the cost of the therapy.

Drug Variables

Whether a drug is useful depends on its ability to produce only the desired effects, with tolerable undesired effects. Thus, from the viewpoint of drug indications, the selectivity of effects is one of the most important characteristics. (*Selectivity* is the ability of a drug to act at specific sites to produce an action, when at the same time the presence of the drug at other sites does not lead to any measurable response.) Selectivity may be inherent to a drug product based on its affinity for a tissue or receptor type. Selectivity can also be influenced or manipulated to the advantage of patients by altering routes of administration or pharmaceutical dosage form. There are also a multitude of factors that influence the decision to use a particular drug regimen. The "STEPS" mnemonic (Preskorn,

1994) helps to organize drug information by level of importance, whether it means searching for reports on MEDLINE, prioritizing reading, or sitting with a patient to decide which treatment to use or drug to prescribe:

S–Safety
T–Tolerability
E–Efficacy
P–Price
S–Simplicity of use

SAFETY. The therapeutic value of the drug is weighed against its inherent risks (i.e., risk-benefit ratio). Historically, this risk-benefit ratio has been determined by the health care provider. Patients who take an active role in their treatment regimen have an increased understanding of their health care needs and the health care system. The seriousness of the disease or illness and the availability of less toxic, more reliable drugs are still taken into consideration.

TOLERABILITY. In part, the drug variables affecting patient tolerability to a drug include (1) the drug's potency (i.e., the absolute amount of drug required to produce a desired effect); (2) the therapeutic index, or the ratio of effective dose to lethal dose (i.e., a smaller therapeutic index infers a drug is relatively more likely to produce toxicity at near-therapeutic doses); (3) maximum effect, or the greatest response possible regardless of the dose given; (4) latency, or the time necessary for the onset of therapeutic effects; (5) peak, or the time it takes for drug effects to reach maximum; and (6) duration of action, or the length of time the drug is effective. Chapters 4 and 5 discuss these variables and more.

EFFICACY. How well does the drug work? In general, efficacy is the ability to produce an effect, usually a specifically desired effect. For example, an efficacious vaccine has the ability to prevent or cure a specific illness.

PRICE. The fundamental objective of managed care is to maximize the quality of care while minimizing costs. Cost limitations are increasing, and cost-effectiveness has become a more critical issue in the day-to-day treatment of patients.

SIMPLICITY OF USE. Drugs can be of great value, particularly when they are taken correctly. Successful therapy requires informed and active patient participation. Therefore, knowledge of the degree to which a patient will follow through with a planned drug regimen influences not only the drug that is ordered but also the dosing, the frequency, and the route of administration. An example is when there is a choice between prescribing two drugs with similar adverse effects but different regimens, such as oral cimetidine 4 times a day, or ranitidine 2 times a day; the twice-daily regimen is more likely to promote adherence. This is particularly true if the patient does not like taking pills or cannot remember to take them at all.

Patient Education

The objective of patient education is to assist the individual to incorporate health-related behaviors into everyday life. The prevention of treatment-associated morbidity, such as might occur if a patient does not take a medication as prescribed, are also important goals of patient education. The void between a patient's knowledge level and what information is needed for adherence is referred to as a *learning deficit*. In order to reduce adverse drug effects, the patient must have knowledge of certain things: the drug's major effects, the time when these reactions are likely to occur, and early signs that a reaction is taking place. Measures used to reduce adverse drug effects include identifying the high-risk patient by obtaining a patient history, ensuring proper administration through patient education, and advising the patient about activities that may precipitate an adverse reaction. Patient education is seen as vital to the successful outcome of drug therapy (see Chapter 9). By educating the patient about the drugs being taken, the health care provider elicits the required level of participation. It is also important to remember that some patients are at an increased risk for nonadherence and may benefit from patient education with ongoing reinforcement: those with conditions that may often be asymptomatic (e.g., hypertension), patients with concurrent medical and mental illness, patients on multiple medications, and older patients.

A large amount of time can be spent in teaching-learning activities as they relate to drug therapies. Adherence is best achieved when both verbal and written information is presented at the appropriate level of understanding. Poor understanding of verbal instructions and written materials remains a major factor in failure to achieve treatment objectives. Further, patients vary greatly in their ability to hear, read, and translate verbal language and written instructions into a meaningful whole. Pay attention to the patient's reading and comprehension abilities.

Evaluation

Evaluation of patient response is an important aspect of drug therapy. After all, evaluation is the process that tells us if the drug therapy worked. Evaluation of patient response is organized around the therapeutic response, adverse effects, accurate self-administration and adherence with therapy, and the patient's satisfaction with prescribed therapy. Evaluating patient response to a drug with more than one application requires that the health care provider know the specific reason the drug is being used.

Evaluation of therapeutic response is accomplished by monitoring physiologic parameters (e.g., vital signs, resolution of infection, serum or urine drug levels, body weight, and serum and urine chemistry values). For example, blood pressure should be monitored for reduction in systolic and diastolic pressures in the patient taking the calcium channel blocker diltiazem to treat hypertension. In contrast, when the same drug is used to treat angina, the patient should be evaluated for decreasing chest pain. Thus knowing the purpose of the drug helps guide the evaluation process. When beneficial responses develop as hoped, ignorance of expected adverse effects might not be so bad. However, when desired responses do not occur, it is essential to identify the situation early, because intervention with an alternative therapy may be needed.

Evaluate any secondary or adverse effects. The responses may be predictable (i.e., dose-related) or unpredictable (i.e., patient sensitivity–related). Dose-related responses result from unknown pharmacologic effects of a drug. Sensitivity-related responses cannot be predicted or foreseen. An allergic reaction is an example of a sensitivity-related response that is unrelated to dosage. Adverse effects are discussed in Chapter 5.

Satisfaction with the treatment regimen is an important consideration that is often ignored or skimmed over when evaluating drug effectiveness. However, patient satisfaction is closely tied to adherence. Dissatisfaction may lead to nonadherence and failure of an otherwise adequate drug regimen. Dissatisfaction can be prevented if therapy is designed around the patient's lifestyle, resources and preferences, and health care needs. Hence patient and family involvement is a necessity.

Methods available to assess the degree of patient adherence and his or her satisfaction with the drug regimen may include pill counts, the review of a drug diary, self-reports, direct observation, assessment of physiologic parameters, and input from other health care workers, family members, or friends. Combining several methods provides for a more accurate assessment. Other assessment and intervention strategies to promote adherence are discussed in Chapter 9.

CONCEPTS AND PRINCIPLES OF PRESCRIBING

The drug order, or the prescription, is a means for communicating treatment plans between the health care provider and the pharmacist. However, even the most carefully written order or prescription becomes useless if it does not clearly communicate the drug regimen.

TYPES OF DRUG ORDERS

Although patients are free to treat themselves with any over-the-counter (OTC) drug available while at home, once they are admitted to a clinical agency, a written drug order is required. A *drug order* is written on an inpatient order sheet found in the patient's medical record. It is filled by the agency's pharmacy or a contract pharmacy. A *prescription* blank is used when patients are discharged and for patients in outpatient or clinic settings. Although the process of ordering drugs has been computerized in recent years, the principles remain the same.

ESSENTIAL COMPONENTS OF DRUG ORDERS

There are several essential components in a drug order or prescription (Fig. 2-2), which are directly related to the "five rights" of drug administration: *right patient, right drug, right dose, right route, and right time.* Ensure that all components of the order are legible and clearly expressed. If there is doubt, the information must be clarified (Table 2-3).

Federal law does not require a particular format to be used when writing prescriptions, nor does it specifically identify what information to include. Some states may require that a prescription be displayed graphically in a specific manner and list a number of required elements.

Regulations for prescribing controlled substances are stringent, and there is additional information that must be included on the prescription blank. Some state laws require the patient's address, telephone number, and age, along with the health care provider's address and telephone number. Federal law requires that the health care provider's Drug Enforcement Administration (DEA) registration number be included for controlled substances. Some states require use of a duplicate or triplicate prescription blank for some or all controlled substances.

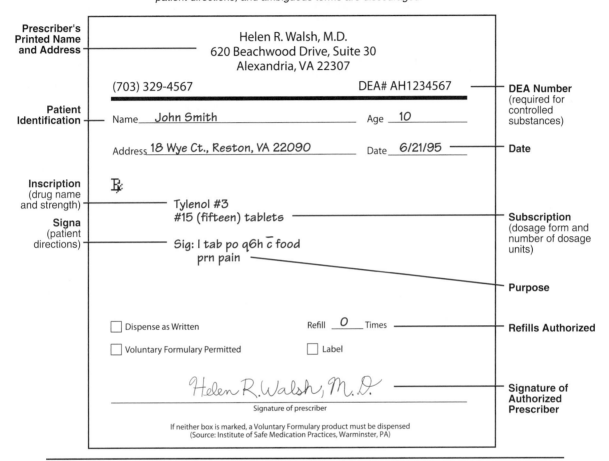

ANATOMY OF A PRESCRIPTION

States may vary in what they require on a prescription. This example was made up to show most types of possible information. Latin terms appear only in the patient directions, and ambiguous terms are discouraged.

Prescriber's Printed Name and Address

Helen R. Walsh, M.D.
620 Beachwood Drive, Suite 30
Alexandria, VA 22307

(703) 329-4567   DEA# AH1234567 — **DEA Number** (required for controlled substances)

Patient Identification — Name John Smith   Age 10

Address 18 Wye Ct., Reston, VA 22090   Date 6/21/95 — **Date**

Inscription (drug name and strength) — ℞

Tylenol #3
#15 (fifteen) tablets — **Subscription** (dosage form and number of dosage units)

Signa (patient directions) — Sig: 1 tab po q6h c̄ food
prn pain

— **Purpose**

☐ Dispense as Written   Refill 0 Times — **Refills Authorized**

☐ Voluntary Formulary Permitted   ☐ Label

Helen R. Walsh, M.D. — **Signature of Authorized Prescriber**
Signature of prescriber

If neither box is marked, a Voluntary Formulary product must be dispensed
(Source: Institute of Safe Medication Practices, Warminster, PA)

FIGURE 2-2 Anatomy of a Prescription. (From Farley, D. [1995]. Making it easier to read prescriptions. *FDA Consumer, 29*(6), 3–4.)

TABLE 2-3 Strategies for Preventing Prescribing Errors

Potential Problem with Drug Orders	Recommended Action
Unusually large dosage or excessive increase in dosage ordered	Check order with health care provider, pharmacist, or literature.
Drug form used in an unfamiliar fashion	
Single order contains more than one drug	
Ambiguous orders, drug names that include numerals	
Multiple tablets or several vials are necessary to prepare single dose	Check all dosage calculations with a peer.
Illegible, incomplete orders	Obtain clear copy of order.
Nonstandard abbreviations or symbols	
Slang names, colloquialisms	Avoid use when transcribing drug orders or writing notes or prescriptions.
Telephone and verbal orders	Do not take or give a telephone or verbal order except in an emergency.
First time patient has taken drug	Read package insert carefully. Double-check for patient allergies.
New drug is added to drug regimen	Check for drug interactions. Commit common interactions to memory.

PRESCRIPTION WRITING

Latin served a worthwhile purpose when it was used, in the 1400s, to write entire prescriptions. Today, Latin still appears in the directions for taking a drug (e.g., *Sig*). On some prescriptions the abbreviation R_x is used; it is Latin for recipe. The cross at the end of the R has been explained as a substitute period. Although the terms *signa* (write) and *signetur* (let it be labeled) are still commonly used (Table 2-4).

TABLE 2-4 The Joint Commission* Official "Do Not Use" List

Do Not Use[†]	Potential Problem	Use Instead
U (unit)	Mistaken for "0"(zero), "4," or "cc"	Write "unit"
IU (International unit)	Mistaken for IV or the number 10	Write "international unit"
Q.D., QD, q.d., qd (daily)	Mistaken for each other	Write "daily"
Q.O.D., QOD, q.o.d, qod	Period after the Q mistaken for "I"	Write "every other day"
Trailing zero (X.0 mg)[‡]	Decimal point can be missed	Write X mg
Lack of leading zero (.X mg)	Decimal point can be missed	Write 0.X mg
MS, MSO_4, $MgSO_4$	Confused for one another	Write "morphine sulfate"
	Can mean morphine sulfate or magnesium sulfate	Write "magnesium sulfate"
ADDITIONAL ABBREVIATIONS, ACRONYMS, AND SYMBOLS (FOR POSSIBLE FUTURE INCLUSION IN THE JOINT COMMISSION OFFICIAL "DO NOT USE" LIST)		
> (greater than)	Confused with each other	Write "greater than"
< (less than)	Mistaken for the number "7" or the letter "L"	Write "less than"
Abbreviations of drug names	Misinterpreted because of similar abbreviations for multiple drugs	Write drug names in full
Apothecary units (e.g., drams, grains)	Unfamiliar to many providers Confused with metric units (e.g., ml, mg)	Use metric units
@	Mistaken for the number "2"	Write "at"
cc	Mistaken for U (units) if poorly written	Write "mL" or "milliliters"
μg	Mistaken for milligrams (mg) resulting in 1000-fold overdose	Write "mcg" or "micrograms"

*The Joint Commission was formerly the Joint Commission on Accreditation of Healthcare Organizations (JCAHO).
†Applies to all orders and all drug-related documentation that are handwritten (including free-text computer entry) or on preprinted forms.
‡*Exception:* A "trailing zero" may be used only where required to demonstrate the level precision of the value being reported, such as for laboratory results, imaging studies that report size of lesions, or catheter and tube sizes. It should not be used in drug orders or other drug-related documentation.

It is good practice to use one prescription pad at a time, securing the remaining pads in a safe location to reduce the possibility of theft. Never sign prescription blanks in advance. Before having prescription blanks printed, review state laws and the practical aspects of use. Consider the dimensions of the prescription blank, the amount of space available to write directions, the location of refill instructions and purpose of the drug, and spaces for names, signature or signatures, and DEA number.

Prescriptions may be written in ink, typewritten, or computer-generated, but they must be signed by the health care provider. Stamped signatures are not considered valid. Federal law mandates that erasable pens not be used to write or sign prescriptions for controlled substances. The ink in erasable pens does not become permanent for approximately 3 days. During this time, it is possible that prescription information could be altered without this being noticed.

In some states, only one drug may be written per prescription blank, and preprinted prescriptions may be forbidden. Preprinted blanks have the drug name, strength, amount, dosage, route, frequency, and use, or some combination of the above information, preprinted on the blank.

Federal law permits an authorized representative, usually a nurse or secretary, to prepare prescriptions (including those for controlled substances) for the health care provider's signature. The patient is not an authorized representative. Avoid ordering greater quantities of a drug than required. Authorized representatives must make sure that the prescription conforms in all essential aspects to the law and regulations. The pharmacist has an equal responsibility to make sure the prescription meets all federal as well as state requirements.

RECORD-KEEPING REQUIREMENTS

Each health care provider must maintain inventories and records of controlled substances listed in Schedules I and II separately from all other records maintained by the provider.

Likewise, inventory and records of controlled substances in Schedules III, IV, and V must be maintained separately or in such a form that they are readily retrievable from the ordinary business records of the health care provider. All records related to controlled substances must be maintained and available for inspection for a minimum of 2 years. Controlled drugs prescribed in the course of practice do not require specific record keeping of the transactions. However, they must be documented in patient records.

A health care provider who administers controlled substances as a part of his or her practice is required to keep records, particularly if patients are charged for the drugs either separately or with other patient services. Providers who dispense controlled substances and who administer the drug (from the same inventory) are also required to keep a record of all transactions. All records, including those for controlled substances, are maintained as part of a patient's file. The records must be made available to a duly authorized DEA official upon request.

Drug transaction records must document inventory of all stock on hand every 2 years. Specific requirements related to taking inventory are found in the 2006 *DEA Practitioner's Manual* available from a DEA field office or online at www.deadiversion.usdoj.gov/pubs/manuals/pract/index.html.

SUBSTITUTIONS

Most states have regulations specifying circumstances under which a pharmacist may substitute a generic drug or a different brand for the prescribed drug. The substitute must be the same chemical entity and must be in the same dosage form as specified in the original prescription. Information about therapeutic equivalencies is identified at the Center for Drug Evaluation and Research (CDER) website (www.fda.gov/cder/ob/default.htm) (Box 2-2). Many states use a formulary system to help in the selection process. Some formularies indicate which drug may be substituted, whereas other

---

BOX 2-2

FDA Therapeutic Equivalence (TE) Ratings

Ratings of Drugs Thought To Be Therapeutically Equivalent Begin with "A"

AA	Products in conventional dosage forms not presenting bioequivalence problems
AB	Products meeting necessary bioequivalence requirements (branded generic drugs)
AN	Solutions and powders for aerosolization
AO	Injectable oil solutions
AP	Injectable aqueous solutions and, in some cases, IV nonaqueous solutions
AT	Topical products

Ratings of Drugs Thought To Be Not Therapeutically Equivalent Begin with "B"

BB	Products requiring further investigation by FDA to determine bioequivalence
BC	Extended-release dosage forms (i.e., capsules, injectables, tablets)
BD	Active ingredients and dosage forms with documented bioequivalence problems
BE	Delayed-release oral dosage forms
BN	Products in aerosol-nebulizer delivery systems
BP	Active ingredients and dosage forms with potential bioequivalence problems
BR	Suppositories or enemas that deliver drugs for systemic absorption
BS	Products having drug-standard deficiencies
BT	Topical products with bioequivalence problems
BX	Drugs for which the data are insufficient to determine therapeutic bioequivalence

FDA, Food and Drug Administration; *IV,* intravenous. Information from the U.S. Department of Health and Human Services FDA's Center for Drug Evaluation and Research (CDER), Office of Pharmaceutical Science, Office of Generic Drugs. *Approved Drug Products with Therapeutic Equivalence Evaluations,* the *"Electronic Orange Book 2006."* Available online: www.fda.gov/cder/ob/default.htm. Accessed February 1, 2007.

---

state formularies may indicate which drug may not be substituted. Review individual state laws. The substitution must be authorized by the health care provider through a variety of means. Authorization is usually noted through a specific statement or abbreviation, such as "dispense as written" (DAW) or "prescribed brand only" (PBO) at the bottom of the prescription.

PRESCRIPTION REFILLS

Always indicate clearly whether a prescription may be refilled. Prescriptions are refilled when authorized on the original prescription or through a verbal order. The most effective method for identifying refills is to indicate a specific number of times it may be refilled. It can be as simple as filling in a blank (e.g., Refill: *2* times), or a series of numbers that can be circled to indicate the refills (e.g., Refill: 0 1 2 3). The absence of refill instructions means that no refills are permitted.

The Food and Drug Administration (FDA) generally discourages the use of the designation "refill PRN") ("as circumstances require," or, as needed) since it is not up to the pharmacist to determine the number of times a prescription is to be refilled. A variation on the PRN theme (e.g., PRN–6 months) may be occasionally seen. In this case, a limit to the number of refills exists. Lifetime refills are unsafe and pointless. In addition, the FDA directs that a prescription is no longer valid when the relationship with the patient is severed, as at the death of the health care provider.

The Durham-Humphrey Amendment (Table 1-4, p. 6) permits pharmacists to take refill orders by telephone for noncontrolled drugs, as well as for controlled substances on

Schedules III and IV. The order must be authorized by the health care provider or a legally authorized representative and recorded by the pharmacist. Because the health care provider cannot delegate decision-making authority to others, the legally authorized representative may only relay the instructions to the pharmacist.

EXPIRED PRESCRIPTIONS

Federal law does not stipulate that a prescription be filled within a specified period after it is written. Some states, however, have established time limits, especially for controlled substances. For example, New York pharmacists will fill a prescription for controlled substances within 30 days of its being written. The pharmacist should question the person who presents a prescription after an extended period since it was written, and the health care provider should be concerned. Encourage patients to have all prescriptions filled within a reasonable time period.

PRESCRIPTION LABELING

Explicit labeling requirements have been established by the Federal Food, Drug, and Cosmetic Act (FFDCA), the Controlled Substances Act, and various state acts. Prescription labels generally include the name and address of the pharmacy, the prescription number, the date the prescription was filled or refilled, and any caution or warning statements, in addition to essential drug components. Information such as the dispensing pharmacist's name or initials, lot numbers, expiration dates, the name of the manufacturer or distributor, and the telephone number for the pharmacy may be required. For controlled substances, caution and warning statements must be included, along with the following federal warning statement for drugs in Schedules I to IV: *"Caution: Federal law prohibits the transfer of this drug to any person other than the patient for whom it was prescribed."*

Some states, such as New York, require a specific label color for controlled substances. Texas law requires that all prescriptions include the intended use of the drug (e.g., for pain), unless the health care provider decides this inclusion is not in the patient's best interest.

PRESCRIPTION COPIES

Patients have the right to request a copy of their prescriptions. However, copies have no legal status and cannot be filled or refilled. Mark copies with a statement such as "Copy–For Information Purposes Only" before giving it to the patient. Without standard consensus on the use of this statement on the prescription copy, there is no guarantee that any other prescription is factual and genuine, and that the prescription has not been filled previously by other pharmacies. There is also no way to absolutely prevent a copy of the prescription from being recognized for the remaining refills. Pharmacists presented with a copy of a prescription should contact the health care provider for authorization to fill or refill the prescription.

OUT-OF-STATE PRESCRIPTIONS

Health care providers may legally write prescriptions only in the states in which they are licensed to practice. A health care provider licensed in at least one state but employed in a federal institution may have prescriptive authority in any federal facility. Nevertheless, whether a pharmacist will fill a prescription written by a health care provider licensed in another state depends on state laws. There is no federal requirement that the prescription be filled in the state in which the health care provider is licensed. The prescription must be valid in the location where it was written.

DRUG SAMPLES

A 1987 amendment to the FFDCA, the Prescription Drug Marketing Act, defines a sample as a drug unit that is not intended for sale, but that is distributed to promote drug sales. Health care providers who receive drug samples have provided a written request to the manufacturer or distributor. A written receipt for the samples must be returned to the manufacturer or distributor.

KEY POINTS

- A variety of health care providers are included in pharmacotherapeutics: physicians and dentists, advanced practice nurses, physician assistants, pharmacologists and pharmacists, pharmacy technicians, and registered respiratory therapists.
- Requisite drug knowledge includes indications, pharmacodynamics, adverse effects and contraindications, pharmacokinetics, dosage regimens, lab considerations, and economic variables.
- Management involves the development of treatment objectives and consideration of treatment options.

- Evaluation of patient response is ongoing. It is organized around therapeutic response, secondary or adverse effects, adherence and accurate self-administration, and the patient's satisfaction with prescribed therapy.
- Patient satisfaction with the prescribed drug regimen promotes adherence with the treatment plan and increases the quality of life in the long term.

Bibliography

Boreham, N., Mawer, G., and Foster, R. (2000). Medical student's errors in pharmacotherapeutics. *Medical Education, 34*(3), 188–193.

Gutierrez, K., and Sciacca, S. (2000). Prescribing behaviors of Colorado advanced practice nurses. *Nurse Practitioner: The American Journal of Primary Health Care, 25*(11), 14–15.

Mantzoukas, S., and Jasper, M. (2005). Reflective practice and daily ward reality: A covert power game. *Journal of Clinical Nursing, 13* (8), 925–933.

Moody, N., Smith P., and Glenn, U. (1999). Client characteristics and practice patterns of nurse practitioners and physicians. *Nurse Practitioner: The American Journal of Primary Health Care, 24*(3), 94–103.

Drug Enforcement Administration. (2006). *Physician's manual.* Washington, DC: Drug Enforcement Administration. Available online: www.deadiversion.usdoj.gov/pubs/manuals/index.html. Accessed February 1, 2006.

Offredy, M., and Townsend, J. (2000). Nurse practitioners in primary care. *Family Practice, 17*(6), 564–569.

Orlander, J., Barber, W., and Fincke, B. (2002). The morbidity and mortality conference: The delicate nature of learning from error. *Academic Medicine: Journal of the Association of American Medical Colleges, 7*(10), 1001–1006.

Mount Sinai School of Medicine. The Lilian and Benjamin Hertzberg Palliative Care Institute. Available online: www.mssm.edu/palliative/. Accessed February 1, 2007.

Parsons, T. (1958). Definitions of health and illness in light of American values and social structure. In E. Jaco, ed. *Patients, physicians, and illness.* New York: The Free Press.

Pearson, L. (2006). The Pearson Report: Part I: Alabama to Michigan. *The American Journal of Nurse Practitioners, 10*(1), entire issue.

Pearson, L. (2006). The Pearson Report: Part II: Minnesota to Wyoming. *The American Journal of Nurse Practitioners, 10*(2), entire issue.

Preskorn, S. (1994). Antidepressant drug selection: criteria and options. *Journal of Clinical Psychiatry, 55*(Suppl A), 6–22, 23–24, 98–100.

Pulcini, J., and Vampola, D. (2002). Tracking NP prescribing trends. *The Nurse Practitioner: The American Journal of Primary Health Care,* 7(10), 641–648.

Schon, D. (1993). *The reflective practitioner: How professionals think in action.* New York: Basic Books.

U.S. Congress, Office of Technology Assessment. (2003). Nurse practitioners, physician assistants, and certified nurse-midwives: A policy analysis. (Health Technology Case Study 37). OTA-HCS-37. Washington, DC: U.S. Government Printing office, December, 1986 (2003 update). Available online: www.wws.princeton.edu/ota/disk2/1986/8615. Accessed February 1, 2007.

World Health Organization. *Palliative care.* Available online: www.who.int/cancer/palliative/en/. Accessed February 1, 2007.

3

Pharmacoeconomics

The study of pharmacoeconomics sometimes resembles the story of the elephant and the blind men, in which each man formed a different belief as to what an elephant was overall according to what he felt when touching only one part of the animal. This chapter is an introduction to the subject; it offers the reader an opportunity to sample the variety and depth of this discipline while beginning to appreciate claims made by researchers in the field. Additional information about pharmacoeconomics is available from resources in the bibliography and through the International Society of Pharmacoeconomics and Outcomes Research.*

In the last decade, pharmacoeconomics has grown from relative obscurity to having a prominent role in the development and application of clinical pharmacology. This is because health care has dramatically changed over this period. Health care's guiding principle was once *"the best that money can buy,"* with little consideration of cost. When a health care provider believed a patient needed treatment, it was ordered and the responsible party paid the bill, whether it was the patient, the insurance company, Medicare, or Medicaid. Pharmaceutical companies even created new products in the belief that health care providers would use them even if the benefits were marginal or the number of adverse effects decreased. Pharmaceutical companies have marketed drugs with "clinically" marginal benefits; furthermore, this process is also supported by the FDA, which does not apply a cost-based analysis of new products seeking approval. Benefits that seem marginal to a health care provider may be statistically significant, and there are also benefits to competition in the market place.

Increasingly, though, the operating principle in health care has changed to *"the best we can afford."* Today's payors of health care services are demanding that new drugs demonstrate benefits worthy of the additional costs. At the same time, employers, insurance companies, and the government are strongly encouraging health care providers to consider the cost-effectiveness as well as the safety and efficacy of their treatment options. In response, pharmacy programs are offering courses and fellowships in pharmacoeconomics, and health science programs are including health care economics in their curricula. In some cases, however, a preferred provider organization (PPO) will develop a formulary of drugs that are indeed cheaper and that have been shown equally efficacious or beneficial, or even superior. Rebates and quick returns also influence formulary decisions. Indeed, it is estimated that

20% of the $400 to $500 million spent by industry to bring a new drug to market is directed toward its economic aspect.

PHILOSOPHICAL BASIS OF PHARMACOECONOMICS

Pharmacoeconomics is the description and analysis of the costs of drug therapy to health care systems and society. This field came about through analysis of the cost-benefit ratios of drugs compared with similar drugs or other therapies. The costs included both financial and quality-of-life measures. It is the means by which cost factors are incorporated into the clinical reasoning for drug therapy.

Cost limitations are increasing, and cost-effectiveness has become a more critical issue in the day-to-day treatment of patients. Pharmacoeconomics was initially concerned only with evaluating drug treatment. However, as the field matures, it is becoming apparent that a complete evaluation of illness treatment must include consideration of non–drug therapies. For example, a thorough analysis of the treatment for depression must include consideration not only of the various antidepressant drugs but also of psychotherapy, a possible adjunct to drug treatment. In keeping with that philosophy, this chapter discusses the evaluation of treatment options in general, not just of drug therapy, although the vast majority of treatment options are pharmaceuticals. There are multiple pharmacoeconomic models, but the important components are the economic, clinical, and humanistic outcomes associated with treatment (or lack of treatment); quality of life and cost are key. The application of pharmacoeconomic modeling to determine the impact of new drug development and reformulation (e.g., combination products) is also a key to the modeling.

Pharmacoeconomic analyses encompass two related but separate philosophies—resource allocation and increased efficiency and profitability. The first is primarily concerned with allocating health care resources between a variety of treatment choices. The second is concerned with increased efficiency of care.

RESOURCE ALLOCATION

In a society with limited resources, it is necessary to have methods that determine an economically feasible and reasonably fair way to allocate resources among the various alternatives. In the mid-1990s, U.S. spending for health care exceeded $1 trillion for the first time, and spending is growing 50% faster than the gross national product. Throughout the world, there are pressures on budgets as policymakers and the public begin to recognize that every dollar spent on health care is $1 no longer available for education, crime prevention, or improvement in the health care infrastructure. Further, much of what we now spend on care may not necessarily

---

*The International Society of Pharmacoeconomics and Outcomes Research; 3100 Princeton Pike, Building 3, Suite E; Lawrenceville, NJ 08648; USA; Tel: 1-609-219-0773; Fax: 1-609-219-0774; URL: www.ispor.org.

improve our health, but in reality yields only small improvements at exorbitant cost. Even the Food and Drug Administration (FDA) and Medicare drug discount plans (there are hundreds of them) do not use cost-effectiveness as a criterion for making what are, in essence, decisions about resource allocation.

The basic question behind allocations in health care has been: *Given a variety of treatment choices and limited resources, which options should we choose?* A common example is whether society is better off spending its limited resources on high-cost drugs that are marginally more effective or that have fewer adverse effects, or whether society would be better off spending its limited resources on existing, less expensive drugs. However, a cheaper therapeutic substitution does not always allow for greater access; it may just mean higher profit. The field of pharmacoeconomics has traditionally focused on society and its choices to provide an optimal mix of services to all patients.

Resource allocation has been the primary concern of government agencies, such as the Health Care Financing Agency, when determining which treatments to fund under Medicare, or the Agency for Health Care Policy and Research (AHCPR), when developing treatment guidelines. Drug companies generally use a policy-making approach when evaluating the cost-effectiveness of its products. Economic studies, on the other hand, are conducted to meet regulatory requirements of the FDA; to convince managed care organizations (MCOs) that their product is more cost-effective than a competitor's; or to determine the potential benefits of pursuing a new product through development or the reformulation of a product as a combination or new delivery formulation.

INCREASED EFFICIENCY

Although resource allocation is useful when determining whether to fund an expensive new treatment, this philosophy provides little guidance to a health care provider or managed care organization trying to determine the most efficient means of treating a patient. Whereas pharmacoeconomics helps determine the best allocation of resources across society, health care providers are concerned with how to treat patients, given that their illnesses must be treated and that there are competing treatments options. One could argue that health care providers want *effective care*, whereas *efficient care* is often driven by payors or the goal of making a profit.

An example might provide a clearer distinction between the philosophies of resource allocation and increased efficiency. It is generally agreed that in treating depression, there is little difference in the efficacy of the various drugs. The differences are in the level of adverse effects and adverse outcomes. One question facing an organization is whether it should pay the additional cost of newer antidepressants that appear to have fewer adverse effects or continue to pay for older drugs that are just as effective, but which have potentially greater adverse effects. One way to answer this question is to conduct a pharmacoeconomic study to determine whether the marginal benefit to be gained by using a new drug is greater than the marginal cost of using an older drug. The answer suggests to the organization how to allocate its limited resources between the various antidepressant drugs.

Yet at the same time, the result of such a study is of little benefit to the health care provider who must choose, from over 20 different drug treatment options and psychotherapy, the option that will best treat the patient for the least total cost. Instead, it is necessary to assess all reasonable treatment options and compare them among each other to make the most efficient choice. Finally, it is possible that a new antidepressant can be cost-effective, from a resource allocation point of view, and still not be the best choice for treating the patient.

PHARMACOECONOMICS AND MANAGED CARE

The term *managed care* refers to an organized delivery system that links health care financing to the delivery of services (www.amso.com/terms.html). The fundamental objective of managed care is to maximize the quality of care while minimizing costs. The term *managed care organization* (MCO) came about in the 1980s to provide an umbrella concept for health management organizations (HMOs) and preferred provider organizations (PPOs), the provider delivery systems that contract with MCO health plans, and the techniques and models used by these organizations in coordinating the delivery of care. And yet, despite the speed at which MCOs are growing, there is no universally accepted definition of their mission, conceptual framework, or services, and a number of permutaions have appeared in the health insurance industry.

MCOs attempt to provide a seamless set of services that stress prevention and primary care. Still, the success of an MCO is based on the ability of the patient's health care provider to spend as little money as possible when providing patient care. This means that the numbers and types of services (e.g., radiologic and nuclear imaging studies) provided to patients must be inexpensive and limited; furthermore, the use of high-tech procedures (e.g., positron emission tomography [PET] scan), newer drugs (e.g., tumor necrosing factor drugs), and even hospitalizations must be carefully planned.

The origins of managed care are often traced back to Dr. Michael Shadid, frequently referred to as a managed care pioneer. In 1929, despite meeting resistance from the American Medical Association and other physicians, he was able to start a rural farmers' cooperative health plan in Elk City, Oklahoma. With help from the Oklahoma Farmers' Union, he succeeded in enrolling several hundred families. Dr. Shadid delivered patient care to these families for a predetermined fee. Also in 1929, Drs. Donald Ross and H. Clifford Loos agreed to provide health care for 2000 workers employed by the Los Angeles Department of Water and Power, as well as their families. Within 5 years, this physician-owned and physician-controlled group practice enrolled a total of 37,000 persons under a low cost prepayment plan.

During World War II, Henry Kaiser, whose name became synonymous with prepaid health care, set up medical programs on the West Coast to provide health services to workers in the shipyards and steel mills. He opened his prepaid health care plans to the public when the war ended with the belief that with prepaid health care plans he could offer cost-effective health care to millions of Americans at prices they could afford.

BOX 3-1

Managed Care Time Line

1917	Prepaid physician services for the lumber industry offered in Western clinic in Tacoma, Washington.
1929	The Baylor plan, a prepaid hospitalization plan, is established by Dr. Justin Ford Kimball at Baylor Hospital in Texas.; it is the first plan to use the Blue Cross logo. A prepaid medical clinic is started by Drs. Donald Ross and H. Clifford Loos for employees of Los Angeles Water and Power. Michael Shadid starts the Rural Farmers' Cooperative Health Plan in Elk City, Oklahoma.
1938	Henry J. Kaiser recruits Dr. Sidney Garfield to establish prepaid clinic and hospital care for his Grand Coulee Dam project in Washington.
1945	Permanente Health Plans opens to the public in California, in addition to serving Kaiser employees.
1973	HMO Act of 1973 is signed into law by President Richard Nixon; it uses federal funds and policy to promote HMOs.
1985	National enrollment in HMOs reaches 19.1 million.
1990	National Committee for Quality Assurance (NCQA) is established.
1991	Health Plan Employer Data and Information Set (HEDIS) 1.0 is released.
1995	National enrollment in HMOs reaches 50.6 million.
1999	National enrollment in HMOs reaches 81.3 million
2000	National enrollment in HMOs declines for the first time, to 80.9 million.
2003	The Medicare Modernization Act establishes health savings accounts, increases payment rates to Medicare Advantage plans, establishes health savings accounts (HSAs), changes the name of Medicare+Choice program to Medicare Advantage, and establishes Part D drug benefit plan.
2004	National enrollment in HMOs is 68.8; national enrollment in PPOs is 109 million.

HMO, Health maintenance organization; *PPO,* participating provider organization.
Adapted from "TimeLine," Managed Care Museum, MCOL, Modesto, CA. Reprinted with permission from MCOL (www.mcol.com) as published in the Managed Care Museum website: www.managedcaremuseum.com. Accessed February 6, 2007.

These prepaid group practices were models for later entities that became known as health maintenance organizations (HMOs) (Box 3-1). HMOs accept responsibility for a specific set of health care benefits offered to patients and provide those benefits through a network of health care providers and hospitals. The limited data that are available suggest that disease state management (DSM) decreases total cost of care because DSM uses Medicare as a basis, which most likely drives profitability downward.

PERSPECTIVES

In attempting to understand pharmacoeconomic concepts and especially when evaluating pharmacoeconomic claims, the single most important issue is *perspective*. Broadly speaking, perspective relates to the focus and orientation of an analysis. The analysis, treatment options, costs, and values chosen for the analysis depend on perspective. For example, a societal perspective could use the average wholesale price of a drug in an analysis. On the other hand, a payor perspective may use the actual cost of that drug to that payor. This is important, because a real difference between the two costs dramatically changes the results and, therefore, the determination of the most cost-effective treatment. It is not uncommon for two separate analyses to reach different conclusions because of diverging perspectives. As will become apparent, there is no correct perspective. Like the approaches to pharmacoeconomic analysis, each perspective has its own advantages and disadvantages.

SOCIETY

From this perspective, the costs and values of treatment are based on the interests of society as a whole. This is because of the early influence of health economics research and the interest of governmental policy-making bodies in regulating and allocating resources across sometimes competing societal interests. It is also the most commonly used type of perspective because pharmaceutical firms try to satisfy the FDA, which, as a governmental regulatory body, tends to favor a societal perspective.

A strong argument can be made that the societal perspective is the only one to use in pharmacoeconomic analyses because it takes into consideration the well-being of all members of society. On the other hand, society is made up of many different values and interests, and it is not always possible to determine which costs and values best reflect the interests of all members. In addition, the societal perspective does not take into account the particular interests and circumstances of individual organizations. In an effort to find a common denominator, the societal perspective could produce results that are not in the best interest of an organization or its patients.

PAYOR

Because this perspective begins with a specific organization and uses its costs as the basis for analysis, it can determine the most cost-effective and efficient treatment choice. Nevertheless, because the costs and values are specific to that organization, it is often difficult to generalize the results to other organizations unless their costs and values are similar, something that is not always true. For example, the cost to a payor (e.g., Blue Cross/Blue Shield or Medicare) equals the charges that are allowed by that payor. This perspective has historically not been used to any great extent, although it is gaining favor as payors demand pharmacoeconomic analyses relevant to their organizations.

HEALTH CARE PROVIDER

The perspective of the health care provider has traditionally focused less on the cost differences between treatment options and more on the differences in effectiveness. This perspective reflects the traditional role of the health care provider as patient advocate. However, this perspective is often closely aligned with the payor perspective, especially when the values of the providers coincide with the interests of MCOs. To determine the provider's cost, it is often necessary to carry out cost-finding exercises using techniques developed by accountants and industrial engineers (e.g., time and motion studies). An example is to calculate the savings to a hospital gained by changing a drug that requires multiple daily doses to a drug that requires once-daily dosing. Studies have looked at the cost savings that result from reducing the need for nursing time, equipment, and so on that accompany multiple daily dose infusions as opposed to once-daily intravenous (IV) or oral drug regimens.

PATIENT

The patient's perspective has occasionally been used in pharmacoeconomic analyses, and a persuasive argument can be made that it should be used more often. Unfortunately, this argument suffers from three major faults. First, there may be significant differences in perspective between various individuals' or groups' interests. Should the interests of patients whose diseases are uncommon be given a lower priority because their disorders are not as prevalent as others? Second, owing to insurance coverage, many patients are divorced from paying directly for the health care resources they consume. This distorts their awareness of the true ratio of costs to benefits. And finally, by its very nature, pharmacoeconomics is population-based rather than individual-based, although this perspective is changing rapidly. There continues to be an inherent conflict between what is in the best interest of the individual and what is in the best interest of a population of patients.

PHARMACOECONOMICS STUDY DESIGNS

There are four basic pharmacoeconomics study designs: (1) cost-benefit analysis; (2) cost-effectiveness analysis; (3) cost-utility analysis; and (4) cost-minimization analysis. Each of these approaches measures costs in dollars, but each measures outcomes (consequences) differently (Table 3-1). It is necessary to understand these basic concepts to follow the

rationale for choices made, to make cost-effective treatment decisions, and to educate and better advise patients.

COST-BENEFIT ANALYSIS

Cost-benefit analysis (CBA) has traditionally been the choice of economists. In CBA, all costs and benefits are valued in monetary terms, generally dollars. If the value (in dollars) is more than the cost (in dollars) the option is cost-beneficial and should be undertaken. Because CBA values everything in a common denominator (i.e., dollars), it allows comparisons to be made between unrelated options. One advantage of CBA is that alternatives for different types of outcomes can be compared.

It is generally possible to assign a value to the costs of an intervention. However, trouble begins when one attempts to evaluate its outcomes. How does one appraise the value of a few days of better health, much less the value of surviving an illness? Because answering this question is plagued with problems, the CBA approach to pharmacoeconomic analysis is rarely used. There are occasional reports of research conducted using this approach, but those studies must be carefully scrutinized.

There are two methods commonly used to estimate a value for this type of question—the human capital approach and the willingness-to-pay approach. The human capital approach presumes that the value of health benefits is equal to the economic productivity that they permit. The cost of a disease includes the costs of lost productivity due to the disease. A person's expected income or an imputed value for non–employment activities (e.g., housework or child care) is used as an estimate of the value of any health benefits for that person. However, earnings may not reflect a person's true worth to society.

The willingness-to-pay method estimates the value of benefits by estimating how much people would pay to reduce their chance of an adverse health outcome. The difficulty with this approach is that what people say they are willing to pay may not correspond with what they actually do when confronted with the choice. The willingness of third parties (e.g., insurers) to pay is also taken into consideration.

COST-EFFECTIVENESS ANALYSIS

Cost-effectiveness analysis (CEA) measures the outcomes of intervention in terms of natural health units: the costs of a

TABLE 3-1 Approaches to Pharmacoeconomic Analysis

Analysis	Costs	Outcomes (Consequences)	Formula
Cost-benefit (CB)	$	$	CB ratio = $ benefit − $ cost
Cost-effectiveness (CE)	$	Natural units (e.g., blood pressure, lipid levels, lives saved, days of illness averted)	$CE\ ratio = \dfrac{\$\ cost}{unit\ of\ effectiveness}$
Cost-utility (CU)	$	Quality adjusted life-years	
Cost-minimization (CM)	$	Equality of outcomes*	$CU\ ratio = \dfrac{\$\ cost}{(\times years)(health\ state)}$

*Assumes a constant outcome (consequence)
Data from Drummond, M., Stoddart, G., and Torrance, G. (1987). *Methods for the economic evaluation of healthcare programmes.* Oxford: Oxford University Press.

treatment option valued in dollars. The value of a CEA is the ratio between a dollar amount and the unit of effectiveness. The simplest form of CEA is based on objective, natural units (such as reduction in blood pressure or lipid levels), the probability of cure, or days of illness averted. The choice of units is determined by what is most relevant to the disease state or treatment in question. The benefit to this approach is that it is often similar to the logic used by health care providers when they make clinical drug decisions.

The CEA ratio depends on the nonmonetary unit chosen, but the advantage is that the investigator is not responsible for assigning a monetary value to health. The disadvantage of CEA is that it becomes difficult to compare unrelated options. The alternatives compared must have outcomes similar enough to be measurable in the same units.

COST-UTILITY ANALYSIS

In cost-utility analysis (CUA), the effectiveness unit is not a natural condition of the disease or a treatment in question, but rather an artificial measure designed to allow for comparisons between different diseases or populations. CUA can take patient preferences into account when measuring health outcomes. The most commonly used utility measures are life-years (LYs) saved, age-adjusted LYs saved, the number of years that a treatment option saves compared with some other option, or quality-adjusted LYs (QALYs), in which the LYs are adjusted to include a preference for the quality of life. The QALY is based on the notion that a year of being healthy is preferable to, and worth more than, a year of illness. For example, 1 year of life in perfect health has a score of 1 QALY. If the health-related quality of life is diminished by disease or treatment, that 1 year of life is worth less than 1 QALY. This method allows for comparisons of mortality and morbidity. In another example, a woman with hypertension dies at age 65 but otherwise would have been expected to live to age 85. Her hypertension is associated with 20 lost LYs. If 100 women die at age 65 (women who also had a life expectancy of 85 years), 20 × 100, or 2000, LYs would be lost. However, death is not the only outcome of hypertension. The disease leaves many people disabled over long periods of time (e.g., as a result of stroke, myocardial infarction, or renal failure). Although the patient remains alert and active, the quality of life has decreased. QALYs take into account the quality of life outcomes of illness. In another example, a disease that reduces the quality of life by one half will take away 0.5 QALYs over the course of 1 year. If the disease affects five people, it will take away 5 × 0.5, or 2.5, QALYs over a period of 1 year. A drug that improves the quality of life by 0.2 for each of the five people will result in the equivalent of 1 QALY if the benefit is maintained over a period of 1 year.

Although there is considerable debate regarding which dimensions should be used as QALY units, the most common are physical functioning, the ability to carry out prescribed roles, and mental health status. A common strategy is to report outcomes along multiple dimensions, but it is unclear whether multiple dimensions are more likely to detect clinical differences than is the use of a single measure. The benefit of CUA is that it allows comparison between unrelated treatment options. The problem is that health care providers or MCOs must apply these utility measures in a meaningful way.

COST-MINIMIZATION AND COST-OF-ILLNESS ANALYSES

Two other common economic analyses are often encountered—*cost-minimization analysis* (CMA) and *cost-of-illness analysis* (CIA). CMA is a variation of CEA in which the outcomes of the possible options are assumed to be equivalent. Although costs are explicitly measured, the consequences are not. One example of a CMA is the measurement and comparison of costs for two equivalent generic drugs. Another example is the measurement and comparison of total costs required for home intravenous antibiotic therapy with the total costs of providing this therapy in the hospital. The strength of CMA depends on the assumption that the outcomes are the same. This evidence is based on previous studies, publications, FDA data, or expert opinion.

CIA measures factors associated with a particular disease including direct costs, like medical services, and indirect costs, such as loss of productivity due to illness or premature death.

ANALYSIS STRATEGIES

Independent of the perspective or approach chosen, there are strategies that can be used to conduct pharmacoeconomic analyses. The choice of strategy depends to some extent on the purpose of the analysis and the expectations of the audience.

CLINICAL TRIALS

The majority of pharmacoeconomic analyses are piggy-backed onto clinical trials evaluating the efficacy and safety of a specific treatment or intervention. The FDA requests that pharmacoeconomic analyses be attached to clinical trials. Economic data are collected as part of the clinical trial and used to determine the cost-effectiveness of the treatment under study.

As the field matures, pharmacoeconomists are realizing the inherent limitation of the clinical trial because of inclusion and exclusion criteria, observational effects, and strict assignment of patients to control and treatment groups. In other words, the results of experimental research do not accurately represent what occurs in the real world. Therefore the results of clinical trials are difficult to generalize to clinical practice settings.

In an attempt to resolve this limitation, some researchers are using open-label clinical trials: a clinical trial conducted without control groups or the blinding of variables normally found in standard clinical trials. Patients and health care providers are allowed to participate in the treatment option of their choosing and even to change treatments if desired. Costs and effectiveness of the interventions are followed, and the results are evaluated to determine the most cost-effective treatment.

The assumption is that an open-label trial more closely mimics what happens in real life. There are fewer limitations than with clinical trials; however, it is still difficult to generalize results beyond the specifics of the open-label trial. In addition, many researchers and health care providers are suspicious of the results of open-label trials because they lack control groups and blinding, the very components needed for unbiased results. Finally, open-label trials are expensive. The expense limits the number of treatment options that can be evaluated at any one time, making it difficult to evaluate more than just a few treatment options.

RETROSPECTIVE DATABASE ANALYSIS

Under the retrospective database analysis approach, a database of clinical and economic information is evaluated using statistical and mathematical methods to determine the relationship between treatment options, outcomes, and costs. The advantage of this approach is that the data are usually readily available and reflect the historical experience of the particular organization.

This approach provides significant results and information to an organization, especially when external factors are properly controlled; however, three limitations must be kept in mind: (1) Data analysis can be technically challenging, especially when there are large, unrelated data sets, and (2) the data may not be accurate. For example, evaluation of current procedural terminology (CPT) coding can be useful, but one must remember that CPT codes are collected to support reimbursement rather than to measure treatment options. The more complicated and strict the reimbursement policies, the more likely that CPT codes will not accurately reflect the real consumption of resources. This is particularly true when significant cost shifting (shifting costs from low-reimbursing patients to higher-reimbursing patients) occurs.

Finally, (3) owing to policies, circumstances, or changes in treatments over time, data may not reflect a fair comparison of all treatment options. For example, some data sets may not include certain drugs (i.e., those drugs not contained in the formulary), or there may be a perception among health care providers that a particular drug should be reserved for sicker patients, thereby distorting the cost of that drug. The limitations to data sets can often be controlled by statistical means, but there is a limit to these types of corrections, especially when subtle biases are not recognized. The net result is that retrospective database analyses provide information with which to make accurate cost-effective determinations but cannot be used exclusively.

MATHEMATICAL MODELING

Mathematical modeling is based on the notion that although it may be impossible or difficult to measure specific phenomena, it is possible to describe the phenomena mathematically. Models can range from simple approximations of what is being measured to much more complex and accurate representations of reality. In pharmacoeconomics, modeling permits an evaluation of the cost-effectiveness of a disease state that would otherwise be impossible to measure through a clinical trial. For example, there are dozens of drugs available for the treatment of primary hypertension, any of which can be used alone or in many different combinations. Only a model could evaluate these combinations of treatment.

A mathematical model begins with a framework that presumes to represent reality. The framework is developed based on assumptions about what really happens in a specific disease state or with a particular treatment. How completely the reader or user of the analysis believes the model depends on the extent of his or her agreement with the assumptions. Experimental or observational data such as cost, efficacy, and adverse effects profile are then used for the variables within the mathematical model, and results are calculated. The results of mathematical modeling include predictions that can be tested. It is this testing of predictions that validates the model's reliability.

The advantage of using a mathematical model is the ability to evaluate questions that cannot be directly analyzed because of complexity or cost. The disadvantage of modeling, especially as the model becomes more complex, is its underlying mathematical nature. A certain degree of comfort and familiarity with mathematical concepts and techniques is required. In addition, developing accurate models is as much an art as a science. Traditionally, mathematical models have not been the preferred means of conducting pharmacoeconomic analyses. However, this attitude may change as more people become familiar with the necessary techniques, MCOs begin to demand more applied pharmacoeconomic analyses, and people realize that some pharmacoeconomic questions can be answered only by mathematical models.

METHODS FOR PHARMACOECONOMIC ANALYSES

Another way to understand pharmacoeconomic analyses is by the method or structure used. Ultimately, the data must be evaluated using one of several methods. For example, during a clinical trial, economic data can be captured that determine the cost-effectiveness of treatment options. However, a pharmacoeconomic method must then be chosen to analyze those data.

DECISION ANALYSIS

A decision analysis is the most common proactive method used. This method reduces the management of an illness into a series of treatment choices to be made by the health care provider. Using this method, a decision tree is created that includes options or decision points from which the health care provider or health care system must choose. Costs and outcomes are assigned to these decisions, and ultimately, the cost-effectiveness for a particular decision is determined. This method can be used in conjunction with clinical trials, databases, or models.

Decision analysis is easy to use, and several computer programs are available to create the decision trees. Unfortunately, as the number of treatment options increases, the number of decision points grows exponentially. Very quickly, a decision tree becomes a decision forest. This growth limits the usefulness of this method when more than a few drug choices must be evaluated.

Consider the management of a sore throat. The treatment options include giving antibiotics to all patients, culturing for strep throat and giving antibiotics to patients with positive cultures, or giving antibiotics to none of the patients. In

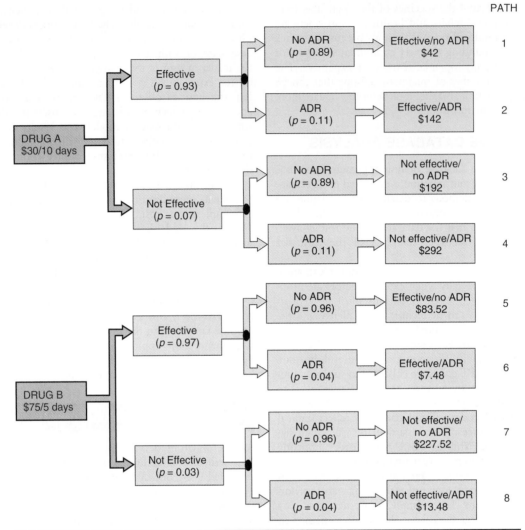

FIGURE 3-1 Decision Analysis Model Comparing Two Drugs. The initial decision point is represented by a square; subsequent decision points at each branch of the model represented by an oval. At each decision point, a probability value is assigned based on the probability (p) of its occurrence. The drug in option B is more specific for the target receptor in the body, is more effective, and produces fewer adverse drug reactions than does option A. However, because drug B is more expensive than drug A, the cost of the added benefits must be analyzed using pharmacoeconomic techniques. This figure was completed using the safety and efficacy values for drugs A and B from Table 3-2. (*ACER,* Average cost-effectiveness ratio; *p,* probability, a decimal fraction between 0 and 1 indicating the likelihood of a particular event occurring in a given period.)

analyses comparing various antibiotics, there would be a branch for each drug under consideration (Fig. 3-1, Table 3-2). Thus, using a decision tree, treatment alternatives, outcomes, and probabilities may be presented graphically and may be reduced algebraically to a single value for comparison (i.e., cost-effectiveness ratio).

SIMULATION MODELING

Simulation modeling is a mathematical method that mimics real inputs and choices made by health care providers. In many ways, this is analogous to mathematical modeling. When properly handled, this method is easy to understand and provides tremendous insight into the choices and

efficiencies of providers in making treatment decisions. At the same time, this approach can be difficult to implement. The results can also be difficult to understand and believe, if the mathematics underlying the simulation is overly obtuse and complex. Despite this problem, simulation modeling remains the approach best able to answer complex questions of cost-effectiveness when the decision involves multiple treatment options.

STATISTICAL ANALYSIS

Statistical analyses are reactive methods best used with large data sets. Descriptive statistics (e.g., means, mediums, standard deviations), inferential statistics (e.g., *t*-test, paired *t*-tests,

TABLE 3-2 Calculating and Comparing Costs

Path	Drug Cost ($)	Culture Cost ($)	Treatment Delay ($)	Cumulative Cost ($)
DRUG A				
1	30	12	–	42
2	30	12	100	142
3	30	12	150	192
4	30	12	250	292

Resultant Cost of Drug A: $ 301.21

Path	Drug Cost ($)	Culture Cost ($)	Treatment Delay ($)	Cumulative Cost ($)
DRUG B				
5	75	12	–	97
6	75	12	100	187
7	75	12	150	237
8	75	12	250	337

Resultant Cost of Drug B:

To calculate the average cost-effectiveness ratios (ACER) for each drug, follow these steps:

1. Multiply the cumulative cost of path 1 by the probability (p) of no adverse drug reaction (or $42 × p value of 0.89 = $37.38). The decimal probability figure is the ratio of the number of ways the outcome may occur to the number of total possible outcomes for the event.
   Repeat calculations for path 2.
   $142 × p value of 0.11 = $15.62

2. Add these two numbers together and multiply by the probability of effective treatment (in this case p = 0.93)
   $37.38 + $15.62 = $53
   $53 × 0.93 = $49.29

3. Repeat steps above for paths 3 and 4 and then add the resultant values:
   Path 3: $192 × 0.89 = $170.88
   Path 4: $292 × 0.11 = $32.12
   $170.88 + $32.12 = $203
   $203.00 × 0.93 = $ 188.79
   Resultant values: $49.29 + $188.79 = $238.08

4. Add the cost of the drug to the resultant value obtained above and divide by the probability of effective treatment
   $238.08 + $30 = $2680.8
   $268.08 ÷ 0.89 = $301.21 = cost of therapy using drug A

5. Repeat this entire process for drug B using paths 5–8 to compare actual costs of drug A to drug B. The process would be continued along the same lines when comparing more than two drugs.

chi-square analysis, etc.), and more advanced inferential techniques, such as regression analysis, factor analysis, and logistic regression, are used to evaluate both the costs and the effectiveness of each treatment option.

Statistical analysis works best when the data already exist, either in a database or as the result of a clinical trial or mathematical model. Statistical evaluation of alternative treatments requires a thorough understanding and modeling of the process that generated the health care provider's and the patient's behaviors, as well as the data collection effort. It is important to go beyond simple univariate statistical analysis to understand how much confidence can be placed in the results (i.e., estimated cost-effectiveness ratio).

Whereas other methods are predictive, statistical methods are descriptive, finding results already inherent in the data. Such statistical analysis looks for relationships within a data set, whereas the other two methods begin with the data and predict (based on assumptions and an analytic framework) the cost-effectiveness. This means that statistical analysis is preferred when the data are extensive and complete.

In order to understand and apply pharmacoeconomic research, health care professionals must be able to critique the quality of that research. Guidelines for research evaluation can help in this process (Box 3-2).

PHARMACOECONOMICS AND FORMULARIES

One of the most effective methods by which MCOs slow the increasing cost of prescription drugs is by using formularies. A formulary is a list of approved prescription drugs covered by a pharmacy benefit plan. Formularies were used originally as cost-control mechanisms but have evolved into effective tools for monitoring and regulating unsafe drug use.

Formularies include brand-name and generic drugs approved by the FDA as safe and effective. When a managed care organization wants to limit the use of a drug for a specific reason (e.g., cost, safety, or efficacy) a formulary allows the flexibility to implement such restrictions. The use of formularies by HMOs increased from 39% in 1989 to 93% in 1997.

There are two basic types of formularies. Restricted formularies limit prescriptions to a preferred list of drugs. For the most part, restricted formularies are used by HMOs to realize cost savings, which in turn help them price their policies below those of PPOs. In contrast, open formularies do not draw on a preferred list of drugs and thus permit the health care provider more freedom when prescribing. Over 90% of formularies used in PPOs and independent provider

BOX 3-2

Points to Consider when Evaluating Pharmacoeconomic Studies

Purpose or objective	Is(are) the purpose(s) and objective(s) clear, well defined, and measurable? Can the objective(s) be answered?
Perspective	What is(are) the perspective(s) of the analysis? Is it appropriate for the given scope of the problem? Does the study clearly identify assumptions used?
Pharmacoeconomic methodology	What pharmacoeconomic tool was used in the study? Is it appropriate for the problem? If so, is it actually what was used?
Design	Does the study describe any competing alternatives? (i.e., Can you tell *who*... did *what*... to *whom*... *where*... and *how often*?) What were the data sources? Does the study provide evidence that treatment effectiveness has been established?
Choices of interventions and alternatives	Does the study identify relevant costs and outcomes for each alternative? Were other appropriate alternatives omitted? Are there alternatives relevant to the perspective and clinical nature of the study? Is there evidence that the effectiveness of alternatives has been established?
Costs and outcomes	Were the costs and outcomes identified and included? Does the perspective chosen relate to costs and outcomes? Are the significant costs and outcomes (e.g., hours of nursing time, number of visits to health care provider, lost work days, life-years gained) measured in appropriate and tangible units? Does the study credibly value costs and outcomes? Does the study take disparities in time into consideration and amend costs and consequences accordingly?
Sensitivity analysis	Does the study use sensitivity analysis? Are the appropriate and relevant variables, costs, and outcomes measured in the appropriate physical units? Does the study justify its choice and use of surveys or other instruments? Are cost ranges for significant variables tested for sensitivity? Do the findings follow the anticipated trend? Does the study concentrate on incremental analysis in terms of costs and consequences of alternatives performed? Does the study apply discounting to multiyear research? If so, were the costs and outcomes discounted to their present value? What justification is provided for the discount rate used?
Sponsorship	Do the sponsors present information in an unbiased manner? Do the sponsors include negative outcomes (failures, adverse drug reactions)? How are they valued?
Results	Was an incremental analysis? Were the appropriate statistical analyses performed? Are all the assumptions and limitations of the study discussed? Does the study present to prospective users all findings of concern?

Adapted from: Drummond, J., Stoddart, G., and Torrance, G. (1987). *Methods for the economic evaluation of healthcare programmes.* Oxford: Oxford University Press; and DiPiro, J., Talbert, R., Yee, G., et al. (2005). *Pharmacotherapy: A pathophysiology approach* (6th ed.). New York: McGraw-Hill.

associations are open formularies. These formularies use a maximum allowable cost per patient to encourage health care providers to order generic drugs.

Drugs within a tiered benefit structure are generally divided into three groups. Generic drugs are in the first tier and generally have the lowest copay. Preferred brand-name drugs are in the second tier, with midrange copays, and nonpreferred brand-name drugs are in the third tier. Third-tier drugs have the highest copay. Yet despite the tiered benefit structure, some drugs require prior authorization (i.e., preapproval by the insurance company) before the pharmacist fills the prescription. The primary purpose for prior authorization is to control the use and overuse of high-priced and non–formulary drugs, thereby decreasing unnecessary cost. Most often prior authorization is needed for drugs with a high toxicity profile, drugs that have a less expensive alternative or those of equal cost that produce rebates to a payor from the company, and drugs newly approved by the FDA.

PHARMACY AND THERAPEUTICS COMMITTEES

A pharmacy and therapeutics committee is generally made up of health care providers, pharmacists, and people with experience in marketing and law whose primary responsibility is to revise a formulary, create and implement drug policies, and provide education for health care providers. Formulary revisions are done frequently, because manufacturers are introducing new drugs at breakneck speed, the addition or deletion of drugs must reflect current standards of care, and the results of clinical research studies often lead to changes in the guidelines for health maintenance and disease management. The committee may add a drug to the formulary unconditionally or set certain restrictions on the new drug to allow inclusion in the formulary.

THE FUTURE OF PHARMACOECONOMICS

The field of pharmacoeconomics and the data it evaluates changes rapidly. Increasingly, several themes are reflected in the literature. These themes include increased pressure on health care providers to consider the economic impact of their decisions on individual patients and on the populations they serve; demands by managed care organizations for pharmacoeconomic evaluations that meet their specific needs rather than the needs of policymakers; and a push toward standardization and guidelines in conducting and reporting pharmacoeconomic evaluations.

KEY POINTS

- The fundamental objective of managed care is to maximize the quality of care while minimizing costs.
- Pharmacoeconomics is defined as a field of study that seeks to identify, measure, and compare the costs and consequences of drug products and services.
- Pharmacoeconomic analyses encompass two related, but separate, philosophies: resource allocation and increased efficiency.
- Thus, the basic question has been: Given a variety of treatment choices and limited resources, which choices should we make?
- One question confronting health care providers and organizations is whether they should pay the additional cost for newer drugs that appear to have fewer adverse effects or continue to pay for older drugs that are just as effective but potentially have more adverse effects.
- There are many different approaches to pharmacoeconomic analysis: CBA, CEA, CUA, and CMA.

- Strategies for conducting pharmacoeconomic analyses include retrospective database analysis and mathematical modeling.
- *Perspective* relates to the focus and orientation of an analysis; the concept includes those of society, the payors, health care providers, and patients.
- The majority of pharmacoeconomic analyses are evaluations piggybacked onto clinical trials being done to evaluate efficacy and safety of an intervention.
- Decision analysis is based on the concept of reducing the disease state management into a series of treatment choices to be made by the health care provider and the patient. This methodology can be used in conjunction with clinical trials, databases, or models.
- Statistical analysis is best used in combination with large data sets. It can also be applied in clinical trials and models when sufficient data are available.

Bibliography

American Medical Specialty Organization. *AMSO Definition of Terms.* Available at www.amso.com/terms.html. Accessed March 10, 2007.

Bootman, J., Townsend, R., and McGhan, W. (Eds.) (1996). *Principles of pharmacoeconomics* (2nd ed.). Cincinnati, OH: Harvey Whitney Books.

Department of Health and Human Services. Office of Disease Prevention and Promotion. (1992). *A framework for cost-utility analysis of government health care program.* Washington, DC: Government Printing Office.

DiPiro, J., Talbert, R., Yee, G., et al. (2005). *Pharmacotherapy: A pathophysiology approach* (6th ed.). New York: McGraw-Hill.

Doubilet, P., Weinstein, M., and McNeil, B. (1986). Use and misuse of the term "cost-effective" in medicine. *New England Journal of Medicine, 314*(4), 253–256.

Drummond, M., Stoddart, G., and Torrance, G. (1987). *Methods for the economic evaluation of healthcare programmes.* Oxford: Oxford University Press.

Feldman, S., Fleischer, A., and Chen, G. (1999). Is prior authorization of topical tretinoin for acne cost effective? *American Journal of Managed Care, 5*(4), 457–463.

Gold, M., Siegel, J., Russell, L., et al. (1996). *Cost-effectiveness in health and medicine.* New York: Oxford University Press.

Grimaldi, P. (1996). Managed care: A glossary of terms. *Nursing Management, 27*(10 Suppl), 5–7.

Heller, B. (1996). Pharmacoeconomics guidelines galore coming. *Drug Topics, 140*(11), 106.

Hoechst Marion Roussel. (1998). *The managed care digest series 1998.* Kansas City, MO: Author.

Kleinke, J. (2000). Just what the HMO ordered: The paradox of increasing drug costs. *Health Affairs, 19*(2), 78–91.

Kaiser Permanente. *History of Kaiser Permanente.* Available on-line: http://newsmedia.kaiserpermanente.org/kpweb/historykp/entrypage.do. Accessed February 6, 2007.

Kozma, C., Reeder, C., and Shultz, R. (1993). Economic, clinical, and humanistic outcomes: A planning model for pharmacoeconomic research. *Clinical Therapeutics, 15*(6), 1121–1132.

Lisi, D. (1997). Ethical issues for pharmacists in managed care. *American Journal of Health-System Pharmacists, 54*(9), 1041–1042, 1045.

Lyles, A., and Palumbo, F. (1999). The effect of managed care on prescription drug costs and benefits. *Pharmacoeconomics, 15*(2), 129–140.

Managed Care Museum. (2005). *History of managed care.* Available on-line: www.managedcaremuseum.com/index.html. Accessed February 6, 2007.

Muirhead, G. (1995). Batty up! Pharmacoeconomics, the rookie, enters game. *Drug Topics, 139*(8), 33–34.

Muirhead, G. (1994). Pharmacoeconomics: A still-fuzzy buzzword. *Drug Topics, 138*(9), 74–75.

Navarre, R. (1999). *Managed care pharmacy practice.* Gaithersburg, MD: Aspen.

Riesenberg, D. (Ed.) (1989). Clinical economics: A guide to the economic analysis of clinical practices. *Clinical Economics, 262*(20), 2879–2886.

Revicki, D., and Kaplan, K. (1993). Relationship between psychometric and utility-based approaches to the measurement of health-related quality of life. *Quality of Life Research, 2*(6), 477–487.

Sanchez, L., and Lee, J. (2000). Applied pharmacoeconomics: Modeling data from internal and external sources. *American Journal of Health System Pharmacists. 57*(2), 146–158.

Sloan, F. (1995). *Valuing health care: Cost, benefits, and effectiveness of pharmaceuticals and other medical technologies.* New York: Cambridge University Press.

Star, P. (1982). *The social transformation of American medicine.* New York: Basic Books.

Tufts Managed Care Institute. (1998). *A brief history of managed care.* Available on-line: www.teacherweb.com/NY/StBarnabas/system/BriefHistMC.pdf. Accessed February 6, 2007.

Wilke, R. (1995). What's all this about pharmacoeconomics? *Business Economics, 30*(2), 26–31.

Pharmaceutics and Pharmacokinetics

4

Rational, safe, drug selection requires choosing among several drugs that may have different mechanisms of action but similar effects. To do so, the health care provider must have knowledge of the pharmaceutic and pharmacokinetic properties of the drug (Box 4-1).

The conceptual model in Figure 4-1 depicts variability in the relationship between the dose of a drug and patient response to that drug. As you know from clinical experiences, you can give the same dose of a drug to two different patients, resulting in very different responses. One patient may not achieve a therapeutic response, while the other has both therapeutic and adverse reactions simultaneously. The model explains that this variability is due to the differences in the four phases of drug action: pharmaceutics, pharmacokinetics, pharmacodynamics, and pharmacotherapeutics. These phases are interrelated and interdependent and as such are not as clearly defined as they might first seem.

PHASES OF DRUG ACTIVITY

PHARMACEUTIC PHASE

In the *pharmaceutic phase* the manufacturer formulates the drug into dosage forms suited for delivery to a site of drug action. Orally administered drugs must undergo *disintegration* and *dissolution* before being absorbed. Once a solid dosage form is in solution in the gastrointestinal (GI) tract or body fluid, it is available for absorption and distribution. Solubility characteristics can be manipulated to delay disintegration and dissolution in the GI tract, or to alter the location where disintegration takes place. By altering solubility characteristics, drug action can be prolonged.

According to the Food and Drug Administration (FDA) *Electronic Orange Book* (http://www.fda.gov/cder/ob/default.htm), "drug products are considered *pharmaceutical equivalents* if they contain the same active ingredient(s), are of the same dosage form, route of administration, and are identical in strength or concentration (e.g., chlordiazepoxide hydrochloride, 5 mg capsules). Pharmaceutically equivalent drug products are formulated to contain the same amount of active

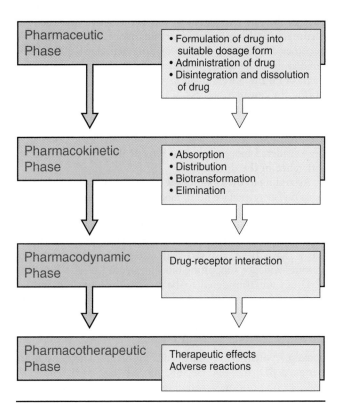

FIGURE 4-1 **Phases of Drug Activity.** During the pharmaceutic phase, the drug enters the body in one form and changes to another in order to be used. In the pharmacokinetic phase, the drug is absorbed into the circulation, distributed to its site of action, biotransformed in the liver or other tissues, and eliminated through the liver or kidneys. The action of the drug on cellular receptors constitutes the pharmacodynamic phase of drug action. The activities taking place within the pharmacodynamic and pharmacotherapeutic phases help determine the proper dosage and dosing schedule.

ingredient in the same dosage form and to meet the same or compendial or other applicable standards (i.e., strength, quality, purity, and identity), but they may differ in characteristics such as shape, scoring configuration, release mechanisms, packaging, excipients (including colors, flavors, and preservatives), expiration time, and, within certain limits, labeling."

Pharmaceutical alternatives are defined as "drug products that contain the identical therapeutic moiety, or its precursor, but not necessarily in the same amount or dosage form or as the same salt or ester. Each such drug product individually meets either the identical or its own respective compendium or other applicable standard of identity, strength, quality, and purity, including potency and, where applicable, content uniformity, disintegration times and/or dissolution rates" (Department of Health and Human Services, 2000: 21 CFR 320.1[c]). In other words the two drugs contain the same

---

BOX 4-1

Principles of Drug Action

Principle 1: Drugs modify existing functions within the body; they do not create function.
Principle 2: No drug has a single action.
Principle 3: Drug effects are determined by the drug's interaction with the body.

active ingredient but have different salts, esters, or complexes of that active ingredient or have different formulations and strengths (e.g., 5 mg of the antihypertensive drug lisinopril as opposed to the 25-mg formulation of lisinopril). This is true for immediate-release and standard-release formulations compared with extended-release drug formulations. Data are generally not available for the FDA to determine the bioequivalence of tablets relative to capsules.

Bioequivalence means the "absence of a significant difference in the rate and extent to which the active ingredient in pharmaceutical equivalents or pharmaceutical alternatives becomes available at the site of drug action when administered at the same dose and under similar conditions" (Department of Health and Human Services, 2000: 21 CFR 320.1[e]) during the research process. If purposeful differences exist in the rate in which the active ingredients become bioavailable at the site of drug action (e.g., certain controlled-release dosage forms; see later section on bioavailablity), the drugs may be considered bioequivalent as long as there is no significant difference in the degree.

According to the *Orange Book* (http://www.fda.gov/cder/ob/docs/preface/ecpreface.htm), bioequivalent drugs carry a designation of AA, AN, AO, AP, or AT depending on the dosage form. The designation AB is used for drugs shown to have actual or potential bioequivalence problems when these problems have been resolved with acceptable in vivo and/or in vitro evidence supporting bioequivalence (see also Box 2-2).

Drugs are considered to be *therapeutic equivalents* only if they are pharmaceutical equivalents and have the same clinical effect and safety profile when given to patients under the conditions specified in the labeling. Drugs not considered to be therapeutically equivalent by the FDA are those with actual or potential bioequivalence problems. These drugs are designed BD, BE, BN, BP, BR, BS, BT, BX, or B. The FDA will take no position in regard to a B drug's therapeutic equivalence without further investigation and review.

Drug Constituents

A drug is made up of one or more active ingredients and various additives (Table 4-1). Active ingredients are responsible for producing desired effects and vary considerably in their

TABLE 4-1 Drug Constituents

Constituent	Form	Example(s)
ACTIVE INGREDIENTS	Alkaloids	atropine, nicotine
	Glycosides	digoxin
	Polypeptides	Insulin
	Salts	morphine sulfate, potassium chloride
	Steroids	estrogen, testosterone, cortisone
ADDITIVES	Binders	dextrose, lactose
	Diluents	Vehicles, fillers
	Disintegrators	Starch
	Dyes	Tartrazine (FD&C Yellow No. 5)
	Flavorings	Cherry, raspberry, licorice syrups
	Fillers	dextrose, lactose, starch
	Lubricants	Hydrogenated vegetable oils, stearates, talc
	Vehicles	Cocoa butter, oils, petrolatum, syrups, water

FD&C, Food, Drugs and Cosmetics Act.

chemical structure. They are categorized based on chemical and physical properties and are used to influence certain properties of the final formulation.

Drug Formulations

Drugs are formulated and administered in such a way as to produce either local or systemic effects. Local effects are confined to one area of the body (e.g., antiseptics, antiinflammatories, local anesthetics). Systemic effects occur when the drug is absorbed and delivered to body tissues by way of the circulatory system.

Drug formulations for local use include aerosols, ointments, creams, pastes, powders, tinctures, and lotions. They can also be formulated as gels, foams, and suppositories for rectal, vaginal, or urethral use. Drug formulations can be administered by douche or as an enema. Sprays, aerosols, gases, and nebulizers are methods for introducing local or systemic drugs, or both, to the respiratory system.

Local drug formulations may be water based (aqueous) or oil based. Water-based formulations are readily absorbed, whereas oil-based formulations are absorbed more slowly. Oil-based drugs are not used in the respiratory tract since the oil may be carried to the alveoli, resulting in lipid pneumonia.

Systemic drug formulations are absorbed into the circulation to affect one or more tissue groups. They can be administered orally, topically, or parenterally, or applied to mucous membranes. Parenterally administered drugs are introduced into the body by any route other than enteral (i.e., intradermal [ID], subcutaneous [subQ], intramuscular [IM], and intravenous [IV] routes). An overview of formulations is seen in Table 4-2. Table 4-3 identifies the absorption speeds of drug formulations.

PHARMACOKINETIC PHASES

The term pharmacokinetics is derived from the Greek words *pharmacon*, meaning "drug" or "poison," and *kinesis*, meaning "motion." The four pharmacokinetic phases of drug absorption, distribution, biotransformation, and elimination, along with the dosage, determine drug concentration at the site of action, the intensity of effects, and the duration of drug action (Fig. 4-2). There are several factors that affect each of the pharmacokinetic processes.

ABSORPTION

For a drug to produce effects, it must be absorbed, that is, transferred from its site of administration (e.g., skin, GI tract, muscle) into the circulation. Absorption must occur before the active ingredients can reach the central circulation, where the drug is then distributed throughout the body. Drugs administered by IV route, those injected into a body space for local effects, topically applied drugs, and drugs administered for their action within the GI tract are exceptions.

Factors influencing the rate and extent of drug absorption into the circulation include dosage form, administration route, age, pregnancy, disease states, food, and other drugs. The rate at which drugs are absorbed determines the onset of effects. In turn, the amount of drug absorbed determines the intensity of effects.

TABLE 4-2 Drug Formulations

SOLID FORMULATIONS

Oral tablets	Contain filler, a binder, a disintegrator, and a lubricant, which influence rate of disintegration. Some contain preservatives, pH stabilizers, coatings, flavorings, or coloring. Bioavailability compromised if tablet poorly compounded.
Buccal tablets	Held in mouth between the cheek and gum until dissolved and absorbed.
Sublingual tablets	Placed beneath the tongue until they are dissolved and absorbed.
Coated tablets	Outside layer usually of sugar or chocolate to make them more palatable.
Effervescent tablets	Contain mixture of sodium bicarbonate and an acidulant, such as citric acid, that generates carbon dioxide when added to water.
Sustained-release tablets	Contain small particles of drug coated with substances that require varying amounts of time to dissolve. Most useful for drugs rapidly biotransformed or eliminated or that would otherwise have to be taken on a more frequent basis. Contain more total drug than single-dose tablets or capsules so irregular absorption may occur. Dosage form not used for drugs with narrow margin of safety (i.e., therapeutic index).
Enteric-coated tablets	Formulated to dissolve in alkaline environment of small intestine rather than acidic environment of stomach. Not used if immediate drug action is desired.
Caplets	Tablets resembling capsules in shape.
Capsules	Gelatin cases enclosing solid drug forms. More easily tampered with after manufacturing than caplets.
Powders	Measured doses of solid drug in powder form. Dissolved in water for administration.
Dusts	Very fine powders applied topically to skin or mucous membranes or inhaled.
Granules	Resemble powders in appearance but particle size is larger. Prepared in bulk or as single-dose packets.
Patches	Drug embedded in the adhesive ring or a central area. Designed to promote gradual absorption through skin.
Pellets, needles	Pellets: small pills or spherical tablets. Needles: long, thin cylinders. Absorb slowly from subcutaneous tissues, muscle, organs after being surgically implanted.
Troches, lozenges	Flat, round, or oval formulations made of drug powder, sugar, and mucilage. Lozenges are designed for oral use; troches used either orally or vaginally.

SEMISOLID FORMULATIONS

Ointments	Soft, fatty substances applied to skin or eyes. May be oil based or water based. Term synonymous with salve, unction, and unguent.
Creams	Less viscous than ointments but more viscous than lotions. Spread easily but tend to hold shape when left undisturbed.
Pastes	Thick, gelatinous substances intended for topical use. Vehicles and fillers include oils, starches, and waxes.
Suppositories	Cone-shaped or cylindrical discs that conform to body cavities such as vagina, rectum, and urethra. Vehicle (e.g., cocoa butter) dissolves at body temperature.
Foams	Combinations of finely dispersed gas bubbles interspersed in liquid. Contraceptive vaginal foams are an example.

LIQUID FORMULATIONS

Solutions	Mixtures of two or more substances dissolved in another substance. Molecules of each solute disperse homogeneously but do not change chemically. Primarily liquids but can be solid, liquid, or gas. Can be administered orally, rectally, topically, by inhalation, or by parenteral routes. Can also be used as sprays or irrigations, or instilled in the nose, eye, or ear.
Elixirs	Clear liquids containing alcohol, water, sweeteners, and flavoring. Usually administered by mouth.
Extracts	Concentrated solutions of active ingredient dissolved or diluted with alcoholic solvent. Strength of extract is several times stronger than crude drug. Fluid extracts are alcoholic solutions of 100% concentration (i.e., each mL of solution contains 1 gram of pure drug).
Tinctures	Alcoholic extracts of vegetable or animal substances administered topically (e.g., tincture of benzoin) or by mouth. Potent drugs dispensed as 10% concentrations; less potent drugs dispensed as 20% concentrations.
Emulsions	Combinations of two liquids, usually oil and water. Oil divides into globules that disperse throughout mixture when shaken. Tend to separate if left undisturbed but can be stabilized by addition of agent that reduces surface tension. May contain oils that are less than palatable.
Liniments	Liquids containing alcoholic, oily, or soapy vehicle. Act as counterirritant when rubbed on the skin.
Lotions	Emollient liquids that are clear solutions, suspensions, or emulsions. Used on the skin.
Suspensions	Combinations of a solid and liquid in which the solid particles do not dissolve. Gels (e.g., aluminum hydroxide gel) and magmas (e.g., milk of magnesia) are viscous suspensions of mineral precipitates in water.
Syrups	Solutions of sugar and water to which a drug is added. Added to drug mixtures to increase palatability. Particularly useful in pediatric formulations.
Oils	Used as vehicles to dissolve other drugs or as the drugs themselves (e.g., castor oil). The viscous, greasy liquids are insoluble in water. Volatile oils evaporate easily, leaving no greasy residue. Fixed oils do not readily evaporate.

There are several physiologic variables affecting the transport of drugs across membranes. In general, the factors include absorptive surface area, contact time with the absorptive surface, concentration gradient, and the extent of presystemic biotransformation.

Transport Mechanisms

In many cases, drug absorption obeys the same pathways as those of nutrients: simple diffusion, carrier-mediated diffusion, pinocytosis, and active transport (Fig. 4-3). These mechanisms allow drugs to penetrate cell membranes to create physiologic effects.

Simple passive diffusion moves drugs from higher to lower concentrations. Absorption occurs as drugs randomly move from high concentrations in the original compartment to areas of lower concentration in another. This mechanism accounts for the absorption of most drugs from the GI tract into the circulation and from the circulation to target cells.

Carrier-mediated diffusion (i.e., facilitated transport) occurs in harmony with concentration gradients. A carrier is needed to move the drug across membranes, but a driving force is not required. Carrier-mediated diffusion is used for physiologic substances such as glucose, certain vitamins, amino acids, and organic acids. Any drug resembling these substances can be transported by carriers. The classic example of carrier-mediated diffusion is dietary vitamin B_{12}. Vitamin B_{12} binds with intrinsic factor in the GI tract to form a complex. The complex is then selectively but passively carried from areas of higher concentrations to areas of lower concentrations.

During *filtration*, small drug molecules move along with fluid through the pores in cell walls. In this manner,

TABLE 4-3 Absorption Speed of Formulations

ABSORPTION SPEED OF ORAL FORMULATIONS	
Fastest	Liquids, syrups, elixirs
↓	Suspensions
	Powders
↓	Capsules
	Tablets
↓	Coated tablets
Slowest	Enteric-coated tablets

ABSORPTION SPEED OF PARENTERAL FORMULATIONS	
Fastest	Intravenous
↓	Intramuscular
	Subcutaneous
↓	Intrathecal
Slowest	Epidural*

*The epidural route is not necessarily the one providing the slowest action. For example, epidural anesthesia for childbirth acts rapidly, since action is local around nerves.

water-soluble drugs and some electrolytes are absorbed through tissue pores (rather than through the lipid matrix of the cells) into systemic circulation. Capillary membrane pores act as barriers only to very large drug molecules.

Pinocytosis involves engulfing the drug particles and moving them across cell membranes. The term pinocytosis is derived from the Greek word *pino,* meaning "I drink," *kytos,* meaning "hollow vessel" (representing cells), and *osis,* meaning "a process." The drug does not have to be dissolved because during pinocytosis, the cell wall invaginates, forms a vacuole for drug transport, breaks off, and moves into the cell. Fat-soluble vitamins such as vitamins A, D, E, and K are commonly transported by pinocytosis.

Active transport moves drug molecules against a concentration gradient using metabolic energy, usually in the form of adenosine triphosphate (ATP). The ATP-drug complex forms on the surface of the cell membrane. The complex carries the drug through the membrane, and then dissociates. The rate of active transport is proportional to drug concentration. When carrier mechanisms become saturated, the transfer rate cannot increase.

The size of drug molecules plays a part in drug transport. For example, urea molecules are small and pass easily across cell membranes. In contrast, glucose molecules are rather large and do not pass easily. Once the concentrations on both sides of the cell membrane are equal, drug movement stops. Thus small, lipid-soluble, nonionized drugs readily cross cell membranes, whereas larger, water-soluble, ionized drugs do not.

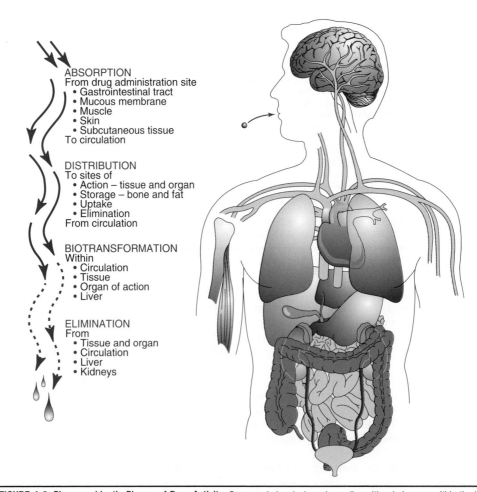

FIGURE 4-2 Pharmacokinetic Phases of Drug Activity. Drugs and chemicals undergo dispositional changes within the body during the pharmacokinetic phase of drug activity.

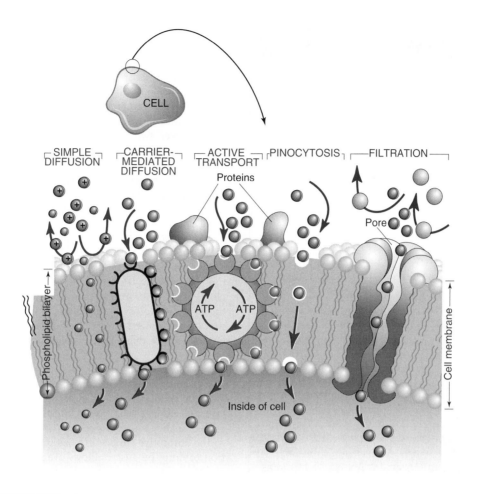

FIGURE 4-3 Transport Mechanisms. The majority of drugs cross cell membranes by simple passive diffusion. Only nonionized (uncharged) lipid molecules diffuse easily. Movement of drug molecules also occurs by carrier-mediated diffusion, active transport, pinocytosis, and filtration.

Factors Affecting Absorption

Bioavailability

Bioavailability, as defined by the FDA, is the rate and extent to which an active drug, or its therapeutic metabolite, is absorbed and becomes available at the site of action (Department of Health and Human Services, 2000: 21 CFR 320.1[a]). In other words, bioavailability is the percentage of drug available (i.e., absorbed) under the curve (following one route of administration) that produces a pharmacologic effect. In general, bioavailability is determined by measuring drug concentration in serum and by assessing the magnitude of response. Bioavailability is rarely calculated by using body fluids other than serum because of the inaccessibility of most fluids other than blood. This means that bioavailability is only half the story; the actual quantity of drug that reaches the site of action is seldom known. The amount of bioavailable drug is dependent on its solubility, chemical structure, size, and polarity (Box 4-2). Bioavailability is influenced by the presence of food within the GI tract. Food reduces the amount of fluid in the GI tract, slowing the dissolution of drugs and thus the absorption rate. In contrast, fasting for more than 12 hours causes vasoconstriction of blood vessels supplying the GI tract, and thus delays the absorption of any drugs that may be present.

Ionization

The movement of a drug by one or more transport mechanisms is influenced by the electrical charge (polarity) of the cell membrane and by the charge on the drug molecule. In order to understand the effect *ionization* has on the absorption of drug molecules, the effect of ionization on solubility must first be understood.

There are two basic rules regarding ionization of drugs: substances of like electric charge repel each other, and unlike forms attract one another. Alkaloids, bases, and metallic radicals are positively charged. Acids and acid radicals are negatively charged. Nonionized (uncharged) drug molecules are usually lipid-soluble and able to cross cell membranes. In contrast, ionized (charged) drug molecules are unable to penetrate lipid cell membranes (Box 4-3). A charge on a drug molecule similar to that of the membrane will delay absorption. Both the dissolution and ionization of drugs are affected by the pH of body solutions.

The ratio of a nonionized drug to an ionized drug is related to two factors: the pH of the aqueous medium in which it is

---

BOX 4-2

Factors Affecting Pharmacokinetic Phases

Absorption
- Bioavailability
- Solubility
- Ionization
- Absorbing surface
- Presystemic biotransformation

Distribution
- Blood flow
- Protein binding
- Tissue binding
- Solubility

Biotransformation
- Age
- Pregnancy
- Disease
- Genetics

Elimination
- Half-life
- Steady state
- Clearance
- Disease states

BOX 4-3

Factors Affecting Drug Movement Across Membranes

- Small, nonionized (uncharged) molecules are lipid-soluble and readily cross cell membranes.
- Large, ionized (charged) molecules are water-soluble and do not readily cross cell membranes.
- High water solubility + high serum protein binding = decreased volume of distribution and increased serum levels.
- High lipid solubility + high serum protein binding = decreased volume of distribution and serum levels.

---

dissolved, and its *pKa value*. The pH of an environment in which exactly half of the drug molecules are charged and the other half are not is called the pKa, or the ionization constant, of a drug. Each acid and base has a characteristic pKa. For example, aspirin (a weak acid) has a pKa value of 3.5. This means that if the pH of the solution in which the aspirin is dissolved is greater than 3.5, the drug will be ionized and relatively insoluble in lipid environments. At pH levels less than 3.5, aspirin will be almost entirely nonionized and lipid-soluble. It will, therefore, readily cross cell membranes.

Because ionization of drugs is pH dependent, drug molecules tend to accumulate on the side of the cell membrane where the pH is most favorable, a phenomenon called *ion trapping*. When an acid drug is in an environment more acidic than its pKa value, it has fewer ionized molecules and thus is more lipid-soluble. For example, aspirin, nonionized in the stomach, crosses cell membranes into plasma. There, where the pH is about 7.4, it becomes ionized and lipid insoluble. Thus, it is trapped in the plasma. Ion trapping is used therapeutically in the treatment of drug overdose and poisoning.

For example, making the urine more alkaline promotes ionization of an acid drug such as phenobarbital (pKa of 7.4) and facilitates its elimination by trapping in the urine.

Basic drugs act in the opposite way. A weak organic base such as codeine will be almost completely ionized when placed in an acid environment. In this form, it is not lipid-soluble and will not be absorbed. When there is a pH difference between two sides of a membrane, basic drugs tend to accumulate on the side that is more acidic. The plasma pH and the pH at the administration site are such that drug molecules have a greater tendency to be ionized in the plasma than at the administration site. Any drug can be absorbed to some extent in both the stomach and the intestines.

▥ Solubility

Solubility refers to the ability of the drug to dissolve and form a solution. To facilitate absorption, the solubility of the drug must be similar to the polar characteristics (i.e., electrical charge) of the absorption site. The more lipid-soluble a drug, the faster it crosses lipid cell membranes. Although a drug may be nonionized in one environment, when it moves to an environment with a different pH, it may become ionized.

▥ Absorbing Surface

Cell membranes determine the speed at which drugs reach systemic circulation. Drug molecules passing through a single layer of cells, as in the case of intestinal epithelium, do so faster than if they must pass several layers of cells. Blood supply to the absorptive surface is a significant factor in the absorption of drugs because it allows drugs to enter the circulation, and then blood flow removes them from that area. In so doing, the body maintains a steady state that encourages absorption and transport of the drug. Blood flow may be increased with local massage, local application of heat, certain metabolic diseases, or the concurrent administration of vasodilator drugs.

The rich blood supply of oral mucous membranes enhances absorption of drugs administered by the sublingual route. In contrast, absorption is delayed from subcutaneous tissues because of poor vascularity. Disease states such as peripheral vascular disease or shock, or the administration of vasoconstrictive drugs, may delay absorption.

It is assumed that the gastric mucosa is a simple lipid membrane permeable to nonionized, lipid-soluble forms of a drug. However, the stomach wall limits absorption to some extent. The surface area of the stomach is relatively small and lacks mucosal villi, and most of its cells are primarily adapted for secretion. Lipid-soluble substances such as ethanol and acid drugs are relatively nonionized at low gastric pH and therefore are absorbed in the stomach because of its rich blood supply. However, because the absorptive surface is small compared with that of the intestine, even acid drugs are significantly absorbed in the intestine.

Delayed gastric emptying slows the absorption of most drugs because it increases transit time to the intestine. High gastric acidity, hot meals, vigorous exercise, pain, and emotion all delay gastric emptying. Many drugs such as morphine, amphetamines, and anticholinergics slow gastric emptying. Gastric emptying time also may be increased by hunger, lying on the right side, ingesting dilute solutions, and mild exercise.

The larger the surface area, the more fully a drug is absorbed. For example, most absorption of orally administered drugs occurs in the small intestine, where many mucosal villi and microvilli provide an extensive surface area. The number of folds in the lining of the small intestine decrease from the proximal to the distal end. Therefore, drugs tend to be absorbed more in the duodenum, less in the jejunum, and least in the ileum. When large sections of the small intestine are diseased or surgically removed, drug absorption decreases. In select cases, a shortened small intestine also causes a decrease in the transit time of substances moving through the intestine.

The rectal route may be used when oral administration of a drug is not possible (e.g., nothing-by-mouth [NPO] status, dysphagia). The rectum, although having a good blood supply, has a limited surface area. Dissolution of drugs occurs slowly with irregular, unpredictable, and incomplete absorption. In addition, many of the drugs formulated for the rectal route are irritating to the fragile, thin mucosa of the rectum. Approximately one half of a rectally administered drug enters the enterohepatic circulation before entering the systemic circulation.

Drugs delivered to the lungs as gases or aerosols are rapidly absorbed because of the rich blood supply, large surface area, and high permeability of alveolar epithelium. Bronchodilator drugs, anesthetics, and the nicotine found in tobacco smoke are examples of substances that may be rapidly absorbed when inhaled.

Few drugs readily penetrate the skin, since it is low in lipid and water content. Absorption of drugs is fostered by suspending the drug in an oily vehicle and rubbing it into the skin. Absorption of the drug is proportional to lipid solubility and the surface area over which it is applied. Because hydrated skin is more permeable than dry skin, dosage forms may be modified or an occlusive dressing used to facilitate absorption. Systemic absorption occurs more readily through abraded, burned, or denuded skin surfaces. Inflammation or other conditions that increase circulation to the skin surfaces also enhance absorption. Body surfaces containing scar tissue generally have poor absorptive surfaces and therefore are not recommended for topical administration of drugs.

Topically applied ophthalmic and otic drugs are used primarily for their local effects. To produce local effects, absorption of the drug through the cornea or the auditory canal is required. Systemic absorption is usually not desired. Ophthalmic and otic drugs are discussed in more depth in Chapters 61 and 62.

Presystemic Biotransformation

Drugs may be biotransformed, usually to inactive metabolites, before reaching the systemic circulation. Orally administered drugs are transformed in the GI tract by acids, digestive enzymes, bacterial action, and enzymes in the cells of the intestinal walls. Venous blood from the GI tract (except the mouth and rectum) passes through the liver via the portal system before entering systemic circulation. Therefore, drugs that are highly cleared by the liver will undergo considerable biotransformation before entering systemic circulation. This phenomenon is known as the *first-pass effect*. Drugs highly cleared by means of the first-pass effect include certain tricyclic antidepressants (e.g., amitriptyline), analgesics (e.g., meperidine, morphine, propoxyphene), and antiarrhythmics (e.g., propranolol). Lidocaine, an anesthetic drug, when taken by mouth is almost completely biotransformed on the first pass through the liver and, therefore, has no pharmacologic effect.

As a general rule, drugs with significant first-pass effects require much larger oral than parenteral doses to achieve the same effects. Variable serum levels occur in the same individual as a result of a large variation in the metabolic activity in the liver. Dosage requirements for drugs that undergo a first-pass effect vary widely between individuals.

DISTRIBUTION

Following absorption, drugs are distributed through circulation to inert plasma and tissue-binding sites, to the site of action, and to the organs of elimination (Fig. 4-4). Several factors influence the distribution of an absorbed drug, including blood flow, protein binding, tissue-binding, and solubility.

Factors Affecting Distribution

Blood Flow

Cardiac output and blood flow influence the time required for a drug to be distributed to body tissues. The uptake of a drug is faster in tissues that are well perfused, such as the kidneys, the heart, the liver, and the brain. The uptake of a drug in poorly perfused tissues, such as muscle and adipose tissue, is slower. High–blood flow areas receive the drug before other body tissues. Unless a drug is given for its effect on the blood itself, drug molecules in the circulation must leave that fluid compartment and cross capillary membranes to reach their site of action. Drug concentrations rapidly equalize between blood and organs with high blood flow and then equalize more slowly within other tissues. For example, a patient who received an IV barbiturate for anesthesia will awaken within a few minutes even though the half-life of the drug is several hours. The rapid response is due to the decline of drug levels in the brain as the drug is redistributed to adipose tissue. It is the redistribution rather than drug elimination that terminates the anesthetic effect.

Protein Binding

Once absorbed, most drugs are bound, to a greater or lesser extent, to various tissues in the body. However, only free, unbound drug is available to cross cell membranes to the site of action. When a bound drug comes off a protein binding site, it is because the concentration around the protein is falling. Accordingly, the release of a drug bound to protein does not necessarily result in an increase in drug action.

Bound drugs are considered pharmacologically inactive because the large molecular size prevents the carrier complex from reaching the site of action. Further, bound drugs cannot be biotransformed or excreted. The exceptions are high–hepatic clearance drugs and those eliminated by renal tubular secretion.

Two independent protein-binding sites have been identified: alpha-1-acid glycoproteins and albumin. Different drugs tend to bind at each site. Basic drugs such as quinidine, meperidine, imipramine, dipyridamole, and chlorpromazine tend to bind to alpha-1-acid glycoproteins for distribution. Acid drugs, on the other hand, bind to albumin, the most abundant plasma protein. Examples of drugs that bind to albumin include warfarin, penicillins, and sulfonamides.

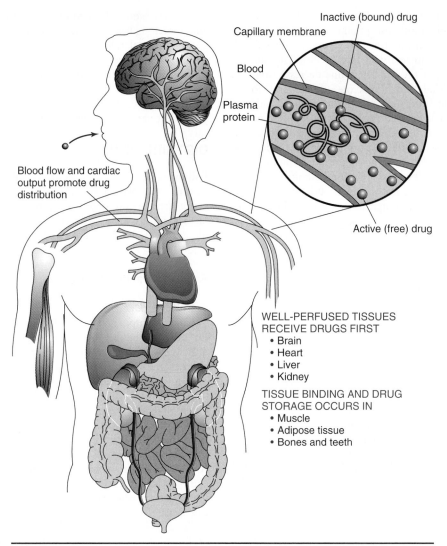

FIGURE 4-4 Drug Distribution. Once absorbed from the administration site, well-perfused tissues receive drug molecules first. Some molecules are reversibly bound to plasma proteins, particularly albumin. Because the drug-protein complex is large, it is trapped in the circulation and serves as a storage site for the drug. The percentage of bound or free molecules depends on the drug itself and the availability of protein-binding sites. Some drug molecules are also bound to tissues such as muscle, adipose tissue, bone, and teeth.

Binding to other plasma proteins occurs to a much smaller extent. A number of disease states alter plasma concentrations of albumin and alpha-1-acid glycoprotein and thus affect drug-protein binding (Table 4-4).

To some extent, plasma protein binding prolongs drug action. The stronger the drug-protein bond, the slower the release of the bonds and the longer the duration of drug action. As drug molecules are released from their bonds, they become free-acting. For example, sulfonamide drugs are highly bound to plasma proteins. To maintain drug equilibrium within the circulation, sulfonamide molecules are slowly released from the proteins and are then free to produce antimicrobial action.

The degree of drug-protein binding is expressed as a percentage. The percentage of protein binding in the circulation depends largely on the chemical nature of the drug. It may range from nearly zero to almost 100%. For example,

warfarin, an anticoagulant, is 99% protein bound. The remaining 1% is free to create pharmacologic effects. As a result, it is necessary to administer the drug only once a day in most cases because of the long duration of action. In contrast, a therapeutic dose of the analgesic acetaminophen is virtually free from protein binding. This permits more drug molecules to reach the site of action.

It should be noted that a patient who has low serum protein levels (i.e., hypoalbuminemia) may have difficulty transporting some drugs. The result of large amounts of unbound drug is an exaggerated effect that could prove hazardous to the patient.

Some proteins are nonspecific in that they are capable of binding with many different drugs at any given time. Several different drugs can compete with one another for the binding sites. If two drug molecules are somewhat equivalent in terms of bonding ability, the one with the stronger protein binding

TABLE 4-4 Plasma Protein Levels in Disease States

Disease States	Albumin Concentration	Alpha-1-Acid Glycoprotein Concentration
Acute infection	Decreases	Increases
Arthritis	Slightly decreases	Increases
Benign tumors	Increases	Varies
Burns	Decreases	Increases
Cirrhosis	Decreases	Varies
Cystic fibrosis	Decreases	Increases
Hepatitis	Slightly decreases	Increases
Inflammatory disease	Decreases	Increases
Liver disease	Decreases	Increases
Myocardial infarction	Decreases	Increases
Neoplastic disease	Decreases	Increases
Nephrotic syndrome	Decreases	Increases
Obesity	No change	Increases
Pregnancy	Decreases	Slightly decreases
Renal failure	Decreases	Increases
Stress or trauma	Varies	Increases
Surgery	Varies	Increases

or the one present in higher concentration will be more extensively bound.

Tissue Binding

Tissue mass determines the amount of drug accumulating outside the vascular space. The amount of drug stored in tissues decreases as the drug concentration in plasma diminishes. The plasma concentration of drug at its site of action is thus sustained, and the pharmacologic effects of the drug prolonged.

The relatively low blood flow to adipose tissue makes this area a stable environment for drug storage, as well as the fact that lipid-soluble drugs have a high affinity for adipose tissue. Even in starvation states, the percentage of body fat can constitute 10% or more of body mass. Barbiturates, antibiotics, anesthetics, and anticoagulants are commonly stored in body fat.

Body fat contains less water than lean body mass, so the amount of body water per kilogram of total body weight is less in an obese person than in a nonobese person. For some drugs, alterations in body makeup that accompany obesity make changes in drug dosages necessary. Drugs that are lipophilic distribute well to fat tissues and as such must often be given in larger doses to achieve the desired results. Drugs that distribute primarily to extracellular fluids (e.g., aminoglycoside antibiotics) may be given to the obese patient in higher doses, but the overall milligram per kilogram dose is lower than that given to a patient of normal weight.

Drugs with an affinity for calcium ions can accumulate in bones and teeth. Tetracycline antibiotics, heavy metals such as lead, radioactive elements such as radium, and environmental pollutants such as fluoride are stored in the bone and may lead to toxicity.

Solubility

Distribution of a drug once it has been absorbed depends on its solubility. Lipid-soluble drugs rapidly cross cellular membranes because of the highly permeable nature of capillary endothelial membranes. Drugs that are insoluble in lipids are limited in their ability to pass capillary endothelial membranes and, therefore, have a restricted distribution.

Barriers to Distribution

The capillary networks of certain endothelial structures act as barriers to drug distribution. The two most significant of these structures are the placental membranes and blood-brain barrier.

Placental Membranes

Nonionized, lipid-soluble drugs readily reach the fetus through maternal circulation. The same factors affecting drug movement across other membranes also determine movement across placental membranes. The long-standing notion that the placenta is a barrier to drugs is inaccurate. Although placental membranes may serve as a means to protect the fetus against potentially harmful drug effects, it is believed that the fetus is exposed to the same drug concentrations as those in the mother or, in some cases, to even higher drug levels. Chapter 6 discusses in more depth the physiologic changes of pregnancy and their influence on pharmacokinetics.

Blood-Brain Barrier

Highly ionized and protein-bound drugs cannot enter the central nervous system (CNS). Only drugs that are very lipid-soluble and poorly bound to plasma proteins are able to cross the blood-brain barrier to produce effects within the CNS. The active transport system of the blood-brain barrier pumps drug molecules out of the brain when diffusion has permitted them to enter.

The blood-brain barrier becomes important in patients with infection. Antimicrobial drugs may be ineffective against CNS infections if they are unable to cross the blood-brain barrier. In select disorders, such as meningitis, the active transport system fails, and large amounts of antibiotics such as penicillin are allowed to remain in the brain.

Volume of Distribution

The actual amount of drug in the body cannot be directly measured; however, an estimate of the concentration of drug in plasma or, sometimes, in the blood can be made. This volume, known as the *volume of distribution* (V_d), describes the amount of fluid necessary to contain the entire drug in the body in the same concentration as that in the blood. One method for calculating the V_d is to divide the amount of drug administered IV by the drug concentration in the plasma 1 hour after the drug is given. Keep in mind that the plasma drug concentration over time, after the administration of a single dose, depends on the rate and extent of drug distribution to the tissues and how readily the drug is eliminated. Thus the formula for calculating the V_d is as follows:

$$V_d = \frac{\text{the amount of drug administered}}{\text{plasma drug concentration}}$$

Many drugs exhibit a V_d far in excess of known body fluid volumes. For lipid-soluble drugs, the V_d is greater than the entire body fluid volume (over 0.6 L/kg). Drugs with extensive tissue binding can have a V_d greater than total body volume (over 1 L/kg).

BOX 4-4

Example of Volume of Distribution

Situation: A 70-kg male has received 500 mcg of IV digoxin. Assuming limited elimination of the drug, the V_d would be calculated as follows:

$$V_d \text{ in liters} = \frac{\text{Amount of drug administered in mcg}}{\text{Plasma drug concentration in mg/L}}$$

$$645 \text{ L} = \frac{500 \text{ mcg digoxin}}{0.775 \text{ mg/L}}$$

Thus: This patient has 9 times the total body fluid volume found in a healthy, 70-kg male (over 0.6 L/kg).

So... the V_d does not represent a real volume but must be thought of as the pool of body fluids that would be required if the drug were distributed equally throughout all portions of the body. In fact, digoxin is relatively hydrophobic, distributing early to muscle and adipose tissue. Only a very small amount of drug is in the plasma.

The V_d and therefore drug concentration is influenced by age, body mass, gender, extent of protein binding, and solubility. Males and females have different percentages of body fat and body water, so drug distribution also differs. Differences in the V_d are also evident during pregnancy, when the fetal-placental membrane unit provides additional tissue storage sites for certain drugs.

High water solubility and high plasma protein binding keep a drug in circulation. This ratio results in a small V_d and high blood levels (see Box 4-4). High lipid solubility and high tissue binding result in a large V_d and lower blood levels. Drugs with a large V_d are spread out to plasma proteins and tissues and are less frequently exposed to elimination, and thus less frequent dosing may be required. A drug with a small apparent V_d is likely contained only within the plasma.

BIOTRANSFORMATION

The term *metabolism*, as originally used, referred to the process by which carbohydrates, proteins, fats, vitamins, and minerals were built into living matter, and by which the living matter is broken down to simpler compounds. Metabolism is the sum total of intracellular chemical changes relating to catabolism and anabolism. However, the chemical changes that drugs undergo do not ordinarily provide new materials or energy. Thus the term *biotransformation* is preferable in the context of drugs. This term more accurately describes the physiochemical reactions that take place and that are not normally considered a part of carbohydrate, protein, fat, vitamin, or mineral metabolism.

A drug that is transformed from an inactive to active state through cleavage by a cellular enzyme is known as a *prodrug*, a precursor to the active compound. Today, prodrugs are widely used to overcome problems of absorption, to improve distribution of drugs that have poor lipid solubility, to increase the duration of action for drugs rapidly eliminated, to circumvent problems of patient noncompliance, and to promote delivery of the drug to a specific site. Examples of prodrugs include levodopa and azarabine, prodrugs of dopamine and azauridine, respectively. Levodopa is readily absorbed after oral administration and is distributed to the CNS. It is converted to dopamine in the basal ganglia. Dopamine is poorly absorbed and is extensively biotransformed so that, if given orally, it would never reach the brain in sufficient concentrations to have a biologic effect. Azarabine, the prodrug of azauridine, is used in anticancer therapy. Given as the prodrug, the formation of azauracil by intestinal microorganisms is blocked, and the toxicity of the drug is thereby reduced.

Mechanisms of Biotransformation

Biotransformation occurs in the plasma, the kidneys, the intestines, and the brain, but by far, the greatest number of transformation reactions occur in the liver. Its enzyme systems function to change lipid-soluble drugs to more polar, less lipid-soluble metabolites, thus fostering elimination and reducing the V_d. The mechanisms of biotransformation are many and varied but can be divided into two primary categories: phase I and phase II reactions (Table 4-5).

Phase I Reactions

The major groups of enzymes that help biotransform drugs during phase I reactions are known as the cytochrome P (CYP) 450 microsomal enzymes. These enzymes are found primarily in the endoplasmic reticulum of the liver. The ancestral cytochrome was probably present more than 1.5 billion years ago. The human genome encodes 57 of these enzymes. Of these, 14 are primarily involved in the metabolism of steroids; 4 oxidize fat-soluble vitamins, and 9 are involved in the metabolism of fatty acids and eicosanoids. Of the CYP450 isoenzymes, 15 are involved in the biotransformation of drugs, with 5 of the 15 accounting for 95% of drug biotransformation (i.e., 3A4, 2D6, 2C9, 1A2, and 2E1). Substrates for the remaining 15 of the 57 CYP450 enzymes are unknown. A substrate is any substance on which an enzyme acts.

Biotransformation of any drug that is a substrate for that particular isozyme (an *enzyme inducer*) will be more rapid, resulting in lower plasma concentrations of the drug. Because of this greater sensitivity, small changes in an amino acid sequence can result in huge changes in substrate specificity for the CYP450 enzymes (Table 4-6). For example, 2C19 is

TABLE 4-5 Biotransformation Processes

PHASE I REACTIONS	
Oxidation	The loss of electrons by an atom. Molecular oxygen serves as the final electron acceptor; usually carried out by a family of isoenzymes called cytochrome P 450 (CYP450)
Reduction	The gain of electrons by an atom
Hydrolysis	The combining of a water with a salt to produce an acid and a base
PHASE II REACTIONS	
Conjugation	The clinically relevant event in conjugation usually involves adding a chemical moiety, like a glucuronide, to an active drug to inactivate it and facilitate its removal from the body, primarily by the kidneys, usually by increasing the water solubility.
Alkylation	A chemical process in which an alkyl radical replaces a hydrogen atom
Acetylation	The introduction of one or more acetyl groups into an organic compound
Methylation	The introduction of a methyl group into a compound

TABLE 4-6 Major CYP450 Isoenzymes and Key Drugs and Drug Classes

Inhibitors	Inducers	Substrates*
ISOENZYME 3A4 (~30%)		
amiodarone	carbamazepine	Antihistamines
Antifungals	dexamethasone	Antiretrovirals
clarithromycin	efavirenz	Benzodiazepines
chloramphenicol	ethosuximide	Calcium channel blockers
ciprofloxacin	nevirapine	HMG CoA reductase inhibitors
delavirdine	phenobarbital	Immune modulators
erythromycin	phenytoin	Macrolides, 6 β-OH steroids
fluoxetine	pioglitazone	
fluvoxamine	rifabutin	
Grapefruit juice	rifampin	
nefazodone	St. John's wort	
norfloxacin	troglitazone	
Protease inhibitors		
quinine		
verapamil		
zafirlukast		
ISOENZYME 2C (<20% primarily 2C9; <5% are 2C19)		
amiodarone	carbamazepine	amitriptyline
cimetidine	phenobarbital	clomipramine
fluconazole	phenytoin	diazepam
fluoxetine	rifampin	imipramine
fluvastatin		losartan
fluvoxamine		phenytoin
isoniazid		omeprazole
metronidazole		Tricyclic antidepressants
omeprazole		warfarin
sertraline		
zafirlukast		
ISOENZYME 1A2 (~15%)		
cimetidine	carbamazepine	theophylline
ciprofloxacin	phenobarbital	Tricyclic antidepressants
clarithromycin	phenytoin	Benzodiazepines
enoxacin	rifampin	warfarin
erythromycin	ritonavir	
norfloxacin	Smoking (polycyclic aromatic hydrocarbons)	
Oral contraceptives		
Selective serotonin reuptake inhibitors (SSRIs)		
zileuton		
ISOENZYME 2D6 (~5%)		
amiodarone	carbamazepine	(No substrates)
cimetidine	phenobarbital	
clomipramine	phenytoin	
codeine	rifampin	
desipramine		
haloperidol		
perphenazine		
propafenone		
quinidine		
SSRIs		
thioridazine		
venlafaxine		
ISOENZYME 2E1 (<10%)		
disulfiram	ethanol	acetaminophen
ritonavir	isoniazid	chloral hydrate
		ethanol
		isoniazid
		ondansetron
		tamoxifen

*A substrate is any substance on which an enzyme acts. Because of the number of drugs considered as substrates, only the drug classes are listed for the 3A4 enzyme. A more complete table can be found at www.drug-interactions.com.

the principal CYP450 enzyme for omeprazole (Prilosec) biotransformation, but a closely related enzyme, 2C9, has no catabolic effect on omeprazole. As a result, there is little meaningful similarity noted in the amino acid sequence of the drug. However, there is some concordance (i.e., the presence of a given trait) between classes of drugs and the CYP450 family that biotransforms them. Similarly, patients whose livers have unusual biotransformation ability may become slow acetylators if they take a drug or food that inhibits the enzyme (an *enzyme inhibitor*). Enzyme induction has three important consequences:

1. The levels of liver enzymes alanine transaminase (ALT) and alkaline phosphatase (alk phos) may rise. This is a manifestation of enzyme induction and does not necessarily mean the liver is being damaged. Bile acid, albumin, cholesterol, and bilirubin measurements also reflect liver function and are more useful indicators of liver damage.
2. The patient may require a dosage increase as the result of increased liver enzyme activity. Increased enzyme activity means, for example, that phenobarbital will be biotransformed more quickly in a patient on long-term therapy than in one who has just started the drug, thus necessitating a dosage increase.
3. Biotransformation of other substances that use the CYP450 system is increased, and therefore these drugs may be less effective. Examples of drugs associated with enzyme induction include benzodiazepines such as diazepam (Valium), the antiepileptic drug carbamazepine (Tegretol), corticosteroids, and beta blockers such as propranolol (Inderal).

Both enzyme induction and inhibition provide a basis for enzyme-mediated drug interactions.

For more information, see the Evolve Resources Bonus Content "Influence of Selected Drugs on Laboratory Values," found at http://evolve.elsevier.com/Gutierrez/pharmacotherapeutics/.

Phase II Reactions

Conjugation, a phase II reaction, forms a covalent bond between the functional group added by the phase I reaction (or, occasionally, some other functional group) and a highly polar molecule derived from within the body. The conjugating agent is ordinarily a carbohydrate, an amino acid, or a substance derived from these nutrients such as glucuronic acid, sulfate, glycine, and acetate. These endogenous substances yield polar molecules that are usually inactive and readily excreted in the urine or bile. However, some conjugates are thought to contribute to hepatotoxic reactions. Drugs associated with hepatotoxicity are identified in Table 4-7.

Factors Influencing Biotransformation

Age

Neonates and infants up to 1 year of age do not have fully developed CYP450-enzyme systems. The combination of poorly developed blood-brain barriers, weak drug-biotransforming activity, and immature elimination mechanisms combine to make the fetus, neonates, and very young children sensitive to the toxic effects of drugs. They are unable to handle either the range or the total quantity of

TABLE 4-7 Major Hepatotoxic Drugs
ANTIMICROBIAL DRUGS
chloramphenicol
isoniazid
nitrofurantoin
Penicillins
Sulfonamides
Tetracyclines
ANALGESICS
acetaminophen
allopurinol
indomethacin
ANTIEMETICS
prochlorperazine
ANTICONVULSANTS
Barbiturates
phenytoin
ANTINEOPLASTICS
chlorambucil
mercaptopurine
methotrexate
CARDIOVASCULAR DRUGS
digoxin
hydralazine
methyldopa
nitroglycerin
DIURETICS
furosemide
PSYCHOACTIVE DRUGS
chlorpromazine
phenelzine
prochlorperazine
trifluoperazine
diazepam

chemicals that adult systems can manage. See Chapter 7 for further discussion of pediatric pharmacotherapeutics.

Similarly, older adults also have a limited capacity to manage drugs. Their limited capacity is related to changes in GI absorption and in the V_d that result from changes in body composition and metabolism, and the use of drugs that decrease renal clearance. With declining functional capacity of body systems, the biotransformation of drugs is reduced. Chapter 8 discusses geriatric pharmacotherapeutics further.

Pregnancy

Chapter 6 further discusses the effect of pregnancy on liver blood flow and the intrinsic activity of biotransformation enzymes.

Disease

Biotransformation rates are directly proportional to the concentration of CYP450 enzymes. If a change occurs in the concentration of an enzyme, there is a proportionate change in the rate of biotransformation. For example, alterations in liver function caused by cirrhosis reduce the production of necessary enzymes, resulting in greater concentrations of drugs typically biotransformed in the liver and thus possible toxicity. Decreased blood flow to the liver, such as occurs with heart failure, decreases the delivery of drug to biotransformation sites in the liver.

Because lipids, proteins, vitamins, and iron are required for the production and function of CYP450 enzymes, poor nutritional states or malnutrition impair enzyme activity; for example, prolonged protein malnutrition impairs biotransformation of barbiturates. A balanced diet fosters biotransformation. Caffeine, ethanol, cruciferous vegetables (e.g., cabbage, cauliflower, broccoli, Brussels sprouts), and charcoal-broiled meats stimulate enzyme induction. Food additives, air pollutants, and insecticides increase or decrease CYP450 enzyme activity. In addition, cigarette smoke contains polycyclic aromatic hydrocarbons that promote enzyme induction. Thus, smokers have considerably higher levels of enzymes that biotransform hepatic and pulmonary drugs.

Genetics

Genetically determined differences also influence the biotransformation of drugs. The differences may be evident in one group of individuals or marginally present or completely absent in another group. One of the most prevalent alterations involves acetylation, a phase II reaction. Half of the U.S. population are *slow acetylators*, an autosomal recessive trait. These persons biotransform drugs more slowly than the rest of the population. As a result, they are more likely to develop toxicity and often require lower dosages (Fig. 4-5). A syndrome resembling lupus erythematosus (characterized by joint pain, arthritis, and pleuritic pain) is more likely to develop in patients who are slow acetylators who are taking drugs such as hydralazine, procainamide, or isoniazid.

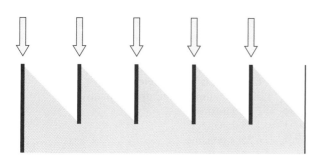

Rapid acetylators

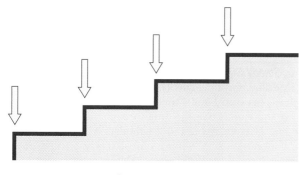

Slow acetylators

FIGURE 4-5 Rapid vs. Slow Acetylators. The pattern typical of rapid acetylators is shown in the upper panel, where the plasma level of the drug is maintained in a certain range over a period of several consecutive doses. Unusually slow biotransformation occurs when a slow acetylator receives the same dose, resulting in elevated plasma levels of the drug.

In another example, a bimodal distribution of drug biotransformation rates is evident in a population of individuals who are considered *rapid acetylators*. These individuals biotransform a drug more rapidly and consequently may develop reactions caused by the increased numbers of metabolites. A classic example of enzyme induction involves CYP450 3A4 and 17α-ethynylestradiol (the estrogen component of oral contraceptives). Ineffectiveness of oral contraceptives occurs with the concurrent use of barbiturates or rifampicin, followed by accelerated clearance of estrogen by the CYP450 3A4 enzyme. Hyperforin, a potent CYP450 inducer found in the herbal product St. John's wort, greatly increases the function of hepatic enzymes that biotransform drugs used for the treatment of acquired immunodeficiency syndrome (AIDS) and for patients undergoing organ transplantation.

Another group of individuals have a genetic defect in the enzyme glucose-6-phosphate dehydrogenase (G6PD) and are more likely to develop drug reactions. Blacks and certain Mediterranean and Asian populations (i.e., Sardinians, Sephardic Jews, Greeks, and Iranians) are more likely to have a G6PD deficiency than other ethnic populations. With the sex-linked incomplete codominant pattern of inheritance, males are more frequently and severely affected. Heterozygous females can exhibit a milder form of the disease. After an initial episode, the disease is usually self-limiting.

ELIMINATION

Elimination refers to the movement of a drug or its metabolites from the tissues back into the circulation and then to the organs of elimination. The organ primarily responsible for drug elimination is the kidneys, but to lesser degrees the GI tract, respiratory system, sweat, saliva, tears, and breast milk also are involved. Efficient elimination depends on proper functioning of the system involved. Lipid-soluble drugs are not eliminated until they have been biotransformed to a more polar compound.

Routes of Elimination

Renal Elimination

Several factors affect the rate of drug elimination through the kidneys. Factors affecting renal elimination include the ability of the heart and blood vessels to deliver an adequate blood supply to the kidneys, the maturity of the kidneys, the presence or absence of kidney disease, and urinary pH. In addition, some drugs (e.g., nonsteroidal antiinflammatory drugs [NSAIDs]) decrease renal blood flow and the glomerular filtration rate, thereby altering the elimination of many other drugs.

The kidneys use glomerular filtration and active tubular secretion to rid the body of unchanged drug molecules and their metabolites. Only free, unbound drug molecules are filtered by the glomeruli. Most drugs passively filter into the tubules, but those bound to plasma proteins are poorly filtered and remain in the plasma. Ionized compounds become trapped in the urine because they do not readily diffuse back across the lipid membranes of tubules into systemic circulation. Large, protein-bound compounds do not pass through the glomeruli. Nonionized, lipid-soluble weak acids and bases, once filtered by the glomeruli, are passively reabsorbed from the proximal and distal tubules.

Drugs that are lipid-soluble or not highly ionized undergo passive reabsorption in the renal tubules. By manipulating urinary pH, the passive reabsorption of a drug can be decreased and elimination enhanced. The effect is greatest for weak acids and bases with pKa values in the range of urinary pH (5 to 8). The administration of systemic alkalizers (e.g., sodium bicarbonate) causes tubular urine to become more alkaline. Tubular urine, also made more alkaline by consuming milk, vegetables, or most fruits, causes weak acids to be rapidly eliminated. The rapid elimination rate occurs because the drug is more ionized and passive reabsorption is decreased. In contrast, high doses of ascorbic acid or ammonium chloride acidify the tubular urine and promote the elimination of basic drugs. Eating cranberries, plums, or prunes makes the urine more acidic, reducing the elimination of weak acids. Alkalinizing or acidifying urine increases the elimination of weak bases.

Biliary Elimination

Although the majority of drugs are eliminated through the kidneys, some are removed through biliary elimination via a phenomenon called *enterohepatic recirculation.* Lipid-soluble drugs present in bile enter the small intestine, where a portion may be reabsorbed, returned to the liver, and again secreted into the bile. The result of significant enterohepatic recirculation is a measurable increase in the plasma concentration of the drug and a delay in elimination.

Elimination by Other Routes

The elimination of gaseous and volatile compounds occurs in the lungs. Drugs administered by inhalation are generally eliminated in their original form (not as metabolites) by this route. Inhaled drugs enter the systemic circulation after passing through alveolar membranes. The rate of drug elimination depends in part on the respiratory rate. For example, deep breathing or exercise increases cardiac output, with a subsequent increase in pulmonary blood flow. Drug elimination is thus fostered. The reverse is also true, if the respiratory rate is impaired.

Drugs taken by breast-feeding women cross epithelial membranes of the mammary glands to be eliminated in breast milk. Breast milk is acidic in nature, and therefore basic compounds such as morphine or codeine reach high concentrations in the milk. Weak acids such as barbiturates, sulfonamides, or diuretics are found in lower concentrations. Although relatively small quantities of any drug pass to the fetus, there is considerable concern about the cumulative effects of drugs on the infant. Because of the potential for a drug to reach the infant, lactating women should check with their health care provider before taking any drug. When the mother's health requires her to take a drug, the risk to the infant can be diminished if the drug is given immediately after breastfeeding.

Small amounts of drug also appear in sweat, saliva, hair, and tears. Although these routes are insignificant in most cases, they may become important if the primary route of elimination is not functional. For lipid drugs to be eliminated in the sweat, they diffuse through the epithelial cells of the sweat glands to the skin surface. Drugs excreted in the saliva are usually swallowed and undergo the same fate as orally administered drugs. Although drug elimination into hair is quantitatively insignificant, it can aid in diagnosis. Some tests for drug abuse involve analysis of hair samples. Arsenic was detected in hair samples

obtained during Napoleon's lifetime but examined 150 years after his death. Some now suggest that he was poisoned.

Factors Influencing Elimination

Half-Life

Half-life (t½) is the time needed to change the amount of drug in the body by one half after absorption and distribution are complete. The concept of half-life is important because it determines the time required to reach steady state (see discussion that follows) and the dosage interval. It takes four to five half-lives to reach steady state concentrations during continuous dosing.

In a practical sense, the body can be thought of as a single compartment equal to the size of the V_d (see Fig. 4-6). However, the organs of elimination can only clear a drug from blood that is in direct contact with the organ. Thus, the time course of a drug in the body depends on both the V_d and the clearance (Cl, which is discussed later in the section under "Clearance"):

$$t_{1/2} = \frac{0.7^* \times V_d}{Cl}$$

Changes in half-life result from changes in either the V_d or clearance; a change in half-life does not necessarily indicate that clearance has changed. Half-life can change solely because of changes in the V_d. Whereas the actual rate of change remains constant, the amount of drug eliminated (or accumulated) is proportional to its concentration. That is, the greater the drug concentration, the faster the change. This phenomenon, known as *first-order kinetics*, applies to most drugs. For example, according to first-order kinetics, a patient with a drug overdose can be expected to eliminate 97% of the original dose after five half-lives (assuming all elimination systems are functional and the elimination rate of the drug is not compromised). To illustrate:

- t_0 = time drug is administered
- t_1 = 50% of administered drug remains
- t_2 = 25% remains
- t_3 = 12.5% remains
- t_4 = 6.25% remains
- t_5 = 3.13% remains

In some cases, elimination (and accumulation) rates are independent of concentration. In these instances, fixed amounts of drugs rather than a proportion are eliminated at a constant rate. This phenomenon is known as *zero-order kinetics*. For example, alcohol is eliminated using zero-order kinetics.

Steady State

In reality, most patients take their drugs on a regular basis, typically between 1 and 4 times daily, and as such are accumulating and eliminating the drug throughout the day. Because the rate of elimination and accumulation is proportional to the concentration, at some point a steady state is reached (Figs. 4-7 and 4-8). With repeated dosing, drugs accumulate in the body until they reach a steady state or until dosing stops. Drug absorption then equals drug elimination during

---

*The constant 0.7 in the formula above approximates the natural logarithm of 2. Since elimination is an exponential process, the time taken for a twofold decrease to occur is proportional to 1n(2).

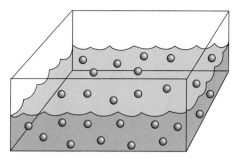

A ONE COMPARTMENT MODEL

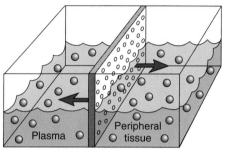

Plasma   Peripheral tissue

B TWO COMPARTMENT MODEL

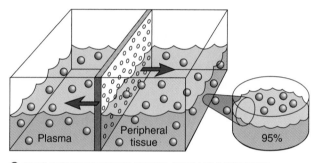

Plasma   Peripheral tissue   95%

C TWO COMPARTMENT MODEL WITH ELIMINATION

FIGURE 4-6 Compartment Models. A, A one-compartment model shows all body tissues and fluids as one compartment. The assumption is that after a dose of drug is administered, it distributes instantaneously to all body areas, much like chemicals added to an aquarium. However, some drugs do not distribute instantaneously to all parts of the body (even after IV bolus administration). **B,** A common distribution pattern is for the drug to distribute rapidly in the blood stream and to highly perfused organs such as the heart, the liver, the lungs, and the kidneys. Then, at a slower rate, the drug is distributed to other body tissues such as fat, muscle, and cerebrospinal fluid. This pattern of drug distribution is represented by a two-compartment model, much like a two-compartment aquarium. Chemicals placed in the first compartment equilibrate rapidly with those of the second compartment. Drugs transfer back and forth between these compartments to maintain equilibrium. The amount of drug in the first compartment declines logarithmically to a new steady state. **C,** When an avenue is created to drain the aquarium (i.e., an elimination route), a more realistic combination of elimination and equilibration results.

the dosing interval. It takes approximately four to five half-lives for plasma drug levels to reach a steady state, with peak and valley (trough) levels remaining constant after each dosing. A practical guide to the time it takes for a drug concentration to reach steady state can be obtained by multiplying the drug's half-life by 5. The result is very close to the time it takes to reach 90% of the steady-state value.

Clearance

Clearance refers to the removal of a drug from the body and is dependent on the integrity of glomerular filtration. Clearance is the most important pharmacokinetic parameter because it determines steady state concentration for a given dosage rate. Physiologically, clearance is determined by blood flow to the organ that biotransforms (e.g., liver) or eliminates (e.g., kidneys) the drug and the efficiency of that organ in removing the drug from the circulation. Because drug elimination takes place in the kidneys, the lungs, the liver, or other structures, it is important to remember the additive characteristic of clearance:

$$Cl_{systemic} = Cl_{kidneys} + Cl_{liver} + Cl_{other}$$

Clearance changes occur when blood flow to organs changes or when the removal ratio changes. Vasodilating drugs such as calcium channel blockers increase blood flow to the liver, whereas hypotension and heart failure reduce blood flow to the liver. Removal ratios increase when enzyme-inducing drugs increase the amount of CYP450 enzymes. Removal ratios decrease when enzyme-inhibiting drugs inhibit CYP450 enzymes or necrosis causes loss of parenchymal tissues.

Rather than estimating renal excretory function using the glomerular filtration rate (GFR), a proxy substrate is used: creatinine. Creatinine is a by-product of muscle metabolism. It is produced at a constant rate in a healthy individual as long as muscle mass remains constant. There is no significant secretion or reabsorption of creatinine, and it is largely eliminated by glomerular filtration. By estimating creatinine clearance, the health care provider also estimates GFR. (See Box 4-5 and Evidence-Based Pharmacotherapeutics box.)

Clearance of a drug from the body depends directly on the apparent V_d and is inversely related to the elimination half-life. The greater the V_d and the shorter the half-life, the faster the clearance and the more frequent the dosing required to maintain steady state. A drug that is slowly removed from the plasma and eliminated through the kidneys has a low clearance rate and requires less frequent dosing. The patient may thus require a change in the frequency of dosing and/or higher doses of a drug, depending on the drug's clearance. Both clearance and half-life vary greatly from one drug to another.

CHRONOTHERAPY

Many body functions such as hormone production, blood pressure, blood clotting, sleep-wake cycles, and response to drugs exhibit a certain rhythm. *Ultracadian rhythms* are shorter than a day. A 90-minute sleep cycle or the millisecond it takes for a neuron to fire are examples of ultracadian rhythms. *Circadian rhythms* last about 24 hours. For example, a circadian variation exists for susceptibility to noxious stimuli, endotoxins, and drugs. Sleep-wake cycles are directed by circadian rhythm. *Infracadian rhythms* are cycles that are longer than 24 hours. A woman's menses usually cycles anywhere from 21 days to 5 weeks. *Seasonal rhythms* influence our reactions and behaviors during particular seasons of the year (e.g., late spring, early fall). Seasonal affective disorder (SAD) causes depression in susceptible individuals during the short days of winter.

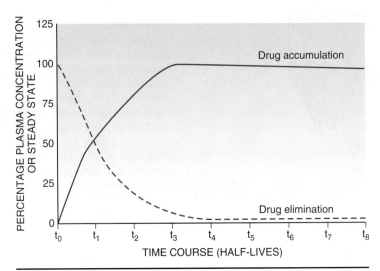

FIGURE 4-7 Time Courses of Drug Accumulation and Elimination. Accumulation is represented by the solid line, which reflects the plasma concentration during a constant-rate IV infusion of a drug. The broken line represents plasma concentration, with elimination after a constant-rate IV infusion reaches steady state.

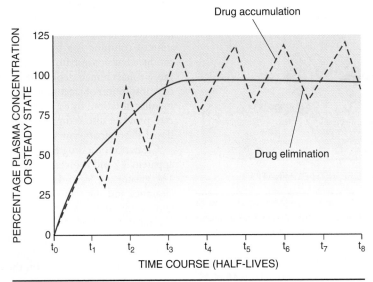

FIGURE 4-8 Relationship Between Dosing Frequency and Plasma Concentration. The rising solid line shows the plasma concentration achieved with a constant-rate IV infusion. The broken line shows the effect of dosing intervals.

BOX 4-5

Cockcroft-Gault Equation for Estimating Creatinine Clearance

$$\text{CrCl}_{\text{est}} \text{ in mL/min} = \frac{[140 - \text{age in years}] \times \text{ideal body weight in kg}}{72 \times \text{serum creatinine in mg/dL}}$$

$$(\text{Multiply the CrCl}_{\text{est}} \text{ by } 0.85 \text{ for women})$$

Serum creatinine is measured by a blood test, with normal values ranging from 0.8 to 1.2 mg/dL. Creatinine clearance is measured by combining this information with a patient's ideal body weight and age. The normal glomerular filtration rate is $120 + 25$ mL/min/1.73 m^2 (rate for males is approximately 5 mL higher; for females, approximately 5 mL lower). Values above 90 are normal for all.

NOTE: Creatinine clearance overestimates GFR in a variety of circumstances because of tubular secretion. This is particularly important at low levels of GFR. With age, GFR tends to fall (to approximately 100 mL/min/1.73 m^2 at age 70), although serum creatinine does not rise much in healthy individuals.

Bodily functions respond to the environment and the rhythms of the solar system that change from night to day and from one season to another; our genetics plays a role in these responses. These rhythms affect the way drugs behave in the body and, subsequently, patient response. The rate of drug absorption, hepatic clearance, half-life, duration of action, and the magnitude of drug effect have all been shown to differ depending on the time of day the drug is administered.

Coordinating these biologic rhythms with medical and pharmacotherapy is referred to as *chronotherapy*. The goal of chronotherapeutics is to match the timing of treatment with the intrinsic timing of illness (Elliott, 2001). Theoretically, the most favorable therapy results when the right amount of drug is distributed to the target organ at the most appropriate time. In contrast, many of a drug's adverse effects can be lessened or eliminated entirely if a drug is *not* given when it is not needed.

Chronotherapy is being studied in relation to diseases such as asthma, arthritis, and cancer and other disorders. For example, chronotherapy for asthma is directed at achieving maximal effects from bronchodilator drugs during the early morning hours, when lung function normally undergoes circadian changes and reaches a low point. Many health care providers believe that unless treatment improves nighttime asthma symptoms, it is difficult to improve the condition's daytime manifestations. Although seldom used today, the long-acting bronchodilator drug theophylline is taken once daily in the evening. Theophylline blood levels thus reach their peak during the early morning hours. For patients with severe persistent asthma who awaken during the night short of breath, a good night's sleep can be a dream come true (Stehlin, 1997).

Chronobiologic patterns have also been noted in patients with osteoarthritis who tend to have less pain in the morning and more toward the evening and nighttime. For these patients, the optimal time for administration of an NSAID such as ibuprofen would be at lunch time or in midafternoon. For patients who have rheumatoid arthritis, the pain is usually worse in the morning and decreases as the day goes on. The administration of corticosteroids and NSAIDs for these patients is timed to ensure that peak serum drug levels coincide with peak pain periods. Thus the best administration time would be after the evening meal.

Antineoplastic therapy may also be more effective and less toxic if the drugs are administered at carefully selected times, for it has been noted that there are different chronobiologic cycles for cancer cells compared with those of normal cells. Assuming this is true, the treatment goal is to time drug administration so that it corresponds with the chronobiologic cycles

EVIDENCE-BASED PHARMACOTHERAPEUTICS

Reliability of Different Formulae to Predict Creatinine Clearance

■ Background
Research studies that evaluate kidney function commonly use a 24 hour urine collection for creatinine clearance (CrCl) to measure glomerular filtration rate (GFR), although the test is often cumbersome and inconvenient for some patients. Using different biomedical means to measure GFR reduces the inconvenience to patients as well as the cost. The most common way to estimate GFR is the Cockcroft-Gault equation although there are other measures that may also be used.

■ Research Article
Verhave, C., Balje-Volkers, C., Hillege, H., et al. (2003). The reliability of different formulae to predict creatinine clearance. *Journal of Internal Medicine, 253*(5), 63–73.

Purpose
The purpose of the study was to determine the relationship between microalbuminuria and cardiovascular and renal disease in the general population.

Design
Cross-sectional cohort study using 8592 subjects, ages 28 to 75 years of age

Methods
This study compared 10 different formulae including the Bjornsson, Hull, Jelliffe-1, Mawer, Salazar-Corcoran, and Cockcroft-Gault formulae with actual measurements of creatinine clearance rates in a large sample of the general population. Study subjects participated in the Netherlands Prevention of Renal and Vascular End-Stage Disease (PREVEND) study. All subjects with microalbuminuria were participants in the cohort. Subjects completed questionnaires; anthropometric measurements were performed and fasting blood samples gathered; and subjects collected 24-hour urine specimens twice during the study. Differences in sexes were compared by a student's t-test or a chi-square test. Differences in microalbuminuria between males and females were compared using the Student's T-test or a chi-square test. A comparison was made of the sums of the individual squared differences between measured CrCl and the formula under study. Scatterplots were used to illustrate the difference between measured CrCl and the formula for each individual subject. To depict the CrCl and the formulae by age, univariate, nonlinear regression analysis was used.

Findings
The formulae used in this study did not provide an accurate measure of CrCl, particularly for male and obese subjects. A reasonably good estimate of CrCl in the overall population and in subjects of specific gender, body mass index, and age were demonstrated by six of the formulae, including the Cockcroft-Gault equation. However, all formulae examined CrCl in the higher ranges and overestimated CrCl in the lower ranges. Further, the age-related decline of CrCl is hard to approximate with a formula.

Conclusions
Formulae that approximate the upper and lower ranges of CrCl in the general population do not offer reliable data and do not adequately estimate the age-related decline in CrCl. There were several limitations to the study: there was an absence of a gold standard for GFR measurement, and the formulae tested were all designed to estimate CrCl instead of the true GFR. Because of the cross-sectional nature of the study, the ability to discuss differences in renal function over time was difficult; and the fact that creatinine in the blood and urine can be measured in different ways limited the study's findings.

■ Implications for Practice
The commonly used Cockcroft-Gault equation is one of the six best formulae for estimating CrCl, but a better approximation of measured CrCl could still be made with less underestimation in the higher ranges and less overestimation in the lower ranges. Future studies may examine the relationship of height to body composition to permit correction of CrCl in relation to body composition.

of tumor cells, thus making the drug more effective against cancer cells and less toxic to normal tissues. Some patients use an implantable infusion pump to administer antineoplastic drugs and thus receive the drugs in the late afternoon or during the night. Adherence to chronotherapeutic principles means that not all patients can receive their antineoplastic drugs first thing in the morning, an otherwise common practice.

What's more, it is believed that scheduling breast cancer surgery to coincide with the last half of the menstrual cycle increases the number of patients who are tumor-free 5 years later. The reason for this effect is that in the first half of the menstrual cycle, estrogen levels are high and progesterone levels are low. However, in the last half of the cycle, progesterone levels rise and estrogen levels fall. It is thought that progesterone may inhibit the production of some enzymes that help cancer to metastasize.

In other examples, patients who received test doses of intradermal histamine experienced the mildest skin response at 11 AM. The most severe responses were noted to occur at 11 PM. Thus, administration of cyproheptadine, an antihistamine, provides 16 hours of relief when it is taken at 7 AM but only 7 hours of relief when taken at 7 PM.

The plasma cortisol rhythm for daytime-active persons typically shows cortisol levels beginning to rise in the latter part of the usual sleep cycle. These levels peak shortly before or just after awakening, irregularly declining throughout the day and evening until minimal levels are reached early in the next sleep cycle. Transplant recipients, for example, are placed on lifetime steroid therapy to augment endogenous cortisol levels and prevent rejection of the donor organ. Under these conditions, the treatment goal is to reinforce intrinsic adrenocortical activity with minimal suppression. In order to achieve this goal, a synthetic glucocorticoid such as prednisone is given after the peak secretion of endogenous cortisol on a daily or alternate-day midmorning schedule.

On the other hand, when the treatment goal is replacement, such as for a person with adrenocortical insufficiency, the steroid is given at a time that mimics natural endogenous rhythm. That is, approximately two thirds of the daily dose would be taken in the morning upon awakening, and the remaining one third before bedtime in the evening.

Patients are more likely to follow a treatment regimen when the drugs are formulated and scheduled for administration according to chronotherapeutic principles. That is, it is possible to optimize desirable effects and minimize undesirable effects, while promoting patient compliance, by reformulating a drug so that absorption into the blood stream is delayed, using a revised dosing schedule, or using programmable infusion pumps that administer the drugs at precise intervals. Although susceptible biologic rhythms are not as well documented in human beings as in animals, research in this area is still rapidly growing. Drugs reformulated to be chronotherapeutic agents are regulated by the FDA.

KEY POINTS

- Pharmacokinetics describes the absorption, distribution, biotransformation, and elimination of drugs in patients requiring drug therapy.
- Simple passive diffusion, filtration, carrier-mediated diffusion, pinocytosis, and active transport are responsible for the absorption of drugs into systemic circulation.
- Factors affecting absorption include bioavailability, solubility, ionization, absorbing surfaces, drug forms, and routes of administration.
- Distribution is influenced by blood flow, the degree of protein and tissue binding, and the affinity of the drug for lipid or aqueous tissues.
- The volume of distribution (V_d) is a proportional constant that relates the amount of drug in the body to the serum concentration. The V_d is used to calculate the loading dose of a drug that will immediately achieve a desired steady state concentration. A large V_d represents a lower blood concentration level of a drug; a small V_d represents a higher blood concentration of a drug.
- Half-life is the time required for serum concentrations to decrease by one half after absorption and distribution are complete. Half-life is important because it determines the time required to reach steady state, and the dosage interval. Half-life is dependent on the values of clearance and the V_d.
- Bioavailability is the fraction of drug absorbed into the systemic circulation after administration.
- Of the CYP450 isoenzymes, 15 are involved in the biotransformation of drugs, with 5 of the 15 accounting for 95% of drug biotransformation (i.e., 3A4, 2D6, 2C9, 1A2, and 2E1).
- Knowledge of a drug's half-life, renal clearance, and steady state assists in determining the frequency of administration and assessing for drug accumulation.
- Age, various diseases and conditions, and genetic variations influence biotransformation, and therefore undertreatment or toxicity is possible.
- Elimination of drugs is primarily through the kidneys and biliary route, but it may also occur through the respiratory system, breast milk, saliva, and tears.
- Chronotherapy considers the patient's biologic rhythms when determining the timing (and sometimes the dosage) of a drug to optimize desired effects and minimize adverse effects.

Bibliography

Aithal, G., Day, C., Kesteven, P., et al. (1999). Association of polymorphisms in the cytochrome P450 CYP2C9 with warfarin dose requirement and risk of bleeding complications. *Lancet, 353* (9154), 717–719.

Bakutis, A. (1983). The P_{450} enzyme system: A key to understanding the metabolism of drugs. *Journal of the American Association of Nurse Anesthetists, 51*(3), 272–274.

Bolt, H., Kappus, H., and Bolt, M. (1975). Effect of rifampicin treatment on the metabolism of oestradiol and 17α-ethynylestradiol by human liver microsomes. *European Journal of Clinical Pharmacology, 85*(1), 301–307.

Department of Health and Human Services. (2000). Bioavailability and bioequivalence requirements. *Federal Register, 21* CFR 320, 188–189. Revised April 1, 2000.

DiPiro, J., Talbert, R., Yee, G., et al. (2005). *Pharmacotherapy: A pathophysiologic approach.* New York: McGraw-Hill.

Elliott, W. (2001). Timing treatment to the rhythm of disease: A short course in chronotherapeutics. *Postgraduate Medicine, 110*(2), 19–29.

Food and Drug Administration-Center for Drug Evaluation and Research. (2002). Preventable Adverse Drug Reactions: A Focus on Drug Interactions, available online: www.fda.gov/cder/drug/drugReactions/default.htm#Drug%20Metabolism). Accessed February 4, 2007.

Food and Drug Administration. (2007). *Electronic orange book.* Available online: www.fda.gov/cder/ob/default.htm, Accessed February 4, 2007.

Hardman, J., and Limbird, L. (2001). *Goodman and Gilman's the pharmacologic basis of therapeutics* (10th ed.). New York: Pergamon Press.

Katzung, B. (2005). *Basic and clinical pharmacology* (9th ed.). New York: Lange Medical Books/McGraw Hill.

Moore-Ede, M., Sulzman, F., and Fuller, C. (1982). Circadian timing of physiologic systems. In M. Moore-Ede and C. Czeisler (Eds.). *The clocks that time us.* Cambridge: Harvard University Press.

Nebert, D., and Russell, D. (2002). Clinical importance of the cytochromes P450. *Lancet, 360* (9340), 1155–1162.

Reinberg, A., Smolensky, M., Labrecque, G., et al (1987). Aspects of chronopharmacology and chronotherapy in children. *Chronobiologia, 14*(3), 303–323.

Rendec, S. (2002). Summary of information on human CYP enzymes: Human P450 metabolism data. *Drug Metabolism Review, 34*(1–2), 83–448.

Smith, R. (1988). The role of metabolism and disposition studies in the safety assessment of pharmaceuticals. *Xenobiotica, 18*(Suppl 1), 89–96.

Stehlin, I. (1997). A time to heal: Chronotherapy tunes in to body's rhythms. *FDA Consumer Magazine, 3* 31:3. Available online: www.fda.gov/fdac/features/1997/397_chrono.html. Accessed February 4, 2007.

Verhave, C., Balje-Volkers, C., Hillege, H., et al. (2003). The reliability of different formulae to predict creatinine clearance. *Journal of Internal Medicine, 253*(5), 63–73.

Wasen, E., Isoaho, R., Mattila, K., et al (2004). Estimation of glomerular filtration rate in the elderly: A comparison of creatinine-based formulae with serum cystatin C. *Journal of Internal Medicine, 256*(1), 70–78.

5

Pharmacodynamics

Pharmacodynamics is the study of the relationship between the concentration of a drug and the response obtained in the patient; in other words, *how the drug acts at various sites in the body*. Most often, the sites of action are receptors on the specific cell, tissue, or organ where the drug initiates a chain of biochemical events that culminate in changes in physiologic functioning of the cell, activity of an enzyme, or of an intracellular protein. Regardless of the drug, or the specific interaction with a receptor, the substance only alters or modifies a cell function or process; it does not create new functions.

DRUG ACTIONS VERSUS DRUG EFFECTS

The difference between drug action and drug effect is important to the understanding of pharmacodynamics. The interaction between a drug and receptor constitutes the *mechanism of action*–how the drug works. Drug action is the means by which the drug initiates the chain of events that leads to an effect.

A patient's responses to a drug's actions represent the *effect*, the observable result of the chain of events. Once a drug reaches the site of action, it produces effects through a nonspecific modification of the cellular environment, or through specific physical and chemical alterations in cell functioning, or both. Drug effects can be seen at nearby physiologic sites or at sites far away from the target organ. The more complex the physiologic processes affected, the more sites the drug may act on to produce an alteration in functioning.

In most cases, the effects are easily recognized and noted as changes in the patient's physiologic state. For example, morphine sulfate minimizes pain and suffering, acetaminophen or aspirin relieves fever, and digoxin slows the heart rate and strengthens its contractions. Figure 5-1 provides a visual representation of the relationships between the pharmacologic effects of a drug and the levels at which it produces therapeutic or toxic effects.

Mechanisms altering a cell's environment range from creating a physical barrier and altering surface tension to lubrication and ionizing radiation. The environment can also be modified by altering osmolality, chemistry, or pH of surrounding body fluids. Drugs modifying a cell's environment do so without physically attaching to cell membranes.

In contrast, alterations in cell functioning occur when a drug structurally interacts with cell components or target tissue. Commonly, the interactions inhibit or support energy metabolism, foster drug transport across cell membranes, or depress membrane function. Specific effects are produced by drug-receptor interactions, drug-enzyme reactions, and

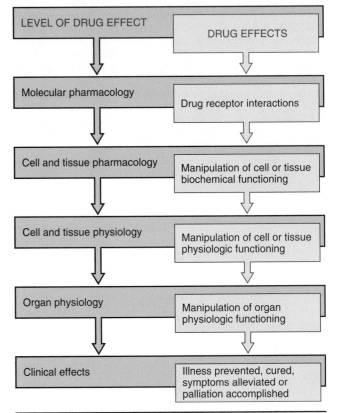

FIGURE 5-1 Comparison of Drug Effects with Level of Effect. A visual representation of relationship between the pharmacologic effects of a drug and the levels at which it produces therapeutic or toxic effects. (From Grahame-Smith, D., and Aronson, J. [1984]. *Oxford textbook of clinical pharmacology and drug therapy.* Oxford: Oxford University Press. Used with permission of Oxford University Press.)

nonspecific drug interactions. Regardless of the target cell, tissue, or process, drug actions accelerate or inhibit cell functioning.

DRUG ACTIONS AND INTERACTIONS

The characteristics of receptors and of the drug-receptor complex are important to the subsequent understanding of pharmacotherapeutics.

RECEPTOR THEORY OF DRUG ACTION

British physiologist John Newport Langley (1878–1925) and German physician immunologist Paul Ehrlich (1854–1915) first proposed that drug actions were mediated by chemical receptors. In 1933, A.J. Clark developed the dose-response theory, which stated that increased response to a drug depends on increased binding of drug to receptors. Several points in Clark's theory turned out to be incorrect: (1) that drug response is proportional to the number of receptors occupied; (2) that all drug-receptor interactions are reversible; (3) that drug binding to receptors represents only a fraction of available drug; and (4) that each receptor binds only one drug. In 1956, R.P. Stephenson presented a modified dose-response theory that is more widely accepted today: (1) drug response depends on both the affinity of a drug for its receptors and the drug's efficacy; (2) maximal response to a drug can be achieved even if fractions of receptors are unoccupied. Thus, there are three important characteristics of receptors to keep in mind:

- Receptors establish the quantitative relationships between dose or concentration of a drug and its effects
- Receptors are responsible for selective drug action
- Receptors mediate the actions of both agonists and antagonists

RECEPTOR TYPES

On a day-to-day basis and under normal homeostatic conditions, receptors interact with cell membranes to serve normal physiologic functions (Box 5-1). Theoretically, it should be possible to synthesize a drug that could alter any physiologic process for which receptors exist. As a general rule, though, if a physiologic process is not regulated through receptors, it is unlikely to be influenced by a drug.

There are several known receptor types: intracellular and transmembranous receptors, ion-gated channels, and G protein–coupled receptors (see Table 5-1). Drugs and receptors combine in a reciprocal manner. Thus, when a drug attaches to a receptor, the resultant complex initiates a biochemical event (Fig. 5-2). A single receptor can react with a number of drugs, provided each drug conforms structurally to the receptor site.

Intracellular and Transmembranous Receptors

Drugs acting at intracellular receptors must be lipid-soluble to cross cell membranes. The highly lipid-soluble steroidal hormones (i.e., glucocorticoids, mineralocorticoids, and sex hormones) bind to receptors in the cytoplasm. The drug-receptor complex then moves into the nucleus, where it affects genetic transcription by binding to DNA sequences near the gene whose expression is stimulated. A delay of 30 minutes to several hours is needed for the synthesis of new

TABLE 5-1 Examples of Receptors

Receptor Type	Receptor Subtype*†	Endogenous Transmitter
Acetylcholine	Nicotinic	Acetylcholine
	Muscarinic (M_1, M_2, M_3, M_4, M_5)	Acetylcholine
ACTH	—	ACTH
Acidic amino acids	NMDA, kainate, quisqualate	Glutamate or aspartate
Adenosine	A_1, A_2	adenosine
Adrenergic	α_1, α_2	epinephrine and norepinephrine
	β_1, β_2, β_3	epinephrine and norepinephrine
Dopamine	D_1, D_2, D_3, D_4, D_5	Dopamine
GABA	A	GABA
	B	GABA
Glucagon	—	Glucagon
Glycine	—	Glycine
Histamine	H_1, H_2, H_3	Histamine
Insulins	—	Insulin
Opioids	μ, μ_1, κ, δ, ε	Enkephalins
Serotonin	$5\text{-}HT_1$, $5\text{-}HT_2$, $5\text{-}HT_3$	5-HT
Steroids	—	Several

*Receptor identification and classification are based in large part on ligand-binding specificity.
†Other receptor subtypes in various stages of documentation have been proposed, especially where no endogenous transmitter is yet defined.
5-HT, 5-Hydroxytryptamine (serotonin); *ACTH*, adrenocorticotropic hormone; *GABA*, gamma-aminobutyric acid; *NMDA*, N-methyl-D-aspartate.

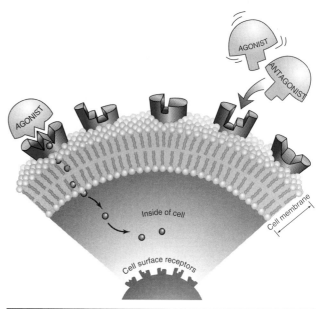

FIGURE 5-2 Drug-Receptor Interactions. *Agonists* with shapes matching an endogenous substance or a drug produce the same response as that of the endogenous substance. The response usually equals or is greater than that of the endogenous substance. Antagonists inhibit or counteract receptor activity through a number of inhibitory actions.

proteins that produce the drug's effects. This is why corticosteroid therapy is used to prevent rather than treat an asthma attack. Similarly, this mechanism is linked to the long-lasting effects seen until new proteins whose formation was stimulated by the drugs are biotransformed.

BOX 5-1

Assumptions About Drug-Receptor Interactions

- All receptors are identical in structure and equally accessible to the ligand.
- The intensity of the ligand-mediated response is proportional to the number of receptors occupied by the ligand.
- The amount of ligand combining with receptors is negligible compared with the amount of ligand to which the receptors are exposed.

Drugs directly affecting genetic transcription include thyroid hormones, vitamin D, and the retinoids—soluble, DNA-binding proteins that regulate the transcription of specific genes (i.e., transmembranous receptors). Nitric oxide, an endogenous substance with an intracellular enzyme, is probably involved in the mechanisms for nitroglycerin and other nitrates.

Ion-Gated Channel Receptors

Channels allow the movement of ions across cell membranes. Drugs bind to ion channel receptors, which then open or close the channel. For example, the antianxiety effects of alprazolam, a short-acting benzodiazepine, are attributed to its binding with a receptor near the GABA receptor, resulting in an increased affinity for GABA. GABA then opens the channels, and the influx of chloride into the cell inhibits neuron depolarization. This mechanism takes milliseconds to complete, so gated channels are frequently the signaling mechanism in the nervous system where information must be rapidly processed.

An initiating stimulus defines the two general categories of ion-gated channels: ligand-binding (or second messenger–gated channels) or voltage-gated channels. Nicotinic cholinergic receptors, the $GABA_A$ receptors for gamma-aminobutyric acid (GABA), and the receptors for excitatory amino acids such as glycine, aspartate, and glutamine are examples of ion-gated channels. Each protein gate is composed of four helical strands. In each strand, the polypeptide chain snakes back and forth across the membrane 6 times. This transmembrane structure is also seen in the voltage-gated potassium, sodium, and calcium channel receptor families, and also in other channel types.

G Protein–Coupled Receptors

Another family of receptors uses distinct glutamyl transpeptidase (GTP) regulatory proteins, known as G proteins, to convey signals to effector proteins. These receptors include those for secondary messengers such as biogenic amines, eicosanoids, and other lipid-signaling molecules, as well as numerous peptid and protein ligands. α- and β-adrenergic receptors use G proteins to affect cell function. G proteins remain active until GTP hydrolyzes to GDP, which does not activate receptors.

A cell can express as many as 20 G protein–coupled receptors, each with distinct specificity for one or several of its half-dozen G proteins. Receptors for multiple drugs can integrate their signals through a single G protein. A receptor can also generate multiple signals by activating more than one effector protein.

RECEPTOR NUMBERS AND RESPONSE

The number of receptor sites available and their affinity for binding determines the magnitude of drug action. It has been suggested that the number of receptor sites available for drug binding at any given time ranges from 2000 to 200,000 per cell. Drug-receptor interactions throughout the body produce widespread and unpredictable effects. If, however, a drug interacts only with specific receptors of highly differentiated cells, the response is much more predictable. To understand the variability in numbers, the concept of down- and up-regulation is helpful.

Down-regulation is seen as a decrease in the sensitivity of receptors to a drug and thus as a loss of effectiveness. For example, down-regulation occurs with repeated use of isoproterenol, a β-adrenergic bronchodilator used in the treatment of asthma. The decreased responsiveness may be due to an actual reduction in the number of receptors, to changes in existing receptors, or both. An increase in dosage or a change of drug may be required to achieve therapeutic effects.

In contrast, *up-regulation* is associated with an increased number of receptors triggered by hormones and neurotransmitters. In other words, the patient's heightened response to the drug exceeds the response seen in most other persons.

Affinity

Affinity is the strength of the attraction of a drug to its receptor sites and is related to the potency and the concentration of drug occupying receptors. Drugs with a high affinity are strongly attracted to receptors and are generally considered potent drugs. For example, a 10-mg dose of morphine sulfate is equivalent to a 1-mg dose of hydromorphone. Therefore hydromorphone is the more potent drug. In other words, drugs with a strong affinity for particular receptors are capable of eliciting a response at lower doses. The reverse is also true. Drugs with low affinity are less strongly attracted to receptors. They are generally weak drugs that require large dosages to elicit a response.

Potency Versus Efficacy

For clinical purposes, it is important to distinguish between a drug's potency and its efficacy. The term *potency* refers to the amount of drug required to produce 50% of the maximal response that the drug is capable of inducing.

The degree to which a drug is able to induce maximal effects as a result of binding to a receptor is referred to as *efficacy* (regardless of how intense the response). This ability can depend on its route of administration and its absorption, distribution, and clearance. In deciding which of two drugs to use for a particular patient, the health care provider must consider the relative efficacy rather than the relative potency; in contrast, potency largely determines the dosage to be used. For example, if drug A reduces blood pressure by 20 mm Hg and drug B reduces blood pressure by 10 mm Hg, drug A has greater efficacy than drug B.

Chirality

In chemistry, chirality refers to the arrangement of molecular components; that is, they have a spatial arrangement making what are called enantiomers, or *isomers*. The shape of a drug must be such that it can interact with receptors. As the mirror image of one another, each isomer is identified by its ability to rotate polarized light to the left, a negative optical rotation (levorotary; counter-clockwise; a [−] isomer), or to the right, a positive optical rotation (dextrorotary, clockwise, a [+] isomer).* For example, the natural flavoring compound carvone is chiral; one form tastes like rye, and the other form tastes like spearmint. The isomers can be distinguished by our taste buds as two separate compounds. A collection of equal amounts of two isomer forms of a chiral molecule is referred to as a racemic mixture or *racemate*. For example, epinephrine is a racemic mixture.

---

*(+) and (−) symbols are now preferred to designate the sign of optical rotation, replacing the previous nomenclature systems dextrorotary and levorotary ("d" or "l"), and "rectus" and "sinister" (R or S).

Isomer pairs can be likened to your hands, and as such, individual members of the isomer pair may not fit equally well into a specific receptor. This is called *stereoselectivity*. In the great majority of cases, one of these isomers will be much more potent than its mirror image companion, reflecting a better fit to the receptor molecule. For example, the commonly used cough suppressant dextromethorphan is a (+) isomer and yet, at usual dosages, dextromethorphan is essentially void of opioid activity. Similarly, dextromethorphan's (−) isomer, levorphanol, is a potent opioid analgesic but also has cough-suppressant properties. In another example, carvedilol is a drug that interacts with adrenergic receptors. It has two isomers. The (−) isomer is a potent beta blocker, 100 times more potent than the (+) isomer at β-receptors. However, both isomers are approximately equipotent as α-receptor blockers. Because enzymes are usually stereoselective, one isomer is often more susceptible than the other isomer to drug-biotransforming enzymes. As a result, the duration of action of one isomer may be quite different from that of the other.

The majority of times, both isomer forms of a drug can be safely used. However, in some cases, one isomer is active and the other is not. For example, in the 1950s thalidomide was used to relieve morning sickness and as a sleep aid. Thalidomide is chiral, and at that time, both isomers were present in the manufactured drug. It soon became apparent that one of the isomers was responsible for its therapeutic effects, whereas the other isomer caused severe birth defects. The drug is now classified as a pregnancy category X agent with restricted access in the United States. To increase the effectiveness of chiral drugs and to reduce possible adverse effects from the "wrong" chiral form, many of today's pharmaceuticals are manufactured as single-isomers. (For more information, see the website www.vioquestpharm.com/chiral/content/what_is_chirality.html.)

Agonists and Antagonists

Agonists combine with receptors to initiate events; that is, they have intrinsic activity that is produced by two different mechanisms. Agonist I drugs bind to the same site as an endogenous substance (e.g., neurotransmitter) to produce a similar response. The response usually equals, or is greater than, that of the endogenous substance. Agonist II drugs bind to different extracellular sites, with no response produced solely in the presence of the agonist. However, an enhanced response is generated when an existing endogenous substance also binds to its site.

Antagonists combine with receptors but do not begin a change in cell function. Occupation of the receptor by the antagonist drug prevents the binding and action of agonists. The effects of antagonists are only visible when they decrease the effect of administered agonists or decrease the action of ongoing, endogenously released ligands. In a sense, antagonists are conceptualized as part of a lock and key mechanism (thanks to Nobel Laureate Emil Fisher, 1852–1919); the key fits into the hole, but because of a different configuration, it cannot be turned. For example, anticholinergic drugs such as atropine prevent acetylcholine from attaching to the acetylcholine receptor. This inhibition stabilizes the receptor in its inactive state, and the actions of acetylcholine are reduced.

Physiologic antagonism is produced when two agonists act at different sites (Fig. 5-3). One drug offsets the effects of the other by producing opposite effects of the same physiologic function. For example, the bronchoconstricting effects of histamine on the respiratory tract can be offset by administering epinephrine.

Physiologic Antagonism

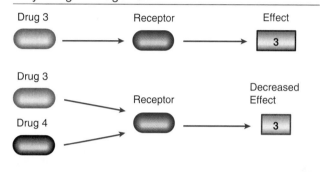

Dispositional Antagonism

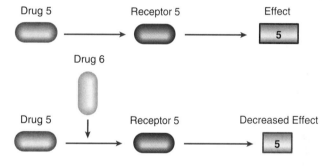

Chemical Antagonism

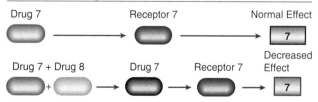

FIGURE 5-3 **Physiologic, Chemical, and Dispositional Antagonism.** Antagonism occurs any time the effect of two drugs is less than the sum of the effects of the drugs acting separately. Drug antagonism causes a diminished therapeutic effect. With *physiologic antagonism,* two agonists acting at different sites counterbalance each other by producing opposite effects on the same physiologic function. *Dispositional antagonism* is the opposite of synergism. It occurs whenever one drug indirectly decreases the amount of a second drug available at its site of action. *Chemical antagonism* occurs when an agonist and an antagonist combine to form an inactive product.

Chemical antagonism occurs when an agonist and an antagonist combine to form an inactive product. For example, the effect of heparin on antithrombin II, prothrombin, and fibrinogen is reduced in the presence of the protein protamine sulfate.

A *competitive antagonist* has affinity for the same receptor sites as that of the agonist drug, binding in a reversible manner. It prevents a response by interfering with the action of the agonist. However, a competitive antagonist does not decrease the maximal response of the agonist drug. Inhibition occurs when the concentration of the antagonist increases without a change in the amount of available agonist. A common example of competitive inhibition is vitamin K, which acts on the same receptors as the oral anticoagulant warfarin. The interaction between vitamin K and warfarin can be reversed by increasing the concentration of the agonist drug (see also Chapter 39).

In contrast to competitive antagonists, *irreversible antagonists* are permanently bound to the receptor. An agonist drug's maximal pharmacologic effect is decreased with these antagonists, because the antagonist drug reduces the number of active receptors. To overcome the antagonist's effects and restore the agonist's maximal pharmacologic effect, new receptor proteins and thus a receptor free of the drug are required to be generated. Environmental pollutants, pesticides, nerve gas, and heavy metals such as lead, mercury, and arsenic are noncompetitive inhibitors.

Dispositional antagonism is the opposite of synergism (see later discussion). It is an alteration in pharmacokinetics of the drug such that less drug reaches the site of action or its presence there is reduced

Partial agonists-antagonists have characteristics of both agonists and antagonists, at times appearing to cause actions and other times to decrease the action of agonists with greater intrinsic activity. At certain concentrations, partial agonists actually can be antagonists.

Selectivity and Specificity

Most drugs interact with several receptors and thus have the ability to produce distinctly different pharmacologic actions. The two factors that determine which drug action will be observed are the *affinity* and the ability to activate the desired receptor *(intrinsic activity).* For drugs to be *selective,* they must preferentially activate one receptor over another. A drug said to be *specific* interacts with one and only one receptor.

It is generally considered good practice to prescribe drugs that are highly selective and specific, because the more selective the drug, the fewer the adverse effects. Likewise, a drug that interacts with many receptors is likely to elicit a wide range and variety of responses.

Dose-Response Curves

Dose-response curves reflect the magnitude of drug action against the concentration (or dosage) of drug required to induce those actions. The receptor affinity, absorption, plasma protein–binding, distribution, biotransformation, and elimination of a drug all affect the dose response curve (Fig. 5-4). It is during this last phase that the next dose of a drug is usually administered. Graded drug dosing usually results in a greater magnitude of response as the dosage is increased. With routine dosing schedules, the serum level of a drug is prevented from dropping below the desired therapeutic range.

A threshold dose is necessary for a given response to be elicited. According to the dose-response curve, an initial low dose usually corresponds with a low response or none at all. Likewise, in most cases, a drug-induced response reaches a plateau rather than indefinitely increasing. Increasing the amount of drug administered often produces undesirable effects to a greater extent than it produces therapeutic effects.

Therapeutic Indices

Dose-response curves are used to generate information about a drug's margin of safety. A drug's *therapeutic index* (TI) expresses its relative safety. TI relates the dose of a drug required to produce a desired effect to that producing an adverse or toxic response. Drugs with a high TI are said to be safe (i.e., to have a wide margin of safety). Those with a low TI are relatively unsafe. They have a narrow margin of safety.

The TI is computed using the following formula, where TD_{50} equals the dose that would be toxic in 50% of patients and ED_{50} equals the dose that produces the desired therapeutic effect in 50% of test animals. In other words: $TI = TD_{50} \div ED_{50}$.

The closer the ratio is to 1, the greater the likelihood of toxicity. For example, digoxin is a cardiac glycoside used in the treatment of heart failure and arrhythmias. In many cases, the TI value for digoxin approaches 1. This means there is an increased risk of toxicity with digoxin than with some other drugs.

Therapeutic indices are derived from animal studies during the developmental phase of a new drug and redefined during clinical trials. Although the TI of a drug in humans is seldom known, clinical trials and accumulated clinical experience often uncover a range of ordinarily effective doses and a different range of possibly toxic doses (given patient comorbidity pharmacokinetics).

Non–Receptor Interactions

Some drugs have little or no structural specificity with receptor sites and yet still elicit a response. Presumably, drugs enter the cell or accumulate in the cell membrane, where they influence chemical or physical functioning. For example, some anesthetics are thought to act by changing membrane dynamics. The following drugs all act without the aid of receptors: chelating drugs such as ethylenediaminetetra-acetate (EDTA), binding calcium, iron, and mercury; alkalinizing drugs with a cation, like sodium; acidifying drugs with a fixed anion; and osmotic diuretics such as mannitol. Vitamins and trace elements influence cell function and therefore are pharmacologically active. Another example of non–receptor drug action is psyllium, a bulk-producing laxative. Psyllium forms a nonabsorbable gel that absorbs water, keeping the stool hydrated and soft.

ADVERSE DRUG REACTIONS

Most people, including health care providers and pharmaceutical manufacturers, refer to a drug's unwanted effects as side effects, implying that the effect in question is insignificant or occurs via a pathway that is to one side of the principle action of the drug. Such implications are frequently erroneous.

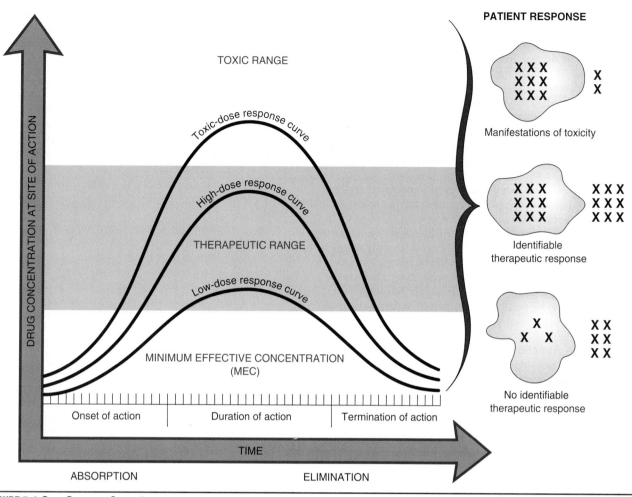

FIGURE 5-4 Dose-Response Curve. Dose-response curves reflect the magnitude of drug action against the concentration (or dosage) of drug required to induce those actions. The ideal drug produces three separate curves that do not overlap: a low dose–response curve, a high dose–response curve, and an adverse- or toxic-effect curve. With adequate distance between the three curves, the possibility of an adverse drug reaction is minimized.

There is no universal scale for describing the severity of an *adverse drug reaction* (ADR). The term ADR is accurate when referring to an unwanted, unpleasant, noxious, or potentially harmful reaction. In general, the expected therapeutic benefits of a drug should outweigh the potential risks of its use. Nonetheless, ADRs are common. Most ADRs are mild, disappearing when the drug is stopped or the dosage changed. Other mild ADRs gradually subside as the body adjusts to the drug. However, some ADRs are more serious and last longer. Numerous studies have been done to determine the incidence of ADRs, which range from 10% to 30% for hospitalized patients and rank fourth to sixth as the most common cause of death in the United States (Kvasz, Allen, Gordon, et al., 2000). Depending on the specific research study read, it is estimated that 3% to 7% of hospital admissions are due to ADRs. For an inpatient, the risk of having at least one ADR increases to 10% to 20%.

The incidence of ADRs also increases with the number of drugs taken. One study showed a 4.2% incidence of adverse reactions in patients taking five or fewer drugs; however, the incidence increased to 24.2% when 11 to 15 drugs are taken and to 45% when 21 or more drugs are taken (Davies, Green, Mottram, et al., 2006).

ADRs occur most often in females, older adults, and patients who have renal disease. Although it is not always possible to predict who will experience adverse effects, knowledge of factors known to increase a patient's risk helps to minimize their occurrence.

TYPE 1 ADVERSE REACTIONS

Many ADRs are an exaggeration of a drug's therapeutic effects—a type 1 reaction. Type 1 reactions are common and usually not serious. Type 1 ADRs may develop, for example, if a patient is unusually sensitive to the drug, when a drug dosage is too high, or if a drug-drug interaction slows biotransformation of the first drug, thus increasing its blood level. For example, a patient taking an antihypertensive drug may feel dizzy or light-headed if blood pressure is lowered too much or too quickly. Weakness, sweating, nausea, and palpitations may result when an antidiabetic drug causes hypoglycemia. Type 1 ADRs are usually predictable, but occasionally cannot be avoided. However, with long-term therapy, such effects persist as troublesome, distressing symptoms that are unresponsive to treatment.

TYPE 2 ADVERSE REACTIONS

For the most part, type 2 ADRs are unpredictable. The term idiosyncrasy is derived from the Greek words *idios,* meaning "one's own," "peculiar," or "distinct," and *synkrasis,* meaning "mixing together." Idiosyncratic reactions, which may consist of unpredictable and unexplainable symptoms, result from extreme sensitivity to a low dose of a drug or extreme insensitivity to high doses of a drug, indicating an abnormal tolerance. Sometimes an idiosyncratic reaction takes on a *paradoxical* response, an effect opposite to that desired.

Although there are many examples of idiosyncratic ADRs, skin rashes (e.g., Steven's-Johnson syndrome), jaundice, and anemia account for the most common ones. Decreases in the white blood cell count, kidney damage, and nerve injury tend to be more serious but typically occur in only a small number of patients. These patients may be allergic or hypersensitive to the drug because of genetic differences in the way their body biotransforms or responds to drugs. Type 2 ADRs can also be precipitated by the secondary actions of the drug and may or may not be dose related.

Cumulative Reactions

Cumulative reactions result when the effects of one drug have not dissipated before the administration of another dose. Cumulative reactions occur most often with drugs whose biologic half-lives are measured in days, weeks, or months, unlike those whose half-lives are measured in hours (whose concentrations fall to ineffective levels long before the drugs disappear from the body). Although they are somewhat unpredictable, cumulative reactions develop when the rate of administration exceeds the rate of biotransformation or elimination. However, toxic symptoms may appear as drug concentrations rise (often owing to continued dosing despite reduced elimination). Cumulative toxicity can progress rapidly, as in the case of ethyl alcohol intoxication, or slowly, as with the slow and insidious poisoning of heavy metals.

Toxic Reactions

Toxic reactions are related to excessive drug levels. In some cases, the effects are an exaggeration of the usual pharmacologic effects. If drug concentration does not exceed a critical level, the effects are usually reversible. The risk of a toxic response is inversely related to the TI of the drug. For example, toxicity with water-soluble vitamins is rarely seen. However, when drugs such as digoxin or insulin, each with a narrow TI, are administered, therapy must be closely monitored and managed to avoid toxicity. Many drugs are not toxic in and of themselves, but toxicity can result through biotransformation; the specific response depends on the rate at which the toxic metabolite is produced and destroyed.

Pharmacogenetic Reactions

Pharmacogenetics is the study of genetic differences in biotransformation. The importance of pharmacogenetics is twofold: investigating and identifying the genetic basis for unusual drug responses, and developing methods for predicting who will react abnormally to drugs. The practical value of pharmacogenetic studies lies in their predictive ability, thereby allowing potentially injurious ADRs to be avoided. As noted in Chapter 4, pharmacogenetic differences result in either increased or decreased intensity of response to a drug, with a longer or shorter duration of action.

Allergic Reactions

Compared to other ADRs, the number and severity of allergic (hypersensitivity) reactions account for as few as 10% of all ADRs and are usually not dose related. Allergic (hypersensitivity) reactions to a drug are difficult to predict and to prevent. For drug-allergic patients, even a small amount of the drug can trigger reactions ranging from the minor and simply annoying to those that are severe and life-threatening.

Although allergies can occur with any route of administration, topical routes present the greatest risk for allergic reactions; the oral route is less likely to result in sensitization. Some drug classes are more likely to cause drug reactions than others, but there is no known way to estimate the allergic potential of any drug. As with most undesirable responses, the health care provider is well advised to limit the number of drugs prescribed.

Contrary to popular belief, allergic reactions do not occur with the first exposure to an antigen. All allergic reactions are the result of an immune system response. An allergic reaction is manifest only after a second or subsequent exposure, and is different from the usual pharmacologic response expected. Because drugs are ordinarily not proteins, they do not, in and of themselves, act as antigens. However, following biotransformation, drugs or their metabolites can combine with endogenous proteins to form reactive compounds.

For example, for a low–molecular weight (LMW) drug to cause an allergic reaction, it or its biotransformed product usually combines with an endogenous protein to form an antigenic complex. The complex stimulates production of antibodies, usually after a latent period of at least 1 to 2 weeks. Subsequent exposures to the antigen result in an antigen-antibody reaction that typically provokes the signs and symptoms of allergy. Dose-response relationships usually are not apparent in the provocation of allergic reactions.

On the basis of the immunologic mechanism in operation, drug allergies may be classified as anaphylactoid or IgE-mediated reactions (type I), tissue-specific reactions (type II), immune complex–mediated reactions (type III), and cell-mediated reactions (type IV) (Table 5-2).

IgE-mediated Reactions

Anaphylactoid reactions are acute, life-threatening events mediated through IgE antibodies. The Fc portion of IgE can bind to receptors on mast cells and basophils. The Fab portion of IgE then binds the antigen, causing the release of various mediators (i.e., histamine, leukotrienes, and prostaglandins). The primary targets of this type of reaction are the gastrointestinal tract (food allergies), the skin (urticaria and atopic dermatitis), the respiratory system (asthma and rhinitis), and the vasculature (anaphylaxis). When severe, the reaction progresses to shock, hypotension, and cardiovascular collapse. Anaphylaxis can occur with all routes of administration but is seen most often following use of parenteral formulations.

TABLE 5-2 Classifications of Allergic Reactions*

Type	Synonyms	Antibody	Effector Cells	Mechanism	Example
I	Anaphylaxis (IgE-mediated)	IgE	Mast cells	Antigen binds with basophils on surface of mast cells and basophils, with release of histamine, leukotrienes, serotonin, and prostaglandins	penicillin, pollens, insect bites, seasonal allergic rhinitis, household cleaning agents
II	Tissue-specific	IgG, IgM	Macrophages in tissues	Antigen binds to allergen on cell membranes; complement system activated with cell destruction	penicillin, methyldopa, sulfonamides, hydralazine, procainamide, quinidine
III	Immune complex–mediated response	IgG, IgM	Neutrophils	Antigen binds to allergen in fluid phase and deposits in small blood vessels; complement system is activated with cell destruction	penicillin, phenytoin, streptomycin, iodides, sulfonamides
IV	Cell-mediated response	Not involved	Lymphocytes; macrophages	Sensitized cells bind to allergen and release lymphokines	tuberculosis skin tests, tumor rejection, graft rejections, rabies vaccination, poison ivy reactions, phenol, benzene products, halothane

*Types I, II, and III allergic responses occur immediately. Type IV responses have a delayed onset.
Adapted from McCance, K., and Huether, S. (2002). *Pathophysiology: The biologic basis for disease in adults and children* (4th ed., p. 230), St. Louis: Mosby.

Tissue-Specific Reactions

Tissue-specific reactions are mediated by both IgG and IgM antibodies and are usually attributed to their ability to activate complement. The major target tissues for this type of reaction are those of the circulatory system. In most cases, the reactions subside a few months after the drug is discontinued.

Immune Complex–Mediated Reactions

Immune complex–mediated reactions result from the deposit of antigen-antibody complexes in the circulation. The complexes deposit in vascular endothelium, causing a destructive, local inflammatory response. This reaction usually lasts 6 to 12 days, subsiding after the offending drug is discontinued. The primary difference between tissue-specific and immune complex–mediated reactions is that the antigen in tissue-specific reactions remains at its normal location on the cell surface, whereas the antigen in immune complex–mediated reactions, being soluble, is released into and circulates in the blood or body fluids.

Cell-Mediated Reactions

Cell-mediated reactions are most often associated with two mechanisms. Either cytotoxic T lymphocytes (T cells) attack and directly destroy cellular targets, or the reaction is mediated by lymphokine-producing T cells. The sensitized T cells release macrophage migration–inhibiting factor, macrophage-activating factor, chemotactic factors, and other substances that attract macrophages and neutrophils to the area. Infiltration by these substances contributes to a local inflammatory response. Tissues are killed by the release of soluble factors such as lysosomal enzymes and toxic oxygen products from macrophages.

TOLERANCE AND DEPENDENCY

Tolerance represents a decreased response to a drug. Clinically, it is seen when the dose of a drug must be increased to achieve the same effects. Tolerance develops to some drug effects more rapidly than to other effects of the same drug. For example, tolerance develops to the euphoria produced by opioids such as heroin, and there is a tendency to increase the dose in order to achieve that same elusive "high." In contrast, tolerance to the GI effects of opioids develops more slowly.

Tolerance is the result of alterations that are (1) related to drug absorption; (2) dispositional (i.e., a reduction in the rate of drug transfer across biologic membranes); (3) pharmacodynamic (i.e., a drug-induced synthesis of CYP450 enzymes after chronic use); (4) cellular (i.e., a decrease in the number of receptors to which a drug attaches or a decrease in the affinity between the receptor and drug); or (5) behavioral (e.g., the alcoholic learns to hide the signs of drinking to avoid being caught by colleagues). Because tolerance does not usually develop to all effects of a drug, the TI of the drug may decrease.

Although tolerance generally develops with prolonged, repeated use of a drug, it may also occur after only one or two doses. Tolerance that develops rapidly is referred to as *tachyphylaxis;* it may be the result of a change in the sensitivity of the target cells. Even with larger dosages of the drug, the patient's initial response cannot be reproduced. Pharmacodynamic tolerance occurs most often with drugs acting on the central nervous system (CNS) to produce changes in mood or behavior.

Drug dependency occurs when a patient needs a drug to function "normally." Clinically, it is detected when cessation of the drug produces withdrawal symptoms. *Psychologic dependence* is characterized by an emotional drive to continue using a drug in order to maintain an optimal sense of well-being. Manifestations of psychologic dependence range from a mild desire for the drug to craving and compulsive use. Craving and compulsivity represent a major problem to the drug abuser because they suggest a loss of control over the drug and its effects.

Physical dependence is described as a resetting of the body's homeostatic mechanisms in response to repeated drug use;

the body adapts to the drug's effects until it can function only in the presence of the drug (e.g., chronic use of laxatives leads to dependence on laxatives to have a normal bowel movement). If the offending drug is abruptly stopped, there is another imbalance, and the body must again go through a process of readjusting to a new equilibrium without the drug. Physical dependence and its concomitant changes in health status do not result from excessive use of all drugs but depend on each drug's properties.

The appearance of a *withdrawal syndrome* is the only real evidence of physical dependence. Withdrawal occurs when a drug is no longer available to a dependent patient. Withdrawal symptoms result not only from removal of the drug of dependence but also from hyperarousal of the CNS caused by absence of the drug. Withdrawal symptoms are characteristic for a given class of drugs and tend to be opposite to the original effects produced by the drug before tolerance developed. For drugs such as alcohol, barbiturates, and opioid analgesics, the physiologic effects of withdrawal are so unpleasant and threatening that they become important factors in continued use of the drug and in motivating drug-seeking behaviors.

Cross-tolerance or *cross-dependence* occurs when tolerance or dependency develops to drugs in the same chemical class. For example, patients use methadone to prevent and/or to relieve symptoms of heroin withdrawal.

DRUG INTERACTIONS

As drug therapy becomes more complex and drugs more potent, beneficial as well as detrimental interactions appear. It is estimated that the average patient receives 6 to 10 different drugs during a hospital stay, and many outpatients are taking 6 to 8 drugs on a somewhat regular basis. Older adults may be taking concurrently as many as 15 to 20 drugs. For the ultimate benefit of the patient, the health care provider must have a working knowledge of potential drug interactions and must share that knowledge and experience.

The term *drug interaction* refers to a change in the magnitude or duration of a response to one drug in the presence of another. Interactions can be related to the pharmacokinetic or pharmacodynamic characteristics of the interacting drugs.

Several mechanisms are involved in drug interactions, but the result is an increase or decrease in the concentration of the drug at the site of action (Box 5-2). The most commonly encountered mechanisms involve poor absorption from the GI tract, displacement of the drug from plasma proteins, or

a very rapid or very slow biotransformation. Interactions increasing therapeutic or adverse drug reactions include additive effects, synergistic effects, and potentiated effects. Interactions resulting in decreased drug effects are generally grouped under the category of antagonism (see earlier discussion).

ADDITIVE EFFECTS

Additive effects occur when two drugs with similar actions are taken (Fig. 5-5). The combined effects of the two drugs are equal to the sum of the effect of each drug given alone. In some cases, combining two drugs at lower dosages produces increased therapeutic effects with a resultant decrease in adverse reactions.

SYNERGISM VERSUS POTENTIATION

Synergism describes the results of two drugs whose combined effects are greater than the sum of those of each drug acting alone (see Fig. 5-4). The term is usually reserved for situations where the two drugs are acting at different sites or have different mechanisms of action. One of the drugs, the synergist, increases the effect of the second drug by altering its absorption, biotransformation, distribution, or elimination. Thus the intensity of effects is increased, or the duration of action prolonged. An example of a common synergistic effect is that produced when penicillin is given concurrently with probenecid. Each drug alone produces its own effect. However, the combination provides penicillin with a longer duration of action than it would have alone, because probenecid inhibits the elimination of penicillin.

Potentiation occurs when a toxic drug is interacting simultaneously with a nontoxic drug to cause increased effects. The

Additive Effect

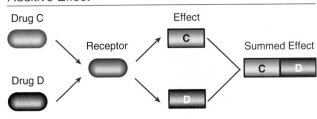

Synergistic Effect

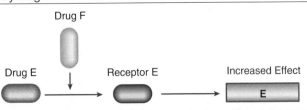

FIGURE 5-5 Additive and Synergistic Effects. *Additive effects* occur when two drugs with similar pharmacologic actions are taken. In some cases, combining two drugs at lower dosages produces increased therapeutic effects with a resultant decrease in adverse reactions. *Synergistic effects* are produced when two drugs whose combined effects are greater than the sum of each individual drug acting alone. The term is usually reserved for situations in which the two drugs act at different sites or have different mechanisms of action.

BOX 5-2

Mechanisms of Drug Interactions

- Acceleration or inhibition of drug biotransformation
- Displacement of plasma protein–bound drug
- Impaired uptake of drug from the gastrointestinal tract
- Altered renal clearance of drug
- Modifications in receptors or blockade of receptor channels
- Changes in electrolyte balance or body fluid pH
- Changes in the rate of protein synthesis

term is often used interchangeably (although not necessarily accurately) with synergism. With potentiation, the first drug may be devoid of an observable effect if given alone but produces a measurable response when combined with a second drug. For example, tyramine is an intermediate product in the conversion of tyrosine, an amino acid, to epinephrine and norepinephrine. In and of itself, tyramine has no pharmacologic effects. However, tyramine is commonly found in a variety of foods and is particularly plentiful in cheese. Patients taking monoamine oxidase–inhibitor drugs such as tranylcypromine (Parnate) are unable to metabolize ingested tyramine. Thus, an ordinarily harmless food is turned into a toxic substance. A sharp rise in blood pressure and, in a few cases, cerebral hemorrhage, has occurred. This response to tyramine is sometimes referred to as the "cheese response" (see Chapter 20).

DRUG-FOOD INTERACTIONS

For the most part, food interactions with drugs occur in three ways: (1) by decreasing the rate or extent of drug absorption; (2) by increasing the rate or extent of drug absorption; or (3) by chemical interactions. Ordinarily, changes in the rate of drug absorption have less significance if only the rate of absorption is affected and not the drug's bioavailability. The underlying mechanisms are highly variable and depend on both on the properties of the drug and the content of the interacting food. For example, tetracycline and fluoroquinolone antibiotics such as levofloxacin, ciprofloxacin, or ofloxacin chelate calcium ions found in milk and milk products, thus reducing bioavailability.*

Food can prevent a drug from being absorbed properly in the small intestine, thus limiting its effectiveness. For example, the bioavailability of the macrolide antibiotic azithromycin is reduced by 43% when taken with food. Similar reactions are seen with erythromycin, isoniazid, penicillins, and zidovudine if taken orally.

On the other hand, the absorption of some drugs is increased in the presence of food. For example, a high-fat meal enhances the absorption of lipophilic drugs such as itraconazole or the benzodiazepines. The absorption of extended-release theophylline, a bronchodilating drug, increases in the presence of a high-fat meal; however, only 40% of the sprinkle formulation is absorbed when taken with meals. Extended-release or controlled-release drugs should be taken apart from meals because of the variability that can exist in absorption.

Some drugs cause depletion of nutrients or minerals found in foods. For example, drugs such as cholestyramine, which is designed to bind bile acid in the GI tract, bind to fat-soluble vitamins (i.e., vitamins A, D, E, and K) and folic acid when taken with food. The result is decreased absorption of these vitamins. Mineral oil used as a laxative acts as a physical barrier, reducing the absorption of the fat-soluble vitamins. Patients who lack adequate nutritional intake are potentially at greater risk for drug-induced vitamin and mineral depletion; however, some drugs are better absorbed when fat is present.

Food also affects biotransformation of some drugs. Grapefruit juice is the classic example since it affects biotransformation of many drugs by specifically inhibiting the CYP450 3A4 isoenzyme. The highest concentrations of extrahepatic CYP450 isoenzymes are found in the distal portion of the villi that line the small intestine. These extrahepatic isoenzymes are responsible for the biotransformation of more than 20 drugs. The result is increased serum concentration of drugs dependent on this enzyme for biotransformation. For example, the bioavailability of felodipine can be enhanced as much as 2 to 3 times in the presence of grapefruit juice.

Food can alter urinary elimination of some drugs. For drugs that are weak bases, consuming grapefruit, orange, or tomato juice raises urinary pH, thus increasing the proportion of non-ionized drug and enhancing systemic reabsorption of the drug. As discussed in Chapter 4, ionizing a drug promotes its water solubility, thereby enhancing elimination into the urine.

DRUG-HERB INTERACTIONS

Until about 150 years ago, all drugs were derived from natural materials. Although the term "herb" suggests something beneficial and with little potential for harm, numerous toxic materials may be used (e.g., foxglove, deadly nightshade, and jimson weed). In addition, herbalists sometimes process herbs, changing them from their original form and isolating active ingredients so that the end products are not "as nature intended." The use of potent and potentially toxic substances and the intentional alteration of natural substances are characteristic of the production of modern herbal remedies. Thus some herbal remedies, when combined with today's drugs, may indeed be beneficial with little potential for harm, whereas others may be toxic in the presence of a drug (see Chapter 11).

DRUG-DISEASE INTERACTIONS

Drugs can affect diseases in various ways, either positively or negatively. Certain diseases and/or conditions change the pharmacokinetics and pharmacodynamic parameters of some drugs, leading to less than ideal therapeutic responses, increased risk for toxicity, physiologic changes, or exacerbation of comorbid conditions. For example, hypothyroidism slows gastric emptying time, thus altering drug absorption. Diseases that reduce plasma albumin levels (e.g., acute infection, burns, nephrotic syndrome, malnutrition, inflammatory diseases, and cystic fibrosis) alter drug distribution and therefore decrease the amount of drug bound to plasma proteins, causing more drug to be free to act at receptors. Cirrhosis impairs hepatic blood flow, synthesis of albumin, and biotransformation of drugs. The use of a prodrug in a patient with hepatic disease potentially reduces the efficacy of the drug. Patients with renal disease may require a downward dosage adjustment to avoid drug accumulation.

VARIABLES AFFECTING DRUG RESPONSE

GENERAL STATE OF HEALTH

Almost all pharmacokinetic and pharmacodynamic principles are formulated using data gathered from healthy individuals.

---

*For further information, see the Evolve Resources Bonus Content "Effect of Foods on Drug Absorption" and "Selected Listing of Drugs Causing Primary Nutrient Malabsorption," found at http://evolve. elsevier.com/Gutierrez/pharmacotherapeutics.

However, drugs are administered to persons in whom a physiologic process is taking place at an abnormal level. The presence of disease contributes to variability in drug response, especially when organs responsible for the absorption, distribution, biotransformation, and elimination of drugs are affected. For example, drugs tend to accumulate in the presence of liver disease. As the liver ceases to function, the rate of biotransformation falls, and drug levels rise. A decrease in dosage levels is required so that drug levels remain below toxic range. Liver disease does not alter plasma levels of drugs that are primarily removed by renal or pulmonary elimination. As with liver disease, kidney disease interferes with the elimination of water-soluble drugs, causing the drugs to accumulate in the body.

LIFE-SPAN CONSIDERATIONS

Pharmacokinetic drug action in infants and that in older adults are different from those in the middle-age group. Infants have a greater proportion of total body water than adults, resulting in expanded distribution and diminished blood levels of water-soluble drugs. Infants and young children also have a low percentage of body fat, thus contributing to increased blood levels of lipid-soluble drugs. A relative lack of gastric acid contributes to an exaggerated absorption of drugs that would normally be inactivated by gastric acid. An exaggerated absorption of drugs normally ionized at a low pH also occurs. Further, an infant's body system lacks the enzymes responsible for drug biotransformation. However, most of the enzyme systems develop quickly, with levels reaching those of an adult 1 to 8 weeks after birth. By the first year of life, the enzyme systems are probably as active as they will ever be. In addition, rapid dehydration caused by immature temperature regulation mechanisms can elevate serum drug levels. The renal elimination of drugs is also reduced in an infant as a result of decreased renal blood flow and a greater volume of distribution. The breastfeeding infant can develop adverse reactions to drugs that pass from the mother and into breast milk (see Chapter 6).

Although numerous physiologic changes that occur during pregnancy affect drug action, the pregnant patient is not necessarily at higher risk for adverse effects. Body water and plasma volume increase by as much as 50% during a normal pregnancy. Therefore, a drug dose is "diluted" compared with what happens in a nonpregnant state. As a result, dosage requirements may increase. This and other factors associated with drug therapy during pregnancy are discussed in depth in Chapter 6. No drug should be given to a woman of childbearing age before it is determined whether or not she is pregnant. A fundamental concept to remember is that the drug will be received by two persons, the mother and the fetus.

On the other end of the age spectrum, older adults are prone to drug interactions as a result of the normal changes of aging and concomitant disease. Alterations in drug absorption, distribution, biotransformation, and elimination are common. A high gastric pH decreases the absorption of drugs normally nonionized at a low pH. Proportional increases in body fat lead to less fat-soluble drug deposition. Reduced body water contributes to higher serum concentrations of water-soluble drugs. Lowered serum albumin levels result in increased amounts of unbound drug, leading to greater drug activity. Further, a reduction in cardiac output and renal blood flow affects the biotransformation and elimination of drugs. All of these changes result in higher drug concentration levels and a greater chance of toxicity (see Chapter 8).

BODY WEIGHT

Body weight is a significant determinant of drug effects. The magnitude of drug response is a function of drug concentration at the site of action. The concentration, in turn, is related to the volume of distribution (V_d) of the drug. As a general rule, a particular quantity of drug might be less effective in a heavier individual, provided renal, hepatic, and cardiovascular functions are adequate. The average adult dose of a drug is calculated on the basis of the amount that will produce a particular effect in half of the population between the ages of 18 and 65 years who weigh approximately 154 pounds (70 kg). The dosage required to obtain a therapeutic effect is roughly proportional to body size. Any variation in effect is minimized when dosages are calculated using kilograms of body weight. The recommended dosages for many drugs are listed in terms of grams or milligrams per kilogram (g/kg or mg/kg) of body weight. Pediatric dosages are most often calculated on the basis of body weight.

SEX AND GENETICS

Sex does not play a significant role in drug action. However, women generally require smaller dosages of drugs than men to produce the same magnitude of response, simply because of lower average weight. For women taking drugs with a narrow TI, the differences in drug response may require a reduction in dosage. There can also be gender-related differences in drug response because of an unequal proportion of lean body mass to fat mass.

An exaggerated response or lack of response to a drug can be the result of genetically determined susceptibility (known as *genetic polymorphism*). Genetic variations may result in abnormal or absent biotransformation enzymes. The abnormality can be harmful or fatal if the drug cannot be transformed and thus exerts toxic effects because of accumulation or prolonged therapy. For example, approximately 8% of the U.S. population lack the CYP450 2D6 isoenzyme and therefore are at greater risk for toxicity from psychoactive drugs, as well as other drugs biotransformed by this enzyme. The biotransformation of isoniazid also shows variability among different people; some are rapid acetylators, others are slow acetylators.

BODY RHYTHMS

Normal body rhythms influence drug action and can, in some cases, lead to adverse drug reactions. Circadian rhythms continue to operate even when external factors that influence behaviors, such as clocks and social and work routines, are removed. For example, cortisol levels normally rise between 8 and 10 AM, decline toward evening, and then rise again in the morning. Human growth hormone and prolactin secretions peak within the first 2 hours after onset of sleep. Thyroid-stimulating hormone is also at maximum levels the first few hours after sleep begins. Thyroid-stimulating hormone levels recede about 3 hours after awakening in the morning. Biologic rhythms must be considered in the interpretation of laboratory results related to drug and hormone levels.

PSYCHOSOCIAL CONSIDERATIONS

Drugs are not always taken or administered as prescribed. *Adherence* (some prefer the term *compliance*) is defined as the extent to which a prescribed care plan is followed (see also Chapter 9, Table 9–2). Doses may be omitted, extra doses taken, or the drug taken at a wrong time. Patients receiving higher than normal dosages for extended periods are at increased risk for adverse effects. On the other hand, patients receiving less than the dose prescribed may have minimal or below minimal effective concentrations of the drug, with therapeutic drug levels never reached.

Failure of the prescribed drug regimen is often a result of *nonadherence* with (or *noncompliance* to) the prescribed plan of care. However, it should be noted that noncompliance defines the problem only from the health care provider's viewpoint. Generated by health care providers, the term denotes deviant behavior when, in reality, the patient may not be aware of the proper dose and regimen, or may have chosen not to take the drug as prescribed for a variety of reasons. One reason for nonadherence is a belief that the drug is no longer needed; this is common with antimicrobial drugs. A patient feels better after 3 to 4 days of therapy and stops taking the drug. The offending organism remains in the body to produce additional signs and symptoms later, perhaps in a newly resistant form. Fears about the drug's adverse effects and of addiction are also possible causes of premature discontinuation of therapy.

Drug misuse, the use of a drug for the wrong purpose, is often the result of inaccurate self-diagnosis. In addition, the administration of a drug in situations in which contraindications are misunderstood or not recognized contributes to drug misuse. The administration of drugs by more than one person, each unaware of the other's actions, and administration of excessive doses based on the false impression that "if a little is good, more is better" are of concern. Patients at greatest risk for ADRs related to compliance or misuse behaviors are those taking drugs with a narrow TI, those taking drugs for which the precise timing of the dosage is important, and those in whom underlying medical conditions are likely to be aggravated by a particular drug.

Further, even with our present-day knowledge of how disease affects normal body functioning, it is difficult to separate pharmacologic effects of drugs from their psychologic effects. Certain symptoms of disease, such as headache, nausea, and even more serious signs, can be brought about by impulses that originate in the cerebral cortex. The degree to which a drug is effective is related to the patient's belief that the substance has desirable powers. A *placebo* is administered specifically for the purpose of satisfying an individual's need for drug dosing. Because the effects obtained from a placebo are determined by psychologic factors rather than physiologic ones, the presence of a placebo response does not suggest that the patient's original problem was imaginary.

DIETARY CONSIDERATIONS

Food in the stomach impairs the absorption of certain drugs. For example, when antacids are taken concurrently with iron preparations, the antacid binds the iron, making it unavailable for absorption. Green leafy vegetables are high in vitamin K.

Their excessive intake decreases the effectiveness of oral anticoagulants such as warfarin. Cabbage, broccoli, charcoal-broiled meats, and caffeine-containing foods stimulate liver enzymes, thereby increasing the rate of drug biotransformation. Drugs can deplete the body of essential nutrients; however, these interactions may go undetected because they are difficult to recognize. An awareness of the patients' nutritional status is important to avoid untoward drug-nutrient interactions.

SMOKING AND ALCOHOL INTAKE

The hydrocarbons in cigarettes induce the CYP450 enzymes, thus altering the biotransformation of certain drugs (e.g., diazepam, propoxyphene, chlorpromazine, amitriptyline). Acute alcohol intake inhibits biotransformation of drugs, thus increasing serum concentrations and increasing the risk for toxicity. It also enhances the pharmacodynamic effects of drugs targeting the CNS (e.g., opioids, antidepressants, antipsychotics, skeletal muscle relaxants), thus causing CNS depression. Chronic alcohol intake, on the other hand, tends to increase CYP450 enzyme synthesis, leading to reduced serum drug concentrations. Long-term alcohol use impairs drug biotransformation by destroying functional liver cells.

ENVIRONMENT

Physical environment affects drug response. For example, environmental temperature affects the action and effects of nitrates and antihypertensives. For example, when used by an individual exposed to high temperatures, these drugs relax peripheral vessels to the extent that excessive vasodilation occurs. Pesticide exposure alters the pharmacokinetics of certain drugs, thereby increasing the risk of adverse effects.

DRUG ADDITIVES AND BIOAVAILABILITY

Variance in onset, peak, and duration of action may lead to adverse effects. Different brands of the same drug can vary in bioavailability because of differences in manufacturing. Therefore, caution must be used when substituting one brand of drug for another, or when changing from a brand name to a generic drug and vice versa. In addition, additives such as buffers, stabilizing agents, or dyes can produce adverse responses in susceptible individuals. When adverse responses to an additive are numerous, the manufacturer may reformulate a drug to remove the offending additive.

Although relatively uncommon, adverse effects have been reported when a drug past its expiration date is administered. Improper storage of drugs contributes to their degradation, rendering some more or less potent.

DOSAGE AND NUMBER OF DRUGS ADMINISTERED

The dosage administered, the formulation, and the route and frequency of administration all modify drug effects. However, the risk of adverse effects increases in direct proportion to the number of drugs the patient takes. These factors all have one thing in common: the effects produced depend on the previous administration of the same or a different drug.

ADMINISTRATION ROUTES AND TECHNIQUES

Drugs are manufactured with specific routes of administration in mind. Administration by routes other than those recommended can cause ADRs. Even use of the recommended routes of administration can cause ADRs at times. A parenterally administered drug does not require absorption through the GI tract before entering systemic circulation. For this reason, drugs administered by this route, especially those given by intravenous (IV) route, reach receptor sites quickly and are more likely to cause adverse responses. Administering an IV drug too rapidly may cause ADRs, because the speed with which a drug is given alters its rate of distribution. Similarly, a drug designed to treat ear problems will cause pain and irritation if administered in the eye.

KEY POINTS

- A fundamental principle of pharmacology states that the intensity of response elicited by a drug is a function of the dose administered. As the dosage of a drug is increased, the proportion of persons experiencing a particular, stated response is also increased.
- Drug action represents the interaction between the drug and the environment, and the interactions between drug and cellular components. The patient's response to drug action represents the effect.
- Drug action occurs at the cellular level; however, drug effects influence total body functioning.
- Receptors are specialized proteins, cell membranes, or enzymes to which drugs display a chemical or biophysical attraction. The stronger the affinity for a receptor, the longer the drug action.
- Drugs are agonists when they interact with a receptor to produce an effect of their own.
- Drugs are antagonists when they interact with a receptor to produce no response of their own. Instead, they impair the receptor's ability to combine with an effector molecule.
- An antagonist is competitive when it combines reversibly with the same sites as the drug and can be displaced from those sites by an excess of the agonist.
- Irreversible antagonist drugs remain tightly bound to receptors. The binding cannot be overcome by increasing the dosage.

- Dose-response curves reflect the magnitude of drug action against the concentration (or dosage) of drug required to induce those actions.
- Therapeutic index, selectivity, and margin of safety all refer to the relationship between a drug's therapeutic and adverse effects.
- Drug idiosyncrasy, toxicity, and allergies are adverse effects considered unusual, in that they occur infrequently. The differences among them influence the subsequent use of a drug.
- Adverse drug reactions are generally categorized as dose related or sensitivity related.
- Variables predisposing the patient to adverse reactions include physiologic and psychosocial factors as well as conditions of administration.
- Drug interaction refers to a change in the magnitude or duration of a response of one drug because of the presence of another drug, food, or herb. In most cases, interactions are related to the pharmacokinetic or pharmacodynamic characteristics of the interacting drugs.
- In addition to pharmacokinetic and pharmacodynamic variables, there are variables that influence a patient's response to drug therapy. The variables include general state of health, life-span considerations, body weight, gender and genetics, body rhythms, psychosocial considerations, dietary considerations, smoking and alcohol intake, environment, drug additives and bioavailability, dosage and number of drugs administered, and the administration routes and techniques.

Bibliography

Bailey, D., Arnold, J., Strong, H., et al. (1993). Effect of grapefruit juice and naringin on nisoldipine pharmacokinetics. *Clinical Pharmacology and Therapeutics, 54*(6), 589–594.

Bailey, D., Spence, J., Munoz, C., et al. (1991). Interaction of citrus juices with felodipine and nifedipine. *Lancet, 337*(8745), 268–269.

Bates, D., Cullen, D., Laird, N., et al. for the ADE Prevention Study Group. (1995). Incidence of adverse drug events and potential adverse drug events: Implications for prevention. *Journal of the American Medical Association, 274*(1), 29–34.

Benjamin, D. (1994). Recognizing and preventing adverse drug reactions. *Drug Therapy, 24*(6), 52.

Beijer, H., and de Blaey, C. (2002). Hospitalizations caused by adverse drug reactions (ADR): A meta-analysis of observational studies. *Pharmacy World & Science, 24*(2), 46–54.

Boston Collaborative Drug Surveillance Program. (1992). 25 years of the Boston Collaborative Drug Surveillance Program: A compilation of abstracts published by the BCDSP 1966–1991. *Hospital Pharmacy, 27*(4), Supp.

Bowden, M. (2003). *Pharmaceutical Achievers*. Philadelphia: Chemical Heritage Foundation.

Chiral Quest. What is chirality? Available online: www.vioquest-pharm.com/chiral/content/what_is_chirality.html. Accessed 10 March 2007.

Davies, E., Green, C., Mottram, D., et al. (2006). Adverse drug reactions in hospital in-patients: A pilot study. *Journal of Clinical Pharmacy and Therapeutics, 31*(4), 335–341.

Davis, L. (1987). Timing is everything. *Hippocrates, 2*(4), 22–25.

Dharmananda, S. (2000). The interactions of herbs and drugs. Available online: www.itmonline.org/arts/herbdrug.htm. Retrieved August 28, 2005.

DiPiro, J., Talbert, R., Yee, G., et al. (2005). *Pharmacotherapy: A pathophysiology approach* (6th ed.). New York: McGraw-Hill.

Guengerich, F. (2003). Cytochromes P450, drugs, and diseases. *Molecular Interventions, 3*(4), 194–204.

Hardman, J., and Limbird, L. (2001). *Goodman and Gilman's the pharmacologic basis of therapeutics* (10th ed.). New York: Pergamon Press.

Kanjanarat, P., Winterstein, A., Johns, T., et al. (2003). Nature of preventable adverse drug events in hospitals: A literature review. *American Journal Health Systems Pharmacists, 60*(17), 1750–1759.

Kenakin, T. (2004). Principles: Receptor theory in pharmacology. *Trends in Pharmacological Sciences, 25*(4), 186–192.

Kvasz, M., Allen, E., Gordon, M., et al. (2000). Adverse drug reactions in hospitalized patients: A critique of a meta-analysis. *Medscape General Medicine, 2*(2), 1–13.

Maehle, A. (2004). "Receptive substances": John Newport Langley (1852–1925) and his path to a receptor theory of drug action. *Medical History, 48*(2), 153–174.

Pratt, W., and Taylor, P. (Eds.). (1990). *Principles of drug action: The basis of pharmacology.* New York: Churchill Livingstone.

Schein, J. (1995). Cigarette smoking and clinically significant drug interactions. *Annals of Pharmacotherapy, 29*(11), 1139–1147.

Shaikh, A. (1985). Application of pharmacokinetic principles in therapeutic drug monitoring. *Journal of Medical Technology, 2*(9), 583–587.

Sigworth, F. (2003). Structural biology: Life's transistors. *Nature, 423* (6935), 21–22.

Stephenson, R. (1956). Modification of receptor theory. *British Journal of Pharmacology and Chemotherapy, 11*(4), 379–393.

Wiffen, P., Gill, M., Edwards, J., et al. (2002). Adverse drug reactions in hospital patients: A systematic review of the prospective and retrospective studies. *Bandolier Extra.* June. Available online: www/jr2.ox.ac.uk/bandolier/extra.html. Accessed February 4, 2007.

FOUNDATIONS

Pharmacotherapeutics for Pregnant and Nursing Women

Perinatal pharmacotherapeutics examines the complex interaction existing between maternal physiologic changes, fetal development, and the placenta. To understand how pregnancy affects pharmacokinetics and pharmacodynamics, it is important to understand the physiologic changes that occur to mother and fetus.

ANATOMIC AND PHYSIOLOGIC VARIABLES

Pregnancy produces striking changes in the physiology of any normal condition that appears in women. From the moment conception occurs, changes begin in a woman's body (Fig. 6-1). The changes are related to several factors: hormonal influences, growth of the fetus inside the uterus, and the mother's physical adaptation to those changes.

REPRODUCTIVE SYSTEM

The most obvious changes associated with pregnancy occur in the reproductive system. The pear-shaped uterus, normally weighing about 60 grams, hypertrophies during pregnancy to a weight of approximately 1000 grams. To support the growing fetus, blood flow increases dramatically from 30 to 40 mL/min to 500 mL/min; uterine vascular resistance decreases, and blood flow to the uterus and placenta is maximized.

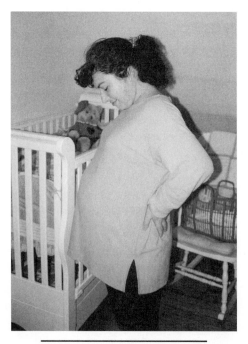

FIGURE 6-1 Photo of Pregnant Woman.

FLUID BALANCE

During pregnancy, total body water increases by 7 to 9 liters in the absence of edema; 40% is distributed throughout the mother, with the remaining 60% distributed to the amniotic fluid, the placenta, and the fetus. Sodium excretion is akin to that of nonpregnant women, indicating that the body senses the physiologic hypervolemia. Pregnancies that do not achieve the expanded plasma volume correlate with poor pregnancy outcomes.

Colloidal osmotic pressure drops as early as 10 weeks' gestation because of decreased concentrations of plasma proteins. This decrease is explained by the concomitant fall in plasma sodium and other associated anions. The fall in osmolarity from nonpregnant values to normal pregnancy levels can be equated to the drop in osmolarity that occurs in a nonpregnant person who quickly drinks a liter of water. The pregnant woman does not respond to the change in osmolarity by water diuresis, suggesting a resetting of the osmoreceptor system to a lower level. This theory is supported by the fact that plasma tonicity, urinary osmolality, and vasopressin levels normally increase after water deprivation and decrease after fluid loading. The osmotic threshold for thirst is also lower.

Given the increase in extracellular fluid during pregnancy, it is not surprising that a considerable amount of sodium is retained. This change is accompanied by an increase in renal tubular reabsorption to prevent maternal sodium depletion. Increases in renin, aldosterone, deoxycorticosterone, human placental lactogen, and estrogen seem to enhance sodium levels.

During a normal pregnancy, circulating levels of renin progressively increase until term, becoming 5 to 10 times higher than in the nonpregnant woman. The elevated levels of renin and angiotensinogen combine to form greater amounts of angiotensin I and II, but the vasoconstriction and associated rise in blood pressure expected in the nonpregnant woman do not occur. Resistance to the pressor effects of angiotensin has been explained in several ways: elevated circulating levels of prostaglandins (which are vasodilatory), an increase in the level of the specific enzyme angiotensinase, and/or a decrease in smooth muscle responsiveness (due to activation of the renal kallikrein-kinin system).

GASTROINTESTINAL SYSTEM

The most fundamental change in the gastrointestinal tract during pregnancy is the increased absorption of the nutrients needed by the developing fetus. Gastric motility and tone are decreased during pregnancy because of the smooth muscle relaxation effects of progesterone. These changes result in delayed gastric emptying, prolonged drug absorption, and lower peak drug concentrations. Decreased gastric acid secretion during the first trimester is thought to result from high levels of placental histaminase and other hormonal influences, particularly estrogen. Later on, the elevated levels of estrogen eventually lead to increases in gastric pH. During the third trimester, gastric acid secretion increases. Reduced gastrointestinal tone also leads to prolonged intestinal transit time, especially during the second and third trimesters.

Despite a 30% to 50% rise in cardiac output during pregnancy, liver size and hepatic blood flow do not change significantly; and in fact, proportionately to the increased cardiac output, the amount of blood arriving at the liver is decreased by about 28% to 35%. Estrogen enhances the production of alpha- and beta-globulins, but the liver's production of albumin and total serum protein levels are reduced by 20%.

Contributing to lower serum albumin levels is the expansion of intravascular volume. The lowered serum albumin levels allow more unbound drug to be available for placental transfer, with the transfer occurring at lower serum drug concentrations than in a nonpregnant state. Albumin-binding capacity is also decreased, mainly because of competition with endogenous factors such as free fatty acids.

Progesterone may be responsible for increased CYP450 enzyme activity in the liver, leading to an increase in liver clearance and the shortened half-life of a drug. However, the responsiveness of the CYP450 system to induction or inhibition by certain drugs does not change as a result of pregnancy.

CARDIOVASCULAR SYSTEM

During pregnancy, the heart enlarges about 12%, the myocardium undergoes some hypertrophy, and the capacity of the heart for blood increases by about 10%. Electrocardiographic changes occur because of a positional shift in the heart but are usually of no clinical significance. The heart rate progressively increases about 15 to 20 beats per minute to maintain cardiac output.

Cardiac output rises in early pregnancy as a result of the increasing heart rate. Later in pregnancy, stroke volume rises by 40 mL above nonpregnant levels, reaching a peak at 20 to 24 weeks of gestation. Distribution of blood flow also changes as cardiac output increases. The most dramatic increase occurs in uterine blood flow, with a change from 50 mL/min to 500 to 700 mL/min. This increase represents 10% to 20% of the cardiac output. The kidneys, the skin, and the breasts also receive higher blood flow. Cerebral and hepatic blood flows remain relatively unchanged.

The blood pressure does not rise despite increases in cardiac output and blood volume. Systolic pressures remain stable or fall slightly, whereas diastolic blood pressure drops more significantly. The changes begin in the first trimester and continue until the middle of pregnancy. At that time, there is a gradual return to prepregnant blood pressure readings. Alterations in blood pressure are probably related to estrogen- and progestin-mediated decreases in systemic vascular resistance.

RENAL SYSTEM

The glomerular filtration rate (GFR) rises 40% to 50% soon after conception. GFR may reach 150% of normal, peaking at 9 to 16 weeks' gestation and remaining relatively stable thereafter. The rise in GFR results in greater elimination of urinary amino acids, glucose, protein, urea, uric acid, potassium, calcium, water-soluble vitamins, creatinine, and certain drugs.

The ability of the kidneys to concentrate and dilute urine remains unchanged in pregnancy. Interestingly, the volume of urine excreted in a 24-hour period remains stable and does not reflect the increase in GFR. Creatinine clearance is increased to 120 to 220 mL/min owing to the elevated GFR. Therefore, values of 100 mL/min or lower in a pregnant woman indicate kidney impairment.

RESPIRATORY SYSTEM

A number of changes take place in the respiratory system, mediated by the mechanical effects of the enlarging uterus, higher oxygen demands, and the stimulant effect of progesterone. There is an estrogen-induced hyperemia of nasopharyngeal mucosa with concurrent edema and greater production of mucus. This leads to a feeling of stuffiness and a greater tendency for epistaxis. Pregnant women should be warned of this normal change and advised against using over-the-counter drugs and nasal sprays in hopes of alleviating symptoms. A normal saline nasal spray may be helpful in reducing some of the discomfort.

The most important biochemical influences on the respiratory system during pregnancy are elicited by progesterone and prostaglandins. Progesterone levels gradually rise from 25 mcg/mL at 6 weeks' gestation to 150 mcg/mL at term. This hormone increases minute ventilation, thereby lowering the carbon dioxide threshold. The increases in ventilation create a state of chronic hyperventilation, resulting in a fall in the partial pressure of arterial carbon dioxide ($PaCO_2$). This important change increases the carbon dioxide gradient between mother and fetus, enabling the fetus to off-load its carbon dioxide to maternal circulation. The maternal response to the falling $PaCO_2$ results in increased renal elimination of bicarbonate, and normal arterial pH is maintained. The sensation of dyspnea felt by 60% to 70% of pregnant women is likely related to reduced $PaCO_2$ levels and a greater sensitivity of the respiratory center to carbon dioxide.

The role of prostaglandins on airway tone during pregnancy is unclear. Prostaglandins E_1 and E_2 act as bronchodilators and may help counteract the structural effect of an elevated diaphragm. Prostaglandin F_2 is a smooth muscle constrictor. Administration of prostaglandin F_2, which has been used for termination of pregnancy or to control postpartum hemorrhage, is contraindicated in women with asthma, because of its potential constrictive effect on the bronchioles. Although prostaglandin F_2 appears elevated throughout pregnancy, higher levels of prostaglandin E have been found only during the third trimester.

ENDOCRINE SYSTEM

Pituitary Gland
The pituitary enlarges in pregnancy because of high circulating levels of estrogen. The higher number of prolactin-producing cells causes enlargement of the anterior pituitary. Prolactin levels increase to initiate DNA synthesis and mitosis of glandular epithelial cells and presecretory alveolar cells in the breast, to ensure lactation.

Thyroid Gland

Maternal adaptations to pregnancy mimic hyperthyroidism, but thyroid function itself does not change. The basal metabolic rate rises as much as 25%, with most of the increase attributed to the metabolic activity of the products of conception. Marked enlargement of the thyroid gland is considered abnormal and requires further evaluation.

Estrogen and human chorionic gonadotropin and the changes in kidney and liver function influence thyroid function. Increases in total thyroxine and triiodothyronine levels begin during the second month of pregnancy, but concentrations of free thyroxine and triiodothyronine remain unchanged. The additional thyroxine-binding globulin binds with thyroxine and triiodothyronine to increase total thyroxine and triiodothyronine.

Thyroid hormones do not cross the placenta. Therefore, fetal thyroid function appears independent of maternal thyroid function. Thyroid-stimulating immunoglobulins may cross the placenta and cause fetal and neonatal hyperthyroidism. The most common cause of hyperthyroidism in pregnancy is Graves' disease. Untreated maternal hyperthyroidism leads to a very poor prognosis for the fetus. In addition, in a euthyroid woman with a history of Graves' disease, thyroid-stimulating immunoglobulins may continue to cross the placenta, leaving the fetus at risk. Neonatal hyperthyroidism is usually temporary, since the half-life of thyroid-stimulating immunoglobulins is approximately 2 weeks.

Parathyroid Glands

Ionized calcium regulates the release of parathyroid hormone. The parathyroid hormone acts directly on bone and the kidneys and indirectly on the intestine to raise serum calcium levels. The ensuing physiologic hyperparathyroidism is probably the result of the body's attempt to supply the fetus with adequate calcium. The fact that ionized calcium levels are only slightly decreased in pregnancy suggests that a new setpoint for the stimulation of parathyroid hormone release exists in pregnancy. Parathyroid hormone levels are low in early pregnancy but progressively rise until delivery.

Pregnancy and lactation cause profound calcium stress, which explains the elevated levels of calcitonin during these times. Calcitonin generally opposes parathyroid hormone and vitamin D, but elevated calcitonin levels inhibit calcium and phosphorus release from bone. This inhibition protects the maternal skeleton from decalcification during times of stress while allowing the renal and intestinal actions of parathyroid hormone to provide the additional calcium needed by the fetus.

Adrenal Glands

Estrogen enhances hepatic synthesis of corticosteroid-binding globulin during pregnancy, resulting in higher levels of free plasma cortisol. The higher levels of free plasma cortisol may be the result of maternal feedback mechanisms resetting themselves to higher levels. The resetting of cortisol levels may be due to tissue refractoriness to cortisol. In this case, higher levels of free plasma cortisol are needed to maintain homeostasis.

Aldosterone levels are significantly increased at 15 weeks' gestation. Higher aldosterone levels provide protection against the natriuretic effect of progesterone, which generally causes a loss of sodium. If sodium is restricted in pregnancy, there is a further rise in aldosterone secretion.

Pancreas

The placenta and the fetus depend on maternal glucose for their primary source of energy. Glucose crosses the placenta by facilitated diffusion, but insulin, owing to its large molecular size, does not cross. The fetal pancreas produces insulin by the tenth to the twelfth week of gestation. Therefore the fetus responds to maternal hyperglycemia by producing excessive amounts of insulin.

The insulin-producing beta cells of the pancreas demonstrate a characteristic hyperplasia during pregnancy. The first half of pregnancy is distinguished by elevated fasting insulin levels despite increased insulin sensitivity. Blood glucose levels are therefore 15 to 20 mg/dL lower after a 12-hour fast than in the nonpregnant state. The lowered glucose levels are attributed to fetal-placental utilization of glucose.

Insulin antagonism emerges during the second half of pregnancy, mediated by the rising levels of placental hormones—estrogen, progesterone, and human placental lactogen. The biphasic effect on glucose metabolism explains why glucose intolerance in pregnancy is often not evident until 24 to 30 weeks of gestation.

MATERNAL PHARMACOKINETIC CONSIDERATIONS

ABSORPTION

The rate and completeness of drug absorption is delayed by high levels of progesterone and subsequent prolonged gastric transit time. Changes in gastric pH, heartburn, and morning sickness, or the treatment of these symptoms with antacids, affect absorption of some orally administered drugs. Increased gastric pH slows the absorption of weakly acidic drugs such as aspirin, and speeds the absorption of weakly basic drugs such as morphine. Decreased gastric tone and motility enhance absorption of lipid-soluble drugs, whereas the bioavailability of slowly absorbed drugs (e.g., digoxin) may be increased. The absorption and peak plasma levels of readily absorbed drugs (e.g., acetaminophen) may be delayed.

DISTRIBUTION

Drug distribution may change because maternal plasma volume increases by about 50%. Water-soluble drugs are diluted, whereas lipid-soluble drugs concentrate in the adipose tissues of the mother and the membrane layers of the fetal-placental unit. Increased body water provides a greater volume in which drugs can be distributed (also known as the volume of distribution [V_d]). However, increased total body water has more profound effects on polar drugs, which are confined to extracellular spaces. The distribution of fat-soluble drugs is influenced by changes in protein and lipid binding. The higher amounts of body fat associated with pregnancy act as reservoirs for fat-soluble drugs and free fatty acids. Free fatty acids compete with some drugs for albumin-binding sites; therefore an elevation in free fatty acids during pregnancy alters drug distribution. Generally, the impact of an increased V_d reduces peak plasma drug concentrations and decreases elimination, resulting in a prolonged half-life. This remains true unless there is a concurrent increase in clearance through biotransformation or elimination.

Plasma albumin, to which most acidic drugs are bound, falls during pregnancy. The consequence of a reduction in plasma proteins is less binding of a given drug and an increased serum concentration of the drug. Basic drugs (e.g., propranolol) tend to bind to alpha-1-acid glycoproteins. Endogenous substances such as free fatty acids compete with drugs for binding sites on both albumin and alpha-1-acid glycoproteins. The resultant larger fraction of unbound drug is more widely distributed, exerts a pharmacologic effect, and is eliminated through biotransformation or elimination.

BIOTRANSFORMATION

Drug biotransformation is heightened by the effects of progesterone. Accompanied by a rise in CYP450 enzymes, liver clearance is increased, elimination accelerated, and drug half-life shortened. The microsomal enzyme system remains sensitive to inhibition as well as stimulation by certain drugs. If hepatic enzymatic processes slow, degradation and biotransformation may be delayed.

Drugs expected to have a shorter half-life ($t_{1/2}$) (e.g., penicillin V; $t_{1/2} = 0.5$ hr) have increased concentrations during labor, when the hepatic clearance of drugs is thought to decrease. Biotransformation also occurs in both the placenta and the fetal liver, although the contribution of the fetal-placental unit is thought to be very small.

ELIMINATION

Increased renal blood flow and glomerular filtration rates result in accelerated clearance of urea, uric acid, and creatinine. Drugs that are excreted unchanged (e.g., gentamicin, digoxin) are cleared in proportion to the creatinine clearance. Serum levels of these drugs are closely monitored to maintain therapeutic levels during pregnancy. Because blood flow through the liver is not appreciably changed in pregnancy, drugs relying solely on hepatic blood flow for clearance are removed at the same rate as in the nonpregnant woman.

Lipid-soluble, nonionized drugs are more likely to be reabsorbed. Drugs that are ionized at the pH of urine are readily excreted. The higher the lipid solubility of a drug, the greater its half-life in pregnancy; and the more polar a drug, the shorter its half-life.

FETAL-PLACENTAL PHARMACOKINETIC CONSIDERATIONS

ABSORPTION

The placenta allows transfer of substances between mother and fetus. The placenta has a high basal metabolic rate, with energy needs supplied predominantly by oxygen and glucose. The placenta transports oxygen and nutrients to the fetus and clears urea, carbon dioxide, and other catabolites produced by the fetus. Gases and some molecules cross the placenta by simple diffusion. Transport depends on the concentration gradient, the size of the molecule, and the surface area available for transfer. Facilitated diffusion transports glucose, the major source of energy for the fetus. This transfer occurs more rapidly than simple diffusion, and it is accomplished by a carrier system in the direction of the concentration gradient. Normally, fetal glucose concentration is approximately 80% of the maternal value. The highest rate of diffusion across placental membranes occurs with substances of low molecular weight, minimal electrical charge, and high lipid solubility.

Essential amino acids and water-soluble vitamins are transferred by active transport. These substances are found in higher concentration in the fetus and are carried across the placenta against the concentration gradient.

Pinocytosis is the ingestion of fluids and solute molecules through the formation of small vesicles. The particles are carried across the membrane virtually intact, to be released on the other side. Complex proteins, immune bodies, small amounts of fat, and viruses travel through the placenta in this manner.

DISTRIBUTION

The effect of drugs on the fetus depends on whether the drug is distributed throughout the body or selectively. Many factors influence placental transfer of drugs, including physiochemical properties, molecular weight and configuration, ionization, lipid solubility, and protein binding.

PROPERTIES OF PLACENTA

The placenta is not an impermeable barrier (Fig. 6-2). It is living tissue that synthesizes a number of peptides, enzymes, and hormones. The placenta usually provides an effective immunologic barrier between mother and fetus but does not act to protect the fetus in the same manner as the blood-brain barrier functions to protect the brain (Table 6-1).

Drug transfer via the placenta is greatest late in gestation. As pregnancy progresses, chorionic villi become more numerous, providing a greater surface area across which diffusion between the two circulations can occur. Near term, the membrane separating maternal and fetal circulation thins considerably, so that fetal capillary endothelium is separated from maternal circulation by a single layer of fetal chorionic tissue. Inflammation, hypoxia, vascular degeneration, or partial separation of the placenta affects drug transfer just as it affects transfer of oxygen and nutrients to the fetus. For example, a woman with diabetes tends to have a larger, thicker placenta, creating a greater distance for molecules to travel before arriving in the fetal circulation.

The placenta contains many of the drug-biotransforming enzymes present in the adult liver. This knowledge might lead one to assume that the placenta would act to protect the fetus from some maternal drugs. However, there is no evidence to suggest the placenta acts as a barrier to any significant degree.

Molecular Weight and Configuration
The placenta permits transfer of drugs with molecular weights of less than 500 grams/mole. Molecules of weights up to 1000 grams/mole, if unbound and nonionized, are usually lipid-soluble and rapidly penetrate the tissues that separate the fetal and maternal circulation. The vast majority of drugs have molecular weights between 100 grams/mole and 500 grams/mole. For example, alprazolam, a benzodiazepine drug used in the treatment of anxiety, has a molecular weight of 308.76 grams/mole.

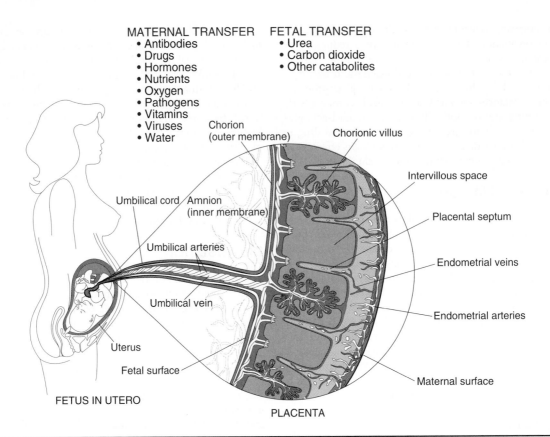

MATERNAL TRANSFER
- Antibodies
- Drugs
- Hormones
- Nutrients
- Oxygen
- Pathogens
- Vitamins
- Viruses
- Water

FETAL TRANSFER
- Urea
- Carbon dioxide
- Other catabolites

FETUS IN UTERO

PLACENTA

FIGURE 6-2 The maternal-fetal unit permits maternal blood to circulate through uterine arteries to intervillous spaces of the placenta and to return to maternal circulation through uterine veins. Fetal blood flows through two umbilical arteries into the placenta and returns through the umbilical vein.

TABLE 6-1 Factors Affecting Placental Transfer of Drugs

Enhance Drug Transfer	Inhibit Drug Transfer
Lipid solubility	Increased diffusion distance
Nonionized substances	High molecular charge
Molecular weight less than 500 grams/mole	High molecular weight
Lack of significant albumin binding	Binding to maternal RBCs and/or proteins
Higher maternal-to-fetal gradient	Binding or altered by placental enzymes
Increased placental blood flow	Decreased placental blood flow
Increased fetal acidity; retains basic drugs	Drugs highly metabolized by mother
Larger surface areas	

RBCs, Red blood cells.

Ionization

The distribution of weak acids and weak bases is somewhat complex. In the blood, a weak acid or weak base distributes to all compartments of the body differently, leading to equilibrium between charged and uncharged forms of the drug in each compartment. In addition, polar substances cross the placenta more slowly than nonionized drugs at a physiologic pH. For example, if a fetus becomes acidotic from prolonged cord compression, a weak base (e.g., amphetamine) diffusing into the fetal compartment will become charged. The charged base does not diffuse passively back into the maternal circulation. The result is a higher concentration of the drug in the acidotic fetus than if the fetus were more alkalotic.

Lipid Solubility and Tissue Binding

Lipid-soluble drugs passively diffuse across the placenta. Small molecules cross at rates dependent on their molecular weight, charge characteristics, and concentration in the maternal blood. Just as drugs bind to plasma proteins, these are removed from circulation and stored in tissue such as bones, teeth, hair, and adipose tissues. Lipid-soluble drugs are stored in adipose tissue. The binding leads to a slight decrease in the amount of free lipid-soluble drugs such as sedatives and hypnotics. When the drug is discontinued, the tissue deposits of drugs are slowly released, resulting in persistent drug effects.

Protein Binding

Circulating plasma proteins are a reservoir for drugs. It is important to remember that only a free drug is able to cross the placenta into the fetal compartment and that many drugs bind to the same proteins. One drug may therefore displace another, resulting in a potentially dangerous increase in free drug concentration.

Maternal-Fetal Blood Flow

Maternal blood pressure, maternal position, fetal cord compression, and uterine contractions influence maternal-fetal blood flow and affect the availability of drugs to the fetus. Maternal blood pressure increases or decreases the amount of unbound drug available to cross the placenta. The left lateral recumbent and sitting positions maximize uterine-placental blood flow. Uterine blood flow is impeded by the standing and supine positions. Any maternal position that does not optimize uterine blood flow decreases the potential for fetal drug exposure.

Fetal Cord Compression and Uterine Contractions

Blood flow through the umbilical cord is an even more important factor in the transfer of freely permeable drugs. Cord compression jeopardizes circulation and hence the delivery of oxygen to and removal of wastes from the fetus. Cord compression thus also affects the delivery of drugs to the fetus. Likewise, uterine contractions impair placental blood flow and thus reduce the transfer of intravenous drugs to the fetal compartment when bolus drug administration coincides with a uterine contraction.

Acid-Base Balance

Weak acids and weak bases result in equilibrium between charged and uncharged forms of a drug, depending on the pH of the substance in which they are dissolved. At a low pH, there is a high concentration of hydrogen ions. In this situation, the nitrogen ion of many weak bases will accept a proton and become charged. Conversely, at a high pH, there is a low concentration of hydrogen ions. In this case, the nitrogen molecule will donate its proton to the solvent and become an uncharged molecule. This fact demonstrates how both maternal and fetal pH values affect the pH gradient.

BIOTRANSFORMATION

Fetal biotransformation of drugs is believed to be minimal. Therefore the fetus must rely on maternal plasma levels to clear a drug from fetal circulation. As maternal serum levels fall, drugs diffuse from fetal circulation into maternal circulation. Highly lipid-soluble barbiturates equilibrate within a few minutes of maternal intravenous injection. On the other hand, dexamethasone takes several hours to equilibrate between maternal and fetal circulations. Consequently, a particular drug may have a profound or a minimal effect on the fetus, as determined by its absorption, distribution, and elimination rates as well as by how long before birth it is administered.

The fetal liver contains the adult complement of enzymes, but the activities of these enzymes at term are only about half those in an adult. In addition, liver enzymes in the fetus are also poorly inducible compared with those in the adult.

The protein content of fetal plasma increases with gestational age. Fetal albumin levels usually exceed maternal levels at time of delivery. A large bound component in the fetus promotes placental drug transfer by promoting the gradient for free drug. The bound component also increases the overall fetal dose after a brief administration of a drug, and thereby prolongs the fetal and, perhaps more importantly, the neonatal effects of a drug given to the mother. Following birth, the neonate must rely on its own limited ability to biotransform and remove a drug from its circulation. Hence, drug action following birth may be prolonged and may have adverse neonatal consequences.

ELIMINATION

Drug metabolites have been found in fetal serum, but because metabolites freely cross the placenta in both directions, it is difficult to prove they are of fetal origin. Drug metabolites themselves may be pharmacologically active and cause adverse effects in the fetus.

A hydrophilic drug may cross the placenta slowly from mother to fetus, but once it reaches the fetus, it undergoes rapid elimination by the kidneys. However, fetal urine voided into the amniotic cavity constitutes a substantial portion of the amniotic fluid. As the fetus goes through the normal process of swallowing amniotic fluid, it ingests the drug or its metabolites that have been excreted in fetal urine. The result is prolonged fetal drug exposure.

Lipid-soluble drugs diffuse back across placental membranes to the mother, who provides the major route of elimination. Metabolites formed by the fetal liver are probably excreted in bile and deposited in meconium.

PHARMACODYNAMICS

A drug demonstrates the same biochemical mechanism of action in all individuals. If a drug normally inhibits the transfer of a substance into a cell, it will do so in persons of any age group. However, the response to the drug varies according to the physiologic changes associated with pregnancy. Consequently, a dosage adjustment may be necessary. The sensitivity of drug receptors is also variable.

Certain factors influence whether a particular drug will have an adverse effect on the fetus. The type and amount of drug, the rate of elimination, distribution in fetal tissue, gestational age, and fetal receptor function affect drug action (Table 6-2). The fetus is most vulnerable during the first trimester. During the preembryonic stage (conception to 14 days following conception), there is little morphologic differentiation. Exposure to teratogens at this time generally has an all-or-nothing effect on the zygote: either the zygote is damaged so severely that it is aborted, or there are no apparent effects.

TERATOGENESIS

A *teratogen* causes abnormal development or function by interfering with embryonic and/or fetal development. It is difficult to establish the teratogenicity of individual drugs because of the ethical implications of such studies. Therefore drug use in pregnancy should be avoided as much as possible. When drugs are necessary, they should be taken at the lowest possible effective dose. The Food and Drug Administration (FDA)

TABLE 6-2 Drugs Contraindicated During Breastfeeding

Drug	Reason(s) for Concern or Reported Effect(s)
Amphetamines*†	Irritability, poor sleeping patterns
bromocriptine	Suppresses lactation; may be hazardous to mother
cocaine*	Cocaine intoxication
cyclophosphamide, cyclosporin,doxorubicin†, methotrexate	Possible immune suppression; unknown effect on growth or association with carcinogenesis; neutropenia
ergotamine	Vomiting, diarrhea, convulsions (dosages used in migraine treatment)
heroin*	Tremors, restlessness, vomiting, poor feeding
lithium	One third to one half therapeutic blood concentration in infant
marijuana*	Only one report in literature; no effect mentioned
nicotine (smoking)*	Shock, vomiting, diarrhea, rapid heart rate, restlessness; decreased milk production
phencyclidine (PCP)*	Potent hallucinogen
phenindione	Anticoagulant; increased prothrombin and partial thromboplastin time in one infant; not used in United States

*The Committee on Drugs strongly believes that nursing mothers should not ingest any of these compounds. Not only are they hazardous to the nursing infant, but are also detrimental to the physical and emotional health of the mother. This list is obviously not complete. No drug of abuse should be ingested by nursing mothers, even though adverse reports are not in the literature.
†Drug concentrates in human milk.
Adapted from American Academy of Pediatrics Committee on Drugs. (2001). The transfer of drugs and other chemicals into human milk. *Pediatrics, 108*(3), 776–789. Used with permission of the American Academy of Pediatrics.

classification system for systemic drug use in pregnancy is based on the level of known risk the drug presents to the fetus (see Box 6-1). The FDA pregnancy categories are usually identified in drug reference books and materials. Drugs on the market before the implementation of the classification system are generally not listed in patient package inserts. The variables associated with teratogenesis are susceptibility, timing, and characteristics of the specific teratogen, mechanism of action, dosage, and manifestation.

Susceptibility

The biochemical and morphologic makeup of an individual embryo affects its particular sensitivity to a teratogenic drug. For example, the response of the human fetus to teratogens such as the rubella virus, thalidomide, and alcohol is variable.

Timing

The timing of drug exposure determines which organ system is affected. The greatest risk for malformations in the fetus is during the period of organogenesis (15 to 60 days after conception). After the first trimester, drugs do not cause gross structural abnormalities but can have toxic effects or affect growth and development. For example, exposure to warfarin sodium during this time can lead to embryopathy (fetal warfarin syndrome), which manifests as developmental delay, neurologic complications (usually hydrocephalus and occasional agenesis of the corpus callosum and meningoencephalocele), midfacial hypoplasia, and various ocular, skeletal, and other defects.

Characteristics of Teratogen

Fetal exposure depends on the characteristics of the teratogen (e.g., lipid permeability, protein binding). Whether a

BOX 6-1

FDA Drug Categories

Category	Description	Examples of Drugs
A	Adequate, well-controlled studies in pregnant women have not shown an increased risk of fetal abnormalities.	Prenatal vitamins, folic acid, thyroid hormone, vitamin B_6
B	No adequate and well-controlled studies in pregnant women or animal studies have shown adverse effect to the fetus.	acyclovir, some antibiotics (e.g., azithromycin, cephalosporins), acetaminophen, aspartame (artificial sweetener), buspirone, bupropion, diphenhydramine, famotidine, lansoprazole, loratidine, metformin, methyldopa, metoclopramide, metronidazole, prednisone, insulin
C or D	Animal studies have shown an adverse effect, and there are no adequate and well-controlled studies in pregnant women.	albuterol, ciprofloxacin, disulfiram, fluconazole, furosemide, inhaled steroids, ketorolac, labetalol, nifedipine, ACE inhibitors, prochlorperazine, pseudoephedrine, sumatriptan, SSRIs, tramadol, trazodone
D	Adequate, well-controlled or observational studies in pregnant women have demonstrated a risk to the fetus. The benefits of therapy may outweigh risk potential.	alcohol, amitriptyline, ACE inhibitors, aspirin, bismuth subsalicylate, diazepam, glyburide, most antineoplastics, lithium, phenytoin, sulfonamides, thiazide diuretics
X	Adequate, well-controlled or observational studies in animals or pregnant women have demonstrated positive evidence of fetal abnormalities. The use of the product is contraindicated in women who are or may become pregnant.	DES, ergotamines, HMG-CoA reductase inhibitors (''statins''), isotretinoin, misoprostol, oral contraceptives, thalidomide, warfarin

ACE, Angiotensin-converting enzyme; *DES*, diethylstilbestrol; *HMG-CoA*, 3-hydroxy-3-methylglutaryl coenzyme A; *SSRIs*, selective serotonin reuptake inhibitors.

teratogen reaches toxic or teratogenic concentrations depends on drug transmission across the placenta, maternal dosage, rate of absorption, maternal homeostatic capabilities, and the physical properties of the drug.

Mechanism of Action

The mechanism of drug action can trigger changes in developing cells. Pathogenesis occurs when cellular damage is caused by secondary interference with cellular interactions or by cell necrosis. For example, acyclovir at high dosages taken at any time during the pregnancy may cause chromosomal breakage.

Dosage

There appears to be a threshold above which toxicity of a particular offending drug occurs. The same or similar teratogenic effects may result from a variety of drugs.

Manifestation

The result of early embryonic exposure is most likely death. Teratogenic events leading to malformation of organs or organ systems most often occur during the period of organogenesis. Later exposures generally lead to functional deficit or growth retardation.

DRUGS AND LACTATION

Breastfeeding is the major form of neonatal nutrition and yet only 39% of all newborns worldwide are breastfed. Approximately 95% of breastfeeding women are taking at least one drug during the first week after delivery. Depending upon the degree of protein binding, ionization, and lipid solubility, almost all drugs transfer to breast milk. Table 6-2 lists drugs that are contraindicated during breastfeeding, along with the reason for concern or the reported effects.

As a general rule, a breastfeeding infant ingests less than 1% to 2% of the total maternal drug dose. Several factors influence drug passage into breast milk. These factors are not unlike those determining the distribution of drugs in the mother. Low–molecular weight drugs penetrate breast milk more easily than high–molecular weight drugs. Only the unbound, free portion of drugs contained within maternal plasma diffuses into breast milk. Drugs that are widely distributed in the maternal body usually do not achieve high concentrations in breast milk. The pH of breast milk has a lower pH than plasma (7.0 versus 7.4, respectively). The lower pH of breast milk may cause organic bases to ionize and become "trapped" in breast milk. Drugs that are highly

fat-soluble can concentrate in breast milk; however, milk fat represents only 3% to 5% of total milk volume. Highly protein-bound drugs enter breast milk poorly, because the concentration of protein in breast milk is only 10% of the concentration in plasma.

Drugs are transported to breast milk via simple diffusion, facilitated diffusion, or active transport. Mammary alveolar epithelium is a lipid barrier with water-filled pores. The pores are most permeable to drugs during the colostrum phase of milk secretion. Drugs enter into the breast in a nonionized, non–protein-bound form. Water-soluble drugs with a molecular weight of less than 200 nanograms pass through the membrane pores. In addition, drugs can enter breast milk through spaces between mammary alveolar cells. For example, milk at the end of a feeding contains considerably more fat than milk produced early in the feeding and may concentrate fat-soluble drugs. The amount of drug transferred to breast milk can be described mathematically using the formula contained in Box 6-2. Drugs leave the breast by diffusion or active transport. Drug-biotransforming capacity of the breast, even if it exists, is not understood.

A listing of drugs that transfer to breast milk was published in 2001 by the Committee on Drugs of the American Academy of Pediatrics. The list identifies drugs contraindicated during breastfeeding, drugs that necessitate temporary cessation of breastfeeding, drugs that should be used with caution during breastfeeding, and drugs that are usually compatible with breastfeeding. Table 6-2 lists drugs contraindicated for use during breastfeeding, along with the reason for concern or the reported effect.

MINIMIZING INFANT DRUG EXPOSURE

Minimizing the risk of potentially harmful drug exposure to the breastfed infant is key. Unfortunately, mothers are often discouraged from breastfeeding when they are taking a drug because of a knowledge deficit about the impact of a specific drug or because of concern over the potential but undefined risk to the infant. When a mother requires a drug that carries minimal hazards for the infant, the health care provider can make the following adjustments to diminish drug effects:

- Avoid sustained-release and long-acting drugs. They are difficult for an infant to excrete, and drug accumulation in the infant is a significant concern.
- Identify the usual rate of absorption and peak plasma levels of the drug, and then schedule drug administration so the least amount possible gets into the milk.

BOX 6-2

Calculating Infant Drug Exposure

Calculation of infant exposure to drugs can be used to help guide safe use. The infant's dose (D_{infant}) received via milk can be calculated using the maternal plasma concentration ($C_{maternal}$), maternal/plasma area under the curve ratio (M/P_{AUC}), and the volume of milk ingested by the infant (V_{infant}).

$$D_{infant}\,(mg/kg/day) = C_{maternal}\,(mg/L) \times M/P_{AUC} \times V_{infant}\,(L/kg/day)$$

From Gardiner, S., and Begg, E. (2001). Drug safety in lactation. MEDSAFE Information for Health Professionals. Prescriber Update No. 21:10–23. Available online: www.medsafe.govt.nz/Profs/PUarticles/lactation.htm. Accessed June 30, 2005.

Having the mother take the drug immediately after breastfeeding is generally the safest for the infant, but keep in mind that this is dependent on the drug.

- Short-acting drugs may never fully equilibrate with milk if the drug is rapidly cleared. In this case, expressing and discarding breast milk after drug administration may not be useful. Using milk that has been expressed before the initiation of drug therapy, if there is a supply available, is a sure way to avoid drug exposure. A mother may also request a temporary supply of milk from a milk bank.
- When possible, a drug that produces the lowest levels of drug in the milk should be used. Drug concentrations in milk decrease by retrograde diffusion; therefore, as maternal serum levels fall, levels of the drug in milk will follow the concentration gradient and also fall.
- See *Drugs in Pregnancy and Lactation*, which is published yearly by the American Academy of Pediatrics, for the latest update of drugs and other chemicals transferred into breast milk and to assist in selection of drugs compatible with breastfeeding.
- Watch the infant for signs of drug reaction (e.g., changes in sleep or feeding patterns, fussiness).

CLINICAL REASONING

Treatment Objectives

Treatment objectives are directed at prevention, cure, alleviation, or palliation. For example, iron supplements are used to prevent iron deficiency anemia. Anticonvulsants prevent maternal seizures, and phenobarbital may be used just before some deliveries in an attempt to prevent severe neonatal intraventricular hemorrhage.

Curative objectives are instituted during pregnancy in the treatment of infection. An antibiotic is chosen on the basis of its effectiveness against the offending organism. The antibiotic of choice would also be one that holds the lowest possible risk to the fetus. In the case of a urinary tract infection or pyelonephritis, for example, failure to treat and cure the infection could lead to preterm labor and subsequent delivery.

Palliation objectives are directed at preventing complications associated with pregnancy. Chronic hypertension requires treatment throughout pregnancy to reduce the risk of complications associated with an elevated blood pressure. Hypertension is one of the leading causes of maternal death and predisposes a pregnant woman to pregnancy-induced hypertension. In addition, chronic hypertension has been linked to intrauterine growth retardation and fetal death. Similarly, a woman with diabetes requires insulin to ensure optimum health for both her and the developing fetus.

Treatment Options

As a rule, some therapies are offered during pregnancy simply to promote maternal comfort, and therefore caution is required. However, well-chosen therapies that provide relief can make a significant difference in how a woman views her pregnancy. The idea is to select a drug identified as safe for use in pregnancy or to substitute one drug for another that is suspected to be teratogenic. The gestational age of the fetus is taken into consideration. The health care provider should consult the FDA pregnancy categories for a listing of drugs safe to administer.

▌▌ *Patient Variables*

In dealing with women of child-bearing age, the health care provider must always be open to the possibility of an unknown preexisting pregnancy. If symptoms require a test that could adversely affect the outcome of a pregnancy, a pregnancy test should be performed. If the woman is indeed pregnant, she and her family or support person should be carefully counseled as to the potential impact of the testing.

Collaboration among and between members of the health care team is the best insurance that appropriate identification and intervention for a woman and fetus or infant at risk will occur. To minimize the risk of drug exposure to mother and fetus, the following administration guidelines should be used:

- Clearly identify the need for any drug used.
- Choose the safest effective drug available.
- Avoid using the newest drugs on the market.
- Use the lowest effective dose possible for the shortest possible time.
- Use topical or local therapy whenever possible.
- Carefully schedule administration times so a breastfeeding mother does not receive the drug before nursing.
- Once-daily drug doses may be taken by a breastfeeding mother before the infant's longest sleep period.

▌▌ *Drug Variables*

ANALGESICS. Minor muscle aches and headaches are common during pregnancy. Acetaminophen is often used short-term during pregnancy. High doses, on the other hand, especially during the first trimester, may result in severe fetal liver damage. Aspirin is commonly ingested by pregnant women. However, aspirin use has been associated with maternal anemia, antepartal and postpartal hemorrhage, and prolonged gestation and labor. Aspirin's effects on the fetus and neonate include intrauterine growth retardation, congenital salicylate intoxication, depressed albumin-binding capacity, and increased perinatal mortality rate. Aspirin taken (even in low doses) during the week before delivery may affect the neonate's clotting abilities.

Opioids should be used cautiously, if at all, in a pregnant woman. When used on a regular basis, opiates induce an intense addiction in both mother and fetus. Pain relief during labor and delivery must be carefully coordinated with the time of delivery and the drug dose to protect the fetus from potentially harmful drug effects. Chapters 16 and 17 discuss analgesia further.

CARDIOVASCULAR DRUGS. Cardiac glycosides are used extensively for the management of heart failure and various supraventricular arrhythmias. Digoxin is the most commonly used cardiac glycoside. No evidence exists of any harmful fetal effects; however, digoxin crosses both the blood-brain barrier and the placenta. At delivery, the serum digoxin concentration in the newborn is similar to the serum concentration in the mother. Because of the expansion of maternal blood volume and the increased GFR, a higher dosage of digoxin is often necessary to maintain therapeutic serum levels as the pregnancy progresses. Chapter 34 discusses cardiac glycosides in more depth.

Secondary uterine effects should be considered in patients receiving cardiac drugs that result in either alpha (uterine contraction) or beta (uterine relaxation) activity. Likewise, women who are taking beta agonists for complications of pregnancy may experience secondary but significant cardiac effects. There is controversy regarding the safety of beta-blocking drugs in pregnancy. No evidence exists to suggest beta blockers are teratogenic, and they can be used for women with hypertension. Chapter 14 discusses sympathetic nervous system drugs in more depth.

Atropine, quinidine, or procainamide can be used to treat arrhythmias during pregnancy without adverse effects on the fetus or newborn. There is a paucity of studies on the use of calcium channel blockers in pregnancy. Antiarrhythmic drugs are discussed in Chapter 36.

Patients requiring anticoagulation during pregnancy because of underlying cardiovascular abnormalities pose a particular problem. A number of complications in both mother and fetus have been recorded with warfarin derivatives, particularly during the first and third trimesters of pregnancy. Heparin is used as an effective therapeutic agent and is the drug of choice if anticoagulation is required. More information about anticoagulants can be found in Chapter 39.

ANTIBIOTICS. Antibiotic choice should be guided by sensitivity testing, with consideration given to maternal and fetal toxicity. Penicillins and cephalosporins are safe in pregnancy; they show no increase in maternal toxicity and have no known fetal toxicity. Oral tetracycline causes staining and deformity of deciduous teeth and inhibition of bone growth in the fetus. Sulfonamides should not be used within 4 weeks of delivery. Sulfonamides and nitrofurantoin can cause hemolysis in patients with glucose-6-phosphate dehydrogenase (G6PD) deficiency. Sulfonamides also can displace bilirubin from its binding sites on albumin; therefore there would be an increase in bilirubin levels. The risk of ototoxicity and nephrotoxicity secondary to aminoglycosides is the same in the pregnant and the nonpregnant woman.

ANTACIDS AND HYPERACIDITY DRUGS. Antacids are used by 50% of pregnant women for heartburn relief. Most antacids containing aluminum, magnesium, and calcium are safe in therapeutic dosages during the second and third trimesters. Sucralfate and histamine₂ antagonists are excellent therapeutic modalities among nonpregnant patients, but their safety during pregnancy is not yet well established. Although the histamine₂ antagonists, such as cimetidine and ranitidine, are FDA category B drugs, their extended use is not recommended. Antacids and hyperacidity drugs are discussed further in Chapter 45.

LAXATIVES. Certain laxatives are not safe for use during pregnancy, when constipation and painful hemorrhoids may appear. Castor oil may initiate premature uterine contractions. Saline laxatives (e.g., magnesium hydroxide) can lead to sodium retention in the mother. Frequent use of lubricants such as mineral oil leads to reduced absorption of fat-soluble vitamins, resulting in neonatal hypoprothrombinemia and hemorrhage. Stimulant laxatives, such as bisacodyl and senna, and stool softeners, such as docusate, are safe during pregnancy. Bulk-forming laxatives (e.g., psyllium) are safe during pregnancy. As a component of patient teaching, the patient should be encouraged to use non–drug measures to alleviate constipation or hemorrhoidal discomfort, such as increasing fluid intake, dietary fiber, and activity, to avoid straining,

Controversy

Perinatal Pharmacotherapeutics—What to Restrict?

Jonathan J. Wolfe

Perinatal drug dosing places the health care provider in uncomfortable territory. It often involves a choice between the best interests of the mother, who can express her needs, and the fetus or neonate, who cannot. Any use of drugs in the later stages of pregnancy and the birth process demands consideration of both parties. At this stage in development, the teratogenicity of drugs is not a significant issue. Developmental defects from drugs are chiefly associated with use in the second trimester of pregnancy. The uncertainty in perinatal drug use focuses rather on the passage of drugs across the placenta and their effect on an emerging child, whose systems for drug biotransformation and elimination are imperfectly developed.

The placenta is not an effective barrier to the transmission of drugs to the fetus. Lipid-soluble, nonionized drugs readily pass across the placenta from the maternal to the fetal circulation. Highly dissociated ionized drugs and those with low lipid solubility pass less easily. In either case, simple diffusion carries drugs across the placenta, and any drug administered to the mother will to some extent be presented to fetal circulation.

Drugs are also transferred from mother to the neonate through breast milk. Here again, the primary concern is that highly lipophilic drugs are carried in the fat content of the milk and are absorbed by the child. A countervailing concern may well be the value of the protective antibodies provided to the newborn through breast milk.

For these reasons, the therapeutic index relationship between blood level to achieve therapeutic effect and blood level associated with toxicity for both mother and fetus or neonate must be considered. Such evaluation lends itself to an interdisciplinary approach. The treatment choice must account for outcomes appropriate to the patient's choice for self and child, the best standard of current practice, and the most current available data about distribution and effects of each drug contemplated.

CLINICAL REASONING

- A patient at 34 weeks of gestation develops a life-threatening gram-positive infection that is responsive to carbenicillin. What interests of mother and fetus are most important here? Are their interests compatible? Is this drug likely to cause significant harm to either party? May treatment reasonably be postponed?

- The same patient is diagnosed with a malignant breast tumor. The oncologist advises immediate excision, followed by combination antineoplastic therapy using 5-fluorouracil and cyclophosphamide. What interests of mother and fetus are most important here? Are their interests compatible? Is this drug likely to cause significant harm to either party? May treatment reasonably be postponed?

- Perinatal analgesia in the past involved use of "twilight sleep" with meperidine and scopolamine. The use of these drugs commonly resulted in neonates with low Apgar scores who required immediate resuscitation involving the use of naloxone. What circumstances might justify this approach to pain management during labor and delivery today? What precautions would you recommend to a mother in the first 24 hours postpartum who wants to breast-feed but has received significant doses of phenobarbital during labor for prophylaxis against a documented seizure disorder?

and to use sitz baths as needed. Laxatives are discussed further in Chapter 46.

ANTIEMETICS. Many antiemetic drugs are linked to increased risk of fetal harm. Diphenhydramine (Benadryl) may cause cleft palate. Trimethobenzamide (Tigan) may produce other congenital anomalies. Prochlorperazine (Compazine) has been linked to an increased risk of cardiovascular and other malformations.

Many antiemetics have the potential for extrapyramidal (and other) adverse effects. With this potential in mind, nausea and vomiting can often be managed with nonpharmacologic practices (e.g., eating small, frequent meals; consuming liquid and dry foods separately; avoiding fried, odorous, spicy, greasy, or gas-forming foods; and keeping crackers or other dry food at the bedside to be eaten in the morning before rising). Antiemetics are discussed further in Chapter 47.

Patient Education

Patient teaching should include the names of the drugs that have been ordered and why. The mother should know the expected duration of the therapy and be advised not to change the dosage or discontinue the drug without consulting the health care provider. The woman should be told about adverse effects that are to be reported as well as what to do if she forgets to take a dose. The addition of any prescription or over-the-counter (OTC) drugs should be approved by the health care provider before use. Special instructions about the timing of drug doses and drug-food interactions should be clarified. Written instructions are helpful as a reference after the patient leaves the office, clinic, or hospital.

Prenatal counseling is beneficial for women with underlying health problems. It provides the opportunity for the health care provider to counsel the woman regarding the potential risks of a drug and to offer an alternative therapy when available. For example, if a woman with chronic hypertension is considering pregnancy and has been taking an angiotensin-converting enzyme inhibitor, she can be switched to a preferred drug, such as methyldopa (Aldomet).

Evaluation

Meticulous, ongoing assessment is essential to achieve optimal perinatal management outcomes. Definitive treatment goals center, in most cases, on prevention and alleviation of potential problems. Understanding the applications, the benefits, and the risks of drugs given during pregnancy and lactation assists the health care provider in safely using drugs and evaluating their effects. Drug therapy may be unavoidable during this period, so it becomes the responsibility of the health care professional to maintain a current knowledge base so as to best respond to the health needs of the pregnant or lactating woman and her infant.

For information on specific drugs and their effects, see the Evolve Resources Bonus Content "Effects of Selected Maternal Drug Ingestion on the Fetus or Neonate," found at http://evolve.elsevier.com/Gutierrez/pharmacotherapeutics/.

KEY POINTS

- Understanding the physical changes of pregnancy as well as the indications for and the risk-benefit ratio of drugs used during pregnancy and lactation assists the health care provider in safely managing drug therapy.
- Maternal factors affecting drug response during pregnancy include reduced tone and motility of the gastrointestinal tract, altered secretion of hydrochloric acid, weight gain, rises in fluid volumes and blood pressure, higher production of plasma proteins such as fibrinogen, and greater competition for plasma protein–binding sites.
- Fetal factors affecting drug response during pregnancy include the fetus's immature hepatic and renal systems, reduced plasma protein–binding sites, umbilical blood flow, immature blood-brain barrier, a high proportion of water to body mass, and placental biotransformation.
- Only free, unbound drug exerts a pharmacologic effect. During pregnancy, the levels of serum albumin are reduced, promoting an increase in the amount of unbound drug. Unbound drugs in the maternal plasma cross the placenta into the fetal compartment.

- Teratogenicity is influenced by the susceptibility of the individual fetus, the timing of use of the offending drug, the characteristics of the teratogen, the mechanism of action that triggers changes in developing cells, the manifestation of the insult, and the dosage of the offending drug.
- The FDA pregnancy classification system for risk factors associated with systemic drug use is based on the level of known risk the drug presents to the fetus.
- When possible, drug therapy for a breastfeeding woman should be delayed until her infant is weaned or is not totally dependent on breast milk for its nutrition.
- When exposure to drugs through breast milk is inevitable, the parents should be taught to monitor the infant and report any changes in levels of activity, changes in behavior or feeding patterns, or skin rashes.
- When drug therapy is unavoidable, it becomes the responsibility of the health care provider to maintain a current knowledge base so as to best respond to the health needs of the pregnant or lactating woman and her baby.

Bibliography

American Academy of Pediatrics Committee on Drugs. (2000). Use of psychoactive medication during pregnancy and possible effects on the fetus and newborn. *Pediatrics, 105*(4), 880–887.

American Academy of Pediatrics Committee on Drugs. (2001). The transfer of drugs and other chemicals into human milk. *Pediatrics, 108*(3), 776–789.

American Academy of Pediatrics. (2005). Breastfeeding and the use of human milk. *Pediatrics, 115*(2), 496–506.

AWHONN, Mattson, S., and Smith, J. (2000). *Core curriculum for maternal-newborn nursing* (2nd ed.). Philadelphia: WB Saunders.

Begg, E., Duffull, S., Hackett, L., et al. (2002). Studying drugs in human milk: Time to unify the approach. *Journal of Human Lactation, 18*(4), 323–332.

Brent, R., Beckkman, D., and Landel, C. (1993). Clinical teratology. *Current Opinions in Pediatrics, 5*(2), 201–211.

Briggs, G., Freeman, R., and Yaffe, S. (2005). *Drugs in pregnancy and lactation: A reference guide to fetal and neonatal risk* (7th ed.). Philadelphia: Lippincott Williams.

Callister, L. (1995). Beliefs and perceptions of childbearing women choosing different primary health care providers. *Clinical Nursing Research, 4*(2), 72–73.

Chan, P., Thomas, D., McKinley, E., et al. (2005). *Outpatient and primary care medicine.* Laguna Hills, CA: Current Clinical Strategies.

Cunningham, F., Leveno, K., Bloom, S., et al. (2005). *Williams's obstetrics* (21st ed.). New York: McGraw-Hill.

Danforth, D., Gibbs, R., Karlan, B., et al. (2003). *Danforth's obstetrics and gynecology* (9th ed.). St. Louis: Lippincott, Williams, & Wilkins.

Dickey, J. (2004). *Managing contraceptive pill patients* (12th ed.). New Orleans: Essential Medical Information Systems.

Gardiner, S., and Begg, E. (2001). Drug safety in lactation. MEDSAFE Information for Health Professionals. Prescriber Update No.21:10–23. Available online: www.medsafe.govt.nz/Profs/PUarticles/lactation.htm. Accessed June 30, 2005.

Hale, T. (2004). Pharmacology review: Drug therapy and breastfeeding: Antidepressants, antipsychotics, antimanics, and sedatives. *NeoReviews, 5*(10), e451-e456.

Hale, T. (2004). Pharmacology review: Drug therapy and breastfeeding: Pharmacokinetics, risk factors, and effects on milk production. *NeoReview, 5*(4), e164-e172.

Howard, C., and Lawrence, R. (2001). Xenobiotics and breast feeding. *Pediatric Clinics of North America, 48*(2), 485–504.

Larimore, W., and Petrie, K. (2000). Drug use during pregnancy and lactation. *Primary Care, 27*(1), 35–53.

McCance, K., and Huether, S. (Eds.). (2002). *Pathophysiology: The biologic basis for disease in adults and children* (4th ed.). St. Louis: Mosby.

Medications in lactation. (2000). Harriet Lane Handbook. St. Louis: Mosby.

O'Dea, R. (1992). Medication use in the breastfeeding mother. *NAACOG's Clinical Issues in Perinatal and Women's Health Nursing, 3*(4), 598–604.

Park-Wyllie, L., Mazzotta, P., Pastuszak A., et al. (2000). Birth defects after maternal exposure to corticosteroids: Prospective cohort study and meta-analysis of epidemiological studies. *Teratology, 62* (6), 385–392.

Porreco, R. (Ed.). (1992). *Contemporary obstetrics for medical students.* Ithaca, NY: Perinatology Press.

Quinn, V., Guyon, A., and Ramiandrazafy, C. (2007). Successfully scaling up exclusive breastfeeding: Lessons from Madagascar. A research brief by the Child Health and Nutrition Research Initiative (CHNRI): An initiative of the Global Forum for Health Research. Available online: www.chnri.org/doc/MADAGASCAR%20FINAL. pdf. Accessed February 5, 2007.

Shaikh, U., and Scott, B. (2005). Extent, accuracy, and credibility of breastfeeding information on the Internet. *Journal of Human Lactation, 21*(2), 175–183.

Scheinfeld, J., and Davis, A. (2005). Teratology and drug use during pregnancy. *eMedicine.* Available online: www.emedicine.com/ med/topic3242.htm. Accessed October 7, 2006.

Spector, R. (1991). *Cultural diversity in health and illness.* Norwalk, CT: Appleton & Lange.

Szeto, H. (1993). Kinetics of drug transfer to the fetus. *Clinical Obstetrics and Gynecology, 36*(2), 246–254.

Wallace, S. (2001). AAP policy addresses transfer of chemicals into breast milk. *AAP News, 19*(3), 104–105.

Webb, R., Howard, L., and Abel, K. (2004). Antipsychotic drugs for non-affective psychosis during pregnancy and postpartum. *The Cochrane Database of Systematic Reviews.* Issue 2. Art. No: CD004411.pub2. DOI: 10.1002/14651858.CD004411.pub2.

United States Department of Health and Human Services. Pregnancy and medications. Available online: www.4woman.gov/faq/pregmed.htm. Accessed September 3, 2005.

University of Washington Clinical Teratology Web. *CARE Northwest counseling and advice on reproductive exposures.* Available online: http://depts.washington.edu/~terisweb/. Accessed October 10, 2005.

7

Pharmacotherapeutics for Children and Adolescents

Children, who are different both from adults and from each other, offer unique challenges in the management of the pharmacokinetic and pharmacodynamic components of drug therapy. Differences in body composition and organ maturation affect drug absorption, distribution, biotransformation, and elimination. Historically, drug studies have been done on adults, and what are felt to be appropriate pediatric drug dosages have been extrapolated from the adult studies and off-label use. Only 20% to 30% of drugs approved by the Food and Drug Administration (FDA) are labeled for pediatric use. The FDA Modernization Act of 1998 required pediatric studies for new drugs and biologic products but was overturned in October 2002 as the result of a lawsuit filed by the Association of American Physicians and Surgeons, the Competitive Enterprise Institute, and the Consumer Alert challenging the FDA's legal authority to require pediatric studies. The Pediatric Research Equity Act (PREA), passed by Congress in December 2003, requires pediatric studies of certain drugs and biologic products for a new indication, dosage form, route dosing regimen, or active ingredient. There were only 58

summaries of medical and clinical pharmacology reviews of pediatric studies listed at the FDA Center for Drug Evaluation and research website as of December 13, 2005.

Factors contributing to the continued lag in extrinsic pharmacokinetic information in children include the resistance of children and their parents to the necessary multiple venipunctures needed to define dose-time-response curves in pharmacokinetic studies and the ethical constraints on clinical research in children. Current best practice relies on our ability to use our best general sense of the pediatric differences in drug absorption, distribution, biotransformation, and elimination as the foundation for understanding and managing pharmacotherapeutics in our pediatric clients (Fig. 7-1).

ANATOMIC AND PHYSIOLOGIC VARIABLES

Crucial for the assessment of a child is a thorough understanding of the anatomic and physiologic differences between children and adults and the clinical significance of these

---

Controversy

Practical and Ethical Issues in Pediatric Clinical Trials

Children have special needs because of their vulnerabilities and stage of growth and development. Health care providers involved in research must be aware of these factors when planning to involve children in research. The child's autonomy should be respected as well as his or her individuality. It is crucial to maintain an awareness of the child's apprehension and fear of medical procedures, as well as of the fundamental differences between adults and children. Consider for a minute, that in 2000, the European Union had about 75 million children and 45,000 pediatricians, but only 12 clinical pediatric pharmacologists. In the United States, the FDA Modernization Act and its successor, the Best Pharmaceuticals for Children Act, provided companies a 6-month patent extension in recognition of adequately conducted pediatric trials.

In 1989, the United Nations General Assembly approved a Convention on the Rights of the Child. The four principles that were articulated are of fundamental importance in pharmaceutical research studies:

- All human rights apply to children without exception.
- All interventions must have the child's best interest as a primary consideration of the highest priority.
- Children have the right to the highest attainable level of health.
- Children have the right to obtain information and the right to respect of their opinion.

Good clinical practice should be based on evidence-based interventions. However, children have been described as "therapeutic orphans" because of the deficit of appropriate studies in their age group. As a result of this deficit, about 50% of drugs used in children's hospitals are not properly licensed for use in children.

CLINICAL REASONING

- One ethical issue pediatric researchers face is the fact that clinical research involves some risk to the subjects. At what point in a drug's development should research in children begin?
- Good clinical practice maintains that a balance be present that ensures that pediatric subjects are properly protected in research studies; the studies are based on good science, well designed, and properly analyzed; and study procedures are properly undertaken and documented. What constitutes a breach in good clinical practice? What if good clinical practices are not followed in pediatric drug research?
- An intellectual age of 7 years has arbitrarily been recommended for including children in the consent process; however, local, state, and federal laws must be considered and not assumed. Although parents are expected to sign the consent documents, should the verbal assent of children suffice, or should they be asked to sign something saying that they have been informed of the risks and assented, or did not dissent?
- Consider the following questions: Can healthy children participate in taste tests of pediatric liquid formulations? How does one define "minimum risk" in terms of venipuncture and sample collection? Should currently well children with cystic fibrosis participate in pharmacokinetic studies of inhaled aerosolized antibiotics? How should investigators handle the need for contraceptives for adolescents involved in therapeutic trials where teratogenesis may be of concern, such as trials of new antiepileptic drugs?

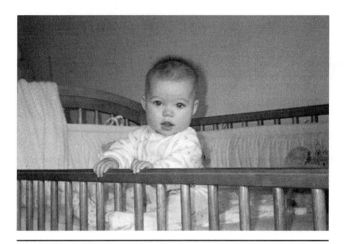

FIGURE 7-1 Developmental differences and changes in children that influence pharmacotherapy:
- Children have a larger body surface area and increased total body water in neonates and infants
- Metabolic rate is 2 times higher than that of an adult
- Of an infant's weight, 25% is muscle mass for injections
- Peripheral circulation less developed
- Cardiac output is dependent on rate, not stroke, until late school-age and adolescence, this makes the heart rate more rapid
- Increased gastric pH; gastrointestinal motility is dependent on maturity of body systems
- Immature hepatic enzyme capacities and activity
- Reduced albumin concentration and plasma protein binding
- Unstable glucose concentrations, unable to concentrate bilirubin
- Ineffective renal concentration of urine before age 12 to 18 months
- Blood-brain barrier not mature until 2 years of age
- Immature immune system

differences. Growth and development proceeds in a logical sequence but at a different rate for different body systems, making generalizations about the use of drugs across the pediatric population impossible.

BODY COMPOSITION AND SIZE

The proportions between height and weight in children differ from those in adults, and significant changes in these proportions occur throughout infancy and childhood. Whereas a child's weight increases about 20 times from birth to adulthood, his or her height only increases about 3.5 times. If the pediatric dose is calculated by adapting an adult dose with the child's weight as a benchmark, an inaccurate dose of drug can be administered.

The body surface area (BSA) offers a more precise way to calculate pediatric drug dosages because it is an accurate reflection of many of the physiologic processes significant in transporting, biotransforming, and eliminating drugs. The physiologic processes influenced by the BSA include the metabolic rate, extracellular fluid and total fluid volumes, cardiac output, and glomerular filtration rate (GFR). The BSA, which is calculated on the relationship between height and weight, is about 7 times greater in

*Available in the Evolve Resources Bonus Content "West Nomogram for estimating body surface area" at URL: http://evolve.elsevier.com/Gutierrez/pharmacotherapeutics/.

adulthood than at birth. A nomogram* or Mosteller's formula below can be used to compute body surface area. Keep in mind that the square root should be taken for the entire equation and not just the numerator. This is a major error that occurs when calculating BSA.

$$BSA\,(m^2) = \sqrt{height\,(cm) \times weight\,(kg) \div 3600}$$

Commercially available charts and devices, such as the Braslow tape, have been developed to assist in a rapid, but accurate, estimation of weight in infants and children in emergent situations to direct appropriate pharmacotherapy. In practice, many drug dosages are based on the child's weight in kilograms, which can be estimated using the following formula: Weight (kg) = 8 + 2(age in years).

FLUID BALANCE

The amount and distribution of total body water (intracellular and extracellular) varies with age. Water, the major constituent of body tissues, is the medium in which solutes are dissolved and all metabolic reactions take place. A premature infant's weight is 86% body water, whereas a full-term neonate's weight is 75% body water. In the immediate postnatal period, as the infant adjusts to a new environment, there is a physiologic loss of body water amounting to 5% of body weight. During the first year of life the proportion of body water decreases to 60% of body weight. The adult male's body weight is 55% water, and the adult female's body weight is 50% water (Table 7-1).

Extracellular and intracellular distribution of total body water start with 45% extracellular fluid and 35% intracellular for the full-term infant. A 1-year-old has 25% to 27% extracellular and 41% intracellular fluid, whereas the adult's percentages are 10% to 15% and 40%, respectively. Males eventually have a greater percentage of body water because of increasing muscle mass. Females, who proportionally have more body fat and less muscle mass as a function of estrogens, have comparatively less body water.

The basal metabolic rate, closely related to the BSA, changes distinctively throughout childhood. Highest in infancy, it progressively decreases to maturity. Infants are particularly susceptible to significant changes in total body water because of their high metabolic rates. The rate of fluid intake and fluid elimination in the infant is 7 times as great, in relation to body weight, as in the adult. Daily water turnover in children involves more than half of the extracellular fluid; in the adult, one fifth of the extracellular fluid is exchanged daily. Because of a child's greater proportion of body fluid, especially in the extracellular compartment, larger mg/kg doses of water-soluble drugs are required in order to achieve therapeutic drug levels.

TISSUE MASS

Skeletal growth and muscle development in healthy children consists of two concurrent processes: the creation of new cells and tissues (growth) and the consolidation of the new tissues into a permanent form (maturation). An infant's muscle mass accounts for approximately 25% of total body weight, compared to 40% in the adult. Composition and size of muscles varies with age as fetal muscle tissue, containing large amounts

TABLE **7-1** Body Weight Composition				
	Components (% of Body Weight)			
Age (Weight)	Extracellular Fluid	Intracellular Fluid	Total Body Water	Fat
Premature infant (1.5 kg)	Not determined	Not determined	85	1
Full-term infant (3.5 kg)	45–47	32–35	70–80	16
1-year-old (10 kg)	25–27	41	58–60	22–24
4-year-old	24	41	60	12
10-year-old	17	41	60	18–20
Adult male	10–15	40	50–60	15

Adapted and used with permission from Bindler, R., and Howry, L. (2005). *Pediatric Drug Guide.* Upper Saddle River, NJ: Pearson Education.

of water and intracellular matrix, changes after birth to accommodate additional cytoplasm. Muscle fibers enlarge, and the amounts of water and intracellular matrix are considerably reduced. Sex differences in muscle size and weight, minor during childhood, become significant with the onset of puberty. Muscle growth during adolescence is a major factor in weight gain, with muscle fibers reaching maximal size at about age 10 years in females and age 14 years in males.

Body fat, approximately 16% of an infant's birth weight, falls to between 8% and 12% between the ages of 1 and 5 years and again increases to 18% to 20% of body weight at about age 10. Premature infants have very little fatty tissue. Fat-soluble drugs, therefore, are not well distributed in an infant's or child's body, leading to a greater blood concentration (and possible toxicity) of the drugs.

HEAD AND NECK

In children, the head, which is larger in proportion to the rest of the body, receives a correspondingly greater percentage of blood. Softer, more pliable skull bones are coupled with weak muscular support of the neck in the young child. The narrowest part of the larynx, which is positioned more anteriorly and cephaloid, is at the cricoid cartilage. A shorter, straighter eustachian tube in the young child, coupled with increased mucus in the eustachian tube during milk consumption, creates a perfect medium for the bacteria that cause ear infections.

RESPIRATORY SYSTEM

The immaturity of the child's respiratory system contributes to the greater number of respiratory illnesses seen in children. Infants, obligate nose-breathers for the first 2 to 4 months of life, need their nasal passages to be kept clear of secretions to prevent respiratory distress. A child's proportionately larger tongue and epiglottis, along with smaller, narrower airways, means that a relatively small amount of mucus or mucosal edema may quickly cause obstruction. The diameter of an infant's trachea approximates that of the infant's little finger. An infant relies primarily on the diaphragm for breathing. The pliable thorax, fewer alveoli in the lungs, and poorly developed intercostal muscles combine to create lower lung compliance in children. Any obstruction of the airway greatly lowers resistance to airflow and increases oxygen requirements as well as the work of breathing.

Physiologic differences in the respiratory tracts of children and adults are reflected in their metabolic rates. Because of

higher metabolic rates and oxygen consumption, children rely on respiratory function to a greater extent than adults. The proportionately larger BSA and respiratory rate of children lead to rapid heat and water loss during infection or fever. Dehydration, and its resulting acidosis, may occur rapidly during the times of decreased oral intake that frequently accompany acute infections in children.

Children are more vulnerable to infections of the respiratory tract than adults, have not had time to develop immunity to most organisms, and are commonly exposed to respiratory tract infections through contact with other children. They also have less compensatory reserve than adults, owing to the size and immaturity of the respiratory tract. Collateral pathways of ventilation are incompletely developed. Children have less elastic and collagen tissue in the lungs, and therefore greater susceptibility to edema. The metabolic rate in infants is approximately 2 times that of adults, thereby increasing the need for oxygen. Anything that raises the metabolic rate contributes to respiratory demands.

CARDIOVASCULAR SYSTEM

Cardiovascular dynamics of the young child change during the transition from fetus to newborn, from newborn to young child, and from child to adult. These dynamics affect the uptake and distribution of drugs.

The heart rate and stroke volume are greater in a child than in an adult. Like respirations and body metabolism, the cardiac output of the newborn is twice as much, in relation to body weight, as that of the adult, or approximately 550 mL/min. The child's circulating blood volume is less than that of the adult. Further, peripheral circulation is poorly developed in the infant, so blood flow to various muscles changes a great deal during the first 2 weeks of life. Peripheral vasoconstriction in response to a cold environment further impedes absorption of subcutaneous and intramuscular injections. There is a greater predictability of drug action by the oral and intravenous routes, making these the administration routes of choice for many drugs.

GASTROINTESTINAL SYSTEM

Gastric absorption depends on the amount, type, osmolality, and pH of gastrointestinal (GI) secretions, as well as GI motility and transit time. The gastric pH ranges from 5 to 8 in neonates, drops to a more acidic pH of 1 to 3 within the first day of life, and reaches adult levels at about 4 months of age.

Irregular peristalsis in young infants contributes to the 6- to 8-hour gastric emptying time in a newborn. Gastric emptying time decreases to that of an adult (i.e., 2 hours) within the first several months of life. Infants, who eat every 2 to 4 hours, have food in their stomachs for much of the day, which can interfere with drug absorption.

Immature liver function in infants and young children affects drug distribution, because fewer plasma proteins, especially albumin, are produced. Therefore less plasma protein is available for drug binding, which results in more free drug, higher drug blood levels, and increased risk for adverse drug reactions and drug toxicity.

RENAL SYSTEM

Drug elimination from our bodies, for the most part, depends upon a functioning renal system. Glomerular filtration, tubular secretion, and tubular reabsorption are the mechanisms the kidney uses to excrete drugs via the urine. Of the three, glomerular filtration is the most common mechanism by which drugs are excreted. In infants the GFR is 30% to 50% of an adult's. Therefore the half-life of drugs cleared by glomerular filtration is increased by 50% in infants.

An infant has fewer tubular cells, shorter tubule length, and smaller rates of tubular blood flow. Renal tubular secretion capacity is subsequently less than an adult's, and the half-life of drugs cleared by tubular secretion is again increased. Tubular secretion reaches adult levels by about 7 months of age.

Tubular reabsorption is the kidney's mechanism to preserve substances coming through the renal tubule. The kidney of a newborn concentrates urine to 1.5 times the osmolality of plasma, instead of 3 to 4 times, as is normally found in an adult. When considering an infant's immature kidneys and marked fluid turnover, one can readily appreciate the increased risk for dehydration, overhydration, and drug toxicity in this age group.

NEUROLOGIC SYSTEM

An infant's nervous system is complete but immature. The number of glial cells and dendrites increases manifestedation until approximately 4 years of age, and myelinization continues throughout childhood. Children younger than 2 years of age have an immature blood-brain barrier and are more susceptible to central nervous system (CNS) drug effects and toxicity. Encephalopathy is a CNS drug toxicity more commonly manifested in this age group.

IMMUNE SYSTEM

Passively acquired maternal IgG antibodies protect most full-term newborns against a variety of infectious agents until the immature immune system mechanisms begin to function between the age of 2 and 3 months. Preterm infants have lower levels of passively acquired antibodies, because the maternal immunoglobulin transfer occurs during the last trimester. The loss of these passively acquired antibodies over the first 3 to 6 months of life dictates the timing of the first childhood immunizations to provide efficacious protection against the communicable diseases. Adult levels of IgG are reached by 7 to 8 years of age. IgM levels, low at birth, rise by 1 week of age and reach adult levels by 1 year.

Manufacture of IgA and IgE, which are not present at birth, begins at 2 weeks of age and reaches adult levels by 6 to 7 years. These differences contribute to the greater number of infectious diseases and altered allergic responses to foreign substances seen during childhood. Childhood allergies are often manifested as insect hypersensitivity, perennial allergic rhinitis, urticaria, and eczema.

PHARMACOKINETIC CONSIDERATIONS

Data on the pharmacokinetics, pharmacodynamics, efficacy, and safety of drugs in infants and children are scarce. Thus drug therapy for a child presents a challenge to the health care provider. Maturational changes provide some guidance in understanding the complex nature of pharmacokinetic principles. A poorly developed blood-brain barrier, weak biotransformational activity, and immature mechanisms for elimination combine to make the fetus and neonate vulnerable to toxic drug effects.

Individualized pharmacokinetic evaluation allows optimization of drug therapy so that benefits may be maximized and risks minimized. The most pressing need in pediatric pharmacotherapy is the formulation of a distinct, rational therapeutic plan, with subsequent individualization of drug dosage based on careful assessment of the patient. There is little doubt that sound pharmacokinetic information can contribute to a more rapid achievement of optimal dosages. Table 7-2 summarizes physiologic factors affecting drug action.

ABSORPTION

Drug absorption depends on the route of administration, disintegration, dissociation, drug concentration, blood flow to the site, and absorptive surface area. The two factors affecting the absorption of drugs from the GI tract are pH-dependent diffusion and gastric emptying time. Both processes are strikingly different in a premature infant, compared with older infants and children and adults. Age-related variables such as delayed gastric emptying time and irregular intestinal motility are examples of mechanisms that affect absorption. The rate of absorption also depends on the specific characteristics of the drug and the child.

Oral Route

Drug absorption via the oral route depends on a number of factors. Drug formulation, the degree of disintegration and dissociation, concentration, blood flow to the site and the absorptive surface area, pH-dependent diffusion, and gastric motility all influence the process.

Absorption of orally administered drugs is often delayed in neonates and young infants, owing primarily to differences in the pH of the GI tract and reduced gastric motility. Immediately after birth, gastric pH is high. By 4 months of age, gastric

TABLE 7-2 Physiologic Factors Altering Pharmacokinetics

Component	Age Group	Physiologic Factor	Comments
Absorption	Neonates, infants, young children	Increased gastric pH	Bioavailability of basic drugs is increased, and bioavailability of acidic drugs is reduced.
	Neonates, infants	Increased gastric emptying time	
	Infants, children	Increased gastric and intestinal motility	Bioavailability is unpredictable.
	Neonates	Decreased bile acids	Bioavailability is reduced.
	Neonate, infants, young children	Little muscle tissue and immature peripheral circulation	Drug absorption is decreased.
Distribution	Neonates, infants	Increased total body water and extracellular fluid	Volume of distribution is increased.
		Reduced albumin concentration and protein binding	Volume of distribution is increased. Concentration of free drug is increased.
	Neonates, infants	Immature blood-brain barrier	Risk for CNS toxicity is increased.
Biotransformation	Neonates, infants	Immature enzyme capacity	Half-life increases, but clearance is reduced.
	Neonates, infants, young children	Faster resting respiratory rate	Metabolism of drugs is more rapid, requiring oxidation.
Elimination	Neonates, infants	Immature glomerular and tubular function	Half-life increases.
	Young children	Increased enzyme capacity	Clearance increases, but half-life is reduced.

CNS, Central nervous system

pH values have reached 50% of the adult value (pH 1 to 3.5), and by 8 months of age, they are thought to reach adult levels. Acidic drugs, such as nalidixic acid, phenobarbital, and phenytoin, are less well absorbed. On the other hand, the absorption of acid-labile drugs (e.g., penicillin) may be enhanced.

Gastric emptying time is 6 to 8 hours in the neonate but reaches that of an adult (about 2 hours) in the first few months of life. Prolonged exposure of certain drugs to gastric contents increases the disintegration of unstable drugs and also delays drug entry into the lower GI tract, thus drug absorption and attainment of peak serum levels are delayed.

Parenteral Routes

Any condition altering muscle growth decreases the number of muscle sites suitable for intramuscular injections. Intramuscular drug absorption may be uncertain because of unpredictable blood flow, decreased muscle tone, lower muscle oxygenation, and vasomotor instability. Repeated injections in the child's few available muscle sites may cause tissue breakdown and poorer absorption of the drug. However, the absorption of drugs administered by the percutaneous route is increased because of an underdeveloped epidermal barrier and greater permeability of the skin.

The intravenous (IV) route is commonly used in pediatric therapy. For some drugs, it is the only effective route. When a drug is administered intravenously, the effect is almost instantaneous, and further control is limited. Most drugs intended for IV administration require a specified minimum dilution and/or rate of infusion.

Intraosseous cannulation provides a reliable method for fluid administration in emergent situations. This route is used temporarily, until venous access sites become available. The flat, anteromedial surface of the tibia, approximately 1 to 3 cm below the tibial tuberosity, is the preferred site. In older children and adolescents, the iliac crest or the sternum are preferred sites. In general, any intravenous drug or fluid can be safely administered by the intraosseous route. Reports of successful administration of catecholamines, calcium, antibiotics, digitalis, heparin, lidocaine, atropine, phenytoin, sodium bicarbonate, neuromuscular blocking drugs, crystalloids, colloids, and blood can be found in the literature.

Topical Routes

The absorption rate of a topically administered drug is not different in a child. However, more of the drug is absorbed in a child because of greater BSA and skin permeability. When occlusive dressings are used, absorption of a topically administered drug is enhanced and the possibility of adverse reactions increased, particularly to steroid creams, salicylic acid, and silver sulfadiazine. Corticosteroids are applied sparingly in children with the goal of preventing absorption that may lead to adrenal suppression.

A few drugs are known for their bioavailability when given rectally, and this avenue provides an alternative to oral or parenteral routes. Rectal administration is generally disliked because of erratic absorption but may be preferred in some cases over intramuscular (IM) injection. Furthermore, acceptance of rectal administration may be culturally influenced. Drugs available in suppository form include acetaminophen, sedatives, antiemetics, and analgesics such as morphine.

DISTRIBUTION

Many age-related differences in drug distribution occur during the first 10 to 12 months of life. The distribution of a drug in children is affected by the changing percentage of body fat, total body water content, total blood volume, and blood flow to target tissues as well as by the physiochemical properties of the drug.

Drug distribution and equilibration rates are faster in children compared with adults. Therefore a larger average dose per kilogram of body weight is needed to reach desired serum concentration levels. The higher the percentage of body water, the more water-soluble drugs are diluted, resulting in a reduction in serum concentration levels. As the percentage of body fat increases with age, so does the distribution of fat-soluble drugs. Therefore the distribution of these drugs is more limited in children than in adults.

Decreased formation of plasma proteins in the immature liver of infants affects drug distribution and results in higher serum drug levels. Factors influencing protein binding include the amount of albumin and/or alpha-1-acid glycoproteins available, the pH of the blood, the binding capacity of the albumin, and other substances in the child's system that compete for binding sites with the available albumin.

The albumin in neonates and infants has a lower binding capacity for certain drugs (e.g., phenytoin, penicillin) compared with the binding capacity of mature albumin. Therefore more unbound drug is free to circulate and act. Thus it is possible that free drug levels will be high enough to produce adverse or toxic effects. To minimize the possibility of toxicity and to compensate for the shorter duration of drug action, it is often necessary to decrease the amount of the drug given and/or lengthen the time between doses.

In contrast, adverse effects may occur when drugs such as salicylates, penicillins, sulfonamides, phenytoin, phenobarbital, and imipramine compete with endogenous substances (e.g., free fatty acids, bilirubin) for the same protein binding sites. Competitive drug binding in the neonate increases the potential for adverse effects from increased concentrations of unbound, unconjugated bilirubin. *Kernicterus* (bilirubin encephalopathy) is a grave condition that can result in brain damage; bilirubin infiltrates the basal ganglia and other areas of the brain and spinal cord. The higher permeability of the blood-brain barrier in children allows this to occur. Any drug that competes with bilirubin for protein binding sites or that inhibits the binding of bilirubin increases the risk. The signs of kernicterus are those of CNS depression or excitation such as decreased activity, lethargy, irritability, and loss of interest in feeding, as well as seizures and gastric or pulmonary hemorrhage.

BIOTRANSFORMATION

Most biotransformation of drugs is accomplished in the liver by microsomal enzymes; however, the activity of the hepatic enzymes is low in the neonate and premature infants. The capacity of an infant's liver to biotransform drugs develops quickly during the first months after birth. The liver's ability to biotransform drugs varies with the enzymes involved. Phase I, nonsynthetic reaction of hydroxylation, is most affected. Slower hydroxylation causes longer plasma half-lives in neonates, so the interval between doses should be increased and/or the daily dose decreased. Examples of drugs hydroxylated during phase I biotransformation include aspirin, meperidine, enalapril, indomethacin, and procainamide, to name a few.

Phase II reactions, such as conjugation with glucuronic acid, are variably reduced. Lower conjugating activity contributes to *hyperbilirubinemia* and the risk of bilirubin-induced encephalopathy. Altered biotransformation processes persist for approximately the first month of life, undergoing a dramatic increase at about 6 months of age. Examples of drugs conjugated during phase II biotransformation include acetaminophen, morphine, lorazepam, sulfonamides, and steroids.

It is almost impossible to predict the effects of maturation on biotransformation solely on the basis of age. Metabolic rates and hepatic drug oxidation remain markedly elevated for the first 2 to 3 years of life. Rates gradually decrease until puberty, when adult levels are reached. The plasma half-lives of diazepam, digoxin, indomethacin, acetaminophen, and phenobarbital appear to be longer in infants.

The first-pass effect has received little attention in pediatric populations but has been demonstrated with a number of drugs. For example, the mean plasma half-life for phenytoin and phenobarbital decreases from 80 hours between birth and 2 days of age to about 15 hours between 3 to 14 days of age, and then declines to 6 hours (approximate adult level) between 14 and 150 days after birth.

Dosages and choice of drug may be altered for an infant with immature liver function or liver disease. For example, when the antimicrobial drug chloramphenicol is inadequately biotransformed, toxic levels are reached, resulting in *gray baby syndrome*. This disorder is characterized by tachypnea, ashen-gray cyanosis, vomiting, loose, green stools, progressive abdominal distention, vasomotor collapse, and perhaps death. Discontinuing the drug as soon as symptoms appear can reverse progression of symptoms.

Body temperature regulation is unstable in children, creating implications for drug action. When infants and toddlers develop an infection, the sudden high temperature increases basal metabolic rates. For each degree (centigrade) the body temperature rises, the metabolic rate increases by approximately 12%. The higher metabolic rate reduces drug half-lives and the duration of therapeutic effects. Antipyretic effects of drugs are short-lived because of this phenomenon.

ELIMINATION

Renal function is lower in infants and small children than in adults. GFR, concentrating and acidifying functions, and tubular function, including secretion and reabsorption, all influence drug action. These factors are reflected in prolonged elimination, increasing the risk for toxicity. Each of the processes matures at a different rate, so the clearance of various drugs may be greater in infants than in older children or adults. There is a disproportionate development of renal filtration and secretion in relation to reabsorption. Full renal function develops in infants by 6 to 12 months of age.

The neonate has glomerular cells at birth, but they are functionally immature. Digoxin, for example, depends on the glomerular filtration rate for elimination. Because of the rapid increase in GFR during the first few weeks of life, the dosage of digoxin may have to be increased to maintain the desired serum drug level.

During the first 6 months of life, an infant has a small number of tubular cells, a shorter tubular length, and a lower tubular blood flow. Drug dosages that depend on the kidneys for elimination must be adjusted to avoid toxic responses. When renal blood flow increases in response to a rise in systemic arterial pressure, intrarenal vascular resistance decreases. This response permits the kidneys to receive a higher percentage of the cardiac output and the circulating drug. Therefore drugs that depend on tubular secretion for elimination, such as the penicillins, have a longer half-life.

Drug elimination is also affected by the urinary pH, because some drugs are more readily eliminated in acid urine and others require basic urine to be excreted. An infant's kidneys are less able to excrete hydrogen ions and reabsorb bicarbonate. As a result, the infant's urine is slightly less acidic than an adult's.

The clearance of drugs is important to pharmacokinetics, primarily because there is little information about drug distribution in children. For example, clearance rates of theophylline are low in infancy but increase fivefold by 4 years of age, and then slowly decline over the years. Theophylline is biotransformed to caffeine in the neonate, whereas adults rapidly biotransform theophylline to inactive metabolites. Both theophylline and caffeine are methylxanthines with similar drug actions. Toxicity can result in the neonate through additive mechanisms.

The net effect of organ immaturity is the potential for drugs to accumulate in the body. Drug dosages may have to be adjusted to maintain a desired serum level and to avoid toxicity.

PHARMACODYNAMIC CONSIDERATIONS

Drugs have the same mechanism of action in all individuals, including children. If a drug normally inhibits the transfer of a substance into a cell, it does so in any age group. The response to the drug, however, varies according to the maturity of the target organ and the specific drug receptors.

CLINICAL REASONING

Treatment Objectives

The primary treatment objective for the pediatric patient is to achieve appropriate outcomes while maintaining therapeutic drug levels and avoiding toxic effects. Other treatment objectives include allaying fears and preventing injury associated with drug regimens. Principles relevant to pediatric pharmacotherapy are identified in Table 7-3.

Treatment objectives also include the avoidance of polypharmacy (limiting the number of drugs prescribed), avoidance of inappropriate drug use (i.e., choosing a particular drug because of wanting to try out a new drug or because samples are available), and enhancement of drug regimen compliance. Specific end points of therapy should be determined so that the dosage can be optimized, irrational combinations

TABLE 7-3 Administration Principles

- Provide explanations using language that is developmentally appropriate or age-appropriate. Ethnic, cultural, and native language of parents and patients should also be considered.
- Keep the time between explanation and administration of drug to a minimum.
- Prepare drugs in advance, keeping needles and syringes out of sight.
- Expect success with positive approaches. Act smoothly and quickly.
- Be honest with the child; involve the child to gain cooperation (e.g., warning that a shot will hurt, emphasizing that drugs are not candy).
- Solicit the parent's help where appropriate.
- Provide distraction for a frightened or uncooperative child.
- Allow the child to express feelings; assure the child that crying is okay.
- Praise the child for doing his or her best.
- Spend time with the child after administering the drug.
- Let the child know he or she is accepted as a person of value.

avoided, and adverse effects minimized. In general, the most efficacious, least toxic, least expensive drug that treats the child's underlying illness (in preference to symptoms) should be chosen.

Treatment Options

▌ Patient Variables

Clearly determine whether the chief complaint is the problem of the patient, the parent(s), or both. Social, educational, and cultural status of the child's parents must be considered. In planning appropriate techniques for drug administration, furthermore, it is imperative to take into consideration the developmental norms for fine motor skills, gross motor skills, feeding behavior, language, and social skills, all of which reduces the risk for physical and psychologic trauma related to drug therapy.

Cultural assessment of the child's and family's health care patterns and beliefs helps to identify and understand factors that may affect proposed treatment plan and adherence. The detail and depth of the assessment depends on the situation and the needs of the child and family. Cultural practices may involve the use of complementary therapies such as "protective devices" (e.g., strings, cords, beads, amulets) to keep the child from harm or illness or to help in the healing process. These devices should be removed only by the patient or family and only when absolutely necessary.

Pediatric pharmacotherapy requires that appropriate dosage regimens be designed to compensate for developmental changes and to optimize therapy at different stages of childhood. The fact that a pediatric dosage cannot be found in current publications and references should be evaluated carefully before any dose is calculated. If a pediatric dosage cannot be found in current drug references, the drug may not be suitable for pediatric use.

Any method devised to calculate drug dosage for children (and adults) provides an estimate only, to be verified or corrected by clinical response and/or measurement of drug concentrations. No universal dosage rule can be recommended. Today, drug manufacturers usually recommend doses expressed in mg/kg of body weight, and generally as ranges rather than fixed doses. There is ample evidence that dosage regimens cannot be based simply on data about body weight or surface area that have been extrapolated from adult data, but must take into consideration that some drug use is also dependent on patient age. Furthermore, bioavailability, pharmacokinetics, efficacy, and adverse effects can differ markedly from patient to patient.

Monitoring therapeutic serum levels is particularly useful in children who have a limited ability to communicate any adverse effects they are experiencing, when the effects of a drug cannot be directly observed, or when the drug has a narrow therapeutic index (e.g., antiepileptic drugs, antineoplastics, theophylline, digoxin).

For further information on drug administration with children and adolescents, see the Evolve Resources Bonus Content at http://evolve.elsevier.com/Gutierrez/pharmacotherapeutics/.

Patient Education

Assessment of the parents' and caregivers' level of understanding and provision of appropriate education is a must. Parents and caregivers must know the name and purpose of the drug; the dosage and concentration, dosing frequency, and route of administration; the length of time the drug is to be administered; and the anticipated effects of the drug. Many parents only know how much (i.e., mL) they are administering. Since most drugs administered are oral liquids and some are available in more than one concentration, it is important also for parents to know which one their child is receiving.

Considerable variation exists in the understanding of the term "teaspoon," causing errors in measurement; therefore the designations teaspoonful or tablespoonful are rarely used today. Drug dosage should be specific and parents provided with proper drug delivery tools. Misinterpretation of the route of administration may occur. For example, ear drops may be prescribed "for the ear" or prescribed to be placed "in the ear." The ability of the parent or caregiver to recognize adverse effects is complicated by the child's lack of language and inability to recognize, understand, and communicate symptoms. Furthermore, the parents' own communication ability must be considered. Educational deficits and native languages other than English may result in otherwise preventable errors. The belief that "if a little is good, more is better" can lead to accidental ingestion and possible overdose.

Adherence with drug regimens is affected by and can even depend on the willingness of others to assist in the child's care. Children's and adolescents' reactions to drug regimens are affected by physical and cognitive abilities, developmental characteristics, environmental influences, past experiences, current relationship with the health care provider and with the parent, and perception of the present situation. Helpful approaches and explanations can increase the potential for compliance. Follow-up by telephone or through a community health nurse may ensure that the drug regimen is accurately implemented.

Stress or fatigue from caring for a sick child may contribute to a drug administration error. In some cases, young or unseasoned parents do not have the experience to ask appropriate questions about a drug to clarify their understanding of the drug regimen. Drug misuse in children has many common causes. The use of multiple drug dispensers (e.g., one each for father, mother, and day-care center personnel) may increase the risk of repeated or missed doses. Drugs prescribed for a previous illness or for a sibling with similar symptoms may be inappropriate for the present illness.

Evaluation

Children are not small adults. Meticulous, ongoing assessment is essential to optimal pediatric drug regimens. Along with an awareness of pediatric physiologic and developmental changes, conscientious attention must be paid to the pharmacokinetics and the pharmacodynamics of the required drugs so that potential complications are avoided or recognized early. Definitive management goals center, in most cases, on prevention and cure. Patient and family education should always be included to promote adherence with drug regimens, drug administration, and drug safety. Available social services may have to be considered.

Applied pediatric pharmacokinetics still has not yet attained the clarity of modern adult drug therapy. Ethical and legal constraints on drug testing in the pediatric population continue to limit the health care provider's knowledge of drug action and response. There is little doubt that sound pharmacokinetic information can contribute to a more rapid achievement of optimal drug dosages for this population of patients. The approach chosen should facilitate a positive experience for the health care provider, the patient, and the family.

KEY POINTS

- Children's body systems grow and develop at different rates; therefore generalizations about the use of drugs in this population are not possible.
- The concept of body surface area is important in pediatrics, because many physiologic functions are proportional to body surface area. Because of a child's greater proportion of body fluid, higher mg/kg doses of certain drugs may be needed to achieve therapeutic drug levels.
- Physiologic differences in the pediatric patient influence drug absorption by oral, parenteral, and topical routes.
- Many age-related differences in drug distribution occur during the first 10 to 12 months of life. Distribution and equilibration rates may be faster in children than in adults.
- Immaturity of the liver in premature infants and neonates reduces the biotransformation of drugs.
- There are significant age-related changes in glomerular filtration rates, tubular secretion, and reabsorption, and thus renal elimination of drugs and their metabolites.
- Drugs have the same mechanism of action in all individuals, including children. The response to the drug, however, varies according to the maturity of the target organ, thereby necessitating a dosage adjustment.

- Clearly determine whether the chief complaint is the problem of the patient, the parent(s), or both.
- Particular attention should be paid to the allergies that are prevalent during infancy and childhood.
- Social, educational, and cultural status of the child's parents must be considered. In planning appropriate techniques for drug administration, furthermore, it is imperative to take into consideration the developmental norms for fine motor skills, gross motor skills, feeding behavior, language, and social skills, all of which reduces the risk for physical and psychological trauma related to drug therapy.
- In general, the least toxic and least expensive drug that treats the underlying cause of the child's illness (in preference to symptoms) should be chosen.
- There are many common causes of drug misuse in the pediatric patient, related to multiple caregivers, misunderstanding of measurement parameters, and the inability of the caregiver to recognize adverse effects.
- Meticulous, ongoing assessment and evaluation are essential to optimize pediatric drug regimens.

Bibliography

Bindler, R., and Howry, L. (2005). *Pediatric drug guide.* Upper Saddle River, NJ: Pearson Education.

FDA, Center for Drug Evaluation and Research. (2005). *Summaries of medical and clinical pharmacology reviews of pediatric studies.* Available online: www.fda.gov/cder/pediatric/Summaryreview.htm. Accessed February 5, 2007.

Gill, D., and Kurz, R. (2002). Practical and ethical issues in pediatric clinical trials. *Applied Clinical Trials,* Available online: www.actmagazine.com/appliedclinicaltrials/article/articleDetail.jsp?id=83744. Accessed February 5, 2007.

Gutierrez, K., and Queener, S. (2003). *Pharmacology for nursing practice.* St. Louis: Mosby.

Hockenberry, M., Wilson, D., and Winkelstein, M. (2005). *Wong's essentials of pediatric nursing* (7th ed.). St. Louis: Mosby.

International Conference on Harmonisation of Technical Requirements for Registration of Pharmaceuticals for Human Use (ICH). (2000). Note for guidance on clinical investigation of medicinal products in the paediatric population. *ICH,* Topic 11, www.ich.org. Accessed February 5, 2007.

Katzung, B. (2004). *Basic and clinical pharmacology.* Chicago: Lange Medical Books/McGraw-Hill.

McCance, K., and Huether, S. (2005). *Pathophysiology: The biologic basis for disease in adults and children* (4th ed.). St. Louis: Mosby.

Turkoski, B., Lance, B., and Bonfiglio, M. (2004). *Drug information handbook for advanced practice nursing* (5th ed.). Hudson, OH: LEXI-COMP.

Youngkin, E., Sawin, K., Kissinger, J., et al. (2005). *Pharmacotherapeutics: A primary care guide.* Upper Saddle River, NJ: Pearson Prentice Hall.

Wechsler, J. (1999). Science, pediatric studies, and surrogates. *Applied Clinical Trials,* June, 28–33.

8

Pharmacotherapeutics for Older Adults

Thirteen percent of the U.S. population is made up of older adults, but they take almost 35% of all prescribed drugs. Seventy-seven million people will be added to this group as the baby boomers age, that is, those born between the years of 1946 to 1964. This means that nearly 1 in 5 people in the United States—20% of the population—will be over age 65 years by the year 2020. Eight million of these persons will be women aged 85 years and older. In 1930, slightly more than 6 million people were older than 65, and the average life expectancy was 60 years. In 1965, the numbers of people over 65 had grown to 20 million, and the average life expectancy was 70 years. Now, life expectancy has reached 75 years. Advances in disease control and health care technologies, reduced infant mortality rates, improved sanitation, and better living conditions have helped increase life expectancy for most Americans.

The management of chronic illness, when one or more drugs may be needed, has potential implications for drug therapy in older adults. Many older adults have at least one chronic condition or disease, and many have several that must be concurrently managed. Comorbid medical and psychiatric illness has also been evaluated in numerous populations of older adults and has various implications for drug use and safety. Chronic illness contributes to self-care limitations in almost half of this population. Approximately one fourth of older adults have difficulty with the activities of daily living. The older the person is, the greater the prevalence of drug therapy and the need for assistance with the tasks of daily living; the likelihood of remaining totally independent declines as well.

Persons over 65 years of age purchase 35% of all prescription drugs and more than 33% of over-the-counter (OTC) drugs sold in the United States, at an annual cost of $3 billion. The average older American residing at home has 11 different prescriptions filled annually; residents of extended-care facilities average 8 prescriptions a year. Of all older adults, 90% take at least one drug daily. Drugs most commonly prescribed are diuretics, potassium salts, histamine$_2$ antagonists, nitroglycerin, insulin, cardiac glycosides, beta blockers, antianxiety drugs, and antihypertensives. The most common OTC drugs purchased by older adults are analgesics, antiinflammatory drugs, laxatives, and antacids (Table 8-1).

THE COMPLEX DYNAMICS OF AGING

A variety of physiologic changes increase the older adult's sensitivity to drugs and drug-induced disease; however, chronologic age is not necessarily related to physiologic age. With aging, there is a gradual decline in many body system functions; some systems are more affected than others. There is a growing awareness that some physiologic changes once

TABLE 8-1 Drugs Commonly Used by Older Adults

Prescription Drugs	Over-the-Counter Drugs
Antianxiety drugs	acetaminophen
Antihypertensives	Analgesics
Beta blockers	Antacids
digoxin	Laxatives
Diuretics	Nonsteroidal antiinflammatory drugs
Proton pump inhibitors	Histamine$_2$ antagonists
Insulin	Antidiarrheals
nitroglycerin	Cough and cold products
Potassium salts	Sleep aids

considered to be inevitable are not evident in physically fit older adults. Indeed, the variations between people of the same age are so great that increased biologic variation is characteristic of this age group. Variation is also highly dependent on the presence of chronic medical and psychiatric illness and chronic use of drugs or other substances known to interfere with physiologic processes such as renal and hepatic function. This is particularly true of physiologic functions that affect drug disposition and response. Therefore each person must be evaluated on his or her own merit.

BODY COMPOSITION

All body cells show age-related changes. Cell numbers gradually decline, leaving fewer functional body cells. The nucleus of each cell appears to enlarge, although there is no discernible

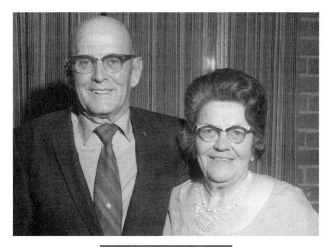

FIGURE 8-1 Older adult couple.

increase in the amount of DNA present. The nucleoli increase in size and number, and there appears to be an increase in RNA. Protoplasmic changes include a rise in protein content but a fall in protein synthesis, an increase in lipids, accumulation of lipofuscin (especially in the fixed cells of nerve tissue and muscle), and glycogen depletion. Lysosomes needed for digestion and breakdown of cellular products accumulate because of either alterations in the rate of protein turnover or deficits in the catabolic process.

Age-related tissue changes are best seen in the extracellular matrix. Elastin, found in tissues associated with body movement (e.g., walls of major blood vessels, heart, lungs, and skin), is reduced and replaced with pseudoelastin. Tissues become less pliable and, ultimately, less efficient. Double chins, elongated ears, and baggy eyelids are obvious manifestations of the loss of elastin. Aortic stenosis may also develop as elastin is replaced with pseudoelastin.

Body fat increases until about age 85 and then decreases. In women, fat and lipids continue to accumulate. In men, there is a steady increase in lipids until age 60, after which there is a gradual decrease. As body fat atrophies, contours gain a bony appearance, with deepening of intercostal and supraclavicular spaces, orbits, and axillae. Skin-fold thickness is significantly reduced in the forearm and on the back of the hands. The loss of subcutaneous fat, responsible for the decrease in skin-fold thickness, causes a decline in the body's natural insulation. This loss makes older adults sensitive to cold and puts them at risk for hypothermia. Many of the lipids are stored in endothelial tissues of arteries, contributing to atherosclerosis.

Bone mass decreases, resulting in a 2-inch loss of height by age 70. The loss in stature is due in part to loss of cartilage and thinning of vertebrae. This change makes long bones seem disproportionately long. Loss of height is as much a result of dehydration of vertebral discs as a loss of bone mass or collapse of the vertebrae. Moreover, the loss of bone mass leaves the older adult susceptible to fractures of the wrist, the hip, and the vertebrae, with all the known physical and psychologic sequelae.

Although the quantity of extracellular fluid remains fairly constant, intracellular volume is decreased, resulting in less overall total body fluid. This change puts the older adult at risk for dehydration and may increase sensitivity to drugs affecting fluid and electrolyte balance.

As with cells and tissues, there is a decrease in the functional capacity of body organs. Physiologic reserves display a linear decline beginning at age 30, especially in cardiac, respiratory, and renal function. As a result, maintenance of homeostasis becomes increasingly difficult. Although changes in these organ systems occur gradually over a long period and are generally insignificant, moderate or severe stressors can precipitate unexpected problems or organ failure.

CARDIOVASCULAR SYSTEM

The efficiency and contractile strength of the myocardium declines with aging, resulting in a 1% per year reduction in cardiac output. Stroke volume decreases by 0.7% yearly. The systolic and diastolic phases of the myocardial cycle are prolonged. Ordinarily, older adults adjust to these changes without much difficulty; however, when unusual demands are placed on the heart (e.g., shoveling snow, running to catch a bus, or having, in general, the effects of a history of coronary artery disease), the changes become more evident. Pulse rates may not reach the levels of younger persons, and tachycardia lasts longer. There is some disagreement among health care providers as to when an elevation in blood pressure becomes hypertension. In some older adults, the blood pressure may remain stable, but tachycardia progresses to heart failure.

Resistance to peripheral blood flow increases by 1% each year. Reduced elasticity of the arteries is responsible for vascular changes to the heart, the kidneys, and the pituitary gland. The rigidity of vessel walls and narrowing of lumens make more force necessary to move blood through the vessels. These changes lead to a higher diastolic blood pressure. There is also a decrease in the ability of the aorta to distend which, in turn, causes a rise in systolic pressure. Vagal tone increases, and the heart becomes more sensitive to carotid sinus stimulation. Reduced sensitivity of the baroreceptors potentiates orthostatic hypotension. The normal changes of aging do not ordinarily influence venous circulation.

RESPIRATORY SYSTEM

Various structural changes in the chest diminish respiratory functioning. In addition, there are reductions in the number of alveoli, diffusion capacity, and elastic recoil of the lungs during expiration. Vital capacity is decreased, but residual volume increases approximately 40% by age 85; thus more energy is required to achieve full respiratory capacity. A slight fall in arterial oxyhemoglobin saturation occurs, and cough efficiency is reduced. With less effective gas exchange and a lack of bibasilar inflation, the older adult is at risk for atelectasis and pulmonary infections.

GASTROINTESTINAL SYSTEM

The gastrointestinal system is altered by the aging process in a number of ways. Natural dentition is usually retained, primarily owing to an increased awareness of, and adherence to, recommended dental hygiene practices. Teeth are meant to last a lifetime; tooth loss is not a normal outcome of growing older but results from poor dental care, diet, and environmental influences. Periodontal disease is the major cause of tooth loss after age 30. Decreased activity of the salivary gland and drier mucous membranes contribute to difficulty swallowing. Lowered esophageal motility and relaxation of the lower esophageal sphincter may occur. Aspiration becomes a risk when these factors combine with a weaker gag reflex and delayed esophageal emptying.

By age 70, the gastric mucosa atrophies, increasing the risk of irritation and ulceration. Mucosal atrophy is thought to be due to changes in the ratio of gastrin-secreting and somatostatin-secreting cells. Somatostatin is a hormone that inhibits gastrin secretion. This change in ratio leads to a diminished ability to secrete hydrochloric acid (i.e., hypochlorhydria). The severity of hypochlorhydria is directly correlated with the extent of atrophy.

Many digestive problems are related to an increased gastric pH and to reduced amounts of hydrochloric acid, pepsin, lipase, and pancreatic enzymes. The pancreas produces normal amounts of bicarbonate, amylase, and trypsin, but there is a decrease in lipase, resulting in subclinical abnormalities in fat absorption. Lowered fat absorption reduces the absorption of fat-soluble vitamins. There is also faulty absorption of vitamins B_1 and B_{12}, calcium, and iron.

Liver cells change in size and character, and hepatic blood flow is decreased. Hepatic protein synthesis is compromised, and there are changes in the microsomal enzyme systems involved in a variety of metabolic pathways.

Intestinal blood flow is decreased, so the absorption of substances actively transported from the intestinal lumen (e.g., some sugars, minerals, and vitamins) may be reduced. The intestinal mucosa atrophies, decreasing its surface area, and the intestinal musculature weakens. Peristalsis is slower, and this may contribute to constipation, particularly when combined with dehydration or decreased oral intake. There are also changes in the integrity of intestinal membranes, and transmembrane shift is a mechanism of aging that can contribute to infection.

RENAL SYSTEM

The creatinine clearance declines approximately 10% each decade after age 40. There is a possibility of protein loss because of decreased cardiac output, subsequently reduced renal blood flow, and lower glomerular filtration rates. Tubular reabsorption is decreased, and a lower threshold for glucose and creatinine clearance develops. As a result, the kidneys are less effective in concentrating urine. At younger ages, the urinary specific gravity is about 1.032, but at age 80, it may be 1.024 (normal range: 1.010 to 1.020). Blood urea nitrogen levels may reach a value of 21.2 mg/dL at age 70 (normal range for persons older than 60 years is 8 to 20 mg/dL).

Urinary frequency and urgency as well as nocturia result in smaller bladder capacities. Nocturia is a consequence of the difficulty in concentrating urine. Although urine leakage is not a normal change of aging, some stress incontinence is common in women because of a weakening of pelvic musculature, particularly in multiparous women, and the decline in estrogen levels with menopause.

Prostatic enlargement occurs in many older men. Approximately 75% of men older than 65 years experience some degree of prostatism, which contributes to urinary frequency. Prostatic enlargement does not always imply a cancerous process.

SENSORY-PERCEPTUAL FUNCTION

The eyes of an older adult reflect a variety of changes that affect functional capacity as well as the ability to protect the self from hazards and to enjoy a high quality of life. The aging eye loses the ability to accommodate and focus for near vision (presbyopia). As a result, many persons older than 40 years require corrective lenses. Lens opacity may develop and is accompanied by a decreased tolerance for glare. A gradual narrowing of the visual field occurs.

Yellowing of the lens and altered color perception make the older adult less able to differentiate the low tone colors of the blues, the greens, and the violets. Depth perception changes, causing problems in judging the height of steps or curbs. Bifocals compound this problem. Adaptation to light and dark takes longer. Sclerosis of the pupillary sphincter and a decrease in pupil size make the pupil less responsive

to light. Further, reabsorption of intraocular fluid is less efficient, increasing the risk for glaucoma. Reduced tear production leads to less lustrous eyes and complaints of dry eyes.

Deterioration of the cochlea and neurons of the higher auditory pathways leads to sensorineural hearing loss (presbycusis), although overall it depends on lifetime noise exposure. Perception of high-pitched sounds such as s, sh, f, ch, and ph is initially impaired, followed by that of the middle and the low frequencies. The change is so gradual and subtle that affected persons may not realize the magnitude of the hearing loss. Stiffening of the cilia combined with the higher keratin content of cerumen causes ear wax to become easily impacted, further decreasing hearing. Presbycusis is typically greater in men than women.

There is some reduction in olfactory senses as sensory cells in the nasal lining decrease in number. The nasal mucosa becomes less moist. A reduction in the number of taste buds alters taste sensations, especially to sweet and salty flavors.

Tactile sensation is reduced, evidenced in the older adult as diminished ability to sense pressure and pain and to differentiate temperatures. The sensory changes can cause faulty interpretation of the environment and increase the risk of harm.

NEUROMUSCULAR SYSTEM

Over the years, the bulk, the strength, and the number of muscle fibers decline. Cartilage decreases, contributing to some discomfort with joint mobility and shortening of the vertebral column. Deep tendon reflexes are sluggish. Muscles become more rigid and easily fatigued. Resting tremors may be present in some people. Bone mass and strength are reduced. Some older adults are at risk for fracture following minimal trauma as a result of physiologic changes in bone integrity or osteoporosis. Bones fracture with less stress than in younger persons. Cartilage decreases, contributing to some discomfort with joint mobility and shortening of the vertebral column.

Beginning around age 30 there is a loss of bone mass in women and men. The average mature woman has 10% to 25% less total bone mass than her male counterpart. Loss of bone mass accelerates considerably following menopause. Annually, women lose as much as 3% of bone mass unless they are on hormone replacement therapy (HRT).

It is difficult to determine with accuracy the impact of aging on the nervous system, because of the system's interdependence with other body systems. Reductions in the total number of nerve cells, cerebral blood flow, and metabolism are seen. Nerve conduction velocity is slowed, leading to slower reflexes and delayed response to multiple stimuli. Kinesthetic sense lessens. Changes in the sleep pattern occur, with stages III and IV of sleep becoming less prominent. The average sleeping time shortens only a minimal amount, although frequent awakening during sleep is common. Many older adults are not aware that sleep changes with aging and will report sleep changes that may not be clinically relevant, or they may self-treat in an attempt to mimic sleep patterns from when they were younger.

ENDOCRINE SYSTEM

The pituitary gland shrinks by 20%, with variable decreases in adrenocorticotropic hormone (ACTH), thyroid-stimulating hormone (TSH), follicle-stimulating hormone (FSH), luteinizing hormone (LH), and luteotrophic hormones. Gonadal secretion declines with age, including gradual decreases in testosterone, estrogen, and progesterone. With the exception of changes in plasma calcium levels or dysfunction of other glands, the parathyroid glands maintain their function throughout life.

With aging, a reduction in T_4 secretion is balanced by a decrease in T_4 clearance, resulting in unchanged circulating T_4 levels. Triiodothyronine (T_3) levels are unchanged until extreme old age, when they decrease slightly. However, T_3 levels are commonly reduced in the setting of illnesses other than those that are thyroid-related because of decreased T_4-to-T_3 conversion. TSH levels are unchanged or minimally changed in healthy older adults. Any decrease in activity reduces the basal metabolic rate, with less thyrotropin secretion and release. Any loss of adrenal function further lowers thyroid activity.

Secretory activity of adrenal glands also decreases. Less aldosterone is produced and excreted in the urine. The secretion of glucocorticoids, 17-ketosteroids, progesterone, androgens, and estrogen, also influenced by the adrenal gland, diminishes. There is insufficient release of insulin by beta cells of the pancreas and reduced sensitivity of insulin receptors, contributing to elevations in blood glucose levels in some patients. Smaller quantities of insulin may make it difficult to maintain a euglycemic state, and prolonged periods of hyperglycemia may occur. Therefore it is not unusual to detect higher blood glucose levels in nondiabetic older adults.

IMMUNE SYSTEM

Serum activity of thymic hormones is almost undetectable in the older adult. A significant decline in cell-mediated immunity occurs, with T cells less able to proliferate in response to antigens. The changes in T cells contribute to a reactivation of varicella-zoster virus (i.e., shingles) and *Mycobacterium tuberculosis* infections. Concentrations of immunoglobulin M (IgM) are lower, whereas those of immunoglobulins A and G (IgA, IgG) are higher. Responses to influenza, parainfluenza, pneumococcus, and tetanus vaccines are less pronounced. Inflammatory defenses decline, and inflammation may be atypical. Older adults do not develop fevers in response to infection as readily as younger individuals.

MENTAL STATUS

The mechanisms involved in plasticity in the nervous system are thought to support cognition, and some of these processes are affected during normal aging. Cognitive functions that rely on the medial temporal lobe and prefrontal cortex, such as learning, memory, and executive function, show considerable age-related decline. More time may be required for older adults to learn new and difficult tasks. It is therefore not surprising that several neural mechanisms in these brain areas also seem to be particularly vulnerable during the aging process.

Long-term memory remains intact. Short-term memory becomes poorer, although there is some controversy as to the extent to which this is true. Altered mental functioning must be evaluated in terms of the older adult's life-long behavioral patterns and potential health problems.

PHARMACOKINETIC CONSIDERATIONS

Older adults respond differently to drug therapy compared to younger adults. Compounding the normal changes of aging on drug action and response are comorbid, chronic disease states (Table 8-2). Drug absorption is the process least affected by physiologic changes of aging. However, age-related changes do have significant implications for changes in drug distribution, biotransformation, and elimination. A summary of the physiologic changes of aging that result in pharmacokinetic alterations is found in Table 8-3.

ABSORPTION

A number of variables affect drug absorption in the older adult. Disorders causing a decreased gastric pH alter the absorption of weak acids and bases. Weak acids (e.g., barbiturates) are more ionized in the gastrointestinal tract and less well absorbed. Weak bases are less ionized and better absorbed. Decreases in gastric motility and in production of trypsin delay or impair drug absorption. Drugs affecting gastric acidity, motility, or trypsin production (e.g., laxatives, antacids, histamine$_2$ antagonists, proton pump inhibitors, anticholinergics, levodopa) can affect the absorption of other drugs. Antacids and other products containing divalent cations as well as bile acid sequestrants are well recognized to decrease absorption of some drugs and nutritional agents. Pain, mucosal edema or stomatitis, diabetes mellitus, and hypokalemia have also been shown to decrease drug absorption.

The age-related decline in cardiac output reduces the perfusion of the gastrointestinal tract by 40% to 50%. Blood flow to the gastrointestinal tract may be altered to maintain coronary and cerebral blood flow. The result is delayed, less thorough absorption, and less reliable removal of drugs and other substances from the intestinal lumen. In turn, however, exercise stimulates circulation and increases drug absorption. Prevention of dehydration, hypothermia, and hypotension promotes drug absorption.

DISTRIBUTION

A small subset of frail older adults experience changes in biotransformation. This population of older adults may not be identified in drug studies of healthy older adults.

TABLE 8-2 Rates of Chronic Illness in Adults*

Illness or Condition	Males and Females Age (yr)			
	18–44	45–64	65–74	>75
Arthritis	61.9	477	1395.2	1014.3
Hypertension	60.1	428.1	704.1	708
Hearing impairments	60.4	266.3	527.1	773.4
Heart conditions	66.2	233.8	480.5	653.5
Visual impairments	33.9	97.4	143.2	216.5
Orthopedic problems	167.7	356.1	348.3	270.4
Diabetes mellitus	15.1	116.3	200.5	214.8

*By age per 1000 male and female population (1996). Covers civilian, noninstitutional population. Adapted from the U.S. National Center for Health Statistics. Vital and Health Statistics. *Statistical Abstract of the US. (2000).* Washington, DC: Bureau of the Census. Conditions classified according to ninth revision of International Classification of Diseases. Based on National Health Interview Survey.

TABLE 8-3 Changes of Aging and Therapeutics

Normal Physiologic Changes	Pharmacotherapeutic Concerns
Reduced long-term and short-term memory in some patients	Higher risk of unintentional nonadherence
Reduced visual acuity	Higher risk of administration errors due to poor vision
Diminished cardiac output and blood flow to organs and tissues	Decreased drug biotransformation and elimination, resulting in longer circulation time
	Potentially decreased absorption of orally administered drugs
	Vaginal and rectal suppositories take longer to dissolve and may be prematurely expelled.
	Decreased biotransformation or elimination of drugs
Altered peripheral vascular tone and reduced baroreceptor activity	Exaggerated effects of antihypertensives and diuretics
Decreased hepatic blood flow and liver mass	Altered biotransformation and detoxification processes; biotransformation time is lengthened, and
Decreased enzymatic activity in liver	both parent drug and active metabolites exert effects for extended periods. Drug toxicity may occur more readily.
Reduced serum albumin	Less availability of albumin for binding; amounts of unbound drug and drug activity both increase
Decreased lean body mass; increased total body fat; decreased total body water	Altered distribution and higher concentration of fat-soluble drugs in adipose tissue; some drugs reach greater peak concentrations with longer half-lives.
	Drier mucous membranes may cause drugs to stick to the oral cavity and cause irritation.
Decreases in tissue elasticity and muscle mass	Poor absorption of drugs with poor sealing of tissues after injection
Higher gastric pH but reduced gastric acid; delayed gastric emptying	Decreased absorption of drugs normally nonionized at low pH (weak acids and bases)
Changes in sensitivity of receptor sites	Increase or decrease in drug activity

Drug distribution and equilibration rates are affected by changes of aging that alter protein binding, volume of distribution, amount of body fat present, and regional perfusion patterns.

Perhaps the most significant factor affecting drug distribution and equilibration is size: older patients are typically smaller than younger patients. An older patient who receives the same dosage as a younger patient has a higher concentration of the drug in the blood because of the older patient's smaller volume.

Total body mass decreases with age along with declines in body water. Total body weight decreases, especially in the "old-old" (older than 75 years), but the ratio of fat to lean body mass is usually greater. Changes in adipose tissue raise tissue drug concentrations and the duration of drug action while lowering plasma concentrations. For example, a highly fat-soluble drug (e.g., diazepam) has a greater volume of distribution and a prolonged distribution phase, leading to an extended half-life. On the other hand, highly water-soluble drugs (e.g., gentamicin) have a smaller volume of distribution. Lowered cardiac output leads to elevated plasma concentrations with less deposition in reservoirs. Older adults are thus at higher risk of drug toxicity; therefore, when treating this population, select drugs with shorter half-lives or extend the interval between doses.

Reduced plasma protein levels can result in higher concentrations of unbound drug, especially when the drug competes with other protein-bound drugs. As a result, more unbound drug circulates, increasing the action of highly protein-bound drugs, but this effect is not always predictable. Moreover, as the amount of unbound drug rises, so does the amount of drug available for biotransformation and elimination. For example, the attraction between albumin and warfarin sodium (an oral anticoagulant) is strong, causing nearly all (99%) of the warfarin in plasma to be bound and leaving only 1% free. Box 8-1 contains a partial listing of these compounds. States of dehydration and hypoalbuminemia require lower dosage levels.

BIOTRANSFORMATION

With aging comes a decrease in hepatic blood flow and, in turn, reduced delivery of drugs for biotransformation.

BOX 8-1

Examples of Highly Protein-Bound Drugs

Acetazolamide	Nortriptyline
Amitriptyline	Phenylbutazone
Cefazolin	Phenytoin
Chlordiazepoxide	Propranolol
Chlorpromazine	Rifampin
Cloxacillin	Salicylates
Digoxin	Spironolactone
Furosemide	Sulfisoxazole
Hydralazine	Warfarin

The relationship between aging and CYP450 enzyme function is complex and depends on the type of reaction and the patient's sex. For example, in the case of the lipid-lowering drug rosuvastatin, the Food and Drug Administration (FDA) requires labeling indicating that drug levels are higher in persons of Asian ethnicity, although a recently published meta-analysis of trials submitted to the FDA found no differences in clinical adverse events according to ethnicity, sex, or age. Oxidative capacity (phase 1) declines with age, with the decline thought to be greater in men than in women. The rate of hepatic conjugation (phase 2) is unaffected by age. However, the effect of aging on oxidation is consistent for drugs with low hepatic extraction rates. Data are less clear about drugs with high extraction ratios, because their rate of biotransformation depends on hepatic blood flow in addition to enzyme activity.

Conditions such as dehydration, hyperthermia, immobility, and liver disease diminish the biotransformation of drugs. As a consequence, the biologic half-life of many drugs is extended, and accumulation and toxicity is a potential problem. Drugs such as morphine, meperidine, propoxyphene, propranolol, lidocaine, warfarin, and benzodiazepines have extended half-lives. Drugs that are normally subject to a considerable first-pass effect (e.g., propranolol) are especially likely to produce exaggerated effects in older adults (see Chapter 4). In addition, patients with chronic medical illness may be treated with a variety of drugs or dietary supplements that can alter the biotransformation or clearance of other agents.

ELIMINATION

The kidneys are primarily responsible for elimination of most drugs. Drugs follow a path through the kidneys similar to that of most constituents of urine. However, with aging the number of functional nephrons falls by as much as 64%, and the glomerular filtration rate (GFR) may fall by nearly 50%. At age 30, the GFR is approximately 140 mL/min/1.73 m^2. The decline continues at an average rate of 8 mL/min/1.73 m^2 every decade. The normal age-related decline in GFR is not reflected in the serum creatinine because of the comparable loss in muscle mass, which lowers the production of creatinine (Evidence-Based Pharmacotherapeutics box). This means that an older patient may not demonstrate high serum creatinine levels until the dysfunction is severe. The change is accompanied by a similar decrease in renal blood flow. Tubular secretory mechanisms and the ability to concentrate urine are diminished. In addition, cardiovascular disease, dehydration, and kidney disease commonly impair renal functioning. Thus the half-life of a drug may be increased by as much as 40%. Because drugs remain in the body longer, adverse and toxic effects are possible. Declines in renal function may be exaggerated by comorbid illness such as chronic hypertension and anemia, which have close associations with chronic kidney disease.

PHARMACODYNAMIC CONSIDERATIONS

The changes of aging are related more to accumulation of pigments and alterations in metabolic processes than to the unresponsiveness of cell receptors. They can be caused by aging organ systems and their role in drug-receptor or drug-organ interactions. Aging reduces tissue responsiveness to drugs in a number of ways. Drug receptor response can be altered because the functional capacity of organs and thus the total number of receptors decline with age, causing any adverse effects to be felt more keenly. The effects of drugs that thwart liver, kidney, or cardiac function may go unnoticed in younger persons but are dangerous to the older adult. In addition, the vitality of control mechanisms is reduced, the maintenance of homeostasis less dynamic, and compensatory responses to primary drug effects less profound. For example, drugs that raise blood pressure often do so in a more profound manner, because the vagal reflex is less efficient in generating a compensatory reduction in cardiac output.

Cardiac glycosides (see Chapter 34) are well known for their narrow therapeutic index in all patients, but older adults are particularly prone to toxicities. Older adults also exhibit reduced pharmacodynamic responsiveness to quinidine but a greater sensitivity to lidocaine. Vascular responses to norepinephrine and cardiac response to isoproterenol and other catecholamines is somewhat diminished (see Chapter 14).

 EVIDENCE-BASED PHARMACOTHERAPEUTICS

Estimating Glomerular Filtration Rate

■ **Background**

Creatinine clearance (CrCl) is a commonly used tool to measure glomerular filtration rate (GFR), but large-scale community-based studies evaluating the prevalence of decreased kidney function in older adults are scarce. Furthermore, there is no marker for GFR ideal for clinical purposes, and the limitations of the currently used tests are magnified in older adults. Serum creatinine levels may be misleading in the older adult, who may have severely compromised renal function despite a serum creatinine level within the normal range.

■ **Research Article**

Wasen, E., Isoaho, R., Matilla, K. (2004). Estimation of glomerular filtration rate in the elderly: A comparison of creatinine-based formulae with serum cystatin C. *Journal of Internal Medicine, 256*(1), 70–78.

Purpose

To estimate the prevalence of decreased kidney function in population of older adults and to evaluate the impact of using alternative markers of GFR, focusing on serum cystatin C and the Modification of Diet in Renal Disease (MDRD) study prediction equation.

Design

Cross-sectional community-based survey of 1246 older adults in Finland, ages 64–100, with a mean age of 74.

Methods

Serum creatinine, cystatin C, and predicted GFR (GFR$_{pred}$) using the Cockcroft-Gault (CG) equation and the MDRD study formula were used to analyze kidney function. Correlations were calculated using Pearson r coefficients, and MDRD, CG, and CG–body surface area (BSA) estimates were compared using a paired t-test. Multivariate linear models were used to assess associations of age, sex, and proteinuria with cystatin C, serum creatinine, and GFR estimates included as continuous dependent variables. Box-and-whisker plots were used to show distribution of markers of renal function across subgroups based on age and health status.

Findings

The Cockcroft-Gault equation yielded 58.6% while the incidence of moderate or severely decreased renal function (as estimated by the MDRD) was 35.7%. Compared with the MDRD, the serum creatinine value, or the estimated GFR from the Cockcroft-Gault equation, the cystatin C measurement showed a greater similarity, including variations across age groups and health status.

Conclusion

The incidence of decreased renal function in older adults varies considerably depending on the formula used. Differences in the metabolism of creatinine among older adults with comorbid conditions and a reliance on the exact calculation of serum creatinine values leave the use of creatinine-based formulae to predict GFR open to discussion. In this setting, cystatin C is a promising alternative.

■ **Implications for Practice**

Regardless of which prediction equation was used, the proportion of normal kidney function in an older adult was small, and the proportion of mildly decreased kidney function was substantial. To what extent mildly reduced kidney function represents pathology, and to what extent normal aging, is unclear.

Therefore, interpret serum creatinine, MDRD formulae, and Cockcroft-Gault equation results cautiously, until longitudinal studies employing different laboratory techniques are done.

Controversy

Drugs and Driving?

Jonathan J. Wolfe

Drug therapy of behavioral disorders opens many doors, particularly for the older adult. It is no longer necessary to accept endogenous depression, panic disorder, or phantom voices as necessary accompaniments to the aging process. The crude chemical straitjackets associated with the early psychotropic drugs are no longer satisfactory. The relatively low cost of phenothiazines, for example, is not a proper argument against the use of more expensive drugs, which enhance the ability to live autonomously.

Operating a motor vehicle is a component of autonomy in most parts of America that reduces dependence on others. However, driving may well be considered separately from activities of daily living that relate to personal care.

Concerns about the older adult's driving may be grouped around two issues. The first, independent of issues of drug prescribing and administration, is a patient's maintenance of the skills and knowledge to safely operate an automobile. No one would argue that the patient whose vision is severely diminished or motor functions importantly impaired has a right to drive that outweighs the risk it may pose to others. The other focus of concern is impairment of driving ability when drugs are used that suppress central nervous system function.

In many cases involving drug therapy, restriction of driving is temporary. When a drug is first introduced into the treatment plan or doses are increased, the patient may experience somnolence, dizziness, or disorientation incompatible with safe driving. Once the sensorium adjusts to higher doses, driving may be appropriate. Permanent loss of driving privileges represents a graver choice. It is, however, necessary for the patient whose skills remain impaired or who requires indefinite use of a centrally acting drug.

CLINICAL REASONING

- Think about your experience as a new driver. Having the car keys opened many opportunities. It also released you from direct parental scrutiny when you were driving alone. What three activities in your daily life would you lose without access to a vehicle?
- Reflect privately on one activity in your adult life that you reluctantly would give up rather than explain or reveal to your family that you could no longer drive.
- What counseling is appropriate for a 72-year-old patient in otherwise good health who is to begin treatment of his anxiety disorder with a short-acting benzodiazepine?
- What is an appropriate response to a concerned adult child who reports that her 85-year-old mother experiences severe postural hypotension from her antihypertensive drug regimen, yet continues to drive on the interstate highway?
- You are asked to present a 30-minute educational program to your state's highway patrol officers. They want you to talk about prescription drugs and driving impairment. What three topics will you discuss?

Orthostatic hypotension caused by antidepressants (see Chapter 20), antipsychotic drugs (see Chapter 21), and antihypertensive drugs (see Chapter 37) is more common in older adults who are volume depleted secondary to diuretic therapy (see Chapter 41). In addition, potassium-wasting diuretics such as furosemide can cause hypokalemia, which potentiates the effects of cardiac glycosides. The incidence of hyperkalemia in older patients taking potassium-sparing diuretics (e.g., spironolactone or eplerenone) is higher, possibly because renal function is impaired. Another example is that of the drugs that inhibit angiotensin-converting enzyme (ACE); hypotension is aggravated in the presence of dehydration.

In the autonomic nervous system, β-adrenergic receptor responses to both agonists and antagonists appear to be blunted. As a result, older adults show diminished response to drugs and increased toxicity to beta blockers. Aging causes a decline in parasympathetic control, which enhances the effects of anticholinergic drugs (see Chapter 15). It also reduces the amounts of neurotransmitters, particularly dopamine and acetylcholine. Reduced dopamine in the brain increases the older adult's risk for the extrapyramidal effects of neuroleptics, metoclopramide, and other drugs.

Central nervous system effects of sedative-hypnotics and antianxiety drugs include paradoxical responses, characterized by restlessness, disorientation, and confusion (see the Controversy box). Dizziness and vertigo are also of concern, in that they often lead to falls and subsequent injury. In contrast, the effects of stimulants such as amphetamines on motor activity are less in the older adult, but their anorexic effects are enhanced.

Several endocrine changes influence drug response. For example, age-related declines in glucose tolerance cause more hyperglycemia than normal in response to a thiazide diuretic.

Moreover, because the response to drug-induced hypoglycemia is reduced, older adults do not seek treatment as early as a younger adult would. For example, gatifloxacin (a fluoroquinolone antibiotic) may precipitate severe hyperglycemia in patients without diabetes, especially in older adults, those with renal insufficiency, and those receiving multiple drugs known to alter glucose metabolism. Discontinuation of gatifloxacin treatment improves glucose homeostasis. In addition, diminished thyroid function decreases the metabolic rate, which in turn slows drug biotransformation.

CLINICAL REASONING

Treatment Objectives

The goal of drug therapy in the older adult is to maintain health status using the fewest drugs possible. Individualize drug dosing to decrease the likelihood of nonadherence, adverse drug reactions, or drug interactions. Weigh the purpose of and need for each drug. Consider the possibility of additive adverse effects when formulating management objectives. Question the use of any contraindicated drugs or those that may exacerbate the older adult's concurrent disease states.

Treatment Options

▮ Patient Variables

Polypharmacy with prescription and OTC drugs is the result of the higher incidence of chronic diseases but also of the prescribing behaviors of multiple health care providers and of poorly coordinated patient management. Polypharmacy results in reduced adherence, higher risks for adverse reactions, greater frequencies of drug interactions, and more frequent or extended hospital stays. Ironically, drug reactions that mimic typical complaints of older patients are often treated with yet another drug. Furthermore, excessive drug use by the older adult inadvertently creates an economically, psychologically, and physiologically costly cycle of events. Keeping these factors in mind, patients should be questioned about any current use of prescribed and OTC drugs, home remedies, herbal treatments or dietary supplements, and vitamins. A listing of the names, the strengths, and how the patient uses each drug should be noted. Include as-needed drugs, especially if the patient reports taking them 1 or more times weekly. Identify the prescriber of the drug(s) during the interview, and check the elicited information against prescription labels. Be sure to obtain a thorough drug history, and document drug allergies, including a description of any allergic response, when it occurred, interventions used, and any sequelae.

Request that older adults bring all drugs they are taking to their appointments. Prescription bottles provide additional information, such as the name of the pharmacy that dispensed the drug. Determine the reason for the use of more than one pharmacy. There are many drugs that should be avoided in older adults (Table 8-4). Because the older adult tends to save leftover drugs, note the expiration dates. After obtaining the patient's permission, dispose of expired drugs, since they carry the potential for ineffectiveness or toxicity.

In addition, ask older adults how they remember to take prescribed drugs, whether they ever forget to take a dose, and if so, what they do about it. Have they ever intentionally discontinued a drug, and if so, why? This information helps evaluate a patient's understanding of and adherence with the drug regimen, as well as its safety. Explore the possibility of physical impairments, memory loss, health or cultural beliefs, financial constraints, or lack of support systems that impair safe drug self-administration.

A variety of assessment instruments may also be used to assess functional abilities such as the CADET, a self-care assessment tool. This tool addressed the patient's level of independence as it relates to communication, ambulation, activities of daily living, elimination, and transfer abilities. The Comprehensive Older Person's Evaluation (COPE) instrument, similar to the CADET, uses categories for cognition, social support, financial considerations, physical and psychologic health, and activities of daily living. A number of other instruments are also available to help assess the patient's functional status. These assessments are vital, particularly for older adults who are living alone or who have multiple limitations; remember, however, that not all older adults are in need of supervision.

Although variations exist, the typical older adult has at least one serious illness or limiting condition and is aware of the increasing frequency of death among his or her peers. These issues, coupled with society's generally negative view of aging, lead to a fear that the person has lost all that remains of youth. The task is not so much to look for new forms of youthfulness but to seek out the meaning of life and the purpose for the

TABLE 8-4 Drugs to be Avoided in Older Adults

Drug	Reasons for Avoiding Use	Type of Support	Comments
Anticholinergics	Arrhythmias, dry mouth and eyes, urinary retention	CS; CT	Avoid if possible
Antihistamines (first-generation)	Sedation, falls, impaired driving	CS, CT	Safer alternatives available
Antipsychotics (first- and second-generation)	Anticholinergic effects, extrapyramidal effects, tardive dyskinesia	CS; CT	Better alternatives available with newer drugs
Barbiturates	Respiratory depression, habituation, falls and hip fractures	CS; CT	Better, safer alternatives available
Benzodiazepines (long-acting)	Falls and hip fractures	CS; CT	Safer alternatives available with shorter duration of action
chlorpropamide (Diabinese)	Overly long action resulting in hypoglycemia	CR	Large CRTs confirm other favorable choices
digoxin (Lanoxin)	Daily doses over 0.125 mg for heart failure have more risk than benefit	HF: small to multicenter CRTs; atrial fibrillation: CRTs show some benefit	Benefits in heart failure and atrial fibrillation; vigilance with clearance and dosing is necessary. Alternatives available for atrial fibrillation
disopyramide (Norpace)	Negative inotrope; high risk for inducing heart failure. Anticholinergic adverse effects	CS, CRTs with other drugs had fewer adverse effects	Other drugs less problematic
dipyridamole (Persantine)	Orthostatic hypotension	CS; case series; some CRTs showed lack of notable hypotension	Newer CRTs for stroke prevention more recent than criteria
meperidine (Demerol)	CNS impairment; toxic metabolite accumulation	CR	Oral meperidine has poor, irregular absorption
meprobamate (Equanil)	Respiratory depression, falls and/or hip fractures, tolerance	CS	Safer alternatives available
pentazocine (Talwin)	CNS impairment; hallucinations	CR; small trials were negative	Avoid high dosages or prolonged use
propoxyphene (Darvon)	CNS impairment with associated fall risk	CR; small and large CRTs	More risk identified, comparative analgesic potency weak
TCAs	Anticholinergic, cardiac toxicity, orthostatic hypotension	CS; CT	Low dose for neuropathic pain is appropriate
trimethobenzamide (Tigan)	Lower potency, extrapyramidal adverse effects	CS; case series; older RT showed efficacy	Very little evidence; other available drugs may be more effective.

CR, Case reports; *CS,* case studies; *CT,* controlled trials; *CRTs,* controlled randomized trials; *HF,* heart failure; *TCAs,* tricyclic antidepressants.
Adapted from: Chutka, D., Takahashi, P., and Hoel, R. (2004). Inappropriate medications for elderly patients. *Mayo Clinic Proceedings, 79*(1), 122–139, with permission.

person's own existence, and adjust to the inevitability of death. The majority of older adults have a calm demeanor and self-assurance and provide satisfying answers to questions. The health care provider must be alert for the occasional person who sounds hopeless and despairing about life at present and in the future. Requests for antianxiety drugs or sedative-hypnotics may help identify the person who has difficulty coping.

Commercial medicine boxes are available that help organize the drugs and allow the patient and caregiver to check if a dose has been taken (see Figure 9–3, p. 113). A labeled egg carton or muffin tin also serves the same compartmentalizing purpose, at much lower cost. Some pharmacists will also make blister packs for patients' monthly drugs.

▥ Drug Variables

Prescribing drugs for an older adult is complex and involves numerous considerations. There are seven basic principles for safe prescribing:
- Start low and go slow.
- Start one (drug), and stop two (if possible).
- Use a drug interactions database to identify possible problems.
- Do not use a drug if the adverse effects are worse than the disease.

- Use as few drugs as possible, choosing non–drug therapies when possible.
- Assess the patient's response frequently.
- Consider drug holidays from time to time.

Ideally, drug regimens are kept simple, with the least frequent administration schedule used. Keeping the number of drugs to a minimum reduces the potential for drug interactions and improves the patient's ability to comply with the drug regimen. Table 8-5 identifies strategies for improving adherence.

Although still somewhat controversial, "drug holidays" may also be considered from time to time. Drug holidays reduce the likelihood that drugs will accumulate to toxic levels, increase mental alertness (in some cases), and provide a cost savings. However, the use of drug holidays requires interdisciplinary support and planning, and thorough assessment of the appropriateness of this strategy. Drugs not usually included in a drug holiday are antibiotics, anticoagulants, anticonvulsants, antidiabetic drugs, and ophthalmic drugs. The health care provider may have overlooked this option and may need to be reminded of the length of time the patient has been using the drug.

Patient Education

Determine the older adult's understanding of the prescribed therapy, and provide the requisite teaching. It is thought that

TABLE 8-5 Strategies for Reducing Nonadherence

Etiology	Possible Solution(s)
Inability to pay for prescribed drugs	• Consider cost of drugs when choosing therapy; use generic when possible. • Minimize number of drugs prescribed; avoid polypharmacy. • Use therapeutic alternatives when possible. • Refer patient to appropriate agency for financial assistance.
Lack of transportation to obtain drugs	• Refer patient to appropriate agency for assistance. • Explore pharmacy delivery or mail-away prescription services.
Forgetfulness	• Advise patient to bring all drugs (prescription and OTC) to each appointment. • Choose a drug with fewest required doses per day. • Use calendars, diaries, drug planners, or dosage containers. • Review drug treatment regimens with family, friends, neighbors, home care personnel.
Confusion surrounding disease, multidrug regimen, or directions or instructions	• Review risks and benefits of adding a drug. • Explore non–drug therapies when appropriate. • Review drugs added by other health care providers; communicate changes in therapy. Provide a portable prescription record that can be taken to other health care providers and pharmacists. • Simplify drug regimen, directions, and instructions; use both generic and brand names on instructions. • Make sure prescriptions are clearly labeled. • Provide written as well as verbal instructions. • Color-code bottles. Use large print materials as needed.
Unable to tolerate adverse effects of drugs	• Adhere to the principles: "Start low and go slow," and "Start one, and stop two," if possible • Closely monitor patient condition. Consider possibility that any new symptoms could represent adverse drug reactions or drug withdrawal. • Consider changing to another drug, or reducing dosage or frequency of administration.
Interference with prescribed drug regimen because of use of self-treatment strategies	• Reassess preferred treatment strategies. • Educate the patient. • Provide large-print handouts to take home.
Overdosing, underdosing, or misusing drug based on perception of need for drug	• Educate patient. • Provide large-print handouts to take home. • Closely monitor patient profile during visits.
Expiration or refilling of prescription or supplies before follow-up	• Closely monitor patient profile. Consider a single appropriate refill (i.e., 30 days) until the patient can get in for an appointment with the health care provider.
Multiple comorbid conditions or fatigue	• Schedule routine follow-up appointments to reevaluate patient condition. • Choose one drug that treats two comorbid conditions, when possible. • Schedule regular blood tests to monitor patient response to diuretics, ACE inhibitors, antiepileptic drugs, anticoagulants, antiarrhythmics, and digoxin. • Stay informed about pharmaceutical innovations (novel new drugs, new diagnostics for predicting drug response, etc.) relevant to disease of older adults.

ACE, Angiotensin-converting enzyme; *OTC,* over-the-counter.

there is no loss of knowledge and little or no loss of vocabulary with aging, although response time is slower than in younger persons. Slower responses may affect new learning. The teaching guidelines in Box 8-2, applicable to all people receiving drug therapy, are particularly useful with the aging population.

Review all drugs with the patient or the family and caregiver, clarifying information as needed. In some cases, complex drug regimens can be simplified by discussing the possible alterations with the health care provider. A homebound, confused, or isolated older adult is less likely to follow a drug regimen properly. The functional assessment obtained during the history and physical exam helps determine whether the older adult needs an adherence aid or a memory cue to take the drugs. In addition, the health care provider should determine whether a family member or a caregiver is available or, if the older adult lives alone, whether it is necessary to locate one. Further, the ability of the patient to obtain necessary drugs should be facilitated when necessary. If the patient is essentially homebound, the use of a pharmacy that delivers can be helpful. Referral to a social worker may be necessary to obtain financial or other forms of assistance.

Many older adults stockpile drugs, and not always in the original containers. Some contain the same drug, differing only in brand or generic name. Others place a current prescription or an OTC drug in a labeled prescription bottle meant for another drug. In addition, the stockpile may contain prescription bottles for family members. Keep in mind that the patient may be sharing drugs with others, or may have received a drug from someone who believed that because it helped him or her, it would also help the patient. Explain to the patient why you are asking questions about the drugs he or she is using. Explanations help alleviate the fear, anger, and resistance that might appear if the patient were questioned without explanation. For the hearing-impaired patient who has good visual acuity, a written explanation may help improve understanding and increase cooperation. An interpreter trained in sign language should be available to the patient as well as the health care provider.

Evaluation

Evaluation involves looking at the overall drug regimen and answering the following questions:

- Were there any recent drug changes? Why were they made?
- Are acute or chronic symptoms improving, or are there new symptoms? Could the symptoms possibly be adverse drug reactions?
- Is the older adult concurrently using other prescription or non–prescription drugs, home remedies, or street drugs?

BOX 8-2

Teaching Guidelines for Older Adults

Do the following for *each* drug taken:

I. Provide both generic and brand names.

II. Explain the purpose for the drug, what it does, and the reason it is prescribed.

III. Describe the color, size, and shape of the dosage form (e.g., tablet, capsule, liquid).

IV. Identify the route of administration (by mouth, inhalation, topical, etc.).

V. Identify the dosing schedule: Consider the following factors:

    A. Patient's activities of daily living schedule (e.g., eating, sleeping, activities)

        i. Specify times of day and associated meals or activities. For example: "Take one tablet at 7 AM when you get up, one at noon with lunch, and one at 5 PM with your dinner."

        ii. Do not assume the number of meals, time of meals, or hours of sleeping.

    B. Should the drug be taken on an empty stomach or with meals?

    C. Can the drug be taken at the same time as other drugs?

    D. Are there any restrictions on alcohol consumption while taking the drug?

    E. If the drug is prescribed on an as-needed basis, how often can it be taken? What signs or symptoms should the patient use to decide whether it can or should be taken?

    F. Indicate what to do if a dose is missed. Should the dose be skipped? Should two doses be taken at the same time?

    G. When the dosage is to be changed after a time, be specific about the instructions. For example, rather than telling the patient, "Take one tablet each day for the next 3 days, then increase to two tablets per day," instruct them as follows: "Take one tablet in the morning each day for 3 days, starting tomorrow, Tuesday, January 15. Then increase to one tablet in the morning and one tablet at night, starting Friday, January 18."

VI. Indicate the length of time the drug should be taken (i.e., a short time for an acute problem as opposed to a prolonged time for a chronic one). Indicate whether the new drug is intended to replace one already being taken or is to be added to current drug regimens.

VII. Describe adverse effects in language recognizable to the patient. Point out what actions the patient should take if symptoms arise, and explain the degree of urgency in reporting them.

VIII. Identify special precautions; for example: "Do not take with drug at the same time as or within 2 hours of your antacid."

IX. Does the drug have to be refrigerated? Should it always be left in its original container? Does the drug have an especially short shelf-life? Is it wise for the patient to request a nonchildproof cap for the drug container, or is a childproof cap warranted? What is the procedure for disposing of drugs that are not current or are expired?

X. Provide instructions on how to refill the prescription: Are the number of refills indicated on the container, and if so, where? This is particularly important for hospitalized patients going home. Give instructions in writing, and review them orally with the patient; encourage the patient to call if he or she has any questions.

XI. When and how should the patient follow up with the health care provider?

- Is there information that has not been reported to the health care provider?
- Are costs or the patient's physical limitations a barrier to safe drug use?
- Have plans for follow-up care been outlined and follow-up done as necessary?

Older adults managing drug regimens at home may misuse drugs in more than one way. They may share drugs with friends or family or save the drugs for use in self-treatment in the future. Furthermore, they may not understand the purpose of the drug and, as a result, may increase their risk of taking duplicate drugs; this situation is a consequence not so much of the aging process as of poor prescribing practices. With the growing availability of generic drugs, the prescriber can choose drugs that are of different colors, sizes, and shapes, to help the patient differentiate them. This possibility exists whether the patient uses the same pharmacy each time or has prescriptions filled at multiple pharmacies.

KEY POINTS

- In general, the changes of aging are related more to accumulation of pigments and alterations in metabolic processes than to the unresponsiveness of cell receptors.
- Signs and symptoms of adverse effects may manifest differently in the older adult and may not become apparent for extended periods.
- In most cases, older adults have less difficulty with absorption than with distribution, biotransformation, and elimination.
- The rate of adverse effects is directly proportional to the number of drugs taken.
- Drug-related problems commonly affect the cardiovascular, central nervous, respiratory, renal, gastrointestinal, endocrine, and musculoskeletal systems.
- Polypharmacy is the result of the presence of multiple disease processes, of the prescribing behaviors of the health care providers, and of poorly coordinated patient care management.

- Polypharmacy raises the risks of adverse effects, drug interactions, and extended hospital stays and reduces the level of patient adherence.
- A major cause of patient nonadherence is lack of understanding of the drug regimen. Cost, memory deficits, physical limitations, and scheduling difficulties also contribute to nonadherence.
- Frequent changing of prescriptions is a common factor in patients' misunderstanding the drug regimen.
- The goal of drug therapy is to maintain the patient on the fewest drugs possible and at an optimal dosage that decreases the likelihood of nonadherence, adverse drug reactions, or drug interactions.
- Prescribing drugs for an older adult involves six basic principles: (1) start low and go slow; (2) start one (drug), and stop two, if possible; (3) do not use a drug if the adverse effects are worse than the disease; (4) use as few drugs as possible using non–drug therapies when able; (5) assess response frequently; (6) consider drug holidays from time to time; and (7) use a drug interaction database to identify possible drug interactions.

Bibliography

Brager, R., and Sloanad, E. (2005). The spectrum of polypharmacy. *Nurse Practitioner, 30*(6), 44–50.

Bushardt, R., and Jones, K. (2005). Nine key questions to address polypharmacy in the elderly. *Journal of the American Association of Physician Assistants, 18*(5), 32–37.

Chutka, D., Takahashi, P., and Hoel, R. (2004). Inappropriate medications for elderly patients. *Mayo Clinic Proceedings, 79*, 122–139.

Curry, L., Walker, C., Hogstel, M., et al. (2005). Teaching older adults to self-manage medications: Preventing adverse drug reactions. *Journal of Gerontology Nursing, 31*(4), 32–42.

Fick, M., Cooper, J., Wade, W., et al. (2003). Updating the Beers criteria for potentially inappropriate medications use in older adults. *Archives of Internal Medicine, 163*(22), 2716–2724.

Food and Drug Administration Center for Drug Evaluation and Research. (2005). FDA public health advisory for Crestor (rosuvastatin). Available online: www.fda.gov/cder/drug/advisory/crestor. htm. Accessed February 5, 2007.

Fulton, M., and Allen, R., (2005). Polypharmacy in the elderly: A literature review. *Journal of the American Academy of Nurse Practitioners, 17*(4), 123–132.

Goulding, M. (2004). Inappropriate medication prescribing for elderly ambulatory care patients. *Archives of Internal Medicine, 164*(3), 305–312.

Kroenke, L., and Pinholt, E. (1990). Reducing polypharmacy in the elderly: A controlled trial of physician feedback. *Journal of the American Geriatric Society, 38*(1), 31–36.

Linnebur S., O'Connell, M., Wessell, A., et al. (2005). Pharmacy practice, research, education and advocacy for older adults. *Pharmacotherapy, 25*(10), 1396–1430.

Meiner, S. (1997). Polypharmacy in the elderly. *Advances for Nurse Practitioners, 5*(7), 27–34.

Pearlman, R. (1987). Development of a functional assessment questionnaire for geriatric patients: The comprehensive older persons' evaluation (COPE). *Journal of Chronic Disease, 40*(Suppl 1), 85S-94S.

Pollow, R., Stoller, E., Forster, L., et al. (1994). Drug combinations and potential for risk of adverse drug reaction among community-dwelling elderly. *Nursing Research, 43*(1), 44–49.

Rameizl, P. (1983). CADET: A self-care assessment tool. *Geriatric Nursing, 4*(12), 377–378.

Shepherd, J., Hunninghake, D., Stein, E., et al. (2004). Safety of rosuvastatin. *American Journal of Cardiology, 94*(7), 882–888.

Statistical Abstract of the United States (2000). Available online:www. census.gov/prod/www/statistical-abstract-us.html. Accessed February 5, 2007.

Wooten, J., and Galavis, J. (2005). Polypharmacy: Keeping the elderly safe. *RN, 68*(8), 44–50.

9

Over-the-Counter Drugs

Knowledge of pharmacotherapeutics takes on growing importance as health care moves out of the institutional setting and into the community. Increasingly, the health care provider is managing the care of patients who are self-administering drugs while residing at home or in community settings. The role of the health care provider is to promote patients' health and support their self-management by educating them about safe, knowledgable drug use and prescribing safely and knowledgably. Knowledge of the patient's health-illness beliefs and practices, religious influences, educational level, sociocultural variables, level of adherence with treatment plans, and family and community support systems is vital to successful pharmacotherapy. A patient's functioning in areas such as vision influences over-the-counter (OTC) drug safety, as do language abilities, since many non–English-speaking patients are unable to get OTC counseling from pharmacists or to obtain products outside of the pharmacy setting.

CONSUMER BUYING PRACTICES

TRENDS IN OTC USE

There are over 600,000 available OTC products, and they are manufactured by some 12,000 companies (Box 9-1). The number of OTC drugs used has increased exponentially, for a number of reasons. The gradual move of some prescription drugs to OTC status continues to gain momentum, making even more drugs even more available; OTC drugs are easily accessible in a free enterprise system. In addition, patients are increasingly engaged in self-diagnosing and self-treatment as the cost of and accessibility to health care has changed. Health care providers promote this trend by encouraging patients to make informed decisions about health care. Thus non–prescription drugs and medical devices such as contraceptives (gels, foams), dental hygiene preparations, home diagnostic products (e.g., pregnancy testing), and monitoring products (e.g., glucometers) continue to constitute a significant portion of OTC purchases.

Over $15.1 billion was spent on OTC drugs in 2004. Of the total sales, 45% of expenditures were made in pharmacies. The remaining expenditures were made in food stores and discount merchandising outlets. With the sales of OTC drugs increasing approximately 8% to 10% annually, the potential for adverse reactions also rises. Like prescription drugs, OTC drugs contain active and inactive ingredients. Active ingredients are those that produce therapeutic effects (e.g., reduce fever), whereas inactive ingredients have no therapeutic effects (e.g., flavorings, coloring, preservatives). As a general rule, the fewer active ingredients contained in an OTC drug, the fewer the potential problems.

BOX 9-1

OTC Facts and Figures*

U.S. retail sales of OTC drugs in 2004 (excluding Wal-Mart) were $15.1 billion (ACNielsen, 2005).

There are approximately 1000 active ingredients used in the more than 100,000 OTC products available in the marketplace today (CHPA, 2001).

Since 1976, almost 80 ingredients, dosages, or indications have made the "switch" from prescription to OTC status. More than 10 medications were introduced during that time directly to the OTC market without having been prescription-only first (CHPA, 2003).

More than 700 medicine products available over the counter today use ingredients and dosages that were available only by prescription less than 30 years ago (CHPA, 2001).

Global OTC product sales totaled $47 billion worldwide in 2001 (IMS Health, 2002).

Using OTC medications to treat common upper respiratory infections saves the U.S. health care system and economy $4.75 billion each year (Northwestern University, 2004).

Of American consumers, 85% think it is important to have access to OTCs to relieve minor medical problems (American Pharmaceutical Association, 2000).

A majority of Americans (87%) believe that OTCs are safe when used as directed (Roper Starch Worldwide, 2001).

Overall, 82% of American women and 71% of American men have used a non–prescription medicine in the last 6 months to treat at least one common health ailment (Roper Starch Worldwide, 2001).

Adults 65 years and older consume 40% of all OTC medicines sold in the United States (American Pharmaceutical Association, 2000).

OTCs save U.S. consumers an average of $20 billion per year in health care costs—taking into account prescription costs, doctor visits, lost time from work, insurance costs, and travel (Kline & Company, 1997).

Of the more than $1.2 trillion spent on health care in 2000 in the United States, over $19 billion paid for non–prescription drugs—less than 2 cents of every health care dollar (CHPA, 2001).

The CPI for OTCs increased only 1.2% from December 2001 over December 2000, less than other segments of the health care industry, including prescription drugs and supplies (6%), and physician and hospital services (3.6% and 7.2%, respectively) (Bureau of Labor Statistics, CPI–All Urban Consumers, 2002).

65% of Americans wish that some of the prescription drugs they take would be made available over the counter (National Consumers League, 2000).

*Most individuals take the necessary precautions, such as reading directions before taking a non–prescription product for the first time (95%), reading labels to choose appropriate OTC medicines (89%), and reading about possible side effects and interactions (91%) (Roper Starch Worldwide, 2001).

CHPA, Consumer Healthcare Products Association: *CPI,* Consumer Price Index; *OTC(s),* Over-the-Counter (drugs). Consumer Healthcare Products Association. (2005). Healthcare Facts and Figures. Available online: www.chpa-info.org/Chpa-Portal/PressRoom/Statistics/OTCFactsandFigures.htm. Accessed February 9, 2007.

Pharmaceutical manufacturers use direct-to-consumer (DTC) advertising to provide information about both OTC and prescription products. This form of advertising promotes patient self-diagnosis, self-treatment, and use of the product. However, DTC advertising creates certain expectations of the health care provider. In addition, pharmaceutical advertising generates a market for OTC drugs while producing a false sense of security about drug safety. For this reason, health care providers must consider the safety as well as the demonstrated cost-effectiveness of OTC drugs when making management decisions.

FACTORS INFLUENCING OTC USE

A number of factors influence consumer buying practices: social pressures that encourage self-reliance and self-responsibility for health, economy of time, and limited resources. Cultural expectations, gender, alternative health care options, education, sophistication, the wide range of OTC products, and the availability of pharmacists all contribute to the trend for self-treatment. When pharmacists are consulted, they often have recommendations for specific OTC drugs. These recommendations include drugs for sore throats, coughs, allergies, diarrhea, hemorrhoids, and yeast and fungal infections (Box 9-2).

OTC drugs and products are purchased most often without professional assistance. Consumers are more inclined to self-treat when they perceive their illnesses to be minor or not amenable to medical interventions, or the cost of medical care to be prohibitive. Consumers may also treat themselves because of distrust of the health care system or its providers.

Symptoms treated by OTC drugs appear to vary with sex and age. Persons younger than 55 years most often treat themselves for symptoms. In contrast, 40% of persons over 65 years of age typically treat themselves for age-related discomforts. Older adults also use more prescription drugs than younger adults.

Figure 9-1 compares women to men in the treatment of certain minor health conditions. In comparison to 71% of

men, 82% of women say they have used non–prescription drugs in the previous 6 months to treat at least one of the common ailments from which they suffer.

BOX 9-2

Problems Amenable to Self-Treatment

Acne
Allergic rhinitis, nasal congestion
Athlete's foot
Bacterial infections (superficial, uncomplicated, topical)
Boils
Burns (minor thermal burns, sunburn)
Calluses, corns, warts
Cold and canker sores
Constipation, flatulence
Contact dermatitis (e.g., poison ivy, poison oak)
Contraception
Coughs and colds, sore throat
Dandruff
Diabetes mellitus (supplies)
Diaper rash
Diarrhea (e.g., traveler's diarrhea)
Dry skin, dry mouth
Dysmenorrhea, premenstrual syndrome
Fever
Halitosis
Head lice
Heartburn, dyspepsia
Hemorrhoids
Insect bites, stings
Insomnia
"Jock itch," prickly heat
Mineral and vitamin deficiencies
Minor aches and pains, headache
Motion sickness
Nausea and vomiting
Sprains and strains
"Swimmer's ear"
Vaginal fungus infection

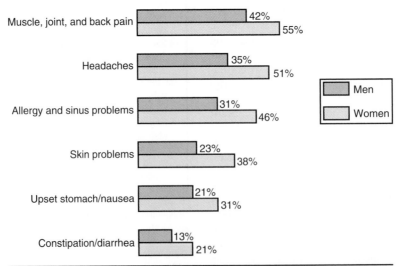

FIGURE 9-1 Self Care Trends as of 2001. (Data from the Consumer Healthcare Products Association Results based on 1505 interviews conducted by telephone by Toper Starch Worldwide from January 8–24, 2001. Margin of error +/−2.6%.)

Self-care strategies are learned early and extend throughout life. Of children less than 2 years of age, 70% have been given OTC drugs at least once, and more than 5 drugs on average are kept on hand by their caregivers. Some families keep as many as 16 different drugs on hand. Over 50% of ambulatory older adults have OTC drugs at home that are not currently being used.

Self-care stems from two important cultural values in U.S. society—independence and freedom of action. The Nonprescription Drug Manufacturers Association (NDMA) emphasizes, however, that self-treatment decisions should include informed, appropriate, and responsible use of OTC products. In addition, the NDMA stresses that responsible self-treatment does not involve the use of prescription drugs without supervision by a health care provider.

OTC drugs have advantages and disadvantages (Table 9-1). In some cases, the consumer does not understand or cannot accurately determine the seriousness of the signs and symptoms he or she is experiencing. In addition, some OTC drugs can relieve the signs and symptoms and yet mask the actual problem. Many OTC drugs contain potentially harmful ingredients (e.g., caffeine, alcohol, phenylpropanolamine). If consumers do not, or cannot, read labels, they remain unaware of the potentially harmful ingredients until problems arise.

Further, partly as a consequence of the proliferation of OTC drugs and other health care products, a growing number of prescription drugs are going unclaimed. A patient visits the health care provider, obtains a prescription, and submits it to the pharmacy for processing. However, the filled prescription is never claimed; in fact, 1 in 5 is not. In many cases, the patient turns instead to OTC drugs and home remedies for symptom relief once the diagnosis is made. Factors contributing to the number of unclaimed prescriptions are the cost of prescription drugs, "forgetting," and an improved condition. Some patients do not want to take the drug or believe that there was a lack of communication with the health care provider. Other patients disagree with a health care provider's assessment and choose not to pick up the prescription.

TABLE 9-1 Advantages and Disadvantages of OTC Drugs

Advantages	Disadvantages
• Promote patient responsibility	• Requires patient self-diagnosis
• Greater availability	• Increased use of anecdotal and/or nonprofessional advice
• Easily accessible and obtainables	• Patient may not be able to read labels, may misread or misunderstand directions
• Free professional advice (RPh) often available	
• Less costly to acquire, because visit to health care provider is not required	• Patient may not ask for or receive professional advice when uncertain about directions
• Generally safe and effective for many conditions when used as directed	• Increased susceptibility to incomplete or exaggerated advertising claims
• Lower cost	• Greater potential for drug-drug and drug-food interactions
	• Higher risk of delay in seeking needed medical attention

OTC, Over-the-counter; *RPh,* registered pharmacist.

LEGISLATIVE CONTROL OF OTC DRUGS

Legislative control of OTC drugs is designed to protect consumers. In 1906, the initial concern of federal legislation on food and drug products was with adulterated products. A 1938 act mandated that all new drugs be proven safe for human use. Although there have been several amendments since, the 1952 Durham-Humphrey amendment was the first to address OTC drugs, thus distinguishing prescription from non–prescription drugs. The act was expanded in 1962 to provide assurance of a drug's safety and its effectiveness for its intended use, and to establish a means of improving communication about the drugs.

In 1972 the Food and Drug Administration (FDA) established the OTC Drug Advisory Review Panel. An advisory review panel was convened and instructed to develop monographs for each therapeutic class of OTC drugs (rather than examining individual products). The panel also set about identifying the circumstances in which an OTC drug is recognized as safe and effective and not mislabeled. Whereas only the active ingredients in OTC drugs are evaluated, prescription drugs are evaluated in their finished dosage forms.

OTC CATEGORIES

According to the OTC Drug Advisory Review Panel, newly introduced OTC drugs are divided into two categories. Category I drugs are *generally recognized as safe and effective* (GRASE). Category II drugs are *generally recognized as safe* (GRAS). A drug classified as GRAS has more relaxed requirements than one classified as GRASE: FDA approval is needed only for the active ingredient rather than for the entire formulation. *Safe* refers to (1) the low potential for harm if the drug is misused and (2) the rarity of major adverse effects when the drug is used as directed. A drug is *generally recognized as effective* (GRAE) (assuming the drug is used as directed) when it provides the intended relief for the majority of the population.

Since the FDA's review of OTC products began in 1972, some ingredients have been removed from the market because they were not safe (e.g., phenacetin). Others have been reclassified as prescription drugs after clinical data revealed serious adverse effects (e.g., hexachlorophene). FDA review also led to the reclassification of some prescription drug ingredients for use in OTC drugs (e.g., ibuprofen and some hydrocortisone creams) (Box 9-3).

DRUG LABELING

Labeling requirements for OTC drugs are strict and specific. Information on the labels must be written clearly so that consumers will be able to read and understand the information, regardless of their reading skills or educational level. Professional labeling in some drug monographs (the written mechanism by which drugs are evaluated by the FDA) provides more information than is otherwise required on an OTC label. Figure 9-2 illustrates a product label that meets FDA labeling requirements (see also Chapter 11).

FDA OTC Drug Classifications

Antacids
Antimicrobials I (GRASE)
Antimicrobials II (GRAS)
Antiperspirants
Bronchodilator and antiasthmatic drugs
Cold, cough, allergy drugs
Contraceptives and other vaginal drugs
Dentifrice and dental care drugs
Hemorrhoidal drugs
Internal analgesics, antipyretics, and antirheumatics
Laxatives, antidiarrheals, emetics, and antiemetics
Miscellaneous external drugs
Ophthalmics
Oral cavity drug preparations
Sedatives, tranquilizers, and sleeping aids
Vitamins, minerals, and hematinics

OTC, Over-the-counter; *GRASE,* generally recognized as safe and effective; *GRAS,* generally recognized as safe.

DRUG PACKAGING

Drug packaging laws came into being in the early 1980s after several reported episodes in the United States of OTC analgesics being poisoned with cyanide. The cyanide was thought to have been added to the analgesic capsules once they reached store shelves. To prevent a recurrence of these problems, drug manufacturers developed sealed, tamper-resistant containers.

The containers usually have an inner seal of aluminum foil, together with a plastic outer ring around the cap or a shrink-sealed full-package plastic wrap. Some drugs are packaged using a unit-dose system.

Health care providers bear a large portion of the responsibility to educate patients about OTC drug safety. Patients should be encouraged to carefully inspect packaging to be sure it is intact before purchase and use, and that the drug is not beyond its date of expiration. A discrepancy between the lot number on the container and the lot number on the outer packaging, as well as breaks, cracks, or holes in the outer wrapping, or other indications that the outer packaging has been disturbed, unwrapped, or replaced may suggest tampering. Distortion or stretching of the shrink-seal, a loose bottle cap, or traces of paper or glue around the outer rim of the container may indicate that the seal has been removed and replaced. Discoloration or disarray of the cotton plug, an overfilled or underfilled bottle, or an unusual appearance of the drug should also alert the consumer to possible tampering.

Tablets are suspect if they do not all appear the same, with the usual size, thickness, color, shine, smoothness, taste, and odor, or if they are not marked with the manufacturer's insignia. Liquids are suspect if they have sediment or a strong odor, or if their usual appearance seems odd. Ophthalmic solutions should have intact protective seals (manufacturers of such products are also required to ensure their sterility). Ointments, creams, and pastes contained in tubes should be properly sealed, and the bottom of the tube crimped and uniform in appearance. Ointments should have a smooth, uniform consistency, and the expiration date should be on the package.

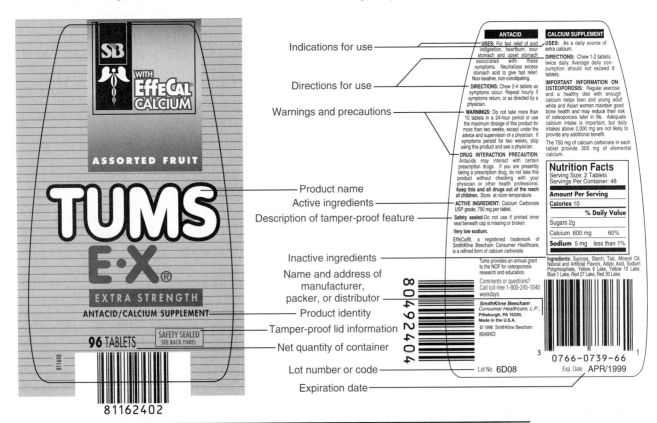

FIGURE 9-2 Labeling Requirements. (Label courtesy of Smith Kline Beecham, Pittsburgh, PA.)

If tampering is suspected, the package should be returned to the pharmacy from which it was purchased. The pharmacy, in turn, will report suspected tampering to the Drug Product Problem Reporting Program. This program is coordinated by the FDA in collaboration with the United States Pharmacopeia and the American Society of Health System Pharmacists.

STORAGE, HANDLING, AND DISPOSAL

STORAGE

Variables affecting drug use in the community differ from those in the hospital. In an institutional setting, the nurse is most often the gatekeeper of the drug supply; in collaboration with colleagues, the nurse determines when and how drugs will be administered. In most cases, there is little input from the patient. Drugs are packaged using a unit-dose system. The standard drug carts or cabinets are equipped with a drawer for each patient's drugs. These individual patient drawers are filled and their contents updated according to orders, by members of the pharmacy staff. Unused and discontinued drugs are returned to the pharmacy for proper disposal. In many hospitals today, a computerized dispensing system is used for dispensing drugs.

In the home setting, the gatekeeper of the drug supply is the patient. Most drugs provided by community pharmacies are dispensed in a single container rather than a unit-dose container, posing a greater risk for misuse or overdosage. Further, any drug remaining after the condition for which it was purchased has improved is commonly saved rather than discarded, increasing the risk of later harm through misuse or reuse.

In the home, drugs should be kept in their original containers to ensure availability of correct directions and to avoid misidentification and unknown expiration dates. Storage in a secure, locked cabinet not located in the bathroom is recommended. Drug storage in the bathroom is not recommended because bathroom cabinets rarely have a lock and are too easily accessible to children. These principles should be followed not only where children live but also where they may visit.

Chemical deterioration of drugs is hastened by heat, moisture and, in some cases, light. Light-sensitive drugs should be stored in their original amber-colored containers and exposure to direct sunlight avoided. To prevent changes caused by moisture, silica gel inserts are packaged with some drugs. Exposure to moisture may dissolve some solid dosage forms. Exposure to heat may melt the waxy base of suppositories and ointments.

Not all drugs are to be stored at room temperature. Some drugs must be refrigerated at temperatures ranging from 35° to 60° F (2° to 15° C), and some drugs must be stored in a freezer. Accidental freezing may alter drug characteristics. Others must be stored where temperatures do not exceed 40° F (4.4° C). Some multidose, injectable drugs and suppositories are stored in airtight containers and refrigerated to protect them from humidity and food residues.

Insulin presents a special storage problem. Bacterial contamination is possible, owing to the multidose container in which insulin is packaged and the prolonged time over which it is used. The potential for contamination of insulin is high; preservatives do not protect against contamination. However, insulin should be administered at room temperature to reduce the risk of lipodystrophy. To decrease these problems, insulin vials currently in use are kept for a period of 1 month or less at room temperature, and any additional vials dispensed are kept refrigerated.

HANDLING

Many drugs are dispensed in containers with childproof caps. Because the caps require complex manipulation, the time required for children to gain access to the drug is prolonged. The caps reduce the potential for accidental ingestion and have lowered the incidence of poisoning in children. However, these childproof caps are difficult for persons with impaired dexterity to use. Standard, easily opened containers are available and can be requested at the time a drug is dispensed. However, special safeguards must be taken to prevent access by children. To maintain the legibility of the label, the patient should pour liquids so that the drug will not spill over the label.

Consumers should be discouraged from borrowing drugs from family members or friends. The money saved by "borrowing" is likely to translate into a much greater expense in the form of ineffective treatment and higher risks of adverse effects and drug interactions. It is also a felony, punishable under the law.

DISPOSAL

Pharmaceutical manufacturers establish expiration dates and print them on the label or package insert of each drug. Expiration dates are only approximations and do not indicate that a drug is at once rendered useless or harmful on that date. However, most drugs at least lose potency over time, and some drugs can become toxic (e.g., tetracycline, acetaminophen).

Patients should be taught to discard drugs according to the following guidelines:

- Aspirin or acetaminophen that smells like vinegar (has become toxic)
- Any drugs in solid dosage form (i.e., pills, tablets, capsules) that are damaged, discolored, softened, or stuck together
- Liquids that have lost their original color, smell, or taste or that have developed gas formations (indicates deterioration)
- Ointments or creams that have changed in odor, color, or consistency
- Any oral drug that is past its expiration date or is more than 2 years old
- Any drug that has not been stored as directed

In years past, outdated or unused drugs were disposed of by flushing them drug down the toilet. A 2002 U.S. Geological Survey (USGS) tested 139 rivers in 30 states (Kolpin, 2002). The report found high levels of toxins from pharmaceuticals in ground water and drinking water sources. Eighty percent of streams sampled by the USGS showed evidence of drugs (e.g., fluoxetine), hormones (e.g., oral contraceptives), steroids, and personal care products such as soaps and perfumes.

As a result, in 2002 the White House Office of National Drug Control Policy (ONDCP), the Department of Health and Human Services (DHHS), and the Environmental Protection Agency (EPA) issued joint guidelines for the proper disposal of unused, unneeded, or outdated prescription drugs (www.systoc.com/newscomments/news/Feb2007/Fed-Guidelines.pdf). These guidelines are designed to reduce the diversion of prescription drugs while also protecting the environment. For proper disposal of prescription drugs, take unused or outdated prescription drugs out of their original containers. Mix the drugs with an undesirable substance (e.g., used coffee grounds, kitty litter) and put them in impermeable, non-descript containers (e.g., empty metal can, resealable milk bottles) to ensure the drugs are not diverted or accidentally ingested by children or pets. Throw the sealed containers in the trash. Flush drugs down the toilet only if the accompanying patient information specifically states that it is safe to do so. In some cases, unused or outdated prescription drugs can be returned to pharmaceutical take-back locations for safe disposal.

The Centers for Disease Control and Prevention recommend disposing of needles, syringes, and vials by placing them in a sturdy container with a tightly fitting lid. The container should be taped closed, double-bagged, and placed with the regular household trash for disposal. Commercially available containers may also be used for disposal. However, some patients are not comfortable with disposal of needles, syringes, and vials at home. In that case, the health care provider or a local hospital or clinic can be contacted to see if the container can be taken where it will be disposed of with other medical waste.

ADHERENCE VERSUS NONADHERENCE

Adherence, that is, how well the patient follows through with a drug regimen, has been a concern of health care providers for decades. Many health care providers assume that once a diagnosis is made and the prescription written, the patient will follow the plan of care. Unfortunately, the effectiveness of drug therapy of any kind is often compromised by lack of adherence by the patient. In many cases, the outcome is often the reason a patient reenters the health care system. One should note, however, that "noncompliance" is a term generated by health care providers and defines the problem from their viewpoint only. Not following the treatment regimen may be regarded as deviant behavior by some, but the patient may see the action as a cautious approach to self-administration of potentially harmful substances. Other reasons for nonadherence by the patient may be a lack of understanding of the need or reason for the drug, the cost of the drug, or the adverse effects it causes.

Nonadherence can arise through either intentional or unintentional actions. The complex medical problems of many individuals and the varied drug regimens that patients are expected to follow lay the groundwork for nonadherence and potential drug interactions. One third to one half of prescription drugs are not taken as directed. As mentioned, some patients fail to pick up the filled prescription or to have the prescription filled at all. Still others stop taking the drug too early in the treatment regimen, leading to treatment failure.

Nonadherence is the most common problem encountered in drug therapy (see also Chapter 5). Over 50% of patients are nonadherent with their drug therapy, which results in poor control of chronic illnesses and sometimes extensive hospitalizations. Older adults are less likely to follow a drug regimen if they are taking five or more drugs, when drug labels cannot be read, or when containers are difficult to open. When the patient's condition does not improve or there is poor control of the illness, it is important for the health care provider to determine the reasons. Sometimes, instead of investigating and resolving the cause of treatment failure, the health care provider simply increases the dosage of the same drug or changes to a new one. Table 9-2 provides examples of cues that may be predictive of nonadherence, along with possible interventions. Questions must be asked that focus on the patient's understanding of the drug, the timing of the drug administration, adverse effects that the patient is experiencing, and any fears the patient may have.

COMMUNITY RESOURCES

COMMUNITY PHARMACISTS

The role of the community pharmacist is growing as a result of the trend toward the use of OTC drugs. The expansion and greater availability of OTC drugs and the likelihood of more sophisticated and technical products provide the impetus for patient and health care provider alike to use the services and expertise of community pharmacists. Before 1972 and the FDA's review of OTC drugs, pharmacists avoided giving patients advice or counseling about health care concerns. Now, this practice is encouraged, and pharmacists' expertise uniquely qualifies them to educate the patient about prescription drugs as well as OTC drugs. Many times, the community pharmacist is the first contact the patient has with a health care professional in regard to a given health concern.

COMPUTER INFORMATION SYSTEMS

According to the American Society for Automation in Pharmacy, more than 90% of U.S. pharmacies use computers to process prescriptions. With a computerized system, a patient's prescribed drug profile can be maintained for a defined number of years. Such systems are an avenue for checking food or drug allergies against each chemical contained in a drug and for any incompatibilities with other drugs the patient is taking. When information about an incompatibility is found, the pharmacist can notify the patient and the health care provider before the drug is dispensed.

Tracking drug regimens through computerized information networks helps provide a safety net, but only to the extent that appropriate information has been provided by the patient. As more and more people engage in self-treatment, the importance of accurate, accessible information cannot be overestimated. It is imperative that the patient communicates information about food and drug allergies, the use of herbs and home remedies, and prescription drugs that may have been dispensed by other health care providers, as well as OTC drugs that are used. Withholding such information from the health care provider and the pharmacist places the patient at risk for harmful drug interactions and reactions and the potential for failure of the management plan.

TABLE **9-2 Promoting Adherence**

Parameter	Factors Related to Nonadherence	Interview Questions	Possible Interventions
Personal health-illness beliefs and practices	Severity of illness not perceived to be as high by patient as by health care provider Denial of problem results in patient's ignoring information Patient is susceptible to actual or potential illness	"How would you describe the severity of your illness?" "Would you describe yourself as healthy or unhealthy?"	Be sure questions asked and information provided are relevant from the patient's perspective.
Beliefs regarding effectiveness of Western health care interventions	Patient does not believe Western health care is effective	"How would you describe the effectiveness of your care?"	Use nonjudgmental, active listening, e.g., ask, "Tell me about your beliefs."
Previous experience with health care system or health care provider	Patient expresses dissatisfaction with past or present interactions	"How do you feel about the care you received?"	Use nonjudgmental, active listening. Avoid false reassurance.
Perception of complexity of management plan	Plan seems difficult to follow, vague, ambiguous, disruptive, or lengthy	"How does the plan of care affect your daily routine?"	Simplify regimen when possible. Adapt it to patient's lifestyle.
Level of trust	Patient lacks trust in health care provider or health care system Health care provider has failed to establish interest and trust	"To what degree do you trust your health care provider?" "What can we do that would foster your trust in us?"	Take a genuine interest in the patient. Follow up on patient responses, requests, and complaints.
Adherence and nonadherence	Patient never intends to adhere to instructions Patient has history of nonadherence	"How do you plan to take your medications?" "How often did you take your medicine for your other illness?"	Acknowledge difficulty with adherence. Explore, with patient, strategies to improve it.
Coping mechanisms	Patient uses denial, does not recognize need for treatment, exhibits repression, or is unable to mobilize energies to cope	Assess for cues such as, "I'm not so ill."	Educate patient about disease, drugs, etc., and effective coping mechanisms.
Patient's self-esteem	Negative self-image	Assess for verbal and/or nonverbal cues, such as, "Don't bother with me; I'm not worth the effort."	Provide resources for counseling relative to the patient's underlying problem.
Economic status	Patient has lower socioeconomic status, is unemployed, lacks health insurance, is homeless, or believes drugs are not worth the cost. Patient believes self-care is a more efficient alternative to high-cost drugs.	"What resources do you have that help you with the cost of your treatment and medicines?"	Investigate situation, and refer patient to appropriate resources for financial assistance. Explore methods to alleviate environmental issues.
Support systems	Patient lacks family or cultural support Patient lives alone	"When you want to talk about a problem, who do you go to?"	Enlist family and friends to assist patient Refer to social services if appropriate
Reading and comprehension abilities	Inadequate and/or inaccessible educational system Patient has limited reading and comprehension skills	Query patient about disease process, drug action, and adverse effects: "Can you tell me what you see on this prescription bottle?" "What directions are on this container?"	Increase sensory exposure with pictures, charts, verbal reinforcement. Assess baseline knowledge and build on that foundation. Use nonjudgmental behaviors. Refer to literacy hotline, local literacy council, or other community service if appropriate.
Physical capabilities to carry out plan of care	Patient physically unable to carry out plan of care Patient faces environmental obstacles	"What kind of problems do you have that make it difficult for you to take your medicine?" "Are you able to reach your medicines and open the containers?"	Assist patient to obtain nonchildproof caps, if appropriate. Explore alternative devices and methods of administration (e.g., automatic injection devices, magnifying glasses).

PUBLICATIONS

There was no information resource for non–prescription drugs until the American Pharmaceutical Association published its first edition of the *Handbook of Nonprescription Drugs* in 1965. The *Handbook of Nonprescription Drugs,* the *United States Pharmacopeia Dispensing Information* (USPDI) compendia, and many lay publications and resource guides are now available to patients. Volume II of the compendia is written specifically for the patient and may be found at most community pharmacies. The *FDA Consumer* is a periodical that focuses on topics related to FDA-regulated products, including food safety, nutrition, prescription and OTC drugs, medical technology, cosmetics, and all of the other products and services under the FDA's jurisdiction. The *FDA Consumer* also provides a behind-the-scenes look at how the FDA uncovers fraudulent and illegal activities. Patients also have easy access to professional resources, many of which are found in local bookstores. Health care providers can recommend publications and help patients evaluate such materials, which vary in accuracy, user-friendliness, and completeness.

WEB-BASED RESOURCES

A 2000 research study by the Pew Commission (Fox & Rainie, 2000) reported the following:

- 48% of consumer respondents noted that the advice they found on the Web improved their self-care; 55% noted that Internet access improved the manner in which they get health information.
- 92% of consumer respondents noted that the information found during an online search was useful, with over 80% noting that they learned new information.
- 47% of consumer respondents who searched for health information for personal use noted that the information found influenced diet and exercise regimens.
- 36% of those searching Web-based resources on behalf of a loved one found the data for which they were searching influenced health care decisions for this person.

The study also found that women were much more likely than men to use health information obtained online and had strong opinions about the benefits of online searches, particularly searches related to the convenience and the wealth of information available. However, these same women were more likely to be concerned about the reliability of information found on online. Women were also more likely than men to search for information on a specific illness, disease, or symptom, or on behalf of a child, and to conduct the search after an appointment with the health care provider. Equal proportions of men and women were found to be seeking information on behalf of a parent or other relative.

Although this 24-hour access to information is convenient, Web-surfers must guard against false, tainted, or misleading data. Sometimes it is difficult to be sure of the quality of the information. Internet information undergoes no quality control, and virtually anyone can publish anything. Centralized control of content is unrealistic, but newer technologies are making it easier for its users to receive only those pages which are appropriate to their needs and that are assessed as relatively reliable. High-quality websites contain a specific set of characteristics that helps to assess the quality of the information (Box 9-4).

CLINICAL REASONING

Assessment

▥▎ *History of Present Illness*

The first step in assessing the patient is to identify the symptoms for which the patient seeks treatment. The health care provider may be seeing the patient in the office or making a home visit as part of a treatment plan initiated after discharge from the hospital or extended care facility. Patients may initially provide incomplete and vague information. The objective is to determine the patient's specific symptoms, review the course of illness, review the plan of care from the discharging facility, and discuss the options for self-care and treatment with the health care provider.

▥▎ *Past Health History*

Information related to the patient's health history is important for effective treatment and drug management.

BOX 9-4

Evaluating Website Information

Questions to ask about websites to help ensure quality and accuracy:
1. Who maintains the online site? What are their credentials?
2. Who is behind the site? Who covers expenses for the site?
3. What is the objective of the online site?
4. Where does the information come from?
5. What process is used to select the information included on the site? How current is the information?
6. How does the site choose links to other sites?
7. Is a membership or a fee required to access the site?
8. What information about you does the site collect, and why?
9. What are your rights and guarantees if you purchase something from the site?
10. Does the site provide information about how to contact the site administrators?

Adapted from A User's Guide to Finding and Evaluating Health Information on the Web. (2007). Available online: www.mlanet.org/resources/userguide.html. Accessed February 9, 2007.

Information to be gathered includes the patient's age, preexisting medical problems, chronic illnesses, drug and food allergies, long-term (more than 2 weeks') use of prescription or OTC drugs and home remedies, and use of vitamins, supplements, nicotine, alcohol, and illicit drugs. Be sure to check previous chart notes to be sure you have an overall picture of the patient.

Several methods can be used to assess adherence with a drug regimen. Patient self-reporting may be inaccurate if the patient has memory problems or is reluctant to admit that the drug was not taken. It is not uncommon, especially with older adults, for the patient to forget about drugs used for self-medication or to store multiple drugs in a single, unlabeled container. The provider should note the drug storage site, which may be unsafe. Exposure to heat, light, and moisture adversely affects most drugs.

Request to see the drugs the patient is taking; have each patient bring to the appointment any prescription, OTC, and herbal remedies used. The patient's ability to read and understand the information on the drug labels and to locate expiration dates, and knowledge about proper disposal of drugs, must be assessed. Many patients have decreased visual acuity, cannot read, or cannot understand the information contained on drug labels or package inserts.

The activities of daily living, including exercise and sleep habits, should be assessed in relation to drug therapy. Some drugs may alter sleep patterns and interfere with the rapid eye movement sleep cycle. The patient may awaken feeling more tired than before going to bed. Diuretics causing frequent urination are best taken when the patient is awake and ambulatory (see Chapter 41). Drugs that alter the patient's level of alertness should be taken at bedtime or when alertness is not required (e.g., not before driving a vehicle or operating machinery). Taking sedating drugs or those likely to cause lightheadedness contributes to an older adult's fall risk, particularly at night. The drug schedule or the activity pattern should be adjusted to minimize the risk of harm to the patient.

COMMUNITY

Physical Exam

The physical exam is directly related to and specific for the health problems being monitored. Physical findings often confirm specific responses to drug therapies. For example, serial blood pressure readings help monitor the effectiveness of antihypertensive drugs. A decrease in the amount of peripheral edema, a loss of weight, or a decrease in blood pressure may provide information about the therapeutic effectiveness of diuretics. A change in the mental status of the patient may provide an early indication of drug toxicity. The patient's physical ability to manage the route of drug administration (i.e., injections, rectal or vaginal suppositories) may affect the patient's adherence with the drug regime. Although many drugs are formulated as sublingual, buccal, and topical rinses, the patient's ability to swallow is necessary for taking oral drugs.

Changes in sensory-perceptual abilities may place patients at higher risk for accidents and injury. In order for the patient to adhere with a drug regimen, the patient must be able to see, read, hear, and comprehend the information. In addition, alterations in taste and smell may affect the patient's ability and willingness to comply with drug or dietary regimens. Decreases in the patient's fine motor function and sensation may create difficulty in preparing and self-administering injectable drugs or in opening drug containers. Gross motor limitations may affect the patient's ability to obtain and self-administer drugs.

Diagnostic Testing

Specimen collection in the community is similar to that in an institutional setting, except that the health care provider must see that the specimen is transported to the lab in a timely fashion. Laboratory protocols should be followed for storage of specimens that cannot be immediately transported to the designated lab. Some specimens, such as those for serum potassium, must be transported with minimum disturbance to ensure accurate test results. All specimens should be collected in appropriate containers to reduce errors and limit the need for repeated procedures.

Life-Span Considerations

Three groups of individuals—pregnant women (see Chapter 6), children and adolescents (see Chapter 7), and older adults (see Chapter 8) often have higher incidences of adverse effects of drug therapy than the general population. Other high-risk patients include those with human immunodeficiency virus or acquired immunodeficiency syndrome (HIV/AIDS), the lactating mother who breastfeeds, patients with end-stage renal disease, and those with cancer. Such high-risk patients require special consideration. Awareness of the patient's physiologic state, disease or illnesses, or sociocultural considerations is necessary for the appropriate assessment and recommendations for treatment.

Moreover, with earlier discharge from acute care settings, many patients are returning home while still in the early recovery period and with limited self-care capabilities. Until a patient is able to manage his or her own care, drug administration is often the responsibility of a family member or other caregiver. Using commercial or homemade pill boxes may be helpful in organizing drugs and thus facilitate adherence.

Drug administration may be the responsibility of supervisory personnel for school-age children or patients living with limited supervision (e.g., group homes). In these situations, the health care provider may have primary care and/or delegatory, educational, and supervisory responsibilities. In some states, the health care provider has the legal power to delegate drug administration activities to nonprofessional staff. In many schools, however, permission must be obtained from the child's parent(s) and the prescribing health care provider for the drug to be administered on the premises.

Psychosocial Considerations

Psychosocial factors affecting the patient provide valuable information to the health care provider. Because of the increasing interest in self-care and the trend toward OTC or non–prescription drug use, the health care provider must understand the factors influencing a patient's treatment choices. Inherent in this understanding is knowledge of the patient's environment, dietary practices, sleeping patterns, and activity levels. Health-illness beliefs and practices, past experiences with the health care system, educational level, religious beliefs, language barriers, support system, and financial resources should also be considered.

DIETARY PRACTICES. A working knowledge of the patient's dietary practices is essential to evaluate the therapeutic effectiveness of drug regimens as well as the risk of drug-food interactions. Most drug-food interactions are not well understood, but such interactions can have dramatic effects on the patient. For example, the patient taking the antibiotic tetracycline with dairy products may receive less benefit from the antibiotic because of its bonding to the calcium ions in the dairy products. Food may also impair absorption of certain drugs. Drugs may also alter nutrient absorption, which can lead over time to vitamin and mineral deficiencies. The health care provider should assess the patient's nutritional status before starting drug therapy, and periodically throughout therapy, to determine the need for dietary or vitamin supplementation.

HEALTH-ILLNESS BELIEFS AND PRACTICES. Patients' health-illness beliefs and practices and their use of the health care system affect adherence with a drug regimen. When confronted with symptoms perceived to be minor or easily controlled, patients often seek self-care remedies or OTC drugs before seeking care from a health care provider. It is only when these attempts do not relieve symptoms, or the problem worsens, that patients seek care from a health care provider. With continued emphasis on individual responsibility for health, the importance of self-care and self-treatment may continue to increase. Individuals who have the greatest trust in contemporary health care practices and technologies are least likely to purchase OTC drugs or to use questionably efficacious products on their own.

Self-treatment is not limited to OTC drugs. Non-Western traditional folk and cultural practices and beliefs are mysterious by Western standards. A patient's use of home remedies and other self-treatment strategies is important to note. The health care provider is in a unique position to acquire information about health and illness practices.

DRUG USE AND MISUSE. The health care provider must be aware of the possibility of drug misuse or drug abuse. The patient's drug history should include use of illicit drugs, alcohol, and nicotine, all of which can significantly influence the effects of other drugs. Though the patient may be hesitant to disclose such information, the health care provider may be the first to detect substance abuse. Chapter 12 discusses substance abuse further.

LANGUAGE DIFFERENCES. The health care provider should consider the patient's health care beliefs and use of non-Western treatments when considering drug options and the patient's potential for adherence. As mentioned previously, ethnic groups often use folk remedies and folk healers because of unfamiliarity with or distrust or dislike of the health care system. Language differences can impair access to health care and may further discourage use of the system. Differences in language may interfere with the health care provider's ability to accurately assess the patient's concerns and symptoms and to educate the patient. The use of non–family interpreters may facilitate an accurate assessment of health care concerns and drug use or abuse.

FAMILY SUPPORT NETWORK. An assessment of the patient's family support network is an important component in understanding the patient. Family living arrangements, the number, ages, and relationships of people in the home, communication patterns, the roles of family members, the power and authority structure of the family, and the presence of a caregiver all affect patient care. To effectively treat the patient, the health care provider must gain the trust of the patient's family.

EDUCATION. Nearly 20% of the U.S. population is functionally illiterate. A subtle approach is necessary to assess a patient's ability to read and comprehend directions for prescribed and non–prescription drug therapy. Patients who are unable to read or comprehend are often ashamed of the deficit and try to compensate by indicating that they understand and will comply. By having the patient read a drug label and explain how the product is to be taken (e.g., times, before or after meals, amount) the health care provider can assess the patient's vocabulary, knowledge of the drug, and comprehension level. The patient's knowledge of the drug may also be assessed through questioning about drug action, adverse effects, and the disease process. The discussion must involve not only the use of the drug but also how and why to read a label.

ECONOMIC FACTORS. The high cost of pharmaceuticals is a commonly acknowledged reason for the patient's lack of adherence with drug regimens. An assessment of the patient's socioeconomic level and the availability of health insurance may provide the health care provider with information that will help in prescribing the most cost-effective drugs for the patient. Assistance programs commonly require a financial needs assessment to determine eligibility. Interpretation of eligibility regulations often becomes the health care provider's responsibility. Many patients regard self-treatment as a more economical alternative, both in time and in money, and may try this approach before seeking care from a health care provider. Astute pharmacists help patients save money by offering less expensive generic drug forms or educating the patient about similarities and differences between products.

Available transportation and pharmacy delivery services may assist patients to obtain needed drugs. Health care providers and pharmacists can furnish information about delivery services to the patient when the cost of transportation or the inability to drive may prevent access to a pharmacy. It is also possible to obtain pharmaceuticals by mail through organizations such as the American Association of Retired Persons (AARP).

Controversy

Why Do We Still Question the Use of Generic Drugs?

Jonathan J. Wolfe

Generic drugs have engendered controversy since their introduction into the American marketplace in the 1960s. The advent of managed care and the use of drug formularies have brought new scrutiny to the growing use of generic drugs as opposed to brand-name products. The question revolves around more than price. Generic drugs initially offered lower price as a reason for their use. However, after a brand-name drug loses its patent protection, its price may be lowered below that of its generic counterpart as a strategy to guard market share.

Initially, concern focused on the efficacy and safety of generic drugs. Now, however, their worth is well established. The *Orange Book** provides documentation of the bioequivalence of generic drug products. The *Orange Book* warns against substitution of generics whose equivalence to the standard brand name product is not established. Within the health care environment, the justice of substitution remains a cogent concern.

Often, patients are the focus of the dilemma. Patients may refuse to accept a generic drug product after years of treatment with a brand-name drug. In other cases, patients who agree to a generic drug substitution may not receive the lower price. A pharmacy benefit company may keep part of the savings and pass on only a small percentage of the reduction to the patient. In addition, the prescription plan manager may receive rebates from drug manufacturers in return for encouraging generic substitution.

CLINICAL REASONING

- When a generic drug has been documented by reliable studies to be equivalent to a well-established brand-name product, what concerns do you have about ordering a generic product when your colleagues write for the brand-name drug?
- There have been product quality problems with drugs from generic manufacturer X. Now your agency hospital has chosen company X as its sole supplier of generic drugs. Under your formulary, you may prescribe a generic equivalent in preference to the brand name as long as the generic is bioequivalent to the brand name. Are you justified in rewriting the order naming the more expensive brand-name product? Is it right for you to give a telephone order for the generic, but to enter the trade name into a patient's records?
- As an advanced practice health care provider, you are a representative on the Pharmacy and Therapeutics Committee at the hospital where you have privileges. What reservations may you properly express about awarding manufacturer X (see preceding question) a new 3-year contract as the hospital's sole supplier of generic drugs?

*The publication, *Approved Drug Products with Therapeutic Equivalence Evaluations* (commonly known as the *Orange Book*), identifies drugs approved on the basis of safety and effectiveness by the Food and Drug Administration (FDA) under the Federal Food, Drug, and Cosmetic Act (the Act). The *Orange Book* is available online: www.fda.gov/cder/ob/default.htm.

MANAGEMENT

Treatment Objectives

In general, prescription and OTC drug therapy is directed at prevention of illness and disease, cure, alleviation of symptoms, or palliation. Prevention of OTC drug–related complications is of primary concern to the health care provider. *Cure* is the relief of the signs and symptoms as well as eradication or elimination of illness. *Supportive therapy* helps alleviate symptoms of certain illnesses, conditions, and diseases that threaten other body systems. The objective of *palliation* is to relieve or alleviate a patient's symptoms; it does not provide a cure.

Treatment Options

Effective health care, whether carried out in an inpatient or home setting, requires communication and collaboration among health care providers. Sharing patient histories with other providers is essential for appropriate follow-up care. Health care providers have a certain liberty in determining or recommending the most effective drug therapy. However, treatment options must recognize that the locus of control belongs with the patient and must promote appropriate and accurate decision making by the patient (see Controversy box).

The patient's drug regimen must be followed closely by the health care provider. By prescribing the minimal number and smallest dose of drugs to achieve the desired effect, the health care provider may encourage the patient's adherence with the drug regimen. Adherence with the prescribed drug regimen is fostered when the patient is included in the plan and feels in control of and knowledgeable about the treatment plan.

Patient Education

Tailoring the drug regimen to the patient's lifestyle helps him or her to remember to take the drugs. Often it is helpful to schedule drug administration to coincide with mealtimes. Patients may also select other specific times during the day when an activity or routine can help "cue" them to take their drugs. The use of egg cartons, muffin tins, or commercially available drug boxes may help the patient organize the drug regimen. Drug boxes can be 7-day organizers but can also be subdivided into several daily-dose compartments (Fig. 9-3). The responsibility for filling the organizers may fall to the health care provider or a caregiver.

A drug diary can help the patient remember whether a particular dose was taken, thus eliminating missed or double doses. However, a diary is disadvantageous in that it requires concerted effort and consistency on the part of the patient or caregiver.

Pill counts are easy to perform and inexpensive. However, they provide no information about the timing of doses, misplaced bottles, dropped pills, or the addition of leftover doses from a previous prescription. One method that has been used to monitor pill counts involves the placement of microprocessors in drug bottle caps. Each time the bottle is opened, the date and time are recorded. This system provides information about the timing of doses and does not rely on the patient's memory. The two disadvantages of the system are that it is based on the assumption that a drug

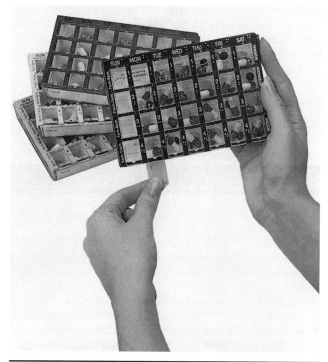

FIGURE 9-3 Commercial Drug Box. Commercially available drug boxes may contain a single compartment or multiple compartments. Some boxes contain just seven divisions, enough for a full week of drugs. Others contain multiple compartments with space available for several doses throughout the day and the week. (Photo courtesy of Apothecary Products, Burnside, MN.)

dose is taken every time the patient opens the bottle, and that the microprocessors are expensive. However, it should be noted that microprocessor systems have largely been replaced by patient self-reports. Self-reports have been shown to correlate with behavior demonstrated by these other systems. Pharmacy records may also be used to monitor patient prescriptions and refills.

Educating the patient requires that the health care provider apply basic principles of teaching and learning. The health care provider must acquire information about the patient such as age, gender, culture or ethnic background, and educational and comprehension level—all of these factors can influence the method and effectiveness of teaching and learning activities. Physiologic factors such as vision or hearing deficits may require alterations in teaching strategies. The health care provider will be more successful in educating the patient when the amount and specific content is tailored to the patient's interest, knowledge base, motivational level, self-care requirements, literacy, and cognitive abilities. The health care provider must remember the key concept that learning and motivation are enhanced by positive reinforcement. Written materials may be helpful but should be appropriate for the patient's reading and comprehension abilities.

In-home teaching allows the health care provider to assess the impact of the home environment on the patient's willingness and ability to learn. Such collaboration within the patient's environment places the locus of control firmly with the patient rather than with the health care provider. Because patients feel more comfortable at home, they may be more receptive and attentive to the information presented. On the other hand, distractions such as telephone interruptions and disruptions by family members may affect the length of teaching sessions in the home setting.

Evaluation

Outcomes criteria are directed toward helping the patient make informed decisions regarding the use of OTCs,

appropriateness of self-care treatments, or concurrent use of Western and non-Western modalities. Evaluating the effects of OTCs would include finding these outcomes: the patient experiences no adverse effects and receives therapeutic effects of the drug. The patient's adherence to an agreed-upon regimen, and improvement or maintenance of health status are long-term outcomes of treatment regimens. Evaluation of the patient's understanding of the drugs involves follow-up care at appropriate intervals.

KEY POINTS

- The number and variety of OTC drugs have exponentially increased, but their use carries risks as well as benefits to the patient.
- The FDA established the OTC Drug Advisory Review Panel in 1972 to ensure that OTC drugs were safe, effective, and not mislabeled.
- The patient's lack of adherence is the most common problem encountered with drug management.
- The OTC drug resources available in the community include pharmacists, computer information systems, publications, and Web-based resources.
- Psychosocial and cultural influences in self-care behaviors and the use of OTC drugs are components vital to the patient database, as is information

about dietary practices, health-illness beliefs, and use of folk medicine, family support, language, financial status, and educational barriers.
- A patient's health-illness beliefs and practices and their use of the health care system affect the patient's adherence with a drug regimen.
- A patient's use of cultural and folk medicine practices must be assessed and incorporated into the plan of care.
- Treatment strategies should recognize that the locus of control belongs with the patient and promote appropriate and accurate decision-making.

Bibliography

American Medical Association. (2004). *Guidelines for physicians for counseling patients about prescription medications in the ambulatory care setting.* Patient education pamphlet.

American Pharmaceutical Association. (2006). *Handbook of nonprescription drugs: An interactive approach to self-care.* (15th ed.). Washington, DC: APha Publications.

Castiel, L. (2003). Self care and consumer health. Do we need a public health ethics? *Journal of Epidemiology and Community Health, 57*(1), 5–6.

Christl, L. (1972). Introduction to non-prescription products. Drug Advisory Review Panel of the Food and Drug Administration. Available online: www.fda.gove/cder/audiences/iact/forum/200609_christl.pdf. Accessed February 9, 2007.

Centers for Disease Control and Prevention. (2005). Syringe disposal. Available online: www.cdc.gov/idu/facts/AED_IDU_DIS.pdf. Accessed February 9, 2007.

Food and Drug Administration. *FDA Consumer Magazine.* Available online: www.fda.gov/fdac/default.htm. Accessed February 10, 2007.

Food and Drug Administration. (2003). *Over-the-counter medicines: What's right for you?* Available online: www.fda.gov/cder/consumerinfo/WhatsRightForYou.htm. Accessed February 9, 2007.

Fox, S., & Rainie, L. (2000). *The online health care revolution: How the web helps Americans take better care of themselves.* Pew Internet and American Life Project: Washington, DCAvailable online:www.pewinternet.org/pdfs/PIP_Health_Report.pdf. Accessed February 9, 2007.

Kolpin, D., Furlong, E., Meyer, M., et al. (2002). Pharmaceuticals, hormones, and other organic wastewater contaminants in U.S.

streams, 1999–2000: A national reconnaissance. *Environmental Science and Technology, 36*(6), 1202–1211.

Medical Library Association. (2006). *A user's guide to finding and evaluating health information on the Web.* Available online: www.mlanet.org/resources/userguide.html. Accessed February 9, 2007.

National Center for Complementary and Alternative Medicine. (2002). *Ten things to know about evaluating medical resources on the web.* NCCAM Publication No. D142, February 19.

National Council on Patient Information and Education. (2005). *Ten ways to be Medwise.* Patient Education Pamphlet. Available online: www.bemedwise.org/ten_ways/ten_ways.htm. Accessed February 9, 2007.

PDR for Nonprescription drugs and dietary supplements. (2005). Montvale, NJ: Thomson PDR.

United States Pharmacopeial Convention. (2005). *USPDI: Drug information for the health care professional* (20th ed.). Rockville, MD: Author.

United States Pharmacopeial Convention. (2005). *Advice for the patient.* Rockville, MD: Mack Printing.

Wilcox, C., Cryer, B., and Triadafilopoulos, G. (2005). Patterns of use and public perception of over-the-counter pain relievers: Focus on nonsteroidal antiinflammatory drugs. *Journal of Rheumatology, 32*, 2218–2224.

Winker, M., Flanagan, A., Chi-Lum, B., et al. (2000). Guidelines for medical and health information sites on the Internet. *Journal of the American Medical Association, 283*, 1600–1606.

10

Vitamins and Minerals

There are approximately 50 known essential nutrients, including vitamins, minerals, essential fatty acids, and amino acids. Thirteen vitamins and 16 minerals are considered essential for human health. *Vitamins* are compounds that indirectly assist other nutrients through the processes of digestion, absorption, metabolism, and elimination. Vitamins have the following defining characteristics: they are organic compounds; they are required in minute amounts for growth and maintenance of health; and they do not serve as sources of energy (i.e., compared with carbohydrates, proteins, and fats). *Minerals*, which are found in body fluids, serve a structural function in the body. Supplemental dosages of minerals and trace elements are determined according to the amount needed to maintain body tissues.

UNIVERSAL CONSIDERATIONS

Reference values on vitamin intake are established by the Food and Nutrition Board of the Institute of Medicine (IOM) of the National Academy of Sciences. The purpose is to provide a good standard for nutrition.

From the 1980s until 2005, the basic standard for nutrition in the United States was the recommended dietary allowance (RDA), issued every 5 years by the Food and Nutrition Board and designed to prevent nutrient deficiencies. Computed along with a significant safety factor, RDA was defined as "the levels of intake of essential nutrients that, on the basis of scientific knowledge, are judged by the Food and Nutrition Board to be adequate to meet the known nutrient needs of practically all healthy persons." For vitamins and minerals about which less is known, safe and adequate daily dietary intakes have been estimated.

In 2005, the RDA was added to dietary reference intakes (DRIs). The DRIs are designed to help prevent chronic diseases that are known to have a dietary component. The DRI has four components: estimated average requirement; recommended dietary allowance; adequate intake; and tolerable upper intake level (Box 10-1).

CLASSIFICATION OF VITAMINS

There are two classes of vitamins: fat-soluble and water-soluble. Vitamins A, D, E, and K make up the group of fat-soluble vitamins (Box 10-2). Each fat-soluble vitamin has a distinct and separate physiologic role. For the most part, these vitamins, chemically related to fats, are absorbed along with other lipids. Efficient absorption requires the presence of bile and pancreatic juice. The vitamins are then transported to the liver via the lymphatics as a part of lipoproteins and stored in various body tissues. Vitamins are not normally eliminated in the urine but rather are stored in body fat.

BOX 10-1

Dietary Reference Intakes

- **Estimated average requirement (EAR):** The intake that meets the nutrient needs of 50% of individuals in any life-stage or sex group. Thus, by definition, the EAR will be insufficient for the other 50%. The definition of EAR implies a median as opposed to a mean, or average. EAR serves as the basis for establishing a recommended dietary allowance (RDA).
- **Recommended dietary allowance (RDA):** The average daily intake necessary to meet the nutrient requirements of 97% to 98% of healthy persons in a specific age or sex group. The RDAs only apply to persons in good health. Because RDAs represent average daily intake, low intake on one day can be offset by high intake on another. The RDAs change for men and women with aging; they typically increase for women who become pregnant or who breastfeed. The RDA is set at 2 standard deviations above the EAR to afford adequate nutrient intake within a specific group.
- **Adequate intake (AI):** The AI is an estimate of the average daily intake that meets nutritional needs. AIs are set with the belief that they will meet the needs of all individuals. For example, the AI for calcium is now 1000 to 1300 mg daily, which observation suggests is adequate to prevent osteoporosis in most otherwise healthy persons. Because AIs are estimates, there is no guarantee that they will be sufficient.
- **Tolerable upper intake level (UL):** The highest daily nutrient intake that is likely to pose no risk of adverse health effects for almost all individuals in the general population. Note that the UL is not a recommended upper limit for intake. It is simply an index of safety. As the intake increases above the UL, the potential risk for adverse effects increases.

Vitamin C and members of the vitamin B complex (thiamine, riboflavin, niacin, pyridoxine, pantothenic acid, biotin, folic acid, and cyanocobalamin) make up the water-soluble group of vitamins. Water-soluble vitamins are not stored in appreciable amounts and are normally eliminated in small quantities in the urine. Thus, a daily supply is desirable to avoid depletion and interruption of normal physiologic functions. Most water-soluble vitamins are ingredients of essential enzyme systems. Many support energy metabolism.

FAT-SOLUBLE VITAMINS

These vitamins have very different functions, which are revealed partly through the symptoms of their deficiency and excess states (Table 10-1).

Vitamin A

Vitamin A is a fat-soluble compound responsible for cell division and differentiation, as well as reproduction, vision quality, and bone growth. Because of its function in helping to

---

BOX 10-2

Classification of Vitamins and Minerals

Fat-Soluble Vitamins
- Vitamin A
- Vitamin B
- Vitamin E
- Vitamin D

Water-Soluble Vitamins
- Biotin (vitamin B$_7$)
- Cyanocobalamin (Vitamin B$_{12}$)
- Folic acid (vitamin B$_9$)
- Niacin (vitamin B$_3$)
- Pantothenic acid (vitamin B$_5$)
- Pyridoxine (vitamin B$_6$)
- Riboflavin (vitamin B$_2$)
- Thiamine (vitamin B$_1$)
- Vitamin B complex
- Vitamin C

Macrominerals
- Calcium
- Chloride
- Magnesium
- Phosphorus
- Potassium
- Selenium
- Silicon
- Sodium
- Zinc

Microminerals
- Chromium
- Cobalt
- Copper
- Fluoride
- Iodine
- Iron
- Manganese
- Vanadium

---

and gastrointestinal tracts. Infection develops when the endothelial linings of these structures are damaged.

Indications

The only indication for vitamin A supplementation is prevention or correction of vitamin A deficiency. It was once thought to enhance resistance to carcinogenesis, possibly by destabilizing lysosomes or enhancing antitumor immunity, or through direct cytotoxic action on abnormal cells. However, it is now clear that vitamin A in the form of beta-carotene supplements does not decrease the risk of cancer or cardiovascular disease. In fact, there is some evidence that persons taking combination vitamin A or beta-carotene supplements have a significantly higher risk of lung cancer and overall mortality. Certain derivatives of vitamin A (e.g., isotretinoin, etretinate) are used topically to treat acne and other dermatologic disorders.

Pharmacodynamics and Pharmacokinetics

Vitamin A has been named *retinol* in reference to its specific function in the retina of the eye. It plays an important role in embryogenesis, spermatogenesis, immunity, growth and development of skeletal and soft tissues, maintenance of the structural and functional integrity of the skin and mucous membranes, and adaptation to dim light. Its effect on protein synthesis and bone cell differentiation makes it necessary for the development of bone, and, through the enamel-forming epithelial cells, it plays a role in the development of teeth. Vitamin A may also play a part in cell membrane regulation as an enzyme cofactor in steroid and mucopolysaccharide synthesis, essential in growth and reproduction. Food sources of vitamin A are identified in Box 10-3.

Beta-carotene is responsible for the deep orange and yellow colors in many fruits and vegetables. These provitamin *carotenoids* are converted to vitamin A with varying degrees of efficiency. They are described in terms of beta-*carotene*. Beta-carotene is split in the cytoplasm of the intestinal mucosal cells into retinyl esters, which are transported via the lymph system to the circulation and then to the liver as a part of chylomicrons and lipoproteins. Retinol-binding protein combines with retinol at the time of mobilization from the liver. The esters are removed from the circulation by the kidneys.

maintain skin integrity, it provides the first line of defense against bacteria and viruses. It also helps regulate the immune system by increasing the production of white blood cells. Vitamin A maintains the retina and the respiratory, urinary,

---

TABLE 10-1 Deficiency and Excess States of Fat-Soluble Vitamins

	Signs and Symptoms of Deficiency States	Signs and Symptoms of Excess States
Vitamin A	Night blindness, xerophthalmia, keratomalacia, blindness (if severe) Dry, scaly skin Deterioration of epithelial tissues Growth retardation Reduced numbers of T cells	Headache, vertigo, blurry vision, bulging fontanelle, seizures Fatigue Anorexia, nausea, vomiting Bone pain Yellowing of skin
Vitamin D	Bone pain Osteomalacia in adults Rickets in children	Weakness, fatigue, lassitude Headache Nausea, vomiting, diarrhea Renal impairment, hypertension
Vitamin E	Nerve degeneration hands and/or feet Lowered lymphocyte count	Headache, blurry vision, fatigue Diarrhea Risk of bleeding
Vitamin K	Petechiae, ecchymosis Hemarthrosis, hematuria Hematemesis, gastrointestinal bleeding	Kernicterus Risk for clots

BOX 10-3

Dietary Sources of Nutrients

Vitamin A
Preformed vitamin A occurs only in foods of animal origin, either in storage areas such as the liver or in association with fat. Rich sources of vitamin A include liver, kidney, fish, liver oils, cream, butter, whole milk, whole-milk cheese, fortified margarine, skim milk, and skim-milk products. Vitamin A precursors (carotinoids) are found in dark green leafy vegetables and red-yellow-orange fruits and vegetables. Deeper colors are associated with higher levels of carotinoids.

Vitamin D
Cholecalciferol (D_3) is found in animal products (e.g., herring, salmon, sardines, shrimp, fish liver oils). Cholecalciferol is also formed in the body when the skin is exposed to sunlight. Vitamin D is found in variable amounts in butter, cream, egg yolks, and liver. Most milk is fortified with 10 mcg/quart of irradiated ergosterol (D_2). Powdered and evaporated milk are also fortified, as are some margarines, butter, certain cheeses, and infant formula. Milk used to make cheese or yogurt may not be fortified.

Vitamin E
Seed oils such as wheat germ oils, corn oil, soybean oil, and sunflower oil are the richest source of vitamin E. Smaller amounts are present in fruits, vegetables, and animal fats. Peanut oil, coconut oil, and fish oils are poor sources of vitamin E.

Vitamin K
Good sources of vitamin K include dark green or leafy vegetables such as kale, turnip greens, spinach, broccoli, cabbage, and lettuce. Cauliflower, tomatoes, fruits, cereals, wheat bran, cheese, egg yolks, and liver contain smaller amounts. Significant amounts of vitamin K are formed by the bacterial flora of the gastrointestinal (GI) tract.

Ascorbic Acid (Vitamin C)
Good sources of ascorbic acid are fresh citrus fruits, leafy vegetables eaten raw, tomatoes, strawberries, cantaloupe, cabbage, green peppers, and potatoes. The ascorbic acid content of fruits and vegetables varies with the conditions under which they are grown and the degree of ripeness when harvested. Refrigeration and quick freezing help retain the vitamin.

Thiamine (B_1)
Dietary sources of thiamine include organ meats, legumes, nuts, whole or enriched grain products, wheat germ, and brewer's yeast.

Riboflavin (B_2)
Dietary sources of riboflavin are milk and milk products, cheddar cheese, cottage cheese, organ meats, eggs, and leafy green vegetables. When flour is milled, 60% of riboflavin is lost; thus most breads and cereals are enriched with riboflavin.

Niacin (B_3)
Niacin is found in meats, legumes, nuts, peanut butter, and whole-grain and enriched-grain products. Tryptophan, a niacin precursor, is also found in protein foods of animal origin.

Pantothenic Acid (B_5)
Good sources of pantothenic acid include liver, kidney, salmon, eggs, legumes, peanuts, whole grains, milk, fruits, vegetables, molasses, and yeast. Much of the pantothenate in meat is lost during thawing and cooking. About half of the pantothenic acid contained in flour is lost in the milling process.

Pyridoxine (B_6)
Pyridoxine is found in meat (especially liver), fish, egg yolks, legumes, nuts, potatoes, whole grains, wheat germ, yeast, prunes, raisins, and bananas.

Biotin (B_7)
Good sources of biotin include liver, kidneys, egg yolk, soybeans, yeast, milk, fish, nuts, and oatmeal. Biotin is also synthesized in considerable amounts by intestinal bacteria.

Folic Acid (B_9)
Good sources of folic acid include liver, kidney beans, lima beans, fresh and dark green leafy vegetables, broccoli, asparagus, spinach, orange juice, white bread, dried beans, and ready-to-eat cereals. Small quantities of folic acid are found in milk, eggs, fruits (except oranges), root vegetables, and most meats. Only 25% to 50% of dietary folic acid is nutritionally available, but intestinal bacteria synthesize large amounts, which add to the daily intake.

Cyanocobalamin (B_{12})
Cyanocobalamin is found in liver, kidney, milk, eggs, fish, cheese, and muscle meats. Some cooked sea vegetables contain cobalamin in the same concentration as beef liver. Well over half of cyanocobalamin (40% to 90%) is lost during pasteurization and evaporation.

The effects of beta-carotene are somewhat different from those of vitamin A. Beta-carotene inactivates single oxygen molecules, which is what makes it an *antioxidant*. It is believed that the protective antioxidant function is carried out by the intact beta-carotene molecule rather than its vitamin A form.

Under normal circumstances, dietary vitamin A is readily absorbed, and 90% is stored in the liver. The remainder is deposited in fat, the lungs, and the kidneys. Hepatic storage of vitamin A peaks in adult life, allowing for a temporarily reduced intake of vitamin A with no significant impact on body functioning. In the absence of vitamin A intake, levels are maintained through mobilization of liver reserves.

▥ *Requirements*
The RDAs for vitamin A were revised in 2002. The new RDAs are slightly lower than the previous ones, which were established in 1989. The new RDAs are recorded in retinol activity equivalents (RAEs), the unit employed to measure vitamin A activity (Table 10-2).

▥ *Deficiency States*
Vitamin A deficiency is generally associated with malnutrition and infectious disease. In almost every infectious disease, vitamin A deficiency is known to occur in greater frequency and severity, and with an increased incidence of mortality. Vitamin A deficiency results in night blindness, xerophthalmia (a dry, thickened condition of the conjunctiva), and keratomalacia (corneal degeneration with keratinization of the epithelium). When the deficiency is severe, blindness may occur (Table 10-1).

Vitamin A deficiency causes characteristic changes in skin texture in which blockage of the hair follicles with plugs of keratin causes the skin to become dry, scaly, and rough, with goose flesh. The changes are first noted on the forearms and the thighs, but in advanced states, the whole body can be involved.

Without vitamin A, the protective barrier of mucous membranes is lost. There is a shrinking, hardening, and progressive deterioration of epithelial tissues and reduced resistance to

DOSAGE
TABLE **10-2** Fat-Soluble Vitamins

Vitamin	Primary and Secondary Prevention*	Toxicity Levels	Comments
Vitamin A	RDAs: Males: 900 RAEs/day Females: 700 RAEs/day	UL: 3000 mcg/day Highly teratogenic during third trimester of pregnancy	1 RAE = 1 mcg of retinol; 12 mcg beta-carotene; 24 mcg α-carotene
Vitamin D	AI: Birth to 50 yr: 5 mcg/day Age 51–70 yr:10 mcg/day Age >71 yr: 15 mcg/day	Not yet determined	1 mcg vitamin D = 40 international units
Vitamin E	RDAs: Age 1–3 yr: 6 mg/day Age: 4–8 yr: 7 mg/day Age 9–13 yr: 11 mg/day Ages >14: 15 mg/day Pregnancy: 15 mg/day Lactation: 19 mg/day	ULs: Age 1–3 yr: 200 mg/day Age 4–8 yr: 300 mg/day Age 9–13 yr: 600 mg/day Age 14–18 yr: 800 mg/day Ages >19 yr: 1000 mg/day Pregnancy, lactation: 1000 mg/day	1.5 international unit = 1 mg of any form of alpha-tocopherol
Vitamin K (phytonadione; vitamin K$_1$)	AI: 10 mg subQ or IM –or– 2.5 to 15 mg/24 hr	Unusual from dietary intake alone	May increase bilirubin levels and risk of kernicterus; risk greater in premature infants

*AI, Acceptable intake; RAEs, retinol activity equivalents; RDAs, recommended daily allowances; subQ, subcutaneously; UL, tolerable upper intake level.

invasion by bacteria, viruses, or parasites. The lack of vitamin A will also reduce the number of circulating T cells as well as their response.

An overgrowth of bone with resultant nerve lesions and growth retardation can occur. The growth retardation is characterized by osteoplastosis, impaired protein synthesis, and loss of appetite.

▌ Excess States

Acute toxicity is associated with single doses of retinol of more than 20,000 to 25,000 mcg in adults; lower dosages produce toxicity in children (i.e., 10,000 mcg). Symptoms include headache, fatigue, weakness, anorexia, nausea, and vomiting. Cerebrospinal fluid pressure increases and may contribute to vertigo, blurred vision, and muscular incoordination. Symptoms disappear weeks or months after the supplement is discontinued.

Chronic hypervitaminosis A in adults occurs when intake exceeds 30,000 mcg daily for several months. Symptoms often include liver toxicity, gastrointestinal discomfort, vomiting, seizures, dry skin, increased intracranial pressure, bone pain, and yellow patches on skin. In females, too much vitamin A can increase the risk of osteoporosis and hip fracture (apparently by blocking the ability of vitamin A to enhance calcium absorption). In children, excess vitamin A may cause bulging of the skull at sites where bone has not yet formed. A bulging fontanelle may be seen in infants. Vitamin A is highly teratogenic during the third trimester of pregnancy; congenital malformations are likely to develop in fetuses exposed to high levels.

Vitamin D

Vitamin D promotes the absorption of calcium and phosphorous, thus helping to form and maintain bone strength. Vitamin D may help maintain a healthy immune system and regulate cell growth and differentiation, the process that determines what a cell is to become. The pharmacology and physiology of vitamin D are discussed in more depth in Chapter 54 in the context of calcium requirements and osteoporosis.

Figure 10-1 illustrates the relationship between vitamin D and calcium.

▌ Requirements

According to the IOM there is insufficient scientific information to establish an RDA for vitamin D. The recommended adequate intake (AI) of vitamin D is that which maintains normal calcium metabolism and bone health (see Table 10-2).

Supplemental vitamin D is not required except for persons who are chronically shielded from sunlight. These are persons who are homebound, who live in sunless areas with high atmospheric pollution, who wear clothing that completely covers the body, or who work at night and stay indoors during the day. Circumstances that require long submarine voyages and living in the Antarctic necessitate a small daily supplement of vitamin D.

▌ Deficiency States

Exposure to ultraviolet (UV) light from the sun triggers vitamin D synthesis in skin. Sunlight exposure from November through February is insufficient to produce significant vitamin D synthesis; however, a twice-weekly exposure (to the face, the arms, the hands, or the back) lasting 10 to 15 minutes without sunscreen is usually enough to provide for the body's requirement of vitamin D. Sunscreen that has a sun protection factor (SPF) over 8 should be used for exposures of longer duration; sunscreen blocks UV rays. Regular use helps reduce the risk for skin cancer and other skin changes associated with excessive sun exposure. Factors affecting UV exposure and therefore the synthesis of vitamin D include the season, geographic latitude, time of day, cloud cover, smog, and use of sunscreen. Complete cloud cover halves the energy of UV rays, and shade reduces it by 60%. Industrial pollution, which increases shade, also decreases sun exposure and may contribute to the development of rickets.

Bones become thin, brittle, or misshapen in the absence of vitamin D. The deficiency, in turn, leads to low serum calcium levels and stimulation of parathyroid hormone (PTH).

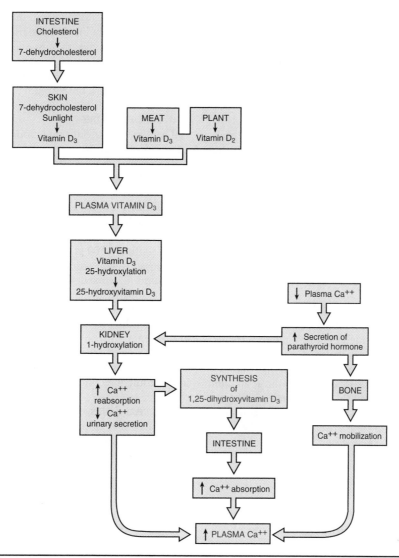

FIGURE 10-1 Vitamin D and Calcium Interactions. Vitamin D is converted in the liver to 25-hydroxyvitamin D_3 (25 [OH] D_3) and to 1,25-dihydroxyvitamin D_3 in the kidneys. Regulation of plasma calcium concentration is controlled by vitamin D and parathyroid hormone (PTH). Vitamin D and PTH regulate plasma calcium concentration by acting on the intestines, kidneys, and bone. (Adapted from Page, C., Curtis, M., Sutter, M., et al. (1997). *Integrated pharmacology* [pp. 496–497]. St. Louis: Mosby. Used with permission.)

Elevated PTH secretion raises serum calcium levels by moving calcium from the bone into serum. In adults, this movement manifests as *osteomalacia*, a condition characterized by decreased bone density and strength. Osteomalacia is more likely to occur during times of increased need for calcium, such as during pregnancy and lactation. In children, this sequence of events produces inadequate mineralization of bones, a condition known as *rickets*. Rachitic bones are unable to withstand ordinary stresses and strains, resulting in the appearance of bowlegs, knock knees, pigeon breasts, and frontal bossing of the skull. Because of vitamin D fortification of foods, rickets is now rare in the United States.

▮ Excess States

Acute *hypervitaminosis D* results from high dosage or prolonged administration of vitamin D. Hypervitaminosis D produces signs and symptoms of hypercalcemia including weakness, fatigue, lassitude, headache, nausea, vomiting, diarrhea, renal impairment, and hypertension. Calcification of soft tissues develops and is most dangerous to the kidneys. High serum calcium is serious in patients with heart failure who are taking digoxin because calcium excess increases the risk of digoxin toxicity. Vitamin D excess may also cause growth retardation for up to 6 months, with the result of permanent stunting. The first step in the treatment of vitamin D excess is to stop the intake.

Vitamin E

Each of the eight forms of vitamin E has its own biologic activity. For example, alpha tocopherol (α-tocopherol) acetate has strong antioxidant activity. The synthetic formulation is labeled "D, L" whereas the natural formulation, which is twice as active as the synthetic formulation, is labeled as "D."

Indications

Vitamin E has both antioxidant properties and properties related to immune-system integrity. Vitamin E appears to prevent cellular and subcellular membranes from deteriorating by scavenging oxygen-containing free radicals (see Box 10-4). The scavenging prevents free radicals from catalyzing peroxidation of the polyunsaturated fatty acids (PUFAs) that constitute structural components of cells. The destruction leads to abnormal cell structure and compromised function. The ability of vitamin E to circumvent such destruction led to the notion that the vitamin may be useful in preventing free radical destruction associated with various disorders (e.g., aging, the effects of environmental toxins, some forms of carcinogenesis).

Some health care providers believe that vitamin E helps reduce menopausal symptoms such as hot flashes, vaginal dryness, and shrinkage. The antioxidant properties of vitamin E have been associated with the healing of chronic resistant dermatitis of the hands.

Pharmacodynamics and Pharmacokinetics

Vitamin E activity in foods is contributed by the *tocopherols* (alpha, beta, tau, delta) and the tocotrienols. Vitamin E resides inside low-density lipoprotein particles that prevent renal elimination of vitamin molecules, and disarms free radicals from within. This activity explains its characteristic as an *antioxidant*. The absorption of vitamin E is inefficient, ranging from 20% to 80%. Vitamin E is stored in the liver and, to a larger extent, in fatty tissues. It is metabolized in the liver, entering the enterohepatic circulation. The metabolites are eventually eliminated in both the urine and feces.

Requirements

In 2000 the RDAs for vitamin E were revised by the Food and Nutrition Board of the IOM to set a tolerable upper level (UL) of intake for any formulation of alpha-tocopherol

---

BOX 10-4

Conditions Thought to be Mediated by Free Radical Damage

Arteriosclerosis	Liver cirrhosis
Autoimmune diseases	Myocardial infarction
Cancer	Nephrotoxicity
Cataracts associated with diabetes	Nutrient deficiencies
Chronic airway limitation	Parkinson's disease
Contact dermatitis	Premature aging
Drug toxicity	Premature retinopathy
Emphysema	Senile dementia and neurologic degeneration
Hypertensive cerebrovascular injury	Thermal injuries
Immune deficiency of aging	Viral infection (including AIDs)
Inflammatory bowel disease	*AIDS,* Acquired immunodeficiency syndrome.
Iron overload disease	

Adapted from Joseph Pizzorno. (1996). *Total Wellness.* Rocklin, CA: Prima. Copyright © 1996 by Joseph Pizzorno. Buy or order at better bookstores or call 800–632–8676 or visit URL: www.primapublishing.com. Used with permission.

(see Table 10-2). Because vitamin E can also act as an anticoagulant and thus may increase the risk of bleeding, the UL is set at the highest dosage that is unlikely to result in bleeding problems.

Breast milk contains a sufficient amount of vitamin E to meet the needs of a breastfeeding infant.

Deficiency States

There are five specific situations in which there is risk of a vitamin E deficiency:

1. Persons who are unable to secrete bile (and therefore unable to absorb dietary fat)
2. Persons who have rare disorders of fat metabolism
3. Persons who have a rare genetic abnormality in the alpha-tocopherol transfer protein (e.g., abetalipoproteinemia)
4. Premature, very low–birth weight infants (birth weights less than 1500 grams or 3 lbs, 4 oz)
5. Persons with a documented zinc deficiency

Vitamin E deficiency is usually characterized by ataxia, sensory neuropathy of hands and feet, and muscle hypertrophy. A deficiency of vitamin E also lowers host resistance by depressing the proliferation of lymphocytes and lowering the antibody response to pathogens, and lowers delayed hypersensitivity reactions. These responses may also have an impact on the immunologic response to cancers, helminthic infestations, and chronic infections.

Excess States

The risk of vitamin E toxicity is fairly low, even at relatively high levels. However, excessive vitamin E may increase the risk of bleeding. It suppresses coagulation and increases prothrombin time and can cause hemorrhage, but at very high dosages (e.g., 500 mg/kg/day). Further, vitamin E–induced bleeding can be controlled by vitamin K, which promotes synthesis of clotting factors.

Signs and symptoms of vitamin E excess include headache, fatigue, blurred vision, and diarrhea. Vitamin E toxicity in preterm infants is characterized by respiratory distress, renal failure, liver disease, ascites, and thrombocytopenia.

Vitamin K

Vitamin K functions as a lipid cofactor in the formation of prothrombin (factor II), proconvertin (factor VII), plasma thromboplastin component (factor IX), and Stuart factor (factor X) in the liver. The cascade theory of blood coagulation is noted in Chapter 39. Vitamin K may also participate in oxidative phosphorylation in the tissues.

Indications

Vitamin K supplementation has two primary indications: (1) the correction or prevention of hypoprothrombinemia and bleeding caused by vitamin K deficiency, and (2) control of hemorrhage caused by overdose with oral anticoagulant, such as warfarin sodium.

Pharmacodynamics and Pharmacokinetics

Vitamin K occurs naturally in two forms: phytonadione (vitamin K_1), which is found in green plants, and menaquinone (vitamin K_2), which is formed as the result of bacterial action in the intestinal tract. Phytonadione and menaquinone are available in water-soluble formulations. Two other forms of vitamin K are produced synthetically: menadiol (vitamin K_4) and the fat-soluble synthetic formulation menadione (vitamin K_3), which is twice as potent as primary food sources of vitamin K_3.

Vitamin K is only absorbed from the upper intestine in the presence of bile and dietary fats. It is incorporated into chylomicrons and lipoproteins, and carried to the liver. Menadiol and menadione do not require bile salts for absorption. None of the forms of vitamin K are stored in large quantities in the body. Vitamin K is metabolized in the liver and eliminated in the urine and feces.

Requirements

Vitamin K requirements have not been precisely defined. In 2002, the Food and Nutrition Board set the dietary AI for adult males at 120 mcg, and for adult females at 90 mcg (see Table 10-2). For most individuals, vitamin K requirements are readily met through dietary sources and through vitamin K synthesis by intestinal bacteria. Vitamin K levels may be low during the immediate postnatal period since bacterial colonization of the gut is not complete until several days after birth.

Deficiency States

Vitamin K deficiency is usually associated with inadequate intake or absorption. Deficiency is common in newborns owing to the lack of dietary intake of vitamin K and the lack of intestinal synthesis of the vitamin during the first week of life. After infancy, deficiency usually results from diseases that interfere with absorption (e.g., biliary tract and gastrointestinal [GI] disorders); in persons who consume large quantities of alcohol, deficiency is related to decreased intake and impaired use. Drug-induced deficiency develops with use of oral anticoagulants or other drugs that act as vitamin K antagonists. Although rare, vitamin K deficiency is also possible as the result of long-term antibiotic use because antibiotics reduce the synthesis of bacteria in the intestine. The signs and symptoms of vitamin K deficiency include petechiae, ecchymosis, bleeding into the joints or muscles, hematemesis, hematuria, GI bleeding, asthenia, and hypovolemic shock.

Excess States

An excess of vitamin K from dietary intake is unlikely to occur. The prothrombin time (PT) and international normalized ratio (INR) values will take 2 to 3 weeks to return to the desired range when a patient has an excess of vitamin K. Excessive amounts of synthetic vitamin K produce kernicterus in an infant. Elevated plasma levels of vitamin K are also seen in patients with hypertriglyceridemia. The water-miscible forms of vitamin K have a much wider margin of safety.

WATER-SOLUBLE VITAMINS

Thiamine

History and Uses

The only indication for thiamine (vitamin B_1) supplementation is treatment and prevention of thiamine deficiency. The active form of thiamine is an essential coenzyme for carbohydrate metabolism. The "antineuritic" vitamin was identified in 1897, but it was not until 1936 that the chemical formula was identified and the vitamin synthesized. The name *thiamine* designates the presence of sulfur and an amino group in the complex molecule.

Pharmacodynamics and Pharmacokinetics

Thiamine, in either its pyrophosphate or triphosphate form, functions as a coenzyme essential for the metabolism of fats, proteins, and nucleic acids; it is most strongly associated with the oxidative decarboxylation of pyruvate, which is involved only with carbohydrate metabolism. Without thiamine triphosphate, pyruvate cannot enter the Krebs cycle, and energy deprivation results. In addition, the triphosphate form is also involved in the oxidative decarboxylation of alpha-keto acids derived from the amino acids methionine, threonine, leucine, isoleucine, and valine. Thiamine triphosphate also functions as an alternate pathway for glucose oxidation. It plays a role in the transmission of impulses on nerve membranes, possibly by promoting sodium influx.

Thiamine is well absorbed from the GI tract and widely distributed to body tissues. It crosses the intestinal membranes by active transport systems in specific areas of the small intestine. Plasma protein binding is minimal. Thiamine is stored to various degrees in the liver and eliminated through the kidneys.

Requirements

Because of the close relationship between thiamine and energy production, the RDA is based on caloric intake (Table 10-3). The RDA for children, adolescents, and adults is 0.5 mg/1000 kcal, with a minimum of 1 mg/day regardless of total intake.

Deficiency States

Thiamine deficiencies are rare in the United States. Severe thiamine deficiency causes beriberi, of which there are two forms. *Wet beriberi* is precipitated by a high carbohydrate intake, along with strenuous physical exertion. It is so named because its primary symptom is fluid accumulation in the legs. Cardiovascular complications of wet beriberi such as palpitations and arrhythmias and high-output heart failure are common and can progress rapidly to circulatory collapse and death. Wet beriberi responds rapidly and dramatically to thiamine replacement therapy. *Dry beriberi* is associated with muscular wasting, energy deprivation, inactivity, and peripheral neuropathy with paralysis of the lower extremities. Recovery can be very slow.

Infantile beriberi, although rare, has been identified in infants fed unusual formulas without adequate thiamine supplementation. Sudden deterioration of the infant occurs accompanied by cyanosis and heart failure.

Alcohol-related thiamine deficiency *(Wernicke-Korsakoff syndrome)* is the third most common cause of dementia in the United States. Wernicke-Korsakoff syndrome is a serious disorder of the central nervous system (CNS) that has neurologic and psychologic manifestations including nystagmus, diplopia, ataxia, and a loss of short-term memory. Immediate parenteral administration of thiamine helps reduce the risk of irreversible brain damage. A deficiency of thiamine also leads to a reduced production of antibodies and increases the risk for infection.

DOSAGE
TABLE **10-3** Water-Soluble Vitamins*

Vitamin	Primary Prevention	Correction of Deficiency	Comments
Thiamine (B₁)	*RDA:* 0.5 mg/1000 kcal with a minimum of 1 mg/day regardless of total intake	*Adults:* 5-10 mg PO 3 times daily –or– 5–100 mg IM or IV 3 times daily *Child:* 10–50 mg PO in divided doses –or– 10–25 mg/day IM or IV	Parenteral administration of higher dosages is reserved for severe deficiency (wet and dry beriberi, Wernicke-Korsakoff syndrome).
Riboflavin (B₂)	*RDA:* 0.4–1.8 mg daily PO	*Adult:* 5–30 mg PO daily in divided doses for several days, then 1–4 mg/day *Child >12 yr:* 3–10 mg/day for several days, then 0.6 mg/1000 calories ingested	Requirements are increased during pregnancy and lactation.
Niacin (B₃)	*RDA:* 10–20 mg daily PO	*Adults:* Up to 500 mg PO daily –or– 50–100 mg IM or subQ 5 or more times daily –or– 25–100 mg IV 2 or more times daily *Child:* To 300 mg PO daily in divided doses	Niacin activity is noted in niacin equivalents (NE). 1 mg of niacin or 60 mg of tryptophan = 1 NE. The nicotinamide formulation is preferred.
Pantothenic acid (B₅)	*RDA:* 4–7 mg/day	None identified	A deficiency is unlikely because of the widespread distribution of the vitamin in foods.
Pyridoxine (B₆)	*Adults:* 2–10 mg daily *Infants <6 mo:* 0.3 mg/day *Infants >6 mo:* 0.6 mg/day should be given to older infants	*Drug-induced deficiency:* 50–200 mg PO, IV, or IM daily for 3 weeks, then 25–100 mg/day *Chronic alcoholism:* 50 mg PO daily for 2–4 weeks *Pyridoxine-dependency syndrome:* 30–600 mg/day IM or IV initially, then 50 mg/day PO for life *Isoniazid overdose (>10 grams):* Amount in mg equal to amount of isoniazid ingested; give 4 grams IV, then 1 gram IM every 30 minutes	A pyridoxine dose of 0.016 mg parallels the intake of 6 grams of protein. Vitamin may be continued indefinitely as long as high dosages are not used.
Biotin (B₇)	*AI:* 30–100 mcg/day	None identified	Data are insufficient at this time to establish RDAs for this vitamin.
Folic acid (B₉)	*RDA:* 400 mcg/day	*UL:* *Adults:* 1000 mcg PO daily *Pregnancy:* 800 mg PO daily	1 mcg folate = 0.6 mcg dietary folate equivalent (DFE) from supplements and fortified foods
Cyanocobalamin (B₁₂)	*RDA:* *Adults:* 0.9–2.4 mcg/day based on age *Infants:* 0.4–0.5 mcg/day	*Adults:* 1–25 mcg/day PO to 100 mcg daily –or– 30 mcg/day IM or subQ for 6–7 days, then 100–200 mcg/month. Doses up to 1000 mcg have been used.	Hydroxocobalamin is better absorbed than cyanocobalamin; it is better absorbed from the GI tract since it does not require intrinsic factor and calcium.
Ascorbic acid (Vitamin C)	50–100 mg/day	*Adults:* 100–250 mg PO, IV, IM, or subQ 1–3 times daily *Child:* 100–300 mg PO, IV, IM, or subQ daily in divided doses	100 mg is recommended for smokers as primary prevention.

*Specific treatment recommendations.
AI, Acceptable intake; *GI,* gastrointestinal; *IM,* intramuscular (route); *IV,* intravenous (route); *PO,* by mouth; *RDAs,* recommended daily allowances; *subQ,* subcutaneously; *UL,* tolerable upper intake level.

▓ Excess States
There are no known toxic effects from thiamine.

Riboflavin

▓ History and Uses
The biologic significance of a yellow-green fluorescent pigment in milk, recognized in 1879 was first understood in 1932. The vitamin was synthesized and named *riboflavin (B₂)* in 1935. Very little is lost in the cooking and processing of foods; however, because it is sensitive to alkali, the common practice of adding baking soda to soften dried peas or beans destroys much of the riboflavin content. Wax-lined paper containers protect milk against riboflavin loss from exposure to sunlight. It may function in the production of corticosteroids and red blood cells, as well as in gluconeogenesis.

▓ Pharmacodynamics and Pharmacokinetics
Riboflavin participates in a number of enzymatic reactions, but in order to do so, it must be converted to one or two active forms: flavin mononucleotide and flavin adenine dinucleotide. It is essential for the completion of several reactions in the energy cycle that produces adenosine triphosphate

(ATP). It is also a component of amino acid oxidases and xanthine oxidase, which are involved in the oxidation of amino acids and hydroxyl acids to alpha-keto acids, and the oxidation of a number of purines.

Riboflavin is well absorbed from the proximal small intestine in the presence of food. Plasma protein binding is minimal. Although riboflavin is stored in small amounts in the liver and kidney, the quantities stored are not sufficient to meet all of the body's needs. Thus riboflavin must be regularly supplied in the diet. Riboflavin is metabolized in the liver to variable degrees and eliminated in the urine, depending on the intake and relative need of the tissues for the vitamin.

▓ Requirements
Riboflavin requirements are based on the amount required to maintain tissue reserves, as well as on urinary elimination, red blood cell riboflavin levels, and erythrocyte glutathione reductase activity (see Table 10-3). Requirements are increased during pregnancy and lactation.

▓ Deficiency States
Riboflavin deficiencies usually occur in combination with deficiencies of other water-soluble vitamins. The deficiency

must exist for several months for signs and symptoms of riboflavin deficiency to appear. Early signs of *ariboflavinosis* include photophobia, lacrimation, burning and itching of the eyes, capillary overgrowth around the cornea, glossitis, angular stomatitis (cracks in the corners of the mouth), and cheilosis (fissuring of the lips). Seborrheic dermatitis, a greasy eruption of the skin in the nasolabial folds, scrotum, or vulva, may appear.

Excess States
There are no known toxic effects for riboflavin.

Niacin

History and Uses
Niacin was identified as a result of the search for the cause and cure of *pellagra*, a disease common in Spain and Italy in the eighteenth century. Recognition of pellagra as a niacin deficiency followed a discovery in 1937 that the pellagrous disease of black tongue in dogs was caused by lack of niacin. Since then it has been established that tryptophan is a precursor of niacin, and tryptophan deficiency is also involved in pellagra. Niacin has been found to reduce migraine headaches, the dizziness of Meniere's disease, and the symptoms of Raynaud's phenomenon to reduce triglyceride levels.

Pharmacodynamics and Pharmacokinetics
Niacin (vitamin B_3) is the generic term for nicotinamide (niacinamide) and nicotinic acid. It is obtained from food and through endogenous synthesis from tryptophan. Niacin is essential for glycolysis, fat synthesis, and tissue respiration. It functions as a coenzyme in many metabolic processes after being converted to nicotinamide, the physiologically active form. Large doses of niacin decrease lipoprotein and triglyceride synthesis by inhibiting the release of free fatty acids from adipose tissue and decreasing hepatic lipoprotein synthesis. It lowers total cholesterol and raises high-density lipoprotein levels (see also Chapter 38). Because niacin is easily converted to niacinamide, it is frequently used therapeutically in that form to avoid the vasodilating effect of nicotinic acid.

The timed-release form of niacin helps reduce hypoglycemic symptoms, especially during withdrawal from sugar. It can also lower blood pressure and improve circulation by dilating blood vessels. Because of this action, some persons experience flushing of the skin similar to that produced by an allergic reaction. This flushing is not harmful and usually disappears within 15 to 20 minutes. However, timed-release niacin must be used with caution because it can cause elevation of liver enzymes, and on rare occasions, it can cause hepatitis in a sensitive individual. Another form of niacin is inositol hexaniacinate, which causes no flushing, liver problems, uric acid elevations, or histamine-induced gastric acid release. It has the same cholesterol-lowering capacity as regular niacin.

The absorption of niacin takes place in the small intestine. Only a small amount of niacin is stored in the body. Excess niacin is eliminated through the kidneys in the urine.

Requirements
Niacin activity is expressed in niacin equivalents (NEs). One mg of niacin or 60 mg of tryptophan equals 1 NE (see Table 10-3). Nicotinamide is the preferred drug, because it is less likely to cause the unpleasant flushing and burning sensations that accompany nicotinic acid therapy.

Deficiency States
Niacin deficiency is most common in persons who have severely inadequate diets with very little protein. Early niacin deficiency manifests as muscular weakness, anorexia, indigestion, and skin eruptions. Severe niacin deficiency leads to pellagra, which is characterized by skin eruptions, dementia, diarrhea, tremors, and sore tongue. The skin is cracked and pigmented, and scaly dermatitis is present in the areas that are exposed to sunlight. Lesions of the CNS lead to confusion, hallucinations, disorientation, and impairment of peripheral motor and sensory nerves. Inflammation of the mucous membranes of the GI tract causes digestive abnormalities. Patient response to treatment becomes observable within 24 hours. In some cases, the CNS manifestations of the deficiency may never respond, most likely because of a previous prolonged state of malnutrition.

Excess States
The large doses of niacin (2 to 6 grams daily) used to treat types I and II hyperlipidemia result in transient flushing, headache, cramps, and nausea and vomiting, as well as increased blood sugar and uric acid levels (see Chapter 38 for more information). Liver function tests reflect hepatic response to excess niacin.

Pantothenic Acid

History and Uses
Pantothenic acid (B_5) is a constituent of acetyl coenzyme A, and as such it is essential to many areas of cellular metabolism. It is present in all plant and animal tissue, hence its name, meaning "widespread."

Pharmacodynamics and Pharmacokinetics
Pantothenic acid is needed to restore normal adrenal function, which can become depleted in times of stress. As a vital constituent of acetyl coenzyme A, it is involved in the release of energy from carbohydrates and in the degradation and metabolism of fatty acids. In addition to functioning in the citric acid cycle, it is involved in the synthesis of cholesterol, phospholipids, steroid hormones, and porphyrin for hemoglobin and choline.

Pantothenic acid is readily absorbed from the GI tract and widely distributed to all tissues. Pantothenic acid is apparently not degraded in the body since the intake and elimination of the vitamin are approximately equal. Approximately 70% of absorbed pantothenic acid is eliminated in the urine.

Requirements
A daily intake of 4 to 7 mg of pantothenic acid is usually adequate (see Table 10-3). A higher intake may be needed in

pregnant or lactating women. The average intake of pantothenic acid in the American diet ranges from 5 to 20 mg/day.

Deficiency States

Because pantothenic acid is so widespread in foods, no deficiency state has been observed. However, a deficiency can lead to depression, fatigue, and insomnia.

Excess States

No serious toxic effects of pantothenic acid are known. However, ingestion of large amounts can cause diarrhea.

Pyridoxine

History and Uses

Pyridoxine (B_6) was identified as a fraction of the vitamin B complex in 1938 and synthesized in 1939. The term vitamin B_6 designates this entire complex of closely related chemical compounds. Pyridoxine is indicated for prevention and treatment of all vitamin B_6 deficiency states (i.e., dietary deficiency, isoniazid-induced deficiency, pyridoxine dependency syndrome).

Pharmacodynamics and Pharmacokinetics

Pyridoxine has three interchangeable forms (pyridoxine, pyridoxal, and pyridoxamine) that serve as coenzymes in many metabolic functions. These three forms convert to the coenzyme pyridoxal phosphate (PLP). The functions of pyridoxine include decarboxylation, transamination, transulfuration, and the conversion of tryptophan to niacin. It is required for glycogenolysis, the synthesis of hemoglobin, and the formation of antibodies. The formation of sphingolipids involved in the development of the myelin sheath surrounding nerve cells is also pyridoxine-dependent. Pyridoxine may also be required for the conversion of linoleic acid to arachidonic acid, as well as for the formation and regulation of neurotransmitters such as epinephrine, norepinephrine, tyramine, dopamine, serotonin, and gamma-aminobutyric acid.

All three forms of pyridoxine are absorbed by mucosal cells of the upper small intestine. They are phosphorylated here to form pyridoxal phosphate and pyridoxamine phosphate. Pyridoxal phosphate is distributed bound to plasma albumin. Some pyridoxine is stored in the body, but a large percentage is eliminated in the urine. Fifty percent of the total body content of pyridoxine is stored in muscle.

Requirements

The RDA for pyridoxine is noted in Table 10-3. Pyridoxine requirements increase as protein intake increases. Pyridoxine intake appears adequate when the vitamin is taken in a ratio of 0.016 mg/g of protein, or 2 times the daily RDA for protein. Additional protein intake during pregnancy and lactation parallel the increased need for pyridoxine. Pyridoxine levels in breast milk correlate with the adequate intake in the maternal diet. The RDAs for children and adolescents are based on average protein intake.

Although these results are considered controversial, up to 500 mg of pyridoxine has been shown effective in the treatment of premenstrual syndrome, and dosages as high as 250 mg have been used for the treatment of carpal tunnel syndrome.

Deficiency States

Although it is relatively rare, pyridoxine deficiency occurs as the result of inadequate intake or impaired absorption. However, there are many drugs that interfere with the metabolism or the performance of pyridoxine, particularly cycloserine, isoniazid, hydralazine, and penicillamine. Signs and symptoms of pyridoxine deficiency include skin and mucous membrane lesions, malaise, depression, and glucose intolerance. Extreme deficiency leads to CNS abnormalities in infants whose formulas do not contain pyridoxine. A deficiency syndrome has been noted in mentally retarded children with an inborn error of pyridoxine metabolism. The inborn error manifests as uncontrollable seizures. Pyridoxine supplementation must be started in the neonatal period to prevent irreversible mental retardation.

Excess States

The risk of toxicity to pyridoxine is low; however, prolonged ingestion of high doses has resulted in severe ataxia and sensory neuropathy. Discontinuation of the drug results in complete recovery within 6 months.

Biotin

History and Uses

Biotin was first isolated in 1936 and synthesized in 1943. It had been previously observed that chicks and rats fed large amounts of raw egg whites developed eczema accompanied by alopecia around the eyes. The chicks and rats were cured by adding egg yolks to the diet, and the corrective factor in the yolk was named vitamin H. Vitamin H was found to be the same as the potent growth factor in yeast called coenzyme R, and the factor was subsequently renamed *biotin*. The vitamin is found in a wide variety of foods, although the exact amounts have not been determined. Biotin is also synthesized by intestinal bacteria.

Pharmacodynamics and Pharmacokinetics

Biotin is involved in metabolic pathways such as gluconeogenesis, fatty acid synthesis, and amino acid catabolism. It assists in the transfer of carbon dioxide from one compound to another, thus playing an important role in carbohydrate, fat, and protein metabolism. Biotin is synthesized in the lower GI tract by bacteria. It is a constituent of a coenzyme for carboxylation and deamination reactions. It is required in the synthesis of fatty acids, the generation of the tricarboxylic acid cycle, and the formation of purines. Biotin is metabolically related to folic acid, pantothenic acid, and cobalamin.

Biocytin, the natural fragment released by degradation, is readily absorbed. Biotin is released during hydrolysis of biocytin and taken up by the muscle, the liver, and the kidneys. It is protein bound in most natural foods. A vegetarian diet may alter the normal flora of the bowel to enhance synthesis of biotin or promote its absorption, or both.

Requirements

The RDA for biotin has not been established because of the lack of knowledge regarding its bioavailability in foods (see Table 10-3). The RDA has been provisionally set at 30 to 100 mcg/day, which appears to meet the needs of most healthy adults.

Deficiency States

The signs and symptoms of biotin deficiency in adults include dermatitis, glossitis, lassitude, depression, hyperesthesia, pallor, anorexia, loss of sleep, muscle pains, and elevated cholesterol levels. In infants under 6 months of age, biotin deficiency appears as seborrheic dermatitis and alopecia. Biotin deficiency is a common disorder in patients receiving total parenteral nutrition (TPN), although there is an inherited form of biotin deficiency (i.e., biotin-dependent multiple carboxylase deficiency syndrome). The antiepileptic drugs primidone and carbamazepine inhibit biotin transport in the intestine, leading to deficiency.

Excess States

No known toxic effects are produced by biotin.

Folic Acid

History and Uses

Folate is a water-soluble B-vitamin. The synthetic form of folate, folic acid, is found in dietary supplements and fortified foods. Adequate dietary or supplemental intake of folate helps DNA replication and may reduce cellular changes that may lead to cancer. Folic acid (B_9) may reverse cervical dysplasia, which in turn helps prevent cervical cancer. It may also be helpful in the prevention of lung cancer and in the prevention and treatment of gum disease and gout. On the other hand, a folate deficiency hinders synthesis of DNA and cell division, resulting in megaloblastic anemia.

Pharmacodynamics and Pharmacokinetics

Folic acid forms coenzymes known as tetrahydrofolates, which are involved in single-carbon transfers during metabolism. Folic acid is essential for the synthesis of the purines guanine and adenine and of the pyrimidine thymine, compounds necessary for DNA and RNA synthesis, and serves as a single-carbon carrier in the formation of heme.

Folic acid is broken down to a monoglutamate form by enzymes from the pancreas and the intestinal mucosa. It is then absorbed by carrier-mediated active transport. A small percentage of folic acid is absorbed by pH-sensitive passive diffusion. During or after absorption, the monoglutamate form of folic acid is changed to methyltetrahydrofolic acid and stored.

Requirements

The 1998 RDA for folate is identified in Table 10-3. The term *dietary folate equivalent (DFE)* is used to compare naturally occurring folate with the more bioavailable synthetic form of folic acid. The RDA for folic acid is equivalent to the average intake of the U.S. and Canadian populations. It has been estimated that 75% of neural tube defects could be prevented by the use of folic acid supplements.

Deficiency States

During home food preparation and processing, 50% to 95% of folic acid is lost. Folate deficiency may be the most common vitamin deficiency in humans. Deficiency results in poor growth, megaloblastic anemia and other blood disorders, elevated blood levels of homocysteine (a blood chemical linked to the clogging of arteries), glossitis, and GI tract disturbances. Low plasma folate and cobalamin levels have been associated with elevated plasma homocysteine levels and an increased risk of heart disease. Some health care providers believe that folic acid deficiency is an independent risk factor for heart disease, unrelated to cholesterol levels, hypertension, or diabetes.

Conditions that increase the body's need for folic acid such as pregnancy, hemolytic anemia, leukemia, Hodgkin's disease, the use of certain drugs (e.g., oral contraceptives, sulfasalazine, hydantoin, barbiturates), and protein malnutrition impair the utilization of folic acid. Excessive alcohol intake impairs the absorption of folic acid or increases its elimination. Low red blood cell folate levels have also been found to enhance the other risk factors for cancer and human papilloma virus infection.

Excess States

Although folic acid supplements are used to correct the anemia associated with vitamin B_{12} deficiency, supplementation does not correct the associated nerve damage. To prevent masking symptoms of a B_{12} deficiency, the dosage of folic acid should not exceed 1000 mcg/day. There are no known toxic effects to folic acid, although dosages of 15 mg have been reported to cause abdominal distention, loss of appetite, nausea, sleep disturbances, and interference with zinc absorption.

Cyanocobalamin

History and Uses

Vitamin B_{12} is called cyanocobalamin because it contains the metal cobalt, which has a blue-green coloration in its natural state. The terms cyanocobalamin and cobalamin are often used interchangeably. Vitamin B_{12} is needed to make DNA and also helps to maintain healthy nerve cells and red blood cells. Cyanocobalamin is essential to the metabolism of all cells, particularly those of the GI tract, the bone marrow, and the CNS. It is required for growth and the metabolism of carbohydrate, proteins, and fats, and is important in the formation of myelin. Along with folic acid, choline, and methionine, cyanocobalamin participates in the synthesis of nucleic acids, purine, and pyrimidines.

Pharmacodynamics and Pharmacokinetics

Cyanocobalamin (B_{12}) is bound to proteins in food. After being released from its peptid bonds by hydrochloric acid in the stomach, B_{12} unites with gastric intrinsic factor to be absorbed by the intestines. The cyanocobalamin–intrinsic factor complex is absorbed in the membranes of the ileum. Calcium is necessary for the transfer to occur. Once absorbed, cyanocobalamin circulates bound to plasma proteins.

The highest concentrations of cyanocobalamin are found in the liver and, to some extent, in the kidney. Enterohepatic circulation recycles cyanocobalamin from bile and other intestinal secretions; thus it may take 5 or 6 years for a deficiency to manifest. Excess vitamin is eliminated in the urine.

Requirements

Vitamin B_{12} deficiencies can be corrected by administering cyanocobalamin, a purified, crystalline form of vitamin B_{12}, either parenterally or orally through a nutritional supplement (if malabsorption is not the primary problem). After the deficiency is corrected, 100 mcg will be required to maintain lifelong health (see Table 10-3). Normal RDAs of cyanocobalamin range from 0.3 mcg/day for infants to 3 mcg/day for adults. This amount provides for substantial body stores in view of the increasing prevalence of achlorhydria, atrophic gastritis, and pernicious anemia in persons older than 60 years of age. Additional cyanocobalamin is recommended during pregnancy and lactation. By increasing vitamin B_{12} intake to 1000 mcg/day, sperm production can increase to over 100 million.

▌Ⅲ Deficiency States

Cyanocobalamin deficiency produces pernicious anemia (also known as megaloblastic anemia). *Megaloblastic anemia* is associated with glossitis, hypospermia, GI disorders, decreased numbers of but abnormally large red blood cells, fatigue, and dyspnea. With severe deficiency, leukopenia, thrombocytopenia, cardiac arrhythmias, heart failure, and infections may occur. Megaloblastic anemia precedes neurologic changes in the majority of patients. Subacute degeneration of cerebral white matter in the brain, optic nerves, spinal cord, and peripheral nerves has been noted. Symptoms include numbness, tingling, and burning of the feet, as well as stiffness and generalized weakness of the legs.

Cyanocobalamin deficiency in the older adult manifests itself in yellow skin tones, resulting from concurrent anemia and jaundice due to ineffective erythropoiesis; a smooth, beefy red tongue and neurologic disorders are also noted. Impaired mentation and depression may also be present, although these findings may also be related to elevated homocysteine levels.

▌Ⅲ Excess States

No toxic effects of cobalamin are known. Dosages as high as 100 mcg/day have been taken without apparent harm.

Ascorbic Acid

▌Ⅲ History and Uses

Scurvy was first described during the Crusades. Early explorers and voyagers were commonly afflicted with it. English sailors have been nicknamed "limeys" since the days when ships were required to carry citrus fruits (lemons, to be precise, despite the name) to prevent scurvy. Still, the specific relationship between scurvy, citrus foods, and ascorbic acid was not established until the twentieth century.

Ascorbic acid (vitamin C) is the most commonly used dietary supplement in the United States. It is essential as a coenzyme or cofactor for collagen formation, and thus is required for wound healing and tissue repair. These collagen tissues include connective tissue, cartilage, bone matrix, tooth dentin, skin, and tendons. It has been associated with the healing of fractures, bruises, pinpoint hemorrhages, and bleeding gums.

▌Ⅲ Pharmacodynamics and Pharmacokinetics

Ascorbic acid plays a part in the metabolism of iron and folic acid, as well as in the synthesis of fats and proteins, the preservation of blood vessel integrity, and resistance to infection. It blocks the degradation of ferritin to hemosiderin, from which iron is poorly mobilized, thus ensuring a more available supply in the form of ferritin. Ascorbic acid is essential in the oxidation of phenylalanine and tyrosine, the conversion of folic acid to tetrahydrofolic acid, and the formation of serotonin and norepinephrine.

The value of ascorbic acid as an antioxidant remains under investigation. There is evidence to suggest that ascorbic acid, as well as vitamin A (particularly beta-carotene and other carotenoids), pyridoxine, and folic acid, protects the body by supporting antioxidant activity. A stable oxygen molecule is essential to life. There are also some unstable oxygen molecules (free radicals) that enable the body to successfully fight inflammation, kill bacteria, and control smooth muscle tone. However, too many free radicals can be generated by exposure to air pollution, cigarette smoke, ultraviolet light, pesticides, and contamination in food, and even from too much exercise. Although the healthy body can more or less control its own production of free radicals, too many free radicals create a problem. They begin to run wild, successfully attacking healthy as well as unhealthy tissues and sometimes resulting in heart disease, various cancers, and many other diseases.

Ascorbic acid is readily absorbed from the small intestine by an active mechanism and diffusion. Of ascorbic acid from foods, 90% is bioavailable to the body when taken in daily quantities between 20 and 120 mg. At very high dosages, bioavailability falls to 16%. Diets high in zinc and pectin may decrease absorption, whereas absorption may be increased in the presence of natural citrus extract. Ascorbic acid is readily taken up by the tissues of the adrenal glands, the kidneys, the liver, and the spleen, appearing in equilibrium with serum levels. Amounts in excess of those needed by the body are eliminated in the urine as oxalic acid or ascorbic acid, or are exhaled as carbon dioxide.

▌Ⅲ Requirements

The minimum RDA of ascorbic acid needed to prevent scurvy is approximately 10 mg daily (see Table 10-3). However, this dosage does not provide for acceptable reserves. The RDA of 60 mg prevents the onset of symptoms for 4 weeks and provides a margin of safety. Regular intake of supplemental vitamin has a strong impact on serum levels of the vitamin, independent of other variables affecting nutritional status. Additional ascorbic acid is necessary for persons under emotional or environmental stress, such as fever, infection, or trauma, or in hot environments. Persons who smoke have lower serum concentrations of ascorbic acid. It is suggested that smokers increase their intake of ascorbic acid to at least 100 mg/day.

▌Ⅲ Deficiency States

Scurvy is rare, although marginal deficiencies may occur in people whose diets are devoid of fruits and vegetables, people who consume excess quantities of alcohol, older adults with very limited diets, critically ill people under chronic stress, and infants fed exclusively cow's milk.

Mild deficiency of ascorbic acid is reflected as irritability, malaise, arthralgia, and an increased tendency to bleed. More severe deficiencies involve most body tissues. The effects include anosmia; gingivitis and bleeding of the gums, skin, joints and other areas; disturbances of bone growth; anemia;

loosening of the teeth; follicular hyperkeratosis; loss of hair; and dry, itchy skin. Because of defects in collagen synthesis, wounds fail to heal and scars of previous wounds may break down. Secondary infections develop in the site of altered skin and mucous membrane integrity. Common psychologic disturbances include hypochondriasis, hysteria, and depression, followed by decreased psychomotor performance. Coma and death may occur if scurvy is not treated.

Elimination of ascorbic acid is increased when the patient is under stress and when the patient has received adrenocorticotropic hormone by injection. This loss is due to high adrenocortical hormone activity. The immunologic activity of leukocytes, the production of interferon, the inflammatory response, and the integrity of the mucous membranes all contribute to resistance to infection. The value of ascorbic acid in the prevention and treatment of the common cold has not been supported.

▓ Excess States

Ascorbic acid is a water-soluble vitamin, so it is not stored in the body—excess is lost primarily through urine. Toxic levels therefore are not accumulated. If extremely large amounts are taken, GI problems may appear, but these will normalize when the intake is cut or reduced. Excessive intake of ascorbic acid may result in diarrhea from the osmotic effect of the unabsorbed vitamin passing through the intestinal tract. Megadoses of ascorbic acid may produce excessive amounts of oxalate and urate in the urine and subsequent renal calculi. Excessive ascorbic acid may also cause retention of iron stores, particularly in blacks who are sensitive to iron.

Although antioxidants contained in foods have been shown to combat the effects of harmful free radicals in physiologic amounts, ascorbic acid and other antioxidants taken in excess of physiologic needs may act as pro-oxidants in some populations. *Rebound scurvy* can be seen when massive doses of ascorbic acid are taken and then suddenly discontinued. For this reason, slowly withdraw high-dose ascorbic acid therapy.

MINERALS AND TRACE ELEMENTS

Minerals (macrominerals) are defined as those requiring a dosage of 100 mg/day. The macrominerals are primarily electrolytes and include calcium, magnesium, potassium, sodium, phosphorus, chloride, and sulfur. If less than 100 mg/day is required by the body, the substance is called a *trace element* or *micromineral*. Trace elements include chromium, cobalt, copper, fluoride, iodine, iron, manganese, molybdenum, selenium, silicon, zinc, and vanadium.

Calcium

Calcium is the most abundant mineral in the body, making up 39% of the total body minerals and 1.5% to 2% of body weight. Ninety-nine percent is found in the bones and teeth. The remaining 1% is in the intravascular fluids and within soft tissues. Approximately half of the calcium contained in intravascular fluids is bound to protein, mostly albumin, and the remaining half is free, ionized calcium. Therefore the total plasma calcium level does not reflect the exact amount of free, active calcium in the body. A more in-depth discussion is found in Chapter 54.

Calcium is needed for the proper function of all cells and tissues. The transmission of nerve impulses, the regulation of cardiac output, and the maintenance of muscle tone require a homeostatic balance of calcium, potassium, and magnesium. Calcium is also a vital cofactor in the conversion of prothrombin to thrombin and in the conversion of fibrinogen to fibrin. Calcium is also essential in the regulation of blood pressure and may help protect against colon cancer. Calcium-rich bones are less susceptible to fracture and osteoporosis.

Very small changes in blood calcium levels profoundly alter many cellular functions, with effects on most body systems. Because of this fundamental role, calcium absorption, distribution, and elimination must be very tightly controlled to maintain a constant concentration of 4.7 to 5.6 mEq/L in the serum.

▓ Requirements

The recommended intake of calcium is between 1000 and 1300 mg daily (Table 10-4). The UL of calcium for adults is 2.5 grams/day. These numbers are associated with the maximum retention of calcium in the body. Factors known to affect the retention of calcium in bones include intermittent rapid growth spurts in children, hormonal balance, exercise, genetics, and the other nutritional components in the diet (e.g., magnesium, potassium).

▓ Deficiency States

Clinical conditions that cause calcium deficiency are many and include changes in dietary habits, GI function, and calcium binding, as well as medical disorders and many drugs. Dietary changes that can cause calcium deficiency include inadequate dietary intake or vitamin D deficiency, or both, or excessive intake of phosphorus, which combines with calcium so that neither mineral is absorbed. Malabsorption of fat in the intestine or diarrhea can also cause a calcium deficiency. There is less ionized calcium available in metabolic alkalosis. Patients receiving multiple transfusions of stored blood are at risk for calcium deficiency, because the calcium is combined with citrate for storage.

Patients with renal failure are at risk for calcium deficiency. Pancreatitis causes the release of lipases into soft tissue spaces so that the free fatty acids that are formed bind with calcium. Burns, Cushing's disease, hypoparathyroidism, inadvertent removal of the parathyroid glands, wounds, alcoholism, tumor lysis syndrome, and liver disease may contribute to calcium deficiency.

A number of drugs can cause hypocalcemia. Magnesium sulfate, colchicine, and neomycin inhibit parathyroid hormone secretion. Aspirin, anticonvulsants, and estrogen alter the metabolism of vitamin D. Phosphate preparations decrease serum calcium levels, and steroids decrease calcium mobilization. Loop diuretics reduce calcium absorption from the renal tubules, and antacids and laxatives decrease calcium absorption.

Calcium deficiency results in *tetany* (twitching around the mouth, tingling and numbness of the fingers, carpopedal spasms, facial spasm, laryngospasm, seizures, and death). Peristalsis is increased, with resultant diarrhea. Arrhythmias, palpitations, weak pulse, and hypotension result from the increase in cell irritability. Decreased myocardial contraction leads to decreased cardiac output. Pathologic fractures can

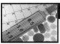

DOSAGE

TABLE 10-4 Selected Minerals

Mineral	Primary Prevention	Dosage Required to Correct Deficiencies	Implications
Calcium	*RDA:* *Adults:* 800–1200 mg PO daily	*Adult:* 1–2 grams PO daily *Child:* 45–65 mg/kg/day PO	Caution: dosages may be expressed in mg, grams, or mEq of calcium depending on formulation.
Phosphorus	*RDA:* *Adults:* 700 mg/day *Child 9–18 yr, pregnant or lactating:* 1250 mg/day	Varies with reason for use. Need for replacement is unlikely. Deficiency is rare.	The average Ca:P ratio should be 1:1.6. Most men get at least 1500 mg and women get more than 1000 mg/day from dietary sources.
Magnesium	*RDA:* *Adults:* 5 mg/kg/day *Child:* 100 mg/day	*Adults:* 200–400 mg/day PO in 3 or 4 divided doses *Child 6–11 yr:* 3–6 mg/kg/day PO in 3–4 doses	Average Ca:Mg ratio should be 4:1.
Iron	*Adults: Fumarate:* 200 mg/day PO; *Gluconate:* 325 mg/day PO; *Sulfate:* 300–325 mg/day PO; *Elemental iron:* 50–100 mg 3 times daily *Child: Fumarate:* 3 mg/kg/day PO; *Sulfate:* 5 mg/kg/day PO; *Elemental iron:* 4–6 mg/kg/day in 3 doses	*Adults: Fumarate:* 200 mg PO 3–4 times daily. CR form may be given twice daily; *Gluconate:* 325–650 mg PO 4 times daily; SR capsules may be given twice daily; *Sulfate:* 300 mg PO 2–4 times daily *Child: Fumarate:* 3–6 mg/kg PO 3 times daily; *Sulfate:* 10 mg/kg PO 3 times daily.	RDA is set at 10 mg/day. Use caution with different formulations: 300 mg of mg of ferrous gluconate = 34.75 mg elemental iron; 200 mg of ferrous fumarate = 65 mg of elemental iron; and 300 mg of ferrous sulfate = 60 mg of elemental iron.
Zinc	*RDA:* *Adults:* 10–15 mg/day; *Pregnant or lactating:* 25–30 mg/day	*UL:* *Adults:* 2.5–4 mg PO daily; an additional 2 mg/day may be needed in catabolic states *Child <5 yr:* 100 mg/kg/day	Doses are expressed in mg of elemental zinc. Zinc sulfate contains 23% zinc. Dosages are individualized based on patient needs.
Copper	*RDA:* *Adults:* 900 mcg/day	*UL:* *Adults:* 10,000 mcg PO daily (10 mg/day)	Median intake of dietary copper in United States is 1 to 1.6 mg/day for adult men and women.
Iodine	*RDA:* *Adults:* 150 mg/day	*UL:* *Adults:* 1100 mcg PO daily (1.1 mg/day)	Median intake of dietary iodine in United States is 240 to 300 mcg/day for men and 190 to 210 mcg/day for women.

AI, Acceptable intake; *CR,* controlled-release; *PO,* by mouth; *RDA,* recommended daily allowances; *SR,* slow-release; *UL,* tolerable upper intake level.

occur secondary to calcium loss from the bone. Patients are also at risk for bleeding, because the intrinsic pathway for blood coagulation is inhibited. Other signs of calcium deficiency include brittle nails, depression, insomnia, and periodontal disease.

Excess States

Excessive calcium intake can cause anorexia, nausea, vomiting, decreased peristalsis, distention, and constipation. The increased calcium level enhances hydrochloric acid, gastrin, and pancreatic enzyme release, and slows GI transit time. Mild to moderate neurologic depression may occur and will manifest as weakness, fatigue, depression, and difficulty concentrating. With severe excess, there is extreme lethargy, depressed sensorium, confusion, and coma.

Arrhythmias, heart block, and cardiac arrest are likely to be due to a shortened repolarization time. Digoxin toxicity contributes to the arrhythmias. Kidney stones are possible because of calcium precipitates. Polyuria occurs because of osmotic diuresis and volume depletion. The kidney's ability to concentrate urine results in polyuria.

Magnesium

Approximately 50% of total body magnesium is found in bone; the other half is found within the cells of body tissues and organs. Magnesium is second only to potassium in concentration in intracellular fluid.

Magnesium helps maintain normal muscle and nerve function, keeps heart rhythm steady, supports a healthy immune system, regulates blood sugar levels, promotes maintenance of normal blood pressure, and helps to keep bones strong. It is also involved in energy metabolism and protein synthesis and used in more than 300 enzymatic reactions in the body. There is an increasing interest in the role of magnesium in preventing and managing disorders such as hypertension, cardiovascular disease, and diabetes.

Calcium and magnesium have complementary roles. Calcium gives bones their strength, whereas magnesium helps them maintain their elasticity to prevent injury. Along with calcium, magnesium moderates the transmission of impulses to nerves and the contraction of skeletal, smooth, and cardiac muscle.

Pharmacodynamics and Pharmacokinetics

Magnesium is responsible for transportation of sodium and potassium across the cell membrane and the synthesis and release of parathyroid hormone. Magnesium is necessary for the conversion of ATP to adenosine diphosphate (ADP) and thus the release of energy. It influences the utilization of sodium, potassium, calcium, and phosphate, and activates enzymes necessary for the metabolism of carbohydrates, proteins, fats, and cyanocobalamin. Magnesium also promotes vasodilation of peripheral arteries and arterioles.

Magnesium is absorbed from the small intestine at the same site as calcium, although the rate of absorption varies from 35% to 45%. Most absorption occurs in the jejunum through simple and facilitated diffusion. The efficiency of absorption varies with the composition of the diet as a whole, the magnesium status of the individual, and the amount consumed in the diet. Magnesium is carried in the plasma as free ions or as a complex with phosphate, citrate, or protein. Maintenance of serum levels depends on absorption, elimination, and transmembranous cation flux rather than on hormonal regulation, as with calcium and phosphorus levels. The kidneys conserve magnesium (especially when intake is low). Reabsorption tends to vary inversely with that of calcium.

Requirements

The RDA for magnesium is 50 to 450 mg daily, although specific recommendations vary with age, sex, and reproductive status (see Table 10-4). Magnesium chloride is 12% magnesium or 9.8 mEq magnesium/gram; magnesium hydroxide is 41.7% magnesium or 34.4 mEq magnesium/gram; magnesium oxide is 60.3% magnesium or 49.6 mEq magnesium/gram.

Deficiency States

Magnesium deficiency is caused by conditions in which there is decreased intake or increased loss; however, magnesium status is difficult to determine, because serum levels remain constant over a wide range of intake levels. Increased calcium or phosphorus intake decreases magnesium absorption from the intestines. Magnesium deficiency is possible in patients with renal disease, those on diuretic therapy, and those who have malabsorption syndrome, hyperthyroidism, pancreatitis, kwashiorkor, diabetes, parathyroid gland disorders, postsurgical stress, and vitamin D–resistant rickets.

Many drugs increase the risk of magnesium deficiency. Excessive amounts of phosphorus (from overuse of antacids) inhibit the intake of magnesium from the intestines. Diuretics and antibiotics interfere with renal handling of magnesium as either a primary action or an adverse effect. The usual offenders are loop, osmotic, and thiazide diuretics, aminoglycoside antibiotics, carbenicillin, amphotericin B, cisplatin, corticosteroids, and cardiac glycosides. The neurologic trauma associated with cocaine abuse has also been linked to magnesium deficiency.

Deficiency of magnesium results in muscle spasm, personality changes, anorexia, nausea, and vomiting. Tetany, myoclonic jerks, athetoid movements, seizures, and coma have also been reported. If the magnesium deficiency continues, parathyroid hormone, calcium, and potassium levels drop and sodium is retained. Neuromuscular changes appear, along with other signs.

Excess States

The signs and symptoms of hypermagnesemia include flaccid paralysis, CNS depression, anesthesia, and even paralysis, especially in patients with renal insufficiency. Cardiac arrest in diastole is possible. There may also be an increased incidence of congenital defects in exposed embryos.

Phosphorus

Phosphorous is a major component of bones and teeth, second only to calcium. Approximately 80% of phosphorus contained in the body is in the form of calcium phosphate crystals ($CaPO_4$). Most of the inorganic phosphorus is contained in two forms: H_2PO_4 and HPO_4.

Pharmacodynamics and Pharmacokinetics

Phosphorus is a component of ATP and cyclic adenosine monophosphate (cAMP), which are essential for energy metabolism and maintaining the structural integrity of cells. It also plays a part in cellular immunity. Phosphorus is needed for phosphorylation and dephosphorylation, which are important steps in the activation and deactivation of many enzymes by cellular phosphatases and kinases. Phosphate is also a buffer in intracellular fluids and the kidneys, where it acts in the elimination of hydrogen ions. Phosphate reacts with hydrogen, releasing sodium in the process. Sodium is reabsorbed under the influence of aldosterone.

Regardless of the form, most phosphorus is absorbed as inorganic phosphate. Phosphorus is hydrolyzed in the intestinal lumen by alkaline phosphatase and released as inorganic phosphate. The acidic environment of the proximal duodenum maintains the solubility of phosphorus and thus its bioavailability.

Phosphorus is eliminated through the kidneys but is reduced in the presence of increased plasma insulin, thyroid-stimulating hormone, growth hormone, and glucagon levels; in metabolic or respiratory alkalosis; and with contraction of extracellular fluid.

Requirements

The RDA for phosphorus approximates that of calcium for all age groups (see Table 10-4). Excessive amounts of phosphorous lower serum calcium levels, particularly if the intake of calcium and vitamin D is insufficient or marginal for some reason.

Deficiency States

Phosphorus deficiency is unlikely, because the element is widely available in a variety of foods. Clinical hypophosphatemia most often results from the long-term administration of intravenous (IV) glucose or TPN without added phosphorus, excessive use of phosphate-binding drugs (see Chapter 44), hyperparathyroidism, the treatment of diabetic ketoacidosis, and alcoholism with or without decompensated liver disease. Premature infants can also develop clinical hypophosphatemia if they are fed unfortified human milk.

The signs and symptoms of hypophosphatemia include muscular weakness, encephalopathy, cardiomyopathy with congestion, hemolytic anemia, ventilatory collapse, and GI and skin hemorrhages.

Excess States

Phosphorus excess is rare but, when present, may cause tachycardia, nausea and diarrhea, abdominal cramps, muscle weakness, and hyperreflexia.

Iron

Nearly three fourths of body iron is in hemoglobin in red blood cells. Hemoglobin is required for transport and use of oxygen by body cells. Iron is also critical for normal brain development and function at all ages. It is also involved in the function and synthesis of neurotransmitters and possibly myelin. ATP cannot be synthesized without adequate iron stores. As a result, some iron-deficient persons become fatigued even when their hemoglobin levels are normal.

Pharmacodynamics and Pharmacokinetics

The absorption of iron from food in the patient with normal hemoglobin values varies considerably, but is estimated to be 5% to 15% under normal circumstances. However, absorption is influenced by several other factors. Iron absorption is increased in the presence of dietary ascorbic acid and gastric acidity. Thus a patient may take iron with a glass of orange juice to hasten absorption.

The rate of iron absorption appears to be under the control of the intestinal mucosa, which accepts amounts dictated by the body's needs. Mucosal transferrin excreted in the bile acts as a shuttle protein in facilitating iron absorption. It picks up iron in the intestine and takes it to the surface of the intestinal cell, releases the iron into the cell, and returns to the intestinal lumen for more iron. Within the mucosal cell the iron may combine with apoferritin to form ferritin for temporary storage within the cell. Once in the mucosal cell, apoferritin and ferritin form a common pool.

Transfer from mucosal cells to the body is slower than uptake and is affected by the size of body stores and the quantity of iron in the diet. The rate at which iron is released into general circulation is regulated by the amount and saturation of transferrin. Two ferric ions are bound to transferrin for transport to the tissues. Current theory suggests that the number of transferrin receptors on a cell membrane can be adjusted to the needs of the individual cell. Deficiencies in dietary iron are reflected first in the saturation of circulating transferrin.

Transferrin is usually saturated to about one third of its total iron-binding capacity (TIBC). If iron is not needed, transferrin remains saturated and less is absorbed from the mucosal cells; the transferrin remaining in the cells is sloughed with the cells at the end of their 2- or 3-day life. Likewise, if iron is needed, the transferrin is less saturated when it reaches the intestinal mucosal cells, and more iron passes from the mucosal cell to the transferrin.

Calcium combines with phosphate, oxalate, and phytate. If this reaction does not take place, iron combines with these substances to produce nonabsorbable compounds. Physiologic states that increase iron absorption include periods of increased blood formation such as pregnancy and growth.

Requirements

Iron formulations vary greatly in the amount of elemental iron they contain (see Table 10-4). Ferrous sulfate, for example, contains 20% iron. Thus, each 300-mg tablet of ferrous sulfate provides about 60 mg of elemental iron. With the usual dosage regimen of one tablet 3 times a day, the daily dose of elemental iron is 180 mg. The need for iron declines after male adolescent growth spurts, but female needs continue to be high until after menopause. Use oral formulations cautiously in patients with peptic ulcer disease and ulcerative colitis, and in patients with allergies to tartrazine. Indiscriminate use may lead to iron overload.

Deficiency States

Iron deficiency is the most common nutritional deficiency and the most common cause of anemia among women and children worldwide. An otherwise adequate diet frequently contains no more than 6 mg of iron per 1000 kcal. The average menstruating female consuming 1800 kcal therefore consumes 10.8 mg of iron, or approximately 73% of the RDA. This appears to meet the needs of 86% of women; however, setting the RDA higher, at 15 mg/day, should meet the needs of all except 5% of menstruating women. Women with high losses generally compensate with an increased rate of absorption. Groups considered at most risk for iron deficiency include infants younger than 2 years of age, female adolescents, pregnant women, and older adults.

Iron deficiency is most often caused by chronic blood loss but can also be aggravated by a diet poor in iron, protein, folic acid and vitamin B_{12}, pyridoxine, and ascorbic acid. Factors that decrease the absorption of iron include the lack of hydrochloric acid in the stomach (achlorhydria) and the use of antacids, which produce an alkaline gastric environment. Further, combining iron with phosphates, oxalates, or phytates in the intestine results in insoluble and nonabsorbable compounds. Increased intestinal motility decreases the absorption of iron by decreasing the contact time with intestinal mucosa. Steatorrhea and other malabsorption disorders also decrease the absorption of iron. T-cell and natural killer–cell concentrations are reduced with iron deficiency, and mitogenic response is muted.

Excess States

Excess iron as well as iron deficiency alters the immune response, which can result in infection. The infection is likely to occur because iron is required by bacteria for growth and reproduction. Iron overload may be caused by hereditary hemochromatosis or transfusion overload. The latter is seen in patients with sickle cell disease or thalassemia major who require transfusions for their anemia. Iron overload in blacks may be linked to a combination of dietary iron intake and the presence of a predisposing gene that is separate from any HLA-linked gene.

Zinc

Zinc helps maintain the health of the eyes, the skin, the hair, and the joints; stabilizes cell membranes against free-radical damage, thereby improving the immune system, it improves reproduction success by increasing the sperm count in males, it reduces menopause-associated depression, and it helps prevent excessive menstrual flow (when taken with choline). Zinc is also an essential component of many enzymes (e.g., alcohol dehydrogenase, DNA polymerase, retinol dehydrogenase). It may help protect the heart from cardiomyopathy and angiopathy. Zinc is also a constituent of the hormone insulin. Zinc supplements help with burn and wound healing, as well as in the treatment of acne and skin disorders. It is one of the several nutrients that are helpful in treating macular degeneration. Zinc has also been used in high doses to treat prostate enlargement.

Pharmacodynamics and Pharmacokinetics

Zinc participates in reactions involving either synthesis or degradation of major metabolites. More than 200 zinc enzymes have been isolated. Zinc is also involved in the stabilization of protein nucleic acid structure and the integrity of cellular organelles, as well as in transport processes, immune function, and expression of genetic information. Zinc is abundant in the nucleus, where it stabilizes DNA and RNA structure and is required for the activity of RNA polymerases important in cell division. Zinc also functions in chromatin proteins involved in transcription and replication. It is thought to be needed for adequate osteoblastic activity; formation of bone enzymes such as alkaline phosphatase; and calcification. Unless bone resorption is taking place, the zinc in bone is not available.

Zinc is poorly absorbed from the GI tract (20% to 30%), although the mechanism is not well understood. A protein-rich meal promotes zinc absorption by forming zinc–amino acid chelates that present zinc in a more absorbable form. It is taken up first by the liver before being redistributed to other tissues. It concentrates in muscle, bone, skin, kidney, liver, pancreas, retina, prostate, red blood cells, and white blood cells. It is highly bound to plasma albumin, although some zinc is transported by transferrin and by alpha$_2$-macroglobulin. Plasma zinc levels drop by 50% in the acute-phase response to injury, probably from sequestration by the liver. Ninety percent of the mineral is eliminated in the feces, with the remainder lost in urine and sweat.

Requirements

A positive zinc balance is attained with intakes of 112.5 mg/day, based on 20% absorption. The zinc density of the American diet appears to be 5.6 to 5.7 mg/1000 calories/day (see Table 10-4). Oral contraceptives may alter zinc distribution; however, there is no evidence available showing that these changes alter the dietary requirement.

Deficiency States

Zinc deficiency is most often caused by a diet high in unrefined cereal and unleavened bread. Acquired zinc deficiency may develop as the result of malabsorption, starvation, or increased loss through urinary, pancreatic, or other exocrine secretions. Patients abusing alcohol and those receiving TPN have developed signs of clinical zinc deficiency because of their underlying disease processes.

The first indication of a zinc deficiency is often hypogeusia (decreased taste acuity). Prolonged zinc deficiency may result in hypogonadism, growth retardation, mental disturbances, anemia, lethargy, diverse forms of skin lesions, delayed wound healing, alopecia, and frequent infections. Testicular function may be adversely affected by a low level of zinc. Depression, as well as anxiety and compulsive states, have been corrected by the administration of 15 to 150 mg of zinc per day.

Excess States

Excess oral ingestion of zinc to the point of toxicity is rare. However, continued supplementation in excess of the RDA will interfere with copper absorption. The most serious form of zinc toxicity is seen in patients with renal failure who are on hemodialysis. The signs and symptoms of overdose include nausea, vomiting, and diarrhea.

Copper

Copper is necessary for the function of the antioxidant enzyme superoxide dismutase as well as for connective tissue maintenance and immune function. Copper is also vital for production of red blood cells, apparently by regulating storage and release of iron for hemoglobin. It also works with vitamin C in the production of collagen and elastin. Copper is essential for correct functioning of the central nervous, cardiovascular, and skeletal systems.

Pharmacodynamics and Pharmacokinetics

Copper is a component of many enzymes. It has well-documented roles in oxidizing iron before it is transported in the plasma and in the cross-linking of collagen necessary for its tensile strength. Through the involvement in copper-containing enzymes, it also has roles in mitochondrial energy production, protection from antioxidants, and synthesis of melamine and catecholamines. Other functions have been suggested but not yet completely defined.

Some copper is absorbed from the stomach, but maximal absorption takes place in the small intestine. The percentage of absorption decreases with increased intake. It is transported bound to plasma albumin. Some copper is stored in the liver as metallothionein or incorporated into ceruloplasmin and secreted back into the plasma for transport to and long-term storage in the cells. Ceruloplasmin is a functional, not a transport, protein. Copper is eliminated via the bile into the intestine and feces. Small amounts of copper are present in urine, sweat, and menstrual blood.

Requirements

Although the RDA for copper has not been established the usual dosage range is 1.5 to 3 mg/day for adolescents and adults (see Table 10-4). This dosage is estimated to be safe and adequate for daily intake.

Deficiency States

Because copper is stored in the liver, copper deficiency is not readily apparent. Copper deficiency is manifested in adults as microcytic hemochromic anemia, followed by neutropenia and leukopenia. Neutropenia and leukopenia are the best early indicators of copper deficiency. Subperiosteal hemorrhages develop, and hair and skin depigmentation appears. There is defective elastin formation. Cerebral and cerebellar degeneration develops, which finally leads to death.

Copper deficiency is also possible as a result of a sex-linked recessive defect called Menkes' disease. Affected infants experience growth retardation, defective keratinization and pigmentation of the hair, hypothermia, degenerative changes in aortic elastin, abnormalities of the metaphyses of long bones, and progressive mental deterioration.

Excess States

Copper toxicity damages the liver, the kidneys, and other organs. Bile contains substantial amounts of copper; thus copper excess is possible with any form of chronic liver disease. Wilson's disease, a rare progressive autosomal recessive disorder, is associated with a defect in copper metabolism and accumulation of copper in the liver. Ceruloplasmin, the alpha$_2$-globulin that transports copper, increases during pregnancy and with the use of oral contraceptives. Serum concentrations of copper in pregnant women are approximately twice those in nonpregnant women. Increased serum copper concentrations can also be found in patients with pellagra, acute and chronic infections, and liver disease. The meaning of these elevations is unknown. This mineral is suspected of being both mutagenic and carcinogenic.

Iodine

The body normally contains 20 to 30 mg of iodine, with more than 75% concentrated in the thyroid gland. The remainder is distributed throughout the body, particularly in the lactating mammary gland, the gastric mucosa, and the blood. Iodine, part of the hormone thyroxine, regulates growth and development, basal metabolic rate, and body temperature. Iodine is used as a supplement during long-term TPN and as an adjunct with other antithyroid drugs in the preparation for thyroidectomy.

▥ Pharmacodynamics and Pharmacokinetics

Iodine is readily absorbed in the form of iodide. It circulates free and in a protein-bound state. Iodine is stored in the thyroid, where it is used to synthesize two hormones: triiodotyrosine (T_3) and thyroxine (T_4). When the hormones are broken down, iodine is conserved if needed and stored in the liver. Selenium is important in iodine metabolism. Elimination of iodine is primarily through the kidneys in urine, although small amounts are eliminated in the feces.

▥ Requirements

The RDA for iodine is 150 mg for adults (see Table 10-4). Larger amounts are needed for children and pregnant or lactating women.

▥ Deficiency States

Iodine deficiency is generally associated with the development of simple goiter, which is an enlargement of the thyroid gland (see Chapter 54). The deficiency may be absolute, particularly in geographic regions where there is suboptimal iodine intake. Iodine deficiency is a preventable cause of mental deficiency *(cretinism)*, especially during pregnancy. Signs and symptoms of iodine deficiency include sluggishness and weight gain.

▥ Excess States

Iodism, or iodine excess, like iodine deficiency, inhibits thyroid function. Enlargement of the thyroid may develop in response to this effect. Acute iodism causes severe damage to the exposed tissues of the GI tract. Chronic iodism is characterized by increased secretions of the respiratory tract, a brassy taste, soreness of oropharyngeal tissues, eye irritations, GI irritation, coryza, sneezing, eyelid swelling, enlargement and tenderness of the parotid and submaxillary glands, bloody diarrhea, fever, anorexia, and depression. Iodism is unlikely with dietary intake but may occur with excessive intake of drugs containing iodine.

Sodium, Potassium, and Chloride

Because they are so closely related in the body, it is convenient to discuss sodium, potassium, and chloride together. Sodium makes up 2% of the total mineral content of the body; potassium, 5%; and chloride, 3%. Although they are distributed throughout the body, sodium and chloride are predominantly extracellular ions, and potassium is predominantly the intracellular ion.

These three ions maintain four important physiologic functions in the body: (1) water balance and distribution, (2) osmotic equilibrium, (3) acid-base balance, and (4) muscular irritability. The sodium-potassium-ATPase pump is important in volume regulation, maintenance of membrane potential (along with calcium), glucose transport, and transport of amino acids such as alanine, proline, tyrosine, and tryptophan.

Sodium assists in regulating osmotic pressure, water balance, conduction of electrical impulses in nerves and muscles, and electrolyte and acid-base balance. It influences the permeability of cell membranes, assists in the movement of substances across cell membranes, and participates in many intracellular chemical reactions. It is found in large quantities in saliva, gastric secretions, bile, and pancreatic and intestinal secretions. Sodium is present in most foods. Proteins contain relatively large amounts, vegetables and cereals contain moderate to small amounts, and fruit contains little to no sodium. The major source of sodium in the diet is table salt that is added to food during cooking, processing, and seasoning. One teaspoon of salt contains 2.3 grams of sodium.

Potassium is present in all body fluids. As an intracellular ion, potassium helps maintain osmotic pressure, fluid and electrolyte balance, and acid-base balance. Along with sodium in extracellular fluid, potassium helps regulate neuromuscular irritability. Potassium is required for conduction of nerve impulses and contraction of skeletal and smooth muscle. It is especially important in activity of the myocardium. Potassium also participates in carbohydrate and protein metabolism. It helps transport glucose into cells and is required for glycogen formation and storage. Potassium is also required for the synthesis of muscle proteins from amino acids and other components. Potassium is present in most foods, including meat, whole grain breads or cereals, bananas, citrus fruits, tomatoes, and broccoli.

Chloride is an ionized form of the element chlorine and is the main anion of extracellular fluid. With sodium, chloride functions to maintain osmotic pressure and water balance. It forms hydrochloric acid in gastric mucosal cells and helps regulate electrolyte and acid-base balance by competing with bicarbonate ions for sodium. Chloride also participates as a homeostatic buffering mechanism in which chloride shifts in and out of red blood cells in exchange for bicarbonate. Most of dietary chloride is ingested as sodium chloride. Foods high in sodium are also high in chloride.

Sodium, potassium, and chloride are readily absorbed from the GI tract and are eliminated through the kidneys in the urine, feces, and sweat.

Other Minerals

▥ Chromium

Chromium potentiates the action of insulin and, as such, influences carbohydrate, protein, and fat metabolism. It is a part of glucose tolerance factor, a biologically active hormone-like compound manufactured in the body that regulates glucose metabolism. It is believed that chromium is related to the high incidence of diabetes in older adults, although research to date has not substantiated this claim. Chromium deficiency may result in insulin resistance, so that elevated insulin levels are required to maintain insulin-dependent functions, as well as function in the presence of normal hormone concentrations being impaired. Consuming large quantities of foods high in refined sugar requires more insulin and, therefore, more chromium. Insulin resistance is recognized as a major independent risk factor for cardiovascular disease.

The required intake of chromium is unknown. The AI is 25 to 35 mcg/day for young adults. An UL has not been established. A precise measurement of chromium content in foods is difficult, because biologically available chromium and inorganic chromium cannot be distinguished from one another. Brewer's yeast, oysters, liver, and potatoes are high in chromium. Seafoods, whole grains, cheeses, chicken, meats, and bran also contain fair amounts of chromium. Dairy products, fruits, and vegetables have little chromium.

Ninety percent of diets are deficient in chromium owing to modern agricultural techniques and the consumption of refined foods. Signs and symptoms of deficiency include anxiety, fatigue, elevated serum cholesterol and triglyceride levels, increased incidence of aortic plaque, corneal lesions, decreased fertility and sperm counts, and glucose intolerance. Supplemental trivalent chromium is believed to improve these symptoms significantly.

Manganese

Manganese is a component of enzymes (e.g., pyruvate carboxylase, glutamine synthetase). It plays a role in oxidative phosphorylation, fatty acid metabolism, and mucopolysaccharide synthesis. Manganese is required for the formation of connective tissues, growth and reproduction, and carbohydrate and lipid metabolism.

Manganese is absorbed throughout the small intestine. Iron and cobalt compete for the same binding sites as magnesium for absorption. Men absorb less manganese than women. The difference in genders may be related to iron status. Manganese is bound to a macroglobulin, transferrin, and transmanganin for transport. Elimination occurs primarily through the feces.

There are insufficient data to set an estimated average requirement (EAR) for manganese. The AI was set based on median intakes reported from the Food and Drug Administration's (FDA's) Total Diet Study (Egan, et al. 2002). The AIs for adult men and women are 2.3 and 1.8 mg/day, respectively. A UL of 11 mg/day was set for adults based on a no-observed-adverse-effects level for Western diets.

Dietary sources of manganese include whole grains, legumes, nuts, tea, fruits, and vegetables. Animal sources, dairy products, and seafood are poor sources of manganese. Substantial amounts are present in instant coffee and tea.

Deficiency of manganese appears to reduce fertility in both sexes. Striking skeletal abnormalities and ataxia characterize the children of deficient mothers. Manganese excess occurs as a result of absorption through the respiratory tract. Excess manganese accumulates in the liver and the CNS, producing parkinsonian symptoms.

Selenium

This nonmetallic chemical forms part of the structure of the antioxidant enzyme glutathione peroxidase. It appears to protect the body from toxic effects of mercury and cadmium. Selenium combines with tocopherol to protect cell membranes and organelle membranes from free-radical lipid peroxidase damage. It facilitates the union between oxygen and hydrogen at the end of the metabolic chain, transfers ions across cell membranes, and aids in immunoglobulin and ubiquinone (i.e., coenzyme Q) synthesis. Adequate intake of selenium reduces menopause-related hot flashes, stimulates the immune response, protects the liver, detoxifies environmental carcinogens and mutagens, and helps cells breathe. Selenium also helps reduce the incidence of heart disease and decreases the risk of cancer, including prostate, colon and breast cancer, with its antioxidant effect. The absorption of selenium occurs in the upper segment of the small intestine. It is transported via albumin and alpha$_2$-globulin.

Food sources of selenium include Brazil nuts, seafood, kidney, liver, meat, and poultry. Fruits and vegetables are low in selenium. Grains vary in selenium content depending on where they were grown and the selenium content of the soil and water.

Selenium deficiency is rare in the United States but is a problem in other locales, most notably China, where soil concentrations of selenium are low. It is thought that selenium deficiency does not by itself cause illness. Instead, it makes the person more vulnerable to illnesses caused by other stressors and contributes to the development of heart disease, hypothyroidism, and a weakened immune system.

Selenium deficiencies have also been linked to reduced male fertility, increased spontaneous abortions, reduced growth rates, and viral epidemics that are normally harmless. A deficiency of selenium reduces glutathione peroxidase activity, causing jaundice in neonates. Deficiency of selenium can also lead to seborrheic dermatitis, dandruff, macular degeneration, low thyroid function, inflammation of the heart muscle, high cholesterol levels, and pancreatic insufficiency. Although animal studies have suggested that high selenium intake protects against certain cancers, in some cases, selenium may be toxic and may actually stimulate tumor growth. The dietary intake at which selenium intake becomes toxic has not been identified.

CLINICAL REASONING

Treatment Objectives

Many people take vitamin and mineral supplements in an effort to promote health and prevent deficiencies and malnutrition. Treatment objectives should center on ingesting appropriate amounts and sources of dietary vitamins and minerals, avoiding megadoses of vitamin supplements and minerals unless recommended by the health care provider, and avoiding symptoms of vitamin or mineral deficiency or excess. The need for vitamin and mineral supplementation is based on the following considerations:

- Daily requirements of the nutrient for healthy individuals
- The nature of the deficiency, disease, or injury
- Body storage of the specific nutrient
- Normal and abnormal losses of the nutrient through the skin, the urinary tract, and the GI tract
- Possible nutrient-drug interactions

Treatment Options

Table 10-5 provides an overview of the signs and causes of malnutrition. Findings of concern that indicate the need for an in-depth assessment to determine a nutritional versus other causes include the following:

- Sudden or unexplained loss of 10% or more of body weight
- Rapid weight loss of more than 2 pounds per week

TABLE 10-5 Physical Signs of Malnutrition

Body Part	Signs of Malnutrition	Deficient Nutrient
Hair	Lacking natural shine, dull, sparse, straight, color changes, easily plucked	Multiple nutrient deficiencies
Face	Malar and supraorbital pigmentation, nasolabial seborrhea, moon face	Riboflavin, niacin, pyridoxine
Eyes	Pale conjunctiva, conjunctiva and corneal xerosis, keratomalacia, redness and fissuring of eyelid corners	Vitamin A, iron
Lips	Cheilosis, angular fissure and scars	Niacin, riboflavin
Tongue	Glossitis	Folic acid, niacin, cyanocobalamin, pyridoxine
	Magenta color	Riboflavin
	Pale, atrophic	Iron
	Filiform papillary atrophy	Niacin, folic acid, cyanocobalamin, iron
Teeth	Mottled enamel	Excess fluoride
Gingiva	Spongy, bleeding, receding	Ascorbic acid
Glands	Thyroid enlargement (goiter)	Iodine
Skin	Follicular hyperkeratosis, xerosis with flaking	Vitamin A, unsaturated and essential fatty acids
	Hyperpigmentation	Folic acid, niacin, cyanocobalamin
	Petechiae	Ascorbic acid
	Pellagrous dermatitis	Niacin
	Scrotal and vulval dermatosis	Riboflavin
Nails	Koilonychia (spoon nails), brittle, ridged	Iron
Musculoskeletal	Frontal and parietal bossing, epiphyseal swelling, craniotabes (soft, thin skull bones in infants), persistently open anterior fontanelle, knock knees or bowlegs, beading of ribs (rachitic rosary)	Vitamin D
Gastrointestinal	Hepatomegaly	Multiple deficiencies
Nervous system	Mental confusion and irritability	Thiamine, niacin
	Sensory loss, motor weakness, loss of position sense, loss of vibratory sense, loss of ankle and knee jerks, calf tenderness	Thiamine
Cardiac	Cardiac enlargement, tachycardia	Thiamine

- Significant weight change (either gain or loss) after age 25
- Height for age is above the 10th percentile, but weight for height is less than the 5th percentile in children
- Excess weight for height (greater than the 95th percentile) in children

Life-Span Considerations

PREGNANT AND NURSING WOMEN. During pregnancy, there should be an increase in all nutrients to meet the physiologic demands of maternal changes and fetal growth. The amount of increase in essential nutrients depends on the woman's general nutritional status before pregnancy, current health status, age and parity, amount of time between pregnancies, height and bone structure, weight, and activity level. If the woman's nutritional status is poor before she becomes pregnant, the additional demands of pregnancy on her body may further compromise her nutritional status. In general, the pregnant woman needs additional folic acid, pyridoxine, ascorbic acid, vitamins A, D, and E, calcium, phosphorus,

iron, zinc, copper, magnesium, and iodine. These nutrients may be supplied with a prenatal vitamin.

For information on specific agents and their effects, see the Evolve Resources Bonus Content "Effects of Selected Maternal Drug Ingestion on the Fetus or Neonate," found at http://evolve.elsevier.com/Gutierrez/pharmacotherapeutics/.

CHILDREN AND ADOLESCENTS. Nutrients likely to be low or deficient in children's diets include calcium, iron, zinc, pyridoxine, magnesium, and vitamin A. Children at nutritional risk include those from deprived families; those from the inner city; homeless children; children with anorexia, poor appetite, and poor eating habits; children with chronic disease (e.g., cystic fibrosis) or liver disease; and those on dietary programs for obesity or who are vegetarians. However, clinical signs of malnutrition in American children are rare.

The American Academy of Pediatrics does not support routine use of vitamin and mineral supplements for normal, healthy children. Parents who desire to give a vitamin and mineral supplement need not be concerned. The quantities of vitamins and minerals contained in supplements do not exceed those of the RDA; however, megadoses should be avoided.

Forty-five percent of bone growth occurs during adolescent growth spurts. Adolescents' need for vitamins A and E, ascorbic acid, pyridoxine, and folic acid are the same as for an adult, but they need additional thiamine, riboflavin, niacin, vitamin B complex, and vitamin D.

OLDER ADULTS. There is growing concern that older adults are particularly deficient in vitamin B_{12}, vitamin B_6, and folate. Further, as lean body mass declines with age, perhaps so does the need for trace elements needed for muscle metabolism. Glucose intolerance associated with aging may suggest the need for additional chromium. Increased calcium is needed owing to bone loss from osteoporosis, hypochlorhydria, and decreased intestinal absorption of calcium. Zinc requirements decline in the older adult, but these patients are in need of additional beta-carotene, vitamin D, vitamin E, ascorbic acid, and cyanocobalamin. Pyridoxine, cyanocobalamin, and folic acid offer protection against elevated homocysteine levels, an independent factor for cardiovascular disease, and certain neurologic deficits.

Lack of transportation, loss of functional ability, immobility, limited income, and living alone may lead to social isolation. Older adults living alone may be deprived of stimulating interaction with others and thus lack incentive to cook and eat meals. Depression frequently accompanies social isolation and the sense of loss experienced with the death of a spouse or friends, retirement, changes in body appearance, impaired vision, and poor physical fitness. Lack of interest in eating and anorexia, common symptoms of depression, result in limited food intake and increased risk of nutrient deficiency.

Drug Considerations

There are many vitamin supplements available over the counter, varying in number, type, and specific ingredients. Some contain a single vitamin, whereas others are combinations of vitamins and minerals. Some persons believe that megadoses of vitamins promote health and provide other beneficial effects. However, there is no evidence to suggest that dosages exceeding those needed for normal body functioning are beneficial, and in fact, they can be harmful in some cases.

Controversy

Dietary Supplements—Some Real Issues

Jonathan J. Wolfe

A patient asks you about a dietary supplement advertised on television. He has internalized the message that older people are healthier if they take this product daily as part of their diet. However, his only income is a fixed pension, and you know that he lives in relative poverty. Buying this dietary supplement will force him to buy less of other types of food, wash his clothes less often, and keep his three-room home colder in winter.

Patients come to their practitioners constantly seeking answers about health issues. Sometimes they are actually asking for a judgment regarding what is important and what is specious. Such requests frequently involve dietary supplementation. Patients are bombarded by recommendations—usually with no scientific grounding, but based in anecdote—that they take a particular vitamin supplement or add a particular food to their diets. Often, the recommendation comes from a source with an economic interest in their decision.

Vitamin supplements are relatively inexpensive and, for the most part, hardly controversial. A multivitamin taken on a daily basis is probably not needed but is not likely to cause harm. In the case of some supplements, however, the issue is not certain. Some are suggested without a known, established recommended dietary requirement (RDA). Some are not standardized or are prepared from materials that are not assayed. Their worth may be impossible to establish. Even the risk of toxicity may be unknown. Some supplements are actually harmful in supraphysiologic doses. This is true particularly of fat-soluble vitamins and nutrients containing metallic elements.

Health care providers are challenged daily to provide guidance in dietary supplementation. The basic guideline that "no one needs vitamins who eats a balanced diet" often fails the test. Patients may have unusual dietary habits, perhaps derived from traditions we do not understand.

CLINICAL REASONING

- What collaboration can you suggest between yourself and dietitians to act as a bridge to cover uncertain areas about dietary supplements?
- What community resources can you find to educate yourself about issues related to dietary supplements?
- Do you perceive sellers of natural products and dietary supplements as adversaries or potential allies?
- What reference should you use to look up interactions between vitamin and other nutritional supplements and your patient's drugs?

For deficiency states, oral vitamin preparations are preferred when possible. They are usually effective, safe, convenient to administer, and relatively inexpensive. If the deficiency involves a single vitamin, that vitamin alone should be taken rather than a multivitamin. However, a multivitamin product may be used because one vitamin deficiency usually does not occur in isolation. Dosages should be titrated as nearly as possible to the amount needed by the body (see Controversy box).

Patient Education

Teach patients that taking a vitamin and mineral supplement each day does not preclude the importance of a well-balanced diet. It is important to counsel the patient to avoid megadoses of vitamins and minerals. No known benefit to health results from ingesting more mineral nutrients than the body needs; some vitamins and minerals are toxic if taken in more than the recommended doses. All vitamins and minerals should be kept out of the reach of young children and should never be referred to as candy.

Evaluation

Treatment effectiveness can be demonstrated through resolution of symptoms of deficiency with no evidence of overdosage.

KEY POINTS

- Vitamin requirements are established by the Food and Nutrition Board of the National Academy of Sciences. RDAs represent 100% of the vitamin intake considered necessary to avoid deficiency.
- Vitamins prescribed by health care providers to prevent or treat deficiencies exert the same physiologic effects as those obtained from foods. Treatment objectives center on ingestion of appropriate amounts and sources of dietary vitamins and minerals, avoidance of megadoses of vitamin supplements and minerals unless recommended by the health care provider, and avoidance of symptoms of vitamin or mineral deficiency or excess.
- Vitamins are divided into two groups: fat-soluble and water-soluble. Fat-soluble vitamins include vitamins A, D, E, and K. Thiamine, riboflavin, niacin, pyridoxine, pantothenic acid, biotin, cyanocobalamin, and folic acid make up the water-soluble vitamins.
- Vitamin A is required for normal vision, growth, bone development, skin, and mucous membranes.
- Vitamin D plays an important role in the regulation of calcium and phosphorus metabolism.
- Vitamin E acts as an antioxidant in preventing destruction of certain fats, including the lipid portion of cell membranes. It may also increase absorption and hepatic storage of vitamin A.
- Vitamin K is essential for blood clotting. It activates precursor proteins found in the liver into clotting factors: prothrombin, proconvertin, plasma thromboplastin component, and the Stuart factor.
- Thiamine (B_1) acts as a coenzyme in carbohydrate metabolism and is essential for energy production.
- Riboflavin (B_2) serves as a coenzyme in metabolism and is necessary for growth. It may function in the production of corticosteroids and red blood cells, and in gluconeogenesis.
- Niacin (B_3) is essential for glycolysis, fat synthesis, and tissue respiration. After conversion to nicotinamide, the physiologically active form, it functions as a coenzyme in many metabolic processes.

- Pantothenic acid (B_5) is essential for cellular metabolism of carbohydrates, proteins, and fats and for synthesis of cholesterol, steroid hormones, phospholipids, and porphyrin.
- Pyridoxine (B_6) serves as a coenzyme in many metabolic processes and functions in the metabolism of carbohydrates, proteins, and fats. It is a part of the enzyme phosphorylase, which helps release glycogen from the liver and muscle tissue.
- Biotin (B_7) is essential to carbohydrate and fat metabolism.
- Folic acid (B_9) is essential for the normal metabolism of all body cells, for normal red blood cells, and for growth.
- Cyanocobalamin (B_{12}) is essential to cellular function, particularly red blood cells and cells of the bone marrow, nervous tissue, and the GI tract; growth; and metabolism of carbohydrates, proteins, and fats.
- Ascorbic acid is an essential coenzyme or cofactor for collagen formation and thus is required for wound healing and tissue repair. It has been associated with the healing of fractures, bruises, pinpoint hemorrhages, and bleeding gums.

- Minerals, which are found in body fluids, serve structural functions in the body. There are 16 essential minerals required by the body to maintain health.
- Calcium is required in the transmission of nerve impulses and in the regulation of heartbeat, maintenance of muscle tone, and formation of bone.
- Calcium and magnesium have complementary roles. Calcium gives bones their strength, whereas magnesium helps them maintain their elasticity to prevent injury.
- Phosphorus aids in bone growth and mineralization of teeth. It is a component of ATP and cAMP, which are essential for energy metabolism, maintenance of cellular integrity, and immune response.
- Nearly three fourths of body iron is in hemoglobin in red blood cells. Hemoglobin is required for transport and use of oxygen by body cells.
- Zinc is a component of many enzyme systems and is necessary for normal cell growth, synthesis of nucleic acids, and the synthesis of carbohydrates and proteins. It may be essential for the use of vitamin A.
- Treatment effectiveness is demonstrated through resolution of symptoms of deficiency with no evidence of overdosage.

Bibliography

Chang, S., Hsiao, L., Shou-Ying, H., et al. (2003). Assessment of vitamin B-6 estimated average requirement and recommended dietary allowance for adolescents aged 13–15 years using vitamin B-6 Intake, nutritional status and anthropometry. *Journal of Nutrition, 133*(10), 3191–3194.

Center for Nutrition Policy and Promotion, United Stated Department of Agriculture. (1992), revised 1996). *Food guide pyramid.* Available online: www.cnpp.usda.gov/. Accessed February 10 2007.

Coppen, A., and Bolander-Gouaille, C. (2005). Treatment of depression: Time to consider folic acid and vitamin B_{12}. *Journal of Psychopharmacology, 19*(1), 59–65.

Dietary Guidelines Advisory Committee, Agricultural Research Service, United States Department of Agriculture (USDA). (2005). *Dietary guidelines for Americans.* HG Bulletin No. 232. Available online: www.health.gov/dietaryguidelines/dga2005/document/. Accessed February 10, 2007.

Egan, S., Tao, S., Pennington, J. et al. (2002). US FDA Total Diet Study: Intake of nutritional and toxic elements 1991-96. *Food Additives and Contaminents, 19*(2), 103–125.

Egan, S., Bolger, P., Carrington, C. (2007). Update of US FDA Total Diet Study food lists and diets. *Journal of Exposure Science and Environmental Epidemiology*, April 4, [Epub ahead of print].

Food and Nutrition Board. Institute of Medicine. (1997). *Dietary reference intakes for calcium, phosphorus, magnesium, vitamin D, and fluoride.* Washington, DC: National Academy Press.

Food and Nutrition Board. Institute of Medicine. (1998). *Dietary reference intakes for thiamin, riboflavin, niacin, vitamin B_6, folate, vitamin B_{12}, pantothenic acid, biotin, and choline.* Washington, DC: National Academy Press.

Food and Nutrition Board. Institute of Medicine. (2000). *Dietary reference intakes for vitamin C, vitamin E, selenium, and carotenoids.* Washington, DC: National Academy Press.

Food and Nutrition Board. Institute of Medicine. (2002). *Dietary reference intakes for vitamin A, vitamin K, arsenic, boron, chromium, copper, iodine, iron, manganese, molybdenum, nickel, silicon, vanadium, and zinc.* Washington, DC: National Academy Press.

Foote, J., Giuliano, A., and Harris, R. (2000). Older adults need guidance to meet nutritional recommendations. *Journal of the American College of Nutrition, 19*(5), 628–664.

Lonn, E., Yusef, S., Arnold, M., et al. (2006). Homocysteine lowering with folic acid and B vitamins in vascular disease. *New England Journal of Medicine, 354*(15), 1567–1577.

Office of Dietary Supplements. NIH Clinical Center. National Institutes of Health. (2005). *Vitamin E.* Available online: http://ods.od.nih.gov/factsheets/. Accessed February 10, 2007.

Suitor, C., and Bailey, L. (2000). Dietary folate equivalents: interpretation and application. *Journal of the American Dietetic Association, 100*(1), 88–94.

U.S. Department of Agriculture, Agricultural Research Service. (2004). *USDA National Nutrient Database for Standard Reference*, Release 16–1. Nutrient Data Laboratory Home Page available online: www.ars.usda.gov/main/site_main.htm?modecode=12354500. Accessed February 10, 2007.

11

Complementary and Alternative Medicine

The roots of modern complementary and alternative medicine (CAM) used to enhance conventional Western medical practice can be traced to early Greek and Chinese treatments. The term *complementary medicine* is defined as that which is *used together* with conventional medical treatments. *Alternative medicine* is that which is *used in place of* conventional medicine.

As a branch of the National Institutes of Health, the National Center for Complementary and Alternative Medicine (NCCAM) is the federal government's lead agency for research on CAM. The center is dedicated to exploring complementary and alternative healing practices (e.g., herbal remedies) in the context of rigorous science, training CAM researchers, and disseminating authoritative information to the public and professionals.

EPIDEMIOLOGY AND ETIOLOGY OF CAM

The use of CAM for health problems has increased dramatically since the 1960s. It is now widespread in the United States, and more health care providers are including some form of CAM in their practice. The results of a national survey conducted at Harvard Medical School found that 1 in 3 Americans visited providers of complementary therapies. In fact, in recent years, more Americans visited health care providers who use CAM than visited primary care providers.

More than 85% of the population worldwide uses botanical preparations as medicine. In most industrialized countries, herbalism is experiencing an unprecedented renaissance. Every third American is thought to use some form of alternative therapy, and use of alternative therapies is more common among well-educated, upper-income, white Americans in the 25- to 49-year-old age range. By and large, CAM is private medicine for which consumers pay substantial amounts from their own pockets. Although Germany leads the market with over $3 billion in annual sales, the United States is second in line for annual sales. The United States is followed by Italy, the United Kingdom, Spain, the Netherlands, and Belgium. Echinacea, ginseng, ginkgo, saw palmetto, St. John's wort, kava kava, and cranberry account for a large portion of these sales.

People use a variety of CAM therapies because they want more control over their health care and health care costs. Often, they are dissatisfied with the attitude of their health care provider, conventional medicine has failed to meet their needs, and they feel an affinity for a natural or holistic approach. Many patients are also attracted to health care providers who uses CAM modalities because they treat the whole person–body, mind, and spirit. Patients find the individualized approach particularly appealing in an age of managed care and impersonal group practices. *Integrative medicine*, a term denoting a combination of mainstream medical therapies and CAM, is using more

evidence-based practice than ever before. This chapter focuses on the remedies, such as herbals and dietary supplements, that are in the mainstream of Western society.

Research on phytotherapy as a modality of complementary medicine is exploding. Medline, the National Institutes of Health's database on health sciences topics, listed over 3700 peer-reviewed journal articles from 1990 to 1997 in the category of medicinal plants. Virtually all contemporary health care providers see patients who routinely use complementary or adjunctive therapies. Yet only 3 in 10 of these patients discuss complementary or adjunctive therapies with their health care provider. This is often due to mistrust of Western medicine and technology. However, most persons who consult alternative providers would probably jump at the chance to consult a physician, advanced practice nurse, or physician assistant who is well trained in scientifically-based medicine but who remains open-minded and knowledgeable about the body's innate mechanisms of healing; the role of lifestyle factors in influencing health; and the appropriate uses of dietary supplements, herbs, and other forms of treatment, from osteopathic manipulation to Chinese and Ayurvedic medicine. In other words, people are looking for guidance through the available therapeutic options, especially in those cases in which conventional approaches are relatively ineffective or harmful.

Education about CAM modalities is a significant, unmet need among health care providers, and education may help alleviate the discomfort providers have when answering patients' questions about CAM. Health care providers who use CAM treatments themselves are much more likely to recommend CAM for their patients than physicians who do not.

CATEGORIES OF CAM

There are five primary categories of CAM, although this chapter focuses primarily on the biologically and pharmacologically based therapies (Table 11-1).

The increased interest in CAM, increasing health care costs, and loss of individualized care led to a major funding increase to a controversial office (controversial within science, at least): the Office of Alternative Medicine (OAM) within the National Institutes of Health (NIH), was awarded a 37.5% budget increase, to $69 million, in the final NIH budget approved by Congress for the fiscal year 2000. The percentage increase was even larger than the whopping 14.7% increase of $2.3 billion added to NIH's overall $17.9 billion. NIH is the main agency for funding biomedical research in the United States, and both it and its growing alternative medicine unit enjoy broad congressional support. The mandate of this federally funded agency is to investigate and evaluate alternative therapies and their effectiveness in relieving suffering, illness, and disease. Although the OAM does not

TABLE 11-1 Categories of CAM

MIND-BODY INTERVENTIONS

Art therapy	Biofeedback
Dance therapy	Guided imagery
Humor	Hypnotherapy
Meditation	Music therapy
Prayer therapy	Psychotherapy
Relaxation, yoga	Support groups

ALTERNATIVE SYSTEMS OF PRACTICE

Acupuncture	Ayurveda
Community-based practices	Environmental medicine
Homeopathy	Latin American rural practices
Native American practices	Naturopathy
Past life therapy	Shamanism
Tibetan medicine	Traditional Chinese medicine

MANIPULATION AND BODY-ORIENTED THERAPIES

Acupressure	Osteopathy
Chiropractic	Prayer
Feldenkrais method	Reflexology
Massage therapy	Rolfing
Meditation	Trager method

DIET, NUTRITION, LIFESTYLE CHANGES

Changes in lifestyle	Diet
Gerson therapy	Macrobiotics
Megavitamins	Nutritional supplements

ENERGY THERAPIES

Bluelight treatment, artificial lighting	Neuromagnetic stimulation
Electroacupuncture	Magnetoresonance spectroscopy
Electromagnetic fields	Therapeutic touch

PHARMACOLOGIC AND BIOLOGIC TREATMENTS

Antioxidizing and oxidizing agents	Chelation treatments
Cell treatments	Metabolic therapies

CAM, Complementary and alternative medicine.
From an undated pamphlet produced by the Office of Alternative Medicine, National Institutes of Health, Bethesda, MD. Categories of CAM. Information also available online: http://nccam.nih.gov/health/whatiscam/. Accessed February 10, 2007.

operate as a referral service, it does serve as a public information clearinghouse, as well as a research training program.

LEGISLATION AND PRODUCT CLAIMS

HEALTH CLAIMS

The FDA determines which health claims may be placed on a product label for a food or dietary supplement. The National Labeling and Education Act (NLEA) of 1990 allows the FDA, after careful review of the evidence, to approve claims placed on food and dietary supplement labels.

NUTRIENT CLAIMS

These claims identify the concentration of a nutrient or dietary substance in the product, using terms such as *free, high,* and *low.* The label is designed so that that the amount of a nutrient in a food can be compared with that contained in another food, using terms such as *more, reduced,* and *lite.*

STRUCTURE AND/OR FUNCTION CLAIMS

Structure and/or function claims identify the role of a nutrient or dietary ingredient in the body. In 1994, the *Dietary*

Supplement Health and Education Act (DSHEA) established a regulatory means for evaluating these claims. Statements may include the mechanism by which a nutrient or ingredient acts to maintain body structure or function; for example, "fiber maintains bowel regularity" or "calcium builds strong bones." A claim may also describe in general terms a benefit to be gained from the nutrient in relation to a nutritional deficiency (e.g., the relationship between iron and anemia), as long as the statement also identifies the prevalence of the disease or condition in the United States.

LABELING ISSUES

In 2000, the FDA issued regulations allowing structure and/or function statements to be made on product labels. Information about therapeutic claims for herbal products can be disseminated as long as the information is not misleading or product-specific and has no product stickers affixed to it. Claims are permitted that do relate not to disease but to health maintenance (e.g., "maintains a healthy gastrointestinal [GI] tract"); also acceptable are non–disease claims (e.g., "helps you to sleep"), and claims for minor symptoms associated with stages of life ("for premenstrual syndrome [PMS] symptoms"). Any statement that uses terms such as "cures," "treats," "prevents," "mitigates," or "diagnoses disease" is subject to drug requirements.

If all of this sounds like semantics, it is. Nonetheless, regardless of what a label says, common sense tells us that people take herbal remedies to prevent and treat disease. However, because the DSHEA does not regulate the accuracy of product labels, there is no assurance that the product actually contains the ingredients listed or in the stated amounts. *Pharmacognosists* (i.e., interdisciplinary scientists who study the physical, chemical, biochemical, and biologic properties of natural drugs, natural drug substances, or potential drugs or drug substances of natural origin; they also assist in the search for new drugs from natural sources) note that consumers of herbal products have less than a 50% chance of receiving a product that is accurately labeled. The product may contain ingredients *not* listed, or it may lack ingredients that *are* listed. In either case, the manufacturer is permitted to sell the mislabeled product. All the DSHEA requires is the following disclaimer: "This statement [i.e., the package label] has not been evaluated by the FDA." **Both consumers** ▲ **and health care providers must remain alert and critical when evaluating claims of herbal supplements** (Box 11-1).

SAFETY ISSUES

Herbs "intended to prevent, alleviate, mitigate, or cure a mental or physical condition in humans or animals, or alter the structure or function of the body" are *drugs* by definition, according to the FDA. Drugs are required by law to provide sufficient information on labels and/or package inserts to enable people to use them properly. Included are (1) description and clinical pharmacology; (2) list of ingredients; (3) list of indications; (4) information on contraindications to use; (5) warnings and precautions; (6) what to do if adverse reactions occur; (7) proper dosage and administration; and (8) what may constitute overdosage. In contrast, over-the-counter (OTC) herbal remedies rarely provide consumers with this important information.

BOX 11-1

Warning Signs of Bogus Scientific Claims

Advise patients and health care providers alike to use caution when reviewing claims for supplements. In the early 1990s, the outcome of court cases regarding adverse effects of supplements relied on the validity of scientific research studies. Decisions were made by jurors who depended on the "expert witness" to provide accurate information and in whom they could believe. However, the expert witnesses could not provide evidence to support the scientific claims that were being made. Jurors were bewildered by technical language they could not understand and that was delivered by persons whose credibility they could not evaluate. The following are warning signs of false claims:

1. *The discoverer attempts to bypass the peer review process while directing the claim to the media and then the public.*
   Research integrity relies on the willingness of investigators to share new ideas, hypotheses, and findings with other investigators. This behavior suggests that the scientific work is unlikely to stand up to close scrutiny by other scientists.
2. *The discoverer indicates that the powerful scientific community is trying to restrain his or her work.*
   The belief here is that members of the research community will go out of their way to suppress discoveries that may shift the balance of wealth and power in society.
3. *The results of purported research is at the very limit of detection.*
   All research studies must recognize there will be some variance in the findings (i.e., statistical variability).
4. *Outcomes of the discovery are supported by anecdotal evidence.*
   The most important discovery of modern medicine is the randomized double-blind test, the means by which we ascertain the validity and reliability of the study's findings.
5. *The discoverer suggests a belief is credible simply because it has lasted for hundreds of years.*
   Much of what is thought of as "alternative medicine" is founded on the belief that because the supplement has endured for centuries its use is valid and reliable.
6. *The scientific breakthrough was uncovered by a lone scientist.*
   Today's breakthroughs are almost always the result of many investigators' work.
7. *The discovery offers a new law of nature that explains the outcomes of the study.*
   A new law of nature that explains some extraordinary outcome must not contradict existing knowledge.

Adapted from Park, R. (2003). The seven warning signs of bogus science. *The Chronicle of Higher Education, 41*(21), B20.

With dietary supplements as well as conventional drugs, the manufacturer is responsible for safety. However, many herbs and alternative medicines have not been adequately studied and may in some cases be toxic. Under the DSHEA, an herbal supplement is considered to be safe until proven hazardous. Further, the burden of proof to the contrary rests with the FDA, not the manufacturer. Research studies of safety are not required because, as previously noted, these products are considered dietary supplements, not drugs. With conventional drugs, the opposite regulations and logic applies: drugs are presumed dangerous until rigorous testing by the manufacturer reveals otherwise.

IMPURITIES, ADULTERANTS, AND VARIABILITY

The DSHEA does not regulate the manufacture of herbal remedies, and therefore impurities and adulterants are commonly found. Also, a lack of uniformity among herbal remedies exists; thus neither do consumers know for sure what a remedy really contains, nor is the package label of help. As a result, the consumer cannot be sure that the product contains the herb mentioned on the label in appropriate amounts, if at all. For example, among the 125 ephedra products analyzed by the FDA, the ephedrine content per dose ranged from undetectable to 110 mg. Some of the products had 6 to 20 additional ingredients. Ephedra, a common ingredient in weight loss products, can cause an increase in blood pressure, tremors, arrhythmias, seizures, strokes, myocardial infarction, and death. Therefore dietary supplements containing ephedra have been banned in the United States since April 2004, after it was determined that ephedra posed an

unreasonable risk to those who used it. In another example, the California Department of Health Sciences examined 243 Asian patented products. They found that 24 contained lead, 35 contained mercury, and 36 contained arsenic—all in levels above those permitted in drugs. Seven of the products were adulterated with undeclared ingredients, including ephedrine, chlorpheniramine, methyltestosterone, and phenacetin.

FORMULATION ISSUES

Bulk herbs are sold loose to be used as teas; however, bulk herbs rapidly loose their potency. Herbs should have a vibrant color and a strong aroma. Leaves and flowers purchased should be as close as possible to whole. Herbs that have been shielded from light and stored in opaque containers to preserve their potency are preferred. The active ingredients of the herb must be water-soluble to be effective in a tea formulation.

Water-based extractions can be used as skin washes, gargles, compresses, and lotions, or diluted as eye baths, douches, and baths. *Teas* are made using 1 oz (25 grams) of a dried herb, or 2 oz (50 grams) of fresh herb, and 500 mL of boiling water. The herb is placed in a pot, the boiling water is poured over the herb, and the pot is covered. The herb should be brewed for 1 to 3 minutes if flowers are used, 2 to 4 minutes if the herb's leaves are used, and 4 to 10 minutes if the bark, roots, or hard seeds of the herb are used. *Decoctions* are brewed from seeds, bark, and roots using the same quantities as for a tea. The herb is placed in a pan, covered with water, and covered with a tight lid. The mixture is allowed to come to a boil and then simmered for 20 to 30 minutes. The mixture is then strained and water added to make 500 mL. Syrups are made from decoctions and reduced slowly over low heat to one third the original amount. Cane sugar or honey is added (2.2 lb or 1 kg) for every 500 mL of decoction. The syrup is then poured into a clean, dark-glass bottle, labeled, and stored in a cool place.

An herbal *compress* is made by soaking a cloth in a warm or cool standard tea solution and is applied directly to an injured area. It is used cold for inflammations and warm for spasms, cramps, muscle tension, joint discomfort, and swellings. Abscesses are treated by alternating hot with cold compresses.

Extracts are the most effective herb forms. Extracts are formulated by pressing the herb and then soaking it in a solvent such as alcohol or water. Evaporation removes excess solvent, resulting in a concentrated liquid. Extracts are ordinarily mixed with a small amount of water before they are taken.

Solid extracts are fluid extracts from which all residual fluid has been removed. The solid residue is then incorporated into a standard oral formulation. Solid extracts are the most concentrated formulations and are preferred by U.S. consumers.

Tinctures are liquid extracts of plants, often in an alcohol base. Tinctures can contain up to 60% alcohol. The good news is that alcohol is a preservative that extends the product shelf life. The bad news is that alcohol can be harmful for some, including recovering alcoholics, alcohol-sensitive individuals, and those taking drugs that block the metabolism of alcohol (the result is an accumulation of acetaldehyde, a toxic metabolite of alcohol). Glycerine-based tinctures are available for those who want or need to avoid alcohol. Glycerites taste better than tinctures, but are often less potent and have shorter shelf lives.

Tinctures are used internally or externally in gargles, douches, compresses, liniments, mouthwashes, and baths. These formulations are stable, convenient, and easy to take and digest. Tinctures are taken by the dropper in a small amount of juice or water. Tinctures are more potent than teas and infusions, and fluid extracts are more potent than tinctures.

Capsules and *tablets* contain powdered or freeze-dried herbs or extracts. Freeze-drying preserves potency better than powdering, which exposes the herb to heat and oxygen. Both powdered and freeze-dried formulations may contain binders and fillers and thus may not be fully absorbed. Capsules and tablet formulations are an option for herbs that have an unpleasant taste.

Ointments are formulated from an extract, tea, pressed juice, or the powdered form of an herb. The herbal substance is added to a salve that is applied to an affected area.

A *poultice* is made of ground or granulated herbs spread onto muslin or other soft cloth. The poultice is warmed and placed over an affected area to relieve inflammation and pain.

STANDARDIZATION OF HERBALS

Standardization involves measuring the amount of certain chemicals in products to try to make different preparations similar to each other. Standardization of herbal formulations requires (1) that cultivation of the raw material be controlled; (2) a standardized production method be used; and (3) chemical analysis be performed to assure homogeneity of plant extracts.

The concentration of active ingredients in herbal crops varies from year to year and from location to location because of differences in sunshine, rainfall, temperature, and soil nutrients; thus the potency of an herb can vary significantly. Herbal remedies are made using a three-step process: (1) an extract is made from the plant's components; (2) the extract is analyzed for one or two known active ingredients; and (3) the extract is diluted or concentrated such that the final product contains a predetermined amount of active ingredients.

To reduce variation and achieve two important benefits, standardization of the product is undertaken. First, it permits accurate dosing; and second, it permits extrapolation of data obtained through clinical trials to the general public. Unfortunately, standardization also has a down side. The extraction process may destroy active compounds, or the process may fail to extract an as-yet unidentified active ingredient, and therefore the extract may have a different spectrum of effects than the intact plant.*

PHYTOMEDICINAL OPTIONS

In botany, an herb is a green plant without a woody stem. In medicine, the term is extended to include any plant, or part of a plant, that can be used to make a remedy. Thus the term *herb* embraces seaweed, ferns, flowers, roots, bulbs, barks, seeds, and leaves, and includes cooking herbs and spices, as well as many fruits and vegetables. Phytotherapy (from the Greek *phyto* for "plant") is the science of using plant-based drugs to treat illness. *Phytomedicines* have a significant history of research and use in clinical settings, most notably in Europe.

Phytomedicines are medicinal products that contain plant materials as their pharmacologically active component. They can be made from whole herb extracts or concentrates of active plant constituents (Fig. 11-1). Phytomedicines occupy the middle ground between drugs and food. At one end of the herbal spectrum are strong remedies that have been used as the source of modern drugs (e.g., poppies used for opium and deadly nightshade for atropine). At the other end of the spectrum are nourishing remedies such as bladderwrack and horsetail, rich sources of vitamins and essential trace minerals. For many phytomedicines, the active ingredients and their mechanism of action have been defined. The scientific basis of phytomedicine is investigated using the same scientific tools as for other drugs, such as double-blind, placebo-controlled clinical trials. Although acidophilus and creatine are not considered to be phytomedicinal products, they are included here because of their popularity. Table 11-2 identifies the herb and the herb's "other" names, and Table 11-3 summarizes adverse effects.

Acidophilus

By definition, a phytomedicine comes from plants; however, acidophilus is a specific type of organism known as the lactobacilli. A discussion of acidophilus is included here only because it is often thought of as an herbal remedy. Acidophilus may contain *Lactobacillus acidophilus*, *Lactobacillus casei*, and/or *Lactobacillus bulgaricus*, bacteria that aid in digestion. Only *L. acidophilus* is the true acidophilus strain, but many producers (mainly in the

---

*For further information, also see the Evolve Resources Bonus Content "Drug-Herb Interactions" found at http://evolve.elsevier.com/Gutierrez/pharmacotherapeutics/.

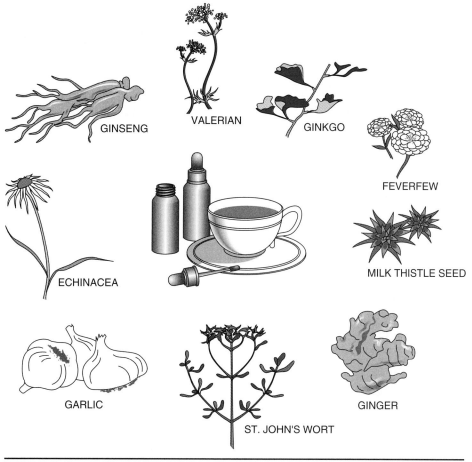

FIGURE 11-1 Components of Selected Phytomedicinals. Phytomedicines are made from flowers, seeds, stems, bark, and roots, and their extracts are commonly used in a variety of phytomedicinals, including tea, capsules, and ointments.

United States) use the term more as a generic name for mixtures of bacteria, one of which is *L. acidophilus*.

L. acidophilus gets its name from *lacto-* meaning "milk," *-bacillus* meaning "rodlike in shape," and *acidophilus* meaning "acid-loving." This bacterium lives best in an acidic environment (pH of 4 to 5 or lower) at a temperature of 45° C. *L. acidophilus* is naturally present in human (and animal) intestines, the oral cavity, and the vagina. It is also contained in foods such as dairy, grains, meat, and fish.

▎ Indications

L. acidophilus is a well-known "probiotic." Literally translated, *probiotic* means "for life." The proper scientific definition of a probiotic is a live microbial feed supplement that beneficially affects those who take it by improving their intestinal microbial balance. *L. acidophilus* helps maintain intestinal health and reduces the risk of vaginal yeast infections and antibiotic-induced diarrhea. Moreover, acidophilus serves as a "natural treatment" against principally harmful organisms (see Pharmacodynamics, next).

▎ Pharmacodynamics

L. acidophilus breaks down food, which in turn produces lactic acid, hydrogen peroxide, and other byproducts that make the environment hostile to other, less desirable organisms. It feeds on some of the same nutrients many other organisms depend on, thus pushing out possibly harmful bacteria in the digestive tract. During digestion, *L. acidophilus* also assists in the production of niacin, folic acid, and pyridoxine, assists in the deconjugation of bile, separates amino acids from bile acids, and absorbs lactose, metabolizing it to lactic acid.

▎ Adverse Effects and Contraindications

Acidophilus may cause gassiness for a few days while the intestines adjust to the bacterial shift. Serious adverse effects include anaphylaxis. Use caution when taking *L. acidophilus* during pregnancy.

▎ Interactions

There are no known drug or drug-herb interactions.

Bilberry

Bilberry *(Vaccinium myrtillus)* is a relative of the blueberry and the cranberry. This shrub produces small, sweet, black berries. It was used by British pilots during World War II to improve night vision.

▎ Indications

The astringent effects of bilberry fruit make it useful in treating inflammation of the mouth and throat, and both the fruit

TABLE 11-2 Supplement Synonyms

Acidophilus	*Lactobacillus acidophilus*
Bilberry	Airelle, bleaberry, black whortles, blueberries, trackleberry, huckleberry hurts, hurtleberry, *Vaccinium frondosum*, whinberry, whortleberry
Black cohosh	Black snakeroot, bugbane, rattleweed, rattleroot, squaw root,* *Cimicifuga*, papoose root, blue ginseng, yellow ginseng, beechdrops, blueberry
Bladderwrack	Kelp, black tang, rockweed, sea wrack, kelp-ware, bladder fucus, cutweed, *Quercus marina*, cutweed, blasentang, seetang, meeriche
Coenzyme Q₁₀	CoQ₁₀, Q₁₀, Vitamin Q₁₀, ubiquinone, ubidecarenone
Cranberry	American cranberry, bog cranberry
Creatine	Creatine citrate, creatine monohydrate, creatine phosphate, squaw root*
Echinacea	Snakeroot, purple coneflower, Sampson root, hedgehog
Feverfew	Altamisa, amargosa, bachelor's button, chamomile grande, featherfew, featherfoil, febrifuge plant, flirtwort, manzanilla, wild chamomile, motherherb, midsummer daisy, mutterkraut, nosebleed, Santa Maria, wild chamomile, wild uinine, *Chrysanthemum parthenium*
Garlic	Garlik
Ginger	Jamaica ginger, African ginger, Cochin ginger, black ginger, race ginger
Ginkgo biloba	Ginkgo, maidenhair tree, golden fossil tree
Ginseng	American ginseng, panax ginseng, san, redberry, five fingers, man root, divine root, root of life, jin-chen, garantoquen
Hawthorn	Mayflower, May tree, quickset, whitethorn, maybush, mayblossom, haw, halves, hagthorn, scouring rush, ladies' meat, bread and cheese tree
Kava kava	Awa, kava pepper, intoxicating long pepper, kao, kava root, malohu, maluk, Maori kava, meruk, milk, pepe kava, sakau, onga, yagona, yangona, yaqona
Milk thistle	St. Mary's thistle, blessed thistle, Our Lady's thistle, silymarin
Saw palmetto	Sabal
St. John's Wort	Spotted St. John's wort, *Hypericum*, klamath weed, touch-and-heal, goat weed, rosin rose
Valerian	Abscess root, blue bells, Jacob's ladder, creeping Jacob's ladder, false Jacob's ladder, Greek valerian, onechte Jacobsladder, polemonie fausse, sweatroot

*The term squaw root can refer to a number of herbs native to North America.

TABLE 11-3 Adverse Effects of Supplements

Remedy	Possible Adverse Effects
Acidophilus	Flatulence
Bilberry	Increases coagulation time
Black cohosh	Increased perspiration, dizziness, nausea, vomiting, visual disturbances, reduced pulse, headaches, stiffness, trembling
Bladderwrack	Hyperthyroidism, tremor, increased pulse rate, elevated blood pressure
Chondroitin	Diarrhea, constipation, stomach pain
Coenzyme Q₁₀	None known
Cranberry	Gastrointestinal (GI) upset, diarrhea (with large amounts of juice)
Creatine	Nausea, vomiting, diarrhea, weight gain
Echinacea	Upset stomach, diarrhea, constipation, skin rash, dizziness
Feverfew	Palpitations, a slightly heavier menstrual flow, colicky abdominal pain, mouth ulcerations, inflamed tongue
Garlic	Allergic reactions, bleeding, diarrhea, irritation of mouth and esophagus, nausea, flatulence, malodorous breath and body, sweating
Ginger	Central nervous system depression, arrhythmias (with large dosages)
Ginkgo biloba	Headache, dizziness, heart palpitations, seizures, skin problems, muscle cramps, restlessness, nausea, vomiting, diarrhea, allergic skin reactions
Ginseng	Headache, nervousness, insomnia, skin rashes, vaginal bleeding, tender breasts, high or low blood pressure, diarrhea
Glucosamine	Alterations in blood glucose levels, heartburn, palpitations, and increased risk for cataract formation; abdominal pain, loss of appetite, vomiting, nausea, flatulence, constipation, diarrhea (rare)
Hawthorn	None known
Kava kava	Headaches, vision disturbances, drowsiness, rash, yellow color to skin, torticollis, oculogyric crisis, choreoathetosis, tremor, blood dyscrasias, hematuria, hepatitis, cirrhosis, liver failure
Milk thistle	Bloating, loose stools, diarrhea (rare)
Saw palmetto	GI upset, decreased libido, headache, back pain (uncommon)
St. John's wort	Dizziness, emotional vulnerability, fatigue, restlessness, sleep disturbances, dry mouth, constipation, photosensitivity, pruritus, weight gain
Valerian root	Headache, nausea, morning headache, blurred vision, excitability, upset stomach

and leaves are used for simple diarrhea. There are preliminary indications that it may be useful in preventing and treating eye conditions such as diabetic retinopathy and night blindness, macular degeneration, glaucoma, and cataracts. It may also be effective for varicose veins and hemorrhoids. The fruit is also helpful in treating scurvy and urinary complaints and, when bruised with the roots and steeped in gin, has diuretic properties valuable in heart failure.

▥ Pharmacodynamics

The active constituents in bilberry are anthocyanosides, bioflavonoids that act as antioxidants. Bilberry is also thought to contain pectin. Pectin is a soluble fiber that counteracts diarrhea by acting as an antioxidant and preventing damage to small blood vessels. It acts by keeping capillary walls strong and flexible, and helps maintain the flexibility of the walls of red blood cells and allows them to better pass through the capillaries. In addition, this herb supports and strengthens collagen structures, inhibits the growth of bacteria, acts as an antiinflammatory, and is thought to have antiaging and antineoplastic effects (in vitro).

▥ Adverse Effects and Contraindications

There are no known adverse effects of bilberry.

▥ Interactions

Bilberry may prolong coagulation time. It should be used with great caution in patients who are concurrently taking aspirin, anticoagulants, antiplatelet drugs, low–molecular weight heparins, vitamin E, fish oils, garlic, or ginger. Bilberry interferes with iron absorption when taken internally.

Black Cohosh

Black cohosh (*Actaea racemosa*), formerly known as *Cimicifuga racemosa*, is a showy plant native to North American forests.

The drug was introduced by Native Americans, who valued it for treating a wide variety of conditions ranging from rheumatism to sore throat and diseases of women. It was also used to stimulate menstrual flow.

Indications

Black cohosh is now used primarily to alleviate menopausal symptoms. In fact, the American College of Obstetrics and Gynecology supports its use for up to 6 months, especially in managing sleep, mood disturbances, and hot flushes. In addition, the German Commission E supports its use for treating dysmenorrhea. Popular lay press claims suggest that it may also be useful for lowering blood pressure and cholesterol levels, as well as for reducing mucus production. It has also been suggested that black cohosh may be helpful for poisonous snake bites.

Pharmacodynamics

The chief constituent of the *Actaea* root is an amorphous resinous substance known as cimicifugin, or macrotin. Other active ingredients include triterpenoid glycosides, isoflavones, and aglycones, which include acteine, isoflerulic acid, oleic acid, palmitic acid, pantothenic acid, phosphorus, racemosin, tannins, and vitamin A. The bitter taste is due to a crystalline substance named racemosin. The drug also contains two resins, together with fat, wax, starch, gum, sugar, and an astringent substance.

A methanol extract of black cohosh contains substances that bind to estrogen receptors. The extract also appears to suppress luteinizing hormone but not follicle-stimulating hormone. This suggests that black cohosh possesses some degree of estrogen-like activity.

Adverse Effects and Contraindications

Because of a risk of spontaneous abortion, black cohosh should not be used during pregnancy.

Interactions

There are few known drug interactions with black cohosh; however, the herb may increase the toxicity of docetaxel (Taxotere) and doxorubicin (Adriamycin), both antineoplastic drugs. It is currently unclear whether toxicity is increased in normal tissues as well as neoplasms. Black cohosh may also have an additive effect on the estrogen-receptor antagonist activity of tamoxifen (Nolvadex), a P-glycoprotein–inhibitor drug used in women who have had breast cancer, but it is highly unlikely at physiologically achievable concentrations. Also do not use the herb in patients taking antihypertensive drugs.

Bladderwrack

Fucus vesiculosis, also known as bladderwrack, is a kind of algae that grows along the coasts of the Atlantic and Pacific Oceans, the North Sea, and the western Baltic Sea. Air-filled bladders keep this algae floating upward in the water. Its long, leathery, olive-green to yellow-brown ribbons are often found on beaches after a storm. Bladderwrack is commonly found in kelp tablets or powders used as nutritional supplements.

Indications

Bladderwrack is thought to have an impact on cholesterol levels and assist in achieving weight loss related to thyroid dysfunction. This herb has also been used to relieve the discomfort of rheumatoid arthritis and is ingested or applied topically to treat joint inflammation.

Bladderwrack has been recommended by some health care providers as a treatment for hypothyroidism, because it contains high concentrations of iodine. However, the amount of iodine contained in bladderwrack is unpredictable, and the herb will only be helpful if the hypothyroidism is caused by an iodine deficiency. Bladderwrack has also been used to treat atherosclerosis and to strengthen immunity, although evidence to support its effectiveness is lacking.

Pharmacodynamics

When taken by mouth, the alginic acid contained in bladderwrack swells upon contact with water, forming a type of seal at the top of the stomach. This mechanism allows it to be used in OTC preparations for the treatment of heartburn. The alginic acid in bladderwrack also has laxative properties.

Adverse Effects and Contraindications

Prolonged ingestion of bladderwrack reduces iron absorption and can lead to anemia. Do not use bladderwrack in persons with heart problems, or during pregnancy and lactation.

Interactions

The isolated fraction of bladderwrack, fucoidin, has 40% to 50% of the anticoagulant activity of heparin, and thus there is a theoretical concern that concurrent use of anticoagulants could increase the risk of bleeding. Bladderwrack has high sodium content, possibly reducing the effect of diuretics, and making its use in patients with sodium restrictions unwise. The high iodine content of bladderwrack may interfere with thyroid hormone replacement therapy and enhance thyroid activity in hypothyroid patients taking lithium.

Coenzyme Q$_{10}$

Coenzyme Q$_{10}$ is a key enzyme in cellular metabolism. It is synthesized in all body tissues and is found in exogenous sources such as organ meats such as heart, liver, and kidney, beef, soy bean oils, sardines, mackerel, and peanuts. For example, 1 lb of sardines, 2 lb of beef, or 2.5 lb of peanuts contain 30 mg of CoQ$_{10}$.

Indications

CoQ$_{10}$ is used as an antioxidant alone or with other drug therapies and nutritional supplements in the prevention and treatment of heart disease, heart failure, hypertension, elevated cholesterol levels, diabetes mellitus, and myocardial damage secondary to administration of antineoplastic drugs, cardiac surgery, breast cancer, and gum disease. CoQ$_{10}$ has also been used to prevent "statin"-induced myopathy, for migraine prophylaxis, and Parkinson's disease. It has several other possible uses: to improve immune system functioning in patients with deficiencies (such as acquired immunodeficiency syndrome [AIDS]) and chronic infections (such as yeast and other viral infections); to enhance fertility by increasing sperm motility; as an adjunct in the treatment for Alzheimer's disease; to reduce damage from strokes; to boost athletic performance; to enhance physical activity in people with fatigue syndromes; and to improve exercise tolerance in those with muscular dystrophy. Even with all of these uses, the most common goal of supplementation is to compensate for large deficiencies of CoQ$_{10}$.

Pharmacodynamics

The synthesis of CoQ$_{10}$ is a multistage process that begins with the amino acid tyrosine. Eight or more vitamins and trace elements are required for synthesis.

The Q and the 10 in CoQ$_{10}$ refer to the chemical groups that make up the coenzyme.

The functional role of coenzymes is to act as transporters of chemical groups from one reactant to another. As an antioxidant, CoQ$_{10}$ plays an important role in the production of energy within the mitochondria. Ubiquinol, the metabolite of CoQ$_{10}$, also serves as an antioxidant, reducing the risk of tissue damage from free radicals. Free radicals are thought to contribute to the aging process as well as the development of a number of health problems, including heart disease and cancer.

Ubiquinol inhibits lipid peroxidation in biologic membranes and in low-density lipoprotein (LDL), and it also protects membrane proteins against oxidative damage. Although ubiquinol does not require vitamin E for its antioxidant activity, it can regenerate the vitamin from its oxidized form, the alpha-tocopheroxyl radical, a process that otherwise relies on water-soluble vitamin C. This interaction with vitamin E is thought to be particularly important for the protection of LDLs and other lipoproteins from oxidative damage. It takes about 3 weeks of daily dosing with CoQ$_{10}$ to reach maximal serum concentrations, which then plateau with continuous daily dosing. CoQ$_{10}$ is distributed to all body tissues including the brain. It is eliminated through the bile.

Adverse Effects and Contraindications

CoQ$_{10}$ has no known adverse effects, contraindications, or toxicity associated with its use.

Interactions

Drugs that lower CoQ$_{10}$ levels include 3-hydroxy-3-methylglutaryl coenzyme A (HMG CoA) reductase inhibitors ("statins") such as atorvastatin, lovastatin, pravastatin, and simvastatin; fibric acid derivatives (specifically, gemfibrozil); and beta blockers (such as atenolol, labetolol, metoprolol, and propranolol).

Coenzyme Q$_{10}$ may help reduce the toxic effects on the heart caused by daunorubicin (Cerebidine) and doxorubicin (Adriamycin), antineoplastic drugs commonly used to treat a variety of cancers. CoQ$_{10}$ supplementation allowed patients taking drugs diltiazem, metoprolol, enalapril, and nitrate to take lower dosages of these antihypertensives.

There have been reports that CoQ$_{10}$ may decrease the effectiveness of orally-administered anticoagulant drugs, leading to a need for higher dosages. Some oral antidiabetic drugs (glyburine, in particular) may lower CoQ$_{10}$ levels.

Cranberry

Cranberry is a common name for several species of low vines that bear small, sour, seedy fruit. The plants, which belong to the same genus as the blueberry, have drooping, pink flowers and small, thick, evergreen leaves. The small, or European, cranberry *(Vaccinium oxycoccos)* grows wild in marshlands of the temperate and the colder regions of Europe and North America. The large, or American, cranberry *(Vaccinium macrocarpon)* is cultivated in the northeastern United States in sand-covered bogs that can be flooded or drained at will. These red berries are used in foods and in herbal products.

Indications

Historically, cranberry fruits and leaves have been used as a urinary deodorizer for people with incontinence, for prevention of urinary catheter blockage, and to heal the skin around urostomy stomas. Cranberry has also been reported to have antioxidant and antineoplastic activity. (See Evidence-Based Pharmacotherapeutics box.)

Pharmacodynamics

The mechanism of action of cranberry is unknown. Cranberry juice is thought to prevent bacteria from embedding in the epithelial layer of bladder lining. It is also thought that cranberry may prevent *Helicobacter pylori* from adhering to the stomach and causing ulcers.

Adverse Effects and Contraindications

There are no known adverse effects of cranberry. However, because of cranberry's high oxalate content, some health care providers recommend avoiding cranberry extract products or excessive consumption of cranberry juice in patients who have a history of kidney stones. Intake of more than 3 or 4 liters of cranberry juice per day often results in GI upset and diarrhea.

Interactions

There are no known interactions with cranberry supplements.

Creatine

Under the 1994 Dietary Supplement Health and Education Act, creatine is classified as a dietary supplement. Also referred to as an ergogenic aid, creatine is supposed to improve the production and use of energy during exercise and/or to enhance recovery after a workout. Creatine supplements are popular among those wishing to bolster their physical strength and endurance. Many athletes use supplements in a relatively safe way, but others are using potentially dangerous—and in some cases, banned—products. Although creatine offers short-term, limited benefits, whether or not it is harmful in the long run has yet to be fully determined. Further, creatine supplements have not been evaluated by the FDA for effectiveness or purity, and there are no regulated manufacturing standards in place for these compounds.

Indications

Creatine is purported to help with athletic performance during quick, high-intensity exercise, to build muscle, and to help produce energy. It must be noted that creatine has no significant effect on the outcomes of aerobic exercise.

Pharmacodynamics

Creatine that is normally present in human muscle comes from two sources, meats and fish. What isn't present in the diet is easily made by the liver and kidneys from a few amino acids (glycine, arginine, and methionine). It is believed that 95% to 98% of the creatine in our body is stored in our

EVIDENCE-BASED PHARMACOTHERAPEUTICS

Cranberries for Urinary Tract Infections

■ Background

Urinary tract infections (UTIs) are among the most common community-acquired and nosocomial infections (see also Chapter 41). *Escherichia coli* are by far the most predominant uropathogen, causing 85% to 95% of uncomplicated UTIs, and over 90% of uncomplicated pyelonephritis in premenopausal women. In the United States, complications resulting from persistent and repeated infections necessitate well over 1 million hospital admissions annually.

Cranberries (particularly cranberry juice) have been used for decades in the prevention and treatment of UTIs. Cranberries contain quinic acid, malic acid, and citric acid, as well as glucose and fructose. Until recently, it was thought that the quinic acid caused large amounts of hippuric acid to be eliminated in the urine, which then acted as an antibacterial agent. Of late, it has been demonstrated that cranberries prevent uropathogenic bacteria (specifically *E. coli*), from adhering to uroepithelial cells of the bladder. Also noted is that cranberries contain two compounds that inhibit adherence of uropathogenic bacteria, fructose, and a polymeric compound of unknown character. Of the many fruit juices containing fructose, only cranberries and blueberries contain this unknown polymeric compound.

■ Research Article

Jepson, R.G., Mihaljevic, L., and Craig, J. Cranberries for preventing urinary tract infections. *The Cochrane Database of Systematic Reviews (Complete Reviews)*. 2004, Issue 1. Art. No. CD001321. DOI: 10.1002/14651858. CD001321.pub2.

Purpose

The purpose of this study was to test whether cranberry juice and other cranberry products are more effective than placebo, no treatment, or any other treatment in the prevention of UTIs in susceptible populations. The primary outcome measures were the number of UTIs as evidenced by catheterized, midstream, or "clean catch" specimens. (The bacteriologic standard for infection is a specimen with greater than 100,000 bacterial colony-forming units /mL [cfu/mL]). The secondary outcomes were adherence to therapy and adverse effects.

Design

All randomized or quasi-randomized controlled trials that included "cranberry juice or derivatives versus placebo," and "treatment or no other treatment for UTIs in susceptible populations" were included in the study. Both parallel group and cross-over designs were included. Each of the subject groups were analyzed separately:

- Subjects with a history of two or more UTIs in the previous 12 months
- Older adult men and women
- Pregnant women
- Subjects needing intermittent catheterization
- Subjects with an indwelling catheter
- Subjects with an abnormality of the urinary tract

Methods

Two investigators independently assessed studies, and a third investigator was consulted for any disagreements. Seven studies met the inclusion criteria (four cross-over and three parallel groups). It was intended that for cross-over studies, the period before the cross-over would be assessed. Relative risks were used as the measure of effect for dichotomous outcomes.

Five of the seven studies evaluated the effectiveness of cranberry juice and cranberry cocktail versus placebo juice or water. Two compared the effectiveness of cranberry capsules versus placebo. An additional two studies had two treatment arms and a control arm; one study randomized subjects to either cranberry-lingonberry juice, *Lactobacillus* GG drink, or no intervention. The other study randomized subjects to cranberry juice, cranberry tablets, or placebo juice. The trials were then subgrouped by the types of subjects: subjects with a history of recurrent lower UTIs, those needing intermittent catheterizations, and older men and women

Findings/Outcomes

	No. of studies	Subjects*	Statistical method	Effect size
Cranberry juice vs. placebo, control	2	191	RR (fixed) 95% CI	0.40–0.97
Cranberry capsules vs. placebo	1	100	RR (fixed) 95% CI	0.27–1.15
Cranberry juice vs. cranberry tablets	1	100	RR (fixed) 95% CI	0.49–2.5
Cranberry products vs. placebo, control	3	241	RR (random) 95% CI	0.4–0.91

*Adverse effects were common in all trials, and dropouts and withdrawals in several of the trials were high.
RR, Relative risk; *CI*, Confidence interval.

Conclusions

There is some evidence that cranberry juice may decrease the number of symptomatic UTIs over a 12-month period in women. Whether or not the juice is effective in children as well as in older men and women is not clear. The large numbers of dropouts and withdrawals from some studies suggest that cranberry juice may not be a tolerable intervention over long periods. The optimal dosage or method of administration to be used remains unclear. Cranberry juice provides significant antiadherence activity against different *E. coli* pathogenic strains commonly found in the urine compared to placebo.

■ Implications for Practice

Additional randomized controlled trials (RCTs) must be done with the following features: use of larger sample sizes, improved designs, use of randomization with placebo controls, inclusion of men, women, and children, and avoidance of heterogenous endpoints.

There are no national guidelines for the use of cranberry juice in the prevention of UTIs. Anecdotally, patients are often advised to use cranberry in the treatment of UTI. Cranberry capsules or tablets may be used, but patient adherence may be poor compared to treatment with cranberry juice.

---

muscles in the form of phosphocreatine. The remaining 2% to 5% is stored in various other parts of the body including the brain, the heart, and the testes. On average, a 160-lb person would have about 120 grams of creatine stored in the body. Ingesting creatine may increase the level of phosphocreatine in the muscles up to 20%.

High-intensity exercise requires that muscles acquire their energy source from a series of reactions involving adenosine triphosphate (ATP), phosphocreatine, adenosine diphosphate (ADP), and creatine. The amount of ATP is relatively constant. ATP provides energy when it releases a phosphate molecule and becomes ADP; it regenerates when phosphocreatine donates a phosphate molecule, which then combines with ADP. Stored phosphocreatine can fuel the first 4 to 5 seconds of high-intensity exercise, but another fuel source must be used to sustain the activity. A good example of an activity for which it might be helpful is football (i.e., 6 seconds of all-out forceful effort, followed by 45 seconds of standing around).

New research has shown that creatine may help buffer lactic acid that builds up and leads to a familiar burning sensation in the muscles during exercise. Basically, the creatine bonds with a hydrogen ion, and that helps delay the build up of lactic acid. More research must be done to see if this point is true.

Adverse Effects and Contraindications

Exercise studies of less than 2 weeks' duration have reported no adverse events associated with creatine use, although no studies have been done to evaluate the safety of long-term use. The short-term adverse effects of creatine include nausea, vomiting, and diarrhea. Creatine often contributes to weight gain because of the osmotic influx of water into the cell. It is possible that the weight gain is related to water retention and not increased muscle mass. Reports of muscle cramps, dehydration, and heat intolerance have been reported as a result of water retention. Symptoms of creatine overdose are not known. Anaphylaxis has been reported.

Interactions

Use creatine with caution in combination with prescription drugs, herbs, or other natural products. In addition, creatine should be used with caution in patients taking a nonsteroidal antiinflammatory drug (NSAID) such as ibuprofen (e.g., Advil, Motrin), indomethacin (Indocin), naproxen (e.g., Aleve, Naprosyn) and others. Interactions with trimethoprim (Bactrim), probenecid (Benemid), and cimetidine (Tagamet) have been reported.

Echinacea

Echinacea (*Echinacea purpurea*) is a member of the daisy family native to the central United States. In addition to *E. purpurea* there are also *E. pallida* and *E. angustifolia*. Echinacea was the most commonly used herb of the Plains Indians and was first introduced into Western medicine about 1871 as a blood purifier and to counteract blood poisoning. Later, it was used for problems ranging from bee stings, rattlesnake bites, and chronic nasal congestion to toothache and leg ulcers.

Indications

At present, the most common use of echinacea is to prevent or moderate symptoms of colds and upper respiratory infections. Either the drug is taken internally to increase the body's resistance to various infections, or it is applied locally for its wound-healing action. It has been approved by the German Commission E to enhance resistance to upper respiratory infections. Topically, echinacea may provide antioxidant protection against ultraviolet A (UVA) and ultraviolet B (UVB) light rays. It is also used topically, more often in Germany, to treat hard-to-heal wounds, eczema, burns, psoriasis, and herpes simplex infections.

Pharmacodynamics

Echinacea also acts as a nonspecific immune system stimulant. Standardized preparations should contain 3.5% echinacoside. The active ingredients of echinacea have been identified as high–molecular weight polysaccharides. Other constituents of echinacea include flavonoids, caffeic acid derivatives (e.g., echinacoside), essential oils, polyacetylenes, alkylamides, and miscellaneous chemicals including resins, glycoproteins, sterols, minerals, and fatty acids. The polysaccharides have been targeted in echinacea as immune-enhancing agents.

Several mechanisms may account for the immune-boosting properties of echinacea. It is thought to stimulate phagocytosis, increase the motility of leukocytes, and increase the number of T cells. Arabinogalactan, one of the plant's polysaccharides, has been shown to activate macrophages to produce tumor necrosis factor and other immune potentiators such as interferon. Echinacea has been shown to help protect the body from infection by stabilizing hyaluronic acid, one component of the ground substance in connective tissue. Hyaluronic acid, a mucopolysaccharide, protects cells and connective tissue from invasion by organisms. Further, echinacea's inhibitory action on lipoxygenase suggests antiinflammatory activity and justifies its use for treating infection.

Adverse Effects and Contraindications

Do not use this herb in persons with systemic autoimmune illnesses including tuberculosis or AIDS, collagen diseases such as lupus erythematosus, multiple sclerosis and other autoimmune diseases, or allergies to the sunflower family.

Interactions

Echinacea may interfere with immunosuppressant drug therapy because of its immunostimulating effects. For that reason, drug interactions can occur with the following immunosuppressants: azathioprine, basiliximab, corticosteroids, cyclosporine, dacliximab, muromonab-CD_3, mycophenolate mofetil, sirolimus, and tacrolimus.

Feverfew

Feverfew (*Tanacetum parthenium*), a short, bushy, perennial, is a member of the daisy family. Because its leaves have a strong fragrance, it was traditionally planted around houses to purify the air. Its yellow flowers and yellow-green leaves resemble those of chamomile. Its name is simply a corruption of the Latin term *febrifugia*, or fever reducer. Historically, the plant was used as an antipyretic.

Indications

Today, feverfew is used to relieve migraine headaches, menstrual pain, asthma, dermatitis, and arthritis. Chewing several leaves a day has proven to be effective in preventing some migraine headaches. Feverfew's sedative property makes it useful in treating hysteria, nervousness, and low spirits, and it is used as a general tonic. It is also purported to be good in syrup form for coughs, wheezing, and breathing difficulties.

Pharmacodynamics

The principal active constituent of feverfew is reported to be parthenoid, a sesquiterpene lactone. The precise mechanism of action of feverfew is not yet fully understood. It is thought that the prophylactic action is due to serotonin (5-hydroxytryptamine [5-HT]) inhibition, possibly via the neutralization of sulphydryl groups on specific enzymes fundamental to platelet aggregation and secretion.

Adverse Effects and Contraindications

There is an occasional report of mouth ulcerations or gastric disturbance with use of feverfew. There is also a concern that feverfew may have additive effects and increase the risk of bleeding with concurrent use of anticoagulant and antiplatelet drugs. Long-term adverse effects are unknown.

Interactions

Because of NSAIDs' effects on prostaglandins, there is a theoretical concern that NSAIDS may reduce the effectiveness of feverfew.

Garlic

Garlic is a common name for several strongly scented herbs of the lily family. Common garlic *(Allium sativum)* has been cultivated since ancient times. Common garlic belongs to the same genus as the onion, the leek, and the shallot. The bulb has a strong characteristic odor and taste, is covered with a papery skin, and may be broken into constituent bulblets, called cloves.

As a medicinal herb, garlic has been used since the earliest days of recorded history. It grows wild almost everywhere in the world, and every culture has recognized its enormous healing powers. To the Greek physician Galen (130 to 200 AD), garlic was known as the great panacea. To the gangs who worked on the great pyramids of Egypt, it was a daily ration given to them to maintain their strength and prevent disease. Because of its supremacy in strengthening immunity, cleansing the blood, and driving out infection, it was championed by the people of central Europe as one of the weapons of choice to combat the depredations of the legendary blood-drinking vampires.

Indications

Garlic is a popular herbal product whose effects are supported by scientific and clinical evidence. Garlic is most commonly used for its antihyperlipidemic, antihypertensive, and antifungal effects, and some believe it has antineoplastic effects. There are insufficient data to draw conclusions regarding garlic's effect on clinical cardiovascular outcomes such as claudication and myocardial infarction. Garlic preparations may have a small, positive, short-term effect on lipid levels; whether effects are sustainable beyond 3 months is not clear. Consistent reductions in blood pressure with garlic have not been supported, and no effects on glucose or insulin sensitivity were found. Promising effects on antithrombotic activity have been reported, but few data are available for a definitive conclusion.

The popular press suggests that garlic may be used also as an anthelmintic, antispasmodic, diuretic, carminative and digestant, and expectorant.

Pharmacodynamics

Garlic bulbs contain an odorless, sulfur-containing amino acid derivative known as alliin. When the bulb is crushed or bruised, alliin comes into contact with alliinase and is converted to allicin, the active ingredient in garlic. The parent substance alliin has no antibacterial properties; however, allicin has potent antibacterial activity against numerous gram-positive and gram-negative organisms. Allicin has a strong garlic odor and is also extremely unstable. In order to obtain the volatile oil from garlic, the bulbs are subjected to steam distillation.

Ajoene is the compound in garlic proposed to act as an antithrombotic agent. Ajoene increases fibrinolysis, the breakdown of fibrin, which slows blood coagulation. The antithrombotic and fibrinolytic actions of garlic have been shown to be at least as potent as aspirin in slowing the blood clotting mechanism. Garlic has also been shown to act like a "statin" to decrease cholesterol synthesis and promote smooth muscle relaxation and vasodilation.

Dried garlic preparations contain neither allicin, the antibacterial component, nor ajoene, the anticoagulant agent. Allicin and ajoene may be present in garlic that has been dried at a relatively low temperature, but it is unstable in the presence of acids. Dried garlic preparations are most effective if they are enteric-coated. Enteric-coated formulations, in which alliinase is destroyed in the stomach, should be more effective (theoretically) than even fresh garlic. Fresh garlic releases its active components primarily in the mouth during chewing, not later in the stomach.

Adverse Effects and Contraindications

Garlic has been reported to affect menses and is a reputed abortifacient, although this information has not been adequately substantiated. There are rare reports of GI upset, changes to intestinal flora, and allergic reactions.

Interactions

Because garlic reduces coagulation, persons taking aspirin or other anticoagulant drugs should avoid eating large amounts of the herb. Garlic may induce the CYP450 2E1 and/or 3A4 isoenzymes, potentially resulting in decreased effectiveness of drugs primarily biotransformed by these enzyme systems.

Ginger

Ginger *(Zingiber officinale)* is a rhizome (underground stem) native to the Orient. The plant has a green-purple flower and resembles an orchid. The family is cultivated widely in the tropics for its showy flowers and useful products, derived mostly from the rhizomes. These products include the flavoring ginger; East Indian arrowroot, a food starch; and turmeric, an important ingredient in curry powder. It continues to be valued throughout the world as a spice.

Indications

Ginger is used as an antiemetic for nausea and vomiting, motion sickness, morning sickness, antineoplastic-induced nausea and vomiting, and/or postoperative nausea and vomiting. The most evidence exists for its use as an antiemetic. Ginger has shown to be effective in the treatment of hyperemesis gravidarum (excessive vomiting during pregnancy), although long-term use during pregnancy is not recommended. Owing to its antiinflammatory actions, other applications of ginger include arthritis, both rheumatoid and osteoarthritis, and muscular pain.

Wild ginger contains the valuable constituent, aristolochic acid. Scientific study shows it to have antiinflammatory, antiviral, and antitumor activity, that it cures warts in some cases, and that it is a broad-spectrum antibacterial and antifungal. Taken orally, aristolochic acid also has contraceptive, spermicidal, and immunostimulant action.

Pharmacodynamics

Between 1% and 4% of the active constituent in ginger is comprised of a volatile oil containing sesquiterpene hydrocarbons, zingiberene, and bisabolene. Pungent oleoresin components of the plant include shogaols and gingerols. These pungent components are thought to be the most pharmacologically active. The antiemetic activity of ginger occurs primarily in the GI tract, although it appears the shogaols and the gingerols may also act on the vestibular impulses to the autonomic centers of the brain. Ginger has not been shown to influence the inner ear or the oculomotor system.

Ginger exerts anticoagulant effects by inhibiting thromboxane production. The sesquiterpene gingerol is responsible for the blood-thinning action of ginger. Ginger has mild antiinflammatory and analgesic effects because of the inhibition of leukotrienes and prostaglandins.

▓ Adverse Effects and Contraindications

Ginger is generally contraindicated in patients with a history of gallstones and should be used by these patients only after consultation with the health care provider. Ginger contains aristolochic acid, a naturally occurring toxin that may contribute to cancer, mutations in human cells, and end-stage renal failure. Ginger should not be used for morning sickness associated with pregnancy, or by nursing mothers.

Health Canada is advising consumers not to use products containing aristolochic acid, which is a naturally occurring toxin that can cause cancer, mutations in human cells, and end-stage kidney failure. The FDA has issued a letter to health professionals that aristolochic acid has been linked to unexplained renal disease.

▓ Interactions

Ginger is contraindicated for use in conjunction with anticoagulants, aspirin, or bilberry, because the risk of bleeding is increased.

Ginkgo

Ginkgo *(Ginkgo biloba)* is the oldest living species of tree. The ginkgo has been preserved as a sacred tree in Chinese temple gardens since ancient times. Botanists long believed that the species would have become extinct without this care, but wild ginkgos have been found in recent years in remote valleys of western China. It can be traced back more than 200 million years to the fossils of the Permian period. It was used medically in China for hundreds of years and is now a popular ornamental tree in parks and gardens throughout the world. The ginkgo tree is hardy, thriving along heavily trafficked streets of major cities.

▓ Indications

Gingko *(G. biloba)* has proven useful for treating dementia, Alzheimer's disease, peripheral arterial occlusive disease, and vertigo and tinnitus of vascular origin.

▓ Pharmacodynamics

The herbal extract of *G. biloba* (GBE) is derived from green-picked ginkgo leaves specifically developed for pharmaceutical purposes. The leaves are extracted with an acetone-water mixture, the organic solvent removed, and the extract processed, dried, and standardized. Standardized preparations of GBE typically contain 24% ginkgo, flavone glycosides, flavonoids (including the bioflavonoids quercetin, kaempferol, and isorhamnetin), and 6% terpene lactones (ginkgolides and bilobalide).

The flavonoids are primarily responsible for GBE's antioxidant activity, particularly in reducing damage to the lipid layer of the cell membrane. The ginkgolides act as platelet-activating factor–antagonists. Platelet-activating factor not only promotes aggregation of blood platelets but also is involved in many of the effects of the allergic response including bronchoconstriction, cutaneous vasodilation, hypotension, and release of inflammatory compounds from phagocytes. It is suggested that GBE and the ginkgolides attach to platelet-activating factor binding sites to reduce these effects. Bilobalide, in action with the ginkgolides, has been shown to increase blood flow in the brain and protect brain tissue from the effects of hypoxia.

▓ Adverse Effects and Contraindications

Unprocessed gingko leaves in any form should be avoided. They contain several potent allergens known as ginkgolic acids. These compounds, which are removed during the processing of GBE, are closely related to urushiol, the chemical that puts the itch in poison ivy. Occasionally, stomach or intestinal upsets, headaches, or allergic skin reactions may occur. Gingko is contraindicated for use during pregnancy and lactation.

▓ Interactions

The risk for bleeding is increased with concurrent use of anticoagulants, antiplatelet drugs (e.g., aspirin, clopidogrel), and other herbals such as bilberry that also decrease platelet aggregation.

Ginseng

Ginseng is a yellowish, radish-like herb with a rich history in Eastern medicine. It is used as a culinary root vegetable in China, particularly in making soup. In China, ginseng has been in continuous use for over 4000 years and has a broad range of medicinal uses. It is expensive and not widely available in the United States.

There are numerous varieties of ginseng, and almost all are cultivated. The most common are *Panax ginseng*, also called Korean, Chinese, or Asian ginseng, and *Eleutherococcus senticosus*, also known as Siberian ginseng. These two types of ginseng are considered the most important species because of the frequency of their use and the amount of research that has been dedicated to them.

References to colors of ginseng indicate how the herb was processed. Red ginseng refers to the ginseng root that has been sterilized and preserved through steam treatment, thus turning it red. White ginseng is the dried root. There are no chemical differences between the red and white varieties.

▓ Indications

Panax ginseng is used primarily to improve psychologic function, exercise performance, immune function, and conditions associated with diabetes. Perhaps the most widely cited reason for using ginseng is its purported ability to help the body compensate for physical and mental fatigue and to improve cognitive function. Students taking ginseng may demonstrate significant improvement in arithmetic and deductive reasoning skills. Athletes use it to increase physical endurance. It enhances cardiovascular response both during and after strenuous physical activity, and enables the body to make better use of its energy stores. Ginseng has been used to improve cardiovascular function and to regulate plasma glucose levels in persons with type 2 diabetes. It is thought to be analogous to the ubiquitous multivitamin tablet. It is also purported to stimulate the immune system, and has been used as an aphrodisiac in healthy men and women.

Pharmacodynamics

A very powerful medicinal herb, ginseng both stimulates and relaxes the nervous system, encourages the secretion of hormones, improves stamina, lowers blood sugar and cholesterol levels, and increases resistance to disease. The ginsenosides that produce these effects are very similar to the body's own natural stress hormones.

Ginseng species differ primarily in their composition and mechanism of action. *P. ginseng* is the most complex, with 13 identified ginsenosides. The interaction of the ginsenosides contributes to ginseng's attribution as an adaptogen. Adaptogens, by definition, must be innocuous and cause minimal disruption of physiologic functioning. Increased vitality and resistance to physical, chemical, or biologic stressors are characteristic of adaptogens. Standardized extracts of the herb contain 4% to 7% ginsenosides.

Because of the interaction of the ginsenosides, which are all contained in small amounts in the root of the plant, the whole root is used in herbal preparations. For example, two ginsenosides in ginseng, Rb_1 and Rg_1, exert different yet harmonizing influences on the body. Rb_1 has a hypoactive effect on blood pressure and a mildly sedative effect, whereas Rg_1 is believed to exert a mildly stimulatory action on the central nervous system (CNS). Its reputation as an aphrodisiac seems to be based on the fact that it relaxes the overly tense person a bit.

Ginseng has an analogous relationship with many of the body's homeostatic control mechanisms, and has several secondary actions on metabolic activity of the body in times of stress, when it may have a modulating effect on the hypothalamic-pituitary-adrenal axis (HPA axis). By inducing secretion of adrenocorticotropic hormone (ACTH), ginseng assists in the production and secretion of adrenal hormones. Ginseng has also shown promise in combating age-related disorders by increasing the life span of cells. It is also thought to stimulate nerve growth factor, which normally becomes deficient with increasing age.

Ginseng has been shown to increase levels of T cells and natural killer cells, and to stimulate production of white blood cells in cancer patients undergoing antineoplastic therapy.

Adverse Effects and Contraindications

Ginseng is contraindicated in patients with known hypertension, asthma, emphysema, fibrocystic breast disease, clotting disorders, or arrhythmias.

Interactions

Ginseng has no reported drug interactions. However, caution is advised with concurrent use of ginseng and warfarin (decreased effectiveness), oral hypoglycemic drugs or insulin (risk for hypoglycemia), monoamine oxidase inhibitors (MAOIs) (phenelzine–insomnia, headache, tremors, and hypomania have been reported), and antihypertensive drugs (ginseng may increase blood pressure). Caffeine used concurrently with ginseng or ginseng mixtures may cause overstimulation and GI distress.

Glucosamine and Chondroitin

Glucosamine is a naturally existing polysaccharide component of cartilage. Chondroitin is a sulfated glycosaminoglycan (GAG) composed of a chain of alternating sugars (N-acetylgalactosamine and glucuronic acid). It is usually found attached to proteins as part of a proteoglycan.

Indications

Glucosamine and chondroitin sulfate are extracellular matrix components of cartilage widely promoted as a remedy for osteoarthritis. Based on human research, there is good evidence to support the use of glucosamine sulfate in the treatment of mild to moderate knee osteoarthritis since its use may allow for reduced doses of NSAIDs.

Pharmacodynamics

The mechanisms by which glucosamine and chondroitin act in relieving arthritis pain and repairing cartilage remain something of a mystery, especially in the absence of quantitative data on the extent to which either substance enters the human circulation after the recommended oral dose. However, we do know a great deal about the biochemistry of the molecules in which these two compounds are found.

Glucosamine is involved in the metabolism of glycoproteins (also known as proteoglycans) and form the ground substance in the extracellular matrix of connective tissue. High–molecular weight proteoglycans contain many different heteropolysaccharide side-chains, including glucosamine, chondroitin, and hyaluronic acid. These substances make up to 95% of the glycoprotein structure. In fact, chemically, these proteoglycans resemble polysaccharides more than they do proteins.

A balance of swelling pressure and the tensile forces of collagen fibers provide the shock-absorbing properties and deformable resilience of glucosamine vital to its function. Hyaluronic acid is important in lubricating articular cartilage.

Adverse Effects and Contraindications

The adverse effects of glucosamine and chondroitin include mild heartburn, epigastric distress, and diarrhea. Glucosamine increases insulin resistance and is thought to significantly decrease the rate of glucose uptake by skeletal muscles. No allergic reactions, including sulfa-allergic reactions, have been reported with glucosamine sulfate.

Interactions

Persons with diabetes who, under advisement by their health care provider, decide to use glucosamine supplements will need to monitor blood glucose levels and adjust the dosages of their antidiabetic drugs accordingly.

Chondroitin has no known drug, nutrient, food or herbal interactions; however, chitosan–a polysaccharide polymer containing more than 5000 glucosamine and acetylglucosamine units–may form complexes with chondroitin sulfate, decreasing its absorption. Chondroitin sulfate should not be used concomitantly with chitosan.

Hawthorn

Hawthorn *(Crataegus oxyacantha)* is a small- to medium-sized tree native to Europe. Other species of hawthorn include *Crataegus monogyna* and *Crataegus pentagyna*. The genus name comes from the Greek *kratos,* referring to the "hardness" of the wood. In Celtic folklore, fairies are said to "hang out" in groves of the small, spiny tree indigenous to the Mediterranean region. The leaves, the blossoms, and the fruits of the plant are used in modern standardized extracts. Much research has been conducted on hawthorn, using proprietary extracts that are not available in the United States. Only leaf and blossom formulations are approved for use in Germany. In Europe, hawthorn berry is the plant medicine of choice for regulation of arrhythmias.

▮▮ Indications

Hawthorn (C. oxyacantha or C. monogyna) may be used in the prevention and management of arrhythmias that lead to myocardial infarction; as protection against toxin-induced arrhythmias; to increase blood flow by slowing and strengthening the heartbeat; and as protection against angina by preventing oxygen deprivation of the heart.

▮▮ Pharmacodynamics

The chemical composition of hawthorn leaves, berries, and blossoms includes oligomeric procyanidins and a mixture of flavonoids. The active constituents of hawthorn include the flavonoids vitexin, quercetin, and rutin, and oligomeric procyanidins. Cardiotonic amines, choline and acetylcholine, purine derivatives, amygdalin, triterpene acids, and pectins are also present.

The highly concentrated flavonoids in hawthorn also exert antioxidant action, mitigating free radical damage to the cardiovascular system by increasing the levels of intracellular vitamin C. The flavonoid quercetin limits oxidation of low-density lipoproteins.

Hawthorn preferentially dilates coronary blood vessels and reduces peripheral vascular resistance, thus lowering blood pressure and the risk of angina. It improves the metabolic processes of the heart through its inotropic (strength of the contraction) and chronotropic (heart rate) actions. In addition, hawthorn inhibits angiotensin-converting enzyme (ACE), which converts angiotensin I to angiotensin II, a powerful blood vessel constrictor. When used to support weight-loss programs, hawthorn berries help reduce water retention by expelling excess salt from the body.

▮▮ Adverse Effects and Contraindications

Hawthorn should not be used for acute angina because of its slow onset of action. It should not be used in children under the age of 12 years, or in the first trimester of pregnancy. It should be used with caution in patients with colitis and peptic ulcer disease.

▮▮ Interactions

Patients taking hawthorn should be carefully monitored by a health care provider, especially in cases where it is combined with cardiac glycosides, beta blockers, or calcium channel–blocking drugs. Overuse can lead to hypotension, arrhythmias, and hypersomnia. No toxic effects or habituation have been noted in hawthorn's long history as a medication.

Kava Kava

Kava is a member of the pepper family and is native to South Pacific islands. Drinks made from kava come from the dried roots of the shrub Piper methysticum, which has been used ceremonially and socially in the South Pacific for hundreds of years, and in Europe since the 1700s.

▮▮ Indications

The FDA has issued a warning that using kava supplements has been linked to a risk of severe liver damage although available studies suggest that kava may be useful in the management of anxiety. The NCCAM-funded studies on kava were suspended after the FDA issued its warning. Early evidence suggests that kava may be equivalent to low-dose benzodiazepine drugs such as diazepam when used for the short-term treatment of anxiety. The effects of kava are analogous to those of the drug buspirone (Buspar), used for generalized anxiety disorder (GAD).

▮▮ Pharmacodynamics

The lactones in kava have been found to have significant analgesic, sedative, anxiolytic, and local anesthetic properties via nonopiate pathways. Despite its properties, kava is not thought to act at opioid, gamma-aminobutyric acid (GABA), or benzodiazepine receptors. This is in stark contrast to the types of drugs that are commonly used for these purposes. Kava lactones are physiologically active, though it is the fat-soluble kava lactones derived from kava resin that have the greatest effect on the CNS. Animal studies show that kava lactones alter neuronal excitation through direct interactions with voltage-dependent ion channels, giving rise to kava's muscle relaxant, anesthetic, anxiolytic, and antiepileptic properties.

▮▮ Adverse Effects and Contraindications

Kava has been associated with damage to the liver ranging from hepatitis, cirrhosis, and liver failure to death. Kava has been linked to several cases of dystonia (abnormal muscle spasm or involuntary muscle movements). Scaly, yellowed skin and weight loss may result from long-term and/or heavy use of kava. The herb is contraindicated for use in pregnant or nursing mothers and in those with liver disorders. Kava use for more than 3 months should be supervised by a health care provider.

▮▮ Interactions

Increased risk of liver damage may occur if kava is taken with drugs that may injure the liver such as anabolic steroids, amiodarone, methotrexate, acetaminophen, and antifungal drugs taken by mouth (e.g., ketoconazole), and in patients with preexisting liver disease or injury. Liver damage can be caused by kava alone. It can be severe, and this has prompted consumer alerts in many countries, including the United States (www.cfsan.fda.gov/~dms/addskava.html); some countries removed kava from the market entirely. Thus close monitoring for liver toxicity is prudent.

Kava's diuretic properties may lead to additive effects when it is taken with diuretic drugs such as acetazolamide, amiloride, and furosemide, or with ACE inhibitors such as benazepril, captopril, lisinopril, quinapril, and ramipril. Further, kava is thought to increase the number of "off" periods in patients with Parkinson's taking levodopa.

Kava may also potentiate the effects of antiepileptic medications, increasing their sedative and cognitive effects. The bottom line is that kava is a CNS depressant and should be used with caution in patients concurrently taking other CNS depressants such as benzodiazepines, barbiturates, alcohol, or levodopa, or the sedative herbal supplements valerian and chamomile.

Milk Thistle

Milk thistle *(Silybum marianum)* is a tall plant with prickly leaves and a milky sap. A member of the daisy family, it is native to the Mediterranean region, but has been naturalized to the eastern United States, California, and other parts of North America. Silymarin, which is obtained from the seeds (fruit) of the plant, is thought to be the active ingredient of the herb. Capsules containing powered or seed formulations of silymarin are used to prepare extracts and infusions (strong teas).

▌ *Indications*

Milk thistle is often associated with its hepatoprotective characteristics. It is typically used to treat cirrhosis, chronic hepatitis, fatty infiltration caused by alcohol or other toxins, and gallbladder disorders. Few studies of the effects of milk thistle on liver disease have been done, and these were small. Promising data have been reported, but results at this time are mixed.

The NCCAM is exploring the use of milk thistle for chronic hepatitis. It is currently in phase II of the study. NCCAM, in conjunction with the National Institute of Diabetes and Digestive and Kidney Diseases (NIDDKD), is preparing additional studies on the use of milk thistle for chronic hepatitis C and nonalcoholic steatohepatitis.

The National Cancer Institute and the National Institute of Nursing Research are examining the herb for use in cancer prevention and to treat patients with complications of human immunodeficiency virus (HIV).

Other treatment claims include lowering cholesterol levels, reducing insulin resistance in people with type 2 diabetes mellitus who also have cirrhosis, and reducing the growth of cancer cells in breast, cervical, and prostate cancers. It has been used to reduce the hepatotoxicity caused by psychoactive drugs such as phenothiazines and in the treatment of overdose of the death cap mushroom *(Amanita phalloides)*.

▌ *Pharmacodynamics*

The active constituent of milk thistle is silymarin, whose highest concentrations are found in the plant's seeds. Silymarin specifically supports the liver by protecting hepatocytes from toxins and stimulating protein synthesis, which increases the ability of liver cells damaged by chronic viral hepatitis B or alcohol use to regenerate. It appears to reverse some liver cell damage (as evidenced with biopsy), increase serum protein levels, and reduce elevated liver function test results. The patient's abdominal discomfort, decreased appetite, and fatigue are also improved with silymarin treatment.

As an antioxidant, silymarin stimulates glutathione production. Glutathione is a powerful endogenous antioxidant, 10 times as powerful as vitamin E.

Dramatic evidence of silymarin's protection of liver cells is its action in cases of ingestion of the death cap mushroom. One of the death cap mushrooms contains phalloidine, one of the quickest and most toxic liver poisons. Phalloidine acts to destroy the outer membrane of liver cells, which can lead to a person's death within 3 to 7 days of eating the mushroom. Silymarin binds to sites on liver cell membranes to make sites unavailable to phalloidine, and the cell membrane is protected from phalloidine damage. Silymarin reverses the organ failure and encephalopathy associated with ingestion of the mushroom.

Silybinin is considered the most important component of silymarin. A strong inhibitory effect of silymarin on leukotriene B_4 by the Kupffer cells partially accounts for the hepatoprotective effects. In addition, silybinin is thought to both inhibit the peroxidase process and stimulate ribonucleic acid synthesis in hepatocytes. Silybinin has also been shown to stabilize the membranes of the hepatocytes by decreasing the turnover rate of membrane phospholipids.

▌ *Adverse Effects and Contraindications*

Milk thistle has been shown in clinical studies to have few adverse effects. Gastrointestinal problems (e.g., nausea, diarrhea, dyspepsia, flatulence, abdominal bloating, abdominal fullness or pain, anorexia, changes in bowel habits) have been reported. Other adverse effects include headache, skin reactions (e.g., pruritus, rash, urticaria, eczema), neuropsychologic events (e.g., asthenia, malaise, insomnia), arthralgias, rhino-conjunctivitis, and impotence.

Allergic reactions to milk thistle tend to occur more often among people who are allergic to plants in the same family (e.g., ragweed, marigold, chrysanthemum, daisy).

▌ *Interactions*

Milk thistle should not be used concurrently with antipsychotic drugs, yohimbine, or male hormones.

Saw Palmetto

Saw palmetto *(Serenoa repens, Sabal serrulata)*, is a shrublike palm tree native to Florida, Georgia, Louisiana, and South Carolina; it is also found in the West Indies. Its fruits were used during the early 1900s as a mild diuretic and to treat chronic cystitis and prostate enlargement.

▌ *Indications*

The efficacy of saw palmetto for the treatment of benign prostatic hyperplasia (BPH) has been substantiated through research. BPH is a nonmalignant abnormal growth of the prostate gland (see also Chapter 43). Saw palmetto reduces the symptoms of BPH; it does not reduce the size of the prostate. BPH affects 50% to 60% of men between the ages of 40 and 60, and over 90% of men older than 80 years of age; it has a significant impact on lifestyle owing to its irritative symptoms and the obstruction of urinary flow it causes. There are also claims by the popular press that it is beneficial in the treatment of asthma and bronchitis, as well as breast enlargement in women.

Saw palmetto helps initiate urine flow and decreases urinary frequency, residual volumes, nocturia, and dysuria. Saw palmetto extract has been favorably compared with the pharmaceutical drug finasteride. However, the saw palmetto extract has fewer adverse effects, including impotence and decreased libido, than finasteride. It is also thought to have antiinflammatory activity, specifically for the prostate.

▌ *Pharmacodynamics*

The active constituents of saw palmetto are derived from the red-brown-black berries, which contain free fatty acids and sterols. The berries are approximately 1.5% comprised of an oil (betasitosterol) that contains saturated (80% to 95%) and unsaturated fatty acids and sterols. A purified liposterolic extract of the berries is used medicinally.

It has been shown to exhibit both dihydrotestosterone binding at the androgen receptor and the enzymatic conversion of testosterone to dihydrotestosterone by the 5-α-reductase enzyme. This action limits the overproduction of testosterone and cellular and prostatic enlargement. The herb has been shown to reduce nocturia and to increase urine flow rates by up to 50%. Saw palmetto may reverse atrophy of the testes and mammary glands and may increase sperm production.

Saw palmetto has also been shown to inhibit both cyclooxygenase and 5-lipoxygenase, thereby contributing to its antiinflammatory and antiedematous effects. The plant has also shown to have spasmolytic activity.

Adverse Effects and Contraindications

The adverse effects of saw palmetto (i.e., sexual dysfunction, fatigue) are primarily related to its antiandrogen actions. Overall, there appear to be few adverse effects or safety concerns with short-term use of saw palmetto, although large-scale and longer-term safety studies have not been performed. Headache and diarrhea are possible. There are some indications that it may have the potential to produce liver toxicity and the risk for pancreatitis. Men with prostate cancer should not use saw palmetto.

Interactions

There are several interactions with saw palmetto. Finasteride and flutamide act to reduce 5-α-reductase and dihydrotestosterone binding to cellular and nuclear receptor sites, respectively. Saw palmetto alters the effects of oral contraceptives and estrogen replacement therapy, although the mechanism for the interaction is unknown. In combination with disulfiram or metronidazole, nausea and vomiting may be induced. The international normalized ratio (INR) level is increased with concomitant use of saw palmetto and warfarin. NSAIDs and saw palmetto may increase the risk of bleeding by inhibiting cyclooxygenase and 5-lipooxygenase.

St. John's Wort

St. John's wort *(Hypericum perforatum)* is an aromatic perennial herb that has gained much popular attention as an antidepressive. The plant is named for Saint John the Baptist because its bright yellow flowers bloom around his birthday, June 24. The plants are characterized by opposite, toothless leaves, generally dotted with blackish spots, which are oil-bearing glands. Mystical properties were attributed to St. John's wort in the Middle Ages, prompting people to place it under their pillows to ward off death. The herb was known to Dioscorides and Hippocrates. The plant is native to Europe but is found throughout the United States.

Indications

St. John's wort is available OTC and is used to support individuals with mild depression and anxiety. **It is not appropriate for patients experiencing severe depression, suicidal ideations, or psychotic behaviors.** It has also been used (rarely) to treat indigestion. Topically, St. John's wort has been used for minor wounds and infections, bruises, muscle soreness, and sprains. The efficacy of St. John's wort as an antidepressant was thought at one time to be comparable to that of imipramine (Tofranil). However, a major study conducted by NCCAM concluded that St. John's wort is ineffective for moderately severe depression. Some compounds of the plant have been shown to have potent antiretroviral activity without serious adverse effects and are being researched in the treatment of AIDS. St. John's wort is also thought to possess antibacterial, antiviral, and wound-healing activity.

Pharmacodynamics

The exact mechanism of action of St. John's wort is unclear. Some health care providers suggest that drug action may be a combination of low-grade MAO inhibition and blockade of the reuptake of norepinephrine and serotonin.

The active ingredient in St. John's wort is thought to be hypericin. When the leaves of the plant are rubbed, a red stain is produced; this stain is hypericin, a photosensitizing substance of the plant.

Adverse Effects and Contraindications

The adverse effects of St. John's wort include feeling tired or sleepy. Abdominal pain and cramping has been reported, along with nausea or vomiting and a rash.

Interactions

St. John's wort induces enzymes in the CYP450 enzyme system that biotransform indinavir (an HIV protease inhibitor) resulting in plasma levels that are subtherapeutic and leading to loss of virologic response and the development of resistance. This finding was so important that the FDA issued a public health advisory in February of 2000, alerting health care professionals of the potential loss of therapeutic effect when the herb was administered to patients concurrently receiving a drug biotransformed by these enzymes. These drugs include those used to treat heart disease, depression, seizures, and certain cancers, or to prevent conditions such as transplant rejection or pregnancy (i.e., oral contraceptives).

Concomitant use of prescription antidepressants, including fluoxetine and MAOIs such as phenelzine and tranylcypromine, is not advised. Other drugs that should not be taken concurrently with St. John's wort include opioids, amphetamines, and OTC cold and flu preparations.

Valerian Root

Valerian root *(Valeriana officinalis)*, or garden heliotrope, is a tall perennial herb whose hollow stem bears leaves with white or reddish flowers. According to legend, the Pied Piper enticed rats from the village of Hamelin with valerian. This vertical rhizome and its numerous rootlets are harvested in the autumn of its second year of growth. It is these parts that possess the volatile essential oil that contains the distinctive and, to some, disagreeable odor. The odor is said to be attractive to rats.

Indications

Valerian *(V. officinalis)* is used as a sedative and sleep aid. Valerian seems to improve the quality of sleep and reduces the time it takes getting to sleep (i.e., sleep latency–even in older persons and poor or irregular sleepers). Morning hangover is rare; however, impaired alertness and information processing may occur. Valerian may also be effective in relieving muscle spasms.

Patients treated with a valerian–lemon balm combination experience no daytime sedation or loss of concentration. Valerian has also been used as adjunctive therapy for benzodiazepine (e.g., diazepam, lorazepam) withdrawal.

▥ *Pharmacodynamics*

The mechanism of action of valerian root appears to be similar to that of benzodiazepines, but valerian root is not addicting. Valerian binds to GABA receptor sites to depress CNS activity. With weak binding of these receptor sites, sedation is caused without adverse effects, addiction, or dependence.

The ingredients responsible for the sedative effects of valerian have been identified. However, because sedation is produced by extracts without what are thought to be the active constituents, it is likely that there are other active constituents that have not yet been identified.

▥ *Adverse Effects and Contraindications*

Withdrawal symptoms following long-term use of valerian may occur.

▥ *Interactions*

In general, valerian should not be used concurrently with other sedative-hypnotic, antianxiety, or antidepressant drugs. Valerian in combination with lemon balm *(Melissa officinalis)* appears to be comparable to the benzodiazepines (e.g., triazolam) in shortening sleep latency and increasing sleep quality. Benzodiazepines are faster-acting; it may take 2 to 4 weeks of valerian use before drug effects are seen.

CLINICAL REASONING

Treatment Objectives

Regardless of the type of therapy used, virtually all CAM therapies share four basic components. They empower the patient to play an integral role in recovering health and wellness, as well as in maintaining it. They encourage a balanced lifestyle, with appropriate rest, sleep, exercise, nutrition, and emotional tranquility. The interventions are directed at the individual rather than at the symptoms. And lastly, CAM therapies recognize that good health is dependent on balance or harmony of all aspects of our lives.

Treatment Options

▥ *Patient Variables*

A directed history is an important assessment tool for health care providers; it should include questions to determine the use of phytomedicines or other complementary modalities, including naturopathic treatment, homeopathic remedies, Chinese herbs, or acupuncture. Ask patients seeking advice on the use of herbal remedies about the following: Why are you interested in taking this product? What allergies, if any, do you have to plant materials? Are you now pregnant or do you plan to become pregnant? When you become pregnant, do you plan to breastfeed? What prescription or OTC drugs are you currently taking?

If the patient reports a symptom, it is important to identify the specific herbal preparation he or she is using to treat it. Many people are not sure what they are using, in part because many OTC preparations are combinations of plant products. Many foreign preparations include herbs about which little is known, particularly Asian and Indian herbs.

Ask patients about the existence of comorbid diseases or conditions and allergies (Box 11-2). At a minimum, the physical exam should include height and weight, blood pressure, pulse, and breath sounds. Further examination will most likely be system-focused, based on the patient's reports. Depending on the herbal remedy used, perform liver function and kidney function tests before and throughout therapy. Allergy skin testing may have to be performed for some patients before the use of herbal remedies.

Factors that influence the choices of cures are bound to cultural beliefs about the causes of illness. Herbal remedies are important aspects of the treatment process for persons of many ethnicities. Contemporary medical practices neither assimilate nor stamp out folk practices. Health care providers, therefore, must learn an effective diplomacy in order to understand and deal responsibly with the cultural beliefs and practices of their patients.

Many people have turned away from conventional therapies because they believe that natural substances such as herbs are safer than synthetic substances. However, patients may not realize the drug properties of herbal remedies. The slogan "all natural" may lead them to believe that all herbal products are safe, because they do not think of them as drugs.

Pregnant and Nursing Women. Pregnant women generally like herbs because of their relative "safety" and lack of adverse effects, although no herbal remedy should be taken during pregnancy without first consulting the health care provider. Herbs contraindicated during pregnancy include angelica, Chinese angelica, comfrey, dang gui (or dong quai), devil's claw, ginseng, lady's mantle, licorice, motherwort, peppermint, sage, thyme, uva ursi, vervain, wild yam, and yarrow. In addition, advise pregnant women to avoid any herbal laxative except dandelion and yellow dock, and any worming herbs except garlic. When a woman is breastfeeding, herbs whose use is contraindicated for infants should also be avoided by the mother. Advise lactating women to avoid sage, which tends to dry up breast milk.

Children and Adolescents. Children respond very well to herbal remedies, but children's illnesses can develop very quickly. An accurate diagnosis from the health care provider

---

BOX **11-2**			
Herbs Frequently Associated with Allergic Reactions			
Angelica	Dandelion	Milk thistle	Rosewood
Arnica	Feverfew	Hops	Royal jelly
Camphor	Gravel root	Hydrangea	Yarrow
Chamomile	Jasmine	Motherwort	Yohimbine
Cowslip	Lavender	Parsley	

Controversy

Unconventional Answers to Illness

Jonathan J. Wolfe

Patients and their caregivers are increasingly interested in unconventional approaches to health promotion and disease treatment. Americans in particular, schooled to be careful consumers and armed with wide stores of uncensored information, often ask whether nontraditional treatments may be tried in their own cases. Some want to avoid painful procedures. Some want a last resort after traditional medicine has failed to produce a satisfactory result.

Mainstream health care providers have begun to accept that treatments other than surgery and drugs may offer real value. This is abundantly clear in the treatment of pain, in which behavioral therapies conclusively offer benefit with minimal cost or adverse effects. Rehabilitation therapy has also advanced rapidly. At present, interest in massage and acupuncture seem to provide evidence of a broader acceptance that adjunctive treatment has value. It seems that the process by which modern Western science–based medicine overcame its rivals may have relegated useful treatments to an obscurity that is now being overcome.

Patients are increasingly demanding these modalities. A fine balance will be required between a request based on some compelling but unreliable anecdote in unrefereed literature and a choice based on experience in controlled conditions.

CLINICAL REASONING

- A 36-year-old man with intractable pain following a lumbar injury and four attempts at surgical restoration tells you that he has received real benefit from drinking six cups of tea made from a natural herb that his wife buys at the local health food store. What is an appropriate response to this statement? What information should you document about the tea, its preparation, and its use? How do you measure this when following his progress?

- A 77-year-old woman has moderate pain from her incurable breast cancer, which has metastasized to her ribs and thoracic spine. She reacts negatively to your suggestion to use a transcutaneous electrical nerve stimulator (TENS) unit and imaging as means to reduce her suffering and limit adverse effects from opioid drugs. What answer is appropriate to her statement, "You are only suggesting this because I am old and poor—and my insurance company doesn't want to spend more on drugs for me!" Will you be able to offer this option to her later? What change in her condition could make such adjunctive treatments proper to offer?

- An orthopedic surgeon in your clinic has become interested in acupuncture and has taken several courses in its use at West Coast hospitals and colleges. Your assistance is requested for a procedure. The surgeon wants you to prep and drape the patient's back, then using aseptic technique, hand her 65 needles that she will insert into points marked on the patient's torso. Is this request proper? Under state law, may you assist in this procedure? What personal reservations do you have about taking an active part in this unconventional treatment? What further information do you need?

should be obtained before beginning a course of an herbal remedy (see Controversy box).

Drug Variables

Compared to conventional drugs, herbal remedies and other dietary supplements are largely unregulated and untested, for both safety and efficacy; and given the issues of inaccurate labeling, product variability, and adulteration, choosing an herbal remedy is largely a guessing game. Many of these remedies have powerful effects, both beneficial and harmful. Nonetheless, reliable information on clinical effects is usually lacking.

Herbs are usually chosen to work in unison with the inherent healing powers of the body. Despite obvious conflicts, herbalism and conventional medicine are not at odds with each other. What one does well, the other tends to do poorly, and vice versa. For example, contemporary medicine treats diseases using drugs that contain isolated compounds. The isolated compounds work well but are often potent and have serious adverse effects. However, for acute conditions, there is no substitute. On the other hand, traditional phytotherapy uses the whole herb. Whole herbs contain hundreds of compounds that may work in concert for a better overall effect than one compound alone could deliver, and yet they are gentler and tend to be safer than isolated drug compounds.

Patient Education

Advise patients that herbs are not regulated in the United States at this time. The vast majority of botanical producers are unlicensed and are not required to demonstrate the efficacy, safety, or quality of their products. Even though they are often promoted as harmless, herbal remedies are by no means free from adverse effects.

Because there are no standards in the United States, formulations vary widely in potency and recommended dosages (Table 11-4). There is no guarantee as to the strength, purity, or safety of the products, and effects may vary. Thus every effort should be made to obtain the highest quality product available; always read product labels. There are a number of ways herbs can be used. The formulation chosen depends on the herb to be used, the purpose for its use and, to some degree, personal preference.

Although most herbs are nontoxic when used at recommended dosages, there are herbs with identified toxic ingredients. These herbs include, for example, arnica, belladonna, hemlock, lily of the valley, and sassafras. Tell patients about the resources that are available to them with information regarding herbal remedies.

Herbal remedies should be taken exactly as instructed on the package label. The adage "if a little is good, more is better" is not correct. For some herbal remedies, a fine line exists between safe dosages and toxicity. Further, self-treatment with herbs is appropriate only for minor, self-limiting conditions. When the decision is made to use an herbal remedy, teach a few cautionary tips:

- Learn about the therapy before beginning a course of it. The more that is known about the efficacy of the remedy, the quality of the herb, and its adverse effects, the safer the remedy may be.

- Do not take herbs casually. Herbs should be used only when the body has a specific need. They should not be used on a regular basis.

TABLE 11-4 Selected Remedies*

Herb	Uses	Comments
Acidophilus†	IBS, UTIs, candidiasis, diarrhea, flatulence, bad breath, antibiotic support	Amount of active cultures in acidophilus products can vary widely. Ideally there should be no fewer than 1 billion organisms per capsule.
Bilberry	Simple diarrhea	Extract is standardized to at least 25% anthocyanosides.
Black cohosh	Menopausal symptoms, PMS	Use for no longer than 6 continuous months. Allow several weeks between uses.
Bladderwrack	Myxedema, lymphadenoid goiter, obesity, rheumatism, rheumatoid arthritis	Used as thyroid stimulant in 1880s; may counter obesity by increasing metabolic rate; since then, it is featured as a weight loss remedy.
Coenzyme Q$_{10}$	Heart failure, concurrently with HMG CoA reductase inhibitors, periodontal disease, cancer, muscular dystrophy, immune dysfunction	Headaches, heartburn, fatigue, diarrhea and skin reactions have been reported with dosages of 600 to 1200 mg per day.
Cranberry‡	Urinary tract infections	Since potency of tablets and capsules may vary, follow the manufacturer's directions whenever available.
Creatine†	Improve athletic performance	Creatine causes muscles to draw water from the rest of your body. Be careful during hot weather, or when you are exercising, or using a hot tub or sauna. Drink extra water while taking creatine.
Echinacea	Nonspecific immune system stimulant	Standardized extract of 4% phenolic compounds; cycled use (8 weeks followed by 1 week rest) is recommended because of the possibility of weakened effects with continued use.
Feverfew	Migraine headaches, menstrual pain, asthma, dermatitis, arthritis	Standardized extract 0.2% parthenolide; continuous use for at least 4 to 6 weeks is recommended.
Garlic	Mild hypertension, anticoagulation antibacterial, antiviral, antifungal agent, reduction of total serum cholesterol and triglyceride levels, prophylaxis for stroke	Formulation should deliver a minimum of 10 mg of alliin or a total allicin potential of 5000 mcg.
Ginger	Dyspepsia, diuretic, dizziness, nausea and vomiting; hyperemesis gravidarum, motion sickness	May aggravate gallstones. Do not use for postoperative nausea or concurrently with bilberry.
Ginkgo biloba	Age-related decline in mental function	Standardized extract of 24% ginkgo flavenoids, 6% terpenoids
Ginseng	Immune system stimulant, erogenic aid	Determine which form of ginseng is being used: Chinese ginseng, Siberian ginseng. Cycled use in 2- to 3-week intervals with a 1- to 2-week rest period is advised for Chinese ginseng and 5- to 7-week rest for Siberian ginseng.
Hawthorn	Hypertension, atherosclerosis, angina, early-stage congestive heart failure	Dosages vary depending on whether the dried berries, leaves, or flowers are used. Use product standardized to 18.75% oligomeric procyanidins and 2.2% flavonoids.
Kava kava	Anxiety	Kava extract is typically standardized to 30% kava lactones. Dosages as high as 800 mg daily have been taken for short periods, but have not been studied over the long term, and safety is not clear.
Milk thistle	Hepatoprotectant	Capsules contain 200 mg of concentrated seed extract representing 140 mg of silybin
Saw palmetto	Benign prostatic hyperplasia	Continuous use for 6 to 8 weeks is recommended before assessing efficacy.
St. John's wort	Mild to moderate depression	Standardized extract of 0.3% hypericin; avoid concurrent use with opioids, amphetamines, OTC cold and flu preparations. Several weeks may pass before improvement is noted.
Valerian root	Insomnia, anxiety	Standardized root extracts should contain 0.5% to 1% valerenic acid.

HMG CoA, 3-Hydroxy-3-methylglutaryl coenzyme A; *IBS*, irritable bowel syndrome; *OTC*, over-the-counter; *PMS*, premenstrual syndrome; *SE*, standardized extract; *UTIs*, urinary tract infections.
*Patients should be advised that herbs are not regulated in the United States at this time. Because there are no standards in the United States, formulations vary widely in potency and recommended dosages. When discrepancies exist the dosage instructions on the product label should be followed.
†Acidophilus and creatine are not herbs; however, because they are used by many persons as a non–prescription remedy, they are included here for the sake of convenience.
‡See also Chapter 43.

- Herbs take longer to work than conventional pharmaceuticals.
- Buy herbs from trusted companies. If possible, ask how and where the herbs are grown and processed. The answer to this question provides the patient with a sense of the quality controls used. Only standardized herbal remedies are recommended.
- Start with a single herb at less than the recommended dose, and carefully monitor the response. This is particularly important for older adults and those with below-average weight for height.
- Avoid herbs entirely if pregnant or lactating.
- Obtain information about potential drug interactions or drug interactions.
- If experiencing adverse effects, stop the herbal remedy immediately and notify the health care provider.

Evaluation

The therapeutic effectiveness of CAM has been determined by patient self-reports and careful research. However, to date only a handful of herbs have been approved by the FDA for selected uses; any book or article touting the benefits of an herbal remedy must be considered in light of the scientific literature on safety. Because the use of CAM is increasing, health care providers must be aware of the different therapies. At each visit, ask the patient about the use of OTC drugs, vitamins and supplements, and herbal products.

KEY POINTS

- Phytotherapy is the science of using plant-based medicines to treat illness. Use of herbal remedies is becoming more widespread among health care providers and the public alike.
- There are a number of ways herbs can be used. The formulation chosen depends on the herb to be used, the purpose for its use and, to some degree, personal preference.
- Any herbal remedy statement that uses terms such as "cures," "treats," "prevents," "mitigates," or "diagnoses disease" is subject to the same regulatory requirements as drugs.

- Under the DSHEA, an herbal supplement is considered to be safe until proven hazardous; the burden of proof rests with the FDA, not the manufacturer. With conventional drugs, drugs are presumed dangerous until rigorous testing by the manufacturer reveals otherwise.
- Patient assessment should include questions about the use of CAM remedies.

Bibliography

Agency for Healthcare Research and Quality. (2000). *Milk thistle: Effects on liver disease and cirrhosis and clinical adverse effects.* Evidence Report/Technology Assessment No. 21. 01; E024. Rockville, MD: Author.

American Society of Pharmacognosy. Should the American Society of Pharmacognosy change its name? Available online: www.phcog.org/societyname.html. Accessed February 10, 2007.

Avins, A., and Bent, S. (2006). Saw palmetto and lower urinary tract symptoms: What is the latest evidence? *Current Urology Reports, 7* (4), 260–265.

Austin, J. (1998). Why patients use alternative medicines: Results of a national study. *Journal of the American Medical Association, 279*(19), 1548–1553.

Blomhof, R. (2005). Dietary antioxidants and cardiovascular disease. *Current Opinion in Lipidology, 16*(1), 47–54.

Bonnar-Pizzorno, R., Littman, A., Kestin, M., et al. (2006). Saw palmetto supplement use and prostate cancer risk. *Nutrition and Cancer, 55*(1), 21–27.

Brace, L. (2002). Cardiovascular benefits of garlic *(Allium sativum L). Journal of Cardiovascular Nursing, 16*(4), 33–49.

Bressler, R. (2005). Herb-drug interactions. Interactions between saw palmetto and prescription medications. *Geriatrics, 60*(11), 32, 34.

Dietary Supplement Health and Education Act of 1994. U.S. Food and Drug Administration Center for Food Safety and Applied Nutrition website. Available online: www.cfsan.fda.gov/~dms/supplmnt.html. Accessed October 10, 2006.

Digiesi, V., Cantini, F., Oradei, A., et al. (1994) Coenzyme Q_{10} in essential hypertension. *Molecular Aspects of Medicine, 15*(Suppl), s257-s263.

Fetrow, C., and Avila, J. (2004). *Professional's handbook of complementary and alternative medicines.* Philadelphia: Lippincott, Williams, & Wilkins.

Food and Drug Administration Public Health Advisory. (2000). NIH Clinical Center study demonstrates dangerous interaction between St. John's wort and an HIV protease inhibitor. Available online: www.fda.gov/cder/drug/advisory/stjwort.htm. Accessed February 10, 2007.

Gardiner, P. (2004). Herbal medicine in the adolescent population: A review of the current literature. *Journal of the American Herbalists Guild, Spring/Summer,* 7–51.

Grossman, L. (2004). The curious case of kava: Why did it take the FDA so long to finally sound the alarm? *Time, 159*(14), 58.

Hespel, P., Maunghan, R., and Greenhaff, P. (2006). Dietary supplements for football. *Journal of Sports Sciences, 24*(7), 749–761.

Hypericum Depression Trial Study Group. (2002). Effect of *Hypericum perforatum* (St. John's wort) in major depressive disorder: A randomized controlled trial. *Journal of the American Medical Association, 287*(14), 1807–1814.

Jepson, R., Mihaljevic, L., and Craig, J. (2004). Cranberries for preventing urinary tract infections. *The Cochrane Database of Systematic Reviews.* 2004, Issue 2. Art. No. CD001321.

Juhn, M. (2003). Popular sports supplements and ergogenic aids. *Sports Medicine, 33*(2), 921–939.

Kiefer, D., and Pantuso, T. (2003). Panax ginseng. *American Family Physician, 68*(8), 1539–1542.

Kligler, B. (2003). Black cohosh. *American Family Physician, 68*(1), 114–116.

Kontiokari, T., Sundqvist, K., Nuutinen, M., et al. (2001). Randomized trial of cranberry-lingonberry juice and *Lactobacillus* GG drink for the prevention of urinary tract infections in women. *British Medical Journal, 322*(7302), 1571–1573.

Lowe, F., and Fagelman, E. (2001). Cranberry juice and urinary tract infections: What is the evidence? *Urology, 57*(3), 407–413.

McAlindon, T., and Biggee, B. (2005). Nutritional factors and osteoarthritis: Recent developments. *Current Opinion in Rheumatology, 17* (5), 647–652.

Messier, S., Loeser, R., Miller, G., et al. (2004). Exercise and dietary weight loss in overweight and obese older adults with knee osteoarthritis: The Arthritis, Diet, and Activity Promotion Trial. *Arthritis and Rheumatism, 50*(5), 1501–1510.

Milk thistle *(Silybum marianum).* In Coates, P., Blackman, M., Cragg, G., et al. (eds.). (2004). *Encyclopedia of dietary supplements.* New York: Marcel Dekker.

Napoli, M. (1998). Herbal remedies: What you see might not be what you get. *Health Facts, 23*(41), 3.

National Center for Complementary and Alternative Medicine. National Institutes of Health. *What is CAM?* Available online: http://nccam.nih.gov/health/whatiscam/. Accessed February 10, 2007.

National Center for Complementary and Alternative Medicine. (2002). *Kava linked to liver damage.* Available online: http://nccam.nih.gov/health/alerts/kava. Accessed February 10, 2007.

Rae, C., Digney, A., McEwan, S., et al. (2003). Oral creatine monohydrate supplementation improves cognitive performance: A placebo-controlled, double-blind cross-over trial. *Proceedings of the Royal Society of London—Biological Sciences, 270*(1529), 2147–2150.

Rhee, S., Gard, V., and Hershey, C. (2004). Use of complementary and alternative medicines by ambulatory patients. *Archives of Internal Medicine, 164*(9), 1004–1009.

Snyderman, R., and Weil, A. (2002). Integrative medicine: Bringing medicine back to its roots. *Archives of Internal Medicine, 162*(20), 395–397.

Sierpina, V., Wollschlaeger, B., and Blumenthal, M. (2003). Gingko biloba. *American Family Physician, 68*(5), 923–926.

Steiger, T. (2002). Complementary and alternative medicine. A primer. *Family Practice Management, 8*(3), 37–42.

Towheed, T., Maxwell, L., Anastassiades, T., et al. (2005). Glucosamine therapy for treating osteoarthritis. *The Cochrane Database of Systematic Reviews.* 2005, Issue 2. Art. No. CD002946.

U.S. Food and Drug Administration (FDA). Center for Food Safety and Applied Nutrition. Available online: www.cfsan.fda.gov. Accessed February 10, 2007.

Wilson, K., Klein, J., Sesselberg, T., et al. (2006). Use of complementary medicine and dietary supplements among U.S. adolescents. *Journal of Adolescent Health, 38*(4), 385–394.

12

Substance Abuse

In modern society the term *drug abuse* has come to mean the misuse of drugs to alter one's mood, to experience a "unique sensation," to alter one's perception of reality, or to attempt to improve one's physical or mental abilities. However, the use of the term is complicated by legal issues and by societal views of drug use, despite the fact that it is a diagnostic term defined by the American Psychiatric Association's *Diagnostic and Statistical Manual*. For example, decades ago it was common in the United States to smoke cigarettes in public. Today, smoking is seen by society as largely unacceptable behavior.

The popularity of drugs of abuse tends to increase and decrease over time as each new generation learns the adverse effects and consequences of particular drugs, or as new drug forms become available. The nation attempts to free its populace from the abuse of illegal substances; nonetheless, each generation has become known for its own prescription drug use and abuse (Fig. 12-1).

CONFUSING TERMINOLOGY

Drug dependence (or substance dependence) refers to a clinical syndrome of drug use that manifests itself as either psychologic or physical reliance on a drug, and it is associated with detrimental effects on the individual or society. A closely related term to drug dependence is *addiction*. According to the World Health Organization (WHO; www.who.int/substance_abuse/terminology/who_lexicon/en/index.html), addiction is defined as the "repeated use of a psychoactive substance or substances to the extent that the user (referred to as an 'addict') is periodically or chronically intoxicated, shows a compulsion to take the preferred substance (or substances), has great difficulty in voluntarily ceasing or modifying substance use, and exhibits determination to obtain psychoactive substances by almost any means." The life of the "addict" may be dominated by substance use to the virtual exclusion of all other activities and responsibilities.

Like drug abuse, drug dependence is a syndrome that has specific diagnostic criteria. However, confusion may occur when referring to the syndrome of drug dependence, because chronic use of the drugs discussed in this chapter can result in either psychologic or physical dependence, or both. For the purpose of this chapter, we will use the terms *drug abuse* and *drug dependence* interchangeably to indicate the misuse of drugs, rather than for the psychologic or physiologic states that occur as a result of chronic drug use (Box 12-1).

Psychologic dependence to a drug is a condition in which there are emotional and mental needs to continue using the drug in order to feel normal and/or to cope with reality. This complex set of feelings and behaviors is reinforced through use and experience with the drug; they make giving up drug use more difficult. Psychologic dependence is often related to the use of the drug to reduce stress, which eventually becomes the only means of stress reduction.

Physical dependence refers to the condition where chronic exposure to a drug alters function sufficiently that physical signs and symptoms occur when the dosage is decreased or the drug discontinued. These signs and symptoms are referred to as an *abstinence syndrome* or as *withdrawal*. Withdrawal symptoms are characteristic of the drug class and are often the opposite of the drug's action. For example, alcohol, a central nervous system (CNS) depressant, produces withdrawal symptoms characterized by hyperactivity. Conversely, when cocaine, a CNS stimulant, is withdrawn, one of the effects is depression and a loss of pleasure. These neurologic rebound effects occur because neurons have adjusted their neurotransmitters to the presence of the drug, or receptor changes have occurred that make postsynaptic neurons more or less sensitive. When the drug is withdrawn, the body lacks the balancing effect of the drug.

The withdrawal symptoms characteristic of alcohol, benzodiazepines, and barbiturates are the most dangerous and require careful monitoring, since individuals vary greatly in their potential for and the range of withdrawal symptoms they experience. Finally, it is important to point out that *cross-dependence* can occur with drugs of a given class (i.e., opioids, which are CNS depressants). This phenomenon is clinically important and the basis for administering methadone to patients dependent on heroin, or for using a standard CNS depressant to detoxify someone physically dependent on these drugs.

In addition to dependence, chronic use of most of the drugs discussed in this chapter results in the development of *tolerance* to the actions of the drugs. Tolerance is defined as the phenomenon whereby repeated use of the drug results in a loss of its effectiveness at the dosage used so that it takes increasing amounts of the drug to achieve the same physiologic or psychologic effects. It is important to point out that the development of tolerance is dependent on the characteristics of the drug, the dosage, and the frequency of administration. In general, there are two types of tolerance: cellular and metabolic. Cellular tolerance refers to the adaptation of individual cells to chronic exposure to drugs; in contrast, metabolic tolerance is where induction of metabolic enzymes results in a more rapid breakdown and thus less drug is available at the site of action.

Cross-tolerance describes the state in which developing a tolerance to one drug also increases the tolerance to a related category of drugs. For example, tolerance to alcohol, a CNS depressant, results in cross-tolerance to other CNS depressants such as benzodiazepines and barbiturates. Because of the potential for cross-tolerance, it is important to obtain a complete drug history of your patient, since tolerance to an

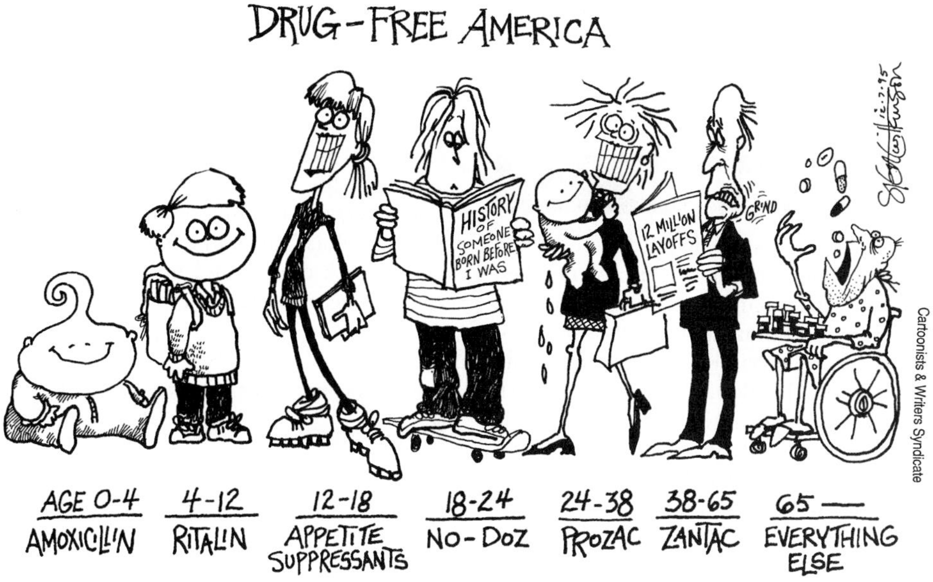

FIGURE 12-1 Drug Use Across American Generations. How we view and use prescription and over-the-counter drugs as a society has an impact on the issue of drug use and abuse. ("Drug-Free America" by Signe Wilkinson, published in the *Philadelphia Daily News,* 1997.)

illicitly used drug can result in cross-tolerance to a drug that is prescribed.

Although there is a correlation between the development of tolerance and physical dependence, they are not produced by the same cellular mechanisms. Furthermore, health care providers should understand that tolerance and physical

dependence will occur with long-term administration of certain drugs to patients. For example, chronic administration of morphine for pain results in tolerance and, perhaps, a need for dosage increase. When the drug is discontinued, the patient will experience a mild withdrawal. These effects are part of the actions of the drug and do not mean that the

---

BOX 12-1

Terms Associated with Substance Abuse

Compulsive drug abuse	Irrational, irresistible, compelling abuse of substances
Cross-tolerance	Tolerance for one drug results in a corresponding tolerance to others with similar chemical make-up. The need for an increased dosage of one carries over to its congeners
Drug abuse	Use of an illegal substance; use of a substance for other than the purpose (or person) for which (or whom) it was prescribed or in amounts larger than prescribed; use of a legal substance in excessive amounts (e.g., alcohol), or use of a substance despite known potential for harm (e.g., tobacco)
Drug addiction	Outdated term for drug dependence
Drug dependence	A human condition that manifests itself as either psychologic or physical reliance on a drug; the drug comes to have a higher value than other, formerly valued things
Drug misuse	Like drug abuse, drug misuse refers to the patient's use of a drug for other than the person or purpose for whom or for which it was prescribed, or in an amount different than prescribed. Term may also be applied to overprescribing and overreliance on drugs by the health care provider rather than other therapies to resolve the patient's problem
Experimental drug abuse	Exploratory use of a substance after which a decision is made to accept or reject continued use
Physical dependence	A condition in which a drug has altered neurons sufficiently so that there will be a physical withdrawal syndrome upon reducing the dose or stopping the drug entirely
Polydrug drug abuse	Use of multiple substances of abuse
Psychic dependence	A psychologic craving for a drug
Recreational or social drug abuse	Use of substances only in social contexts; most often alcohol, marijuana, cocaine, and caffeine
Situational drug abuse	Use of a drug to assist in task accomplishment
Street drug	An illegal drug with no guarantee of purity, or a legally prescribed drug sold on the street illegally
Tolerance	A condition in which it is necessary, after repeated administration of a drug, to increase the dose in order to achieve the same effect

patient has a drug abuse problem. Indeed, a common misconception that interferes with adequate drug therapy for pain is that long-term use of opioids will result in dependency. The development of a dependence syndrome after the chronic therapeutic use of drugs is rare and is usually associated with a preexisting drug dependence problem.

EPIDEMIOLOGY OF SUBSTANCE ABUSE

Psychoactive substance use poses a significant threat to the health and the social and economic fabric of families, communities, and nations. The extent of worldwide substance use is estimated at 2 billion alcohol users, 1.3 billion smokers, and 185 million drug users. The burden of these three substance categories varies across the globe. The disease burden in "disability-adjusted-life-years" (DALYs) is significantly higher in Europe and the western Pacific than in Africa and the eastern Mediterranean regions. Also, the share of the burden for the different substances varies; tobacco is the largest burden in Europe and Southeast Asia, whereas alcohol poses the largest burden in Africa, the Americas, and the western Pacific.

Rates of illicit drug use varied significantly among the major racial and ethnic groups in 2003. The rate was highest among Native Americans or Alaska Natives (12.1%), persons reporting two or more races (12%), and Native Hawaiians or Other Pacific Islanders (11.1%). Rates were 8.3% for whites, 8% for Hispanics, and 8.7% for blacks. Asians had the lowest rate at 3.8%. Young Native Americans also tend to use more marijuana and inhalants.

The prevalence of marijuana, alcohol, and cocaine use over the life span is higher in men than in women. Men tend to obtain drugs illicitly, whereas women are more likely to abuse prescription drugs. Heroin use by blacks decreased in the 1970s, only to be replaced by cocaine and crack. Crack use among blacks peaked in 1988. Hispanics are less likely than whites or blacks to use stimulants or hallucinogens, but as a group, they have a longer history of abuse, arrests for use and distribution, and incarcerations, and they are slower in seeking treatment.

There is a 20% to 30% incidence of alcohol abuse among older adults, which frequently masks other health problems. Whites were more likely than any other racial or ethnic group to report current use of alcohol in 2003. An estimated 54.4% of whites reported use in the past month. The rates were 44.4% for persons reporting two or more races, 43.3% for Native Hawaiians or Other Pacific Islanders, 42% for Native Americans or Alaska Natives, 41.5% for Hispanics, 39.8% for Asians, and 37.9% for blacks. The Jewish population has a low rate of alcohol abuse, most likely because they tolerate the drug poorly.

Of the homeless in the United States–approximately 2 million people each year–30% have alcohol abuse problems, and 40% have abuse problems with other substances. Thus the incidence and prevalence of substance use problems is significant. Prison populations have doubled since the 1970s as a result of substance abuse–related convictions. In addition, two thirds of the populations who abuse alcohol have other psychiatric disorders. Over 50% of traffic fatalities involve alcohol, with 80% of the fatalities occurring between 8 PM

and 4 AM. Alcohol has been linked to 40% of all reported assaults and 30% of forcible rapes and cases of child molestation.

The economic cost of substance abuse is significant. Accordingly, health insurance coverage for substance abuse has more limitations than for other illnesses or disorders. The use of alcohol by those responsible for operating automobiles, airplanes, or other high-powered equipment has resulted in loss of life and property, and has been blamed for disastrous effects on the environment (e.g., oil and chemical spills). Airline pilots, air traffic controllers, train engineers, ship pilots, truck drivers, and nuclear power plant operators who abuse drugs also place the populace at risk for accidents and injury.

AT-RISK POPULATIONS

Drug dependency is a brain disease. Although initial drug use might be voluntary, drugs of abuse have been shown to alter gene expression and brain circuitry, which in turn affect human behavior. Once dependency develops, these brain changes interfere with an individual's ability to make voluntary decisions, leading to compulsive drug craving, seeking, and use.

WAR VETERANS

Vietnam veterans have had a much larger problem with substance abuse than Gulf War veterans or veterans of World War I, World War II, or the Korean War. There are no statistics available at this time for the Afghanistan and Iraq conflicts. There are various reasons for this situation. Vietnam bordered the so-called Golden Triangle for opiate production and use, which included Myanmar (formerly Burma), Laos, and Thailand. Thus access to drugs of abuse was easy. Also, World War II and the Vietnam Wars were fought during a period when laws against these substances were not as stringently enforced as they are today. A legal substance, alcohol, remains at the heart of the greatest substance abuse problem for veterans. Over 100,000 veterans are treated annually in veteran's administration health care facilities for problems related to alcohol abuse.

PEOPLE WITH CHRONIC PAIN

People with chronic pain are a diverse group, especially with respect to drug abuse. Few health care providers deny appropriate analgesia to those suffering from terminal cancer; neither would they freely give analgesics to people they suspect are drug seeking and using a physical condition as an excuse to obtain drugs. Yet, there is a large middle ground that is difficult for the health care provider to assess. These are the individuals with chronic headaches, back or neck pains, fibromyalgia, and so forth. On the one hand, pain relief is important and humane (see also Chapter 16). On the other hand, the health care provider does not want to be an unwitting enabler to a potential drug abuse problem. Unfortunately, because patients with chronic pain do not meet official diagnostic criteria for drug abuse or dependence, the diagnosis is often overlooked in this population.

ATHLETES

Since the time of the original Greek Olympiad, athletes have used substances to enhance their performance. Today's athletes are tempted to use anabolic steroids to enhance their muscle bulk, and amphetamines to enhance confidence and performance. Athletes also perceive other substances, such as erythropoietin, and blood transfusions as giving them an edge in competition. Erythropoietin, a hormone produced by the kidney, increases red blood cell production (see Chapter 44) and, along with blood transfusions, (the so-called "blood doping") is used to increase the oxygen-carrying capacity of the blood.

ADOLESCENTS

Adolescents tend to use alcohol as their primary substance of choice. Fifteen percent of adolescents have a definable problem with alcohol. However, fewer than 1% of adolescents who use alcohol or drugs are truly dependent on these substances. Still, substance abuse is often associated with risky sexual behavior in heterosexual as well as gay and lesbian interactions. Many substances break down inhibitions and increase desire, so that the use of safe sex techniques and safe drug administration become secondary to immediate gratification. Consequently, drug abuse clinics are witnessing a larger number of substance abusers who are positive for human immunodeficiency virus (HIV).

OLDER ADULTS

Fifteen percent of community-based older adults are dependent on alcohol, but as many as 44% of older adults in inpatient medical and psychiatric facilities abuse alcohol. Individuals who have a dual diagnosis are more likely to become substance abusers than the rest of the population. A surprising discovery is that the highest rate of alcoholism for any professionally defined group is found among American Nobel laureates for literature. Of 10 laureates to date, 50% have abused alcohol.

HEALTH CARE PROVIDERS

Researchers have long recognized the strong correlation between stress and substance abuse, particularly in prompting relapse. Although exposure to stress is a common occurrence for many health care providers, it is also one of the most powerful triggers for relapse to substance abuse in dependent individuals, even after long periods of abstinence. Given the recent increase in man-made and natural disasters in this country and abroad, and their tragic human aftermath, our awareness of the effects of stress in increasing vulnerability to substance abuse must be especially keen.

Health care providers over 40 years of age typically abuse alcohol alone, whereas providers younger than 40 years of age tend to use other drugs, either alone or in combination with alcohol. The most common substances abused by health care providers include opioids, benzodiazepines, alcohol, and tobacco. The incidence of substance abuse by health care providers is in line with that of the general population. However, injectable drugs are more likely to be used by providers working in acute care settings. Pharmacists tend to abuse multiple orally administered drugs, with CNS stimulants being most common. Nitrous oxide use by dentists is common. Anesthesiologists and nurse anesthetists may use fentanyl or its analogues.

COMMONLY ABUSED SUBSTANCES

The drugs discussed in this chapter can be categorized into four groups: CNS stimulants, CNS depressants, hallucinogens, and inhalants. Obviously these drugs have diverse pharmacologic and toxicologic effects, yet all have the capacity to produce dependence based on their euphoric and positive reinforcing actions. The major characteristics suggesting substance abuse are summarized in Box 12-2. Many of these drugs have prescribed clinical uses (e.g., opioids, CNS depressants, and some CNS stimulants); some are legally obtainable for recreational use (e.g., nicotine, alcohol); and others are illegal (e.g., LSD, cannabis). Regardless, they all have the potential for chronic abuse resulting in dependency.

CNS STIMULANTS

Nicotine

Tobacco continues to be the substance causing the most health damage globally. According to WHO estimates (www. who.int/substance_abuse/facts/tobacco/en/index.html), there are around 1.1 thousand million smokers in the world among approximately one third of the global population, those aged 15 and over. Among industrialized countries where smoking has been common, smoking is estimated to cause over 90% of lung cancer in men and about 70% of lung cancer among women. Worldwide, it is estimated that tobacco causes about 8.8% of deaths (4.9 million) and 4.1% of DALYs (59.1 million). Unless current trends are reversed, that figure is expected to rise to 10 million deaths per year by the 2020s or early 2030s, with 70% of deaths occurring in developing countries.

Although consumption is leveling off and even decreasing in some countries, worldwide more people are smoking, and those who do use nicotine are smoking more cigarettes. Substantially fewer cigarettes are smoked per day per smoker in developing countries than in developed countries. However, this gap is fast narrowing, and unless effective tobacco control measures take place, daily cigarette consumption in developing countries is expected to increase as economic development results in increased real disposable income.

Nicotine dependency is widely confirmed as the basis of the smoking habit. Nicotine has no therapeutic use but is of pharmacologic interest and toxicologic importance, since it is contained in some prescription drugs and over-the-counter (OTC) products. Nicotine improves memory, especially long-term memory, and increases the accuracy and speed of information processing. Other benefits include a reduction of tension and anxiety and an increase in pain threshold. Perhaps it is the reduction of tension and anxiety that was responsible for its use by some Native Americans in the peace pipe.

In spite of the above-mentioned benefits, tobacco has been shown to cause heart disease, stroke, emphysema, and lung cancer. It can produce complications in pregnancy including

BOX 12-2

Characteristics Suggesting Substance Abuse

Substance	Characteristics
Alcohol	Arrhythmias, idiopathic cardiomyopathy, coma
	Behavioral problems in infants, fetal alcohol syndrome
	Cirrhosis, pancreatitis, splenomegaly
	Conflicts with legal system (DUI, family violence, MVAs)
	Depression, social isolation
	Eating disorders, malnutrition, gastritis
	Headaches, neurologic problems
	House fires
	Hypersexuality
	Hypertension
	Hypothermia
	Unexplained accidents, changes in behavior, suicide attempt
Amphetamines	Anxiety, sleep disorders
	Conflicts with legal system (MVAs, violence)
	Hypersexuality
	Malnutrition
	Membership in high-risk population group
	Mood swings, unexplained changes in behavior, psychoses
	Multiple skin disorders (infections, ulcerations)
	Needle marks and bruises on the arms
Barbiturates	Suicide attempt, coma
	Depressed responses
	Endocrine imbalances
	Hypotension
Benzodiazepines	Anxiety
	Suicide attempt, coma
Caffeine	Arrhythmias
	Eating disorders, sleeping disorders
	Headaches
	Hyperactivity
	Hypertension
Cocaine	Conflicts with legal system (MVAs, violence)
	Epistaxis, defects of nasal septum
	Headaches
	Hypersexuality, impotence
	Masculinization
	Mood swings
	Behavior problems in infants (when consumed by the mother)
Hallucinogens	Conflicts with legal system (MVAs, violence)
	Disorientation, fear of surroundings
	Unexplained accidents, suicide attempts
	Psychosis, mood swings, unexplained changes in behavior
Inhalants	Burns around mouth, nose; epistaxis
	House fires
	Mood swings, social isolation
	Respiratory difficulty, suffocation
Opioids	Malnutrition
	Multiple skin disorders (infections, ulcerations)
Anabolic steroids	Conflicts with legal system (violence)
	Depression, mood swings
	Hypertension
	Masculinization, impotence
	Growth retardation in children

DUI, Driving (while) under the influence; *MVAs*, motor vehicle accidents.

low birth weight, prematurity, and fetal injury. Some health care providers claim that any use of tobacco is substance abuse.

▥ *Pharmacodynamics*

Nicotine is the chief alkaloid in tobacco. It first stimulates and then depresses the CNS, with the responses being dose related. In general, small doses stimulate, whereas large doses depress. Stimulation occurs as a result of norepinephrine release from the sympathetic nervous system and acetylcholine from the parasympathetic nervous system (Fig. 12-2). The depression that follows tends to last longer than stimulant effects. The depressant effects of nicotine are related to curare-like action on skeletal muscle.

▥ *Pharmacokinetics*

Nicotine enters the body through inhalation, by injection, from the chewing or snuffing of tobacco, and by absorption through the skin by means of nicotine patches or gum. It is readily absorbed from the gastrointestinal (GI) tract, the mucous membranes of the respiratory tract, and the skin. The average cigarette provides 0.05 to 2.5 mg of nicotine. Nicotine reaches the brain much more rapidly through its most common route, inhalation (7 seconds), than if it is injected. Nicotine is biotransformed in the liver, with a half-life of 2 hours.

A genetic variation that decreases CYP 2A6 enzyme function lessens the tendency for a person to become dependent on nicotine. Persons lacking this genetic variant are more likely to become dependent on nicotine. A better understanding of the role this enzyme plays in the development of nicotine dependency would help in developing more effective intervention strategies.

There are several drug interactions with nicotine. Table 12-1 provides an overview of the interactive drugs. Nicotine increases the biotransformation of some drugs, resulting in reduced blood levels. Insulin dosages may have to be increased in the nicotine-using patient. Nicotine also decreases cardiac output and diuresis.

▥ *Effects and Adverse Effects*

Regular use of tobacco products causes nicotine to accumulate in the body. Whether the source of nicotine is cigarettes, cigars, pipes, or chewing tobacco, the nicotine contained in tobacco products is readily absorbed into the lungs and the circulation.

Nicotine increases dopamine levels in the body, which in turn affects the limbic and reticular activating systems of the CNS. Research is evaluating the role of the β_2 subunit of the nicotinic receptor as the component required for nicotine dependency to develop. Without this molecule, the properties of nicotine that provide positive reinforcement for use do not develop.

A person dependent on nicotine will have withdrawal symptoms within 24 hours of stopping use. Symptoms of withdrawal include fatigue, irritability, insomnia, dizziness, loss of coordination, difficulty concentrating, hunger, constipation, flatus, and stomach pain. Psychomotor and cognitive function is impaired as well. The adverse effects of nicotine are reflected in Figure 12-2.

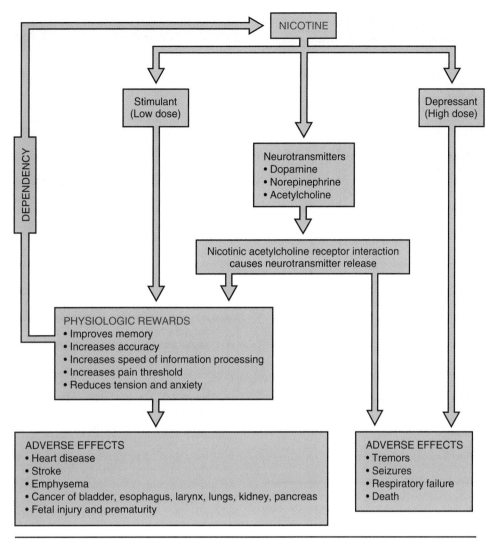

FIGURE 12-2 Addictive Effects of Nicotine. The algorithm follows the sequence of events leading to the physiologic rewards as well as adverse effects of nicotine addiction.

The risk of giving birth to a stillborn or premature infant or an infant of low birth weight or of having chronic bronchitis, emphysema, reactive airway disease, lung cancer, cardiovascular disease, and premature menopause increases with each exposure to tobacco products. Conduct disorders have been reported in female children of mothers who smoked during pregnancy.

▌ *Overdose and Withdrawal*

Acute signs and symptoms of nicotine toxicity most often involve the CNS, cardiovascular, and GI systems. There may be confusion or cold sweats. Fainting, hypotension, tachycardia, prostration, and collapse have been noted. Increased salivation, nausea, vomiting, diarrhea, and abdominal cramps may become apparent.

Smoking cessation produces withdrawal symptoms such as craving (which peaks at 24 to 48 hours), irritability, weight gain, restlessness, sleep disturbance, dullness, impaired judgment, inability to concentrate, fatigue, depression, and GI upset. Withdrawal symptoms from chronic nicotine use are similar to the changes seen with withdrawal from alcohol, amphetamines, cocaine, and opioid analgesics.

Caffeine

Caffeine is probably the world's most widely used psychoactive substance. It is found in many beverages, foods, and OTC and prescription drugs. It has been estimated that 7 million kg of caffeine are consumed annually in the United States. Coffee is consumed in every country of the world and is a mainstay of most offices in the United States and Europe. As many as 30% of coffee drinkers say they "couldn't do without it" and are probably mildly dependent on the substance. Tolerance develops rapidly. The basis for the popularity of all caffeine-containing beverages has been the ancient belief that the beverages had stimulant and antisoporific actions that elevate mood, decrease fatigue, and increase the capacity for work.

▌ *Pharmacodynamics*

The action of caffeine is similar to other stimulants such as the amphetamines and cocaine. Caffeine increases cyclic adenosine monophosphate (cAMP) levels by blocking phosphodiesterase, the enzyme responsible for degradation of cAMP. It also antagonizes the central neurotransmitter adenosine at receptor sites.

TABLE 12-1 BAC Levels and Effects

BAC	Effects
0.02–0.03 e.g., 1 drink	Light euphoria and loss of shyness Relaxed, lightheaded
0.04–0.06	Euphoria Behaviors exaggerated; emotions intensified Improved sense of well-being, relaxation, lowered inhibitions Minor impairment of reasoning and memory, lowering of caution
0.07–0.09*	Euphoria Slight impairment of balance, speech, vision, hearing, reaction times Judgment and self-control reduced Caution, reason and memory impaired False perception of functional level
0.10–0.125 e.g., 5 drinks	Euphoria Significant impairment of motor coordination and loss of judgment Speech slurred; balance, vision, hearing, and reaction times impaired
0.13–0.15	Euphoria lessens and dysphoria appears Gross motor impairment, lack of physical control, loss of balance Blurry vision; judgment and perception severely impaired
0.16–0.19	Dysphoria predominates Nausea may appear
0.20–0.29 e.g., 12 drinks	Mental, physical and sensory functions severely impaired Needs help to stand, walk Nausea and vomiting possible; gag reflex impaired Increased risk of asphyxiation from aspiration and of serious injury
0.30–0.39	Loss of physical orientation Deep sleep, difficulty awakening
Over 0.40	Onset of coma, death from respiratory arrest

*Legal impairment in most states at 0.08 BAC. Some users may become intoxicated at a much lower BAC level than that noted. One drink is equal to 3–4 oz of wine or champagne (12% alcohol), 8–12 oz of beer (4% alcohol), or 20–30 mL of 90-proof spirits (45% alcohol).
BAC, Blood alcohol content.
Adapted from the National Institute on Drug Abuse. Available online: www.drugabuse.gov/infofacts/workplace.html); OSHA Health and Safety Services, Inc. Available online: www.ohsinc.com; and *The Police Notebook*, Oklahoma Police Department. Available online: www.ou.edu/oupd/legalst.htm.

▥ Pharmacokinetics

Caffeine is well absorbed from the GI tract and distributes to all body compartments, including breast milk. Peak plasma levels are achieved 50 to 75 minutes after consumption. It is biotransformed in the adult liver to theophylline and theobromine. In the neonate, only a small portion is biotransformed to theophylline. The elimination half-life of caffeine is 6 hours in adults and 36 to 144 hours in the neonate. The adult half-life value is reached by age 4 to 6 months. In adults, caffeine's metabolites are eliminated by the kidneys, with 1% to 2% eliminated unchanged. In neonates, caffeine is also eliminated by the kidneys, but with 85% eliminated unchanged.

▥ Effects and Adverse Effects

Although much of the populace does not consider caffeine a drug, it does produce many long- and short-term therapeutic and adverse effects on body systems (Box 12-3). Although all levels of the CNS are affected by caffeine, the standard dose

BOX 12-3

Caffeine's Actions and Effects

- Stimulates release of norepinephrine, which improves mental alertness; increases capacity for intellectual activities; aggravates schizophrenia
- Decreases motor reaction time to both visual and auditory events
- Tasks requiring delicate muscular coordination and accurate timing or arithmetic skills decline
- Constricts cerebral blood vessels, resulting in reduced blood flow and oxygen tension in the brain
- Stimulates myocardium, increasing both heart rate and cardiac output; large amounts slow heart rate, cause vasoconstriction, and increase respiratory rate
- Causes esophageal sphincter to relax, contributing to reflux
- Secretion of pepsin and hydrochloric acid are increased
- Stimulates release of epinephrine, leading to increased glucose metabolism and the formation of lactate; as lactate levels rise, so do anxiety and panic
- Increases renal blood flow and glomerular filtration by decreasing reabsorption of sodium and water in proximal tubules
- Limits body's absorption of calcium; kidneys flush out essential vitamins and minerals
- Reduces voluntary muscle fatigue
- Increases metabolic rate, inhibits uterine contractions, and increases plasma and urinary catecholamine levels
- Produces bladder irritation and frequent urination
- Implicated in fibrocystic breast disease
- Combined with ergotamine, caffeine promotes absorption of ergotamine and enhances pain relief

needed for stimulant effects is 200 mg, or the equivalent of two cups of strong coffee or three cans of soft drink.

A withdrawal syndrome including increased irritability, headache, and increased weakness has been reported when users who ingest more than 600 mg of caffeine per day decrease their consumption.

Signs of overdose include agitation, confusion, insomnia, irritability, nausea, vomiting, tinnitus, sensitivity to pain or touch, increased urination, abdominal pain, and muscle twitching. Seizures are possible. Tachycardia and palpitations are noted in some patients. Death from caffeine has been known, but only after doses of around 10 grams, the same as 50 to 100 cups of coffee.

Amphetamines

A public health issue of great concern has been the use of amphetamines, methylenedioxymethamphetamine (MDMA), and other psychostimulants. Although amphetamine-type stimulants (ATSs) have been available and used for many years, in the last decade or so their manufacture, trafficking, and use have been increasing in many countries. The use of MDMA and other amphetamine analogues is a relatively new international phenomenon. In many countries the use of these drugs is widespread. Health risks and other problems associated with ATS use are poorly understood. This lack of understanding presents obstacles to prevention, treatment, and policy responses.

Amphetamines are a favorite drug of abuse across a wide range of age groups. Amphetamines were used by the military in World War II to heighten alertness, eliminate fatigue, strengthen endurance, and produce euphoria. Prescription amphetamines such as dextroamphetamine have been used for short periods in weight-control programs to suppress appetite and to treat narcolepsy. Amphetamine dependency is common among such diverse groups as truck drivers, students, and athletes, who have used the drugs for increased energy, alertness, or endurance.

Methamphetamine use has risen in popularity, and it is readily available and cheaper to produce than cocaine. Profit margins for the producer and for the dealer are thus greater, and so is the desire for new recruits. Children as young as 11 years of age have become dependent on it. The price varies according to its purity. The purest form of methamphetamine is used for smoking.

Pharmacodynamics

Amphetamines alter brain receptors for dopamine, norepinephrine, and serotonin. It also appears that the major mechanism by which amphetamines produce the effects that reinforce its use is their capacity to release newly synthesized dopamine and norepinephrine from intraneuronal stores. Dextroamphetamine is said to have the fewest peripheral adverse effects.

Amphetamine and related compounds raise the blood pressure by causing the body to release epinephrine, postpone the need for sleep, and can reverse, partially and temporarily, the effects of fatigue. Amphetamines enhance mental alertness and the ability to concentrate, and also cause wakefulness, euphoria, and talkativeness. When the drugs wear off, a long period of sleep ensues, often followed by hunger and depression, which can lead to further use of amphetamines.

Pharmacokinetics

Oral doses of amphetamines are absorbed from the GI tract and concentrate in the brain, the lungs, and the kidneys. They are biotransformed in the liver and eliminated via the kidneys. The half-life of metabolites varies with changes in urinary pH. A urine pH of 7 extends the half-life of amphetamines to 20 hours. In contrast, a pH of 5 reduces the half-life to 5 or 6 hours. Thus the higher the urinary pH, the longer the half-life.

Effects and Adverse Effects

The subjective effects of amphetamines, like those of all centrally active drugs, are dependent on the user, the environment, the amount of drug used, and the route of administration. Amphetamines increase sociability in the early phases of use but tend to substitute for sociability in later phases. Moderate doses taken orally commonly result in elevation of mood, a sense of increased energy and alertness, reduced need for sleep, decreased appetite, and improved task performance. They do not create extra physical or mental energy but rather promote expenditure of present resources, sometimes to the point of unsafe fatigue. The fatigue often goes unrecognized since users continually engage in vigorous activity that is perceived as exhilarating and creative. Some manufacturers combine a CNS stimulant such as dextroamphetamine with a CNS depressant such as amobarbital in an attempt to minimize overstimulation.

The effects of amphetamines on the cardiovascular system are profound. Tachycardia, chest pain, hypertension, and dyspnea contribute to a panic state because these signs and symptoms are also those of myocardial infarction. To cope with these effects, the individual often uses CNS depressants ("downers").

Amphetamines increase self-esteem to the point of grandiosity. Heavy users can develop amphetamine psychosis, which is characterized by aggression, delusions of persecution, depression, paranoia, euphoria, and fully formed visual and auditory hallucinations. Some users become wordy and long-winded. Some health care providers suggest that these symptoms are associated with sleep deprivation, which in and of itself leads to psychologic disturbance. The paranoid rages of amphetamines are associated with violent and unpredictable behavior. Grandiosity coupled with rage can be deadly. Amphetamines are responsible for some of the most audacious crimes. The saying "speed kills" is true in at least one context: amphetamines trigger violent actions as well as pose a threat from toxic overdose.

Overdose and Withdrawal

Abrupt cessation of amphetamines after long-term use, or even after a binge of a few days, is commonly followed by depression, anxiety, and craving for the drug. These feelings are soon followed by general fatigue and a need for sleep. Upon awakening, there is compulsive overeating (hyperphagia), continued sleepiness, depression, and anhedonia (lack of interest in usual activities). Mood returns to normal over a period of days, although the dysphoria and anhedonia may persist for weeks in some cases. Although these responses meet the criteria for a withdrawal syndrome, there are no obvious physiologic disruptions that require gradual withdrawal of the drug.

Acute intoxication from amphetamines and amphetamine-like drugs is more likely to occur in the neophyte user. Acute symptoms include dizziness, tremor, irritability, confusion, hallucinations, chest pain, palpitations, hypertension, sweating, and arrhythmias. Amphetamines can produce panic attacks, extreme paranoia, and death. Death is usually preceded by elevated body temperature, seizures, and shock.

Cocaine

Cocaine and its derivative "crack" cocaine provide an example of both the globalization of substance use and the cyclical nature of drug epidemics. Cocaine use dates back to at least 500 AD. Spanish explorers noted that the people of Peru chewed the leaf of a certain plant because it seemed to give them energy and a sense of well-being. These explorers introduced the coca leaf to Europeans.

The main alkaloid of the coca leaf, cocaine, was isolated from the leaves of the plant *Erythroxylon coca* about 1860. Cocaine was then used in patent drugs, beverages, and "tonics" in developed countries in Europe and North America and in Australia until the early 1900s. Laws restricting the availability of cocaine saw a decrease in consumption in these countries until the 1960s. Since that time, cocaine use has become popular among certain groups of young people in some developed countries and in the producer countries of South America.

Pharmacodynamics

Cocaine, an alkaloid, is ingested orally, chewed, snorted, taken intravenously, administered topically, and smoked.

COMMUNITY

The effects of cocaine have been linked directly to its action on cortical cells and to the alteration of central catecholamine levels. Cocaine inhibits the reuptake of norepinephrine at adrenergic synapses, which accounts for some of its central and peripheral effects. In the CNS, it potentiates neurotransmission of norepinephrine, dopamine, and serotonin. The reabsorption of neurotransmitters is blocked, leaving circuits open that would otherwise close. The sequence of events associated with cocaine dependency is shown in Figure 12-3. The resulting effects depend on the dosage and the concentration in the blood.

Freebasing is the process for extracting cocaine from its hydrochloride salt. Freebase-cocaine (crack) contains impurities that were used to extract the cocaine base. Bicarbonate is one of these. When it is heated, the trapped bicarbonate is released, producing a crackling sound, hence the name crack. By extracting and concentrating the cocaine, stronger effects are produced.

Pharmacokinetics

Cocaine is readily absorbed from its various routes of entry. It is biotransformed in the liver and has a very short half-life. Effects last 5 to 15 minutes after nasal or buccal absorption. To maintain CNS stimulation over longer periods, cocaine must be inhaled or injected every 15 to 30 minutes. Cocaine metabolites may be detected in the urine for 24 to 36 hours after use.

Effects and Adverse Effects

At low concentrations, there is a general arousal of the sympathetic nervous system and an increase in motor activity. It makes the user more alert and active; however, at moderately increased concentrations, heart rate and blood pressure increase, body temperature rises, and pupils dilate. High concentrations result in seizures. When cocaine causes sudden death, it is usually the result of ventricular fibrillation, myocardial infarction, stroke, or respiratory arrest. Perforation of the nasal septum and bleeding occurs when cocaine is snorted. Pulmonary effects include wheezes and rhonchi.

Cocaine use causes liver damage, especially when the cocaine user also uses barbiturates. The combination of the metabolites of the two substances produces a liver toxin. Still, although the specific mechanism is unclear, cocaine use alone also damages the liver. It is uncertain whether this is due to the drug itself or to the impurities associated with it. Chronically inhaled cocaine causes lung damage by constricting local blood vessels. In addition, impurities from solvents (e.g., kerosene) left behind in the freebasing procedure contribute to the damage.

The incidence of violence attributed to cocaine users is partially attributed to paranoia and increased motor activity. Cocaine psychosis consists primarily of hallucinations and misperceptions.

Chronic cocaine abuse results in arrhythmias, weight loss due to anorexia, paranoia, and liver and pulmonary damage. In addition, the user experiences unusual tactile sensations such as so-called "cocaine bugs." This is a sensation of insects crawling all over the body. Lesions, scratches, and ulcerations of the skin result when the user attempts to get rid of the "bugs."

Abrupt withdrawal from cocaine results in what many users call anguish, an extreme restless irritability. So intense is this feeling that the user attempts to ameliorate the effect by taking more cocaine, in addition to opioids such as heroin. "Speedballs" are just such a combination of cocaine and heroin. Withdrawal from cocaine produces changes in electroencephalogram patterns and disruption of sleep cycles.

CNS DEPRESSANTS

Alcohol

Alcohol has been used at social events and in religious ceremonies from the earliest recorded history. It is the substance of choice for those prone to substance abuse. Its only competitor in contemporary times is caffeine. Most societies accept alcohol use as normal and unremarkable and do not view alcohol as a drug, unless its use is excessive. Although there are many problems associated with alcohol abuse, there are benefits from low to moderate alcohol use.

Despite the fact that alcohol abuse has occurred for thousands of years, many of the varied health effects have been discovered only fairly recently. With long-term use, alcohol contributes to traumatic outcomes that kill or disable at a relatively young age, resulting in the loss of many years of life

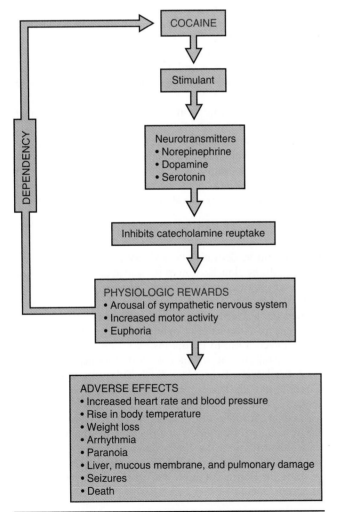

FIGURE 12-3 Addictive Effects of Cocaine. The algorithm follows the sequence of events leading to the physiologic rewards as well as adverse effects of cocaine addiction. A similar action occurs in the peripheral nervous system.

to death or disability. There is increasing evidence that in addition to the amount of alcohol consumed, the pattern of the drinking is relevant to health outcomes. Overall, there is a causal relationship between alcohol consumption and more than 60 types of disease and injury. Alcohol is estimated worldwide to cause 20% to 30% of esophageal cancer, liver cancer, cirrhosis, epilepsy, motor vehicle accidents, and homicide.

Pharmacodynamics

It has been suggested that alcohol affects the brain by interacting with specific protein constituents of brain cell membranes, but the exact mechanism is unclear. The major inhibitory neurotransmitter gamma-aminobutyric acid (GABA) has been implicated. The GABA receptor recognizes not only GABA but also barbiturates and benzodiazepines; when these latter bind to neurons, effects similar to those of alcohol are produced. The amino acid glutamate and its N-methyl-D-aspartate (NMDA) receptor, another neurotransmitter system, mediate many of the acute effects of alcohol and the characteristic behaviors of dependency. Glutamate appears to be the primary excitatory neurotransmitter and is stimulated by alcohol.

Alcohol's depressant action and effects result from inhibition of the depression of the limbic system, which creates the "high" often associated with alcohol intake. However, as the depression worsens, sedation increases, a deep sleep ensues, and coma can result (see Table 12-1). Alcohol also causes peripheral cutaneous vasodilation, which reduces body temperature. Saliva and gastric juices are stimulated by alcohol, which can lead to gastritis with continued use. Alcohol also increases diuresis, partly as a result of the increased fluid intake but also because it blocks ADH secretion from the pituitary. The blockade results in reduced reabsorption of body water, a build-up of uric acid, and the risk for gout and gouty arthritis.

Pharmacokinetics

Although small quantities of alcohol are absorbed in the stomach, most absorption takes place in the duodenum, primarily by diffusion. The absorption rate increases with the concentration of alcohol consumed. The absorption rate decreases as the alcohol restricts blood supply to the stomach. The presence of food or milk also slows the absorption of alcohol. Alcohol is uniformly distributed to all body tissues in the same ratio as water.

Ninety-five percent of alcohol is oxidized in the liver by the enzyme alcohol dehydrogenase, first to acetaldehyde and then to acetic acid, CO_2, and water. Oxidation is the rationale for using disulfiram (Antabuse) in the treatment of alcoholism. Disulfiram inhibits alcohol dehydrogenase, which results in the accumulation of acetaldehyde and the symptoms that make alcohol intake an undesirable activity (Box 12-4).

Although the rate of metabolism differs with acute or chronic ingestion and other factors, it is generally about 10 mL/hour. This is the amount of alcohol contained in 3 to 4 oz of wine or champagne (12% alcohol), 8 to 12 oz of beer (4% alcohol), or 20 to 30 mL of 90-proof spirits (45% alcohol). The blood alcohol content (BAC) noted with social drinking follows zero-order kinetics, meaning there is a constant rate of 7 to 10 grams per hour, the equivalent to one drink per hour (Table 12-2). Alcohol not oxidized is eliminated via the lungs and the kidneys. Large quantities of alcohol damage renal epithelium and alter urinary elimination.

Effects and Adverse Effects

Alcohol has a very simple molecular structure. This makes it easy for it to cross almost every biologic membrane and affect almost every organ. The effects depend on the amount consumed, the number of years during which it has been consumed, and genetic factors. Table 12-3 summarizes alcohol's effects and adverse effects.

Overdose and Withdrawal

Alcohol withdrawal of mild to moderate severity is characterized by tremors, restlessness, agitation, insomnia, and other signs and symptoms. Signs and symptoms of severe withdrawal involve those noted but also include seizures, hallucinations, and delirium tremens (DTs). Intervention for the withdrawal syndrome usually involves use of antianxiety drugs (i.e., benzodiazepines) (see also Chapter 19). The primary purpose of short-term benzodiazepine therapy is to permit the patient to participate in a rehabilitation program. Long-term use of antianxiety drugs should be avoided because they, too, can be abused. Other treatment measures for withdrawal include vitamins, nutritional therapy, and symptomatic measures.

Long-term drug therapy for chronic alcoholism involves disulfiram (Antabuse). Disulfiram blocks the action of aldehyde dehydrogenase, allowing acetaldehyde to accumulate. **Accumulation of acetaldehyde in the blood produces a ▲ complex of highly unpleasant symptoms referred to hereinafter as the _disulfiram-alcohol reaction:_** flushing, throbbing in the head and neck, respiratory difficulty, nausea, copious vomiting, sweating, thirst, chest pain, palpitation, dyspnea, hyperventilation, tachycardia, hypotension, syncope, marked uneasiness, weakness, vertigo, blurred vision, and confusion. In severe reactions, there may be respiratory depression, cardiovascular collapse, arrhythmias, myocardial infarction, acute heart failure, unconsciousness, convulsions, and death. The severity of the reaction is proportional to the amount of alcohol ingested and the dosage of disulfiram taken. The reaction lasts as long as alcohol is present in the circulation, which may be a few minutes to several hours. Further, use of prescription or OTC drugs containing alcohol precipitates a disulfiram-like reaction. Table 12-4 provides a brief list of the concentration of alcohol in selected OTC drugs.

Disulfiram should be used with caution in patients tak- ▲ ing phenytoin (Dilantin) and its congeners, since the concomitant administration of these two drugs can lead to phenytoin intoxication. Before administering disulfiram to a patient on phenytoin therapy, a baseline phenytoin serum level should be obtained. Serum phenytoin levels should be determined on different days for evidence of an increase or to ascertain a continuing rise in serum levels of the drug. Increased phenytoin levels are treated with the appropriate dosage adjustment.

Opioids

Naturally occurring drugs (e.g., morphine, codeine), semisynthetic drugs (e.g., hydromorphone, oxymorphone), and synthetic derivatives (e.g., meperidine, levorphanol, propoxyphene,

---

BOX 12-4

Disulfiram

Indications

Disulfiram is an aid in the management of selected patients with chronic alcoholism who want to remain in a state of enforced sobriety so that supportive and psychotherapeutic treatment may be applied to the best advantage. It is not a cure for alcoholism, but discourages drinking. Treatment may continue for years.

Pharmacodynamics

Disulfiram inhibits acetaldehyde dehydrogenase, thereby interfering with the metabolism of alcohol. Following disulfiram intake, the concentration of acetaldehyde occurring in the blood may be 5 to 10 times higher than that found during metabolism of the same amount of alcohol alone.

Pharmacokinetics

Disulfiram is well absorbed from the GI tract and eliminated from the body 1 or 2 weeks after the last dose of drug is taken. It is biotransformed in the liver and is a CYP 2C9 enzyme inhibitor. Elimination is primarily in the urine, with 5% to 20% eliminated unchanged through the feces and the lungs.

Adverse Effects and Contraindication

Common reactions that occur during the first 2 weeks of therapy include drowsiness, rash, peripheral neuropathy, impotence, headache, acne, metallic taste, or disulfiram-alcohol reaction. Alcohol taken concurrently with disulfiram results in anxiety, confusion, weakness, diaphoresis, flushing of the face, headache, blurry vision, a sensation of choking, dyspnea, chest pain, nausea, and vomiting. These effects begin within 10 minutes of alcohol intake and last for 1 hour or more. The longer a patient uses disulfiram, the more sensitive he or she becomes to alcohol.

Advise patients to stop taking the drug and contact the health care provider if they experience any of the following: weakness, dizziness or loss of coordination; severe diarrhea or vomiting; allergic reaction (i.e., swelling of lips, tongue, or face; shortness of breath; closing of the throat; or hives); seizures; extreme tiredness; dark urine; jaundice; or large appetite changes.

More serious reactions include arrhythmias, cardiovascular collapse, heart failure, respiratory depression, seizures, optic neuritis, hepatitis, psychosis, and coma.

Disulfiram is contraindicated for use in patients who have had alcohol intake within 12 hours of starting drug therapy, who have psychosis or severe coronary artery disease, who use metronidazole or paraldehyde, or who are pregnant. Caution is warranted if the patient has comorbid disorders such as diabetes mellitus, seizure disorder, hypothyroidism, or impaired renal or liver function.

Drug Interactions

- Alcohol: disulfiram-alcohol reaction
- Warfarin: prolongation prothrombin (PT) time
- Isoniazid: ataxic gait and marked mental status changes
- Bupropion: interference with dopamine-norepinephrine system
- Amitriptyline, amphetamines, methylphenidate, cocaine: inhibition of biotransformation of disulfiram

Dosage

- 500 mg daily PO with a full glass of water for 1 to 2 weeks
- Average maintenance dose: 250 mg daily (range: 125 to 500 mg)

Lab Considerations

- Baseline and follow-up ALT, AST, and GGTP in 10 to 14 days
- Complete blood count and a metabolic panel (e.g., SMA-12) test should be done every 6 months

Patient Teaching

- Do not take disulfiram for at least 12 hours after drinking alcohol. Do not drink alcohol while taking disulfiram. Common substances such as mouthwash contain alcohol and must be avoided for safety.
- It takes as long as 14 days to recover from the effects of disulfiram because of the slow rate of restoration of aldehyde dehydrogenase. Alcohol consumed within the 14-day period can be dangerous.
- Flushing, tachycardia, nausea, thirst, chest pain, vertigo, and low blood pressure may occur when alcohol is ingested during disulfiram therapy.
- Carry an identification card that states you are taking disulfiram.
- **Be aware of the alcohol content of common products such as cough and cold medicines, mouthwashes, tonics, sauces, fermented vinegars and some sauces, and other food products. Alcohol in these products can also cause a reaction.**
- Tell your health care provider (or dentist) that you are taking disulfiram before taking an antibiotic or before having surgery.
- Avoid drugs such as metronidazole or oral hypoglycemic agents, because these drugs may cause a disulfiram-like reaction.
- Disulfiram increases the absorption rate and the toxicity of lead and nickel in the blood and the accumulation of lead and nickel in the brain. Avoid disulfiram if you are likely to encounter lead in the environment.
- Do not come in contact with or breathe the fumes of products that may contain alcohol including paint thinners, solvents, stains, and lacquers. Use caution when applying or using products that may contain alcohol including aftershaves, mouthwashes, colognes, perfumes, and antiseptics.
- Symptoms of a disulfiram overdose include nausea, vomiting, dizziness, loss of coordination, numbness and tingling, and seizures. Seek emergency medical attention.

ALT, Alanine transaminase; AST, aspartate transaminase; GGTP, gamma glutamyl transpeptidase; PO, by mouth; SMA, sequential multiple analysis.

---

methadone) are classified as opioids if they act at opioid receptors and have actions similar to morphine. The most potent and highly abused opioid is the semisynthetic compound heroin, although a number of other opioids are also widely misused. Over 5 million people in the United States use opioid analgesics for nonmedical purposes. Approximately 3 million of these report using heroin, with 500,000 being dependent on the drug. Of heroin abusers, 80% are in their mid-20s. The largest populations of heroin abusers are found in New York, with Los Angeles holding second place. The opioids as analgesics are discussed in Chapter 16.

In general, opioids are self-administered by intravenous (IV) or subcutaneous (subQ) route or through smoking to produce feelings of peace and contentment. Most opioid-dependent individuals agree that initial injection of heroin produces a rush or thrilling sensation followed by "coasting" or a drowsy state. In nontolerant persons, opioids produce sedation and sleep. Tolerance develops to these effects and to the euphoric actions of these drugs.

Both physical and psychologic dependence can develop during periods of continuous opioid use; the degree of dependence varies with the individual and with the amount and

DRUG INTERACTIONS

TABLE 12-2 Drug Interactions of CNS Depressants and Stimulants

Drug	Interactive Drugs	Interaction
CNS DEPRESSANTS		
Alcohol	Antianxiety drugs, antihistamines, antidepressants, antipsychotics, opioids, sedative-hypnotics	Additive CNS depression
	Salicylates	Additive GI irritation and bleeding
	Nitrates, nitroglycerine	Additive vasodilation leading to hypotension and syncope
	phenytoin	May increase or decrease liver metabolism
	chlorpropamide, disulfiram, metronidazole	Inhibits aldehyde dehydrogenase, leading to accumulation of acetaldehyde and a disulfiram reaction
CNS STIMULANTS		
Caffeine	CNS stimulants	Increases CNS stimulation
	MAO inhibitors	Increases risk of severe hypertension and arrhythmias
Nicotine	acetaminophen, caffeine, oxazepam, pentazocine, propranolol, propoxyphene, theophylline	Increases biotransformation of interactive drug
	Adrenergic agonists and blockers, catecholamines, cortisol	Increases plasma levels of interactive drug
	furosemide	Reduces cardiac output and diuretic effects of furosemide
	Insulin	Decreases effects of interactive drug

CNS, Central nervous system, *GI,* gastrointestinal.

frequency of drug administered. When opioids are discontinued, there is a predictable set of withdrawal symptoms that occur. Early on, individuals experience rhinorrhea, increased salivation, and lacrimation; yawning and stretching are common behaviors. Loss of appetite, dilated pupils, tremor, and gooseflesh (so called "cold turkey") follows. At peak withdrawal, patients are restless and have nausea, diarrhea, muscle cramps, twitching, and tremors. This syndrome lasts 3 to 5 days but may be followed by extended periods of craving, insomnia, and weakness. Although the withdrawal syndrome is very uncomfortable, it is not life threatening (compared to other CNS depressants; see next section). Nonetheless, it is important to detoxify patients who are dependent on opioids, as part of a treatment program to break the cycle of dependency.

Opioid withdrawal can be treated in several ways. Methadone is a long-acting cross-dependence opioid that is administered once daily to prevent withdrawal symptoms. The use of methadone as a replacement drug has long been the treatment of choice; however, recent data suggest that this approach may increase the likelihood of relapse to opioid use (see Controversy box). Other alternatives are the alpha-adrenergic agonist clonidine, which can be used to relieve specific symptoms rather than to substitute for the opioid, and buprenorphine, a mixed opioid agonist-antagonist, given over 5 to 8 days.

Overdose and Withdrawal

Acute overdose of opioids produces CNS depression, respiratory depression, and pinpoint pupils. Fatal overdose often

TABLE 12-3 General and Adverse Effects of Alcohol

- Increases salivary secretion and gastric acid production (small quantities); large quantities of alcohol inhibit gastric acid secretion and prostaglandin activity, thus contributing to the risk of gastritis and malnutrition.
- Deficiencies in thiamine (B_1), niacin (B_3), pyridoxine (B_6), folic acid (B_9), cyanocobalamin (B_{12}), iron, ascorbic acid (C), and vitamins A, D, and K
- Protein and zinc deficiencies, resulting in night blindness, susceptibility to infection and injury, and slowed wound healing
- Irritation of GI tract, precipitating inflammation of the esophagus, the stomach, and the duodenum.
- Vomiting may result in mucosal tears and bleeding at the esophagogastric junction (Mallory-Weiss syndrome)
- Increases risk of cancer of the tongue, the mouth, the oropharynx, the esophagus (tenfold), and the liver
- The liver stores fat instead of burning it for fuel, resulting in steatosis (fatty liver), alcoholic hepatitis, and cirrhosis; cirrhosis results in portal hypertension and esophageal varices
- Acute and chronic pancreatitis with intractable abdominal pain; splenomegaly results in pancytopenia
- Anemia results from nutritional deficits and bleeding
- Decreased WBCs increase risk of immunosuppression and the risk of infections, especially mycobacterial infections and pneumonia
- Suppresses ADH, resulting in increased urinary output and dehydration
- Hypocalcemia from loss of calcium in urine and low magnesium levels increase risk for tetany, fracture, and osteoporosis
- Hypoglycemia results from interference with gluconeogenesis
- Altered production of sex hormones, resulting in reduced fertility, impotence, and amenorrhea; disinhibitory effects increase risk for sexually transmitted diseases, including HIV
- Reduced vasomotor responses in medulla result in peripheral vasodilation, which reduces core body temperature and increases the risk of hypothermia
- Idiopathic cardiomyopathy and arrhythmias result in heart failure refractory to cardiac glycosides
- Asymptomatic, transient elevations of creatine kinase to frank rhabdomyolysis

ADH, Antidiuretic hormone *GI,* gastrointestinal; *HIV,* human immunodeficiency virus; *WBCs,* white blood cells.

TABLE 12-4 Alcohol Content of Select OTC Drugs

Over-the-Counter Drug	Content (%)
Terpin hydrate with codeine	40
Listerine mouthwash	26.9
NyQuil LiquiCaps	25
Halls	22
Romilar cough formula	20
Comtrex	20
Formula 44 Multi-Symptom Cough & Cold Relief	20
Scope mouthwash	18.9
Cepacol throat lozenges	15
Tylenol Multi-Symptom Cough	10

OTC, Over-the-counter.

Controversy

Methadone: To Use or Not To Use, That is the Question

Methadone has been used effectively for more than 40 years as a treatment for heroin dependency. Its use is not without controversy, however. The drug acts by blocking heroin's effects without creating a "high," eliminates withdrawal symptoms, and relieves the craving associated with opioid dependency.

Defenders assert that it is an effective adjunct for an individual determined to stay away from drugs. Detractors claim that its use simply substitutes one drug of abuse for another, that therapy often requires indefinite maintenance, and that detoxification is often followed by a return to heroin.

Nonetheless, methadone has been used for decades, although no clinical consensus has been reached about the most effective daily dose. Many clinics do not adjust dosages according to the needs of patients. Instead, they administer fixed doses. One clinic may use doses of 25 mg per day for all patients; others may administer daily doses of 60 mg. Federal regulations require that a clinic receive a special exemption to provide patients with doses greater than 100 mg per day, but no contemporary studies have examined the effectiveness of daily doses greater than 80 mg.

CLINICAL REASONING

- What are the potential health hazards that the use of controlled substances poses? Are these the same hazards posed by using methadone?
- What social problems are generated by the unregulated use of controlled substances?
- Should tax monies be required to pay for drug rehabilitation for substance abusers?
- Is the threat to society related to the use and abuse of these substances sufficient to warrant government intervention in areas many would reserve to the individual?

---

occurs by accident because it is not known how much of the drug that is injected is actual opioid. Death from overdose is usually secondary to respiratory arrest or pulmonary edema.

Withdrawal from opioids without medical supervision is called "going cold turkey" because the skin is cold and the piloerection resembles a plucked turkey. There may be a crawling sensation of the skin. Histamine release is responsible for the sweating, the itching, and the dilation of superficial blood vessels, especially of the face, the neck, and the upper thorax. The individual takes on a flushed appearance. Muscle spasms, especially of the back and limbs, result in kicking motions, and hence the phrase "kicking the habit." Yawning, sweating, rhinorrhea, hot flashes, nausea, vomiting, abdominal cramps, tachypnea, and tachycardia can also be present.

Administration of the "pure" opioid antagonists naloxone (Narcan) (short-acting) or naltrexone (Vivitrol) (longer-acting) to an overdosed patient rapidly reverses the coma and respiratory depression of opioids (see Box 16–2 in Chapter 16 for more information regarding opioid antagonists). Since naloxone has little significant action on its own, and since it reverses opioid toxicity but not that of alcohol, barbiturates, or other CNS depressants, it can be used to differentiate overdose with opioids from that of other CNS depressants. There are two caveats with the use of naloxone, however. First, it is relatively short-acting, so more than one dose may be required. Second, caution should be exercised when administering pure antagonists to opioid-dependent individuals, since the drugs can precipitate withdrawal.

Opioid overdose can be managed with the administration of an opioid antagonist (see Chapter 16) and respiratory support. Clonidine (Catapres), a sympatholytic antihypertensive (see Chapter 37), is used in the management of opioid withdrawal. It stimulates α_2 receptors in the brain, resulting in reduction in sympathetic outflow and a decrease in peripheral vascular resistance, heart rate, and blood pressure. At present, it is under investigation for relieving symptoms of acute drug withdrawal. Clonidine patches take 2 to 3 days to reach peak effect, which is often too late to manage the worst effects of opioid withdrawal. The tablet formulation offers a rapid and more easily titrated treatment modality.

The clinical efficacy of clonidine is limited by its sedative and hypotensive effects. Extremely close supervision is necessary to monitor for adverse effects and possible dosage manipulation by the patient.

Barbiturates

Barbiturates were popular in the 1960s and 1970s for the treatment of seizure disorders, anxiety, and insomnia. They were also used to treat the unwanted effects of illicit drug use. Barbiturates can cause dependency and life-threatening withdrawal syndrome, and even a slight dosage excess can lead to coma and death. Barbiturates are used less frequently today, and illegal use has declined.

The incidence and prevalence of the nonmedical use of barbiturates exceeds that of the opioids. Opioid users frequently take barbiturates, benzodiazepines, and other sedative-hypnotics to augment the effects of weak illicit heroin, or to produce psychologic effects when they have become tolerant to prescribed opioids. The short-acting barbiturates such as pentobarbital (Box 12-5) or secobarbital are preferred over longer-acting drugs such as phenobarbital. Most users take the drugs by mouth, but a few inject barbiturates by IV or intramuscular (IM) route. Abusers who inject the tablet or capsule forms of barbiturates by IV can develop serum hepatitis, septicemia, pulmonary emboli, papilloma, bacterial endocarditis, tetanus, and various skin rashes. Because barbiturates are highly alkaline sclerosing agents, these persons can be identified by the large abscesses that spread over the injection sites.

The amount of barbiturate used varies considerably, but an average dose of 1.5 grams of a short-acting drug is not uncommon. Some persons use as much as 2.5 grams daily over several months. Because tolerance develops to most of the actions of barbiturates, there may be no apparent signs of long-term use. For the patient taking barbiturates on a regular basis, the only manifestation of abuse may be rebound insomnia and some anxiety when the drug is stopped. For persons attempting to

---

BOX 12-5

Street Names of Commonly Abused Substances

Central Nervous System Depressants

amobarbital	Blues, blue devils, blue angels, blue heavens, bluebirds, blue velvet
barbiturates	Barbs, reds, red birds, phennies, tooies
chlordiazepoxide	Green and whites, libs, roaches
codeine	Schoolboy, robo, romo, syrup
fentanyl	Apache, China girl, China white, dance fever, friend, goodfella, jackpot, murder 8, TNT, Tango and Cash
flunitrazepam (Rohypnol)	Forget-me pill, Mexican Valium, R2, Roche, roofies, roofinol, rope, rophies
gamma-hydroxybutyrate (GHB)	Georgia home boy, grievous bodily harm, liquid ecstasy
heroin	Boy, brown sugar, doojee, dope, H, hairy, Harry, horse, junk, noise, pee, scag, shit, skid, skunk, smack, TNT, white horse
hydrocodone with acetaminophen	Vike, Watson-387
morphine	M, Miss Emma, monkey, white stuff
opium	Big O, Black stuff, block, gum, hop, poppy, tar, hop, pin, yen, skee, wen shee
oxycontin	Oxy, OC, killer
pentobarbital	Nembies, yellow jackets, yellowbirds, yellows, Mexican yellows
phenobarbital	Barbs, goof balls, purple hearts
secobarbital	Seccy, red birds, red devils, reds, F-40, lily, pink ladies
tuinal	Tooeys, rainbows, double trouble, F-66, gorilla pills

Central Nervous System Stimulants

amphetamine (racemic)	Bennies black beauties, crosses, hearts, LA turnaround, speed, truck drivers, uppers
amphetamine complex	Black beauty, black Cadillacs
cocaine	Bump, C, candy, crack, Carrie, Cecil, Charlie, coke, crystal blow, dope, flake, girl, gold dust, happy dust, heaven dust, joy powder, lady, snow, rock dream, nose candy, rock, snow, toot
dextroamphetamine	Christmas trees, dexies, hearts, oranges, spots, wedges
methylphenidate	JIF, MPH, R-ball, Skippy, the smart drug, vitamin R
methamphetamine	Chalk, crank, Chris, Christine, crystal, fire, glass, go fast, ice, meth, speed, whites, X crank
methylenedioxyamphetamine (MDA)	Love drug
methylenedioxymethamphetamine (MDMA)	Adam, clarity, ecstasy, Eve, lover's speed, peace, spots, X, XTC, STP
Nicotine	Cigarettes, cigars, smokeless tobacco, snuff, spit tobacco, bidis, chew

Hallucinogens

Cannabis (marijuana)	Acapulco gold, ace, ashes, baby, broccoli, grass, dope, ganja, herb, hemp, jive, joint, Mary Jane, pot, THC, weed, Panama red, MJ, loco weed, Texas tea, Sweet Lucy, blunt, joints, reefer, sinsemilla, skunk, many others
Hash, hashish	Black hash (hashish containing opium), black Russian (potent, dark hashish), boom, chronic, gangster, hash, hash oil, hemp
ketamine	Cat valiums, K, special K, super K, vitamin K
lysergic acid diethylamide (LSD)	Acid, barrels, battery acid, Berkeley blood, big D, chief, black magic, blue acid, blue dots, blue heaven, California sunshine, cube, chocolate chips, cupcakes, domes, Hawaiian sunshine, HCP, micro dots, peace tablets, purple haze, purple ozone, squirrels, strawberry field, sugar, window pane
mescaline	Bad seed, big chief, cactus buttons, peyote, pink wedge, white light, mescal, half moon
phencyclidine (PCP)	Angel dust, boat, dummy dust, embalming fluid, flying saucers, hair hog, killer week, love boat, mist, peace pill, rocket fuel, sheets, hog, Shermans, super grass, tranq, whack
psilocybin	God's flesh, magic mushroom, purple passion, shrooms

Other

Anabolic steroids	Arnolds, gear, gym candy, roids, juice, pumpers, stackers, weight trainers
Inhalants	Laughing gas, poppers, snappers, whippets

---

maintain a state of intoxication, the acute and chronic effects resemble those of alcohol. Such a person shows a general sluggishness, difficulty thinking, faulty judgment, poor comprehension and memory, a narrow attention span, and is emotionally labile. There is also an exaggeration of basic personality traits. Slurring and a slowness of speech are noted; quarrelsome behaviors and moroseness are common. The person may have an unkempt appearance, laugh or cry without provocation, and maintain hostile, paranoid, and suicidal ideations. Toxic doses of barbiturates lead to stupor and respiratory depression.

Long-term use of short-acting barbiturates results in both drug disposition alterations and pharmacodynamic tolerance. Although there may be considerable tolerance to the sedative and intoxicant effects of barbiturates, the lethal dose is not much different than that in persons who do not abuse the drugs. Consequently, acute barbiturate poisoning may be accidentally or deliberately superimposed on chronic intoxication. Cross-tolerance to other barbiturates is common.

Barbiturates increase the biotransformation of other drugs by increasing microsomal enzyme activity. The combination of amphetamines and barbiturates produces greater euphoria than either type of drug alone. Hence concurrent use of barbiturates with other drugs can be problematic. Specific and efficient antidotes to offset barbiturate overdoses are not available. Individuals dependent on barbiturates should not abruptly stop the drug because of the risk of withdrawal syndrome.

In its mildest form, the withdrawal syndrome from short-acting barbiturates may consist only of electroencephalogram (EEG) changes, rebound increases in rapid-eye-movement (REM) sleep, insomnia, and anxiety. Somewhat greater degrees of dependency result in tremulousness, weakness, GI disturbances, and orthostatic hypotension that may last from 3 to 14 days. These symptoms leave the patient unable to get out of bed.

When the withdrawal syndrome is severe, there may be symptoms of psychosis that progress to confusion, delirium, hallucinations, and tonic-clonic seizures. Seizure activity is more common in withdrawal from barbiturates than from alcohol withdrawal. The number of seizures can vary from a single episode to status epilepticus. Agitation and hyperthermia lead to exhaustion, cardiovascular collapse, and death.

With longer-acting barbiturates, withdrawal symptoms may not begin until the second or third day and peak more slowly. Anxiety rises with time, and frightening dreams may be succeeded by refractory insomnia. Persecutory visual hallucinations generally start at the same time that clouding of the senses begins. Full-blown delirium is manifested in disorientation to time and place. Once the delirium starts, even the administration of large doses of barbiturate may not suppress it immediately. This is true also of the delirium that develops during alcohol withdrawal. The reason for the irreversibility is unclear. The withdrawal syndrome, even if it is left untreated, usually clears by the eighth day. Barbiturates are discussed further in Chapter 19.

Benzodiazepines

Benzodiazepines are widely prescribed antianxiety drugs used for reducing stress and tension and for sleep disorders. The discovery of benzodiazepines in the 1950s was exciting, because although they produced sedating and euphoric effects, they were thought to be less lethal than opioids or barbiturates. Moreover, these drugs did not appear to promote dependency in people who were not already predisposed. It takes ingestion of larger doses of benzodiazepines, for longer periods of time, to produce the life-threatening problems of the barbiturates. Today, benzodiazepines are rarely primary drugs of abuse; nonetheless, they are commonly abused.

Use of a benzodiazepine for other than sedative-hypnotic purposes is estimated to occur in 11% of the population each year. Approximately 37% of prescriptions for controlled substances are for benzodiazepines. This translates to about one prescription for every two adults. Of this figure, 80% report drug use for less than 4 months, 5% used the drug from 4 to 11 months, and 15% used the drug for 12 months or longer. Nearly two thirds of benzodiazepine abusers are female. Older adults tend to be overrepresented in these figures, and they tend to use the drug on a chronic basis.

Benzodiazepines reduce fear and anxiety and produce euphoria, which explains their potential for abuse. However, individuals who abuse benzodiazepines often combine them with alcohol or barbiturates because of the enhanced effects. However, the consequences can be tragic.

The euphoric effect of benzodiazepines depends on the drug's onset of action. As a group, benzodiazepines are slower to produce adverse effects than alcohol or barbiturates, but diazepam is biotransformed the most quickly and, consequently, has the greatest potential for abuse. Lorazepam and alprazolam are the next most likely benzodiazepines to be abused. Oxazepam, prazepam, and clorazepate are the least likely to be abused. The prescription benzodiazepines most often abused include diazepam, alprazolam, triazolam, and chlordiazepoxide. Recently, there have been increasing reports of drug dependency to clonazepam. Chapter 19 discusses the benzodiazepines in more depth.

As with other CNS depressants, acute overdose of benzodiazepines causes sedation, gait disturbances, stupor, and respiratory depression, but these drugs are less potent than barbiturates. Tolerance develops to the sedative actions of these drugs. Benzodiazepines act at specific receptor sites in the CNS; however, administering flumazenil blocks the depressant action of these drugs. Although not as labile as the short-acting barbiturates, long-term use of benzodiazepine results in physical and psychologic dependence.

Withdrawal symptoms include tremors and anxiety, with a potential for seizures that can be avoided by gradual reduction of the dosage over a relatively long time period.

Persons on concurrent methadone maintenance may experience a boost with simultaneous use of benzodiazepines. The theory is that both methadone and benzodiazepines compete for oxidation sites. Thus there are higher levels of methadone in the blood and the brain.

HALLUCINOGENS

Although a number of different classes of drugs alter perception of reality and can produce hallucinations, for the purpose of this chapter we will subdivide the drugs into general hallucinogens (D-lysergic acid diethylamide, mescaline, psilocybin, and MDMA); cannabinoids (marijuana, hashish); and dissociative anesthetics (phencyclidine, ketamine). See Box 12-5 for common street names of these drugs. At present, these drugs have no medical uses, with the exception of the cannabinoids, which are used to decrease the nausea associated with antineoplastic therapy, and in glaucoma to help reduce intraocular pressure.

In general, these drugs are abused out of the desire to alter thought processes and induce unique experiences. Indeed, high doses of these drugs produce altered sensations, disorientation, delusions, and frank hallucinations. As with other drugs, tolerance develops to the effects. In addition, persons taking these drugs chronically can develop a psychologic dependence. This is particularly true for the cannabinoids, since they often are self-administered, with much greater frequency than other drugs of this class.

Several factors influence the response to hallucinogens. Among these factors are dosage, personality of the individual, the expectation the person has in using the drug, and the immediate environment and social setting in which the drug is used. Because many of the hallucinogens make a person highly suggestible, the environment and people in it, and especially the "guide" who is making the suggestions, are very important.

Cannabis

Cannabis is by far the most widely cultivated, trafficked, and abused illicit drug. Marijuana, hashish, and hemp are the three better known cannabinoids. Of the three, marijuana is the most widely used in the United States and, in fact, is the most widely used illicit drug in the world. Approximately 20 million individuals in the United States are current users. Approximately one third of the U.S. population 12 years or older reported that they have tried the drug, and close to 9% used it in the past year. Of the world population, 2.5%, or about 147 million people, consume cannabis annually, compared with 0.2% who use cocaine and 0.2% who use opiates. Half of all drug seizures worldwide are cannabis seizures. The geographic spread of those seizures is also global, covering practically every country of the world.

Marijuana is derived from the *Cannabis sativa* plant, the same plant that produces *hemp,* the fiber used in rope, carpets, sails, linen, and clothes. The seed is used as bird seed. Marijuana is produced from the dried leaves and the flowering tops of the plant and contains over 400 different chemicals, 61 of which are cannabinoids. There are 11 tetrahydrocannabinoids (THC), of which Δ-9-THC is the most psychoactive. Marijuana typically contains about 1% to 6% THC. However, cannabinoids vary greatly from plant to plant and even in different parts of the same plant. No two plants are identical in chemical composition.

Part of the controversy over marijuana use concerns its therapeutic effects, not to mention its legal or illegal status. Marijuana has been used as an antiemetic in cancer therapy. Marijuana reduces intraocular pressure in patients with glaucoma. It has antidepressant effects and is used with some success for this purpose in Great Britain. Native South African women smoke it to reduce the pain of childbirth. Unlike opioids, marijuana does not suppress respiration. It is also a muscle relaxant, which helps decrease the pain of muscle spasms. Dronabinol (Marinol), a synthetic THC product, is used in the management of cancer-associated nausea and vomiting and to stimulate the appetite of patients with acquired immunodeficiency syndrome (AIDS). Marinol is a Schedule III drug. Marijuana has also been used as an antihistamine, a bronchodilator, and an antiseizure drug.

It is speculated that people enjoy smoking marijuana because of its effect on the limbic system in the brain. This is the system that is activated in sexual arousal and orgasm. The aftereffects of this type of arousal seem to be indolence, a personality trait associated with marijuana use.

Marijuana can be smoked, mixed with tobacco, used in a water pipe, or eaten alone or in foods, or it can be mixed with phencyclidine (PCP). The effects noted are based on the user's expectations and past experiences with the drug, and the pharmacodynamics of the drug itself. Inhalation of the smoke results in rapid absorption of THC into the blood stream. Blood levels decline slowly over 2 to 3 hours. If it is ingested in food, effects occur 30 minutes to 2 hours later, with an average duration of action of about 6 hours. THC is stored in body fat, which accounts for its detection in urine months after cessation of use. Because it is stored in body fat, weight reduction results in its release back into the blood stream. Biotransformation to metabolites takes place in 1 to 4 hours to the metabolites 8,11-dihydroxy-THC and 11-hydroxy-Δ-9-THC.

It is also speculated that marijuana alters the lipid membrane in all neurons, which may account for its wide range of effects and its nonspecificity and unpredictability. The responses can range from euphoria to paranoia and from sedation to hallucinations. Loss of orientation to time and space, lack of motivation, increased appetite, and dry mouth are commonly experienced.

Because marijuana users inhale more deeply than cigarette smokers, more tar builds up in the lungs from each cigarette. This is balanced by marijuana users' smoking fewer cigarettes. However, when marijuana and tobacco are combined, the lung damage is greatly increased. Marijuana is also thought to reduce the ability of the alveolar macrophages in the lungs to remove debris and combat bacteria. Hence users have a higher incidence of respiratory problems. It also affects the immune system in a more general manner by reducing T cell counts.

Long-term use decreases libido and increases impotence. This may be due to chemicals that reduce the quantity of testosterone and lower the sperm count. Initially, marijuana can be an aphrodisiac, perhaps because the slowing of time makes the pleasure of sex seem to last longer. The longer-term effect is reduced interest in sex. If marijuana is used during pregnancy, fetal toxicity and organ malformations may occur. In the cardiovascular system, marijuana use produces tachycardia.

Marijuana use is detectable by a number of signs and symptoms, among them reddening of the eyes. There is a sweet odor about the user, similar to the burning of rope. There may be an appearance of intoxication but with no smell of alcohol, and yellowish stains on the fingertips from smoking the joint closer to the fingers than is customary with cigarettes. Excessive laughter is not uncommon. The ability to engage in skilled tasks, such as driving, is reduced or disrupted. Abusers tend to drop out of school or be excessively absent.

Hashish and Hashish Oil

The Middle East, North Africa, and the Pakistan-Afghanistan regions are the primary sources of hashish. Hashish is composed of the THC-rich resins of the *C. sativa* plant. The resin is collected, dried, and readied for use in pipes. Hashish reaching the United States in the 1990s contained 5% THC.

In contrast, hashish oil usually contains 15% THC. According to the Drug Enforcement Administration (DEA; www.dea.gov/pubs/abuse/7-pot.htm), hashish oil is produced using a solvent to remove the cannabinoids from the plant. The color and odor of the extracted oil varies depending on the solvent used. One or two drops of hashish oil on a cigarette equates to a single marijuana cigarette.

Lysergic Acid Diethylamide (LSD)

Lysergic acid diethylamide (LSD) is the most potent and highly studied hallucinogen. It is one of the most powerful psychoactive substances known. LSD was originally synthesized in 1938 by Dr. Albert Hoffman. Using LSD for its hallucinogenic effect became fashionable in the 1960s with persons like Timothy Leary, who persuaded many American students to "turn on, tune in, and drop out" (DEA, www.usdoj.gov/dea/pubs/abuse/8-hallu.htm).

Mild euphoria and increased empathy are produced by 10 mcg of LSD. A minimal psychedelic dose is 50 to 100 mcg, and doses of 400 to 500 mcg elicit maximal psychedelic effects. Because very small amounts are needed and because it is odorless and colorless, it is stored in an amazing variety of ways. It can be painted onto the fingernails or stored in blotters or as dried droplets on paper.

In general, LSD produces increased empathy and euphoria and decreased inhibitions, as well as kaleidoscopic hallucinations. Synesthesia is common; this is a phenomenon involving sensory crossover, such as seeing sounds or hearing colors. There is a loss of identity and "cosmic merging," a sort of self-reflection in which long-repressed material comes to the surface. LSD is not physically addicting, and there is no evidence that it is teratogenic, despite earlier speculations to the contrary. However, whether it produces a "good trip" or a "bad trip" is unpredictable and seemingly dependent on personality traits of the user and variations in dosage and environment at the time of use. Panic, paranoia, and terrifying visions are among the more frequently encountered symptoms or effects of LSD, especially during a bad trip.

The CNS receptor for LSD has not been identified at this time. The compound seems to affect multiple transmitter systems. LSD is rapidly absorbed. It is biotransformed in the liver with elimination in the feces. The half-life of LSD is approximately 2 hours. There is a cross-tolerance of LSD with mescaline and psilocybin. The potency of LSD can be conceptualized by noting that it takes 6000 times as much mescaline to produce a comparable psychedelic effect.

There is a potential for the user to experience unexpected "flashbacks" days, months, or more than a year after using LSD. This syndrome is called *persisting perception disorder* and involves a recurrence of some part of the initial drug experience. It is more often associated with long-term drug use, but it can occur in infrequent users. Finally, the use of LSD and other potent hallucinogens can precipitate psychotic episodes in persons with underlying disease.

Although symptoms of LSD use can be treated with sedatives, caution is advised when treating a person having a bad trip. Because it is difficult to know which drug the patient is on, the decision to use other drugs to reverse toxicity can be risky. For example, administering antipsychotic drugs to patients on some hallucinogens can cause seizures. For a bad trip, talking the subject down in a safe, friendly environment is often successful.

Peyote and Mescaline

Mescaline comes from the peyote and the San Pedro cacti, and its effects, although not as strong as LSD, are similar. Mescaline belongs to a family of compounds known as phenethylamines, making it quite distinct from other major hallucinogens—LSD, psilocybin, harmaline, and dimethyltryptamine (DMT)—which all belong to the indole family.

In the United States, peyote is illegal for all but members of the Native American Church, and it is seldom seen in the psychedelic underground. Apparently there is even becoming a shortage for the Native American population,

since the cactus grows at a very slow rate. A typical peyote "button" may require 20 years to reach 2 inches in diameter. For many years, peyote has been harvested much faster than it can grow.

Mescaline, the major psychoactive ingredient in peyote cactus buttons, is short-acting. Like LSD, mescaline acts as an agonist at serotonin receptors. Mescaline alters the senses and causes visual hallucinations, but is much less potent than peyote. Acute administration produces nausea, diaphoresis, and tremors. It also causes pupil dilation, dizziness, vomiting, tachycardia, sensations of warm and cold, sweating, headaches. Some visions can cause nightmares that give rise to psychosis.

Although derived from the peyote cactus, mescaline was named in honor of the mescal bean, a red seed that comes from an evergreen shrub. The active substance in this seed, the alkaloid cytosine, is related to nicotine. The hallucinogenic dose of mescaline is about 300 to 500 mg (about half a bean) with effects lasting about 12 hours. A whole bean might kill. More recently, the wearing of a red bean has come to be a symbol of loyalty to traditional Native American cultural values. Both peyote and mescaline are Schedule 1 agents.

3,4-Methylenedioxymethamphetamine (MDMA)

3,4-Methylenedioxymethamphetamine (MDMA, "ecstasy") gained popularity as a drug of abuse in the1980s. In 2000, 2 million tablets of MDMA were smuggled into the United States each week.

MDMA has been used by some as a "date-rape" drug because it causes euphoria and sexual arousal while boosting tactile sensations. Because MDMA causes damage to 5-hydroxytryptamine–containing neurons, long-term cognitive impairment and psychiatric disturbances can result. Blurry vision, muscle tension and tremors, nausea, increased blood pressure and heart rate, sleep disturbances, anxiety, paranoia, and hypothermia have been reported. As with other hallucinogens, users can develop psychologic dependence to this drug. High doses result in *malignant hyperthermia*, a syndrome that includes high fever, renal failure, and cardiovascular collapse.

The tablets, frequently manufactured in clandestine laboratories, may contain 80 to 100 mg of MDMA. Pharmacologic effects are usually seen 30 to 45 minutes after ingestion, with maximal effects noted in 60 to 90 minutes. The duration of action of MDMA is 4 to 6 hours. MDMA is a Schedule I agent.

Phencyclidine (PCP)

Phencyclidine (phenylcyclohexyl piperidine, PCP), also known as "angel dust," is derived from a genus containing more than 30 similar chemical substances, all of them dissociative anesthetics (see Chapter 18). Classification of this substance is difficult because the effects range beyond those of simple hallucinogens. PCP acts on the limbic system, the hippocampus, and on cholinergic and dopaminergic neurotransmitters to produce hallucinogenic as well as a host of other effects.

A helpful mnemonic device for remembering the eight cardinal signs of PCP intoxication is the acronym *"red danes"*: *r*ed skin, *e*nlarged pupils, *d*elusions, *d*issociations, *a*mnesia, *n*ystagmus, *e*xcitement, and dry *s*kin. PCP also produces a subjective "high," a staggering gait, slurred speech, and numbness of the extremities. The heart rate and blood pressure are elevated, and there is hypersalivation, fever, and seizure activity. Depending on the dose, users may have a blank stare, changes in body image, and/or disorganized thoughts, and they may display catatonic rigidity, hostile and bizarre behaviors, and overpowering strength. The combination of delusions and overpowering strength requires that special precautions be taken for staff and patient safety when it becomes necessary to restrain the patient. However, with increasing dosage, analgesia becomes more profound and anesthesia, stupor, or coma may occur, although the eyes may remain open.

PCP is a generally psychoactive substance, but because it affects many areas, there is no one antidote. Consequently, treatment should be focused on specific presenting symptoms. Haloperidol has been effective for PCP psychosis. Diazepam is used to help prevent seizures, but it is not useful for PCP psychosis. It merely delays its presentation by modulating downward the dopaminergic effects while blocking the breakdown of the PCP. The patient's psychosis may appear to be controlled well enough to allow the patient to be transferred from the emergency room to a psychiatric unit, only to have the psychosis reappear. Atonic bladder and ileus that accompany PCP use can be treated with physostigmine. Because of the dissociative anesthetic effects of PCP and the paranoia and irritability it often precipitates, care should be taken to avert the possibility of self-injury or injury to others. Because of the irritability that additional stimuli may elicit in the patient, "talking down" is contraindicated in favor of a quiet room that is free from provocation.

Biotransformation of PCP occurs primarily in the liver, and it is eliminated in the urine with nearly half of the agent unchanged. The half-life of PCP ranges from 10 hours to 4 days.

PCP may be taken by oral, IV, or IM routes, by smoking, as a vaginal douche, or as a rectal enema. The most rapid effects are obtained by the IV route or by smoking. Mild intoxication occurs with 0.5 mg of PCP and severe intoxication with about 20 mg; chronic users may ingest up to 1 gram in 24 hours.

Ketamine

Ketamine is a rapid-acting, dissociative general anesthetic whose pharmacokinetic profile is similar to that of PCP. As with PCP, patients taking ketamine are detached from their pain and their surroundings. Like MDMA, ketamine has also been used by some as a "date-rape" drug. Those who abuse ketamine may add the drug to marijuana or tobacco to be smoked.

The effects of ketamine taken orally or intranasally become evident in 10 to 15 minutes and are gone in about 1 hour. After IV use, the effects are seen within minutes, but their effects are also short-lived. Effects of oral or intranasal administration are seen in 15 minutes but are gone in 1 hour.

The effects of low doses of ketamine include euphoria, vertigo, slurred speech, slow reaction times, and ataxia. There is less confusion and irrational or violent behaviors with ketamine compared with PCP. High doses cause muddled thinking, vivid visual hallucinations, and an altered body image. Even higher doses produce analgesia, amnesia, and coma.

Inhalants

Parents are concerned about their children's use of alcohol, tobacco, or drugs but are often unaware of the risks associated with household products. Understanding which household products are likely to be abused and the harm they can use, and recognizing the signs and symptoms of their use can help parents prevent inhalant abuse. Inhalants are most often used by preteens between 10 and 12 years of age. Research has indicated that the younger the age of first use of alcohol, cigarettes and marijuana, the more likely the use, and the higher the lifetime use, of inhalants (Siqueira and Crandall, 2006).

Household products commonly found in the home that can be abused include spray paint and paint products, cleaning fluids, lighter fluid, dust removers, and whipped cream canisters; they may be deliberately used to produce intoxicating effects similar to that of alcohol. It is thought that approximately 1000 substances are misused in this manner (Table 12-5). The lost cost, easy accessibility, and ease of transport and concealment make inhalants one of the first substances abused by children and adolescents. The rates of misuse ordinarily decline with age.

For whatever reasons, certain job types and locales produce higher numbers of inhalant abusers: shoe making, petroleum refining, service stations, bicycle repair shops, chemical plants, and health care providers with access to anesthetics. Inhalants are also used when other hallucinogenic substances are unavailable.

There are various methods for abusing inhalants. Some are "huffed," that is, they are orally inhaled from a rag soaked in the desired liquid. Teachers have found cleaning fluids placed on shirt sleeves or head and wrist bands that enable students to continually inhale fumes without being noticed. Others have found users inhaling chemicals through the nose, referred to as "sniffing"; sometimes an agent is sprayed into a paper or plastic bag and then inhaled. One of the most dangerous methods is to sniff the abusive substance with a plastic bag placed over the head (referred to as "bagging"). Group use is popular when this method is adopted, in part because the sniffer may pass out and die of aspiration, asphyxiation, or heart failure before help can be summoned. Some products are heated on a stove top, hotplate, or by other means and the fumes inhaled with a towel over the head. Still others (e.g., lighter fluid and nail polish) may be mixed in a soft drink or beer. "Fire breathing" is another dangerous route of entry for aerosols, butane lighter fluids, or propane. These substances are sprayed directly into the mouth.

Once inhaled, the extensive capillary surface of the lungs allows rapid absorption of the substance, and blood levels peak rapidly. The intoxicating effects of solvent abuse and inhalants are intense and short-lived but vary with age and weight, personality characteristics, and the environmental circumstances in which the substance is used. Users describe various pleasant effects within seconds or minutes after inhalation. These effects begin with intoxication, euphoria, sensation of flying, sensation of the ground moving, delusion of great strength, giddiness, loss of inhibitions, and dream states, and progress to sometimes less pleasant effects such as depersonalization and paranoia. Hallucinations of various types can occur: auditory, tactile (e.g., a sensation of crawling insects or being pricked with needles, or of being touched by human hands or animals), olfactory, and visual (e.g., gory wounds, savage animals). Users report distortion in perceptions of time and space. Solvents can also produce erotic visual hallucinations. Other effects include numbness of the

TABLE 12-5 Inhalants

Category	Active Chemical	Effects
Acrylic paint	Methylethyl ketone	Intoxicant
Adhesives	Hydrocarbons, aromatic hydrocarbons	Intoxicant
Aerosols	Fluorinated hydrocarbons, propane, isobutane, isopropanol, xylene, ethanol	Intoxicant
Amyl nitrite	Aliphatic nitrites	Intoxicant, enhances orgasm
Anesthetics	Halothane, chloroform, ether	Intoxicant, causes euphoria
Antifreeze	Ethyl glycol, methanol, isopropanol	Intoxicant
Cement cleaners	Toluene and toluene mixtures	Intoxicant, similar to opioids
Correction fluid	Trichloroethylene, trichloroethane, chloroform, methylchloroform, amyl acetate	Intoxicant, causes euphoria
Degreasers	Isopropanol, benzene, ketones, n-butyl acetate, xylene, methylethyl ketone	Intoxicant
Dry cleaning solvents, spot removers	Trichloroethylene, trichloroethane petroleum distillates, perchloroethylene	Intoxicant
Fingernail-polish remover	Acetone, alcohol, aliphatic acetates	Intoxicant
Fire extinguishers	Bromochlorodifluoromethane	Intoxicant
Foam dispensers	Nitrous oxide	Intoxicant, causes giddiness
Gasoline	Aliphatic and aromatic hydrocarbons	Intoxicant
Glue	Naphtha, petroleum distillates, acetone, polyvinyl chloride, benzene, hexane, heptanes	Intoxicant
Household cleaners	Chlorine, trichloroethane	Intoxicant
Lighter fluid	Butane, naphtha, aliphatic hydrocarbons	Intoxicant
Nitrous oxide	Nitrous oxide	Intoxicant, causes giddiness
Paint thinners, removers, lacquers	Benzene, naphthalene	Intoxicant hallucinogen
Printing ink	Ketones	Intoxicant
Refrigerant	Freon	Intoxicant
Room deodorizers	Amyl nitrite, butyl nitrite, isobutyl nitrite, isoamyl nitrite	Orgasm enhancers, causes giddiness
Shoe polish, spray	Isopropanol	Intoxicant
Spray paint (especially metallic gold or silver)	Ketones	Euphoriant
Tape head cleaner	Butyl nitrite, aliphatic nitrite	Intoxicant
Whipped cream dispensers	Nitrous oxide	Euphoriant, intoxicant

face and the extremities, dental pain, confusion, insomnia, muscular cramps in calves and sides, a buzzing noise and dizziness, anxiety, delusion of demonic possession, urge for self-mutilation, self-tattooing, tremors, hypersensitivity to noise, chest pain, and dysuria. Hallucinations during intoxication differentiate inhalant intoxication from that of alcoholic and sedative intoxication.

Inhalant use may be suspected if the abuser has a rash around the nose or mouth or if wheezing is heard. The odor of paint or solvents on clothes or skin is sometimes also a sign of inhalant abuse. Inhalants also depress respirations and blood pressure. Many users complain of headaches and nausea and slurred speech, and a loss of motor coordination can be seen. Renal damage is possible from sniffing glue and paint thinner. Liver damage is possible with the use of solvents such as toluene and trichloroethylene. Attention deficit disorders, diminished nonverbal communication skills, and memory impairment have been reported, as have deaths resulting from heart failure, asphyxiation, and aspiration.

The apparent lack of societal concern about inhalant abuse can be attributed to various factors, including underreporting due to reluctance to involve the children and the difficulty in detecting the substances used. It is often believed that because most of the children who experiment with inhalants do so only briefly, adults' and society's time and energy would be better spent combating other, more major, drug problems. However, it may not be understood that experimentation is sometimes fatal, with children dying after the first dose. Death is attributed not only to the toxicity of the substances themselves but also to the method of administration.

Another reason for the paucity of information about this problem is the possibility that a general alarm might result in an increase in experimentation rather than the intended, opposite effect. Such was the case in the early 1960s, when a national alarm sounded concerning the toxic effects of glue sniffing. The result was an increase of such activity, leading in many instances to experimentation with other substances.

OTHER SUBSTANCES OF ABUSE

Anabolic Steroids
Anabolic steroids are synthetic analogues of the male hormone testosterone and are not to be confused with glucocorticoids, or "steroids," which are described further in Chapter 56. Although anabolic steroids may be legally prescribed, illicit use far exceeds legitimate use. These steroids are called anabolic because of their ability to convert nutrients into tissue mass, especially muscle tissue. The desired effects include increased strength, lean body mass, and aggressiveness, and enhanced athletic performance. It is still uncertain whether or not the increase in athletic ability is due to the steroid itself or the belief of the user that it is effective. Anabolic steroids are discussed further in Chapter 57.

Adolescents recognize that prominent athletes are abusing steroids in an attempt to enhance their athletic performance. A 2003 study by the Center for Disease Control and Prevention (CDC) of U.S. high school students found that 6.1% reported having abused steroids, showing a 10-year increasing trend. The drugs are commonly injected, creating in a risk of HIV transmission among needle sharers.

Androgenic steroids accentuate secondary male characteristics in both males and females. Both genders show mood swings, aggressiveness (so called "roid rages"), depression, and psychosis. In addition, there is an arrest of bile secretion, cellular damage to the liver, and an increased risk of cancer. Endocrine system changes occur in the form of decreased glucose tolerance. The cardiovascular system may be affected by an overall increase in cholesterol, especially high-density lipoproteins, and an increase in blood pressure. Increased blood pressure and cardiac workload can lead to heart failure or pulmonary edema. There is also some evidence that steroids may increase the incidence of Wilms' tumor (nephroblastoma) of the urinary tract.

When taken by children before growth is complete, androgenic steroids produce premature closure of the epiphyseal growth plates at the ends of the long bones, thus resulting in a short stature. Some users experience muscle tears or stress. There are some immunologic changes, including a decrease in immunoglobulin A (IgA).

If the patient is using androgenic steroids, he or she may also be taking human growth hormone, which is not detectable by current urine testing methods. The desired effects of growth hormone include tissue building, faster repair of injured tissue, and the conversion of fats to lipids to increase energy. Undesirable effects include development of diabetes, muscle weakness, and cardiac muscle problems.

Erythropoietin use and blood doping are methods used to increase energy by increasing the oxygen-carrying capacity of the blood to increase endurance. Erythropoietin, a hormone that stimulates red blood cell production (see Chapter 44), and blood transfusion (so-called doping) are used by some athletes to produce additional red blood cells. Both practices are unequivocally disapproved by sports officials and governing bodies like the International Olympics Committee. However, their use is also not detectable by current testing methods.

Nutmeg

Nutmeg *(Myristica fragans)* and mace (the covering of nutmeg) also belong in this category. Nutmeg abuse is common among prison inmates in the United States. The oral ingestion of the equivalent of two nutmegs produces, after a latency of several hours, leaden feelings in the extremities and a sense of depersonalization and unreality. Agitation and apprehension are common. Dry mouth, thirst, rapid heart rate, and a red, flushed face are common and may mimic atropine poisoning (see Chapter 15 for more information about adverse effects of atropine and other anticholinergics). Both nutmeg and mace contain the hallucinogenic compound myristicin, which is structurally similar to mescaline.

Sassafras contains safrole, which is similar to myristicin. The harmala alkaloids are hallucinogens that produce a trance with intense imagery. These alkaloids are present in *Peganum harmala,* the seeds of which are chewed in India for their intoxicant effect. Catnip *(Nepeta cataria)* contains the hallucinogen nepetalactone, and the Mexican morning glory seed *(Rivea corymbosa)* and its American cousin, the morning glory seed *(Ipomoea),* are other examples of plants containing natural hallucinogens. Panacea tea, available in health food stores, is made from morning glory seeds.

CLINICAL REASONING

Treatment Objectives

The ultimate goal of all drug abuse treatment is to enable the patient to achieve lasting abstinence, but the immediate goals are to reduce drug use, improve the patient's ability to function, and minimize the medical and social complications of drug abuse. Treatment objectives for the patient with an overdose are primarily symptomatic and supportive. The aim of treatment is usually to support vital functions until the drug is biotransformed and eliminated from the body.

Treatment Options

Although the principles of treatment remain similar, treatment options vary depending upon the substance the patient is abusing, the extent of the dependence, the patient's incentive to stop the abuse, the depth of the commitment to stop, and the support structure available to the patient (Table 12-6). There are several types of drug abuse–treatment programs. Short-term methods last less than 6 months and include residential therapy, medication therapy, and drug-free outpatient therapy. Longer-term treatment may include, for example, outpatient methadone maintenance treatment for opiate dependency and residential therapeutic community treatment.

Many rehabilitation programs attempt to teach the patient new ways to interact, drug-free. In particular, patients are generally encouraged or required not to associate with friends who still use the addictive substance. Twelve-step programs encourage those with substance abuse to not only stop using alcohol or other drugs, but also to examine and change habits related to their dependency. Many programs emphasize that recovery is a permanent process without a culmination. Whether moderation is achievable by persons with a history of abuse remains a controversial point, but it is generally considered unsustainable. Even for legal drugs such as alcohol, complete abstention is also emphasized rather than attempts at moderation, which may lead to relapse.

TABLE 12-6 Principles of Drug Abuse Treatment

1. No single treatment is appropriate for all individuals.
2. Treatment must be readily available.
3. Effective treatment attends to multiple needs of the individual, not just his or her drug use.
4. At different times during treatment, a patient may develop a need for medical services, family therapy, vocational rehabilitation, and social and legal services.
5. Remaining in treatment for an adequate period of time is critical for treatment effectiveness.
6. Individual and/or group counseling and other behavioral therapies are critical components of effective treatment for addiction.
7. Medications are an important element of treatment for many patients, especially when combined with counseling and other behavioral therapies.
8. Addicted or drug-abusing individuals with coexisting mental disorders should have both disorders treated in an integrated way.
9. Medical detoxification is only the first stage of addiction treatment and by itself does little to change long-term drug use.
10. Treatment does not have to be voluntary to be effective.
11. Possible drug use during treatment must be monitored continuously.
12. Treatment programs should provide assessment for HIV/AIDS, hepatitis B and C, tuberculosis and other infectious diseases, and counseling to help patients modify or change behaviors that place them or others at risk of infection.
13. Recovery from drug addiction can be a long-term process and frequently requires multiple episodes of treatment.

HIV/AIDS, Human immunodeficiency virus/acquired immunodeficiency syndrome.
From the National Institute on Drug Abuse. Principles of drug abuse treatment. Available online: www.nida.nih.gov/Drugpages/DrugsofAbuse.html. Accessed March 17, 2007.

Patient Variables

Changing views of substance abuse will continue to create gray areas where the justification for drug testing and the necessity for treatment are unclear. Overall, interventions for the substance abuser should include maintenance of existing body system function along with adequate nutritional support. A multidisciplinary team approach will assist the patient to make the biologic and psychosocial adjustments necessary to successfully eliminate use of substances.

LIFE-SPAN CONSIDERATIONS

Pregnant and Nursing Women. When considering the effects of substance abuse on the perinatal period, the primary concerns are the health of the mother and preventing or curtailing complications to the fetus. If the mother continues to abuse drugs throughout her pregnancy, neonatal complications and the potential for her to neglect or abuse her child are increased.

The effects of substance abuse on mothers and unborn infants have been studied intensely, although many questions remain unanswered. It is safe to say that the fetus is exposed to virtually all of the substances the mother consumes. It is unknown which effects are the direct results of the substances themselves, and which are related to indirect consequences such as the mother's general health, her prenatal nutrition status, or her general lifestyle and living conditions. Drugs with high lipid-solubility are particularly dangerous to the fetus, because they penetrate the fetal blood more easily through simple diffusion.

For information on specific agents and their effects, see the Evolve Resources Bonus Content "Effects of Selected Maternal Drug Ingestion on the Fetus or Neonate," found at http://evolve.elsevier.com/Gutierrez/pharmacotherapeutics.

Children and Adolescents. Children exposed to severe stress may be more vulnerable to drug abuse. A number of clinical and epidemiologic studies show a strong association between psychosocial stressors early in life (e.g., parental loss, child abuse) and an increased risk for depression, anxiety, impulsive behavior, and substance abuse in adulthood.

There is a general consensus among health care providers, social workers, and others that the more risk factors children or adolescents have in their life, the higher the likelihood of their becoming substance abusers. Childhood physical abuse has proven to be a strong predictor of young adults' current substance abuse problems. However, having a significant number of risk factors does not predict a child's inevitable development of substance abuse or other problem behaviors. Many children and adolescents in high-risk, dysfunctional families and circumstances grow up relatively unscathed. The presence of preventive and buffering factors in their lives more than makes up for the dysfunctional aspects (Table 12-7).

Older Adults. The recorded rates of alcohol and drug abuse in the elderly are low, but there is increasing concern that the actual rates may be higher and undetected. The expectation of low abuse rates in this population results in the problem of health care providers not asking the appropriate questions during an assessment. Conventional wisdom holds that because alcoholism begins at younger ages and results in a reduced life expectancy, few alcoholics survive to become older adults. One theory holds that the reason so few opioid-dependent individuals are reported between the ages of 35 and 45 is that there is "a maturing out"; that is, they die, or they become debilitated and are treated for something else, just get tired of their dependency and manage to stop using the substance, or know how to manage it so well that they do not come to the attention of the health care provider. If they are still abusing at middle age and beyond, they are probably obtaining the substances via OTC and prescription drugs. Loneliness, depression, and isolation that are seen in many older adults can contribute to the potential for current substance abuse, even by those who have not abused drugs in the past.

Community Variables

Measures that prevent development of alcohol and drug abuse should be explored. Although there are problems with trying to prevent a condition for which causes are essentially unknown, community-wide and individual measures may be helpful. Most efforts aimed toward preventing substance abuse are directed toward reducing the drug supply, often by law enforcement agencies. Legislative intervention often takes a parallel approach to such efforts—essentially, initiatives to decrease the demand for drugs. Because these efforts involve changing attitudes, the task is likely to be very difficult but more effective in the long run.

Encourage individuals to take personal responsibility for drinking alcohol and taking mind-altering drugs. Prescribe drugs appropriately, using mild-altering drugs in limited amounts and for limited periods. Promoting non–drug measures when they will likely be effective, educating patients about drugs that are prescribed, participating in drug education programs, and recognizing patients who are at risk for substance abuse as early as possible are all approaches that contribute to reducing the incidence and prevalence of this health care problem.

Also encourage parents to model appropriate behaviors by minimizing their own drug use and avoiding smoking. Children are apt to use a drug if their parents hold a generally permissive attitude about drug use, if either parent uses mild-altering drugs, and if either parent is a heavy drinker or smoker.

Drug Variables

Drug therapy is relatively controversial for the management of patients with substance abuse, for several reasons. First, specific antidotes are available only for benzodiazepines and opioids. Second, there is a high risk of merely substituting one abused substance for another. Third, there are significant drawbacks to giving CNS stimulants to reverse the effects of CNS depressants, and vice versa. However, there are some clinical indications for pharmacotherapy. These indications include disulfiram as a deterrent for chronic alcohol abuse, methadone maintenance for opioid drug–dependence, symptomatic treatment of acute drug toxicity or overdose, and treatment of withdrawal syndromes.

During the acute phase of withdrawal, it is important that the health care provider monitors the patient frequently for challenges to the patient's vital processes. Ensuring adequate respiratory, cardiac, and circulatory function is a priority. It is important to know what substances the patient is withdrawing from to anticipate the characteristics of the withdrawal.

TABLE 12-7 Factors Related to Substance Abuse

Risk Factors for Substance Abuse	Preventive Factors for Substance Abuse
INDIVIDUAL FACTORS	
• Rejected by peers in elementary grades	• Informed about risks associated with substance abuse and use
• Thinks most friends use substances of abuse	• Displays negative attitudes and behaviors toward substances and substance use
• Unable to defy peer pressure at older ages	• Bonds to prosocial culture
• Genetic vulnerability, psychologic disorders	• Views parents, teachers, doctors, law enforcement officers and other adults as allies
• Low self-esteem, loner, rebellious	• Comfortable in social situations
• Inappropriate or ineffective coping responses	• Involved with same-age peers in alternative activities
• Violent and/or aggressive behaviors, impulsive	• Strong sense of well-being and self-confidence
• Rejects social activities, cultural, values, religion	• Has positive plans for the future
• Early sexual activity, teen pregnancy	
• Begins using substances at a young age	
• Early antisocial behavior	
• Poor academic performance	
PEER FACTORS	
• Negative norms and expectations reinforced by peer group	• Peers involved in substance-free activities
• Inappropriate sexual activity among peers	• Peers disapprove of alcohol and other drug use
FAMILY FACTORS	
• Family history of alcohol or other substance abuse ("Get me a beer, would you?")	• Parents are nurturing, consistent, and supportive of each other
• Family dysfunctional, spend little time together	• Education is valued and encouraged: parents are actively involved
• Parents lack knowledge of whereabouts of teens, who they're with and where they go	• Has and develops positive coping strategies
• Lack of clear rules, expectations, and consequences of alcohol and drug use or abuse	• Expectations and limits regarding drug and alcohol use are clear
• Parents inconsistent about expectations and limits of behavior	• Supportive relationships with caring adults beyond immediate family
• Frequent family conflicts and abuse	• Shares family responsibilities, including chores and decision making
• Unemployment	
SCHOOL FACTORS	
• Lacks clear expectations regarding academic and personal behavior	• School responsive to students' needs
• Lacks commitment or sense of belonging at school	• School fosters active involvement of students, parents, and community
• Large numbers of students are academically unsuccessful	• School provides leadership and decision making opportunities for students, parents, community
• Parents and community members not actively involved	• Encourages and expects goal-setting, academic achievement and positive social development
COMMUNITY AND SOCIETAL FACTORS	
• Alcohol and other drugs readily available	• Opportunities exist for community involvement
• Inconsistent enforcement of laws and ordinances	• Religious affiliations reflected in community
• Community norms are unclear or encourage use	• Laws and ordinances are consistently enforced
• Residents have little sense of "connection" to community	• Informal social control
• Neighborhood in disorganization	• Policies and norms encourage nonuse of drugs
• Rapid turnover in neighborhood populations	• Community service opportunities available for youth
• High unemployment, economically deprived	• Resources (housing, health care, child care, jobs, recreation, etc.) are available
• Residents at or below the poverty level	• Comprehensive risk-focused programs available
• Lack of strong social institutions	• Programs for parents of children and adolescents
• Lack of monitoring youths' activities	• Early childhood and family support programs
• Inadequate media portrayals	• Widely supported community prevention efforts exist
• Pro-use messages	

Maintain patient safety and reduce environmental stimuli while the patient is in the acute withdrawal phase. Regularly monitor cardiovascular, respiratory, and neurologic functions, mental status, and behavior. Check lab reports, when available, for abnormal liver function tests, indications of anemia, and abnormal white blood cell or electrolyte counts. Hypocalcemia, hypomagnesemia, and acidosis are common in alcohol abusers. In addition, monitor drug and alcohol blood levels.

Patient Education

The best intervention for substance abuse is primary prevention. Educational programs are available in the elementary and secondary classrooms as well as public service announcements in the media. Because substance abuse and child abuse and neglect are correlated, it is important to educate parents not only about the effects of substance abuse but also about successful parenting techniques. Educating parents about the clues of substance abuse in their child is important, as well as enlightening parents about role-modeling behaviors that promote respect for moderation or abstinence and for healthy ways to resolve conflict.

Responsibility for recovery and optimal health is placed on the patient once physiologic and psychologic stability has been established. This is often a long-term process and involves the attainment of patient self-awareness and self-acceptance. Education, along with support and encouragement regarding changes in lifestyle, plays a significant part in the patient's recovery. Self-help groups such as Alcoholics Anonymous, Synanon, Alateen, Alanon, and others educate the public about the dangers of substances.

Once the patient has passed the acute stage of withdrawal, treatment is focused on prevention of relapse. The path to abstinence is divided into several options. Support networks such as Alcoholics Anonymous have been effective. Behavioral approaches, marital and family counseling, and hypnosis have been tried with varying degrees of success.

Many patients find smoking extremely difficult to stop, given the positive benefits of continuing and the very unpleasant withdrawal symptoms experienced on attempting withdrawal. Advise patients that nicotine patches, gum, aversion therapy, behavior modification, the substitution of other activities (especially physical activities), and avoidance of activities associated with smoking are all interventions that have proved successful.

Evaluation

The patient bears the burden of stopping drug abuse, and the health care provider must make and proceed on the assumption that the patient in treatment wants to stop. It is important to convey the attitude that the patient will succeed. Many health care providers who have worked with patients trying to reform become cynical. The cynicism is a natural outcome of repeated disappointments, when highly motivated patients are unable to remain drug-free after completing drug treatment programs. In addition, patients who abuse drugs generally will do or say anything to obtain the drugs. This includes lying and manipulation of the health care team. Any health care provider who has ever been misled by a patient does not want to repeat the experience. Yet, if the health care provider presumes that the patient will fail, this expectation may be conveyed to the patient and unwittingly contribute to its fulfillment. The recovering patient needs all possible resources available in order to stop the abuse, and an environment that has firm limits but one with a "can do" approach is one such resource. Health care providers who work with patients who abuse substances walk a delicate line. It requires great skill and the willingness to appear gullible from time to time.

Although the approach is optimistic, the health care provider can look for some clues in the patient that would raise the possibility for success. The patient who accepts responsibility for choices made and does not blame external situations for the drug abuse has a better chance of success. The patient increases the likelihood for successful recovery if, after the acute withdrawal phase has passed, there is a willingness to accept the discomfort of the emotional withdrawal of the substances without seeking or demanding immediate relief. The chance of success is increased if the patient resists the temptation to think too soon that recovery has taken place. This means accepting the harsh reality that the substance and its abuse have pervaded the person's life space, and that as recovery evolves, the problems that were shielded by the substance abuse still remain. The process of confronting those problems extracts an emotional toll for which preparation is needed. If the patient substitutes a comfortable support system for the drugs, the chances for success are even greater.

Evaluating the effectiveness of interventions for substance abuse involves the patient's and the family's responses to the management plan. Some health care providers believe that management is considered successful when the patient is clean and sober. This means that the patient abstains from illegal drug use, and abstains from alcohol completely or drinks alcohol in moderation. It also means that the patient uses prescription drugs according to directions and for the condition for which they were prescribed, and that illicit use of drugs is stopped. Success for some patients may be defined as diminishment of the undesirable adverse effects of the substance abused. If so, success might be defined in terms of the patient not engaging in high-risk behaviors.

KEY POINTS

- There are four main categories of abused substances in the United States: sedatives, stimulants, hallucinogens, and anabolic steroids.
- A number of populations are at risk for substance abuse: adolescents, older adults, health care providers, dual-diagnosis psychiatric patients, Vietnam veterans, individuals with chronic pain, and athletes.
- Commonly abused CNS depressants include alcohol, opioids, benzodiazepines, and barbiturates.
- Commonly abused CNS stimulants include amphetamines, cocaine, caffeine, and tobacco.
- Assess for substance abuse or misuse even if the patient comes for treatment for another problem.
- Substance abuse affects growth and development, contributes to school dropout rates and gang membership, can result in violence and death, and is a catalyst for sexual promiscuity, teen pregnancy, and sexually transmitted disease.

- The ultimate goal of all substance abuse treatment is to enable the patient to achieve lasting abstinence, but the immediate goals are to reduce drug use, improve the patient's ability to function, and minimize the medical and social complications of drug abuse.
- Treatment options vary depending on the substance abused, the extent of the dependence, the patient's incentive to stop the abuse, the depth of the commitment to stop, and the support available to the patient.
- The patient bears the burden for halting drug abuse. Health care providers must assume the patient in treatment wants to stop and proceed with this assumption.
- The best "treatment" for substance abuse is primary prevention.
- Responsibility for recovery and optimal health is placed on the patient, once physiologic and psychologic stability has been established.
- Evaluating the effectiveness of interventions for substance abuse involves the patient's and the family's responses to the management plan.

Bibliography

Cami, J., and Farre, M. (2003). Drug addiction. *New England Journal of Medicine, 349*(10), 975–986.

Drug Enforcement Administration. (2006). *Fact 3: Illegal drugs are illegal because they are harmful.* Available online: www.usdoj.gov/dea/demand/speakout/03so.htm. Accessed March 17, 2007.

Drug Enforcement Administration. (2006). *Fact 4: Smoked marijuana is not scientifically approved medicine. Marinol, the legal version of medical marijuana, is approved by science.* Available online: www.usdoj.gov/dea/demand/speakout/04so.htm. Accessed March 17, 2007.

Drug Enforcement Administration. (2006). *Fact 5: Drug control spending is a minor portion of the U.S. budget. Compared to the social costs of drug abuse and addiction, government spending on drug control is minimal.* Available online: www.usdoj.gov/dea/demand/speakout/04so.htm. Accessed March 17, 2007.

Drug Enforcement Administration. (2006). *Fact 6: Legalization of drugs will lead to increased use and increased levels of addiction. Legalization has been tried before, and failed miserably.* Available online: www.usdoj.gov/dea/demand/speakout/06so.htm. Accessed March 17, 2007.

Galvin, D., Miller, T., Spicer, R., et al. (2007). Substance abuse and the uninsured worker in the United States. *Journal of Public Health Policy, 28*(1), 102–117.

Hobbs, W., Rall, T., and Verdoorn, T. (2001). Hypnotics and sedatives: Ethanol. In Hardman, J., and Limbird, L. (Eds.). *Goodman and Gilman's the pharmacologic basis of therapeutics.* (10th ed.). New York: McGraw-Hill.

Korsten, T., and O'Connor, P. (2003). Management of drug and alcohol withdrawal. *New England Journal of Medicine, 34*(8), 1786–1795.

Lo, C., and Cheng, T. (2007). The impact of childhood maltreatment on young adult's substance abuse. *The American Journal of Drug and Alcohol Abuse, 33*(1), 139–146.

National Institute on Drug Abuse. (2006). *Substance abuse.* Available online: www.nida.nih.gov. Accessed March 17, 2007.

Proceedings of the Community Epidemiology Work Group. (2006). *Epidemiological trends in drug abuse.* National Institute on Drug Abuse. NIH Publication No. 06-5281A.

Siqueira, L., & Crandall, L. (2006). Inhalant use in Florida youth. *Substance Abuse, 27*(4), 27–35.

Substance Abuse and Medical Health Services Administration. *Results from the 2002 National Household Survey on Drug Use and Health: National Findings.* Office of Applied Studies. NHSDA Series H-22, DHHS Publication No. SMA 03-3836. Rockville, MD. Available online: www.samhsa.gov/oas/nhsda/2k2nsduh/Resluts.htm#fig3.3. Accessed March 17, 2007.

Swotinsky, R. (Ed.). (1992). *The medical review officer's guide to drug testing.* New York: Van Nostrand Reinhold.

Williams, C., and Woodcock, K. (2000). Do ethanol and metronidazole interact to produce a disulfiram-like reaction? *The Annals of Pharmacotherapy, 34*(2), 255–257.

World Health Organization. Addiction. In *Lexicon of alcohol and drug terms.* Available online: www.who.int/substance_abuse/terminology/who_lexicon/en/index.html. Accessed February 10, 2007.

World Health Organization. (2002). Tobacco. Available online: www.who.int/substance_abuse/facts/tobacco/en/index.html. Accessed February 10, 2007.

COMMUNITY

13

Poisonings

A poison is defined as "any substance that causes injury, illness, or death, especially by chemical means" (American Heritage Dictionary, 2000). Poisons may be a solid, liquid, spray, or gas formulation. Exposure may be accidental or intentional; contact may be from ingestion, inhalation, or topical exposure.

POISONINGS

EPIDEMIOLOGY AND ETIOLOGY

According to the American Association of Poison Control Centers (AAPCC), more than 2 million poison exposures are reported annually: that is 1 exposure every 15 seconds. An additional 2.1 million go unreported. More than 100,000 poisonings result in hospitalization annually, with about 20% of the cases resulting in death. The cost of treatment for poisonings totaled over $3 billion dollars in the 1990s, and even more during the years of 2000 and beyond.

Over 90% of poison exposures occur in the home. Poisonings occur in persons of all ages; however, the incidence is highest among young children. Of the reported exposures in the United States, 52.7% occurred among children younger than 6 years of age. The most common poisonings come from household products (e.g., cosmetics and personal care products, cleaning products, OTC analgesics, plants).

For adults, the most common toxicant exposures are pain relievers, sedatives, cleaning products, and antidepressants (Box 13-1). The drug classes commonly associated with nonaccidental poisonings include amphetamines, antidepressants, barbiturates, benzodiazepines, opioids, analgesics, and cocaine. Approximately 76% of these exposures are intentional and lead to death. Some 90% of nonaccidental poisonings are caused by fewer than 20 of the 600,000 different drugs in the health care arena.

The toxicity of a chemical substance is determined by the interactions of the specific substance with food and other drugs, the dose, susceptibility of the individual, biologic and genetic factors, and the route of contact.

CLINICAL REASONING

Treatment Objectives

Interventions for patients who have overdosed on drugs or ingested foreign substances center on three major objectives: supporting the patient's vital functions; preventing absorption of and/or eliminating the toxicant; and preventing or managing complications. The acronym *SIRES* is an aid to remembering the essentials of care:
- *S*tabilize the patient.
- *I*dentify the toxic substance.

BOX 13-1

Examples of Poisons

Drugs
- Inotropics
- Antiarrhythmics
- Anticoagulants
- Antidiabetic drugs
- Analgesics
- Tranquilizers
- Cough and cold drugs
- Iron supplements
- Antianxiety drugs

Household Products
- Drain cleaners
- Oven cleaners
- Toilet bowl cleaners
- Windshield cleaners
- Furniture polish
- Lamp oil
- Pesticides
- Gasoline
- Kerosene
- Antifreeze

Personal Care Items
- Mouthwash
- Permanent wave solutions
- Hair removal products
- Nail glue remover
- Nail primer

Plants
- Wild mushrooms
- Philodendron
- Dieffenbachia
- Pokeweed
- Holly berries
- Foxglove

Environmental Poisons
- Carbon monoxide
- Lead paint

- *R*everse its effects and manage any complications.
- *E*liminate the substance from the body.
- *S*upport the patient and significant others (physically and psychosocially).

▌ *Patient Variables*

LIFE-SPAN CONSIDERATIONS
Children. Drugs specifically packaged for children generally contain small quantities to reduce the likelihood of serious

harm if the entire package were consumed. For example, baby aspirin is packaged in containers of 36 or fewer tablets. Child-resistant containers are a further means of protection. However, even with these safety factors, the majority of pediatric poisonings involve accidental ingestion by children younger than 6 years. Toddlers between the ages of 2 and 3 years are the most common victims of accidental prescription drug poisoning, and 25% of all the solid prescription drugs involved in poisonings are enclosed in child-resistant containers. In addition, most accidentally ingested drugs are stored in ordinary containers or improperly used child-resistant containers; many are in no containers at all. Although the Poison Prevention Packaging Act (PPPA) of 1970 resulted in a 65% decrease in the ingestion of household products (e.g., antifreeze, lye), prescription drug ingestion by children has declined only 36%.

Accidental ingestions of analgesics and antipyretics are the leading causes of pediatric poisoning emergencies. Other substances commonly ingested are flavored chewable vitamins, household cleaners and polishes, plants, cosmetics, pesticides, paints and solvents, and petroleum products.

Adolescents and Adults. Though pediatric poisonings constitute the majority of calls to poison control centers, adolescent and adult poisonings more often result in serious morbidity and mortality. A high percentage of these poisonings are related to drug abuse or suicide attempts. Men aged 20 to 39 years account for 70% of all drug abuse–related emergency room visits. Cocaine and heroin or morphine are involved in more than one third of the deaths. Because of the growing prevalence of street drug–abuse, it may be difficult to distinguish a suicide attempt from a recreational overdose.

Older Adults. Although older adults make up approximately 12% of the population, they use 40% of all prescription drugs. Further, 25% of suicides reported each year in the United States involve older adults. Poisonings in older adults related to polypharmacy and suicide attempts are common. It is estimated that the average older adult has 11 prescriptions filled per year. An average of 8 drugs is administered to each nursing home resident. The combination of increased drug use, declining organ function, and the potential for depression raises the risk of poisoning and drug toxicity in this population.

Treatment Options

When overdose of a drug or ingestion of a toxicant occurs, the poison control center should be contacted. Information that must be available when contacting the center includes the following:
- Generic, trade, or chemical name of the substance, if known
- Purpose, or how the substance was meant to be used
- Physical appearance of the substance
- Odor, color, texture, and any distinguishing characteristics of the substance
- Label statements related to "poison" content or flammability
- Quantity ingested
- Time of ingestion

The time of ingestion is important, because the elapsed time since ingestion helps determine the treatment strategies to be used. Recognize, however, that approximately 50% of the information gathered during a poisoning crisis may be inaccurate.

The bottle containing the drug should be kept so that necessary information can be obtained. **If the amount of an ingested liquid is not known, an assumption is made that the largest amount that could have been taken was consumed.** As a general rule, a small child swallows approximately 5 mL at a time, a 10-year-old approximately 10 mL, and an adult approximately 15 mL. Saving the emesis or the stool is often helpful in identifying the substance and may provide some clue to how much was ingested. Depending on the specific poisoning, assessment includes not only the patient but household members as well.

In their assessment of the patient, health care providers include a history or present thoughts of suicide, homicide, or the intent for either (including the immediacy of acting on a plan), and previous incidents of poisonings or ingestion of foreign substances. An assessment of the patient's present drug regimen including prescription and over-the-counter (OTC) drug use, and any use of herbs, is also needed.

▥ *Toxidromes*

Toxidromes, the clinical manifestations of ingestion, are helpful in determining the ingredients ingested (Box 13-2). Become familiar with the clinical manifestations of specific drug ingestions and overdoses, but also assess breath odor, respiratory rate, the presence of dyspnea or cyanosis, changes in pulse rate, the appearance and odor of any vomitus, and any abnormalities of stool and urine to confirm a suspicion of drug overdose or ingestion. Other findings to consider include evidence of burns around the lips and mouth, discolored gums, hypodermic pricks, pustules, or scars on the exposed and accessible surfaces of the body. Signs of nervous system involvement include excitement, muscular twitching, delirium, dysarthria, pupillary constriction or dilation, an elevated or subnormal temperature, stupor, and coma. Coma related to drug overdose is categorized as follows:
- *Grade I*–Patient asleep but easily aroused, reacts to painful stimuli; deep tendon reflexes (DTRs) intact; pupils equal and react to light, ocular movements present; vital signs stable
- *Grade II*–Vital signs stable; pupils slightly dilated but reactive; pain response absent; DTRs depressed
- *Grade III*–Vital signs stable; pupillary reflexes and DTRs absent
- *Grade IV*–Respirations and circulation depressed

The key principle in the management of patients who have experienced poisonings is to "treat the patient, not the poison." This principle is important, because treatment for most poisonings is symptomatic and supportive in nature. The first priority is to stabilize the patient before treating the poisoning. Once the patient is stable, treatment options and interventions can be explored (see Box 13-2). Emotional support of the patient and others is crucial.

The most reliable information about poisoning emergencies is available through the network of regional poison control centers. These centers were established to provide current and comprehensive management guidelines to the general public and health care providers. Although several references on toxicity and the treatment of poisoning are

Common Toxidromes

The common clinical manifestations of toxic ingestion are listed here according to the type of substance ingested.

Anticholinergics, Atropine, Scopolamine
- Agitation
- Coma
- Delirium
- Dilated pupils
- Dry, beet-red skin
- Hallucinations
- Hyperthermia
- Tachycardia

Barbiturates, Sedative-Hypnotics, Tranquilizers
- Ataxia
- Drowsiness
- Hypotension
- Slurred speech (without alcohol breath odor)

Organophosphates (Cholinergics), Mushrooms
- Involuntary defecation, urination
- Lacrimation
- Miosis
- Pulmonary congestion
- Salivation
- Seizures

Opioids
- Coma
- Hypotension
- Miosis
- Respiratory depression

Salicylates
- Fever
- Hyperglycemia
- Hyperventilation
- Mixed respiratory alkalosis and metabolic acidosis

Tricyclic Antidepressants
- Anticholinergic signs and symptoms
- Arrhythmias (prolonged QRS interval)
- Coma
- Seizures

Poison Control Centers

★ ★ ★ ★ 1-800-222-1222 ★ ★ ★ ★

The American Association of Poison Control Centers (AAPCC) has launched a nationwide number for access to the 62 U.S. poison control centers. The number is routed to the local poison center serving the caller, based on the area code and exchange of the caller. The number is available 24 hours a day, 7 days per week in all 50 states, the District of Columbia, the U.S. Virgin Islands, and Puerto Rico. Go to the website for information on state poison control centers: www.aapcc.org/. A list of state poison control centers may be found in the Evolve Resources Bonus Content at http://evolve.elsevier.com/Gutierrez/pharmacotherapeutics/.

Support Vital Functions

Treatment for most poisonings and complications is symptomatic and supportive. In all cases of poisoning, speed in treatment is essential, but a deliberate pace and calm thinking will avoid hasty decisions that may result in ineffective, if not harmful, treatment. Support vital functions such as respirations, circulation, and acid-base and fluid-electrolyte balances. Ensure that supplemental oxygen and suction equipment are readily available. Implement basic and advanced life support as warranted by the patient's condition. A ventilator may be kept on hand in case the patient needs ventilatory assistance. Cardiac monitoring may be necessary, because many poisoning substances precipitate rhythm disturbances. Establish a large-bore intravenous line for all patients with actually or potentially unstable vital signs or a decreased level of consciousness. Arterial blood gas specimens may be drawn for the patient who arrives in respiratory distress or who has ingested a poisoning substance that may alter acid-base balance.

Patients who arrive with a decreased level of consciousness will receive an intravenous dose of the opioid antagonist naloxone (see Chapter 16) and the benzodiazepine antagonist flumazenil (see Chapter 18). A positive response to the usual dose of naloxone or flumazenil indicates the presence of opioids or benzodiazepines, respectively. These two drugs thus serve not only as potential treatment for narcotic or benzodiazepine overdose but also as useful diagnostic aids.

It is important to monitor the patient's response after receiving these drugs. Both naloxone and flumazenil are short-acting, so the patient's level of consciousness may again decrease once therapeutic effectiveness of the drug declines. Repeated administration of the antagonist may be necessary until the patient recovers sufficiently.

Identify the Poison

Correct sampling of appropriate body fluids, prompt reporting of the results, and the number of substances listed on the analysis profile all contribute to effective diagnostic testing and subsequent management. Toxicology screens are used to diagnose, assess the prognosis of, and manage acute poisoning, particularly in uncooperative or comatose patients. However, toxicology screening is time-consuming, expensive, often unreliable, and no substitute for patient assessment

available, the most up-to-date information on both human and animal poisonings is provided by *Poisondex*. Developed in conjunction with the Rocky Mountain Poison and Drug Centers in Denver, Colorado, *Poisondex* is reviewed and updated every 3 months. This detailed toxicology database is designed to identify and provide information to poison control centers and health care providers on chemical composition, toxicity, and medical management of over 750,000 drugs, household chemicals, industrial and environmental toxins, and biologics (including plant and animal toxins). *Poisondex* also provides a visual reference (e.g., drug color, shape, imprinted symbols) to facilitate identification of manufactured and street drugs. All regional poison control centers accept calls 24 hours a day, 7 days a week, 365 days a year. Many also have "800" numbers. The database may be purchased through Micromedex (www.micromedex.com/products/poisindex/) (Box 13-3).

and good clinical judgment. Reliability of results depends on precise communication between the laboratory and the health care provider about the drugs under suspicion. The plasma levels of a few toxins may influence the plan of care (e.g., acetaminophen, carbon monoxide, ethylene glycol, iron, lithium, methanol, salicylates, theophylline). For others, however, there is a poor correlation between plasma drug levels and toxicity (e.g., tricyclic antidepressants). The interpretation of toxicology results should take into account the patient's clinical status, the time elapsed since exposure, and the potential for delayed toxic effects. For example, therapeutic levels of acetaminophen 4 to 8 hours after ingestion are associated with little risk of hepatotoxicity, but the same level obtained more than 16 hours after ingestion indicates a high risk of hepatotoxicity.

▓ Prevent Further Absorption

By preventing further absorption of the poison, serum levels are reduced and there is a reduction in morbidity and mortality. When the poison has been ingested, there are several options available for treatment: giving activated charcoal, gastric lavage and aspiration, whole bowel irrigations, and catharsis, although using cathartic drugs is not advisable. The "universal antidote," a mixture of burnt toast, magnesium oxide (milk of magnesia), and tannic acid (tea), is ineffective and, in some instances, may even be harmful. If the exposure is topical, surface decontamination is used. The most effective method for removal of ingested toxins is usually the most natural one—inducing vomiting as soon as possible. However, it should be noted that there are many contraindications to use of the method, and thus it is rarely used today.

ACTIVATED CHARCOAL. Activated charcoal is the favored method for poison removal from the gastrointestinal tract since it detoxifies ingested toxic substances and irritants. Activated charcoal absorbs large molecules that contain a carbon atom. Substances in this category include the salicylates, opioids, barbiturates, benzodiazepines, phenothiazines, digoxin, atropine, and penicillin. Small molecules or molecules lacking a carbon atom are poorly absorbed. Poorly absorbed substances include alcohols and glycols, chlorine, iodine, caustics and corrosives, heavy metals, and petroleum distillates. The charcoal may also serve as a stool marker to indicate when gastrointestinal absorption of the ingested poison has ended. The occasional adverse effects are diarrhea, gastrointestinal discomfort, and intestinal gas.

The desired dose of activated charcoal in an adult is 30 to 100 grams given as a slurry (30 grams in at least 8 oz of water), or 12.5 to 50 grams in an aqueous or sorbitol suspension. If dosing is based on body weight, the dose is 1 gram/kg or, otherwise calculated, approximately 5 to 10 times the amount of poison ingested. Pediatric doses range from 25 to 50 grams. Because charcoal absorbs antidotes as well as the poison and thereby counteracts their benefits, antidotes should not be given immediately before, with, or shortly after the administration of activated charcoal.

Activated charcoal is usually administered as a single oral dose. For poisons that are slowly absorbed or that undergo enterohepatic recirculation, sequential doses can be beneficial. There is no upper limit to the amount that may be given.

Further, the mixture need not be removed from the stomach after ingestion. No known adverse effects to activated charcoal have been identified.

GASTRIC LAVAGE. Gastric lavage should only be done in life-threatening cases, and then only if less than 60 minutes has elapsed since ingestion of the poison. Contraindications to gastric lavage include ingestion of caustic substances; seizures (because of the risk of injury from the procedure and possible aspiration of stomach contents); ingestion of high-viscosity petroleum distillates; significant arrhythmias; and bloody emesis.

Gastric lavage is carried out using a large-bore orogastric tube (number 36 or 42 French for adults and number 22 to 28 French for children) with the patient in a left side–lying, head-down position. Large-bore tubing is needed because smaller diameters impede the flow and aspiration of lavage fluid. Gastric contents should be aspirated and sent to the lab for toxicology analysis before lavage. Lavage is done using multiple instillations of 150 to 200 mL of tap water or saline solution for adults, and 50 to 100 mL of solution for children under age 5. Larger fluid volumes should be avoided because of the risk of pushing stomach contents into the small intestine. Lavage should be continued until 10 to 12 washes have been done or until gastric contents are clear. For patients who are unresponsive, an endotracheal tube with the cuff inflated should be inserted to protect the airway before the lavage.

HYPEROSMOLAR LAXATIVE. Hyperosmolar laxatives such as polyethylene glycol, which contains a balance of electrolytes, are used for whole-bowel irrigations. This solution fosters passage through the intestine of poisons such as iron, lithium, and lead, as well as sustained-release products, thereby minimizing absorption (see also Chapter 46). These drugs act quickly and have little toxicity. Hyperosmolar laxatives should be avoided in patients who have bloody vomitus; an ileus, obstruction, or bowel perforation; or peritonitis. There are no data to support the use of cathartics, which hasten the passage of the poison through the intestine. Therefore these drugs are seldom recommended today.

ENHANCE RENAL ELIMINATION. Drugs that alter urinary pH accelerate removal of organic acids and bases from the body through ion trapping (see Chapter 4). Because of the buffer systems in blood, drugs such as sodium bicarbonate and ammonium chloride (see Chapter 49) have a relatively small effect on the pH of blood but a significant effect on urinary pH. Sodium bicarbonate makes urine alkaline, which in turn decreases the passive resorption of acids such as aspirin and phenobarbital. Ammonium chloride acidifies the urine, which promotes the elimination of bases such as amphetamines and phencyclidine.

SURFACE DECONTAMINATION. Removing poisons from topical surfaces usually consists of first aid for the system involved. Topical exposures should be treated by immediately flooding the body parts that came in contact with the poison with water. A shower including shampooing is the best strategy. Clothing removal should be accomplished while the patient is in the shower, to prevent exposure of the health care provider or others. The flooding should be followed with gentle soap-and-water washes and thorough rinsing. Health care personnel performing surface decontamination should take precautions to avoid personal exposure to the poison.

Treatment of ocular exposure involves flushing the eye(s) with water or normal saline for up to 20 minutes. The eyelids should be held open to facilitate thorough washing of the eyes. Eye drops and other chemicals should be avoided after flushing. A follow-up ophthalmic exam should be scheduled as soon as possible.

Non-Drug Methods. Other methods used to block or eliminate toxins from the system include peritoneal dialysis, hemodialysis, hemoperfusion, and exchange transfusions. These methods are not universally effective and are used much less commonly, but they can be life-saving in certain circumstances. These non–drug methods are most effective when the binding of poisons to plasma proteins is low and serum levels of the poison are high.

Peritoneal dialysis is reasonably simple and takes little staff time. Hemodialysis, on the other hand, is more difficult and time-consuming for staff, but about 20 times more effective than peritoneal dialysis. Dialysis is often effective when the usual supportive or corrective measures do not suffice in preventing further organ damage, and when biotransformation or elimination routes are damaged, blocked, or otherwise dysfunctional. The usefulness of dialysis depends on the pharmacokinetics of the substance. Drugs not amenable to removal by dialysis are diazepam, digoxin, doxycycline, phenothiazines, propoxyphene, and zidovudine.

Hemoperfusion strips a poison from binding sites on plasma proteins. It is accomplished by passing blood over a column of charcoal or absorbent resin. If the affinity of the resin for a particular poison is high, this procedure is very effective. The primary disadvantage to hemoperfusion is loss of platelets. When the poison is strongly bound to plasma proteins, exchange transfusions may be an effective method of removal.

Specific Antidotes

Antidotes or antagonists may be used in selected cases for management or diagnosis of the toxin (Table 13-1). An antidote may produce significant improvement initially, but the half-life of the toxic substance may be longer than that of the antidote. For example, naloxone is a potent antagonist used in opiate overdose. Initially, the patient may respond rather quickly but, as the naloxone wears off, the patient may become obtunded.

Treatment of Complications

CNS Stimulation. CNS stimulation may require sedation. In patients who have pure amphetamine poisoning, chlorpromazine or a benzodiazepine may be used. To terminate seizures and prevent their reoccurrence, a benzodiazepine (e.g., diazepam) is given slowly by intravenous (IV) route, or IV or intramuscular (IM) phenobarbital is given. Ideally, phenytoin is avoided. Oxygen saturation should be closely monitored. Refractory seizures, although rare, necessitate general anesthesia.

Severe CNS Depression. Severe CNS depression necessitates circulatory and ventilatory support. Endotracheal intubation and, rarely, a tracheostomy may be necessary. In suspected or known cases of opioid poisoning, naloxone should be used in repeated dosages. Stimulant drugs are ineffective, and their use is generally contraindicated.

Cerebral Edema. Cerebral edema in poisoning is common as a result of sedatives, carbon monoxide, lead, and other CNS depressants. A 20% mannitol solution is given

TABLE 13-1 Specific Antidotes

Poison and/or Overdosed Substance	Antidote(s)	Other Chapters
acetaminophen	acetylcysteine (Mucomyst)	17
Anticholinergics and antimuscarinics (atropine, scopolamine), tricyclic antidepressants	physostigmine (Antilirium)	15, 20
Benzodiazepines	flumazenil (Romazicon)	19
Beta blockers	isoproterenol (Isuprel), glucagon	36, 37
Calcium channel blockers	calcium chloride	36, 37
Carbon monoxide	Oxygen	—
Cholinergics and acetylcholinesterase inhibitors (e.g., organic phosphates, insecticides, nerve gases, carbamates)	atropine, pralidoxime (2-PAM)	15
cyanide, nitroprusside sodium	amyl nitrate, then sodium nitrite, then sodium thiosulfate	35
digoxin, digitoxin, oleander, foxglove	digoxin immune Fab (Digibind, Digidote)	34
ethylene glycol	fomepizole	—
heparin	protamine sulfate	39
ferric iron	deferoxamine (Desferal)	10
Insulin-induced hypoglycemia	Glucagon, 50% dextrose	53
Mercury, arsenic, lead, other heavy metals*	dimercaprol (BAL in oil), edetate calcium disodium (calcium ethylenediaminetetraacetic acid [EDTA]), penicillamine, succimer (Chemet)	—
Methanol, ethylene glycol	ethanol	—
methotrexate and other folate antagonists	leucovorin (Wellcovorin)	33
Opioids and opioid derivatives	naloxone (Narcan)	16
warfarin, salicylates	vitamin K (phytonadione)	39

*Characteristics of a desirable heavy metal antagonist include (1) high affinity for a toxic metal; (2) low affinity for essential endogenous metals such as magnesium and zinc; (3) the ability to reach storage sites for heavy metals; (4) high activity at physiologic pH; (5) formation of chelates that are less toxic than the metal; and (6) formation of chelates that are readily eliminated.

slowly by IV over 30 to 60 minutes. Corticosteroids such as dexamethasone may be given by IV drip. Intracranial monitoring with hyperventilation to alter the degree of cerebral edema is used less frequently. Induction of a barbiturate coma with cerebral edema because of hypoxic events is no longer recommended.

RENAL AND HEPATIC FAILURE. Renal failure, if present, may require a form of dialysis. Hepatic failure may warrant transplantation in some patients.

Patient Education

Educating the general population about poison prevention is vital. Ideally, primary prevention activities occur before poison exposure; however, in many cases, the awareness of poisoning potential comes after an exposure. Patient readiness to learn often peaks immediately after a poisoning has taken place. The combined efforts of poison control centers and health care providers have had a significant impact on the frequency of certain categories of drug poisonings, most notably aspirin poisoning.

Prevention of accidental drug ingestion involves teaching about the appropriate storage of drugs so that children do not gain access to them. Parents or guardians of small children must survey their homes for hazardous substances stored in unsafe locations. Even alcoholic beverages must be safely stored, because fatal poisonings have occurred in young children who ingested relatively small amounts of alcohol.

Keeping all drugs in their original containers prevents confusion as to the contents. Furthermore, families should be cautioned that toxic substances must not be stored in food containers. Household cleaners and other toxic substances should be kept in original, well-marked containers and stored in a location inaccessible to children. The telephone numbers of the poison control center and the health care provider should be readily available.

Childproof caps delay, even if they don't totally prevent, children's indiscriminate drug ingestion. Graphic symbols such as "Mr. Yuk," an ugly, green-faced, scowling image, were placed on labels of poisoning substances in years past to alert adults and children to the potential hazards. However, research has shown that such symbols did more to attract children to the poison than to keep them away. Poisonous plants should not be kept in homes where there are small children.

Evaluation

Patient outcomes vary with the specific poison and the interventions instituted. In addition, health care providers can evaluate the effectiveness of a plan of care by implementing epidemiologic methods that help identify drug-related problems. For example, poison prevention programs can be implemented at the primary prevention level, early diagnosis and screening for drug abuse at the secondary prevention level, and rehabilitation and restoration efforts at the tertiary prevention level.

KEY POINTS

- The local poison control center should be contacted when an overdose of a drug or an accidental ingestion of poisons is suspected.
- Children younger than 6 years of age are at highest risk for accidental drug poisonings.
- Adolescent and adult poisonings often result in serious morbidity and mortality.
- Distinguishing between a suicidal drug overdose and recreational drug use may be difficult.
- A complete accounting of the suspected poison is needed, including the name of the substance (if known), the quantity consumed, and the time of ingestion.
- Toxidromes—the clinical manifestations of ingestion—and toxicology testing are helpful in determining the exposure.

- The key principle in the treatment of poisonings is to "treat the patient, not the poison." Treatment for most poisonings is symptomatic and supportive.
- Treatment focuses on supporting vital functions, identifying the poison, administering specific antidotes, preventing further absorption of and eliminating the poison, and managing complications.
- Basic and advanced life support protocols should be used as warranted by the patient's condition.
- Drugs and procedures used to reduce further absorption of the poison include activated charcoal, ipecac syrup, lavage and aspiration, hyperosmolar laxatives, enhancing renal elimination, surface decontamination, and non–drug methods.
- Patient education emphasizes primary prevention; however, patient readiness to learn often peaks immediately after a poisoning has taken place.

Bibliography

American Academy of Clinical Toxicology. Available online: www.clintox.org/. Accessed February 10, 2007.

American Association of Poison Control Centers. Available online: www.aapcc.org/. Accessed February 10, 2007.

The American Heritage Dictionary of the English Language. (4ᵗʰ ed.) (2000). Boston: Houghton Mifflin. Available online: www.bartleby.com/61/. Accessed 21 March 2007.

Centers for Disease Control and Prevention. National Center for Environmental Health Fact Sheet. Available online: www.cdc.gov/nceh/. Accessed February 10, 2007.

Flomenbaum, N., Goldfrank, L., Hoffman, R., et al. (2006). *Toxicologic emergencies.* (8ᵗʰ ed.). New York: McGraw Hill.

Litovitz, T., Klein-Schwartz, W., White, S., et al. (2001). 2000 annual report of the American Association of Poison Control Centers Toxic Exposures Surveillance System. *American Journal of Emergency Medicine, 19*(5), 337–396.

Manoguerra, A., Cobaug, D., and Members of the Guidelines for the Management of Poisonings Consensus Panel. (2005). Guidelines on the use of ipecac syrup in the out-of-hospital management of ingested poisons. *Clinical Toxicology, 43*(1), 1–10.

Picket, J. (Ed.) (2000). American Heritage Dictionary. Boston: Houghton Mifflin.

Sympathetic Nervous System Drugs

Virtually all bodily functions are influenced by drugs altering neuronal regulation. Drugs influencing the sympathetic and parasympathetic nervous systems have important roles in the treatment and management of many disorders. Some drugs are purposely designed to alter nervous system functioning, and others alter the nervous system as an adverse effect. For this reason a basic understanding of nervous system physiology is key to understanding how and why these drugs produce the effects they do. Thus, the beginning section of this chapter provides a review of the anatomy and physiology of the autonomic nervous system, and is followed by how pharmacotherapeutics is applied to them. Because our purpose here concerns drug therapy, and not physiology, not every aspect of peripheral nervous system physiology will be addressed. Instead, the discussion is limited to those aspects of peripheral nervous system physiology that have a direct bearing on the ability to understand these drugs.

FUNCTIONAL ORGANIZATION OF THE NERVOUS SYSTEM

The nervous system has two primary divisions, the central nervous system (CNS) and the peripheral nervous system (PNS) (Fig. 14-1). The CNS is divided into the brain and the spinal cord. The PNS is divided into the somatic nervous (motor) system and the autonomic nervous system (ANS).

AUTONOMIC NERVOUS SYSTEM

The ANS has two divisions: the parasympathetic nervous system (PSNS) and the sympathetic nervous system (SNS) (Fig. 14-2). These divisions act primarily below the level of consciousness to regulate internal body functions necessary for life, particularly the involuntary actions of smooth muscles, the myocardium, and glands. The parasympathetic and sympathetic nerve fibers have both "preganglionic" and "postganglionic" nerve cells. The fibers converge at the ganglion, where acetylcholine (ACh) transfers the nerve impulse across the synapse to a second neuron. In turn, a second neurotransmitter is released that continues the transfer of impulses. Thus the actions of ANS drugs can be understood and classified in terms of their ability to mimic or modify the actions of the neurotransmitters.

Parasympathetic Nervous System

The PSNS counterbalances activity of the SNS through seven regulatory functions that bear particular significance to drug therapy. Specifically, stimulation of the appropriate PSNS nerves causes (1) slowing of the heart rate; (2) increased gastric secretion; (3) bladder emptying; (4) emptying of the bowel; (5) focusing of the eye for near vision; (6) constriction of the pupil; and (7) contraction of bronchial smooth muscle. How the PSNS accomplishes these activities is based on the functions of PSNS receptors. The PSNS drugs are further discussed in Chapter 15.

Structural Arrangement

As is seen in Figure 14-3, in the ANS there are two neurons leading from the spinal cord to effector cells. The synapse between neurons occurs within the ganglion, a cluster of nerve cell bodies. The neurons leading from the spinal cord to parasympathetic ganglia are predictably referred to as preganglionic neurons. Neurons leading from the parasympathetic ganglia to effector cells are known as postganglionic neurons. This structural arrangement offers two general sites at which drugs can act: (1) the synapses between preganglionic and postganglionic neurons, and (2) the junctions between postganglionic neurons and effector cells (Table 14-1).

PSNS Receptors

ACh activates two different receptor types, muscarinic (M) and nicotinic (N). Muscarinic receptors are primarily found on all organs regulated by the PSNS (i.e., organs innervated by postganglionic parasympathetic neurons). Muscarinic receptors are also found on sweat glands. There are three types of muscarinic receptors: M_1, M_2, and M_3. M_1 receptors are typically found in CNS neurons, sympathetic postganglionic neurons, and some presynaptic sites. M_2 receptors are found in the myocardium, smooth muscle, and some presynaptic sites. M_3 receptors are found in exocrine glands and vessels of the smooth muscle and the endothelium.

The nicotinic N (N_N) receptors are found on the cell bodies of all postganglionic neurons of the PSNS and SNS systems. N_N receptors are also located on cells of the adrenal medulla. N_M receptors are found in the neuromuscular end plates of skeletal muscles. Activation of ACh receptors causes the movement of sodium (Na^+) into the cell and the movement of potassium (K^+) out of the cell. This reciprocal movement results in depolarization of postsynaptic neurons and the creation of a new action potential.

Were it not for receptor subtypes, a drug acting on *cholinergic receptors* (i.e., neurons that synthesize and release ACh) at one site would alter activity of cholinergic receptors at all other sites. The existence of receptor subtypes for a particular neurotransmitter makes possible a selectivity in drug actions that could not otherwise be achieved if all of the receptors for the transmitter were the same.

Life Cycle of PSNS Neurotransmitters

All preganglionic neurons of the PSNS (and the SNS) release ACh as their neurotransmitter. The synthesis of ACh begins with the interaction of two precursors: acetylcoenzyme A (CoA) and choline. ACh is stored in neuronal vesicles to be released later

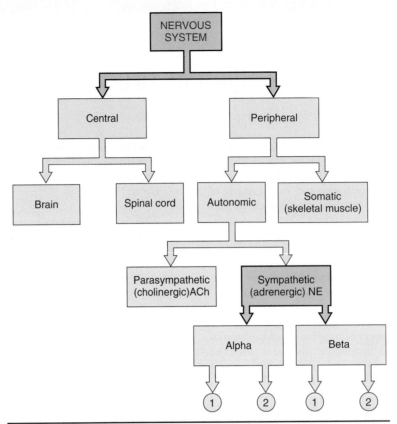

FIGURE 14-1 The Sympathetic Nervous System in Relation to the Entire Nervous System. (Redrawn from Lilley L., Harrington S., and Snyder J. (2005). *Pharmacology and the Nursing Process.* (4th ed.). St. Louis: Mosby.)

in response to an action potential. The ganglionic neurons of the PSNS also release ACh as their neurotransmitter.

Following release, ACh binds to N_N, N_M, or M receptors located on the postjunctional cell. This binding to receptors increases the permeability of the membrane to sodium and potassium ions, resulting in depolarization of nerve fibers and excitation or inhibition of neural, muscular, or glandular activity. However, the opposing membrane across the synapse contains the enzyme acetylcholinesterase (AChE), an enzyme that breaks down ACh in a few milliseconds to acetate and choline. Any remaining ACh diffusing across the synapse is almost immediately degraded by nonspecific enzymes in the blood or tissues. Uptake of choline into cholinergic nerve terminals completes the life cycle of ACh. Note than choline (an inactive substance), and not the active neurotransmitter (ACh), is taken back up for reuse.

PSNS drugs and toxic agents can interfere with the ACh life cycle at several points. Several of the drugs act by inhibiting AChE, leading to the accumulation of ACh in the synapse.

Sympathetic Nervous System

The SNS is responsible for the body's "fight or flight" response that is needed to cope with life's stressors (e.g., fear,

extremes of physical activity). In addition, the SNS has two other primary functions: management of the cardiovascular system and regulation of body temperature. Stimulation of the SNS causes blood pressure and the heart rate to rise and thereby causes blood to be shunted to skeletal muscles rather than the gastrointestinal (GI) tract, the kidneys, and the skin; there is dilation of the pupils and bronchioles, with glycogenolysis in the liver and lipolysis in adipose tissue. A sensation of cold is brought on by the shunting of blood away from the skin. By initiating these responses, the SNS accomplishes three homeostatic objectives: (1) maintenance of blood flow to the brain; (2) redistribution of blood flow during exercise; and (3) vasoconstriction, primarily to compensate for blood loss.

The SNS helps to control body temperature by regulating blood flow to the skin; sympathetic nerves increase or decrease heat loss by dilating or constricting cutaneous vessels. Sympathetic neurons of the sweat glands encourage diaphoresis, thereby helping the body to cool. Piloerection (i.e., erection of hair) promotes heat conservation.

SNS drugs produce their effects by altering body functions under SNS control. Such drugs are used primarily for their effects on the heart, blood vessels, and the lungs. Drugs that alter cardiovascular function are used to treat hypertension,

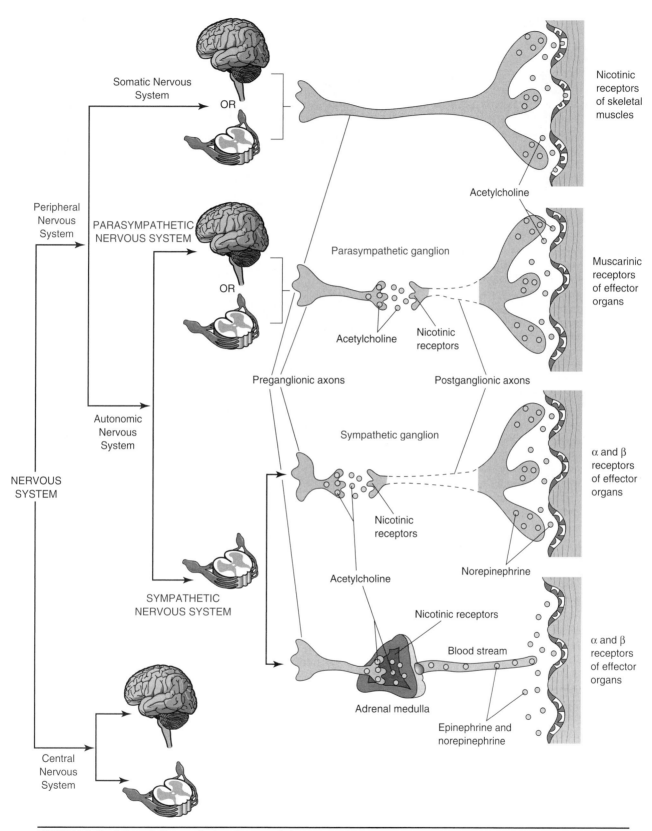

FIGURE 14-2 The Autonomic Nervous System. Parasympathetic neurons originate in the craniosacral regions of the spinal cord. Preganglionic fibers are long and travel to ganglia located close to or in the walls of effector organs. Postganglionic fibers are short. Sympathetic neurons originate in the thoracolumbar region of the central nervous system (CNS). Preganglionic fibers are short, terminating in ganglia adjacent to the spinal cord. Postganglionic fibers are long, traveling some distance through effector cells to reach effector organs.

SYMPATHETIC NERVOUS SYSTEM

PARASYMPATHETIC NERVOUS SYSTEM

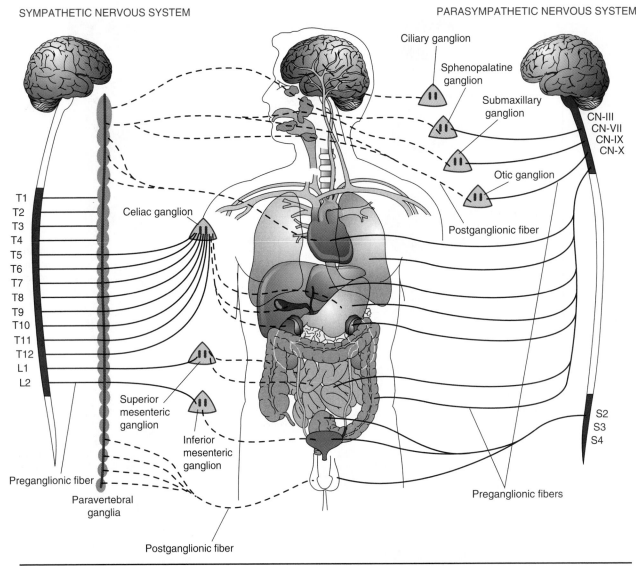

FIGURE 14-3 Components of the Autonomic and Somatic Nervous Systems. All preganglionic nerves release acetylcholine (ACh). The ACh interacts with nicotinic receptors of the postganglionic sympathetic and parasympathetic nerves, the adrenal medullae, or skeletal muscle within the somatic system. ACh is released by postganglionic parasympathetic nerves to act on muscarinic receptors. Norepinephrine (NEPI) is released from postganglionic sympathetic nerves to act on α or β receptors of effector organs (smooth muscle, cardiac muscle, glands). The preganglionic fiber that innervates adrenal medullae without synapsing at a ganglion releases NEPI and epinephrine (EPI) directly into the circulation to the effector organs.

heart failure, angina, and other disorders. Drugs affecting the lungs are used primarily to treat asthma.

Structural Arrangement

The anatomic arrangement of the SNS is similar to that of the PSNS; and like the PSNS, the SNS employs two neurons leading from the spinal cord to organs under its control. The junction of these neurons is in the ganglion. Neurons leading from the spinal cord to the sympathetic ganglia are known as preganglionic neurons. Neurons leading from the ganglion to effector cells (or organs) are known as postganglionic neurons.

The cells of the adrenal medulla are similar to other sympathetic ganglion neurons in that they are innervated by a preganglionic fiber and upon stimulation release epinephrine

(EPI). However, they differ from other postganglionic neurons in two important ways: (1) postganglionic neurons of the adrenal medulla do not send projections to a specific target tissue where the neurotransmitter is released. Instead, these specialized quasi-neurons (i.e., adrenal chromaffin cells) release EPI into the circulation, where it acts on a variety of tissues; (2) the chromaffin cells synthesize norepinephrine (NEPI) like other sympathetic ganglia, but most of the NEPI (80% to 85%) is biotransformed to EPI. Thus the transmitter released by the adrenal medulla when a patient is under stress is primarily EPI.

SNS Receptors

There are five major adrenergic receptors: *alpha-1* (α_1) and *alpha-2* (α_2) receptors; *beta-1* (β_1) and *beta-2* (β_2) receptors;

TABLE 14-1 Effector Responses to ANS Impulses

Effector Cells	SNS Receptor	SNS Response to Receptor Stimulation	PSNS Receptor	PSNS Response to Receptor Stimulation
CARDIOVASCULAR				
SA node	β_1	Increased rate	M	Decreased rate; vagal arrest possible
Atria	β_1	Increased strength of contraction; increased conduction velocity	M	Decreased contractility and shortened AP duration
AV node	β_1	Increased automaticity and conduction velocity	M	Decreased conduction velocity, AV block possible
His-Purkinje system	β_1	Increased automaticity and conduction velocity	M	Little effect
Ventricles	β_1	Increased contractility, conduction velocity, automaticity, and rate of idioventricular pacemakers	M	Slightly decreased contractility
VASCULATURE				
Coronary arterioles	α_1, α_2, β_2	Constrict, dilate*	—	Usually dilate but with endothelial damage constrict
Cerebral arterioles	α_1	Slightly constrict	—	Dilate
Pulmonary arterioles	α_1, β_2	Constrict, dilate*	—	Dilate†
Abdominal viscera arterioles	α_1, β_2, D	Constrict, dilate§	—	—
Renal arterioles	α_1, α_2, β_1, β_2	Constrict, dilate‡	—	—
Systemic arterioles	α_1, α_2, β_2	Constrict, dilate	—	—
Systemic veins	α_1, β_2	Constrict, dilate	—	—
LUNGS				
Trachea, bronchi	β_2	Relax	M	Constrict
GI TRACT				
GI motility, tone	α_1, α_2, β_2	Decreased	M	Usually increased
GI sphincters	α_1	Relax	M	Usually relax
Gallbladder and ducts	β_2	Relax	M	Contract
Liver	α_1, β_2	Glycogenolysis, gluconeogenesis	M	Glycogen synthesis
Islets of Langerhans	α_2	Decreased secretion	M	—
	β_2	Increased secretion	M	—
Fat cells	β_3	Lipolysis	—	—
GENITOURINARY TRACT				
Renin secretion	α_1	Decreased	—	—
	β_2	Increased	—	—
Detrusor muscle	β_2	Usually relaxes	M	Usually contracts
Trigone and sphincter	α_1	Contract	M	Relax
Ureter motility and tone	α_1	Increased	—	—
Pregnant uterus	α_1	Contracts	—	Variable
	β_2	Relaxes	—	Variable
Nonpregnant uterus	β_2	Relaxes	—	Variable
Male sex glands	α_1	Ejaculation	M	Erection
EYES				
Radial muscle of iris	α_1	Mydriasis	—	—
Iritic sphincter	β_2	—	M	Miosis
Ciliary muscles	β_2	Accommodation (relaxation)	M	Miosis for near vision
GLANDS				
Posterior pituitary	β_1	Antidiuretic hormone secretion	—	—
Pineal gland	β	Melatonin synthesis	—	—
Salivary gland secretion	α_1, β	Potassium and water	M	Increased
	β	Amylase	M	Potassium and water
Lacrimal gland secretions	α	Slight	M	Increased
Airway and GI tract secretions	α_1, β_2	Decreased	M	Increased
Sweating	—	—	M	Increased*

M = Not a direct innervation; however, vasodilation may occur in response to muscarinic agonists.
*Dilation predominates in situ because of metabolic autoregulatory phenomena.
†This is an exception to the rule that norepinephrine is the postganglionic neurotransmitter at all sympathetic postganglionic nerve endings.
‡Cholinergic vasodilation at these sites is of questionable physiologic significance.
§Above the usual concentration of physiologically released, circulating epinephrine, beta-response (vasodilation) predominates in vessels of skeletal muscle and the liver, alpha responses (vasoconstriction) in vessels of other abdominal viscera. Mesenteric and renal vessels also contain specific D receptors, activation of which causes dilation.
The α_1 receptor has been further subdivided into (α_{1A}, (α_{1B}, and α_{1D} subtypes. There are claims that the α_{1A} receptor would be specific for smooth muscle of the prostate. Its blockade with an antagonist causes relaxation, thus facilitating urinary flow in patients with benign prostatic hyperplasia (BPH).
ANS, Autonomic nervous system; AP, action potential; AV, atrioventricular; D, dopamine (receptor); GI, gastrointestinal; M, muscarinic; PSNS, parasympathetic nervous system; SA, sinoatrial; SNS, sympathetic nervous system;
Adapted from Hardman, J., and Limbird, L. (2005). *Goodman & Gilman's the pharmacologic basis of therapeutics.* (10th ed.) New York: McGraw-Hill; and Gutierrez, K. (1999). *Pharmacotherapeutics: Clinical decision making in nursing.* Philadelphia: WB Saunders.

and dopamine (D) receptors. α_1 Receptors are found on postsynaptic cells (particularly smooth muscle), whereas α_2 receptors are found on presynaptic nerve terminals, platelets, lipocytes, and smooth muscle. β_1 Receptors are found in postsynaptic cells, especially of the heart, lipocytes, the brain, and the presynaptic sympathetic and parasympathetic nerve terminals. β_2 Receptors appear in the postsynaptic cells of the smooth muscle of the bronchioles, the arterioles, the myocardium, and various other visceral organs.

Dopamine (NOTE: abbreviation *D* is used in text for dopamine receptors, and the word *dopamine* is used when the substance is meant) is generally thought of as an excitatory transmitter produced by the decarboxylation of DOPA. Dopamine is the direct precursor in the synthesis of NEPI and is also a neurotransmitter in the CNS. In the periphery, the D_1 and D_5 receptors are located in the vasculature of the kidneys and are of clinical significance. Stimulation of these two receptors produces adenylcyclase and increased cyclic adenosine monophosphate (cAMP), resulting in dilation of renal blood vessels and enhanced renal perfusion.

Other D receptors found in the CNS are also of great therapeutic significance. The functions of these receptors are discussed in Chapters 21 and 26.

▥ Life Cycle of SNS Neurotransmitters

The principal neurotransmitters of the SNS are NEPI, EPI, and dopamine. NEPI is released by almost all postganglionic neurons of the SNS. The only exception is the postganglionic sympathetic neurons that innervate sweat glands, which use ACh as their neurotransmitter. EPI is released by the adrenal medulla.

EPI and NEPI are formed from phenylalanine and tyrosine (Fig. 14-4). The liver produces tyrosine from phenylalanine by the action of the enzyme phenylalanine hydroxylase. A series of actions at catecholamine-secretion neurons convert tyrosine to dopamine, then to NEPI and, finally, to EPI. The final step in synthesis takes place within vesicles, where NEPI is then stored before release. Following release, NEPI binds to adrenergic receptors on effector cells or organs. NEPI interacts with postsynaptic α_1 and β receptors, and with presynaptic α_2 receptors. Transmission is halted by the reuptake of NEPI back into nerve terminals.

NEPI removal is distinctive in two respects from that of ACh, whose effects are terminated by enzymatic degradation rather than reuptake. Reuptake of NEPI into vesicles accounts for the recovery of 50% to 80% of the secreted neurotransmitter. Any remaining neurotransmitter is degraded by monoamine oxidase (MAO), an enzyme found in mitochondria of most cells, or catechol-*O*-methyltransferase (COMT). COMT is found in the cytoplasm of most cells and in large concentrations in the kidneys and the liver.

More or less every step in the life cycle of NEPI can be changed by SNS drugs. There are drugs that alter synthesis, storage, and release of NEPI. There are also drugs that act at adrenergic receptors to mimic or block the effects of NEPI. In addition, there are drugs that inhibit the reuptake of NEPI and the intensity of neurotransmission (e.g., tricyclic antidepressants and cocaine); and drugs that inhibit MAO with the subsequent breakdown of NEPI (e.g., transdermal selegiline [Emsam]), thereby causing an increase in the amount of transmitter available for release.

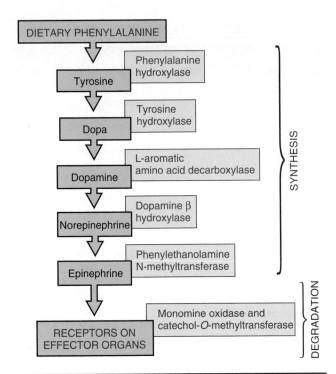

FIGURE 14-4 Life Cycle of Sympathetic Nervous System Neurotransmitters. Dietary phenylalanine is converted to tyrosine with the aid of the enzyme phenylalanine hydroxylase, which in turn is converted to DOPA with the aid of tyrosine hydroxylase. Additional enzymes continue the conversion to dopamine, norepinephrine, and finally, epinephrine. Monoamine oxidase (MAO) and catechol-*O*-methyltransferase (COMT) enzymes act to degrade catecholamines in the synapse, and a portion of the catecholamines go on to interact with receptors on effector organs.

PHARMACOTHERAPEUTIC OPTIONS

Adrenergic Agonists

Alpha and Beta Agonists
- dopamine (Intropin, ◆ Revimine)
- epinephrine (Asrelin)
- norepinephrine (Levophed)

Beta Agonists
- dobutamine (Dobutrex)
- isoproterenol (Isuprel)

▥ Indications

Adrenergic agonists are used in the treatment of a wide variety of illness and conditions. Their selectivity for either α or β receptors and their affinity for certain tissues or organs determine how they are most commonly used.

Vasoactive Indications. In general, adrenergic agonists are used to increase blood pressure in patients with severe hypotension, to reverse anaphylactic shock, and to minimize bleeding at a superficial operative site (in conjunction with local anesthetics). Note, however, that drugs other than catecholamines have also been used for these purposes including phosphodiesterase III inhibitors (e.g., amrinone, milrinone), naloxone, nitric oxide synthase inhibitors, calcium sensitizers, and vasopressin. Common vasoactive adrenergics include dopamine, EPI, NEPI, and isoproterenol.

Isoproterenol, used cautiously, can be a temporary treatment measure for patients with symptomatic bradycardia or heart block for whom an external pacemaker is not readily available. It can also be used in patients with refractory torsades de pointes unresponsive to magnesium sulfate, and for patients with overdose from beta blockers (see Chapter 37).

NEPI is similar to EPI in many respects. Unlike EPI, NEPI does not activate β_2 receptors; nonetheless, NEPI can elicit all the responses EPI can (except those that are β_2-mediated). It is rapidly removed from the synapse by MAO or COMT. Despite its similarities to EPI, NEPI has limited clinical indications. The only recognized uses are for hypotensive states and cardiac arrest.

Currently, there is insufficient evidence to promote the use of dopamine as a first-line drug for the treatment of shock because regional hemodynamics, oxygen transport variables, and functional parameters of improved organ perfusion are not improved in a sustained manner and may be impaired. Dopamine is a second-line drug (after atropine) for symptomatic bradycardia.

Dobutamine, a nonselective beta agonist, may be used to improve cardiac output in patients with heart failure. The drug has also been shown to increase stroke volume and left ventricular stroke work index, and thus cardiac index and dissolved oxygen without increases in pulmonary arterial occlusion pressure (PAOP). It is also used in the treatment of heart failure after cardiac surgery and in patients awaiting transplantation.

RESPIRATORY INDICATIONS. Selected adrenergic agonists have an affinity for receptors located in the respiratory tract and are classified as bronchodilators. They tend to preferentially stimulate β_2 receptors rather than α receptors and cause bronchodilation. Of the two subtypes of beta agonists, these drugs are predominantly more attracted to receptors on the bronchial tree and in uterine and vascular smooth muscles, rather than β_1 receptors on the heart. Thus, common bronchodilators used in the treatment of asthma and bronchitis include albuterol, bitolterol, epinephrine, formoterol, isoetharine, levalbuterol, metaproterenol, pirbuterol, salmeterol, and terbutaline. See Chapter 50 for further discussion of beta agonists.

Some adrenergic agonists are used to constrict dilated arterioles and bring about a reduction in nasal blood flow, thus reducing congestion. These drugs include EPI, ephedrine, naphazoline, oxymetazoline, phenylephrine, and tetrahydrozoline. Chapters 51 and 52 discuss alpha-1 agonists in relation to topical nasal decongestants.

OPHTHALMIC INDICATIONS. Some of the adrenergics are used to treat eye disorders and act much the same way as nasal decongestants, except that they act on the vasculature of the eye, stimulating α receptors located on arterioles in the eye to temporarily relieve conjunctival congestion. The ophthalmic adrenergic drugs include EPI, naphazoline, phenylephrine, and tetrahydrozoline.

Adrenergics can also be used to reduce intraocular pressure and to cause mydriasis (pupillary dilation), characteristics that make them helpful in the treatment of open-angle glaucoma. They stimulate α and β_2 receptors, or both. Examples of two adrenergics used for this purpose are EPI and dipivefrin. Chapter 61 discusses ophthalmic drugs and their uses in more detail.

Pharmacodynamics

Because most body tissues possess both α and β receptors, drug effects depend largely on the drug's ability to activate specific receptors (Fig. 14-5), the number of receptors available, and the patient's physiologic state. Some drugs act on both α and β receptors (nonselective), whereas others are more discriminating, acting only on specific receptor subtypes (selective). Table 14-2 identifies the receptor selectivity of the adrenergic drugs.

EPI, a potent stimulant of both α and β receptors, is nonselective. It is one of the most potent vasopressor drugs known. EPI exerts a direct stimulation on myocardial tissues, increasing the strength of ventricular contraction (positive inotropic action), increasing heart rate (positive chronotropic action), and causing vasoconstriction in many vascular beds (particularly in the precapillary resistance vessels of skin, mucosa, and kidneys), along with marked constriction of veins.

Keep in mind that various vascular beds respond differently, resulting in significant redistribution of blood flow. The primary vascular action of EPI is exerted on smaller arterioles and precapillary sphincters, although veins and large arteries also respond. There is a markedly decreased cutaneous blood flow with injected epinephrine, constricting precapillary vessels and small venules. Cutaneous vasoconstriction accounts for the marked decrease in blood flow to the hands and feet. Blood flow to skeletal muscles is increased in part as a result of the powerful β_2 vasodilator action that is only partially counterbalanced by a vasoconstrictive action on α receptors also present in the vascular bed.

EPI has a number of influences on metabolic processes. It elevates glucose and lactate concentration in blood. Insulin secretion is inhibited through an interaction with α_2 receptors and is enhanced by activation of β_2 receptors. Glucagon secretion in the pancreas is enhanced by action on the alpha cells of the pancreatic islets (see Chapter 53). EPI also decreases the uptake of glucose by peripheral tissues, in part as a result of its effects in insulin secretion, but also perhaps owing to direct effects on skeletal muscle. The ability of EPI to stimulate glycogenolysis in most tissues involves β receptors. In addition, EPI raises the concentration of free fatty acids by stimulating β receptors in fat cells. The result is activation of triglyceride lipase, which accelerates the breakdown of triglycerides to form free fatty acids and glycerol.

NEPI is a combined alpha and beta agonist, differing from EPI only in its lack of a methyl substitution in the amino group; however, it primarily produces vasoconstriction via its more prominent alpha effects on all vascular beds, thus increasing systemic vascular resistance. NEPI generally produces either no change or mild increase in cardiac output. Both EPI and NEPI are direct agonists on effector cells and are equipotent in stimulating β_1 receptors. Their actions differ primarily in the ratio of their effectiveness in stimulating α_1 and β_1 receptors. At low doses, NEPI primarily stimulates β receptors, to cause peripheral vasodilation with an increase in heart rate and myocardial contractility. As the infusion rate is increased, alpha-vasoconstrictive effects become more prominent. For example, at the high infusion rates used in septic shock, EPI predominantly produces alpha effects with increases in systemic vascular resistance and mean arterial pressure; thus its clinical utility is limited.

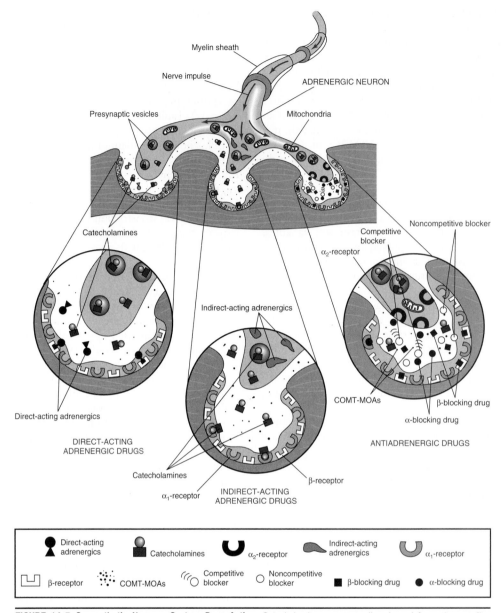

FIGURE 14-5 Sympathetic Nervous System Drug Action. Catecholamines are normally released from storage sites within adrenergic neurons upon arrival of a nerve impulse. Most adrenergics directly mimic the activity of these neurotransmitters on α or β receptors. Indirect-acting adrenergics act by first triggering the release of the neurotransmitter from presynaptic vesicles. The neurotransmitters, in turn, activate α and β receptors. Antiadrenergic drugs (i.e., alpha and beta blockers) are receptor-specific or nonspecific and act through noncompetitive or competitive blockade of the neurotransmitter at receptor sites. The neurotransmitters are degraded by monoamine oxidase (MAO) or catechol-*O*-methyltransferase (COMT) in the synapse.

TABLE **14-2 Receptor Selectivity**	
Drug	**Receptors Activated**
epinephrine	α_1, α_2, β_1, β_2
norepinephrine	α_1, α_2, β_1
isoproterenol	β_1, β_2
dobutamine	β_1
dopamine	α_1, β_1, D

The primary pharmacologic action of dobutamine is as a beta agonist at both β_1 and β_2 receptors. Dobutamine's actions do not appear to be the result of NEPI release from sympathetic nerve endings, nor are they exerted through dopaminergic receptors.

Dopamine has dose-related activities at renal D receptors and at α_1 and β_1 receptors. Unfortunately, the dose-response relationship has not been confirmed in critically ill patients.

In patients with septic shock, there is a great overlap of hemodynamic effects even at low doses.

Isoproterenol is a potent but nonselective beta agonist. It has powerful effects on both β receptors and almost no action at α receptors. An intravenous (IV) infusion of isoproterenol lowers peripheral vascular resistance, primarily in skeletal muscle, but also in renal and mesenteric vascular beds, bringing about a fall in diastolic pressure. Systolic pressure may remain unchanged or may rise, although mean arterial pressure typically falls. Positive inotropic and chronotropic action increases cardiac output in the face of diminished peripheral resistance. Isoproterenol relaxes almost all smooth muscle when the tone is high; this action is most pronounced in bronchial and GI smooth muscle.

Pharmacokinetics

The pharmacokinetics of adrenergic agonists varies with the specific drug; however, because most are given parenterally, onset of drug action ranges from immediately to 30 minutes later, with peak effects seen in minutes (Table 14-3). The duration of action for adrenergic agonists is short, often averaging minutes rather than hours. Many adrenergic agonists are partially biotransformed by MAO. The remaining drug is biotransformed in the liver and eliminated through the kidneys.

Adverse Effects and Contraindications

The most common unwanted adverse effects of alpha agonists are headache, restlessness, excitement, insomnia, and euphoria. Their adverse cardiovascular effects include vasoconstriction, hypertension, tachycardia, and palpitations or arrhythmias. Their effects on the GI tract include anorexia, dry mouth, nausea, vomiting, and changes in taste (rare).

The adverse effects of beta agonists include headache, mild tremors and nervousness, dizziness, and insomnia. Unwanted effects on the cardiovascular system include increased inotropic effects (increased heart rate), palpitations and arrhythmias, and fluctuations in blood pressure. Patients with underlying coronary artery disease may complain of angina. Sweating, nausea, vomiting, and muscle cramps are also possible. A paradoxical bronchospasm is sometimes noted with excessive use of adrenergic agonist inhalers.

General contraindications to the use of adrenergic agonists include arrhythmias, angina pectoris, hypertension, hyperthyroidism, cerebrovascular disease, narrow-angle glaucoma, and hypersensitivity to the drug or any component. Adrenergic agonists are also contraindicated in combination with local anesthesia of distal areas (i.e., fingers, toes, ears, nose, and penis) because of the potential for tissue damage and sloughing from vasoconstriction. Avoid adrenergic agonists during the second stage of labor, because they may delay progression. Use the drugs with caution in patients with anxiety, insomnia, and psychiatric disorders because of their stimulant effects on the CNS, and in older adults because of their cardiac- and CNS-stimulating effects.

Drug Interactions

There is an increased risk of cardiac arrhythmias and pressor responses when adrenergic agonists are used in the presence of general anesthetics, digoxin, antihistamines, cocaine, MAO inhibitors, thyroid hormones, and xanthines (Table 14-4). A number of other drugs cause increased bronchodilation, which can be helpful in patients with underlying respiratory disorders. Because of the variety of drugs that interact with adrenergic agonists, the health care provider is advised to check for interactions before administering the drug.

Dosage Regimen

The dosage of adrenergic agonists depends on the specific drug and its use. For example, IV dopamine is used to maintain renal perfusion at a dosage range different from that used to increase peripheral vascular resistance (Table 14-5). EPI, on the other hand, can be given by subcutaneous (subQ), intramuscular (IM) or IV route, with each route requiring different dosages. The dosage of many of these drugs is titrated based on the patient's response.

Lab Considerations

Adrenergic agonists can cause a transient decrease in serum potassium concentrations when administered via nebulizer or in higher than recommended concentrations. Beta agonists can decrease serum potassium levels; however, hypokalemia is rare at recommended dosages. EPI may cause an increase in blood glucose and serum lactic acid concentrations.

For more information, see the Evolve Resources Bonus Content "Influence of Selected Drugs on Laboratory Values," found at http://evolve.elsevier.com/Gutierrez/pharmacotheraupeutics.

PHARMACOKINETICS
TABLE **14-3 Adrenergic Agonists**

Drug	Route	Onset	Peak	Duration	t1/2
ALPHA AND BETA AGONISTS					
dopamine	IV	1–2 min	10 min	Duration of infusion	2 min
epinephrine	IV	Immed	20 min	20–30 min	UA
	SubQ	6–12 min	20 min	<1–4 hr	
	IM	6–12 min	20 min	<1–4 hr	
	IT	3–5 min	UA	1–3 hr	
norepinephrine	IV	Rapid	Immed	1–2 min	UA
BETA AGONISTS					
dobutamine	IV	1–2 min	10 min	Duration of infusion	2 min
isoproterenol	IV	Immed	UA	Duration of infusion	1–2 min

IM, Intramuscular; *Immed*, immediate; *IT*, intratracheal; *IV*, intravenous; *t₁/₂*, elimination half-life; *subQ*, subcutaneous; *UA*, unavailable.

DRUG INTERACTIONS

TABLE **14-4** Drug Interactions of Adrenergic Agonists

Interactive Drugs	Interaction
General anesthetics, digoxin	Increases risk of arrhythmias
Anticholinergics	Increases bronchial relaxation and mydriasis
Tricyclic antidepressants	Increases pressor response with IV epinephrine
Antihistamines, doxapram, methylphenidate, cocaine	May increase pressor and mydriatic effects; risk for arrhythmias, seizures, acute glaucoma
Ergot alkaloids	Increases vasoconstriction and extremely high blood pressure
MAO inhibitors	Increases risk of arrhythmias, respiratory depression, acute hypertensive crisis, seizures, coma, and death
Thyroid hormones	Increases adrenergic effects and possible arrhythmias
Xanthines	Enhances bronchodilating effect, excessive CNS stimulation, arrhythmias, emotional disturbances, insomnia
Beta blockers	Decreases bronchodilating effect of adrenergic agonist
Antihypertensives, phentolamine	Decreases pressor effects of adrenergics
Antipsychotic drugs (those with alpha-blocking activity)	Blocks vasopressor effects of epinephrine

CNS, Central nervous system; *IV,* intravenous; *MAO,* monoamine oxidase.

DOSAGE

TABLE **14-5** Adrenergic Agonists

Drug	Use(s)	Dosage	Implications
ALPHA AND BETA AGONISTS			
dopamine	Maintain renal perfusion	*Adult:* 0.5–3 mcg/kg/min IV *Child:* 5–20 mcg/kg/min IV, based on desired response	Correct hypovolemia with volume expanders before initiating dopamine therapy. Increase infusion rate as needed. Extravasation may cause tissue necrosis and sloughing.
	Improve cardiac output	*Adult:* 2–10 mcg/kg/min IV *Child:* 5–20 mcg/kg/min IV, based on desired response	
	Increase peripheral vascular resistance	*Adult:* 10 mcg/kg/min IV *Child:* 5–20 mcg/kg/min IV, based on desired response	
epinephrine	Anaphylaxis	*Adult & Older Adult:* 0.3–0.5 mg IM or subQ every 15–20 min, based on response *Child:* 0.01 mg/kg every 15 min for 2 doses, then every 3 hr, based on desired response. Maximum single dose: 0.5 mg	Assess breath sounds, respiratory pattern, and BP before giving and during time of peak drug effects. Observe patient for tolerance and paradoxical or rebound bronchospasm.
	Severe or refractory hypotension	*Adult:* 0.01–1 mcg/kg/min IV *Child:* 0.1–4 mcg/kg/min IV	
	Cardiopulmonary resuscitation	*Adult:* 1 mg IV every 3–5 min up to 0.1 mg/kg every 3–5 min *Child:* 0.01 mg/kg of a 1:10,000 solution IV. Subsequent doses 0.1 mg/kg of a 1:1000 solution every 3 to 5 min	Monitor BP, pulse, ECG, respiratory rate, hemodynamic parameters, and urinary output frequently during use. Notify health care provider if chest pain, arrhythmias, heart rate over 100 beats/min or hypertension develops.
norepinephrine	Cardiogenic shock and ischemic heart disease	*Adult:* 0.5 to 1 mcg/min initially by IV infusion. Range: 2–12 mcg/min depending on BP *Child:* 0.1 mcg/kg/min up to 1 mcg/kg/min, depending on BP	Drug of last resort. Correct hypovolemia with volume expanders before starting therapy. Do not give in same IV line as alkaline solutions. Prevent extravasation.
ALPHA AGONISTS			
phenylephrine	Hypotension associated with shock	*Adult:* 100–180 mcg/min IV initially. Maintenance: 40–60 mcg/min or 2–5 mg subQ or IM every 10–15 min. Initial dose not to exceed 5 mg	Monitor BP every 2–3 min until stabilized and every 5 min thereafter during IV administration. Monitor ECG continuously. Prevent extravasation.
isoproterenol	Management of heart block and shock	*Adult:* 10 mg SL initially, with dose adjusted as needed. Range 5–50 mg or 0.5–5 mcg/min IV infusion. *Child:* 5–10 mg SL. Not to exceed 30 mg/day, more than 3 doses/day, or more often than every 3–4 hr, or 0.1 mcg/kg/min IV initially. Adjust dose based on response. Range: 0.1–1 mcg/kg/min	Monitor BP, pulse, ECG, respiratory rate, hemodynamic parameters, and urinary output during use. Notify health care provider if chest pain, arrhythmias, heart rate over 100 beats/min, or hypertension develops. Adjust dosage to keep heart rate under 110 beats/min.
	Cardiac standstill	Adult: 20–60 mcg IV initially, followed by 10–200 mcg as bolus or 5 mcg/min continuous infusion	Monitor BP, pulse, ECG, respiratory rate, hemodynamic parameters, and urinary output. Notify health care provider if chest pain, arrhythmias, heart rate over 100 beats/min, or hypertension develops.

BP, Blood pressure; *ECG,* electrocardiogram; *ET,* endotracheal(ly); *IM,* intramuscular(ly); *IV,* intravenous(ly); *SL,* sublingual(ly); *subQ,* subcutaneous(ly).

Adrenergic Blocking Drugs

Alpha Blockers

- phenoxybenzamine (Dibenzyline)
- phentolamine (Regitine); ◆ Rogitine
- tamsulosin (Flomax)
- tolazoline (Priscoline)

The nonselective alpha blockers have extremely limited clinical use. Tolazoline is occasionally used in the treatment of pulmonary hypertension in newborns. Phentolamine and phenoxybenzamine are sometimes used in the management of hypertension associated with pheochromocytoma, a tumor of the adrenal medulla. Pheochromocytoma tumors secrete large amounts of EPI or NEPI into circulation, placing the patient at risk for increases in blood pressure great enough to cause stroke. Phentolamine and phenoxybenzamine are effective in controlling blood pressure until the adrenal medulla tumor can be removed. Adverse reactions limit their usefulness for other purposes.

Selective alpha blockers are much more useful than non-selective drugs. The most useful responses to alpha blockers result from blockade of α_1 receptors on blood vessels; they are used in the treatment of hypertension (see Chapter 37), Raynaud's disease, and symptomatic benign prostatic hyperplasia (BPH), a condition whereby an enlarged prostate gland causes symptoms of urinary hesitancy and retention. Tamsulosin, a peripherally-acting selective drug, acts on the bladder more than it affects blood vessels and so is used only in the treatment of BPH. The alpha-blocking drugs such as doxazosin (Cardura), prazosin (Minipress), terazosin (Hytrin), and alfuzosin (Uroxatral) are discussed in Chapter 43.

The most serious adverse reaction to alpha blockers is orthostatic hypotension, caused by blockade of α_1 receptors in venous vasculature, which reduces muscle tone in the venous wall. α_1-Receptor blockade results in vasodilation and a reduction in blood pressure. The baroreceptors sense the blood pressure reduction and, in an attempt to restore normal blood pressure, initiate a reflex increase in heart rate. The tachycardia may be due in part to blockade of presynaptic α_2 receptors on sympathetic neurons.

Beta Blockers

Although beta blockers are considered SNS antagonists, they are most often used in the management of cardiovascular disorders such as hypertension, tachyarrhythmias, angina pectoris, heart failure, hypertrophic subaortic stenosis, and migraine prophylaxis, and for the prevention of myocardial infarction. Other uses of beta blockers include glaucoma (e.g., betaxolol, levobunolol, metipranolol, and timolol), pheochromocytoma, tremors (e.g., propranolol), and the symptoms of hyperthyroidism.

Beta blockers act by competing with the neurotransmitters EPI and NEPI for β receptor sites (Fig. 14-5). Nonselective beta blockers block both β_1 and β_2 receptors; selective beta blockers block either β_1 or β_2 receptors. These nonselective and selective beta-blocking drugs are discussed further in Chapter 36 in relation to their use as antiarrhythmic drugs; in Chapter 37 in relation to their use in hypertension, in Chapter 34 in relation to inotropes, and in Chapters 50, 51, 52, and 61 in relation to their use in respiratory and ophthalmic disorders.

These drugs are contraindicated for use in patients with decompensated heart failure or obstructive airway disease, acute bronchospasm, some forms of valvular heart disease, bradyarrhythmias, and heart block. Use them with caution in patients with any form of lung disease or with underlying compensated heart failure. Also, be cautious when using the drugs in patients with diabetes or severe liver disease. Do not abruptly discontinue beta blockers in patients with cardiovascular disease.

Beta blockers cause additive myocardial depression and bradycardia when used with other drugs that also have these effects (e.g., cardiac glycosides, certain antiarrhythmics). They antagonize the therapeutic effects of bronchodilating drugs and may alter insulin requirements in patients who have diabetes. Cimetidine, a histamine$_2$ antagonist, decreases the biotransformation of beta blockers, thus increasing its effects.

CLINICAL REASONING

Treatment Objectives
The desired objectives for the use of adrenergic drugs are to (1) correct hemodynamic imbalances and (2) increase cardiac output, blood pressure, peripheral circulation, and urinary output.

Treatment Options

Patient Variables
LIFE-SPAN CONSIDERATIONS

Pregnant and Nursing Women. Dopamine is preferable if blood pressure support is needed in the pregnant woman, because at low doses it not only increases cardiac output and arterial blood pressure but also improves renal perfusion. Dopamine may decrease uterine blood flow and should be used once it has been demonstrated that volume replacement is sufficient. Ephedrine is valuable to counteract hypotension from epidural or spinal anesthesia if fluids are ineffective.

Children and Adolescents. The safety and efficacy of many of the adrenergic drugs has not been established for children. Watch children closely for excessive CNS stimulation, irritability, palpitations, tachycardia, and chest pain.

Older Adults. Because of the changes of aging, older adults are more sensitive to drugs. For this and other reasons, it is important to monitor the older adult for excessive CNS and cardiac stimulation. Many older adults needing treatment with adrenergic drugs also have underlying comorbid conditions such as hypertension, peripheral vascular disease, and heart disease. Monitor these patients carefully before, during, and after use of adrenergic drugs. Use caution with the older adult because of the risk of reduced renal function secondary to the changes of aging and other comorbid disorders.

Drug Variables
The health care provider must decide on the choice of drug, treatment end points, and the safe and effective

dosages of adrenergic drugs to be used. In general, SNS agonists are rapid-acting and have short duration of action, and as such can be given as continuous infusions. Careful monitoring and calculation of infusion rates is advised, because dosing adjustments are made frequently, and varying admixtures and concentrations are used in volume-restricted patients.

In critically ill patients, faulty adrenergic receptor activity may result in resistance to exogenous catecholamine administration. This "desensitization" is often characterized by hyporesponsiveness of myocardial and vascular tissues to high dosages of vasopressors and inotropes. Prolonged contact of vascular endothelial tissue to vasopressor drugs (e.g., alpha agonists) or catecholamines may result in reduced response. Increased endogenous catecholamine concentrations have been reported in critically ill and endotoxemic patients, suggesting an acquired β receptor defect and desensitization of β receptors and alteration in voltage-sensitive calcium channels. Although the problem may reside in decreased β receptor activity or density, in patients with septic shock, catecholamine concentrations are even higher; thus abnormalities in β receptor function are greater and, accordingly, entail reductions in myocardial cyclic monophosphate concentrations. The receptor dysfunction may be explained by defects distal to the receptor site, such as uncoupling of the β receptor from adenyl cyclase or a dysfunction in the regulatory G protein unit of the adenyl cyclase system.

Because α and β receptor derangements vary among patients, as well as in a given patient during a bacteremic insult, dosages of catecholamines vary during the insult. For these reasons, dose adrenergic drugs to clinical end points and not to arbitrary maximal dosages.

NEPI is often started after vasopressor dosages of dopamine, alone or in combination with dobutamine, fail to achieve desired goals. Dosages of dopamine and dobutamine may be kept constant or the drugs stopped altogether; or, in some cases, dopamine is kept at low dosages for renal protection. It may be more reasonable to use NEPI, because it is more potent than dopamine and more effective at increasing mean arterial pressure. A clinically significant increase in mean arterial pressure is generally accompanied by an increase in systemic vascular resistance. In contrast to dopamine, NEPI generally does not cause an increase in heart rate, owing to decreased stimulation of myocardial β receptors.

Overall, data suggest that NEPI should be reconsidered as the vasopressor of choice in patients with septic shock because of its multiple benefits, which include the following: decreased mortality; attenuating inappropriate vasodilation and low global oxygen extraction; lessening of myocardial depression at unchanged or increased cardiac output and increases in coronary blood flow; improving renal perfusion

pressures and renal filtration; improving splenic perfusion; and reducing the likelihood that the drug (compared with other vasopressors) will cause tachycardias and tachyarrhythmias.

Dobutamine may temporarily improve cardiac output and renal blood flow, ameliorate symptoms, and relieve sodium and water retention in patients with uncompensated heart failure who are refractory to maximal oral therapy with angiotensin-converting enzyme (ACE) inhibitors. Dobutamine has relatively more inotropic and chronotropic effects on the heart compared to isoproterenol. The explanation for this useful selectivity is not clear. It may be due in part to relatively unchanged peripheral vascular resistance. In equivalent inotropic dosages, dobutamine enhances automaticity of the sinus node to a lesser degree than isoproterenol; however, the improvement in atrioventricular and intraventricular conduction is similar for the two drugs. Dobutamine has limited long-term use in heart failure because it must be administered by IV route and because of the tendency for its efficacy to decline over 48 to 72 hours.

Dobutamine is the preferred drug for patients with low output states in the setting of an acute myocardial infarction. In contrast to dopamine, dobutamine has much less α-related vasoconstriction activity but equal positive inotropic effects. Thus, in equal doses, dobutamine tends to lower pulmonary capillary wedge pressure (PCWP), whereas dopamine tends to increase it. Dobutamine is also associated with fewer arrhythmias. Patients with atrial fibrillation who are to be treated with dobutamine may require rate control before being given dobutamine, since the drug facilitates atrioventricular (AV) conduction.

EPI is included in advanced cardiac life support (ACLS) protocols such as those used to manage asystole and ventricular fibrillation that are unresponsive to electric cardioversion. It increases cardiac output but redistributes blood flow away from the kidney and splenic circulations toward skeletal muscle.

Patient Education

Adrenergic drugs are most often used in emergency situations, and the extent of patient teaching depends on the patient's awareness and clinical status. Advise patients to notify the health care provider if they develop chest pain, dizziness, insomnia, weakness, or tremor, or sense an irregular heartbeat while receiving adrenergic drugs.

Evaluation

The desired outcome of drug therapy with adrenergic drugs is to correct hemodynamic imbalances and to increase cardiac output, blood pressure, peripheral circulation, and urinary output.

KEY POINTS

- Sympathetic nervous system agonists stimulate sympathetic nervous system activity. These drugs are also referred to as sympathomimetic or adrenergic agonists and are divided into five groups: alpha-1 and alpha-2, and beta-1 and beta-2 agonists and antagonists, and D agonists and antagonists.

- EPI activates α_1, α_2, β_1, and β_2 receptors; NEPI activates α_1, α_2, and β_1 receptors; isoproterenol activates β_1 and β_2 receptors; dobutamine activates β_1 receptors; and dopamine activates α_1, β_1, and D receptors.

- The choice of drug, dosage, and route of administration depend largely on the reason for use.
- Indications for adrenergic agonists stem primarily from their effects on the heart, blood vessels, and the bronchi. They are most often used in the emergency management of acute shock; to reverse anaphylactic shock; to increase blood pressure in severe hypotension; to reduce bleeding at the operative site in conjunction with local anesthetics; to treat asthma attacks; and to increase cardiac output in acute decompensated heart failure.

- Beta blockers are the cornerstone therapy for hypertension, heart failure, and coronary artery disease, and have many other pharmacotherapeutic uses.
- Selective alpha-1 blockers are useful in the management of hypertension, Raynaud's disease, and symptoms of BPH.
- Adverse effects of adrenergic agonists are essentially extensions of therapeutic effects. The adverse effects include nervousness, restlessness, insomnia, tremors, headache, tachycardia, arrhythmias, angina, and hypertension.

Bibliography

Bernardin, G., Kisoka, R., Delporte, C., et al. (2003). Impairment of beta adrenergic signaling in healthy peripheral blood mononuclear cells exposed to serum from patients with septic shock: Involvement of the inhibitory pathway of adenyl cyclase stimulation. *Shock, 19*(2), 108–112.

Bonow, R. (2005). ACC/AHA clinical performance measures for adults with chronic heart failure: A report of the American College of Cardiology/American Heart Association task force on performance measures. *Journal of the American College of Cardiology, 46* (6), 1144–1178.

Braunwald, E., Fauci, A., Kasper, D., et al. (2005). *Harrison's principles of internal medicine.* (15th ed.). New York: McGraw-Hill.

Cummins, R. (2003). *ACLS Provider Manual.* Dallas: American Heart Association.

DiPiro, J., Talbert, R., Yee, G., et al. (2005). *Pharmacotherapy: A pathophysiologic approach.* (6th ed.). New York: McGraw-Hill.

Goldman, L., and Ausiello, D. (ed.). (2005). *Cecil textbook of medicine* (22nd ed.). Philadelphia: WB Saunders.

Gutierrez, K., and Queener, S. (2003). *Pharmacology for nursing practice.* St Louis: Mosby.

Hardman, L., and Limbird, L. (2001). *Goodman and Gilman's the pharmacological basis of therapeutics.* (10th ed.). New York: McGraw-Hill.

Martin, C., Viviand, X., Leone, M., et al. (2000). Effect of norepinephrine on the outcome of septic shock. *Critical Care Medicine, 28*(8), 2758–2765.

Minneman, K., and Wecker, L. (2005). *Brody's human pharmacology: Molecular to clinical.* (4th ed.). Philadelphia: Mosby.

Sharma, V., and Dellinger, R. (2003). The International Sepsis Forum's controversies in sepsis: My initial vasopressor agent in septic shock is norepinephrine rather than dopamine. *Critical Care, 7*(1), 6–8.

AUTONOMIC NERVOUS

15

Parasympathetic Nervous System Drugs

The parasympathetic nervous system functions to conserve energy. As discussed in the previous chapter, postganglionic nerves release acetylcholine (ACh), which activates muscarinic cholinergic receptors on exocrine glands, smooth muscle, and cardiac muscle to produce parasympathetic responses. Stimulation of this system leads to decreased heart rate, blood pressure, and respiration, increased secretions, and miosis. ACh, the primary parasympathetic nervous system neurotransmitter, is synthesized from choline and acetyl coenzyme A with the assistance of the enzyme choline acetyltransferase (Fig. 15-1).

PHYSIOLOGY OF PARASYMPATHETIC NEUROTRANSMISSION

The large pyramidal cells of the motor cortex, the cells of the basal ganglia, preganglionic neurons, and the motor neurons are major sources of ACh. The neurotransmitter is also released from postganglionic sympathetic nerves, where it stimulates muscarinic receptors located on sweat glands and some blood vessels. ACh is also released from neurons throughout the central nervous system, where it acts on both muscarinic and nicotinic receptors (for definition and discussion of these receptor types, see Chapter 14).

The effects of ACh on muscarinic cholinergic receptors, which belong to the class of G protein–coupled receptors, include increased salivary secretion, gastric motility, and gastric acid secretion. As with other body systems, there is a checks-and-balances system that prevents normal functions from proceeding uncontrolled. The key to the balance mechanism is acetylcholinesterase, an enzyme that breaks down ACh.

Drugs affecting the parasympathetic nervous system mimic, antagonize, or prolong the actions of ACh at muscarinic receptors. These drugs are often referred to as *parasympathomimetics*, or *cholinergics*, and are used to increase the motility of the gastrointestinal (GI) and urinary tracts and to reduce intraocular pressure in patients with glaucoma. All actions of ACh and its congeners at muscarinic receptors can be blocked by atropine, an anticholinergic drug.

Both the parasympathetic and sympathetic nervous systems use ACh as a neurotransmitter, as does the neuromuscular junction and innervation to the adrenal medullae. The receptors that mediate responses of these nervous systems' responses to ACh are referred to as nicotinic receptors. In fact, the nicotinic receptor has become the prototype for other ligand-gated ion channels, which include the receptors for certain inhibitory amino acids such as gamma-aminobutyric acid (GABA) and glycine, and certain serotonin (5-HT$_3$) receptors.

In contrast to muscarinic receptors, nicotinic receptors are ligand-gated ion channels. Nicotinic acetylcholine receptors are stimulated by both ACh and the alkaloid nicotine. Activation of the nicotinic receptors always causes a rapid increase in cellular permeability to sodium (Na$^+$) and calcium (Ca^{++}), leading to depolarization and excitation. Nicotinic effects include tachycardia, elevated blood pressure, and peripheral vasoconstriction. However, rapid biotransformation of ACh weakens these effects.

A number of conditions can be treated with parasympathetic nervous system drugs, including urinary retention, dementia of the Alzheimer's type, peptic ulcer disease, irritable bowel syndrome, and Parkinson's disease. To understand the use of these drugs in the treatment of some of these disorders, a brief explanation of each disorder is appropriate.

DEMENTIA OF THE ALZHEIMER'S TYPE

EPIDEMIOLOGY AND ETIOLOGY

There are approximately 4.5 million people in the United States living with Alzheimer's disease, a form of dementia. One in 10 of us have at least one family member suffering from Alzheimer's. Dementia involves progressive deterioration in cognition (usually memory), language, calculation abilities, visual-spatial perception, judgment, the ability to abstract, and personality. Dementia of the Alzheimer's type (DAT) makes up at least 50% of all dementias. The prevalence of DAT doubles for every 5 years a person lives beyond the age of 65. DAT occurs in 10% to 15% of people over 65 years of age, in 19% of people older than 75, and in 47% of people older than 85. The lifetime risk for the disease is approximately 25.5% for men and 32% for women. The differences in risk correlate with the longer life span of today's women. Within the next 50 years, as many as 16 million men and women in the United States are expected to develop DAT.

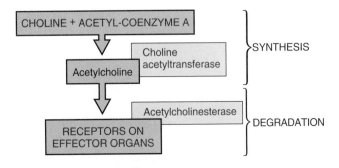

FIGURE 15-1 Acetylcholine synthesis combines choline with acetyl coenzyme A and is degraded by the enzyme acetylcholinesterase.

The familial form of DAT affects less than 10% of patients, usually has an onset before age 65, and is accompanied by gene mutations on three chromosomes. In the more common late-onset form of DAT, inheritance of the E4 allele of the apolipoprotein E gene on chromosome 19 may be involved (E4 allele is much less of a risk factor for blacks and Hispanics). Although there is no obvious inheritance pattern, there is a greater risk of developing DAT if a first-degree relative has the condition.

The exact etiology of DAT has not been identified. At least four chromosomes are involved in some forms of familial DAT. The lack of 100% concordance in identical twins suggests that environmental, metabolic, and other factors may also play a role. It is believed that DAT may be associated with aluminum intoxication, disordered immune function, and viral infection; however, these factors have not been proven. Female sex, head trauma, lack of education, and myocardial infarction have been linked to DAT, but the associations are weak. Although some risk factors for DAT (e.g., age, family history) are not modifiable, efforts to reduce the incidence of head trauma and cardiovascular disease may reduce the incidence of DAT and other types of dementia. To date, there is no cure for DAT.

PHYSIOLOGY AND PATHOPHYSIOLOGY

Neurofibrillary tangles and neuritic plaques characterize DAT. The remnants from disintegration of dendrite branches and axon terminals result in neuritic plaques. The plaques are clumps of beta amyloid protein that accumulate around the brain's nerve cells and eventually cause them to die. The orderly arrangement of neurons normally found in the brain is lost.

The neurofibrillary tangles are twisted strands of another protein (called *tau*) that form within the cells. Although the structural changes begin in small areas of the brain, axonal spread allows transmission to other areas of the brain. The more areas of the brain that are affected, the more severe the symptoms.

The hippocampus is the first area of the brain to be affected by DAT. Short-term memory requires a functional hippocampus. Impairment of the hippocampus is correlated with mild memory loss, one of the first signs of DAT. Neurofibrillary tangles and neuritic plaques are also seen in the raphe nuclei within the cerebellum. The raphe nuclei secrete serotonin, a neurotransmitter responsible for mood control. Lower than normal levels of serotonin can result in depression. Depression superimposed on top of DAT further impairs cognitive function. Antidepressant drugs may improve the depression but will not change the course of the disease. In some cases, the adverse effects of the antidepressant drugs compromise the patient's condition to an even greater extent.

The most recent speculations about the cause of DAT implicate insulin. It appears that insulin concentrations in the brain drop dramatically in early DAT and continue to fall as the disease progresses. It is thought that this may contribute to the cell death and tangles characteristic of DAT. Another hallmark of DAT, low levels of ACh, is also directly linked to the loss of insulin, all of which suggests that DAT may be associated with diabetes.

PHARMACOTHERAPEUTIC OPTIONS

Cholinesterase Inhibitors

◆ donepezil (Aricept); ✦ Aricept
◆ galantamine (Razadyne); ✦ Razadyne
◆ rivastigmine (Exelon); ✦ Exelon
◆ tacrine (Cognex)

▌ Indications

Donepezil, galantamine, rivastigmine, and tacrine are approved for the treatment of cognitive impairment in mild to moderately severe DAT (mini-mental state exam [MMSE] scores of 10 to 26).

▌ Pharmacodynamics

Cholinesterase inhibitors act as competitive and reversible inhibitors of acetylcholinesterase. Although the precise mechanism is unclear, the drugs are thought to exert therapeutic effects by enhancing cholinergic function. This is accomplished by increasing the concentration of ACh through reversible inhibition of its hydrolysis by cholinesterase. The effects of cholinesterase inhibitors may lessen as the disease process advances and fewer cholinergic neurons remain functionally intact. Cognitive improvement is generally modest, with a sustained cognitive benefit of 6 to 9 months followed by a gradual decline thereafter. There is no evidence that these drugs alter the course of the underlying dementia process.

▌ Pharmacokinetics

The pharmacokinetics of cholinesterase inhibitors are identified in Table 15-1. The drugs are rapidly absorbed from the GI tract following oral administration. Food decreases the absorption of tacrine 30% to 40%. Although drug effects are often noted within 6 weeks, noticeable improvement in cognitive function may take 18 to 24 weeks. Further, plasma drug concentrations are two thirds lower in patients who smoke. It is theorized that smoking increases the rate of drug biotransformation in the liver.

▌ Adverse Reactions and Contraindications

Common adverse effects of donepezil include insomnia, fatigue, dizziness, confusion, ataxia, somnolence, tremor, agitation, depression, and difficulty in problem solving. Adverse effects on the GI tract include anorexia, nausea, vomiting, dyspepsia, abdominal pain, and diarrhea. Donepezil-induced hepatotoxicity is possible, although the type of liver dysfunction it induces is less severe than that seen with tacrine. Donepezil is contraindicated for use in patients with hypersensitivity to the drug, in pregnancy, and in women who are breastfeeding. Use it with caution in patients who have sick sinus syndrome, GI bleeding, seizures, or asthma.

A relatively small percentage of patients will note the common adverse effects of galantamine: anorexia, nausea, vomiting, diarrhea, and weight loss. Occurring less often are constipation, agitation, confusion, anxiety, hallucination, back pain, peripheral edema, asthenia, chest pain, urinary incontinence, upper respiratory infection, bronchitis, coughing, hypertension, and purpura. There are no statistically significant differences related to dose or sex in the rate of adverse effects. Galantamine is contraindicated for use in patients with known hypersensitivity to the drug or to excipients used in the formulations.

The common adverse effects of rivastigmine include anorexia, nausea, vomiting, diarrhea, and abdominal pain. Dizziness, fatigue, weight loss, tremors, asthenia, somnolence, and confusion have been reported. In some patients sialorrhea is a problem. Serious reactions include seizures,

AUTONOMIC NERVOUS

PHARMACOKINETICS

TABLE 15-1 Selected PSNS Drugs

Drug	Route	Onset	Peak	Duration	PB (%)	t½
CHOLINESTERASE INHIBITORS						
donepezil	PO	Varies	2–4 hr	24 hr	96	7–8 hr
galantamine	PO	60 min	2–4 hr	24 hr	18	7 hr
galantamine ER	PO	UA	4.5–5 hr	24 hr	18	7 hr
rivastigmine	PO	UA	1 hr*	10 hr*	40	1.5 hr
tacrine	PO	UA	1–2 hr	4–8 hr	55	2–4 hr
NMDA RECEPTOR ANTAGONIST						
memantine	PO	UA	3–7 hr	UA	45	60–80 hr
ANTICHOLINERGICS						
atropine	PO, subQ	30–90 min	1–2 hr	4–6 hr	Mod	2.5 hr
	IM	30 min	1–1.6 hr	Brief	Mod	2.5 hr
clidinium	PO	60 min	UA	3 hr	UA	UA
dicyclomine	PO, IM	60 min	60–90 min	4 hr	UA	9–10 hr
glycopyrrolate	PO	50 min	60 min	8–12 hr†	UA	0.6–4.6 hr
	IM	20–40 min	30–45 min	2–7 hr	UA	0.6–4.6 hr
	IV	10–15 min	UA	2–7 hr	UA	0.6–4.6 hr
hyoscyamine	PO, IM	5–30 min	30–60 min	4–12 hr	Mod	3.5 hr
	IV	2 min	15–30 min	4–12 hr	Mod	3.5 hr
propantheline	PO	30–60 min	2–6 hr	6 hr	UA	3–4 hr
scopolamine	TD	4 hr	24 hr	3 days	Low	9 hr
	PO, IM	30–60 min	60 min	4–6 hr	Low	UA
	IV	10 min	20–60 min	2 hr	Low	UA

*Referring to peak and duration of anticholinesterase activity of rivastigmine.
†The antisecretory effects of glycopyrrolate last up to 7 hours. Vagal blockade lasts 2–3 hours.
IM, Intramuscular; *mod,* moderate; *PB,* protein binding; *PO,* by mouth; *PSNS,* parasympathetic nervous system; *subQ,* subcutaneous; *t½,* half-life; *TD,* transdermal patch; *UA,* unavailable.

urinary obstruction, bradycardia, hypotension, and respiratory depression. Rivastigmine is contraindicated for use or is to be used with caution in patients with cardiovascular disease, asthma or chronic obstructive pulmonary disease (COPD), peptic ulcer disease, sick sinus syndrome, and bradycardia.

Common adverse effects of tacrine include diarrhea, loss of appetite, clumsiness or unsteadiness, nausea, and vomiting. The cholinergic action of tacrine increases gastric secretions and can be problematic for patients with peptic ulcer disease. Agitation and hallucinations are seen in a small percentage of patients. These adverse effects may be particularly troublesome if the patient has a history of behavioral problems. The major adverse effect of tacrine is elevation of alanine transferase (ALT). The degree of elevation of this liver enzyme determines the possibility of increasing the dosage or continuing the drug, or both. Because of its cholinergic effects, use tacrine cautiously in patients with GI obstruction, urinary tract obstruction, asthma, or cardiac disease.

▥ Drug Interactions

Drug interactions of cholinesterase inhibitors are noted in Table 15-2. Concurrent use of theophylline and other cholinesterase inhibitors increases the risk of toxicity of cholinesterase inhibitors. Succinylcholine used concurrently with cholinesterase inhibitors increases the risk of neuromuscular blockade. Donepezil specifically decreases the effects of anticholinergics, and there is an increased risk of GI bleeding with concurrent use of nonsteroidal antiinflammatory drugs. Cholinesterase-inhibiting drugs reverse the paralysis associated with the use of nondepolarizing neuromuscular blocking drugs.

▥ Dosage Regimen

Table 15-3 provides an overview of cholinesterase inhibitor dosages. Dosages must be titrated if therapy is interrupted for several days or longer. There are no appreciable differences in pharmacokinetics when extended-release formulations are given with food rather than during a fasting state.

▥ Lab Considerations

Serum drug levels of donepezil, galantamine, and rivastigmine are not measured. Regularly obtain blood counts and ALT values for patients taking donepezil.

N-methyl-ᴅ-aspartate (NMDA) Receptor Antagonist
◆ memantine (Namenda)

Memantine is the first drug of this class and has been approved as a noncompetitive N-methyl-ᴅ-aspartate (NMDA) receptor antagonist. Its action is related to the activity of glutamate, a specialized neurotransmitter in the brain that is associated with storing, processing, and retrieval of information. It also plays an important role in learning and memory by stimulating NMDA receptors on nerve cells to accept a controlled amount of calcium. In contrast, excessive amounts of glutamate can allow too much calcium into the nerve cells. The resulting overstimulation of NMDA receptors can cause cell death.

Memantine's mechanism of action is different than that of cholinesterase inhibitor drugs which have been used in the past for the treatment of Alzheimer's. In contrast to cholinesterase inhibitors, which temporarily increase levels of ACh in the synapse, memantine blocks NMDA receptors, thereby creating a partial blockade to excess glutamate.

Memantine is rapidly and completely absorbed following oral administration. The drug undergoes little biotransformation,

DRUG INTERACTIONS
TABLE 15-2 Selected PSNS Drugs

Drug	Interactive Drugs	Interaction
CHOLINESTERASE INHIBITORS		
donepezil, galantamine, rivastigmine, tacrine	Cholinesterase inhibitors, theophylline	Increases effects and risk for potential toxicity of interactive drug
	Antimuscarinics	Decreases effects of both drugs
	NSAIDs	Increased risk of NSAID-induced gastropathy
	cimetidine	Decreases biotransformation of tacrine
	succinylcholine	Exaggerates neuromuscular blockade
	nicotine	Decreases blood levels of tacrine
	Neuromuscular blockers	Decreases effect of neuromuscular blocker
NMDA RECEPTOR ANTAGONIST		
memantine	Carbonic anhydrase inhibitors, sodium bicarbonate	Reduces elimination of memantine
ANTIMUSCARINIC DRUGS		
atropine, dicyclomine, hyoscyamine, scopolamine	Antacids	Decreases absorption of antimuscarinic drug
	Antihistamines, amantadine, antiparkinsonian drugs, disopyramide, histamine$_1$ antagonists, gluthethimide, meperidine, MAO inhibitors, procainamide, quinidine, tricyclic antidepressants	Additive antimuscarinic effects
	Wax matrix potassium chloride	Increases risk of mucosal lesions from antimuscarinic drug
scopolamine	Alcohol	Additive CNS depression

CNS, Central nervous system; *GI*, gastrointestinal; *MAO*, monoamine oxidase; *NSAIDs*, nonsteroidal antiinflammatory drugs; *PSNS*, parasympathetic nervous system.

with the majority of the drug eliminated unchanged in the urine. The dosage is identified in Table 15-3.

The most common adverse effects of memantine include dizziness, headache, confusion, cough, constipation, and hypertension. Although rare, back pain, nausea, fatigue, anxiety, peripheral edema, arthralgias, and insomnia have been reported. Memantine is not recommended for use in patients with severe renal impairment. There are no known lab value considerations.

CLINICAL REASONING

Treatment Objectives

The treatment goal for the patient with DAT is to slow the cognitive deterioration that inevitably occurs. Drug therapy may allow the patient to enjoy an independent lifestyle for longer and postpone the burden on family and significant others. An extended period of dependency carries enormous implications for family functioning and caregiver burnout, and placement in a skilled health care facility incurs considerable financial strain.

Treatment Options

▌ Patient Variables

Compliance with drug therapy is usually enhanced with once-daily dosages. Galantamine, rivastigmine, and donepezil require once-daily dosing, whereas tacrine must be administered 4 times daily. The patient's ability to understand and comply with administration schedules is an important factor. Tacrine interacts with a variety of drugs commonly taken by older adults. Further, the ability of the patient, the family, and significant others to comply with treatment regimens and lab work schedules is very important. Tacrine therapy may not be a safe therapy if the patient does not have the ability or the resources to comply.

LIFE-SPAN CONSIDERATIONS. DAT is a disorder of late middle to old age. The gene most commonly associated with DAT is found on chromosome 21, the same chromosome responsible for Down syndrome. Most individuals with Down syndrome begin exhibiting changes in brain structure similar to those associated with DAT by 20 years of age. By the time these individuals reach 40 years of age, they may begin showing symptoms of DAT. The common manifestations of DAT are identified in Table 15-4.

▌ Drug Variables

Each of the cholinesterase inhibitors has demonstrated benefit in DAT, slowing the rate of decline relative to placebo and sustaining higher levels of function. Early diagnosis and treatment is correlated to less cognitive decline, at least in the short term.

Tacrine and donepezil carry a significant risk of hepatotoxicity, thus requiring regular monitoring of liver function. Tacrine also has the potential to cause clumsiness and unsteadiness. This may be particularly problematic for older individuals, who are not as steady on their feet as the young.

Patient Education

Advise patients, family, and significant others to contact the health care provider who is prescribing cholinesterase-inhibitor drugs before taking any new prescribed or over-the-counter medication. Also, instruct them to tell all health care providers, including dentists, about the drugs being taken.

The patient, family, and significant others need to understand that drug therapy does not cure DAT and that the drugs prescribed may not be effective for all patients. In addition, explain the risk of liver enzyme elevation, and reinforce the necessity of stopping treatment if the ALT reaches dangerous levels. It is possible to restart the drug after liver function test values return to normal. Stopping treatment can be devastating

DOSAGE
TABLE **15-3 Selected PSNS Drugs**

Drug	Indications	Dosage	Implications
CHOLINESTERASE INHIBITORS			
donepezil	Mild to moderate DAT	*Adult:* 5 mg PO daily at HS. May increase to 10 mg daily after first 4–6 wk	Notify health care provider if surgery is required, because exaggerated muscle relaxation may occur if succinylcholine type of drugs is used concurrently.
galantamine		*Adult:* ER formulation: 8 mg PO daily. Increase to 16 mg/day after 4 wk. May increase to 24 mg/day after another 4 wk	Retitrate dosage if therapy is interrupted for several days or longer.
rivastigmine		*Adult:* 1.5 mg PO twice daily initially. After 2 wk, may increase to 3 mg twice daily if tolerated. May increase after 2 wk to 4.5–6 mg twice daily as tolerated	Give with food in divided doses morning and evening.
tacrine		*Adult:* 10 mg PO 4 times daily initially for 6 wk; 20 mg 4 times daily for 6 wk if needed. Increase to 30 mg 4 times daily for 6 wk, and then maintain at 40 mg 4 times daily if needed.	Use and titration must be accompanied by evaluation of ALT levels. Teach caregivers the signs and symptoms of liver disease.
NMDA RECEPTOR ANTAGONIST			
memantine	Moderate to severe DAT	*Adult:* Initiate at 5 mg PO once daily. Increase by 5 mg every wk. Recommended target dose: 20 mg daily in 2 divided doses	Drug can be taken with or without food. Minimum recommended interval between dose increases is 1 week.
ANTICHOLINERGIC DRUGS			
atropine	Treatment of bradycardia and bradyarrhythmias Preoperatively to decrease secretions and block cardiac vagal reflexes Adjunctive treatment of IBS Reversal of cholinesterase-inhibitor drug	*Adult:* 0.5–1.0 mg by IV push. Repeat every 3–5 min as needed to max of 3 mg *Child:* 0.02 mg/kg by IV push every 5 min. Minimum single dose is 0.1 mg, and max single dose is 0.4 mg/kg. *Adult:* 0.4 to 0.6 mg IV or IM 30 to 60 min preoperatively *Child >5 kg:* 0.01–0.02 mg/kg/dose to max of 0.4 mg/dose preoperatively *Child <5 kg:* 0.02 mg/kg/dose 30–60 min preoperatively *Adult:* 0.4–0.6 mg PO every 4–6 hr *Child:* 0.01 mg/kg to max dose of 0.4 mg/kg *Adult:* 0.6–1.2 mg for each 0.5–2.5 mg of neostigmine –or– 10–20 mg of pyridostigmine currently with cholinesterase inhibitor	Doses less than 0.5 mg in adults may cause paradoxical bradycardia. Intense flushing of the face and trunk occurs 15–20 min after IM administration. This response is not harmful. Instruct patient that oral rinses, sugarless gum or candy, and frequent oral hygiene help relieve dry mouth. Caution patients that atropine impairs heat regulation—strenuous activity in hot environment may cause heat stroke. Instruct patients with BPH that drug may cause urinary hesitancy and retention. Changes in urinary stream characteristics should be reported to health care provider.
clidinium	Adjunct in IBS	*Adult:* 2.5–5 mg PO 3–4 times daily before meals and at HS *Older Adult:* 2.5 mg PO 3 times daily before meals	Administer 30 min to 1 hr before meals for better absorption.
dicyclomine	Irritable bowel syndrome	*Adult:* 10–20 mg PO 3–4 times daily to max of 160 mg/day *Child >2 yr:* 10 mg PO 3–4 times daily Adjust dose as tolerated. *Child 6 mo-2 yr:* 5–10 mg PO 3–4 times daily. Adjust dose as tolerated.	Do not use subQ or IV. Separate administration of dicyclomine and antacids by 2–3 hr. Give 30–60 min before meals. Bedtime dose should be administered at least 2 hr after last meal.
glycopyrrolate	Control of secretions during surgery Adjunct to NM blockade reversal	*Adult:* 4.4 mcg/kg IM 30–60 min preoperatively. Not to exceed 0.1 mg/kg IV intraoperatively as needed. *Child: <2 yr:* 4.4–8.8 mcg/kg IM 30–60 min preoperatively *Child >2* yr: 4.4 mcg/kg IM *Children intraoperatively:* 4 mcg/kg IV, not to exceed 0.1 mg 0.2 mg IV per each 1 mg neostigmine or each 5 mg pyridostigmine	The antisecretory effects of glycopyrrolate last up to 7 hr. Vagal blockade lasts 2–3 hr.
hyoscyamine	Management of IBS	*Adult, child >12 yr:* 0.125–0.5 mg PO 3–4 times daily –or– 0.375 mg twice daily as ER capsule *Child <2 yr:* 12.5–45 mcg/kg every 4 hr as needed *Child 2–10 yr:* 31–125 mcg/kg every 4 hr	Give before meals and at HS. Other formulations are available, but the concentrations are not the same. Avoid mistakenly substituting one for the other. Administer 30–60 min before meals. Bedtime dose should be given at least 2 hr after last meal.
propantheline	Antisecretory or antispasmodic drug	*Adult:* 15 mg PO 3 times daily with 30 mg at HS *Older adults:* 7.5 mg PO 3–4 times daily *Child:* 0.375 mg/kg PO 4 times daily	Administer 30 min before meals. Bedtime dose should be given at least 2 hr after last meal of the day.
scopolamine	Preoperatively to decrease secretions and block cardiac vagal reflexes	*Adult, child >12 yr:* 0.2–0.6 mg IM, subQ, or IV 30–60 min before anesthesia *Child 8–12 yr:* 0.3 mg IM or subQ 45 min before anesthesia *Child 3–8 yr:* 0.2 mg IM or subQ 45 min before anesthesia *Child 7 mo-3 yr:* 0.15 mg IM or subQ 45 min before anesthesia *Infants 4–7 mo:* 0.1 mg IM or subQ 45 min before anesthesia	Assess patient for urinary retention. May act as stimulant in presence of pain, producing delirium if used without morphine or meperidine.

ALT, Alanine transaminase; *BPH,* benign prostatic hyperplasia; *ER,* extended-release; *HS,* bedtime; *IBS,* irritable bowel syndrome; *IM,* intramuscular(ly); *IV,* intravenous(ly); *NM,* neuromuscular; *PSNS,* parasympathetic nervous system; *subQ,* subcutaneous(ly);

TABLE 15-4 Manifestations of DAT

Stage	Impairment	Manifestations
Stage 1	No impairment (Normal function)	Unimpaired; no memory problems
Stage 2	Very mild cognitive decline (may be normal age-related changes or earliest signs of Alzheimer's disease)	Memory lapses, especially in forgetting familiar words or names or the location of keys, eyeglasses, or other everyday objects. These problems are not evident during examination or apparent to friends, family or co-workers.
Stage 3	Mild cognitive decline: (early-stage Alzheimer's can be diagnosed in some, but not all, individuals with these symptoms) *EEG, CT, MRI:* Essentially normal *PET scan:* Hypometabolism and hyperperfusion of bilateral parietal lobe	Friends, family, or co-workers notice deficiencies. Problems with memory or concentration are measurable. Common difficulties include following: • Word- or name-finding problems noticeable to family or close associates • Decreased ability to remember names when introduced to new people • Performance issues in social or work settings noticeable to family, friends, or co-workers • Reading a passage and retaining little material • Loses or misplaces valuable objects • Decline in ability to plan or organize
Stage 4	Moderate cognitive decline (mild or early-stage Alzheimer's disease)	Overt deficiencies in the following areas: • Decreased memory of personal history, or recent or current events • Difficulty performing mental arithmetic (e.g., counting backward from 100 by 7s) • Decreased ability to perform complex tasks such as marketing, planning dinner, paying bills, managing finances • Subdued and withdrawn, especially in socially or mentally challenging situations
Stage 5	Moderately severe cognitive decline (moderate or midstage Alzheimer's disease) *EEG:* Slowing of background rhythm *CT and MRI:* Normal or ventricular dilation and enlargement of sulcus *PET scan:* Hypometabolism and hypoperfusion of parietal and frontal lobes	• Major gaps in cognition and memory • Unable to recall details such as current address, telephone number, or name of college or high school attended • Confusion about the date, day of the week, or season • Worsening difficulty performing mental arithmetic (e.g., counting backward from 40 by 4s; from 20 by 2s) • Requires assistance with day-to-day activities (e.g., dressing) • Requires little assistance eating or toileting • Usually retains substantial knowledge about self and knows own name and names of spouse or children
Stage 6	Severe cognitive decline (moderately severe or midstage Alzheimer's disease) *EEG:* Diffusely slow *ECT and MRI:* Ventricular dilation and enlargement of sulcus *PET scan:* Hypometabolism and hypoperfusion of parietal and frontal lobes	Memory difficulties continue to worsen, significant personality changes emerge, and affected individuals need extensive help with customary daily activities. At this stage, individuals may demonstrate the following: • Loses most awareness of recent experiences, events, and surroundings • Generally recalls own name but recall imperfect • Occasionally forgets name of spouse or primary caregiver; usually able to distinguish familiar from unfamiliar faces • Needs help dressing; without supervision, may make such errors as putting pajamas over daytime clothes or shoes on wrong feet • Normal sleep-waking cycle disrupted • Needs help handling details of toileting (i.e., wiping and disposing of toilet tissue properly and flushing the toilet) • Increasing episodes of urinary or fecal incontinence • Significant behavioral and personality changes including suspiciousness and delusions (e.g., believing that caregiver is an impostor); hallucinations (seeing or hearing things that are not really there); or compulsive, repetitive behaviors such as hand-wringing or tissue shredding • Tends to wander and become lost
Stage 7	Very severe cognitive decline (severe or late-stage Alzheimer's disease)	• Unable to respond to environment; ability to speak and control of movement lost • Unable to recognizable speech, although words or phrases may occasionally be uttered • Requires help eating and toileting; general incontinence of urine • Ability is lost to walk without assistance, to sit without support, to smile, and to hold the head up. Reflexes abnormal, and muscles rigid. Swallowing is impaired.

Adapted from the work of Barry Reisberg, MD, Clinical Director of the New York University School of Medicine's Silberstein Aging and Dementia Research Center.
CT, Computed tomography scan; *EEG,* electroencephalogram; *MRI,* magnetic resonance imaging; *PET,* positron emission tomographic scan.

to these individuals if the drug was noticeably effective; pre-therapy cognitive levels may not be reached once the drug is restarted. Clearly explain this fact.

Evaluation

The effectiveness of cholinesterase-inhibitor therapy is tracked according to the patient's ability to perform activities of daily living. The degree of supervision needed and the relative safety in performing tasks are evaluated. Many health care providers use the MMSE as an objective measure of cognitive functioning. However, MMSE results are subjective in nature and are only as functional as the patient. The health care provider must assess the reliability of the testing based on patient status, and will have to depend on the family and significant others as the condition progresses for information about the patient's cognition.

Controversy

Clinical Trials Involving Alzheimer's Disease Patients

Sally Schnell

During new product development, most drugs are initially tested on healthy volunteers to determine adverse effects and safe dosages. After safe dosages have been established, the drug is tested on individuals suffering from the targeted disease. It is at this point that the ethics surrounding the inclusion of patients with cognitive impairment comes into play.

One school of thought posits that a patient who is not cognitively competent to give consent to participate should not be included in such a trial. This belief assumes that if the patient cannot express his or her wishes, no one else should presume to do so. Adherence to this perspective would effectively block further trials for the products designed to treat dementia of the Alzheimer's type.

The opposite perspective counters that if a competent significant other understands the risks and benefits of the trial and consents to enrollment, the patient should be allowed to participate. This point of view assumes that the significant other knows the patient's wishes and will act in his or her best interest.

CLINICAL REASONING

- Who should decide on participation in clinical trials if the patient is not competent to make the decision?
- How much risk is acceptable?
- Is it acceptable to force a confused patient to undergo necessary testing or monitoring of the clinical trial?
- Is mathematical modeling an acceptable substitute for long-term, randomized, placebo-controlled trials in demented patients?

CASE STUDY — Dementia of the Alzheimer's Type

ASSESSMENT

History of Present Illness	HW is a 74-year-old female who is worried about memory difficulties over the last 6 months. She is accompanied at this visit by two of her daughters, who agree that their mother is experiencing significant impairment of memory and judgment. HW's daughters also state that she does not maintain her personal hygiene and diet as well as she used to. They state she has lost 10 pounds in the last 6 months. HW blames her hygiene and diet issues on the pain she has in her hips and knees from arthritis. HW has three younger siblings. Her oldest sister died in a skilled nursing facility after spending 4 years there with a diagnosis of DAT.
Past Health History	HW's medical history is unremarkable except for her arthritis, for which she regularly takes ibuprofen. She denies use of alcohol or tobacco.
Life-Span Considerations	HW wants to remain independent in her own home and gets upset whenever the topic of changing her living environment comes up. HW may have less effective hepatic function owing to the changes of aging.
Psychosocial Considerations	The daughters live within 15 minutes of HW. They will no longer allow her to supervise the grandchildren alone, a situation that causes HW a great deal of frustration. HW has a few close friends, all of whom are about her age. She still drives locally, but her daughters are concerned about her safety. HW has Social Security as her main source of income and Medicare as her primary insurance. She has selected a Medicare pharmacy plan but knows little about what drugs will be covered.
Physical Exam Findings	VSS. Weight down 10 pounds from 6 months ago. HW ambulates independently but slowly with the help of a walker. She is expressionless and has a flat affect.
Diagnostic Testing	Head MRI reveals moderate cortical atrophy; otherwise within normal limits. CBC, chemistry panel, thyroid function studies, folate and B_{12} levels, RPR, and ESR are within normal limits. MMSE score 3 months ago was 29, today MMSE score is 22. Unable to illustrate 10:50 on clock drawing.

DIAGNOSIS: DAT

MANAGEMENT

Treatment Objective	1. Slow the rate of cognitive deterioration as much as possible. 2. Allow HW to function as independently as possible.
Treatment Plan	**Pharmacotherapy** • Galantamine, 8 mg daily each morning. Increase by 8 mg every 4 weeks to 24 mg each morning as tolerated.

Continued

CASE STUDY Dementia of the Alzheimer's Type—Cont'd

Patient Education

1. Teach HW and daughters the importance of not stopping galantamine without talking with her health care provider, since her baseline cognition function may decline and not return to the same level as when she was taking the drug.
2. Use cognitive reminder methods (e.g., calendars, drug boxes, clocks) to help HW with activities of daily living (ADLs).

Evaluation

1. Evaluate patient's ability to perform ADLs and decide the degree of supervision needed and the relative safety in performing tasks.
2. Use family reports and the MMSE as objective measures of cognitive functioning.
3. Arrange for physical therapy and occupational therapy to do an initial home safety evaluation.

CLINICAL REASONING ANALYSIS

Q1. How do you know when to start a cholinesterase inhibitor drug for HW?

A. Sometimes it is difficult to know; however, essentially it should be started when all other causes of cognitive decline have been ruled out (e.g., vascular dementia, multi-infarct dementia, Parkinson's, brain tumors, normopressure hydrocephalus, drug reactions, substance abuse, depression, nutritional). A cholinesterase inhibitor is usually started as soon as noticeable cognitive decline is noted. In HW's case, I would start the drug now, because her cognition has declined rather dramatically in the last 3 months according to the clock drawing and the MMSE score.

Q2. Why did you choose galantamine over donepezil or tacrine?

A. Donepezil and tacrine have an estimated period of effectiveness of 24 months, whereas with galantamine the estimated period before cognitive decline becomes noticeable again is 36 months. Further, tacrine and donepezil have been associated with hepatotoxicity and require frequent liver function tests, which add significantly to the cost of therapy.

Q3. Generally speaking, it is better to give her a once-daily drug rather than something she has to take more than once a day, right?

A. You are correct in saying that once-daily dosing is an easier regimen; and galantamine is given just that way. Donepezil is taken once daily, also, but tacrine must be taken 4 times daily. If her pharmacy insurance does not cover galantamine, we will use donepezil instead. The dosing frequency of tacrine and its adverse effects preclude using this drug unless we have no other choice.

IRRITABLE BOWEL SYNDROME

Theoretical causes of irritable bowel syndrome (IBS; i.e., spastic colon, irritable colon, mucous colitis) range from fear and anxiety to depression, foods, drugs, toxins, and colonic distention. Contributing factors include diverticular disease, caffeine and other gastric stimulants, and lactose intolerance. IBS is a functional disorder whose exact cause is unknown. It is the most common digestive disorder in the United States, although reliable data are unavailable. Irritable bowel disease affects 15% to 20% of the population, with two thirds of the cases involving women. Most patients who report symptoms are between the ages of 35 and 40 years. The symptoms include a change in bowel habits, with abdominal pain and distention. There may be alternating periods of constipation and diarrhea, with cramping and abdominal discomfort. Belching and increased flatus are also noted.

PHARMACOTHERAPEUTIC OPTIONS

Anticholinergics

◆ atropine
◆ clidinium (Quarzan)
◆ dicyclomine (Antispas, Bentyl, Byclomine, others); ◆ Bentylol, Formulex
◆ glycopyrrolate (Robinul)
◆ hyoscyamine (Anaspaz, Cystospaz, Levsin, Levsinex Timecaps); ◆ Levsin
◆ propantheline (Pro-Banthine); ◆ Propanthel
◆ scopolamine (Transderm Scop); ◆ Buscopan, Transderm-V

▌▌ *Indications*

There are many uses for anticholinergic (i.e., muscarinic cholinergic antagonist) drugs. Atropine is the best known and has the most uses. Atropine is used to reverse toxicity associated with cholinesterase-inhibitor drugs and to treat cardiac arrhythmias. Atropine, clidinium, dicyclomine, hyoscyamine, and propantheline are often used in the treatment of IBS. These drugs are discussed in more depth in Chapter 46.

Glycopyrrolate may be used preoperatively to inhibit salivation and excessive respiratory secretions. Glycopyrrolate is also used as an adjunct to reverse the secretory and vagal actions of cholinesterase inhibitors used to treat nondepolarizing neuromuscular blockade (see later sections on Neuromuscular Blockade and Reversal of Neuromuscular Blockade).

EVIDENCE-BASED PHARMACOTHERAPEUTICS

Cholinesterase Inhibitor Treatment for Dementia of the Alzheimer's Type

■ Background
Dementia of the Alzheimer's type (DAT), the most common cause of late-life dementia, causes progressive cognitive and functional decline over the years. A deficit in brain cholinergic function contributes to the cognitive impairments of DAT. Even though cholinesterase inhibitors have demonstrated efficacy in studies lasting 3 to 6 months, there is a scarcity of information about use in long-term therapy.

■ Research Article
Raskin, M., Peskind, E., Truyen, L., et al. (2004). The cognitive benefits of galantamine are sustained for at least 36 months: A long-term extension trial. *Archives of Neurology, 61,* 252–256.

Purpose
Determining the long-term benefits of cholinesterase inhibitor treatment for DAT would require a multiyear, placebo-controlled clinical trial. Further, ethical considerations preclude long-term placebo use. Therefore, a less direct approach was used to determine if patients with DAT given a cholinesterase inhibitor for multiple years manifest more gradual cognitive decline than would be predicted using a mathematical model derived from observations of DAT patients followed by longitudinally predating the introduction of cholinesterase inhibitor.

Design
Over a 12-month period this double-blinded, placebo-controlled trial examined cognitive function and adverse effects in subjects (N = 194) with mild to moderate DAT. This study was preceded by subject participation in either of two double-blind, placebo-controlled, multicenter galantamine trials that used continuous an open-label extension for a total original trial of 12 months.

Methods
Cognition was analyzed as changes from baseline scores on the Alzheimer's Disease Assessment Scale (ADAS). Because the ADAS is an 11-item cognitive subscale (ADAS-cog/11) and is the most common measure of cognition in DAT clinical trials, it is possible to compare ADAS-cog/11 score changes observed over time in DAT patients treated continuously with cholinesterase inhibitor.

Decline in cognition in the galantamine-treated subjects was compared with DAT patients who received a placebo and with the mathematically-predicted decline in untreated patients over 36 months. Cognitive decline of patients who completed the entire 36-month trial (N = 119) was also compared with that of patients who withdrew for any reason during the long-term open-label extension (N = 75). Within groups, comparisons of the changes from baseline or the initial visit were performed using the paired t-test.

Findings
Patients treated continuously with galantamine for 36 months increased a mean +/− standard error (SE) of 10.2 +/− 0.9 points on the ADAS-cog/11—a substantially smaller cognitive decline (approximately 50%) than that predicted for untreated patients. Patients who stopped galantamine therapy before the end of the 36 months declined at a similar rate before discontinuation as those who completed the study. Eighty percent of subjects who were continuously treated with galantamine exhibited cognitive benefits as compared with predicted benefits for the untreated patients (Mean ≠ SE, 76.1 ≠ 0.52 vs. 74.1 ≠ 0.52 years; p = 0.19).

Conclusions
Galantamine use for at least 36 months seems to be an effective, safe, and well-tolerated intervention for patients with mild to moderate DAT.

■ Implications for Practice
Although these results suggest long-term positive effects on cognitive decline, the conclusions should be interpreted with caution, because study outcomes are limited owing to the lack of biologic indicators of disease progression and the absence of a true long-term placebo-controlled group. Given the ethical considerations, more convincing randomized, placebo-controlled studies of the disease-modifying effects of cholinesterase inhibitors for patients with DAT are still needed for long-term effects to be truly known.

⫶ Pharmacodynamics

Anticholinergic drugs block the action of ACh at postganglionic muscarinic receptor sites located in smooth muscle, secretory glands, the central nervous system (CNS), sinoatrial (SA) and atrioventricular (AV) nodes, and cardiac muscle. Some muscarinic antagonists enhance pain relief by relieving gastric distress caused by gastric spasm and hyperperistalsis. Excessive hydrochloric acid secretion and gastric motility associated with peptic ulcer disease can be partially reduced by decreasing vagal stimulation.

⫶ Pharmacokinetics

The pharmacokinetics of selected anticholinergic drugs are identified in Table 15-1. The onset of drug action for most of these drugs ranges from 5 minutes for hyoscyamine to as long as 90 minutes for atropine. The duration of drug action ranges from 3 hours to 3 days, depending on the specific drug.

⫶ Adverse Effects and Contraindications

The adverse effects and contraindications associated with anticholinergic drugs are many. The drugs produce a high incidence of adverse effects such as dilated pupils, dry mouth and skin, flushing, thirst, tachycardia, and urinary retention.

Because of their tendency to decrease gastric motility, avoid the use of anticholinergic drugs in cases in which delayed gastric emptying increases the patient's level of discomfort. All anticholinergic drugs suppress perspiration, thus contributing to the possibility of overheating. Atropine, dicyclomine, or hyoscyamine may result in extrapyramidal symptoms.

Anticholinergics are contraindicated for use in patients with known hypersensitivity, narrow-angle glaucoma, hemorrhage, tachycardia due to thyrotoxicosis, cardiac insufficiency, and myasthenia gravis. Pediatric patients and older adults are more susceptible to the adverse effects of these drugs than are younger individuals.

Use anticholinergic drugs with caution in patients with urinary tract pathology, those at risk for GI obstruction or GI atony, patients with toxic megacolon, and those with chronic renal, hepatic, pulmonary, or cardiac disease. These drugs are considered to belong in pregnancy category C.

⫶ Drug Interactions

Concurrent use of antacids and anticholinergics results in decreased absorption of the anticholinergics. Table 15-2 lists other drug classes that act synergistically with anticholinergic drugs, thereby increasing their action. Among the more commonly used drugs with anticholinergic effects are antihistamines, procainamide, meperidine, and tricyclic antidepressants. Concurrent use of anticholinergic drugs with ketoconazole or levodopa may cause decreased absorption and efficacy of the anticholinergic drug. Wax matrix formulations of potassium chloride should be used cautiously with atropine because of the risk of mucosal lesions.

Simultaneous use of ethanol or CNS depressants and scopolamine results in increased CNS depression. Stress this interaction to patients who use the scopolamine patch for motion sickness prophylaxis. Even moderate use of alcohol while using the patch may result in significant CNS depression.

▥ Dosage Regimen

The dosages of anticholinergic drugs are identified in Table 15-3. Because of the many uses of anticholinergic drugs, the health care provider must carefully check drug references for appropriate dosages. When using atropine for treatment of bradycardia and bradyarrhythmias, remember that doses of less than 0.5 mg can actually cause bradycardia. The maximum cumulative adult dose of intravenous (IV) atropine is 3 mg. Children's dosages of atropine are calculated based on body weight or square meters of body surface.

▥ Lab Considerations

Serum drug levels are not required with anticholinergic drugs. Dicyclomine and glycopyrrolate should not be used 24 hours before the pentagastrin and histamine gastric acid secretion tests. Dicyclomine acts as an antagonist to these other drugs. Glycopyrrolate may cause decreased uric acid levels in patients who have gout or hyperuricemia. Propantheline may cause elevated antinuclear antibody (ANA) titers, a condition that is usually asymptomatic and reversible.

CLINICAL REASONING

Treatment Objectives

The goal of treatment for the patient with IBS is to diminish the motility of the GI tract. When atropine is administered as an antidote to acetylcholinesterase-inhibitor toxicity, the objective is to reestablish the effect of the acetylcholinesterase.

Treatment Options

▥ Patient Variables

LIFE-SPAN CONSIDERATIONS

Pregnant and Nursing Women. Atropine, hyoscyamine, and the transdermal form of scopolamine cross the placenta. IV administration of atropine or hyoscyamine can result in fetal tachycardia. There have been isolated reports of fetal malformations associated with dicyclomine administration. Retrospective studies did not confirm the association. Parenteral administration of scopolamine during labor may cause CNS depression in the neonate. Owing to a reduction in clotting factors dependent on vitamin K, administration of parenteral scopolamine can contribute to neonatal hemorrhage. All of these factors make the use of these drugs in pregnant women a risk-versus-benefit decision. If the drugs are administered, closely monitor both the mother and fetus or neonate.

All of the anticholinergic drugs have the capacity to inhibit lactation. Atropine and hyoscyamine cross into breast milk. Infants are very sensitive to anticholinergics. Again, in the population of nursing mothers, the anticholinergics must be used judiciously. If long-term use is necessary, the mother must be counseled about the advisability of breastfeeding.

Children and Adolescents. In a hot environment, the decrease in perspiration caused by anticholinergics may result in the body temperature's reaching dangerous levels. Dicyclomine syrup used in infants under 3 months old may contribute to respiratory distress. The parenteral form of hyoscyamine contains benzyl alcohol as a preservative. Do not use this form in neonates or very young infants.

Older Adults. Any patient taking an anticholinergic may experience excitement, agitation, drowsiness, or confusion. In the older adult, these adverse effects occur more frequently and with greater severity. Memory impairment associated with an anticholinergic is due to inhibition of ACh action. The behavioral effects may be severe in patients with underlying cognitive dysfunction. Further, as a result of the changes of aging, these individuals are particularly prone to the constipation, dry mouth, and urinary retention that may accompany use of anticholinergics. Use anticholinergics cautiously in this population, because many older adults may have undiagnosed glaucoma.

▥ Drug Variables

Many patients find the adverse effects of anticholinergic drugs difficult to tolerate. These adverse effects are very similar among drugs in this class; therefore, switching to a different anticholinergic may not provide relief.

Hyoscyamine is more potent than atropine in the treatment of IBS. It also comes in a variety of formulations and strengths, which helps to individualize therapy and promote patient compliance. Scopolamine has an increased risk for adverse CNS effects compared with other anticholinergics. It is used primarily in the perioperative setting. Controversy exists as to whether or not transdermal scopolamine has the ability to decrease postoperative nausea and vomiting.

Patient Education

Instruct patients, family, and significant others that anticholinergic drugs may have undesirable adverse CNS effects. Encourage the patient to refrain from driving or other potentially dangerous activity until the effect of the drug is known. Encourage the patient to report dizziness, agitation, or disorientation to the health care provider. Dosage adjustment may be required.

Warn individuals who take anticholinergics about the risk of overheating in hot environments as a result of decreased perspiration. This is particularly pertinent to children and older adults, who may experience significant increases in body temperature. Prolonged use of anticholinergics decreases salivary flow and contributes to dental disorders. Tell patients to notify their dentist that they are taking anticholinergics. Decreased salivation makes patients more prone to dental caries, oral candidiasis infections, and periodontal disease. Encourage the use of sugarless hard candy and regular consultation with a dentist. Constipation may be lessened with increases in activity and fluid and fiber intake. Encourage the patient to consult the health care provider before beginning to use laxatives.

Evaluation

Successful treatment using an anticholinergic drug is determined by relief or decrease of symptoms. Patients with IBS should expect less muscle spasm and abdominal discomfort. The frequency or amount of diarrhea may not be greatly affected.

STIMULATION AND BLOCKADE OF GANGLIONS

Ganglionic Stimulants

With the exception of nicotine gum and transdermal nicotine patches, there are no therapeutically useful ganglionic stimulant drugs. However, it is important that they be understood because of their toxic effects. Nicotine is used in smoking cessation programs. The gum, transdermal, and puffed formulations provide a source of nicotine for the nicotine-dependent patient who is attempting smoking cessation.

Ganglionic stimulants activate nicotinic receptors at ganglionic sites rather than at the effector organs such as muscle. Thus stimulation occurs as a result of norepinephrine release from sympathetic fibers and ACh release from parasympathetic fibers. These actions generate nerve impulses down postganglionic fibers to produce specific effects on smooth muscle, cardiac muscle, and glands. Nicotine stimulates the CNS, particularly the respiratory, vomiting, and vasomotor centers in the medulla oblongata. Large doses of nicotine cause tremors and seizure activity. The curare-like effects of nicotine on diaphragmatic nerve endings contribute to the risk of respiratory failure and death. The heart rate slows but later may increase above normal, with arrhythmias noted. Small peripheral blood vessels may first constrict, only to dilate with a resultant fall in the blood pressure. Nicotine also has an antidiuretic effect. Nicotine is further discussed in Chapter 12.

Ganglionic Blockers

The only remaining use for ganglionic blockers such as mecamylamine (Inversine) in hypertension is for the initial control of blood pressure in patients with acute dissecting aortic aneurysm and for managing uncomplicated malignant hypertension. Ganglionic blockers are ideal for these purposes, because they not only reduce blood pressure but also inhibit sympathetic reflexes. Thus they reduce the rate of the rise of pressure at the site of the aneurysm.

Mecamylamine reduces arterial blood pressure by diminishing autonomic outflow to the heart and vascular smooth muscle at the level of the thoracolumbar autonomic ganglia. Arteriolar and venous smooth muscle tone is thus reduced. Venous dilation promotes peripheral pooling of blood and diminishes venous return to the heart. Arteriolar dilation decreases total peripheral resistance and organ vascular resistance. Autonomic inhibition of the heart results in diminished cardiac reflexes.

Mecamylamine is completely absorbed from the GI tract. It has a gradual onset of action of 0.5 to 2 hours, with effects lasting 6 to 12 hours and elimination unchanged in the urine. The rate of renal elimination is markedly influenced by urinary pH. Alkaline urine reduces the elimination of the drug, whereas acidic urine promotes renal elimination.

Mecamylamine interferes with parasympathetic as well as sympathetic function. The adverse effects include orthostatic hypotension; an inability to focus vision for near sight (accommodation); drying of secretions in the eyes, the mouth, and the stomach; paralytic ileus; retention of urine; and failure of erection and ejaculation. Mecamylamine readily penetrates the brain to produce syncopal episodes, paresthesias, weakness, fatigue, sedation, tremor, choreiform movements, mental aberrations, and seizure activity. These adverse effects occur with large doses and may be worsened in patients with renal insufficiency. Glossitis, anorexia, nausea, and vomiting are possible. Do not use mecamylamine in patients with mild, moderate, or labile hypertension. Also, it may be unsuitable for uncooperative patients. The drug is contraindicated for use in patients with coronary insufficiency or recent myocardial infarction. Mecamylamine crosses the blood-brain and placental barriers and is distributed in breast milk (FDA pregnancy category C).

Patients receiving antibiotics and sulfonamides should not receive ganglionic blockers. The action of mecamylamine is potentiated by anesthesia, other antihypertensive drugs, and alcohol.

Mecamylamine therapy is usually started with one 2.5-mg tablet twice a day. Adjust this initial dosage in daily increments of 2.5 mg, at intervals of no less than 2 days, until the desired blood pressure response occurs (i.e., dosage below that which causes signs of mild postural hypotension). The average total daily dose of mecamylamine is 25 mg, given in three divided doses. Patients may develop a partial tolerance and thus require an increased dosage. Hypertensive levels return if ganglionic blockers or other potent antihypertensive drugs are suddenly discontinued. In patients with a history of malignant hypertension, the return to hypertension may occur abruptly, causing a fatal stoke or heart failure.

NEUROMUSCULAR BLOCKADE

Neuromuscular blockers are most frequently used in the operating room, primarily as an adjunct to general anesthesia to facilitate endotracheal intubation and to relax skeletal muscle during surgery. More recently, health care providers in intensive care units and emergency rooms have found them useful in the management of respiratory problems. Neuromuscular blockers commonly are classified by type of block produced (depolarizing versus nondepolarizing), chemical structure, or duration of action (ultra–short-acting, short-acting, intermediate-acting, or long-acting). However, to help the reader understand neuromuscular blockade, a brief review of physiology follows.

No muscle stays completely relaxed. So long as the patient is conscious, muscles remain slightly contracted. This condition is called *tonus*. When a muscle contracts, a nerve impulse is sent from the brain and spinal cord through a motor neuron to muscle cell membranes at a communication point called the *motor endplate*. The space between the nerve and the muscle membrane is known as the *neuromuscular junction*. The neuromuscular junction is composed of the axon, the presynaptic motor nerve terminals, the synaptic cleft, and the postsynaptic motor endplate membranes (Fig. 15-2). Nerve impulses arriving at the motor neuron evoke liberation of ACh stored in presynaptic vesicles. ACh release occurs through the calcium-dependent process of exocytosis. ACh

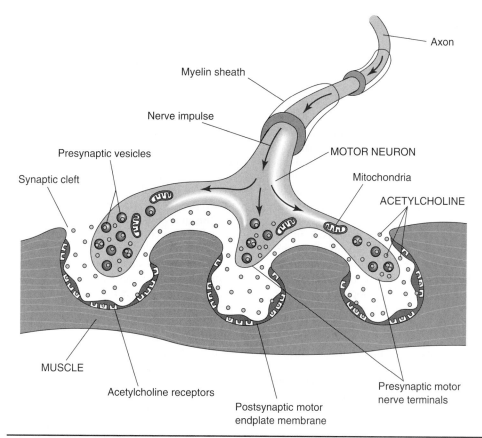

FIGURE 15-2 The term *neuromuscular junction* refers to the axon terminal of a motor neuron together with the motor endplate. Distal ends of axon terminals expand into bulblike structures called *presynaptic motor nerve terminals*. The structures contain vesicles that store neurotransmitters (e.g., ACh and norepinephrine). Presynaptic motor nerve terminals come into close approximation with the muscle fiber. Direct-acting cholinergics stimulate cholinergic receptors in postsynaptic membranes that are innervated by parasympathetic neurons (see Chapter 43). They mimic the action of acetylcholine. Cholinesterase-inhibitor drugs act primarily by shielding ACh from acetylcholinesterase. The blocking effects result in accumulation of ACh at all sites where it is liberated. Anticholinergic drugs block the action of ACh at postganglionic sites.

diffuses across the synapse to reversibly bind to cholinergic receptors located on the postsynaptic motor endplate. One molecule of ACh binds to each of two sites on a single cholinergic receptor to induce the ion channel to open. Once the channel opens, sodium ions flow through, causing depolarization of the muscle cell. The degree of depolarization is proportional to the number of receptors occupied. After depolarization of the endplate, ACh binds to acetylcholinesterase, where it is hydrolyzed to acetate and choline. Calcium released from the sarcoplasmic reticulum binds to troponin C (a complex of muscle proteins), uncovering myosin-binding sites on actin. Cross-linkages form between actin and myosin, resulting in contraction of skeletal muscle.

Sustained muscle contraction demands an endless series of action potentials. The generation of action potentials results in repeated release of ACh. In turn, there is repeated stimulation of cholinergic receptors on the motor endplate. Repeating cycles of depolarization and repolarization result in sufficient release of calcium from the sarcoplasmic reticulum to sustain the contraction. If the motor endplate remains depolarized, the stimuli for calcium release stop. There is an immediate reuptake of calcium by the sarcoplasmic reticulum, and muscle contraction ceases.

PHARMACOTHERAPEUTIC OPTIONS

Nondepolarizing Neuromuscular Blockers
- atracurium (Tracrium)
- cisatracurium (Nimbex)
- doxacurium (Nuromax)
- gallamine (Flaxedil)
- metocurine (Metubine Iodide)
- mivacurium (Mivacron)
- pancuronium (Pavulon)
- pipecuronium (Arduan)
- rocuronium (Zemuron)
- tubocurarine; ◆ Tubarine
- vecuronium (Norcuron)

Depolarizing Neuromuscular Blocker
- succinylcholine chloride (Anectine, Quelicin, Sucostrin)

▌ Indications
There are limited uses for nondepolarizing neuromuscular blockers. Neuromuscular blockers are not sedatives or analgesics. They do not affect consciousness or pain perception. They are used most often to produce muscle relaxation during

endotracheal intubation and surgical procedures, and to facilitate mechanical ventilation. Some drugs have been used as an adjunct during electroconvulsive therapy (ECT). Tubocurarine has been used to diagnose myasthenia gravis. Another use of nondepolarizing blockers is in the management of tetanus, a potentially fatal bacterial infection.

Intubation generally involves the use of neuromuscular blockers, because laryngeal stimulation is associated with reflex closure of vocal cords and hypoxemia if intubation is unsuccessful. Neuromuscular blockers are used during intraabdominal and intrathoracic procedures to prevent reflex muscle contraction and to permit surgical exposure and effective wound closure. Reflex muscle responses can be suppressed by high concentrations of a volatile anesthetic, but this practice results in circulatory depression.

Neuromuscular blockers are used for patients requiring mechanical ventilation for three primary reasons. They promote ventilation by reducing or eliminating spontaneous breathing efforts. They reduce oxygen consumption in patients with severely compromised cardiopulmonary function. Lastly, neuromuscular blockers reduce motor activity that may disturb vascular catheters, access tubes, and surgical dressings.

Neuromuscular blockers also prevent the intense muscle contracture and rigidity associated with tetanus that causes serious systemic problems (e.g., electrolyte imbalances owing to muscle damage). They also aid in mechanical ventilation of the patient when needed.

Succinylcholine is the most commonly used depolarizing drug. It is used primarily to produce muscle relaxation during endotracheal intubation, ECT, endoscopy, and other short procedures.

▥ Pharmacodynamics

ACh must bind to nicotinic receptors for normal neuromuscular transmission to occur. Nondepolarizing neuromuscular blockers compete with ACh for binding to nicotinic receptors on the motor endplate. Thus muscle relaxation lasts as long as the quantity of drug at the neuromuscular junction is adequate to deter receptor occupation by ACh. Muscle strength can be restored by increasing the amount of ACh at the neuromuscular junction or by increasing drug elimination from the body.

Although nondepolarizing drugs paralyze all skeletal muscles, the paralysis affects muscles in a specific and predictable sequence. Small, rapidly moving muscles of the eyes, the face, and the neck are affected first. Muscles of the limbs, the abdomen, and the trunk are affected next, followed by the intercostal muscles and the diaphragm. Muscle weakness rapidly progresses to flaccid paralysis. Typically, recovery from drug-induced paralysis occurs in reverse order from the induction sequence.

Like ACh, succinylcholine binds to receptors at the motor endplate to produce depolarization. However, unlike ACh, succinylcholine remains receptor bound for several minutes, and muscles do not respond to the subsequent release of ACh. Succinylcholine is biotransformed by plasma cholinesterase, and the postjunctional cholinergic membrane repolarizes. Repolarization and further muscle contractions are inhibited as long as an adequate concentration of drug remains at receptor sites. Histamine is released, which may contribute to hypotension.

▥ Pharmacokinetics

As a class these drugs are poorly absorbed from the GI tract and therefore must be administered parenterally. Muscular paralysis develops in minutes following IV administration. Peak effects are reached in 2 to 10 minutes, with the duration of effective paralysis lasting 45 minutes to hours (Table 15-5). Complete recovery may take several hours.

Pancuronium, vecuronium, and rocuronium are biotransformed in the liver. Atracurium and mivacurium are broken down in the plasma. The majority of the nondepolarizing

PHARMACOKINETICS

TABLE 15-5 Selected NM Blockers

Drugs	Onset	Time to Maximum Paralysis	Duration of Effective Paralysis*	Time to Spontaneous Recovery†	PB (%)	t½
LONG-ACTING NONDEPOLARIZING DRUGS						
doxacurium	5 min	4–10 min	100 min	Hours	30	99 min
metocurine	1–4 min	6 min	25–90 min	Hours	55	3.6 hr
pipecuronium	2.5–3 min	3–5 min	60–120 min	Hours	UA	1.7 hr
tubocurarine	1 min	2–5 min	35–60 min	Hours	40–45	2 hr
INTERMEDIATE-ACTING NONDEPOLARIZING DRUGS						
atracurium	2–2.5 min	5 min	30–40 min	60–70 min	82	20 min
cisatracurium	1–2 min	5–7 min	22–63 min	60–70 min	UA‡	20
gallamine	1–2 min	3–5 min	15–30 min	—	16	2.5 hr
pancuronium	30–45 sec	3–4.5 min	35–45 min	60–120 min	15	2 hr
rocuronium	1 min	1.8 min	31 min	13 min	30	1.4 hr
vecuronium	1 min	3–5 min	15–30 min	45–60 min	27	31–80 min
SHORT-ACTING NONDEPOLARIZING DRUG						
mivacurium	2.5 min	3.3 min	26 min	6–8 min	UA	2 hr
ULTRA–SHORT-ACTING DEPOLARIZING DRUG						
succinylcholine	0.5–1 min	1–2 min	4–10 min	—	30	2–8 min

*Duration of effective paralysis varies with dosage. Figures presented are for an average adult dose administered as a single IV injection.
†Spontaneous recovery from paralysis can take a long time. Reversal of nondepolarizing drug effects is accomplished by administering a cholinesterase inhibitor.
‡Protein binding for cisatracurium has not been successfully studied owing to its rapid degradation at physiologic pH.
NM, Neuromuscular; *PB*, protein binding; *t½*, half-life; *UA*, unavailable.

neuromuscular blockers are eliminated unchanged in the urine. The half-life of nondepolarizing neuromuscular blockers ranges from 20 minutes to 4 hours.

Succinylcholine is well absorbed intravenously and is widely distributed into extracellular fluid. It crosses the placenta in small amounts. The onset of skeletal muscle relaxation occurs in 30 seconds to 1 minute, with peak paralysis noted in 1 to 2 minutes. Paralysis lasts from 4 to 10 minutes. Ninety percent of the drug is biotransformed by pseudocholinesterase in the plasma. Ten percent is eliminated unchanged by the kidneys. The half-life of succinylcholine is unknown, although some claim the half-life to be around 1 minute.

▌ *Adverse Effects and Contraindications*

The principal adverse effects of nondepolarizing neuromuscular blockers are on the cardiovascular and respiratory systems. The underlying physiologic mechanisms for the adverse cardiovascular effects are identified in Table 15-6. Neuromuscular blockers cause hypotension through partial ganglionic blockade and histamine release. Ganglionic blockade decreases sympathetic tone of arterioles and veins, with subsequent vasodilation. Histamine release also promotes vasodilation. Ganglionic blockade is common with metocurine and tubocurarine. Metocurine, tubocurarine, and atracurium cause histamine release and thus a drop in blood pressure. Blockade of muscarinic receptors results in tachycardia, yet bradycardia, arrhythmias, and cardiac arrest can result. However, the mechanism that underlies these latter effects is unclear.

Paralysis of intercostal muscles and the diaphragm leads to respiratory arrest. Overadministration of drugs, an accumulation of active metabolites, and end-organ damage or dysfunction can result in short-term persistent paralysis that lasts from hours to days. The paralysis is clearly drug-based. Long-term persistent paralysis lasts from days to weeks and is characterized by muscle and nerve degeneration.

Contraindications to nondepolarizing neuromuscular blockers include hypersensitivity to this class of drugs or to bromides (only pancuronium and vecuronium) and iodides or iodine (only gallamine and metocurine). Products containing benzyl alcohol should be avoided in neonates.

Cautious use of nondepolarizing drugs is warranted in patients with dehydration, electrolyte imbalance, or underlying cardiovascular disease (because of an increased risk of arrhythmias). Situations in which histamine release may occur (e.g., asthma, allergic conditions) could be problematic. Closely monitor older adults and patients with impaired renal function, which can lead to decreased elimination of gallamine, metocurine, pancuronium, and tubocurarine. Hepatic disease reduces biotransformation of vecuronium. Shock related to prolonged paralysis from gallamine, metocurine, and tubocurarine has been noted. Cautious use is also warranted in patients with low plasma pseudocholinesterase levels associated with anemia, dehydration, the use of cholinesterase inhibitors or insecticides, severe liver disease, or pregnancy.

The safety of use during pregnancy or lactation or in children has not been established for most agents. Exercise extreme caution when using neuromuscular blockers for patients with myasthenia gravis or myasthenic syndromes. Patients with myasthenia gravis, an autoimmune disorder characterized by antibodies to the nicotinic ACh receptor, are extremely sensitive to nondepolarizing neuromuscular blockers.

Most adverse effects of succinylcholine are extensions of pharmacologic effects. The adverse effects include bronchospasm and apnea, hypotension, arrhythmias, bradycardia, hyperkalemia, tachyphylaxis, and muscle fasciculations. The risk of myoglobinemia and myoglobinuria is increased in children. Malignant hyperthermia is the most life-threatening adverse effect of succinylcholine.

Muscle fasciculations that occur as a result of drug action often result in postoperative myalgias. Some 10% to 70% of patients complain of neck, shoulder, and back pain 12 to 24 hours after administration. The discomfort can persist for several days.

AUTONOMIC NERVOUS

TABLE **15-6 Physiologic Causes of CV Adverse Effects***

Drugs	Histamine Release	Ganglionic Blockade	Vagolytic Activity
LONG-ACTING NON-DEPOLARIZING DRUGS			
doxacurium	None	None	None
metocurine	Slight	Weak	None
pancuronium	Slight	None	Increased
pipecuronium	None	None	None
tubocurarine	Moderate	Weak	Decreased
INTERMEDIATE-ACTING NON-DEPOLARIZING DRUGS			
atracurium	Slight	None	Minimal effect
cisatracurium	None	None	Minimal effect
gallamine	High dose only	None	Increased
rocuronium	None	None	Increased
vecuronium	None	None	None
SHORT-ACTING NON-DEPOLARIZING DRUG			
mivacurium	Slight	None	Slightly increased
ULTRA–SHORT-ACTING DEPOLARIZING DRUG			
succinylcholine	Slight	Stimulated	Increased or decreased

*Histamine release is related to the dose and speed of administration. CV effects can be lessened by minimizing the dose and increasing IV administration time. The histamine response can be minimized by pretreating the patient with histamine$_1$ and histamine$_2$ antagonists.
CV, Cardiovascular.

Succinylcholine is contraindicated for use in patients with hypersensitivity to the drug or to parabens, and in patients with pseudocholinesterase deficiency. Continuous infusion of succinylcholine is contraindicated in children and neonates. Succinylcholine raises intraocular pressure and is absolutely contraindicated for use in patients with glaucoma.

A history of malignant hyperthermia, of pulmonary, renal, or liver impairment, or of myasthenia gravis or myasthenic syndromes warrants cautious use of succinylcholine. Use it with caution in older adults or debilitated patients, in the presence of electrolyte disturbances, and in patients receiving cardiac glycosides.

▥ Drug Interactions

Drug interactions with nondepolarizing drugs are many and occur at the terminal, synapse, or motor endplate of the nerve, and sometimes at more than one site. Table 15-7 provides an overview of key interacting drugs. The intensity and duration of paralysis may be prolonged if the patient has been pretreated in some fashion with succinylcholine (see the discussion of depolarizing drugs), inhaled general anesthesia, aminoglycosides and certain other antibiotics, quinidine, procainamide, beta blockers, potassium-losing diuretics, and magnesium. Most neuromuscular blockers are incompatible with barbiturates and sodium bicarbonate. High-dosage antibiotics may intensify or produce neuromuscular blockade on their own. They should not be admixed.

Concurrent administration of succinylcholine with cholinesterase inhibitors (i.e., echothiophate, isoflurophate, demecarium eye drops) reduces pseudocholinesterase activity and intensifies paralysis. The intensity and duration of paralysis can be prolonged in the presence of anesthetics, aminoglycoside antibiotics, cimetidine, polymyxin B, colistin, clindamycin, lidocaine, quinidine, procainamide, beta blockers, lithium, cyclophosphamide, phenelzine, potassium-losing diuretics, and magnesium. There is an increased risk of adverse cardiovascular reactions with opioids and cardiac glycosides.

▥ Dosage Regimen

The dosage regimen for nondepolarizing neuromuscular blockers depends on the purpose for their use (Table 15-8). Standard dosing according to body weight alone often results in overadministration of neuromuscular blockers. Maintenance doses differ from those administered initially and are titrated to patient response. Many of the drugs are administered as a continuous IV infusion. Although tubocurarine can be administered by intramuscular (IM) route, the preferred route is IV. The IM route can be used for infants and other patients who do not have venous access devices.

Succinylcholine dosing hinges on the reason for its use. However, a test dose followed by assessment of respiratory function is needed before administration. Additional doses are dependent on response. Continuous IV infusion is not recommended for children or neonates.

▥ Lab Considerations

The sustained depolarization produced by succinylcholine is associated with potassium leakage from muscle along with a slight increase in serum potassium concentrations. In patients with recent burns, spinal cord injuries, and myopathies, however, succinylcholine can lead to sudden hyperkalemia and cardiac arrest.

CLINICAL REASONING

Treatment Objectives

Neuromuscular blockers should be administered only by health care providers skilled in their use. There are three clinical outcomes of muscular relaxation: no evidence of spontaneous patient movement, some patient movement but no spontaneous respirations, and movement and spontaneous respirations. When the desired clinical outcome is no spontaneous movement, peripheral nerve stimulation is necessary to reduce the risk of excessive blockade.

Treatment Options

▥ Patient Variables

The preference for one neuromuscular blocker over another depends on the patient's end-organ dysfunction, the route of drug biotransformation and elimination, and the duration of therapy. The onset and duration of paralysis

DRUG INTERACTIONS
TABLE 15-7 Selected NM Blockers

Drug	Interactive Drugs	Interaction
NONDEPOLARIZING DRUGS		
Nondepolarizing drugs as a class	Cholinesterase inhibitors	Reversal of NM blockade
	Aminoglycoside antibiotics, clindamycin, colistin, polymyxin B, beta blockers, lidocaine, inhaled general anesthetics, opioid analgesics, magnesium, MAO inhibitors, potassium-losing diuretics, procainamide, quinidine, succinylcholine	Additive NM blockade, apnea, respiratory depression
DEPOLARIZING DRUG		
succinylcholine	Local anesthetics, cimetidine	Prolonged apnea
	Cholinesterase inhibitors, eye drops	Reduced pseudocholinesterase activity and intensify paralysis
	Cardiac glycosides, opioids	Increased risk of adverse cardiovascular effects

MAO, Monoaminse oxidase; *NM,* neuromuscular.

DOSAGE

TABLE **15-8 Selected NM Blockers**

Drug	Use(s)	Dosage	Implications
LONG-ACTING NONDEPOLARIZING DRUGS			
doxacurium	Skeletal muscle paralysis and facilitation of intubation; facilitation of compliance during mechanical ventilation	*Adult:* 50 mcg/kg IV initially, followed 60–100 min later by 5–10 mcg/kg, repeated as necessary. May need up to 80 mcg/kg for prolonged effect, 25 mcg/kg for succinylcholine-assisted intubation *Child 2–12 yr:* 30–50 mcg/kg IV initially	Maintenance doses may be required more frequently in children than in adults.
metacurine	Adjunct to ECT	*Adult:* 150–400 mcg/kg IV initially. Additional doses of 0.5–1 mg every 30–90 min *Adjunct to ECT:* 1.75–5.5 mg IV	Relaxation from initial dose averages 60 min. Administer supplemental doses as needed.
pancuronium	Skeletal muscle paralysis and facilitation of intubation and mechanical ventilation	*Adult or Child >1 mo:* 40–100 mcg/kg initially. Incremental doses of 10 mcg/kg may be given every 20 min to maintain paralysis	Relaxation for mechanical ventilation: 15 mcg/kg. Monitor for prolonged drug effects beyond the time needed or anticipated by drug use. Supportive care may be needed.
pipecuronium	Skeletal muscle paralysis and facilitation of intubation and mechanical ventilation	*Adult:* 70–85 mcg/kg (if given following recovery from succinylcholine; decrease dose to 50 mcg/kg if longer paralysis is desired). Additional doses of 10–15 mcg/kg may be required for maintenance *Child 1–14 yr:* 57 mcg/kg IV initial dose *Infant 3 mo-1 yr:* 40 mcg/kg IV initial dose	Dosage reduction recommended with concurrent use of inhaled anesthetics. Dosage determined on basis of IBW in obese patients and may require adjustments in patients with renal impairment. Recommended only for procedures lasting less than 90 min.
tubocurarine	Diagnosis of myasthenia gravis; adjunct to ECT	*Adult:* 6–9 mg initially IV followed by 3–4.5 mg after 3–5 min if needed. Additional doses of 0.165 mg/kg as needed *Infant or Child:* 500–600 mcg/kg IV *Neonates—4 wk:* 250–500 mcg/kg initially; additional increments at one fifth to one sixth of the initial dose may be given. *Mechanical ventilation:* 16.5 mcg/kg with subsequent doses as necessary *Adjunct to ECT:* 165 mcg/kg IV. Initial doses should be 3 mg less than calculated dose. *Diagnosis of myasthenia gravis:* 4–33 mcg/kg IV	When drug is used for diagnosis of myasthenia gravis, profound myasthenic symptoms may occur. Do not use any solution that has developed a faint color.
INTERMEDIATE-ACTING NONDEPOLARIZING DRUGS			
atracurium	Skeletal muscle paralysis and facilitation of intubation and mechanical ventilation	*Adult or child >2 yr:* 0.4–0.5 mg/kg initially IV, followed by continuous infusion of 2–15 mcg/kg/ min. Dosage is 0.25–0.35 mg/kg if given after steady-state anesthesia achieved with enflurane or isoflurane, –or– 0.3–0.4 mg/kg following succinyl choline *Child 1 mo-2 yr:* 0.3–0.4 mg/kg initially (while under halothane anesthesia)	Do not use before induction of unconsciousness. Bradycardia during anesthesia is common.
cisatracurium		*Adult:* 0.15 mg/kg initially IV, followed by 0.03 mg/kg every 40–50 min based on response to sustain NM blockade. Continuous IV infusion under nitrous oxide, oxygen, and opioid anesthesia: 1–2 mcg/kg IV. Max dose: 1.6 mg/kg *Child 2–12 yr:* 0.1 mg/kg IV. For NMB maintenance in ICU: 3 mcg/kg/min IV infusion; titrate to response	This relatively new drug is primarily used for short procedures.
gallamine		*Adult or Child:* 1 mg/kg (not to exceed 100 mg/dose) initially, and then 0.5–1 mg/kg may be given 30–40 min later if needed	Dose cautiously in patients weighing <5 kg. Monitor patient for increased heart rate
rocuronium		*Adult:* 0.6 mg/kg IV for rapid-sequence ET intubation. Maintenance: 0.1–0.2 mg/kg. Continuous IV infusion: 0.01–0.012 mg/kg/ min, with a range of 4–16 mcg/kg/min *Child:* 0.6 mg/kg for intubation. Maintenance dose: 0.075–0.125 mg/kg IV. Continuous IV infusion: 0.012 mg/kg/min	Dosages are not different in obese and nonobese patients when calculated on their actual body weight
vecuronium		*Intubation of Adult or Child >10 yr:* 80–100 mcg/kg (60–85 mcg/kg if given after steady-state anesthesia achieved, or 40–60 mcg/kg after succinylcholine-assisted intubation and anesthesia). Wait for disappearance of succinylcholine effects (or 50–60 mcg/kg during balanced anesthesia). Maintenance: 10–15 mcg/kg 25–40 min after initial dose, then every 12–15 min as needed –or– as a continuous IV infusion at 0.8–1.2 mcg/kg/min	Doses of 150–280 mcg/kg have been used in some patients for intubation. Prolonged NM blockade has been reported. Monitor patient during recovery, and provide supportive care.

Continued

AUTONOMIC NERVOUS

DOSAGE
TABLE 15-8 Selected NM Blockers—Cont'd

Drug	Use(s)	Dosage	Implications
SHORT-ACTING NONDEPOLARIZING DRUG			
mivacurium	Skeletal muscle paralysis and facilitation of intubation; facilitation of compliance during mechanical ventilation	*Adult:* 150–200 mcg/kg IV initially, then 100 mcg/kg as bolus doses every 15 min or as a continuous infusion at 9–10 mcg/kg/min. Start at 4 mcg/kg/min if infusion is begun at same time as initial dose. Infusion rates vary: 1–20 mcg/kg/min *Child 2–12 yr:* 200 mcg/kg IV initially. May be repeated as needed or continued as an infusion at 14 mcg/kg/ min. Average range: 5–31 mcg/kg/min	Do not use before unconsciousness has been induced.
ULTRA–SHORT ACTING DEPOLARIZING DRUG			
succinylcholine	Skeletal muscle paralysis; adjunct to ECT	*Test dose in Adult:* 0.1 mg/kg IV; then assess respiratory function *Short procedures in Adult:* 0.3–1.1 mg/kg, with additional doses dependent on response *Short Procedure in Child:* 1–2 mg/kg, with additional doses dependent on response *Prolonged Procedures in Adult:* 0.6 mg/kg initially, then 0.04–0.07 mg/kg as necessary *ECT in Adult:* 10–30 mg IV 1 min before shock. Further individualization of dose may be required.	Continuous IV infusion not recommended in children or neonates for short procedures. Continuous IV infusion is preferred in adults for prolonged procedures. Monitor patient for histamine release and resultant hypotension and flushing.

ECT, Electroconvulsive therapy; *ET,* endotracheal; *IBW,* ideal body weight; *ICU,* intensive care unit; *IV,* intravenous; *NM,* neuromuscular; *NMB,* neuromuscular blockade.

should be equivalent to that dictated by the procedure. Relatively short procedures (e.g., intubation) require a short-acting agent. Bolus administrations of intermediate-acting or long-acting drugs are used for longer procedures (e.g., radiologic scans or dressing changes). Lengthy procedures may require intermittent doses of long-acting drugs or continuous infusions of short-acting or intermediate-acting drugs.

Because the ability to interact with the paralyzed patient is lost, physical examination of the patient cannot be accurately performed; identifying changes in mental status or the presence of anginal pain, seizures, or peritonitis is difficult when the patient is paralyzed. Some health care providers advocate stopping neuromuscular blockade every 24 hours to reassess the patient and evaluate the need for continued paralysis. However, reversing the paralysis may result in deterioration of the condition that required the paralysis.

Patients requiring mechanical ventilation are at risk for respiratory distress syndrome. Signs of impending distress include desaturation with movement, rising peak inspiratory pressures, and difficulty maintaining adequate blood gas values despite sedation. Many times, drug-induced paralysis prevents or minimizes the risks of further complications.

Hyperkalemia may develop after a dose of succinylcholine in patients with burns, intraabdominal abscess, or trauma, or in patients confined to bed. Use atracurium with caution in patients with asthma or allergies because of the likelihood of histamine-induced bronchospasm. Avoid long-term administration of steroid-based neuromuscular blockers (e.g., pancuronium, pipecuronium, and vecuronium) in patients with severe renal failure (because of accumulation of active metabolites). Of the currently available neuromuscular blockers, doxacurium, pipecuronium, cisatracurium, and vecuronium are essentially devoid of clinically significant cardiovascular effects. These are the drugs of choice for patients with unstable cardiovascular profiles (Box 15-1).

BOX 15-1

Factors Altering Responses to Neuromuscular Blockers

Potentiating Factors	Antagonizing Factors
Acidosis	Alkalosis
Aminoglycosides, lincomycin, neomycin, polymyxins, tetracyclines, vancomycin	aminophylline
	Burns
Benzodiazepines, midazolam	Hypercalcemia,
Beta blockers	hyperkalemia
Calcium channel blockers	Pregnancy
Corticosteroids	ranitidine
droperidol, lithium	
Hypocalcemia, hypokalemia, hypothermia	
magnesium sulfate	
Neuromuscular disease	
nitroglycerin, procainamide	
phenytoin	
Potassium-wasting diuretics	

Nondepolarizing drugs are safe to use in patients susceptible to malignant hyperthermia. The depolarizing drug succinylcholine can trigger malignant hyperthermia and is absolutely contraindicated for use in susceptible patients.

▓ Drug Variables

The drug of choice is influenced by the mode of administration. Long-acting neuromuscular blockers are usually given by intermittent injection. Short-acting or intermediate-acting drugs are suited for bolus injection or continuous infusion. Continuous infusion provides stable blockade for extended periods. Even though continuous infusions are more convenient, patients must be closely monitored to avoid excessive dosing. Intermittent doses of short-acting or intermediate-acting drugs may be used for short-term paralysis. However, long-term use of this technique is inconvenient and permits wide fluctuations in the degree of blockade. On the other hand, this mode allows for assessment of patient movement before each dose is given, which minimizes the risk of unintentional overdose. If a drug or its metabolite accumulates, the time between doses can be lengthened. The single disadvantage is simple: dosing based on patient movement contradicts the original purpose of the neuromuscular blockade.

In determining which nondepolarizing blocker to use, take into consideration the patient's history and physical exam results, as well as the drug's characteristics. Tubocurarine causes the greatest amount of histamine release and ganglionic blockade compared with other neuromuscular blockers. As a result, the risk of hypotension is relatively high. Doxacurium is essentially devoid of adverse cardiovascular effects. Pipecuronium does not cause histamine release and does not produce vagal blockade. It is relatively free of adverse cardiovascular effects. Age has no effect on pipecuronium's duration of paralysis.

Atracurium's organ-independent biotransformation makes it attractive for patients with multiple organ system failure. Gallamine causes histamine release in high doses. Other intermediate-acting neuromuscular blockers cause slight or no histamine release and no ganglionic blockade. Gallium, pancuronium, and rocuronium can cause tachycardia by blocking vagal input to the heart. Like gallamine, pancuronium can cause tachycardia through its vagolytic effects. Vecuronium does not produce ganglionic or vagal blockade and does not cause histamine release; thus cardiovascular effects are minimal.

Mivacurium causes cutaneous flushing secondary to histamine release. Other cardiovascular effects are minimal. Its duration of blockade at equipotent doses is 2 times greater than that of atracurium or vecuronium.

Succinylcholine causes large amounts of histamine to be released and stimulates ganglionic blockade. It may increase or decrease vagolytic activity.

Patient Education

Explain all procedures to the patient receiving neuromuscular blockers, particularly when they are used without general anesthesia. Remember, consciousness is not affected when these drugs are used alone. Routinely remind the patients why they are paralyzed and that the paralysis is only temporary. Reassure them that communication abilities and movement will return as the drug wears off. Also reassure patients that they will be monitored closely during the period of paralysis.

Muscle fasciculations during the initial phase of succinylcholine action account for patient complaints of muscle pain. A small dose of a nondepolarizing agent may be used before succinylcholine is administered to decrease the severity of muscle fasciculations and the resultant myalgia. Administer sedatives (e.g., lorazepam and midazolam) or analgesics (e.g., morphine, alfentanil, and fentanyl) concurrently when prolonged therapy is required. Reassure the patient that the discomfort, although unpleasant, is expected and temporary. The discomfort can persist for several hours or days.

Evaluation

The effectiveness of therapy with neuromuscular blockers is demonstrated by adequate suppression of the twitch response when it is tested with peripheral nerve stimulation and subsequent muscle paralysis.

Increased blood pressure and heart rate, diaphoresis, and lacrimation during a painful procedure (e.g., endotracheal tube suctioning) may indicate inadequate sedation and analgesia. The ability to assist or impede ventilator breaths, gagging, or coughing during suctioning indicates that the patient is inadequately paralyzed or sedated. Conversely, failure to produce a physiologic response during stimulation may indicate that the levels of sedation and/or analgesia are excessive.

Because the patient will be awake but will not appear to be, ensure that conversations taking place in the patient's presence contain only what is suitable for the patient to hear. A sign should be placed on the patient's bed to alert visitors that the patient is in a drug-induced paralysis. Take care to ensure patient comfort (e.g., frequent mouth care, frequent repositioning, and bathing) when these drugs are used for prolonged periods. Protect the patient's corneas with ocular lubricants (e.g., artificial tears), because the eyelids will remain open. If a patient will be paralyzed for extended periods, a special bed should be used to minimize pressure areas. Implement physical therapy and anticoagulation, which are considered to help maintain range of motion of joints and minimize the risk of deep vein thrombosis.

Check vital signs and temperature every hour during neuromuscular blockade. Close monitoring of intake and output is necessary to predict drug excretion and end-organ function. In addition, neurologic signs (including pupillary reaction) must be monitored closely. Devastating neurologic events are often difficult to recognize because of the drug-induced muscular paralysis.

Closely monitor respirations during periods of peak drug activity. Intubation and ventilation equipment should be readily available because all neuromuscular blockers can cause respiratory arrest. An Ambu bag and mask must always be kept at the patient's bedside. All ventilator alarms must be kept on. Patients also benefit from pulse oximetry and end-tidal carbon dioxide (CO_2) monitoring. Decreasing oxygen saturation or increasing CO_2 tension may indicate that patients are not being effectively ventilated and oxygenated. Ensure that anticholinesterase drugs are readily available to reverse respiratory depression. Remember, reversal agents are not effective for succinylcholine-induced respiratory depression.

Malignant hyperthermia has been associated with the use of succinylcholine. Determine whether or not there is a patient or family history of this disorder before its use. Monitor the patient throughout administration for signs that malignant hyperthermia may be developing. Signs of malignant hyperthermia include development of tachycardia, tachypnea, hypercapnia, jaw muscle spasm, lack of laryngeal relaxation, and hyperthermia. Monitor the heart rate and rhythm and blood pressure throughout the duration of the therapy.

Monitor Peripheral Nerve Stimulation

The extent of neuromuscular blockade is objectively assessed using peripheral nerve stimulation before and after treatment. Peripheral nerve stimulation is particularly helpful for patients who exhibit pharmacokinetic and pharmacodynamic characteristics predisposing them to prolonged paralysis. Failure to monitor blockade can result in an unintentional overdose.

▦ Reversal of Neuromuscular Blockade

Reversal of neuromuscular blockade is possible only with nondepolarizing drugs. The reversal drugs act at the neuromuscular junction to decrease the natural metabolism of acetylcholine and overcome the competitive block. The anticholinesterase drug (e.g., neostigmine, pyridostigmine, and edrophonium) is combined with a muscarinic receptor antagonist (e.g., atropine or glycopyrrolate) to prevent cardiac arrest and bronchospasm due to excess stimulation of muscarinic receptors.

Muscle tone returns either spontaneously with the discontinuation of the drug or after administration of an anticholinesterase reversal drug. Spontaneous return of muscle tone is permitted when the drug was used to facilitate intubation and mechanical ventilation. Reversal drugs are used to return muscle tone and respirations after surgical procedures. Reversal drugs are also used when a patient is weaned from mechanical ventilation and when immediate reversal of the neuromuscular blockade is needed. Spontaneous patient movement usually begins within 1 hour of discontinuation or reversal of the drug activity.

Check the gag reflex and the ability to swallow before administering oral drugs or food to a patient recovering from neuromuscular blockade to reduce the possibility of aspiration. Monitor the respiratory rate, depth, and adequacy during the period of recovery. Note changes in heart rate and blood pressure as indications for supplemental drugs.

KEY POINTS

- The treatment objective for Alzheimer's disease is to slow the progress of the dementia. The disease is not curable. Cholinesterase inhibitor drugs are used most often.
- Cholinesterase inhibitors act primarily by shielding ACh from degradation by the enzyme acetylcholinesterase. This results in accumulation of ACh at all sites where ACh is liberated.
- Although effective in reducing the cognitive dysfunction associated with Alzheimer's disease, some cholinesterase inhibitors carry a significant risk of liver dysfunction and require frequent monitoring of ALT levels.
- Irritable bowel syndrome may be treated with anticholinergic (muscarinic cholinergic inhibitor) drugs to reduce cramping. Anticholinergic drugs block the action of ACh at postganglionic receptor sites located in smooth muscle, secretory glands, the CNS, the SA and AV nodes, and cardiac muscle.
- Significant adverse effects of anticholinergics (e.g., dry mouth, blurred, vision, urinary retention) may decrease patient compliance.
- With the exception of nicotine there are no therapeutically useful ganglionic stimulant drugs. Ganglionic stimulants activate nicotinic cholinergic receptors at ganglionic sites rather than at effector organs such as muscle. Stimulation occurs as the result of norepinephrine release from sympathetic fibers and ACh release from parasympathetic fibers.
- Ganglionic blockers effectively prevent the autonomic nervous system from participating in body responses by blocking all transmission in the autonomic nervous system. The only remaining use of ganglionic blockers in hypertension is for the initial control of blood pressure in

patients with acute dissecting aortic aneurysm and in patients with uncomplicated malignant hypertension.
- Neuromuscular blockers are used for endotracheal intubation and surgical procedures, and to facilitate mechanical ventilation. Some drugs have been used as adjunctive agents during ECT. Tubocurarine can be used to diagnose myasthenia gravis.
- The primary differences in neuromuscular blockers are potency and duration of action. The degree of blockade required to facilitate patient management varies from patient to patient.
- Three clinical outcomes exist for neuromuscular blockade: no evidence of spontaneous patient movement; some patient movement but no spontaneous respirations; and movement and spontaneous respirations.
- Peripheral nerve stimulation monitoring is needed when the clinical objective is no patient movement, so as to reduce the risk of excessive blockade that may result from overdose.
- Reversal of nondepolarizing neuromuscular blockade is accomplished by administration of an anticholinesterase drug (e.g., neostigmine, pyridostigmine, edrophonium). There is no reversal agent for succinylcholine. Adequate reversal is noted when the patient can lift his or her head off the bed for at least 5 seconds.
- The health care provider has an essential role as patient advocate to ensure that every paralyzed patient, regardless of age, is adequately medicated with analgesics and sedatives. Neuromuscular blocking drugs should never be used as a substitute for analgesics and sedatives.

Bibliography

Abramowicz, M. (1997). Donepezil (Aricept) for Alzheimer's disease. *The Medical Letter on Drugs and Therapeutics, 39*(1002), 53–54.

Bender, K. (2005). Slowing the progression of Alzheimer's disease: The role of cholinesterase inhibitors. Supplement to *Consultant, 45*(3), 51–59.

Braunwald, E., Fauci, A., Kasper, D., et al. (2005). *Harrison's principles of internal medicine.* (15th ed.). New York: McGraw-Hill.

Collins, V. (1996). *Physiologic and pharmacologic bases of anesthesia.* Baltimore: Williams & Wilkins.

DiPiro, J., Talbert, R., Yee, G., et al. (2005). *Pharmacotherapy: A pathophysiologic approach.* (6th ed.). New York: McGraw-Hill.

Geldmacher, D. (1997). Donepezil (Aricept) therapy for Alzheimer's disease. *Comprehensive Therapy, 23*(7), 492–493.

Goldman, L., and Ausiello, D. (Eds.). (2005). *Cecil textbook of medicine* (22nd ed.). Philadelphia: WB Saunders.

Gutierrez, K., and Queener, S. (2003). *Pharmacology for nursing practice.* St. Louis: Mosby.

Hardman, L., and Limbird, L. (2001). *Goodman and Gilman's the pharmacological basis of therapeutics.* (10th ed.). New York: McGraw-Hill.

Karlawish, J., Casarett, D., Bioethics, J., et al. (2005). The ability of persons with Alzheimer disease (AD) to make a decision about taking an AD treatment. *Neurology, 64*(9), 1514–1519.

Larson, E., Shadlen, M., Want, L., et al. (2004). Survival after initial diagnosis of Alzheimer disease. *Annals of Internal Medicine, 140*(7), 501–509.

Martin, C., Viviand, X., Leone, M., et al. (2000). Effect of norepinephrine on the outcome of septic shock. *Critical Care Medicine, 28*(8), 2758–2765.

Minneman, K., and Wecker, L. (2005). *Brody's human pharmacology: Molecular to clinical.* (4th ed.). Philadelphia: Mosby.

Raskin, M., Peskind, E., Truyen, L., et al. (2004). The congnitive benifits of galantamine are sustained for at least 36 months: A long–term extension trial. *Archives of Neurology, 61(2), 252–256.*

Small, G., Ercoli, L., Silverman, D., et al. (2000). Cerebral metabolic and cognitive decline in persons at genetic risk for Alzheimer's disease. *Procedures of the National Academy of Science USA, 97*(11), 6037–6042.

AUTONOMIC NERVOUS

Opioid Analgesics and Related Drugs

The most popular definition of pain is put forth by Margo McCaffery, a widely recognized authority. According to McCaffery, *"Pain is whatever the person says it is, existing whenever he says it does"* (1999, p. 16). This definition requires that the patient be seen as the authority on his or her pain and the only person who can define the experience. Pain components span a three-level hierarchy: it has a sensory-discriminative component (e.g., location, intensity, quality), a motivational-affective component (e.g., depression, anxiety), and a cognitive-evaluative component (e.g., thoughts concerning the cause and significance of the pain). Pain is thus a combination of sensory, emotional, and cognitive factors; however, physical pathology does not necessarily have to be present for a patient to experience pain. Indeed, pain is the primary and sometimes, in the absence of other physical complaints, the sole symptom that causes people to see a health care provider.

The principal objective of pain management is not only to decrease pain to a tolerable level but also to improve a patient's level of functioning. Opioids, which are derived from the opium poppy, accomplish this objective in many cases. However, the importance and scope of effective pain management go well beyond alleviating patient suffering. Poorly managed pain significantly diminishes quality of life for all persons. Acute pain is associated with psychologic disturbances and changes in autonomic nervous system function.

PAIN

EPIDEMIOLOGY AND ETIOLOGY

Ninety percent of Americans ages 18 and older reported feeling pain at least once a month, and 42% of adults indicated that they experience pain at least once a day according to a 1999 Gallup survey (Blizzard, 2005). Some 75 million Americans have persistent pain, and at least 9% of the U.S. adult population is estimated to suffer from moderate to severe nonmalignant pain. Back pain is one of the most common pain complaints, second only to headache. Pain can also result from central or peripheral nervous system disorders, musculoskeletal damage, vascular disease, inflammation, or malignancy.

Treating patients with persistent pain can prove to be particularly challenging. A study conducted for The American Pain Society (1999) found that 47% of participants with moderate, severe, or very severe pain had chosen to see a different health care provider at least once since their first medical visit for pain relief. Participants attributed their change in provider to still having too much pain (42%), the provider's lack of knowledge about pain treatment (31%), the provider's not taking the pain seriously enough (29%), and the provider's unwillingness to treat their pain aggressively (27%). Women, minority groups, persons with cancer, and older adults, especially those living in a nursing home, have a heightened risk for receiving inadequate pain assessment and treatment.

PATHOGENESIS

Pain begins when pain fibers are stimulated. Painful stimuli can be mechanical (i.e., stretching of organs or pressure), thermal (i.e., heat or cold), or chemical (e.g., ischemia or inflammation). Pain can be present even in the absence of disease or a pathologic condition. Psychogenic pain, although not related to physiologic dysfunction, is pain nonetheless. Pain syndromes can be divided, based on their attributes, into nociceptive, neuropathic, psychogenic, mixed, or idiopathic forms.

Nociceptive Pain

The physiologic process of transmitting pain signals within the central nervous system (CNS) is called *nociception*. Nociceptors are simply free nerve endings found under the epidermis within deep tissues, muscles, tendons, and subcutaneous tissue. Nociceptors are unevenly distributed throughout the body, which accounts for variations in relative sensitivity to pain. Peripheral nociceptors are located at the distal ends of afferent sensory neurons. Some peripheral nociceptors may have a small amount of myelination or may have no myelination at all.

Mechanical, thermal, or chemical factors stimulate nociceptive nerve fibers, which in turn transmit impulses first to the spinal cord and then to the brain (Fig. 16-1). This transmission process is referred to as *transduction*. Many different substances are active in transduction including potassium, hydrogen, histamine, serotonin, and prostaglandins.

Transmission occurs when activated nociceptors send impulses to the CNS by way of specialized nerve fibers (Fig. 16-1). Known as A-sigma fibers, these are relatively large, and myelinated, which allows them to transmit pain impulses much more rapidly than the smaller, unmyelinated C fibers. A-sigma fibers transmit sharp, stinging, cutting, and pinching sensations, whereas C fibers transmit dull, aching, and burning sensations. Rapid transmission along A-sigma fibers allows a person to localize the pain quickly and withdraw from a potential source of injury. Pain signals transmitted by C fibers are of longer duration, are poorly localized, and tend to cause more distress for the patient.

Pain *perception* takes place once pain impulses are recognized within the cerebral cortex as painful. Pain perception is not necessarily related to the degree of tissue damage. Pain perception may be altered or *modulated* by the administration of drugs, by initiating other stimuli (such as rubbing a painful area), or by the release of endogenous endorphins within the body.

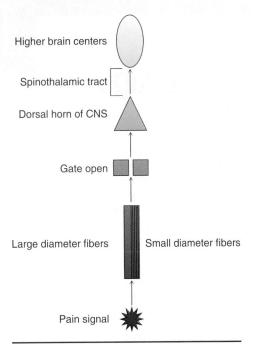

Higher brain centers

Spinothalamic tract

Dorsal horn of CNS

Gate open

Large diameter fibers   **Small diameter fibers**

Pain signal

FIGURE 16-1 **Gate Control Theory of Pain.** Pain signal is transmitted through small fibers to higher brain centers for interpretation. Transmission of a pain signal can be attenuated by stimulating large fibers (i.e., pressure, counter-irritant, electrical stimulation). (From Melzak, R. (1982). Recent concepts of pain. *Journal of Medicine, 13*(3), 147–160.)

Numerical Rating Scale (NRS)

0	1	2	3	4	5	6	7	8	9	10
No pain					Moderate pain					Worse possible pain

Visual Analog Scales (VAS)

No distress	Unbearable distress

No pain	Pain as bad as it could possibly be

Adjective Rating Scales (ARS)

No pain	Little pain	Medium pain	Large pain	Worse possible pain
None	Annoying	Uncomfortable	Dreadful	Agonizing

FIGURE 16-2 **Examples of Pain Assessment Instruments.** Numerical rating scales (NRS), visual analogue scales (VAS), and adjective rating scales (ARS) can be used to assess pain intensity and affective distress. The tools quantify the pain. Visually impaired or confused patients may have difficulty using the scales.

The *pain threshold*, which is the lowest intensity of stimulus that is perceived by the patient as pain, is essentially the same for all people as long as the central and peripheral nervous systems remain intact. However, the threshold may vary among different persons according to a number of physiologic and psychosocial factors (e.g., age, gender, disease or condition, fatigue, insomnia, anxiety, the meaning of the pain, past experiences with pain, depression, isolation, religious beliefs, cultural expectations). *Pain tolerance,* on the other hand, is different for each person and varies according to many subjective factors. In reality, pain tolerance refers to the amount of pain the patient is willing to endure. Only the patient can identify what a tolerable level is, not the health care provider (Fig. 16–2).

Interpretation of pain based on a patient's behavior is cumbersome because the amount of pain and responses to pain differ from person to person. Objective findings can be divided into three categories: sympathetic responses, parasympathetic responses, and behavioral responses. Although these responses are not diagnostic in and of themselves, they provide clues to the cause of the pain. Sympathetic responses seen with minimal to moderate pain intensity include tachycardia, increased blood pressure and respirations, skeletal muscle tension, dilated pupils, and diaphoresis.

Parasympathetic responses are seen with intense, severe pain, or with deep pain. Objective manifestations include pallor, decreased blood pressure and heart rate, nausea and vomiting, weakness, prostration, and loss of consciousness.

Objective behavioral responses to pain include a guarded, rigid position. The patient's facial expression is drawn.

The patient may cry, appear frightened, and be restless. Moaning, sighing, grimacing, clenching of the jaws or fist, and withdrawal from others may be noted.

Psychologic effects of unmanaged or undermanaged pain include fear, helplessness, anxiety, anger, and frustration, which lead to decreased thoracic movement; further, the normal sigh (yawn) is abolished, and there is increased splinting and a reduction in lung compliance, lung volumes, and lung capacities that leads to atelectasis. As a result, there is often decreased mobility and an increased risk of thromboembolism. Untreated or undermanaged pain exaggerates the catecholamine response and is manifested as increased systemic vascular resistance, increased myocardial oxygen demand, and the potential for arrhythmias and hypertension.

Emotional and psychologic components of pain are intertwined with perceptual and reflex components; but more important is the meaning of the pain to the patient. Pain perception and reactions are based heavily on expectations and learned responses. Some of these responses are culturally derived. Psychosocial factors influencing pain perception include anxiety, feelings of powerlessness, and ineffective coping mechanisms (Box 16-1). In addition to personality and other factors that cannot be changed (e.g., age and sex), variables that influence pain experiences include insomnia, fatigue, fear, anger, sadness, depression, mental isolation, introversion, and past experiences with pain. Factors tending to increase pain thresholds include relief of symptoms, sleep, rest, and elevation of mood, as well as use of empathy, diversion, analgesics, antianxiety drugs, and antidepressants. A particularly important factor influencing severe, chronic pain is its significance to the patient as an actual or potential loss, along with its associated loss of personal control and autonomy.

Types of Pain

Nociceptive pain is typically classified as somatic (i.e., arising from skin, bone, muscle, or connective tissues) or visceral

BOX 16-1

Psychosocial Factors Influencing Perception of Pain

Increases Pain	Decreases Pain
Sadness, depression	Happiness
Fatigue	Rest
Anger	Diversion
Discomfort	Relief of symptoms
Insomnia	Sleep
Anxiety	Sympathy
Fear	Understanding; relational support

(i.e., arising from internal organs). It can be short-lived, resolving over a short time (acute), or long-lasting and relentless (chronic). *Acute pain* usually is the result of direct tissue injury, has an immediate onset, and resolves when the damaged tissue heals, usually in 3 months or less. Acute pain often stimulates the sympathetic nervous system, with increases in blood pressure and pulse and the occurrence of nausea, sweating, and pallor. Patients with acute pain can usually locate their pain within a single area and tend to use descriptors such as throbbing, stabbing, gnawing, sharp, or aching when describing their pain. Acute unrelieved pain increases cardiac workload and oxygen demands and subsequently increases the risk for myocardial infarction. Severe unrelieved pain may also cause splinting and inadequate respiratory expansion and can be a predisposing factor for pneumonia, especially in postoperative patients. Examples of acute nociceptive pain include sprains and fractures, burns, tension headaches, and unstable angina. Without intervention, acute nociceptive pain may progress to acute neuropathic pain or a chronic nociceptive pain.

Visceral pain is caused by stimulating receptors located in viscera. Visceral pain caused by obstruction of a hollow organ is poorly localized because most organs do not contain nociceptors. This pain is described as sharp, stabbing, or throbbing when the capsules surrounding viscera are involved but can also be described as a cramping and gnawing sensation of varying intensity.

Neuropathic pain is caused by injury to nerves. The injury may be due to disease (e.g., diabetes, fibromyalgia), infection, trauma, surgery, injury from tumor growth, or antineoplastic or radiation therapy. Neuropathic pain is not completely understood, and is thought to be due to changes in CNS processing of nociceptive input. Many patients have allodynia, which is pain in response to a stimulus that would not ordinarily be painful.

Referred pain is present at a location away from its point of origin. For example, an obstructed bile duct may produce pain near the right scapula, whereas pain from a hip injury may be referred to the knee. This phenomenon occurs because nerve signals from different parts of the body travel along the same pathways going to the spinal cord and the brain.

Ischemic pain is caused by loss of blood flow to tissues in a particular part of the body. Failure to perfuse the area causes tissue hypoxia and damage, leading to release of inflammatory mediators and chemicals that stimulate nociceptors. Angina is an example of pain due to ischemia.

Cancer-related pain can have many different causes. Tumors can compress or obstruct vital organs, resulting in visceral pain. Cancers may also infiltrate nerve fibers, causing neuropathic pain. Adverse effects of certain cancer therapies, such as antineoplastic or radiation therapy, may indirectly cause pain. This type of pain may cause further physical and emotional distress for the patient because of fear that the disease is worsening.

The patient's psychologic state contributes significantly to pain perception and associated suffering. In some cases, evidence that the pain itself is sustained by psychologic factors can be inferred. This phenomenon is known generically as *psychogenic pain*. When reasonable inferences about the sustaining pathology of a pain syndrome cannot be made, it is best to refer to the pain as *idiopathic*.

Chronic pain persists for 6 months or more or beyond the expected healing time after the initial tissue injury. The pain may be continuous or recurrent. Chronic pain is not always accompanied by sympathetic nervous system activity, because the nervous system becomes desensitized to the noxious pain stimulus. Examples of chronic pain include gastritis, pancreatitis, gout, osteoarthritis, sickle cell anemia, and low back pain.

PHARMACOTHERAPEUTIC OPTIONS

Analgesics are usually divided into two classes on the basis of their clinical effectiveness: (1) opioid agonists and agonist-antagonist analgesics, and (2) nonopioid analgesics. In general, opioid analgesics are used to relieve severe central pain, whereas nonopioid analgesics are given for peripheral pain. The nonopioid analgesics are discussed in Chapter 17.

Opioid Analgesics

- codeine; ✦ Paveral
- fentanyl (Fentanyl Oralet, Sublimaze, Duragesic)
- hydrocodone (Duocet, Hycodan, Hydrogesic, Vicodin, Lortab ASA); ✦ Robidone, Lortab
- hydromorphone (Dilaudid, Dilaudid-HP)
- levorphanol (Levo-Dromoran, Levorphan)
- meperidine (Demerol)
- methadone (Dolophine, Methadose)
- morphine sulfate (Duramorph, MS, MSIR, MSO, MS Contin, Roxanol); ✦ Statex, Epimorph, Morphine HP, Morphitec, M.S.S.
- oxycodone (Oxicodone, Percocet, Tylox, Percodan, others); ✦ Supeudol, Oxycocet, Endocet, Endo-dan, Oxycodan
- oxymorphone (Numorphan)
- propoxyphene (Darvon, Darvocet, Wygesic, Darvon Compound-65); ✦ Novo-Propoxyn, 642, Darvon-N with ASA, Darvon-N Compound, 692, others

▮ Indications

The primary use of opioid analgesics is to relieve moderate to severe acute or chronic pain of various etiologies. Opioids are the mainstay of treatment for pain from traumatic injuries, burns, and biliary or renal colic, as well as for cancer-related pain and pain related to postoperative states. Opioids are also used for many chronic pain syndromes including osteoarthritis, pancreatitis, sickle cell anemia, and low back pain. Other uses for opioids include the treatment of acute pulmonary edema, as an obstetric analgesic during labor and delivery, and for pain relief during invasive diagnostic procedures. A handful of the opioids (e.g., alfentanil, fentanyl, sufentanil) are most often used as adjuncts to general anesthesia. Morphine is the standard by which other opioids are measured, although they all share certain desirable and certain undesirable characteristics. Morphine acts as a reducer of preload in patients with myocardial infarction (MI).

Pharmacodynamics

The pharmacologic action of opioid analgesics is similar to those of their parent compound–morphine. Opioids provide pain relief by activating specific opioid receptors found on the surface of pain-transmitting nerves, and thus blocking the nerve from sending the pain transmission signal. Five major categories of opioid receptors are known: mu (μ), kappa (κ), sigma (σ), delta (Δ), and epsilon (ε) (Table 16-1). The principal opioid receptors μ, Δ, and, κ each produce analgesia when activated. σ Receptors have been implicated in psychomimetic and dysphoric adverse effects, and possibly in dilation of the pupil.

μ Receptors have been further subtyped as $μ_1$ receptors, which are supraspinal and mediate analgesia, and $μ_2$ receptors, which mediate respiratory depression. Enkephalins and endorphins are endogenous ligands for these receptors, and morphine is an exogenous ligand. The $μ_1$ receptor is morphine-selective.

The two major metabolites of morphine, morphine-3-glucuronide (M3G) and morphine-6-glucuronide (M6G), are neurotoxic. Both metabolites are water-soluble and are cleared through the kidneys. M3G is found in significantly higher quantities and appears to antagonize the beneficial effect (i.e., to relieve nociceptive pain) of morphine. M6G has analgesic properties, making it considerably more potent than its parent drug on a milligram-to-milligram basis. Poor pain control and the risk for toxicity increases when M3G and M6G accumulate in the body.

Spinal and supraspinal analgesia are mediated by Δ receptors along with dysphoria, psychomimetic effects (e.g., hallucinations), and respiratory and vasomotor stimulation. These receptors have been subtyped as $Δ_1$ and $Δ_2$ and are thought to be relatively unimportant in terms of analgesia. κ Receptors

mediate pentazocine-like spinal analgesia, sedation, miosis, respiratory depression, and dysphoria.

$κ_1$ Receptors mediate spinal analgesia; $κ_3$ receptors mediate supraspinal analgesia, and the function of $κ_2$ receptors is unknown. Activation of these receptors is thought to cause a sedating analgesia with reduced risk of dependency and respiratory depression.

Effectively all of the analgesia-inducing opioids on the market today activate the μ opioid receptors in the brain and the spinal cord. Activation of the μ opioid receptors by morphine and other opioids blocks the pain signal from transmitting along nerve cells from the pain source to the brain. The feeling of pain is lessened, but oftentimes serious adverse effects (e.g., sedation, decreased respiratory function, dependency) can result from the use of opioid analgesics. Because of the potential for tolerance and dependency, drugs that activate μ opioid receptors are regulated under the Controlled Substances Act and policed by the Drug Enforcement Administration (DEA).

In proof-of-concept studies conducted in both humans and animals, morphine was reported effective in providing pain relief when applied locally to inflamed tissues such as skin, joints, and eyes. These results present the possibility of creating analgesics that will activate opioid receptors in the inflamed area, without activating the opioid receptors of the CNS. Consequently, the adverse CNS effects associated with opioid analgesics would be prevented. In other preclinical studies, peripheral μ agonists have demonstrated efficacy in inflammatory pain models. Peripheral κ agonists have also shown efficacy in preclinical models of visceral and inflammatory pain. Serious adverse CNS effects could be potentially averted with the use of peripheral analgesics, because these drugs are engineered to have limited ability to cross the blood-brain barrier at therapeutic doses.

Pharmacokinetics

Opioids are variably absorbed from mucosal surfaces of the nose and the gastrointestinal (GI) tract as well as from intramuscular (IM) and subcutaneous (subQ) injection sites. Rectal absorption can be erratic. Opioids are distributed to the lungs, the liver, the kidneys, and the spleen. Skeletal muscle and fatty tissues act as storage sites, although opioid concentrations in brain tissue are less than that of other areas. Slow penetration of the opioid to brain sites and an effective first-pass effect influences the onset, the peak, and the duration of drug action (Table 16-2).

The onset of analgesia is rapid by most routes. Highly lipid-soluble drugs generally have a more rapid onset of action. The duration of action varies with the route of administration, the dosage, and patient characteristics; with the exception of sustained-release formulations, most have a duration of action of 4 to 6 hours. Protein binding varies from 33% for morphine to 90% for methadone, with variable half-lives. Opioids are converted to metabolites to be excreted in the urine.

Adverse Reactions and Contraindications

The adverse effects of opioids are all direct consequences of receptor activation. The effects are largely due to the preponderance of opioid receptors in the medulla and peripheral

---

TABLE 16-1 Opioid Receptors and Effects

Receptor	Clinical Effects	Opioid/Endogenous Peptide
Mu (μ)	Euphoria Physical dependence Respiratory depression Supraspinal analgesia	morphine meperidine methadone codeine fentanyl levorphanol buprenorphine
Kappa (κ)	Miosis Sedation Spinal analgesia Respiratory depression	morphine pentazocine
Delta (Δ)	Dysphoria Hallucinations Respiratory stimulation Vasomotor stimulation	Enkephalins Endorphins
Sigma (σ)	Dysphoria Hallucinations Respiratory stimulation Vasomotor stimulation	pentazocine

PHARMACOKINETICS

TABLE 16-2 Opioids, Opioid Agonist-Antagonists, and Opioid Antagonists

Drug	Route	Onset	Peak	Duration	PB (%)	$t_{1/2}$
POTENT AGONISTS						
fentanyl	TD	Up to 24 hr	12–24 hr	48–72 hr*	79–87	13–22 hr
	IM	7–15 min	20–30 min	1–2 hr	79–87	13–22 hr
	IV	1–2 min	3–5 min	1–2 hr	79–87	1.5–6 hr
hydromorphone	PO	15–30 min	30–60 min	4 hr	UA	2–3 hr
	IM†	15 min	30–60 min	4–5 hr	UA	2–3 hr
	IV	10–15 min	30–60 min	2–3 hr	UA	2–3 hr
	subQ	30 min	30–90 min	4 hr	UA	2–3 hr
levorphanol	PO	10–60 min	90–120 min	4–5 hr	40–50	12–16 hr
	IM	UA	60 min	4–5 hr	<50	12–16 hr
	IV	Immed	<20 min	6–8 hr	<50	12–16 hr
	subQ	UA	60–90 min	6–8 hr	<50	12–16 hr
meperidine	PO, subQ	15 min	60–90 min	2–4 hr	60–80	3–4 hr
	IM	10–15 min	30–50 min	2–4 hr	60–80	3–4 hr
	IV	1 min	5–7 min	2 hr	60–80	3–4 hr
methadone	PO	30–60 min	2–4 hr	6–8 hr (acute); 24–48 hr (chronic)	90	15–40 hr
	IM	10–20 min	60–120 min	4–5 hr	90	15–40 hr
	IV	10–20 min	30–60 min	3–4 hr	90	22–48 hr†
morphine	PO	60 min	60–120 min	4–5 hr	33	2–3 hr
	IM	10–30 min	30–60 min	4–5 hr	33	2–3 hr
	IV	5–10 min	20 min	2–3 hr	33	2–3 hr
	subQ	10–30 min	50–90 min	4–5 hr	33	2–3 hr
	EP	15–60 min	5–10 min	24 hr	—	—
oxymorphone	IM	10–15 min	30–90 min	4- 6 hr	33	2–3 hr
	IV	5–10 min	15–30 min	3–6 hr	33	2–3 hr
	subQ	10–20 min	UA	3–6 hr	33	2–3 hr
MILD TO MODERATELY POTENT OPIOID AGONISTS						
codeine	PO, subQ	30–40 min	60–120 min	4 hr	50	2.5–4 hr
	IM	10–30 min	30–60 min	4 hr	50	2.5–4 hr
hydrocodone	PO	10–30 min	30–60 min	4–6 hr	UA	3.8 hr
oxycodone	PO	10–15 min	60–90 min	3–4 hr	<50	2–3 hr
propoxyphene	PO	15–60 min	120 min	4–6 hr	78	6–12 hr
POTENT OPIOID AGONIST-ANTAGONISTS						
butorphanol	IM	10 min	30–60 min	3–4 hr	96	2.5–4 hr
	IV	Immed	4–5 min	3–4 hr	80–83	2.5–4 hr
buprenorphine	IM	15 min	60 min	6 hr‡	96	2–3 hr
	IV	Immed	<60 min	6 hr	96	2–3 hr
nalbuphine	IM, subQ	<15 min	60 min	3–6 hr	<30	2–5 hr
	IV	2–3 min	30 min	3–4 hr	<30	2–5 hr
pentazocine	PO, subQ	15–30 min	60–90 min	3 hr	60	2–3 hr
	IM	15–20 min	30–60 min	2–3 hr	60	2–3 hr
PURE OPIOID ANTAGONISTS						
naloxone	IM, subQ	15 min	UA	45 min	50	60–90 min in adults; 3 hr in neonates
	IV	1–2 min	UA	20–60 min§		
naltrexone	PO	5–60 min	UA	Varies‖	21	4–13 hr¶
NONOPIOID ANALGESIC						
tramadol	PO	lt;60 min	2–3 hr	4–6 hr	20	6.3 hr for active drug; 7.4 hr for metabolite

*Duration of action of fentanyl patch after the patch is removed.
†Duration of action and half-life of methadone's active metabolites with repeated dosing; may be even longer in older adults, and in patients with renal dysfunction. Extended half-life is not related to analgesic effects.
‡Respiratory-depressant effects of buprenorphine occur 1–3 hr after IM injection.
§Duration of action of naloxone varies with dose administered and route of administration.
‖Duration of action of naltrexone is dose dependent. 25 mg blocks effects of IV heroin for up to 24 hours, whereas a 100- to 150-mg dose lasts 48–72 hr, respectively.
¶Half-life of naltrexone's metabolites.
EP, Epidural; *IM*, intramuscular; *immed*, immediate; *IV*, intravenous; *PB*, protein binding; *PO*, by mouth; *subQ*, subcutaneous; $t_{1/2}$, half-life; *TD*, transdermal; *UA*, unavailable.

nervous system. The incidence and severity of adverse effects increase as the dosage increases.

CNS EFFECTS. Opioids cross the blood-brain barrier to alter pain perception, thus explaining the CNS effects seen with the drugs. Adverse CNS effects vary from drowsiness to sleep to unconsciousness, as well as decreased mental and physical activity. In addition, headache, dizziness, confusion, dysphoria, unusual dreams, hallucinations, and delirium can result. Opioids reduce the ability to make accurate judgments, to operate machinery, and to drive.

CARDIOVASCULAR EFFECTS. In a supine patient, therapeutic doses of morphine or the synthetic opioids have very little effect on blood pressure and cardiac rate or rhythm. However, some patients experience orthostatic hypotension. The orthostatic hypotension is due to the direct dilating action of some opioids (e.g., morphine) on peripheral blood vessels, which reduces the capacity of the cardiovascular system to respond to gravitational changes. This effect occurs more commonly with some opioids (e.g., morphine) than others (e.g., fentanyl). Therefore, opioids are used with caution in patients who are volume-depleted, because hypotensive effects are more pronounced. Increasing blood volume decreases the orthostatic changes.

GASTROINTESTINAL EFFECTS. A common adverse effect of opioids is constipation. Constipation is caused by diminished peristaltic contractions in the small and large intestines and a delay in passage of gastric contents through the duodenum. There is also decreased lower GI smooth muscle tone and glandular secretion, and increased water reabsorption from the intestines. Tolerance does not develop to constipation as it does to the other adverse effects of opioids, such as respiratory depression.

Biliary colic may occur, since smooth muscle contraction increases the pressure within the biliary ductal system (although it happens less frequently with meperidine than with morphine). In susceptible persons, opioids stimulate the chemoreceptor trigger zone (CTZ) in the medulla, especially in low doses, to produce nausea and vomiting. Tolerance to nausea and vomiting may develop with continued treatment.

GENITOURINARY EFFECTS. Ureteral spasm, spasm of urinary sphincters, urinary retention or hesitancy oliguria, antidiuretic effects, and a reduced libido have been noted with opioid use. Urinary retention is especially problematic in patients who have prostatic hypertrophy. Opioids also tend to prolong labor and produce respiratory depression in the neonate.

⚠ RESPIRATORY EFFECTS. **Therapeutic dosages of opioids can cause respiratory depression.** Low doses primarily depress depth, whereas higher dosages also depress respiratory rate. Medullary depression is due to both the drug's action on the respiratory center in the medulla and to its ability to suppress the medulla's response to carbon dioxide levels. Respiratory depression is noted roughly 7 minutes after intravenous (IV) administration, 30 minutes after an IM injection, and 90 minutes after a subQ injection. Depressant effects can last from 4 to 5 hours. Respiratory depression is the most common cause of death from opioids, although there really is no upper limit on drug dosage (ceiling effects) (Box 16-2).

⚠ **The clinically observable signs of morphine's respiratory-depressant effects and its ability to increase cerebrospinal fluid pressure may be exaggerated in the patient experiencing head injury, other intracranial lesions, or a preexisting elevation in intracranial pressure. On the other hand, the adverse effects resulting from opioid use may also conceal any signs of further pressure increases. In such cases, morphine use must proceed with caution and only when deemed necessary.**

Tolerance develops to the respiratory-depression effects of opioids. A patient in whom tolerance has developed may experience only slight effects after receiving doses that could cause serious or fatal respiratory depression in patients who are opioid-naïve, that is, who have not received opioids in the past. Accumulated drug, especially in patients with liver or renal failure or underlying heart disease, or in the older adult, can cause overdose. Note that equianalgesic doses of opioids produce sedative and respiratory-depressant effects comparable to those of morphine.

Most opioid analgesics were designed to be as effective as morphine but less sedating, and to produce less depression and dependence. However, efforts in this direction have been less than successful. In contrast to the problematic multisystem adverse effects seen with opioids, on the other hand, they do have an adverse effect that is clinically useful: they exhibit antitussive activity. The antitussive activity of opioids is discussed in Chapter 52.

OTHER EFFECTS. Severe hypersensitivity reactions to opioids are rare; however, when present, they usually appear as urticaria or a skin rash. Some patients have itching or wheal formation at the injection site, but this effect is usually a local, histamine-mediated response. Anaphylaxis is rare. All opioids except meperidine cause pupillary constriction. Some patients may have blurred vision, dry eyes, and lens opacities. Opioids also stimulate the release of antidiuretic hormone, prolactin, and human growth hormone.

DRUG TOLERANCE AND DEPENDENCY. Although tolerance and physical dependence can develop when an opioid is used for pain relief, addiction does not necessarily follow.

Tolerance to opioids develops quickly depending on the dose, the dosing frequency, and how consistently the drug is used over an extended period. Tolerance to the adverse effects of opioids (i.e., respiratory depression, CNS depression, nausea and vomiting) normally develops within the first 5 to 7 days of continuous use. Tolerance is characterized by a shorter duration of pain relief, a decrease in peak analgesic effect, and an increase in the amount of opioid needed to relieve the pain. Increasing the dosage or lengthening the time between doses reduces the likelihood of tolerance, although there are other reasons for drugs to become less effective (e.g., worsening tissue damage).

The need to increase the opioid dosage for reasons other than physical adaptation to a drug is known as *pseudotolerance*. There are a number of causes for pseudotolerance including (1) the worsening of the patient's health care problem; (2) changes in opioid formulation; (3) a new pathologic problem; (4) drug interactions; (5) drug-food interactions; (6) an increase or decrease in physical activity; (7) psychologic dependence; and (8) nonadherence with therapy.

Physical adaptation of the body to a drug is referred to as *physical dependence*. Signs and symptoms of withdrawal appear when a person who is physically dependent on an opioid stops using the drug. Withdrawal symptoms include a characteristic mix of CNS and autonomic nervous system (ANS) responses such as tactile hallucinations, irritability, sleeplessness, restlessness, yawning, tremor, and joint and muscle pains. Anorexia, nausea, vomiting, diarrhea, dehydration, abdominal cramps, ketosis, weight loss, distorted vision, and photophobia may also plague the individual. Peak severity of withdrawal symptoms occurs 36 to 72 hours after the last dose of opioid, with symptoms gradually waning over 2 to 5 weeks. Withdrawal episodes persisting for months have been documented. Withdrawal is not usually life-threatening in an otherwise healthy individual.

BOX 16-2

Treatment of Opioid Toxicity

Naloxone

Indications

- Opioid antagonist of choice to reverse respiratory and CNS depression due to suspected opioid excess
- Used in management of refractory circulatory shock, although not FDA-approved for such use

Pharmacodynamics

- No pharmacodynamic activity of its own; works only in the presence of an opioid
- High affinity for μ receptors, acts to competitively displace opioids, endorphins, and enkephalins already present and to block further binding

Pharmacokinetics

- Readily absorbed from IM and IV injection sites with rapid onset of action
- Duration of action depends on the dose and the route of administration
- Plasma half-life of naloxone 60 to 90 minutes with excretion through the kidneys

Adverse Effects

- Intense nausea, vomiting, and occasionally elevated blood pressure and tachycardia
- Opioid withdrawal within a few minutes to 2 hours

Dosing Regimen

- *Adults:* 0.4–2 mg by IV or IM route every 2 to 3 minutes PRN.
- *Children >22 kg:* 2 mg/dose; if no response, may repeat every 2–3 minutes PRN.
- *Children <22 kg:* 0.1 mg/kg, if no response, may repeat every 2–3 minutes PRN.
- *Naloxone by continuous infusion:* Dilute 2 mg of naloxone in 500 mL. Supplemental doses may be given by IM or subQ route to provide longer lasting effects. If there is no response, dosage may be increased to 100 mcg/kg.

Evaluation

- Patients receiving opioids for longer than 1 week are remarkably sensitive to the effects of naloxone. Titrate dose to avoid withdrawal, seizures, and severe pain.
- Lack of significant response suggests symptoms may be due to a disease process or to another, nonopioid, CNS depressant.

Naltrexone

Indications

- FDA-approved only for opioid-dependent patients; candidates must be detoxified before using naltrexone
- Unlabeled uses: eating disorders and treatment of postconcussion syndrome

Pharmacodynamics

- A pure antagonist with no agonist action; competitively inhibits the effects of opioids by binding at the opioid receptor sites
- Produces withdrawal symptoms but prevents the euphoria associated with opioid use; does not reduce craving for the drug

Pharmacokinetics

- Rapidly absorbed when taken by mouth but undergoes significant first-pass effects; bioavailability 5% to 40%
- Onset occurs in 20 to 30 minutes; peak concentrations in 1 hour; duration of action is dose dependent
- Half-life of parent drug is 4 hours; half-life of metabolite is approximately 13 hours
- Excretion via kidneys; small portion eliminated in stool

Adverse Effects

- Precipitates withdrawal syndrome, edema, hypertension, palpitations, phlebitis, shortness of breath, anxiety, depression, disorientation, dizziness, and headache
- Anorexia, nausea, vomiting, diarrhea or constipation, thirst, dose-dependent hepatocellular damage, decreased libido, delayed ejaculation, and urinary frequency

Dosing Regimen

- *Adults:* 25 mg orally with additional 25 mg 1 hour later if no signs of withdrawal are present; then 50 mg daily
- A 50-mg dose of naltrexone blocks the effects of 25 mg of IV opioid (e.g., heroin) for up to 24 hours
- A 100- to 150-mg dose produces antagonistic effects for 48 to 72 hours; 50 to 150 mg/per day can be given depending on patient need

CNS, Central nervous system; *FDA*, Food and Drug Administration; *IM*, intramuscular; *IV*, intravenous; *subQ*, subcutaneous.

A psychologic compulsion to use a substance is known as *pseudo-addiction*. It is characterized by an ongoing craving for the psychologic effects of an opioid. Euphoria and hallucinations are produced by opioids with an affinity for both μ and σ receptor sites.

A *pseudo-dependency* exists when a person who has severe unrelenting pain is preoccupied with acquiring pain relief. Pursuit of opioids is ordinarily the direct result of inadequate pain assessment, use of the wrong opioid, substitution of a drug from another analgesic class when an opioid is required, or use of a dosing frequency that is too drawn out.

CONTRAINDICATIONS. **All opioids should be used with extreme caution in patients having an acute asthmatic attack, patients with chronic obstructive pulmonary disease or cor pulmonale, patients who have a substantially decreased respiratory reserve, and patients with preexisting respiratory depression, hypoxia, or hypercapnia. In such patients, even the usual therapeutic doses of opioids may decrease respiratory drive while simultaneously increasing airway resistance to the point of apnea.**

Furthermore, opioids are contraindicated for use or must be used very cautiously in people with liver or kidney disease, and in persons with a previous hypersensitivity reaction. Also use caution when prescribing these drugs in patients with head injuries, increased intracranial pressure, adrenal insufficiency, Addison's disease, alcoholism, undiagnosed abdominal pain, urethral stricture, and prostatic hyperplasia or hypertrophy. Because of the potential for neonatal respiratory depression, opioids are used with caution during labor and delivery.

Drug Interactions

Opioids interact with other CNS depressants such as alcohol, anesthetics, barbiturates, and sedative-hypnotics to enhance CNS depression (Table 16-3). Constipation and urinary retention may result from concurrent use of tricyclic antidepressants, phenothiazines, and anticholinergic drugs.

Controversy

Administering Opioids to Chemically Dependent Patients

The World Health Organization (WHO) made pain management a priority among its programs for the 1990s. The WHO makes it clear that the needs of patients for diagnosis and treatment far exceed health care resources, particularly in developing nations. This is particularly so for serious diseases such as cancer. However, the WHO suggests that treatment of pain is a reasonable goal and one that can be achieved using inexpensive, orally administered agents, if opioid drugs form the mainstay.

In the United States, people affected by terminal diseases associated with unhealthy lifestyles comprise a particularly hard-to-treat subgroup. Many patients suffering the severe, deep abdominal pain associated with terminal acquired immunodeficiency syndrome (AIDS) require pain relief that can be achieved only with opioids. However, these patients often have a long-standing history of substance abuse that includes intravenous injection of heroin and other opium derivatives.

Contemporary thinking strongly suggests that patients in pain have almost no risk for developing opioid dependence. Such patients may paradoxically exhibit pseudoaddiction if health care providers use subtherapeutic doses of opioids. The central question then concerns the relative risks and benefits of using strong opioids (e.g., morphine, hydromorphone, methadone) in people who have a history of drug dependence. Indeed, a patient who is actively dependent on drugs may have such severe pain that it is only relieved by opioid drugs.

The challenge facing the health care provider is to decide whether an opioid constitutes effective therapy for a particular patient. If it does, a plan must be devised to provide the patient with the opioid on a regular basis while minimizing the likelihood that psychologic dependence will reemerge.

CLINICAL REASONING
* What is the role of pain management in preventing substance abuse?
* Does the patient who has a history of substance abuse have the same right to opioid therapy as the patient who has never become dependent?
* Does the patient who has a history of substance abuse pose any special risk for renewed dependence during opioid therapy?
* Does the patient who has a history of substance abuse pose any special risk to the health care provider and members of the health care team?

The paralyzing effects of neuromuscular blockers are enhanced in the presence of opioids. Smoking and nicotine use decrease the analgesic effects of opioids. Concurrent use of diuretics can result in additive orthostatic hypotension. Cimetidine inhibits the biotransformation of opioids, leading to increased risk for respiratory and CNS depression.

▥ *Dosage Regimen*

Opioids are administered by mouth or by IM, subQ, or IV routes (Table 16-4). They may also be given as suppositories (although rectal absorption can be erratic), by the epidural route, directly into the spinal cord (intrathecally), and transdermally. Transdermal drug delivery systems allow the problem of fluctuating drug levels associated with intermittent dosing to be avoided. For example, a fentanyl transdermal patch delivers 25 to 100 mcg of fentanyl per hour for a period of 72 hours. **The patient's 24-hour requirement of currently used oral or parenteral opioid must be calculated before calculating the dosage of transdermal fentanyl.**

▥ *Lab Considerations*

Elevated biliary tract pressure associated with opioid use may cause increases in plasma amylase and lipase. Accurate determination of the values may be unreliable for 24 hours in the presence of opioids.

For more information, see the Evolve Resources Bonus Content "Influence of Selected Drugs on Laboratory Values," found at http://evolve.elsevier.com/Gutierrez/pharmacotherapeutics.

Mixed Opioid Agonists-Antagonists
◆ butorphanol (Stadol, Stadol NS)
◆ buprenorphine (Buprenex)
◆ nalbuphine (Nubain)
◆ pentazocine (Talwin, Talwin NX)

▥ *Indications*

Mixed opioid agonists-antagonists are used for moderate to severe pain. Butorphanol, buprenorphine, and nalbuphine are used for patients who have a true hypersensitivity to meperidine or who are intolerant to morphine. Butorphanol, nalbuphine, and pentazocine have been used for analgesia during labor, as sedation before surgery, and as a supplement in balanced anesthesia.

▥ *Pharmacodynamics*

Combination agonist-antagonists activate one type of opioid receptor while simultaneously blocking another type (Fig. 16-3). However, they produce fewer adverse effects than true opioids and have little antitussive action. These drugs alter the perception of and response to painful stimuli while producing generalized CNS depression. They have partial antagonist properties that can result in opioid withdrawal symptoms in physically dependent patients. Pentazocine tablets contain naloxone, which has no pharmacologic activity when taken by mouth.

▥ *Pharmacokinetics*

Absorption of opioid agonist-antagonists readily occurs with parenteral formulations. Some variation exists in the pharmacokinetic properties, depending on the formulation (see Table 16-2). The drugs are distributed to most body tissues, including the placenta and breast milk. Opioid agonists-antagonists are biotransformed in the liver and excreted in the urine.

▥ *Adverse Reactions and Contraindications*

Adverse effects of opioid agonist-antagonists are less common than reactions to true opioids. Common adverse effects include nausea, vomiting, lightheadedness, sedation, and euphoria. Visual hallucinations, disorientation, dysphoria, and confusion can also occur. As with true opioids, respirations are depressed with initial doses but do not worsen with dosage increase. Insomnia and disturbed dreams can develop, especially with nalbuphine and pentazocine. Anticholinergic effects (e.g., dry mouth, blurred vision, constipation, and urinary retention) are common. Hypertension is especially problematic with nalbuphine. Hypersensitivity reactions to opioid

DRUG INTERACTIONS

TABLE 16-3 Selected Opioids, Opioid Agonist-Antagonists, and Opioid Antagonists

Drug	Interactive Drugs	Interaction
OPIOIDS		
Opioids	Alcohol, anesthetics, antianxiety drugs, antihistamines, barbiturates, sedative-hypnotics	Enhances CNS depression, respiratory depression, and hypotension
	Tricyclic antidepressants, phenothiazines, anticholinergics	Severe constipation and urinary retention
	cimetidine	Inhibits opioid biotransformation leading to increased respiratory and CNS depression
	MAOIs	CNS excitation, severe hypotension or hypertension
	pentazocine	Precipitates opioid withdrawal in dependent patients
	Skeletal muscle relaxants	Additive respiratory depression
meperidine	MAOIs	Additive CNS depression with hypotension and respiratory depression, or CNS stimulation with hyperexcitability and seizures
methadone	Hydantoins	Induces biotransformation of methadone
propoxyphene	carbamazepine	Decreases biotransformation and increases serum concentrations of interactive drug
	Naltrexone	Withdrawal symptoms
OPIOID AGONIST-ANTAGONISTS		
buprenorphine, butorphanol	MAOIs	Increases CNS and respiratory depression, hypotension
nalbuphine	Antihistamines	
pentazocine	Antidepressants, sedative-hypnotics	Additive CNS depression
	Opioids	Decreases effectiveness of interactive drug
OPIOID ANTAGONISTS		
naloxone, naltrexone	Opioids	Withdrawal symptoms
NONOPIOID ANALGESIC		
tramadol	Alcohol, CNS depressants	Additive CNS depression
	MAOIs	Increases tramadol concentrations
	carbamazepine	Increases tramadol biotransformation

CNS, Central nervous system; *MAOI*, monoamine oxidase inhibitor.

agonist-antagonists are possible. Parenteral use of pentazocine may lead to severe, potentially fatal reactions including pulmonary emboli, vascular occlusion, ulceration, and abscess. These drugs precipitate withdrawal symptoms in patients who are physically dependent on a pure opioid.

Drug Interactions

Decreased effectiveness of a true opioid drug may occur in the presence of an opioid agonist-antagonist. Additive CNS depression may result when opioid agonists-antagonists are taken concurrently with other CNS depressants (see Table 16-3). Concurrent use of monoamine oxidase inhibitors (MAOIs) with opioid agonists-antagonists result in unpredictable reactions including, but not limited to, increased CNS and respiratory depression and hypotension. Antihypertensive drugs and other drugs that lower blood pressure can exacerbate opioid-induced orthostatic hypotension.

Dosage Regimen

Dosages of opioid agonists-antagonists vary with the specific use and route of administration (see Table 16-4). Switch patients receiving more than 100 mg of pentazocine to a true opioid. The initial dose of opioid agonists-antagonists may have to be reduced to 25% of the usual dose in the presence of MAO inhibitors.

Lab Considerations

Agonist-antagonists can cause elevated serum amylase and lipase levels. Accurate determination of these levels may be unreliable for 24 hours in the presence of opioids.

Nonopioid Analgesic

◆ tramadol (Ultram)

Tramadol is a centrally-acting, nonopioid drug unrelated to either the opioids or the nonsteroidal antiinflammatory drugs (NSAIDs). It predominantly binds to μ receptors and is used for mild to moderately severe pain. Tramadol is particularly beneficial for patients who are in acute pain but for whom an opioid is not an option and an NSAID may introduce unnecessary risks (e.g., GI upset and bleeding).

Tramadol is rapidly absorbed, with peak serum levels reached in 2 hours. The duration of action persists for 4 to 6 hours. Tramadol is biotransformed by CYP 2D6 in the liver to *O*-demethy tramadol, its active metabolite, with 30% eliminated in the urine. The half-life of tramadol is 6.3 hours for the active drug, and 7.4 hours for its metabolite. It is designated by the Food and Drug Administration (FDA) as a pregnancy class C drug with unknown safety during lactation.

The common adverse effects of tramadol include dizziness and vertigo, nausea, constipation, headache, and somnolence. Occurring less often are vomiting, pruritus, CNS stimulation (nervousness, anxiety, agitation, tremors, euphoria, mood swings, and hallucinations), asthenia, diaphoresis, dyspepsia, and dry mouth. Unlike opioids, tramadol poses little risk for tolerance and abuse; however, tolerance and dependence can occur with prolonged use. Visual disturbances and urinary retention and frequency are rare. Overdosage results in respiratory depression and seizures. Cumulative effects and prolonged duration of action may occur in patients with impaired liver or kidney function.

DOSAGE

TABLE 16-4 Selected Opioids, Opioid Agonist-Antagonists, and Opioid Antagonists

Drug	Use(s)	Dosage	Implications
POTENT OPIOID AGONISTS			
Transdermal fentanyl	Chronic pain	*Adult:* 25 mcg/hr after assessment of 24-hr opioid requirement for opioid-naïve patient, older adults, and patients on low doses of morphine or morphine equivalent	Not recommended for postoperative, mild, or intermittent pain. Additional short-acting opioids should be used for breakthrough pain until conversion from other opioids is successful.
hydromorphone	Moderate to severe pain	*Adult:* 2 mg PO every 3–6 hr. Increase to 4 mg PO every 4–6 hr –*or*– 1–2 mg IM or subQ every 3–6 hr if needed. Increase to 3–4 mg every 4–6 hr –*or*– 0.5–1 mg IV every 3 hr	Initial IV bolus of 2 times the hourly rate in mg may be given, with subsequent breakthrough boluses of 50% to 100% of the hourly rate in mg.
levorphanol	Moderate to severe pain	*Adult >50 kg:* 4 mg PO every 6–8 hr –*or*– 2 mg subQ or IV every 6–8 hr –*or*– 1–2 mg subQ 90 min before surgical procedure *Adults, child <50 kg:* 0.04 mg/kg PO every 6–8 hr –*or*– 0.2 mg/kg subQ or IV every 6–8 hr	Use with extreme caution in patients receiving MAO inhibitors. Not for use in children.
meperidine	Moderate to severe pain, obstetric analgesia, preoperative sedation, adjunct to anesthesia	*Adult:* 50–150 mg PO, IM or subQ every 3–4 hr –*or*– 15–35 mg/hr by IV infusion *Child:* 1–1.8 mg/kg PO, IM, or subQ every 3–4 hr. Not to exceed 100 mg/dose	**Not to be confused with morphine or hydromorphone—fatalities have occurred.** Local irritation possible with repeated subQ administration. **Do not use in renal failure. May precipitate tremors, myoclonus, or seizures.**
methadone	Severe pain; suppression of opioid withdrawal symptoms	*Adult >50 kg: As Analgesic:* 2.5–5 mg PO every 3–4 hr as analgesic –*or*– 2.5–10 mg IM or subQ every 6–8 hr; *For Detoxification:* 15–40 mg PO, IM, or subQ daily *Adult, child <50 kg:* 0.2 mg/kg PO every 6–8 hr –*or*– 0.1 mg/kg IM or subQ every 6–8 hr	Diskettes (dispersible tablets) are dissolved and used for detoxification and maintenance treatment only. May be given with food or milk to minimize GI irritation.
morphine	Moderate to severe pain, pulmonary edema, myocardial infarction	*Adult >50 kg:* 10–30 mg PO, PR every 3–4 hr PRN –*or*– equivalent dose every 8–12 hr as CR formulation once 24-hr opioid requirement is determined –*or*– 5–10 mg IM, IV, or subQ every 3–4 hr –*or*– 0.8–10 mg/hr for continuous IV infusion after bolus of 15 mg *Adult, child <50 kg:* 0.15–0.3 mg/kg PO every 3–4 hr –*or*– 0.1 mg/kg IM, IV, or subQ every 3–4 hr	Larger doses may be required for chronic therapy. IV infusion rates vary greatly; up to 440 mg/hr have been used. Usual range: 80 mg/hr.
oxymorphone	Moderate to severe pain	*Adult:* 1 to1.5 mg IM or subQ every 3–6 hr PRN –*or*– 0.5 mg IV every 3–6 hr PRN –*or*– 5 mg PR every 4–6 hr PRN	Suppositories should be stored in the refrigerator
MILD TO MODERATELY POTENT OPIOID AGONISTS			
codeine	Mild to moderate pain	*Adult:* 15–60 mg PO, IM, IV, or subQ every 4–6 hr PRN *Child 6–12 yr:* 0.5–1 mg/kg PO, IM, or subQ every 4–6 hr PRN. Max: 60 mg/dose	When combined with nonopioid analgesics (i.e., aspirin or acetaminophen): #2 = 15 mg codeine, #3 = 30 mg codeine, and #4 = 60 mg codeine.
hydrocodone	Moderate to severe pain	*Adult:* 5 to 10 mg PO every 4–6 hr *Child:* 0.2 mg/kg PO every 3–4 hr	APAP or ASA content may limit doses used, thus preventing max recommended dosage of opioid from being exceeded. Advise patient not to take additional APAP or ASA.
oxycodone	Moderate to severe pain	*Adult:* 5–10 mg PO every 3–4 hr PRN. CR tabs every 12 hr –*or*– 10–40 mg per rectum every 3–4 hr *Child < 50 kg:* 0.05–0.15 mg/kg to 5 mg/dose every 4–6 hr PRN	May be given with food or milk to minimize GI irritation. CR tablets should be taken whole, not crushed, broken, or chewed. Empty CR-matrix tablets may appear in stool.
propoxyphene	Mild to moderate pain	*Adult:* 65 mg hydrochloride PO every 4 hr –*or*– 100 mg napsylate every 4 hr PRN. Not to exceed 390 mg/day as hydrochloride –*or*– 600 mg/day as napsylate	Weak analgesic; most effective when used with NSAIDs or APAP
OPIOID AGONIST-ANTAGONISTS			
butorphanol	Moderate to severe pain, analgesia during labor, preoperative sedation, adjunct to anesthesia; migraine headache	*Adult:* 2 mg IM every 3–4 hr PRN (range 1–4 mg) –*or*– 1 mg every 3–4 hr IV PRN (range 0.5–2 mg) –*or*– 1 mg IM or IV every 4–6 hr for older adults –*or*– 1 mg (1 spray) intranasally in 1 nostril every 3–4 hr. May repeat in 60–90 min	May precipitate withdrawal in opioid-dependent patients. Instruct on proper use of nasal spray formulation. Use with extreme caution in patients taking MAO inhibitors.
buprenorphine	Moderate to severe pain	*Adult:* 0.3 mg every 4–6 hr PRN. May repeat initial dose after 30–60 min	0.6-mg doses should be given only by IM in deep, well-developed muscle.
nalbuphine	Moderate to severe pain, obstetric analgesia, preoperative sedative, adjunct to anesthesia	*Adult:* 10 mg IM, subQ, or IV every 3–4 hr. Single dose not to exceed 20 mg. TDD not to exceed 160 mg –*or*– 0.3–3 mg/kg over 10–15 min as adjunct to anesthesia	Coadministration with nonopioid analgesic may have additive effects and permit lower doses. Administer deep IM into well-developed muscle.
pentazocine	Severe pain, obstetric analgesia, preoperative sedative, adjunct to anesthesia	*Adult:* 50–100 mg PO every 3–4 hr. Not to exceed 600 mg/day –*or*– 30 mg subQ, IM, or IV every 3–4 hr as needed. Max: 30 mg/dose IV –*or*– 60 mg/dose IM or subQ. Not to exceed 360 mg/day subQ, IM, or IV.	Change to opioid agonist if >100 mg needed. Reduce dosage by 25% to 50% in patients taking MAO inhibitors to minimize unpredictable adverse reactions. Not recommended for prolonged use or as first-line therapy.

OPIOID ANTAGONISTS			
naloxone	Opioid-induced CNS depression; management of refractory circulatory shock (unlabeled)	*Adult:* 0.4–2 mg IV or IM every 2–3 minutes PRN. *Child >22 kg:* 2 mg/dose. If no response, may repeat every 2–3 min. *Child <22 kg:* 0.1 mg/kg. If no response, may repeat every 2–3 min.	IV route preferred. May be given by IV infusion at rate adjusted to patient response.
naltrexone	Management of opioid or alcohol dependence	*Adult:* Must be opioid-free for 7–10 days before starting drug. 50 mg/day PO –or– 100 mg every other day – or– 150 mg every third day.	A 50-mg dose blocks effects of 25 mg of IV opioid (e.g., heroin) up to 24 hr. A 100- to 150-mg dose blocks effects for 48 to 72 hr. Analyze UA for opioids and follow with naloxone challenge before giving naltrexone.
NONOPIOID ANALGESIC			
tramadol	Moderate to moderately severe pain	*Adult:* 50–100 mg every 4–6 hr. Max: 400 mg/day. Max >age 75 yr: 300 mg/day.	Increase dosing interval to every 12 hr for doses exceeding 200 mg.

APAP, acetaminophen; *ASA,* aspirin; *CR,* controlled-release; *GI,* gastrointestinal; *IM,* intramuscular; *IV,* intravenous; *MAO,* monoamine oxidase; *NSAIDs,* nonsteroidal antiinflammatory drugs; *PO,* by mouth; *PR,* per rectum; *PRN,* as needed; *subQ,* subcutaneous; *TDD,* total daily dose; *UA,* urinalysis.

Alcohol and other CNS depressants may increase CNS-depressant effects, respiratory depression, and hypotension. MAO inhibitors increase the concentration of tramadol. Carbamazepine increases the biotransformation of tramadol, decreasing serum concentrations.

Tramadol may increase serum creatinine and liver function test results and decrease hemoglobin and protein values.

CLINICAL REASONING

Treatment Objectives
It is important that patients have realistic expectations regarding pain relief. As mentioned, the goal is to improve patients' level of functioning; they should not expect to have 100% of their pain relieved 100% of the time. Often patients believe the health care provider is going to make all of the pain go away. This is a particularly unrealistic expectation for patients with chronic pain conditions.

Treatment Options
Once the underlying cause of pain has been identified and interventions do not, or cannot, alleviate the discomfort, pain management should begin promptly and aggressively. If the underlying cause cannot be identified, start therapy but maintain an awareness of the patient's symptoms so as not to mask a diagnosis (e.g., abdominal pain associated with perforation of a gastric ulcer). Management is directed at eliminating the pain as much and as quickly as possible, using the lowest possible dose to achieve adequate pain control while minimizing adverse effects.

Adjunctive therapies are many and varied (Fig. 16-4). Provide the patient an opportunity to use available adjunctive therapies, if they wish, before initiating maintenance opioid therapy. Cognitive-behavioral strategies include relaxation, distraction, imagery, and biofeedback. Physical agents such as massage or the application of heat and cold or transcutaneous electrical nerve stimulation (TENS), when available, are also effective for some patients. These strategies can be used alone or in concert with systemic analgesics and other adjunctive drug measures.

▦ *Patient Variables*
Provide opioid analgesia for chronic pain around the clock or by continuous infusion rather than on an as-needed basis. It has been well established that a pro re nata (PRN; as needed) regimen is not effective for pain management and should be avoided. Further, a PRN order is not recommended because it requires the patient to communicate the presence of pain and the need for the drug. In addition, a PRN schedule promotes delays in drug administration and subsequent periods of inadequate pain relief. The best strategy, and the one that helps prevent progression of chronic pain syndrome, is the appropriate and adequate treatment of acute pain.

Severe pain leads to intense emotional distress, and therefore drug therapy for the associated anxiety may be helpful (see Chapter 19). The benzodiazepines diazepam and lorazepam are usually the drugs of choice, providing effective antianxiety coverage over a long period. Considering the additional mild amnestic effects provided, concurrent administration of a benzodiazepine may be beneficial in some patients. In other patients, particularly the older adult, benzodiazepines can cause distress and confusion. Special caution is in order when opioids are used with other CNS depressants or in patients who have emphysema, bronchial asthma, or any other limitations of respiratory gas exchange, and in patients who have the potential for abusing the drug. Many health

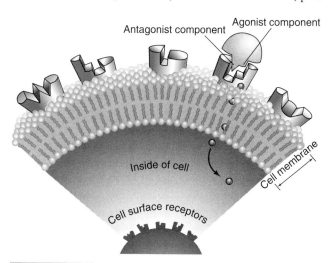

FIGURE 16-3 Agonist-Antagonist Drug–Receptor Interactions. Combination agonist-antagonists activate one type of opioid receptor while simultaneously blocking another type. These drugs alter the perception of and response to painful stimuli while producing generalized central nervous system depression.

CENTRAL NERVOUS

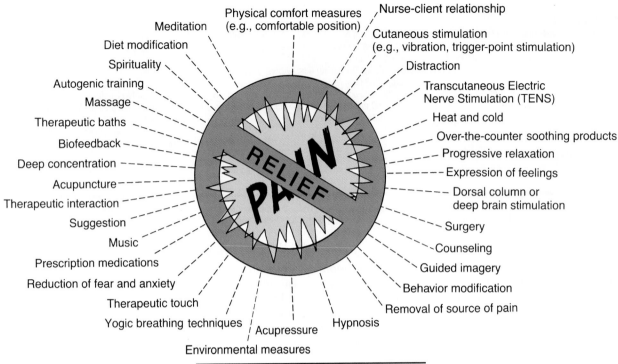

FIGURE 16-4 Adjunctive Pain Management Strategies.

care providers use a "controlled substances contract" similar to the one in Box 16-3 when prescribing an opioid for long term use.

Postoperative pain serves no useful purpose. When they are comfortable, patients are better able to turn, cough, and deep breathe and implement other activities that promote recovery. Postoperative pain management leads to earlier ambulation with decreased risk of deep vein thrombosis and pulmonary embolism, and pneumonia (see Case Study).

BOX 16-3

Informed Consent Contract for Controlled Substances

Opioids, tranquilizers, and certain drugs used for sleep are controlled substances. They are very useful but have a high potential for misuse and abuse and are therefore closely controlled by the health care provider and local, state, and federal government regulations.

I understand that the primary treatment goal is to improve my ability to function and/or to work. In consideration of that goal, and that I am being given potent drug(s) to help me reach that goal, I agree to help myself by adhering to the following conditions:

1. I am responsible for my drug(s):_____. If the prescription or the drug is lost, misplaced, or stolen, or if I use it up sooner than prescribed, I understand that it will not be replaced.

2. I will not request or accept controlled substances from any other health care provider or individual while I am receiving such drug(s) from _____. To do so endangers my health and may also be illegal. The only exception is if it is prescribed while I am admitted to a hospital.

3. I understand that refills of my controlled substances will only be made in person and only once each month during a scheduled office visit during business hours. Refills will not be approved at night, on weekends, or holidays.

4. I understand that I am responsible for taking my drug(s) in the dose prescribed and for keeping track of the amount remaining. Refills will not be approved if I use up my drug supply sooner than expected or if I suddenly realize that I will "run out tomorrow" and need an "emergency supply" of my drug(s).

5. I understand that if I violate any of the above conditions, my controlled-substance prescriptions and/or treatment may be ended immediately. If my violation involves obtaining controlled substances from another individual, as described above, I may also be reported to my primary health care provider, local medical facilities, and local, state, and federal government authorities.

I have been informed about the adverse effects of my controlled substance by my heath care provider including, but not limited to the following: physiologic effects or tolerance (need for more medicine to achieve the same pain relief), dependence (withdrawal will occur if I stop the medicine abruptly), and addiction (abnormal psychologic dependence), which is rare in patients with pain; constipation, lethargy, decreased sex drive and potency, diminished short-term memory, and an overall decrease in concentration- and problem-solving abilities.

Patient Signature:_____   Provider Signature:_____
Date:_____   Date:_____

CASE STUDY   Postoperative Analgesia

ASSESSMENT

History of Present Illness	AB is a 24-year-old female who was involved in a motor vehicle accident. She was sent to surgery from the ER for splenectomy. It is now 3 days later, and she has undergone an open reduction and internal fixation of an open leg fracture. AB is now 12 hours postop, and reporting thirst and feeling weak and "out of it," but that her left side and leg hurt "somethin' awful." She has had three doses of meperidine, 100 mg IV, since surgery; the last dose was given 3 hours ago but without providing much relief. She refuses to cough or deep breathe, and is lying very still and rigid. She is becoming more irritable and communicates in yes or no answers only. She occasionally answers questions inappropriately. She also refuses to use the overhead trapeze because of pain from her abdominal incision and does not move unless someone turns her. Patient reports pain level of 9 out of 10. She reports her pain has been at this level since she came out of surgery.
Past Health History	AB's records show a history of IV crack use and hepatitis B since age 19, but apparently she has been drug-free for the last 3 months. She has been in and out of drug abuse treatment programs since age 21. She admits to smoking 1 to 1½ packs of cigarettes a day for the past 8 years.
Life-Span Considerations	AB admits the sense of responsibility appropriate for her age has been lacking in her. She has little impulse control and has lacked the ability to implement realistic goals or to develop a career and has been unable to enter into mature, intimate relationships. Since she has been in a substance abuse program, she has been working on these age-appropriate behaviors.

AB is reluctant to ask for pain medication, afraid that she will once again become "addicted" and that the nurses will think "bad" of her for asking. She admits to searching for the "meaning of life." AB recently returned to work after leaving the drug treatment program. She is not eligible for health insurance through her employer for another 3 months. A social worker has been contacted to explore financial alternatives with AB. It is anticipated that AB will be off work for approximately 3 to 4 months during rehabilitation. |
| Physical Exam Findings | *Temp:* 99.6° F; *BP:* 140/92; *Pulse:* 128; *Respirations:* 28 and shallow. Urinary output over 50 mL/hr. Skin cool and clammy. Breath sounds with crackles in lower lobes. Abdominal and leg dressings are dry and intact. DP and PT pulses 2+ bilaterally. Tremors of hands noted and patient irritable. |
| Diagnostic Testing | CBC with differential and electrolytes WNL. Wound cultures negative. |

DIAGNOSIS: Open reduction and internal fixation open leg fracture

MANAGEMENT

Treatment Objectives	1. Prevent and alleviate pain. 2. Minimize anxiety, fear, and learned responses that may augment pain and pain-related behaviors.
Treatment Plan	**Pharmacotherapy** • Change from IM meperidine to morphine PCA. • Morphine per PCA 1 mg/hr with a lock-out time of 6 minutes. Initial dose to be preceded by a bolus of 15 mg. Dosage to be titrated based on patient response. Duration of treatment approximately 72 hours; then switch equianalgesic dose of hydrocodone and then to a combination of NSAIDs and opioid oral preparation by discharge. • Use adjunctive pain management strategies; these include massage, biofeedback, and Yogic breathing exercises, guided imagery, cutaneous stimulation, and physical comfort measures (e.g., positioning). • Monitor for signs and symptoms of respiratory depression, constipation, and other adverse reactions. **Patient Education** 1. Advise as to reason for side rail use and calling for assistance when changing position. 2. Change positions slowly to minimize orthostatic hypotension. 3. Stress importance of participation in physical therapy, increased food and fiber in diet, and use of opioids as needed. 4. Instruct to avoid alcohol and smoking upon discharge.

Continued

CENTRAL NERVOUS

CASE STUDY Postoperative Analgesia—cont'd

Evaluation
1. Pain level has reduced to 2 to 3 out of 10.
2. Mental status and irritability have improved.
3. Constipation has been prevented.
4. Patient demonstrates decreased behavioral manifestations of pain or discomfort.
5. There is increased participation in the usual activities of daily living.

CRITICAL REASONING ANALYSIS

Q1. Aren't you afraid that by giving her drugs for pain, her addiction will come back?
A. Even persons who have been dependent on opioids should expect to have their pain managed. When opioids are used for "legitimate" pain, the risk of dependency is quite low.

Q2. Shouldn't AB have intermittent dosing rather than using the PCA, because of her past history of substance abuse?
A. PCA with morphine provides more constant and uniform analgesia, avoids first-pass effects in the liver, provides the patient with a sense of control over her pain, reduces the likelihood of overdose and respiratory depression, and may reduce CNS irritability secondary to the meperidine metabolite, normeperidine. AB's ability to control the administration of pain medication promotes her sense of control, and therefore postoperative pain management is improved. Because of the lock-out on the PCA machine and the appropriate demand-dosing regimen, she is unlikely to receive too much analgesia. The basic principle is to dose around the clock

Q3. What effect will AB's history of hepatitis have on her pain relief?
A. AB's history of hepatitis may alter the first-pass effect of orally administered opioids. It is likely that it will have no effect unless she has actual inflammation of the liver.

Q4. Is AB's fear of once again becoming addicted part of the reason she is so irritable and refusing to participate in her care?
A. That is possible, but there are several possible explanations. One explanation for her irritability relates to normeperidine, the metabolite of meperidine. High-dose meperidine can cause CNS stimulation (i.e., tremors, seizures) as a result of the metabolite's accumulation. Another cause is simply fear: fear of recurrent dependency, outcomes of hospitalization, and other psychosocial issues. Irritability may also be a reflection of poorly controlled pain.

Nausea and vomiting can occur because of the action of opioids on brainstem centers. Changing the type of opioid used may stop the adverse effect, or the addition of an antiemetic drug may help. However, it is important to note that patients quickly develop a tolerance to nausea and vomiting. No patient should be denied pain relief because of this effect. Instead, he or she should simply receive treatment for the nausea and vomiting until it subsides.

Use caution in prescribing opioids in patients with severe burns. A common cause of respiratory arrest in burned patients is excessive analgesia. Generally, agitation in a burned patient is interpreted as hypoxia, hypovolemia, or pain unless proved otherwise. Use small IV doses of opioid analgesics when needed. Drugs given by other routes are absorbed erratically in the presence of shock and hypovolemia.

LIFE-SPAN CONSIDERATIONS

Pregnant and Nursing Women. The gate-control theory of pain transmission has two important implications for childbirth. First, pain can be controlled by tactile stimulation; and, second, pain is modified by the use of activities that affect the CNS, such as back rubs, effleurage, suggestion, distraction, and physical conditioning.

Pain during the first stage of labor is, for the most part, related to dilation of the cervix. During the second stage of labor, pain is related to distention of the vagina and perineum and pressure on adjacent structures. Uterine contractions and cervical dilation as the placenta is expelled produce pain during the third stage of labor. The absence of crying or moaning during labor does not necessarily mean the woman is not in pain. On the other hand, crying or moaning does not necessarily mean that pain relief is desired.

For information on specific agents and their effects, see the Evolve Resources Bonus Content "Effects of Selected Maternal Drug Ingestion on the Fetus or Neonate," found at http://evolve.elsevier.com/Gutierrez/pharmacotherapeutics.

Children and Adolescents. In general, pain in children younger than 5 years of age is difficult to assess. Contributing to the difficulty are level of language development and comprehension; the confounding variables of anxiety, fear, or loneliness; the lack of a good understanding of pain phenomena; and the relative lack of valid and reliable pain assessment instruments. Infants may cry and display muscular rigidity and thrashing behaviors. Preschoolers can be aggressive or verbally complain of discomfort. School-age children express pain verbally or behaviorally, often by displaying regression behaviors. Adolescents are often reluctant to admit that they are uncomfortable or need help.

Pain experiences of children are also influenced when the child observes the expression of pain in another child or their parent. Such observation can result in anxiety and negative social modeling that leads children to act much like the person in pain. Conversely, if the child views another child or adult coping well with the painful situation, pain expression and acting-out behaviors can be reduced.

Older Adults. Population studies have suggested that painful experiences occur 2 times more often in persons over 60 years of age as compared with younger individuals. Among institutionalized older adults, the prevalence may well be over 70%. Indeed, more than 80% of older adults suffer various forms of arthritis, and most will have acute pain at some time during the course of their disease.

The widespread belief that aging increases the pain threshold is a myth. In addition, pain is often harder to assess in older patients because of such obstacles as cognitive impairment, delirium, and dementia. Whether behavioral observations (agitation, restlessness, groaning) are sufficiently sensitive and specific for pain assessment among demented older adults remains uncertain. Also, visual, hearing, and motor impairments impede the use of some assessment instruments. Preliminary reports suggest that older adults with moderate to severe cognitive impairment can reliably report acute pain when it occurs or with prompting. Pain recall and integration of the pain experience over time may be less reliable, however.

Physiologic as well as psychologic and cultural changes associated with aging cause pain to be perceived differently in this population. Institutionalized older adults are often stoic about pain. In addition, older adult patients often have altered presentations of common illnesses such as the so-called silent myocardial infarctions and painless intraabdominal emergencies.

Older adults, especially the frail and those over age 75, are at particular risk for both too much and too little pain management, although age-related responses are variable. Older adult patients experience a higher peak and longer duration of drug action than younger counterparts. Age-related changes in drug distribution and elimination make the older adult more sensitive to sedation and respiratory distress.

Opioids are effective for the management of acute pain in older adults. Cheyne-Stokes respirations are not unusual in the older adult during sleep. This respiratory pattern need not prompt discontinuance of an opioid unless it is associated with unacceptable levels of arterial oxygen desaturation (less than 85%).

Drug Variables

Relative potency estimates are used to select the appropriate starting dose, to change the route of administration, or to change from one opioid to another. The time course to pain relief depends on the drug dose, the blood level achieved, pain severity, and the patient's threshold for pain. Caution is warranted when selecting dosages to be certain that excessive CNS and respiratory depression is avoided (see the Evidence-Based Pharmacotherapeutics box).

Management of mild to moderate pain begins with NSAIDs unless otherwise contraindicated (see Chapter 17). NSAIDs decrease levels of inflammatory mediators that are generated at the pain site. Although NSAIDs may be insufficient to control pain when used alone, they have profound dose-sparing effects and serve a function in reducing the adverse effects of opioids. Furthermore, the use of an NSAID as an adjuvant to opioids can provide a more complete analgesia then opioid-induced analgesia alone. Although it is plausible that NSAIDs also act within the CNS in contrast to the opioids, they neither cause sedation or respiratory depression nor interfere with bowel or bladder function.

Moderate to severe pain can be managed initially with an opioid. The requisite conditions for rational opioid therapy have several components. Knowledge of drug indications for acute and chronic pain, mechanism of action, the relationships between drug action and potentially serious adverse effects, the variability among patients with regard to pharmacokinetics, and the variability between patient and disease condition as it relates to the magnitude of effects are just a few. Drug selection, dose, route, and treatment regimen are also based on anticipated pain. That is, drug therapy should correspond with the overall pain syndrome. Using the placebo-effect potentially present in all patients and reducing sensory input that aggravates pain provides the most effective and complete pain relief. Agonist-antagonists are not recommended for prolonged use, as first-line therapy for acute or cancer pain, or for chronic (nonmalignant) pain.

Morphine is the standard for opioid therapy. If it cannot be used, another opioid such as hydromorphone may be substituted. There are no clinically apparent differences between hydromorphone and other opioids. Hydromorphone has an advantage over morphine in that it can be administered in smaller volumes of fluid because of its higher potency. Oxycodone is as potent as morphine ,and although it can be used alone, it is commonly used in combination with nonopioid analgesics such as acetaminophen (APAP) or aspirin (ASA).

Codeine has more of a stimulant effect on the CNS than morphine. The stimulatory effect is due to the formation of the metabolite norcodeine. Codeine salts are well absorbed orally and have a higher bioavailability than morphine. This is because codeine has the lowest oral-parenteral dose ratio of all injectable opioids. Furthermore, codeine is less likely to cause dependency compared with morphine, but at equianalgesic dosages it induces greater histamine release than morphine. The greater histamine release increases the risk of vasodilation, hypotension, bronchoconstriction, and urticaria.

Meperidine, sometimes called the "opioid to avoid," binds to both μ and κ receptors and is less potent than morphine. Although most of its effects are similar to those of morphine, high-dose meperidine causes CNS stimulation (i.e., tremors, seizures) as a result of the accumulation of normeperidine, its metabolite. The patients at most risk for CNS toxicity are older adults, those with renal insufficiency or who receive high doses for an extended period, and patients with a history of seizures.

Methadone is a potent analgesic, has a long duration of action (upon repeated dosing), and is much cheaper than many long-acting morphine formulations (MS Contin, Oxy-Contin) used for long-acting pain relief. It may also provide pain control in patients whose pain was not controlled with other opioids. The long biologic half-life of methadone probably accounts for the mild, but prolonged, withdrawal syndrome if drug use stops abruptly.

Fentanyl is available in parenteral formulations, as a transdermal patch, and as a lollipop for oral administration. The transdermal patch may be as effective as sustained-release morphine, but the drug is not recommended for acute pain management because of the kinetic characteristics of the delivery system and the fact that the dosage is more difficult

EVIDENCE-BASED PHARMACOTHERAPEUTICS

Management of Acute and Chronic Pain

■ Background
For years, morphine has been the gold standard for the management of advanced cancer pain. For these patients, hydromorphone, an alternative to morphine, may be recommended. The efficacy and potency of hydromorphone are less well understood.

■ Research Article
Quigley, C. Hydromorphone for acute and chronic pain. *The Cochrane Database of Systematic Reviews.* 2002, Issue 1. Art. No. CD003447. DOI: 10.1002/14651858.CD003447.

Purpose
The purpose of this study was to investigate available evidence as to the effectiveness of hydromorphone in the management of acute and chronic pain.

Design
A total of 43 randomized, controlled studies of subjects ($N = 2725$) treated for acute or chronic pain with hydromorphone were analyzed. Subjects ($N = 645$) in 11 of the studies had cancer-related chronic pain, whereas in the other 32 studies ($N = 2080$), subjects had acute pain. Hydromorphone was compared with other opioids (i.e., fentanyl, morphine, meperidine, oxycodone, sufentanyl), with bupivicaine, and with itself. Different formulations of hydromorphone were used (oral, intravenous, intramuscular, subcutaneous, spinal routes). Data-gathering included searches of electronic databases and hand-searching of relevant journals.

Methods
Using concealment strategies, the validity of each study for inclusion in the review was assessed and a grade assigned. An investigator-developed checklist was used to assess blinding. Meta-analysis was not possible because a low-quality score was found in over half the studies analyzed. The diverse nature of the studies did not permit the combining of data and results.

Findings
Based on the examination of the limited number of valid trials, there are few differences between hydromorphone and morphine in relation to analgesia produced, adverse effects, and subject preference for one drug over another. Most of the valid studies had small numbers of subjects, precluding identification of any true differences between hydromorphone and morphine.

Conclusions
The issue of equianalgesic ratios and drug effectiveness between hydromorphone and morphine in subjects with acute and chronic pain was not resolved. The valid studies suggest efficacy of hydromorphone appears to be dose-related. The adverse effects of hydromorphone are comparable to those of other μ-receptor agonists.

■ Implication for Practice
Evidence from this review does not support the notion that hydromorphone is more efficacious compared with morphine in the management of moderate to severe cancer-related pain. There is a need for high-quality, head-to-head studies comparing hydromorphone, morphine, and other opioids in terms of analgesia effectiveness in adults and children alike.

---

to titrate. The patches are designed to deliver a near-constant rate of drug to the upper skin layers at the rates of 25, 50, 75, and 100 mcg/hr. It has the advantage of a 72-hour dosage frequency but should be used only after the patient has first been stabilized on a regularly dosed opioid. However, fentanyl is the drug of choice for epidural administration because of its faster onset of action.

Because of fentanyl's lipid-solubility, it is easier to titrate than epidural morphine. Epidural fentanyl produces less nausea and vomiting and itching than epidural morphine. There is a greater incidence of late respiratory depression from epidural morphine because of its longer duration of action and its active metabolites. Further, monitoring for up to 24 hours is necessary for patients who have received epidural morphine. This is in contrast to epidural fentanyl, in which monitoring is necessary for only about 4 hours.

Butorphanol, buprenorphine, and nalbuphine are less likely to cause respiratory depression than morphine because they are partial agonists. However, if morphine (as with any other opioid) is properly titrated, there is little (if any) clinical difference between these drugs in regard to respiratory depression. Buprenorphine has a slightly longer duration of action than morphine but is more expensive. There is agonistic activity at therapeutic dosages on the μ receptors, which produces analgesia; at higher dosages, the agonist-antagonist drugs produce antagonistic activity, diminishing the analgesic effects and, in some cases, precipitating withdrawal syndrome. These opioid agonist-antagonists were originally thought to have less abuse potential than true opioid agonists. However, butorphanol and pentazocine reportedly have contributed to dependence.

ROUTE CONSIDERATIONS. Determining the best route for opioid administration may be difficult. The route of choice for opioids is oral, if the patient tolerates oral intake. Oral formulations are also convenient and inexpensive; they are the mainstay of treatment for the ambulatory patient. The oral route is as effective as parenteral routes (although it does not have as quick an onset) when the drug is used in appropriate dosages.

The parenteral route of choice for opioids is IV. It is suitable for titrated bolus or continuous administration, including use with patient-controlled analgesia (PCA). The disadvantage to an IV route is that it requires continual monitoring, and there is a significant risk of respiratory depression with inappropriate dosing. In contrast, PCA provides steady levels of analgesia and less respiratory depression, and is popular with patients and nursing staff alike. It does require special infusion pumps and staff education to be effective.

IM injections have been the standard parenteral administration route in the past, but absorption is unreliable and the injections are painful. This route is generally avoided as much as possible. When a low-volume continuous infusion is needed and IV access is difficult or impossible, the subQ route is preferable to the IM. However, as with IM injections, subQ injections are painful and have long absorption rates. Avoid the subQ route when long-term repetitive dosing is needed.

Epidural and intrathecal administration routes are suitable in some circumstances and provide good analgesia. With these routes, there is a significant risk of respiratory depression. The respiratory depression is sometimes delayed in onset and necessitates careful monitoring, the use of infusion pumps, and a specially educated staff.

PATIENT-CONTROLLED ANALGESIA. PCA permits intermittent self-administration of opioids. The PCA method provides constant and uniform analgesia by avoiding the potentially wide variations in serum drug levels associated with infrequent IM or IV administration. In addition, PCA provides patients with a sense of control and, more often than not, results in use of lower amounts of a drug compared to conventional IM or IV administration. The potentially addictive aspects of opioid infusions are negligible.

PCA begins with setting pump parameters. The PCA unit operates under two modes: demand dosing, in which a fixed dose is taken intermittently, or constant-rate infusion plus demand dosing. A loading dose is determined, along with a background infusion rate, the dose to be administered per demand, the lockout interval (i.e., the minimum time between demand doses), and the maximum total dosage received over a specified time interval (e.g., a demand dose of 1 mg of morphine with a lockout time of 5 to 10 minutes).

For the patient using a PCA unit with morphine, 1 mg per bolus with a lockout time of 6 minutes is recommended. Some health care providers believe that 1 to 2 mg/hour permits a postoperative patient to sleep through the night. However, using a bolus with a baseline infusion may increase the amount of opioid used, along with adverse effects, without improving pain relief. Reassess the patient every 1 to 2 hours, and if the pain is not well managed, increase the bolus dose by 25% to 50%. If pain relief from the bolus is adequate but the duration of pain relief is too short, the lockout time should be decreased.

For the patient using PCA with meperidine, a starting dose of 10 mg per bolus with a lockout time of 6 minutes is recommended. However, using a bolus along with a baseline infusion increases the risk of seizures. As for those receiving morphine via PCA, the patient receiving meperidine should be reassessed every 1 to 2 hours and the dosage adjusted 25% to 50% if pain is uncontrolled. Again, if pain relief from the bolus is adequate but the duration of pain relief is too short, reduce the lockout time.

Consider the use of PCA with developmentally normal children aged 7 years and older. However, keep in mind that a steady-state drug level is necessary for a drug to be continuously effective. Interruption of an around-the-clock schedule can cause resurgence of pain as blood levels of the drug decline.

Assess blood pressure, pulse, and respiratory rate before and periodically during administration of an opioid. If the respiratory rate falls below 10 breaths per minute, the patient's level of sedation should be assessed. Physical stimulation may be sufficient to prevent significant hypoventilation, although an opioid antagonist may be required.

EQUIANALGESIA. It is sometimes necessary to change to a different opioid or to change the route by which it is administered. This practice is known as *equianalgesia*. By estimating the relative potency of the opioids, the health care provider can determine the proper dosage and administration route. However, clinical judgment must always be used to arrive at the appropriate route, dosage, and dosage conversion.

Be aware that different equianalgesic tables may show different equivalencies (Table 16-5). Another potential problem is the difficulty in understanding the conversions needed to use equianalgesia, particularly when the drug, the route, and the dosage all change at the same time. Nonetheless, these tables can be safely used as long as the health care provider adheres to the following seven caveats:

1. *Treat the patient, not the table:* Available drug formulations may not match the calculated dose. In these situations, begin with a dose lower than the calculated dose. For example, if the calculated dose minus 25% (to account for incomplete cross-tolerance) is 10 mg but the available formulation is a 4-mg tablet, start with an 8-mg dose, or two tablets.

2. *Use one equianalgesic table:* With the regular use of the same equianalgesic table, the potential for calculation errors is reduced and the comfort of the health care provider increased, in relation to drug and dosage conversions.

3. *Know the drugs and the patient under consideration:* Equianalgesia dosages of certain opioids vary based on whether the patient is opioid-naïve or someone who uses opioids chronically.

4. *Start conservatively, titrating to effect:* A patient may have become tolerant to one opioid, but the equianalgesia drug to be used may be more potent than expected at recommended dosages. For this reason, the *calculated* equianalgesic dosage of the new drug is lowered 30% to 50% to avoid overshooting the patient's analgesic needs. Titrate the dose as needed. Frequent reevaluation of the patient and the pain level is useful in determining when dosage increases are needed.

5. *Calculate dosage based on 24-hour usage:* Equianalgesic tables ordinarily include *per dose* equivalencies. Establish the patient's total opioid use in the previous 24 hours, calculate the equianalgesic dosage of the new drug, subtract 25%, and divide by the number of desired doses per day.

6. *Don't forget rescue doses:* Despite around-the-clock dosing regimens, it may still be necessary for rescue doses to be readily available. A rescue dose is ordinarily 15% to 20% of the total daily dosage.

7. *Request assistance:* Request that another health care provider review the equianalgesic treatment plan, as well as the dosing calculations, to reduce the risk for error (Quinn, 2002).

Placebos have little use today in pain management. Placebo effects can be seen with all drugs; illness and the related behaviors provide some degree of secondary gain. Further, a positive response to a placebo does not mean that the patient's pain is not real, that the patient is faking the pain, or that the patient is imagining some illness or symptom. Likewise, a positive response to opioids or other analgesics allows no judgment one way or the other about the patient's pain.

The World Health Organization (WHO) recommends the following a three-step approach when managing a patient in pain:

Step 1: Use maximum dosages of NSAIDs (e.g., aspirin, ibuprofen, adjuvants). Go on to step 2 if the pain persists.

Step 2: Use a less potent opioid (e.g., codeine) along with adjuvant therapies. Go on to step 3 if the pain persists.

Step 3: Use a more potent opioid (i.e., morphine, oxycodone, hydromorphone, fentanyl) and adjuvants. Morphine is the gold standard and should be the considered a first-line step 3 drug for all patients, including older adults.

TABLE 16-5 Equianalgesia Dosing Data for Opioid Analgesics

Drug	Approximate Equianalgesic Oral Dose	Approximate Equianalgesic Parenteral Dose	Recommended Starting Dose (Adult >50 kg Body Weight)		Recommended Starting Dose (Child, and Adult <50 kg Body Weight)	
			Oral	Parenteral	Oral	Parenteral
OPIOID AGONIST						
morphine*	30 mg every 3–4 hr (around-the-clock dosing) 60 mg every 3–4 hr (single dose or intermittent dosing)	10 mg every 3–4 hr	30 mg every 3–4 hr	10 mg every 3–4 hr	0.3 mg/kg every 3–4 hr	0.1 mg/kg every 3–4 hr
codeine†	130 mg every 3–4 hr	75 mg every 3–4 hr	60 mg every 3–4 hr	60 mg every 2 hr IM or subQ	1 mg/kg every 3–4 hr‡	Not recommended
hydromorphone* (Dilaudid)	7.5 mg every 3–4 hr	1.5 mg every 3–4 hr	6 mg every 3–4 hr	1.5 mg every 3–4 hr	0.06 mg/kg every 3–4 hr	0.015 mg/kg every 3–4 hr
hydrocodone (Lorcet, Lortab, Vicodin, others)	30 mg every 3–4 hr	UA	10 mg every 3–4 hr	UA	0.2 mg/kg every 3–4 hr	UA
levorphanol (Levo-Dromoran)	4 mg every 6–8 hr	2 mg every 6–8 hr	4 mg every 6–8 hr	2 mg every 6–8 hr	0.04 mg/kg every 6–8 hr	0.02 mg/kg every 6–8 hr
meperidine (Demerol)	300 mg every 3–4 hr	100 mg every 3 hr	Not recommended	100 mg every 3 hr	Not recommended	0.75 mg/kg every 2–3 hr
methadone (Dolophine, others)	20 mg every 6–8 hr	10 mg every 6–8 hr	20 mg every 6–8 hr	10 mg every 6–8 hr	0.2 mg/kg every 6–8 hr	0.1 mg/kg every 6–8 hr
oxycodone (Roxicodone, Percocet, Percodan, Tylox, others)	30 mg every 3–4 hr	UA	10 mg every 3–4 hr	Not available	0.2 mg/kg every 3–4 hr‡	UA
oxymorphone* (Numorphan)	UA	1 mg every 3–4 hr	UA	1 mg every 3–4 hr	Not recommended	Not recommended
OPIOID AGONIST-ANTAGONIST						
buprenorphine (Buprenex)	UA	0.3–0.4 mg every 6–8 hr	UA	0.4 mg every 6–8 hr	UA	0.004 mg/kg every 6–8 hr
butorphanol (Stadol)	UA	2 mg every 3–4 hr	UA	2 mg every 3–4 hr	UA	UA
nalbuphine (Nubain)	UA	10 mg every 3–4 hr	UA	10 mg every 3–4 hr	UA	0.1 mg/kg every 3–4 hr
pentazocine (Talwin, others)	150 mg every 3–4 hr	60 mg every 3–4 hr	50 mg every 4–6 hr	Not recommended	Not recommended	UA

*For morphine, hydromorphone, and oxymorphone, rectal administration is an alternate route for patients unable to take oral agents, but equianalgesic doses may differ from oral and parenteral doses because of pharmacokinetic differences.
†Caution: Codeine doses above 65 mg often are not appropriate because of diminishing incremental analgesia with increasing doses along with continually increasing constipation and other adverse effects.
‡Caution: Doses of aspirin and acetaminophen in combination opioid-NSAID formulations must also be adjusted to the patient's body weight.
NSAID, Nonsteroidal antiinflammatory drug; *UA*, unavailable.
From the U.S. Department of Health and Human Services. (1992). *Clinical practice guidelines. Acute pain management: Operative or medical procedures and trauma* (AHCPR 92–0032). Rockville, MD: Author.

Malignant Cancer Pain. When opioids are needed for cancer pain, the primary consideration is patient comfort, not preventing drug dependency. With disease progression and the development of drug tolerance, larger doses and increased dosing frequency may be necessary. Consider using potent opioids when initiating management of malignant cancer pain; potent opioids provide immediate relief, and the dosage can be slowly reduced until pain relief is achieved at a lower dosage.

Methadone is increasingly being used in treatment of chronic pain. It does require slow, careful dose titration.

Many of the studies have been done on patients with cancer and demonstrate that methadone may offer relief for patients unable to achieve adequate relief from or who cannot tolerate other opioids. The drug's long half-life and potency makes titration difficult and frequently causes oversedation and toxicity.

Nonmalignant Chronic Pain. Evolving changes in the chronic pain paradigm include choosing a treatment most appropriate for the pain condition. Since the early 1990s, health care providers have been encouraged to treat chronic intractable nonmalignant pain with opioids. There has been an emphasis on using sustained-release opioids whenever the pain lasts 12 hours or more during a 24-hour period. The reason for advocating sustained-release opioids was primarily to provide more consistent pain relief and decrease the risk of abuse, which is thought to be greater with short-acting opioids. In addition, it is believed that opioids are to be titrated to the dosage necessary to adequately control pain. The upper limit is determined only by adverse effects.

Breakthrough pain is quite common in persons with chronic pain, with current estimates of its incidence as high as 90% in patients with some forms of chronic pain. The personal burden of breakthrough pain can be quite high, and there is a strong association with impaired daily functioning, demoralization, and generally poor medical outcomes. Poorly managed breakthrough pain has significant socioeconomic considerations, since these patients are also more likely to utilize health care resources than patients without breakthrough pain, to have more pain-related hospitalizations and emergency department visits, and to experience increased direct and indirect treatment costs.

For the patient with nonmalignant chronic pain, it may be appropriate to bypass some of the more conservative steps to more quickly provide pain relief (Box 16-4). The better the understanding of pain mechanisms, the more likely that we will be able to match the most effective treatment to patient needs. In particular, patients with breakthrough pain have unique needs and are not best served by being lumped into the same treatment approach as patients with chronic persistent pain.

Patient Education

Teach patients to take their opioid analgesic as directed. Although this principle applies to all drugs, it is particularly important with opioids because of potentially serious adverse effects and because analgesics may mask or enable the patient to tolerate pain for which medical attention would otherwise be required. Advise patients not to save leftover prescriptions for use with other disorders and not to let anyone else take their prescription drugs.

Teach the patient the importance of avoiding concurrent use of alcohol and other CNS depressants without first checking with the health care provider. It is suggested that patients not keep their opioid at the bedside to prevent inadvertent overdose.

Teach patients to change positions slowly to minimize any orthostatic hypotension, particularly if they are also taking antihypertensive drugs or diuretics. Teach hospitalized patients the reasons for raising the side rails on the bed after they have received an opioid. Side rails promote safety by serving as a reminder to stay in bed or to call for assistance.

Many patients report an allergy to codeine because of a history of nausea; nausea is not a sign of true allergy, but rather the result of GI irritation. Instruct the patient to take the opioid analgesic with small amounts of food to reduce the potential for nausea.

Constipation can be prevented, or at least minimized, by consuming high-fiber foods such as whole grain cereals, fruits, and vegetables; drinking 2 to 3 quarts of fluids daily; and remaining as active as possible. A stool softener such as ducosate sodium may be taken daily. Bulk-forming drugs such as psyllium (see Chapter 46) are effective for most patients, as long as adequate hydration is maintained. Cancer experts recommend a bowel regimen that includes stimulant laxatives in addition to the stool softener (e.g., senna and docusate). Institute a bowel program for patients receiving an opioid for longer than 24 hours (Box 16-5). Assess bowel sounds on a regular basis.

Patients provided with instructions about coping with pain (instruction on turning, coughing, deep breathing, and ambulation) during the preoperative period report less pain, use fewer analgesics, and have shorter hospital stays than patients who did not receive instruction.

Evaluation

Evaluation of the therapeutic effectiveness of opioids depends in part on the reason for their use. Patients may provide a verbal statement of pain relief, demonstrate decreased behavioral manifestations of pain or discomfort, and increase participation

---

BOX 16-4

Key Points for Opioid Use for Nonmalignant Chronic Pain

- A single health care provider should take primary responsibility for treatment and for dispensing opioids.
- Patients should provide informed consent before initiation of therapy (see Box 16-3).
- Only after all reasonable attempts at analgesia with other analgesics have failed should opioid maintenance therapy be considered.
- A patient's history of substance abuse should be a relative contraindication to opioid therapy.
- Administer opioid analgesics on an around-the-clock or time-contingent basis rather than on a PRN basis.
- Failure to even partially reduce pain should provoke concerns about the viability of continued opioid therapy.
- Allow patients to temporarily increase drug dosages when needed.
- Exacerbations of pain that are not effectively managed by temporary, small increases in dosage are best managed on an inpatient basis;

thus dosage increases can be closely monitored and the return to baseline dosing achieved.
- Monitor for drug effectiveness, adverse reactions, and signs of drug misuse or abuse. Prescribe the opioid only after the patient has been seen. Most patients with nonmalignant pain should be seen monthly and opioid refills written as appropriate.
- Tapering and a discontinuance of opioid therapy should follow objective evidence of uncontrolled increases in dosage, acquisition of drugs from other health care providers, drug hoarding, or other unusual behaviors.
- Proper documentation of pain assessment and opioid use is essential! Documentation should also include the degree to which pain relief was obtained, adverse effects that appeared, and the patient's functional capacity and any aberrant behaviors.
- Make note of any gains in the patient's physical and social functioning, which are usually a sign of improved analgesia.

PRN, As needed.

Adapted from Portenoy, R. (1996). Opioid therapy for chronic nonmalignant pain: A review of the critical issues. Reprinted from *Journal of Pain Symptom Management. 11*(4), 203–217. Copyright ©1996, with permission from the U.S. Cancer Pain Relief Committee.

CENTRAL NERVOUS

BOX 16-5

Treatment of Opioid-Induced Constipation

All patients on opioid therapy require an individualized bowel regimen. The following regimen is but one example of the many available. Begin with step 1, continuing the course of treatment for the duration of opioid therapy.

- **Step 1**: Docusate, 100 mg twice daily; plus 1 tablet of senna once or twice daily
- **Step 2**: Docusate, 100 mg twice daily; plus 2 tablets of senna twice daily
- **Step 3**: Docusate, 100 mg twice daily; plus 3 tablets of senna twice daily
- **Step 4**: Docusate, 100 mg twice daily; 4 tablets senna twice daily; plus lactulose, 15 mL twice daily

- **Step 5**: Docusate, 100 mg twice daily; 4 tablets senna twice daily; plus lactulose, 15 mL twice daily, plus sodium phosphate or oil retention enema; if no results, add a high-colonic tap-water enema
- **Step 6**: Docusate, 100 mg twice daily; 4 tablets senna twice daily; plus lactulose, 30 mL twice daily
- **Step 7**: Docusate, 100 mg twice daily; 4 tablets senna twice daily; plus lactulose, 30 mL 4 times daily

Rule out impaction with digital rectal examination, or bowel obstruction with abdominal radiographs, when there is clinical suspicion of their presence. Rectal disimpaction must be accomplished before treating constipation with an oral laxative regimen.

From *Treatment of Opioid-Induced Constipation.* Sinai Onsite Health. Palliative Care Center. Available online: www.sinaionsitehealth.org/palliative/pdf/paincardv20011.pdf. Accessed December 24, 2005.

in the usual activities of daily living. There may be a decrease in blood pressure and pulse rate, and slower and deeper respirations. The frequency of pain evaluation is based on knowledge of how quickly the drug works. Additional benefits are gained when earlier mobilization, shortened hospital stays, reduced cost, and improved quality of life are realized.

It is crucial that both the desired and the adverse effects of opioid therapy be monitored and the results documented. The most frequent cause of legal action against health care providers is failure to document the rationale for the initial and continuing use of opioids and the resulting outcomes.

KEY POINTS

- Pain perception is activated by pain-specific receptors (nociceptors) in peripheral tissues.
- Acute pain is short-term, generally lasting only for the duration of tissue damage. Chronic pain is pain that lasts longer than 6 months.
- Somatic pain originates in cutaneous tissues and is well defined, localized, and of low to moderate intensity.
- Visceral pain arises from body organs. Because there are few nociceptors in body organs, pain sensations are diffuse and poorly localized.
- Neuropathic pain is related to injury or damage to nerve fibers in the periphery or damage to the CNS.
- The primary treatment objective in pain management is to eliminate the pain as much and as quickly as possible using the least potent drug and the lowest possible dose to achieve adequate pain control while minimizing adverse effects.
- Effective pain management also results in earlier mobilization, shortened hospital stay, reduced cost, and improved quality of life.
- Management of mild to moderate pain should begin with NSAIDs unless otherwise contraindicated.

- Moderate to severe pain is best managed with an opioid.
- Adjunctive drug therapy may include capsaicin, caffeine, adrenergic agonists, tricyclic antidepressants, carbamazepine, phenytoin, and hydroxyzine.
- The preferred method of treatment for chronic pain is to use long-acting formulations on a scheduled basis and provide patients with short-acting formulations for breakthrough pain.
- Naloxone is the antagonist of choice if an antidote is required to reverse opioid-induced respiratory depression or coma.
- Teach patients to take their opioid as directed because of potentially serious adverse effects and because analgesics may mask or enable the patient to tolerate pain for which medical attention is required.
- Avoid alcohol and other CNS depressant drugs when taking opioid analgesics.
- Assess pain relief through verbal statements of pain relief, a decrease in behavioral manifestations of pain or discomfort, and an increase in participation in the usual activities of daily living.

Bibliography

American Medical Association. (2005). *Pain management–Pathophysiology of pain and pain assessment:* Available online: www.amacmeonline.com/pain_mgmt/module01/. Accessed December 24, 2005.

American Pain Society. (1999). *Chronic pain in America: Roadblocks to relief. Survey Highlights.* Roper Starch Worldwide Inc: [telephone survey]. Available online:www.ampainsoc.org/links/roadblocks/ Accessed December 24, 2005.

Gordon, D., Dahl, J., Miaskowski, C., et al, and American Pain Society Quality of Care Task Force. (2005). Improving the quality of acute and cancer pain management. *Archives of Internal Medicine,* 165(14), 1574–1580.

International Association for the Study of Pain. *Definition of pain.* Available online: www.iasp-pain.org. Accessed December 8, 2005. (Membership required.)

Jackson, K., and Stanford, L. (2003). *Opioid use in clinical practice.* Available online: secure.pharmacytimes.com/lesson/2003,08-02.asp. Accessed February 20, 2007.

McCaffery, M., and Pasero, C. (2004). *Pain: Clinical manual.* (2nd rev. ed.). Philadelphia: Mosby.

McCaffery, M. (1994). How to use the new AHCPR cancer pain guidelines. *American Journal of Nursing, 94*(7), 42–47.

McCaffery, M., and Ferrell, B. (1991). Patient age: Does it affect your pain-control decisions? *Nursing, 21*(9), 44–48.

McCaffery, M., and Ferrell, B. (1994). Nurses' assessment of pain intensity and choice of analgesic dose. *Contemporary Nurse, 3*(2), 68–74.

Melzak, R. (1982). Recent concepts of pain. *Journal of Medicine, 13*(3), 147–160.

Melzak, R. (1987). The short form McGill pain questionnaire. *Pain, 30*(2), 191–197.

Melzak, R., and Wall, P. (1992). *The puzzle of pain.* New York: Basic Books.

National Institutes of Health. (2005). An update of NIH pain research and related program initiatives. Subcommittee on Health, Committee on Energy and Commerce, United States House of Representatives, 12/8/2005. Available online: www.hhs.gov/asl/testify/t051208a.html. Accessed December 8, 2006.

Ortho-McNeil Pharmaceutical. (1997). Product information: Ultram. Raritan, MT: Author.

Pain management issues. (2004). Copiscope: Bi-Monthly Newsletter of COPIC Insurance Company. No. 119, 5–6. Available online: www.callcopic.com/resources/custom/PDF/secure/colorado-copi-scope/issue-119-may-2004.pdf. Accessed February 20, 2007.

Pain management still tender issue at hospitals—care and compassion can make a difference. Blizzard, R. (Ed., (2005). *Gallup Poll.* Available online:poll.gallup.com/content/default.aspx?=;18484&pg=1 Accessed February 20, 2007.

Portenoy, R. (1996). Opioid therapy for chronic nonmalignant pain: A review of the critical issues. *Journal of Pain Symptom Management, 11*(4), 203–217.

Quinn, T. (2002). Converting opioid analgesics, Part I: Use of equianalgesic tables. *Pain Relief Connection, 1*(6), 3–4Revised 7/16/2003. Available online:www.massgeneral.org/painrelief. Accessed April 8, 2007.

World Health Organization. (1996). *Cancer pain relief: With a guide to opioid availability.* (2nd ed.). Washington, DC: Author.

World Health Organization. (1990). Cancer pain relief and palliative care: Report of a WHO expert. *Committee Technical Report Series,* No. 804. Washington, DC: Author.

CENTRAL NERVOUS

17

NSAIDs, DMARDs, and Related Drugs

Inflammation, pain, and fever are common symptoms of many health-related conditions. These symptoms help the body provide a level of protection by increasing awareness of the injured site and, possibly, by temporarily restricting movement. There are many therapeutic classes of medications used in the management of the inflammation, pain, and fever associated with a variety of medical conditions. This chapter specifically addresses the following drug classes:

- Nonsteroidal antiinflammatory drugs (NSAIDS), the prototype of which is aspirin
- Cyclooxygenase inhibitors (COX-2 inhibitors), the prototype of which is celecoxib
- Disease-modifying antirheumatic drugs (DMARDs), the prototype of which is methotrexate
- Tumor necrosis factor (TNF) blockers, the prototype of which is etanercept
- Interleukin-1 (IL-1) blocker, the prototype of which is anakinra
- Antigout drugs, the prototype of which is allopurinol

Although not an antiinflammatory drug by mechanism, acetaminophen is included in this chapter because of its extensive use as an analgesic and antipyretic. Corticosteroids, a powerful class of antiinflammatory drugs are discussed in Chapter 56.

The drugs discussed in this chapter relieve symptoms and contribute to a patient's comfort and quality of life; they do not cure the underlying disorder producing the symptoms. To understand the actions of these drugs, an understanding of inflammation is needed.

PATHOGENESIS OF INFLAMMATION

Inflammation is a local reaction to tissue injury that can be caused by any number of factors. Exogenous factors include physical (e.g., surgery, heat, trauma, foreign bodies), chemical, and biologic factors (i.e., viruses, bacteria, parasites, fungi). Endogenous factors (e.g., inflammatory mediators, antigens, antibodies) often enter the picture in response to exogenous damage.

Inflammation and infection often coexist. As a result, the terms are often confused. Under normal circumstances, infection is always accompanied by inflammation. However, not all inflammation involves an infection. Inflammation is not a pathophysiologic mechanism; however, whenever cells or body tissues are injured or killed, there is a striking but nonspecific response by adjacent tissues, as well as changes in vessel wall permeability and infiltration of white blood cells. The inflammatory process is beneficial in promoting removal of dead cells, microorganisms, debris, and exudate. The body uses inflammation to limit the extent and severity of injury (Fig. 17-1).

TYPES OF INFLAMMATION

There are two broad categories of inflammation: acute inflammation and chronic inflammation. *Acute inflammation* develops in immediate response to tissue damage. Acute inflammation results in typical signs of inflammation: pain, redness, warmth, and swelling. It is an immediate response to stressors. This type usually resolves entirely in 8 to10 days, if complications do not interfere with healing. However, acute inflammation sometimes develops into the chronic form. *Chronic inflammation* involves the same signs as acute inflammation, which persists for weeks, months, or even years, commonly as a result of the immune response being triggered. Chronic inflammation is common in immune system–mediated diseases such as atherosclerosis and rheumatoid arthritis.

Acute Inflammation

Chemical Response

The inflammatory response is similar regardless of cause. Events in the process include chemical responses, vascular responses, and cellular responses. Prostaglandins (PGs), leukotrienes (LTs), and thromboxanes (TXAs) are chemical mediators released by activated granulocytes, lymphocytes, and macrophages. These three mediators are primary participants in all inflammatory processes. Other chemical mediators associated with inflammation include histamine, serotonin, cytokines, calcitonin gene–related peptide (CGRP), nitric oxide (NO), oxygen radicals, enzymes, and more.

Histamine is the first mediator released to be widely distributed through the body. It is released in large amounts from mast cells and basophils during degranulation. Histamine's actions are mediated by histamine$_1$ (H$_1$) receptors, whose stimulation results in venous vasodilation. If the area of vasodilation is near the body surface, the skin takes on a reddened appearance. As proteins leak through capillary walls into interstitial tissues, colloidal osmotic pressure rises and edema results. The mediators released and the pressure of fluid and cellular exudate on nerve endings contribute to pain. Histamine release also causes increased mucus production and bronchial constriction.

The inflammation process relies on arachidonic acid, a polyunsaturated omega-6 fatty acid that is metabolized to a series of PGs. There are nine types of PGs, designated by the letters A to I (NOTE: *PG* is written *Pg* when in combination with additional letter type). The degree of saturation of the side chain of each is designated by the subscript 1, 2, or 3. PgE$_2$, PgF$_2$, and PgI$_2$, as well as TXA$_2$, are transiently present at the site of injury, and are extraordinarily potent. PGs produce more erythema than histamine, and evidence suggests that PgE$_2$ sensitizes pain receptors to bradykinin. Aspirin and other NSAIDs block the synthesis of PGs through

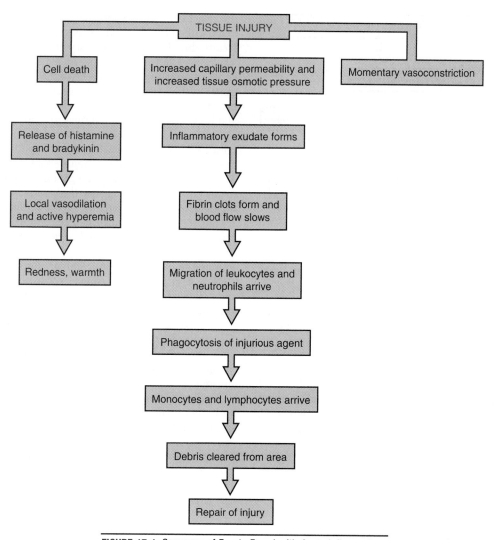

FIGURE 17-1 Sequence of Events Found with Acute Inflammation.

inhibition of COX enzymes, thereby inhibiting the inflammatory process. The functions of other arachidonic acid metabolites are listed in Table 17-1.

PGs contribute to vasodilation and increased vascular permeability and are thought to be responsible for the pain associated with inflammation. PGs arise from the cyclooxygenase (COX) metabolic pathway (Fig. 17-2). COX-1 mediates PGs that primarily maintain the integrity of the gastrointestinal (GI) mucosa and protect the surface of epithelial cells. COX-2 induces proinflammatory PGs, which cause the stiffness, swelling, and pain that accompany an illness or injury.

Like PGs, LTs are mediators synthesized by mast cells. LTA_4, LTB_4, LTC_4, LTD_4, and LTE_4 are generated along the lipoxygenase pathway. These LTs are acidic, sulfur-containing lipids that produce effects like that of histamine: smooth muscle contraction, increased vascular permeability, and neutrophil and eosinophil chemotaxis. LTB_4 is a potent chemotactic that causes granulocytes to aggregate. LTs are thought to be important in the later stages of the inflammatory response because they produce slower and more prolonged responses than histamines.

TABLE 17-1 Arachidonic Acid By-Products

By-product	Functions and Effects
PgD_2	Bronchoconstriction
PgE_1, PgE_2	Hyperalgesia (along with bradykinin and histamine)
	Increases permeability of vasculature (along with bradykinin and histamine)
	Vasodilation
	Increases activity of gastrointestinal smooth muscle
PgI_2	Vasodilation
	Bronchodilation
	Inhibits platelet aggregation
PgD_2	Platelet aggregation and brain function
$PgF_{2\alpha}$	Increases uterine contraction
	Bronchoconstriction
TXA_2	Platelet aggregation
	Vasoconstriction
	Bronchodilation
LTB_4	Chemotaxis
LTC_4, LTD_4, LTE_4	Bronchoconstriction
	Vasodilation

LT, Leukotriene (various subtypes indicated by additional letters, subscripts); *Pg-*, prostaglandin (various subtypes indicated by additional letters, subscripts); *TXA*, thromboxane.

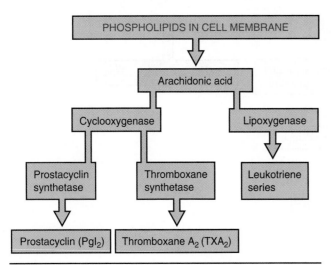

FIGURE 17-2 Synthesis of Prostaglandins and Leukotrienes from Arachidonic Acid, Simplified.

Nitrous oxide (NO) prolongs the inflammatory response by increasing neutrophils, monocytes, and eosinophil counts. This process prolongs the inflammatory response, thus protecting the injured site from further damage. NO also inhibits leukocyte adhesion to vascular endothelial tissues and the epithelium of the bronchial tree.

Oxygen radicals are the most destructive of all cell enzymes or toxins. Oxidizing radicals include hydroxyl ions (OH^-), superoxide (O_2^-) and hydrogen peroxide (H_2O_2). They are formed as the result of an enzyme system present on neutrophil plasma membranes. With these oxidizing agents, neutrophils are capable of synthesizing and attacking microorganisms and increasing vascular permeability.

⦚ Vascular Response

Disorders of cellular aggregation play an important role in the pathogenesis of various inflammatory disease processes because of platelet adhesion to injured endothelium during the early stages of clot formation. Capillary vasoconstriction causes tissue hypoxia and acidosis that lasts from 2 seconds to 5 or 10 minutes in acute inflammation. The degree of vasoconstriction depends on the extent of vascular injury. Following vasoconstriction there is a period of arteriolar vasodilation. An increased blood volume raises hydrostatic pressure within vessels, causing fluid to move into surrounding tissues and contributing to edema.

Platelets move to the injury site, adhering to exposed vascular collagen. The intrinsic clotting cascade is stimulated, and a fibrin meshwork forms. Platelets release a number of growth factors, and a fibrin clot forms within several minutes, with the remaining blood becoming thick and slowing circulation. At the same time, venous capillaries become more permeable, allowing more fluid to leak into surrounding tissues. Fibrin is deposited in lymphatic channels, causing blockage of the system. The lymphatic blockage localizes the area of inflammation from the surrounding tissues and delays the spread of toxins.

⦚ Cellular Response

Neutrophils migrate through vascular endothelium into tissues by a process called *chemotaxis*. Neutrophils are lured to

the area by bacterial toxins, degenerative products of inflammation, the C_{5a} complement fragment, and other substances. Neutrophils begin phagocytosis by producing collagenases, which break down dead tissue. At the same time, they release endogenous pyrogen that travels to the temperature-regulating center in the hypothalamus. Fever results, vessels dilate, more blood reaches the periphery, the patient becomes diaphoretic, and body temperature is returned to a normal range.

However, during febrile states, biochemical mediators are released from macrophages in the hypothalamus, and the thermostatic mechanism is adjusted to a higher set point. The mediators are both endogenous and exogenous. The major endogenous pyrogen is the proinflammatory cytokine interleukin-1 (IL-1). There are 14 known interleukins. IL-1 is released by almost all nucleated cells. It activates growth and function of neutrophils, lymphocytes, and macrophages, and promotes the release of additional mediators influencing the immune response. IL-6 and TNF are also endogenous pyrogens. IL-6 is produced by many cell types including phagocytes. It mediates the acute phase response, enhances B-cell production and differentiation to antibodies, and stimulates megakaryocyte production. TNF is released primarily by macrophages and T cells to help regulate immune response. TNF action is almost identical to those of IL-1. TNF and IL-1 are involved in fever production and other systemic effects of inflammation.

Known exogenous pyrogens include microorganisms and their endotoxins, and certain drugs (e.g., bleomycin and colchicine, and a few corticosteroids). Bacterial endotoxins cause release of PGs and endogenous pyrogens from neutrophils. Other arachidonic acid metabolites may also be involved in the production of fever. The reason aspirin does not reduce body temperature in patients without a fever is that no pyrogen is present to stimulate PG synthesis.

⦚ Outcomes of Acute Inflammation

The end result of inflammation is determined by the extent of tissue injury and the agent causing the damage. There are three possible outcomes of inflammation, based on the extent of tissue injury and the agent causing the damage:

1. *Complete resolution:* Tissues are capable of regeneration. This does not ordinarily occur.
2. *Scarring of connective tissues (fibrosis):* Healing begins within the first 24 hours after injury. At this point, connective tissue is formed that bridges the gap caused by injury, and the process of angiogenesis (i.e., the formation of new vessels that carry nutrients to healing tissues) begins. If healing is delayed or not complete, a scar will form.
3. *Chronic inflammation:* Chronic inflammation results when the inflammatory process continues for an extended period (e.g., days, months, or years). With prolonged capillary permeability, neutrophils accumulate in the affected area. As they release their lysosomes and oxidizing agents, the surrounding tissues also become inflamed and in time are replaced with scar tissue.

⦚ Outcomes of Chronic Inflammation

Little is known about the mediators of chronic inflammation. However, macrophage dominance and the appearance of fibroblasts and lymphocytes signal the beginning of a chronic cellular response such as that seen in rheumatologic diseases. Macrophages are necessary for tissue healing because of their functions in phagocytosis and debris removal. The macrophages produce a variety of chemical mediators. Proteases help remove foreign protein from the site of injury. Tissue thromboplastin from macrophages facilitates hemostasis and stimulates the fibroblast activity necessary for healing. Because chronic inflammation involves proliferation of fibroblasts, the risk of scarring and deformity is greater than with acute inflammation. In some instances, granulation tissue replaces normal supporting connective tissue elements or the functional parenchymal tissue of the involved structure.

Systemic Manifestations of Inflammation

Systemic signs and symptoms of inflammation vary depending on the cause and extent of tissue damage. Localized symptoms (redness, warmth, swelling, pain, and in some cases, loss of function) occur with both acute and chronic inflammation. Depending on the severity of tissue injury and the patient's vulnerability, localized inflammation can lead to systemic involvement. Fever is omnipresent in severe inflammation, assuming the immune system launches a response. Other systemic manifestations of inflammation include headache, loss of appetite, lethargy or malaise, and weakness. In severe cases, systemic responses to inflammation include acute respiratory distress syndrome (ARDS), disseminated intravascular coagulation (DIC), and damage to vascular endothelium resulting in shock, multiple organ system failure (MOSF), and often death. The terms *systemic inflammatory response syndrome (SIRS)* or *the shock cascade* are used to refer to these extreme inflammatory responses.

Leukocytosis and increased erythrocyte sedimentation rates (ESRs) also occur with systemic involvement. Note that a low neutrophil count is frequently interpreted as a sign of chronic, rather than acute, inflammation.

PHARMACOTHERAPEUTIC OPTIONS

Antiinflammatory drugs are the most widely prescribed and the most common over-the-counter (OTC) drugs used today. It is important to clearly understand their indications for use, drug action, adverse effects, drug interactions, and care implications. There is clear evidence to support the benefit of these drugs in the management of a variety of inflammatory conditions; however, their use must be balanced against the potential risk they pose. Serious and, at times, fatal consequences have occurred as a result of failure to recognize drug actions. This statement notwithstanding, antiinflammatory drug use is often based more on tradition and empirical results than a clear understanding of drug action.

Nonsteroidal Antiinflammatory Drugs

Antiinflammatory drugs are organized into two groups, the steroidal or the nonsteroidal drugs. In the United States, 70 million prescriptions are written annually for an NSAID, one of the most widely used classes of drugs. By custom, the NSAID class is further divided into those that are nonselective COX inhibitors and those that selectively inhibit

TABLE 17-2 Chemical Classifications of NSAIDs

Drug Class	Drug Examples
NONSELECTIVE COX INHIBITORS	
Salicylic acid derivatives	aspirin (Aspergum, ASA, Bayer Aspirin, Ecotrin, Empirin, others); ◆ Apo-ASA, Arthrisin, Astrin, Headstart, Riphen, others
	choline-magnesium salicylates (Tricosal, Trilisate)
	choline salicylate (Arthropan)
	diflunisal (Dolobid)
	magnesium salicylate (Doan's Pills, Magan, Mobidin); ◆ Back-ese
	salsalate (Dilsalcid, MonoGesic, Salicylic Acid, others)
	sodium salicylate (Uracel)
Para-aminophenol derivative	acetaminophen (Tylenol, (Datril, Tempra, Tylenol); ◆ Apo-Acetaminophen, Tempro, Tylenol
Heteroaryl acetic acids	diclofenac (Voltaren), ketorolac (Toradol), tolmetin (Tolectin); ◆ Novo-Tolmetin
Arylpropionic acids	ibuprofen (Advil, Motrin, Excedrin IB, Midol IB, others); ◆ Actiprofen, Apo-Ibuprofen, Novo-Profen
	fenoprofen (Nalfon)
	flurbiprofen (Ansaid)
	ketoprofen (Actron, Orudis, Oruvail); ◆ Orudis-E, Orudis KT
	naproxen (EC-Naprosyn, Naprosyn, Aleve, Anaprox; ◆ Apo-Naproxen, Naprosyn-E, Apo-Napro-NA, Synflex
	oxaprozin (Daypro)
Acetic acid derivatives	etodolac (Lodine)
	indomethacin (Indocin); ◆ Apo-Indomethacin, Indocid, Nu-Indo
	ketorolac (Toradol)
	nabumetone (Relafen)
	sulindac (Clinoril); ◆ Apo-Sulin, Novo-Sundac
Enolic acids	piroxicam (Feldene, Nu-Pirox); ◆ Apo-Piroxicam, Novo-Pirocam
	meloxicam (Mobic)
Anthranilic acids (fenamates)	meclofenamate (Meclofen)
	mefenamic acid (Ponstel)
SELECTIVE COX-2 INHIBITORS	
Diaryl-substituted pyrazoles	celecoxib (Celebrex)

COX, Cyclooxygenase; *NSAIDs*, nonsteroidal antiinflammatory drugs.

COX-2 (Table 17-2). With chronic use, the annual risk of serious complications from NSAIDs is 1% to 4%.

▌ Indications

NSAIDs as a class of nonopioid analgesics exert analgesic, antipyretic, and antiinflammatory effects. Thus these drugs are used for a variety of conditions to reduce pain, fever, and inflammation (Table 17-3). In the past, NSAIDs were the initial drug of choice in the treatment of rheumatoid arthritis, but they are now adjuncts for some patients. Aspirin, as the prototype salicylate NSAID, is used as prophylaxis for myocardial infarctions and strokes (see Evidence-Based Pharmacotherapeutics).

▌ Pharmacodynamics

Despite differences in chemical class, the NSAIDs have the same mechanisms of action. Blocking PG synthesis by

TABLE 17-3 NSAID Indications

Condition or Purpose	acetaminophen*	aspirin	diflunisal	salsalate	fenoprofen	flurbiprofen	ibuprofen	indomethacin	ketoprofen	naproxen	oxaprozin	etodolac	ketorolac	nabumetone	sulindac	tolmetin	meclofenamate	mefenamic Acid	diclofenac	piroxicam
Abort a migraine						X				X							X	X		
Acute gout			X					✓		✓		X			X					X
Adherence								✓												
Advancing age, in general															✓					
Alcohol abuse								✓												
Ankylosing spondylitis						X		✓		✓		X							✓	
Anticoagulation therapy																✓			✓	
Antihypertensive therapy		✓													✓					
Aspirin allergy, polyps, asthma	✓					✓														
Aspirin, patient intolerance of							✓													
Bursitis, tendinitis						X		✓		✓		X			✓					
Closure of persistent PDA								X†												
Cluster headache								X												
Diuretic use															✓					✓
Dysmenorrhea, primary						X	✓	X	✓	✓								✓		X
Fever	✓	✓		✓		X	✓			✓		✓	✓							
Heart failure															✓					✓
Juvenile RA					X		X		X	✓									X	
Lithium use		✓													✓					
Menorrhagia																	X			
Mild to moderate pain	✓	✓	✓	✓	✓	✓	✓		✓			✓	✓				✓	✓‡	X	
Osteoarthritis			✓		✓	✓	✓	✓	✓	✓	✓	✓		✓					✓	✓
Prophylaxis: dysmenorrhea						X		X	X	X										
Polyhydramnios								X												
PMS										X								X		
RA		✓	✓	✓	✓	✓	✓	✓	✓	✓	✓	✓	X	✓	✓	✓	✓		✓	✓
Resistant acne vulgaris							X§													
Sunburn					X	X	X	X‖	X	X							X	X	X	

✓ = Food and Drug Administration (FDA)-labeled uses.
X = Non–FDA-labeled uses.
*Acetaminophen is not an NSAID, but is included here because of its use as analgesic and antipyretic.
†Intravenous indomethacin is FDA-approved for this indication.
‡Mefenamic acid may be used to treat mild to moderate pain if used for less than 1 week.
§Ibuprofen may be used along with tetracycline for the treatment of persistent acne vulgaris.
‖Topical indomethacin may be used to prevent as well as treat sunburn.
PDA, Patent ductus arteriosis; PMS, premenstrual syndrome; RA, rheumatoid arthritis.

inhibiting COX-1 and COX-2 enzymes is thought to be the principle mechanism by which NSAIDs relieve pain and inflammation. To appreciate the differences between the COX inhibitors, a basic understanding of COX enzymes is needed.

The COX-1 enzyme is involved in routine body functions such as generation of protective prostaglandins to promote gastric blood flow and bicarbonate generation. The COX-1 enzyme is found in gastric mucosa, vascular endothelial cells, platelets, and renal collecting tubules, and thus COX-1–generated PGs also participate in hemostasis and renal blood flow.

In contrast, the COX-2 enzyme is not ordinarily found in most body tissues, but is rapidly induced by inflammatory mediators, local injury, and cytokines (i.e., interleukins, interferon, and TNF). COX-1 blockade occurs with nonspecific NSAIDs and is potentially undesirable; they can cause GI ulcerations and an increased risk of bleeding due to inhibition of platelet aggregation. On the other hand, COX-2 inhibition is desirable, because it lacks such toxicities while still providing antiinflammatory and analgesic effects. However, caution is warranted here, since COX-2 inhibition does not eliminate risk entirely, but simply decreases it; the COX-2 inhibitor can lose enzyme specificity and pose a risk for both GI and renal problems.

Nonspecific NSAIDs and COX-2 inhibitors demonstrate mechanistic differences. NSAIDs penetrate the enzyme's active site for both COX-1 and COX-2 to block entry of the enzyme's usual substrate, arachidonic acid. The nonspecific NSAIDs include, for example, aspirin, ibuprofen, and naproxen. These drugs block the action of both COX-1 and COX-2 enzymes. In contrast, COX-2 inhibitors are much more potent at inhibiting COX-2; they interact in a time-dependent fashion within the active site of COX-2. This high-affinity binding to COX-2 provides excellent COX-2 inhibition and has no effect on COX-1.

The mechanism and the extent of antiplatelet effects differ between aspirin and other NSAIDs. When aspirin is absorbed, the acetyl portion of the compound dissociates, binding irreversibly to platelet COX. The binding prevents the synthesis of TXA_2, and thus platelet aggregation is inhibited. A single dose of aspirin (325 mg or less) acetylates circulating platelets within a few minutes, but the effects are irreversible for the life span of the platelet, about 7 to 10 days. In contrast, acetylated salicylates

EVIDENCE-BASED PHARMACOTHERAPEUTICS

NSAIDs and Myocardial Infarction

■ Background

Although nonsteroidal antiinflammatory drugs (NSAIDs) are popular among patients and health care providers alike as over-the-counter and prescription analgesics, their use is plagued with problems of gastrointestinal upset and bleeding. To help combat these adverse effects, three receptor-specific cyclooxygenase (COX) inhibitors—rofecoxib (Vioxx), valdecoxib (B extra), and celecoxib (Celebrex)—were developed. Although they are as effective as traditional NSAIDs in managing musculoskeletal pain and acute joint inflammation, as well as in minimizing GI upset and bleeding, concerns about the drugs' cardiovascular safety has arisen. Rofecoxib was removed from the market in 2004 after the Vioxx Gastrointestinal Outcomes Research (VIGOR) study found a much higher risk of rofecoxib-associated myocardial infarction (MI) compared with naproxen (Aleve). Removal of valdecoxib followed in 2005. Since then, questions remain as to whether or not the increased risk of MI is a class effect applicable to the remaining COX-2 inhibitor, celecoxib.

■ Research Article

Hippisley-Cox, J., and Coupland, C. (2005). Risks of myocardial infarction in patients taking cyclooxygenase-2 inhibitors or conventional nonsteroidal antiinflammatory drugs: Population-based, nested, case-control analysis. *British Journal of Medicine, 330*(7504), 1–7.

Purpose

The primary objective of this study, carried out between 2000 and 2004 in primary care settings, was to establish the relative risk for MI in patients taking naproxen (Aleve) and the selective COX-2 inhibitor rofecoxib. The study also examined the risk for MI in patients (1) with and without preexisting coronary heart disease and (2) who were and were not taking aspirin.

Design

This study used a population-based, nested, case-controlled design with data obtained from 367 general practices that contribute to the United Kingdom's QRESEARCH database and that are located throughout each health authority and health board in England, Wales, and Scotland.

Methods

Investigators from the University of Nottingham, United Kingdom, conducted a population-based study using control subjects matched by age, calendar time, sex, and practice (N = 86,349). A cohort of patients between the ages of 15 and 100 years with a first MI (N = 9218) were included. All prescriptions for NSAIDs were identified for each case and control subject used in the 3 years before the date of the MI. Comorbidities, drugs, and other confounding variables were adjusted for, using multivariate analyses. A 95% confidence interval (CI) for the odds ratios were set for the COX-2 inhibitors rofecoxib (Vioxx) and celecoxib (Celebrex), and for naproxen (Aleve), ibuprofen, diclofenac, and other COX-1 inhibitors. Odds ratios (ORs) were amended for comorbidities such as diabetes, hypertension, coronary artery disease, osteoarthritis and rheumatoid arthritis, and obesity. Other variables included smoking status, aspirin, selective serotonin reuptake inhibitors (SSRIs), and HMG coenzyme A reductase inhibitors (i.e., statins). The numbers-needed-to-harm for patients over 65 years of age were calculated (rofecoxib, 695; diclofenac, 521; and 1005 for ibuprofen).

Findings

There was a significantly increased risk of MI associated with rofecoxib (adjusted OR 1.32, 95% CI 1.09–1.61) compared with subjects (1) who did not use the drug within the previous 3 years; (2) with current use of diclofenac (OR 1.55, 95% CI 1.39–1.72); and (3) with existing use of ibuprofen (OR 1.24; 95% CI 1.11–1.39). An increased risk for MI was associated with naproxen and other selective and nonselective NSAIDs. These risks were significant at p < 0.05 for current use and significance at <0.01 in testing for trends. No significant interactions were found between COX-1 drugs and aspirin use, or between COX-1 drugs and coronary artery disease.

Conclusions

This study suggests, regardless of the many confounding variables, in the study that use of rofecoxib, diclofenac, and ibuprofen were associated with an increased incidence of MI. There is no evidence to support MI risk reduction and the current use of naproxen.

■ Implications for Practice

This study has significant implications for pharmacotherapy and public health given the prevalent use of NSAIDs, particularly in older adults. Although observational studies are subject to confounding variables that cannot be fully controlled, sufficient trepidation exists about the use of NSAIDs and cardiovascular risk that reexamination of all NSAIDs would be wise. The results of complete meta-analysis may help to resolve decision-making issues about which NSAIDs are safest and yet effective for patients with musculoskeletal pain.

(e.g., diflunisal, salsalate) bind reversibly with platelet COX, so their antiplatelet effects exist only while the drug is present in the serum. For this reason, many of the NSAIDs are not used for antiplatelet activity. Chapter 39 discusses antiplatelet drugs.

꘡ Pharmacokinetics

As active drugs, NSAIDs exhibit several pharmacokinetic similarities, including high absorption, oral bioavailability, and high protein binding (except for sulindac and nabumetone, which require hepatic conversion for activity). NSAIDs penetrate joint fluids, reaching about 60% of serum levels. The most important difference in NSAIDs is a serum half-life ranging from 1 hour for tolmetin to 50 hours for piroxicam, which affects dosing frequency and, potentially, adherence with therapy (Table 17-4).

Elimination of NSAIDs largely depends on hepatic biotransformation, with a small fraction of active drug being excreted through the kidneys. The elimination of free drug in the urine depends on both the dose and the urinary pH.

More than 30% of a salicylate is eliminated unchanged in alkaline urine, whereas the amount eliminated in acidic urine can be as low as 2%. Because of different chemical properties, some NSAIDs have substantial biliary (bile ducts, gallbladder) excretion (e.g., indomethacin, sulindac).

꘡ Adverse Effects and Contraindications

The risk factors for adverse effects to NSAIDs are identified in Box 17-1. Aspirin hypersensitivity is neither an immune response, nor is it dose related. It may be due to blockade of the COX pathway and activation of the lipoxygenase pathway. The result is an accumulation of LTs (specifically, LTC_4, LTD_4, and LTE_4). The highest incidence of hypersensitivity is seen in middle-aged patients with a history of asthma or nasal polyps. Symptoms of hypersensitivity include rhinitis with profuse watery secretions, bronchial constriction, hypotension, vasomotor collapse, and coma.

NSAIDs are generally well tolerated; however, in a small percentage of patients, adverse GI events can occur. Aspirin

PHARMACOKINETICS
TABLE 17-4 Selected NSAIDs

Drug	Route	Analgesic Action			Antirheumatic Action		PB (%)	t½
		Onset	Peak	Duration	Onset	Peak		
NONSELECTIVE COX INHIBITORS								
acetylsalicylic acid	PO	15–30 min	1–3 hr	3–6 hr	—	—	90–91	2–3 hr; 15–30 hr*
choline-magnesium salicylates	PO	5–30 min	1–3 hr	3–6 hr	—	—	25–60*	2–3 hr; 15–30 hr*
choline salicylate	PO	5–30 min	1–3 hr	3–6 hr	—	—	UA	2–3 hr; 15–30 hr*
diclofenac sodium	PO	60 min	2–3 hr	4–6 hr	—	—	99	1.2–1.8 hr
diflunisal	PO	1 hr	2–3 hr	8–12 hr	—	—	UA	8–12 hr
etodolac	PO	30 min	1–2 hr	4–8 hr	—	—	99	6–8 hr
fenoprofen	PO	30 min	1–2 hr	4–6 hr	2 days	2–3 wk	99	2–3 hr
flurbiprofen	PO	60 min	1.5 hr	4–6 hr	—	—	>90	5.7 hr
ibuprofen	PO	30–60 min; 7 days†	1–2 hr	4–6 hr	<7 days	1–2 wk	90–99	1.8–2.5 hr
indomethacin	PO	0.5–2 hr	1–2 hr	4–6 hr	<7 days	1–2 wk	99	4.5 hr
ketoprofen	PO	30 min	0.5–2 hr	4–8 hr	—	—	99	2–4 hr
ketorolac	PO	Varies	30–60 min	4–6 hr	—	—	99	2.4–8.6 hr
	IM	5–10 min	30–90 min	4–8 hr	—	—	99	5–6 hr
magnesium salicylate	PO	5–30 min	1–3 hr	3–6 hr	—	—	UA	2–3 hr; 15–30 hr*
meclofenamate	PO	Days	2–3 wk	Days	Few days	2–3 wk	>99	40 min-2 hr
mefenamic acid	PO	Varies	2–4 hr	6 hr	—	—	90	2–4 hr
nabumetone	PO	1–2 hr	5 hr	24–48 hr	—	—	99	24 hr
naproxen	PO	1–2 hr	2–4 hr	7–12 hr	<14 days	2–4 wk	99	10–20 hr
oxaprozin	PO	60 min	3–6 hr	24–48 hr	<7 days	—	>99	26–92 hr
piroxicam	PO	15–30 min	3–5 hr; 7–12 days‡	24–48 hr	7–12 days	2–3 wk	99	30–80 hr
salsalate	PO	5–30 min	1–3 hr	3–6 hr	—	—	UA	2–3 hr; 15–30 hr*
sodium salicylate	PO	5–30 min	1–3 hr	3–6 hr	—	—	UA	2–3 hr; 15–30 hr*
sulindac	PO	60 min	2–4 hr	7–16 hr	<7 days	2–3 wk	93–98	7–8 hr; 16 hr§
tolmetin	PO	Rapid	0.5–1 hr	6–8 hr	<7 days	1–2 wk	99	1–1.5 hr
COX-2 INHIBITOR								
celecoxib	PO	45 min	3 hr	97	11.2 hr	45 min	97	4–8 hr
OTHER								
acetaminophen	PO	30–60 min	—	Low; 25–50¶	1–4 hr	15–30 min	1–1.5 hr	4–6 hr
	ER	UA	—					
	SUP	30–60 min	—					
capsaicin	Top	Varies	1–2 wk	2–4 wk	NA	NA	UA	UA

*Protein binding and the half-life of low-dose and high-dose salicylates, respectively.
†The onset time of ibuprofen's analgesic and antiinflammatory effects, respectively.
‡Peak blood levels and days to therapeutic effects respectively for piroxicam.
§Half-life of sulindac metabolites.
¶Protein binding of acetaminophen is low at therapeutic dosages; is 20% to 50% at toxic levels.
ER, Extended-release formulation (oral); *IM,* intramuscular; *PB,* protein binding; *t₁/₂* elimination half-life; *PO,* by mouth; *SUP,* suppository; *Top,* topical; *UA,* unavailable.

and other salicylates do not produce sedation, physical dependence, or tolerance like opioid analgesics. Nausea and vomiting sometimes occurs through stimulation of the chemoreceptor trigger zone in the medulla. Daily use of 4 to 5 grams of aspirin can cause 3 to 8 mL/day of blood loss compared with 0.6 mL/day loss in non–aspirin users. Non-acetylated salicylates are typically associated with less ulceration.

Salicylate doses of 1 to 2 grams/day decrease urate elimination, thus raising serum urate levels *(hyperuricemia)*. Midrange doses of 2 to 3 grams/day usually do not alter urate elimination. Doses exceeding 5 grams/day actually lower plasma urate levels, thus improving gout; however, such large doses generally are not tolerated.

In July 2005 the Food and Drug Administration (FDA) ▲ issued letters to manufacturers of all prescription and OTC NSAIDs requesting them to revise labeling to include a boxed warning highlighting the potential for increased risk of cardiovascular events and the well-described, serious, potentially life-threatening GI bleeding associated with their use. Patients taking rofecoxib (Vioxx) had more thrombotic events compared with patients taking naproxen in the

BOX 17-1

Risk Factors for NSAID Adverse Effects

- Alcohol intake
- Over age 60
- Female sex
- Duration of treatment
- Increased dosage
- Type of NSAID used
- Multiple NSAID use
- Corticosteroid use
- History of previous ulcer
- Comorbid cardiovascular condition

NSAID, Nonsteroidal antiinflammatory drug.

Vioxx Gastrointestinal Outcomes Research study (VIGOR), which led to the labeling change and the product's subsequent withdrawal from the market. Celecoxib labeling, in addition to the general labeling that applies to all NSAIDs, also contains safety data from long-term treatment trials.

Contraindications to NSAID use include peptic ulcer disease, GI or other bleeding disorders, hyperuricemia, hypersensitivity, or impaired renal or hepatic function. Also avoid salicylates in patients who have an allergy to tartrazine (a food additive, FD&C [the designation for food coloring according to the Food, Drugs, and Cosmetics Act] Yellow No. 5), and in patients with a vitamin K deficiency, because of their antiplatelet effects. Aspirin use for fever in patients with high cell turnover (i.e., cancer patients) is contraindicated because of the potential for uric acid build-up. Aspirin may also reduce the function of white blood cells because of its cellular inhibitory effects.

NSAID use places a fetus at risk for oligohydramnios, a deficiency of amniotic fluid. The deficiency is secondary to a decrease in fetal urine elimination. There is also a theoretical risk of premature closure of the ductus arteriosus in utero. Thus NSAIDs are generally contraindicated during pregnancy and also during lactation. Since the pharmacologic target of NSAIDs is COX, and since COX-2 is active in the ovaries during follicular development, its inhibition is thought to cause luteinized unruptured follicle syndrome, an anovulatory condition characterized by clinical signs of ovulation in conjunction with the absence of actual follicular rupture and ovum release.

Patients with the triad of asthma, aspirin-induced allergy, and nasal polyps are at increased risk for hypersensitivity reactions. At high doses, NSAIDs stimulate the respiratory center in the medulla, increasing the rate and depth of respirations. Hyperventilation leads to respiratory alkalosis, with toxic doses directly depressing the respiratory center to cause metabolic acidosis.

Drug Interactions

Since NSAIDs bind to plasma proteins, they may be displaced by or may displace other plasma-bound drugs such as warfarin, methotrexate, digoxin, cyclosporine, oral antidiabetic drugs, and sulfa drugs (Table 17-5). This interaction can enhance either therapeutic or toxic effects of either drug.

The effects of uricosuric drugs can be blocked in the presence of aspirin. Aspirin competes with the organic renal transport system to increase penicillin G concentration. The concurrent use of an ACE-inhibiting drug (i.e., ACE-inhibitor or angiotensin-receptor antagonist), an NSAID or COX-2 inhibitor, and a thiazide diuretic increases the risk of renal impairment. This increased risk includes use in fixed-combination products containing more than one class of drug. Combined use of these drugs makes increased monitoring of serum creatinine mandatory. Exercise caution when using a combination of drugs from these three classes, particularly in older adults and those with preexisting renal impairment.

Dosage Regimen

As with all other drugs, NSAID dosages vary considerably depending on the age of the patient, the patient's medical condition, the route of administration, and the condition treated (Table 17-6). Dosage regimens for severe and chronic inflammatory disorders such as rheumatic fever and rheumatoid arthritis are significantly greater than those needed for analgesia or fever reduction. Treatment regimens are also more rigorous and prolonged.

Lab Considerations

Salicylates can cause elevated alanine aminotransferase (ALT), aspartate aminotransferase (AST), and alkaline phosphatase levels, especially when plasma salicylate concentrations exceed 25 mg/100 mL. Levels often return to normal despite continued drug use or dosage reduction. If severe abnormalities persist or active liver disease develops, discontinue salicylate use, and use caution with the drug in the future. Monitor hepatic function before and periodically during long-term therapy. Hepatotoxicity is more likely to occur in patients with rheumatic fever, systemic lupus erythematosus (SLE), juvenile arthritis, or preexisting hepatic disease (Table 17-7).

Monitor serum salicylate levels and hematocrit periodically in patients undergoing prolonged high-dose therapy. Salicylates prolong bleeding time, and in large dosages prolong prothrombin (PT) and international normalized ratio (INR) values. In addition, salicylates can cause false-negative urine glucose test results when using enzymatic glucose testing methods (e.g., Clinistix and Tes-Tape), and false-positive urine glucose test results when using the copper sulfate method (e.g., Clinitest). However, they have no effects on testing modes used for blood glucose monitoring. They also alter the results of serum uric acid, urine vanillylmandelic acid, protirelin-induced thyroid-stimulating hormone, and urine hydroxyindoleacetic acid determinations, as well as radionuclide thyroid imaging. Salicylates can cause serum potassium and cholesterol values to fall. Like salicylates, other NSAIDs can cause prolonged bleeding times that persist for some time following discontinuation of therapy.

For more information, see the Evolve Resources Bonus Content "Influence of selected Drugs on Laboratory Values," found at http://evolve.elsevier.com/Gutierrez/pharmacotherapeutics.

Acetaminophen
Indications

Acetaminophen (Tylenol) is a nonopioid, non-NSAID analgesic used in the treatment of fever and mild pain. Unlike NSAIDs, it has no antiinflammatory properties but it is discussed within this drug class because its mechanism of action is similar to that of NSAIDs.

Pharmacodynamics

The analgesic effect of acetaminophen occurs through PG and COX inhibition in the central nervous system (CNS), but because it lacks peripheral PG inhibitory action, it is a weak antiinflammatory drug. For this reason, it is not helpful in treating inflammatory disorders such as rheumatoid arthritis. The antipyretic action of acetaminophen results from direct action on the hypothalamus to cause increased vasodilation and sweating and therefore a reduction in fever.

Pharmacokinetics

Acetaminophen is well absorbed when taken by mouth and well distributed to all body tissues (see Table 17-4). The manner in which acetaminophen is biotransformed depends on the dosage. At low dosages, most of the drug is biotransformed

DRUG INTERACTIONS
TABLE 17-5 Selected NSAIDs

Drug	Interactive Drugs	Interaction
NONSTEROIDAL ANTIINFLAMMATORY DRUGS		
Salicylates in general	Alcohol, corticosteroids	Increases ulcerogenic effects of salicylates and corticosteroids
	Anticoagulants	Increases risk of bleeding
	Corticosteroids	Decreases plasma salicylate levels
	methotrexate	Increases effects and toxicity of methotrexate, leading to pancytopenia
	probenecid, sulfinpyrazone	Aspirin decreases the uricosuric effects of interacting drugs
	Antacids, citrates, mannitol, sodium bicarbonate	Increases excretion of salicylates
	penicillin G	Increases serum concentration of interactive drug
	Sulfonylureas	Enhances hypoglycemic effects of interacting drug
	zidovudine	Metabolism of interactive drug inhibited
	Aminoglycosides, bumetanide, cisplatin, etracrynic acid, furosemide vancomycin	Increased risk for ototoxicity when given with salicylates
	spironolactone	Decreases effectiveness of interactive drug
	acetazolamide	May cause acetazolamide intoxication
NSAIDs in general	cefamandole, cefotetan, plicamycin	Induces hypoprothrombinemia or inhibit platelet aggregation
	acetaminophen, gold products	Increases risk of renal toxicity
	ACE inhibitors, beta blockers	Reduces antihypertensive effects
	cimetidine, ketorolac	Increases serum concentrations of NSAID
	Hydantoins, nifedipine, sulfonylureas, verapamil	Displaces interactive drug with increased incidence of adverse effects
	Antihypertensives, bumetanide, furosemide	Decreases effects of interactive drug
	Alcohol, dextran, corticosteroids, oral anticoagulants, penicillins, sulfinpyrazone, valproates, anticoagulants, thrombolytics	Increases risk of GI ulceration, bleeding
	Insulins, oral hypoglycemics	Increases risk of hypoglycemic effects of interactive drug
	lithium	Increases lithium concentrations
	methotrexate	Decreases tubular secretion of interactive drug leading to toxicity
	zidovudine	Inhibits biotransformation of interactive drug leading to toxicity
Indomethacin	Anorexiants	May cause hypertension
COX-2 INHIBITORS		
Celecoxib	metoprolol	Increased plasma concentrations of interactive drug
	ACE inhibitors, loop diuretics, thiazide diuretics, chlorthalidone, ethacrynic acid	Decreased antihypertensive and natriuretic effects
	chlorothiazide, clopamide, indapamide, metolazone, torsemide	Decreased diuretic and antihypertensive efficacy
	aspirin, fluvoxamine, nefazodone, paroxetine, sertraline, venlafaxine	Increases risk of bleeding
	diltiazem	Loss of blood pressure control
	fluconazole	Increases celecoxib plasma concentrations
	lithium	Increases plasma concentrations and risk of toxicity
OTHERS		
Acetaminophen	Alcohol, hepatotoxic substances	Additive effects with increased risk of toxicity for acetaminophen
	Oral anticoagulants	Increases risk of hypoprothrombinemia and bleeding
	Barbiturates, carbamazepine, hydantoins, rifampin, sulfinpyrazone	Increases risk of hepatotoxicity and decreased therapeutic effects of interactive drug
	aspirin	Increases risk of adverse renal effects
	diflunisal	Increases acetaminophen levels and increases the risk of hepatotoxicity with chronic concurrent use
Capsaicin	ACE inhibitors	Increases incidence of cough with capsaicin use

ACE, Angiotensin-converting enzyme; *GI*, gastrointestinal; *NSAID*, nonsteroidal antiinflammatory drug.

into inactive compounds. A small fraction is converted to a toxic metabolite that can harm the liver. Fortunately, the toxic metabolite usually undergoes rapid conversion to a nontoxic form. When an overdose of acetaminophen is ingested, a large quantity of the toxic metabolite is produced. The capacity of the liver to detoxify the metabolite is exceeded, and hepatic injury results.

Adverse Effects and Contraindications

The adverse effects of acetaminophen are relatively few, but they can be serious. Renal tubular necrosis (analgesic nephropathy) was the basis for removing the other para-aminophenol, phenacetin, from the market. Acetaminophen is a related drug, and the lifetime risk of nephropathy increases with the cumulative intake of 1000 tablets. The risk of acetaminophen hepatotoxicity increases with as little as 4 grams/day in the presence of ethanol or fasting, or both. Ethanol induces hepatic mixed-function oxidase metabolism, shifting the reaction toward the more toxic metabolite. Fasting moves biotransformation of acetaminophen from one set of metabolic pathways to others by reducing the required precursor molecules. Cautious use of acetaminophen is warranted in patients with severe hepatic disease, renal disease, chronic alcohol abuse, and malnutrition.

Drug Interactions

Drug interactions with acetaminophen are many (see Table 17-5). Chronic concurrent acetaminophen use with

DOSAGE

TABLE 17-6 Regimen for Selected NSAIDs

Drug	Use(s)	Dosage	Implications
NONSELECTIVE COX INHIBITORS			
acetylsalicylic acid	Fever, pain, headache, dysmenorrhea	*Adult:* 325–975 mg PO every 3–4 hr PRN	**Risk of Reye's syndrome in children with viral illnesses**
	Rheumatic fever	*Adult:* 3600–7800 mg PO daily in 3–4 divided doses *Child:* 80–100 mg/kg/day PO in divided doses; not to exceed 130 mg/kg/day	Take with food.
	Rheumatoid arthritis	*Adult:* 3600–5400 mg PO daily in divided doses	Take with food.
	TIAs	*Adult:* 1–3 grams PO daily in divided doses	Doses may be as low as 325 mg/day in patients who are intolerant of higher doses.
	Prophylaxis TIA, recurrent MI or CVA	*Adult:* 300–325 mg PO daily as single dose	Dosages as low as 81 mg/day are effective for stroke prevention.
choline-magnesium trisalicylate	Fever, rheumatoid conditions	*Adult:* 2–3 grams PO daily in 2–3 divided doses *–or–* 1500 mg PO twice daily *Child >37 kg:* 2.2 grams/day in 2 divided doses *Child <37 kg:* 50 mg/day in 2 divided doses	Strength expressed in mg salicylate: 500-mg tab = 650 mg aspirin; 750-mg tab = 975 mg aspirin; 1000-mg tab = 1300 mg aspirin
choline salicylate	Fever, rheumatoid arthritis	*Adult:* 435–669 mg PO every 3 hr *–or–* 425–870 mg PO every 4 hr *–or–* 870 to1305 mg every 6 hr PRN *Adult:* Antiinflammatory: 4.8–7.2 grams PO daily in divided doses	Each teaspoon contains 870 mg choline salicylate and 650 mg aspirin. 435 mg of choline salicylate is equivalent to 325 mg of aspirin.
diclofenac	Ankylosing spondylitis	*Adult:* (Sodium formulation) 100–125 mg PO daily in 25-mg doses 4 times daily and at bedtime	Patients with asthma, aspirin-induced allergy, and nasal polyps are at increased risk of hypersensitivity reactions. May take first 1–2 doses on empty stomach for more rapid onset.
	Osteoarthritis	*Adult:* (Sodium or potassium formulation) 50 mg PO 2–3 times daily *–or–* 75 mg PO twice daily of sodium formulation	**Do not confuse sodium and potassium formulations.**
	Rheumatoid arthritis	*Adult:* (Sodium or potassium formulation) 50 mg PO 3–4 times daily *–or–* 75 mg twice daily of sodium formulation	**Do not confuse sodium and potassium formulations.**
	Dysmenorrhea, analgesia	*Adult:* 100 mg PO 3 times daily initially; not to exceed 200 mg PO during first 24 hr *–or–* 150 mg/day on subsequent days	Take as soon as possible with onset of menses; prophylaxis has not been shown effective.
diflunisal	Mild to moderate pain, osteoarthritis	*Adult:* 500–1000 mg initially PO followed by 250–500 mg PO every 8–12 hr	Not indicated for fever. Takes up to 2 wk for therapeutic effects to be reached.
etodolac	Osteoarthritis	*Adult:* 400 mg PO initially 2–3 times daily *–or–* 300 mg PO 3–4 times daily; adjust dose based on patient response. Range: 400–1200 mg/day	For rapid effect, administer 30 min before or 2 hr after meals.
	Mild to moderate pain	*Adult >60 kg:* 400 mg initially PO, then 200–400 mg PO every 6–8 hr; not to exceed 1200 mg/day *–or–* 20 mg/kg in patients <60 kg	Food slows but does not reduce the extent of absorption.
fenoprofen	Mild to moderate pain, rheumatic conditions, dysmenorrhea	*Adult:* 300–600 mg PO 3–4 times daily; not to exceed 3.2 grams/day	Patients with asthma, aspirin-induced allergy, and nasal polyps are at increased risk of hypersensitivity reactions.
flurbiprofen	Rheumatic conditions, dysmenorrhea, mild to moderate pain (unlabeled)	*Adult:* 200–300 mg PO daily in 2–4 divided doses; not to exceed 300 mg/day *–or–* 100 mg/dose *Child:* 50 mg PO every 4–6 hr as needed	Patients with asthma, aspirin-induced allergy, and nasal polyps are at increased risk of hypersensitivity reactions.
ibuprofen	Rheumatic conditions	*Adult:* 300–800 mg PO 3–4 times daily; not to exceed 3600 mg/day *Child 6 mo to 12 y:* 20–40 mg/kg/day PO in divided doses; not to exceed 50 mg/kg/day	Higher dosages not recommended. For rapid initial effect, give 30 min before or 2 hr after meals. Prophylaxis for dysmenorrhea not shown to be effective. Therapeutic response may develop over several wk.
	Fever, mild to moderate pain, dysmenorrhea	*Adult:* 200–400 mg PO every 4–6 hr PRN; not to exceed 1200 mg/day *Child:* 5 mg/kg PO; not to exceed 40 mg/kg/day. May repeat every 4–6 hr	
indomethacin	Rheumatic conditions, bursitis, tendinitis, ankylosing spondylitis	*Adult:* 25–50 mg PO 2 to 4 times daily *–or–* 75 mg of ER capsule 1–2 times daily; not to exceed 200 mg *–or–* 150 mg of SR capsule/day. *Child:* 1.5–2.5 mg/kg/day PO, PRN in 3–4 divided doses; not to exceed 4 mg/kg/day *–or–* 150–200 mg/day	Single bedtime dose of 100 mg may be used. Multiple drug interactions. Use with caution and in patients with history of peptic ulcer disease.
	Acute gouty arthritis	*Adult:* 100 mg initially, then 50 mg PO 3 times daily until pain subsides	

Continued

CENTRAL NERVOUS

DOSAGE
TABLE **17-6** Regimen for Selected NSAIDs—Cont'd

Drug	Use(s)	Dosage	Implications
ketoprofen	Rheumatic conditions	*Adult:* 150–300 mg PO daily in 3–4 divided doses *–or–* 200 mg once daily as ER form	Coadministration with opioid may produce additive analgesia thus permitting lower opioid doses.
	Dysmenorrhea, mild to moderate pain	*Adult:* 25–50 mg PO every 6–8 hr	
ketorolac	Short-term pain management	*Adult <65 yr:* Initially 20 mg PO, followed by 10 mg every 4–6 hr PRN; not to exceed 40 mg/day *–or–* 60 mg IM single dose *–or–* 30 mg every 6 hr *–or–* 30 mg IV single dose *–or–* 30 mg IV every 6 hr. Not to exceed 120 mg/day *Adult >65 yr –or– <50 kg –or– with renal failure:* 10 mg PO every 4–6 hr PRN; not to exceed 40 mg/day *–or–* 30 mg IM single dose *–or–* 15 mg IM every 6 hr *–or–* 15 mg IV single dose *–or–* 15 mg IV every 6 hr; not to exceed 40 mg/day	Always give initial ketorolac therapy IM or IV. Oral therapy should be used as a continuation of parenteral therapy. Duration of ketorolac by all routes should not exceed 5 days.
magnesium salicylate	Fever, rheumatic conditions, mild to moderate pain	*Adult:* 325–1300 mg PO daily in 3–4 divided doses	Therapeutic response in arthritis may take up to 2 wk.
meclofenamate	Rheumatoid conditions, mild to moderate pain, dysmenorrhea	*Adult:* 200–400 mg PO daily in 3–4 divided doses *–or–* 50–100 mg PO every 4–6 hr *–or–* 100 mg PO 3 times daily for up to 6 days	Wear sunscreen and protective clothing to reduce risk of photosensitivity reactions. Patients with asthma, aspirin-induced allergy, and nasal polyps are at increased risk of hypersensitivity reactions.
mefenamic acid	Moderate pain	*Adult:* 500 mg PO initially followed by 250 mg PO every 6 hr PRN; not to exceed 1 wk of therapy	Arrange for periodic ophthalmologic examination during long-term therapy.
nabumetone	Rheumatic conditions	*Adult:* 1 gram PO daily as a single daily dose *–or–* divided doses twice daily; may increase to 2 grams/day	Use lowest effective dose during chronic therapy.
naproxen	Rheumatic conditions, ankylosing spondylitis	*Adult:* 250–500 mg PO twice daily to maximum of 1500 mg/day for 6 mo *–or–* 375–500 mg ER form PO daily *–or–* 275–550 mg twice daily to maximum of 1650 mg/day *Child:* 10 mg/kg/day PO in 2 divided doses	Do not confuse with naproxen sodium. Use for shortest duration possible. Monitor blood pressure. Caution patient to wear sunscreen and protective clothing to reduce risk of photosensitivity reactions.
	Mild to moderate pain	*Adult:* 250–500 mg PO twice daily Max: 1250 mg/day acute or 1 gram/day maintenance	Use lowest effective dose for the shortest treatment duration possible.
	Gout	*Adult:* 750 mg PO initially, then 250 mg PO every 8 hr	Use lowest effective dose for the shortest treatment duration possible.
	Dysmenorrhea	*Adult:* 500 mg PO initially, then 25 mg every 6–8 hr Max: 1250 mg/day acute or 1 gram/day maintenance	Use lowest effective dose for the shortest treatment duration possible.
oxaprozin	Osteoarthritis	*Adult:* 1.2 grams PO daily Max: 1.8 grams/day	Use lowest effective dose for the shortest treatment duration possible. Monitor BP.
piroxicam	Rheumatic conditions	*Adult:* 10–20 mg/day as single dose *–or–* 2 divided doses	Begin with 10 mg/day initially for older adults.
	Dysmenorrhea (unlabeled use)	*Adult:* 40 mg PO initially, then 20 mg/day	—
salsalate	Rheumatic conditions	*Adult:* 1.5 g PO twice daily *–or–* 750 mg PO 4 times daily; not to exceed 4 grams/day	Reduce dose in older adults. Use lowest effective dose for shortest treatment duration. Monitor BP.
sulindac	Rheumatic conditions, acute gouty arthritis, bursitis	*Adult:* 150–200 mg PO twice daily; not to exceed 400 mg/day	Food slows but does not reduce extent of absorption. Tablets may be crushed and mixed with food or fluids.
tolmetin	Rheumatic conditions	*Adult:* Initially 400 mg PO 3 times daily followed by maintenance of 600–1800 mg/day in 3–4 divided doses; not to exceed 2000 mg/day *Child >2 yr:* Initially 20 mg/kg followed by maintenance of 15–30 mg/kg/day in 3–4 divided doses; not to exceed 30 mg/day	
COX-2 INHIBITOR			
celecoxib	Osteoarthritis, ankylosing spondylitis	*Adult:* 200 mg PO daily *–or–* 100 mg twice daily Max: 400 mg/day	Use lowest effective dose for shortest treatment period. Avoid use if severe renal disease is present. Monitor BP.
	Rheumatoid arthritis	*Adult:* 100–200 mg PO twice daily	
	Dysmenorrhea	*Adult:* 200 mg PO twice daily	
	Acute pain	*Adult:* 400 mg PO initially for one dose, then 200 mg PO twice daily.	

OTHERS			
acetaminophen	Fever, headache, myalgia, neuralgia, mild to moderate pain	*Adult:* 325–1000 mg PO every 4–6 hr PRN –or– 1300 mg every 8 hr as ER tablets; not to exceed 4 grams/day –or– 2.6 grams/day PO for chronic use – or– 325–650 mg PR every 4 hr PRN; not to exceed 6 suppositories/24 hr *Child:* 10–15 mg/kg/dose every 4–6 hr as needed. Max: 5 doses/24 hr	**Children may repeat doses 4–5 times daily; maximum of 5 doses/24 hrs.** Avoid alcohol. Acute hepatic necrosis occurs with doses of 10–15 grams. Doses over 25 grams are usually fatal. Consult health care provider if fever lasts over 3 days or if >103° F (39.5° C). ▲
capsaicin	Peripheral neuropathy	*Adult:* Apply to affected areas 3–4 times daily	**Avoid getting drug in eyes or on broken or irritated skin surfaces** ▲

*Hepatotoxicity is more likely to occur in patients with rheumatic fever, systemic lupus erythematosus (SLE), juvenile arthritis, or preexisting hepatic disease.
†Risk of GI distress associated with etodolac, ketorolac, and oxaprozin is not fully established.
BP, Blood pressure; *CVA,* cardiovascular accident; *ER,* extended release; *GI,* gastrointestinal; *IM,* intramuscular; *IV,* intravenous; *MI,* myocardial infarction; *NSAID,* nonsteroidal antiinflammatory drug; *PO,* by mouth; *PRN,* as needed; *SR,* sustained release; *TIA,* transient ischemic attack.

NSAIDs increases the risk of renal injury. Diflunisol increases acetaminophen blood levels; and the use of other hepatotoxic drugs, including alcohol, increases the risk of hepatotoxicity with chronic concurrent use. High-dose, chronic use of acetaminophen (over 2 grams/day) increases the risk of bleeding in the presence of warfarin.

▌ Dosage Regimen

Acetaminophen is available as chewable tablets, granules, extended-release tablets, solutions, liquids, elixirs, and suppositories. The dosage varies from formulation to formulation (see Table 17-6). Children's dosing is weight based (e.g., 10 mg/kg). Caution is warranted when using Tylenol Infant's Drops, because it is a concentrated solution. Be sure to read labels closely to reduce the risk of overdose.

▌ Lab Considerations

Acetaminophen interferes with Chemstrip G, Dextrostix, and Visidex II home blood glucose monitoring systems. The effects vary with the testing method. Falsely decreased values may be noted when measured with glucose–oxidase-peroxidase methods but probably not with the hexokinase–glucose-6-phosphate dehydrogenase method. Increased serum bilirubin, lactic dehydrogenase (LDH), liver function tests, and PT and INR times may indicate hepatotoxicity.

Capsaicin (Zostrix; ✦ Zostrix)

Capsaicin is a topical analgesic used for the temporary management of pain due to rheumatoid arthritis and osteoarthritis. It is effective for pain associated with neuralgias (e.g., shingles or diabetic neuropathy). Postmastectomy pain and

TABLE 17-7 Relative Potential for NSAID-Induced Toxicities

NSAID	GI Distress	Nephrotoxicity	Hepatotoxicity*	Cardiotoxicity
NONSELECTIVE COX INHIBITORS				
acetylsalicylic acid	+	++	++	
celecoxib				++
choline salicylates	+			
diclofenac	++	++		++
diflunisal	+++			
etodolac	+†			
fenoprofen	++	+++		
flurbiprofen	+++	++		
ibuprofen	++	++		++
indomethacin	+++	++		
ketoprofen	+++			
ketorolac	†			
magnesium salicylate	+			
meclofenamate	++			
mefenamic acid		++		
nabumetone	+	+		
naproxen	++	++		+
oxaprozin	†			
piroxicam	+++	+		
salsalate	+			
sulindac	+++	+		
tolmetin	++	+		

*Hepatotoxicity is more likely to occur in patients with rheumatic fever, systemic lupus erythematosus (SLE), juvenile arthritis, or pre-existing hepatic disease.
†Risk of GI distress associated with etodolac, ketorolac, and oxaprozin is not fully established.
+, Considered least toxic, mild, usually no change in drug therapy is required; ++, Frequent incidence of GI adverse effects, may need to add cytoprotective drug to treatment regimen; +++, Considered most toxic; often requires withdrawal of the drug; no information available for areas without designation.
GI, Gastrointestinal; *NSAID,* nonsteroidal antiinflammatory drug.

reflex sympathetic dystrophy syndrome have also responded to application of capsaicin, although it is not approved for these uses by the FDA. Capsaicin is thought to act by depleting or preventing the reaccumulation of substance P, which is responsible for transmitting pain impulses from peripheral sites to the CNS.

The onset of drug action occurs in approximately 1 to 2 weeks, with peak effects noted in 2 to 4 weeks. For patients with head and neck neuralgias, it may take up to 6 weeks for peak effects to be reached. The duration of action of capsaicin is unknown, as are the biotransformation, the elimination route, and the half-life.

Capsaicin's adverse effects are few, but include cough and transient burning at the site of application. Contraindications include hypersensitivity to capsaicin, hot peppers, or components used in the formulation. Do not use capsaicin near the eyes or on broken skin. Safe use during pregnancy or lactation, and in children, has not been established.

Pain relief lasts only as long as capsaicin is used regularly. Advise the patient that any burning usually disappears after the first few days of use but can continue 2 to 4 weeks or longer. Also advise patients that burning is increased by heat, sweating, bathing in warm water, humidity, and clothing. Decreasing the number of daily applications will not lessen the amount of burning but may reduce the degree of pain relief obtained and may prolong the period of burning.

Instruct the patient with herpes zoster not to apply capsaicin cream until the lesions have completely healed. In addition, tell patients to discontinue capsaicin and to notify the health care provider if pain persists longer than 1 month or worsens, or if signs of infection are present.

CLINICAL REASONING

Treatment Objectives
The overall objectives for patients receiving NSAIDs depend on the reason for their use; however, in general they include reducing pain and inflammation while preserving function and quality of life. The treatment objective for fever is to return body temperature to a normal range and increase the patient's comfort.

Treatment Options

▌ Patient Variables
As discussed in Chapter 16, non–drug therapies are available that may correct the underlying cause of the pain; these should be given a full and fair trial before deciding on a drug therapy. Adjunctive therapies include cognitive-behavioral strategies such as relaxation, distraction, imagery, and biofeedback. Massage, the application of heat and cold, or transcutaneous electrical nerve stimulation is also effective for some patients. These strategies can be used alone or in alliance with systemic analgesics and other adjunctive drug measures.

For reasons not clearly understood, patients often respond better to one NSAID than another; and some patients tolerate one NSAID better than another. Thus, to optimize therapy, treatment trials with more than one NSAID may be necessary.

Because aspirin is such a familiar drug, many patients are suspicious of its efficacy. Consequently, if compliance is to be achieved, an attempt must be made to persuade patients that aspirin is, in fact, an effective drug. In some cases, using a prescription formulation may convince the patient that aspirin is indeed a genuine, effective drug.

LIFE-SPAN CONSIDERATIONS. The risk of NSAID-related complications is higher in older adults, patients with a prior history of cardiovascular disease or bleeding ulcers, patients with rheumatoid arthritis, or those taking anticoagulants or prednisone. The risk also increases with dosage increases, long-term use, concomitant use of other NSAIDs or steroids, and comorbid disease.

Pregnant and Nursing Women. If the patient is of child-bearing age, determine whether she is pregnant or nursing before using an NSAID. Some NSAIDs are teratogenic, and still others have not been studied during pregnancy. It is clear that any drug or chemical administered to the mother is capable to some extent of crossing placental membranes to reach the fetus. Of greater concern is whether the rate and extent of drug transfer are sufficient to result in significant concentrations in the fetus. The notion that the placenta is an impermeable barrier must be discarded.

For more information, see the Evolve Resources Bonus Content "Effects of Selected Maternal Drug Ingestion on the Fetus or Neonate," found at http://evolve.elsevier.com/Gutierrez/pharmacotherapeutics.

Drug therapy in a pregnant woman presents unique problems for the health care provider. Not only must maternal pharmacologic mechanisms be taken into account, but also the fetus must always be kept in mind as a potential recipient of the drug (see Chapter 6). Consult the FDA pregnancy classification system when assessing potential use of an NSAID.

Children and Adolescents. In general, assessing the discomfort in children younger than age 5 years is difficult because of the varying levels of language development and comprehension. However, it is not impossible. Infants may cry and display muscular rigidity and thrashing behaviors. Toddlers and preschoolers may be aggressive or complain verbally of discomfort. School-age children express discomfort verbally or behaviorally, often with regression to behaviors used at younger ages. Adolescents are often reluctant to admit they are uncomfortable or need help.

Children and adolescents who have influenza or chicken ▲ pox should abstain from the use of salicylates because of the epidemiologic relationship between aspirin use in children and adolescents and *Reye's syndrome*. Although rare, it is a fatal disorder that carries a mortality rate of 20% to 30%. Reye's syndrome is often the sequela of varicella and other viral infections. Salicylates may precipitate or worsen this disorder, but there is no unequivocal proof at this time that aspirin is a major factor. Reye's is characterized by encephalopathy, hepatic damage, and other serious problems. Acetaminophen can be used for fever reduction and minor pain relief. It is the drug of choice for the child with febrile illness and older adults with impaired renal function (see Controversy box).

Older Adults. Older females are most likely to experience the adverse GI effects of NSAIDs. These persons also easily

Controversy

Salicylates and Reye's Syndrome: When to Use Aspirin?

Jonathan J. Wolfe

Reye's syndrome is a serious disease involving malignant elevation of intracranial pressure. Untreated, the syndrome leads directly to irreversible brain damage or even death. Most troubling to the health care provider is the reality that Reye's syndrome is frequently an iatrogenic disease. Use of salicylates, particularly aspirin, in febrile children has been linked to the onset of Reye's syndrome. It is for this reason that "baby aspirin" has been banned from use in the United States.

Interventions required to manage Reye's syndrome are expensive. Patients are admitted to the intensive care unit (ICU) to allow vigilant observance of vital signs. They may require risky invasive procedures in order to survive, including induction of coma with barbiturates and the placement of an intracranial pressure monitoring device.

Clearly, prevention is the best solution for aspirin-induced Reye's syndrome. The treatment for flulike symptoms (aches, low-grade fever, and headache) in children is acetaminophen. The drug is cheap, universally available, and conveniently formulated in many strengths and dosage forms. It is difficult to imagine a reason to use any other antipyretic or analgesic in this susceptible patient population.

CLINICAL REASONING

- At what age does a patient no longer display a significant risk for developing Reye's syndrome if treated with aspirin?
- Is it possible to establish definite divisions among minor patients according to calendar age (e.g., infant, child, adolescent)? Is such an arbitrary classification possible for any drug?
- What about the time and effort expended in assigning blame when Reye's syndrome manifests itself in a patient?
- What is the ethical responsibility of a health care provider who has inadvertently administered aspirin to a febrile 10-year-old who later is seen with what appears to be Reye's syndrome?
- What safeguards ought to be in place within a health care system to prevent the use of hazardous therapies of any kind in vulnerable patient populations?
- What needs do you identify in a parent who has unknowingly administered aspirin to a child who is subsequently admitted to the intensive care unit for management of Reye's syndrome?

develop sodium and fluid retention, which exacerbates other medical problems such as heart failure. Because the older adult commonly has reduced serum protein levels, drugs that are normally highly protein bound (such as NSAIDs) have increased free fraction of drug at typical doses and may produce increased toxicity. Older adults often do not complain of pain, and experience a higher peak and a longer duration of drug action than their younger counterparts. Keep in mind the patient's functional health literacy.

Drug Variables

If noninflammatory mechanisms (e.g., headache or muscle aches) are thought to be causing mild pain symptoms, acetaminophen is effective and inexpensive and produces little, if any, GI toxicity. Acetaminophen's advantage in the management of discomfort and fever is that it produces minimal GI irritation compared with NSAIDs and that it has no effect on bleeding times, uric acid levels, or respirations. However, it can cause toxicity in selected patients. The lifetime risk of nephropathy from acetaminophen increases when 5000 tablets have been taken.

Given the similar efficacy of nonspecific NSAIDs and COX-2 inhibitors, toxicity and cost play major roles in determining the drug chosen for a given patient. There are no predictive measures for selection of which NSAID a patient may respond to; about 60% of patients will respond to any single NSAID. All NSAIDs reduce inflammation, pain, and edema and improve movement when used in sufficient dosages. Management of mild to moderate inflammation and pain begins with an NSAID, unless otherwise contraindicated. NSAIDs relieve symptoms rather quickly but do not retard the progression of disease.

Naproxen is 20 times more potent than aspirin, whereas ibuprofen, fenoprofen, and aspirin are roughly equipotent in this action. Indomethacin has a high incidence of adverse effects and drug interactions, and therefore therapy should

not begin with this drug in most clinical situations. (The exception is for the treatment of acute gout; see later discussion.) Further, do not start pain management with piroxicam, because its long half-life does not allow the flexibility of rapid dosing. Use piroxicam for maintenance therapy only.

NSAIDs can be used in combination with other drugs (i.e., opioids) to provide more effective analgesia than either drug class alone. When used in combination for treatment of pain, NSAIDs have pivotal opioid dose-sparing effects and can be used to reduce the adverse effects of opioids. If a trial of a regularly scheduled, maximum-dose NSAID is not effective, a combination of an NSAID with an opioid (e.g., aspirin with oxycodone) may be effective. Although it is likely that NSAIDs also act within the CNS, they neither cause sedation or respiratory depression nor interfere with bowel or bladder function.

When monitoring the efficacy of a NSAID, it is important to assess symptoms once an adequate trial period has been achieved. The onset of antiinflammatory drug action occurs in about 7 days for ibuprofen, tolmetin, diclofenac, and ketoprofen, and in 14 days for sulindac, flurbiprofen, naproxen, and piroxicam. Increase the dosage if initial drug dosages are not effective by the end of this period. If maximum dosages are also not effective in a similar period, prescribe a different NSAID.

There is no clear evidence that NSAIDs vary in their ability to cause GI distress, nephrotoxicity, and hepatotoxicity. Trends suggest that the least GI-toxic NSAIDs are usually enteric-coated aspirin, ibuprofen, and salsalate. The most GI-toxic drugs are indomethacin, tolmetin, ketoprofen, and meclofenamate.

All NSAIDs have the potential to cause nephropathy. Sulindac, piroxicam, nabumetone, and tolmetin generally have the least toxic effects on the kidneys. Drug-induced nephrotic syndrome has been reported with use of indomethacin, ibuprofen, naproxen, fenoprofen, sulindac, and tolmetin. Fenoprofen has been implicated in 71% of the cases of nephrotic syndrome. Heart failure and kidney failure can be worsened with NSAID use.

CENTRAL NERVOUS

When changing drug therapies, there is little evidence that choosing a drug from another NSAID class significantly benefits the patient. It is sufficient to merely switch to another drug. Sustained-release NSAIDs appear to be as effective as regular-release forms, but long-term study is needed before definitive declarations can be made about efficacy and toxicity. The decision about which drug to use is based on potential toxicities, concomitant disease, and cost.

Evidence suggests that H_1 antagonists (e.g., cimetidine, ranitidine, famotidine), antacids, and sucralfate do not prevent NSAID-induced ulcers (see Chapter 45). However, use of high-dose proton pump inhibitors has been shown effective in evidence-based studies. Misoprostol, a PgE_1 analogue, acts on PgE_2 receptors to increase mucus formation and decrease gastric acid secretion. As a cytoprotective drug, misoprostol is helpful in reducing GI irritation from NSAIDs, but it is expensive, and there is no firm evidence that it prevents ulcer complications and death. Because misoprostol stimulates uterine contractions, the drug is absolutely contraindicated in pregnancy.

When a rapid initial effect is desired, NSAIDs are taken 1 hour before or 2 hours after meals. To reduce the risk of esophageal irritation caused by NSAIDs lodging against the lining of the esophagus, a full glass of fluid or other food should be taken. Even though food delays drug absorption and decreases peak plasma levels of some of the drugs, it is probably safer to take them with food. Advise the patient to remain upright for 15 to 30 minutes after taking the drug.

Pain relief provided by NSAIDs is subject to a ceiling effect. In other words, higher-than-recommended dosages may not necessarily provide additional therapeutic benefit in the treatment of pain unrelated to inflammation. Thus the patient who omits a scheduled dose should not double the next dose but should resume the usual dosing schedule. Once pain is controlled, the average daily dosage is decreased by 25% every 1 to 2 weeks until the minimum effective dose is reached. Once-daily or even as-needed dosing may be all that is required.

SALICYLATE TOXICITY. Although uncommon, salicylate toxicity may occur. The health care provider should be aware of symptoms and signs and treatment of salicylate toxicity (Box 17-2). Measure plasma salicylate concentrations when large doses of salicylates are used for antiinflammatory effects. Chronic administration of large doses saturates a major metabolic pathway, thereby slowing drug elimination, prolonging serum half-life, and causing drug accumulation. Drug accumulation can also occur with intentional overdose. Remain aware of symptoms and signs and treatment of salicylate toxicity.

ACETAMINOPHEN TOXICITY. In recommended dosages, acetaminophen is usually well tolerated; however, toxicity can occur with both acute and chronic ingestion. The health care provider should be aware of the signs and symptoms and treatment of acetaminophen toxicity (Box 17-3). Fortunately, liver damage related to acetaminophen overdose can be minimized by administering acetylcysteine. Although most effective when given shortly after acetaminophen ingestion, acetylcysteine can still provide significant protection when administered up to 24 hours after the poisoning has occurred.

Patient Education

To fully participate in treatment, the patient must know the nature and time course of expected beneficial drug effects.

BOX 17-2

Salicylate Toxicity

Definition
Systemic disorder caused by acute and/or chronic ingestion of salicylate containing drugs.
- *Mild toxicity:* Plasma salicylate levels of 40 to 70 mg/dL (chronic administration of 150–250 mg/kg/day)
- *Moderate toxicity:* Plasma salicylate levels of 70 to 150 mg/dL
- *Severe to lethal toxicity:* Plasma salicylate levels above 150 mg/dL (doses exceed 250 mg/kg/day)

Incidence
- Children and adults of any age; over 73% of cases are in children over age 5 and adults
- Males = females

Risk Factors
Dehydration, conditions causing respiratory or metabolic acidosis, extremes of age (very young and older adults), mental illness, history of previous toxic ingestions or suicide attempts, concurrent poisoning with other substances, concurrent use of acetazolamide

Signs and Symptoms
- **Early***: Tinnitus* secondary to vasoconstriction of auditory microvasculature or to increased pressure within the labyrinth and effects on cochlear hair cells, headache, nausea and vomiting, dizziness, and dimness of vision. *High-frequency hearing loss* is correlated with salicylate concentration but is reversible by stopping drug. *Hyperventilation* is attributable to direct CNS-stimulating effects on respiratory centers and from CO_2 generated by uncoupling of oxidative phosphorylation. Initially, *respiratory alkalosis* during first 3 days is compensated by enhanced renal elimination of sodium and potassium bicarbonate.
- **Late:** Without intervention, *respiratory alkalosis* is followed by metabolic acidosis as respiratory efforts weaken and CO_2 builds up.

Management
- Reduce salicylate levels by reducing absorption and promoting elimination (gastric lavage, activated charcoal).
- Correct hypovolemia, dehydration, and acid-base and electrolyte imbalances with IV fluids.

Prognosis
Complete recovery with early therapy. Noncardiogenic pulmonary edema possible, including the development of acute respiratory distress syndrome (ARDS) if not promptly treated with hemodialysis, peritoneal dialysis, or exchange transfusions.

CNS, Central nervous system; *IV,* intravenous.

BOX 17-3

Acetaminophen Toxicity

Definition

Excessive intake of acetaminophen. Plasma concentration over 200 mcg/mL.
- Toxic doses in children: 150 mg/kg or greater
- Toxicity from therapeutic use (rare): Occur with ingestion of 150 mg/kg/day for several days, or about double recommended maximum therapeutic dose (90 mg/kg/day)

Incidence
- Occurs in children and adults at any age
- Approximately 31% of exposures are in children under 6 years of age.

Risk Factors
- Age less than 6 years
- Concurrent oral poisoning with other substances
- Psychiatric illness
- History of previous toxic ingestions or suicide attempts
- Regular ingestion of large amounts of alcohol
- Lifetime risk of neuropathy from acetaminophen increases when 5000 tablets have been taken.

Signs and Symptoms
- *2 to 4 hr after ingestion:* Nausea, vomiting, sweating, pallor
- *24 to 36 hr after ingestion:* Symptoms lesson, patient's condition improves, but levels of toxic metabolites continue to rise

- *2 to 7 days after ingestion:* Hepatic damage as evidenced by RUQ pain, jaundice, confusion, stupor; AST, ALT, and LDH elevations; increased prothrombin time (PT) and INR and decreased blood sugar levels. Hepatic damage may be permanent.

Management
- Empty stomach of its contents by inducing emesis or by thorough lavage.
- Liver damage from toxic metabolite of acetaminophen can be minimized by timely use of acetylcysteine (Mucomyst), a sulfhydryl compound that scavenges free radicals. Most effective when administered as soon as possible after overdose. If administered 15 to 24 hr after ingestion, incidence of severe liver damage increases to 85%.
- The initial loading dose of acetylcysteine is 140 mg/kg, followed by 70 mg/kg every 4 hr for up to 17 doses. Follow package instructions for dilution of product. Mix with juice, cola, or water to increase the palatability.
- Acetylcysteine has an extremely unpleasant odor (rotten eggs), which may itself induce vomiting. If vomiting interferes with oral administration, the drug can be given through a nasogastric or orogastric tube.
- Therapy is discontinued when acetaminophen blood levels indicate low risk of hepatotoxicity.

ALT, Alanine transaminase; *AST,* aspartate transaminase; *INR,* international normalized ratio; *LDH,* lactate dehydrogenase; *RUQ,* right upper quadrant.

With this information, the patient can help monitor and evaluate treatment outcomes. Although analgesic and antipyretic effects may become evident in a short time, in some cases, weeks or months may be required before beneficial antiinflammatory effects are known. As previously discussed in Chapter 16, teaching non–drug measures for concomitant pain relief enhances success with drug therapy. Teach that acetaminophen is an effective aspirin substitute for pain or fever but not for inflammation or to prevent heart attack or stroke.

OTC and prescription drugs containing aspirin are potential sources of salicylates and may contribute to toxicity (Table 17-8). Similarly, there are many OTC products containing acetaminophen, most with 500 mg of drug per tablet or capsule. Teach patients to read labels carefully to avoid doubling of aspirin or acetaminophen doses.

Just as patients must know when and how to take their drug, they must also know when to stop. Instruct patients to discontinue the NSAID when symptoms subside. However, in some patients, longer treatment courses may be required. Inform patients self-managing their NSAID therapy of the importance of periodic measurements of white blood cell, hemoglobin, and hematocrit levels, electrolytes, blood pressure, and stool guaiac to assess for safety.

Advise patients on chronic aspirin therapy to discontinue their NSAID-based therapy at least 5 half-lives before the procedure; at this point, approximately 97% of the drug will be eliminated. Most health care providers will err on the longer side because of protein binding and redistribution.

A woman of child-bearing age or one who intends to become pregnant while using an NSAID should be instructed to consult her health care provider. These drugs may interfere with maternal and infant blood clotting and prolong the duration of pregnancy and parturition, and may have teratogenic effects. If the mother intends to breastfeed, consultation with the health care provider is warranted since many of these drugs are detected in breast milk and are cleared slowly from the body of an infant.

The patient with comorbid disorders (e.g., gastritis, ulcers, bleeding disorders, diabetes, gout, renal insufficiency, comorbid cardiovascular disease) or any of the risk factors mentioned in Table 17-1, or one who is on anticoagulant therapy, should discuss the addition of NSAIDs to the treatment regimen with the health care provider. Advise the patient with hypertension to use effervescent aspirin products with caution because of their high sodium content.

Because fever is an important body defense mechanism in fighting infection, drug therapy may not be needed unless the fever is particularly high (i.e., more than 101.5° F) or is accompanied by other uncomfortable signs and symptoms. Pain is not usually associated with the common cold, so analgesic-antipyretic drugs are used only for their fever-relieving characteristics. If acetaminophen use is required for more than 2 to 3 days, the health care provider should be contacted for further evaluation of the fever.

As with any drug, teach patients to store NSAIDs in a closed, childproof container and to keep them out of the reach of children. It is wise to never call aspirin or other drugs "candy," because aspirin is a common cause of drug overdose in children. Further, advise the patient to discard any drug beyond its expiration date. In the case of salicylate tablets, a vinegar-like odor is a sign of salicylate deterioration.

Advise patients to avoid alcohol intake while taking NSAIDs; alcohol intake produces synergistic effects with NSAIDs, thus increasing the risk of GI distress and bleeding.

TABLE 17-8 OTC and Prescription Formulations Containing Salicylates and Salicylate-Like Compounds*

EXAMPLES OF OTC PREPARATIONS CONTAINING SALICYLATES

Alka-Seltzer Effervescent tablet	Buffets II tablets
Alka-Seltzer Plus Cold Medicine	Buf-Tabs
Anacin and Anacin Maximum Strength tablets	Carma Arthritis Strength tablets
Arthralgen tablets	Cope tablets
Arthritis Pain Formula	Doan's pills
Arthritis Strength Bufferin tablets	Ecotrin tablets
Arthropan liquid	Emagrin tablets
A.S.A. Enseals	Empirin tablets
Ascriptin tablets	Excedrin tablets and caplets
Ascriptin A/D tablets	Maximum Bayer aspirin
Ascriptin Extra-Strength tablets	Mobigesic tablets
Aspergum	Momentum tablets
Bayer Aspirin tablets	Pepto-Bismol tablets and liquid
Bayer Children's Aspirin tablets	St. Joseph aspirin for adults
Bayer Children's Cold tablets	St. Joseph Cold tablets for children
Bayer Timed Release 8-Hour caplets	Stanback powder
BC Tablet and powder	Trigesic
Bufferin Arthritis Strength tablets	Vanquish caplets

EXAMPLES OF PRESCRIPTION PREPARATIONS CONTAINING SALICYLATES

Ascriptin with Codeine tablets	Lanorinal tablets
Axotal tablets	Magan tablets
Buff-A Comp tablets and capsules	Magsal tablets
Buff-A Comp No. 3 tablets (with codeine)	Mobidin tablets
Darvon Compound pulvules	Norgesic and Norgesic Forte tablets
Darvon Compound-65 pulvules	Percodan and Percodan-Demi tablets
Disalcid capsules	Robaxisal tablets
Easprin	Soma compound
Empirin with Codeine tablets	Synalgos-DC capsules
Equagesic tablet	Talwin Compound tablets
Fiorinal tablets	Trilisate tablets and liquid
Fiorinal with Codeine	

*Not a complete listing. Other products may also contain aspirin, salicylates, and salicylamides.
OTC, Over-the-counter.

Some patients experience drowsiness and dizziness while taking NSAIDs. Caution them about performing tasks that require alertness. Further, aspirin should not be taken concurrently with vitamin C–containing products (e.g., orange juice), because it may contribute to increased gastric acidity and thereby decrease the rate of absorption.

Encourage the patient to report hearing changes, because bilateral hearing loss of 30 to 40 decibels can occur with prolonged use of a salicylate. Reassure the patient that hearing usually returns to normal within 2 weeks after treatment is stopped.

Instruct patients hypersensitive to salicylates to avoid these and other NSAIDs. Advise the patient with nasal polyps to avoid using acetylated salicylates (e.g., aspirin) for self-treatment of minor aches and pains since these drugs may trigger an acute asthma attack. Nonacetylated salicylates may be used cautiously.

Evaluation

NSAID treatment effectiveness is evaluated through patient reports of increased comfort and range of motion, increased mobility, and the ability to perform activities of daily living. Redness, warmth, edema, and pain are reduced or absent. If the drug is being used for its antipyretic effects, the patient's temperature will be within the normal range. Because the health care provider has information about which activities were most impaired by the problem, this information can also be used as an indicator of improvement.

Evaluation of any drug therapy should always include both the drug and disease or symptom outcomes, and both short- and long-term benefits and risks. NSAID treatment effectiveness is evaluated through patient reports of increased comfort and range of motion, increased mobility, and the ability to perform activities of daily living. Redness, warmth, edema, and pain are reduced or absent. If the drug is being used for its antipyretic effects, the patient's temperature will be within the normal range. Because the health care provider has information about which activities were most impaired by the problem, this information can also be used as an indicator of improvement.

RHEUMATOID ARTHRITIS

Rheumatoid arthritis (RA) is characterized by joint stiffness, damage, and pain. Symptoms are most intense in the morning and abate as the day goes on. The joints become warm, tender, and swollen. In addition to joint damage, RA has systemic manifestations including fever, weakness, fatigue, weight loss, thinning of the skin, scleritis, corneal ulcers, and nodules under the skin and periosteum. A particularly severe

CASE STUDY | Disease-Modifying Antirheumatic Drugs

ASSESSMENT

History of Present Illness	MJ is a 35-year-old female who comes to town today requesting assistance with managing her rheumatoid arthritis. She was diagnosed 5 years ago when the arthritis affected her left hand and gradually began affecting both. She has used salicylates and other NSAIDs in the past several months with varying degrees of success. MJ reports she usually gets along fine by balancing rest and exercise, and by using indomethacin several times a day for inflammation and pain.
Past Health History	ROS is unremarkable except for a gastric ulcer 5 years ago, which was treated with antibiotics and acid-reducers. She denies drug or food allergies, or history of renal, hepatic, or GI bleeding.
Life-Span Considerations	MJ's husband died during the Iraq war. They have no children. She decided to stay in the family ranch home, which is 50 miles from the nearest town. The distance causes MJ a great deal of distress because it is painful to drive into town. She wants to remain as independent as possible despite her need for assistance with daily activities.
Psychosocial Considerations	MJ's husband managed their 1000-acre cattle ranch until his entry into the Marines. She has not yet started receiving survivor benefits from the military. MJ has a limited income and would prefer to "spend my money on good food rather than on expensive medicine for my joints." She has catastrophic health care insurance only, lacking coverage for office visits.
Physical Exam Findings	*Temp:* 99.4° F. *Pulse;* 80 beats/min. Early subcutaneous nodules over MCP joints, mild bilateral ulnar drifting. Joints warm with mild edema.
Diagnostic Testing	Radiographic report from previous health care provider reveals arthritic changes bilaterally. CBC, UA, renal function, and liver function tests within normal limits. ESR was elevated with RF and ANA positive.

DIAGNOSIS: Rheumatoid arthritis

MANAGEMENT

Treatment Objectives	1. Reduce pain and inflammation while maintaining existing joint function. 2. Preserve quality of life and ability to carry out activities of daily living.
Treatment Options	**Pharmacotherapy** • Stop indomethacin. • Methotrexate, 5- to 10-mg test dose. If no reaction, start methotrexate, 2.5 mg PO every 12 hours for three doses, then 7.5 mg weekly. • Folic acid, 1 mg PO daily • Start diclofenac, 50 mg PO 2 to 4 times daily until desired response from methotrexate is achieved. • Adjunctive pain management strategies to include joint rest, Yogic breathing exercises, guided imagery, cutaneous stimulation, and physical comfort measures (e.g., positioning). **Patient Education** 1. Do not have immunizations without approval by health care provider. 2. Avoid aspirin and alcohol during methotrexate therapy. 3. Promptly report fever, sore throat, signs of local infection, unusual bruising or bleeding, onset of dry cough, dyspnea, or fever. 4. Good oral hygiene. Keep well hydrated. Take drugs with food. **Evaluation** 1. Pain and inflammation are reduced and existing joint function is maintained. 2. Quality of life is preserved with moderate ability to carry out activities of daily living.

CLINICAL REASONING ANALYSIS

Q1. **Why are you using an antineoplastic drug to treat MJ? She doesn't have cancer.**

A. It is now the standard of care for RA. Approximately 70% to 75% of patients respond favorably to methotrexate. Starting therapy early helps prevent irreversible joint damage and minimizes the toxicity associated with NSAIDs and steroids. Although DMARDs, such as methotrexate, have no immediate analgesic effects, methotrexate can control symptoms and has been shown to delay and possibly stop disease progression.

Continued

CENTRAL NERVOUS

CASE STUDY   Disease-Modifying Antirheumatic Drugs—Cont'd

Q2. **Why did you start the methotrexate yourself? Shouldn't MJ have seen a rheumatologist to order the methotrexate?**
A. Because of the distance into town, I contacted the only rheumatologist in town and asked for assistance. MJ, the rheumatologist, and I had a teleconference. After reviewing her case and seeing the exam findings and previous x-ray films, he recommended the methotrexate therapy. She will see me once a month and the rheumatologist every 4 weeks. I will monitor her BUN and creatinine levels, liver function tests, and CBC and contact the rheumatologist if MJ or I have concerns.

Q3. **How often does MJ need the blood tests?**
A. Ordinarily the liver function tests and CBC are done monthly and the BUN and creatinine every 3–4 months. One mg of folic acid daily helps to minimize adverse reactions such as anemia, leukopenia, thrombocytopenia, and stomatitis. Although methotrexate may inhibit folic acid metabolism, it does not seem to affect the efficacy of the drug.

Q4. **Why did you tell her not to use aspirin or drink alcohol while taking the diclofenac?**
A. Aspirin and alcohol in combination with diclofenac increase the risk of GI bleeding. She was told to take the drug with food to minimize the risk for GI bleeding.

---

manifestation of RA is vasculiltis. Some patients have periods of spontaneous remission.

EPIDEMIOLOGY AND ETIOLOGY

Pharmaceutical companies and the media have both recently paid an increasing amount of attention to diseases associated with aging, RA among them. Despite the attention paid to the issue, estimates of the prevalence of RA vary widely. RA has a worldwide distribution and affects all ethnic groups. The disease can occur at any age, but its prevalence increases with age; the peak incidence is between the fourth and sixth decades. RA affects 2.1 million Americans, women more than men (2.5:1).

There are no reports of clustering in space or time that would support an infectious cause, and no environmental factors that precipitate disease onset have been identified. Factors associated with RA include the possibility of infectious triggers, genetic predisposition, and autoimmune response. CD4+ T cells stimulate the immune cascade, leading to cytokine production such as TNF-alpha (TNF-α) and IL-1.

PATHOPHYSIOLOGY

Chronic inflammation of the synovial tissue lining the joint capsule results in the proliferation of this tissue. The inflamed, proliferating synovial tissue characteristic of rheumatoid arthritis is called *pannus*. The pannus invades cartilage and bony surfaces, eventually producing erosions of bone and cartilage and ultimately leading to total joint destruction. Damage to the cartilage is caused by enzymes released from the pannus and by proinflammatory enzymes and chemicals produced by the inflammatory response within the synovial space. Factors initiating the inflammatory response are presently unclear; however, once the articular cartilage has been totally destroyed and ankylosis occurs, the inflammatory response subsides. The progression of joint destruction is depicted in Figure 17-3.

The joint destruction is associated with an autoimmune attack of the joint tissues. During the attack, mast cells, macrophages, and T cells produce cytokines and cytotoxins, compounds that promote inflammation and joint destruction. The cytokines of greatest interest are TNF, IL-1, IL-6, interferon-gamma, platelet-derived growth factor, and granulocyte-macrophage colony stimulating factor.

PHARMACOTHERAPEUTIC OPTIONS

Disease-modifying Antirheumatic Drugs

Disease-modifying antirheumatic drugs (DMARDs) have antiinflammatory properties as well as the ability to slow disease progression. Although not members of a single drug family, the DMARDs all suppress the body's overactive immune system in some way, thereby controlling a key aspect of many systemic inflammatory based disease conditions (e.g., rheumatoid arthritis, systemic lupus erythematosus) Slow-acting antirheumatic drugs (SAARDs), such as hydroxychloroquine and aurothioglucose, are a subclass of the DMARDs. Onset of the effects of SAARDs is slow; it takes 3 to 5 months before effects are noted. For this reason, these drugs are often used in combination with rapid-acting NSAIDs. Biologic response modifiers are also considered DMARDs but are discussed in Chapter 32.

In the past, treatment for rheumatoid arthritis was simple: (1) start with an NSAID (e.g., aspirin, ibuprofen, celecoxib); (2) if symptoms are not controlled with an NSAID, add a DMARD (e.g., methotrexate) and continue the NSAID until the DMARD takes effect; (3) provide a short course of corticosteroids, if needed, while responses to the DMARD are developing; and (4) supplement treatment any time symptoms flare. In this traditional regimen, DMARDs were used only if the NSAIDs did not control symptoms. Today, however, aggressive treatment of rheumatoid arthritis is used early in therapy to delay joint degeneration, symptomatology, and loss of quality of life. Recall that NSAIDs provide symptomatic relief; they do not retard disease progression. DMARD dosages are identified in Table 17-9.

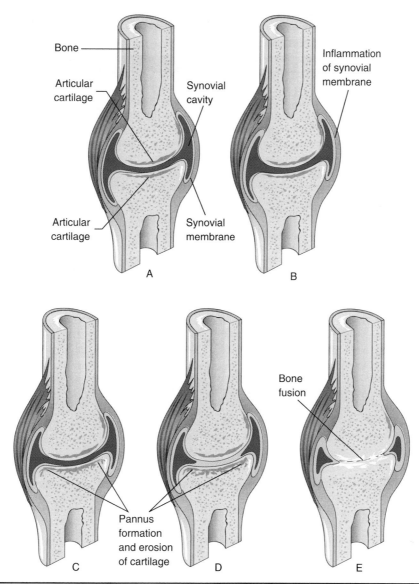

FIGURE 17-3 Progressive Joint Destruction of Rheumatoid Arthritis. A, Healthy joint; **B,** Synovial membrane inflammation; **C,** Formation of pannus; **D,** Worsening pannus formation; cartilage continues to degenerate; **E,** Total destruction of joint resulting in alkylosis.

Methotrexate

▌▎ Indications

Methotrexate (MTX; Trexall and Rheumatrex Dose Pack) is the current first-line drug in the management of rheumatoid arthritis. It is used to relieve symptoms of severe arthritis and, in some cases, produce a prolonged remission. In cases where multiple drugs are needed for treatment, methotrexate is normally the baseline drug to which other pharmacologic options are added.

▌▎ Pharmacodynamics

MTX has an affinity for tissues with high rates of cellular proliferation such as neoplasms, bone marrow, hair matrix, and psoriatic lesions. This accounts for its success in selected patients with recalcitrant psoriasis, in addition to malignant neoplasms. MTX also has immunosuppressive activity and at lower doses has been used in the treatment of RA and SLE.

MTX is a folic acid antagonist. The result is inhibition of DNA synthesis and cell reproduction. It is structurally similar to folic acid and acts by reversibly inhibiting dihydrofolate reductase, the enzyme that reduces folic acid to tetrahydrofolic acid. This inhibition ultimately interferes with the synthesis of DNA and cell reproduction and slows disease progression.

▌▎ Pharmacokinetics

Small doses of MTX are absorbed from the GI tract; larger doses are incompletely absorbed. MTX is actively transported across cell membranes to be widely distributed. The drug crosses the placenta and enters breast milk in low concentrations. MTX is eliminated mostly unchanged by the kidneys (Table 17-10).

DOSAGE
TABLE **17-9** Regimen of Selected DMARDs

Drug	Use(s)	Dosage	Implications
adalimumab	Moderate to severe rheumatoid arthritis resistant to conventional therapy	*Adult:* 40 mg subQ once every 2 wk when given with methotrexate	Monitor for infection. Expensive: annual cost $18,000
anakinra	Moderate to severe rheumatoid arthritis resistant to conventional therapy	*Adult:* 100 mg subQ daily	Injection site reactions may occur during first 4–6 wk of therapy. Monitor for infection.
azathioprine	Severe, erosive rheumatoid arthritis unresponsive to conventional therapy	*Adult:* 1 mg/kg/day PO for 6–8 wk; increase dose by 0.5 mg/kg every 4 wk until desired response or 2.5 mg/kg/day reached; decrease by 0.5 mg/kg every 4–8 wk to minimum effective dosage	May be administered with or after meals or in divided dose to minimize nausea.
auranofin	Progressive rheumatoid arthritis resistant to conventional therapy	*Adult:* 6 mg/day PO in 1–2 divided doses; may increase to 9 mg/day in 3 divided doses if no improvement occurs after 6 mo	Take with meals. Contains 29% gold.
aurothioglucose	Progressive rheumatoid arthritis resistant to conventional therapy	*Adult:* 10 mg IM first wk; 25 mg IM weeks 2–3; 25–50 mg/wk until improvement or toxicity occurs. Max: 1 gram total. Maintenance: 25–50 mg every 2 wk for up to 20 wk, then every 3–4 wk *Child ages 6–12 yr:* 2.5 mg first wk; 6.25 mg in weeks 2–3; 12.5 mg weekly until a total of 200–250 mg has been given. Maintenance: 6.25–12.5 mg every 3–4 wk	Never give by IV route. Patient to remain recumbent for 15 min after injection. Closely monitor for nitritoid or allergic reaction. Injections may be followed by joint pain for 1–2 days. Contains 50% gold.
etanercept	Severe rheumatoid arthritis; ankylosing spondylitis; JRA	*Adult:* 50 mg subQ 1–2 times weekly *Child 4–17 yr:* 0.4 mg/kg twice weekly to maximum of 25 mg	Injections are given 3–4 days apart. Expensive: 12-month course of therapy is about $15,500.
gold sodium thiomalate	Progressive rheumatoid arthritis resistant to conventional therapy	*Adult:* 10 mg IM initially; 25 mg IM 1 wk later, followed by 25–50 mg IM weekly until improvement or toxicity occurs; then 25–50 mg IM every 2 wk up to 20 wk, then every 3–4 wk. Max: 1 gram total. *Child:* 10 mg IM initially followed 1 wk later by 1 mg/kg every 2 wk up to 20 wk, then every 3–4 wk	History of previous mild reaction: Start with initial dose of 5 mg, increasing by 5–10 mg weekly or monthly until a dose of 25–50 mg is reached.
hydroxychloroquine	Severe rheumatoid arthritis and systemic lupus erythematosus	*Adult:* Initially 400–600 mg PO daily. Maintenance: 200–400 mg/day *Child:* 3–5 mg/kg/day; not to exceed 7 mg/kg/day or 400 mg/day	May require up to 6 mo for full benefit to be noted. Take with food or meals. 200 mg of hydroxychloroquine sulfate = 155 mg of hydroxychloroquine base.
infliximab	Moderate to severe rheumatoid arthritis resistant to conventional therapy	*Adult:* 200–400 mg per treatment based on body weight; give at 0, 2, and 6 wk, then every 8 wk	Monitor for infection. Expensive: $14,000-$37,000/year depending on dosage and administration schedule.
leflunomide	Rheumatoid arthritis	*Adult:* 10–20 mg PO daily. Start with 100 mg PO daily for 3 days —or— 10 mg PO every other day	Monitor LFTs and CBC at baseline and monthly for 6 months, then every 6–8 wk if stable.
methotrexate	Rheumatoid arthritis resistant to conventional therapy	*Adult:* Initially 7.5 mg PO weekly (2.5 mg PO every 12 hr for 3 doses); not to exceed 20 mg/wk	Therapy preceded by 5- to 10-mg test dose. Dosage decreased once desired response is obtained. Monitor LFTs.
D-penicillamine	Rheumatoid arthritis resistant to conventional therapy	*Adult:* 125–250 mg/day PO as single dose; may be slowly increased up to 1000–1500 mg/day	Monitor 24-hr urinary protein levels every 1–2 wk in patients with moderate proteinuria. Monitor liver function tests every 6 mo during first 18 mo of therapy.
sulfasalazine	Rheumatoid arthritis; treatment of ankylosing spondylitis	*Adult:* 0.5–1 gram/day for 1 wk; increase by 500 mg/wk to max of 3 grams/day *Child:* 10 mg/kg/day PO; may increase by 10 mg/kg/day at weekly intervals; range 30–50 mg/kg/day. Max: 2 grams/day	May cause yellow-orange discoloration of urine, skin. May be necessary to take drug even after symptoms relieved.

CBC, Complete blood count; *DMARD,* disease-modifying antirheumatic drug; *IM,* intramuscular; *IV,* intravenous; *JRA,* juvenile rheumatoid arthritis; *LFTs,* liver function tests; *PO,* by mouth; *subQ,* subcutaneous.

▥ *Adverse Effects and Contraindications*

Common adverse effects of MTX include stomatitis, anorexia, nausea, vomiting, and hepatotoxicity. Anemia, leukopenia, thrombocytopenia, and neuropathy are also fairly common; pulmonary fibrosis can occur and is life threatening. Use MTX with caution in patients with creatinine clearance rates lower than 60 mL/min. Cautious use is also warranted in patients with active infections and decreased bone marrow reserve, in older adults, and in patients with chronic debilitating illnesses.

MTX is contraindicated during pregnancy and lactation, and in patients with liver disease, immunodeficiency syndromes, or preexisting blood dyscrasias. Since MTX is a folic acid antagonist, the teratogenic effects of MTX therapy during the first trimester can be severe, including spontaneous abortion. If either the male or the female partner have undergone

PHARMACOKINETICS

TABLE 17-10 Selected DMARDs

Drug	Route	Onset	Peak	Duration	PB (%)	$t_{1/2}$
DMARDs						
adalimumab	subQ	UA	3.1–4.6 hr	UA	UA	2 wk
anakinra	subQ	UA	UA	UA	UA	4–6 hr
azathioprine	PO	6–8 wk	3 mo	UA	UA	3 hr
auranofin	PO	3–6 mo*	2–4 mo*	6 mo	60	26 days; 40–128 days†
aurothioglucose	IM	6–8 wk*	1–2 mo	6 mo	85–95	3–26 days; 40–128 days†
etanercept	subQ	UA	UA	UA	UA	170–230 hr
gold sodium thiomalate	IM	6–8 wk*	1–2 mo	6 mo	85–95	14–10 hr; 168 hr‡
hydroxychloroquine	PO	Rapid	1–2 hr	Days-wk	45	72–120 hr
infliximab	IV	Rapid	UA	UA	UA	8–9.5 days
leflunomide	PO	UA	UA	UA	UA	>14 days
methotrexate	PO/IM	4–7 days	7–14 days	21 days	50	2–4 hr
D-penicillamine	PO	1–3 mo	UK	1–3 mo	UA	60 min
sulfasalazine	PO	Varies	1.5–6 hr§	UA	UA	8.4–10.4 hr

Note: Occasionally, products are reformulated to add or remove salicylates.
*Peak blood levels and antiinflammatory effects of gold salts.
†Half-life of gold salt in the blood and tissues, respectively.
‡Half-life of a single dose of gold sodium thiomalate; 14–40 hours by the third dose, and up to 168 hours after the eleventh dose.
§Peak effects of enteric coated sulfasalazine occur in 3–12 hours.
DMARD, Disease-modifying antirheumatic drug; *IM,* intramuscular; *IV,* intravenous; *PB,* protein binding; *PO,* by mouth; *subQ,* subcutaneous; $t_{1/2}$, elimination half-life; *UA,* unavailable.

MTX therapy, pregnancy should be avoided for a minimum of 3 months for males, and at least one ovulatory cycle for females. The safety and effectiveness of MTX in children has only been established for antineoplastic therapy and poly-articular juvenile rheumatoid arthritis (JRA).

▥ Drug Interactions

Many drug interactions are associated with MTX (Table 17-11). Additive toxicity can occur with concurrent use of other hepatotoxic and nephrotoxic drugs. MTX decreases antibody response to live virus vaccines and increases the risk of adverse effects.

▥ Lab Considerations

MTX may cause elevated serum uric acid concentrations. Obtain complete blood count (CBC) and differential values before and frequently throughout therapy. Monitor renal and hepatic function before and throughout therapy.

Etanercept
▥ Indications

Etanercept (Enbrel) is the first of a new class of drugs known as tumor necrosis factor (TNF) blockers. Etanercept quickly reduces the signs and symptoms of RA, inhibits the progression of structural damage, and improves physical function in patients with moderately to severely active RA. The drug is also used in patients with moderate to severe JRA who have not responded to one or more of the DMARDs. NSAIDs, MTX, corticosteroids, or analgesics may be continued during treatment with etanercept.

▥ Pharmacodynamics

Etanercept inhibits binding of TNF-α and TNF-β to TNF receptors on the cell surface, rendering TNF biologically inactive. Etanercept also modulates biologic responses

regulated by TNF, including the appearance of molecules responsible for leukocyte migration and serum levels of cytokines.

▥ Pharmacokinetics

Etanercept is well absorbed following subcutaneous administration. With repeated dosing there is a twofold to sevenfold increase in peak serum concentrations. Pharmacokinetic parameters do not vary between adult men and women or with age. Clinical responses generally appear within 1 to 2 weeks after the start of therapy and nearly always occur by 3 months.

▥ Adverse Effects and Contraindications

One third of patients have injection site reactions. Headache, rhinitis, dizziness, pharyngitis, cough, asthenia, and dyspepsia occur in about 20% of patients. Pyelonephritis, cellulitis, osteomyelitis, wound infections, leg ulcers, septic arthritis, diarrhea, and upper respiratory infections such as bronchitis and pneumonia occur in more than 38% of patients. Serious adverse effects such as heart failure, hypertension and hypotension, pancreatitis, GI hemorrhage, and dyspnea occur but are rare. The incidence of abdominal pain and vomiting is higher in children than adults.

Rare cases of demyelinating disorders such as optic neuritis and multiple sclerosis have been reported with etanercept. Blood dyscrasias, including fatal cases of aplastic anemia, have also been noted. A cause-and-effect relationship has not been established between etanercept and these disorders.

Etanercept should not be given to patients with any localized or chronic infection. Closely monitor patients who develop new infections while taking etanercept. Etanercept should be used with caution in patients who have a condition that predisposes them to infection (e.g., diabetes). Prospective patients should have a chest x-ray exam and tuberculin skin test to rule out latent tuberculosis before starting treatment.

CENTRAL NERVOUS

DRUG INTERACTIONS
TABLE 17-11 Selected DMARDs

Drugs	Interactive Drugs	Interaction
adalimumab	Live virus vaccines	Increases risk of acquiring or transmitting infection following immunization
anakinra	TNF blockers	Increases incidence of neutropenia, resulting in severe infections
azathioprine	Antineoplastics, cyclosporin, myelosuppressive drugs Allopurinol Live virus vaccines	Additive myelosuppression Inhibits release of azathioprine, increasing toxicity Decreases antibody response and increases risk of toxicity
Gold salts	Antineoplastics, radiation therapy	Additive myelosuppression
hydroxychloroquine	D-penicillamine Digoxin Urinary acidifiers	Increases risk of hematologic toxicity Increases risk of digoxin toxicity Increases renal excretion of hydroxychloroquine
infliximab	Live virus vaccines	Increases risk of acquiring or transmitting infection following immunization
leflunomide	ibuprofen, diclofenac, rifampin warfarin	Increases concentration of leflunomide Increases warfarin effects
methotrexate	High-dose salicylates, NSAIDs, oral hypoglycemics, phenytoin, tetracyclines, probenecid, chloramphenicol Hepatotoxic drugs Nephrotoxic drugs Live virus vaccines asparaginase	Increases risk of methotrexate toxicity Increases risk of hepatotoxicity Increases risk of nephrotoxicity Decreases antibody response to interactive drug Decreases effects of methotrexate
D-penicillamine	Immunosuppressive drugs, antineoplastics, gold salts Iron supplements digoxin	Increases risk of adverse hematologic effects Decreases absorption of penicillamine Decreases serum levels of digoxin
sulfasalazine	Salicylates glyburide, tolbutamide, warfarin acetaminophen Beta blockers, cardiac glycosides cyclosporine	Decreases effectiveness of sulfasalazine Increases effectiveness of interacting drug Increases risk of hepatotoxicity Reduces serum concentrations of interactive drug Additive nephrotoxicity and reduced plasma concentrations of interactive drug

DMARD, Disease-modifying antirheumatic drug; *NSAID*, nonsteroidal antiinflammatory drug; *TNF*, tumor necrosis factor.

▮▮ Drug Interactions

There are no known drug interactions with etanercept. Nonetheless, live virus vaccines should be avoided because of the risk of acquiring or transmitting infection following immunization.

▮▮ Lab Considerations

Monitor erythrocyte sedimentation rates or C-reactive protein levels, CBC with differential, and platelet counts for evidence of infection and sepsis.

Infliximab
▮▮ Indications

Infliximab (Remicaid) is the second TNF blocker approved for treatment of RA in combination with methotrexate for reducing signs and symptoms, inhibiting the progression of structural damage, and improving physical function in patients with active RA that is moderate to severe.

▮▮ Pharmacodynamics

Infliximab neutralizes the biologic activity of TNF-α by binding with high affinity to the soluble and transmembrane forms of TNF-α, and inhibits binding of TNF-α with its receptors. Infliximab does not neutralize TNF-β (lymphotoxin a), a related cytokine that uses the same receptors as TNF-α. Despite their similar effects, etanercept and infliximab are structurally different; whereas the former is composed of two TNF receptors, the latter is a TNF antibody. In one study, inhibition of progression of structural damage was observed at 54 weeks and maintained through 102 weeks (Maini et al., 1998).

▮▮ Pharmacokinetics

There is a linear relationship between the dose of infliximab administered and the maximum serum concentration. No systemic accumulation of infliximab occurs with continued repeated treatment. Development of antibodies to infliximab increases infliximab clearance. Clinical responses generally appear within 1 to 2 weeks after initiation of therapy.

▮▮ Adverse Effects and Contraindications

The common adverse effects of infliximab include headache, nausea, fatigue, fever, and infusion reactions. Pharyngitis, vomiting, pain, dizziness, bronchitis, rash, rhinitis, coughing, pruritus, sinusitis, myalgias, and back pain have been reported in less than 10% of patients. In patients with heart failure, infliximab may increase the risk of hospitalizations and mortality, hence the drug should be avoided in these patients. Multiple sclerosis has developed in patients receiving infliximab.

▮▮ Drug Interactions

As with etanercept, there are no known drug interactions with infliximab. Nonetheless, avoid live virus vaccines because of the risk of acquiring or transmitting infection following immunization.

Lab Considerations

Monitor erythrocyte sedimentation rates or C-reactive protein levels, CBC with differential, and platelet counts for evidence of infection, including bacterial sepsis, invasive fungal infections, and reactivation of latent tuberculosis. Accordingly, do not give the drug to patients with a history of chronic infections, and temporarily suspend treatment if an acute infection develops. Prospective patients should have a chest x-ray exam and tuberculin skin test to rule out latent tuberculosis before starting therapy.

Adalimumab

Indications

Adalimumab (Humira) is the third TNF-blocking drug approved for treatment of RA. Like infliximab, it is a monoclonal antibody that binds to and thereby neutralizes TNF. The drug is indicated for adults with moderate to severe RA who have not responded adequately to one or more DMARDs. In these patients, adalimumab reduces symptoms and slows the progression of joint damage. It may be used alone or in conjunction with MTX or other DMARDs.

Pharmacodynamics

As a monoclonal antibody, adalimumab, like etanercept and infliximab, has immunosuppressant actions. It binds specifically to TNF-α and blocks its interaction with the p55 and p75 cell-surface TNF receptors. Adalimumab also modulates biologic responses that are induced or regulated by TNF, including changes in the levels of adhesion molecules responsible for leukocyte migration.

Pharmacokinetics

The bioavailability of adalimumab is 64% when given subcutaneously. The pharmacokinetics of adalimumab is linear over the dose range of 0.5 to 10 mg/kg following a single intravenous (IV) dose. The systemic clearance of adalimumab is approximately 12 mL/hr. The mean terminal half-life was approximately 2 weeks.

Adverse Effects and Contraindications

Adalimumab is generally well tolerated. The most common adverse effects include injection-site reactions and headache. Allergic reactions occur in approximately 1% of patients. The drug has been associated with neurologic injury (i.e., numbness, tingling, dizziness, disturbed vision, and leg weakness), but very rarely.

Drug Interactions

As with etanercept and infliximab, there are no known drug interactions with adalimumab. Nonetheless, avoid live virus vaccines because of the risk of acquiring or transmitting infection following immunization.

Lab Considerations

As with the other TNF blockers, monitor erythrocyte sedimentation rates or C-reactive protein levels, CBC with differential, and platelet counts for evidence of infection, including bacterial sepsis, invasive fungal infections, and reactivation of latent tuberculosis. Accordingly, do not give the drug to patients with a history of chronic infections, and temporarily suspend treatment if an acute infection develops. Prospective patients should have a chest x-ray exam and tuberculin skin test to rule out latent tuberculosis before starting therapy.

Leflunomide

Indications

Leflunomide (Arava) is a relatively new immunomodulator that not only decreases the pain and swelling of arthritis but may also decrease damage to joints and long-term disability. Leflunomide is used to treat the symptoms of RA and may also be combined with MTX therapy. It may take several weeks before improvement in joint pain and swelling is noted. The drug can be used in combination with NSAIDs and low-dose corticosteroids if needed. Use with other DMARDs has not been studied.

Pharmacodynamics

Leflunomide interferes with the formation of DNA. It acts by reducing synthesis of pyrimidine by inhibiting dihydroorotate dehydrogenase, thus acquiring antiinflammatory and antiproliferative properties.

Pharmacokinetics

Leflunomide is well absorbed following oral administration, with 99% of the drug bound to plasma proteins. Leflunomide is extensively biotransformed by CYP 2C9 enzymes to active metabolites in the liver and the GI tract, with elimination in the feces. It is unknown if it is excreted in breast milk. Safety and efficacy has not been established in children younger than 18 years.

Adverse Effects and Contraindications

Diarrhea is the most common adverse effect of leflunomide; it occurs in approximately 20% of patients but often improves with time or responds to antidiarrheal drugs. The dosage of leflunomide may have to be reduced if diarrhea is not relieved. Less common adverse effects include nausea or dyspepsia, rash, or hair loss. As seen in fewer than 10% of patients, the drug can cause abnormal liver function test results or decreased blood cell or platelet counts. Transient thrombocytopenia and leukopenia rarely occur. Leflunomide is contraindicated during pregnancy (FDA pregnancy category X).

Drug Interactions

Leflunomide can inhibit the biotransformation of certain NSAIDs (e.g., ibuprofen, diclofenac), causing serum levels to rise. In addition, leflunomide can intensify hepatic toxicity caused by other hepatotoxic drugs, such as MTX, and therefore should not be used in combination. Leflunomide increases the effects of warfarin.

Cholestyramine, tolbutamide, and rifampin interfere with the action of leflunomide: rifampin, an antitubercular drug, can elevate leflunomide levels by as much as 40%, whereas cholestyramine or activated charcoal can rapidly decrease leflunomide levels. There are no known food or herbal interactions.

Lab Considerations

Leflunomide may increase serum levels of AST and ALT.

Anakinra

Indications

Anakinra (Kineret) is the first member of a new class of DMARDs known as interleukin-1 (IL-1)–receptor blockers. It has been approved for patients with moderate to severe active RA who have not responded to therapy with one or more older DMARDs (e.g., MTX). In clinical trials, anakinra was more efficacious than placebo at reducing the signs and symptoms of RA and reducing disease progression. Responses to anakinra plus MTX were greater than those produced with MTX alone. The drug may be combined with most other DMARDs but not with the TNF blockers (e.g., etanercept, infliximab).

Pharmacodynamics

Anakinra is a recombinant, nonglycosylated form of the human IL-1 receptor antagonist (IL-1Ra), a naturally occurring compound that blocks access of IL-1 to its receptors. Blocking IL-1 receptors suppresses inflammation and joint destruction.

Pharmacokinetics

Anakinra yields peak plasma levels in 3 to 7 hours when given subcutaneously (see Table 17-10). The drug is eliminated in the urine primarily as metabolites. The terminal half-life in patients with normal renal function is 4 to 6 hours.

Adverse Effects and Contraindications

Although usually mild, injection site reactions (i.e., pruritus erythema, rash, pain) have caused patients to discontinue the drug. Headache, nausea, diarrhea, and abdominal pain are possible, but rare. Upper respiratory infections, sinusitis, influenza-like symptoms, and cellulitis have been reported.

Drug Interactions

Like the TNF blockers, anakinra increases the incidence of neutropenia, resulting in severe infections. For this reason, do not combine the drug with TNF blockers; do not give it to patients with active infection, and stop the drug if the patient develops an acute infection. Avoid live virus vaccines because of the risk of acquiring or transmitting infection following immunization (see Table 17-11).

Lab Considerations

Obtain neutrophil counts at the start of anakinra therapy, monthly for the first 3 months of treatment, and then every 3 months through the first year of treatment. Without neutrophil counts, neutropenia may go undetected.

Hydroxychloroquine

Indications

Hydroxychloroquine (Plaquenil; ♣ Plaquenil) is classified as an antiarthritic and antimalarial drug. Traditionally, the drug was reserved for patients who were unresponsive to NSAIDs. Today, the drug is prescribed earlier in the management of severe RA and SLE in an attempt to induce remission. Its use in the treatment of malaria is discussed in Chapter 30.

Pharmacodynamics

The precise antiinflammatory mechanism of action of hydroxychloroquine is unknown; it binds to DNA and inhibits phospholipid metabolism, rheumatoid factor, acute phase reactants, and many enzymes.

Pharmacokinetics

The drug is well absorbed and widely distributed following oral administration. Hydroxychloroquine has a delayed onset of action (see Table 17-10); full therapeutic effects take 3 to 6 months to be noted. Partial biotransformation takes place in the liver, with a portion of the drug eliminated unchanged in the urine. There is some indication that the drug enters breast milk.

Adverse Effects and Contraindications

There are many adverse effects of hydroxychloroquine, but the most common include nausea, vomiting, diarrhea, corneal changes, pruritus, and bleaching of the hair. The most serious adverse effects are irreversible retinal damage leading to blindness, agranulocytosis, and aplastic anemia. Visual loss is directly related to drug dosage. Because retinal damage is progressive and may continue even in the absence of continued drug use, discontinue therapy at the first sign of retinal changes. Fatalities have occurred with the ingestion of even three or four tablets of hydroxychloroquine, so the drug should be kept out of children's reach.

Drug Interactions

There is increased risk of hepatotoxicity when hydroxychloroquine is administered concurrently with other hepatotoxic drugs (see Table 17-11). It may increase the risk of hematologic toxicity when concurrently taken with penicillamine. The patient's risk for dermatitis increases when the drug is used with other drugs known to cause dermatologic toxicities. Serum digoxin levels may be increased, and urinary acidifiers increase the renal elimination of hydroxychloroquine.

Sulfasalazine

Indications

Sulfasalazine (Azulfidine; ♣ PMS Sulfasalazine, Salazopyrin, SAS-500) has been used for years to treat ulcerative colitis, and is now used in treating the synovitis of RA.

Pharmacodynamics

The drug is split by colonic bacteria into two component parts—sulfapyridine and 5-aminosalicylic acid. 5-Aminosalicylic acid is poorly absorbed, whereas sulfapyridine (the active component) is biotransformed in the liver by acetylation. The results are antiinflammatory and antibacterial effects.

Pharmacokinetics

The time of drug onset varies, with variable peak drug action (see Table 17-10). Fifteen percent of sulfasalazine is eliminated unchanged in the urine and the remainder as metabolites.

Adverse Effects and Contraindications

The frequent adverse effects of sulfasalazine are dose dependent and include nausea and diarrhea. Occasionally, hypersensitivity reactions, rash, urticaria, pruritus, fever, and anemia have occurred. Other adverse effects include tinnitus, dizziness, urinary and intestinal obstruction, stomatitis, thrombocytopenia, a yellow-orange skin discoloration, headache, and depression. Life-threatening adverse effects include Stevens-Johnson syndrome, hematologic toxicities, hepatotoxicity, and nephrotoxicity, although they rarely occur. Use caution when giving sulfasalazine to patients with renal failure and to women who are pregnant or lactating. It is specifically contraindicated for patients with allergies to sulfinpyrazone or other pyrazoles; peptic ulcer disease and symptoms of other GI inflammation; and blood dyscrasias.

▥ Drug Interactions

Drug interactions of sulfasalazine include decreased effectiveness with salicylates (see Table 17-11). Increased drug effects are noted with antidiabetic drugs (i.e., tolbutamide and glyburide) and warfarin. There is an increased risk of hepatotoxicity when sulfasalazine is used concurrently with acetaminophen.

▥ Lab Considerations

Urinary glucose tests using the Benedict method may be falsely elevated. Periodic monitoring of liver function and hematologic activity is necessary.

D-Penicillamine
▥ Indications

D-Penicillamine is an analogue of the amino acid cysteine and is a chelator of heavy metals. It is used in the management of progressive RA unresponsive to conventional therapy. It is also used for prophylaxis and treatment of copper deposition in Wilson's disease and in the management of recurrent cystine calculi. D-Penicillamine has been used as an adjunct in the treatment of heavy metal poisoning, although it has not been approved for such use by the FDA.

▥ Pharmacodynamics

There is conflicting data as to whether D-penicillamine prevents joint erosion in patients affected by RA. The antirheumatic effect of D-penicillamine is related to reducing the conversion of monocytes to macrophages. It reduces immunoglobulin synthesis by monocytes and lymphocytes, inhibits polymorphonuclear leukocytes, and inhibits T-cell function. It may protect tissues from damage by oxygen radicals.

▥ Pharmacokinetics

D-Penicillamine is well absorbed following oral administration, although its oral bioavailability is decreased in the presence of food, antacids, and iron supplements. The onset of antirheumatic effects occurs 1 to 3 months after administration, with duration of action from 1 to 3 months (see Table 17-10).

▥ Adverse Effects and Contraindications

The most common adverse effects of D-penicillamine include anorexia, oral ulcerations, epigastric pain, nausea, vomiting, diarrhea, and altered taste perception. Bone marrow depression, proteinuria, and a generalized pruritus have been noted. Polymyositis and a myasthenic syndrome are

life-threatening adverse effects. More than 25% of patients taking penicillamine will have to discontinue the drug because of adverse effects within the first 12 months of therapy.

▥ Drug Interactions

Drug interactions are relatively few but potentially serious. When used with antineoplastic or immunosuppressive drugs, penicillamine increases the risk of adverse hematologic effects (see Table 17-11). D-Penicillamine in combination with iron supplements or digoxin decreases drug absorption and serum digoxin levels. Daily requirements for pyridoxine (vitamin B_6) may be increased.

▥ Lab Considerations

Perform CBC with differential, platelet counts, and urinalysis (especially for protein and cells) every 2 weeks during the first 6 months of therapy and monthly thereafter, and after any increase in dosage. Monitor 24-hour urinary protein levels every 1 to 2 weeks in patients with moderate proteinuria. Perform liver function tests every 6 months during the first 18 months of therapy.

Azathioprine
▥ Indications

Azathioprine (Imuran) is a cytotoxic immunosuppressive drug used in the treatment of severe, active, erosive RA unresponsive to more conventional therapy. It is not recommended for initial DMARD therapy. The antiarrhythmic effects of azathioprine are equivalent to those of gold salts and penicillamine. In addition to its use in arthritis, azathioprine is used to prevent organ rejection in patients receiving kidney transplants.

▥ Pharmacodynamics

As a purine agonist, azathioprine antagonizes purine metabolism, with inhibition of DNA and RNA synthesis. The benefits result from suppression of cell-mediated immunity and altered antibody formation.

▥ Pharmacokinetics

Azathioprine is readily absorbed following oral administration. The onset of antiinflammatory effects occurs in 6 to 8 weeks, with peak action noted in 4 months (see Table 17-10). The duration of antiinflammatory action is unknown. Azathioprine is biotransformed to the active metabolite mercaptopurine.

▥ Adverse Effects and Contraindications

When used in dosages appropriate to the management of immune-based inflammatory diseases, the most common adverse effects of azathioprine are fever, chills, anorexia, nausea, vomiting, and hepatotoxicity. Leukopenia, anemia, pancytopenia, and thrombocytopenia have also been noted. Serum sickness can be life threatening. Azathioprine is teratogenic; do not use it during pregnancy. The drug may pose a small risk of malignancy.

▥ Drug Interactions

Drug interactions include additive myelosuppression with antineoplastics, cyclosporin, and myelosuppressants (see

Table 17-11). Allopurinol inhibits the biotransformation of azathioprine, thus increasing the risk of toxicity. Reduce the dosage of azathioprine by 25% to 33% with concurrent use of allopurinol. Like other DMARDs, azathioprine decreases the antibody response to live virus vaccines and increases the risk of adverse effects.

ⅲ Lab Considerations

Baseline and ongoing monitoring should include a CBC with differential, platelet count, and liver function tests for the first several months of therapy, then biweekly for the second and third months. If lab values remain stable, monitoring frequency can be decreased to monthly. Azathioprine decreases serum and urine uric acid, and plasma albumin levels. A leukocyte count lower than 3000/mm^3 or a platelet count below 100,000/mm^3 may warrant a reduction in dosage or a temporary interruption in therapy. Decreased hemoglobin levels may suggest bone marrow suppression. Although hepatotoxicity is rare when azathioprine is used to treat arthritis, elevations in alkaline phosphatase, bilirubin, AST, ALT, and amylase concentrations may occur. Elevated liver function test values are reversible on discontinuation of azathioprine.

Gold Salts
ⅲ Indications

Gold salts administered by intramuscular (IM) route were, until the 1990s, the most often used DMARDs. Gold compounds are rarely used now because of their adverse effects and very slow onset of action. Gold salts relieve pain and stiffness associated with RA and, for some patients, may arrest the progression of joint degeneration; however, they do not reverse damage that has already occurred. Symptomatic improvement is seen in 60% to 70% of patients, and about 15% go into remission.

Aurothioglucose (Solfanol) is most effective early in the course of RA in both adults and children. Gold sodium thiomalate is effective in the treatment of RA when given by IM route. Oral gold-based therapies have not been shown to be as effective as injection-based therapy.

Gold sodium thiomalate (Myochrysine) is used in initial and maintenance treatment of adult RA. Auranofin (Ridaura) has been used also as an alternative or adjunct to corticosteroids in treating pemphigus and systemic lupus, and for patients with psoriatic arthritis who do not tolerate or respond to NSAIDs; however, gold compounds have not been approved for use in these conditions by the FDA.

ⅲ Pharmacodynamics

The precise mechanism of action of gold salts is still unknown, but they appear to decrease concentrations of rheumatoid factor and immunoglobulins, which are the primary elements causing joint damage. Suppression of T-lymphocyte activity by gold compounds due to inhibition of adenylyl cyclase may also play a role. It is also thought that gold salts are taken up by macrophages, followed by inhibition of phagocytosis and activity of lysosomal enzymes. The dominant effect is suppression of the synovitis in active rheumatoid disease.

ⅲ Pharmacokinetics

Orally administered auranofin is 20% to 25% absorbed from the GI tract. Aurothioglucose and gold sodium thiomalate are rapidly absorbed following IM injection. The onset of antiinflammatory drug action takes 6 to 8 weeks for IM formulations, and 3 to 6 months for orally administered drugs. Gold salts are widely distributed, concentrating in arthritic joints more than in uninvolved joints. They are also distributed in breast milk. Sixty percent to 90% of gold salts are eliminated by the kidneys for up to 15 months. Up to 40% is eliminated in the feces. The half-life of gold salts in the blood is 3 to 26 days; however, in tissues, the half-life ranges from 40 to 128 days (see Table 17-10).

ⅲ Adverse Effects and Contraindications

Gold has several toxicities that limit its use. Between 15% and 20% of patients must discontinue gold salt treatment because of adverse effects. The most common adverse effects of gold salts are a metallic taste, stomatitis, and diarrhea accompanied by abdominal pain and cramping. Oral formulations cause less mucocutaneous and renal toxicity than IM formulations. Some patients develop a rash, dermatitis, or dizziness. Although thrombocytopenia is a possible adverse effect, aplastic anemia and agranulocytosis are more important concerns. Interstitial pneumonitis, ulcerative colitis, fibrosis, and acute nephrotic syndrome are reported in patients taking aurothioglucose. Renal toxicity, manifested as proteinuria, occurs frequently. Adverse effects also have been reported that affect the dermatologic, GI, hematologic, immunologic, musculoskeletal, neurologic, ophthalmic, renal, reproductive, and respiratory systems.

Toxicity and overdose become evident as a rapid decrease in hemoglobin, a white blood cell count below 4000/mm^3, eosinophil count above 5%, granulocyte counts lower than 1500/mm^3, or a platelet count under 100,000 to 150,000/mm^3.

ⅲ Drug Interactions

Additive bone marrow toxicity may develop when gold salts are used in conjunction with other myelosuppressive drugs (e.g., antineoplastics). Combined use of gold salts with radiation therapy also contributes to myelosuppression (see Table 17-11).

Gold salts are contraindicated for use in patients with hypersensitivity to gold, in patients with severe hepatic or renal dysfunction, and in patients who have a history of heavy metal intoxication. Cautious use of gold salts is warranted in patients with a history of colitis, exfoliative dermatitis, uncontrolled diabetes mellitus, tuberculosis, heart failure, systemic lupus erythematosus, and recent radiation therapy. Do not use gold salts in debilitated patients or in women who are pregnant or lactating.

ⅲ Lab Considerations

Serum levels are of no value in predicting therapeutic response to gold salts. A decrease in circulating immune complexes may indicate a favorable response in patients with RA. Frequent laboratory testing and close observation of the patient is required to monitor for gold toxicity. Monitor hematologic status and liver and kidney function before and periodically throughout therapy with gold salts. Obtain a urinalysis for protein before each injection. Because these drugs may cause thrombocytopenia, leukopenias, and anemia, obtain a CBC and platelet values every 2 to 4 weeks.

CLINICAL REASONING

Treatment Objectives

Recent emphasis has been placed on aggressive treatment early in the disease course of RA. The primary objective of DMARD therapy is to improve and maintain functional status, slow the degeneration of tissues, and thereby improve quality of life and the patient's ability to carry out activities of daily living. Provide an early referral to a rheumatologist. The rheumatologist should coordinate care with other health care professionals including nurses, counselors, and occupational and physical therapists.

Treatment Options

Rest, occupational and physical therapy, use of assistive devices, weight reduction, and surgery are the most useful types of non–drug therapies for RA.

▥ Patient Variables

Of patients with rheumatic disorders, 70% to 80% follow a cyclic course of remissions and exacerbations. About 10% of patients have one to two acute exacerbations and then achieve a long-lasting remission for several years. Another 3% to 10% of patients have progressively inflammatory, painful disorders with no remission. These persons generally respond poorly to drug treatment. During remission, use the lowest dosage of an NSAID that is effective to maintain control. Thus it is important to know the onset time of antiinflammatory drug action. About 10% of RA patients will not respond to any NSAID.

▥ Drug Variables

An effective DMARD should control the active synovitis and constitutional features of RA and prevent joint erosions and damage. DMARDs cannot heal erosions or reverse joint deformities. The American College of Rheumatology (ACR) recommends early diagnosis and treatment of RA, because studies show that early use of DMARDs slows joint damage. DMARDs should be prescribed when the diagnosis is made—before there is radiographic evidence of erosive changes. The ACR recommends that DMARD use start within 3 months of diagnosis for all patients who have ongoing joint pain, morning stiffness, or other signs of active RA, regardless of possible treatment with NSAIDs. DMARDs may retard the progression of arthritis but are more toxic than NSAIDs and require more vigorous monitoring.

Approximately 70% of rheumatologists use three-drug combinations to induce remission of rheumatoid arthritis. Despite the availability of newer DMARDs, the most common combination is MTX, sulfasalazine, and hydroxychloroquine. Many rheumatologists consider MTX the first-line drug among the DMARDs since it interferes with DNA synthesis, which prevents cell replication, and suppresses the immune reaction in the body. MTX is the fastest acting of the DMARDs, with therapeutic effects seen as early as 3 to 6 weeks. However, experience with MTX remains relatively limited, and long-term risk of toxicity is not yet clear. In the past, liver biopsy has been recommended to monitor the presence and extent of hepatotoxicity. The question as to when, or if, to biopsy the liver of patients on long-term MTX therapy remains controversial. The decision to biopsy should be made on an individual basis and determined by previous hepatic disease, length of time on and dosage of MTX, and other risk factors. Many health care providers recommend a liver biopsy after a cumulative MTX dose of 1.5 to 2 grams, or once every 2 to 3 years. Table 17-12 provides an overview of relative GI, renal, and hepatic toxicity for DMARDs.

Sulfasalazine may be an initial choice more often in patients with reactive arthritis. Sulfasalazine has similar efficacy to gold and penicillamine, although comparative trials have not been sufficient to demonstrate differences. It is thought to retard progression of joint deterioration and may be superior to hydroxychloroquine in this regard. It may have comparable efficacy to parenteral gold salts but with less toxicity. Adverse GI effects can be minimized by using enteric-coated formulations and by dividing the daily dosage. Some health care providers note that sulfasalazine is as effective as IM gold salts and causes less toxicity. Approximately 50% of patients on sulfasalazine develop adverse effects, and in the majority of cases, these occur within the first 4 months of therapy.

According to the ACR, when the highest dosage of one DMARD does not work within 3 months, it should either be replaced by, or used in combination with, a new DMARD. DMARD selection will depend on the stage of disease,

TABLE 17-12 Relative Potential for DMARD-Induced Toxicities

Selected DMARDs	GI Distress	Nephrotoxicity	Hepatotoxicity
anakinra	+	−	−
auranofin	+++	+	+
aurothioglucose	+	++	+
azathioprine	++	0	++
cyclophosphamide	++	0	0
gold sodium thiomalate	+	++	+
hydroxychloroquine	++	0	0
infliximab	++	−	−
leflunomide	++	−	−
methotrexate	+++	0	++
D-penicillamine	++	++	+
sulfasalazine	++	++	++

+++, Considered the most toxic, often requires withdrawal of the drug; +, considered the least toxic, usually no change in drug therapy required; 0, no toxicity documented.
DMARD, Disease-modifying antirheumatic drug; *GI*, gastrointestinal.

comorbid conditions, and the patient's response to previous therapies. Some patients need more than one DMARD to control their arthritis. For other patients, even a combination of DMARDs will not prevent the joint damage that ultimately requires surgery. The ACR also recommends that rheumatologists be consulted when combination therapy is being considered or whenever a primary care provider is unsure about any aspect of arthritis diagnosis or treatment.

As noted, NSAIDs are the initial drugs of choice. Aspirin or another salicylate is often chosen first because of reduced cost. If the adverse effects of salicylates are intolerable, one of the newer, nonacetylated salicylate NSAIDs may be chosen. If rheumatic symptoms cannot be controlled with an NSAID, a DMARD is warranted. Because therapeutic effects are delayed, continue therapy with an NSAID until the DMARD has produced an adequate response. Corticosteroids are commonly used as bridge therapy until DMARDs begin to take effect; they rapidly relieve symptoms but do not retard the progression of RA. Because of the toxicity, corticosteroids (Chapter 56) are usually reserved for short-term therapy.

Patient Education

To fully participate in treatment of RA, the patient must know the nature and time course of expected beneficial drug effects. Teach patients who are self-administering their DMARD therapy of the importance of blood work so as to monitor hematologic, renal, and liver function tests as well as treatment effectiveness. With this information, the patient can help monitor and evaluate treatment outcomes.

As with all other drugs, inform patients of the signs and symptoms of allergic and other adverse drug reactions and advise them of appropriate actions to take should these occur. Some DMARDs are formulated as injectables. Instruct patients as to the importance of proper storage and disposal of the drug container and the syringe and needle.

Evaluation

The primary outcome of DMARD therapy is evaluated as a decrease in symptoms, an improvement and maintenance of functional status, and a slowing of tissue degeneration. An improvement in the patient's quality of life and ability to carry out activities of daily living indicates treatment goals are met.

GOUT

EPIDEMIOLOGY AND ETIOLOGY

Gout is one of the oldest known diseases and affects people of all ages. It was mentioned in the medical literature as early as 2000 years ago. Gout, or gouty arthritis, is a systemic disorder whereby urate crystals (the end product of purine metabolism) deposit in joints and other body tissues, resulting in inflammation. Primary gout, the most common, is inherited as an X-linked trait, meaning that males are affected through female carriers. Approximately 5 million people in the United States have gout, with about 25% having a family history of gout. Of patients with gout, 85% to 90% are middle-aged and older men, and postmenopausal women. The peak onset of gout is between the ages of 30 and 40 years.

Secondary gout is caused by another disease or condition, or by drugs, that produce elevated serum uric acid levels

(Box 17-4). Renal insufficiency, certain antineoplastic drugs, and diuretics reduce elimination of uric acid, whereas multiple myeloma and some other cancers cause an increase in uric acid production. The end result is an imbalance between production and elimination that leads to uric acid accumulation. Typically, uric acid concentrations above 7 mg/dL are associated with an increased risk of gout. Treatment goals should be a target 6 mg/dL or below.

PATHOPHYSIOLOGY

There are four stages of primary gout: an asymptomatic hyperuricemia, acute gout, intercritical gout, and chronic gout. In *asymptomatic hyperuricemia,* there are no obvious signs and symptoms, thus the patient is usually unaware of the elevated serum uric acid levels.

Acute gout occurs as a result of an inflammatory response to deposits of sodium urate crystals in the synovium and other body tissues. There is local infiltration of tissues by granulocytes, which phagocytize urate crystals. The lactate production is high in synovial fluids, thus favoring a local decrease in pH that fosters further deposition of urate crystals. Although PGs may be implicated in the pain and inflammation of gout and gouty arthritis, there is no evidence that they contribute to its pathogenesis.

With an acute attack the patient has excruciating pain and inflammation in one or more small joints. Of all patients with gout, 75% have inflammation of the metatarsophalangeal joint of the great toe as an initial manifestation.

BOX 17-4

Drugs and Diseases Contributing to Gout

- aspirin
- bumetanide (Bumex, Edecrin)
- chlorothiazide (Diuril)
- chlorthalidone (Hygroton)
- cyclosporine (Sandimmune, Neoral)
- ethacrynic acid
- furosemide (Lasix)
- hydrochlorothiazide (HydroDiuril, Oretic)
- levodopa
- metolazone (Mykrox, Zaroxolyn)
- nicotinic acid (Niacin)
- pyrazinamide (PZA)
- torsemide (Demadex)
- Alcoholism
- Anemia
- Diabetes
- Down syndrome
- Heart failure
- Immobility due to bed rest
- Kidney dysfunction
- Leukemia, lymphoma
- Lung cancer, smoking
- Obesity
- Psoriasis
- Severe illness or injury
- Starvation
- Thyroid disorders
- Untreated high blood pressure

Intercritical gout takes months or years to develop. The term is used to describe the periods between attacks. After the first attack, patients usually experience a complete remission of symptoms. If the gout is not treated, however, symptoms almost always recur. Recurrence has been reported at 62% within a year, 78% within 2 years, and 93% within 10 years.

Chronic gout appears after repeated bouts of acute gout. Deposits of urate crystals develop within major organ systems, particularly the kidneys, and under the skin. Tophi, the chalky deposits of urate, typically form around the joints in cartilage and bone, and in bursae, subcutaneous tissues, and the external ear (particularly the pinna). Kidney stones of urate crystals are more common in patients with chronic gout.

PHARMACOTHERAPEUTIC OPTIONS

Antigout Drugs

- allopurinol (Lopurin, Zyloprim)
- colchicine (Colsalid); ✤ Novo-Colchicine

▌ Indications

Allopurinol is effective for the treatment of both primary hyperuricemia and secondary gout related to hematologic disorders or antineoplastic therapy. It is generally used in severe chronic forms of gout characterized by hyperuricemia not readily controlled with uricosuric drugs, tophaceous deposits, gouty nephropathy, renal urate stones, and impaired renal function.

Colchicine is a unique antiinflammatory drug effective only against gouty arthritis. It provides dramatic relief from acute gout and is effective for prophylaxis, especially when there are frequent attacks. It also been used in the treatment of skin disorders including psoriasis and Behçet's syndrome (a multisystem illness characterized by lesions of the oral mucosa, the genitalia, the eyes, and the skin). It has been approved as an orphan drug to arrest the progressive neurologic disability caused by multiple sclerosis.

▌ Pharmacodynamics

An *antigout* drug acts to reduce the inflammatory process or to prevent the synthesis of uric acid. Allopurinol inhibits the terminal stages of uric acid synthesis. Both allopurinol and its primary metabolite, alloxanthine, are inhibitors of xanthine oxidase. Inhibition of this enzyme accounts for the major drug effects of allopurinol, a reduction of urates.

In contrast to allopurinol, colchicine is a particularly effective antigout drug, probably because of its effect on the mobility of granulocytes. It binds to microtubular proteins to interfere with function of mitotic spindles, and inhibits the migration of granulocytes to the inflamed area. The inhibition reduces the release of lactic acid and proinflammatory enzymes during phagocytosis. In other words, it breaks the cycle leading to inflammation. Colchicine also inhibits the release of histamine from mast cells and the secretion of insulin from beta cells of the pancreas.

▌ Pharmacokinetics

Antigout drugs have paradoxical effects on uric acid levels. Depending on the dosage, they can either decrease or increase elimination of uric acid. Decreased elimination ordinarily occurs with low dosages, whereas increased elimination is observed at higher dosages.

Allopurinol is rapidly absorbed following oral administration, with peak plasma concentrations reached in 30 to 60 minutes (Table 17-13). Neither allopurinol nor its metabolite plasma concentrations correlate well with therapeutic or toxic effects.

Colchicine is absorbed from the GI tract, undergoing enterohepatic recirculation where reabsorption may occur. It is distributed to and concentrates in white blood cells. Biotransformation of colchicine takes place in the liver, with elimination in the feces. Small amounts of colchicine are eliminated in the urine.

▌ Adverse Effects and Contraindications

Allopurinol's most common adverse effect, hypersensitivity, can occur after months or years of use. Pruritus or an erythematous or maculopapular eruption characterizes the reaction. Occasionally, the lesions are exfoliative, urticarial, or purpuric. Fever, malaise, and muscle aches are present. Transient leukopenia or leukocytosis and eosinophilia are rare but may necessitate stopping the drug. Other undesirable adverse effects include headache, drowsiness, nausea and vomiting, vertigo, diarrhea, and GI upset, but their appearance usually does not necessitate stopping treatment. Allopurinol use is contraindicated in patients who have had serious

PHARMACOKINETICS
TABLE 17-13 Gout Drugs

Drug	Route	Onset	Peak	Duration	PB (%)	t₁/₂
ANTIGOUT DRUGS						
allopurinol	PO	30–60 min; 24–48 hr*	1.5–4.5 hr; 1–3 wk†	18–30 hr; 1–2 wk‡	UA	1–2 hr; 18–30 hr§
colchicine	PO	20 min	0.5–2 hr	9 days	UA	20 min; 60 hr‖
URICOSURIC DRUGS						
probenecid	PO	30 min	2–4 hr	5–8 hr	75	4–9 hr
sulfinpyrazone	PO	30 min	1–2 hr	4–6 hr	98–99	2.2–3 hr

*Onset times of allopurinol in the blood and therapeutic onset, respectively.
†Peak blood levels and therapeutic effects of allopurinol.
‡Allopurinol's duration of action with effects lasting 1–2 weeks.
§Allopurinol's half-life and half-life of metabolites, respectively.
‖Half-life of colchicine in plasma and in white blood cells, respectively.
PO, By mouth; *PB*, protein binding; *t₁/₂*, elimination half-life; *UA*, unavailable.

adverse reactions, nursing mothers, and children, except those who have a malignancy or certain inborn errors of purine metabolism.

Colchicine's most common adverse effect reflects drug action on rapidly proliferating epithelial cells of the GI tract, especially in the jejunum. Nausea, vomiting, diarrhea, and abdominal pain are common and the earliest signs of colchicine overdose. There is a latent period of several hours or more between drug administration and onset of symptoms. This interval is not altered by dose or route of administration. For this reason and because of individual variation, adverse effects may be unavoidable during the initial course of therapy. However, if the patient remains relatively consistent in his or her response to the drug, toxicity can be minimized or avoided during subsequent courses of therapy. The adverse GI effects may be almost completely avoided if colchicine is given by IV route.

Colchicine produces a temporary leukopenia that is soon replaced by leukocytosis. Long-term use of colchicine increases the risk of agranulocytosis, aplastic anemia, myopathy, and alopecia. Azoospermia has also been noted. Use of the drug is contraindicated in patients who have severe GI disorders or creatinine clearance rates below 10 mL/min. Use it with caution in older adults and in patients who have creatinine clearance rates of 10 to 50 mL/min. Safe use during pregnancy and lactation and in children has not been established.

▥ Drug Interactions

Allopurinol interferes with hepatic inactivation of other drugs including oral anticoagulants (Table 17-14). It is thought there is an increased risk of skin rash with concurrent administration of ampicillin. Hypersensitivity reactions have been reported in patients with compromised renal function who receive allopurinol and thiazide diuretics. Concurrent use of allopurinol and theophylline preparations leads to an increased concentration of theophylline's active metabolites. In contrast, colchicine has few drug interactions, although it may cause a reversible malabsorption of vitamin B_{12}.

▥ Dosage Regimen

A slow upward titration of allopurinol dosage is recommended to prevent or minimize the risk of sudden elimination of large amounts of uric acid through the kidneys (Table 17-15).

Gout prophylaxis with colchicine depends on the frequency and severity of attacks. Give colchicine 3 days before and 3 days after surgery in patients with gout. This approach greatly reduces the very high incidence of acute attacks precipitated by operative procedures. Colchicine may be used intermittently with 3 days between courses to decrease the risk of toxicity.

▥ Lab Considerations

Serum uric acid levels usually decrease 2 to 3 days after the start of allopurinol therapy. Monitor blood glucose levels in patients receiving antidiabetic drugs, because it may cause hypoglycemia secondary to the decrease in insulin production. Perform hematologic, renal, and liver function testing before and periodically throughout therapy, especially during the first few months. Allopurinol can cause elevations in alkaline phosphatase, bilirubin, AST, and ALT levels. A decreased CBC and platelet level may suggest bone marrow depression. Elevated blood urea nitrogen (BUN), creatinine, and creatinine clearance levels suggest nephrotoxicity. These values are usually reversed by stopping therapy. Colchicine interferes with the results of urinary 17-hydroxycorticosteroid concentrations.

Uricosuric Drugs

◆ probenecid (Benemid, Probalan)
◆ sulfinpyrazone (Anturane); ✦ Anturan, Apo-Sulfinpyrazone, Novo-Pyrazone

▥ Indications

The use of probenecid and sulfinpyrazone for the mobilization of uric acid in chronic gout is well established. Probenecid was developed in response to a specific need. When penicillin was first developed, it was in short supply, and the rapid renal elimination of the antibiotic thus had a practical significance. Researchers subsequently found an organic acid that depresses tubular secretion of penicillin. The oral administration of probenecid together with penicillin G results in higher, more prolonged serum concentrations of the antibiotic than when penicillin is given alone. The increase in plasma concentration is at least twofold and sometimes much greater.

▥ Pharmacodynamics

In contrast to antigout drugs, *uricosuric* drugs increase the rate of uric acid secretion, thus reducing plasma uric acid

DRUG INTERACTIONS
TABLE **17-14 Gout Drugs**

Drugs	Interactive Drugs	Interaction
ANTIGOUT DRUGS		
allopurinol	theophylline	Increases concentrations of theophylline's metabolites
	Thiazide diuretics	Hypersensitivity reactions in patients with compromised renal function
	Oral anticoagulants	Increases effects of interactive drug
colchicine	Vitamin B_{12}	Reversible malabsorption of interactive drug
URICOSURIC DRUGS		
probenecid	Sulfonamides	Increases concentration of sulfonamide in serum
sulfinpyrazone	probenecid	Additive effects to that of interacting drug
	Salicylates	Antagonizes effects of salicylates
	Oral hypoglycemics	Inhibits metabolism of oral hypoglycemic

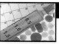

DOSAGE

TABLE 17-15 Regimen of Gout Drugs

Drug	Uses	Dosage	Implications
ANTIGOUT DRUGS			
allopurinol	Prophylaxis for gouty arthritis	*Adult:* 100 mg PO daily initially; increase weekly based on serum uric acid level; not to exceed 800 mg/day; doses over 300 mg/day should be given in divided doses. Maintenance: 100–200 mg PO 2–3 times daily; doses less than 300 mg can be given as single daily dose.	Take with milk or meals. Alkaline ash diet may be ordered. Large doses of alcohol decrease drug's effectiveness.
colchicine	Acute gouty arthritis	*Adult:* 0.5–1.2 mg PO, then 0.5–0.6 mg every 1–2 hr –or– 1–1.2 mg every 2 hr until relief, diarrhea, or total cumulative dose of 6 mg is reached *Prophylaxis:* 0.5–0.6 mg PO daily; may be used 3 times daily or 1–4 times weekly –or– 2 mg IV initially, then 0.5 mg every 6 hr –or– 1 mg every 6 hr until relief or cumulative dose of 4 mg is reached	If surgery is planned, give 3 times daily for the 3 days before the procedure and the 3 days after the procedure. Other regimens may use lower doses.
URICOSURIC DRUGS			
probenecid	Prophylaxis for recurrent gouty arthritis	*Adult:* 250 mg PO twice daily for 1 wk; increase to 500 mg twice daily; then may increase by 500 mg/day every 4 wk based on response; not to exceed 3 grams/day *Child ages 2–14 yr:* Initially 25 mg/kg, then 10 mg/kg	Not used to treat gouty arthritis but rather for prevention. In acute attack, continue at full dosage along with colchicine or NSAID.
sulfinpyrazone	Chronic gout	*Adult:* 100–200 mg PO twice daily; may increase to 800 mg/day	Regulate dose by checking serum uric acid levels.

IV, Intravenous (route); *NSAID,* nonsteroidal antiinflammatory drug; *PO,* by mouth.

concentrations. Probenecid and sulfinpyrazone inhibit the tubular reabsorption of urate, thereby increasing urinary elimination of uric acid, decreasing serum uric acid levels, and retarding urate deposition. In addition, probenecid inhibits tubular reabsorption of most penicillins and cephalosporins. Sulfinpyrazone also inhibits PG synthesis, which prevents platelet aggregation, but it lacks analgesic and antiinflammatory activity.

▌ Pharmacokinetics

Probenecid is a highly soluble benzoic acid derivative that is completely absorbed after oral administration. Biotransformation takes place in the liver, with less than 10% of the drug eliminated unchanged in the urine (see Table 17-13). Like probenecid, sulfinpyrazone is well absorbed following oral administration.

▌ Adverse Effects and Contraindications

Probenecid is well tolerated by most patients. Some degree of GI irritation is noted in a small percentage of patients. Serious hypersensitivity reactions are rare. Nephrotic syndrome has been reported. A large overdose of probenecid results in CNS stimulation, seizures, and death from respiratory failure.

GI irritation occurs in about 10% to 15% of patients receiving sulfinpyrazone. Hypersensitivity reactions do occur, usually consisting of a rash with fever, but they occur less frequently than with probenecid. There is inhibition of hematopoiesis. Sulfinpyrazone is contraindicated in patients with allergies to phenylbutazone or other pyrazoles, and in patients with blood dyscrasias or a history of peptic ulcer disease. Sulfinpyrazone is used with caution in patients with renal failure or in women who are pregnant or lactating.

▌ Drug Interactions

Probenecid increases the concentration of sulfonamide in the blood, to some degree. The uricosuric action of sulfinpyrazone is additive to that of probenecid but is mutually antagonistic to that of salicylates (see Table 17-14).

▌ Dosage Regimen

The dosage of probenecid depends on the objectives of therapy. In the treatment of chronic gout, 250 mg are given twice daily for 1 week, after which 500 mg are given twice daily (see Table 17-15).

Sulfinpyrazone is given in two divided doses for a daily total of 200 to 400 mg. The dosage can be gradually increased to a maintenance dosage of 400 mg/day over a period of 1 week, if needed. The dosage is regulated by monitoring serum uric acid concentrations.

▌ Lab Considerations

Probenecid can cause false-positive results in copper sulfate urine glucose tests (e.g., Clinitest). Use glucose oxidase methods (e.g., Keto-Diastix, Tes-Tape) to monitor urine glucose. Monitor CBC, serum uric acid levels, and renal function before and routinely throughout long-term therapy. There are no significant laboratory considerations for sulfinpyrazone.

Newer Drugs for Gout

Febuxostat (TMX-67) is the first new drug for gout in 40 years. It offers an alternative to allopurinol in the management of gout symptoms, and appears to be twice as effective as allopurinol in lowering uric acid concentrations. This new drug has a different chemical structure; it works like allopurinol but is a non–purine selective inhibitor of xanthine oxidase.

PEG-uricase is a poly (ethylene glycol) conjugate of recombinant porcine uricase (urate oxidase) for the treatment of patients with severe gout or chemotherapy-induced hyperuricemia for whom conventional therapy is contraindicated or has been ineffective. The manufacturer initiated phase 3 clinical testing during the first quarter of 2006.

CENTRAL NERVOUS

CLINICAL REASONING

Treatment Objectives

The treatment objectives for gout include decreasing pain and inflammation associated with acute attacks and preventing recurrent attacks. For control of hyperuricemia, the goal is to reduce plasma uric acid concentrations to less than 6 mg/dL or lower, although uricosuric or allopurinol drug therapy is usually not started during an acute attack since it can precipitate an ongoing attack. It is important to note that an acute attack of gout is often self-limiting; however, short-course therapy has been demonstrated to be beneficial in relieving symptoms.

Treatment Options

▥ Patient Variables

It is well known that alcohol intake and starvation diets contribute to gout attacks. Because the pKa of uric acid is 5.6 and the solubility of the nonionized form is very low, maintaining a large output of alkaline urine minimizes intrarenal deposition. This precaution is essential during the early weeks of treatment, when uric acid elimination is large, especially in patients with a history of renal disease associated with urate stones or gravel.

In patients who do not respond to uricosuric drugs because of impaired renal function, allopurinol is especially helpful. For patients with gouty nephropathy, allopurinol offers an additional advantage over uricosuric drugs in that their daily elimination of uric acid is reduced rather than increased. Neither the antigout drugs nor allopurinol alter the course of the disease or supplant the use of colchicine and NSAIDs in its management.

▥ Drug Variables

Acute Gout. Several strategies are used to counter acute gout attacks, although drug therapy is the primary modality. Colchicine or corticosteroids are effective for symptoms. However, the initial drug of choice is the NSAID indomethacin, an acetic acid derivative. Indomethacin is usually better tolerated than colchicine. Patients benefit more from indomethacin than from colchicine, including those for whom therapy was delayed several days after onset of an acute attack. This is true even though colchicine has been the initial drug of choice in the past. Other NSAIDs have also been used (e.g., ibuprofen, naproxen, ketorolac) with apparently similar efficacy, but experience is much less extensive to date. The other NSAIDs can be used if the patient cannot tolerate indomethacin.

Use a full dosage of indomethacin (50 mg 3 times daily) until a significant response occurs, usually in 2 to 3 days. The dosage can then be reduced to 25 mg 3 times daily, with therapy continued for an additional 7 to 10 days until the attack has fully resolved. If there has been no response after 24 hours of treatment, try an alternative drug.

Corticosteroids (e.g., prednisone) are used when indomethacin or other NSAIDs are not effective, or when the patient is intolerant. They are the initial drug of choice in patients with hypersensitivity to aspirin or for the patient with renal failure. Prednisone is given in full dosage (for 3 to 4 days) and then tapered by 5 mg/day over the next week. Consider intraarticular injections of corticosteroids if only the knee or ankles are affected.

Use colchicine for patients who have a history of heart failure, active peptic ulcer disease, or severe hypertension. Pain, swelling, and redness usually abate within 12 hours and are completely gone in 48 to 72 hours. Fewer than 5% of patients fail to obtain relief with colchicine even when it is given within the first hours of an attack. The disadvantage to colchicine is a high incidence (80% to 100%) of diarrhea. If colchicine is used, give it for 1 day only, and then start again on day 7 if prophylaxis is required. This is because colchicine is eliminated slowly, its toxicity is dose related, and it has a long duration of action.

Chronic Gout. Allopurinol therapy is a rational approach for chronic gout because most patients are underexcreters of uric acid. Overproduction of uric acid is a contributing factor in some patients and is characteristic of many cases of secondary hyperuricemia. In two thirds of patients, probenecid and sulfinpyrazone cause uric acid to be eliminated at a rate exceeding that of formation. Although IV administration of these drugs can cause a fivefold to sevenfold increase in urate excretion, regular use of an oral drug for patients with tophaceous gout approximately doubles the daily elimination of urates. In such patients, new tophi formation is prevented, and there is a gradual reduction and even disappearance of old tophi.

Indeed, acute attacks may increase in frequency or severity during early months of therapy, when urate is being mobilized from affected joints. Therefore, therapy with uricosuric drugs should not be initiated during an acute attack but may be continued if already started.

Patient Education

Increasing fluid intake is one of the best measures to prevent urate stone formation. It also helps dilute the urine and prevent formation of sediment. Instruct patients taking uricosuric drugs to maintain oral intake sufficient to ensure a daily urinary output of at least 2 L. This may require 3000 mL of fluid intake per day. Instruct patients to limit their intake of alcohol.

Uric acid is less likely to form stones in alkaline urine. Advise the patient to increase the intake of alkaline ash foods such as citrus juices and fresh fruits (except cranberries, plums, and prunes), milk, buttermilk, cream, almonds, chestnuts, and coconuts, and all vegetables (except lentils and corn). (For more information, see the Evolve Resources Bonus Content "Alkaline Ash and Acid Ash Foods" found at http://evolve.elsevier.com/Gutierrez/pharmacotherapeutics.) For this reason, furthermore, sodium bicarbonate, potassium citrate, or other alkalinizing drugs may be prescribed concurrently with probenecid.

Whether or not dietary restriction of purines should be recommended is controversial. Some health care providers advocate a strict low-purine diet; others believe limiting protein foods is sufficient. Still others do not believe that dietary restrictions affect treatment outcomes. However, if purine restriction is recommended, instruct the patient to avoid organ meats, roe, sardines, scallops, anchovies, broth and consommé, and mincemeat.

Advise the patient to avoid alcohol and all forms of aspirin and diuretics. Teach patients that excessive physical or emotional stressors also exacerbate the disease, and emphasize stress management techniques.

Evaluation

Treatment effectiveness is demonstrated by a decrease in the pain and swelling of affected joints, a decrease in serum uric acid levels, resolution of tophi, and a subsequent decrease in the frequency of attacks. Several months of continuous therapy may be required before maximum benefits are apparent.

KEY POINTS

- Inflammation is a nonspecific response occurring with tissue injury. Chemical mediators cause vasodilation, increased capillary permeability, chemotaxis of white blood cells, and fever.

- Treatment options for the short-term management of fever, mild to moderate pain, and inflammatory disorders in adults include NSAIDs. Acetaminophen acts to reduce fever and mild to moderate pain. NSAIDs are much safer than glucocorticoids and most DMARDs.

- NSAIDs are not used in children and adolescents who have viral infections or chicken pox, owing to the risk of Reye's syndrome.

- NSAIDs act quickly to reduce symptoms but do not prevent tissue injury and do not delay progression of chronic inflammatory conditions.

- Dosages of NSAIDs used for RA are much higher than the doses used to relieve pain or fever.

- DMARDs are used in progressive rheumatoid disorders unresponsive to conventional therapies to delay disease progression and reduce joint destruction; onset of effects is delayed.

- NSAIDs and DMARDs are contraindicated or should be used with caution in patients with hypersensitivity, extensive heart disease, a history of peptic ulcer disease, liver disease, or renal insufficiency.

- Acetaminophen should be avoided or used with caution in patients with hepatic disease.

- Acute gout occurs as a result of an inflammatory reaction to deposits of sodium urate crystals, the end product of purine metabolism, in the synovium and other body tissues.

- Chronic gout appears after repeated bouts of acute gout with deposits of urate crystals developing within major organ systems and under the skin.

- Treatment options for gout include antigout drugs such as allopurinol and colchicine, uricosuric drugs such as probenecid and sulfinpyrazone, and the NSAID indomethacin.

- Increasing fluid intake prevents urate stone formation for patients with gout, and uric acid is less likely to form stones in alkaline urine.

- Treatment effectiveness can be demonstrated by a decrease in the pain and swelling of affected joints, a decrease in serum uric acid levels, resolution of tophi, and a subsequent decrease in the frequency of attacks.

Bibliography

American College of Rheumatology. (2005). *Understanding your treatment options—recommendations for managing RA.* Available online: www.ra.com/ra/rastore/cgi-bin/ProdSubEV_Cat_200702_NavRoot_300.htm. Accessed March 8, 2007.

American College of Rheumatology Subcommittee on Rheumatoid Arthritis Guidelines. (2002). Guidelines for management of rheumatoid arthritis. *Arthritis and Rheumatism, 46*(2), 326–346.

American College of Rheumatology Committee on Clinical Guidelines. (1996b). Guidelines for monitoring drug therapy in rheumatoid arthritis. *Arthritis and Rheumatism, 39*(5), 723–731.

Arthritis Foundation. (2003). *Pocket primer on the rheumatic diseases: A guide to diagnosis, treatment options and more for physicians.* Atlanta: Author.

Chen, M., Lam, B., Kanaoka, Y., et al. (2006). Neutrophil-derived leukotriene B₄ is required for inflammatory arthritis. *Journal of Experimental Medicine, 203*(4), 837–842.

Drug Digest. (2005). *Disease-modifying antirheumatic drugs.* Available online: www.drugdigest.org/DD/PrintablePages/Comparisons/1,20038,32–4,00.html. Accessed March 8, 2007.

eMedicine. (2005). Rheumatoid arthritis overview. Available online: www.emedicinehealth.com/articles/37138–1.asp. Accessed March 8, 2007.

Fries, J., Williams, C., and Bloch, D. (1991). The relative toxicity of nonsteroidal antiinflammatory drugs. *Arthritis and Rheumatism, 34*(11), 1353–1360.

Goldstein, J. (2004). Challenges in managing NSAID-associated gastrointestinal tract injury. *Digestion, 69*(Suppl 1), 25–33.

Griffin, M., Piper, J., Daugherty, J., et al. (1991). Nonsteroidal antiinflammatory drug use and increased risk for peptic ulcer disease in elderly persons. *Annals of Internal Medicine, 11*(4), 257–263.

Hardman, J., Limbird, L., and Gilman, A. (Eds.). (2001). *Goodman and Gilman's the pharmacologic basis of therapeutics.* (10th ed.). New York: McGraw-Hill.

Hippisley-Cox, J., and Coupland, C. (2005). Risks of myocardial infarction in patients taking cyclooxygenase 2 inhibitors or conventional nonsteroidal antiinflammatory drugs: Population-based, nested, case-control analysis. *British Journal of Medicine, 330* (7504), 1–7.

Klippel, J. (2001). *Primer on the rheumatic diseases.* (12th ed.). Atlanta: Arthritis Foundation.

Levy, M., Spino, M., and Read, S. (1991). Colchicine: A state of the art review. *Pharmacotherapy, 11*(3), 196–211.

Magnani, A., Palmisani, E., Sala, I., et al. (2005). Review for the generalist: Update on biologic therapies for pediatric rheumatic diseases. *Pediatric Rheumatology Online Journal.* Available online: www.pedrheumonlinejournal.org/july-august05/PDF/Biologics_new%20pdf%20format.pdf. Accessed March 8, 2007.

Maini, R., Breedveld, F., Kalden, J., et al. (1998). Therapeutic efficacy of multiple intravenous infusions of anti-tumor necrosis factor a monoclonal antibody combined with low-dose weekly methotrexate in rheumatoid arthritis. *Arthritis and Rheumatism, 41*(9), 1552–1563.

Matsumoto, A., and Bathon, J. (2005). *Rheumatoid arthritis treatments.* Johns Hopkins Arthritis Website. Available online: www.hopkins-arthritis.som.jhmi.edu/rheumatoid/rheum_treat.html. Accessed March 8, 2007.

Maxwell, S., and Webb, D. (2005). COX-2 selective inhibitors—important lessons learned. *Lancet, 365*(9458), 449–451.

Medicinenet. 2006. COX-2 Inhibitors. Available online: www.medicinenet.com/cox-2_inhibitors/article.htm. Accessed March 9, 2007.

Perneger, T., Whelton, P., and Klag, M. (1994). Risk of kidney failure associated with use of acetaminophen, aspirin, and non-steroidal antiinflammatory drugs. *New England Journal of Medicine, 331* (25), 1675–1679.

Rindfleisch, J., and Muller, D. (2005). Diagnosis and management of rheumatoid arthritis. *American Family Physician, 72*(6), 1037–1047, 1049–1050.

Savient Pharmaceuticals Initiates Patient Dosing for Puricase(R) Phase 3 Clinical Study; Company on track for BLA filing in late 2007. (2006). Bioscreening Industry News. Available online: www.bioscreening.net/2006/06/19/savient-pharmaceuticals-initiates-patient-dosing-for-puricaser-phase-3-clinical-study-company-on-track-for-bla-filing-in-late-2007/. Accessed September 9, 2006.

Suarez-Almazor, M., Belseck, E., and Spooner, C. (2000). Penicillamine for treating rheumatoid arthritis. *The Cochrane Database of Systematic Reviews.* 2000, Issue 4. Art. No. CD001460. DOI: 10.1002/14651858.CD001460.

Wilcox, C., Shalek, K., and Cotsonis, G. (1994). Striking prevalence of over-the-counter nonsteroidal antiinflammatory drug use in patients with upper gastrointestinal bleeding. *Archives in Internal Medicine, 154*(1), 42–46.

Anesthetics

18

The term *anesthesia* is derived from the Greek word *anaisthesia* (*an*, "without"; *aisthesis*, "feeling") and denotes a loss of sensation with or without loss of consciousness. Such drugs have been used since 1842 when diethyl ether was first used. Four years later, a Boston dentist demonstrated the use of ether to relieve pain during surgical procedures. Modern-day surgical procedures would be impossible without anesthetics to block the emotional and physical pain that otherwise would be experienced by the patient.

The ideal anesthetic induces anesthesia smoothly and rapidly and allows prompt recovery after administration. The ideal drug would also possess a wide therapeutic index and be devoid of adverse effects. Unfortunately, no single anesthetic, when used alone, is capable of achieving these desirable effects without some disadvantages. Today, the modern practice of general anesthesiology involves the use of multidrug therapies, taking advantage of the favorable properties of each individual drug while attempting to reduce their potential for adverse effects. This chapter introduces the concept of regional anesthetic, conscious sedation, and general anesthetic states; a discussion is included of the types of anesthetics, the signs and stages of anesthesia, and the pharmacodynamics and the pharmacokinetics of the different drugs.

PHARMACOTHERAPEUTIC OPTIONS

Infiltrative Anesthetics

Infiltrative anesthesia (i.e., local anesthesia) is produced in a limited area by infiltration by a local anesthetic. Local anesthesia does not result in loss of consciousness. Box 18-1 identifies the various routes. Local anesthetics are available in a wide range of formulations including solutions, ointments, gels, creams, powders, lozenges, suppositories, sprays, and ophthalmic solutions.

▥ Pharmacodynamics

Most local anesthetics fall into one of two groups: esters or amides. Both provide anesthesia and analgesia by reversibly blocking sodium channels. Their site of action is believed to be the intracellular parts of the channel. This slows the rate of depolarization of the nerve action potential; thus propagation of the electrical impulses needed for nerve conduction is prevented. Repolarization returns sodium channels to a resting state. The transmembrane gradients are maintained by the sodium-potassium–adenosine triphosphatase (Na^+-K^+-ATPase) pump.

▥ Pharmacokinetics

Local anesthetics include esters and amides. An ester linkage (-COO-) is relatively unstable. The linkage is broken by hydrolysis in solution and, following injection, in the plasma by pseudocholinesterase. Because they are broken down in the plasma, ester types of local anesthetics are relatively nontoxic if this process is rapid, as with procaine and chloroprocaine, but in such cases their duration of effect is also brief. The exception is the patient who has a pseudocholinesterase deficiency, in which the biotransformation may be prolonged as well as the risk of toxicity increased. In contrast, amide linkages (-NHC-) are much more stable. They are not broken down in plasma but must be biotransformed by the liver.

The amount of local anesthetic reaching a nerve depends on the proximity of the injection to the nerve. Lipid solubility, protein binding, and pKa characteristics influence the potency, the onset, and the duration of action. The smaller and more lipophilic the drug, the faster the interaction with sodium channel receptors. Potency is positively correlated with lipid solubility as long as the drug remains sufficiently water-soluble to diffuse to the site of action. Lidocaine, procaine, and mepivacaine are more water-soluble than tetracaine, etidocaine, and bupivacaine; thus the latter drugs are more potent and have longer durations of action. They also bind more extensively to proteins and will displace or are displaced from these binding sites by other drugs. In the case of chiral drugs (e.g., bupivacaine), one isomer is moderately more potent than the other, in most cases. The addition of an adrenergic drug (e.g., epinephrine) to a local anesthetic slows systemic absorption of the drug by one third, prolongs the anesthetic effect, increases the intensity of blockade, and reduces surgical bleeding.

As weak bases with pKa values (8 to 9) above physiologic pH (7.4), most local anesthetics in normal tissues are primarily in their ionized form. Local anesthetics whose pKa is close to the physiologic pH will have the fastest onset of action. Only the nonionized lipid-soluble form diffuses through tissues and crosses nerve membranes. Once inside the cell, the ionized form blocks the sodium channel. See Table 18-1 for a summary of the pharmacokinetics of local anesthetics.

▥ Adverse Effects and Contraindications

The primary adverse effects of local anesthetics are allergic reactions and systemic toxicity. Although rare, allergic reactions can be life threatening. An allergy to novocaine does not predict that the patient is also allergic to lidocaine, because novocaine is an ester whereas lidocaine is an amide. Esters are more allergenic than amides because of the metabolite para-aminobenzoic acid (PABA). True allergy to an amide anesthetic is rare; rather, adverse reactions are usually to the preservative methylparaben. Local reactions include erythema, urticaria, edema, and dermatitis. Systemic reactions include generalized erythema, urticaria, edema, bronchoconstriction, hypotension, and cardiovascular collapse. Treatment is symptomatic and supportive. Cutaneous reactions may

BOX 18-1

Routes of Local Anesthesia

Local Infiltration

Local infiltration anesthesia is produced by injecting the drug into the intracutaneous and subcutaneous tissues surrounding an incision, wound, or lesion. Lidocaine is commonly used. The drug blocks only peripheral nerve stimulation at its origin. However, caution must be used to avoid infiltrating the drug into a vein. Once a local anesthetic becomes systemic, the risk of cardiovascular collapse or seizures increases.

Field Block

A field block is a series of injections made around an operative field, forming a barrier between the incision and the nervous system. By injecting the drug around a specific nerve or group of nerves, the sensory input to a localized area is obstructed. This is in contrast to infiltration anesthesia, in which only the area of the incision is injected. This type of anesthesia is used for thoracic procedures, herniorrhaphy, dental procedures, and plastic surgery. Again, care must be taken to avoid inadvertent intravenous (IV) administration.

Peripheral Nerve Block

Peripheral nerve blocks (e.g., axillary block, interscalene block, cervical block) desensitize individual nerves or nerve plexuses rather than all local nerves. The nerves most commonly blocked are those of the brachial plexus and the intercostal, sciatic, and femoral nerves. Onset and duration of the block are related to the drug used, its concentration and volume, and the presence or absence of epinephrine. Drugs commonly used in peripheral nerve blocks include lidocaine, bupivacaine, and chloroprocaine. The addition of epinephrine to the anesthetic is not recommended for digital blocks of the fingers, the toes, the ears, the nose, and the penis, owing to the risk of peripheral ischemia. Complications of peripheral nerve blocks are usually caused by inadvertent intravascular injection or an overdose of the local anesthetic. Nerve damage from trauma produced by the needle or compression from the volume of local anesthetic is rare.

Spinal Anesthesia

Spinal anesthesia is one of the older and most valuable of regional anesthesia techniques. It is the most efficient of blocks, in that a small quantity of local anesthetic injected into the spinal subarachnoid space causes widespread blockade of spinal nerves. Spinal anesthesia can be used for almost any procedure performed below the level of the diaphragm (e.g., herniorrhaphy, appendectomy, hysterectomy).

A spinal needle is usually inserted in the L_2-L_3, the L_3-L_4, or the L_4-L_5 interspace. Autonomic nerves are the first affected and the last to recover. Blockade affects nerve fibers in the following sequence: touch, pain, motor, pressure, and proprioceptive fibers. The patient experiences a loss of sensation and paralysis of first the toes, then the feet and legs, and finally the abdomen. Recovery is in the reverse order.

Different levels of block are required for different operations: upper abdomen (T_5-T_6), lower abdomen (T_8-T_9), kidneys (T_8), bladder (T_{10}), lower limbs (T_{12}), and perineal region (S_1). Sympathetic fibers are blocked by low drug concentrations and, depending on the drug, may be anesthetized two to six segments higher than sensory fibers. Similarly, the level of sensory anesthesia may be two dermatomes higher than that of motor blockade, which requires the highest concentration of anesthetic (Fig. 18-1).

Epidural Anesthesia

The epidural space lies within the spinal canal but outside the dura mater. An anesthetic injected into the epidural space spreads both up and down the spinal canal, blocking spinal nerves as they run from the spinal cord to their respective intervertebral foramina. All motor, sensory, and autonomic nerve functions are affected. Much like spinal anesthesia, spinal nerves supply specific dermatomes in the body, and therefore different levels of blockade are required for different surgical procedures.

Epidural blockade begins quickly and is most intense at the level of the injection, diminishing as it moves inferiorly and superiorly. This means that needle and catheter insertion should be as close to the dermatomal level of the surgical procedure as possible, with the concentration of the anesthetic dictating the intensity of the blockade. Surgical epidural anesthesia usually requires intense blockade. The most commonly used drugs include lidocaine (with or without epinephrine), bupivacaine, and chloroprocaine.

Intravenous Regional Anesthesia

Intravenous regional anesthesia (i.e., Bier's block) produces anesthesia of the upper and lower extremities. Its use is based on the notion that if the circulation to a limb is occluded and the injection of local anesthetic is made into a vein distal to that occlusion, the drug will reach the capillaries by retrograde flow and enter the extravascular space. Here it comes in contact with nerve endings, and paralysis of the limb below the tourniquet is achieved for the duration of the circulatory occlusion. At present, lidocaine without additives is the only drug approved for IV regional anesthesia.

The primary complications of IV regional anesthesia are toxicity due to accidental deflation of the cuff and tourniquet pain. Once the cuff is pressurized, a sudden deflation below arterial pressure increases plasma levels of the drug as it moves into systemic circulation; toxicity can result. A nonelastic bandage should be wrapped around the cuff once it has been inflated to avoid accidental slippage.

---

respond to an antihistamine (see Chapter 51). More severe reactions may respond to epinephrine and systemic glucocorticoids such as methylprednisolone. Bronchoconstriction is treated with epinephrine, and hypotension is managed with fluids and vasopressors, such as phenylephrine, or inotropic drugs like dopamine.

Systemic absorption is greatest when an intratracheal route of administration is used, followed by intercostal nerve block; absorption is intermediate for epidural block, and least for brachial plexus block, subarachnoid, and subcutaneous sites, respectively. Manifestations of central nervous system (CNS) toxicity include numbness of the tongue, lightheadedness, visual disturbances, muscular twitching, seizures, and coma. CNS toxicity is worsened by hypercapnia. The risk of cardiovascular toxicity is increased in the presence of acidosis, hypoxia, pregnancy, and hyperkalemia, which all reduce myocardial contractility, increase vasodilation, and contribute to arrhythmias.

Drug Interactions

Because of their localized use, drug interactions to local anesthetics are rare.

Benzocaine

Benzocaine (Lanacane, Solarcaine) is formulated as a dental wax, cream, gel, liquid, lotion, ointment, solutions, and spray. This ester has been approved by the FDA as a treatment for congestive and serious acute otitis media and otitis externa; for denture stomatitis; for toothaches and painful teething; and for pain associated with insect bites, minor cuts and scrapes, and minor skin irritations; approval also extends to its use as a lubricant for nasogastric and endoscopic intubation, as well as

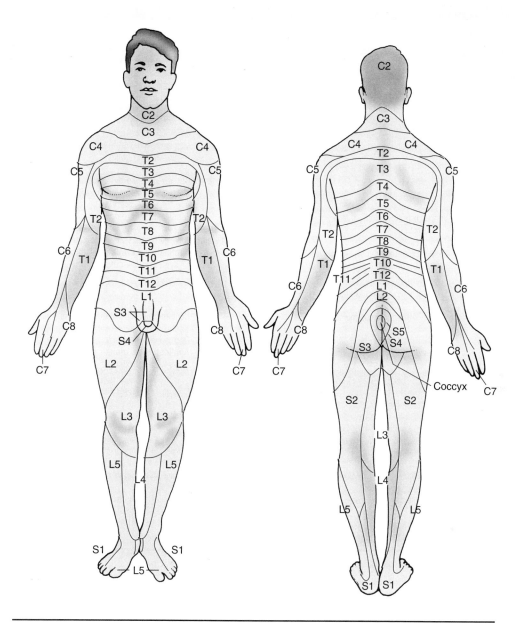

FIGURE 18-1 Dermatomes. (Redrawn from Ignatavicius, D., Workman, M. [2006]. *Medical-surgical nursing: A nursing process approach* [5th ed., p. 930]. Philadelphia: Saunders. Used with permission.)

for urinary catheters, proctoscopes, and vaginal specula. It can also be used as a topical anesthetic for all accessible mucous membranes (except the eyes) during surgical or other procedures of the ear, the nose, the mouth, the pharynx, the larynx, the trachea, the bronchi, and the esophagus. Use very little benzocaine spray, and that with caution, since this drug may cause methemoglobinemia; maintain a healthy respect for the spray's effects on mucous membranes. Use of the drug is contraindicated in patients with sensitivity to ester anesthetics.

Ethyl Chloride

Ethyl chloride (Chloroethane) is a skin refrigerant. It is used topically for pain related to injections and minor surgical procedures (e.g., toe nail removal) and for transient relief of certain minor sports injuries. It is also used for myofascial pain.

Skin areas adjacent to the site of use should be covered with petrolatum before use of ethyl chloride.

Some health care providers believe not only that the thawing process after use is painful, but also that freezing tissues delays healing and increases the risk for infection. Changes in skin pigmentation may also occur with ethyl chloride. Exercise caution when using ethyl chloride since inhalation can cause CNS depression and fatal coma.

EMA-Max

EMA-Max contains 4% lidocaine cream in a liposomal matrix. It is FDA-approved for the temporary relief of pain from minor cuts and abrasions, and has been used to provide dermal analgesia before a chemical peel. EMA-Max is applied for 15 to 40 minutes to intact skin without a dressing. The

PHARMACOKINETICS
TABLE 18-1 Local Anesthetics

Drug	Uses	Onset	Duration	Comments
TOPICAL PREANESTHETICS				
benzocaine	Skin and mucus membranes	<5 min (peak)	15–45 min	Contraindicated in patients sensitive to ester anesthetics
ethyl chloride	Skin	Instant	1–2 sec	Freezing may lower local resistance to infections and delay healing.
EMLA (2.5% lidocaine and 2.5% prilocaine)	Used with occlusion for closed wounds	1 hr (peak)	1–2 hr after removal	Variable effectiveness depending on duration of application
lidocaine	Iontophoresis*	10 min at depth of 1–2 cm	15 min	May burn skin if used with high DC current. Depth of anesthesia greater than EMLA
4% lidocaine–0.1% epinephrine–0.5% tetracaine (LET)†	Open wounds	20–30 min	UA	Dosage: 4 mg/kg to a total of 280 mg (7 mL = 280 mg) Maximum lidocaine dosage: 3–5 mg/kg
70% lidocaine–70 mg tetracaine	Venous access; superficial skin procedures	30 min (peak)	UA	Formulated as a patch; avoid simultaneous or sequential patches.
pramoxine 1%	Topical (anal)	Fast	15–45 min	For external use only; also available OTC
tetracaine	Skin, mucus membranes, tracheobronchial tree	3–8 min (peak)	UA	**Application to broken or inflamed skin increases risk of systemic toxicity.** ▲
ESTERS				
chloroprocaine 0.5%-1%	Local infiltrate, nerve block, spinal	6–12 min	0.25–0.5 hr	Contraindicated for use in patients sensitive to ester anesthetics
cocaine	Topical skin and mucus membranes	2–5 min (peak)	0.5–1 hr	Contraindicated for systemic or ophthalmic use and in patients with cholinesterase deficiency
procaine 0.5%-1%	Local infiltrate, nerve block, spinal	Fast	0.5–1 hr	Dose varies depending on use.
tetracaine	Spinal	15 min	2–3 hr	**Application to broken or inflamed skin increases risk of systemic toxicity.** ▲
AMIDES				
bupivacaine 0.25%	Local infiltrate, nerve block, epidural, spinal	5 min	2–4 hr	Dosage: 2.5 mg/kg to a total of 175 mg total (50 mL)
etidocaine 0.5%-1%	Local infiltrate, nerve block, epidural	3–5 min	3–7 hr	Produces profound motor blockade
lidocaine 0.5%-2%	Local infiltrate, nerve block, spinal, epidural, topical, IV regional	<2 min	0.5–1 hr	Most versatile, most frequently used local because of potency, rapid onset, moderate duration, and efficacy
lidocaine with epi 1:100,000–1:200,000	Local infiltrate	<2 min	3–12 hr	Dosage: 4 mg/kg to a total of 280 mg (25 mL 1%; 50 mL 0.5%)
mepivacaine 0.5%-1%	Local infiltrate, nerve block, epidural, spinal	3–5 min	0.75–1.5 hr	Dosage: 4 mg/kg to a total of 280 mg (14 mL 2%; 28 mL 1%)
prilocaine 1.5%-2%	Local infiltrate, nerve block	2 min	2–6 hr	Dosage: 7 mg/kg to a total of 500 mg (25 mL 2%; 50 mL 1%). Large dosages increase the risk for methemoglobinemia.
ropivacaine	Local infiltrate, nerve block, epidural, spinal	1–15 min	2–6 hr	Less potent and shorter-acting than bupivacaine

*Iontophoresis, DC current applied to electrodes over anesthetic. Drug not FDA-approved at this time for preanesthesia purposes.
†LET replaces combination of tetracaine, adrenalin, and cocaine (TAC).
EMLA, Eutectic mixture of local anesthetic; *epi,* epinephrine; *IV,* intravenous; *OTC,* over the counter; *UA,* unavailable.

drug is also being used for many dermatologic procedures, although the FDA has not approved it for such purposes. Safe use on mucous membranes has not been evaluated.

Eutectic Mixture of Local Anesthetic (EMLA) Cream
EMLA is an emulsion mixture of the local anesthetics lidocaine 2.5% and prilocaine 2.5% in a ratio of 1:1 by weight. It is indicated for topical use on normal intact skin. It may be used on genital mucous membranes for superficial minor surgeries and as pretreatment for infiltration anesthesia. EMLA can be used in healthy, full-term neonates before circumcision. The drug is applied to the penis 1 hour before the procedure.

The emulsion formulation allows the drug to penetrate dermal layers of the skin more effectively than single-component creams. Anesthetic effects reach a depth of 3 mm after a 60-minute application, and 5 mm after a 120-minute application. To facilitate absorption, EMLA cream is covered with an occlusive dressing.

Local effects at the application site include pallor and blanching, redness, a rash, swelling, itching, and changes in the ability to feel hot or cold. These mild adverse effects usually disappear within 1 to 2 hours. Serious adverse effects may occur (e.g., methemoglobinemia) if EMLA is left on the skin for prolonged periods, or when applied over larger than recommended surface areas. EMLA is contraindicated in patients with known sensitivity to amide anesthetics or other ingredients contained in the product.

Eutectic Mixture of Local Anesthetic (EMLA) Patch
Like the EMLA cream previously discussed, this newest patch anesthetic is an emulsion mixture of the local anesthetics lidocaine 75% and tetracaine 75%. It is for use on intact skin to provide local dermal anesthesia for superficial venous access and superficial dermatologic procedures such as excisions, electrodessication, and shave biopsies of skin lesions. The patch, applied for about 30 minutes, generates a mild warming that enhances delivery of the local anesthetics.

CENTRAL NERVOUS

BOX 18-2

Advantages and Disadvantages of Regional Anesthesia

Advantages

Airway maintenance—Ability to have patient conscious to maintain own airway. Likelihood of aspiration reduced. Presence of anesthesiologist unnecessary

Smooth recovery—Many procedures do not require the same degree of care that is necessary with unconscious patient. In most cases, local anesthesia is still present at end of procedure, and patient will be awake and rational when pain eventually appears.

Postoperative analgesia—In many cases it is possible to continue local anesthesia for hours or days (e.g., epidural).

Reduces surgical stress—Modification of surgical stress is greatest when local anesthesia is continued 1 to 2 days postoperatively.

Earlier discharge—Outpatient and same-day surgery patients are usually ready for discharge the same day.

Disadvantages

Patient wants to sleep. Does not preclude use of regional anesthesia, which can be combined with light general anesthetic.

Restlessness seen frequently in semiconscious patient with severe pain after general anesthesia. Systemic toxicity possible if inadvertently given by IV route or an overdose is inadvertently given. Some degree of practice and skill required for best results.

Some blocks require up to 30 minutes or more to be fully effective. Some surgeries unsuitable for local anesthesia.

Analgesia may not always be totally effective. Patient may require additional analgesics, or a light general anesthetic.

Small risk but definite evidence of prolonged nerve damage. Widespread sympathetic blockade results in hypotension when using certain techniques (e.g., spinal or epidural blockade).

It is not known if the drugs contained in the EMLA patch are biotransformed in the skin. Lidocaine is rapidly biotransformed in the liver. Tetracaine undergoes rapid hydrolysis by plasma esterases.

Reported adverse effects include erythema, blanching, edema, and abnormal sensations. These reactions are generally mild, resolving shortly after treatment. Use of the EMLA patch is contraindicated in patients with a known history of sensitivity to lidocaine, tetracaine, or local anesthetics of the amide or ester type. It is also contraindicated in patients with PABA sensitivity. The patch should be used with caution in patients receiving class I antiarrhythmic drugs (e.g., tocainide, mexiletine), since the systemic toxic effects are thought to be additive and potentially synergistic with lidocaine and tetracaine. The drug is pregnancy category B.

Lidocaine-epinephrine-tetracaine (LET)

LET is safe and more cost-effective than the combination of topical tetracaine-adrenaline-cocaine (TAC), and has essentially replaced it. Sodium metabisulfite has been added to the product to improve the stability of epinephrine. Both the gel and solution formulations are safe down to 2 years of age.

LET is ineffective on intact skin and slightly less efficacious for extremity lacerations. Approximately 5% of patients do not achieve anesthesia when the gel formulation of the drug is used in the treatment of face or scalp lacerations. Infiltrative anesthesia may be used when adequate anesthesia is not achieved; the maximal lidocaine dosage of 3 to 5 mg/kg of lidocaine should not be exceeded.

The general rule of thumb is to avoid use of local anesthetics containing epinephrine in the fingers, the toes, the ears, the nose, and the penis. Lengthy constriction of arterioles in these end-arteriolar areas may lead to tissue death and gangrene. Also, the gel formulation of LET is more effective on mucous membranes because it stays within the wound. Increased absorption of the drug occurs when used in contaminated or complex wounds, and in wounds of 6 cm or larger.

Chloroprocaine

Chloroprocaine (Nesacaine) is a short-acting ester anesthetic. Because chloroprocaine antagonizes mu (μ) receptors, its duration of action is short-lived. It is ineffective topically and is not recommended for intravenous (IV) regional anesthesia because of its association with a high incidence of thrombophlebitis. Occasional cases of severe back pain have occurred after epidural anesthesia with chloroprocaine. Contributing factors to the pain include a preservative, disodium edetate (EDTA); use of volumes greater than 20 mL; and the low pH of the solution. Persistent neurologic damage or prolonged sensory or motor deficits have been reported after accidental spinal anesthesia with large doses of sodium bisulfite or methyl paraben–containing solutions. Chloroprocaine should not be used for spinal anesthesia.

Cocaine

Cocaine is a long-acting ester anesthetic and a particularly strong stimulant of the cerebral cortex. The drug is commonly used to densensitize the eye and the mucous membranes of the nose, the mouth, and the urethra. It is known to inhibit the reuptake of norepinephrine at adrenergic synapses, which may account for some of its central and peripheral effects. It potentiates neurotransmission of norepinephrine, dopamine, or serotonin in the CNS and blocks the reabsorption of neurotransmitters, leaving circuits open that would otherwise close. Cocaine is discussed as a drug of abuse in Chapter 12.

Procaine

Procaine (Novocain, others) is used for nerve blocks and local and spinal anesthesia. Procaine's rapid onset of action and short duration depends on the type of block, the concentration, and the individual patient. Procaine is a weakly toxic ester because of rapid plasma hydrolysis. However, it is hydrolyzed to PABA, which is responsible for the allergic reactions in some patients.

Tetracaine

Tetracaine (Pontocaine) is a potent, long-acting ester primarily used for spinal anesthesia. Its longer duration of action compared to that of other esters is due to the much slower rate of hydrolysis by plasma cholinesterase. High plasma levels can cause seizures and cardiovascular collapse because of decreased peripheral vascular resistance and myocardial depression.

Bupivacaine

Bupivacaine (Marcaine, Sensorcaine) is a long-acting amide local anesthetic capable of profound blockade, with separation of sensory anesthesia and motor function. Although bupivacaine is useful for infiltration, peripheral nerve blocks, and spinal anesthesia, its major advantage appears to be its use in epidural analgesia for labor. Compared with other amides, inadvertent IV injection of bupivacaine is associated with a greater risk of cardiotoxicity. This is because of the slower recovery from cardiac sodium channel blockade and greater depression of myocardial contractility and cardiac conduction.

Etidocaine

Etidocaine (Duranest) is also a long-acting amide with a rapid onset of action. Dosages high enough to achieve sensory anesthesia produce profound motor blockade. This characteristic limits its use in obstetrics and for postoperative pain relief. It has been used for local anesthesia, peripheral nerve block, and epidural anesthesia.

Lidocaine

Lidocaine (Xylocaine) was the first amide to be introduced. This drug remains the most versatile and most frequently used local anesthetic because of its potency, rapid onset, moderate duration, and topical anesthetic activity. Lidocaine remains the only approved drug in the United States for IV regional anesthesia. It may also be used topically, for peripheral nerve block, and for spinal or epidural anesthesia. *Iontophoresis* is a method of delivering lidocaine through a drug-soaked dressing using a mild electric current (DC) whose source is placed on top of the anesthetic. It is intended for use over a small surface area. Some patients find the mild electrical sensations of iontophoresis painful. Anesthesia of the affected area to a depth of 2 cm appears within 10 minutes and lasts about 15 minutes. The effectiveness of iontophoresis equates to that of EMLA, but it remains underutilized.

Mepivacaine

Mepivacaine (Carbocaine, Polocaine) is similar to lidocaine in potency and speed of onset, but it has a slightly longer duration of action and lacks vasodilator activity. This amide is used for infiltration, peripheral nerve blocks, and epidural anesthesia. It is especially useful for brachial plexus blocks when large volumes of drug are given. High plasma levels, such as occur with paracervical blocks, produce uterine vasoconstriction and a decrease in uterine blood flow. In addition, the biotransformation of mepivacaine is prolonged in the fetus and newborn, and therefore the drug is generally not used in obstetric anesthesia.

Prilocaine

Prilocaine (Citanest) is equipotent to lidocaine, but has a longer duration. This amide is less toxic than lidocaine and undergoes rapid hepatic biotransformation to orthotolidine, which oxidizes hemoglobin to methemoglobin. If the dose exceeds 600 mg, there may be sufficient methemoglobin to cause cyanosis since oxygen-carrying capacity of the red cell is reduced. This unique propensity of prilocaine to cause dose-related methemoglobinemia limits its usefulness. It is also useful for infiltration, peripheral nerve blockade, and epidural anesthesia.

Ropivacaine

Like many of the other local anesthetics, ropivacaine (Naropin) is used for local anesthesia, nerve block, and epidural and spinal anesthesia. The onset of action is similar to that of bupivacaine. Potency and duration of sensory blockade appear similar for both drugs, but ropivacaine is less potent and shorter-acting on motor fibers. Ropivacaine appears less cardiotoxic than bupivacaine.

CONSCIOUS SEDATION

Conscious sedation, also known as procedural sedation and analgesia (PSAA), reduces patient awareness, memory, and the discomfort associated with unpleasant diagnostic or therapeutic procedures while preserving the protective airway reflexes and spontaneous respirations. Depth of sedation and analgesia are titrated with the selective use of combinations of opioids and benzodiazepines administered by IV route. The most commonly used drugs for conscious sedation include midazolam and fentanyl or lorazepam.

Proper monitoring of respirations is needed during procedures using conscious sedation, because sedation is a continuum ranging from light to deep sleep. Qualified providers of conscious sedation include anesthesiologists, certified registered nurse anesthetists (CRNAs), other physicians, dentists, and oral surgeons. The monitoring health care provider should have no other responsibilities during the procedure and should remain with the patient at all times.

PHARMACOTHERAPEUTIC OPTIONS

Benzodiazepine and Opioid Combinations

Fentanyl and midazolam are safe and effective for conscious sedation, titrate easily, and have a rapid onset and a short duration of action. Because midazolam has no analgesic properties, it is used primarily for its sedative, amnestic, and anxiolytic properties. Fentanyl, an opioid, is added for its analgesic effects (see Chapters 16 and 19).

Midazolam is ordinarily administered by IV route for a rapid onset of action and is generally preferred over other benzodiazepines for conscious sedation. It can be given as continuous IV infusion, has the shortest half-life of the available benzodiazepines, is biotransformed in the liver to inactive metabolites, and is eliminated through the kidneys. Yet, even with its short half-life, widespread distribution can result in prolonged sedation, particularly in the presence of liver or kidney dysfunction. It is a pregnancy category D drug.

Fentanyl is a synthetic opioid (see also later section under General Anesthesia, and Chapter 16). It should not be used alone for conscious sedation because it is a pure analgesic. (A pure analgesic in one whose effectiveness is limited by its dose-related ceiling effects.) Given by IV route, the time to onset of action is 1 to 2 minutes; its duration of action is approximately 30 to 60 minutes. The rapid redistribution of the drug from the CNS contributes to its short duration of action. Fentanyl is biotransformed by the liver and primarily eliminated via the biliary tract. It is a pregnancy category C drug.

The major disadvantages of midazolam and fentanyl for conscious sedation are the risks for respiratory and cardiac depression. Twenty-five percent of patients develop some degree of respiratory depression; for this reason give the drugs slowly rather than as a bolus. The advantage of this combination of drugs is that both have antagonists (i.e., flumazenil and naloxone, respectively) that can be used to reverse their effects.

GENERAL ANESTHESIA

General anesthesia is a controlled, reversible loss of consciousness and sensation. Physiologically, the alterations result in four classic states: *hypnosis* (unconsciousness), *analgesia* (insensibility to pain), *amnesia* (loss of memory), and *muscle relaxation* (relaxation or paralysis of skeletal muscle).

General anesthetics fall into two primary categories: inhaled and injected. Inhaled anesthetics are volatile liquids or gases that are vaporized in oxygen and inhaled to induce anesthesia. Injected anesthetics are administered by IV route. Injected anesthetics are used to induce or maintain general anesthesia, to induce amnesia, and as adjuncts to inhaled anesthetics. These adjunctive drugs commonly include barbiturates (e.g., thiopental, methohexital) and benzodiazepines (e.g., midazolam, lorazepam), opioids (e.g., fentanyl, sufentanil), propofol, and neuromuscular blocking drugs (e.g., succinylcholine, vecuronium). Use of the minimum dose of each drug to achieve the desired level of anesthesia is referred to as balanced anesthesia.

PHARMACOTHERAPEUTIC OPTIONS

Barbiturates

Intravenous anesthesia, as we know it today, had its beginnings in 1934 when thiopental sodium was introduced. The patient undergoes an extremely rapid induction, with unconsciousness occurring about 30 seconds after initial IV administration. These drugs are potent enough to be used alone for minor procedures such as dental extractions or pelvic exams. Injected drugs used for induction or maintenance of anesthesia are identified in Table 18-2, along with their advantages and disadvantages.

Thiopental sodium

Thiopental sodium (Pentathol) is an ultra–short-acting barbiturate that depresses the CNS and induces hypnosis and anesthesia, but not analgesia. It is used for induction of general anesthesia and as a supplement to regional anesthesia. It may also be used as an anticonvulsant and to reduce elevated intracranial pressure. The drug produces some anterograde amnesia, and airway reflexes are heightened. Thiopental is associated with respiratory depression and hemodynamic effects, including a decrease in systemic vascular resistance, arterial pressure, cardiac output, and coronary perfusion pressures. Marked hypotension can occur in a hypovolemic patient. Although histamine release is rare, anaphylaxis with cardiovascular collapse has been reported. Thiopental is contraindicated for use in patients who have porphyria (a genetic disorder characterized by disturbance in porphyrin metabolism with resultant gastrointestinal, neurologic, and psychologic symptoms).

The onset of drug action following an induction dose occurs in 10 to 15 seconds, with duration of action of 5 to

TABLE 18-2 Injected Anesthetics

Drugs	Advantages	Disadvantages
BARBITURATES		
thiopental sodium	Rapid induction; cerebral vasoconstrictor	Venodilation with decreased blood pressure, increased heart rate; laryngospasm; bronchospasm; hypotension with hypovolemia; vasospasm with intraarterial injection; tissue necrosis with subQ route; no skeletal muscle relaxation; shivering; anaphylaxis, contraindicated with porphyria
methohexital	Most rapid induction	Involuntary muscle movement, seizures
BENZODIAZEPINES		
midazolam	Useful for conscious sedation; IV route provides fastest onset. Does not have active metabolites. Has antagonist that can be used to reverse effects if needed.	Prolonged effects may be seen with renal or hepatic dysfunction.
OPIOID		
fentanyl	Useful for conscious sedation. Short duration of action. Has antagonist that can be used to reverse effects if needed.	Cannot be used alone for conscious sedation
MISCELLANEOUS DRUGS		
etomidate	Minimal changes in blood pressure, heart rate; respiratory stability; no histamine release	Myoclonic movement; pain with injection; transient adrenocortical depression
ketamine	Profound analgesia; bronchodilator; hemodynamic support	Increased skeletal muscle tone, blood pressure, heart rate, cerebral blood flow, metabolic oxygen requirements, intracranial pressure, salivary gland secretion; delirium, hallucinations
propofol	Hypnosis; rapid induction; clear-headed, rapid emergence; less nausea, vomiting	Hypotension, tachycardia, or bradycardia; clonic-myoclonic movement on emergence; pain on injection; sexual illusions

IV, Intravenous; *subQ*, subcutaneous.

15 minutes. Recovery from a small dose is rapid, but high lipid solubility and slow elimination result in cumulative drug effects after repeated bolus injection or infusion.

Methohexital Sodium

Methohexital sodium (Brevital) produces a rapid, ultra–short-acting anesthesia. Methohexital does not produce analgesia and has no muscle relaxant properties. This barbiturate depresses the sensory cortex, decreases motor activity, alters cerebellar function, and produces dose-dependent drowsiness, sedation, and hypnosis. These effects are mediated by enhancing gamma-aminobutyric acid (GABA), a major inhibitory transmitter in the CNS. Methohexital is associated with a more rapid return to consciousness, making it especially useful in outpatient anesthesia.

Methohexital may produce excitement in older adults and children, and in other patients in the presence of pain. Induction is associated with involuntary skeletal muscle movement and respiratory depression. Pretreatment with opioids reduces the incidence of excitatory phenomena. Cardiovascular adverse effects are secondary to decreased myocardial contractility and peripheral vasodilation. Adverse reactions are rare but may include laryngospasm, bronchospasm, emergence delirium, nausea, emesis, hiccups, skeletal muscle hyperactivity, and shivering. Extravascular injection causes tissue necrosis, and an accidental intraarterial injection may result in gangrene. An inadvertent injection is managed with an arterial injection of 10 mL of 1% procaine, 40 to 80 mg of papaverine, or local infiltration of phentolamine (2.5 to 5 mg) to produce vasodilation. Methohexital is contraindicated for use in patients with porphyria and must be used with caution in patients with status asthmaticus.

Opioid Antagonists

Opioid receptors are classified as μ_1, μ_2, Δ, κ, and σ. Drug interaction at μ_1 receptors provides analgesia, whereas μ_2 receptor interaction is associated with adverse effects including respiratory depression, decreased heart rate, physical dependence, and euphoria. Δ Receptor stimulation is associated with modulation of μ receptor activity. κ Receptor stimulation leads to analgesia, sedation, respiratory depression, and miosis. Dysphoria, hypertonia, tachycardia, and tachypnea result from σ receptor stimulation.

Alfentanil

Alfentanil (Alfenta) is a potent opioid analgesic. Small doses are used for analgesia, whereas large doses may be used for induction and maintenance of inhaled anesthesia. Alfentanil produces a deep level of analgesia and attenuates the hemodynamic response to surgical stress. Like most opioids, it reduces sympathetic tone and may produce bradycardia because of stimulation of the vagal nucleus in the medulla. This is especially true when it is used in combination with nonvagolytic neuromuscular blockers or if an anticholinergic has not been given. Induction doses produce respiratory depression and reduce blood pressure secondary to peripheral vasodilation. Hypotension and bradycardia are seen more often with alfentanil than with either fentanyl or sufentanyl. Extreme bradycardia may be treated with atropine. Repeated doses or continuous infusions do not result in a significant accumulation. Alfentanil does not produce clinically significant changes in cerebral blood flow (CBF), cerebral metabolic rate ($CMRO_2$), or intracranial pressure.

Fentanyl

Fentanyl (Sublimaze) is a potent lipid-soluble opioid agonist with an analgesic potency 75 to 125 times that of morphine. Fentanyl may be used for induction or analgesia or as a supplement to other drugs. It may be added to spinal or epidural blocks and can be used postoperatively in patient-controlled analgesia. Cardiovascular stability is generally maintained, but in high doses, such as those formerly used in cardiac surgery, fentanyl can cause bradycardia and chest wall rigidity. Respiratory depression with fentanyl is dose dependent, is potentiated by other CNS depressants, and may last longer than analgesia.

Remifentanil

Remifentanil (Ultiva) is a pure agonist at μ receptors with little binding to others. This characteristic of the newest opioid makes it extremely useful for induction and maintenance of general anesthesia, monitored anesthesia care, and postoperative analgesia. The use of remifentanil as part of monitored anesthesia care effectively provides patient comfort and analgesia during placement of local or regional anesthetic blocks. It can be rapidly titrated to provide patient comfort without sedation, and careful titration is associated with an adequate respiratory rate. It is associated with hemodynamic stability and is well tolerated.

Although remifentanil is not considered suitable as the sole drug used for induction of anesthesia, it is well tolerated in combination with nitrous oxide, thiopental, or propofol. Remifentanil is an ester and is therefore biotransformed by both plasma and tissue esterases. It has an onset of action of approximately 1 minute, similar to that of alfentanil. However, termination of opioid effect is extremely rapid, making this the first truly titratable opioid.

Circulating esterases are responsible for biotransformation of remifentanil. The short duration of remifentanil action is preserved in patients with a deficiency of pseudocholinesterase activity and in patients taking drugs that inhibit plasma pseudocholinesterase (e.g., echothiophate). The pharmacokinetics of remifentanil in patients with impaired hepatic or renal function appears to be unchanged.

Remifentanil's effects on CBF and $CMRO_2$ are similar to those of alfentanil. When given in opioid-equivalent dosages, hemodynamic responses are similar to those with the other opioids. The most profound cardiovascular depression is seen after the first dose of remifentanil. The maximal cardiovascular depression can be mostly prevented by premedication with glycopyrrolate. Although use of remifentanil is associated with nausea and vomiting, the incidence is no higher than that seen with alfentanil. The incidence of muscle rigidity, which is also comparable to that seen with alfentanil, may be prevented by slow infusion or slow injection of bolus doses over 60 to 90 seconds.

Emergence from remifentanil-based anesthesia is swift and predictable. Because of its short duration of action, which is otherwise desirable, inadequate postoperative analgesia may result. A transition must be made from remifentanil to some other, longer-acting analgesic for surgeries that result in significant pain. In select patients who have been maintained intraoperatively with infusions of this opioid, the infusion of remifentanil can be continued into the immediate postoperative setting. The use of this drug postoperatively should be under the direct supervision of an anesthesia provider.

Sufentanyl

Sufentanyl (Sufenta) is an analogue of fentanyl with 5 to 7 times the analgesic potency. Cardiovascular effects are similar to those of fentanyl. Like other opioids, sufentanyl may produce a dose-dependent bradycardia, which is sufficient to decrease cardiac output. Respiratory depression is due to a decrease in response of the respiratory centers in the brainstem to carbon dioxide. Skeletal muscle rigidity sufficient to interfere with ventilation may occur at higher doses. Sufentanyl has no clinically significant effects on CBF or intracranial pressure, but it does cause a decrease in the $CMRO_2$.

Miscellaneous Injectables
Etomidate

The CNS depression caused by etomidate (Amidate), an imidazole compound, is thought to be due to its action at the GABA receptors. Although etomidate lowers $CMRO_2$, CBF, and intracranial pressure, cerebral perfusion pressure is well maintained because of the drug's minimal effects on systemic blood pressure. It neither produces analgesia nor triggers malignant hyperthermia (MH) and is not generally associated with histamine release, so allergic reactions are rare. Therapeutic doses have minimal effect on myocardial contractility, cardiac output, and peripheral circulation. Myoclonic movement occurs in about one third of patients during induction and is due to a lack of subcortical suppression of extrapyramidal activity. Etomidate is rapidly biotransformed by the liver.

The most desirable quality of etomidate is that it has few to no hemodynamic effects and maintains a neutral cardiovascular adverse effects profile. There is a 3% to 5% incidence of respiratory depression and hypoxia, although patients usually respond well to supplemental oxygen. In rare instances, patients have required assisted ventilation. Emergence nausea and vomiting have been reported. Adrenocortical suppression lasting 4 to 8 hours may occur after a single induction dose, although the significance of this effect is thought inconsequential.

Propylene glycol is a preservative of etomidate. IV injection is associated with pain on injection and, on occasion, thrombophlebitis. Pain is more likely if the drug is injected into small veins.

This drug should be used with caution in patients with epilepsy. Myoclonus may be reduced by pretreating with a benzodiazepine or opioid. Although intraocular pressure is reduced, eye movements may be problematic for surgical procedures on the eye. Hypersensitivity to etomidate or its ingredients contraindicates use. Cautious use is warranted during pregnancy; it is a category C drug.

Propofol

Since its introduction in 1989, propofol (Diprivan) has been approved for monitored anesthesia care, neuroanesthesia, and cardiac and pediatric anesthesia, and for sedation in intensive care units. Propofol produces rapid induction of anesthesia with minimal excitatory effects. Its rapid onset and the rapid, clear-headed emergence from it make the drug very attractive.

Sedation occurs on a continuum from minimal to deep sedation and to anesthesia. Although a reduced incidence of postoperative nausea and vomiting is also attractive, there is inconsistency of opinion regarding propofol's role in perioperative emesis (see Controversy box).

Propofol is rapidly cleared from the body. Compared with thiopental, recovery is more rapid, and there is less nausea and vomiting during recovery. It reduces nausea and vomiting in high-risk patients and has been effective as a long-term infusion for refractory postoperative nausea. It is believed the drug may have direct antiemetic effects. Subhypnotic doses of propofol may be used in the postanesthesia care unit to treat postoperative nausea and vomiting, particularly if it is not of vagal origin.

Induction doses of propofol may lead to apnea and hypotension secondary to slight myocardial depression and a decrease in systemic vascular resistance. There is minimal change in heart rate. Venodilation also contributes to the 15% to 30% decrease in blood pressure that is occasionally seen. Hypotension is especially likely in older adults or in hypovolemic or high-risk patients who have received other CNS depressants.

Even with dosages commonly used for induction anesthesia, propofol can cause significant cardiac and respiratory depression. The effects of propofol are unpredictable, accumulate with prolonged infusion, and are more pronounced than those seen with midazolam, etomidate, and thiopental. Propofol is eliminated through the biliary tree but clearance can be prolonged in patients who have liver disease.

There have been rare reports of seizures and *opisthotonos* (a form of spasm in which the head and the heels are bent backward and the body arched). These effects occur most often during emergence or in the postoperative period. Propofol-induced dyskinesias in Parkinson's disease have also been reported. A possible association between propofol and development of postoperative pancreatitis has been reported. Sexual illusions and disinhibition are observed during propofol sedation. To avoid complications of misconduct, it is advisable to have a third party in the room at all times when this drug or any drug with central effects is given. Anaphylaxis has been occasionally seen.

Ketamine

Although it is rarely used today, ketamine (Ketalar) can be used as pretreatment, for sedation or analgesia, or for induction and maintenance of anesthesia. Ketamine is a phencyclidine derivative that produces rapid dissociative anesthesia owing to a functional and electrophysiologic dissociation between the thalamoneocortical and limbic systems of the CNS. Analgesic effects of ketamine may be due to its effect at central and spinal opiate receptors. The unique clinical anesthetic state of catalepsy is observed with this drug. Eyes remain open with a slow nystagmic gaze, whereas corneal and light reflexes remain intact; vocalizations may occur. Varying degrees of hypertonus and occasional purposeful movements unrelated to painful stimuli are noted in the presence of adequate surgical anesthesia. The determination of the adequacy of anesthesia is based on noting the presence or absence of purposeful responses to noxious stimuli.

Ketamine generally preserves airway patency and respiratory function. Laryngeal reflexes are normal or slightly enhanced. It is a mild respiratory depressant. Salivary and tracheobronchial secretions are increased, and a prophylactic antisialagogue (a drug that inhibits the flow of saliva) is required. Ketamine causes bronchodilation and has been used in the treatment and emergency intubation of pediatric patients with status asthmaticus.

A major feature that distinguishes ketamine from other IV anesthetics is stimulation of the cardiovascular system. It may produce myocardial depression; however, central sympathetic stimulation, neuronal release of catecholamines, and inhibition of neuronal uptake of catecholamines usually override the direct myocardial depressant effects of the drug. Hemodynamic effects include increases in systemic and pulmonary artery pressure, heart rate, and cardiac output. This advantage makes ketamine a good choice in patients with hemodynamic compromise from hypovolemia or cardiac tamponade. Critically ill patients with catecholamine depletion may respond

Controversy

Appropriateness of Increased Utilization of Propofol in Anesthesia

Jonathan J. Wolfe

Propofol, a novel anesthetic, offers apparent advantages over other intravenous (IV) drugs for the induction and maintenance of anesthesia. The patient stands to receive superior anesthesia with less stressful induction, maintenance, and emergence. There is a smoother and more predictable onset of anesthesia as well as rapid recovery from anesthesia. The drug also causes a reduced incidence of perioperative nausea and vomiting. Surgical and anesthesia teams can anticipate less likelihood of patient hazard, a situation likely to promote both confidence and performance. If drug response were the only issue, propofol might quickly replace IV barbiturates and volatile anesthetics.

However, propofol carries a far higher price tag than traditional anesthetics. Most rapid-acting barbiturates and inhaled drugs are available at reduced prices, simply because several generic forms of them are readily available on the market. Propofol is a patented product with a single manufacturer. Therefore it is likely to retain a higher purchase price. A surgical department may face little difficulty deciding to adopt propofol for high-risk cases, such as cardiac surgery, in which a reduction in adverse effects is desirable regardless of price. However, the decision to make the drug broadly available may result in far greater problems.

CLINICAL REASONING

- Does a hospital have an obligation to provide the advantages of propofol anesthesia to all patients, based on the right each person has to equal protection from adverse effects during treatment?
- Would an outpatient surgery center be justified in adopting propofol as its usual and customary drug for induction and maintenance of anesthesia, and charging higher prices to its patients and their insurance carriers, if its fewer adverse effects permitted better facility utilization and hence higher net profits for the surgery center?
- After you have discussed an anesthesia plan using thiopental sodium for induction, a competent and well-informed patient refuses to sign the consent forms. This person instead demands that the plan be changed to propofol induction, which the patient considers to be so far superior that thiopental is not an option. The case is elective and of low risk. Your department's procedures clearly indicate that as a cost-containment matter, propofol is not to be used. How will you respond to this patient?

---

to ketamine with unexpected reductions in blood pressure and cardiac output. Ketamine does not cause histamine release.

The incidence of psychic disturbances with ketamine ranges from 5% to 30%. Postanesthetic psychic sensations have been noted, with alterations in mood and body image, dissociative or extracorporeal experiences, floating sensations, vivid dreams or illusions, or delirium. Although these sensations generally occur immediately upon awakening, flashbacks several weeks later have been reported. Factors associated with a higher incidence of reactions include age, sex, and current personality disorders. Females have a higher incidence of psychic disturbances than males, and 24% to 34% of reactions occur in patients over 16 years of age. There is a decreased incidence of emergence reactions when ketamine is used in conjunction with sedative-hypnotics or when it is used with benzodiazepines. Ketamine is usually a poor choice for patients with a history of psychiatric illness.

It should be used with caution in patients with severe hypertension, ischemic heart disease, or aneurysms, and in patients with intracranial hypertension. It should also be used cautiously in chronic alcoholics or in acutely intoxicated patients.

Reversal Drugs

Opioid agonist-antagonists bind to μ receptors, where they produce limited or no response. They do, however, provide partial agonist action at Δ and κ opioid receptors. Cautious use of reversal drugs is warranted since effects of the original drug may last longer than those of the reversal drug. Patients who receive a reversal drug may appear recovered only to have the sedation return once the action of the reversal drug has worn off.

Neuromuscular Blockers

Neuromuscular blockers (NMBs) are one of the most frequently used classes of drugs in surgical suites. They are used primarily as an adjunct to general anesthesia to facilitate endotracheal intubation and to relax skeletal muscles during surgery. More recently, health care providers in intensive care units and emergency rooms have found them useful in managing respiratory problems. NMBs commonly are classified by type of block produced (depolarizing versus nondepolarizing), chemical structure (steroidal compound, acetylcholine derivative, isoquinoline derivative, or benzylisoquinolinium ester), or duration of action (ultra–short-acting, short-acting, intermediate-acting, or long-acting).

In essence, these drugs block the transmission of nerve impulses to muscle fibers (Fig. 18-2). They produce temporary paralysis of voluntary muscles, including muscles that control respirations. NMBs are given by IV route to facilitate intubation, relax muscles in the surgical field, ease laryngospasms, and relax muscles for controlled mechanical ventilation.

Succinylcholine

Succinylcholine (Anectine, Quelicin, Sucostrin) is the most commonly used depolarizing neuromuscular blocking drug. It is used to secure an airway emergently or under a rapid intubation sequence. It is also used for muscle relaxation during electroconvulsive therapy (ECT), endoscopy, and other short procedures.

Like acetylcholine (ACh), succinylcholine binds to cholinergic receptors at the motor endplate to produce depolarization. However, unlike ACh, succinylcholine remains receptor-bound for several minutes as a result of deactivation by acetylcholinesterase, and muscles do not respond to the subsequent release of ACh. After a few minutes, succinylcholine is biotransformed by plasma cholinesterase, and the postjunctional cholinergic membrane repolarizes. Repolarization and further muscle contractions are inhibited as long as adequate concentrations of drug remain at receptor sites. Histamine is released, which may contribute to hypotension. Like the nondepolarizing drugs, depolarizing drugs have no analgesic properties.

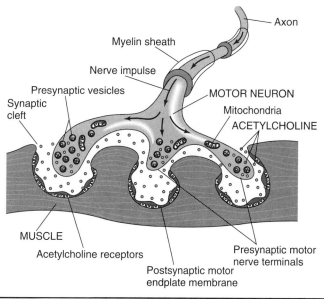

FIGURE 18-2 Neuromuscular Junction. Axon terminals of a motor neuron together with the motor endplate make up the neuromuscular junction.

Succinylcholine is well absorbed with IV administration, and widely distributed into extracellular fluid. It crosses the placenta in small amounts. Ninety percent of the drug is biotransformed by pseudocholinesterase in the plasma; 10% is eliminated unchanged in the kidneys.

Most adverse effects of succinylcholine are an extension of pharmacologic effects. The adverse effects include bronchospasm and apnea, hypotension, arrhythmias, bradycardia, hyperkalemia, tachyphylaxis, and muscle fasciculations. The risk of myoglobinemia and myoglobinuria is increased in children. MH is the most life-threatening adverse effect of succinylcholine.

Muscle fasciculations often result in postoperative myalgia. Neck, shoulder, and back pain are complained of by 10% to 75% of patients within 12 to 24 hours after administration of succinylcholine. The discomfort can persist for several hours or days. Succinylcholine is contraindicated in patients with hypersensitivity to the drug or hypersensitivity to parabens, and in patients with pseudocholinesterase deficiency. A continuous infusion of succinylcholine is contraindicated in children and neonates. Succinylcholine raises intraocular pressure and thus is absolutely contraindicated in patients with glaucoma.

A history of MH or pulmonary, renal, or liver impairment or of myasthenia gravis or myasthenic syndromes warrants cautious use of succinylcholine. It should also be used with caution in older adults or debilitated patients, patients with electrolyte disturbances, and patients receiving cardiac glycosides.

Concurrent administration of succinylcholine with cholinesterase inhibitors (e.g., echothiophate, isoflurophate, demecarium eye drops) reduces pseudocholinesterase activity and intensifies paralysis (Table 18-3). The intensity and duration of paralysis may be prolonged by pretreatment with general anesthetics, aminoglycoside antibiotics, cimetidine, polymyxin

DRUG INTERACTIONS
TABLE 18-3 Selected Anesthetics

Drug	Interactive Drug	Interaction
IV ANESTHETICS		
midazolam, propofol	Alcohol, antihistamines, antihypertensives, nitrates, Sedative-hypnotics	Additive CNS depression and increased risk of hypotension
midazolam	Calcium channel blockers, erythromycin, ketoconazole, itraconazole	Increases midazolam levels, sedation, respiratory depression
NEUROMUSCULAR BLOCKERS		
succinylcholine	Aminoglycosides, Beta blockers, Cardiac glycosides, cimetidine, clindamycin, colistin, cyclophosphamide, Inhaled anesthetics, lidocaine, lithium, magnesium, Opioids, phenelzine, polymyxin B, Potassium-losing diuretics, procainamide, quinidine	Increases risk of cardiovascular reactions
INHALED ANESTHETICS		
Inhaled drugs	Alcohol, ketamine, nitrous oxide, tetrahydrocannabinol	Potentiates effects of inhaled anesthetics
	Alcohol, aminophylline, Amphetamines, Barbiturates, Benzodiazepines, cocaine, fentanyl, morphine, naloxone, sufentanil, Phenothiazines, tetrahydrocannabinol	Sensitizes myocardium to ventricular arrhythmias; raises level of hypercapnia required to stimulate ventilation; depresses ventilatory responses to hypercapnia; antagonizes effects of inhaled anesthetics

CNS, Central nervous system; *IV,* intravenous.

CENTRAL NERVOUS

B, colistin, clindamycin, lidocaine, quinidine, procainamide, beta blockers, lithium, cyclophosphamide, phenelzine, potassium-losing diuretics, and magnesium. There is an increased risk of adverse cardiovascular reactions with opioids or cardiac glycosides.

Succinylcholine dosing hinges on the reason for its use, with additional doses dependent on patient response. Avoid continuous IV infusion for children or neonates. For prolonged procedures in adults, the dose is titrated to patient response and the degree of paralysis required.

The sustained depolarization induced by succinylcholine is associated with potassium leakage from muscle. There is also a slight increase in serum potassium concentrations. In patients with recent burns, spinal cord injuries, and myopathies, however, succinylcholine can lead to sudden hyperkalemia and cardiac arrest.

Nondepolarizing Neuromuscular Blockers

▥ Indications

Nondepolarizing NMBs, such as those identified in Table 18-4, are used most often to produce muscle relaxation during endotracheal intubation and surgical procedures, and to facilitate mechanical ventilation. NMBs are used for intubation, because laryngeal stimulation is associated with reflex closure of the vocal cords and hypoxemia if the intubation is unsuccessful. NMBs also are used during intraabdominal and intrathoracic procedures to prevent reflex muscle contraction and to permit surgical exposure and effective wound closure. Reflex muscle responses can be suppressed by high concentrations of a volatile anesthetic, but this practice results in circulatory depression.

Some NMBs have been used as an adjunct during ECT for patients in status asthmaticus who need ventilatory assistance and in the management of tetanus, a potentially fatal bacterial

infection. Tubocurarine has been used to help diagnose myasthenia gravis.

▥ Pharmacodynamics

ACh must bind to nicotinic receptors for normal neuromuscular transmission to occur. Thus nondepolarizing NMBs compete with ACh at nicotinic receptors on the motor endplate. Muscle relaxation lasts as long as the quantity of drug at the neuromuscular junction is adequate to deter receptor occupation by ACh. Muscle strength can be restored by increasing the amount of ACh at the neuromuscular junction or by increasing elimination of the drug from the body.

Although nondepolarizing NMBs paralyze all skeletal muscles, the paralysis affects muscles in a predictable sequence. Small, rapidly moving muscles of the eyes, face, and neck are affected first. Muscles of the limbs, abdomen, and trunk are affected next, followed by intercostal muscles and the diaphragm. Muscle weakness rapidly progresses to flaccid paralysis in the absence of attention to patient response. Recovery from drug-induced paralysis occurs in reverse order from the induction sequence. NMB drugs have no analgesic properties.

▥ Pharmacokinetics

These drugs as a class are poorly absorbed from the gastrointestinal (GI) tract and therefore must be administered parenterally. Muscular paralysis develops in minutes after IV administration. Complete recovery may take several hours.

Pancuronium, vecuronium, and rocuronium are biotransformed in the liver. Atracurium and mivacurium are broken down in the plasma. The majority of NMB drugs are eliminated primarily in an unchanged form in the urine.

▥ Adverse Effects and Contraindications

The principal adverse effects of nondepolarizing NMBs are on the cardiovascular and respiratory systems. The underlying

PHARMACOKINETICS

TABLE 18-4 Selected Neuromuscular Blockers

Drugs	Onset	Time to Maximum Paralysis	Duration of Effective Paralysis*	Time to Spontaneous Recovery†	PB (%)	$t_{1/2}$
LONG-ACTING NONDEPOLARIZING DRUGS						
doxacurium (Nuromax)	5 min	4–10 min	100 min	Hours	UA	99 min
metocurine (Metubine Iodide)	1–4 min	6 min	25–90 min	Hours	55	3.6 hr
pipecuronium (Arduan)	2.5–3 min	3–5 min	60–120 min	Hours	UA	1.7 hr
tubocurarine	1 min	2–5 min	35–60 min	Hours	40–45	2 hr
INTERMEDIATE-ACTING NONDEPOLARIZING DRUGS						
atracurium (Tracrium)	2–2.5 min	5 min	30–40 min	60–70 min	82	20 min
cisatracurium (Nimbex)	1–2 min	5–7 min	20–60 min	60–70 min	UA	UA
gallamine (Flaxedil)	1–2 min	3–5 min	15–30 min	—	16	2.5 hr
pancuronium (Pavulon)	30–45 sec	3–4.5 min	35–45 min	60–70 min	15	2 hr
rocuronium (Zemuron)	1 min	1.8 min	30 min	13 min	30	1.4 hr
vecuronium (Norcuron)	1 min	3–5 min	15–30 min	45–60 min	27	31–80 min
SHORT-ACTING NONDEPOLARIZING DRUG						
mivacurium (Mivacron)	2.5 min	3.3 min	25 min	6–8 min	UA	2 hr
ULTRA–SHORT-ACTING DEPOLARIZING DRUG						
succinylcholine (Anectine, others)	0.5–1 min	1–2 min	4–10 min	—	UA	UA

PB, Protein binding; $t_{1/2}$, half-life; UA, unavailable.
*Duration of effective paralysis varies with dosage. Figures presented are for an average adult dose administered as a single intravenous (IV) injection.
†Spontaneous recovery from paralysis can take a long time. Recovery from nondepolarizing drugs may be accelerated by administering a cholinesterase inhibitor (see Chapter 15).

TABLE 18-5 Causes of Adverse Cardiovascular Effects*

Drugs	Histamine Release	Ganglionic Blockade	Vagolytic Activity
LONG-ACTING NONDEPOLARIZING DRUGS			
doxacurium	None	None	None
metocurine	Slight	Weak	None
pipecuronium	None	None	None
tubocurarine	Moderate	Weak	Decreased
INTERMEDIATE-ACTING NONDEPOLARIZING DRUGS			
atracurium	Slight	None	Minimal effect
cisatracurium	None	None	Minimal effect
gallamine	High dose only	None	Increased
pancuronium	Slight	None	Increased
rocuronium	None	None	Increased
vecuronium	None	None	None
SHORT-ACTING NONDEPOLARIZING DRUG			
mivacurium	Slight	None	Slight increase
ULTRA–SHORT-ACTING DEPOLARIZING DRUG			
succinylcholine	Slight	Stimulates	Increase or decrease

*Histamine release is related to the dose and the speed of administration. Cardiovascular effects can be lessened by minimizing the dose and increasing the intravenous (IV) administration time. The histamine response can be minimized by pretreating the patient with histamine$_1$ and histamine$_2$ antagonists.

physiologic mechanisms for the cardiovascular adverse effects are identified in Table 18-5.

Overadministration of drug, an accumulation of active metabolites, and end-organ damage or dysfunction can result in short-term persistent paralysis that lasts from hours to days. Paralysis of intercostal muscles and the diaphragm leads to respiratory arrest. Long-term persistent paralysis lasts from days to weeks and is characterized by muscle and nerve degeneration.

Contraindications to nondepolarizing NMBs include hypersensitivity to this class of drugs and to bromides (only pancuronium and vecuronium) and iodides or iodine (only gallamine and metocurine). Products containing benzyl alcohol should be avoided in neonates.

Nondepolarizing drugs must be used cautiously under many circumstances, including in patients with underlying cardiovascular disease (because of an increased risk of arrhythmias), dehydration, or electrolyte imbalance. Situations in which histamine release may occur (e.g., asthma, allergic conditions) could be problematic. Older adults and patients with impaired renal function (leading to decreased elimination of gallamine, metocurine, pancuronium, and tubocurarine) should be monitored closely. Hepatic disease reduces the biotransformation of vecuronium, and therefore the drug should also be used with caution. Shock related to prolonged paralysis from gallamine, metocurine, and tubocurarine has been noted.

Cautious use is also warranted in patients with low plasma pseudocholinesterase levels in association with anemia, dehydration, the use of cholinesterase inhibitors or insecticides, severe liver disease, or pregnancy. Extreme caution should be exercised when NMBs are used for patients with myasthenia gravis or myasthenic syndromes. A patient with myasthenia gravis, an autoimmune disorder characterized by antibodies to the nicotinic receptor, is extremely sensitive to nondepolarizing NMBs. Safe use during pregnancy or lactation or in children has not been established for most of these drugs.

Drug interactions with nondepolarizing drugs are many. Drug interactions may occur at the nerve terminal, the synapse, or the motor endplate, and sometimes at more than one site. Table 18-3 provides an overview of key interacting drugs. The intensity and duration of paralysis may be prolonged if the patient has been pretreated in some fashion with succinylcholine (see the discussion of depolarizing drugs), inhaled general anesthesia, aminoglycosides and certain other antibiotics, quinidine, procainamide, beta blockers, potassium-losing diuretics, and magnesium. Most NMBs are incompatible with barbiturates and sodium bicarbonate. High-dose antibiotics may intensify or produce neuromuscular blockade on their own. They should not be admixed with NMBs.

The majority of these drugs are dosed based on micrograms per kilogram (mcg/kg) or milligram per kilogram (mg/kg) of body weight. Standard dosing according to body weight alone often results in overadministration of NMBs. Maintenance doses in the operating room are guided by the use by the anesthesia provider of a nerve stimulator and are titrated to patient response. Many of the drugs can be administered by continuous IV infusion. The health care provider is cautioned to check dosage regimens closely before administering the drug.

Inhalational Anesthesia

The four stages of inhalational (i.e., general) anesthesia are known as Guedel's signs. The signs were described in 1920 based on observations of a patient receiving diethyl ether, which has a slow onset of central action owing to its high solubility in blood. The distinctive signs of each of the four stages are usually obscured by the relatively rapid onset of action of many IV and inhaled anesthetics compared with diethyl ether and the fact that respiratory activity is controlled mechanically with muscle relaxants. In addition, the use of other drugs during the preoperative or intraoperative period can also alter the clinical signs of anesthesia. Box 18-3 provides a summary of the four stages.

Pharmacodynamics

Inhalational anesthetics, such as those identified in Table 18-6, produce a dose-dependent CNS depression caused by

---

BOX 18-3

Stages of Inhaled General Anesthesia

- *Stage I anesthesia* (i.e., induction) depresses the cortical areas of the brain and is characterized by loss of response to verbal commands and loss of consciousness. The patient may be drowsy or dizzy, or may experience auditory or visual hallucinations.
- *Stage II anesthesia* (i.e., excitement) begins with loss of consciousness and extends through the loss of eyelid reflexes. There is a transient increase in autonomic nervous system activity, with hyperreflexia, random motor activity, exaggerated orotracheal reflexes, and irregular respirations. The patient may appear to struggle at this stage.
- *Stage III anesthesia* (i.e., surgical anesthesia) produces a profound depth of anesthesia. Neurologic depression provides a motionless patient. Respirations are shallow but regular, and there is no blink or gag reflex. Surgical stimuli fail to produce reflex motor withdrawal, and there are less intense cardiovascular, respiratory, and neuroendocrine responses. When surgery is complete and anesthesia withdrawn, the patient moves backward through each of these three stages.
- *Stage IV anesthesia* is characterized by even deeper and more profound anesthesia, evidenced by apnea and cardiovascular collapse. These signs reflect overdose and the toxic effects of high concentrations of potent inhalational drugs. Death rapidly ensues without full circulatory and respiratory support.

---

inhibiting synaptic transmission, with effects noted in the CNS, cardiovascular, respiratory, renal, hepatic, and GI systems and the uterus. There is a dose-dependent reduction in cerebral metabolism, with an increase in CBF and intracranial pressure. The degree of cerebral vasodilation varies with the specific drug, but the effects occur within minutes of administration. If necessary, an induced state of hypocapnia can be used to help prevent further increases in cerebral blood flow and intracranial pressure.

Inhaled anesthetics sensitize the heart to the dysrhythmic actions of catecholamines, increasing the risk of ventricular ectopy, tachycardia, or ventricular fibrillation. Halothane is more sensitizing than isoflurane, which, in turn, is more sensitizing than enflurane.

All inhaled anesthetics produce an effective bronchodilation in unconscious patients. In conscious patients, only halothane and sevoflurane are not irritating to the airways. The bronchodilation facilitates ventilation in patients with bronchospastic diseases. Further, because the drugs cause the laryngeal and pharyngeal reflexes to be obtunded, intubation is facilitated. However, the patient is at increased risk for aspiration and aspiration pneumonitis if gastric contents are present.

Inhaled anesthetics decrease renal blood flow and the glomerular filtration rate. This effect can be offset by adequate prehydration. There is also a dose-dependent reduction in hepatic blood flow. The greatest effect is noted with halothane.

The smooth muscle of the GI tract relaxes in the presence of inhaled anesthetics. The drugs decrease gastric, jejunal, and colonic motility. There is also a dose-dependent relaxation of uterine smooth muscle, which can result in uterine bleeding following delivery.

The combined use of inhalation anesthetics, opioids, benzodiazepines, anticholinergics, and muscle relaxants mask many of the signs of the depth of anesthesia. Although it is possible to monitor exhaled concentrations and thus site concentrations of inhalation drugs through mass spectrometry, it is not possible to routinely monitor plasma concentrations of IV drugs.

Sensory input obtained through the CNS can originate from somatic or visceral tissues. The patient must be conscious to perceive pain. Low concentrations of inhaled or IV anesthetics can eliminate recall or awareness of pain but still allow movement. The concentration of anesthetic required to eliminate somatic motor responses is higher than that needed to induce unconsciousness and eliminate perception of pain. The respiratory motor response to noxious stimuli can involve an increase in tidal volume and respiratory rate.

Although many advances have been made in the administration of anesthesia, the measurement of the depth of anesthesia is not precise. Depth of anesthesia is often measured by somatomotor reflexes or a change in those parameters controlled by the autonomic nervous system. When the somatomotor reflex is assessed, the patient moves away from the site of stimulation. Autonomic changes may include changes in cardiovascular or respiratory parameters. More elaborate but complex attempts to estimate the neuroendocrine response to pain can be made by analyzing plasma catecholamine

---

TABLE 18-6 Inhaled Anesthetics

Drug	Advantages	Disadvantages
desflurane (Suprane)	Decreased $CMRO_2$; uterine relaxation; rapid induction and emergence; no organ toxicity	Increased CBF; coughing; excitation during inhalation induction; trigger for MH; hypertension, arrhythmias; respiratory depression, apnea; nausea, vomiting, ileus
enflurane (Ethrane)	Decreased $CMRO_2$; bronchodilator; less myocardial sensitization to catecholamines; no coronary steal; uterine relaxant	Increased CBF; seizure activity on EEG; hypotension, arrhythmias; respiratory depression, apnea, nausea, vomiting; occasional renal dysfunction; trigger for MH
halothane (Fluothane)	Decreased $CMRO_2$; good induction agent for children; bronchodilator; uterine relaxant	Increased CBF, decreased BP, heart rate, arrhythmias; respiratory depression, apnea; nausea, vomiting, ileus; hepatic dysfunction; trigger for MH
isoflurane (Forane)	Decreased $CMRO_2$; uterine relaxation; no organ toxicity; less myocardial sensitization to catecholamines	Trigger for MH; coronary steal, hypotension, tachycardia; apnea or respiratory depression; nausea, vomiting, ileus
nitrous oxide	Amnesia and analgesia; rapid onset and recovery	Incomplete anesthetic; low potency, diffusion hypoxia, expansion in closed gas spaces; postoperative nausea and vomiting
sevoflurane (Ultane)	Decreased $CMRO_2$; rapid induction for emergencies; minimal respiratory irritation	Not stable in soda lime, biotransformed; trigger for MH; increased CBF

BP, Blood pressure; *CBF,* cerebral blood flow; *CMRO2,* cerebral metabolic rate of oxygen; *EEG,* electroencephalogram; *MH,* malignant hyperthermia.

concentrations or monitoring cerebral cortical electrical responses by electroencephalograph or specialized, evoked potentials. Esophageal motility measurements have been used to assess the adequacy of the depth of anesthesia. A relatively new development in measuring depth of anesthesia is a cerebral function monitor or bispectral index. Four electrodes are placed on the head, and ranges are reported on a digital readout. The bispectral index is illustrated in Box 18-4.

Pharmacokinetics

The term *pharmacokinetics* refers to the rate of change in an anesthetic's concentration within the body and its component organs, tissues, and fluids, as well as the drug's absorption, distribution, biotransformation, and elimination within the biologic system. The effectiveness of an anesthetic depends on the concentration at the effect site. The concentration or therapeutic window for IV anesthesia is determined by the plasma concentration and the biotransformation of the drug. In contrast, an inhaled anesthetic moves from a vaporizer outside of the body to within the body as a result of partial pressure differences between compartments. In the gas phase, which exists between the vaporizer and the alveoli, the anesthetic concentrations and the partial pressure are equal. However, once the anesthetic enters the circulation, the brain, and other tissues, concentration and partial pressure are a function of solubility.

Unopposed ventilation produces a very rapid change in alveolar concentration of an inhaled anesthetic. However, this effect is opposed by absorption or uptake of the anesthetic. The alveolar concentration that is obtained with a given anesthetic is the result of a balance between the delivery of

anesthetic by ventilation and the removal of anesthetic by absorption.

Uptake is the product of three factors: solubility, cardiac output, and the alveolar-to-venous anesthetic partial pressure difference. Solubility is defined by the blood-gas partition coefficient. The coefficient represents the capacity of the blood to hold anesthetic and determines the amount of anesthetic taken up by the blood. If cardiac output is large, uptake will be larger. Alveolar-to-venous anesthetic partial pressure difference is the driving pressure that pushes anesthetic from the alveoli into the blood. If the gradient is large, absorption will be large.

The arterial-to-venous partial pressure difference is a function of tissue absorption. Uptake of the anesthetic by tissues is determined by the same three factors that determine absorption from the lungs: solubility, cardiac output, and the alveolar-to-venous anesthetic partial pressure difference. Body tissues are divided into four groups: highly perfused (liver, brain, kidney, heart, endocrine glands), moderately perfused (muscle, skin), mildly perfused (fat and bone marrow), and poorly perfused (tendons, ligaments, bone). Absorption of an anesthetic is fastest in the highly perfused, vessel-rich group of tissues and slowest in the mildly and poorly perfused groups of tissues.

The anesthetic effect of inhalation anesthetics is achieved by inhalation of the drug, uptake by the blood, and delivery to target tissue sites within the nervous system. Although these drugs are usually added after an IV induction with a barbiturate (e.g., pentathol), some patients are anesthetized by inhalation of the vapor. Anesthetic requirements (i.e., percent concentration) for inhalation drugs are judged in terms of the *minimum alveolar concentration* (MAC). MAC is defined as the concentration of an anesthetic vapor (at 1 atmosphere) that prevents skeletal muscle movement in 50% of patients given a painful stimulus (e.g., surgical skin incision).

The determination of MAC is made only after the drug has evenly distributed itself throughout the body. Although MAC can serve as a guide for the required concentration, it is influenced by many physiologic and pharmacologic factors. The addition of nitrous oxide to inhaled drugs lowers the MAC, as does the addition of other CNS depressants. Table 18-7 lists other factors that alter the MAC.

In addition to MAC, there are two other, related terms that are important to understand. MAC-BAR represents the "minimum alveolar concentration" necessary to "block the adrenergic response" to skin incision. It can be expressed as either

---

BOX 18-4

Bispectral Index (BIS) Range Guidelines

BIS*	Clinical Endpoints and Sedation Range	Clinical Situation
100	Awake	• Awake or resting state; conscious-sedation • Response to vigorous stimulation during surgery • Emergence from general anesthesia
70	Light hypnotic effects	• Short procedures requiring deep sedation or light anesthesia • Very low probability of recall
60	Moderate hypnotic effects	• Maintenance range during general surgical procedures • Unconscious
40	Deep hypnotic effects	• High-dose opioid anesthesia • Procedures where deep anesthesia is required • Barbiturate coma • Profound hypothermia
0	EEG suppression	

*Table adapted from Aspect Medical Systems, Inc. (1996). *BIS range guidelines* (Appendix I) (p. 9). Natick, MA: Author. Used with permission.

NOTE: BIS values and ranges assume that the EEG is free of artifacts that can affect its performance, i.e., ECG and EMG artifacts.

ECG, Electrocardiogram; *EEG,* electroencephalogram.

TABLE 18-7 Factors Affecting MAC

Reduced MAC	Increased MAC	No Effect
Advanced age	Hyperthermia	Duration of anesthesia
Hypoxemia, hypothermia	Hyperthyroidism	Sex
Hypotension	ethanol (chronic)	Hypocapnia, hypercapnia
Pregnancy	Monoamine oxidase inhibitors	Hypertension
ethanol (acute), other CNS depressants		
Acidosis		

CNS, Central nervous system; *MAC,* minimal alveolar concentration.

MAC-BAR$_{50}$ or MAC-BAR$_{95}$. MAC-BAR values exceed the requirements for ablation of skeletal muscle movement with surgical stimulation. Blocking the adrenergic response requires a greater depth of anesthesia than preventing movement. The advantages and disadvantages of today's drugs are summarized in Table 18-6.

▥ Adverse Effects and Contraindications

Of the complications associated with anesthesia, aspiration, pulmonary dysfunction, and MH are among the most serious. Inhalation of gastric fluid or gastric contents fluid in patients with depressed airway reflexes may result in aspiration pneumonitis or airway obstruction. The effects range from undetectable changes in respiratory status to sudden death, depending on the amount aspirated and its acidity. The reported incidence of aspiration pneumonitis is about 1.4 to 6 per 10,000 patients, although 40% to 80% of patients scheduled for elective surgery may be at risk based on gastric pH and volume. Patients with gastroesophageal reflux disease (GERD) are at a greater risk, as are the following: obese patients; patients with diabetes, peptic ulcer disease, stress or pain, or trauma; patients who have been premedicated with an opioid; ambulatory surgery patients; older adults; children; and pregnant women. The risk is also higher than average for patients undergoing emergency esophageal, upper abdominal, and emergency laparoscopic surgery. The effects tend to be more severe if the pH of gastric contents is less than 2.5 and the volume is greater than 0.4 mL/kg of body weight.

The clinical signs of aspiration include tachypnea, wheezing, bronchospasm, tachycardia, hypotension, hypoxia, and pulmonary edema. The chest x-ray study may show lobar consolidation, but an immediate change may not be noted. Arterial blood sampling generally reveals a low PaO$_2$.

Treatment of aspiration pneumonitis involves correction of arterial hypoxemia with supplemental oxygen. Tracheal intubation and positive-pressure ventilation with end-expiratory pressure may be required if hypoxemia persists despite supplemental oxygen administration. Bronchoscopy may be required to remove the foreign material, and bronchodilators may be required for poor pulmonary compliance. Treatment with steroids remains controversial, and antibiotics are recommended only if sputum cultures indicate development of a bacterial infection.

Postoperative pulmonary dysfunction may be due to hypoventilation. Residual effects of anesthetics in the absence of respiratory stimulation and poor patient positioning may lead to inadequate ventilatory drive. Residual neuromuscular blockade may also be responsible. Supplemental oxygen, reversal of drug effects or intubation, and positive-pressure ventilation may be required.

MH is a life-threatening disorder of skeletal muscle that is believed to be due to decreased calcium reuptake by the sarcoplasmic reticulum with increased resting intracellular calcium levels. It usually occurs within 30 minutes after induction of anesthesia. Although the classic case of MH most often occurs in the operating room, it can also occur within a few hours in the postanesthesia care unit.

The early symptoms of MH are characterized by unexplained increases in expired carbon dioxide concentration, hypoxemia, acidosis, tachypnea, cyanosis, hyperkalemia, unstable blood pressure (BP), and myoglobinuria. Tachycardia

is one of the first signs of MH. Muscle rigidity is usually seen first in the masseter muscles of the jaw and may occur in the chest or extremities. Elevation in body temperature is usually a late sign and results from a hypermetabolic state of the skeletal muscle. Body temperature elevation results in an oxygen consumption of 2 to 3 times normal. If MH is not treated, the temperature may rise 1° C every 5 minutes. Temperatures of 109° F to 111° F (42.8° to 44° C) have been reported. The patient develops a rosy, flushed appearance owing to the increased metabolism, which produces body heat. This heat causes vasodilation, and the skin may become mottled or cyanotic. There can be premature ventricular contractions or ventricular tachycardia on an ECG.

Susceptibility to MH is an autosomal dominant hereditary trait, which very often is initiated by a pharmacologic trigger, most often succinylcholine. The incidence of MH is estimated to be 1 in every 15,000 pediatric surgical cases and 1 in every 50,000 adult surgical cases. Approximately 50% of children of MH-susceptible parents are at risk. It is more frequent in males and in patients with muscular abnormalities such as ptosis, strabismus, and kyphoscoliosis. At one time, the mortality rate was 70%, but this has now decreased to 10% with early recognition and treatment with a drug called dantrolene (Dantrium). Dantrolene is discussed further in Chapter 23.

▥ Drug Interactions

There are many drug interactions with inhaled anesthetics (Table 18-3). Drugs that potentiate the effects of inhaled anesthetics and thus decrease the amount of anesthetic drug required include alcohol (in acute alcohol intoxication), ketamine, nitrous oxide, and tetrahydrocannabinol (marijuana). Aminophylline sensitizes the myocardium to ventricular arrhythmias when it is used in conjunction with an inhaled anesthetic. Opioids (e.g., morphine, fentanyl, sufentanyl) raise the level of hypercapnia required to stimulate ventilation, and sedative-hypnotics (e.g., benzodiazepines, barbiturates, phenothiazines) may depress the maximal ventilatory response to hypercapnia. Hypercapnia is the build-up of carbon dioxide in the blood.

Drugs that antagonize the effects of inhaled anesthetics and thus increase the amount of anesthetic required include the amphetamines, cocaine, and naloxone; chronic alcohol and chronic tetrahydrocannabinol intoxication have the same effect.

CLINICAL REASONING

Treatment Objectives

The objectives for anesthetic therapy center around relief of anxiety, sedation, amnesia, analgesia, little or no emesis, aspiration prophylaxis, reduction of oral secretions, facilitation of induction, and reduction of anesthesia requirements. Almost all therapeutic and diagnostic procedures performed will require analgesia; some will require both sedation and analgesia; a few will require sedation only.

Treatment Options

▥ Patient Variables

Many variables influence the patient's physiologic and psychologic response to surgery and general anesthesia. These variables include the patient's physical and mental state, the extent of disease and comorbid disorders, the magnitude of the specific procedure, and preoperative psychologic and physiologic preparations. When these variables are considered collectively, they reveal the degree of surgical risk. Fears that the patient may express concerning anesthesia should be addressed.

A preoperative assessment that begins with the patient's general state of health, concurrent drug use, and allergies should be elicited. For example, antibiotics (e.g., aminoglycosides), when used with some NMB drugs, increase the risk of postoperative respiratory depression. Antianxiety drugs lower blood pressure and increase the risk of shock. They also potentiate the effects of opioids and barbiturates. Thiazide diuretics contribute to potassium depletion. Chronic corticosteroid use impairs adrenal cortex function and thus impairs physiologic response to the stress of anesthesia and surgery. Antidepressants such as monoamine oxidase inhibitors can cause hypertensive crisis when combined with anesthetics. Antiparkinsonian drugs can cause hypotension or hypertension when combined with anesthetics. The use of illicit drugs and alcohol abuse increase the patient's tolerance to opioids.

Specific information about comorbid conditions, past surgical and anesthetic history, and, particularly, information about family history of MH should be elicited. Patient statements regarding a history of asthma and previous anesthesia problems in themselves or in family members are of special interest to the health care provider. Question the patient carefully about smoking habits and alcohol use. Serious neurologic conditions, such as uncontrolled epilepsy or severe Parkinson's disease, increase surgical risk.

LIFE-SPAN CONSIDERATIONS

Pregnant and Nursing Women. The physical changes of pregnancy have an impact on the choice of anesthesia techniques and drugs to be used. When using anesthesia in pregnant women, the objective is to provide maternal anesthesia without stimulating uterine activity or precipitating preterm labor. The choice of anesthesia should be made with the consideration of maintaining uteroplacental perfusion and preventing preterm labor.

In general, less anesthesia is required during a gravid state because of physiologic, anatomic, and hormonal changes associated with pregnancy. There is a more rapid loss of consciousness and protective airway reflexes at lower inspired concentration of IV and inhalation anesthetics. The nasal and respiratory tract mucosa becomes edematous and hyperemic during pregnancy, thus making intubation difficult. Furthermore, the pressure of the fetus on the stomach increases the risk of regurgitation and aspiration pneumonitis, thus patients should be premedicated with sodium bicitrate and a histamine$_2$ antagonist to decrease gastric acidity.

Halogenated gases decrease uterine resting tone, uterine muscle tension, and spontaneous uterine activity. Deep anesthesia can lead to significant decreases in maternal cardiac output and BP, leading to decreased uterine blood flow. Endogenous catecholamine release from inadequate general anesthesia or airway manipulation can also decrease uterine blood flow. Uterine blood flow is also reduced in the presence of ultra–short-acting barbiturate induction drugs. Neonatal depression can result from placental transmission of IV or inhaled drugs.

The objectives of anesthesia in the pregnant woman are the achievement of maternal anesthesia without stimulating uterine activity or precipitating preterm labor, as well as the maintenance of uteroplacental perfusion and prevention of preterm labor.

Children and Adolescents. Halothane was commonly used in pediatric patients because it could be given by mask, was well tolerated, was less pungent than some of the other drugs, and produced less airway limitation and laryngospasm. Sevoflurane for induction by mask has largely replaced halothane in the United States. Ketamine can be used and is particularly helpful in developmentally disabled children. Regional anesthesia is sometimes used as an adjunct to general anesthesia to provide for pain management during the postoperative period.

When intubation is used for infants, bradycardia results rather than the tachycardia commonly found in adults. Therefore, short procedures may be carried out using a mask rather than intubating the child. The bradycardic response is the response of a mature parasympathetic nervous system in the presence of an immature sympathetic innervation. Atropine is commonly used preoperatively in children to manage the bradycardia.

Older Adults. There are minimal physiologic alterations with regional anesthesia in the older adult. Regional anesthesia permits rapid recovery and postoperative analgesia. It also reduces the risk of cardiovascular complications and postoperative confusion. The effects of spinal anesthesia are prolonged in the older adult, and hypotension may be pronounced. In contrast, epidural anesthesia has less impact on BP and cardiovascular status. Musculoskeletal changes associated with aging may make administration of spinal anesthesia or epidural anesthesia difficult.

Inhalation requirements are lower in the older adult because MAC values decrease by 4% per year after age 40. However, drug biotransformation and clearance are delayed, necessitating lower doses of barbiturates, benzodiazepines, and opioids to be used. Moreover, the older adult is at risk of hypothermia owing to the decreased proportion of body fat. It may be difficult to ventilate an edentulous patient, and arthritis may restrict the cervicospinal region and inhibit intubation.

▥ Drug Variables

With increased national attention on health care and health care costs, anesthesia providers have had to become more conscious of their choice of anesthetic techniques and drugs. Compared with general anesthesia, regional or local anesthesia generally results in significant savings in hospital costs. This is in part due to shorter hospital stays and reduced need for critical care services. Significant savings are also achieved in the proper selection of anesthetic drugs.

The decision as to which type of anesthetic to use is made largely by the anesthesia provider (when appropriate) in consultation with the patient and the health care provider. The anesthetics to be used are determined with consideration of the following variables:

- Age of the patient, level of anxiety, and general physical condition
- Drug allergies and the presence of comorbid disease
- Physical status
- Patient preference (e.g., regional versus spinal versus general anesthesia)
- Patient history of previous adverse reactions to anesthesia

- Magnitude of specific surgical procedure and its duration
- Technical intricacies of the procedure
- Outpatient versus inpatient status

In choosing a local anesthetic drug and the appropriate concentration, the factors to be considered include the specific nerves to be blocked, the onset time or latency, and the required duration of action. Small nerves are in general much easier to block than large ones. Thus nerve endings and small cutaneous nerves are easily and quickly blocked by low concentrations of drugs given by infiltration. Large nerves with thick perineurium are much more difficult to block and require high drug concentrations. In general, motor fibers are the most difficult to block, followed by sensory and autonomic fibers in descending order. However, there is evidence that the small C fibers can be relatively resistant to local anesthetics.

All local anesthetics have a common molecular structure and a similar mechanism of action. There are many drugs available that differ to a greater or lesser extent in regard to potency, time to effect or latency, duration of effect, and toxicity. Thus the choice of drug will be primarily influenced by individual patient requirements. Clearly, the duration should outlast the operation or procedure. Thereafter, optimal duration will depend on the relative desirability of postoperative analgesia as opposed to a speedy return to full function. The duration of action of most local anesthetics varies from 30 minutes to 180 minutes or longer. Moreover, increasing the dose gives a longer duration of action. The duration can be increased by using a local anesthetic containing epinephrine. When very prolonged anesthesia is required, an indwelling catheter may be used and repeat injections of local anesthetic made as required.

Spinal anesthesia offers many advantages. First, it is relatively safe while providing excellent muscle relaxation. It does not cloud the patient's consciousness or alertness and can be used for patients who have recently eaten; this is advantageous because the patient will be awake to maintain the airway if vomiting occurs. However, spinal anesthesia can evoke several physiologic responses that result in complications if it is not properly managed.

Compared with spinal anesthesia, epidural anesthesia requires a larger dose of anesthetic, a larger needle for insertion, and a more subtle technique for entry into the appropriate space. The flexibility of the epidural route has advantages in a variety of surgical procedures. There is a decreased incidence of headache, and the segmental block can be focused on the area of the surgery. The onset of drug action is gradual and is associated with fewer hemodynamic changes than spinal anesthesia. Compared to inhalational anesthesia, the autonomic response is decreased.

The disadvantages of epidural anesthesia are that it cannot be used in patients with coagulopathy, sepsis, spinal anomalies, or elevated intracranial pressure, in patients who are hemodynamically unstable, or in patients with advanced respiratory disease. High blocks can weaken the cough reflex. Inadvertent puncture of the dura with a 17- to 18-gauge epidural needle can cause a postdural puncture headache. This headache is significant in about 50% of patients and can be incapacitating. Treatment is the same as that used for spinal headaches.

Absolute contraindications to the use of spinal or epidural anesthesia include patient refusal, infection at the puncture site, uncorrected hypovolemia, and coagulation or anatomic abnormalities. Relative contraindications to the use of spinal or epidural anesthesia include bacteremia, preexisting neurologic conditions, and patients receiving minidose anticoagulation therapy. Contraindications to peripheral nerve blocks include patient refusal or objection to being awake, local infection at the block site, coagulopathy, and preexisting peripheral vascular disease.

The relative safety of regional versus general anesthesia has been debated and remains a matter of controversy. Epidural anesthesia and analgesia appear to play a positive role in decreasing cardiovascular and pulmonary morbidity and the stress response. The incidence of thromboembolus is reduced, and there may be a reduction in blood loss as well with some regional techniques.

Most adults prefer an IV induction, whereas children may elect to be anesthetized by inhalation. The choice of induction drug is often made according to patient stability and the preference of the anesthesia provider. For example, ketamine or etomidate may be better tolerated than thiopental or propofol in a hypovolemic trauma patient. In contrast, ketamine would not be a choice in a stable patient with coronary artery disease because of its tendency to cause tachycardia. Tachycardia in these patients increases myocardial oxygen demand and decreases myocardial oxygen supply. These changes lead to myocardial ischemia.

The newer IV anesthetics (e.g., etomidate) are associated with rapid induction and emergence with minimal risk of organ toxicity. IV drugs also have a rapid onset and short duration, and can be used intraoperatively and postoperatively. Newer IV drugs have minimal cardiovascular effects, have no hepatic or renal toxicity, have less potential for MH, and are compatible with epinephrine. Further, IV drugs are not associated with pollution of the operating room by anesthetic gases.

The decision as to which anesthesia to use for maintenance is usually based on the route of administration. Inhalation drugs can be administered as the sole drug with 100% oxygen. Although newer induction drugs such as propofol are more expensive, they actually reduce overall hospital costs when used appropriately and when hospitals change protocols to permit earlier discharge.

Patient Education

The patient scheduled for any procedure requiring anesthesia must give informed consent before the procedure is performed. Teach patients to ask questions about anesthesia before surgical or diagnostic procedures where conscious sedation will be used. The questions may include those listed in Box 18-5.

The patient or legal guardian is to be informed about potential risks, complications, and anesthesia alternatives. Patients should be advised in general about the anesthesia technique to be used. The expected outcome and the likelihood that the chosen anesthetic will be effective should be addressed.

The procedure for obtaining signed consent varies from state to state and according to the policy of the health care agency. Emancipated minors (children who are younger than 18 but because of marriage or other circumstances are independent of the family) may give consent. Children under legal

---

BOX 18-5

Questions to Ask Before Anesthesia

- Will a well-educated, skilled health care provider be dedicated to monitoring me during conscious sedation?
- Will this health care provider monitor my breathing, heart rate, and blood pressure?
- Will oxygen be available, and will the oxygen content of my blood be monitored?
- Are personnel who will be present educated in advanced cardiac life support?
- Is resuscitation equipment immediately available and accessible on-site in the event of an emergency?
- Will a trained and skilled provider stay with me during my recovery period and, if so, for how long?
- Should a friend or family member take me home, or can I drive myself?

American Association of Nurse Anesthetists. *Conscious sedation: What patients should expect.* Available online: www.anesthesiapatientsafety.com/patients/safety/sedation.asp. Accessed March 24, 2007.

---

age (18 in most states) who are not emancipated must have consent from their parents or legal guardian. In some cases, a court order may be needed to permit the use of anesthesia and surgery to take place.

Advise patients who are receiving regional anesthesia that the sensation and movement in the area will return once the effects of the drug have worn off.

Reassure patients receiving general anesthesia that their vital physiologic functions will be continually monitored until the effects of the drugs have dissipated. They will be kept warm and have their BP, heart rate, oxygenation status, and comfort level monitored.

Evaluation

The evaluation of local anesthetic effectiveness is determined most often simply by patient statements that there is no sensation in the area. Optimal conscious sedation and analgesia is achieved when the following can be said of the patient:

- Is not anxious or afraid
- Maintains consciousness
- Independently maintains his or her airway
- Retains protective reflexes (swallow and gag)
- Responds to physical and verbal commands
- Is cooperative during the procedure
- Has minimal changes in vital signs
- Experiences acceptable pain relief
- Has mild amnesia for the procedure
- Recovers to preprocedure status safely and promptly

The effectiveness of inhaled anesthesia is demonstrated by a patient who has a rapid induction, adequate sedation, amnesia, and analgesia for the procedure, a reduction of oral secretions, little or no emesis or aspiration, and a reduction in anesthesia requirements.

Essential requirements are vigilance by the health care provider and the ability on the part of individuals administering sedation and analgesia to recognize and intervene in the event that complications or undesired outcomes arise. The key to effective anesthesia is the use of appropriate techniques and anesthetic levels for the procedure and rapid emergence free of complications.

KEY POINTS

- Local anesthesia includes topical anesthesia, local infiltration, field block, peripheral nerve block, spinal or epidural anesthesia, and IV regional anesthesia.
- Regional anesthesia produces a loss of painful sensation in only one region of the body by blocking painful stimuli at their origin, along the afferent neurons, or along the spinal cord.
- IV anesthetics are used for rapid induction, with unconsciousness occurring about 30 seconds after the initial IV administration. IV anesthesia is most commonly used for induction before inhaled drugs are used.
- Inhaled anesthesia produces widespread depressive effects of the CNS. This physiologically altered state classically results in hypnosis, analgesia, amnesia, and muscle relaxation.
- Inhaled anesthesia produces a dose-dependent CNS depression with effects noted in the CNS, cardiovascular, respiratory, renal, hepatic, and GI systems and the uterus.
- The most serious complications of general anesthesia are aspiration pneumonitis, pulmonary dysfunction, and malignant hyperthermia.

- Drugs used for general anesthesia include barbiturates, nonbarbiturates, opioid agonists, opioid agonist-antagonists, antagonists, and liquid and gaseous inhalation agents.
- There are many drug interactions with inhaled anesthetics. Drugs that potentiate the effects of inhaled anesthetics require decreased amounts of the anesthetic drug. There are also drugs that antagonize the effects of inhaled anesthetics and thus increase the amount of anesthetic required.
- Treatment objectives for anesthetic therapy include relief of anxiety, sedation, amnesia, analgesia, little or no emesis, aspiration prophylaxis, reduction of oral secretions, facilitation of induction, and reduction of anesthesia requirements. When using anesthesia in the pregnant woman, the objective is to provide maternal anesthesia without stimulating uterine activity or precipitating preterm labor, while maintaining uteroplacental perfusion.
- Anesthesia effectiveness includes use of appropriate techniques and anesthetic levels for the procedure and rapid emergence free of complications.

Bibliography

Bahn, L., and Holt, K. (2005). Procedural sedation and analgesia: A review and new concepts. *Emergency Medical Clinics of North America, 23*(2), 503–517.

Bridenbaugh, P. (2005). Office-based anesthesia: Requirements for patient safety. *Anesthesia Progress, 52*(3), 86–90.

Brown, T., Lovato, L., and Parker, D. (2005). Procedural sedation in the acute care setting. *American Family Physician, 71*(1), 85–90.

Hardman, J., Limbird, L., and Gilman A. (Eds.). (2001). *Goodman and Gilman's the pharmacologic basis of therapeutics.* (10th ed.). New York: McGraw-Hill.

Katzung, B. (2004). *Basic and clinical pharmacology.* (9th ed.). New York: Lange Medical Books/McGraw-Hill.

Kleiber, C., Sorenson, M., Whiteside, K., et al. (2002). Topical anesthetics for intravenous insertion in children: A randomized equivalency study. *Pediatrics, 110*(4), 758–761.

Kundu, S., and Achar, S. (2002). Principles of office anesthesia: Part I. Infiltrative anesthesia. *American Family Physician, 66*(1), 91–95.

Kundu, S., and Achar, S. (2002). Principles of office anesthesia: Part II: Topical anesthesia. *American Family Physician, 66*(1), 99–102.

Michelsen, L., and Hug, C. (1996). The pharmacokinetics of remifentanil. *Journal of Clinical Anesthesia, 8*(8), 679–682.

Salem, G. (2004). Regional anesthesia for office procedures: Part II. Extremity and inguinal area surgeries. *American Family Physician, 69*(4), 896–900.

Schilling, C., Bank, D., Borchert, B., et al. (1995). Tetracaine, epinephrine [adrenalin], and cocaine [TAC] versus lidocaine, epinephrine, and tetracaine [LET] for anesthesia of lacerations in children. *Annals of Emergency Medicine, 25*(2), 203–208.

Waring, T., Baron, T., Hirota, W., et al. (2003). Guidelines for conscious sedation and monitoring during gastrointestinal endoscopy. *Gastrointestinal Endoscopy, 58*(3), 317–322.

19

Antianxiety and Sedative-Hypnotic Drugs

The universal human emotion called *anxiety* is experienced along a spectrum of intensity. At one end of the spectrum is mild apprehension, which produces increased awareness and anticipation, such as a runner might experience before a race. At the other extreme, however, anxieties block awareness of surroundings, cloud judgment, and can lead to panic with complete disintegration of coping abilities. Anxiety arises from many sources. It can be a normal reaction to stress, the adverse effect of drugs or disease processes, or a distinct psychologic condition (Box 19-1).

Anxiety and impaired sleep patterns are common complaints, and the drugs used for treatment widely prescribed. Emotionalism (i.e., the tendency to display emotion freely or to rely on or place too much value on emotion; an undue display of emotion) and anxiety are common enemies of sleep and the most common cause of impaired sleep patterns. The distinction between antianxiety (i.e., anxiolytic, minor tranquilizer), sedative, and hypnotic drugs is most often a matter of dosage. Some drugs relieve anxiety in low doses but induce sleep at higher doses. Therefore a single drug can be considered an anxiolytic at one extreme and a hypnotic at the other.

Among the many neural signals involved in regulation of levels of arousal, including anxiety and sleep, are the neurotransmitters gamma aminobutyric acid (GABA) and serotonin (5-hydroxytryptamine, or 5-HT). Receptors for these substances are found in the cell membranes of neurons in regions of the central nervous system (CNS) associated with these functions. Therefore, drugs acting at receptors for GABA or serotonin have important effects on anxiety and sleep. *Sedation* refers to a state of calm and reduced activity, and drugs that cause it are called *sedatives*. Sedation is generally accompanied by relief of anxiety, termed an *anxiolytic* effect. The medical term for sleep is *hypnosis* (not to be confused with the stage-show phenomenon), and drugs that induce or facilitate sleep are called *hypnotics*. Drugs that produce any of these effects are called sedative-hypnotics; those used in the treatment of anxiety are called *anxiolytics*.

ANXIETY, SLEEP, AND OTHER DISORDERS

EPIDEMIOLOGY AND ETIOLOGY

Anxiety

Anxiety has no gender, social, or economic boundaries, although it tends to be more common in women. Common to the shared human experience, this emotion arises from many sources. As has been previously stated, anxiety is experienced along a spectrum of intensity from a mild adaptive response to the environment to a severe, disabling disease condition. The health care provider must determine both the severity and the etiology of the anxiety to provide proper treatment. An anxiety disorder is defined as an illness that prevents an individual from coping and that can disrupt daily life. Although the anxiety arising from the stresses of everyday life is not an indication for treatment with drugs, anxiety disorders often are. The various anxiety disorders and their characteristic elements are identified in Table 19-1. Table 19-2 identifies the various levels of anxiety.

Approximately 7 million Americans are estimated to have *generalized anxiety disorder (GAD)*. This disorder is one of chronic and exaggerated worry and tension persisting for more than 6 months and without a recognized cause. People with this disorder are unable to relax and have trouble falling or staying asleep. They may have physical symptoms such as trembling, twitching, muscle tension, headaches, irritability, sweating, or hot flushes. They are easily startled and may have frequent urination or defecation. The overall impairment associated with GAD is usually mild; people with this disorder do not feel restricted in social situations or in their jobs. The disorder commonly begins in childhood or adolescence. It is more common in women than in men and tends to run in

---

BOX 19-1

Causes of Anxiety and Insomnia

Diseases or Conditions
- Angina
- Arrhythmias
- Asthma
- Chronic obstructive pulmonary disease
- Chronic painx, fatigue
- General anxiety disorder
- Heart failure
- Hyperthyroidism
- Hypoglycemia
- Hyponatremia
- Irritable bowel syndrome
- Liver failure
- Migraine headaches
- Mitral valve prolapse
- Myocardial infarction
- Obsessive compulsive disorder
- Gastroesophageal reflux disease
- Panic disorders
- Phobias
- Posttraumatic stress disorder
- Rheumatic disorders
- Seizure disorders

Drugs
- Amphetamines
- Anticholinergics
- caffeine
- cocaine
- Corticosteroids
- ephedrine
- epinephrine
- Hallucinogens
- levodopa
- pseudoephedrine
- theophylline
- Thyroid hormones

TABLE **19-1 Elements of DSM-IV-TR–Defined Anxiety Disorders**

Disorder	Symptoms
Panic disorder (with or without agoraphobia): A discrete period of intense fear or discomfort, in which four (or more) of the symptoms listed in next column developed abruptly and reached a peak within 10 minutes	Palpitations or rapid heart rate Diaphoresis, chills or hot flushes Tremors Sensations of shortness of breath or smothering Choking sensation Chest pain or discomfort Nausea or abdominal distress Dizziness, unsteadiness, lightheadedness, or faintness Feelings of unreality (derealization) or of being detached from oneself (depersonalization) Fear of losing control or going crazy; fear of dying Paresthesias
Agoraphobia (without panic disorder): Anxiety about being in places or situations from which escape might be difficult (or embarrassing), or in which help may not be available in the event of having an unexpected or situationally predisposed panic attack or paniclike symptoms	Recurrent unexpected panic attacks (see above) At least one of the attacks was followed by 1 month (or more) of the following: 　Persistent concern about having additional attacks 　Worry about the implications of the attack or its consequences 　Significant changes in behavior related to the attacks 　Attacks are not related to the direct physiologic effects of a substance (e.g., drug of abuse) or a general medical condition (e.g., hyperthyroidism)
Social phobia: A marked and persistent fear of one or more social or performance situations in which the person is exposed to unfamiliar people or to scrutiny of others	Immediate anxiety when confronted by stimulus Persistent fear of public scrutiny Awareness that the fear may be unreasonable
Specific phobia: A marked and persistent fear that is excessive and unreasonable, cued by the presence or anticipation of a specific object or situation (insects, flying, tight spaces, seeing blood) Formerly known as simple phobia	Immediate anxiety if stimulus is present Avoidance of situations if stimulus is present or anticipated Persistent fear of a discrete stimulus
Obsessive-compulsive disorder: *Obsessions:* Recurrent and persistent thoughts, impulses, or images experienced at some time during the disturbance as intrusive and inappropriate and that cause marked anxiety or distress *Compulsions:* Repetitive behaviors or mental acts that the person feels driven to perform in response to an obsession, or according to rules that must be applied rigidly	Intentional, repetitive behaviors that help to block or blunt the anxiety of obsessive thoughts Compulsive acts are disruptive, time-consuming, and usually unwanted 　Resisting the compulsion causes further anxiety
Posttraumatic stress disorder (PTSD): Person experienced, witnessed, or was confronted with an event or events involving actual or threatened death or serious injury, or a threat to the physical integrity of others	Ability to function normally is greatly impaired Intense anxiety surrounding recollection of event Often related to death of others or imminent threat of death to self Person had an experience outside range of usual human experience Intrusive and unwanted recollections of the event Nightmares and sleep disturbances Thoughts or situations related to the event vigorously avoided
Generalized anxiety disorder (GAD): Excessive anxiety and worry occurs more days than not for at least 6 months, regarding two or more life circumstances, events, or activities	Person finds it difficult to control the worry (e.g., personal safety, finances) Restlessness or feeling keyed up or on edge Easily fatigued Difficulty concentrating or mind going blank Irritability Muscle tension Difficulty falling or staying asleep, or restless unsatisfying sleep
Anxiety (not otherwise specified)	Anxiety present but does not fit into specific category

Data from the American Psychiatric Association. (2000). *Quick reference to the diagnostic criteria from DSM-IV-TR.* Washington, DC: Author.

families. The symptoms tend to diminish with age, although they can affect the patient's quality of life and relationships.

Panic Attack

An extreme variant of anxiety is seen in *panic disorder*, a sudden episode of terror that happens more than twice. A panic attack can occur with any anxiety disorder but is characterized by chest pain, heart palpitations, shortness of breath, dizziness, feelings of unreality, and fear of dying. These attacks usually come on abruptly and last from 2 to 10 minutes. The person may develop a phobia (see next section) based on where the attacks have occurred—for instance, an elevator. Depression and alcoholism are other conditions that may accompany panic disorder. Women are more commonly affected than men, and the condition usually begins in young adults, although it can appear at any age. It is estimated that between 3 and 6 million Americans have panic attacks. Patients ordinarily seek treatment for panic attacks when the attacks are affecting the patient's quality of life and social and occupational functioning.

Phobias

A *phobia* is any fear experienced to an intense and irrational degree. *Agoraphobia* is the extreme state of panic disorder and occurs in about one third of cases. In agoraphobia the individual fears being in any situation that might provoke a panic attack and may be housebound as a result. Phobias can be very specific so that a certain object or situation is feared, such as flying, confining spaces, specific animals, or

TABLE 19-2 Signs and Symptoms of Anxiety

Anxiety Level	Characteristics of Anxiety Level
Mild anxiety	Appears calm Perceptual field broadens; perceptual abilities intensified Learning and critical thinking abilities enhanced Able to connect feelings, thoughts, and actions Focuses on present problems; cause-and-effect relationships identified
Moderate anxiety	Appears tense and restless Perceptual field narrows; perceptual abilities restricted to immediate situation Able to attend to stimuli if they are pointed out Alertness reaches its highest, most efficient level Uses ego defense mechanisms
Severe anxiety	Appears tense with increased respirations, blood pressure, and pulse Perceptual field significantly reduced Learning and critical thinking abilities reduced Unable to connect feelings, thoughts, and actions Able to focus on small aspect of problem of environment Behaviors directed at immediate relief of anxiety
Panic level	Demonstrates symptoms of helplessness, hopelessness, rage Behaviors directed at gaining or maintaining control Perceptual field distorted; details scattered, spinning Physiologic response includes hypertension, and hyperventilation is possible Learning and critical thinking abilities nonexistent

water. Specific phobias affect about 1 in 10 persons. Childhood phobias are common and usually outgrown. Phobias that persist usually begin in adolescence or adulthood, and only about 20% disappear with time.

Social phobia, a discrete form of *social anxiety*, is a fear of being painfully embarrassed in a social setting. People with social phobia see themselves as incompetent in public. Fear of public speaking is a common social phobia. Some social phobias involve fear of specific public areas, such as restrooms, restaurants, or public phones. It is important to differentiate between social phobias and having a shy personality.

Obsessive-Compulsive Disorder

Obsessive-compulsive disorder (OCD) affects 1 in 50 people, occurring equally in men and women. OCD is characterized by anxious thoughts (obsessions) and rituals (compulsions) that cannot be controlled; the behaviors are performed in an effort to relieve anxiety about the obsession. The anxious thoughts include persistent and unwelcome images, and the rituals are driven by an urgent need to perform repetitive acts over and over. Most people have some behavior patterns that are necessary for comfort. However, when rituals become distressing, take 1 hour or more a day, and interfere with daily life, they are viewed as constituting OCD. OCD usually begins in teens or early adulthood, but about one third of cases begin in childhood. The progression of OCD is highly variable. It may increase or decrease over time and can be accompanied by depression or other anxiety disorders.

Posttraumatic Stress Disorder

Posttraumatic stress disorder (PTSD) is a disabling condition that can follow a terrifying event. Memories of the ordeal come flooding back, with persistent frightening thoughts and nightmares, leaving the individual emotionally numb even to loved ones. Events that lead to PTSD include war, kidnapping, rape or other violent personal attacks, and serious accidents or natural disasters. In many cases, traumatized persons have flashbacks. Individuals who develop PTSD experience the symptoms for more than 1 month beginning within 3 months of the trauma. PTSD can occur at any age, including childhood. Between 5 and 6 million Americans are believed to have PTSD. Persons with this disorder may also abuse alcohol or other substances and be depressed or anxious. Some substance abuse is an attempt to "self-medicate," and some is the result of a separate substance abuse disorder, a symptom of a comorbid condition, or both. Severe symptoms include easy irritability and violent outbursts so that the individual cannot have a normal social life or hold a job.

Sleep Disorders

If fear, anxiety, and panic are at one end of the scale of physiologic states of arousal for humans, sleep is at the other end of this scale. Sleep is defined as a period of rest in which physiologic activities and consciousness are diminished and voluntary physical activity is absent. As with fear and anxiety, sleep is a normal physiologic response. Unlike anxiety, however, sleep is a necessary part of the usual cycle of daily living. Sleep is thought to result from decreased activity in the reticular-activating system, which consists of neuronal pathways in the brainstem and midbrain where incoming signals from the senses (light, sound, smell, touch, taste, and balance) and viscera are collected, processed, and passed on to higher brain centers. Typically sleep occupies about 8 hours of a 24-hour day, although persons may differ widely in the normal amount of sleep required. Sunlight is a major factor that sets the biologic clock for sleep.

Normal sleep has two major components: rapid eye movement (REM) sleep and non-REM (NREM) sleep. *REM sleep* is characterized by fast brain waves, eye movements, and metabolic and temperature changes. The body is physiologically active during REM sleep, so the heart rate is increased, breathing is irregular, stomach acid is secreted, and the clitoris or the penis may become erect. However, muscles lose their tone during REM sleep, so only the mind and autonomic nervous system are active during this stage. Because dreaming occurs exclusively during REM sleep, this time is also called *dreaming sleep*. Some believe that during the REM sleep period, we integrate emotionally meaningful experiences. *NREM sleep* is subdivided into four stages based on brain wave patterns. REM and NREM sleep cycle over a 90- to 100-minute period with four to five periods of NREM sleep per sleep period (Box 19-2). Although REM sleep is associated with dreams, night terrors and sleep walking occur during NREM sleep. Older adults tend to spend less time in stages III and IV of NREM sleep, and they are more easily aroused by sounds. Children spend more total time in stages III and IV of NREM sleep. Box 19-2 summarizes the sleep stages.

Impaired sleep can result in many problems, ranging from an occasional "bad day" to complete disruption of family, work, and social activities. Many physiologic and psychologic changes occur as a result of sleep deprivation. Stress hormones from the adrenal cortex increase in the serum and contribute to the possibility of hallucinations. Reflexes slow, and

BOX 19-2

Summary of Sleep Stages

Stage	Characteristics	Percentage (%) of Time
Stage 1	*Light NREM:* Dreamlike state; lasts a few minutes	2%-5%
Stage 2	*Lighter NREM:* Fragmented thoughts, lasts 15–20 minutes	50%
Stage 3	*Deep NREM:* Cerebral metabolism of glucose, respiratory rate, heart rate, and blood pressure are reduced; starts 35–40 minutes after falling asleep; lasts 40–70 minutes	5%
Stage 4:	*Deeper NREM:* Very difficult to awaken person; may be very groggy when awakened; dreaming about daily events; sleepwalking or bedwetting may occur	10%-15%
REM sleep	Starts 90 minutes after falling asleep; lengthens towards the end of the night; cycles at intervals of 90–100 minutes, 4 to 6 times per night	25%-33%

NREM, Non–rapid eye movement, *REM,* rapid eye movement.

muscle coordination decreases. Equilibrium and muscle strength may be lost, with nystagmus and ptosis appearing. Respiratory efforts may diminish, and arrhythmias may appear. Sleep deprivation is associated with bizarre behavior and temporary neuroses or psychoses. Mental agility decreases, memory fails, attention span is limited, and sense of reality is distorted.

Although the body attempts to establish a normal equilibrium between REM and NREM sleep periods, deep sleep takes priority over dreaming sleep when there has been prolonged sleep deprivation. Deep sleep needs are met first, after which dreaming needs will be met. The outcomes of sleep deprivation can be relieved by 12 to 14 hours of sleep characterized by increased REM sleep periods. Ten days of such sleep are usually required to counteract 4 to 5 days of sleep deprivation.

▥ *Insomnia*

Insomnia is defined as the inability to either get to sleep, or to maintain sleep. Like anxiety, sleep problems do not appear to vary across countries, or cultures either. It is estimated that over one third of people in the United States have some form of sleep disorder. Persons of higher socioeconomic classes are more likely to seek and receive treatment, for insomnia than those of lower socioeconomic classes. However, there appears to be a preponderance of cases in lower socioeconomic groups. The female-to-male ratio for insomnia is 2:1.

Insomnia is a symptom of physical or mental distress that may be transient, short-term, or chronic. Of the reported cases the following is known:

- 30% to 35% are due to psychiatric illness
- 15% to 20% are psychophysiologic in nature (e.g., imbalances in neurotransmitters)
- 10% to 15% are due to alcohol or drug use, which may affect how patients are treated
- 10% to 15% are due to periodic limb movement disorder (i.e., restless leg syndrome)
- 5% to 10% are due to sleep apnea syndrome (e.g., obstructive sleep apnea, central sleep apnea).
- 5% to 10% are due to medical illness

Hospitalized patients commonly experience disrupted sleep both from their underlying illnesses or conditions and as a result of the treatments they must receive to alleviate their problems. The incidence of impaired sleep among hospitalized patients is reported to range from 27% to 76%. Impaired sleep may be secondary to situational and environmental stressors, associated with the illness itself, or related to preexisting health problems. In any case, the disorder disrupts sleep, and in turn, the decreased sleep worsens the disorder.

Sleep disorders are caused by sleep deprivation, a state in which overall sensory input is decreased, or by sensory overload, or both. With sensory deprivation, there is an overall reduction in stimuli. Patients respond by becoming more sensitive to the stimuli present around them. In contrast, sensory overload is defined as a state in which the degree and nature of sensory input exceed the patient's level of tolerance. Regardless of the cause, the patient is left distressed and in a state of hyperarousal with impaired cognition and problem-solving abilities.

Treatment of insomnia involves assessment of physical problems, drug use and history, and sleep habits (Box 19-3). Emotionalism and anxiety are common enemies of sleep and the most common cause of impaired sleep patterns. People who are depressed often awaken early and cannot go back to sleep. Chronic alcoholism, hyperthyroidism, heart or kidney failure, and pregnancy are commonly accompanied by insomnia. Pain of arthritis or muscle aches can make sleep difficult, as can respiratory problems and urinary tract problems. More than half of people older than 65 years of age have difficulty falling asleep or have excessive sleepiness during the day. Many drugs disrupt sleep, including decongestants and beta blockers and drugs used to treat high blood pressure.

PATHOGENESIS OF ANXIETY AND SLEEP DISORDERS

Three primary structures thought to play interactive roles in the generation of emotions are the reticular activating system, the limbic system, and the hypothalamus (Fig. 19-1). The reticular activating system is a network of neurons extending from the spinal cord through the medulla oblongata and the pons to the thalamus and the hypothalamus. It receives impulses from ascending sensory pathways, evaluates the significance of the impulses, and decides which impulses to transmit to the cerebral cortex. It excites or inhibits motor nerves controlling both reflex and voluntary movement. Stimulation of these neurons produces wakefulness and mental alertness, whereas depression causes sedation and loss of consciousness.

The receptors in these areas and other regions of the CNS are thought to constrain anxiety. It is believed that benzodiazepine (BZD) receptors located in the brain play a role to inhibit anxiety and moderate sleep. The inhibitory neuroregulator GABA has been studied in relation to its anxiety-inhibiting properties. BZD_1 receptors are thought to be involved with sleep

BOX 19-3

Sleep History Questions*

- What type of work do you do? Is there shift work involved? Which shift?
- What time are you getting to bed and getting up? Are there variations between weekdays and weekends? Any recent changes?
- What is the subjective quality of sleep (i.e., soundness, restorativeness)?
- How much daily sleep is needed to feel ideally alert and energetic throughout the day? Are drugs required?
- How often is that amount of sleep obtained, compared to the nightly average?
- What were your sleep habits during childhood and other major periods in life? What were the attitudes at home toward sleep? What was the subjective quality of sleep in those periods?
- Is there difficulty getting to sleep, staying asleep, or awakening earlier? If so, what is the effect on daily functioning? Are there daytime symptoms related to poor sleep? Is so, what?
- Is sleepiness during waking hours a problem? Is the problem worsening? Is it impossible to resist falling asleep during the day? Are there episodes of muscle weakness with laughter? Snoring? Intermittent period of snoring or gagging? Leg movements in sleep? Any other troublesome events in sleep?
- Do you take a daytime nap? If so, how long?
- What is the likelihood of dozing while reading? Watching TV? Sitting, inactive, in public place? As a passenger in car for 1 hour without a break? Sitting and talking with someone? After lunch? Stopped in traffic?
- What drugs or alcohol is used before 6 PM? After 6 PM?
- When do you exercise? If you don't, why?
- Any general emotional and physical problems? How are these treated?
- What are your sleep hygiene practices? Bathing? Eating before bedtime? Drinking before bedtime? Bed and pillow comfort? Sleep environment? Room temperature? Noise level? Light? TV or computer in bedroom?

*Adapted from the National Institutes of Health, National Heart, Blood, and Lung Institute, National Center on Sleep Disorders Research. (2006). Guide to selected publicly available sleep related data resources. Available online: www.nhlbi.nih.gov/about/ncsdr/research/sleep-datasets-july-06.pdf. Accessed March 28, 2007; Bailes, S., Libman, E., Baltzan, M., et al. (2006). Brief and distinct empirical sleepiness and fatigue scales. *Journal of Psychosomatic Research, 60*(6), 605–613; and Johns, M. (1991). A new method for measuring daytime sleepiness: the Epworth Sleepiness Scale. *Sleep, 14*(6), 540–545.

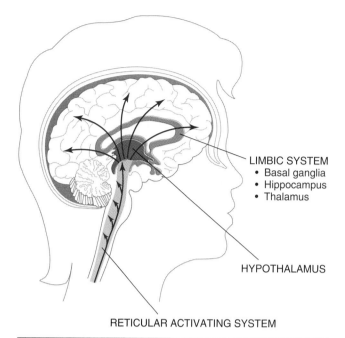

FIGURE 19-1 Structures of Emotion. Three primary structures thought to play interactive roles in the generation of emotions are the reticular activating system (RAS), the limbic system, and the hypothalamus.

Anxiety is a complex emotion and is experienced in many ways, because it has many origins; thus it must be properly diagnosed and categorized. The best management plans result when the health care provider has a complete understanding of the patient's diagnosis. The fourth edition of the *Diagnostic and Statistical Manual of Mental Disorders* (DSM-IV-TR) differentiates types of anxiety. In the structure of the DSM-IV, anxiety is viewed in one of four ways: as the primary problem, as the result of a situation, as resistance to thoughts, or as the reliving of a traumatic event. Proper diagnosis of the patient with an anxiety disorder allows the health care provider to initiate a therapeutic plan with the proper goals.

PHARMACOTHERAPEUTIC OPTIONS

Benzodiazepines

SHORT- TO INTERMEDIATE-ACTING BENZODIAZEPINES

- alprazolam (Xanax); ♣ Apo-Alpraz, Novo-Alprazol, Nu-Alpraz
- clonazepam (Klonopin); ♣ Rivotril
- lorazepam (Ativan); ♣ Apo-Lorazepam, Novo-Lorazem
- oxazepam (Serax); ♣ Apo-Oxazepam, Novoxapam, Oxpam, Zapex
- temazepam (Restoril)
- triazolam (Halcion); ♣ Apo-Triazo, Gen-Triazolam, Novo-Triolam, Nu-Triazol

LONG-ACTING BENZODIAZEPINES

- chlordiazepoxide (Librium, Libritabs, Mitran); ♣ Apo-Chlordiazepoxide
- clorazepate (Tranxene); ♣ Apo-Clorazepate, GenXene, Novo-Clopate
- diazepam (Valium); ♣ Apo-Diazepam, Diazemuls, Vivol
- estazolam (Prosom)
- flurazepam (Dalmane); ♣ Apo-Flurazepam, Novo-Flupam, Somnol

BENZODIAZEPINE-LIKE DRUGS

- eszopiclone (Lunesta)
- zaleplon (Sonata)
- zolpidem (Ambien)

mechanisms. BZD$_2$ receptors are associated with cognitive, memory, and sensory functions.

The limbic system of the brain involves the thalamus, the hypothalamus, the basal ganglia, and other structures. The function of the limbic system is to regulate emotions, such as pleasure, fear, anger, and sadness. It also regulates behaviors such as aggression, laughing, and crying. Physiologic changes in blood pressure, heart rate, respiration, and hormone secretion occur in association with emotions and behaviors.

The hypothalamus has extensive neuronal connections with higher and lower levels of the CNS and the pituitary gland. It continually collects information about the internal environment of the body, helping to maintain homeostasis by making physiologic adjustments in cardiovascular and gastrointestinal systems, levels of fluid and electrolytes, endocrine functions, and other body systems.

Indications

Benzodiazepines (BZDs) are widely used for both their sedative effects in the treatment of diverse anxiety disorders and for their hypnotic effects in the treatment of insomnia. Table 19-3 provides a listing of Food and Drug Administration (FDA)–approved uses of BZDs. The most frequently prescribed drugs in this class are lorazepam and alprazolam (see Evidence-Based Pharmacotherapeutics).

Pharmacodynamics

BZDs have a characteristic chemical structure that increases the inhibitory action of GABA (Fig. 19-2). They do so by binding at the GABA receptor sites. In this way, the BZDs strengthen the inhibitory effects on neurons in the region of the brain that plays a role in fear, anxiety, and arousal. The result is muscle relaxation (spinal cord), antianxiety and emotional effects (limbic-cortex area), ataxia (cerebellum), and anticonvulsant activity (brainstem).

Eszopiclone, zolpidem, and zaleplon, though chemically unlike BZDs, are thought to act in a similar manner but at different subtypes of BZD receptors. Eszopiclone and zaleplon produces effects very similar to those of the BZDs. The (−)isomer of eszopiclone displays considerable activity at both alpha-1 and alpha-3 GABA receptor subtypes. This isomer has a 1000 times greater binding affinity for GABA$_A$ receptors than the (+)isomer. However, zolpidem appears to act through a different subset of receptors to cause BZD-like sedation but only weak muscle relaxation and antiseizure effects.

Pharmacokinetics

BZDs are administered by a variety of routes for different purposes and indications. Ordinarily the more rapidly absorbed the BZD, the more prompt and intense the onset of action (Table 19-4). The drug companies have played up the idea that BZDs should be separated on the basis of onset of action and short versus long half-lives. There is theoretical benefit in looking at them this way—especially the half-life issue and the older adult population (see Life-Span Considerations section).

Some parenterally administered BZDs are highly lipid-soluble and therefore are widely distributed in body tissues, easily crossing the blood-brain barrier to be widely distributed in the CNS. With repeated dosing, the drugs accumulate in body fluids and tissues. Saturation of storage sites permits greater serum concentrations and longer durations of action. The accumulation of drug in storage sites also accounts for the prolonged action of BZDs after they have been discontinued.

TABLE 19-3 FDA-Approved Uses for Antianxiety-Sedative–Hypnotic Drugs

Drugs	Anxiety	Insomnia	Alcohol Withdrawal	Seizure Disorder	Muscle Spasm	Preop Med	Panic Disorder
SHORT-TO INTERMEDIATE-ACTING BZDS							
alprazolam		X					X
clonazepam	X			X			X
eszopiclone		X					
lorazepam	X	X	X	X		X	X
oxazepam	X		X				
temazepam		X					
triazolam		X					
zaleplon		X					
zolpidem		X					
LONG-ACTING BZDS							
chlordiazepoxide	X		X			X	
clorazepate	X		X	X			
diazepam	X	X	X	X	X	X	X
estazolam		X					
flurazepam		X					
ATYPICAL ANXIOLYTIC							
buspirone	X						
OTHER SEDATIVE-HYPNOTICS							
chloral hydrate		X	X				
eszopiclone		X					
melatonin		X					
meprobamate	X						
ramelteon		X					
zaleplon		X					
zolpidem		X					
SHORT-ACTING BARBITURATES							
pentobarbital		X				X	
secobarbital		X		X		X	
INTERMEDIATE-ACTING BARBITURATES							
butabarbital	X	X				X	
LONG-ACTING BARBITURATES							
phenobarbital		X		X		X	

BZDs, Benzodiazepines; *FDA,* Food and Drug Administration.

EVIDENCE-BASED PHARMACOTHERAPEUTICS

Use of Antidepressants in the Treatment of Generalized Anxiety Disorder

■ Background

Anxiety disorders, such as general anxiety disorder (GAD), are prevalent in the United States, with antianxiety drugs (e.g., benzodiazepines and benzodiazepine-like drugs) the mainstay of treatment. Occurring in two thirds of patients, major depression is most common comorbid condition. Research done over the last 2 decades, however, suggests that antidepressants are as efficacious as antianxiety drugs in treating GAD (see also Chapter 20).

■ Research Article

Kapczinski, F., Lima, M., Souza, J., et al. Antidepressants for generalized anxiety disorder. *The Cochrane Database of Systematic Reviews.* 2003, Issue 2. Art. No. CD003592. DOI: 10.1002/14651858.CD003592.

Purpose

This study was undertaken to evaluate use and effectiveness of antidepressants for the treatment of GAD.

Design

Fifteen randomized, controlled studies of subjects with GAD were used for the metaanalysis. Nonrandomized studies containing subjects who had a dual diagnosis of GAD and another psychiatric syndrome were not included in the analysis.

Methods

Eight of the 15 trials used commonly accepted means for diagnosing GAD. Six trials were eliminated; two additional studies used open-label techniques but no control group; two studies included subjects with dual diagnoses; and one other study used subjects who were in the process of stopping long-term BZD therapy. One of the studies used children and adolescents diagnosed with GAD; these results were analyzed separately from the other analyses. Estimates of the relative risks, mean differences, and the numbers needed to treat (NNT) were included in the analyses. Subjects dropping out of the study or who died were shown as having no improvement.

Findings

Imipramine, venlafaxine, and paroxetine were found to be more efficacious than a placebo for the treatment of GAD. Five subjects need to be treated for one person with GAD to benefit from treatment using an antidepressant (NNT = 5.5). Subject numbers who were lost to follow-up did not differ between antidepressants.

Conclusions

Evidence suggests that certain antidepressants are well tolerated and efficacious compared with placebo in treating GAD. No evidence was found to conclude that certain antidepressants were superior to others in the treatment of GAD.

■ Implications for Practice

The studies examined in this study varied in terms of quality and methodology. Nonetheless, additional randomized, placebo-controlled trials evaluating antidepressants in the treatment of GAD should help to uncover which drugs should be used and for which patients. The efficacy of antidepressants in treating children and adolescents diagnosed with GAD should be explored.

Protein binding is reduced in patients with cirrhosis and renal insufficiency and in newborns, and these patients often have impaired biotransformation of BZDs as well, making a reduction in dosage important.

Chlordiazepoxide, clorazepate, diazepam, and flurazepam are transformed by the liver to active metabolites that have clinical effects beyond their stated duration of action. Patients with liver failure may not be able to transform the compounds, so this effect may not be seen in 100% of patients; the low protein state in these patients may result in higher, more prolonged serum levels. Conversely, alprazolam, lorazepam, oxazepam, temazepam, triazolam, and zolpidem are transformed into weak or inactive metabolites and therefore are less likely to accumulate. Elimination of BZD and non–BZD-like drugs varies somewhat, but essentially it occurs eventually via the kidneys.

Zaleplon and zolpidem are also readily absorbed, but bioavailability is only about 30% and 70%, respectively, because of first-pass biotransformation by the liver. Both drugs are rapidly cleared from the circulation by a combination of hepatic biotransformation and renal elimination.

▥ Adverse Effects and Contraindications

To one degree or another, BZDs rely on CNS depression to relieve symptoms of anxiety. Adverse reactions common with BZDs include daytime sedation, ataxia, dizziness, and headaches. Tolerance usually develops to these adverse effects. Use BZDs with caution in patients with a history of substance abuse. Unfortunately, tolerance also develops to the antiseizure effect of BZDs as well, limiting their usefulness in the chronic treatment of seizure disorders. Less common adverse effects of BZDs include blurred or double vision, hypotension, tremor, amnesia, slurred speech, urinary incontinence, and constipation.

There is a risk of developing hyperbilirubinemia and neutropenia. These results can reflect a number of disorders (e.g., fatty liver, hepatitis B, cholecystitis, physiologic hyperbilirubinemia, pancreatic cancer) that may require withdrawal of the BZD. Evaluate the patient for other disorders that cause jaundice.

BZDs are contraindicated in hypersensitive patients or in patients with an allergy to specific ingredients. The potential for respiratory depression caused by BZDs can lead to problems in patients with sleep apnea or chronic obstructive pulmonary disease. Fatal overdosage is rare with oral BZDs unless taken with alcohol or other CNS depressants.

▥ Drug Interactions

By far the most significant drug interaction is the potential for excessive depression when combined with other CNS-depressant drugs (Table 19-5). The interaction with alcohol is particularly marked and important because of the widespread social use of this drug. The combination of BZDs and alcohol produces marked incoordination and motor impairment. Combining BZDs with other CNS-depressant drugs, including alcohol, may also lead to life-threatening respiratory depression.

Concurrent alcohol ingestion with a BZD or other sedative-hypnotics may result in death. The ultra–short-acting BZDs (e.g., triazolam) administered by intravenous (IV) route,

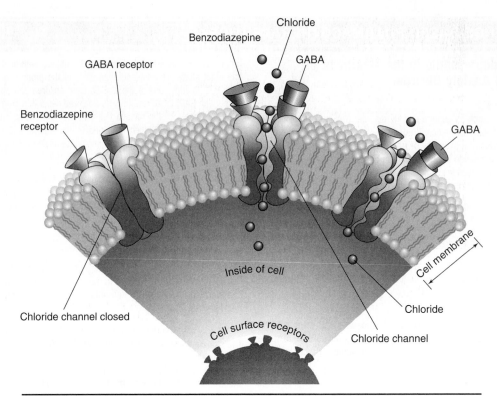

FIGURE 19-2 Schematic Model of GABA Receptor–Chloride Channel Complex for BZD Action. The channel exists in an open or closed configuration. Equilibrium between open and closed states of the chloride channel is altered by the presence of GABA. The channel is opened by GABA. The inward flow of chloride ions hyperpolarizes neurons, reducing their ability to fire. Thus GABA is an inhibitory neurotransmitter. Binding of a BZD to the chloride channel complex prolongs the time the channel remains open.

or in overdose, may lead to apnea and subsequent death. The very young and older adults are more likely to experience the CNS-depressant effects of BZDs compared with other age groups. Significant hypotension and occasionally cardiac or respiratory arrest are associated with IV administration of BZDs compared with other routes of administration.

A number of drugs and other substances are known to interfere with the hepatic biotransformation of many BZDs, thus prolonging their half-lives and leading to increased plasma levels. These include fluvoxamine, ketoconazole, nefazadone, and grapefruit juice. Cimetidine (but not ranitidine, famotidine, or nizatidine) reduces the plasma clearance of BZDs, which in turn leads to increased plasma concentrations of some drugs. Cigarette smoking or any nicotine use decreases the effectiveness of BZDs.

⫼ Dosage Regimens

Keep initial dosages of BZDs and BZD-like drugs as low as possible, and increase only after evaluating effectiveness (Table 19-6). Intramuscular (IM) and IV formulations are available for severe anxiety episodes, preoperative apprehension, and control of acute seizure activity. The non-BZDs

eszopiclone, zolpidem, and zaleplon are administered in once-daily doses at bedtime as needed for short-term (i.e., 7 to 14 days) management of insomnia.

⫼ Lab Considerations

Perform periodic blood counts and liver function testing for patients on long-term BZD therapy. Bilirubin, AST, ALT, and 17-ketosteroid levels are increased in the presence of chlordiazepoxide. Radioactive iodine uptake is decreased. False-positive results have been noted with the Gravindex pregnancy test.

For more information, see the Evolve Resources Bonus Content "Influence of selected Drugs on Laboratory Values," found at http://evolve.elsevier.com/Gutierrez/pharmacotherapeutics.

Atypical Anxiolytic

◆ buspirone (BuSpar)

⫼ Indications

Buspirone is the first of a class of antianxiety drugs called axapirones. Buspirone is only approved for patients with GAD. In addition, it may be a viable option for anxious

PHARMACOKINETICS
TABLE **19-4** Antianxiety and Sedative-Hypnotic Drugs

Drug	Route	Onset	Peak	Duration	PB (%)	t½*	BioA (%)
SHORT- TO INTERMEDIATE-ACTING BZDS							
alprazolam	PO	15–60 min	1–2 hr	6–12 hr	71–100	12–15 hr	80
clonazepam	PO	20–60 min	1–2 hr	6–12 hr	85	18–50 hr	UA
eszopiclone	PO	Rapid	1 hr	6–8 hr	52–59	6 hr	UA
lorazepam	PO	15–45 min	2 hr	12–24 hr	85	12–16 hr	90
	IM	15–30 min	60–90 min	>48 hr	85	12–16 hr	90
	IV	5–15 min	15–20 min	4 hr	85	12–16 hr	100
oxazepam	PO	45–90 min	3 hr	6–12 hr	97	10–25 hr	92
temazepam	PO	30 min	2–3 hr†	UA	96	4–18 hr	80
triazolam	PO	15–30 min	3 days‡	UA	91	1.6–5.4 hr	44
zaleplon	PO	Rapid	1 hr	6–8 hr	45–75	1 hr	UA
zolpidem	PO	1.5 hr	2 hr	6–8 hr	UA	2–3 hr	UA
LONG-ACTING BZDS							
chlordiazepoxide	PO	30–60 min	0.5–4 hr	12–24 hr	95	9–34 hr	UA
	IM	15–30 min	1–2 hr	UA	95	9–34 hr	UA
	IV	1–5 min	UA	0.25–1 hr	95	9–34 hr	100
clorazepate	PO	30–60 min	1–2 hr	To 24 hr	High	48 hr	UA
diazepam	PO/IM	15–45 min	1–2 hr	12–24 hr	98	20–80 hr	85–100
	IV	1–3 min	15–30 min	12–24 hr	98	20–80 hr	100
estazolam	PO	15–30 min	2 hr	6–8 hr	UA	10–24 hr	UA
flurazepam	PO	15–45 min	0.5–1 hr	7–8 hr§	97	2.3 hr†	UA
ATYPICAL ANXIOLYTIC							
buspirone	PO	7–10 days	40–90 min‖	UA	95	2–4 hr	90
OTHER SEDATIVE-HYPNOTICS							
chloral hydrate	PO/SUP	30–60 min	1 hr	4–8 hr	35–41¶	8–10 hr	UA
meprobamate	PO	<1 hr	1–3 hr	6–12 hr	UA	6–16 hr	UA
ramelteon	PO	Rapid	0.5–1.5 hr	6–8 hr	70	1–2.6 hr††	1.8
SHORT-ACTING BARBITURATES							
pentobarbital	PO	10–15 min	3–4 hr	3–4 hr	**	15–48 hr	UA
secobarbital	PO	10–15 min	3–4 hr	3–4 hr	**	15–40 hr	UA
INTERMEDIATE-ACTING BARBITURATES							
butabarbital	PO	45–60 min	6–8 hr	3–4 hr	**	34–42 hr	UA
LONG-ACTING BARBITURATES							
phenobarbital	PO	>60 min	10–12 hr	10–12 hr	**	80–120 hr	UA

*Half-life of active metabolites: *Flurazepam:* Half-life of active metabolite may be 30–100 hr for desalkylflurazepam, and for the metabolite *N*-1-hydroxyethylflurazepam, 2–4 hr. *Quazepam:* Half-life of metabolites is increased in the older adult—half-life for 2-oxoquazepam is 39 hr and for *N*-desalkylflurazepam is 70–75 hr. *Prazepam:* Half-life of active metabolite desmethyldiazepam with multidosing is 30–100 hr; for oxazepam, it is 5–15 hr.
†Effectiveness of temazepam may be demonstrated for up to 35 days with daily administration.
‡Triazolam's maximum hypnotic response. Has a reported range of effectiveness of 1–42 days.
§Flurazepam reportedly effective for up to 28 days.
‖Peak serum levels of buspirone may be reached 40–90 minutes after oral dosing; however, it may take 7–10 days for relief of anxiety to be noted.
¶Half-life of the chloral hydrate metabolite.
**Barbiturate binding to plasma proteins is a function of lipid solubility.
††Mean half-life of the short-acting, intermediate-acting, and long-acting barbiturates is dependent on the dose.
BioA, Bioavailability; *BZDs,* benzodiazepines; *IM,* intramuscular; *PB,* protein binding; *PO,* by mouth; *SUP,* suppository formulation; *t½,* half-life; *UA,* unavailable.

patients with chronic obstructive pulmonary disease or sleep apnea, because no respiratory depression occurs with this drug. In fact, some patients may experience an increase in their resting respiratory rate. Buspirone does not have the associated adverse effects of sedation, drowsiness, or motor retardation.

▦ *Pharmacodynamics*
Unlike other sedative-hypnotic drugs in common use today, buspirone has no effect on GABA$_A$ receptor sites, nor does it potentiate BZD receptor binding. It is thought to selectively antagonize 5-hydroxytryptamine-1 (i.e., serotonin, 5-HT$_{1A}$) receptors in the CNS and may produce action at dopamine (D$_2$) receptors.

Although buspirone has antianxiety activity comparable to that of BZDs, it has no significant antiseizure or muscle relaxant

activity, and may produce less sedation as well. However, an anxiolytic effect may not be evident for up to a week after therapy with buspirone is begun, and may not be maximal for a month.

▦ *Pharmacokinetics*
Buspirone is well absorbed, but because of extensive first-pass biotransformation it has a bioavailability of only 4%. Absorption is enhanced in the presence of food. The drug is rapidly biotransformed by the liver and so has a relatively short plasma half-life (less than 3 hours).

▦ *Adverse Effects and Contraindications*
Over 10% of patients taking buspirone will experience dizziness. Fewer than 10% of patients have drowsiness, extrapyramidal symptoms, serotonin syndrome, confusion, nervousness,

DRUG INTERACTIONS

TABLE **19-5** Antianxiety and Sedative-Hypnotic Drugs

Drug	Interactive Drugs	Interaction
BZDS		
Benzodiazepines	cimetidine, digoxin, erythromycin, fluoxetine, isoniazid, ketoconazole, metoprolol, oral contraceptives, propranolol, propoxyphene, valproic acid, zidovudine	Increases plasma half-life of BZD, particularly alprazolam; increases risk of digoxin toxicity
	phenytoin	Increases concentration of interactive drug
	levodopa	Decreases plasma concentration of interactive drug; decreases effectiveness of oxazepam
	Barbiturates, rifampin, theophylline, tobacco	Increases biotransformation of BZDs, decreasing their effectiveness
	Alcohol, anesthetics, antihistamines, opioids, phenothiazines, tricyclic antidepressants	Additive CNS depression
lorazepam	probenecid	Decreases biotransformation of lorazepam
eszopiclone, zaleplon, zolpidem	CNS depressants, opioids, other sedative-hypnotics	Additive CNS depression
NON-BZDS		
buspirone	MAO inhibitors, cimetidine	Increases buspirone effect; potential for toxicity
OTHER SEDATIVE-HYPNOTICS		
chloral hydrate, meprobamate	Alcohol, antihistamines	Additive CNS depression
ramelteon	Antiarrhythmics, antidepressants, azole antifungals, barbiturates, carbamazepine, celecoxib, cimetidine, delaviridine, estrogens, imatinib, macrolide antibiotics, methoxsalen, phenytoins, protease inhibitors, quinolones, rifampin, tacrine, ticlopidine, zileuton	Biotransformation of ramelteon inhibited leading to increased serum levels
BARBITURATES		
Barbiturates	Alcohol, antihistamines, opioids	Additive CNS depression
	chloramphenicol, cyclosporine, dacarbazine, glucocorticoids, oral contraceptives, sedative-hypnotics, tricyclic antidepressants, quinidine, warfarin	Induces CYP450 enzymes to increase biotransformation of interactive drugs
	acetaminophen	Increases risk of hepatotoxicity to interactive drug
	divalproex, valproic acid	Decreases biotransformation of phenobarbital, increasing sedation
	cyclophosphamide	Increases risk of hematologic toxicity

BZDs, Benzodiazepines; *CNS,* central nervous system; *MAO,* monamine oxidase.

DOSAGE

TABLE **19-6** Antianxiety and Sedative-Hypnotic Drugs

Drugs	Uses	Dosage	Implications
SHORT- TO INTERMEDIATE-ACTING BZDS			
alprazolam	Anxiety disorders, panic attacks, adjunct treatment of depression	*Adult:* 0.25–0.5 mg PO 2–3 times daily. Max: 4 mg daily	Not for use under 18 yr of age. Begin with 0.25 mg 2–3 times daily for older adults or debilitated patients.
clonazepam	Prophylaxis of seizures, sedation, uncontrolled leg movements during sleep (unlabeled use)	*Adult:* 0.25–0.5 mg 3 times daily. May increase by 0.5–1 mg every third day. Maintenance: Not to exceed 20 mg/day. *Child <10 years of age or <30 kg:* Initial daily dose 0.01–0.03 mg/kg/day 2–3 times daily, not to exceed 0.05 mg/kg/day; increase by no more than 0.25–0.5 mg every third day until therapeutic levels are reached; not to exceed 0.2 mg/kg/day	Therapeutic serum concentrations are 20–80 mcg/mL. Missed doses should be taken within 1 hr or omitted. Do not double dose. **Abrupt withdrawal can cause tremors, nausea, vomiting, abdominal and muscle cramps, and status epilepticus.** ▲
eszopiclone	Insomnia	*Adult:* 2 mg initially at HS. Max: 3 mg	Reduce dose if concurrent use with a strong CYP 3A4 inhibitor
lorazepam	Anxiety, insomnia, preoperative sedation, preantineoplastic antiemetic in children	*Adult: Anxiety or sedation:* 1–10 mg PO in 2–3 divided doses; usual dose 2–6 mg/day in divided doses. *Insomnia:* 2–4 mg PO at HS PRN	Prolonged high-dose therapy may lead to psychologic or physical dependence. Initial dose not to exceed 2 mg in debilitated patients.
oxazepam	Anxiety, insomnia, alcohol withdrawal	*Adult:* 10–30 mg PO 3–4 times daily.	Taper drug at completion of therapy. **Sudden cessation may lead to withdrawal symptoms.** ▲
temazepam	Short-term management of insomnia	*Adult:* 15–30 mg PO at HS PRN	Reduce dosage for older adults and debilitated patients.

triazolam	Short-term management of insomnia	*Initial:* 0.125–0.5 mg PO at HS	CYP450 3A4 substrate
zaleplon	Short-term management of insomnia	*Adult:* 5–10 mg PO at HS PRN	Avoid taking with high-fat meal.
zolpidem	Short-term management of insomnia	*Adult:* 5–10 mg PO at HS	Start older adults, debilitated patients, or those with hepatic impairment on 5 mg.
LONG-ACTING BZDS			
chlordiazepoxide	Anxiety, alcohol withdrawal	*Adult: Anxiety:* 5–25 mg PO –or– 25–50 mg IM, IV 3–4 times a day. *Withdrawal:* 50–100 mg PO, IM, or IV, repeated until agitation is controlled, up to 400 mg/day *Child >6 yr of age:* 5–10 mg PO 2–4 times daily	Metabolites active for up to 100 hr
clorazepate	Anxiety, alcohol withdrawal	*Adult: Anxiety:* 15–60 mg PO once daily. *Withdrawal:* 7.5–15 mg PO 2–4 times daily; then 15 mg PO 2–4 times daily on first day; then gradually taper off. Max: 90 mg/day	May be given as a single dose of 11.25–22.5 mg at bedtime for anxiety. For older adults or debilitated patients, give 7.5–15 mg daily.
diazepam	Anxiety, alcohol withdrawal	*Adult: Anxiety:* 2–10 mg PO 2 to 4 times daily –or– 15–30 mg PO (SR) daily –or– 2–10 mg IM or IV every 3–4 hr PRN. *Withdrawal:* 10 mg PO 3–4 times daily first 24 hr; then decrease to 5 mg PO 3–4 times daily *Child >6 yr of age:* 0.1–0.8 mg/ kg/day PO divided every 6–8 hr for anxiety	Metabolite active for up to 200 hours. Monitor closely for excessive sedation. Extremely cautious use in children.
estazolam	Short-term management of insomnia	*Adult:* 1–2 mg PO at HS.	Assess sleep patterns before and throughout therapy.
flurazepam	Insomnia	*Adult:* 15–30 mg PO at HS	Reduce dosage in older adults and debilitated patients.
ATYPICAL ANXIOLYTIC			
buspirone	Anxiety	*Adult:* 10–15 mg PO 2–3 times daily. May increase by 5 mg/day every 2–4 days to max of 60 mg daily. Usual dose 20–30 mg daily	May take up to 2 wk for onset of action. Monitor patients closely during initial phase.
OTHER SEDATIVE-HYPNOTICS			
chloral hydrate	Short-term sedative-hypnotic	*Adult: Anxiety-sedation:* 250 mg PO 3 times daily; 325 mg rectally 3 times daily. *Insomnia:* 0.5–1 gram PO or rectally at HS *Child: Anxiety-sedation:* 8.3 mg/kg PO or rectally up to 500 mg 3 times daily. *Insomnia:* 50 mg/kg PO or rectally at HS, up to 1 gram	If suppository is too soft for insertion, chill in refrigerator for 30 minutes or run under cold water before removing foil wrapper.
meprobamate	Anxiety	*Adult:* 1.2–1.6 grams PO daily in 2–3 divided doses –or– 0.8–1.6 grams in 2 divided doses as SR capsules; not to exceed 2.4 grams daily *Child 6–12 yr:* 25 mg/kg/day in 2–3 divided doses	Use smallest effective dose. May cause psychologic or physical dependence.
ramelteon	Insomnia	*Adult:* 8 mg PO 30 min before HS	Avoid taking with high-fat meal.
BARBITURATES			
butabarbital	Short-term sedation and sleep induction	*Adult: Sedation:* 15–30 mg PO 3–4 times daily *Hypnosis:* 50–100 mg PO at HS	Do not increase dose. Avoid other CNS depressants.
pentobarbital	Short-term sedation, hypnosis	*Adult: Sedation:* 20 mg PO 3–4 times daily. *Hypnosis:* 100 mg PO –or– 150–200 mg IM –or– 100 mg IV to total of 500 mg *Child: Sedation:* 2–6 mg/kg/day PO, IM –or– 50 mg IV –or– 2 mg/kg rectally 3 times daily	Half-life 15–50 hr. CYP450 activity unknown. Supervise ambulation and transfer of patients after administration.
phenobarbital	Preoperative sedation, hypnosis	*Adult: Sedation:* 30–120 mg/day PO, IM, or IV 2–3 times daily. *Hypnosis:* 100–320 mg PO, IM, or IV at HS *Child: Sedation:* 2 mg/kg PO 3 times daily	CYP 2C9 (primary); 2E1 substrate. Half-life: 79 hr. Taper dosage gradually to minimize risk of seizures.
Secobarbital	Short-term hypnosis; preoperative sedation	*Adult: Hypnosis:* 100–200 mg IM –or– 50–250 mg IV *Sedation:* 1.1–2.2 mg/kg IM 10–15 min preoperatively	Half-life: 28 hr. CYP450 activity unknown

HS, Bedtime; *IM*, intramuscular (route); *IV*, intravenous (route); *PO*, by mouth; *PRN*, as needed; *SR*, sustained release.

lightheadedness, excitement, anger, hostility, and headache. The drug produces little sedation or impairment and appears to lack the potential for abuse and dependence.

Because bioavailability of buspirone is greatly reduced and plasma half-life is normally very short, exercise caution using buspirone in patients with significant liver disease or impairment. Monitor for elevated liver function test results because of the risk for hepatotoxicity. It has a low potential for abuse and does not cause withdrawal effects when abruptly discontinued. Safe use in pregnancy and use in children younger than 18 years of age has not been established.

▮ Drug Interactions

Drugs that compete for the hepatic enzymes responsible for biotransformation of buspirone may greatly enhance its bioavailability. This may result in much higher plasma levels after a typical oral dose and therefore an increase in the incidence of adverse effects. Erythromycin and itraconazole may increase peak plasma levels of buspirone fivefold through this mechanism. Administration of buspirone to patients taking monoamine oxidase (MAO) inhibitors has been reported to provoke significant increases in blood pressure.

CENTRAL NERVOUS

Other Sedative-Hypnotics

◆ chloral hydrate (Aquachloral); ◆ Novo-Chlorhydrate, PMS-Chlorate Hydrate
◆ melatonin
◆ meprobamate (Meprospan, Miltown, Trancot); ◆ Apo-Meprobamate
◆ ramelteon (Rozerem)

▌ Indications

Chloral hydrate is one of the oldest hypnotics and is well tolerated by older adults. It is occasionally used for preoperative sedation but is no longer employed to induce hypnosis or to treat anxiety or sleep disorders.

Meprobamate has been used for relief of anxiety and muscle tension. However, because of the risk for tolerance, physical dependency, severe withdrawal reactions, and life-threatening toxicity, it has fallen from favor. It is used much less frequently than BZDs or buspirone.

Melatonin is a nonprescription over-the-counter (OTC) herbal product used for treatment of insomnia and jet lag. It is widely available in health food stores and is used in self-treatment of insomnia, jet lag, and a wide variety of disorders. In some patients, melatonin has been shown to decrease both the severity and duration of jet lag symptoms. It has been recommended that the drug be taken once daily at bedtime beginning 3 days before the flight and continuing for 3 days after arrival at the destination. Some providers feel that the herb seems to be most helpful when flying from west to east, but to date there is no research available to support this contention.

Ramelteon, the newest hypnotic drug, has been approved by the FDA for use in patients who have difficulty getting to sleep, rather than staying asleep.

▌ Pharmacodynamics

The precise mechanism underlying the sedative-hypnotic action of chloral hydrate and meprobamate is unknown; however, best evidence points to an action through $GABA_A$ receptors. Chloral hydrate is biotransformed to trichloroethanol, which is thought to be responsible for its CNS effects. Meprobamate also acts in the CNS by blocking neuron impulses between the cerebral cortex and the thalamus. Its primary actions are global CNS sedation and skeletal muscle relaxation.

Melatonin is made from bovine pineal glands, but it can also be synthesized in the laboratory. Melatonin is normally synthesized in the pineal gland from tryptophan. In healthy individuals, endogenous melatonin increases rapidly in the evening, peaks after midnight, and declines toward morning. The rise in endogenous melatonin may help entrain the circadian rhythm of sleep and body temperature to the external world. In contrast, melatonin's role in gonadal function is uncertain, at least in humans. There is only scant evidence that an abnormality in melatonin secretion causes illness; hence there are few data to support the use of melatonin as replacement therapy. However, ramelteon acts as a melatonin (MT) receptor agonist, binding to MT_1 and MT_2 receptors to induce sleep.

▌ Pharmacokinetics

All of these drugs are orally bioavailable and subject to extensive hepatic biotransformation. Chloral hydrate is rapidly absorbed when taken orally. The drug is converted to an active metabolite (trichlorethanol) in the liver; the half-life

of the metabolite is 8 to 10 hours. The metabolite exerts the pharmacologic effects (see Table 19-4).

Meprobamate is well absorbed following oral administration and is widely distributed. The onset and peak action profile of the sustained-release formulation is unknown. Meprobamate is biotransformed in the liver.

When taken 2 hours before bedtime, melatonin is thought to decrease the time needed to fall asleep by an average of 14 minutes. It was also noted to decrease the time awake after onset of sleep by 24 minutes and to improve sleep efficiency (total time asleep as a percentage of time in bed) from 75% to 83%. It does not appear to increase total sleep time.

Ramelteon has a rapid onset of action, with peak levels reached relatively quickly.

▌ Adverse Effects and Contraindications

The most common adverse effects of chloral hydrate are excessive sedation, nausea, vomiting, diarrhea, and flatulence. Administer it in capsule form, or advise patients to take it with food, because of its unpleasant taste. The development of tolerance is possible, as well as physical and psychologic dependency. A hangover, disorientation, headache, irritability, dizziness, and incoordination are possible.

The most common adverse effects of meprobamate are drowsiness and ataxia. Blurred vision, hypotension, anorexia, nausea, vomiting, and diarrhea have been noted. Carisoprodol (Soma), a centrally-acting skeletal muscle relaxant (see Chapter 23) is biotransformed to meprobamate. Given the popularity of carisoprodol with some health care providers, it is not surprising that an unrecognized meprobamate withdrawal syndrome can occur after abrupt cessation of carisoprodol therapy. Exercise caution when using meprobamate in patients with hepatic dysfunction or severe renal impairment and in patients who may be suicidal or who have been addicted to drugs in the past. Dosage reduction is recommended for older adults. It is contraindicated in patients with hypersensitivity to any of its components, in comatose patients or those with preexisting CNS depression, and in patients with uncontrolled severe pain. Safe use in pregnancy and in children has not been established.

There have been no reports of toxicities or serious adverse effects with melatonin, but no long-term studies of the herb have been conducted. The adverse effects of melatonin appear to include abdominal cramping, decreased alertness, circadian rhythm disruption, daytime fatigue, transient depression, dizziness, drowsiness, headache, irritability, and dysphoria in depressed patients.

The relatively large doses of melatonin available OTC may be associated with adverse effects such as hypothermia, seizures in children with existing neurologic disease, or gynecomastia. There are no controlled studies to suggest that a more physiologic dosage (i.e., about 0.3 mg) would avoid these adverse effects, but experience suggests a lower dosage would minimize the risk.

Ramelteon is contraindicated for use in patients receiving fluvoxamine since the combination inhibits biotransformation of ramelteon, thereby increasing its serum levels.

▌ Drug Interactions

As with other BZDs and related drugs, the CNS depression caused by these drugs is greatly enhanced in the presence of other CNS depressants. The list of drug interactions with ramelteon is extensive. Table 19-5 provides an overview.

▥ *Dosage Regimen*

The dosage of chloral hydrate depends on the diagnosis, the age of patient, the route of administration, and the purpose and goal of therapy. It is available as capsules and suppositories in a variety of dosages.

Keep initial doses of meprobamate as low as possible, and increase only after measuring clinical effects. Begin treatment for frail older adults or debilitated patients at lowered doses, and increase doses more slowly if needed. Therapeutic plasma levels are between 6 and 12 mcg/mL; toxic levels are over 60 mcg/mL. Meprobamate must be tapered carefully, because abrupt discontinuation can precipitate potentially dangerous withdrawal reactions. Overdose is marked by severe hypotension, coma, and potential respiratory collapse. Care consists of hemodynamic support and, possibly, mechanical ventilation in severe cases.

The safety and efficacy of OTC melatonin has not been established, and because the concentrations of active ingredients may vary widely between products, no dosage recommendations have been established.

Ramelteon should be taken about 1 hour before sleep. Advise patients taking it to avoid high-fat meals.

Barbiturates

As a class of drugs, barbiturates were once widely used for the treatment of insomnia and anxiety disorders. However, these drugs have now been largely replaced by BZDs and others that are just as effective and not as dangerous. Barbiturates are structurally similar compounds that act at the level of the presynaptic and postsynaptic membranes throughout the CNS. It is unclear at which level the sedative-hypnotic action takes place. The tables within this chapter include information on the barbiturates.

Barbiturates present several important problems that severely limit their usefulness as sedative hypnotics. Most importantly, these drugs produce excessive depression of the CNS, including coma and potentially lethal respiratory depression. This danger is compounded by their low therapeutic index and short-term efficacy, and the fact that the depression is greatly enhanced in the presence of other CNS depressants. Other serious adverse effects of barbiturates include hypersensitivity reactions (i.e., skin rash, exfoliative dermatitis, and urticaria), sore throat, fever, edema, serum sickness, apnea, bronchospasms, and Stevens-Johnson syndrome (although rare). Prolonged use of high doses of barbiturate can lead to tolerance and physical or psychologic dependence. Withdrawal syndrome can occur and is at times fatal. Chapter 25 discusses the use of barbiturates as antiepileptic drugs.

CLINICAL REASONING

Treatment Objectives

The treatment goal of drug therapy is to reduce the patient's anxiety, return the patient to a normal level of functioning with a minimum of adverse effects, and improve quality of life. Helping the patient develop effective coping skills to deal with some aspects of the anxiety and to prevent secondary

disorders such as depression or substance abuse is also an important goal. Finally, treatment goals also include preventing relapse or recurrence of the anxiety.

Treatment goals for the patient with impaired sleep are directed at promoting sleep in the short term (i.e., 1 to 4 days). Thus, daytime disruptions such as fatigue, impaired work performance, and transient mood disturbances may be lessened. Sleep can be supported for up to 3 weeks while a patient is learning alternative, behavioral techniques (e.g., eliminating daytime napping, instituting relaxation exercises) to promote sleep.

Treatment Options

There are no specific guidelines as to when to initiate drug therapy for anxiety or impaired sleep; although drug therapy is ordinarily initiated after the patient has failed non–drug therapies. Good sleep hygiene practices improve daytime alertness and reduce the risk of sleep disorders. Table 19-7 provides an overview of simple practices that help ensure a restful night's sleep (see Controversy).

Drug therapy is usually considered when non–drug treatment modalities have been unsuccessful, if the patient is suicidal, or if symptoms of anxiety are severe, persistent, and recurrent enough to disrupt the patient's daily life. Greater response rates occur with combined behavioral and drug therapy.

Because sleep disturbances may signal an underlying physical and/or psychiatric disorder, institute treatment of insomnia only after a careful and thorough patient evaluation. Sedative-hypnotics are the primary drugs used for insomnia, although antidepressants (Chapter 20) or antihistamines may also be helpful (Chapter 51). Note, however, that typically patients can become tolerate to chronic use of antihistamines. Given in adequate dosages, all sedative-hypnotics reduce anxiety and promote sleep; the key is to determine the minimal dosage that will do both with few to no adverse effects. It is important to match the patient's need for the drug with the aspect of anxiety and sleep that is disturbed (i.e., getting to sleep as opposed to staying asleep). If the patient has a problem getting to sleep, use a quick-onset BZD that has a short half-life; if the patient is having problems staying asleep; use a BZD with an intermediate half-life (e.g., temazepam).

A chronic, fluctuating clinical course of anxiety raises difficult concerns regarding long-term treatment goals. There have been several studies describing GAD as a chronic illness. However, few long-term efficacy studies have been conducted, and the efficacy of drug therapy after 6 months is unknown. Employ the lowest effective dosage for the shortest period of time, and periodically attempt discontinuation. A selective serotonin reuptake inhibitor (SSRI) antidepressant drug can be used long-term for maintenance.

Do not use antianxiety and sedative-hypnotic drugs in place of analgesics for the patient in pain. Pain alters the patient's response to hypnotic drugs, causing an increased incidence of disorientation and paradoxical excitement. Analgesics are discussed in Chapters 16 and 17.

▥ *Patient Variables*

How a person with anxiety or an impaired sleep pattern appears to the health care provider when seeking care is important. Because anxiety is a normal human response, a basic task is determining whether a patient is suffering from an abnormal anxiety response or reacting to the normal stress of life. The

CENTRAL NERVOUS

TABLE 19-7 Strategies for Good Sleep

Poor sleep hygiene is one of the most common problems encountered in our society. All of us stay up too late and get up too early. We interrupt our sleep with drugs, caffeine, chemicals, and work, and we overstimulate ourselves with late-night activities such as television. Strategies that help us get to sleep and stay asleep include the following:

- Obtain adequate exposure to natural daylight every day.
- Obtain regular exercise, but not within 1 hour of bedtime.
- Adhere to the same bedtime and awaken at the same time each day, including weekends or days off from work or school.
- Avoid taking a nap during the day.
- Assign a "worry period" early in the day, so that issues are dealt with before bedtime.
- Avoid alcohol, caffeine, and heavy, spicy, or sugary foods 3 to 4 hours before bedtime. Warm milk and foods high in the amino acid tryptophan, such as bananas, turkey, and milk, may help.
- Establish a regular bedtime routine (e.g., meditation, yoga, warm bath, brushing teeth), allowing at least 1 hour to wind down before bedtime.
- Use the bedroom only for sleep and sexual activity. Don't use the bed or bedroom as an office, workroom, or recreation room.
- Remove the television from the bedroom. Simply turning it off is not sufficient.
- Block out all distracting light and noise. Keep the bedroom as dark as possible.
- Keep the bedroom at a comfortable temperature and leave it that way. It is better for the bedroom to be slightly cooler—losing body heat has been shown to help the onset of deep sleep.
- Use comfortable bedding and pillows.

A word about getting up during the night:
For various reasons, most people awaken once or twice during the night. If you find you are unable to go back to sleep *within 15–20 minutes, do not* remain in the bed. Get out of bed. Leave the bedroom. Sit in the dark, read (although some experts suggest turning the light on to do so stimulates your daytime internal clock), have a light snack, do some quiet activity, or take a bath. Generally you will be able to go back to sleep 20 minutes or so later. Do not perform challenging or engaging activity such as office work, housework, and so forth.

A word about television:
Watching television before bedtime is often a bad idea. Many people fall asleep with the television on. Television viewing is an engaging medium that tends to keep people up. Do not put or keep a television in the bedroom. At the appropriate bedtime, turn off the television (which is, of course, not in the bedroom), perform your prebedtime rituals, and go to bed. Some people find that a radio helps them go to sleep. Since radio is a less engaging medium than TV, this is usually a good idea.

---

patient can help by identifying how severely his or her life at home, work, or school is affected by the anxiety level. High anxiety levels or panic states are associated with feelings of intense fear and doom. Include the patient's usual sleep habits and quality of sleep in the initial assessment (see Box 19-3).

Anxiety and impaired sleep are frequently associated with medical problems. Perform a thorough physical exam with an eye toward discovering the underlying causes of the anxiety. Pay attention to the patient's pulse rate, blood pressure, and respiratory rate. Observe for diaphoresis, restlessness, or trembling, because these manifestations are often hallmarks of anxiety. In addition, assess for visible signs of fatigue and

lack of sleep, such as reddened eyes, lack of coordination, drowsiness, and irritability. Table 19-2 summarizes the signs and symptoms of anxiety (see Case Study).

Baseline laboratory values may be appropriate to determine underlying causes of the anxiety or impaired sleep. If endocrine abnormalities are suspected, a thyroid screen or a glucose tolerance test is indicated. A toxicology screen is called for if drug ingestion or withdrawal from illicit drugs is suspected. There are also a number of anxiety assessment tools that can be used to assess the extent of the anxiety.

The primary diagnostic test for sleep disorders is polysomnography. Patients may be referred to a sleep center for an

---

Controversy

Appropriate Use of Antianxiety Drugs

Jonathan J. Wolfe

Antianxiety drugs are among the most commonly prescribed in the United States. They have progressed from early drugs such as meprobamate (which is still popular with some health care providers and patients) to those with far greater clinical finesse. The discovery of benzodiazepines (BZDs) produced new possibilities in treating personality disorders. The progression to shorter-acting drugs with enhanced potency (e.g., alprazolam) has opened pathways to more appropriate dosing regimens for special populations, particularly older adults.

However, each drug class comes with a definable set of adverse effects. In some cases, improved pharmacokinetic profiles (e.g., shorter half-life) allow use of BZDs in patients who could not tolerate previous drugs. In many cases, vigorous marketing ploys promote wider use of drugs, simply because earlier safety concerns have been met by triumphs of drug discovery.

There is a tendency in some health care settings to overuse antianxiety drugs, although it may be done with the best intentions. In every case,

the autonomy and dignity of the patient require that we ask whether antianxiety drugs are the proper therapy.

CLINICAL REASONING

- What concerns would you have if a 63-year-old woman who is the principal caregiver for her 82-year-old mother asked about getting a prescription for diazepam? The daughter states, "Mother is just driving me around the bend talking all the time about things that happened 60 years ago!" Remember that BZDs are to be used with caution in the older adult population. Also, Medicare Part D won't pay for BZDs.
- What role would a BZD properly play in long-term treatment of an older adult male with a 50-year history of alcohol abuse?
- At what point in the treatment of a sleep disturbance would an antianxiety drug play a proper role?
- Depression and anxiety are often unappreciated facets of the existential suffering of dying patients. What benefit might a patient in hospice care, whose physical pain is well controlled with other therapies, derive from judicious use of an antianxiety drug?

CASE STUDY | Sedative-Hypnotics

ASSESSMENT

History of Present Illness	RD is a 25-year-old veteran presenting to the primary clinic with a complaint of feeling nervous, not being able to concentrate, and not being able to get to sleep at night. He reports sleeping 4 to 5 hours per night because of his busy school schedule. He has occasional feelings of suffocating or blacking out. Occasionally, he is unwilling to leave his home for fear that something terrible will happen. He has tried taking diphenhydramine for sleep, but it dries out his mouth too much, and he feels hung over the next day. He relates that anxiety attacks and insomnia started soon after learning he would be deployed to Iraq but have increased in frequency and intensity since he returned and was discharged 3 months ago. RD currently sees a social worker once a week for counseling. He sustained injuries to his left leg while in Iraq and now has a permanent disability.
Past Health History	RD reports overall good health (except for his leg) with no cardiovascular or pulmonary problems. He has a five pack/year smoking history. He has been abstinent from alcohol for the past 4 months, with heavy use in the past. RD uses marijuana about twice a week but reports using no other illicit drugs.
Life-Span Considerations	RD married before going to Iraq. Since his return he has been taking classes to earn a real estate sales license. RDs wife is working many hours to help with household expenses while RD is in school. RD is worried about his ability to complete coursework because of difficulty concentrating and fatigue from not sleeping. He is using military education benefits to change career fields. RD's knee injury is service-connected, and therefore he is eligible for treatment at the local Veterans Administration Hospital.
Physical Exam Findings	VS: 37° C-90-22. *BP:* 146/85. He was well groomed and articulate but rarely made eye contact with the interviewer. He positioned himself so that the door to the exam room was in his sight at all times. Lungs clear to auscultation. Heart rate and rhythm regular. Noticeable limp; walks with cane. The remainder of the physical exam was unremarkable.
Diagnostic Testing	EKG NSR, unchanged from previous tracing. FSBS: 98 mg/dL. Thyroid levels within normal limits. Toxicology screen negative for illicit substances.

DIAGNOSIS: Anxiety and insomnia secondary to posttraumatic stress disorder

MANAGEMENT

Treatment Objectives	Minimize frequency and intensity of anxiety and insomnia to allow RD to assume his normal daily regimen with minimal sedation.
Treatment Plan	**Pharmacotherapy** • lorazepam 0.5 mg orally every 6 to 8 hours PRN for anxiety (#15 only with no refills) • ramelteon 8 mg at HS PRN for sleep **Patient Education** 1. Take ramelteon 30 minutes before bedtime. 2. Avoid concurrent use with other CNS depressants (no alcohol or marijuana). 3. Avoid taking drug with or immediately after a high-fat meal. 4. Keep symptom diary and bring to follow-up visit in 2 weeks. 5. Keep appointments with social worker. **Evaluation** Frequency and intensity of anxiety should lessen and improve his sleep, allowing him to concentrate better and cope with daily activities.

CLINICAL REASONING ANALYSIS

Q1. Why did you choose lorazepam rather than diazepam?
A. I chose lorazepam rather than diazepam because lorazepam is rapid-acting with a relatively short half-life. The problem with diazepam is that although diazepam is also rapid-acting, it has an active metabolite that can lead to excess sedation. Further, RD expressed a desire not to feel excessively sedated. He believes that mental alertness is vital not only to his safety but also to his studies.

Continued

CASE STUDY   Sedative-Hypnotics—Cont'd

Q2. Why did you choose ramelteon rather than zolpidem to help RD sleep? I heard that zolpidem is the best?

A. Zolpidem appears to be more efficacious as a hypnotic, with little development of tolerance, compared with BZDs; and zolpidem's effects are not augmented by small amounts of alcohol. However, a hangover effect, dizziness, and a drugged feeling has been reported with zolpidem, and it is for short-term use only. The primary disadvantage of zolpidem is that it can cause anterograde amnesia if not taken at a time when RD would have a full 8 to 9 hours of sleep. In contrast, ramelteon is the first and only nonscheduled prescription drug for insomnia. It is not a controlled substance and has been approved for long-term use. Although there isn't much clinical postmarketing data, ramelteon is indicated for patients who have trouble getting to sleep rather than staying asleep.

Q3. Aren't you worried about RD abusing the ramelteon?

A. Persons with insomnia tend to show therapy-seeking rather than drug-seeking behaviors, and the majority of persons with insomnia use prescribed hypnotics appropriately, without evidence of abuse. Nevertheless, we need to use caution with prescribing a hypnotic for RD because of his history of substance and alcohol abuse. Ramelteon has not been shown, at least in animal studies, to produce rewarding effects with use. Furthermore, discontinuance of ramelteon did not produce withdrawal signs.

Q4. Why did you tell RD to not take his ramelteon with a high-fat meal?

A. High-fat meals delay the absorption of ramelteon.

---

overnight assessment of any nocturnal hypoxia or sleep apnea. Depending on the cause of the sleep disorder, a variety of other studies may be performed.

Patients may initially be reluctant to start on antianxiety medicine. They may fear feeling sedated or worry about becoming dependent. With prolonged BZD therapy, tolerance occurs to the sedating effects but not to the anxiolytic effects. Initial and maintenance doses of BZDs must be individualized.

All drugs have benefits and risks associated with onset, duration, and adverse effects. The nature and severity of symptoms, the patient's medical history, and liver and kidney function, as well as other drugs used concomitantly by the patient, guide the health care provider in the selection of the most appropriate drug. There is no one "best drug."

LIFE-SPAN CONSIDERATIONS

Pregnant and Nursing Women. Pregnancy brings enormous changes to a woman's body. She must deal with alterations in body image, hormone fluctuations, the role change of becoming a mother, and normal worries about the health of her child. The potential for anxiety and sleep disturbances as a normal response or as a pathologic adjustment is apparent. The antihistamine diphenhydramine is the only drug available to treat sleep disorders during pregnancy; however, if the child is born prematurely to a mother who has been receiving diphenhydramine, there is a risk of retinal detachment.

Temper your response to the pregnant patient with consideration for fetal safety. The first trimester has the greatest risk of fetal damage from drugs. Unless benefits greatly outweigh risks, avoid antianxiety drugs during this time. In addition, drugs used during the third trimester or during breastfeeding can lead to withdrawal symptoms in neonates, floppy baby syndrome, or poor sucking response. Consider non–drug therapies first.

If antianxiety drugs are used before delivery, the neonate will need to be thoroughly assessed for possible withdrawal symptoms or other potential adverse effects such as retardation or physical anomalies.

Children and Adolescents. Developmental stereotypes often lead to underestimating the prevalence of anxiety disorders in children and adolescents. In fact, anxiety disorders are more prevalent than attention deficit disorders in this age group. Children can have so-called adult anxiety disorders, as well as disorders specific to children such as separation anxiety, overanxious behavior, and stranger anxiety that do not ordinarily require treatment. Children rarely have a pure anxiety disorder but instead display multiple symptoms, making diagnosis more challenging. Explore the likelihood of substance abuse or sexual abuse. A full psychiatric review of the family is important, because children with overanxious parents often learn similar behaviors.

The use of BZDs in children is controversial at best. Drug therapy can decrease most symptoms but does nothing to solve the underlying cause of anxiety. Most authorities agree that, most especially in children, drug therapy should not be a first-line treatment for anxiety or sleep disorders. Behavioral, cognitive, or family therapies or psychotherapy should be initiated first. Some drugs are contraindicated for use in children under specific ages and require cautious use in all instances. Furthermore, children are more susceptible to withdrawal problems owing to the drugs' faster clearance rate in this group.

Older Adults. The adjustments needed to cope with the multiple losses of independence, health, and family, which are so often encountered in older adults, contribute to anxiety. Many emotional dilemmas of the older adult can mimic or have an overlay of anxiety. Dysfunctional grieving, Alzheimer's disease, and confusion can all bear a striking resemblance to anxiety. The older adult can show somatic or behavioral symptoms similar to those noted in a younger patient, but may use social withdrawal more frequently as a coping mechanism. A careful geropsychiatric evaluation will help define actual pathology and allow a definitive diagnosis of anxiety or sleep disorder to be made.

Decisions to use antianxiety or sedative-hypnotic drugs in an older adult must be made only after careful evaluation of significant factors. First, rule out diseases or drug-induced confusion. Delirium is a true medical emergency with a potential for lethal outcome. Delirium is often accompanied by a hyperadrenergic state, making it closely resemble anxiety or, more commonly, psychosis. In many cases, delirium has been misinterpreted as a psychotic state rather than an anxiety state, thus delirium is an important differential diagnosis of anxiety or even insomnia. Second, use short-acting drugs with short half-lives to help prevent accumulation. Carefully monitor the patient for signs of confusion, sedation, or ataxia during the early phase of therapy. Keep initial doses as low as possible, and increase slowly. Older adults are at risk for injury because they often react more strongly to the sedative effects of antianxiety drugs. Thus they are at greater risk for falls and subsequent hip fractures. Careful attention to elimination pathways helps in selecting drugs that are safe for older adults or for those with hepatic or renal impairment.

Older adults are more likely to experience the typical adverse effects of BZDs to a disabling degree. Moreover, older adults do not readily biotransform BZDs because of age-related changes in liver function, so the drug persists 2 to 3 times longer. In theory, drug compounds whose activity depends on their transformation into active metabolites should be rapidly eliminated in the older patient with lower liver function; the transformation in the liver does not occur, and the parent compound is eliminated via the kidney. However, whereas patients with normal liver function are in effect receiving a minimum of two drugs (e.g., diazepam and its metabolite desmethyldiazepam), those with impaired livers are only receiving one drug (in our example, just diazepam). If the full therapeutic effect of the drug *depends* upon the presence of active metabolites, the dose would have to be increased to derive the same effect, not decreased—although this may never occur in clinical practice. On the other hand, the lack of proteins synthesized by the lower-functioning liver results in more unbound drug being available at any dosage level, thus increasing the effect and potentially causing toxicity. This suggests that the dose in the patient with liver failure be reduced, *not* because of decreased biotransformation in the liver or hepatic elimination, but because of increases in free drug caused by the decrease in plasma proteins. In patients with renal insufficiency or disease, drug elimination is reduced and the risk of accumulation increases with repeated dosing.

Patients with anxiety levels bordering on panic can be expected to have minimal perception of the reasons for their distress. Lower anxiety levels can translate into patients having a heightened awareness of their condition. Dosages of antianxiety drugs can be proportionately adjusted to modulate higher or lower anxiety levels.

Older adults, who often suffer from insomnia, have lower serum concentrations of melatonin. People who are blind often have irregular sleep cycles and may have free-running (not 24-hour) rhythms of melatonin production.

▮▮ Drug Variables

ANXIETY. BZDs have been first-line drugs for treatment of anxiety disorders for over 40 years. Their popularity is the result of a combination of pharmacologic actions and their safety profile (Box 19-4). Dosages of BZDs for panic disorders tend to be higher than those used for other anxiety diagnoses. Highly potent BZDs are recommended for panic attacks (i.e.,

---

BOX 19-4

Comparison of Benzodiazepines

Advantages	Disadvantages
Anxiolytic properties at relatively low dosages; can use for daytime anxiety and for insomnia with one dose.	Dependence and discontinuance problems can occur even at therapeutic dosages
Sedative-hypnotic effects at higher doses	Dependency and discontinuance problems more likely with high-potency drugs compared with short-acting BZDs
Greater margin of safety between anxiolytic action and sedation	Potency compounds on several consecutive nights; interdose rebound anxiety and early morning anxiety (with high potency compounds)
Higher ratio of median dose producing lethality to median effective dose (LD_{50}:ED_{50})	
Rarely associated with death from overdose alone	

Drugs with Long $t_{1/2}$

Less frequent dosing; lack of interdose rebound anxiety and insomnia; can be used for insomnia and daytime anxiety with a single dose; withdrawal problems less severe	Accumulation (problem in older adults); greater risk for next day sedation after used for insomnia

Drugs with Short $t_{1/2}$

No accumulation; less daytime drowsiness after repeated nightly use as hypnotic	More frequent dosing; rebound insomnia (especially after use of high potency compounds on several consecutive nights); interdose rebound anxiety and early morning anxiety (with high potency compounds)

---

clonazepam or alprazolam). BZDs are best prescribed for motivated patients with acute exogenous anxiety in response to a time-limited stressor.

Evidence suggests there is marked improvement in about 35% of patients in whom BZDs are used, moderate improvement with residual symptoms in about 40%, and no improvement in about 25%. However, the drugs are intended for episodic, short-term, adjunctive therapy to relieve specific symptoms. Their use on a long-term basis can lead to significant withdrawal problems when discontinued (even at therapeutic doses). Clinical experience has shown that concurrent psychotherapy reduces the time needed for drug therapy, and improved response rates may occur with combined behavioral and drug therapy.

The BZDs differ little in their pharmacologic properties, but are significantly different in potency, their ability to cross the blood-brain barrier, and their half-lives. High-potency BZDs such as alprazolam and clonazepam have a strong affinity for BZD receptors. The rate of absorption from the GI tract after oral administration determines the onset and intensity of drug action. Patients exhibiting high levels of anxiety will benefit from a drug with a rapid onset. Although some patients with anxiety may benefit from a long-acting BZD once daily at bedtime (e.g., diazepam), these drugs cause daytime sedation and motor impairment; thus an intermediate-acting BZD (e.g., lorazepam or oxazepam) is preferred, because rebound and hangover effects may be avoided. Often these patients are started on a higher dose, with the dosage being decreased as anxiolytic effects become evident. Alprazolam, chlordiazepoxide, and diazepam have shown efficacy in these instances.

Alprazolam is the only BZD specifically approved for panic disorders. It has a relatively rapid onset and very weak metabolites, and is well tolerated in terms of sedation. Its shorter half-life may be preferred in cases in which drug accumulation could be a problem. With proper dosing and close monitoring, adverse effects are relatively predictable and controlled with dosage adjustments.

Alprazolam is rapidly cleared from the system when discontinued. Abruptly stopping alprazolam results in rebound CNS excitation and seizures. If cost is a major issue, high-dose diazepam or lorazepam can be used in place of alprazolam. Diazepam and chlordiazepoxide are similarly rapid in their onset, but they have active metabolites that can cause increased sedation if they accumulate. Most adverse effects appear early in therapy and decrease after a patient has adjusted to the drug.

Buspirone may be considered first-line therapy if the patient is newly diagnosed, when chronic anxiety is present with symptoms of GAD, and when there is an absence of acute precipitants. It appears to dampen anxiety rather than extinguish it. Buspirone may be an appropriate choice if sedation or psychomotor or cognitive impairment would be dangerous. Buspirone may also be appropriate for patients with a history of substance abuse and those with personality disorders. It has not been approved for obsessive-compulsive disorders. The disadvantage of buspirone is that therapeutic effects are delayed for up to 4 weeks. BZDs, on the other hand, produce effects almost immediately. Clinical experience suggests that patients who have previously responded to BZDs may not respond as well to buspirone. Patients report less dramatic effects on somatic symptoms with buspirone than the effects seen with BZDs.

INSOMNIA. Persons with insomnia tend to show therapy-seeking rather than drug-seeking behavior, and the majority of persons with insomnia use prescribed hypnotics appropriately, without evidence of abuse. Nevertheless, BZDs are intended for short-term use only, with the goal of resetting the body's internal clock. Use BZDs cautiously in patients with a history of alcohol or substance abuse.

As noted previously, it is important to match the patient's need for a sleep aid with the aspect of their sleep that is disturbed. Patients with difficulty staying asleep require a drug with a longer duration of action, so the decision should be based on the half-life of the drug. Unlike BZDs, which tend to suppress sleep stages III and IV (deep sleep) and REM sleep, the non-BZDs eszopiclone, zolpidem, and zaleplon have little effect on the relative amount of sleep in each stage. Use a drug with a rapid onset such as zaleplon if the difficulty is falling asleep; it is the best choice given its quick onset of action and clean adverse effect profile.

Zolpidem differs from the BZDs in a number of ways. Zolpidem appears to be more efficacious as a hypnotic, with little development of tolerance. It does not interfere with sleep stages III and IV. Zolpidem does not decrease REM sleep. Short-term use of these drugs is not associated with significant tolerance or physical dependence, and withdrawal symptoms

are minimal or absent. Thus the abuse potential is relatively low. However, like the BZDs, zolpidem is classified as a Schedule IV controlled substance. Synergistic effects with BZDs and alcohol have been observed. The safety of the drugs in overdosage is not as clear as that of oral BZDs, but no fatalities have been reported with these drugs alone. In contrast to BZDs, these drugs lack antianxiety, muscle relaxant, and antiepileptic activities.

The disadvantages of zolpidem are that it is more expensive than the BZDs and can cause *anterograde amnesia,* an inability to remember events that occur for a period after drug administration; thus they must be taken at a time when the patient will be able to spend the following 8 to 9 hours asleep. Problems have been identified with vivid dreams, nightmares, and rebound insomnia. A hangover effect, dizziness, and a drugged feeling have been reported with zolpidem, although in doses of 5 to 20 mg, the drug did not impair memory or other mental functions the day after use.

Other non-BZD drugs have been used in the management of insomnia. These include the sedating antidepressant trazodone (Desyrel), tertiary tricyclic antidepressants such as amitriptyline (Elavil) and doxepin (Sinequan), and newer antidepressant agents such as nefazodone (Serzone) and mirtazapine (Remeron) (see also Chapter 20). Not only do the non-BZDs produce a more normal sleep pattern than BZDs, but they are also less likely to result in next-day drowsiness, because their durations of action are shorter than even the short-acting BZDs.

A key feature making BZDs particularly advantageous over other hypnotic drugs is their wide therapeutic index (Box 19-5). Even at relatively high dosages, BZDs are unlikely to produce notable respiratory depression in patients with normal pulmonary function (unless taken with other CNS depressants). Nevertheless, respiratory depressant effects of BZDs may become significant in patients with pulmonary disease, and therefore use of these drugs is contraindicated in this setting.

All BZDs differ in their pharmacokinetics, profile of adverse effects, and capacity to cause rebound insomnia and dependence. BZDs with a short duration of action (e.g., triazolam) can cause daytime anxiety and rebound insomnia. Anterograde amnesia appears to occur more often with triazolam than with other BZDs.

BZDs help the patient get to sleep more quickly and stay asleep for a longer period compared to a placebo. However, the sleep pattern produced is not entirely normal, because more time is spent in NREM sleep at the expense of REM sleep. In contrast, *rebound insomnia* is defined as a worsening of at least one of the following parameters, compared to the time before starting treatment: (1) sleep latency, the time until the patient falls asleep; (2) nocturnal awakenings; and (3) total sleep time. Drugs associated with moderate or severe rebound insomnia include triazolam, midazolam, and zopiclone. Rebound insomnia is most apparent when high-potency, short-acting BZDs are abruptly stopped. Longer-acting BZDs (and zolpidem) are less likely to cause rebound effects. Alprazolam is a short- to intermediate-acting drug, but it is not recommended for use as a hypnotic because it can be especially difficult to discontinue.

Lorazepam, oxazepam, and temazepam are equally effective in the treatment of transient situational and short-term insomnia, although data are sparse on the use of lorazepam

BOX 19-5

Benzodiazepine Antagonist

Drug: flumazenil (Romazicon)

Indications
Effective in reversing sedation or overdose effects of BZDs

Pharmacodynamics
Acts as a competitive antagonist at the GABA-BZD receptor complex

Pharmacokinetics
Onset: 1–2 minutes after IV administration
Peak: 6–10 minutes
Duration: Depends on dosages of BZD and of the flumazenil; resedation may occur as a result of incomplete gastric emptying of previously administered BZDs
Protein binding: 50%
Half-life: 40–80 minutes
Elimination: Primarily hepatic; administration of food during a flumazenil infusion increases drug clearance and may decrease the effect of flumazenil

Adverse Effects
- May precipitate acute withdrawal syndrome and seizures in BZD-dependent person
- Dizziness, headache, fatigue, nausea, vomiting
- Agitation, emotional lability, confusion, somnolence, sleep disorders
- Abnormal, blurred vision; altered hearing
- Arrhythmias, chest pain, hypertension

Contraindications
- Cautious use is necessary with a mixed CNS-depressant overdose, because effects of other drugs may emerge when BZD effect is removed.
- May increase ICP and risk of seizures in patients with head injury.
- Safe use during pregnancy and lactation has not been established.
- Contraindicated in patients with hypersensitivity to flumazenil or BZDs, in patients receiving BZDs for life-threatening medical conditions, and in patients with serious tricyclic antidepressant overdosage.

Drug Interactions
- No significant drug interactions.
- Does not antagonize other drugs active at GABA sites, such as alcohol, barbiturates, opioids, or general anesthetics.

Dosage
Adults: 0.2 mg IV over 30 seconds. If no response is noted, 0.5 mg is given over 30 seconds until a total of 3 mg is administered.

BZDs, Benzodiazepines; *GABA,* gamma-aminobutyric acid; *ICP,* intracranial pressure; *IV,* intravenous.

---

and oxazepam as hypnotics. As with other high-potency, short-acting BZDs, lorazepam is associated with worse rebound effects than the less potent, longer-acting drugs. This factor may not be relevant if the drugs are used for just a few nights. Triazolam is useful for the short-term (i.e., less than 2 weeks) management of stress-related insomnia when it is important to avoid daytime sleepiness.

BENZODIAZEPINE WITHDRAWAL. The development of withdrawal syndrome ordinarily results from cessation of (or reduction in) BZD use that has been heavy and prolonged. The BZDs with short half-lives increase the risk for withdrawal symptoms. BZDs are viewed by some as one of the most difficult drugs to stop (see Box 19-6). Unless the withdrawal process is slow and purposeful, the withdrawal symptoms usually stop patients from completing the taper process. The goal here is to attain a slow but steady decline of BZD serum concentrations to permit the brain to recover without adverse events taking place.

Long-term use of BZDs results in fewer GABA receptors in the brain and a decline in GABA function resulting in hyperexcitability of the CNS. Hyperexcitability is the underlying cause of most withdrawal symptoms, the severity of which varies depending on the dosages used and their duration of use. Recovery of normal brain function takes time, not unlike the slow but sure recovery after major surgery.

⚠ **Common symptoms of BZD withdrawal include elevated pulse rate, fatigue, ataxia, blurry vision, hyperreflexia, depression, and nausea. Frequently there will also be irritability, anxiety, insomnia, and muscle aches. Confusion, delirium, psychoses, and seizures are rare but possible.**

Collaborate with the patient in developing plans for retreating from BZD use, remembering that the patient is ultimately in control of the manner in which this occurs. The health care provider provides guidance and prescriptive advice, but the patient must do the work.

Jointly develop a dosage reduction schedule for the initial stages of retreating from BZD use, making sure the patient has a copy of the schedule. Discuss the importance of flexibility in the schedule so that the dosage tapering rate can be changed if needed. There may be times when tapering has to stop for a time; the schedule can be restarted at a later point, depending on how the patient is doing, and the schedule revised if needed. Advise the patient not to expect a "quick fix." In some cases the patient may need to be hospitalized for detoxification. This monitored approach usually includes a moderately rapid withdrawal but is generally considered to be safe. Psychologic support is ordinarily available during a monitored withdrawal.

Patient Education

Successful antianxiety and sedative-hypnotic therapy depends on a close alliance between patient and health care provider. Patients must be taught that antianxiety and sedative-hypnotic drugs are useful for short-term relief from anxiety and to promote sleep. They are not a solution to stress. Drug therapy is most effective as an adjunct, combined with other intervention modalities (see Table 19-7). Any critical decisions or judgments that are required of the patient should be made before sedative-hypnotic drugs are prescribed. The validity of legal documents may come into question if they are signed while the patient is under the influence of any CNS-depressant drug.

Advise the patient that BZDs may cause drowsiness at the start of therapy. Activities requiring mental alertness (e.g., driving or using power tools) should be avoided in the early stages of therapy. Also instruct the patient to avoid alcohol, sleep-inducing OTC drugs, and other CNS depressants while taking sedative-hypnotic drugs. Dangerous drug combinations are more likely to be identified when the patient purchases all drugs from the same pharmacy. Most pharmacists maintain

BOX 19-6

Characteristics of BZD-Dependent Persons

People who have become dependent on therapeutic doses of benzodiazepines (BZDs) usually have several of the following characteristics:

1. They have taken benzodiazepines in prescribed "therapeutic" (usually low) doses for months or years.
2. They have gradually come to "need" benzodiazepines to carry out normal, day-to-day activities.
3. They have continued to take benzodiazepines although the original indication for prescription has disappeared.
4. They have difficulty in stopping the drug, or reducing dosage, because of withdrawal symptoms.
5. If on short-acting benzodiazepines (e.g., alprazolam), they develop anxiety symptoms between doses, or get craving for the next dose.
6. They contact the health care provider regularly to obtain repeat prescriptions.
7. They become anxious if the next prescription is not readily available; they may carry their tablets around with them and may take an extra dose before an anticipated stressful event or a night in a strange bed.
8. They may have increased the dosage since the original prescription.
9. They may have anxiety symptoms, panic attacks with or without agoraphobia, insomnia, depression, and increasing physical symptoms despite continuing to take the drug.

Ashton, H. (2006). Benzodiazepine dependence—typical characteristics. Web4Health. Available online: web4health.info/en/answers/bio-benzo-dependence.htm. Accessed March 28, 2007.

drug profiles on patients, monitoring records for inappropriate or potentially dangerous drug interactions.

Patients who take sedative-hypnotics can develop amnesia about their use. Teach patients to store the antianxiety drug far enough away from the bedroom so that they are alert before taking another dose. It is thought that many cases of overdose arise from repeated doses taken by the patient during waking periods. In some cases, it may be necessary to place the drug supply under the supervision of a second person.

Because antianxiety and sedative-hypnotic drugs are used for adjunctive therapy, it is important that patients stay in close contact with their health care provider. Dosages and administration times may have to be adjusted in the early stages of treatment. Also, advise patients to inform you or another health care provider of any increase in sedation, lethargy, or difficulty staying awake after initial therapy has been established. In many cases, education about sleep hygiene practices (e.g., reducing caffeine intake, changing sleep habits, or pain relief) might be more appropriate than using a sedative-hypnotic drug. Early-morning wakening is one of the biologic features of depression; thus, an antidepressant may be appropriate (see Chapter 20).

Instruct the patient not to increase the dosage or to abruptly stop a BZD. When tapering begins, most drugs can be safely decreased by 10% per day. The patient will need to be monitored for the early onset of withdrawal symptoms. If withdrawal symptoms appear or anxiety increases, halt the tapering until the patient stabilizes.

Evaluation

Evaluating the efficacy of antianxiety and sedative-hypnotic drugs can be problematic because the essential characteristics of anxiety and insomnia cannot be adequately reproduced. Cognition, communication, and social relationships are difficult to assess objectively. However, clinical improvement should be evaluated, and patients should report a decrease of anxiety or insomnia. They will note better concentration and fewer tendencies toward distraction. The sense of dread and negative anticipation is lessened, and they begin to gain an insight into the reasons they are anxious. Further, there should be no symptoms of dependency.

When impaired sleep is the problem, the patient should report a decrease in symptoms. Daytime disruptions such as fatigue, impaired work performance, and transient mood disturbances may be lessened. The patient should report that he or she is learning alternative behavioral techniques (e.g., eliminating daytime napping or practicing relaxation exercises) to promote sleep. Failure of insomnia to remit after 7 to 10 days of treatment suggests the presence of an underlying primary psychiatric and/or medical condition that should be diagnosed and treated. Referral to a sleep disorder center may be appropriate.

Be alert in the outpatient setting to patients who request prescription refills on an increasingly frequent basis; this behavior may suggest improper use, abuse, or a knowledge deficit about the hazards of continued use of the drug. Some cases of chronic overdose arise because the patient receives prescriptions from more than one health care provider, each of whom is unaware of the others' prescriptions. Encourage patients to use one pharmacy, which permits tracking of all drugs used, even if provided by a different health care provider. Evaluate patients carefully for possible depression and suicidal ideations. Suicide is always a potential with use of psychoactive drugs.

KEY POINTS

- Anxiety and impaired sleep patterns have no social, economic, racial, or gender boundaries. Up to 11% of Americans suffer from some form of identifiable anxiety, and one third of the population has impaired sleep during any given year.

- Anxiety can arise from three distinct sources: as a response to a medical condition, from faulty neuroregulation in the brain, and from an identifiable psychiatric condition.
- Antianxiety drugs are not intended to relieve everyday stresses or the occasional case of impaired sleep patterns.

- Assessment of the level of anxiety a patient is experiencing is vital in allowing the care provider to intervene at the appropriate level.
- Use of the DSM-IV-TR categories assists the health care provider in identifying a patient's anxiety disorder, thus allowing greater specificity of treatment.
- First-line drugs used to treat anxiety and impaired sleep patterns are BZDs. All have different half-lives, onsets of action, and elimination pathways. Non-BZD drugs are also used to treat anxiety and impaired sleep pattern disorders. Barbiturates are seldom used as sedative-hypnotics.
- Whenever an antianxiety or sedative-hypnotic drug is started, the next step is to plan a tapering program.
- Successful initial therapy is evidenced by a decrease in the physical manifestations of anxiety or impaired sleep patterns.

Bibliography

American Psychiatric Association. (2000). *Diagnostic and statistical manual of mental disorders.* (4th ed., text revision [DSM-IV-TR]). Arlington, VA: Author.

Benca, R. (2005). Diagnosis and treatment of chronic insomnia: A review. *Psychiatric Services, 56*(3), 332–343.

Brody, T. (2005). *Human pharmacology: Molecular to clinical.* (4th ed.). St. Louis: Mosby.

DiPiro, J., Talbert, R., Yee, G., et al. (2005). *Pharmacotherapy: A pathophysiologic approach.* (6th ed.). New York: McGraw Hill.

Doran, C. (2003). *Prescribing mental health medicine: The practitioner's guide.* London: Routledge.

Fricchione, G. (2004). Generalized anxiety disorder. *New England Journal of Medicine, 351*(7), 675–682.

Gutierrez, K., and Queener, S. (2003). *Pharmacology in nursing practice.* St. Louis: Mosby.

Hardman, J., Limbird, L., and Gilman, A. (Eds.). (2001). *Goodman and Gilman's the pharmacologic basis of therapeutics.* (10th ed.). New York: McGraw-Hill.

Hobson-DuPont, J. (2006). *The benzo book.* New York: Harper Collins.

Keltner, N., and Folks, D. (2005). *Psychotropic drugs.* (4th ed.). St. Louis: Mosby.

Laudon, M. (2003). Subjective assessment of the effects of CNS-active drugs on sleep by the Leeds Sleep Evaluation Questionnaire. *Human Psychopharmacology: Clinical and Experimental, 18*(1), 570–577.

Longo, L., and Johnson, B. (2000). Addiction: Part I: Benzodiazepines, side effects, abuse risks, and alternatives. *American Family Physician, 61*(7), 2121–2128.

Mendelson, W. (2005). A review of the evidence for the efficacy and safety of trazodone in insomnia. *Journal of Clinical Psychiatry, 66*(4), 469–476.

National Center on Sleep Disorders Research (NCSDR). Available online: www.nhlbi.nih.gov/about/ncsdr.

National Sleep Foundation. (2005). *Myths—and facts—about sleep.* Available online: www.sleepfoundation.org/.

Rosenberg, R., Caron, J., Roth, T., et al. (2005). An assessment of the efficacy and safety of eszopiclone in the treatment of transient insomnia in healthy adults. *Sleep Medicine, 6*(1), 15–22.

Scharf, M., Erman, M., Rosenberg, R., et al. (2005). A 2-week efficacy and safety study of eszopiclone in elderly patients with primary insomnia. *Sleep, 28*(6), 720–727.

Swainston, H., and Keating, G. (2005). Zolpidem: A review of its use in the management of insomnia. *CNS Drugs, 19*(1), 65–89.

Thase, M. (2005). Correlates and consequences of chronic insomnia. *General Hospital Psychiatry, 27*(2), 100–112.

Walsh, J. (2006). Insights into the public health burden of insomnia. *Sleep, 29*(2), 142–143.

CENTRAL NERVOUS

20

Antidepressant and Antimania Drugs

Depression and mood disorders are underrecognized and undertreated public health and psychiatric problems. Mood disorders are so prevalent, in fact, that nearly 15% of the population of the United States will have a serious episode sometime in their lives. Mood disorders tend to be chronic in many individuals, requiring prolonged and, in some cases, lifelong treatment with drugs. Depression is at least 5 times more common than bipolar disorder (manic-depression).

DEPRESSION

EPIDEMIOLOGY AND ETIOLOGY

Depression is characterized by feelings of sadness, despair, disinterest in surroundings or pleasurable activities, and discouragement lasting over 2 weeks. Profound depression may be an isolated illness, such as major depressive disorder, or a symptom of another psychiatric disorder such as schizophrenia (see Chapter 21). A diagnosis of depression includes both depressive (unipolar) as well as manic-depressive states (bipolar). Although the recurrence rate of *unipolar depression* is high, it is approximately half the rate of those with bipolar disorder. With *bipolar* disorder, episodes of depression alternate with periods of mania.

Major depression is prevalent in Western industrialized nations (2% to 3% for males; 4% to 9% for females). Almost half of these patients have a history of one or more non–mood disorders. Men have a 7% to 12% lifetime risk for the disorder, and the life time risk for women is 20% to 25%.

Patients with major depressive disorder have substantial physical, psychologic, and occupational disabilities, including loss of work time. These patients have more physical illnesses than other patients seen in primary care settings, and their use of health care resources is greater. Depression is second only to suicide and accidents in mortality rates. A large percentage of persons who commit suicide (70%) have visited their primary care provider with mood or somatic complaints within 4 to 6 weeks of their suicide. Of patients with untreated recurrent major depression, 15% die of suicide. The U.S. mortality rate associated with depression is estimated to be 30,000 to 35,000 suicides per year.

Risk Factors
Major depressive disorder is twice as likely to occur in women, with a peak onset between the ages of 20 to 40 years. If there is a family history of major depression, an individual has 1.5 to 3 times the risk of having this disorder than the general population. Although the cause and effect are unknown, it is likely that depression leads to the separation and divorce. Depression is also more likely to be reported in unmarried

men. Again, the cause is unknown; however, it is theorized that men who are depressed are less able to fulfill the role of suitor. Depression is more likely in married women than in unmarried women; perhaps women with chronic low self-esteem settle for abusive and dysfunctional mates.

There is also an increased risk in women during the last trimester of pregnancy, the first 3 months after childbirth, and during the onset of menopause. These findings suggest that fluctuations in sex hormones are important triggers for depression. The presence of comorbid disorders contributes to the incidence; examples are diabetes; pituitary, adrenal, or thyroid disorders; occult malignant diseases; and neurologic, autoimmune, and nutritional deficiencies. The risk of depression also increases if the patient has had prior suicide attempts, is currently engaged in drug or alcohol abuse, or if there have been multiple stressful life events occurring within a short period of time.

Types of Depression
The *Diagnostic and Statistical Manual of Mental Disorders IV (DSM-IV-TR)* describes several types of depression. *Major depression* implies a prominent and relatively persistent depressed or dysphoric mood that usually interferes with daily functioning (nearly every day for at least 2 weeks). *Primary dysthymia* (formerly called endogenous depression) has no identifiable cause. *Secondary dysthymia* (formerly called exogenous or reactive depression) may be precipitated by a number of factors such as environmental stress, adverse life events, drugs, or concurrent disease states. Regardless of the type of depression, they all share common symptoms of varying degrees and durations (Box 20-1).

Depression also can be categorized as an adjustment disorder with depressed mood, substance-related mood disorder, dementia with depressed mood, depressive disorder due to a general medical condition, and depressive disorder not otherwise specified. This last category might include depression associated with premenstrual syndrome or any other disorder that does not meet the full criteria for the previously mentioned forms of depression.

PATHOPHYSIOLOGY

Although it is not clearly understood, the pathophysiology of depression can be viewed from any number of hypotheses (Box 20-2). Mood disorders such as depression are thought to arise as a result of changes in the levels of the neurotransmitters serotonin and norepinephrine and, to a lesser extent, dopamine. Serotonergic neurons originating in the median raphe and terminating in the cortex and limbic system appear to be most involved in the regulation of mental and emotional states (Fig. 20-1). Serotonin influences functions such

---

BOX 20-1

Common Symptoms of Depression*

- Fatigue or loss of energy
- Subjective reports or observation by others of a depressed, sad, irritable, or empty mood most of the day
- The presence of anhedonia; a noticeably declining interest or pleasure in all, or almost all, activities of daily living (e.g., appearance, work, sexual activities)
- A decrease or increase in food consumption; considerable weight loss (when not dieting) or weight gain (e.g., a change of more than 5% of body weight in a month).

- Insomnia or hypersomnia
- Observable psychomotor agitation or retardation; not simply subjective feelings of restlessness, or of slowing down
- A self-perception of worthlessness or excessive or inappropriate guilt
- Self-reports of indecisiveness or a reduced ability to concentrate as observed by others
- Persistent thoughts of death, suicidal ideation, or suicide attempt

*According to DSM-IV criteria, a major depressive episode includes at least 5 of the above 9 symptoms (with at least one of the symptoms being depressed mood or loss of interest or pleasure).

American Psychiatric Association. (2000). *Diagnostic and statistical manual of mental disorders* (4th ed., text revision [DSM-IV-TR]). Washington, DC: Author.

BOX 20-2

Selected Hypotheses of Depression

Psychodynamic Hypothesis
Involves difficulties with the formation and maintenance of self-esteem

Cognitive Hypothesis
Views depression as the consequence rather than the origin of negative or distorted thinking

Genetic Hypothesis
Suggests there is a dominant gene with incomplete penetrance (a hereditary condition in persons who have the dominant or double recessive gene)

Neuroendocrine Hypothesis
Suggests there is a functional or absolute deficiency in neurotransmitter release (i.e., norepinephrine, serotonin, or dopamine) and neurohormone activity involving hypothalamic functioning

Serotonin Hypothesis
Suggests there is a functional or absolute deficiency in the neurotransmitter serotonin

Permissive Hypothesis
Suggests diminished levels of serotonin gives "permission" for a superimposed deficiency of norepinephrine to manifest as depression

Dysregulation Hypothesis
Suggests noradrenergic and serotonergic postsynaptic receptors become hypersensitive because of homeostatic dysregulation of neurotransmitters

Beta-Adrenergic Receptor Hypothesis
Suggests depression results from increased beta-adrenergic receptor sensitivity

---

as anxiety, sexual behavior, appetite, aggression, pain, obsessions, emesis, learning, aversion, psychosis, vasoconstriction, migraine, sleep, suicidal ideation, and circadian rhythms. At least 14 subtypes of serotonin receptors are known.

PHARMACOTHERAPEUTIC OPTIONS

Drugs used for the treatment of depression are derived from several chemical groups and have been available for approximately 60 years. First-generation antidepressants include tricyclic antidepressants (TCAs) and monoamine oxidase inhibitors (MAOIs). Second-generation antidepressants include selective serotonin reuptake inhibitors (SSRIs) and several miscellaneous drugs. The newer drugs, although they are chemically different from TCAs, are similar in their pharmacologic actions and antidepressant effectiveness.

Selective Serotonin Reuptake Inhibitors
- citalopram (Celexa, generic)
- escitalopram (Lexapro)
- fluoxetine (Prozac, Sarafem, generic)
- paroxetine (Paxil, Pexeva)
- sertraline (Zoloft, generic)
- trazodone (Desyrel, generic)

▌▌▌ *Indications*
TCAs were the mainstay of antidepressant therapy until the introduction of the SSRIs in 1988. Fluoxetine was the first SSRI released for use in the United States. It has been used by over 21 million patients worldwide and is effective in treating depression. Fluoxetine is also approved for the treatment of major depressive disorder, obsessive-compulsive disorder (OCD), bulimia nervosa, and panic disorder. Paroxetine is FDA-approved for use in major depression, OCD, panic disorder, social anxiety disorder, generalized anxiety disorder (GAD), and posttraumatic stress disorder (PTSD). Sertraline has received approval for use in major depression, OCD, panic disorder, PTSD, premenstrual dysphoric disorder, and social anxiety disorder. Escitalopram has also received approval for GAD. Fluvoxamine is only approved for the treatment of OCD. Although trazodone has been approved for major depressive disorders, it is used more often for insomnia because of its highly sedative adverse effect. SSRIs are also used in the treatment of obesity, chronic pain,

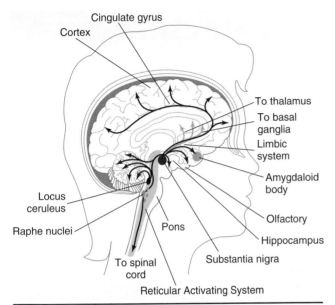

Cingulate gyrus
Cortex
To thalamus
To basal ganglia
Limbic system
Amygdaloid body
Locus ceruleus
Raphe nuclei
Pons
Olfactory
Hippocampus
Substantia nigra
To spinal cord
Reticular Activating System

FIGURE 20-1 Three neurotransmitter pathways have been mapped in the brain—norepinephrine, serotonin, and dopamine. Most norepinephrine-containing neurons are located in the locus ceruleus of the pons and the midbrain. Serotonin is found in the nuclei of the raphe. Norepinephrine and serotonin pathways are illustrated by the black arrows. Dopamine pathways are found in the substantia nigra region and follow the red arrows.

fibromyalgia, migraine, attention deficit/hyperactivity disorder (ADHD), aggression, and impulsivity (see Evidence-based Pharmacotherapeutics).

▌ *Pharmacodynamics*

Serotonin is known to modulate mood, emotion, sleep, and appetite and thus is implicated in the control of numerous behavioral and physiologic functions. Decreased serotonin neurotransmission has been proposed to play a key role in the etiology of depression. The concentration of synaptic serotonin is controlled directly by its reuptake into the presynaptic terminal, and thus drugs blocking serotonin transport have been successfully used for the treatment of depression. The SSRIs are potent blockers of serotonin reuptake, with weak affinity for norepinephrine or dopamine blockade. They have limited affinity for α_1, α_2, β-adrenergic, gamma-aminobutyric acid (GABA), histamine, and cholinergic receptors.

▌ *Pharmacokinetics*

SSRIs are well absorbed when taken by mouth. Like the TCAs, their onset, peak, and duration of action range from 1 to 4 weeks, and they may require up to 12 weeks for complete effectiveness (see Table 20-1). SSRIs are distributed throughout the body, cross placental membranes, and have been found in breast milk. The half-lives of SSRIs are prolonged in patients with hepatic impairment because they

---

EVIDENCE-BASED PHARMACOTHERAPEUTICS

Continuation of SSRI Therapy versus Therapy with TCAs

■ Background
Selective serotonin reuptake inhibitors (SSRIs) are generally considered superior to tricyclic antidepressants (TCAs) in terms of their adverse effects profiles. For this reason, the SSRIs have largely replaced TCAs as first-line drug therapy for depression. Further, the SSRIs are thought to have better stop-out rates (i.e. fewer people stopping therapy) than TCAs and heterocyclic antidepressant drugs. It is important to compute the stop-out rates for these two drug classes in order to have a better understanding of the relative tolerability of these drugs.

■ Research Article
Barbui, C., Hotopf, M., Freemantle, N., et al. Treatment discontinuation with selective serotonin reuptake inhibitors (SSRIs) versus tricyclic antidepressants (TCAs). *The Cochrane Database of Systematic Reviews.* 2000, Issue 4. Art. No. CD002791. DOI: 10.1002/14651858.CD002791.

Purpose
The purpose of this study was to evaluate the tolerability of SSRIs in relation to stop-out rates compared to TCAs and heterocyclic antidepressant drugs.

Design
A review of 136 parallel-group, randomized, controlled studies comparing SSRIs with TCAs or heterocyclic antidepressants in subjects treated for depression.

Methods
Two investigators independently evaluated and extracted data from the 136 studies, and a third investigator assessed instances of disagreement.

The Cochrane Collaboration Depression, Anxiety and Neurosis Controlled Trials Registers, MEDLINE, and EMBASE were searched, as well as specialty journals, government documents, bibliographies, conference abstracts, and previous systematic reviews. Pharmaceutical company representatives were also contacted for information.

Findings
Fewer subjects stopped SSRI therapy compared to the TCA-heterocyclic group (OR 1.21, 95% CI 1.12- 1.30). There were statistically significant differences between the SSRIs and the older and newer TCAs in relation to total stop-outs. No significant differences favoring SSRIs were noted when they were compared with heterocyclic antidepressants. According to the study's analysis, the less-than-desirable adverse effects profile of the older TCAs explained the differences in stop-outs, but not for ineffectiveness.

Conclusions
Overall, subjects taking SSRIs will probably continue antidepressant therapy compared with subjects taking TCAs and heterocyclic drugs. Although SSRIs are thought to be advantageous to the TCAs in relation to the total number of subjects who discontinued therapy, this advantage was fairly small.

■ Implications for Practice
The results of this analysis are based on short-term, randomized, controlled trials and may not generalize to clinical practice. This has implications for pharmacoeconomic models, some of which may have overvalued the difference between stop-out rates with SSRIs compared to TCAs. There is a need for larger, high-quality, head-to-head studies comparing the SSRIs and other classes of antidepressants in terms of tolerability and likelihood of stopping therapy.

SSRIs, Selective serotonin reuptake inhibitors; *TCAs,* tricyclic antidepressants.

PHARMACOKINETICS

TABLE 20-1 Antidepressant and Mood-Stabilizing Drugs

Drug	Route	Onset	Peak	Duration	PB %	t½	BioA%
SELECTIVE SEROTONIN REUPTAKE INHIBITORS (SSRIs)							
citalopram	PO	1–4 wk	4 hr	1–2 wk	80	35 hr	80
escitalopram	PO	1–4 wk	5 hr	1–2 wk	56	35 hr	80
fluoxetine	PO	1–4 wk	6–8 hr	24–48 hr	95	1–3 days; 5–7 days*	>90
paroxetine	PO	1–4 wk	3–7 hr	24 hr	90	21 hr	>90
sertraline	PO	1–8 wk	6–8 hr	24 hr	98	26 hr	>90
trazodone	PO	1–2 wk	0.5–2 hr	8 hr	90	5–9 hr	UA
SEROTONIN–NOREPINEPHRINE REUPTAKE INHIBITORS (SNRIs)							
amoxapine	PO	1–6 wk	2–4 hr	16–24 hr	90	8 hr	UA
duloxetine	PO	2 hr	6 hr	24–48 hr	>90	8–17 hr	~90
venlafaxine	PO	4 days-6 wk	2–4 hr	6–8 hr	27	5 hr	>90
TRICYCLIC ANTIDEPRESSANTS (TCAS)							
amitriptyline	PO	2–3 wk	2–6 wk	18–24 hr	>90	10–50 hr	UA
	IM	2–3 wk	2–6 wk	Days-weeks	>90	10–50 hr	UA
clomipramine	PO	2–6 wk	2 hr	12–24 hr	96	21 hr	UA
desipramine	PO	2–6 wk	4–6 hr	24 hr	90	UA	UA
doxepin	PO	2–3 wk	6 wk	18–24 hr	>90	8–24 hr	UA
imipramine	PO, IM	1–2 hr	2–6 wk	Weeks	>90	8–16 hr	86
nortriptyline	PO	2–3 wk	6 wk	18–24 hr	>90	18–28 hr	UA
protriptyline	PO	2–6 wk	24–30 hr	12–24 hr	>90	>67 hr	UA
trimipramine	PO	2–6 wk	2 hr	8–16 hr	>90	UA	UA
MONOAMINE OXIDASE INHIBITORS (MAOIs)							
isocarboxazid	PO	1–4 wk	2–6 wk	2 wk	UA	UA	UA
phenelzine	PO	1–4 wk	2–6 wk	2 wk	UA	24–48 hr	UA
tranylcypromine	PO	Days	2–3 wk	3–5 days	UA	UA	UA
MISCELLANEOUS ANTIDEPRESSANTS							
bupropion	PO	1–4 wk	2 hr	6–12 hr	80	14 hr	UA
maprotiline	PO	2–6 wk	8–24 hr	18–24 hr	88	>51 hr	UA
mirtazapine	PO	2–6 wk	1.5 hr	12–24 hr	85	20–40 hr	50
nefazodone	PO	2–6 wk	48 hr	12–24 hr	99	2–4 hr	20
MOOD STABILIZERS							
carbamazepine	PO	1–2 wk	1.5 hr; 4–5 hr; 12 hr‡	8–12 hr	76; 57†	8–29 hr	UA
lamotrigine	PO	4–6 wk	1–4 hr	8–12 hr	55	25–33 hr	98
lithium	PO	1–2 wk	0.5 hr; 1–3 hr; 3–4 hr‡	6–12 hr	0	20–27 hr	UA
valproic acid	PO	4 days-2 wk	1–4 hr	8–12 hr	90–95	6–16 hr	UA

*Half-life of fluoxetine is 1–3 days, and the half-life of the metabolite norfluoxetine is 5–7 days.
†Protein binding of carbamazepine in adults and children, respectively.
‡Time to peak effects of tablets or capsules, syrup, and extended-release forms of carbamazepine, respectively.
BioA, Bioavailability; *IM*, intramuscular; *PB*, protein binding; *PO*, by mouth; $t_{1/2}$, half-life; *UA*, unavailable.

---

inhibit the CYP450 system. The majority of these drugs are eliminated through the urine.

▌▌ Adverse Effects and Contraindications

SSRIs are not without adverse effects. They tend to produce excitation rather than sedation (20%). These effects have been referred to as "energizing or activating" adverse effects. Although there is reduced risk of orthostatic hypotension, tachycardia, heart block, blurred vision, and dry mouth, the adverse effects of SSRIs are similar to those of other antidepressants: nausea, insomnia, sexual dysfunction (anorgasmia), ejaculatory disturbances, and decreased libido. There have been reports that antidepressants, including SSRIs, make patients "less sensitive" to the needs of others, outside of sexual contact. Most adverse effects tend to be mild and well tolerated, and in some cases quickly disappear after 1 to 2 weeks of treatment. Rare adverse effects may include hyponatremia, suicidality, and increased bleeding times. Disturbance of sexual function does not go away, a disturbing aspect of antidepressant drug therapy.

SSRIs are contraindicated in patients with hypersensitivity to the drug or its ingredients, and they should not be used by patients with narrow-angle glaucoma or immediately after a myocardial infarction. In the past, it was thought that the SSRIs were relatively safe during pregnancy, but recent studies indicate that they may not so benign after all. Additionally, exercise caution when using these drugs in older patients and those with preexisting cardiovascular disease. Children and adolescents need to be especially monitored for increased suicidality, which has been reported to occur in these populations.

▌▌ Drug Interactions

All SSRIs are absolutely contraindicated for concomitant use with MAOIs. The combination of SSRI and MAOI may result in a severe serotonergic syndrome, which is characterized by autonomic instability, rigidity, hyperpyrexia, widely fluctuating vital signs, stuporous rigidity, and possibly death (Table 20-2).

DRUG INTERACTIONS
TABLE 20-2 Antidepressant and Mood-Stabilizing Drugs

Drug	Interactive Drugs	Interaction
SELECTIVE SEROTONIN REUPTAKE INHIBITORS		
SSRIs as class of drugs	MAOIs	Increases risk of serotonergic syndrome
	Antifungals, macrolide antibiotics, cimetidine	Increases plasma levels of citalopram
	carbamazepine	Decreases plasma levels of citalopram
	metoprolol	Increases metoprolol plasma levels
paroxetine	risperidone	Increases risperidone concentration enough to cause EPS
fluoxetine, sertraline	Alcohol, CNS depressants	Increases CNS depressant effects
	digoxin, highly protein-bound drugs, warfarin	Displaces interactive drug from binding sites
	MAOIs	Risk of serotonergic syndrome
	phenytoin	Increases phenytoin concentration and risk of toxicity
trazodone	Alcohol, CNS depressants	Increases CNS depression
	Antihypertensives	Increases effects of antihypertensives
	digoxin, phenytoin	Displaces interactive drug from binding sites
	ketoconazole, indinavir, ritonavir	Increases concentrations and toxicity of trazodone
SEROTONIN-NOREPINEPHRINE REUPTAKE INHIBITORS		
duloxetine	Quinolone antibiotics, fluoxetine, quinidine, paroxetine	Increases concentration of duloxetine
	warfarin	Increases concentration of warfarin
	MAOIs	Increases risk of serotonergic syndrome
	thioridazine	Increases risk for ventricular arrhythmias
	Alcohol	Increases risk of hepatic injury
venlafaxine	MAOIs	Increases risk for serotonin syndrome
	St. John's wort	Increases sedative-hypnotic effects
TRICYCLIC ANTIDEPRESSANTS		
TCAs as class of drugs	Alcohol, antihistamines, barbiturates, opioids	Additive CNS depression
	MAOIs	Increases risk of serotonin syndrome
	Anesthetics	Tachyarrhythmias
	Anticoagulants	Increases effects of anticoagulant
	Anticonvulsants	Increases seizure risk
	Antipsychotics, aspirin, cimetidine, disulfiram, methylphenidate, oral contraceptives, phenothiazines, phenylbutazone, phenytoin, SSRIs, glucocorticosteroids, thyroid hormones	Increases effects of TCA
MONOAMINE OXIDASE INHIBITORS		
MAOIs as class of drugs	Amphetamines	Increases effects of MAOI
	Adrenergics, antihypertensives, cocaine, cough and cold remedies, ephedrine, methylphenidate, phenylephrine, TCAs, SSRIs, trazodone	Hypertensive crisis
	meperidine	Hyperpyrexia
	Antiepileptics	Increases CNS depression
	Insulin, sulfonylureas	Increases effect of interactive drugs
MISCELLANEOUS ANTIDEPRESSANTS		
amoxapine	clonidine, MAOIs	Hyperpyrexia, hypertension, seizures, death
	Antihypertensives	Decreases effects of antihypertensive
	Alcohol, antihistamines, opioids, sedative-hypnotics	Additive CNS depression
	Adrenergic drugs, anticholinergics	Additive effects of interactive drugs
	cimetidine, fluoxetine, phenothiazines, oral contraceptives	Increased levels of interactive drugs
	disulfiram	Transient delirium
bupropion, maprotiline	levodopa, MAOIs	Increases risk of adverse reactions to interactive drug
	Alcohol, antidepressants, benzodiazepines, phenothiazines	Increased risk of seizures with cessation of drug use
	MAOIs	Hyperpyrexia, seizures, hypertension, death
	Antihypertensives	May prevent antihypertensive effects
	Alcohol, antihistamines, clonidine, opioids, sedative-hypnotics	Additive CNS depression
	Phenothiazines	Increases risk of seizures
	Adrenergics, decongestants, vasoconstrictors	Additive adrenergic effects, increases risk of adverse cardiovascular reactions
	Anticholinergics, antihistamines, atropine, disopyramide, haloperidol, phenothiazines, quinidine	Additive anticholinergic effects
	cimetidine, fluoxetine, oral contraceptives	Increases levels of maprotiline
nefazodone	alprazolam, triazolam	Increases serum levels of interactive drug
MOOD STABILIZERS		
carbamazepine	diltiazem, erythromycin, propoxyphene, verapamil	Increases serum levels of interactive drugs
	MAOIs	Hyperpyrexia, hypertension, seizures, death if interactive drug taken within 2 weeks
		Decreases effects of interactive drug

	Anticoagulants, antiepileptics, barbiturates, benzodiazepines, doxycycline, felbamate, glucocorticoids, oral contraceptives, phenytoin, quinidine	
	acetaminophen, dextropropoxyphene, isoniazid	Increased risk of hepatotoxicity
	cimetidine, diltiazem, verapamil	Increases serum levels of carbamazepine
lamotrigine	carbamazepine, phenobarbital, phenytoin, valproic acid	Decreases lamotrigine levels
lithium	Neuromuscular blockers	Prolongs action of NMB
	Amphetamines, calcium channel blockers, carbamazepine, haloperidol, molindone	Increases risk of neurotoxicity
	ACE inhibitors, amiloride, chlorpromazine, diuretics, fluoxetine, methyldopa, NSAIDs, probenecid	Increases risk of lithium toxicity
	aminophylline, caffeine, digoxin, phenothiazines, sodium bicarbonate, sodium chloride, theophylline, urea	Decreases effects of lithium
	chlorpromazine	Decreases effects of chlorpromazine
	Antithyroid drugs, potassium iodide	Hypothyroid effects may be additive
valproic acid	carbamazepine	Decreases level of valproic acid
	Aspirin, NSAIDs, cefamandole, cefaperozone, cefotetan, heparin, thrombolytics, warfarin	Increases risk of bleeding
	Barbiturates, primidone	Decreases biotransformation of interactive drug
	Alcohol, antihistamines, antidepressants, opioids, MAOIs, sedative-hypnotics	Additive CNS depression
	phenytoin	Increases or decreases effects of interactive drug
	chlorpromazine, felbamate	Increases valproic acid levels

ACE, Angiotensin-converting enzyme; *CNS*, central nervous system; *EPS*, extrapyramidal symptoms; *MAOIs*, monoamine oxidase inhibitors; *NMB*, neuromuscular blocker; *NSAIDs*, nonsteroidal antiinflammatory drugs; *SNRIs*, serotonin-norepinephrine reuptake inhibitors; *SSRIs*, selective serotonin reuptake inhibitors; *TCAs*, tricyclic antidepressants.

◼ Dosage Regimen

Dosage regimens for the treatment of depression vary from drug to drug (Table 20-3). Use the appropriate resources and references when prescribing SSRI antidepressants. Pay close attention to cardiovascular, hepatic, and renal status, particularly in the young and the elderly. Employ lower doses of paroxetine and fluoxetine in patients with renal impairment, because increased concentrations may occur.

◼ Lab Considerations

Monitor the complete blood count (CBC) and differential before and throughout the course of therapy, with attention to leukopenia, anemia, thrombocytopenia, or increased bleeding times when warranted. Proteinuria and a mild increase in aspartate transaminase (AST) levels may occur during sensitivity reactions to fluoxetine. It may cause hypoglycemia and hyponatremia in some patients. Slight, clinically insignificant decreases in leukocyte and neutrophil counts may occur with trazadone.

Serotonin-Norepinephrine Reuptake Inhibitors

◆ duloxetine (Cymbalta)
◆ venlafaxine (Effexor, Effexor SR, Effexor XL)

Duloxetine

Duloxetine, a serotonin-norepinephrine reuptake inhibitor (SNRI), is one of the newer antidepressants on the market. It has been approved for the treatment of major depressive disorder characterized by persistent, prominent dysphoria (occurring nearly every day for at least 2 weeks) and manifested by four of eight symptoms (change in appetite, changes in sleep patterns, increased fatigue, impaired concentration, feelings of guilt or worthlessness, anhedonia, psychomotor agitation or retardation, or suicidal tendencies).

The exact mechanism of action of duloxetine is unknown, but it is thought to inhibit the reuptake of serotonin and norepinephrine at central nervous system (CNS) presynaptic membranes. Duloxetine has no activity at dopaminergic, adrenergic, cholinergic, or histaminergic receptors. It does not inhibit monoamine oxidase (MAO).

Duloxetine is well absorbed when taken orally. There is a median 2-hour lag before absorption begins. Duloxetine undergoes extensive biotransformation, but the circulating metabolites have not been shown to contribute significantly to pharmacologic activity. Most of a duloxetine dose (about 70%) appears in the urine as metabolites; about 20% is excreted in the feces.

Frequent adverse effects of duloxetine include nausea, dry mouth, constipation, and insomnia. Occasionally dizziness, fatigue, diarrhea, somnolence, anorexia, diaphoresis, and vomiting may occur. Although rare, blurry vision, erectile dysfunction, delayed or failed ejaculation, anorgasmia, anxiety, decreased libido, and hot flashes have been reported. Duloxetine may increase serum levels of AST, alanine transaminase (ALT), and bilirubin. It is a pregnancy category C drug. Safety and efficacy have not been established in children.

Venlafaxine

Venlafaxine is a phenylalanine compound structurally unrelated to other antidepressants. In addition to depression, venlafaxine is approved for the treatment of GAD, panic disorder, and social anxiety disorder. It strongly inhibits the reuptake of both serotonin and norepinephrine but has no significant cholinergic, histaminergic, or adrenergic receptor action. It is a weak inhibitor of dopamine reuptake.

Venlafaxine is well absorbed following oral administration, but undergoes extensive first-pass biotransformation. Of the parent compound, 56% is converted to its active metabolite O-desmethylvenlafaxine (ODV). The primary route of elimination is via the kidneys.

Venlafaxine has an adverse effect profile that includes nausea (especially in high or rapidly increased dosages), somnolence, nervousness, constipation, abnormal ejaculation or orgasm, dizziness, sweating, and fatigue. Venlafaxine is weight-neutral compared to the other antidepressants. Venlafaxine is also associated with sustained blood pressure increases of 1 to 7 mm Hg in some patients. This dose-related adverse effect occurs in about 13% of patients taking more than 300 mg/day. Only 3% of patients experience an

CENTRAL NERVOUS

DOSAGE
TABLE 20-3 Antidepressant and Mood-Stabilizing Drugs

Drug	Uses(s)	Dosage	Implications
SELECTIVE SEROTONIN REUPTAKE INHIBITORS (SSRIs)			
citalopram	Depression, diabetic neuropathy, OCD, dementia, smoking cessation, alcohol abuse	*Adult:* 20 mg PO daily initially. May increase in 20-mg increments at intervals of no less than 1 wk to max of 60 mg/day *Older Adult: hepatic impairment:* 20 mg PO daily. Titrate to 40 mg only for nonresponding patients.	Should not be used within 14 days before or after MAOI therapy. Not recommended in children under age 18 yr.
escitalopram	Depression	*Adult:* 10 mg PO daily; may increase to 20 mg after 1 wk	Should not be used within 14 days before or after MAOI therapy. Not for children under age 18 yr.
fluoxetine	Depression, obesity, OCD	*Adult:* 20 mg PO daily. Increase after 2–4 wk to max of 20–80 mg. Give doses over 20 mg/day twice daily	Use lower doses in older adults and those with renal impairment. Safety and efficacy not established in children.
paroxetine	Depression, panic disorder, OCD	*Adult:* 20 mg PO daily. Increase in 2–4 weeks to max of 20–50 mg PO daily	Should not be used within 14 days before or after MAOI therapy.
sertraline	Depression, panic disorder, OCD	*Adult:* 50 mg PO daily in single dose in AM or PM. Increase weekly to 200 mg PO as needed depending on response.	Should not be used within 14 days before or after MAOI therapy.
trazodone	Depression, chronic pain, insomnia	*Adult:* 150 mg PO daily in 3 divided doses. Increase by 50 mg PO every 3–4 days until desired response occurs. Do not exceed 400 mg as outpatient or 600 mg as hospitalized patient. *Older Adult:* 75 mg PO daily in divided doses initially. May be increased every 3–4 days *Child 6–18 yr:* 1.5–2 mg/kg/day in divided doses. Increase every 3–4 days up to 6 mg/kg/day.	A larger dose may be given at HS to decrease daytime drowsiness and dizziness.
SEROTONIN-NOREPINEPHRINE REUPTAKE INHIBITORS (SNRIs)			
amoxapine	Depression	*Adult:* 100–150 mg PO daily in divided doses. Increase to 200–300 mg by end of first week. Max: 300 mg daily as outpatient and 600 mg daily in divided doses as inpatient *Older Adult:* 25 mg PO 2–3 times daily initially. Increase to 50 mg PO 2–3 times daily.	Once optimal dose is achieved, may give as single HS dose.
duloxetine	Depression	*Adult:* 40 mg PO daily in divided doses Max: 60 mg/day	Should not be used within 14 days before or after MAOI therapy.
venlafaxine	Depression	*Adult:* 75 mg PO in 2–3 divided doses. Increase slowly to maximum of 225 mg/day until desired effect is achieved.	Safety and efficacy not established in children or older adults.
TRICYCLIC ANTIDEPRESSANTS			
amitriptyline	Depression, chronic pain	*Adult:* 30–100 mg PO daily as single dose at HS –or– in divided doses. Increase gradually to 150–300 mg PO daily –or– 20–30 mg IM 4 times/day *Older Adult:* 25 mg PO at HS. Increase to up to 10 mg PO 3 times daily and 20 mg at HS. Not to exceed 100 mg/day *Child 6–12 yr:* 1–5 mg/kg PO daily in divided doses *Child >12 yrs:* 10 mg PO 3 times daily and 20 mg PO at HS. Increase slowly to 100 mg PO as single dose at HS.	Dosage increases should be made at HS because of sedation. Titration may take weeks to months. IM route for short-term use only.
clomipramine	OCD, depression, panic disorder, bulimia, neurogenic pain Off-label use: cataplexy with narcolepsy	*Adult:* 25 mg PO 3 times daily. Increase as tolerated to 100 mg during first 2 wk. Max: 250 mg PO daily *Child >10 yr:* 25 mg PO initially. Gradually increase as tolerated during first 2 wk to max of 3 mg/kg or 100 mg, whichever is smaller.	Once maximum dose is reached, give at HS to minimize sedation. Titrate to lowest effective dose. Effectiveness after 10 wk has not been documented.
desipramine	Depression, cocaine withdrawal, eating disorders	*Adult:* 100–200 mg PO daily as single or divided doses. Increase gradually to maximum of 300 mg. *Older Adult:* 25–100 mg PO daily initially. Not to exceed 150 mg daily *Child 6–12 yr:* 1–5 mg/kg/day in divided doses	Not recommended for children <12 yr. Maintenance: At reduced dosage for at least 2 mo after desired response achieved.
doxepin	Depression, chronic pain	*Adult:* 25–150 mg PO daily as single dose at HS –or– 2–3 divided doses. Gradually increase to 300 mg.	Single dose should not exceed 150 mg.
imipramine	Depression, enuresis	*Adult and Child: Depression:* 25–50 mg PO 3- 4 times daily –or– 100 mg IM daily in divided doses. Not to exceed 300 mg/day *Older Adult:* 25 mg PO at HS initially. Increase to 100 mg daily in divided doses. *Child 6–12 yr:* 10–30 mg PO daily in 2 divided doses *Child >12 yr:* 25–50 mg PO in divided doses. Not to exceed 100 mg daily *Enuresis:* 25 mg PO 1 hr before HS. Increase by 25 mg at weekly intervals PRN to 50 mg in child <12 yr; in child >age 12 yr, increase at weekly intervals PRN to 75 mg.	Total daily dose may be given at HS.
nortriptyline	Depression, chronic pain	*Adult:* 25 mg PO 3–4 times daily. Increase to 150 mg PO daily. *Child >12 yr or Older Adult:* 30–50 mg PO as single divided doses	Not recommended in children <18 yr.

protriptyline	Depression, OSA	*Adult:* 15–40 mg PO 1–4 times daily. Increase to 60 mg PO if required. Max: 60 mg daily. *Child >12 yr or Older Adult:* 5 mg PO 3 times daily. Increase gradually if necessary.	Make changes in dosage with morning dose. Not for children <12 yr. Monitor cardiovascular system if dosage exceeds 20 mg daily.
trimipramine	Depression associated with sleep disorders, peptic ulcer disease, dermatologic disorders	*Adult:* 75–100 mg PO daily in divided doses. Increase to150–200 mg as needed. Maintenance: 50–150 mg PO as single dose at HS *Older Adult:* 50 mg PO with gradual increases up to 100 mg PO daily. *Child >12 yr:* 50 mg PO daily. Gradually increase to 100 mg PO daily.	Reduce dosage to lowest effective dose after satisfactory response. Continue for 3 mo to lessen possibility of relapse.

MONOAMINE OXIDASE INHIBITORS

isocarboxazid	Atypical depression	*Adult:* 20–60 mg PO daily in divided doses. Increase by 10 mg/day every 2–4 wk.	**Patient should be cautioned verbally and in writing to avoid foods containing tyramine.**	⚠
phenelzine	Atypical depression, panic attacks	*Adult:* 15 mg PO 3 times daily. Increase to 60–90 mg/day in divided doses, reduce to smallest effective dose. *Older Adult:* 15 mg PO daily with slow dose titration *Panic Attacks:* 15 mg PO daily, increase over 2 wk to 15 mg 3–4 times daily	**Patient should be cautioned verbally and in writing to avoid foods containing tyramine.**	⚠
tranylcypromine	Atypical depression	*Adult:* 30 mg PO daily in divided doses initially. Increase after 2 wk by 10 mg/day at 1- to 3-wk intervals up to 60 mg/day *Older Adult:* 2.5–5 mg/day initially. Increase every 3–4 days up to 45 mg/day *Panic Attacks:* 10 mg PO daily initially. Increase over 2 wk to 20–30 mg day.	**Advise patient verbally and in writing to avoid foods containing tyramine.**	⚠

MISCELLANEOUS ANTIDEPRESSANTS

bupropion	Depression	*Adult:* 100 mg PO twice daily. Increase after 3 days to 100 mg 3 times daily; after 4 wk of treatment, increase to 450 mg PO in divided doses.	Wait 6 hr between dosages of 300 mg/day, or at least 4 hr between doses of 450 mg/day. No single dose should exceed 150 mg.
maprotiline	Depression, bipolar disorder	*Adult:* 25–75 mg PO daily as outpatient; 100–150 mg PO daily as impatient. Increase by 25 mg daily to 150–225 mg PO as outpatient; by 25 mg daily to 300 mg PO as inpatient. *Older Adult >age 60 yr:* 50–75 mg PO daily for maintenance	Do not use within 14 days before or after MAOI therapy. Not for children <18 yr. Maintenance: Lowest effective level
mirtazapine	Depression	*Adult:* 15 mg PO at HS; may increase by 15 mg/day every 1–2 wk to maximum of 45 mg/day *Older Adult:* 7.5 mg at HS; increase by 7.5–15 mg/day every 1–2 wk to maximum of 45 mg/day	Do not use within 14 days before or after MAOI therapy. Not for children <18 yr.
nefazodone	Depression	*Adult:* 100 mg PO twice daily. Increase weekly up to 600 mg/day in divided doses. *Older Adult:* 50 mg PO twice daily. Increase weekly as patient needs dictate.	Do not use within 14 days before or after MAOI therapy. Not for children <18 yr.

MOOD-STABILIZING DRUGS

carbamazepine	Seizures Off label: bipolar disorder	*Adult:* 10–20 mg/kg/day PO initially. Usually started at 200 mg PO 2–3 times daily. Increase at 4- to 5-day intervals. Maintenance: 800–1200 mg PO daily	Induces its own biotransformation. Many drug interactions. Check list before using.
lamotrigine	Long-term maintenance therapy of bipolar disorder	*Adult:* 25 mg PO daily initially. May double dose after weeks 2, 4, and 5. Target dose: 200 mg/day	Decreased dosage may be effective in patients with significant renal impairment. Reduce dosage over at least 2 wk (approximately 50%/wk) when discontinuing the drug.
lithium	Bipolar disorder	*Adult:* 300–600 mg PO initially 3 times daily; increase at weekly intervals to 900–1200 mg PO twice daily. Maintenance: 300 mg 3–4 times daily *–or–* 600 mg twice daily. Max: 2400 mg daily *Child:* 0.4–0.5 mEq/kg/day in 2–3 divided doses	300 mg lithium carbonate contains 8 to 12 mEq lithium. Dosage listed is for tablets or capsules. The dosage for SR formulations is different.
valproic acid divalproex	Bipolar disorder, acute mania	*Adult and Older Adult:* 750 mg PO daily in divided doses. Max: 60 mg/kg/day	Give in divided 150 mg doses once daily.

HS, Bedtime; *IM,* intramuscular (route); *MAOI,* monoamine oxidase inhibitor; *OCD,* obsessive compulsive disorder; *OSA,* obstructive sleep apnea; *PO,* by mouth; *PRN,* as needed.

increase in blood pressure at a dosage less than 100 mg. Venlafaxine use is acceptable in hypertensive individuals if their hypertension is well controlled on antihypertensive drugs. Venlafaxine use is contraindicated in patients taking MAOIs.

Reduce the dosage of venlafaxine by 25% in patients with renal impairment and by 50% in patients on dialysis. A 50% reduction in dose is recommended for patients with liver impairment.

Tricyclic Antidepressants

◆ amitriptyline (Elavil, Endep); ♣ Levate, Meravil, Novo-Triptyn
◆ clomipramine (Anafranil)
◆ desipramine (Norpramin, Pertofrane)

- ◆ doxepin (Adapin, Sinequan); ◆ Novo-Doxepin, Triadapin
- ◆ imipramine (Tofranil, others); ◆ Apo-Imipramine, Impril, Novo-Pramine
- ◆ nortriptyline (Aventyl, Pamelor)
- ◆ protriptyline (Vivactil); ◆ Triptil
- ◆ trimipramine (Surmontil)

Indications

Although less commonly used today, TCAs are still used as first-line drugs in the treatment of major depression. They elevate mood, increase activity and alertness, decrease morbid preoccupation, improve appetite, and normalize sleep patterns. TCAs have also been used for the treatment of chronic pain syndromes (amitriptyline, doxepin, imipramine, and nortriptyline), neuropathy, migraine headache, attention deficit disorder, and enuresis (imipramine). Doxepin has been used for panic disorders. TCAs eliminate panic attacks in about 75% of patients. Anticipatory anxiety and phobic avoidance behaviors are not affected.

Pharmacodynamics

Tricyclic antidepressants contain a 3-ring structure and differ structurally and pharmacologically from other currently available antidepressants (e.g., SSRIs, MAOIs).

Antidepressant drugs appear to work by blocking presynaptic reuptake of serotonin and norepinephrine (Fig. 20-2). Thus there is an increased amount of these neurotransmitters in the synapse, prolonging and intensifying their effects. Such action is consistent with the monoamine hypothesis of depression, which asserts that depression stems from a deficiency in monoamine-mediated neurotransmission. If that is true, drugs that increase the effects of monoamines should reduce symptoms of depression. The relative ability of individual TCAs to block the reuptake of serotonin and norepinephrine are summarized in Table 20-4.

Note that blockade of neurotransmitter reuptake by itself does not fully explain the therapeutic effectiveness of the TCAs. This statement is based on the observation that clinical responses of antidepressants and the neurotransmitter

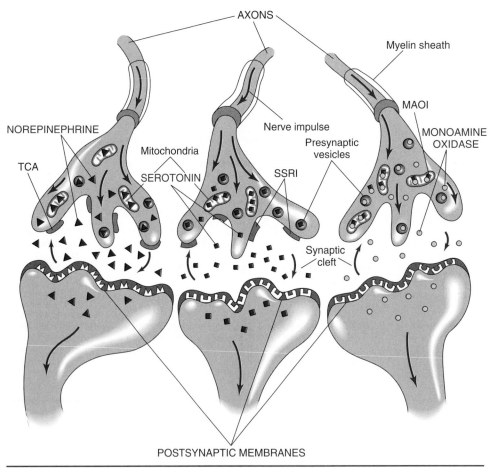

FIGURE 20-2 Pharmacodynamics of Antidepressant Drugs. Normally, norepinephrine, serotonin, and MAO are released from storage sites within the adrenergic nerve by arrival of a nerve impulse. Norepinephrine is metabolized within the nerve by MAO or by catechol-O-methyltransferase (COMT) in the synapse. Most norepinephrine is taken back into the nerve and stored. TCAs block the reuptake of norepinephrine in the synapse. SSRIs inhibit the reuptake of serotonin and minor amounts of norepinephrine from the synapse. SNRIs inhibit the reuptake of serotonin and norepinephrine from the synapse. MAOIs preferentially block the reuptake of MAO, norepinephrine, and serotonin at the mitochondria level rather than in the synapse. *MAO,* Monoamine oxidase; *MAOIs,* monoamine oxidase inhibitors; *SNRIs,* serotonin-norepinephrine reuptake inhibitors; *SSRIs,* selective serotonin uptake inhibitors; *TCAs,* tricyclic antidepressants.

TABLE 20-4 Potency of Neurotransmitter Blockade

Drug and Class	Serotonin	Norepinephrine	Anticholinergic	Dopamine	Sedation
TRICYCLIC ANTIDEPRESSANTS (TCAs)					
amitriptyline	+2	+3	+3	0	+3
desipramine	0	+5	+1	0	+1
doxepin	+3	+2	+3	0	+4
imipramine	+3	+2	+4	0 to +1	+3
nortriptyline	+2	+3	+3	0	+2
protriptyline	+2	+3	+3	0	+1
trimipramine	+3	+2	+4	0	+4
SELECTIVE SEROTONIN REUPTAKE INHIBITORS (SSRIs)					
citalopram	+3	+2	0	0	0
escitalopram	+3	+2	0	0	0
fluoxetine	+4	+3	0	0	*
paroxetine	+4	+3	+1	0	+1
sertraline	+4	+2	0	0	*
trazodone	+2	0	0	0	+3
SEROTONIN-NOREPINEPHRINE REUPTAKE INHIBITORS (SNRIs)					
amoxapine	+3	+3	+2	0	+2
duloxetine	+1	+1	+	0	+1
venlafaxine	+1	+1	+1	0 to +1	+2
MONOAMINE OXIDASE INHIBITORS (MAOIs)					
isocarboxazid	†	†	0	0	+2
phenelzine	†	†	0	0	+2
tranylcypromine	†	†	0	0	+2
MISCELLANEOUS ANTIDEPRESSANTS					
bupropion	‡	‡	+2	+1	*
maprotiline	+1	+3	+3	0	+3
mirtazapine	+2	0	+2	0	+1
nefazodone	+4	0	0	0	+2

*Fluoxetine, sertraline, and bupropion produce moderate stimulation, not sedation.
†MAOIs do not block the uptake of transmitter. Instead they increase the intraneuronal stores at norepinephrine, serotonin, and dopamine.
‡Bupropion primarily inhibits reuptake of dopamine rather than norepinephrine or serotonin.
+5 strongest response; 0, none.

blockade do not occur in the same time frame. In other words, the drugs block transmitter uptake within a few hours of administration, whereas relief of depression may take several weeks to develop. Therefore, it appears that an intermediary response must be occurring between the onset of the blockade and the onset of therapeutic response. What composes this intermediate response is not clear.

One theory, the biogenic amine dysregulation theory of depression, suggests that noradrenergic and serotonergic postsynaptic receptors become hypersensitive because of homeostatic dysregulation of neurotransmitters. Antidepressant treatment may reverse this phenomenon over a period of a few weeks, explaining the delay in efficacy.

▮ Pharmacokinetics

As noted in Table 20-1, the majority of TCA antidepressants are well absorbed when taken by mouth and widely distributed throughout the body. Effective relief of depression is achieved within 2 to 6 weeks, in most patients. Most of the drugs are extensively biotransformed in the liver with enterohepatic recirculation and secreted into gastric juices. Some of the drugs are biotransformed to active metabolites. TCAs are thought to cross the placenta and enter breast milk.

▮ Adverse Effects and Contraindications

TCAs are used less often than SSRIs because of the magnitude of the adverse effects and the extreme toxicity of the TCAs in the suicide-prone older adult population. Orthostatic hypotension is the most serious of the common adverse effects and is due in part to blockade of α_1 receptors on blood vessels. Cardiovascular effects of TCAs are rare in the absence of overdosage or preexisting cardiac impairment. These drugs affect the heart by decreasing vagal influence secondary to the muscarinic blockade and by acting directly on the bundle of His to slow conduction. Both mechanisms increase the risk of arrhythmias (premature atrial and ventricular contractions); ST segment depression, flattened or inverted T waves, and a prolonged QRS may be noted on electrocardiogram. Heart failure can be worsened. Tricyclic antidepressants are contraindicated in patients with third-degree heart block.

Anticholinergic adverse effects are often the most disturbing. By blocking cholinergic receptors, an array of anticholinergic effects is possible. These include blurred vision, worsening of narrow angle glaucoma, photophobia, dry mouth, constipation, urinary retention (particularly in older adults and those with dementia and pseudodementia), sinus tachycardia, and mental clouding.

Drowsiness, muscle tremors or twitches, paresthesias, fatigue, weakness, and seizures may occur with overdose or in patients with known seizure disorders. In addition, hallucinations, delusions, and activation of schizophrenic or manic states are possible. TCAs have been associated with successful suicides.

Adverse gastrointestinal (GI) effects include nausea, vomiting, and heartburn, as well as weight loss or weight gain. TCAs can also cause sexual dysfunction, which is manifested as decreased libido, reduced arousal, and impaired orgasm.

▥ Drug Interactions

Many drug interactions occur with TCAs (see Table 20-2). The drug groups that commonly interact with TCAs include MAOIs, direct-acting and indirect-acting sympathomimetic drugs, and CNS depressants.

▥ Dosage Regimen

Although tricyclic antidepressants have been administered in up to four divided doses throughout the day, the drugs are long-acting, and the entire daily dosage may be administered orally at 1 time (see Table 20-3). Administration of single daily doses may improve patient compliance. Administration of the entire daily dose at bedtime may promote sleep, reduce daytime sedation, and possibly reduce the awareness of other adverse effects. Patients who experience insomnia and stimulation from the drugs may receive the entire daily dose in the morning.

▥ Lab Considerations

Amitriptyline causes an increase in AST, ALT, and serum alkaline phosphatase concentrations. Doxepin can cause elevated serum sodium levels. Imipramine and nortriptyline may cause alterations in blood glucose levels.

Monoamine Oxidase Inhibitors (MAOIs)

◆ isocarboxazid (Marplan)
◆ phenelzine (Nardil)
◆ selegiline transdermal system (Emsam); ✦ Apo-Selegiline, Novo-selegiline
◆ tranylcypromine (Parnate)

▥ Indications

Four MAOIs are approved for use in the United States: selegiline transdermal, isocarboxazid, phenelzine, and tranylcypromine. These drugs are considered second- or third-line antidepressants for most patients. Because their use can be hazardous, they are reserved for patients who have not responded to TCAs, SSRIs, newer drugs, or electroconvulsive therapy (ECT). However, for patients with atypical depression, MAOIs may be the drugs of first choice. MAOIs have also been used with some success in the treatment of panic disorder, bulimia, obsessive-compulsive disorders, and agoraphobia.

▥ Pharmacodynamics

MAOIs exert their effects primarily on organ systems influenced by sympathomimetic amines and serotonin. By nonspecifically and irreversibly inhibiting intraneuronal MAO_A and MAO_B, the amount of norepinephrine and serotonin available is increased (see Fig. 20-2). The increased transmission that results from these supranormal quantities is thought key to relief of depression. Eighty-five percent of MAO must be degraded to produce an antidepressant effect.

Phenelzine produces irreversible inhibition of intraneuronal MAO. Recovery of irreversible inhibition is a slow process, requiring synthesis of new enzyme. Hence the effects of irreversible inhibitors persist for about 2 weeks after the drug is withdrawn. In contrast, tranylcypromine produces reversible inhibition. Recovery from reversible inhibition is more rapid, occurring in 3 to 5 days. These drugs inhibit not only MAO but other enzymes as well, and they interfere with the hepatic biotransformation of many drugs.

▥ Pharmacokinetics

The onset of MAOI therapeutic activity ranges from 1 to 4 weeks. Peak serum levels and duration of action are variable (see Table 20-1).

▥ Adverse Effects and Contraindications

The most common adverse effect associated with MAOI drugs is orthostatic hypotension. Restlessness, insomnia, anorexia, constipation, nausea, vomiting, dry mouth, urinary retention, impotence, drowsiness, headache, rash, dizziness, and weakness have also been noted. Other adverse effects include increased perspiration, urinary frequency, weight gain, flushing, increased appetite, numbness, paresthesias, tremor, myoclonic jerks, hyperreflexia, and muscle spasm.

Adverse effects of MAOIs are dose dependent for the most part; however, they cause severe hypertension when taken with foods containing large amounts of tyramine (Box 20-3). Following ingestion of tyramine, there is a rapid displacement and release of norepinephrine from noradrenergic neurons, resulting in severe hypertension. The hypertensive crisis is the most serious adverse effect of MAOIs and is potentially fatal. Severe headache, nausea, vomiting, sweating, neck stiffness and soreness, and mydriasis also occur. Intracranial hemorrhage can result, which may lead to death. Tranylcypromine produces greater CNS stimulation than phenelzine, perhaps because of its close structural similarity to amphetamine.

▥ Drug Interactions

A number of drugs must be avoided when taking MAOI therapy. Most drug interactions occur with the indirect-acting sympathomimetic drugs (e.g., cough and cold drugs, asthma drugs, phenylephrine, ephedrine, and amphetamine). The interactions are secondary to inhibition of hepatic MAO (see Table 20-2).

▥ Dosage Regimen

Titrate the initial oral adult dosages of phenelzine and tranylcypromine to the patient needs and tolerance (see Table 20-3).

The initial dosage of selegiline transdermal system is 6 mg/24 hr. The transdermal patch should be applied each day to dry, hair-free skin on the upper torso, the upper thigh, or the outside upper arm. A modified diet is only indicated at the higher dosages of 9 mg/24 hr and 12 mg/24 hr.

▥ Lab Considerations

Serum glucose levels may decrease in the presence of MAOIs.

Miscellaneous Antidepressants

◆ bupropion (Wellbutrin, Wellbutrin SR, Wellbutrin XL)
◆ maprotiline (generic)
◆ mirtazapine (Remeron, Remeron Sol Tab)
◆ nefazodone (generic)

Bupropion

Bupropion is used in the treatment of depression, often in conjunction with psychotherapy. The mechanism of action

BOX 20-3

Tyramine-Restricted Diets

General Information
- Tyramine-restricted diets are designed for patients taking monoamine oxidase (MAO) inhibitors, drugs that have been reported to cause hypertensive crisis when taken concurrently with tyramine-rich foods. These include foods in which aging, protein breakdown, and putrefaction are used to increase flavor. As little as 5 to 6 mg of tyramine can produce a response, and 25 mg is a dangerous amount.
- Food sources of other pressor amines such as histamine, dihydroxyphenylalanine, and hydroxytyramine are also avoided.
- Avoid over-the-counter (OTC) drugs such as decongestants, cold remedies, and antihistamines.

Foods to Be Avoided
- *Cheeses:* New York State cheddar, Gruyere, Stilton, Emmentaler, Brie, Camembert, processed American
- *Other aged cheeses:* Blue, Boursault, brick, cheddars, Gouda, mozzarella, Parmesan, Romano, Roquefort
- *Wines, beers, and ales:* All on-tap beer, Chianti, domestic nonalcoholic beer, Riesling, sauternes, sherry, vermouth
- *Yeast and yeast products:* Homemade bread, yeast extracts such as soup cubes, canned meats, and marmite

- *Meat:* Aged game, beef and chicken liver, canned meats with yeast extracts, any meats marinated over 24 hours
- *Fish* (salted dried): Cod, herring, pickled herring
- *Other:* Anchovies, broad bean pods, chocolate, cream (especially sour), dates, dried figs, eggplant, nuts, overripe fruit, raisins, salad dressing, sauerkraut, soy sauce, vanilla, yogurt

Foods to Consume Cautiously
- Avocado (fresh)—maximum one per day
- Aspartame-containing foods and beverages—not more than 3 servings per day
- Chocolate candy—up to 4 oz per day
- Cottage cheese or cream cheese, fresh—up to 4 oz per day of each
- Monosodium glutamate (MSG) in prepared foods, snack foods, Chinese foods—minimize use
- Processed American cheese, fresh—up to 2 oz per day
- Raspberries—not more than 1½ oz per day
- Sour cream—up to 4 oz per day
- Soybean paste or tofu—not more than ½ oz per day
- Yogurt—8 oz fresh, refrigerated, or frozen

---

is unknown, but it is thought to be primarily a weak blocker of norepinephrine. Bupropion has mild dopaminergic actions and does not inhibit MAO. It is also used to treat sexual dysfunction related to SSRI treatment and as an aid for smoking cessation and in the management of ADHD. The anticholinergic adverse effects of TCAs make bupropion a more appealing option for depression.

Bupropion is rapidly absorbed, with peak plasma concentrations occurring within 2 hours. Bupropion is widely distributed throughout the body. Bupropion has two active metabolites, each with longer elimination half-lives than the parent compound. Bupropion is biotransformed in the liver, with elimination in the feces following a biphasic decline (see Table 20-1).

Common adverse effects of bupropion include agitation, anxiety, restlessness, insomnia, and weight loss. It has a significant incidence of seizures, approximately 4 times that of any other antidepressant. It is specifically a concern in patients with a history of seizures, head injury, anorexia, or bulimia (i.e., related to electrolyte imbalance), and those who are taking other drugs that lower the seizure threshold.

Bupropion is contraindicated for concurrent use with MAOI drugs. It should be used with caution in patients taking gingko biloba and those with alcohol intake, since it increases the risk for seizure activity.

The initial adult dosage of immediate-acting bupropion is 2 to 3 times daily. The dosage may be increased after 3 days if needed. After the fourth week of therapy, the dosage may be increased to its maximum if necessary. The extended-release formulation of bupropion is dosed once daily. Dosage may be increased after 4 days to 300 mg/day if needed. Equally spaced dosing intervals reduce the risk of seizures (see Table 20-3).

Maprotiline

Maprotiline is a tetracyclic antidepressant with chemical properties similar to TCAs. It blocks only the reuptake of norepinephrine at the synapse, not serotonin. It retains some anticholinergic properties.

Maprotiline is slowly absorbed from the GI tract, with peak plasma concentrations reached 8 to 24 hours after administration (see Table 20-1). It is biotransformed in the liver to the active metabolite desmethylmaprotiline. One third of the drug is eliminated in the feces and two thirds in the urine.

Although maprotiline has the same adverse effects profile as that of TCAs, there is a higher risk of seizures, even in patients with no known seizure disorder. Seizures are most likely to occur when recommended doses are exceeded. Avoid concurrent administration of other drugs known to lower the seizure threshold. There are a multitude of drug interactions (see Table 20-2).

Mirtazapine

Like maprotiline, mirtazapine has a tetracyclic molecular structure and is chemically unrelated to SSRIs, TCAs, and MAOIs. The role of mirtazapine in treating depression is similar to that of the TCAs. Although its exact mechanism of action is unknown, it is a selective alpha-2–receptor antagonist affecting both norepinephrine and serotonin activity. It also blocks 5-hydroxytryptamine-2 (5-HT$_2$) and 5-hydroxytryptamine-3 (5-HT$_3$) receptors, and thus is not associated with the nausea, sexual dysfunction, nervousness, diarrhea, or insomnia that is relatively common with the use of SSRIs.

Mirtazapine is rapidly absorbed following oral administration and has a half-life of 20 to 40 hours. Peak plasma concentrations are reached 2 hours after an oral dose. It has a bioavailability of 50% and is eliminated predominantly in the urine (75%) and feces (15%). Women demonstrate a significantly longer half-life than men (37 hours versus 26 hours). Clearance is reduced by 30% in patients with hepatic impairment and by 30% to 50% in those with moderate to severe renal impairment. Clearance in older adult men is

CENTRAL NERVOUS

40% lower, whereas in older adult women, it is only reduced by 10%.

Mirtazapine's adverse effects profile includes weight gain and sedation, both of which are related to its affinity for histamine$_1$ receptors. It also has moderate peripheral alpha-1 antagonist activity, which is associated with orthostatic hypotension. There have been rare cases of reversible agranulocytosis with mirtazapine.

Nefazodone

Nefazodone is structurally similar to trazodone, a weak SSRI, but is most helpful in the treatment of depression characterized by prominent anxiety and sleep disturbances. It acts in a manner similar to trazodone but has potent, postsynaptic serotonin receptor blockade while simultaneously inhibiting presynaptic serotonin and norepinephrine reuptake. It also antagonizes α_1 receptors.

Nefazodone is rapidly and completely absorbed after oral administration, but it has a bioavailability of only 20% (see Table 20-1). Nefazodone is subject to an extensive first-pass effect. The half-life is dose dependent, increasing from 1 hour at 50 mg to 2.4 hours at 300 mg. After multiple doses of 200 to 300 mg, the elimination half-life is increased to 3 to 4 hours.

Common adverse effects of nefazodone include headache, nervousness, insomnia, drowsiness, anxiety, tremor, dizziness, and lightheadedness. GI effects may include anorexia, altered taste, nausea, vomiting, dry mouth, dyspepsia, and constipation. Postural hypotension is also possible. Sweating, rash, and pruritus have also been noted. Because nefazodone lacks significant anticholinergic and antihistaminic activity, reports of blurry vision, urinary retention, and weight gain are relatively infrequent.

Cases of life-threatening liver failure (1 per 250,000 to 300,000 patient years) have been reported in the United States in patients treated with nefazodone. Concurrent administration of another highly protein-bound drug may cause increased free concentrations of the other drug or of nefazodone, possibly resulting in adverse events. Initial sedation sometimes limits nefazodone's usefulness and tolerability. Smaller doses, slower titration, or daily late-day dosing may be used to help patients through an initial period of sedation. Before initiating nefazodone therapy, conduct a washout period of 4 to 5 days for paroxetine and sertraline and several weeks for fluoxetine.

CLINICAL REASONING

Treatment Objectives

The ultimate goal in acute-phase (0 to 12 weeks) treatment of depression is achieving symptomatic remission and full return of psychosocial functioning. The prevention of relapse and recurrence is the essential goal of the continuation and maintenance phases of treatment.

Objectives for the patient with chronic depression include reducing the likelihood of relapse or recurrence. To accomplish these objectives, several issues must also be addressed: rapid stabilization of mood, establishment of euthymia (normal mood), and establishment of normal sleep and eating patterns; prevention of suicide or self-injurious behaviors; education concerning the course of depression, its biologic basis, and potential for recurrence; and drug management. This is necessary for both the patient and any significant others.

Treatment Options

Depression remains an extremely stigmatized medical disorder. There are widespread misconceptions about the cause, the treatment, the degree of suffering and impairment caused by depression, and even about its existence. Depression may be erroneously regarded as merely feeling blue or a character weakness, or something the patient can recover from quickly. For this reason, many individuals are reluctant to take drugs or fear discussing the illness with their families, friends, or employers.

Patients also fear becoming dependent on antidepressants and misunderstand the need for daily dosing. Often they do not accept the idea that they have to depend on a drug, especially on a long-term basis, to help them manage something they feel they should be naturally and inherently able to manage. Some patients refer to antidepressants as "happy pills," suspecting that they will induce euphoria, which they do not. (See the Case Study–Antidepressants.)

Unipolar depression can present as a single episode but more often, in vulnerable individuals, it tends to recur. Therefore it is important to determine if the patient has a history of depression. A personal or family history of depression, bipolar disorder, substance abuse, violence, panic, attention deficit disorder, OCD, anorexia or bulimia, anxiety, or suicide attempts are all potentially important factors to note before therapy is started.

▦ Patient Variables

Diagnosis of depression is made on the basis of DSM-IV criteria, after other treatable causes of depressive-like illness are ruled out. Testing used to rule out other diseases includes CBC; liver, thyroid, and renal function testing; urinalysis; and electrolyte, vitamin B$_{12}$, and folate levels. Various screening tools and depression scales are available to assist in making or confirming a diagnosis of depression. Among those most commonly used are the Beck Depression Inventory and the Hamilton Depression Scale. The Zung Self-Rating Depression Scale is a simple screening instrument that can be used in any outpatient setting.

Seriously consider the patient's past experience with antidepressants and current preferences, when making the decision for an antidepressant. A patient's past response tends to predict future response. Another factor to consider is the perception of the efficacy and adverse effects of the drug, either in the patient or in family members. There is a high incidence of suicide associated with depressive disorders; therefore question the patient directly about suicidal thoughts and impulses and his or her personal history of suicide attempts. As a result of their narrow therapeutic index, TCAs have been used as a lethal means of suicide.

LIFE-SPAN CONSIDERATIONS

Pregnant and Nursing Women. An adjustment reaction with depressed mood is known as postpartum or maternal depression, or the so-called baby blues, occurring in at least 50% of all women. It is a short-lived, early-onset disorder characterized by mild depression, anxiety, crying episodes, headache, fatigue, and irritability. It is more severe with first births and seems related to the rapid alterations of estrogen,

CASE STUDY   Antidepressants

ASSESSMENT

History of Present Illness	MG is a 42-year-old white female with complaints of sad mood, intermittent crying, hypersomnia, and lack of appetite. She has decreased energy, focus, and concentration. She reports feeling hopeless and helpless, has anhedonia, and vague suicidal ideations. These patterns have persisted for 8 weeks. MG has a history of mild depression but denies receiving drug therapy. She has a workout routine to help with much-needed weight loss but has not had the energy to follow through with her trainer.
Past Health History	She reports no drug or alcohol abuse. She is a nonsmoker. There is a family history of depression, Alzheimer's disease, and alcoholism. She has a history of a head injury 4 years ago secondary to a fall but takes no seizure drugs.
Life-Span Considerations	MG is a healthy middle-aged woman. She is in a supportive, consistent relationship with a husband of 17 years. MG is gainfully employed in a responsible, executive position. Her degree of compliance is judged to be adequate, although she leads a very busy life, has a hectic schedule, and frequently travels on business. MG has an insurance plan with a formulary that covers most of the antidepressants.
Physical Exam Findings	VSS: *BP:* 110/76. *Height:* 5'6". *Weight:* 190 pounds. Otherwise unremarkable.
Diagnostic Testing	Blood chemistry normal, including thyroid function tests

DIAGNOSIS: Major depression

MANAGEMENT

Treatment Objectives	1. Achieve symptomatic remission and full return of psychosocial functioning 2. Reestablish normal sleeping, eating, and ADL patterns. 3. Prevent relapse and recurrence of depressive symptoms.
Treatment Plan	**Pharmacotherapy** venlafaxine XR 37.5 mg PO daily during first week of therapy; 75 mg daily during second week; then titrate dosage based on patient response to a maximum of 225 mg/day. **Patient Education** 1. Common adverse effects including the drug-induced excitation that may occur in the first 2 weeks of therapy. The excitation usually disappears within those first 2 weeks. 2. Follow up in office in 2 weeks or sooner if needed. 3. Continue venlafaxine for at least 6 months following full remission of depressive symptoms. 4. Antidepressants are not dependency-producing but do need to be tapered down to avoid withdrawal symptoms. 5. Do not stop therapy without first contacting the health care provider to avoid withdrawal symptoms. 6. Drug-induced excitation usually disappears within the first 2 weeks of therapy. If drowsiness occurs, avoid tasks that require alertness until response to drug is established. 7. Health care provider and family are to monitor for worsening depression, suicidal thoughts during initial months of therapy, and with any dosage changes. 8. Carry medical alert identification. **Evaluation** 1. Sleep, eating, and activity patterns have returned to normal. Suicide ideations no longer present. 2. Energy levels, concentration, and ability to focus have improved. 3. The patient and family express knowledge and some degree of acceptance of depression, and they demonstrate an awareness of the nature, course, and treatment of depression.

CLINICAL REASONING ANALYSIS

Q1. There are so many different classes of antidepressants. How do you know which antidepressant to use for MG?

A. All of the classes of antidepressants are effective in treatment of major depression, with similar efficacy, and all of the antidepressants have roughly equal response rates. The decision about which drug to use is based on recommendations from the Texas Implementation of Medication algorithm, which suggests that an SSRI, sustained-release bupropion, nefazodone, venlafaxine, or mirtazapine be used during initial treatment of major depression without psychotic features.

Continued

CASE STUDY Antidepressants—Cont'd

Q2. I've heard that venlafaxine causes excitation. Is that why you chose it over another SSRI?

A. First of all, venlafaxine is an SNRI, not an SSRI. Because venlafaxine inhibits reabsorption of serotonin as well as nor-epinephrine, it can indeed cause excitation. This early response to the drug usually resolves within the first 2 weeks, but it is important to warn the patient about the effect. Because of venlafaxine's excitation possibility, it may also give MG a boost and reduce her hypersomnia a bit.

Q3. According to the Redbook's wholesale drug prices, the TCAs are cheaper than venlafaxine. Why did you not choose a TCA?

A. MG has had vague suicidal ideations. Because of the long-half life of most TCAs, a suicidal attempt by overdose can be lethal. Additionally, venlafaxine XR has a relatively rapid onset of action, requires once-daily dosing, and has a half-life of 5 hours, compared to the half-life of TCAs whose half-lives range from 18 to more than 67 hours.

Q4. When we did our psychiatric rotation, we saw a number of patients taking MAOIs. Could we have used one of them?

A. Yes, we could have, although I refer patients in need of an MAOI to the psychiatric or mental health professionals who work with them regularly. MAOIs are also not practical, owing to their problematic adverse effects and considerable dietary restrictions, which may be difficult or impossible to follow given MGs business, travel, and hectic life. Further, newer drugs do not require the close monitoring that older agents do. Lack of frequent laboratory monitoring should enhance compliance and safety, which are concerns because of her unpredictable work and travel schedule.

---

progesterone, and prolactin levels after delivery. Women with histories of mood disorders are especially vulnerable during the postpartum period.

Children and Adolescents. Clinical manifestations of depression vary across the life span, but in essence, they are developmentally specific. The clinical presentation of depression in children and adolescents can differ from that in adults and generally varies with the age and developmental stages of the child. Younger children may exhibit behavioral problems (e.g., social withdrawal, aggressive behavior, apathy, sleep disruption, weight loss); adolescents may show somatic complaints, self-esteem problems, rebelliousness, poor performance in school, or patterns of risky or aggressive behaviors.

Risk factors for depression can be genetic, environmental, and psychosocial. If one parent has a depressive disorder, the risk of depression for the offspring is 27% to 29%. If both parents are affected, the risk increases to 74% to 76%. Psychosocial factors play a part in putting children at risk for depression. Early trauma, self-blame, rigid family dynamics, disturbance in mother-child relationships, or unresolved loss have been reported precursors to depression. Other contributing factors include loss of self-esteem, learning disabilities, chronic illness, or physical deformity.

During infancy, the manifestations are noted as biologic and deprivation syndromes. During early childhood (3 to 4 years of age), abnormal motor activity is most notable, with more observable episodes of sadness during the ages of 5 to 8 years. During late childhood (9 to 12 years of age), low self-esteem and disappointment with self are characteristic; girls are more likely to suffer from depression than boys at this age. In adolescence, depression heralds much the same signs and symptoms as those of an adult but may also manifest as anorexia nervosa, somatization disorders, and looking at options in an inflexible all-or-none manner.

Limited data are available to date from studies evaluating various antidepressant drugs in children and adolescents, and many of these studies have methodologic limitations. However, there is some evidence that a child's response to antidepressants may differ from that seen in an adult. Use caution in extrapolating data from adult studies when making treatment decisions for children and adolescents. Results of several studies evaluating TCAs in preadolescent and adolescent patients with major depression indicate a lack of overall efficacy in this age group. Based on the lack of efficacy data regarding use of TCAs and MAO inhibitors in this population and because of the potential for life-threatening adverse effects associated with their use, many experts consider SSRIs the drugs of choice when antidepressant therapy is indicated for the treatment of major depressive disorder in children and adolescents.

The FDA notes that, whereas efficacy of fluoxetine has been established in children and adolescents, efficacy of newer antidepressants (i.e., citalopram, fluvoxamine, mirtazapine, nefazodone, paroxetine, sertraline, venlafaxine) was not conclusively established in clinical trials. Also, the FDA states that use of antidepressants may increase the risk of suicidal thinking and behaviors. Thus, when considering an antidepressant for a child or adolescent, the health care provider must balance the clinical need with the risk of increased suicidality.

Parents or guardians must deliberate four important considerations when their child is prescribed an antidepressant: (1) the risk of suicidal thoughts or actions; (2) the need and the means to prevent suicidal thoughts or actions in their child; (3) the need to watch for warning signs of suicide if the child is taking an antidepressant; and (4) the benefits and risks to their child in using antidepressants.

Older Adults. The response to antidepressants in older adults is similar to that in younger adults, but depression in older

Controversy

Antidepressants for Adolescents: Good or Bad?

According to the Centers for Disease Control and Prevention, suicide is the third leading cause of death among people ages 15 to 24 years. Major depression and bipolar disorder were present in over 90% of these suicides. Controversy surrounds the treatment of depression in young people since many of these deaths may have been preventable.

In September of 2004, the Food and Drug Administration (FDA) ordered black box warnings for antidepressants, as well as other product labeling changes and a drug guide pertaining to pediatric suicidality. Nonetheless, the results of several recent studies concluded that not treating the adolescent or young adult for depression may be a worse threat to their safety and that FDA-imposed black box warnings on antidepressants may be delaying or inhibiting treatment. Although only fluoxetine is approved by the FDA for the treatment of pediatric depression, the following drugs were also affected:

amitriptyline (Elavil)
amoxapine (Asendin)
bupropion (Zyban, Wellbutrin)
clomipramine (Anafranil)
chlordiazepoxide/amitriptyline
    (Limitrol)
citalopram (Celexa)
desipramine (Norpramin)

doxepin (Sinequan)
duloxetine (Cymbalta)
escitalopram (Lexapro)
fluoxetine (Prozac, Sarafem)
fluvoxamine maleate (Luvox)
imipramine (Tofranil, Tofranil-PM)
isocarboxazid (Marplan)
maprotiline (Ludiomil)

mirtazapine (Remeron)
nefazodone (Serzone)
nortriptyline (Aventyl, Pamelor)
olanzapine, fluoxetine (Symbyax)
paroxetine mesylate (Pexeva)
paroxetine HCL (Paxil)
phenelzine (Nardil)
perphenazine, amitriptyline (Etrafon,
    Triavil)

protriptyline (Vivactil)
sertraline (Zoloft)
tranylcypromine (Parnate)
trazadone (Desyrel)
trimipramine (Surmontil)
venlafaxine (Effexor)
selegiline (Emsam)

CLINICAL REASONING

- What concerns do you believe underlie the decision to use a potent antidepressant drug in treating major depression or bipolar disorder?
- Given the black box warnings on the above list of drugs, what support can you provide to a concerned parent whose child has been prescribed an antidepressant?
- Under what circumstances would you decide to withdraw antidepressant therapy in an adolescent?
- Would your willingness to prescribe an antidepressant vary with the age of your patient (child vs. adolescent vs. postpartum female vs. older adult)?

---

adults is often not recognized and not treated. Of all suicides, 23% involve older adults. In older adults with major depression, TCAs (e.g., amitriptyline) appears to be as effective as SSRIs (e.g., fluoxetine, paroxetine, sertraline) but may cause more overall adverse effects than the SSRIs. Older adults appear to be more susceptible to adverse effects of MAO inhibitors (e.g., episodes of hypertension, malignant hyperthermia) than younger patients, and these adverse effects are associated with increased morbidity in older patients because they have less compensatory reserve to cope with serious adverse reactions. Further, older adults appear to be especially sensitive to anticholinergic, cardiovascular, and sedative effects of TCAs, as well as susceptible to the orthostatic hypotension they often cause. The low incidence of anticholinergic effects associated with SSRIs compared with TCAs is a potential advantage, since some of these effects (e.g., constipation, dry mouth, confusion, memory impairment) may be particularly troublesome in these patients. Some health care providers feel that SSRIs may be preferred for treating depression in older adults, in whom the orthostatic hypotension associated with TCAs may result in injuries related to falls. Still, despite the fewer cardiovascular and anticholinergic effects associated with SSRIs, these drugs have no advantages over TCAs with regard to incidence of hip fractures. In addition, there is little difference in the rates of falls between nursing home residents receiving TCAs and SSRIs. Therefore all older adults receiving either type of antidepressant should be considered at increased risk and appropriate measures taken to prevent falls.

Patients with dementia of the Alzheimer's type (Alzheimer's disease, presenile or senile dementia) often manifest depressive symptoms such as depressed mood, appetite loss, insomnia, fatigue, irritability, and agitation. Most experts recommend that patients with dementia of the Alzheimer's type and depressive symptoms be considered for drug therapy even if they fail to meet the criteria for a major depressive syndrome. The goals of such therapy are to improve mood, functional status (e.g., cognition), and quality of life. Although patients may demonstrate only depressed mood, the possibility of more extensive depressive symptomatology should be considered. Patients should be monitored carefully for indices of major depression, suicidal ideation, and neurovegetative signs, since safety measures (e.g., hospitalization for suicidal ideation) and more vigorous and aggressive therapy (e.g., relatively high dosages, multiple drug therapies) may be needed in some patients.

If drug therapy is initiated for depressive symptoms in patients with Alzheimer's disease, an SSRI such as fluoxetine, paroxetine, or sertraline is recommended for first-line therapy because of the favorable adverse effects profile of these drugs in this population compared with other currently available antidepressants. Available evidence and experience with the use of antidepressants in patients with dementia of the Alzheimer's type and associated depressive manifestations indicate that depressive symptoms (including depressive mood alone and with neurovegetative changes) in such patients are responsive to antidepressant therapy. In some patients, cognitive deficits may partially or fully resolve during antidepressant therapy, but the extent of response will be limited by the degree of cognitive impairment that is related to depression. In a controlled study comparing paroxetine and imipramine in patients with coexisting depression and dementia, both drugs were found to be effective; however, paroxetine was better tolerated (fewer anticholinergic and serious adverse effects).

Drug Variables

Barring contraindications to drug therapy, antidepressant drugs are first-line treatment for major depressive disorders in the following circumstances:

- Depression is moderate to severe.
- Psychotic, melancholic, or atypical features are present.
- Psychotherapy by a trained, competent, psychotherapist is not available.
- Maintenance treatment is planned, and the patient has shown a positive prior response to treatment.

Optimizing antidepressant drug therapy is not trivial; it requires an understanding of the antidepressant being used, as well as close follow-up of patient response. Treatment should be individualized; the most appropriate strategy for a particular patient is determined by clinical factors such as severity of depression (i.e., mild, moderate, severe), presence or absence of certain psychiatric features (e.g., suicide risk, catatonia, psychotic or atypical features, alcohol or substance abuse or dependence, panic or other anxiety disorder, cognitive dysfunction, dysthymia, personality disorder, seasonal affective disorder), and concurrent illness (e.g., asthma, cardiac disease, dementia, seizure disorder, glaucoma, hypertension). Demographic and psychosocial factors as well as patient preference also are used to determine the most effective treatment strategy.

Although use of psychotherapy alone may be considered initially for patients with mild to moderate major depressive disorder, combined use of antidepressant drug therapy and psychotherapy may be useful for patients with moderate to severe major depressive disorder who have psychosocial concerns, interpersonal problems, or a comorbid disorder. In addition, combined use of antidepressant drug therapy and psychotherapy may be beneficial in patients who have a history of poor compliance or only partial response to adequate trials of either antidepressant drug therapy or psychotherapy alone.

Antidepressant drug therapy can be used alone for initial treatment of patients with mild depression (if preferred by the patient) and usually is indicated alone or in combination with psychotherapy for initial treatment of patients with moderate to severe major depression (unless ECT is planned).

ECT is not generally used as initial treatment of uncomplicated major depression, but is recommended as first-line treatment for severe major depression that includes psychotic features, catatonic stupor, severe suicidality, food refusal leading to nutritional compromise, or other situations when a rapid antidepressant response is required. ECT also is recommended for patients who have previously shown a positive response or a preference for this treatment modality, and it can be considered for patients with moderate or severe depression who have not responded to or cannot receive antidepressant drug therapy.

In certain situations involving severely depressed patients unresponsive to adequate trials of monotherapy with several individual antidepressant drugs, adjunctive therapy with another drug (e.g., buspirone, lithium), or the addition of a second antidepressant (e.g., bupropion) has been used. However, combination therapy is associated with an increased risk of adverse effects, usually requires dosage adjustments, and should be undertaken only after careful consideration of the relative risks and benefits.

Most clinical studies have shown that antidepressant effects of usual dosages of TCAs in patients with major depression are comparable to those of usual dosages of SSRIs, or other antidepressants (Fig. 20-3). Studies comparing the TCAs have not conclusively demonstrated superiority of one drug over another. The onset of action of TCAs appears to be comparable to that of SSRIs, although there is some variability in the data reported by different studies.

Because response rates in patients with major depression are similar for most currently available antidepressants, the drug choice for a given patient depends primarily on other factors such as potential adverse effects, safety or tolerability of the adverse effects, psychiatric and medical history, patient or family history of response to specific therapies, patient preference, quantity and quality of available clinical data, cost, and relative safety in the event of acute overdose. No single antidepressant can be recommended as optimal for all patients because of substantial heterogeneity in individual responses and in the nature, likelihood, and severity of adverse effects. In addition, patients vary in the degree to which certain adverse effects and other inconveniences of drug therapy (e.g., cost, dietary restrictions) affect their preferences.

Because of differences in the adverse effects profile between TCAs and SSRIs, particularly in relation to anticholinergic effects, cardiovascular effects, and weight gain with TCAs, SSRIs may be preferred in patients in whom such effects are not tolerated or are of potential concern. The decreased incidence of anticholinergic effects associated with SSRIs compared with TCAs is a potential advantage, since TCAs may be discontinued early in unusually sensitive patients. Furthermore, some anticholinergic effects may become troublesome during long-term TCA therapy (e.g., persistent dry mouth may result in tooth decay). Although the action of MAO inhibitors is not anticholinergic, many of their adverse effects resemble anticholinergic symptoms. Certain adverse GI effects (e.g., nausea, anorexia) or CNS effects (e.g., anxiety, nervousness, insomnia, weight loss) appear more often with SSRIs than with other antidepressant drugs, and alternatives may be preferred in patients who cannot tolerate these effects or when these effects are a concern.

TCAs and MAO inhibitors have the capacity to induce weight gain. In overweight or obese patients and/or patients in whom the increase in appetite, carbohydrate craving, and weight gain associated with TCA therapy may be undesirable (e.g., pose a potential hazard to the patient's health, result in possible discontinuance of or noncompliance with therapy), some health care providers feel that other drugs (e.g., SSRIs) may be preferred since they possess anorectic and weight-reducing properties. However, the possibility that some patients with concurrent eating disorders or those who may desire to lose weight may misuse such drugs for their anorectic and weight-reducing effects should be considered.

RISK FOR SUICIDE. **Antidepressants have been implicated** ▲ **in worsening depression and the appearance of suicidality in selected patients** (see **Box 20-4**). An increased number of deaths related to suicide in children and adolescents

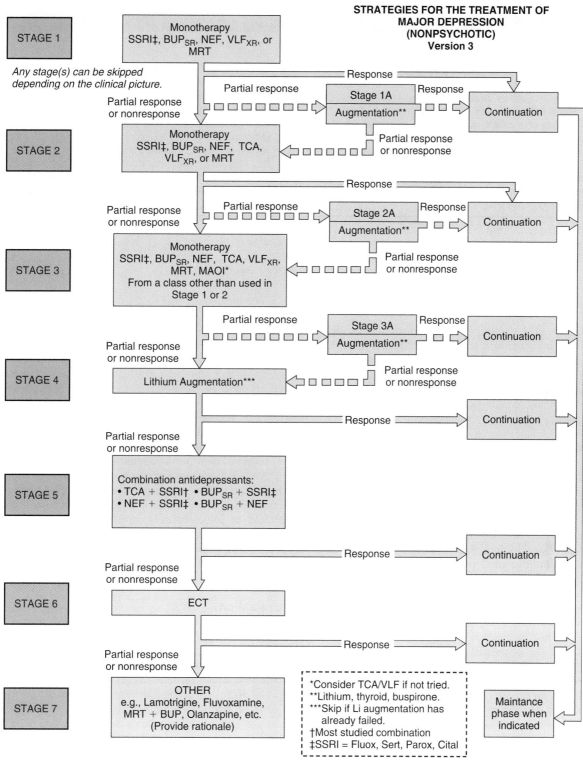

STRATEGIES FOR THE TREATMENT OF
MAJOR DEPRESSION
(NONPSYCHOTIC)
Version 3

STAGE 1 — Monotherapy SSRI‡, BUP_SR, NEF, VLF_XR, or MRT

Any stage(s) can be skipped depending on the clinical picture.

STAGE 2 — Monotherapy SSRI‡, BUP_SR, NEF, TCA, VLF_XR, or MRT

STAGE 3 — Monotherapy SSRI‡, BUP_SR, NEF, TCA, VLF_XR, MRT, MAOI* From a class other than used in Stage 1 or 2

STAGE 4 — Lithium Augmentation***

STAGE 5 — Combination antidepressants:
• TCA + SSRI† • BUP_SR + SSRI‡
• NEF + SSRI‡ • BUP_SR + NEF

STAGE 6 — ECT

STAGE 7 — OTHER e.g., Lamotrigine, Fluvoxamine, MRT + BUP, Olanzapine, etc. (Provide rationale)

*Consider TCA/VLF if not tried.
**Lithium, thyroid, buspirone.
***Skip if Li augmentation has already failed.
†Most studied combination
‡SSRI = Fluox, Sert, Parox, Cital

SSRI, selective serotonin reuptake inhibitor; BUP_SR, sustained release bupropion; NEF, nefazodone; VLF_XR, extended release venlafaxine; MAOI, monoamine oxidase inhibitor; MRT, mirtazapine; TCA, tricyclic antidepressant; ECT, electroconvulsive therapy

FIGURE 20-3 Treatment Strategy for Major Nonpsychotic Depressions. (Redrawn from Texas Implementation of Medication Algorithm (TIMA), Major Depressive Disorder, Non-psychotic Algorithm. (2006 Update). Available online: www.dshs.state.tx.us/mhprograms/TIMA.shtm. Accessed June 27, 2007.)

BOX 20-4

Black Box Warning Information About Antidepressants

- Carefully monitor patients receiving antidepressants for possible worsening of depression or suicidality. Monitoring is crucial with the onset of therapy and with any increase or decrease in dosage. At this time the FDA is lacking data that indicate antidepressants directly cause deterioration of a patient with depression or suicidal thoughts. A decline in the patient's condition may be associated with a comorbid condition or drugs used in the treatment of those conditions.
- Antidepressants may induce mania in patients with bipolar disorder. Screen patients to determine their risk factors (e.g., family history of bipolar disorder, depression, and suicide) for bipolar disorder before starting antidepressant therapy.

- Adolescents and adults undergoing treatment for depression or other psychiatric illnesses who display one or more of the following symptoms are at increased risk for worsening depression and suicidality: insomnia, anxiety, agitation, panic attacks, hostility, and impulsiveness. The antidepressant drug should be stopped if these symptoms of bipolar disorder have an abrupt onset, are severe, or which were not part of the patient's initial symptomatology.
- Determine what interventions, including discontinuing or modifying the current drug therapy, are indicated. If a decision is made to stop treatment, taper these drugs off slowly rather than abruptly discontinuing therapy.

FDA, Food and Drug Administration.
Adapted from Strong, C. (2004). FDA requests warning statement about risks for antidepressants. *Neuropsychiatry Reviews, 5*(2). Available online: www.neuropsychiatryreviews.com/apr04/npr_apr04_FDAwarn.html. Accessed March 31, 2007.

---

prompted the FDA to require a black box warning for all antidepressants. It is unknown at this time whether the black box warning also applies to adults. Because the risk of suicidality may persist until substantial remission of depression occurs, close supervision of patients is recommended. TCAs may produce potentially life-threatening cardiotoxicity following overdosage.

Patient Teaching

Reinforce the importance of compliance with the treatment regimen, especially when drug therapy is first started, because a lag time of 2 to 12 weeks may pass before the patient feels substantial benefit. Also, warn patients at the start of therapy that it is common to have to titrate, augment, or change drugs if sufficient response is not obtained or if adverse effects limit the use of a specific drug. Patients should be warned not to abruptly discontinue antidepressant therapy because of either withdrawal-like symptoms or the risk of recurrent depression symptoms. Treatment of first-episode depression in remission should continue for at least 9 months to 1 year. Recurrent depressions may require longer treatment durations.

Teach patients to avoid alcohol and other CNS depressants while taking the antidepressant. Patients receiving MAOIs should also avoid over-the-counter (OTC) drugs, as well as foods or beverages containing tyramine, during therapy and for at least 2 weeks after therapy has been discontinued (see Box 20-3). Warn patients verbally and in writing that if signs or symptoms of hypertensive crisis occur, they are to proceed immediately to an emergency care center. Warning signs include intense, pounding headache, sweating, flushing, rapid heartbeat, dizziness, faintness, chest pain, and neck stiffness.

Inform the patient that drowsiness or dizziness may occur with certain antidepressants. Caution the patient to avoid driving or operating machinery or other activities that require alertness until response to the drug is known. Patients should also be informed about the possibility of hypotension (dizziness, light-headedness) and be advised to sit or lie down if this occurs.

Advise the patient that dry mouth, urinary retention, or constipation may occur with some of the antidepressants. Frequent mouth rinses, good oral hygiene, and sugarless candy or gum may diminish the dry mouth. An increase in fluid intake, fiber, and exercise may prevent constipation. Instruct the patient to notify you or another health care provider if these adverse effects occur.

Treatment of depression with drugs alone is not optimal therapy. Emotional support and traditional psychotherapy can complement and reinforce responses to antidepressants. Therefore, provide patients with the resources and information necessary to pursue additional therapy.

A medical alert bracelet or necklace should be worn at all times by the patient taking MAOIs. Those extending hospitality to a patient taking MAOIs and restaurant personnel should be informed of dietary restrictions. MAOI therapy is usually withdrawn for at least 2 weeks before the use of anesthetics; however, advise the patient to notify the surgeon or the dentist of their drug regimen before treatment or surgery.

Evaluation

Indications that drug therapy has been successful include resolution of depression and restoration of euthymia (without invoking mania), resolution of a psychotic process if those symptoms were initially present (coadministration of an antipsychotic drug is generally required), and a therapeutic, nonproblematic physiologic response to the drug. If adverse effects develop, they are tolerable, not life threatening, and do not jeopardize compliance or interfere with the activities of daily living. Sleep, eating, and activity patterns return to normal. Suicidality resolves. The patient and family express knowledge and some degree of acceptance of depression, and they demonstrate an awareness of the nature, course, and treatment of depression.

Furthermore, the patient has a means of accessing ongoing care and drug therapy and actually does access it. When appropriate, the patient is aware of psychosocial supports and rights as a disabled person under the Americans with Disabilities Act. Further, the patient expresses a desire to stop concomitant use of alcohol and street drugs.

Carefully monitor blood pressure during initiation of drug therapy with MAOIs to evaluate orthostatic hypotension or a pressor response. Discontinue MAOIs immediately if a hypertensive crisis occurs; treat the patient with an alpha-blocking drug such as IV phentolamine. This intervention lowers blood pressure and resolves the intense headache. Fever may be treated with external cooling.

Caution must be exercised in changing between classes of drugs, especially when MAOIs are being started or discontinued. Half-lives of other drugs and the biologic changes that occur in response to MAOIs, and the continuing potential for severe drug interactions, even once a drug is discontinued, are major considerations. This is particularly true with drugs having long half-lives (e.g., fluoxetine in succession with MAOIs or TCAs).

BIPOLAR DISORDER

EPIDEMIOLOGY AND ETIOLOGY

Bipolar disorder (previously known as manic-depressive disorder) is a mood disorder characterized by expansive emotional states, flights of ideas, hyperactivity, destructive behaviors, and psychotic processes. It consists of periods of depression, alternating with mania, usually separated by periods of near-normal, euthymic functioning. Bipolar disorder affects at least 3 million people in the United States. It disrupts relationships, careers, and families, contributing to billions of dollars in direct and indirect costs, and a number of deaths by suicide or recklessness.

PATHOPHYSIOLOGY

Mania is thought to be caused by dysregulation of some of the same neurotransmitters that cause depression (i.e., serotonin, norepinephrine, dopamine, and perhaps an excitatory neurotransmitter, glutamate). In theory, if a relative lack of neurotransmitters contributes to depression, then a relative excess may contribute to what appears to be an opposite mood state of mania.

Forms of Bipolar Disorder

▓ Hypomania

Hypomania is an expansive, energized portion of the mood cycle, characterized by disturbances in speech, cognition, judgment, self-concept, and behavior lasting at least 4 days. Accompanying this mood are other disturbances such as inflated self-esteem, flights of ideas, distractibility, increased involvement in goal-directed activity, or psychomotor agitation. Another symptom of hypomania is excessive involvement in pleasurable activities that have a high potential for painful consequences. Hypomania may progress in some individuals to full mania, which is characterized by a more amplified and sustained version of hypomania, as well as delusions or hallucinations.

▓ Mania

A full *manic* mood state lasts at least a week and is accompanied by the other characteristics already noted. The disturbance is severe enough to cause significant impairment in social or occupational functioning. The mood is often euphoric, and at least initially, it has an infectious quality. It is characterized by unceasing, indiscriminate enthusiasm and may be intrusive. However, the mood may be consistently irritable or labile, alternating between euphoria and irritability. In some cases, hospitalization is required.

It is common for a person in a manic state to give advice to anyone encountered, write letters, or communicate with government officials or company presidents, offering direction. Patients with mania may believe they have a special relationship with famous people or religious figures, including God. They may dress in loud clothing or wear excessive makeup or jewelry, or extreme hairstyles. There is almost invariably a decreased need for sleep, or the person may not sleep for days at a time. Manic speech is typically loud, pressured, tangential, nonstop, rapid, and difficult to interrupt. Irritable manics are critical and cutting. Racing thoughts cannot be stopped or slowed down. While acutely manic, they frequently engage in reckless and dangerous activities such as excessive, inappropriate, or unprotected sex; make poor business investments and decisions; and go on buying sprees. These activities are all pursued despite the painful consequences the acts may cause. The patient's appetite is usually decreased, or at least the person is unable to devote any time to eating. Many thousands of calories may be expended while the patient is engaged in frantic activity, and it is common for him or her to lose weight during a manic episode. The person also does not recognize illness and resists treatment, often adamantly. Hallucinations or delusions must be present, and are the defining characteristics that delineate hypomania from full mania.

▓ Mixed Mania

Mixed mania is characterized by a concurrent blend of mania and depression. It is estimated that approximately 40% of all patients with mania present with a mixture of depressed mood and hyperactivity. They report feeling dysphoric, depressed, and unhappy yet exhibit the characteristic energy associated with mania. This state is often complicated by concomitant substance abuse. It is very common to find bipolar patients (as well as psychiatric patients with any other type of mood or thought disorder) attempting to self-medicate with drugs and alcohol. Alcohol, heroin, benzodiazepines, marijuana, and sedative-hypnotics impart a sense of calmness to manic patients. Cocaine and amphetamines may be used by depressed patients to feel more energized or euthymic.

Bipolar patients may cycle only a few times within a lifetime, or they may cycle once or twice a year. Patients with rapid-cycling bipolar disorder may have four or more distinct, complete cycles within a year. Some patients with ultrarapid cycling describe almost constant, quick, up-and-down cycling.

PHARMACOTHERAPEUTIC OPTIONS

Mood-Stabilizing Drugs

- carbamazepine (Tegretol, Epitol); ✦ Apo-Carbamazepine, Mazepine, Novo-Carbamaz
- lithium (Duralith, Eskalith, Lithane, Lithonate, Lithotabs); ✦ Carbolith, Lithizine
- lamotrigine (Lamictal)
- valproic acid (Depakene, Depakote)

CENTRAL NERVOUS

Indications

Lithium is the first-line drug used for symptomatic control of bipolar disorders. Its beneficial effects were first noted in 1949. However, because of concerns about toxicity, it was not approved for use in the United States until 1970. At present, carbamazepine and valproic acid are used for patients who fail to respond to lithium or who cannot tolerate lithium's adverse effects. Carbamazepine and valproic acid drugs are most often used for the treatment of rapid-cycling bipolar disorder. Lamotrigine is indicated for the maintenance treatment of bipolar depression. Second-generation antipsychotic drugs, such as valproic acid, are often used alone or in combination when patients can not tolerate or respond to other first-line treatments (see Chapter 21).

Carbamazepine was first used during the 1960s for the treatment of trigeminal neuralgia and various convulsive disorders, including temporal lobe epilepsy. In the late 1960s, a series of worldwide investigations found that carbamazepine exerts potent antimania effects. At present, it is not FDA-approved for the treatment of mania, but nonetheless it is commonly used for this purpose both alone and in combination with other drugs. Carbamazepine is effective treatment for acute mania and for bipolar prophylaxis. During acute mania, it is ordinarily used in conjunction with an antipsychotic drug (see Chapter 21). The success rate is about 60% when carbamazepine is used in patients who have failed lithium therapy.

In 1966, the mood-stabilizing effects of valproic acid were first described. As scrutiny of the compound moved through early studies, it became clear that valproic acid consistently demonstrated some additional degree of efficacy in comparison with other drugs and improved the baseline symptoms of mania. Valproic acid was also originally used as an antiepileptic drug, and in 1995 was approved for the treatment of mania.

Lamotrigine is recommended in combination with another mood stabilizer if a patient had a recent and/or severe manic episode; in all other patients it can be used as monotherapy. Lamotrigine was also originally indicated as an antiseizure medication, and in 2003 it was also approved for maintenance treatment of bipolar depression.

Pharmacodynamics

The exact mechanism of action of mood-stabilizing drugs is unknown. It is thought that carbamazepine and valproic acid act by reducing the amount of neurotransmitters at the synapse or by increasing the levels of GABA, an inhibitory neurotransmitter. Lithium may impart some antidepressant effect by enhancing β-receptor activity. Its antimania properties may be related to its ability to dampen the brain's response to glutamate.

Carbamazepine has antimanic, anticholinergic, antidepressant, and sedative properties, and it is structurally related to imipramine and other TCAs. Although its mechanism of antimania action is unknown, early research focused on its ability to inhibit kindling. *Kindling* represents a process in which increasing behavioral and convulsive responses occur in response to repetition of the same stimulus, repeated over time. Some type of antikindling mechanism may be integral to its therapeutic and prophylactic effects in mania.

Lamotrigine's mechanism of action includes inhibition of glutamate and sodium channels in the neurons, which may account for its antiseizure and possibly mood-stabilizing properties.

Pharmacokinetics

Lithium is completely absorbed within the GI tract in 1 to 2 hours. It is widely distributed to many tissues and body fluids, crossing placental membranes and entering breast milk in low concentrations. It is excreted unchanged by the kidneys (see Table 20-1).

The absorption of carbamazepine is slow, but it is almost completely absorbed from the GI tract. It is biotransformed in the liver.

Valproic acid is rapidly and well absorbed from the GI tract. The divalproex sodium formulation is enteric-coated, so absorption is delayed by 1 to 4 hours. The presence of food in the stomach significantly slows the rate but not the extent of absorption. It is rapidly distributed to plasma and extracellular fluids, crossing the blood-brain barrier and placental membranes and entering breast milk. Valproic acid is 90% to 95% protein bound at serum concentrations of 50 mcg/mL. With serum concentrations of 50 to100 mcg/mL, the percentage of protein binding is 80% to 85%. Further, the free fraction becomes larger, increasing the concentration gradient to the brain. It is primarily biotransformed in the liver, with minimal amounts excreted unchanged in the urine.

Adverse Effects and Contraindications

Lithium has a narrow therapeutic index and a potential for lethal toxicity. The adverse effects of lithium are further categorized into those that occur at therapeutic levels and those likely to occur at toxic levels. Several responses occur early in treatment at levels that are within the therapeutic range (i.e., below 1.5 mEq/L) and then usually resolve. These responses include GI effects (e.g., anorexia, nausea, bloating, and diarrhea) and transient headache, fatigue, confusion, memory impairment, and muscle weakness in 30% of patients. Thirst and polyuria are experienced early in treatment by 30% to 50% of patients. In 50% to 70% of cases, the thirst and polyuria continue with chronic lithium use.

Drug-induced fine hand tremors may be noted that interfere with writing and other motor skills. The tremors are worsened by stress, fatigue, and certain drugs such as caffeine, antidepressants, or antipsychotics. They can be reduced with the concurrent use of propranolol, a beta blocking drug, and by dose reduction, use of divided doses, or the use of sustained-release formulations.

Although it is usually a benign state, hypothyroidism is sometimes associated with a lithium-induced goiter. Synthetic thyroid hormone replacement is often required to restore a euthyroid state. Renal toxicity has been associated with degenerative changes in the kidney and most often is a problem in older adults.

Mild benign leukocytosis (15,000 to 20,000/mcL) and dermatologic reactions such as psoriasis, acne, folliculitis, and alopecia have been reported with lithium use. These problems usually respond to a dosage reduction or discontinuation. Lithium is a teratogen, and its use is discouraged during the first trimester of pregnancy. Cardiovascular abnormalities, including Ebstein's anomaly, are known to occur in the fetus. The primary abnormality in Ebstein's anomaly is of the tricuspid valve, the valve that lies between the right atrium and the right ventricle. Although there is free flow of blood forward across the tricuspid valve to the right ventricle, the deformed tricuspid valve allows a large amount of blood to flow backwards from the right ventricle to the right atrium when the right ventricle contracts.

The most serious adverse effect of lithium is toxicity (i.e., serum levels exceeding 1.5 mEq/L). The risk of toxicity is related to the magnitude and duration of exposure and individual susceptibility. Severe toxicity is associated with myoclonic jerks, seizures, impaired consciousness, coma, and ultimately death. Renal failure and nephrogenic diabetes insipidus (in 20% to 40% of patients) are common consequences of lithium therapy. A portion of patients with nephrogenic diabetes insipidus will have a persistent concentrating defect long after lithium use is discontinued. Although toxicity usually resolves without complications once dosages are lowered or stopped, some patients die, and others develop persistent neurologic disability. The most common cause of lithium accumulation in compliant patients is sodium depletion and dehydration, which reduces the volume of distribution of lithium and increases serum levels.

The adverse effects of carbamazepine primarily include drowsiness and ataxia. Other adverse effects include blurred vision, blood pressure alterations, urinary hesitancy and retention, rashes, urticaria, and photosensitivity. The most severe effects include heart failure, pneumonitis, hepatitis, aplastic anemia, agranulocytosis, and thrombocytopenia. Leukopenia, leukocytosis, and eosinophilia may be noted. Carbamazepine and valproic acid are also known teratogens and should be avoided during pregnancy, especially during the first trimester.

Valproic acid is most commonly associated with indigestion, nausea, and vomiting. Hepatotoxicity is the most serious adverse effect. Other adverse effects include drowsiness, sedation, headache, dizziness, ataxia, and confusion. Anorexia, increased appetite, diarrhea, and constipation are noted in some patients. Prolonged bleeding times, leukopenia, and thrombocytopenia can occur. Increased serum ammonia levels, which can lead to mental status changes (confusion, delirium, encephalopathy), have been known to occur with valproic acid use in some children and adults.

Lamotrigine is most commonly associated with headaches, dizziness, sedation, and nausea. Rapid dosage increases have been associated with skin rashes. Also, as with carbamazepine, there is a risk for Stevens-Johnson syndrome, which may be life threatening. Patients should be instructed to contact a physician if a skin rash develops while taking these medications.

Drug Interactions

Of the top 200 drugs prescribed in the United States in 2004, at least 25% interact with lithium, 42% interact with carbamazepine, and 5% interact with valproic acid (see Table 20-2). Thiazide and loop diuretics, potassium-sparing diuretics, amiloride, and nonsteroidal antiinflammatory drugs (NSAIDs) (except aspirin) create a definite reduction in renal elimination of lithium and an increased risk for toxicity. An especially problematic combination may be lithium, carbamazepine, and diuretics, because these drugs dramatically alter normal renal function and fluid and electrolyte balance.

Lamotrigine is significantly affected by other medications that inhibit or induce hepatic enzymes known as CYP 3A4. For example, valproic acid dramatically decreases the metabolism of lamotrigine, thus requiring an every-other-day dosing schedule for the first 2 weeks of treatment and slow titration afterwards. On the other hand, carbamazepine significantly increases the breakdown of lamotrigine and decreases the risk for inducing adverse effects.

Dosage Regimens

Lithium is initially taken 3 times daily (see Table 20-3). The dosage is adjusted at intervals of 5 to 7 days, as needed and tolerated. Start older adults or debilitated patients at lower dosages. Lithium levels should be monitored once or twice weekly during the acute manic phase, until serum concentrations have stabilized and the patient's condition improved. Desirable lithium levels generally fall in the range of 1 to 1.5 mEq/L for acute mania and 0.5 to 1 mEq/L for maintenance regimens. Serum drug levels are measured approximately 10 to 12 hours after the previous dose. Levels of 1.5 to 2.5 mEq/L represent moderate lithium toxicity, whereas levels of 2.5 to 3.5 mEq/L indicate severe toxicity. Levels above 3.5 mEq/L are usually fatal. Even when lithium is immediately discontinued, a week or more of vigorous hydration may be required before levels drop substantially.

Treatment of lithium toxicity is directed at preventing further absorption and enhancing elimination of the drug from the body. Gastric lavage is warranted in acute overdose. Mild toxicity can be treated with hydration to increase urine output. Severe toxicity should be treated with hemodialysis, especially if renal function is impaired.

Lithium drug concentrations in children, adolescents, older adults, those with chronic illnesses, and especially those with any renal involvement should be maintained at lower levels. Lithium levels should be reevaluated every 2 to 3 months during long-term therapy and more frequently in older adults, because they are more prone to dehydration, hypothyroidism, and CNS toxicity.

Carbamazepine is usually taken 2 to 3 times daily at the start of therapy and the dosage increased every 4 to 5 days or until a clinical response occurs, adverse effects prohibit further increases, or desired blood levels are reached. The oral suspension may produce higher peak serum concentrations and should be initiated at smaller, more frequent dosages spread out over the day.

Doses of valproic acid are given 2 to 3 times per day, with dosages increased over 2 to 3 days to achieve the desired effect and blood levels, or until adverse effects prohibit further increases.

If a patient is taking valproic acid, the starting dosage of lamotrigine is 12.5 to 25 mg every other day for 2 weeks and then daily for 2 weeks; then increase by 25 mg to 50 mg every 1 to 2 weeks until the usual maintenance dosage is reached (100 to 400 mg/day in divided doses). Otherwise, in the absence of a liver enzyme inhibitor, lamotrigine may be started at 50 mg/day and increased by 50 mg every 2 weeks until the maintenance dosage is reached.

▥ *Lab Considerations*

Carbamazepine may cause elevated AST, ALT, serum bilirubin, blood urea nitrogen (BUN), serum protein, and urine glucose levels, and these parameters should be monitored at least yearly. Thyroid function test values and serum calcium concentrations may be decreased. Further, carbamazepine may cause false-negative results for pregnancy tests that use methods identifying the presence of human chorionic gonadotropin.

Dose-related elevations in lactate dehydrogenase (LDH) and aminotransferases may occur with valproic acid. It can also interfere with the accuracy of thyroid function tests, and produce false-positive results in urine ketone tests. Occasionally, liver function tests, including serum bilirubin, may show increases and values should be monitored at least yearly.

CBCs, chemistry profiles, and liver function tests should be done at least yearly in patients on lamotrigine.

CLINICAL REASONING

Treatment Objectives

Treatment objectives for the patient with bipolar disorder are to correct the neurotransmitter imbalance through the appropriate use of drugs and to return the patient to an optimal level of functioning. The resolution of mood disorders is not conceptualized in terms of a cure but rather in terms of treatment, maintenance of remission, and prevention of relapse. Thus, rapid stabilization of mood, reestablishment of normalized sleep patterns, prevention of self-injurious acts, and long-term stabilization are necessary. Untreated or inadequately treated bipolar disorder tends to become more serious over time and more difficult to arrest.

Treatment Options

Because bipolar disorder is a lifelong, unremitting, chronic medical and psychiatric disease characterized by multiple relapses, it is common for patients not to adhere to complex or demanding drug regimens. Furthermore, patients with bipolar disorder are often oblivious to their mood cycling, even though those around them are acutely aware of the situation. They may actively resist treatment and may be particularly reluctant to have the euphoric, energized periods of mania controlled. Patients with mania are frank about missing their highs, and this factor contributes to their discontinuing drug therapy. Patients with bipolar disorder may also be actively self-treating painful mood states with alcohol, street drugs, or prescription drugs such as benzodiazepines, opioids, and sedative-hypnotics. The patient and the health care provider may remain unaware of the underlying disorder until the other substances are removed.

It may be particularly difficult for bipolar patients who lack family, social support, easily accessible community caregivers, structured housing or day programs, or financial resources to consistently comply with therapeutic regimens. On the other hand, many patients with bipolar disorder respond very favorably to treatment and continue to live extremely productive lives. They may be very successful in their careers and personal lives, particularly if their energy and creativity can be constructively harnessed. (See Case Study–Mood-Stabilizing Drugs.)

Patient Variables

Conduct a careful analysis of the patient's medical health, as well as concomitant drug use, before initiating a trial of any mood-stabilizing drug. The decision to use a particular drug for a particular patient is, of course, based on accurate diagnosis.

Before initiating therapy with mood-stabilizing drugs, obtain baseline renal and thyroid function, white blood cell count with differential, serum electrolytes, and glucose levels. It is important to establish that a woman is not pregnant. If there is any possibility of pregnancy, obtain a serum human chorionic gonadotropin pregnancy test. In addition, liver function tests, bilirubin, urinalysis, and BUN should be routinely performed for patients taking carbamazepine and valproic acid and lamotrigine. For the second-generation antipsychotics, metabolic parameters (weight, glucose, lipids) should be routinely assessed every 3 months for the first year and then yearly afterwards.

LIFE-SPAN CONSIDERATIONS

Pregnant and Nursing Women. A decision to use mood-stabilizing drugs during pregnancy must be weighed against the risk of untreated bipolar disorder and the efficiency and teratogenic risk of the proposed drug. If therapy is continued during pregnancy, it should be carefully monitored, as physiologic and pathologic complications of pregnancy (e.g., increased glomerular filtration rate, sodium retention, edema, and hypertension) can alter blood concentrations in the newborn. ECT may be a safer strategy for controlling mania in a pregnant woman. Drug therapy may be resumed after delivery to reduce risk of relapse.

Children and Adolescents. The occurrence of true mania in children is somewhat unusual, and it may be difficult to differentiate from ADHD, depression, oppositional defiant disorder, or other problems that are more common in children. Careful evaluation should be undertaken by qualified child experts in assessing psychiatric, psychologic, medical, and neurologic bases for behavior resembling bipolar disorder.

Lithium, carbamazepine, and valproic acid have been used in children, but extensive studies of the relationship of age, effects, adverse effects, and long-term effects have not been conducted. Lithium may decrease bone formation and density in children by altering parathyroid hormone concentrations. Lithium is also deposited in bone, replacing calcium, an effect that is more pronounced in immature bones.

Valproic acid places children under the age of 2 years at greater risk for serious or fatal hepatotoxicity. The risk of hepatotoxicity increases with the concurrent use of antiepileptic drugs, and in patients with complex medical problems. Carbamazepine is likely to induce behavioral changes in children.

Older Adults. Older adults are at much the same risk for mood disorders as other population groups. Physical or mental illness contributes to acute confusion in older adults, and although temporary and reversible, can sometimes be mistaken for mood disorders. Delirium is a medical emergency, however, although it can be mistaken for mania or psychosis. Many disorders cause delirium, for example, conditions or illnesses limiting blood flow and oxygen to the brain, pneumonia, chemicals, comorbid conditions, poisonings, fluid and electrolyte imbalances, and acid-base disturbances. Urinary tract infections or pneumonia may trigger delirium in persons with preexisting brain damage (e.g., prior strokes, dementia).

CASE STUDY Mood-Stabilizing Drugs

ASSESSMENT

History of Present Illness	SN is a 36-year-old female with complaints of frequent, rapid mood fluctuations for the past several years. She reports at least four complete mood cycles per year. She has been on lithium in the past, but its effects seemed to wear off over time. When depressed, she has feelings of irritable mood, crying, hopelessness, helplessness, insomnia, decreased appetite, and weight loss. She loses interest in usually pleasurable activities and is unable to care for her 12-year-old son. She has made a suicide attempt by ingestion of large amounts of alcohol, benzodiazepine tranquilizers, and aspirin. When her mood is elevated, she feels alternatively euphoric and irritable; she may not sleep for several days at a time; she has engaged in reckless activities; and she exercises poor judgment in relationships, sexual encounters, and care of her child. She tends to wear excessive makeup and jewelry when manic, and spends large amounts of money and charges her credit cards beyond their limit.
Past Health History	SN's health history is unremarkable. She smokes one pack per day of cigarettes and drinks alcohol primarily when manic, but also occasionally while depressed. She has one child by vaginal delivery. She has no known allergies and no renal, hepatic, or coagulation problems. She is taking oral contraceptives.
Life-Span Considerations	Although she is a single parent, SN expresses interest in having another child before age 40. SN lives on emergency assistance from the state because she has been unable to maintain employment owing to her mood lability, poor judgment, and need to care for her child. She has a tenth-grade education. Her potential for compliance is judged to be fair to good. She is highly motivated to control her mood cycling so she can be a better parent, complete her education, and start a career. SN has a pharmacy plan through her emergency assistance entitlement program.
Physical Exam Findings	Vital signs within normal limits. Underweight woman with no physical stigmata. Otherwise the exam was unremarkable.
Diagnostic Testing	SN meets DSM-IV criteria for rapid-cycle bipolar disorder.

DIAGNOSIS: Rapid-cycle bipolar disorder

MANAGEMENT

Treatment Objectives	1. Correct the neurotransmitter imbalance contributing to depression. 2. Return the patient to optimal level of functioning.
Treatment Plan	**Pharmacotherapy** divalproex 750 mg PO daily in divided doses. Titrate rapidly to desired clinical effect or trough plasma levels of 50–125 mcg/ml. Maximum dosage: 60 mg/kg/day **Patient Education** 1. Do not abruptly stop therapy after long-term use; doing so may precipitate seizures. 2. Drowsiness usually disappears with continued therapy. Avoid tasks that require alertness until response to drug is established. 3. Carry medical alert identification. 4. Inform health care provider if nausea, vomiting, lethargy, weakness, loss of appetite, abdominal pain, yellowing of skin, or unusual bruising or bleeding occurs. 5. Monitor closely for suicidal ideations and/or plans. **Evaluation** 1. SN reports taking the drug regularly and keeping follow-up appointments with her health care provider. 2. Compare symptoms with treatment compared to previous symptoms. There should be an increased ability to concentrate; relaxed facial expressions; less irritability, crying, feelings of hopelessness, and helplessness; improved sleep patterns, improved appetite, and weight gain. She returns to pleasurable activities and is providing effective care for her 12-year-old son. 3. Liver function tests, CBC, and platelets are within normal limits. There is no evidence of bruising or bleeding, or seizure activities.

Continued

CASE STUDY — Mood-Stabilizing Drugs—Cont'd

CLINICAL REASONING ANALYSIS

Q1. Why did you choose divalproex rather than lithium for SN's rapid-cycling bipolar disorder?

A. Lithium, carbamazepine, and valproic acid are effective in various forms of bipolar disorder, although lithium is less efficacious than divalproex and has a narrow therapeutic index. Divalproex, on the other hand, is most effective for rapid-cycling disorders, and SN has at least four full mood cycles per year, which constitutes rapid bipolar cycling.

Q2. The literature says that lithium is the drug of choice for bipolar disorder. Shouldn't we be using evidence from the literature to make a decision?

A. Yes and no. Evidence-based decisions are all well and good, but we still need to consider the patient as an individual. Since treatment of bipolar disorder is essentially lifelong and subject to continued cycles and relapse, even with an ongoing drug regimen, the better drug for SN is divalproex. Further, divalproex has a wide therapeutic index, and we do not have to regularly monitor her thyroid function as we would with lithium. Divalproex has consistently demonstrated some additional degree of efficacy in comparison with other drugs, improves baseline symptoms of mania, and is enteric-coated. Carbamazepine may cause anorexia, and SN is already thin and has an appetite disturbance. In addition, the patient reports failure of lithium therapy in the past—we don't know if it really failed, or whether she just quit taking it; but either way, she did not recover and remain stable while on lithium in the past. Even if the lithium did work, but she was not compliant, there was a reason for the noncompliance—and either is unacceptable. The other consideration is that she stopped lithium because she lost her "high" from the mania. This should be determined, if possible, because it could predict failure of this new therapy as well.

Q3. But aren't valproic acid and divalproex the same thing? Couldn't we use valproic acid instead?

A. They are similar drugs, but the advantage is that most patients tolerate divalproex sodium better than valproic acid. The disadvantage is that divalproex is more expensive than valproic acid. In this "public assistance" patient, this is an important consideration—especially if she does not like "feeling normal" and is looking for a reason to go off the therapy.

Lastly, antidepressant and antimania drugs increase the risk for falls and hypotensive responses.

For these reasons, Congress passed the comprehensive Nursing Home Reform Act in 1987 (Box 20-5). This legislation requires that restraints be used only to ensure safety of a nursing home resident or other residents and then only upon a written order from the health care provider. The duration and circumstances of the use of restraints must be clearly specified in the patient record. The use of as-needed (PRN) orders is limited, and documentation is required of efforts to discontinue the drug or at least reduce the dosage of an antipsychotic drug.

▥ Drug Variables

Tricyclic antidepressants have been used to treat the depressive phase of bipolar disorder, but they do not prevent and may precipitate hypomania or manic attacks in patients with this disorder. Tricyclic antidepressants appear to be associated with response rates equivalent to or poorer than other antidepressants (e.g., SSRIs, bupropion) although TCA response rates are superior to placebo, and also may carry a greater risk of precipitating hypomania or manic episodes in patients with bipolar disorder than other classes of antidepressants.

Base the decision to use a mood-stabilizing drug, at least in part, on the particular variety of mania present. In acute mania, there is typically a lag time of 5 days to 3 weeks before first-line drugs effectively manage the problem.

Since antidepressant drugs may precipitate manic states in vulnerable individuals, manage patients with bipolar disorder with mood-stabilizing drugs alone, whenever possible, unless there is a clear need for the addition of antidepressants to the regimen.

The only drugs approved for the maintenance or prevention of bipolar symptoms are lithium, lamotrigine, olanzapine, and aripiprazole. However, valproic acid may be used as an adjunct that can be tapered and stopped as the mania subsides and primary drugs become effective (see Chapter 21). The second-generation antipsychotics approved for acute mania include risperidone, quetiapine, olanzapine, and aripiprazole.

Antipsychotic drugs are used during acute mania to treat psychotic processes, as well as to provide a margin of calmness and safety for patients who are clearly out of control. There is some evidence that newer antipsychotic drugs such as clozapine, olanzepine, and risperidone have mood-stabilizing properties as well as antipsychotic properties. Because long-term use of antipsychotic drugs carries a risk of tardive dyskinesia and metabolic syndrome, use antipsychotic drugs for bipolar disorder only when they are absolutely necessary and then only with caution and in the lowest effective doses. Tardive dyskinesia is chronic disorder of the nervous system characterized by involuntary jerky movements of the face, the tongue, the jaws, the trunk, and the limbs, usually developing as a late side effect of prolonged treatment with antipsychotic drugs.

Anxiolytic drugs (see Chapter 19) such as the benzodiazepines may also be effective adjuncts in the management of acute mania. Benzodiazepines are helpful in controlling agitation, hyperactivity, anxiety, and sleeplessness associated with mania. They also offer the advantage of a more rapid antimanic response by restoring normal sleep patterns, imparting a

---

BOX 20-5

Legislative Guidelines on Psychoactive Drug Usage

The following use of psychoactive drugs must be justified in patient records of nursing home residents:

- Continuous use of hypnotic drugs for more than 30 days
- Use of two or more hypnotic drugs at the same time
- Hypnotic or anxiolytic drugs administered in excess of listed maximum doses
- Use of neuroleptic drugs in dementia unless the condition is associated with psychotic or agitated features that are subjectively disturbing to the patient or lead to agitated or dangerous behavior that interferes with patient safety or care
- Use of antipsychotics purely to control anxiety, wandering, restlessness, or insomnia

- Use of antipsychotics for less than 3 days unless to control acute episodes of agitation
- Use of two or more antipsychotic drugs at the same time
- Use of anticholinergic therapy with antipsychotic drugs in the absence of extrapyramidal symptoms
- Neuroleptic drugs administered in excess of listed maximum dosages

In addition, federal guidelines require periodic monitoring for tardive dyskinesia (using the Abnormal Involuntary Movement Scale [AIMS] assessment tool) in recognition of the older adult's vulnerability to this disorder when taking antipsychotic drugs. Patients must be provided with drug holidays, gradual dose reductions, and behavioral management in an effort to discontinue the drugs.

Office of the Inspector General, Department of Health and Human Services. (2001, November). *Psychotropic drug use in nursing home supplemental information: 10 case studies.* (OEI - 02–00–00491). Available online: www.oig.hhs.gov/oei/reports/oei-02-00-00491.pdf. Accessed March 31, 2007.

---

calming effect, and eliminating or minimizing the need for exposure to antipsychotic drugs.

Lithium is the drug of choice for euphoric, classic, milder forms of mania, but it is less likely to be effective for patients with dysphoric mania, psychotic mania, rapid-cycling bipolar disorder, or comorbid drug and alcohol abuse, or for patients who have had three or more episodes of mania. Lithium may also require up to 3 to 4 weeks to exert its full antimanic effect. Older adults usually require lower lithium dosages, lower serum concentrations, and more frequent monitoring than younger patients. The rate and effectiveness of renal clearance may be decreased, as well as the volume of distribution, because of the normal changes of aging. Lithium may be more toxic to the CNS in the aging population, even when serum lithium levels are within the therapeutic range. There is also a propensity to develop lithium-induced goiter and clinical hypothyroidism. Polyuria and polydipsia may be more pronounced in the older adult.

Carbamazepine may be considered an alternative drug, although it is not FDA-approved for mania. Carbamazepine has a narrow therapeutic index, interacts with a large number of commonly prescribed drugs, and has many potential adverse effects. Carbamazepine may promote confusion or agitation in the older adult. It may also cause atrioventricular heart block, syndrome of inappropriate antidiuretic hormone secretion (SIADH), and bradycardia. For younger patients and older adults, valproic acid is the safest, most effective drug for most types of mania. It is efficacious in controlling mania either alone or in conjunction with other mood stabilizers.

For older adults taking valproic acid, start therapy with lower daily doses and maintain at lower serum concentrations that are still within the therapeutic range. Valproic acid is likely to be more effective in rapid-cycling or ultra–rapid-cycling mania (up to 20% of bipolar disorders), mixed states (up to 40% of episodes), mania in the older adult, episodes of mania associated with alcohol or substance abuse, personality disorders, and secondary mania (i.e., nonpsychiatric medical condition). Mania from corticosteroids is a possibility but, when present, is an adverse effect and is usually treated with

dosage reduction rather than addition of a mood-stabilizing drug. However, caution is warranted if using valproic acid for patients who abuse alcohol because of the potential for worsening liver damage. Older adults tend to have increased free drug concentrations, lowered clearance, and a reduced capacity to biotransform drugs.

Most patients tolerate divalproex sodium better than valproic acid. To change a patient from valproic acid therapy to divalproex therapy, initiate divalproex at the same total daily dosage and dosing schedule as valproic acid. Once the patient is stabilized, an administration schedule of 2 to 3 times daily may be attempted. A good correlation between daily dosage, serum level, and therapeutic effects has not been established. Treatment of valproic acid overdose is supportive and is aimed at facilitating elimination by ensuring adequate urinary output. Gastric lavage is usually of little use because of rapid drug absorption.

When mood-stabilizing drugs are used in combination with each other, CNS toxicity and adverse effects such as ataxia, clouded sensorium, and sedation may occur. These adverse effects may occur even when all drugs are within therapeutic range. This is true for patients of all ages, but particularly for older adults or those on complicated drug regimens.

ECT is sometimes employed in the treatment of both depression and mania. Although the mechanism of action is unknown, it may be related to its ability to normalize neurotransmitter production, raise the seizure threshold, or decrease amygdaloid kindling. ECT may be a realistic alternative for those who are pregnant or who are unresponsive to or unable to tolerate first-line drugs or who need rapid remission of acute mania owing to suicidal ideation. Normal mood can then be supported by drug therapy, if indicated.

Patient Teaching

Warn patients to promptly report any deterioration of sleep ▲ **pattern promptly, because often it is the first warning sign of an impending episode of hypomania or mania.**

The patient and family require education about the course of the illness, its symptoms, and its management. Reinforce the importance of compliance with the drug regimen. Make patients aware, however, that even with complete adherence to therapy, they may have periods of relapse. Sleep hygiene, a regular daily routine, cognitive-behavioral therapy, group therapy, and family support are all factors that optimize functioning. Patients may choose, for example, to avail themselves of information from drug manufacturers, advocacy groups, and state and local chapters of the National Alliance for the Mentally Ill (NAMI), and to participate in employee assistance programs. Families also require information and support because the disorder makes an impact on the entire family system and its roles, relationships, responsibilities, finances, and parenting. Assist the patient to understand that the illness does have to be an important focus of life, but not the only focus, and that resuming as normal, productive, and stable a life as possible is vital.

Patients also require education concerning their drug regimen, adverse effects, and discontinuation of the drug, as well as situations that require contact with the health care provider. Include information about drug interactions, especially drugs provided by nonpsychiatric health care providers and any OTC drug. In the case of lithium, information concerning potential toxicity and fluid and electrolyte balance is important. Also include the necessity of maintaining adequate hydration and salt in the diet, especially during periods of illness, fever, vomiting, diarrhea, or profuse sweating. Fluids should be increased during periods of hot weather to prevent dehydration.

Evaluation

Indications that drug therapy and any other measures employed in the management of bipolar disorder have been effective include the resolution of mania or hypomania, the establishment of euthymia (normal mood), the resolution of psychotic or dysphoric symptoms (if they were present), and a therapeutic, nonproblematic physiologic response to the drug. If adverse effects develop, they are tolerable, non–life-threatening, and noncompromising, and do not compel the patient to discontinue the drug.

The patient and family should be able to express an understanding of the disorder and demonstrate an awareness of its nature, course, and treatment, as well as have some degree of acceptance. Document that the patient has a means of accessing prescribed drugs and ongoing care and actually uses them. Many of the pharmaceutical manufacturers have compassionate use programs available for those who are uninsured or who cannot afford their drugs. A list of drug programs can be found on the Internet at www.needymeds.com.

Assess lithium drug concentrations once or twice weekly during the acute manic phase until serum concentrations have stabilized and the patient's condition has improved, and then every 2 to 3 months during long-term therapy and more frequently in older adults. Lithium levels must be monitored for safety as well as effectiveness; see the earlier Dosage Regimen section for desirable serum levels, particular precautions to be taken in certain populations, and appropriate interventions in the case of toxicity or overdose.

KEY POINTS

- Depression arises as a result of changes in the neurotransmitters serotonin, norepinephrine, and, to a lesser extent, dopamine.

- The ultimate goal in acute treatment of depression is achieving symptomatic remission and full return of psychosocial functioning. The prevention of relapse and recurrence is the essential goal of the continuation and maintenance phases of treatment. Objectives for chronic depression include reducing the likelihood of relapse or recurrence.

- TCAs, SSRIs, SNRIs, MAOIs, and a variety of miscellaneous antidepressants are useful in treating depression. Drug variables to consider include the specific type of depression, short- and long-term adverse effects, and the concomitant use of other, nonpsychiatric, drugs.

- Patient variables to consider include type of depression, compliance and noncompliance, financial resources, age, and state of renal and hepatic functioning.

- Patients should be advised that a period of 2 to 12 weeks may pass before they notice substantial benefit from drug treatment.

- Patients using MAOIs should be advised to avoid OTC drugs, and foods or beverages containing tyramine, to minimize the risk of hypertensive crisis.

- Effectiveness of therapy can be demonstrated by the resolution of depression and the restoration of euthymia without evoking mania.

- Bipolar disorder affects at least 3 million people in the United States.

- Bipolar disorders can occur in three forms: hypomania, full mania, and mixed mania.

- Mania is thought to be caused by a relative excess of the same neurotransmitters whose relative deficiency causes depression (i.e., serotonin, norepinephrine, and dopamine).

- Mania may first appear in childhood or adolescence or may emerge in early adulthood. A family history of bipolar disorder is common.

- Treatment objectives for the patient with bipolar disorder are to correct the neurotransmitter imbalance through the appropriate use of drugs and to return the patient to an optimal level of functioning. The resolution of mood disorders is not conceptualized in terms of a cure but rather in terms of treatment, maintenance of remission, and prevention of relapse.

- Mood-stabilizing drugs used in the treatment of bipolar disorders include carbamazepine, lithium, and valproic acid or divalproex sodium and lamotrigine.

- The patient and serum drug levels should be closely monitored for evidence of toxicity.

- Patients should be taught that treatment of bipolar disorder is lifelong in most cases, and they should be informed of the drug regimen, adverse effects, situations that require contact with the health care provider, and any OTC drugs that should be avoided.

- Indications that drug therapy employed in the management of bipolar disorder has been effective include the resolution of mania or hypomania, the establishment of euthymia (normal mood), the resolution of psychotic or dysphoric symptoms (if they were present), and a therapeutic, nonproblematic physiologic response to the drug.

Bibliography

Agency for Healthcare Research and Quality: U.S. Preventive Services Task Force now finds sufficient evidence to recommend screening adults for depression, Press Release, Rockville, MD. May 20, 2002. Available online: www.ahrq.gov/news/press/pr2002/deprespr.htm. Accessed March 31, 2007.

Angst, J., Gamma, A., Sellaro, R., et al. (2003). Recurrence of bipolar disorders and major depression: A life-long perspective. *European Archives of Psychiatry and Clinical Neuroscience, 253*(5), 237-240.

American Psychiatric Association. (2000). *Diagnostic and statistical manual of mental disorders.* (4th ed., text revision [DSM-IV-TR]). Washington, DC: Author.

Anderson, I. (2001). Meta-analytical studies on new antidepressants. *British Medical Bulletin, 57*(1), 161-178.

Anonymous. (2003). Are SSRIs safe for children? *Medical Letter on Drugs and Therapeutics, 45*(W1160A), 53-54.

Emslie, G., Hughes, C., Crismon, M., et al. (2004). A feasibility study of the childhood depression medication algorithm: The Texas Children's Medication Algorithm Project (CMAP). *Journal of the American Academy of Child and Adolescent Psychiatry, 43*(5), 519-527. Available online: www.medscape.com/medline/abstract/15100558. Accessed March 31, 2007.

Food and Drug Administration. (2005 Jan 16). Medication guide: About using antidepressants in children or teenagers. Rockville, MD. Available online: www.fda.gov/cder/drug/antidepressants/MG_template.pdf. Accessed March 31, 2007.

Food and Drug Administration. (2004 Oct 15). Public health advisory: Suicidality in children and adolescents being treated with antidepressant medications. Rockville, MD. Available online: www.fda.gov/cder/drug/antidepressants/SSRIPHA200410.htm. Accessed March 31, 2007.

Hardman, J., Limbird, L., and Gilman, A. (Eds.). (2001). *Goodman and Gilman's the pharmacologic basis of therapeutics.* (10th ed.). New York: McGraw-Hill.

Holden, C. (2004). Psychopharmacology: FDA weighs suicide risk in children on antidepressants. *Science, 303*(5659), 745.

Joffe, R., Levitt, A., Sokolov, S., et al. Treatment failures in depression: A systematic approach for family practitioners. *PsycheDirect.* Hamilton, Ontario: Department of Psychiatry and Neurobehavioral Science, McMaster University. Available online: www.psychdirect.com/depression/d-treatmentfailure.htm. Accessed March 17, 2006.

Keltner, N., and Folks, D. (2001). *Psychotropic drugs.* St. Louis: Mosby.

Katona, C., Hunter, B., and Bray, J. (1998). A double-blind comparison of the efficacy and safety of paroxetine and imipramine in the treatment of depression with dementia. *International Journal of Geriatric Psychiatry, 13*(2), 100-108.

Lantz, M., Giambanco, V., and Buchalater, E. (1996). A 10-year review of the effect of OBRA-87 on psychotropic prescribing practices in an academic nursing home. *Psychiatric Services, 47*(9), 951-955.

Neal, C., Lattimore, K., Donn, S., et al. (2005). Selective serotonin reuptake inhibitor (SSRI) use during pregnancy and effects on the fetus and newborn: A meta-analysis. *Journal of Perinatology, 25*(9), 595-604.

Office of the Inspector General, Department of Health and Human Services. (2001, November). Psychotropic drug use in nursing homes. (OEI -02-00-00490). Available online: www.oig.hhs.gov/oei/reports/oei-02-00-00490.pdf. Accessed 31 March 2007.

Office of the Inspector General, Department of Health and Human Services. (2001). Psychotropic drug use in nursing home supplemental information: 10 case studies. November. (OEI -02-00-00491). Available online: www.oig.hhs.gov/oei/reports/oei-02-00-00491.pdf. Accessed March 31, 2007.

Reynolds, C., Drew, M., Pollock, B., et al. (2006). Maintenance treatment of major depression in old age, *New England Journal of Medicine, 354*(11), 1130-1138.

Strong, C. (2004, April). FDA requests warning statement about risks for antidepressants. *Neuropsychiatry Reviews, 5*(2). Available online: www.neuropsychiatryreviews.com/apr04/npr_apr04_FDAwarn.html. Accessed 31 March 2007.

Strakowski, S., DelBello, M., and Adler, C. (2001). Comparative efficacy and tolerability of drug treatments for bipolar disorder. *CNS Drugs, 15*(9), 701-718.

Suppes, T., Dennehy, E., Hirschfeld, R., et al. (205). The Texas implementation of medication algorithms: Update to the algorithms for treatment of bipolar I disorder. *Journal of Clinical Psychiatry, 66*(7), 870-886.

CENTRAL NERVOUS

21

Antipsychotic Drugs

Interactions between the neurobiologic and endocrine systems strongly influence human functioning and behavior. Psychosis is a disruptive mental state in which an individual struggles to distinguish the external world from his or her internally generated perceptions. Psychosis develops when these connections become dysregulated. The word *psychosis* invokes images of bizarre behaviors, loss of control, and disconnection from reality. Although such psychotic behavior is associated primarily with schizophrenia, it may also be noted with other physical and psychiatric disorders (Box 21-1).

Throughout much of the twentieth century, there was little success in the treatment of these disorders. However, in the 1950s, an accidental discovery of the antipsychotic properties of the antihypertensive drug chlorpromazine changed the course of treatment and the entire field of psychiatry. Since then, newer drugs have proven even more useful in the management of psychoses, and research is ongoing. Over the past decade, new evidence has demonstrated that primary psychotic disorders have neuroanatomic and physiologic features that are indeed different and out of balance.

Antipsychotic drugs assist in managing symptoms of psychosis including thought disorders, hallucinations, bizarre behaviors, agitation, and hyperactivity. The drugs do not cure psychoses but do ease many of the most distressing symptoms. Although the evolution of new antipsychotic drugs has lagged considerably behind that of antianxiety drugs (see Chapter 19) and antidepressants (see Chapter 20), promising drugs have appeared in the market place in recent years. Antipsychotic drugs are used to manage a variety of disorders including schizophrenia, schizoaffective and schizophreniform disorders, delusional disorders, acute mania, depressive psychosis, and substance-induced psychosis. The primary use of antipsychotic drugs remains the management of schizophrenia, although atypical antipsychotic drugs are also recommended for maintenance therapy in patients with severe bipolar disorder.

SCHIZOPHRENIA

EPIDEMIOLOGY AND ETIOLOGY

Schizophrenia is a chronic mental illness prevalent in 1% of the population, with no differentiation by sex. Onset is most often in young adulthood; males tend to be diagnosed between the ages of 15 and 24 years, whereas females are often diagnosed between the ages of 24 and 34. There is no association between schizophrenia, socioeconomic status, or ethnicity. However, the disorder is so all-pervasive that the affected individual often cannot continue as a productive member of society and suffers a tendency to drift downward in socioeconomic status.

The exact etiology of schizophrenia is unknown. Alterations are recognized in dopamine transmission, as well as anatomic brain differences such as enlarged ventricles. There appears to be a genetic link, with a high concordance rate among blood relatives. Past hypotheses about poor mothering have generally been discarded as newer etiologic models focusing on biochemistry are proposed.

PATHOPHYSIOLOGY

The psychosis pathway reflects dysfunction of limbic system structures (i.e., hippocampus, anterior cingulate, and amygdala) in which the neurotransmitter dopamine is found. It has been hypothesized that excess dopamine causes psychotic symptoms. The limbic area may be hyperresponsive, or in an effort to modulate the overactivity, the frontal areas of the brain become hyporesponsive to dopamine. The end results are dysregulation and deficits in information processing.

Schizophrenia influences perception, thought content and process, affect, and day-to-day functioning. The behavioral manifestations can be grouped into positive, negative, and cognitive symptoms (Box 21-2). *Positive symptoms* are behaviors existing in addition to or outside the range of usual human responses (e.g., hallucinations and delusions). *Negative symptoms* are behaviors that are lessened or diminished compared to what is typical of a healthy individual (e.g., flat affect, poverty of speech). The distinction between positive and negative symptoms is important because different psychotropic

---

BOX 21-1

DSM-IV Criteria for Schizophrenia and Psychotic Disorders

1. A continuous disturbance lasting at least 6 months
2. Two or more of the following symptoms lasting for a significant portion of the last month:
   - Delusions
   - Hallucinations
   - Disorganized speech
   - Catatonic or grossly disorganized behaviors
   - Negative symptoms
3. One or more areas of social or occupational dysfunction
   - Work
   - Interpersonal relationships
   - Self-care

Data from the American Psychiatric Association. (2000). *Diagnostic and statistical manual of mental disorders*. (4th ed., Text Revision [DSM-IV-TR]). Washington, DC: Author.

BOX 21-2

Symptoms of Schizophrenia

Positive Symptoms
- Agitation, combativeness, rage
- Delusions, hallucinations, feelings of unreality, terror
- Hyperactivity, insomnia
- Negativism
- Neologisms, racing thoughts
- Paranoia, sensitivity to environmental stimuli

Negative Symptoms
- Amotivation, anhedonia, lack of spontaneity
- Blunted affect, apathy, emotional withdrawal, poor rapport
- Disheveled appearance, poor hygiene

Cognitive Symptoms
- Attention deficits, memory deficits
- Concrete thinking, inability to change cognitive set
- Inability to concentrate, slowed thought processing
- Lack of judgment, insight
- Information processing deficits, word salad

drugs tend to affect each group of symptoms differently. Psychotropic drug therapy is used to manage many of these symptoms. Note, however, that the adverse effects of these drugs can mimic the psychosis itself.

The cognitive symptoms, which may also be listed among the positive and negative symptoms, seem to be the least responsive to drug therapy. Examples of cognitive disturbances include looseness of association, tangentiality, circular thought process, and use of *neologisms* (words that have a meaning known only to the patient).

The person suffering from schizophrenia also demonstrates psychomotor and affective disturbances. Affective disturbances associated with schizophrenia include an overall reduction in emotional responsiveness, flat affect, *anhedonia* (loss of interest in normally pleasurable activities), abnormal emotions, and inappropriate responses. Psychomotor disturbances may include impulsivity, overexcitement, aggression, automatic obedience, *echopraxia* (stereotyped imitation of the movements of another person), stupor, or catalepsy (characterized by lack of response to external stimuli and by muscular rigidity, so that the limbs remain in whatever position they are placed).

PHARMACOTHERAPEUTIC OPTIONS

Several different terms have been used to categorize antipsychotic drugs. The traditional antipsychotic drugs were developed between 1950 and 1990 and have strong neuroleptic (a "tranquilizer" used to treat psychotic conditions when a calming effect is desired) properties. With the advent of newer drugs that do not have the same effects and that influence different neurochemical pathways, the terms *novel* or *atypical antipsychotics* came to be used. However, as newer drugs are developed and the mechanisms of action of antipsychotics are further delineated, the more accepted current terminology has become the *first-generation antipsychotics* and *second-generation antipsychotics*.

First-Generation Antipsychotic Drugs

- chlorpromazine (Thorazine)
- fluphenazine (Prolixin); ◆ Modecate
- haloperidol (Haldol); ◆ Peridol
- loxapine (Loxitane); ◆ Loxapac
- mesoridazine (Serentil)
- molindone (Moban)
- thioridazine (Mellaril); ◆ Thioridazine

First-generation antipsychotics (i.e., phenothiazines) are often thought of according to potency and chemical structure and are roughly equivalent with respect to their effect on symptoms. The *phenothiazines* are tricyclic molecules. Three subtypes of phenothiazines are identified: aliphatics, piperidines, and piperazines. Phenothiazines with aliphatic side chains (e.g., chlorpromazine) tend to be low-potency compounds. Piperidine substitutions impart anticholinergic properties and have a lower incidence of extrapyramidal symptoms (EPS) (e.g., thioridazine, mesoridazine). Piperazine phenothiazines (e.g., perphenazine, trifluoperazine, fluphenazine) are among the most potent antipsychotics.

The thioxanthenes class of antipsychotics is chemically similar to phenothiazines. The butyrophenones represent a class of extremely potent antipsychotic drugs. Of these, only haloperidol is currently approved for psychiatric use in the United States.

Dopamine-2 (D_2) antagonist drugs were the principal means of treating psychosis for more than 40 years, yet they were not particularly effective in improving negative and cognitive symptoms. Nonetheless, the approach based on potency relative to D_2 has proven useful. For example, 100 mg of chlorpromazine results in the same clinical levels of D_2 antagonism as 2 mg of haloperidol. Drugs 1 to 4 times as potent as chlorpromazine are designated as low potency; those 20 times or more as potent are designated as high potency. Several drugs do not fit into the high- or low-potency categories and are placed in an intermediate-potency category.

▥ Indications

Schizophrenia is the most common indication for these drugs; they are used to suppress the symptoms associated with acute psychosis. They are also useful in the treatment of disorders such as schizoaffective disorder, severe mania or the acute manic phase of bipolar disorder, drug-induced psychosis, delusional disorders, Tourette's syndrome, and Huntington's chorea. In addition, some antipsychotic drugs possess antiemetic effects and may be used to treat severe nausea.

▥ Pharmacodynamics

Positive symptoms of schizophrenia are affected by blocking D_2 receptors in the mesolimbic area of the brain. Clinical effectiveness is seen when 60% to 70% of these receptors are blocked. Blocking D_2 receptors in the chemoreceptor trigger zone (CTZ) of the medulla and the peripheral blockade of vagal influences in the gastrointestinal (GI) tract produce antiemetic effects. Blocking D_2 receptors in the nigrostriatal pathways, however, creates EPS (see discussion that follows).

Other neurotransmitter systems are also affected by these drugs, and they cause many other adverse effects. Anticholinergic effects are caused by partial blockade of acetylcholine (ACh). Orthostatic hypotension results from antagonism of the alpha-adrenergic system. Alpha blockade produces sedation and raises the pain threshold. Drowsiness and weight gain result from the partial antagonism of histamine.

Pharmacokinetics

Phenothiazine drugs are well absorbed when they are taken orally and parenterally, although bioavailability is variable. They are lipophilic, readily entering the central nervous system (CNS) and most other body tissues. In addition, many antipsychotic drugs are highly bound to plasma proteins. Phenothiazines are biotransformed in the liver, with a portion of the metabolites eliminated via the kidneys. Thirty percent to 50% of the administered dose of phenothiazine passes through the GI tract unchanged. Each first-generation antipsychotic drug has specific pharmacokinetic properties (Table 21-1).

Adverse Effects and Contraindications

First-generation antipsychotics are associated with a wide variety of undesired, adverse effects that affect multiple body systems (Table 21-2). The adverse effects are drug-specific but include neurologic responses such as sedation, extrapyramidal reactions, tardive dyskinesia, seizures, and neuroleptic malignant syndrome (including diaphoresis, muscular rigidity, and hyperpyrexia; see discussions that follow). Anticholinergic effects such as dry mouth and eyes, hypotension, changes in electrocardiogram (ECG) tracings, sexual dysfunction, allergic responses, dermatologic effects, neuroendocrine effects, hematologic effects, and urinary effects also occur.

Sedation is an adverse effect of all antipsychotics, but the degree of sedation is related to the specific drug, the dose, and the individual patient. Sedation usually occurs with initial administration of the drug and is experienced for the first few days of therapy. After several weeks of treatment the patient develops a tolerance to the sedative effects.

Extrapyramidal symptoms (EPS) are among the most uncomfortable and debilitating adverse effects of antipsychotic drugs. These neuromuscular movement disorders are divided into early-onset and late-onset types. Early-onset symptoms include acute dystonia (impairment of muscular tone), parkinsonism, and akathisia (i.e., motor restlessness with a feeling of muscular quivering, an urge to move about constantly, and an inability to sit still). The primary late symptom is tardive dyskinesia. EPS wax and wane over time and disappear during sleep. The symptoms can be aggravated by emotional stress.

Acute dystonia develops early in treatment, with 90% of patients developing symptoms by the fourth day of treatment. These involuntary tonic contractions of skeletal muscles manifest as severe spasms of the tongue, the face, the neck, or the back. *Oculogyric crisis* (movement of the eyeball about the anteroposterior axis) and *opisthotonos* (a form of spasm in which the head and heels are bent backward and the body arched), carpopedal spasms, and dorsiflexion of the toes may also occur as part of the disorder. Dystonia can occur at any age, but is more common in patients under 35 years of age.

PHARMACOKINETICS

TABLE 21-1 Antipsychotics

Drugs	Route	Onset	Peak	Duration	t½	Chlorpromazine Equivalent
FIRST-GENERATION (TYPICAL) ANTIPSYCHOTICS*						
chlorpromazine	PO, IM	30–60 min	2–4 hr	4–6 hr; 10–12 hr†	23–37 hr; 10–40 hr†	100
fluphenazine	PO, IM	60 min	2–4 hr	6–8 hr	13–56 hr	2
haloperidol	PO	Erratic	3–5 hr	8–12 hr	21–26 hr	2
	IM	15–30 min	15–20 min	4–8 h§	21–24 hr	2
loxapine	PO	30 min	2–4 hr	12 hr	8–30 hr;12 hr‖	10
	IM	15–30 min	15–20 min	12 hr	8–30 hr, 12 hr‖	10
mesoridazine	IM	UA	4–7 days‡	UA	UA	50
molindone	PO	Erratic	30–90 min	24–36 hr	6.5 hr	10
perphenazine	PO	Erratic	2–4 hr	6 hr	9–21 hr	10
	IM	10 min	1–2 hr	6 hr	9–21 hr	10
thioridazine	PO	Erratic	2–4 hr	8–12 hr	9–30 hr	100
thiothixene	PO	Slow	1–3 hr	12 hr	34 hr	5
trifluoperazine	PO	UA	2–4 hr	12–24 hr	3–40 hr	5
SECOND-GENERATION (ATYPICAL) ANTIPSYCHOTICS						
aripiprazole	PO	UA	2 wk	UA	75 hr; 18 hr¶	UA‡‡
clozapine	PO	UA	1–6 hr**	4–12 hr	9–17 hr	UA‡‡
olanzapine	PO	UA	4–5 hr	UA	21–54 hr	UA‡‡
quetiapine	PO	Rapid	1.5 hr	UA	4–10 hr	UA‡‡
risperidone	PO	UA	2 hr	UA	3–24 hr††	UA‡‡
ziprasidone	PO	UA	4 hr	UA	5–10 hr	1:5

*Potency ratio compared with 100 mg of chlorpromazine.
†Chlorpromazine's duration of action for oral and extended-release formulations, respectively. The half-life for parent drug and metabolite hydroxychlorpromazine, respectively.
‡Steady state of mesoridazine with chronic dosing. Full therapeutic effects may take 6 weeks to 6 months to become evident.
§Haloperidol's antipsychotic effects may persist for several days.
‖Loxapine's half life when given IM.
¶Aripiprazole's half-life for rapid metabolizers and slow metabolizers, respectively.
**Peak antipsychotic effects of clozapine are reached in several weeks.
††Half-life of risperidone for extensive metabolizers is 3 hours; 24 hours for the metabolite 9-hydroxyrisperidone. The half-life of risperidone is 20 hours and 30 hours for 9-hydroxyrisperidone for slow metabolizers.
‡‡Chlorpromazine equivalents are not relevant with second-generation antipsychotics; therefore no chlorpromazine equivalents are identified for the second-generation drugs.
IM, Intramuscular; *PB*, protein binding; *PO*, by mouth; *t½* half-life; *UA*, unavailable.

TABLE 21-2 Adverse Effects of Antipsychotics

Drug	EPS Effects	Prolactin Elevation	Weight Gain	Glucose Abn	Lipid Abn	Prolonged QT	Sedation	Low BP	Anticholinergic Effects
FIRST-GENERATION (TYPICAL) ANTIPSYCHOTICS									
chlorpromazine	+	0	+++	0	0	0	+++	+++	++
fluphenazine	+++	0	+	0	0	0	+	+	+
haloperidol	+++	+++	+	0	0	0	++	0	0
loxapine	+++	0	+	0	0	0	++	++	++
mesoridazine	+	0	+++	0	0	0	+++	++	++
molindone	++	0	+	0	0	0	++	+	++
perphenazine	+++	0	+	0	0	0	+	+	0 to +
thioridazine	+	++	+++	+?	+?	+++	+++	+++	+++
thiothixene	+++	0	++	0	0	0	+	+	+
trifluoperazine	+++	0	0	0	0	0	+	+	+
SECOND-GENERATION (ATYPICAL) ANTIPSYCHOTICS									
aripiprazole*	0§	0	0	0	0	0	+	0 to +	0
clozapine	0§	0	+++	+++	+++	0	+++	+++	+++
olanzepine‡	0	0	+++	+++	+++	0	+	+	++
quetiapine†	0 to +§	0	++	++	++	0	++	++	0
risperidone	+	+++	++	++	++	+	+	0 to +	0
ziprasidone	0 to +§	+	0 to +	0	0	++	0	0 to +	0

0, No risk or carries little risk of adverse effect; +, mild, or occasionally causes adverse effects at therapeutic dosages; ++, sometimes causes adverse effects at therapeutic dosages; +++, frequently causes adverse effects at therapeutic dosages; ?, data too limited to rate with confidence.
*Aripiprazole also causes headache and nausea
†Also causes agranulocytosis, seizures, and myocarditis.
‡Also carries risk for development of cataracts.
§Except possibly for akathisia.
BP, Blood pressure; *EPS,* extrapyramidal symptoms (include acute dystonia, parkinsonism, and akathisia).

Men under age 50 are twice as likely to experience the disorder as women.

Dystonia may be seen in some patients even after a short course of phenothiazines for nausea and vomiting. Health care providers prescribing these drugs for nausea and vomiting are often caught off guard with respect to the dystonia. Dystonia is a very frightening experience, and the patient rushes to the acute care setting for emergent treatment. The three treatments for dystonia are oral drugs, injections of botulinum toxin, and surgery. These treatments can be used individually, in combination, or along with adjunctive therapies such as physical therapy, speech therapy, and psychotherapy.

Parkinsonism is usually dose related and characterized by bradykinesia (the unpredictable slowing down and loss of spontaneous and automatic movement), a mask-like facies, drooling, tremors, cogwheel rigidity, and a shuffling gait. These symptoms, virtually the same as those seen with idiopathic Parkinson's disease, occur within the first month of antipsychotic therapy.

Akathisia is best described as the patient's subjective experience of restlessness. Akathisia generally occurs within the first 2 weeks of treatment. It occurs equally across age groups and is seen twice as often in women.

Tardive dyskinesia (TD) is a chronic disorder of the nervous system characterized by involuntary jerky movements of the face, the tongue, the jaws, the trunk, and the limbs, usually developing as a late side effect of prolonged treatment with antipsychotic drugs; it usually appears more than a year after treatment and can affect any muscles of control. **TD shows itself as involuntary oral-buccal movements of the mouth, lips, and tongue, and may be accompanied by *choreiform* (rapid, involuntary) limb movements. Lip smacking, cheek puffing, and lateral jaw movements are the most commonly described triad of symptoms**. Many cases are mild and do

not get worse. In some cases, the condition is lifelong. Severe, disabling forms of the disorder occur in both adults and children, often resulting in malpractice payments to the patient.

A few of the more severe cases have resulted in hefty, court-ordered malpractice payments. A mentally retarded man developed TD after receiving antipsychotic drugs at an Iowa state institution and won a $760,000 lawsuit; a Michigan woman who had been treated with the drugs after two psychotic episodes was awarded over $1 million because several psychiatrists failed to diagnose TD and continued to administer antipsychotic drugs in the face of severe abnormal movements and the woman's objections; and a Midwest Veterans Administration hospital was ordered to pay nearly $2.2 million in damages to a man who was not regularly monitored by physicians while taking antipsychotic drugs that led to severe TD. In a 2000 court case, a jury in the circuit court of Philadelphia awarded $6.7 million to a patient afflicted with TD caused by risperidone.

The exact mechanism for TD is unknown, and at present, there is no specific treatment other than stopping the drug. Because of an up-regulation of D_2 receptors induced by a blockade by antipsychotics, dopaminergic hypersensitivity remains the most accepted hypothesis of tardive dyskinesia. For example, olanzapine has a higher affinity and striatal occupancy rate for D_2 receptors than clozapine, thus leading to greater up-regulation and hypersensitivity of these receptors. Another theory is that genetic traits produce a susceptibility to developing TD when an individual is exposed to particular drugs. Interestingly, the symptoms may become more severe for several weeks after the drug is withdrawn. Drugs associated with TD are identified in Box 21-3.

Anticholinergic effects, including peripheral and CNS symptoms, occur secondary to cholinergic blockade. The

BOX 21-3

Drugs Associated with Tardive Dyskinesia

Tricyclic Antidepressants
- alprazolam (Xanax)
- amitriptyline (Elavil)
- amoxapine
- clomipramine (Anafranil)
- desipramine (Norpramin)
- imipramine (Tofranil)
- nortriptyline (Pamelor)
- trimipramine (Surmontil)

Antidepressants
- bupropion (Wellbutrin)
- buspirone (Buspar)
- fluoxetine (Prozac)
- trazadone (Desyrel)

Antiepileptic Drug
- carbamazepine (Tegretol)

First-Generation (Typical) Antipsychotics
- chlorpromazine (Thorazine)
- fluphenazine (Prolixin)
- haloperidol (Haldol)
- loxapine (Loxitane)
- molindone (Moban)
- pimozide (Orap)
- perphenazine (Trilafon)
- prochlorperazine (Compazine)
- promethazine (Phenergan)
- protriptyline (Vivactil)
- trifluoperazine
- thioridazine
- thiothixene (Navane)

Second-Generation (Atypical) Antipsychotics
- aripiprazole (Abilify)
- clozapine (Clozaril)
- mesoridazine (Serentil)
- olanzapine (Zyprexa)
- risperidone (Risperdal)
- quetiapine (Seroquel)
- ziprasidone (Geodon)

MAO Inhibitor
- selegiline (Eldepryl)

Prokinetic Drug
- metoclopramide (Reglan)

symptoms include dry mouth and eyes, blurred vision (due to ciliary muscle paresis), constipation, urinary hesitancy and retention (related to increased sphincter tone, which in turn requires more fluid to initiate the detrusor contraction), and disrupted thermoregulation. Urinary retention may lead to incontinence and enuresis.

There are two primary *adverse cardiovascular effects* with the use of antipsychotics. Orthostatic hypotension is related to alpha-receptor blockade, which inhibits reflex vasoconstriction. The inhibition, in turn, causes peripheral pooling of venous blood. Orthostatic hypotension is common during the first hours or days of treatment. ECG changes include flat T waves and increased QT and PR intervals.

Patients taking antipsychotic drugs experience a *reduction in seizure threshold*. This is especially true with low-potency antipsychotics and is problematic in patients who have a preexisting seizure disorder, abnormal electroencephalogram (EEG), or other pathologic CNS conditions. Patients often develop tolerance to this adverse effect. In some cases, lowering the dose of the antipsychotic drug or increasing the dose of the anticonvulsant drug may be necessary.

Sexual dysfunctions include disturbances in ejaculation (delayed or blocked), prolonged erection, impotence, decreased libido, and changes in the quality of orgasm or the ability to experience orgasm. The exact mechanism for these effects is unknown. The adverse effects on sexual dysfunction are possibly related to endocrine influences, the calcium channel–blocking effects of the drugs, or alpha-adrenergic effects.

Allergic responses have been reported and include a maculopapular rash of face, neck, upper chest, and extremities; erythema multiforme; and localized or generalized urticaria. Five percent to 10% of patients on antipsychotic therapy develop the maculopapular rash. Dermatologic adverse responses of photosensitivity or pigmentary skin changes are rare.

Neuroendocrine effects often associated with first-generation antipsychotics include amenorrhea, galactorrhea, and gynecomastia (rare). These effects are related to increased prolactin levels, which in turn are secondary to dopamine blockade.

Adverse hematologic effects include transient leukocytosis and eosinophilia. These specific transient changes are of little clinical consequence. However, agranulocytosis, although rare with first-generation antipsychotics, requires changing the class of antipsychotic used.

The antipsychotic drugs are generally contraindicated or use in older adults and debilitated patients and are not recommended for children younger than 12 years of age owing to their susceptibility to EPS and adverse neuromuscular effects. Do not use these drugs to treat persons with hepatic, renal, or cardiovascular disorders. In addition, phenothiazines have a relative contraindication for use in patients who have severe CNS depression, coma, subcortical brain damage, or seizure disorders, or who are taking antiepileptic drugs. Although first-generation antipsychotics are not thought to possess abuse potential, abrupt discontinuation can cause withdrawal symptoms. Within a few days of terminating the drug, symptoms such as headache, nausea and vomiting, excessive salivation, diarrhea, and insomnia may develop. Tapering of the drug is advised.

▌▌▌ Drug Interactions

Most other psychotropic drugs and drugs that affect the CNS influence the effectiveness of first-generation antipsychotics and the incidence of adverse drug responses (Table 21-3). When possible, avoid drugs that interfere with the absorption, biotransformation, distribution, or elimination of phenothiazines. In addition, any drugs that potentiate therapeutic effects predispose the patient to drug toxicity.

▌▌▌ Dosage Regimen

The dosage regimen for phenothiazines varies with the individual drug. Many of the drugs can be given on a once-daily basis once the patient's condition is stable, thus enhancing the potential for patient adherence (Table 21-4).

DRUG INTERACTIONS
TABLE 21-3 Antipsychotics

Drug	Interactive Drugs	Interaction
FIRST-GENERATION (TYPICAL) ANTIPSYCHOTICS		
chlorpromazine, fluphenazine, mesoridazine, thioridazine	Antihypertensives, nitrates, alcohol, antidepressants, antihistamines	Additive hypotension
haloperidol	MAO inhibitors, opioids, sedative-hypnotics, general anesthetics	Additive CNS depression
	phenobarbital	Decreases effectiveness of chlorpromazine
	lithium	Increases risk for encephalopathy, increases excretion of lithium
	Antacids, absorbent antidiarrheals	Decreases absorption of chlorpromazine
	Antithyroid drugs	Increases risk of agranulocytosis
	bromocriptine, levodopa	Decreases antiparkinsonian activity
	epinephrine, norepinephrine	Decreases vasopressor response to interactive drug
	guanethidine	Decreases antihypertensive effects
	Beta blockers	May increase response to chlorpromazine
	Antihistamines, TCAs, quinidine, disopyramide	Increases risk of anticholinergic effects
molindone	phenytoin, tetracycline	Decreases absorption of interactive drug
perphenazine	Alcohol	Additive CNS depression
trifluoperazine	Phenothiazines, metrizamide	Increases potential for seizures
	Barbiturates	Increases risk of neuromuscular excitation and hypotension
	Antihypertensives	Decreases effect of interactive drug
SECOND-GENERATION (ATYPICAL) ANTIPSYCHOTICS		
aripiprazole	Alpha-1 antagonists, carbamazepine	Increases or decreases CYP 2D6 and 3A4 enzymes
clozapine	Bone marrow suppressants	Agranulocytosis worsens
	Anticholinergics	Increased anticholinergic effects
	Antiepileptic drugs	May diminish efficacy of clozapine
	Antihypertensives	Increases hypotensive effect
	cimetidine	Increased therapeutic or toxic effects of clozapine
	CNS depressants	Additive effect
	epinephrine	Severe hypotension
	Protein-bound drugs	Potentiates clozapine or other drug
	phenytoin, mephenytoin, ethotoin	Decreases therapeutic effects of clozapine
olanzapine	carbamazepine	Decreases serum levels of olanzepine by 50%
	Nicotine and smoking	Decreased plasma level of olanzapine
	cimetidine	Inhibits biotransformation of olanzapine
	CNS depression	Increases absorption of olanzapine
	Alcohol, diazepam	Orthostatic effect of olanzapine is increased
	Drugs inhibiting CYP450 enzymes, fluvoxamine	Inhibits biotransformation of olanzapine
	levodopa	Antagonizes levodopa
quetiapine	cimetidine	Reduces clearance of quetiapine
	lorazepam	Reduces clearance of lorazepam
	ketoconazole, other azoles	Increases serum levels of quetiapine
	thioridazine	Increases clearance of quetiapine
risperidone	carbamazepine, clozapine	Increases biotransformation of risperidone
	Drugs inhibiting CYP 2D6 enzyme pathway	Increases serum levels of risperidone
	levodopa	Decreases antiparkinsonian effects of levodopa
	Alcohol, antihistamines, opioids, sedative-hypnotics	Additive CNS depression

CNS, Central nervous system; *MAO,* monoamine oxidase; *TCAs,* tricyclic antidepressants.

▌▌ Lab Considerations

Before initiation of antipsychotic therapy, obtaining a baseline ECG is indicated, especially for patients over 40 years of age. Serial cardiac monitoring is warranted in patients with cardiac disease. Transitory elevations in liver enzymes may occur after initiation of drug therapy; perform baseline liver function tests to provide for comparison over time. Older adults, those with comorbid conditions, or patients on multi–drug therapies have increased potential for hepatotoxicity and should be carefully monitored.

A baseline complete blood count (CBC) is useful in evaluating transient hematologic responses to therapy and in monitoring for agranulocytosis. Clinical signs or symptoms of an infection during the first 3 months of treatment suggest agranulocytosis, a potentially fatal disorder that needs further investigation.

Second-Generation Antipsychotic Drugs

- ◆ aripiprazole (Abilify); ◆ Abilify
- ◆ clozapine (Clozaril); ◆ Clozaril, Leponex
- ◆ olanzapine (Zyprexa); ◆ Zyprexa
- ◆ quetiapine (Seroquel); ◆ Seroquel
- ◆ risperidone (Risperdal); ◆ Risperdal
- ◆ ziprasidone (Geodon)

▌▌ Indications

The second-generation (atypical) antipsychotic drugs were approved for use in the United States during the 1990s.

CENTRAL NERVOUS

DOSAGE
TABLE 21-4 Antipsychotics

Drugs	Use(s)	Dosage	Implications
FIRST-GENERATION (TYPICAL) ANTIPSYCHOTICS			
chlorpromazine	Acute and chronic psychoses, particularly when accompanied by increased psychomotor activity	*Adult:* Initial: 100 mg PO *–or–* 0.25 mg IM every 30–60 min until control is achieved (usually 2–3 doses) or patient does not tolerate drug. Maintenance: 300–400 mg/day as single daily dose *–or–* 100 mg 3 times daily. Max: 2000 mg/day *Child >6 mo:* 0.55 mg/kg PO every 4–6 hr *–or–* 0.55 mg/kg IM every 6–8 hr PRN *Child 6 mo to 5 yr:* Not to exceed 40 mg/day *Child 5–12 yr:* Not to exceed 75 mg/day	**Administer by deep IM; do not give by subQ. Keep patient recumbent for at least 30 min after IM use to minimize hypotensive effects.** Administer oral doses with full glass of water to minimize GI irritation. May color urine pink or reddish brown.
fluphenazine	Acute and chronic psychoses	*Adult:* Enanthate: 0.5–10 mg PO initially *–or–* 2.5–5 mg IM every 30–60 min until control achieved (usually 2–3 doses) or patient becomes intolerant. Maintenance: 15 mg PO daily as single dose. Max: 60 mg PO daily Decanoate: 12.5–25 mg IM or subQ every 1–3 wk.	IM doses can be increased up to 100 mg; however, experience is limited with doses greater than 75 mg/2 wk.
haloperidol	Psychoses, Tourette's syndrome, hyperactivity	*Adult:* Initial: 5–10 mg PO *–or–* 2.5-mg IM every 30–60 min until control achieved (usually 2–3 doses) or patient becomes intolerant. Maintenance: 15 mg PO as single dose *–or–* 0.5–5 mg PO 2–3 times daily. Max: 100 mg PO daily *–or–* 2–5 mg IM every 1–8 hr; not to exceed 100 mg/day *Child:* 0.05–0.15 mg/kg/day PO	Consider switching to different antipsychotic drug or adding concurrent use of BZD once initial 20-mg dose has been reached. IM maintenance doses can be increased up to 500 mg. Experience is limited with doses over 300 mg/mo.
loxapine	Psychoses, management of depression and anxiety associated with depression (unlabeled use)	*Adult:* Initial: 10–25 mg PO twice daily *–or–* 12.5–50 mg IM every 4–6 hr as needed. Increase in 2 wk based on response. Maintenance: 100 mg PO daily in divided doses. Max: 150 mg daily *Adolescents:* Initial dose 10 mg twice daily. Max: 100 mg daily	Severely ill patients may require up to 50 mg/day initially, then maintenance doses up to 250 mg/day.
mesoridazine	Schizophrenia, behavioral problems in mental deficiency and chronic brain syndrome	*Adult:* Initial: 25–50 mg PO 2–3 times daily *–or–* 25 mg IM. Repeat in 30–60 min if needed. Maintenance: 75–400 mg/day PO *–or–* 25–400 mg/day IM	Do not change dosage in chronic therapy more often than weekly. Avoid prolonged exposure to sun. May color urine pink or reddish brown.
molindone	Acute and chronic psychoses	*Adult:* Initial: 50–75 mg/day PO. Increase to 225 mg/day in 3–4 divided doses. Maintenance: 5–15 mg PO 3–4 times daily. Moderate symptoms: 10–25 mg PO 3–4 times daily. Severe symptoms: 225 mg/day	Use lower doses and increase dosage more gradually for older adults. Pink or reddish brown urine is common, as well as yellowing of the skin and eyes.
perphenazine	Psychoses	*Adult:* Initial: 2–16 mg PO 2–4 times daily. Not to exceed 64 mg/day PO *–or–* 5–10 mg IM. May repeat every 6 hr. Not to exceed 15–30 mg/day IM *Child >12 yr:* 8 mg/day in divided doses	Keep patient recumbent at least 30 min following IM administration to minimize hypotensive effects.
thioridazine	Acute and chronic psychoses	*Adult:* Initial: 50–150 mg PO twice daily. Maintenance: 300–400 mg PO daily as single dose. Max: 800 mg daily	Risk of pigmentary retinopathy with doses exceeding 800 mg/day
thiothixene	Psychoses	*Adult:* Initial: 10–15 mg PO *–or–* 4–10 mg IM every 30–60 min until control achieved (usually 2–3 doses) or patient becomes intolerant. Generally 2–5 mg 3 times daily. Maintenance: 30 mg PO daily in single dose. Max: 60 mg/day	Avoid prolonged exposure to sun. May color urine pink or reddish brown Discontinue drug if creatinine and BUN become abnormal or if WBC count is depressed.
trifluoperazine	Psychoses	*Adult:* Initial: 2–5 mg PO twice daily *–or–* 1–2 mg IM every 4–6 hr. Maintenance: 15–20 mg/day PO. More than 6 mg/day IM is rarely needed.	Avoid prolonged exposure to sun. May color urine pink or reddish brown. Stop drug if creatinine and BUN abnormal or WBC count is depressed.
SECOND-GENERATION (ATYPICAL) ANTIPSYCHOTICS			
aripiprazole	Schizophrenia	*Adult:* 10–15 mg PO initially once daily. May increase up to 30 mg/day.	Improves and achieves target goals in schizophrenia
clozapine	Unresponsive schizophrenia	*Adult:* Initially 12.5–25 mg PO once daily to twice daily. Increase by 25–50 mg/day over 2 wk to 300–450 mg/day. Increase by up to 100 mg/day once or twice weekly. Max: 900 mg/day	Drug lowers seizure threshold. Transient fevers may occur during first 3 wk of use. Monitor WBC weekly during therapy and 4 wk after stopping the drug.
olanzapine	Psychoses	*Adult:* Initial: 5–10 mg PO daily. Increase to 10 mg daily within several days, adjusting by 5 mg/day; thereafter at weekly intervals. Max: 20 mg/day	Avoid prolonged exposure to sun. Avoid extremes in temperature since drug impairs body temperature regulation. Monitor patient for NMS.
quetiapine	Psychoses	*Adult:* 25 mg twice daily initially. Increase by 25–50 mg 2–3 times daily on second or third day to target of 300–400 mg in 2–3 divided doses.	Cardiovascular monitoring required for older adults taking more than 20 mg/day.
risperidone	Psychoses	*Adult:* 1 mg PO twice daily. Increase by third day to 3 mg twice daily. Maintenance: 4–6 mg/day. Max: 16 mg/day	Further increments of 1 mg twice daily may be made at weekly intervals.
ziprasidone	Psychoses	*Adult:* 80–160 mg/day in divided doses	5 times more potent than chlorpromazine. There is little experience with ziprasidone overdosage at this time.

BUN, Blood urea nitrogen; *BZD*, benzodiazepine; *IM*, intramuscular (route); *NMS*, neuroleptic malignant syndrome; *PO*, by mouth; *PRN*, as needed; *subQ*, subcutaneous (route); *WBC*, white blood count.

These phenothiazines are also indicated as first- or second-line drugs (except for clozapine) in the treatment of schizophrenia and other psychotic disorders. They have also been used as adjuncts in the management of mania and borderline personality disorder. Because of the adverse effects and monitoring required for clozapine, its use is limited to patients who are nonresponsive to management with first-generation drugs.

▌ Pharmacodynamics

Second-generation antipsychotics appear to have different receptor interactions than their predecessors. Aripiprazole is a partial agonist at D_2 and 5-hydroxytryptamine-1A ($5-HT_{1A}$) receptors. Partial agonist activity presumably "cools" hyperdopaminergia in limbic areas, decreases dopamine activity in hypodopaminergic sites, and does not cause significant blockade in motor and hypothalamic pathways.

Aripiprazole is also a $5-HT_2$ receptor antagonist and thus in theory provides some protection from EPS and hyperprolactinemia, as well as some improvement of cognitive negative symptoms. The drug also blocks α_1 receptors, which may account for occasional episodes of orthostatic hypotension.

Clozapine selectively binds to D_1 and D_4 receptor sites in the cortical and limbic regions of the brain, with less effect in the nigrostriatal region. It is preferentially more active at limbic than at striatal dopamine receptors, which may account for the relative lack of EPS. Clozapine influences $5-HT_2$ receptors, as well as blocking the reuptake of norepinephrine.

Olanzapine blocks D_1, D_2, D_3, and D_4 receptors. It has a high affinity for 5-HT receptors, as well as binding muscarinic and H_1 receptors, but has less affinity for α_1 receptors. Clinical response takes weeks to months.

Risperidone resembles high-potency first-generation antipsychotics, although its mechanism is unclear. Its antipsychotic action is thought to be the antagonism of both D_2 and $5-HT_2$ receptors. Hypothetically, by blocking D_2 receptors in the mesolimbic area, positive symptoms are improved; by blocking $5-HT_2$ receptors in the cortex, negative symptoms are improved. It is also an antagonist to D_1, D_4, histamine, ACh, and α_1 receptors.

▌ Pharmacokinetics

All second-generation antipsychotics are well absorbed when taken by mouth, with variable availability, and are biotransformed in the liver. The majority of metabolites are inactive and eliminated in the urine, with a small amount eliminated through the feces (see Table 21-1).

▌ Adverse Effects and Contraindications

The adverse effects of second-generation antipsychotics fall into many of the same categories as the first-generation drugs but with some distinct differences (see Table 21-2). These drugs cause sedation, whereas others have EPS or anticholinergic adverse effects, or both. Other adverse effects include agitation, headache, insomnia, nausea, rhinitis, salivation, and weight gain. On the other hand, the relative incidences of adverse effects are different than those of first-generation drugs. This is one reason second-generation drugs are used more frequently.

Since their introduction, a clearer picture of the adverse effects of second-generation antipsychotic drugs have emerged. Some are similar to the older drugs, but newer ones

unique to these drugs have been identified. Adverse effects of second-generation drugs include weight gain, hyperglycemia including the development of type 2 diabetes mellitus, hypercholesterolemia, ECG abnormalities (prolonged QT intervals), increased risk for cerebrovascular accidents in older adults with dementia, sexual dysfunction, and possible development of neuroleptic malignant syndrome (NMS).

The risk for type 2 diabetes has been linked to three specific drugs. The manufacturers of aripiprazole, risperidone, and quetiapine have each added warnings indicating an increased risk of high blood sugar or type 2 diabetes in patients taking these drugs. In addition, risperidone has a warning that there may be an increased risk of stroke among older adults taking this drug.

Although uncommon, all second-generation antipsychotic drugs can cause neuroleptic malignant syndrome. **Neuroleptic** ▲ **malignant syndrome (NMS) is a potentially lethal hypodopaminergic adverse effect of high-potency antipsychotic drugs.** Onset usually appears within the first 2 weeks of therapy. Risk factors for NMS are many but primarily include use of high-potency antipsychotic drugs, dehydration, young adulthood, male sex, nonschizophrenic illness, and prolonged use of restraints. Coadministration of lithium, a mood-stabilizing drug, or withdrawal from anticholinergic drugs, alcoholism, organic brain syndrome or previous brain injury, or iron deficiency may contribute to its onset.

Criteria for NMS include hyperthermia (sometimes to 108° F), muscle rigidity, and the presence of five of the following: (1) stupor, (2) tremors, (3) tachycardia, (4) incontinence, (5) unstable blood pressure, (6) metabolic acidosis, (7) tachypnea or hypoxia, (8) elevation of creatinine phosphokinase (caused by muscle rigidity and subsequent rhabdomyolysis), (9) diaphoresis or sialorrhea, (10) leukocytosis, and (11) exclusion of other central and systemic causes of hyperthermia.

Death from NMS can result from a number of problems caused by hyperthermia including, but not limited to, aspiration pneumonia, pulmonary emboli, renal failure, disseminated intravascular coagulation (DIC), renal failure, and unexpected cardiopulmonary arrest. Patients may recover but will continue to be at high risk for recurrent episodes of NMS if antipsychotic drugs are once again prescribed.

▌ Drug Interactions

Drug interactions of second-generation antipsychotics are similar in many ways to those of first-generation drugs in that there is additive CNS depression with the concurrent use of alcohol, antihistamines, opioids, and sedative-hypnotics. Anticonvulsants and antiparkinsonian drugs are most affected by interaction with second-generation antipsychotic drugs (see Table 21-3).

▌ Dosage Regimen

The dosage regimens for second-generation antipsychotics are identified in Table 21-4.

▌ Lab Considerations

Additional monitoring is required because of the risks unique to second-generation antipsychotics. Obtain vital signs, a fasting lipid profile, and fasting blood glucose level, as well as a hemoglobin A_{1c} before treatment, at 3 months, and then annually. Monitor the patient's body mass index

(BMI), waist circumference, and blood pressure; mental status; the presence of abnormal involuntary movements (AIMs); and orthostatic blood pressure changes for 3 to 5 days after starting therapy or increasing dosage. Weight should be assessed before treatment, at 4, 8, and 12 weeks, and then at quarterly intervals. Consider titrating to a different antipsychotic drug if the patient has a weight gain of 5% or more from baseline.

In addition to the baseline lab studies done for patients taking antipsychotics, those receiving clozapine must have weekly blood monitoring. The weekly white blood cell (WBC) count for the patient taking clozapine must be $3500/mm^3$ or greater for therapy to continue. A differential count is warranted if the granulocyte count is greater than $1500/mm^3$. If the WBCs fall below $2000/mm^3$ or the granulocyte count is less than $1500/mm^3$, clozapine must be discontinued and the patient hospitalized in isolation for observation. Hematologist, internist, and infectious disease consultations are warranted. If the patient is to continue clozapine therapy, follow-up includes monitoring of absolute neutrophil count (ANC) for the first 6 months, then every 2 weeks for 6 months. If the WBC stabilizes, monitoring may continue on an every-4-week regimen. For patients in whom the drug is discontinued, the WBCs and the ANC are assessed every week for 4 weeks. Other lab monitoring is drug-specific.

CLINICAL REASONING

Treatment Objectives

The primary treatment objective for schizophrenia and other psychoses is to diminish psychotic behaviors, thus preventing harm to the patient or others, improving thought disorders, reducing the duration of inpatient hospitalization, and preventing or decreasing the severity of future exacerbations. Accomplishing these objectives permits the patient to participate more fully in psychotherapy and other non–drug treatment modalities, and allows the patient to attain a higher level of functioning. However, in so doing, the safety and functioning of the patient are key foci.

Treatment Options

Antipsychotic drugs are the primary treatment modality for patients with psychoses. Whether the patient is hospitalized, is participating in a community-based outpatient program, or is residing at home, little improvement can be made without the drugs (see Evidence-based Pharmacotherapeutics).

Nonadherence is a major reason that antipsychotic drugs are not more effective in keeping persons with schizophrenia out of the hospital. Nonadherence accounts for about 50% of all relapse. In addition, relapse from nonadherence may be more severe or dangerous than relapse occurring while on antipsychotic drugs. Persistent nonadherence may worsen the overall course of the schizophrenic illness, and eventually make the person less likely to respond to drug therapy. Prescribing health care providers frequently do not detect or ask about nonadherence and are not always good at recognizing when patients stop their drugs. In fact, some health care providers may not recognize nonadherence until the person becomes psychotic and starts hallucinating.

▥ Patient Variables

Initial assessment of baseline functioning and mental status is imperative to manage psychosis with antipsychotic drugs. This is particularly important because drug therapy is aimed at treating symptoms and behaviors. What specific behaviors are noted? When did the psychotic behaviors begin? Was there an identifiable precipitating situation, event, or element linked to the onset of behaviors? Have the symptoms ever occurred before? If so, what was the treatment? Has the patient been treated with antipsychotic drugs in the past? Family members and others may be interviewed if patient interaction fails to provide the necessary information.

Although it may be difficult to perform a full physical exam on a person who is psychotic, it is vital to establish baseline parameters. Keep in mind that many of the adverse effects noted with antipsychotic therapy have physical manifestations. In addition, because virtually all of the antipsychotic drugs rely on the liver for biotransformation, identification of potential preexisting hepatic disorders is needed. Perform a neurologic exam also. Record the results of the CBC, liver function tests, and the ECG. These baseline values are used as a measure of patient response to drug therapy, as well as to avert severe adverse effects. No specific ongoing monitoring of blood levels of first-generation antipsychotic drugs is mandated at this time. However, ongoing monitoring of the CBC and the ANC is mandatory if the patient is receiving clozapine, because of the potential for agranulocytosis.

Adverse effects of many of the antipsychotic drugs may interfere with patient functioning, and some of the adverse effects seen with the atypical antipsychotic drugs can be lethal. Support and education help in the day-to-day management of the patient with psychosis.

Patients with schizophrenia should receive drug therapy unless there are compelling contraindications. The adverse effects profile depends on the actual drug and the person's response. Age and sex influence the patient's responses to antipsychotic drugs. Young men tend to be particularly susceptible to EPS or dystonic reactions. Therefore it is best to avoid the high-potency drugs (e.g., haloperidol) in these patients. Older adults tend to have a greater number of chronic health conditions influencing their responses. Haloperidol may be chosen for older adults and for patients with cardiovascular or seizure disorders. Haloperidol is a high-potency antipsychotic with low anticholinergic effects. It produces less sedation and orthostatic hypotension than loxapine or thiothixene. However, it does produce a higher incidence of acute EPS and dystonic reactions. In addition, some adverse effects occur more frequently in women, whereas others occur more frequently in men. Fluphenazine is similar to haloperidol, and if it is less expensive, it may be chosen over haloperidol for older adults and for those with comorbid cardiovascular or seizure disorders. In most cases, antipsychotics are not recommended for children under 12 years of age.

In some cases, the concurrent use of a benzodiazepine (BZD; e.g., lorazepam; see Chapter 19) and an antipsychotic drug can be effective. For example, lorazepam permits control of agitation and decreases the need for initial high doses of antipsychotics, which in turn decreases the likelihood of adverse effects. Further, lorazepam can be administered

EVIDENCE-BASED PHARMACOTHERAPEUTICS

Antipsychotic Drug Therapy

■ Background

Antipsychotic drugs have become the cornerstone of treatment for schizophrenia. The first-generation (typical) antipsychotic drugs are high-affinity antagonists of dopamine D_2 receptors that are most effective against psychotic symptoms but have high rates of neurologic adverse effects, such as extrapyramidal symptoms (EPS) and tardive dyskinesia. The introduction of second-generation (atypical) antipsychotic drugs promised enhanced efficacy and safety. The second-generation drugs differ pharmacologically from first-generation drugs in their lower affinity for dopamine D_2 receptors and greater affinities for other neuroreceptors, including those for serotonin and norepinephrine.

Although studies indicate that second-generation drugs are similar to first-generation drugs in reducing psychotic symptoms and that they produce few neurologic effects, the evidence of their superior efficacy has been neither consistent nor robust, with the exception of clozapine, which repeatedly has been shown effective in patients whose schizophrenia is unmanageable with other drugs but has severe adverse effects and monitoring requirements that limit its use. The second-generation drugs appear more efficacious than first-generation drugs in reducing negative symptoms (e.g., lack of emotion, interest, and expression), possibly owing to the absence of EPS or other secondary causes of negative symptoms (e.g., depression) rather than to direct therapeutic effects.

■ Research Article

Lieberman, J., Stroup, S., McEvoy, J., et al. for the Clinical Antipsychotic Trials of Intervention Effectiveness (CATIE) Investigators. (2005). Effectiveness of antipsychotic drugs in patients with chronic schizophrenia. *New England Journal of Medicine, 353*(12), 1209–1223.

Purpose

The purpose of the CATIE study was to evaluate the use and efficacy of current antipsychotic drugs including the following: (1) a comparison of effectiveness of second-generation antipsychotics with a first-generation antipsychotic, (2) a comparison of effectiveness among the second-generation antipsychotics, and (3) a cost-effectiveness analysis of the second-generation antipsychotics. The basic hypotheses were that (1) there are overall differences among antipsychotic medications (olanzapine, quetiapine, risperidone, and perphenazine); (2) there are differences between the second-generation antipsychotic drugs olanzapine, quetiapine, and risperidone; (3) there are differences between the first-generation antipsychotic perphenazine and olanzapine, quetiapine, and risperidone; and (4) there are differences between ziprasidone and the other antipsychotic olanzapine, quetiapine, risperidone, and perphenazine.

Design

The study was designed as a double-blind, controlled, randomized treatment trial divided into three major phases. In phase 1, patients were randomized into one of five treatment groups: (1) olanzapine, (2) quetiapine, (3) risperidone, (4) ziprasidone, or (5) perphenazine. Perphenazine was chosen as the comparator first-generation antipsychotic in this study because of its relatively favorable safety profile. Drug dosages were flexible and ranged from one to four capsules daily based on the investigators' judgment.

In phase 2, subjects who discontinued phase 1 were then allowed to choose enrollment into one of two pathways. If discontinuation was due to lack of efficacy, patients were randomized either to open-label clozapine or to a double-blinded second-generation drug that was available but not assigned in phase 1 (olanzapine, quetiapine, or risperidone). If discontinuation was due to lack of tolerability, double-blinded randomization to ziprasidone or another second-generation drug that was available but not assigned during phase 1 (olanzapine, quetiapine, or risperidone) occurred.

Phase 3 included subjects who discontinued phase 2 but who were allowed to choose another open-label treatment from the following: aripiprazole, clozapine, fluphenazine, olanzapine, perphenazine, quetiapine, risperidone, ziprasidone, or a combination of any of these drugs. This open-label treatment phase allowed the patient and health care provider to select treatment based on the subject's experience with phase 1 and phase 2 study drugs as well as their previous experiences with first and second-generation antipsychotics.

Methods

Subjects ($N = 1493$) ages 18 to 65 (mean age 40.6 years; 74% males) were recruited at 57 U.S. sites and randomized to receive olanzapine (7.5 to 30 mg/day), perphenazine (8 to 32 mg/day), quetiapine (200 to 800 mg/day), risperidone (1.5 to 6.0 mg/day), or ziprasidone (40 to 160 mg/day) for up to 18 months. The primary objective was to identify in a quantitative fashion differences in the overall effectiveness of these five treatments.

Of the subjects, 60% were white, 35% black, and 5% from other groups; 12% were of Hispanic origin. Eighty-five percent of subjects were unemployed. Baseline factors associated with the metabolic syndrome including hypertension, body mass index (BMI), hyperlipidemia, and type 1 or type 2 diabetes were matched between groups.

The primary outcome measure for CATIE was all-cause treatment discontinuation with a major secondary outcome being reason for discontinuation (efficacy, tolerability, patient decision). This was chosen as the primary measure because it is a discrete outcome and because changing drug therapy is a common problem in the treatment of schizophrenia. This measure was also practical in that it combined both patients' and health care providers' judgment of efficacy, safety, and tolerability into a single global effectiveness measure.

Secondary outcomes included the specific reasons for discontinuing treatment (e.g., lack of efficacy or the development of intolerable adverse effects such as weight gain, EPS, or sedation as judged by the health care provider). Scores on the Positive and Negative Syndrome Scale (PANSS) and the Clinical Global Impression (CGI) scale were also evaluated at months 1, 3, 6, 9, 12, 15, and 18. Other secondary outcomes included psychopathology, safety, service utilization and costs, neurocognitive effects, treatment adherence, comorbid conditions, quality of life, substance use, and violence.

Because of the multiple treatments arms and the unequal number of subjects per group, attention to statistical analyses was necessary, including adjustments for multiple comparisons and a corresponding increase in the definition of statistical significance.

Findings

Seventy-four percent of subjects (i.e., 1061 of the 1432 subjects) stopped the drug during the 18 months of the study, some after the first dose of the drug. Sixty-four percent of subjects received olanzapine, 75% received perphenazine, 85% quetiapine, 74% risperidone, and 79% ziprasidone. Less than half of the subjects reached maximal dosages of the antipsychotic drugs used allowable in the study. Only 40% of subjects were treated with the maximal allowable doses of olanzapine, risperidone, and perphenazine, 44% received the maximal dosage of quetiapine, and 48% received the maximal dose of ziprasidone.

Seventy-four percent of subjects discontinued phase 1 of the study with a median of 6 months and a mean of 8.3 months. Subjects taking olanzapine used the drug considerably longer before discontinuing treatment compared with subjects taking quetiapine (p < 0.001) or risperidone (p = 0.002). This was not the case for subjects taking perphenazine (p = 0.021) or ziprasidone (p = 0.028). Olanzapine was associated with undesirable metabolic effects or weight gain whereas perphenazine was stopped because of EPS.

Subjects treated with olanzapine gained an average of 2 lb/month, and a larger percentage of olanzapine-treated subjects gained 7% or more of their baseline body weight than those treated with the other drugs (30% vs. 7% to 16% in the other groups, p < 0.001). Olanzapine also had the greatest increase in hemoglobin A_{1c} levels, total cholesterol, and triglyceride levels compared with other study drugs. Ziprasidone was associated with improvements in each of those metabolic parameters. More patients

Continued

CENTRAL NERVOUS

EVIDENCE-BASED PHARMACOTHERAPEUTICS—Cont'd

discontinued perphenazine as a result of EPS than any of the other drugs (8% vs. 2% to 4% for the other drugs, p = 0.002). Subjects taking olanzapine or quetiapine were less likely to report insomnia (16% and 18%, respectively, vs. 24% to 30% for the other drugs). Quetiapine was associated with more urinary hesitancy, dry mouth, and constipation relative to other drugs (31% vs. 20% to 25% for the other drugs).

All study drugs showed significant improvements in PANSS scores over time. Scores were greatest for olanzapine, but this advantage diminished over time. This was also true for mean change in CGI severity. Even though olanzapine showed the greatest improvement initially, other drugs reached similar changes in scores later in the study.

Overall, patients treated with olanzapine were significantly less likely to be hospitalized than patients on the other drugs (p = 0.001), but hospitalizations per person-years of exposure to each drug showed no difference among the drugs.

Results confirm previous findings that TD is associated with older age, longer duration of antipsychotic treatment, and treatment with an anticholinergic drug. In addition, TD patients had higher ratings of psychopathology as measured by the PANSS, more EPS, and more akathisia. Although stimulant abuse and/or dependence were significantly associated with TD, neither diabetes mellitus nor hypertension predicted TD.

Conclusions

CATIE is the largest, longest, and most comprehensive trial ever conducted investigating the effectiveness of antipsychotic drugs in the management of schizophrenia. Olanzapine was the most effective antipsychotic drug of those tested in relation to discontinuation rates; however, olanzapine was associated with greater increases in weight and elevations in glucose and lipid metabolism. The efficacy of the first-generation antipsychotic drug perphenazine appears to be similar to that of quetiapine, risperidone, and ziprasidone.

■ Implications for Practice

The CATIE trial addressed many of the questions that health care providers face when treating patients with schizophrenia, in particular the unacceptably high rate of drug discontinuation in patients with schizophrenia. The need for safer, more effective, and more tolerant therapies remains an area in which new research is vital. Data from this trial will assist health care providers in making educated decisions about treatment of schizophrenia by providing detailed adverse effects and efficacy profiles in a diverse number of patients with schizophrenia for many of the currently used drugs. How clinicians, patients, families, and policymakers evaluate the trade-offs between efficacy and side effects, as well as drug prices, will determine future patterns of use.

---

parenterally, which may be helpful for patients who are unwilling to take oral formulations. Other drugs that may be used for adjunctive therapy include carbamazepine, lithium, and valproic acid.

For the otherwise healthy young patient with psychosis, loxapine may be useful. Loxapine is a medium-potency antipsychotic drug that produces less sedation, has moderate anticholinergic activity, and causes less orthostatic hypotension than does chlorpromazine or thioridazine. It also has a lower incidence of acute extrapyramidal or dystonic reactions than higher-potency drugs such as haloperidol and fluphenazine.

If sedation of the patient is desired, chlorpromazine may be chosen. It produces sedation and orthostatic hypotension more than the medium-potency or high-potency drugs. However, it has a low incidence of acute EPS and dystonic reactions. Thioridazine can also be used, although there is no parenteral form of this drug available.

LIFE-SPAN CONSIDERATIONS

Pregnant and Nursing Women. Determine if there is a previous history of psychosis that may be complicated by a pregnancy. During the first trimester, the woman normally feels some ambivalence about the pregnancy, even if it was planned. Discuss these feelings with the woman, because she may otherwise feel the need to hide the negative feelings, thinking they are abnormal. The ambivalence usually ends by the beginning of the second trimester. Treatment of psychosis during pregnancy is complicated, because many of the antipsychotic drugs are pregnancy category C drugs.

Children and Adolescents. The term *childhood schizophrenia* is no longer used when discussing mental disorders of childhood. Normal children adapting to life experiences exhibit symptoms that in an adult would be characteristic of mental illness. Psychotic behaviors generally appear after 5 years of age. Psychotic behavior in an adolescent may have been obvious from childhood, or it can be triggered by a developmental crisis. Some health care providers believe that an individual

must at least reach the developmental stage of adolescence before the diagnosis of schizophrenia can be made.

An adolescent is not a miniature adult, but a developing person within a family system. The adolescent's needs are not those of an adult, but those of an individual in an emotional and often confusing world. Therefore collect information from the parents and the adolescent about the history and progress of the illness. Observations of parent-adolescent interactions and the effectiveness of those interactions with the environment should be documented. In addition, the extent to which an adolescent can distinguish the self from the environment can help ascertain whether or not he or she can distinguish between reality and fantasy, as can the determination of any self-mutilation or aggressive behaviors. The adolescent may be unaware of anything but a growing sense of unhappiness, but asking for help is developmentally inconsistent with the internal drive for mastery and control. Until recently, seeking professional help also carried social stigma.

Older Adults. An older adult's sense of self and security is threatened when adapting to various personal changes of aging. Changes in physical status, loss of the significant other, hospitalization, or movement to an assisted living or long-term care facility have a profound effect on the older adult's sense of independence. Uncharacteristic behaviors may emerge or existing personality traits exaggerated when a person is confined, is in a crisis state, or is receiving treatment and drugs.

▥ Drug Variables

The indications for first- and second-generation antipsychotic drugs are the same. The choice of drugs depends on the tolerance of the patient. Overall, the greatest distinctions between antipsychotic drugs are in their adverse effects profiles. High-potency drugs require smaller dosages to produce an effect, cause less sedation and orthostatic hypotension, and produce fewer anticholinergic effects (see Table 21-4). However, they tend to have a higher incidence of early EPS. When adverse effects become too disturbing to the patient, drug therapy is often stopped. Thus selection of an antipsychotic drug is based on the patient's and family members' previous therapeutic response to a specific drug, differences in adverse effects, and cost. Despite the wide variety of available antipsychotic drugs, there are no convincing data that one antipsychotic drug is necessarily more effective than another.

Thirty percent of patients with stable psychoses do not adhere to their drug therapy. The relapse rate for patients not on drug therapy approaches 60%. For most patients treated with first-generation drugs, prescribe a dosage close to the "EPS threshold" (i.e., the dosage that will induce EPS adverse effects) that results in the least possible rigidity detectable on physical exam. Second-generation antipsychotic drugs can generally be prescribed at dosages that are therapeutic but that will not cause EPS.

Maintain the therapeutic dose of a drug for at least 4 to 6 weeks at standard dosage, and evaluate the patient's response before considering the use of a different drug. Because first-generation antipsychotics tend to have a slow onset of action, the direct correlation between dose and therapeutic effectiveness is difficult to judge. If improvement is seen at 4 weeks, therapy is continued for an additional 2 weeks and the patient reevaluated. The duration of therapy depends on the patient's specific diagnosis. However, in schizophrenia, maintenance therapy is usually needed to maintain patient functioning.

Further, there is no evidence suggesting that higher doses of antipsychotic drugs are likely to improve psychosis more quickly. Higher dosages increase the risk of adverse effects and should be avoided. Allow several days to weeks for patient response before increasing the dosage. In controlled, nonagitated patients, begin at low dosages and increase every 2 weeks to minimize adverse effects and to increase the patient's acceptance of drug therapy. Once the patient is tolerant of the adverse effects, a full dosage of the drug can be given at bedtime (except for loxapine).

In some cases the patient is provided with an order for an as-needed (PRN) BZD during the initial titration of the antipsychotic to a maintenance dosage. If frequent doses of the BZD or antipsychotic are needed, maintenance doses of the antipsychotic drug may be increased more often than every 2 weeks. BZDs are not intended for long-term maintenance; taper off their use within the first few weeks as the patient becomes less agitated. Tapering therapy usually starts after the first week of therapy.

Two oral dosing strategies are used for maintenance treatment: intermittent targeted treatment and continuous minimal dosing. The goal of the *intermittent targeted treatment* strategy is to reduce total drug exposure; the drug is administered only when there are active symptoms. The goal of *continuous minimal dosing* is the avoidance of relapse by providing a continuous coverage at a much lower dosage than during the acute episodes. Dosage reduction may be considered once the patient has been stabilized for a 3- to 6-month period.

Long-acting parenteral antipsychotics are recommended for patients unable to manage daily-dosage regimens and for the patient on maintenance therapy who is likely to be nonadherent. Depot formulations, for instance of haloperidol or fluphenazine, can be used. Typically, antipsychotic drugs are first given orally for at least 1 to 2 weeks before the patient is switched to a depot formulation. The depot form is administered, and the oral dosage is tapered. At this time, no specific guidelines for tapering the oral dose have been developed. Tapering is handled on an individual basis, remaining cognizant that the steady state of the parenteral formulations is not achieved for several weeks.

A calculated nonloading maintenance dose of the decanoate form may also be administered during tapering-off periods. For example, a patient has been receiving a 30-mg/day oral dose of fluphenazine. A parenteral dose of 10 to 15 times that would be calculated for a monthly dose—that is, the month's total amount is 300 mg. This, in turn, is broken into two doses of 150 mg (administered every 2 weeks). The previous oral dose is reduced over a period of 4 months, pending the development of adverse effects. If adverse effects develop, the reduction of the oral dose is accelerated.

Another protocol for initiating a depot regimen has been used with haloperidol decanoate. Once the patient has been stabilized on the oral form, a parenteral loading dose equal to 20 times the oral dose is administered during the month. The initial maximum dosage is seldom above 100 mg, with the remaining amounts administered in the next weeks. Oral haloperidol is discontinued when the full loading dosage has been reached. The maintenance dose (50% of the loading dose) is achieved by tapering the loading dose downward by 25% each month for 2 months. Thus, if the patient has been receiving 10 mg/day orally, a loading dose of at least 200 mg IM would be indicated, administered as 100 mg for the first dose and 100 mg for the second, 7 days later. With the administration of the second 100-mg dose, oral haloperidol would be discontinued. Replace parenteral therapy with oral therapy when the patient is able and willing to comply with a therapeutic regimen.

Patients who respond to treatment should be permitted a gradual reduction in dosage to allow for a drug holiday and to determine the need for ongoing therapy. In addition, to better manage symptoms and adverse effects, it is common to administer antipsychotic drugs as a single daily dose, which is generally given at bedtime. The drug can also be given in a split-dose regimen, with one third of the total daily dose taken in the morning and two thirds at bedtime.

Patient Education

Teach the patient and support individuals who assist the patient (e.g., family or assisted living supervisor) about the psychotic disorder, its possible etiologies, the associated behaviors, and the importance of drug therapy in managing symptoms so as to minimize the risk of relapse. Because some symptoms subside before others, it is helpful to educate the patient and members of the support system about which behaviors are likely to change first and how long after initiation of treatment the change will take place.

Information about possible adverse effects is needed so the patient does not become anxious when they develop; many of the effects will subside in a few weeks. Also, it is imperative to instruct the patient and members of the support system about early- and late-onset adverse effects and how they might be managed. Patients often worry that varying the dosage may exacerbate symptoms. Ongoing reinforcement is especially important given the cognitive effects of schizophrenia and other psychoses. Advise the patient taking chlorpromazine, mesoridazine, thiothixene, or trifluoperazine that it may color the urine pink or reddish brown. Yellowing of the skin and eyes is common with molindone. Caution patients taking trifluoperazine to avoid prolonged exposure to the sun to minimize photosensitivity reactions.

The adverse effects may be managed by the concurrent administration of another drug. Teach the patient that chewing sugarless gum assists in relieving dry mouth. Frequent rinsing with cool water also refreshes a dry mouth. Teach the patient to change positions slowly to avoid experiencing the hypotensive effects of the drug.

Give the patient drug-specific instructions about withdrawal. In addition, caution patients not to take over-the-counter (OTC) drugs containing interactive ingredients (e.g., antacids and drugs containing alcohol).

Advise the patient to carry medical alert identification containing information about the antipsychotic regimen and to inform all health care providers (e.g., nurses, health care providers, dentists, physical therapists, etc.) about it. By doing so, it is possible to monitor for therapeutic effects and adverse drug effects and interactions.

Evaluation

The effectiveness of antipsychotic therapy is demonstrated by a decrease in the severity of psychosis and diminished symptoms. A decrease in agitation should be noted within hours of initiating therapy, and significant improvement should be seen within 24 to 48 hours. Sleep disturbances should improve within days, hallucinations within weeks, and thought disorders within 1 to 2 months. Negative symptoms such as anhedonia and restricted or blunted affect take weeks to months to improve. In some cases, negative symptoms may not improve at all. Some patients require 8 to 12 weeks of therapy at typical doses before a full response is noted.

Monitor patients regularly, watching for early symptoms of relapse. Note if the patient has had an adequate period to adjust to the antipsychotic drug and its dosage, and whether or not the patient is taking the drug as prescribed. The biggest mistake health care providers make is to change drug therapy too quickly. Determine if the patient's negative symptoms are related to parkinsonian syndrome or to untreated major depression, and intervene accordingly. The antipsychotic drug that provides the best therapeutic results with the fewest adverse effects is the most effective option. If a positive response is seen but intolerable adverse effects develop, the dosage can be lowered. If dosage reduction is ineffective, the drug can be stopped and the patient switched to an alternative drug; monotherapy is recommended. There is no therapeutic advantage in combining different classes of drugs.

A trial of clozapine is appropriate for patients who have not responded clinically to two antipsychotic drugs, one of which was a second-generation drug. Clozapine is also appropriate for patients whose behaviors or suicidal thoughts have not responded to other treatment. Depending on the type of residual symptoms (e.g., cognitive, positive, negative, mood symptoms, aggression), consider adding another antipsychotic, an antiepileptic drug, or a benzodiazepine.

Consider hospitalization for patients who pose a serious threat to self or others or who are unable to provide self-care, and those in need of constant supervision. Legal proceedings may be required for patients resistant to inpatient care when hospitalization or supervised care is clearly indicated.

Monitor outpatients on a weekly basis for signs of decompensation. There is a 50% relapse rate at 6 months, even for patients on drug therapy. One year after therapy is discontinued the relapse rate is approximately 70%. If therapy is continued, only 40% of patients relapse. As a rule, after the first episode of decompensation, the patient is treated continuously for 1 year. After a second episode, he or she is treated continuously for at least 3 years. With a third episode of decompensation, consider treating the patient for at least 5 years before attempting a drug holiday. Remember, the risk of developing TD increases with the length of therapy and the patient's age.

Controversy

Diagnostic Approach to Schizophrenia

Some health care providers argue that current methodologies used to diagnose schizophrenia are flawed because they rely on an unprovable conjecture (i.e., there is a clear difference between mental illness and mental health). Psychologist Richard Bentall (*Madness Explained*, 2004) states that psychoses are present in many people who never develop symptoms or who need medical attention. There is also a contention that using symptoms to make a diagnosis of schizophrenia is like using unstable scaffolding to paint a house.

The diagnostic approach to schizophrenia has also been contested in general by those against the movement to recognize and treat psychiatric symtoms and disorders under the health care umbrella. They argue that by categorizing specific thoughts and behaviors as an illness, social control of persons society finds objectionable is permitted. They feel that categorizing certain thoughts and behaviors as a medical problem, rather than a social issue, is discriminatory.

CLINICAL REASONING

- The *DSM-IV-TR* is considered by many to be the definitive work on psychiatric diagnoses. Given the controversy just described, what factors would you consider before refilling a prescription for an antipsychotic drug for patient who was diagnosed by another health care provider?
- How would you respond to a colleague who agrees with the perspective of the antipsychiatry movement that classifying specific thoughts and behaviors as an illness allows for social control of persons?

Extracted from Tsuang, M., Stone, W., and Faraone, S. (2000). Toward reformulating the diagnosis of schizophrenia. *American Journal of Psychiatry, 157*(7), 1041–1050; and Bentall, R. (2004). *Madness explained: Psychosis and human nature.* New York: Penguin Global.

KEY POINTS

■ Schizophrenia affects perception, thought content and process, affect, and day-to-day functioning. The behavioral manifestations can be grouped into positive, negative, and cognitive symptoms.

■ The exact etiology of schizophrenia is unknown, but it is thought to be related to biologic alterations in dopamine transmission and anatomic differences in the brain.

■ Antipsychotic drugs help in managing symptoms of psychosis, including thought disorders, hallucinations, bizarre behaviors and agitation, and hyperactivity.

■ First-generation antipsychotic drugs block dopamine receptors in post-synaptic nerve tissues and in the CTZ of the medulla.

■ Second-generation drugs act at one or more dopamine sites at the cortical and limbic regions of the brain, with less effect in the nigrostriatal region.

■ First- and second-generation drugs have different adverse effects profiles. Those of second-generation antipsychotics are related to hyperglycemia and the development of type 2 diabetes mellitus, hyperlipidemia, NMS, and risk of stroke.

■ There are many drug interactions with antipsychotics. Be sure to check for interactions before prescribing.

■ The primary treatment objectives for the patient with schizophrenia are to diminish psychotic behaviors, thus preventing harm to the patient or others, improving thought disorders, reducing duration of inpatient hospitalization, and preventing or decreasing future exacerbations.

■ Maintenance drug therapy is valuable in preventing psychotic relapse, recurrence, and rehospitalization.

■ Therapeutic dosages should be maintained for at least 4 to 6 weeks, and the patient's response should be evaluated before use of a different drug is considered.

■ Dosage is individualized based on patient response and tolerance to adverse effects. No evidence suggests that higher doses of antipsychotic drugs are likely to improve psychosis more quickly; in fact, high doses of antipsychotics increase the risk of adverse effects and should be avoided.

■ The intermittent targeted treatment strategy reduces total drug exposure by administering the drug only when there are active symptoms. Continuous minimal dosing helps prevent relapse by providing continuous coverage at a much lower dosage than during acute episodes.

■ Patient teaching includes information about illness, drug actions, interactions, anticipated therapeutic effects, adverse effects, and administration regimen.

■ The effectiveness of antipsychotic therapy is demonstrated by a decrease in the severity of psychosis and diminished symptoms.

Bibliography

American Psychiatric Association. (1995). Practice guideline for psychiatric evaluation of adults. *American Journal of Psychiatry, 152* (11 Suppl), 63–80.

American Psychiatric Association. (2000). *Diagnostic and statistical manual of mental disorders.* (4th ed., Text Revision [DSM-IV-TR]). Washington, DC: Author.

Rosenbaum, J., Arana, G., Hyman, S., et al. (2005). *Handbook of psychiatric drug therapy.* Philadelphia: Lippincott, Williams, & Wilkins.

Bentall, R. (2004). *Madness explained: Psychosis and human nature.* New York: Penguin Global.

Brier, A. (1995). Serotonin, schizophrenia and antipsychotic drug action. *Schizophrenia Research, 14*(3), 187–202.

Chandron, G., Mikler, J., and Keegan, D. (2003). Neuroleptic malignant syndrome: Case report and discussion. *Journal of the Canadian Medical Association, 169*(5), 439–442.

Ereshefsky, L. (1999). Pharmacologic and pharmacokinetic considerations in choosing an antipsychotic. *Journal of Clinical Psychiatry, 60* (Suppl 10), 20–30.

Erhart, S., Marder, S., and Carpenter, W. (2006). Treatment of schizophrenia negative symptoms: Future prospects. *Schizophrenia Bulletin, 32*(2), 234–237.

Freedman, R. (2005). The choice of antipsychotic drugs for schizophrenia. *New England Journal of Medicine, 353*(10), 1286–1288. (Editorial.)

Garhol, J. (2006). Schizophrenia. PsychCentral. Available online: www.psychcentral.com/psypsych/Schizophrenia. Accessed June 27, 2007.

Harvey, P., Koren, D., Reichenberg, A., et al. (2006). Negative symptoms and cognitive deficits: What is the nature of their relationship? *Schizophrenia Bulletin, 32*(2), 250–258.

Keltner, N., and Folks, D. (2005). *Psychotropic drugs.* (4th ed.). St. Louis: Mosby–Year Book.

Laughren, T., and Levin, R. (2006). Food and Drug Administration perspective on negative symptoms in schizophrenia as a target for a drug treatment claim. *Schizophrenia Bulletin, 32*(2), 220–222.

Lieberman, J. (2007). Effectiveness of antipsychotic drugs in patients with chronic schizophrenia: Efficacy, safety and cost outcomes of CATIE and other trials. *Journal of Clinical Psychiatry, 68*(2), e04.

Miller, D., McEvoy, J., Davis, S., et al. (2005). Clinical correlates of tardive dyskinesia in schizophrenia: Baseline data from the CATIE schizophrenia trial. *Schizophrenia Research, 80*(1), 33–43.

Motsinger, C., Perron, G., and Lacy, T. (2003). Use of atypical antipsychotic drugs in patients with dementia. *American Family Physician, 67*(11). Available online: www.aafp.org/afp/20030601/2335.html. Accessed June 27, 2007.

National Center for Policy Analysis. (2006). Antipsychotic Rx: Doctors prescribe more to children. March 21. Available online: www.ncpa.org. Accessed June 27, 2007.

National Guideline Clearing House. (2004). *Practice guideline for the treatment of patients with schizophrenia.* (2nd ed.). Arlington, VA: American Psychiatric Association. Available online: www.guideline.gov/. Accessed June 27, 2007.

National Guideline Clearing House. (2001). Practice guideline for the treatment of patients with borderline personality disorder. American Psychiatric Association. *American Journal of Psychiatry, 158*(10 Suppl), 1–52.

National Institutes of Mental Health. (2005). Schizophrenia. Available online: www.nlm.nih.gov/medlineplus/schizophrenia.html. Accessed June 27, 2007.

National Institutes of Mental Health. (2003). Childhood-onset schizophrenia: An update from the National Institute of Mental Health. Available online: www.nimh.nih.gov/publicat/schizkids.cfm. Accessed June 27, 2007.

PsychopharmInfo. Available online: www.psychopharminfo.com/. Accessed June 27, 2007.

Rosenheck, R. (2006). Outcomes, costs, and policy caution: A commentary on the Cost Utility of the Latest Antipsychotic Drugs in

Schizophrenia Study (CUtLASS 1). *Archives in General Psychiatry, 63*(10), 1074–1076.

Seaman, M. (2004). Gender differences in the prescribing of antipsychotic drugs. *American Journal of Psychiatry, 161*(8), 1324–1333.

Tsuang, M., Stone, W., and Faraone, S. (2000). Toward reformulating the diagnosis of schizophrenia. *American Journal of Psychiatry, 157*(7), 1041–1050.

Verdoux, H., and van Os, J. (2002). Psychotic symptoms in non-clinical populations and the continuum of psychosis. *Schizophrenia Research, 54*(1-2), 59–65.

Wahlbeck, K., Cheine, M., Essali, A., et al. (1999). Evidence of clozapine's effectiveness in schizophrenia: A systematic review and meta-analysis of randomized trials. *American Journal of Psychiatry, 156*(7), 990–999.

Central Nervous System Stimulants

22

Central nervous system (CNS) stimulants increase excitability in different regions of the brain, inducing arousal and increasing motor function, and resulting in increased alertness, decreased fatigue, and decreased appetite.

CNS stimulants are classified based on their major effects. Psychomotor stimulants (e.g., amphetamines) primarily stimulate the cerebral cortex. Anorexiants suppress the appetite center and are used to treat exogenous obesity. The term anorexiant is composed of the Greek *an,* meaning "not, without," and *orexis,* meaning "appetite;" and *analeptikos,* meaning "restorative, strengthening." The analeptics (e.g., caffeine) affect centers in the medulla and brainstem and are used in the treatment of severe respiratory depression.

NARCOLEPSY

EPIDEMIOLOGY AND ETIOLOGY

Narcolepsy is a chronic neurologic disorder caused by a disturbance of the rapid eye movement (REM) sleep cycle. Patterns of REM sleep disturbances are particular to an individual; they begin subtly and sometimes change drastically as time progresses. Typically, REM sleep occurs approximately 45 minutes to 1 hour after the onset of sleep, but patients with narcolepsy experience REM almost immediately. It is estimated that narcolepsy affects one in every 2000 Americans, or more than 135,000 individuals. Narcolepsy is the third most common primary sleep disorder diagnosed, preceded in prevalence by obstructive sleep apnea and periodic limb movement disorder. Although narcolepsy is found in familial clusters, evidence suggests that the disorder occurs independently in individuals and thus is not inherited. Narcolepsy commonly begins in adolescence or young adulthood but can first manifest itself as early as the age of 2 years or as late as middle age. Men and women are equally affected.

Factors associated with the development of narcolepsy include disease, tumor growth, and trauma to parts of the brain involved in REM sleep. Alterations in the patient's diet and sleep schedule, toxin exposure, infections, stress, and hormonal changes produce direct or indirect effects on the brain, thus contributing to narcolepsy.

PATHOPHYSIOLOGY

The cause of narcolepsy remains unknown, although progress is being made to better understand its pathogenesis and identify the genes associated with the disorder. There has been research linking narcolepsy with multiple alleles (i.e., variant human lymphocyte antigen [HLA] complexes) found near chromosome 6. The HLA complex comprises a number of genes that regulate parts of the immune system.

ATTENTION DEFICIT HYPERACTIVITY DISORDER

Attention deficit hyperactivity disorder (ADHD) is one of several problems that include attention deficit disorder without hyperactivity, minimal brain dysfunction, and hyperkinesias. Diagnosis depends on patient symptoms. This section discusses ADHD because it is representative of the others.

EPIDEMIOLOGY AND ETIOLOGY

ADHD is characterized by an inability to concentrate and sustain attention and control impulsive behaviors. Symptoms must be present for 6 months before a diagnosis can be made. It is estimated that 4.4 million youth ages 4 to 17 years have been diagnosed with ADHD by a health care provider, and 2.5 million youth in that age range are receiving drug therapy for the disorder. Studies have shown that male sex, low socioeconomic status, and young age are associated with the prevalence of ADHD. The male-to-female ratio for the disorder is greater in clinical studies than in community studies, which suggests that females with ADHD are less likely to be referred for services than males (see Case Study).

ADHD is the single most common chronic psychiatric disorder in children who seek treatment from primary care providers and mental health professionals. Because other disorders (e.g., anxiety, learning disorders, depression) may cause similar symptoms, a diagnosis of ADHD must be made with care. There are three types of ADHD: combined inattentive, hyperactive, and impulsive (80% of patients); predominantly inattentive (10% to 15%); and predominantly hyperactive and impulsive (5%).

Although ADHD was initially seen as a disorder of childhood, a growing number of affected adults are being identified. Health care providers do not routinely screen for ADHD in adults, and therefore the disorder is underrecognized, underdiagnosed, and undertreated. The longitudinal course of ADHD and its prevalence in adulthood is controversial, but research supports the persistence of this condition into adulthood. Data suggest that 70% of children with ADHD continue to manifest symptoms in adulthood. Genetic studies have shown a 92% concordance in monozygotic twins and a 33% concordance in dizygotic twins. First-degree relatives are at greatest risk for ADHD.

Although there is no known etiology of ADHD, it is likely heterogeneous. A substantial body of research implicates a range of neurobiologic factors, including genetics. Much research has focused on the neuropsychologic and neurobiologic substrates. Early theories emphasized abnormal patterns of arousal or of sustained attention. Subsequent studies shifted the focus to an impairment of abilities involved in forward planning or to difficulties with response inhibition. Difficulties in these domains are consistent with

CASE STUDY   Central Nervous System Stimulants

ASSESSMENT

History of Present Illness	CB is a 15-year-old adolescent boy with difficulty concentrating, short attention span, irritability, and hyperactivity. His parents report that he has been in good health since his last checkup. CB has an inability to follow parent and teacher directives, distractibility, poor social skills, poor academic performance, and low frustration tolerance. His parents confide that he has a difficult time playing on the playground and with friends because he does not follow the rules. His teacher indicates that CB tends to be disruptive in class and frequently gets into arguments. CB's teacher suggested that he be evaluated by a health care provider for possible ADHD.
Past Health History	CB has no known allergies. He had the typical childhood illnesses, but no major health problems. There is a history of risky behaviors that have resulted in injuries. At age 6, CB climbed a large tree in the yard and fell, resulting in a dislocated shoulder. He has had "near misses" when crossing roads without looking both ways for traffic, and rides his bicycle forgetting to wear his helmet. His parents report that his impulsiveness seems to be progressing, and they are afraid injury will result.
Life-Span Considerations	CB's lack of self-control negatively affects social skills and interactions with peers. Despite CB's poor academic performance, his teachers agree with his parents that he is an intelligent child. CB is an only child. His parents have tried to compensate for his lack of friends, but when CB is seen hanging around his parents, other children are quick to tease him and label him a "loser" or a "mommy's boy."
Psychosocial Considerations	Inability to control behavior makes CB unpredictable; his few friends have been in trouble with the law several times for drug violations. CB's father is a technical advisor in a large information systems company, and CB's mother works part-time as a customer service representative at a nearby retailer. The family has conveyed that they have both the means and desire to provide CB with the necessary help and support to manage this problem.
Physical Exam Findings	*Weight:* 125 lb. *Height:* 5′6″. *BP:* 100/70. PE findings are within normal limits.
Diagnostic Testing	CB performed several psychologic tests, including testing his ability to focus his attention and perform motor tasks. Hematologic and chemistry testing were normal.

DIAGNOSIS: Attention deficit hyperactivity disorder

MANAGEMENT

Treatment Objectives	1. Control impulsive behaviors; minimize risk of injury 2. Increase ability to attend and focus 3. Improve academic and social skills
Treatment Plan	**Pharmacotherapy** • Initial titration with immediate-release methylphenidate, 5 mg PO twice daily for 1 week. • methylphenidate ER (Methylin ER), 10 mg PO each morning beginning week 2 of treatment

CRITICAL REASONING ANALYSIS

Q1. I see you decided to use methylphenidate ER rather than using a transdermal formulation of amphetamine or dextroamphetamine. What factors did you consider in choosing the drug?

A. Methylphenidate reduces the overactivity, impulsivities, and inattentiveness of ADHD patients and improves academic performance, social functioning, and occurrence of on-task behavior. Methylphenidate is the most commonly used, although the amphetamines are equally as effective. The few studies to date comparing methylphenidate with amphetamines in ADHD found that methylphenidate ER is as effective as amphetamines for children in a classroom setting with continued benefit into the evening home environment. This response suggests minimal rebound, and it is generally preferred by parents, counselors, and teachers over amphetamines. Neither drug should be used for "problem children" who do not meet the diagnostic criteria for ADHD.

Continued

CASE STUDY Central Nervous System Stimulants—Cont'd

Q2. I know some of CB's peer group have been "snorting" their short-acting methylphenidate. Would it be helpful to use the long-acting form of methylphenidate instead?

A. Perhaps. Once-daily dosing is all that is needed for the long-acting formulation, which makes it more convenient and also provides less access to the drug during or after school hours. The long-acting formulation of methylphenidate is less likely to produce a "high" if it was snorted than the shorter-acting formulations.

Q3. What if methylphenidate ER does not help control his symptoms?

A. Stimulants work in slightly different ways, so one may work better than another. If CB does not improve with one psychomotor stimulant, another can be tried. We can titrate the dose upward if CB shows minimal improvement clinically. The goal is to find a drug that gives CB the maximum response with the minimum dosage.

---

neuroimaging research, which suggests structural and functional abnormalities in the prefrontal structures and basal ganglia regions. Abnormalities in these regions of the CNS are the foundation for motor response inhibition and executive functions.

PATHOPHYSIOLOGY

The pattern of neuropsychologic deficit in patients with ADHD is thought to be related to dysregulation of frontal-subcortical circuits. The frontal-subcortical circuits control executive functions such as inhibition, working memory, set-shifting, interference control, planning, and sustained attention. Structural and functional neuroimaging studies show that patients with ADHD have a small reduction in volume in these regions. However, other studies suggest that aberrant frontal-subcortical circuitry is not sufficient to explain the pathophysiology of the disorder.

Neurologic research focusing on dopamine brain-imaging seems to implicate the dopamine and norepinephrine neurotransmitter system in frontostriatal circuitry. Studies also indicate that neurochemical etiologies are a plausible cause of the disorder, in that many patients with ADHD respond to drugs that affect the dopamine and norepinephrine neurotransmitter system in frontostriatal circuitry.

EXOGENOUS OBESITY

EPIDEMIOLOGY AND ETIOLOGY

Recent data indicate that 34% of American women and 28.1% of American men are obese. Obesity is defined as a body mass index (BMI) of 30 or above. The BMI is the ratio of the weight in kilograms to height in square meters. The normal range for both men and women is a BMI of 18.5 to 24.9. An individual with a BMI of 25 to 29.9 is overweight. The desirable percentage of fat to lean body mass in men is 9% to 18% of total body weight, and the ideal for women is between 18% and 28%.

Obesity is a refractory problem in the United States. Before the U.S. industrial revolution, obesity was rare. In more recent times, however, obesity has been recognized as a national health problem and is especially prevalent among the poor and the lower economic classes. Data from the National Center for Health Statistics show that 30% of U.S. adults aged 20 years and older—that is, over 60 million people—are obese;

however, this problem is not isolated to adults. The percentage of young people who are overweight has dramatically increased since 1980. Among children and teenagers aged between 6 and 19 years, 16% (over 9 million young people) are considered overweight. African-American women are twice as likely to be obese as Caucasian women.

PATHOPHYSIOLOGY

Obesity is classified as either exogenous or endogenous. Exogenous obesity is defined as an imbalance between caloric intake and caloric needs. Endogenous obesity is secondary to another physical problem such as diabetes or an endocrine disorder. The underlying problem in endogenous obesity must be treated before the problem of obesity can be resolved. Obesity is associated with several different conditions including diabetes, cardiovascular disease, hypertension, hyperlipidemia, back problems, and strokes.

Studies suggest that the resting metabolic rate of people who are obese may be slower from the beginning. Other studies suggest that children who are obese have an increased number of fat cells (hyperplasia), not just larger fat cells (hypertrophy). Thus adults who were obese as children have up to 3 times as many fat cells as those who were of normal weight as children, which may have made it easier for those children to develop obesity as adults. Persons who become obese later in life do not have an increased number of fat cells; rather, their fat cells become much larger.

PHARMACOTHERAPEUTIC OPTIONS

Psychomotor Stimulants

◆ amphetamine, dextroamphetamine (Adderall); ♣ Adderall
◆ benzphetamine (Didrex)
◆ dexmethylphenidate (Focalin)
◆ dextroamphetamine (Dexedrine, Dextrostat)
◆ methamphetamine (Desoxyn)
◆ methylphenidate (Concerta, Metadate, Methylin, Ritalin)
◆ modafinil (Provigil); ♣ Alertec

Indications

Patients who are potential candidates for psychomotor stimulants are those with narcolepsy or excessive daytime sleepiness (EDS) and intermittent manifestations of REM sleep at times when a person would normally be awake. Patients with REM manifestations that include cataplexy, sleep paralysis, and hypnagogic hallucinations are also candidates for psychomotor stimulants. However, psychomotor stimulants, specifically, and CNS stimulants, in general, should not be used to combat fatigue or delay sleep. Amphetamine and methylphenidate are the first-line drugs in the management of ADHD. These drugs aid in the management of maladaptive behavior, increase cognition, and have the potential for memory enhancement.

Pharmacodynamics

Amphetamines produce CNS-stimulant activities in addition to the peripheral alpha and beta actions common with indirect-acting adrenergic drugs. The powerful stimulating action of amphetamines is related to the release of amines from storage sites in nerve terminals. The stimulant, anorectic effect of amphetamines and a portion of the locomotor-stimulating actions are mediated by the release of norepinephrine. The anorectic action of amphetamines is likely centered in the lateral hypothalamic feeding center. However, tolerance to the effects of appetite suppression rapidly develops. Some aspects of locomotor activity and stereotypic behaviors induced by amphetamines are probably related to the release of dopamine from dopaminergic nerve terminals. Disturbances in perception and overt psychotic behavior result with high doses of amphetamines. These effects are due to the release of serotonin (5-hydroxytryptamine; 5-HT) from tryptaminergic neurons and of dopamine from the mesolimbic system.

Pharmacokinetics

Psychomotor stimulants are rapidly absorbed after oral administration. The time to onset of drug action averages 1 to 2 hours, with a duration of action of 4 to 10 hours (Table 22-1). Biotransformation is by the liver. The plasma half-life varies from 7 to 34 hours depending on urinary pH. Alkaline urine (as with consumption of cranberry juice) promotes reabsorption and prolongs drug action. The more acidic the urine, the faster the rate of drug elimination. Amphetamines cross the placental membranes and enter breast milk.

Adverse Effects and Contraindications

As a drug class, psychomotor stimulants cause CNS excitation; hence their adverse effects are numerous. Tachycardia, irritability, nocturnal sleep disturbances, tremor, restlessness, psychosis, seizures, arrhythmias, anorexia, drug tolerance, and dependency are all associated with stimulants. They have a high potential for tolerance and abuse (Chapter 12), particularly with prolonged therapy. Periodically interrupt therapy and reevaluate the patient's condition to determine if continued use of the drug is needed.

The adverse gastrointestinal (GI) effects of amphetamines are unpredictable but include dry mouth, a metallic taste, anorexia, nausea, vomiting, diarrhea, and abdominal cramps. If enteric activity is pronounced, amphetamines may cause relaxation and delay transit of intestinal contents. If the gut is already relaxed, the opposite effect may be seen.

Psychomotor stimulants are contraindicated for use in patients with cardiovascular disease (e.g., hypertension, angina, arrhythmias) or hyperthyroidism. They are also contraindicated for use in patients who are anxious or agitated and in patients who have asthenia, psychopathic personalities, or a history of homicidal or suicidal tendencies. Do not give psychomotor stimulants to patients with glaucoma. Amphetamines in general have teratogenic effects; avoid their use during pregnancy. Uterine response varies, but usually there is an increase in uterine muscle tone.

PHARMACOKINETICS

TABLE 22-1 Selected CNS Stimulants

Drug	Route	Onset	Peak	Duration	PB (%)	$t_{1/2}$
PSYCHOMOTOR STIMULANTS						
amphetamine, dextroamphetamine	PO	1–2 hr	3 hr	4–10 hr	UA	7–34 hr*
benzphetamine	PO	Rapid	UA	4 hr	UA	6–12 hr
dexmethylphenidate	PO	Rapid	1–2 hr	3.5–5.5 hr	UA	2 hr
dextroamphetamine	PO	1–2 hr	2 hr	2–10 hr	UA	10 hr; 6.8†
methylphenidate	PO	Rapid	1–3 hr	4–6 hr; 8 hr+	UA	1–3 hr
methamphetamine	PO	1–2 hr	4–6 hr	2–10 hr	UA	10 hr; 7 hr‡
modafinil	PO	Rapid	2–4 hr	UA	UA	15 hr§
ANOREXIANTS						
diethylpropion	PO	Rapid	UA	4 hr	UA	4–6 hr
phendimetrazine	PO	Rapid	4–6 hr	4 hr	UA	2–10 hr
phentermine	PO	UA	UA	4 hr	UA	UA
sibutramine	PO	Rapid	3–4 hr	12.5–22 hr	UA	14–16 hr
ANALEPTICS						
caffeine	PO	15 min	15–45 min	UA	UA	3–4 hr
doxapram	IV	20–40 sec	1–2 min	5–12 min	UA	2–4 hr

*Depends on the acidity of the urine. If pH is less than 5.6, the half-life is 7 to 8 hr. Alkalinization of the urine increases the half-life, with a range between 18.6 and 33.6 hr. Every unit increase in urinary pH increases the plasma half-life by an average of 7 hr.
†Dextroamphetamine and methamphetamine: half-life in children is 6.8 hr.
‡Methylphenidate: duration of action is 8 hr with extended-release formulations.
§Modafinil: 15 hr after multiple doses.
IV, Intravenous; *PB*, protein binding; *PO*, by mouth; *UA*, unavailable; $t_{1/2}$, half-life.

Psychomotor stimulants are not recommended for treatment of ADHD in children under the age of 6 years, or as anorexiants in children less than 12 years old. When used, dose carefully, and closely monitor the child. The effects of long-term use are unknown, although suppression of height and weight has been reported as a result of appetite suppression. Psychomotor stimulants may exacerbate symptoms in children with psychosis or Tourette's syndrome.

Exercise caution when using psychomotor stimulants in the older adult. As with most other drugs, the slowed biotransformation and elimination associated with aging increase the risk of accumulation and toxicity. Older adults are likely to experience anxiety, nervousness, insomnia, and mental confusion from excessive CNS stimulation. Although studies indicate that CNS stimulants reduce fatigue in patient populations receiving advanced and palliative care, there still are no evidence-based guidelines for dosing.

Drug Interactions

Psychomotor stimulants change insulin requirements, and therefore caution is required when these drugs are used in patients who have diabetes (Table 22-2). Amphetamines decrease the effects of antihypertensives and should not be used in combination with monoamine oxidase (MAO) inhibitors. Death results from hypertensive crisis or cerebral hemorrhage.

Dosage Regimen

Dosages of psychomotor stimulants are tailored to patient needs and symptoms (Table 22-3). Many of the psychomotor stimulants are available as extended-release or resin complex formulations, so the patient need take only one dose per day. Although these formulations are convenient, do not use them in the initial or subsequent titrations of the drug. The extended-release or resin-complex formulations are used only when the titration-determined daily dose is equal to, or exceeds, the dose of the extended-release formulation.

Lab Considerations

No specific lab monitoring is required of patients taking psychomotor stimulants. Serum drug levels are seldom measured. Obtain a complete blood count before the start of therapy. Leukopenia and anemia have been seen with methylphenidate. Check urine catecholamines before and during methylphenidate therapy to reveal any increased dopamine levels.

Anorexiants
- diethylpropion (Tenuate)
- phendimetrazine (Bontril)
- phentermine (Adipex-P, Inoamin)
- sibutramine (Meredia)

Indications

All anorexiants are used in the short-term management of obesity. Ordinarily, pharmacotherapy for obesity is only effective when combined with behavioral modifications. They are intended as adjuncts to other therapies, such as behavior modification, exercise, and calorie restrictions. Anorexiant use should not exceed 6 to 12 weeks; however, sibutramine may be prescribed up to 2 years. Tolerance to the anorectic effect usually occurs within that time.

Pharmacodynamics

Anorexiants are compounds similar to amphetamines. Their mechanism of action leading to appetite suppression is unknown, but they may stimulate the satiety center in the hypothalamus. It is also thought that they act in the CNS to cause release of catecholamines from nerve terminals.

Pharmacokinetics

Anorexiants are rapidly absorbed when taken orally. Table 22-1 summarizes the pharmacokinetics of selected anorexiants. Although there are wide individual variations, metabolites are excreted in the urine within 2 hours of administration. Acidic urine increases the elimination; alkaline urine decreases the rate of elimination.

Adverse Effects and Contraindications

Because of CNS-stimulant actions, the most frequently reported adverse effects of anorexiants include palpitations, tachycardia, restlessness, dizziness, insomnia, weakness, fatigue, and drowsiness. Less frequently reported effects include depression, confusion, allergic skin rashes, and psychosis. Arrhythmias, dyspnea, pulmonary hypertension, hypertension, malaise, euphoria, vomiting, diarrhea, rash, and menstrual irregularities are less common. Centrally-acting weight loss drugs have a contributory relationship with cardiac dysfunction including valvular heart disease.

Drug Interactions

As with the amphetamines, there are many drug interactions with anorexiants. Table 22-2 provides an overview of selected drug interactions. Do not administer anorexiants to patients who have been on MAO inhibitors within the previous 14 days. The beneficial effects of antihypertensives can be blocked by anorexiant drugs.

Dosage Regimen

Dosages of anorexiant drugs are individualized based on the drug prescribed (see Table 22-3). Anorexiants are for short-term use and only as an adjunct to other weight loss therapies. When tolerance develops, the drug is discontinued. Do not increase the dosage to achieve the same therapeutic effect.

Lab Considerations

Urine and serum drug levels of CNS stimulants and anorexiants are only marginally helpful because of the wide individual variations in individual therapeutic responses. The health care provider's observations of the patient, the patient's weight, and patient self-reports are the most useful means for evaluating drug efficacy and treatment success.

Analeptics
- caffeine (Caffedrine, NoDoz, Quick Pep, Vivarin, Pep-Back)
- doxapram (Dopram)

Indications

Although caffeine is not ordinarily used in the management of medical disorders, it does stimulate the cerebral cortex to increase alertness and decrease fatigue. It is used by many persons as an aid to stay awake. Caffeine has been used

DRUG INTERACTIONS

TABLE 22-2 Selected CNS Stimulants

Drug	Interacting Drug	Interaction
PSYCHOMOTOR STIMULANTS		
amphetamine, dextroamphetamine, methamphetamine	Urinary acidifiers (ammonium chloride, ascorbic acid, potassium or sodium phosphates)	Decreases serum concentrations, resulting in lower efficacy of amphetamines
	Urinary alkalizers (antacids, sodium bicarbonate)	Increases serum concentrations, potentiating the actions of amphetamines
	TCAs	Enhances the activity of tricyclic or sympathomimetic drugs; effects of cardiovascular effects are potentiated
	MAO inhibitors	Increases SNS effects, resulting in headaches and other signs of hypertensive crisis (fatal)
	Antihistamines	Counteracts sedative effects of antihistamines
	Antihypertensives	Antagonizes blood pressure–lowering effects of antihypertensives
	haloperidol	Inhibits CNS effects
	Insulin	Changes insulin requirements
	lithium carbonate	Inhibits anorectic and stimulatory effects
	meperidine	Potentiates analgesic effects of meperidine
	phenytoin	Synergistic anticonvulsant action
methylphenidate	Anticonvulsants (phenobarbital, phenytoin, primidone)	Inhibits the biotransformation of anticonvulsants
	Coumarin anticoagulants	Inhibits the biotransformation of coumarin anticoagulants
	MAO inhibitors	Results in hypertensive crisis
	Vasopressor drugs	Increases pressor effects
	SSRIs	Inhibits the biotransformation of SSRIs
	TCAs	Inhibits the biotransformation of TCAs
modafinil	clomipramine	Potentially increases levels of clomipramine with patients with narcolepsy
	cyclosporine	Dosage adjustment for cyclosporine may be needed
	dextroamphetamine, methylphenidate	Delays absorption by 1 hour
	triazolam	Elimination half-life of triazolam decreases by approximately 1 hour
	warfarin	Caution advised: monitor INR levels
sibutramine	MAO inhibitors	In combination with serotonergic drugs, serious, fatal reactions may occur.
ANOREXIANTS		
diethylpropion	Insulin	Reduces insulin requirements
	MAO inhibitors	Results in hypertensive crisis
	Phenothiazines	Concurrent use antagonizes anorectic effects of diethylpropion
phendimetrazine, phentermine	Urinary acidifiers (ammonium chloride, ascorbic acid, potassium or sodium phosphates)	Decreases serum concentrations, resulting in less appetite suppression
	Alcohol	Increases CNS effects such as dizziness, fainting, confusion
	Urinary alkalizers (antacids, sodium bicarbonate)	Increases serum concentrations, potentiating the actions of appetite suppressant
	TCAs	Hypertension, cardiac arrhythmias
	Antihypertensives	Hypotensive effects may be decreased
	Appetite suppressants	Increases prevalence of abnormal cardiac valve function
	CNS stimulants	Increases CNS effects
	halothane	Produces arrhythmias
	Insulin	Reduces insulin requirements
	MAO inhibitors	Potentiates SNS effects of appetite suppressants (hypertensive crisis)
	Phenothiazines	Antagonizes anorectic effects of the appetite suppressant
	SSRIs	Increases prevalence of cardiac valve dysfunction
	Thyroid hormones	Increases CNS effects
	Vasopressors	Potentiates vasopressant effects
ANALEPTICS		
doxapram	CNS stimulants	Additive CNS stimulation
	SNS drugs, MAO inhibitors	Increases pressor effects
caffeine	ciprofloxacin, cimetidine, oral contraceptives, disulfiram	Increases caffeine concentrations and may enhance adverse effects
	Smoking	Decreases effects of caffeine
	aspirin, phenobarbital	Increases biotransformation of interacting drugs

CNS, Central nervous system; *INR,* international normalized ratio; *MAO,* monoamine oxidase; *SNS,* sympathetic nervous system; *SSRI,* selective serotonin reuptake inhibitor; *TCA,* tricyclic antidepressant.

as an adjunct to analgesic formulations; it also may be used in conjunction with supportive measures to treat respiratory depression related to CNS-depressant overdose.

Doxapram is used occasionally to stimulate respirations and to hasten arousal in patients experiencing apnea or drug-induced CNS depression (i.e., postanesthesia).

▥ *Pharmacodynamics*

Caffeine increases the calcium permeability in sarcoplasmic reticulum, promotes the accumulation of cyclic adenosine monophosphate (AMP), and blocks adenosine receptors. It stimulates the CNS, cardiac activity, secretion of gastric acid, and diuresis.

DOSAGE
TABLE 22-3 Selected Central Nervous System Stimulants

Drug	Use(s)	Dosage	Implications
PSYCHOMOTOR STIMULANTS			
amphetamine, dextroamphetamine	Narcolepsy	*Adult:* 10–60 mg PO daily in single or 2 divided doses. Maximum: 60 mg daily *Child 6–12 yr:* 5 mg PO daily. Increase by 5 mg weekly based on response. *Child ≥ 12 yr:* 10 mg PO daily. Increase by 10 mg weekly based on response.	Give initial dose on awakening. Give divided doses at 4- to 6-hr intervals. Reduce dosage, if ADRs are intolerable. Give last daily dose early enough not to interfere with night's sleep. Monitor blood pressure.
	ADHD	*Adult:* 5–60 mg PO daily in divided doses *Child >6 yr:* 5 mg PO 1–2 times daily. Increase by 5 mg weekly based on response. *Child 3–5 yr:* 2.5 mg PO daily. Increase by 2.5 mg weekly based on response.	Initial dose should be taken on awakening. Give divided doses at 4- to 6-hr intervals.
benzphetamine	Exogenous obesity	*Adult:* 25–50 mg PO daily midmorning or midafternoon. Max: 50 mg 3 times daily	Avoid late-afternoon administration. Safety and efficacy have not been established for children <12 yr.
methamphetamine	Exogenous obesity	*Adult:* 5 mg PO 2–3 times daily before meals	Adjust dose individually; use smallest possible dose to achieve desired effect. Do not use to combat exhaustion or fatigue.
	ADHD	*Child >6 yr:* 5 mg PO 1–2 times daily. Increase by 5 mg weekly based on response. Maintenance: 20–25 mg PO daily	Do not use as substitute for sleep or as anorexiant in children <12 yr. Reevaluate need for drug on regular basis.
	Narcolepsy	*Adult:* 10 mg PO 2–3 times daily before meals. Max: 60 mg daily	Do not use for normal fatigue states.
modafinil	Narcolepsy	*Adult:* 200 mg PO daily	Not recommended for children <16 yr of age.
ANOREXIANTS			
diethylpropion	Exogenous obesity	*Adult:* 25 mg PO 3 times daily. May give additional 25 mg in midevening if needed.	Use with calorie restriction. Prolonged therapy and use in children is contraindicated.
phendimetrazine	Exogenous obesity	*Adult:* 35 mg PO 2–3 times daily. Max: 70 mg 3 times daily	Use with calorie restriction. Prolonged therapy and use in children is contraindicated.
phentermine	Exogenous obesity	*Adult:* 8 mg PO 3 times daily or 15–37.5 mg 1 hr before breakfast	Take split doses 1 hr before meals. Not for children <12 yr.
sibutramine	Exogenous obesity	*Adult:* 10 mg PO once daily; titrate to 15 mg after 4 wk if needed.	Safety and efficacy in children <16 yr have not been established.
ANALEPTICS			
caffeine	Aid in staying awake, adjunct to analgesics, respiratory effects of CNS depression	*Adult:* 100–200 mg PO every 3–4 hr PRN. ER formulation: 200 mg PO every 3–4 hr. *Respiratory depression:* 500–1000 mg IM. Do not exceed 2.5 g/day.	May be given by IV route in severe emergent situation. Safety and efficacy in children have not been established.
doxapram	Drug-induced CNS depression	*Adult:* 0.5–1 mg/kg IV repeated at 5-min intervals. Repeat every 1–2 hr until patient awakens. Initiate infusion at 5 mg/min. Once response is seen, 1–3 mg/min is satisfactory.	If no response, continue supportive measures and repeat priming dose in 1–2 hr.

ADRs, Adverse drug reaction; *CNS,* central nervous system; *ER,* extended-release; *IM,* intramuscular (route); *IV,* intravenous; *PO,* by mouth; *PRN,* as needed.

CENTRAL NERVOUS

Doxapram excites peripheral carotid chemoreceptors to cause an increase in tidal volume and a slight increase in respiratory rate. This stimulation also results in pressor effects.

Pharmacokinetics
Caffeine is biotransformed in the liver and excreted in the urine (see Table 22-1). It crosses the placental membranes and passes into breast milk.

Doxapram is given by intravenous (IV) route, with the onset of drug action in 20 to 40 seconds and peak effects noted in 1 to 2 minutes. Its duration of action is 5 to 12 minutes. It is biotransformed in the liver and excreted in the urine. The half-life of doxapram is approximately 2 to 4 hours.

Adverse Effects and Contraindications
The adverse CNS effects of caffeine most often include insomnia, restlessness, excitement, tachycardia, and diuresis.

Headaches, light-headedness, nausea, vomiting, diarrhea, and abdominal pain also have been reported. Caffeine withdrawal is manifest as anxiety, increased muscle tension, and headache. Caffeine is generally contraindicated for use in patients with a history of depression, duodenal ulcers, and diabetes mellitus, as well as in lactating women.

Adverse effects of doxapram most often include increased reflexes and increased blood pressure. Laryngospasm, bronchospasm, and seizures have been reported and can be life threatening. Other, less common effects include headache, dizziness, disorientation, hyperactivity, diaphoresis, and flushing. Nausea, vomiting, and diarrhea can be troublesome. Use of doxapram is contraindicated in the presence of epilepsy, head injury, cerebrovascular accident, severe hypertension, flail chest, pneumothorax, acute asthma, and pulmonary fibrosis. It is to be used cautiously during pregnancy and lactation.

⫶⫶ Drug Interactions

There are increased CNS effects when caffeine is taken with cimetidine, oral contraceptives, disulfiram, and ciprofloxacin. Caffeine decreases the absorption of iron if it is taken with, or 1 hour after, coffee or tea. The effects of caffeine are also diminished if it is taken while the patient is smoking (see Table 22-2).

Doxapram produces increased effects when it is given to patients who have also received halothane, cyclopropane, or enflurane anesthetics. Delay treatment with doxapram for at least 10 minutes after the anesthetic has been discontinued. The pressor effects of doxapram are increased if the drug is given with MAO inhibitors or adrenergics.

⫶⫶ Dosage Regimen

The likelihood of potentiating CNS activity increases as the dosage of caffeine reaches 250 mg or more (e.g., 2 to 3 cups of coffee). The usual adult intake of caffeine is 100 to 200 mg orally every 3 to 4 hours as needed (see Table 22-3). When using a time-release formulation, 200 mg every 3 to 4 hours is recommended. If caffeine is used to counteract respiratory depression, 500 to 1000 mg of caffeine and sodium benzoate by intramuscular (IM) route is used. It may be given by IV route in a severe emergent situation, but the dosage should not exceed 2.5 grams/day.

Doxapram is given intravenously with a priming dose of 2 mg/kg. The dose may be repeated in 5 minutes, if necessary, and then every 1 to 2 hours until the patient awakens, or if relapse occurs. It also may be given by intermittent IV infusion at a rate of 1 to 3 mg/min.

⫶⫶ Lab Considerations

Caffeine, when used for its pharmacologic effects, may cause falsely elevated readings of serum urate and urine vanillylmandelic acid (VMA), resulting in a false diagnosis of pheochromocytoma or neuroblastoma. There are no known laboratory test interferences with doxapram.

CLINICAL REASONING

Treatment Objectives

The major treatment objective for the patient with narcolepsy is to combat somnolence, to restore a normal sleep-wake cycle when possible, and aid in restoring normal function.

For the patient with ADHD, treatment is directed toward correction of cognitive and behavioral problems. The categories of effective interventions include behavior modification, educational modifications, and stimulant drug therapy. The drugs are appropriately used together as multimodal therapy.

For patients who are overweight or obese, the goal in using an anorexiant is to reduce and stabilize the patient's weight at a more desirable level. Pharmacotherapy for overweight or obese individuals is reasonable only for those who have a BMI of 30 or greater. The BMI may not necessarily be within normal limits, but reduction in weight of even a few pounds significantly lowers the risk of major health problems. Advise patients with a BMI less than 30 to consider self-help and behavioral programs over pharmacotherapy.

Treatment Options

⫶⫶ Patient Variables

Some patients with narcolepsy respond well to nonpharmacologic therapies if their symptoms are not too severe. Others require drug therapy to remain alert throughout the day. Although the psychomotor stimulants are effective for many patients, they are not effective for all (see Controversy box).

The decision to start and continue drug treatment for ADHD is difficult. Not all children who exhibit signs of ADHD should be treated with psychomotor stimulants. The decision regarding drug therapy depends in part on societal expectations and demands. Before beginning drug treatment, carefully evaluate the motivation of parents and teachers in seeking treatment for the child with ADHD. Because drug therapy is intended as an

---

Controversy

Long-Term Safety and Effectiveness of CNS Stimulants

The use of CNS stimulants has become commonplace for treatment of ADHD in children and adolescents. In fact, CNS stimulants are often prescribed for the treatment of adults with ADHD. However, there are few published data directly pertinent to the long-term drug safety and effectiveness of CNS stimulants for adults with ADHD (see also Evidence Based Pharmacotherapeutics). Of the more than 2500 published controlled clinical trials, fewer than 20 focus on persons over the age of 18 years.

Amphetamines entered the market more than 100 years ago as over-the-counter decongestants. Methylphenidate entered the market in 1958 as a treatment for narcolepsy but was not approved for ADHD until 1968. Less than 20 trials and nearly 50 years later there remains a research and practice gap in the safety and effectiveness of CNS stimulants within the adult population.

The American Heart Association (AHA) has found that finely tuned stimulant drugs for ADHD are cardiac-neutral, and the AHA does not recommend special monitoring of children and adolescents. There are as yet no similar guidelines for adults who take stimulant drugs.

Clinical experience consistently finds that persons who have high blood pressure experience further blood pressure increase even

with well-refined stimulant doses. However, if the hypertension is controlled before the start of ADHD medication, the first-line stimulant drugs may be used but should be monitored at every follow-up assessment.

CLINICAL REASONING

- What evidence is there to support the use of CNS stimulants for ADHD within the adult population?
- What are the ethical considerations of prescribing CNS stimulants for adults with ADHD? Should there be a set of mandated clinical guidelines that all health care providers use when treating the adult with ADHD?
- Should CNS stimulants be used for the older adult with heart disease, and what dosage guidelines are available, if any?
- You are seeing a new patient who comes with a request for immediate-release methylphenidate for his ADHD. What is your perspective on the use of immediate-release formulations versus the longer-lasting formulations? Would you comply with the patient's request?

adjunct to other modalities, an evaluation of the patient's interest and ability to comply with therapy should be determined; however, drug therapy is not warranted if symptoms are mild.

The health care provider has many options in the management of ADHD because the choice of a drug for a particular patient is pragmatic. The drug of choice is the one best expected to target the symptoms. Whatever the drug chosen, titrate the dosage for 1 month and evaluate the results. If the first drug is not effective, a second may be tried. It is not unusual to try three different types of stimulants before finding one that is effective. When pharmacotherapy is used, employ periodic drug holidays to assess the need for continued use of the drug. In no case should treatment continue for more than 1 school year without reevaluation.

For patients in need of weight loss, evaluate motivation carefully before starting drug therapy. The unmotivated or ambivalent patient is unlikely to adhere to even the most excellent and well-thought out program. The psychologic effects of yet another failure often outweigh the benefits of any short-term weight loss that may be obtained through drug therapy. A patient with a history of drug abuse may not be a candidate for psychomotor stimulants.

Amphetamines and anorexiants are used widely in the treatment of obesity; however, the wisdom of this strategy is at best questionable. (Some states prohibit the use of amphetamines for weight reduction.) Weight loss secondary to amphetamine use is almost entirely due to reduced food intake and only in small measure to increased energy expenditure. Do not provide amphetamines when overeating is the result of psychologic factors, since they are ineffective under these circumstances. Further, continuous weight reduction is not usually observed in obese individuals without dietary restrictions.

When health care providers consider pharmacotherapy in the treatment of obesity, it is usually after the patient has exhausted other therapies first, and when the patient has a BMI greater than 30. Amphetamines are usually the first choice as an adjunct to other therapies in the treatment of obesity; however, they have a multitude of adverse effects and a great risk for dependence, abuse, and tolerance. Anorexiants are amphetamine-like drugs. Drugs for obesity should be used in the short term and only as an adjunct to other therapies intended to increase exercise while decreasing caloric intake.

LIFE-SPAN CONSIDERATIONS. Narcolepsy, ADHD, and obesity frequently begin in early adult life. The impact of the disorders on the patient's interpersonal relationships can be devastating, whether they occur in the perinatal, pediatric, or geriatric populations. Changes in self-image and self-esteem may be present and can be identified with sensitive questioning.

Narcolepsy is a lifelong disease that tends to worsen with aging. Symptoms seem to improve in some women after menopause.

Early identification of ADHD in affected children is important, since the characteristics of the disorder significantly interfere with the normal course of emotional and psychologic development. In an attempt to cope with attention deficit, many of these children develop maladaptive behavior patterns that are a deterrent to psychosocial adjustment. Their behavior evokes negative responses from others, and repeated exposure to negative feedback adversely affects the child's self-concept, especially in boys. About half the children with ADHD also have learning disorders. Most of these children have average or above-average intelligence, and they are often very creative.

Birth weight offers no clue to the detection and prediction of childhood obesity. However, there is a high correlation in childhood adiposity with both parental adiposity and children's daytime activity levels.

▮▮ Drug Variables

Clinical experience has shown that lack of response to one psychomotor stimulant does not necessarily mean that another agent will not be effective. Because CNS stimulants work through slightly different mechanisms and at different sites, one drug may provide improved efficacy over another. However, it is important not to use psychomotor stimulants for an extended period, because they are intended to be an adjunct to other therapies, not a substitute for them.

ATTENTION DEFICIT HYPERACTIVITY DISORDER. Pharmacotherapy itself does not correct ADHD; it only makes the patient more receptive to treatment (see Evidence-based Pharmacotherapeutics box). The drug therapies used in ADHD are stimulants with dopaminergic and adrenergic effects. Stimulants symptomatically improve ADHD core symptoms as well as the associated features including aggression, social interaction, and academic productivity. The majority of patients with ADHD will respond to either amphetamines or methylphenidate if the health care provider is attentive to the different drugs and dosages.

Catecholamines may be involved in the control of ADHD at the level of the cerebral cortex. They increase attention span and the expression of goal-oriented behaviors while decreasing impulsiveness, distractibility, hyperactivity, and restlessness. Overall, behavior becomes more tolerable to self, parents, and teachers. However, the calming effect of amphetamines in children is not understood, and the long-term efficacy of both drugs is limited. Methylphenidate, although a psychomotor stimulant, is structurally distinct from the amphetamines, but its pharmacologic effects and abuse potential are similar. Consequently, methylphenidate can be considered an amphetamine in all but name and structure. Dextroamphetamine is the only psychomotor stimulant approved for ADHD in children aged 3 years and older.

ANOREXIANTS. The use of prescription-only appetite suppressants has been shown to significantly increase weight loss relative to placebo. Recent research indicates an average weight loss of 3 to 4.5 kg over a period of 1 year. The long-term safety of appetite suppressants has not been demonstrated, and patients tend to regain their weight when the drugs are discontinued. These drugs also may interfere with the effectiveness of behavioral interventions.

Patient Education

CNS stimulants such as coffee, tea, chocolate, cola drinks, cocaine, yerba mate, betel, mescaline, and peyote are used in various cultures in modern-day society. Advise patients that continuous use and abuse of CNS stimulants may result in the potential development of drug tolerance and dependency.

Patients taking a psychomotor stimulant, anorexiant, or analeptic require thorough education about their disorder, the purpose and expected outcomes of drug therapy, adverse effects, and the importance of follow-up. Instruct the patient not to increase the dosage of the prescribed drug or abruptly

🔍 EVIDENCE-BASED PHARMACOTHERAPEUTICS

Methylphenidate for Adults with Attention Deficit Hyperactivity Disorder

■ Background

Methylphenidate (Ritalin) is one of the first-line treatments of ADHD. This drug reduces the overactivity, impulsivities, and inattentiveness of ADHD patients and improves academic performance, social functioning, and the likelihood of on-task behavior. Many studies have assessed the efficacy of methylphenidate for treating ADHD in childhood and adolescents. Metaanalyses of these studies show the effect to be robust and statistically significant. However, no meta-analyses of methylphenidate responses for adults with ADHD are documented.

■ Research Article

Faraone, S., Spencer, T., Aleardi, M., et al. (2004). Meta-analysis of the efficacy of methylphenidate for treating adult attention-deficit/hyperactivity disorder. *Journal of Clinical Psychopharmacology, 24*(1), 24–29.

Purpose

The purpose of this study was to estimate the effect size of methylphenidate therapy in adults and to determine if features of the study design influenced the estimate of drug efficacy.

Design

A meta-analysis of six randomized, double-blind studies using placebo controls was analyzed. Subjects treated with methylphenidate (*N* = 140) and those treated with a placebo (*N* = 113) were evaluated. Four studies used crossover designs, and two used parallel designs. All but one study included predominantly male subjects with a mean age range of 27 to 40 years. The effect sizes for each study were determined using different tools.

Methods

The meta-analysis analyzed the comparisons of double-blind studies of methylphenidate for adult ADHD. The studies reviewed all used DSM-III, DSM-III-R or DSM-IV diagnostic criteria. Studies had to include the means and standard deviations of either change scores or end-point scores for the drug and placebo groups. Testing of potential bias was conducted using statistical measures for publication bias.

Findings

The larger effect sizes of methylphenidate are linked to the health care providers' rating of outcomes and higher dosages of the drug. The mean daily doses were 44 mg (0.63 mg/kg/day or higher) for the low-dose group and 70 mg (1.05 mg/kg) for the high-dose group. The effect size for crossover studies was greater than the effect size for parallel studies, but the difference was not significant. The mean effect size was significant at 0.9.

Conclusions

Evidence from this study supports the notion that methylphenidate is effective in treating adults diagnosed with ADHD, and is analogous to the evidence found in studies of children and adolescents. This meta-analysis provides further assurance to health care providers that the diagnosis of ADHD can be validly applied in adulthood.

■ Implications for Practice

There are few studies of ADHD in adults treated with methylphenidate compared with studies of children and adolescents (see also Controversy). The sample size of this meta-analysis is quite small, indicating the need for additional controlled trials.

---

stop therapy without consultation. Abrupt cessation of high-dose therapy may cause extreme fatigue and mental depression.

Inform the patient that these drugs may impair judgment. Caution the patient to use extra care when driving or operating machinery and to avoid the use of alcohol.

Instruct the patient with narcolepsy to document the frequency and character of attacks. They may be able to counteract the effects of daytime sleepiness using a number of adjuncts or substitutes for pharmacotherapy. The strategies may include frequent short walks or other forms of exercise, avoiding large meals and caffeinated beverages, eating before important meetings, and taking short naps throughout the day.

Parents should periodically monitor a child's height and report any growth inhibition that occurs. They also should report any adverse effects such as tachycardia, loss of appetite, abdominal pain, or weight loss.

Many commercial programs and support groups are available to the patient with narcolepsy, ADHD, or obesity. Encourage the patient to follow through with behavior modification therapies and exercise regimens.

Evaluation

Success of narcolepsy treatment is evaluated according to the patient's ability to stay alert and functional throughout the day. Some patients with severe narcolepsy may not overcome fatigue and sleepiness even with CNS stimulants. In this case, success is measured by improved functioning.

Treatment success for the patient with ADHD is determined by the patient's marked improvement in behavior and cognition and in the ability to focus and attend. It is estimated that drug-related improvements occur in 60% to 90% of children taking CNS stimulants. Teacher ratings of children with ADHD who are actively treated with drug therapy reflect improvements in behavior and attention span. In any case, closely monitor the child so that the smallest effective dosage can be used. Evaluation of adults with ADHD is similar.

Effectiveness of anorexiant therapy is demonstrated by a decrease in appetite and a subsequent decrease in weight.

KEY PONITS

- Psychomotor stimulants (e.g., amphetamines) primarily stimulate the cerebral cortex; anorexiants suppress the appetite center, and analeptics (e.g., caffeine) affect centers in the medulla and brainstem.

- Narcolepsy is a chronic, genetically-based, neurologic sleep disorder caused by a disturbance of the REM sleep cycle. It is the third most common diagnosis within primary sleep disorders.

■ ADHD is the single most common chronic psychiatric disorder that causes children and families to seek treatment from primary care providers and mental health professionals. Data suggest that up to 70% of children with ADHD continue to manifest symptoms in adulthood.

■ Exogenous obesity is defined as an imbalance between caloric intake and caloric needs. Endogenous obesity is secondary to another physical problem such as diabetes or an endocrine disorder.

■ Patient assessment should elicit any history of cardiovascular disease, hyperthyroidism or hypothyroidism, or depression or other psychiatric illness before starting any CNS stimulant.

■ The motivation of the patient who is a candidate for psychomotor stimulant therapy and the ability of the patient to follow through with the plan of care should be determined.

■ The major treatment objective for the patient with narcolepsy is to combat somnolence, to restore a normal sleep-wake cycle when possible, and to aid in the restoration of normal functioning.

■ The treatment objective for ADHD is to make the patient more amenable to treatment and to aid in the correction of the associated cognitive and behavioral problems.

■ The treatment objective for the overweight or obese patient is to reduce and stabilize the patient's weight at a more desirable level. The BMI may still not necessarily be within normal limits, but may be reduced sufficiently to lower the risk of major health problems.

■ Psychomotor stimulants can be used in the management of narcolepsy, ADHD, and obesity.

■ First-line drugs for patients with narcolepsy and ADHD include amphetamines and methylphenidate. These drugs increase the availability of dopamine and norepinephrine in the brain.

■ All anorexiants are used as adjuncts to other therapies, such as behavior modification, exercise, and calorie restrictions, in the short-term treatment of obesity.

■ Patients who take psychomotor stimulants require thorough teaching about their disease, drug therapy, adverse effects, and the importance of follow-up.

■ The patient should be instructed not to increase the dosage of the prescribed drug, or abruptly stop therapy without consulting the health care provider.

■ Treatment success for the patient with narcolepsy is measured by the patient's ability to stay alert and functional throughout the day.

■ ADHD treatment success is demonstrated by a marked improvement in behavior and cognition and in the ability to focus and attend.

■ Effectiveness of anorexiant therapy is demonstrated by a decrease in appetite and a subsequent decrease in weight.

Bibliography

Biederman, J., and Faraone, S. (2005). Attention-deficit hyperactivity disorder. *Lancet*, *366*(9481), 237–248.

Centers for Disease Control and Prevention. (2005). Overweight and obesity. Available online:www.cdc.gov/nccdphp/dnpa/obesity/index.htm. Accessed April 7, 2007.

DeNisco, S., Tiago, C., and Kravitz, C. (2005). Evaluation and treatment of pediatric ADHD. *The Nurse Practitioner*, *30*(8), 15–23.

Littner, M., Johnson, S., and McCall, W., et al. (2001). Practice parameters for the treatment of narcolepsy: An update for 2000. *Sleep*, *24*(4), 451–466.

National Center on Birth Defects and Developmental Disabilities. (2005). Attention-deficit/hyperactivity-disorder. Available online: www.cdc.gov/ncbddd/adhd/. Accessed April 7, 2007.

National Institute of Neurological Disorders and Stroke. (2005). Narcolepsy Fact Sheet. Available online:www.ninds.nih.gov/Disorders/narcolepsy/detail_narcolepsy_pr.htmAccessed April 7, 2007.

National Women's Health Information Center. (2003). *Frequently asked questions about health problems in African-American women.*

Washington, DC. U.S. Department of Health and Human Services, Office on Women's Health.

Rappley, M. (2005). Attention deficit-hyperactivity disorder. *New England Journal of Medicine*, *352*(2), 165–173.

Siegel, J., Badr, S., and Krieger, C. (2005). When sleep is the enemy. *Patient Care for the Nurse Practitioner*. Available online:www.patient-carenp.com/pcnp/article/articleDetail.jsp?id=144631. Accessed April 7, 2007.

Vignatelli, L., D'Alessandro, R., and Candelise, L. Antidepressant drugs for narcolepsy. *The Cochrane Database of Systematic Reviews*. Issue 3. Art. No. CD003724. DOI: 10.1002/14651858.CD003724.pub2.

Volkmar, F. (2005). Toward understanding the basis of ADHD. *American Journal of Psychiatry*, *162*(2), 1043–1044. [Editorial.]

Zeman, A., Britton, T., and Douglas, N., et al. (2004). Narcolepsy and excessive daytime sleepiness. *British Medical Journal*, *329*(7468), 724–728.

Zhaoping, L., Maglione, M., and Tu, W., et al. (2005). Meta-analysis: Pharmacologic treatment of obesity. *American College of Physicians*, *142*(7), 532–546.

CENTRAL NERVOUS

23

Skeletal Muscle Relaxants

The neuromuscular system is controlled by a complex interrelationship between the central nervous system (CNS) and the skeletal muscles. Many disorders of the neuromuscular system result in muscle tone imbalances. Although the exact mechanisms of many neuromuscular disorders are not understood, physical and drug therapy provides clues to the pathways and medical management.

Deep tendon reflexes (DTRs) are used to assess the integrity of the neuromuscular system. The muscle contractions are elicited by a quick tap of a reflex hammer to the muscle's tendon insertion. The strength of the reaction, calibrated from 0 to +4, gives the health care provider a wealth of information. A normal reaction (+2) demonstrates that neuromuscular synapses are operative and muscle fibers can contract. It also indicates that the spinal cord, the dorsal root ganglion, and extrapyramidal and pyramidal systems are functional. Abnormal reactions indicate neuromuscular disorders.

SPASM VERSUS SPASTICITY

EPIDEMIOLOGY AND ETIOLOGY

Spasms are sudden, violent, painful, involuntary contractions of a muscle or group of muscles. Most muscle spasms are related to local injury of muscles, joints, tendons, or ligaments. Specific trauma-related causes of spasms include whiplash injuries, cervical root syndrome, herniated discs, and lower back pain syndrome (Table 23-1). Bursitis, myositis, neuritis, dislocations and fractures, muscle strains from excessive stretching or overuse, and sprains from joints with stretched or torn ligaments can result in spasms, as well. Although hypocalcemia or epileptic seizure activity also produces spasms, the discussion in this chapter is limited to spasm resulting from musculoskeletal injury.

In contrast to spasm, *spasticity* involves resistance to stretching by a muscle because of abnormally increased tension. The increased muscle tone or contractions cause stiff, awkward movements. Spasticity is considered permanent and, without the assistance of physical and drug therapy, frequently progresses to disabling contractures. Disorders of the CNS such as closed head injuries, cerebral palsy, multiple sclerosis, and cerebrovascular accident (stroke) are common causes of spasticity. Two thirds of patients with multiple sclerosis have moderate to severe spasticity. Patients with spinal cord trauma, spinal tumors, poliomyelitis, hemiplegia, paraplegia, quadriplegia, and tetanus also may experience spasticity.

PATHOPHYSIOLOGY

Spasms

A delicate balance between musculoskeletal movement and body posture allows the execution of fine and gross motor skills. The hierarchy controlling this balance includes the motor cortex and upper motor neurons (UMNs), extrapyramidal and pyramidal systems, basal ganglia, cerebellum, descending brainstem circuitry, spinal cord, and lower motor neurons (LMNs) (Fig. 23-1). Feedback from the muscle fibers, muscle and tendon joint afferents, and the thalamus helps complete the information loop that regulates movement and posture.

Motor neurons in the ventral regions of the brainstem and the spinal cord are directly responsible for motor function. Action potentials from motor neurons are conducted directly to nerve terminals in muscle fibers that form synapses called *neuromuscular junctions* (NMJs). Acetylcholine (ACh) is released from the nerve terminals and stimulates nicotinic receptors on the muscle, producing contraction. A deficiency in synaptic activity at the NMJ causes myasthenia gravis (see Chapter 26). A number of drugs block nicotinic receptor activation and serve as neuromuscular blockers; they are discussed in Chapter 18.

The stretch reflex maintains muscle tone (Fig. 23-2). Muscle tone is described as normal, *hypotonic* (less than normal), *flaccid* (absent), or *hypertonic* (excessive, rigid, spastic, tetany). LMNs in the ventral horn link spinal cord reflexes to muscles. When the motor neuron axon or cell body is damaged, a pattern of hyperexcitability develops that can produce multiple contractions of the muscle. These muscle spasms can be mild or severe, and acute or chronic. Muscle spasms may also be *clonic*, characterized by alternate contraction and relaxation, or *tonic*, sustained contractions of striated muscle. Depending on their location, spasms can be aggravated by movement, sneezing, coughing, or straining. Muscle atrophy may develop as a consequence of motor neuron lesions.

TABLE 23-1 Comparing Etiologies of Spasm and Spasticity

	Spasm	Spasticity
Definition	Sudden, violent, painful, involuntary contractions of a muscle or group of muscles	Increased muscle tone or muscle contractions that cause stiff, awkward movement
Mediator	LMNs	UMNs
Etiology	Cervical root syndrome	Cerebrovascular accident, CHI
	Bursitis, overuse syndromes	Hemiplegia, paraplegia, quadriplegia
	Dislocation, fracture	Multiple sclerosis
	Epilepsy	Poliomyelitis
	Herniated disc	Spinal cord trauma or tumor
	Hypocalcemia	Tetanus
	Myositis, neuritis	Cerebral palsy
	Sprains, strains	
	Whiplash injuries	

CHI, Closed head injury; *LMNs;* lower motor neurons; *UMNs,* upper motor neurons.

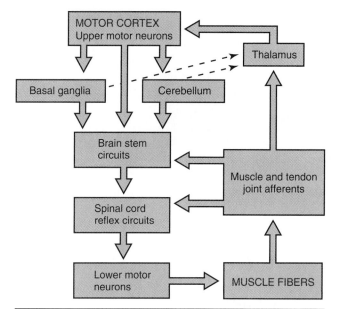

FIGURE 23-1 Algorithm of Neural Pathways Controlling Motor Function. The hierarchy of neuromuscular control begins in the motor cortex and moves through motor neurons and the spinal cord to direct muscles, and ends in feedback information that helps regulates movement and posture. Damage or injury to lower motor neurons (LMNs) results in the development of hyperexcitability or spasms. Damage or injury to upper motor neurons (UMNs) causes a spastic paralysis and hyperreflexia because the spinal reflex remains intact below the level of the lesion. (Adapted from Porth, C. [1994]. *Pathophysiology: Concepts of altered health states.* [4th ed., p. 1029]. Philadelphia: JB Lippincott. Used with permission.)

Spasticity

In contrast to spasm, *spasticity* is a velocity-dependent increase in the passive stretch resistance of a muscle or muscle group. *Clonus,* flexor spasms, mass reflexes, and a positive Babinski's sign are identifiable signs of spasticity. *Hypertonus* results from either an increase in excitatory influences or a decrease in inhibitory influences. As a result, the stretch reflex is augmented and muscle fibers may lengthen in an exaggerated way (see Fig. 23-2).

Spasticity does not develop immediately after neural injury occurs. Therefore severity may vary throughout the progression of the disorder. A gradual increase in muscle tone triggers increases in resistance until tone is suddenly reduced, resulting in a very painful *clasp-knife* phenomenon (a motion similar to the sudden closing of a jackknife). Urinary tract infections, decubitus ulcers, and other painful stimuli can exacerbate spasticity.

Two types of spasticity have been identified. *Spinal spasticity* is characterized by a discernible loss of inhibitory influences. Hyperactive DTRs, clonus, primitive withdrawal reflexes, and a flexed posture are present. In contrast, *cerebral spasticity* produces hypoactive DTRs, increased muscle tone, or inappropriate posture. Ordinarily, there are no primitive withdrawal reflexes or flexed postures with cerebral spasticity. *Dystonia* or disordered muscle tone also may be present in individuals with cerebral spasticity.

PHARMACOTHERAPEUTIC OPTIONS

Centrally Acting Drugs
◆ carisoprodol (Soma, Rela)
◆ cyclobenzaprine (Flexeril); ◆ Flexeril

◆ metaxalone (Skelaxin)
◆ methocarbamol (Robaxin, Marbaxin); ◆ Robaxin
◆ orphenadrine (Norflex, Banflex); ◆ Norflex

Indications
As a rule of thumb, drugs used to treat acute spasm do not relieve spasticity, and vice versa. Centrally acting skeletal muscle relaxants are used primarily for muscle spasms that do not promptly respond to other forms of therapy. They do not completely stop spasms, but they reduce the severity. Patients with pain related to flexor spasms benefit the most.

Carisoprodol, cyclobenzaprine, metaxalone, and methocarbamol are used for spasms related to musculoskeletal pain. Cyclobenzaprine is also used with some effectiveness in the management of fibrositis syndrome, although it is not FDA-approved for such use. Methocarbamol is also used as an adjunct in the treatment of tetanus. Orphenadrine has been used in the management of quinine-resistant leg cramps.

Diazepam, an antianxiety drug discussed in Chapter 19, is effective in relieving spasticity associated with spinal cord injury, multiple sclerosis, and cerebral injury, and in treating muscle spasms. Relatively high dosages are required to relieve muscle hyperactivity.

Pharmacodynamics
The exact mechanism of action for centrally acting skeletal muscle relaxants is unknown. Drug action is thought to result from CNS depression of the brainstem, the thalamus, the basal ganglia, and the spinal cord. Skeletal muscle relaxants also block nerve impulses that cause increased muscle tone and contraction. It is unclear whether pain relief is secondary to use of skeletal muscle relaxants or occurs as a result of the sedative effects, muscular relaxation, or placebo effects.

The mechanism of action of carisoprodol is also not well understood. Considered an interneuronal blocking drug, carisoprodol is chemically related to meprobamate, an antianxiety drug. Carisoprodol depresses excitatory and inhibitory neuron activity affecting muscle stretch reflexes. There are no known peripheral or autonomic effects. In contrast, cyclobenzaprine is structurally and pharmacologically related to tricyclic antidepressants (see Chapter 18); however, antidepressant effects are thought to be minimal. Cyclobenzaprine acts at the level of the brainstem rather than the spinal cord to reduce muscle tone and hyperactivity. Loss of muscle function does not occur.

Pharmacokinetics
The pharmacokinetics of selected skeletal muscle relaxants are identified in Table 23-2. Most drugs are readily absorbed from the gastrointestinal (GI) tract following oral administration. Most skeletal muscle relaxants are biotransformed in the liver and eliminated via the kidneys.

Adverse Effects and Contraindications
The use of centrally acting skeletal muscle relaxants is almost always associated with some degree of sedation, drowsiness, light-headedness, ataxia, and dizziness that can lead to falls. Use caution with patients who have preexisting comorbid conditions that produce weakness, ataxia, or light-headedness. Other adverse effects and contraindications are drug-specific.

CENTRAL NERVOUS

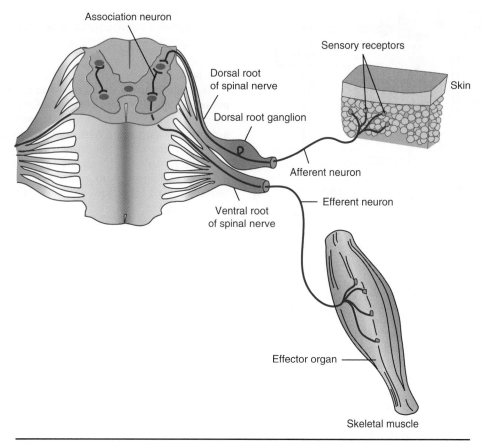

FIGURE 23-2 **Reflex Arc.** The stretch reflex maintains muscle tone. When communication between sensory receptors and muscles is broken, a pattern of hyperexcitability develops that produces multiple contractions or spasms. (From Black, J., and Matassarin-Jacobs, E. [1997]. *Medical-surgical nursing: Clinical management for continuity of care.* [5th ed., p. 701]. Philadelphia: WB Saunders.)

PHARMACOKINETICS
TABLE 23-2 Skeletal Muscle Relaxants

Drug	Route	Onset	Peak	Duration	PB (%)	$t_{1/2}$	BioA (%)
CENTRALLY ACTING DRUGS							
carisoprodol	PO	30 min	4 hr*	4–6 hr	UA	8 hr	UA
cyclobenzaprine	PO	60 min	3–8 hr	12–24 hr	93	12–24 hr	UA
metaxalone	PO	60 min	2 hr†	4–6 hr	30	2–3 hr	UA
methocarbamol	PO	30 min	2 hr	3–6 hr	UA	1–2 hr	UA
orphenadrine	PO	60 min	3 hr‡	8 hr	UA	14 hr	UA
PERIPHERALLY ACTING DRUGS							
baclofen	PO	Hours to weeks	2–3 hr	8 hr	30	2.5–4 hr	UA
botulinum toxin type A	IM	Rapid	UA	3–4 mo	NA	UA	100
dantrolene	PO	1 hr§	5 hr	6–12 hr	>90	6–9 hr	70
quinine	PO	Varies	1–3 hr	6–8 hr	70–90	4–21 hr	UA
tizanidine	PO	30 min	1–2 hr	3–6 hr	30	2.5 hr	40

*Peak drug activity for 350 mg dose of carisoprodol.
†Peak drug activity for 800 mg of metaxalone.
‡Peak drug activity for 50 mg of orphenadrine.
§Time for dantrolene to reach blood levels; therapeutic effect may take 1–2 wk.
BioA, Bioavailability; *IM,* intramuscular; *NA,* not applicable; *PB,* protein binding; *PO,* by mouth; *$t_{1/2}$,* half-life; *UA,* unavailable.

Headaches, sleepiness, and visual disturbances are common. Nausea, vomiting, constipation, and diarrhea have been associated with carisoprodol, cyclobenzaprine, methocarbamol, and orphenadrine. Cyclobenzaprine has significant anticholinergic activity (e.g., dry mouth, urinary retention, blurred vision) and produces alterations in the sense of taste. Increased excitability, nervousness, and irritability have been associated with carisoprodol, metaxalone, and orphenadrine.

Do not use carisoprodol in patients with a history of porphyria. An autosomal dominant trait, porphyria disturbs the metabolism of porphyrin, any of a group of nitrogen-containing organic compounds that occurs in the protoplasm and forms the basis of respiratory pigments. Carisoprodol increases the synthesis of porphyrin, thereby exacerbating symptoms.

▥ Drug Interactions

Muscle relaxants taken concurrently with alcohol, benzo-diazepines, or other CNS depressants results in additive depression and possible toxicity (Table 23-3). The combination of propoxyphene and orphenadrine results in confusion, anxiety, tremors, and additive hypoglycemia. A dosage reduction or discontinuance of one or both drugs is warranted.

▥ Dosage Regimen

The dosage regimen for centrally acting skeletal muscle relaxants varies with the individual drug (Table 23-4).

▥ Lab Considerations

A reducing substance in the urine of patients receiving metaxalone may cause false-positive results for glucose determination using a cupric sulfate (Benedict's solution, Clinitest, Fehling's solution) but does not interfere with glucose tests using glucose oxidase (Clinistix, Diastix, TesTape). These tests

DRUG INTERACTIONS
TABLE 23-3 Skeletal Muscle Relaxants

Drug	Interactive Drug	Interaction
CENTRALLY ACTING DRUGS		
baclofen, cyclobenzaprine, methocarbamol carisoprodol	Alcohol, antihistamines, CNS depressants, MAOIs	Increases CNS depression; increases risk of hepatotoxicity with combination of chlorzoxazone and alcohol
cyclobenzaprine	Phenothiazines	Potentiates anticholinergic effects
	MAOIs	May precipitate hypertensive crisis
orphenadrine	propoxyphene	Increases confusion, anxiety, tremors; additive hypoglycemia
PERIPHERALLY ACTING DRUGS		
baclofen	Alcohol, antihistamines, CNS depressants, MAOIs	Increases CNS depression; increases risk of hepatotoxicity with combination of alcohol
dantrolene	Alcohol, CNS depressants	Increases CNS depression
	Estrogens	Increases risk of hepatotoxicity
	Calcium-channel blockers	Increases risk of ventricular fibrillation
quinine	digoxin	Increases digoxin levels
	Anticholinergic drugs	Increases vagolytic effects
	Cholinergic drugs	Antagonizes cardiac effects
	Anticonvulsants, barbiturates, rifampin	Increases metabolism of quinine, thus decreasing efficacy
	CAIs, chronic antacid use, sodium bicarbonate	Decreases renal elimination quinine, thus increasing toxicity
	Neuromuscular blockers	Increases effectiveness of neuromuscular blockers
	warfarin	Increases hypoprothrombinemic effects
Tizanidine	Alcohol	Additive CNS depression
	Contraceptives, acetaminophen	Decreases clearance of tizanidine
	Antihypertensives	Additive hypotension
	Tricyclic antidepressants, MAOIs	Fever, convulsions

CAIs, Carbonic anhydrase inhibitors; *CNS,* central nervous system; *MAOIs,* monoamine oxidase inhibitors.

DOSAGE
TABLE 23-4 Skeletal Muscle Relaxants

Drug	Indication(s)	Dosage Regimen	Implications
CENTRALLY ACTING DRUGS			
carisoprodol	Muscle spasm caused by inflammation and trauma	*Adult:* 350 mg PO 3–4 times daily PRN	Take the last dose at HS. Not used for children <12 yr, older adults, and those with hepatic or renal impairment.
cyclobenzaprine	Muscle spasm caused by inflammation and trauma	*Adult:* 10 mg PO 3 times daily PRN. Range: 20–40 mg in divided doses. Maintenance: Not to exceed 60 mg/day	**Do not use longer than 2–3 wk.** Safe use in children <15 yr not established. **Not effective for spasticity associated with cerebral palsy or cerebral cord disease.**
metaxalone	Muscle spasm caused by inflammation and trauma	*Adult:* 800 mg PO 3–4 times daily PRN	Safe use in children has not been established.
methocarbamol	Muscle spasm caused by inflammation and trauma	*Adult:* 1.5 grams PO 4 times daily PRN for 2–3 days (up to 8 grams/day) Maintenance: 750 mg PO every 4 hr –or– 1 gram 4 times daily –or– 1.5 grams 3 times daily	Safe use in children has not been established.
	Adjunct for tetanus	*Adult:* 1–2 grams IV. Total initial dose 3 grams. May repeat every 6 hr PRN up to 24 grams/day in divided doses. *Child:* 15 mg/kg IV every 6 hr	IV route may be used until NG tube is inserted; then change to oral formulation.
orphenadrine	Muscle spasm caused by inflammation and trauma	*Adult:* 100 mg PO twice daily –or– 60 mg IM, IV every 12 hr	Safe use in children has not been established.

Continued

DOSAGE
TABLE **23-4** Skeletal Muscle Relaxants—Cont'd

Drug	Indication(s)	Dosage Regimen	Implications
PERIPHERALLY ACTING DRUGS			
baclofen	Multiple sclerosis, cerebral palsy, spinal cord insults, CVA	*Adult:* 5 mg PO 2–3 times daily initially. Increase by 15 mg/dose every 3–7 days until desired response is achieved. Maintenance: Usually does not exceed 80 mg/day	If benefits are not evident after a trial period, gradually withdraw drug. Dosage for children has not been determined. Dosage reduction needed in older adults and those with renal impairment.
botulinum toxin type A	Blepharospasm, spasticity caused by muscle sclerosis, stroke, brain injury, or spinal cord injury	*Adult:* 1.25–2.5 units/site every 3 mo. Max: 200 units or 30 days' cumulative dose	Pharmacoeconomic consideration: 100-unit powder for solution costs approximately $560.
dantrolene	Multiple sclerosis, cerebral palsy, spinal cord insults, CVA	*Adult:* 25 mg PO daily. Increase by 25 mg 2–4 times daily PRN. Maintenance: Not to exceed 400 mg/day *Child:* 0.5 mg/kg twice daily. Increase by 0.5–3 mg/kg 2–4 times daily. Maintenance: Not to exceed 100 mg 4 times daily	Maintain each dosage level for 4–7 days to evaluate response before increasing. Discontinue drug after 45 days if benefits are not evident.
	Prevention of malignant hyperthermia	*Adult and Child:* 4–8 mg/kg/day PO in 3–4 divided doses for 1–2 days preoperatively. Last dose 3–4 hr before scheduled surgery	Adjust dosage to recommended range to prevent drowsiness and excessive GI irritation.
	Malignant hyperthermic crisis	*Adult and Child:* 1 mg/kg IV. May repeat up to cumulative dosage of 10 mg/kg, followed by 4–8 mg/kg/day PO in 4 divided doses for 1–3 days to prevent recurrence.	Dosage is for adults and children.
quinine	Nocturnal leg cramps	*Adult:* 260–300 mg PO at HS	May be taken after evening meal and at HS.
tizanidine	Relief of spasticity	*Adult:* 4 mg PO every 6–8 hr. Single dose not to exceed 8 mg. Increase slowly by 2–4 mg to optimal response. Not to exceed 36 mg daily	Safe use in children has not been established. Not recommended in pregnancy. Use low dose in older adults.

CVA, Cerebral vascular accident; *GI,* gastrointestinal; *HS,* bedtime; *IM,* intramuscular (route); *IV,* intravenous (route); *NG,* nasogastric; *PRN,* as needed; *UMN,* upper motor neuron.

are outdated but are still used in some patient care environments. Methocarbamol can cause false increases in urinary 5-hydroxyindoleacetic acid (using nitrosonaphthol reagent) and vanillylmandelic acid (VMA) (Gitlow method) levels.

Peripherally Acting Drugs

◆ baclofen (Lioresal); ◆ Alpha-Baclofen
◆ botulinum toxin type A (Botox)

◆ dantrolene (Dantrium); ◆ Dantrium
◆ quinine (Quinamm, Quiphile); ◆ quinine sulfate
◆ tizanidine (Zanaflex); ◆ tizanidine (Zanaflex)

▥ *Indications*

Baclofen is most effective in relieving spasticity caused by spinal cord injury and is less effective in relieving spasticity from brain damage (see Controversy box). It is taken orally

---

Controversy

Intrathecal Baclofen in Cerebral Palsy

Jonathan J. Wolfe

Cerebral palsy presents difficult challenges to the patient, the family, and the health care provider. One of its cruelest manifestations is painful spasticity. The pain related to this element of the disease easily qualifies as malignant, for it causes intense and long-term suffering while serving no useful physiologic purpose. The patient and all concerned already know that the disease is serious, with poor prognosis.

Early attempts to use baclofen, marketed as baclofen tablets, met with indifferent success. Concern about drug effects properly limited daily doses and approved durations of therapy. Even patients who were aided by baclofen therapy frequently could not sustain therapeutic levels because of the adverse effects at high dosages. Difficulties in swallowing large numbers of tablets were remedied only imperfectly by preparation of extemporaneous oral liquid formulations.

Because baclofen is a peripherally-acting skeletal muscle relaxant, investigation of direct injection into the intrathecal space offered a reasonable focus for research. Results in a significant number of patients indicated that baclofen administered via this route is of genuine value. A parenteral formulation without preservatives for intrathecal injection came to market as an orphan drug under federal Food and Drug Administration (FDA) guidelines.

Therapy with intrathecal baclofen requires a trial of the drug by bolus injection. Continuous treatment requires surgical placement of a programmable infusion pump that is refilled periodically thereafter. Treatment exposes the patient to all the hazards of lumbar puncture, intrathecal catheter placement, and use of an implanted pump. Treatment is also quite expensive.

CLINICAL REASONING

- Do you feel that a patient with the spasticity of cerebral palsy must "fail" on oral baclofen therapy before being considered for intrathecal therapy?
- What education is appropriate for a minor child and the family members to ensure proper informed consent to intrathecal baclofen therapy?
- What education is appropriate for an autonomous adult patient to ensure proper informed consent to intrathecal baclofen therapy?
- What, if any, problems do you perceive given the fact that the company sponsoring baclofen as an intrathecal injection is also a leading manufacturer and marketer of implanted programmable infusion pumps?
- What reservations would you have in evaluating continuing education materials about intrathecal baclofen therapy that were provided by the corporate sponsor of the drug? Would FDA requirements for such materials answer your reservations?

CASE STUDY   Centrally Acting Skeletal Muscle Relaxants

ASSESSMENT

History of Present Illness	SK is a 37-year-old man with complaints of low back pain described as "knifelike burning." The pain radiates from the lumbar region to the right midbuttock and hip. He is unable to sit or stand comfortably. "Any movement hurts." He was helping to unpack and transfer oversize library books to high shelves when the pain occurred.
Past Health History	SK denies history of neuromuscular, musculoskeletal, renal, or peptic ulcer disease. He has a history of acute intermittent porphyria. No weight gain or loss in the past year. Routine exercise regimen limited to walking to and from his car and the library. Denies taking any other drugs or consuming alcohol on a regular basis.
Life-Span Considerations	SK is single. Has degree in library science and works at the university library. In his spare time he watches videos and "veges out." Describes his lifestyle as that of a "couch potato." Carries health insurance through the university that also includes a pharmacy plan. Workers' compensation is available through his employer.
Physical Exam Findings	*Height:* 5'9". *Weight:* 255 lbs. *VS:* 132/88 98° F-120-24. SK is pacing in exam room, holding right lower back and hip. Muscle firmness and tenderness noted from L_4-S_3 on palpation, and tautness of sacrospinalis and gluteal muscles. Straight leg raises aggravate low back pain. Severe discomfort when toe walking. He is unable to twist or bend at the waist without obvious discomfort. Muscle tone increased on affected side. Abdomen soft, flat, nontender. No CVA tenderness.
Diagnostic Testing	KUB, flat plate films of lower back, CT scan, and MRI are all WNL. CBC, electrolytes, BUN, creatinine, and urinalysis are WNL.

DIAGNOSIS: Low back pain with spasms

MANAGEMENT

Treatment Objectives	1. Improve functional state and minimize discomfort. 2. Help patient return to work as soon as possible. 3. Establish normal muscle tone and function.
Treatment Plan	**Pharmacotherapy** • ibuprofen 600 mg PO 3 times daily with food for 10 days • metaxalone 800 mg PO 3 to 4 times daily PRN for 2 weeks **Patient Education** 1. Take metaxalone on empty stomach to facilitate absorption. 2. Learn, and use, proper body mechanics when bending or lifting. 3. Continue applying ice packs to affected area for 20 minutes every 4–6 hours. 4. Keep regular appointments with the physical therapist for next 2 weeks. 5. Use caution driving when taking metaxalone. No alcohol intake is advised. 6. Begin weight loss and exercise program once back pain is relieved. **Evaluation** SK is more comfortable, with improvement in functional abilities, muscle tone, and function. He has returned to work and is using proper body mechanics when moving objects.

CLINICAL REASONING ANALYSIS

Q1. Why didn't you tell him to do back exercises instead of prescribing a skeletal muscle relaxant?
A. Systematic reviews and randomized controlled trials have found neither significant differences between back exercises and conservative treatments for pain or disability, nor that back exercises increase pain and disability. The best therapy is to do both: stay active and use NSAIDs.

Q2. I expected you to order a skeletal muscle relaxant first, but you gave him a prescription for ibuprofen. Why?
A. Research has shown that nonsteroidal antiinflammatory drugs (NSAIDs) increase overall performance after 1 week and reduce the need for additional analgesics compared with placebo.

Continued

CENTRAL NERVOUS

Q3. **You considered using carisoprodol and cyclobenzaprine for SK but then ordered metaxalone. Why was that?**
A. There is a trade-off between the benefits and the harm that skeletal muscle relaxants may produce. Systematic reviews have found that muscle relaxants improve symptoms, including pain and muscle tension, and increase mobility compared with placebo. In reality there is no significant difference in outcomes among the various muscle relaxants. Metaxalone and cyclobenzaprine are less likely to alter muscle function compared with carisoprodol, but cyclobenzaprine is contraindicated in patients with a history of porphyria, which SK has.

or administered directly into the thecal space so it has direct exposure to the spinal cord, thereby reducing the severe spasticity of multiple sclerosis and the spasticity of childhood cerebral palsy. Intrathecal administration produces less sedation than high doses of orally administered baclofen. Baclofen also has been used in the management of trigeminal neuralgia (tic douloureux), although this use has not been approved by the FDA. It is also used in the management of detrusor sphincter incoordination associated with spinal cord disease.

Botulinum toxin type A is used to treat spasticity caused by muscle sclerosis, stroke, brain injury, or spinal cord injury, and as an adjunct therapy in cerebral palsy. It has recently been approved for reduction of facial wrinkles.

Dantrolene is most useful for the patient whose spasticity causes pain or discomfort or limits functional rehabilitation. In addition to the spasticity caused by spinal cord injury, dantrolene relieves the spasticity of stroke, cerebral palsy, and multiple sclerosis, for which other drugs have limited effectiveness. Dantrolene is also used in the management of preoperative and intraoperative malignant hyperthermia.

Quinine has been used for the relief of nocturnal leg cramps, although it has generally been replaced by more effective, less toxic drugs. It has also been used alone and with pyrimethamine and sulfonamides (or with an oral tetracycline) for the treatment of chloroquine-resistant *Plasmodium falciparum* malaria (Chapter 30).

Tizanidine is used for chronic or intermittent management of increased muscle tone associated with spasticity, especially that related to spinal cord injury or multiple sclerosis.

▥ *Pharmacodynamics*

Baclofen was developed as an oral analogue of the inhibitory transmitter gamma-aminobutyric acid (GABA). Although the underlying mechanisms are not well understood, observations of CNS neurons suggest that baclofen acts as an inhibitory neurotransmitter at the spinal level. It also reduces pain in patients with spasticity by inhibiting the release of substance P in the spinal cord.

Botulinum inhibits ACh release from nerve endings, thus reducing neuromuscular transmission and local muscle activity. It acts as a neurotoxin.

Dantrolene is unique in that it reduces muscle contractility by 75% to 80% by inhibiting calcium release from the sarcoplasmic reticulum. The blockage of calcium release is not complete, and contraction is never completely abolished. The effects are more noticeable in fast-contracting muscle fibers and depend on the frequency of nerve stimulation. Single-twitch contractions are more affected than tetanic contractions. Dantrolene does not possess GABA-like actions.

Dantrolene reduces both monosynaptic- and polysynaptic-induced muscle contractions.

Quinine, a naturally occurring substance from the bark of the cinchona tree, resembles salicylates in its analgesic properties. It exerts curare-like skeletal muscle relaxation.

Tizanidine reduces spasticity by increasing presynaptic inhibition of motor neurons.

▥ *Pharmacokinetics*

The onset of baclofen is long, ranging from hours to weeks. Peak action times range from 1 to 4 hours. Although therapeutic serum levels are not routinely measured for patients on skeletal muscle relaxants, the level of baclofen ranges from 80 to 400 mcg/mL (see Table 23-2).

In contrast to baclofen and other peripherally active drugs, the absorption of dantrolene from the GI tract is slow and incomplete. Nonetheless, absorption is thought to be sufficient to provide dose-related plasma concentrations. It takes approximately 1 hour to raise blood levels, but therapeutic effects can take 1 to 2 weeks to be achieved. Peak action is reached in 5 hours, with a duration of action of 6 to 12 hours. Dantrolene is highly protein bound when given in a 100-mg dose and has a mean half-life of 6 to 9 hours.

Serum concentrations of dantrolene and its metabolites are not significantly different after a 400-mg dose than concentrations obtained after a single oral dose of 100 mg. This finding does not appear to be related to enzyme induction, but rather to capacity-limited absorption or protein binding. Dantrolene is almost entirely biotransformed by the liver, with its metabolites eliminated in the urine. The therapeutic range for dantrolene is 300 to 1100 mcg/mL for 100-mg doses.

Botulinum toxin type A has minimal to no systemic absorption. The action of the drug on CYP450 is unknown at this time, as are the half-life and elimination patterns.

The onset of quinine action varies when taken by mouth. Peak action is reached in 1 to 3 hours, with a duration of action of 6 to 8 hours. The bioavailability of quinine is unknown, but it is 70% to 90% protein bound, with a half-life of 4 to 21 hours in the healthy or convalescing patient. Serum drug concentrations vary.

Tizanidine is extensively biotransformed in the liver, with 60% of the drug eliminated in the urine. It acts as a CYP 1A2 substrate.

▥ *Adverse Effects and Contraindications*

Baclofen is relatively well tolerated; however, its more common adverse effects include transient drowsiness, vertigo, confusion, sleepiness, increased weakness, and nausea. Less common effects include headache, fatigue, nasal congestion, abdominal pain, anorexia, diarrhea or constipation, dysuria, urgency, urinary incontinence, and, in males, sexual dysfunction. Ataxia, insomnia, slurred speech, muscle stiffness, increased excitability, ankle edema, hypotension, tachycardia, and weight gain are also possible adverse effects.

Severe adverse effects of baclofen rarely appear, but they include syncope, chest pain, dark urine, auditory and visual hallucinations, and tinnitus. Neuropsychiatric signs and symptoms (e.g., euphoria, depression, accommodation disorders, and paresthesias) are also rare but may be difficult to discern from those of the underlying disease. An overdose of baclofen appears as visual disturbances (blurred vision, diplopia), vomiting, seizures, respiratory difficulties, and severe muscle weakness. There are no absolute contraindications to baclofen therapy other than hypersensitivity.

The common adverse effects of botulinum toxin type A depend on the injection site but generally include dysphagia, ptosis, vertical ocular deviation, headache and neck pain, dry eyes, punctate keratitis, cough and a flulike syndrome, dizziness, muscle weakness, injection site pain or irritation, xerostomia, vision and speech disturbances, and a rash. Do not use the drug in patients with hypersensitivity to the drug or to albumin; in patients with neuromuscular disease, myasthenia gravis, amyotrophic lateral sclerosis, a motor neuropathy, or heart disease; or in patients who lack adequate neck-muscle mass to hold up their heads.

Dantrolene and quinine may cause dizziness, headache, confusion, euphoria, tachycardia, blurred vision, nausea, vomiting, diarrhea, pruritus, and urticaria. In addition, dantrolene may cause muscle weakness and fatigue, speech disturbances, nervousness, depression, insomnia, seizures, erratic blood pressure readings, photophobia, urinary frequency or retention, nocturnal diuresis, and erectile dysfunction. Prolonged use of dantrolene at high doses can cause hepatitis, hepatomegaly, and hepatic necrosis. The most serious adverse effect of dantrolene is an idiosyncratic or hypersensitivity-mediated injury to the liver. When injury does occur, it ordinarily appears 3 to 12 months after the start of therapy. It is seen most often in women with multiple sclerosis.

Quinine can cause ototoxicity, tinnitus, anxiety, acute asthmatic episodes, fever, angina, and rash. Leukopenia, thrombocytopenia, agranulocytosis, hemolytic anemia, and hypoprothrombinemia are of major concern. Toxic levels are reflected as hypotension, hypothermia, seizures, cardiovascular collapse, coma, and death.

Tizanidine can produce hypotension, sedation, hallucinations, somnolence, asthenia, dizziness, and dry mouth. With long-term use, bradycardia and prolonged QT intervals may occur.

Drug Interactions

Benzodiazepines are the most commonly used drugs that interact with skeletal muscle relaxants (see Table 23-3). In women older than 35 years of age, concurrent use of dantrolene with estrogen replacement therapy increases the potential for hepatotoxicity. Verapamil and other calcium channel blockers increase the risk of ventricular fibrillation and cardiovascular collapse when administered in conjunction with intravenous (IV) dantrolene.

Quinine increases digoxin levels, antagonizes the cardiac effects of cholinergic drugs, and adds to the vagolytic effects of anticholinergics. The biotransformation of quinine is increased in the presence of anticonvulsants, barbiturates, and rifampin. Renal elimination of quinine is decreased by carbonic anhydrase inhibitors, sodium bicarbonate, and chronic antacid use. Warfarin may increase the hypoprothrombinemic effects.

Dosage Regimens

Determination of the optimal dosage for skeletal muscle relaxants requires careful titration. Almost all skeletal muscle relaxants can be administered orally, and some by intramuscular (IM) or IV routes (see Table 23-4).

Lab Considerations

Serum drug levels for skeletal muscle relaxants are not ordinarily required; however, they may be desirable if the drugs are used on a long-term basis. In general, skeletal muscle relaxants produce mild elevations in aspartate aminotransferase (AST), alkaline phosphatase, and blood glucose levels. Monitor liver function tests and creatinine levels for the patient taking dantrolene, quinine, or tizanidine on a regular basis. In addition, obtain a complete blood count to monitor the hematologic impact of therapy on the patient taking quinine (see Case Study–Peripherally Acting Skeletal Muscle Relaxants).

CLINICAL REASONING

Treatment Objectives

The decision to treat spasms and spasticity is based on the cause and issues of pain and mobility. Skeletal muscle relaxants are used to minimize or stop unwanted spasm and spasticity, with the ultimate goal of establishing normal muscle tone and function. In addition, effective treatment regimens improve activity tolerance, range of motion, strength, and mobility.

The potential impact of spasticity on the patient's physical condition, functional status, and adaptation to disability is significant. Desired outcomes of interventions for spasticity can be realistic or unrealistic; unrealistic expectations may lead to disappointment. Effective ongoing contact between the patient, caregivers, and health care providers about realistic treatment goals is vital in developing effective management plans. Realistic goals that are commonly developed for the management of spasticity include the following:

- Alleviate the signs and symptoms of spasticity.
- Lessen exposure to irritating stimuli, the frequency of spasms, and pain.
- Enhance gait, hygiene, activities of daily living, and/or ease of care.
- Diminish problems related to with passive function (i.e., functions required of another person), such as bathing, dressing, feeding, and transfers.
- Improve voluntary active motor function (i.e., behaviors and functions under the patient's control), such as reaching for, grasping, moving, and releasing an object.

Treatment Options

Perceived susceptibility to disease and its seriousness influences the plan of care. Many of the skeletal muscle relaxants have unpleasant or undesirable adverse effects; therefore the likelihood of compliance is a concern. There is no completely satisfactory intervention that will alleviate spasm and spasticity. Most spasms are self-limiting, responding rapidly to rest and physical measures. Physical measures include rest,

CASE STUDY   Peripherally Acting Skeletal Muscle Relaxants

ASSESSMENT

History of Present Illness	DL is a 40-year-old woman with a 10-year history of multiple sclerosis. She is now complaining of reduced strength and mobility; increased cutaneous, flexor, and extensor spasms; and pain that started 1 month ago. The spasms disturb her sleep. States that she is unable to carry out routine activities of daily living and her daily ROM exercises as before. She used a cane until recently but now must use a walker. She denies recent illness, infection, unusual stress, or trauma.
Past Health History	DL has been taking alternate-day low-dose prednisone for the past year, with general improvement in symptoms. She was actively employed until the recent change in her health status. She usually follows a prescribed exercise regimen and by record is a motivated patient. Until this visit, the exercise regimen has kept DL from taking drugs for her MS. DL is postmenopausal; takes estrogen-progesterone daily. There are no known food or drug allergies.
Life-Span Considerations	DL is single and lives alone and, overall, copes well with her disease. She works as secretary-receptionist. Her family and employer are emotionally supportive. She most fears incapacitation and has a sense of powerlessness from real and perceived losses. She has changed jobs several times in past 3 years because of the MS and now perceives her financial, physical, and social independence as threatened. DL is interested in the theater and arts and attends shows on a regular basis with a theater group. She has health insurance with an HMO but no pharmacy coverage. She is worried that if she changes jobs again she will lose her coverage.
Physical Exam Findings	*Height:* 5'4". *Weight:* 125 lbs. *VS:* 122/72 98° F-72-20. Extensor and flexor spasms and clonus are noted. DTRs are exaggerated. DL has an unsteady gait and 1+/5 borderline muscle strength bilaterally.
Diagnostic Testing	CBC, electrolytes, BUN, and creatinine are WNL. CSF reflects slightly elevated WBCs and cell and protein counts. EMG reflects slow-wave activity compared to exam 2 years ago. Repeat CT scan shows increased density in the white matter with MS plaques.

DIAGNOSIS: Multiple sclerosis

MANAGEMENT

Treatment Objectives	1. Minimize severity of spasticity. 2. Improve activity tolerance, ROM, strength, and mobility. 3. Maintain existing system functioning.
Treatment Plan	**Pharmacotherapy** • Baclofen 5 mg PO 3 times daily initially. May increase by 15 mg/day every 3–7 days until desired response achieved. Maintenance dose usually does not exceed 80 mg/day. **Patient Education** 1. Drowsiness usually diminished with continued therapy. Avoid tasks that require alertness or motor skills until response to drug is established. 2. Do not abruptly stop the drug. 3. Avoid taking alcohol and other CNS depressants without first checking with the health care provider. 4. Follow up in the office in 72 hours. **Evaluation** DL currently has minimal spasticity, improved activity tolerance, ROM, strength, and mobility. The functions of other body systems are normal (i.e., no constipation, incontinence of urine or stool).

CLINICAL REASONING ANALYSIS

Q1. We learned in pharm class that people with MS can take either baclofen or dantrolene. Why did you choose to use baclofen?

A. There are several reasons. Baclofen is useful with flexor and extensor spasms and spasticity of spinal origin, all of which DL has. Further, it is preferred in patients with borderline strength, which DL also has right now. Baclofen produces no direct relaxation in peripheral muscle strength, although it can produce annoying muscle weakness and alterations in gait in susceptible patients. Dantrolene also relieves spasticity, but its major use is in nonmobile patients.

Q2. I heard you tell DL that drowsiness is an adverse effect of baclofen. Does the drowsiness ever go away?
  A. Yes, the drowsiness goes away with continued therapy, although it may continue for a small number of patients. For some patients it takes 2 to 3 weeks, and in others a bit longer. She should be advised, though, to avoid taking alcohol and other CNS depressants without first checking with the health care provider, and to avoid driving until her response to the drug is known.

Q3. The record shows that DL takes estrogen and progesterone daily. Is that part of the reason you ordered baclofen instead of dantrolene for DL?
  A. Yes, it is. DL is over 35; and because of the hormones she takes, she is at increased risk for blood clots, but she also has an increased risk for hepatotoxicity if we use dantrolene. Hepatotoxicity is less of a concern with baclofen.

application of cold or warm compresses, whirlpool baths, and physical therapy. Physical therapy interventions include stretching, strengthening, range of motion exercises, assistive-adaptive devices, and hydrotherapy.

▌ Patient Variables

When obtaining the history of present illness, it is important to elicit information about the cause, as well as the effects, of the spasm or spastic state. Is the injury or illness interfering with employment or leisure-time activities? When did the symptoms occur in relation to activities? What activities or situations aggravate or alleviate the discomfort? What has been used for self-treatment, and how effective was the treatment?

Pain is the prominent symptom of muscle spasm and is usually aggravated by movement. Therefore assessment should include the subjective descriptions of the discomfort or pain. Identify the location of the spasm or spasticity as precisely as possible, as well as the intensity, the duration, and any precipitating factors. Also consider the potential for secondary gain related to spasms.

Assess the patient with spasticity for pain and impaired functional abilities (e.g., eating, dressing, and bathing). Determine whether the spasticity interferes with joint and muscle mobility, as well as the ability for self-care. Also elicit the factors contributing to the development of spasticity.

The clinical presentation of spasm and spasticity depends on the location of the injury in the neuromuscular system. For this reason, the physical exam includes an assessment of DTRs and muscle strength, range of motion of joints, gait, balance, coordination, and dexterity. Note the muscle size, tone, and symmetry, and the presence of tremor, spasms, or spasticity. In patients with spasms, muscle firmness and tenderness may be noted over the affected area and are accompanied by limited movement and guarding. DTRs may be hyperactive. Adduction contractions can cause difficulties with personal hygiene, particularly of the perineal and axillary regions.

There are no definitive testing methods for spasms. An electromyelogram (EMG) is helpful to confirm nerve damage associated with spasticity. Magnetic resonance imaging is useful in detecting abnormalities of the spine or lesions in the gray or the white matter of the brain. Radiography assists in determining the presence of fractures, dislocations, bony spurs, and soft tissue swelling, and the presence of foreign objects that may be causing the spasm.

The psychologic response to spasms or spasticity is determined by the cause of the disorder, severity of symptoms, and the impact of those symptoms on lifestyle. Chronic or recurrent spasm and spasticity cause the patient to fear incapacitation if the symptoms cannot be managed effectively.

Consider the potential for secondary gain associated with the patient's illness or condition. The illness or condition affects and is affected by the patient's emotional response. Emotional distress associated with spasm and spasticity can manifest as sleep disturbances, restlessness, irritability, decreased appetite, and loss of interest in daily activities. The perceived vulnerability and associated powerlessness complicate the plan of care for some patients. The sense of powerlessness stems from real and perceived losses. Losses may include employment and financial security, role status, physical or social independence, and control of home environment.

LIFE-SPAN CONSIDERATIONS

Pregnant and Nursing Women. Do not use skeletal muscle relaxants during pregnancy unless the anticipated benefits outweigh the risks. Most skeletal muscle relaxants cross placental membranes. Less is known about the presence of skeletal muscle relaxants in breast milk

Children and Adolescents. Skeletal muscle relaxants are not ordinarily used in children, with the exception of children with spinal cord injuries or cerebral palsy. Most drugs are not recommended for children under age 5 years, and others are not recommended until age 12 years.

Older Adults. Spasms and spasticity are not uncommon in older adults. All skeletal muscle relaxants have adverse effects that alter the functional abilities of an older adult. If dizziness or weakness is exacerbated, caution is warranted to prevent falls or injuries.

▌ Drug Variables

The health care provider has several factors to review when considering use of a muscle relaxant drug. Patients wishing to continue their activities of daily living may benefit from using a more potent muscle relaxant but one with less-sedating properties. Patients often overlook the benefits of skeletal muscle relaxants in reducing spasticity because the sedative and relaxant properties of other drugs enhance well-being. When choosing a muscle relaxant, the health care provider also considers dosage, time to onset, duration of action, adverse effects, and the route of administration.

CENTRAL NERVOUS

Spasms. Drug therapy for spasms usually involves two groups of drugs, skeletal muscle relaxants and nonsteroidal antiinflammatory drugs (NSAIDs) (Chapter 17). Characteristics of the ideal skeletal muscle relaxant include a high degree of efficacy (for specific spasm or spasticity patterns), minimal adverse effects, and no clinically significant drug interactions. The drug should be formulated in oral as well as IV dosage forms, with the oral dose exhibiting a minimal first-pass effect.

A reasonable half-life that promotes infrequent dosing and a positive correlation between drug effectiveness and plasma concentrations are ideal. However, few drugs possess all of these characteristics. Because no studies indicate that any one skeletal muscle relaxant has superiority over another, drug selection is largely based on the preference of the health care provider and the patient's response (see Evidence-Based Pharmacotherapeutics box).

EVIDENCE-BASED PHARMACOTHERAPEUTICS

Noninvasive Treatments for Nonspecific Low Back Pain

■ **Background**

The management of nonspecific acute and chronic low back pain (LBP) varies significantly among health care providers. Traditional interventions for LBP include instructions for the patient to stay active, use of nonsteroidal antiinflammatory drugs (NSAIDs), muscle relaxants, and lumbar supports; back schools; use of progressive relaxation techniques, cognitive therapies, and exercise and physical therapy strategies; and use of antidepressants. Even with all of these interventions there is no evidence supporting their use in the long-term management of nonspecific low back pain.

■ **Research Article**

van Tulder, M., Koes, B., and Malmivaara, A. (2006). Outcome of non-invasive treatment modalities on back pain: An evidence-based review. *European Spine Journal, 15*(Suppl 1), S64–81.

Purpose

The purpose of this literature review of randomized and/or double-blind, controlled studies was to determine the effectiveness of pharmacotherapy and non–drug therapies in the management of acute, subacute, and chronic LBP.

Design

The studies chosen for inclusion in this large-scale review were obtained by searching Medline and Embase from their inception; searching the

Cochrane Central Registry of Controlled Trials; and screening the references found in study reports; and through personal communication with the original study investigators. This macro–meta-analysis was carried out by two independent reviewers using methodologic quality assessment and data extraction techniques in reviewing the randomized, controlled trials. Criteria necessary for inclusion in the study included the following: (1) concealment allocation strategies were used; (2) randomization was apparent; (3) baseline characteristics were similar; (4) the study and its outcomes were blinded to subjects and health care providers alike; (5) there was adequate adherence to interventions; (6) outcome assessments had identical timing; (7) the number of withdrawals and subjects lost to follow-up were adequate; and (8) there were intention-to-treat analyses. The criteria were scored as positive, negative, or unclear.

Methods

Both qualitative ("best-evidence synthesis") and quantitative (statistical pooling) analyses were carried out on the 76 studies included in the metaanalysis. Statistical pooling was avoided with studies lacking sufficient data points, those for which data were sparse or of poor quality, or those in which the data were too heterogenous or not discussed. In these situations, various levels of evidence were used to examine subjects, interventions, outcomes, and methodologic qualities of the original studies. Both qualitative and quantitative analyses were used when subsets of available studies provided sufficient data for inclusion in a macro–meta-analysis (e.g., some studies reported standard deviations and others did not).

Findings

Intervention Acute Low Back Pain	Summary of Results
NSAIDs vs. placebo (18 studies)	There was conflicting evidence whether NSAIDs are more efficacious than placebo in providing pain relief for acute LBP. There were dichotomous data on global improvement, but pooled RR data suggest a statistically significant benefit in favor of NSAIDs compared with placebo.
Benzodiazepine vs. placebo (2 studies)	There was limited evidence to suggest IM diazepam followed by PO diazepam for 5 days is more efficacious than placebo for short term LPB pain relief and better overall improvement. Strong evidence suggested tetrazepam is more effective than placebo for short-term pain relief and providing overall improvement in patients with chronic LBP.
Nonbenzodiazepines vs. placebo (8 studies)	One study demonstrated that IV injection of orphenadrine is more effective than placebo for acute pain. Three studies had strong evidence to suggest that PO nonbenzodiazepines are more effective than placebo for short-term pain relief and global efficacy.
Antispasticity drug vs. placebo (2 studies)	Strong evidence supported the notion that antispasticity muscle relaxants are more effective than placebo for short-term pain relief and reduction of spasm after 4 days.
Advice to stay active vs. bed rest or exercise (5 studies)	Activity significantly improved functional status and reduced sick leave time after 3 weeks compared with bed rest for 2 days. There was significant pain reduction with activity. One study showed no significant differences between activity and bed rest in terms of pain intensity and functional disability.
Bed rest vs. advice to stay active vs. other treatments (7 studies)	Studies suggested small but significant differences favoring the subject remaining active. There were significant differences in the amount of sick leave used in favor of remaining active. Strong evidence to suggest that bed rest is less effective than advice to stay active in reducing pain and functional status and reducing the back-to-work time.
Exercise vs. no treatment vs. usual other interventions (13 studies)	Pooled data suggest there are differences in short-term pain relief with treatment compared with no treatment. There is conflicting evidence suggesting no difference is obtained regarding pain relief, functional outcomes, and short-term or intermediate- or long-term follow-up with exercise or no treatment vs. other conservative treatments.
Back schools vs. control group vs. placebo (5 studies)	There was conflicting evidence on effectiveness of back schools vs. control group vs. placebo regarding pain, functional status, and return to work.

Cognitive-behavioral therapy vs. traditional care (1 study)	There was reduced pain and perceived disability after 9–12 months compared with traditional care.
Multidisciplinary treatment programs for subacute LBP vs. control group with usual care (2 studies)	The multidisciplinary group of subjects returned to work 10 weeks sooner compared with the control group's return to work at 15 weeks.
Spinal manipulation vs. sham therapy (2 studies)	Spinal manipulation had statistically significant and clinically important short-term improvement in pain compared with sham therapy. Functional improvement was not statistically significant but was clinically important.
Spinal manipulation vs. other therapies (12 studies)	Spinal manipulation had statistically significant and clinically important short-term improvement in pain compared with other therapies thought to be unsafe or ineffective. Functional improvement was not statistically significant but was clinically important.

Chronic Low Back Pain

NSAIDs vs. placebo (5 studies)	One small study suggests that naproxen sodium decreased pain more than placebo after 14 days of treatment. COX-2 inhibitors decreased pain and improved function compared with placebo at 4 and 12 weeks of therapy, but the efficacy was small.
Antidepressants vs. placebo (10 studies)	Antidepressants significantly increased pain relief compared with placebo but no significant difference was found in functioning.
Benzodiazepine vs. placebo (3 studies)	There was strong evidence that tetrazepam is more effective than placebo for short-term treatment of chronic LBP and for providing overall improvement. There is moderate evidence to suggest that tetrazepam is more effective than placebo for short-term relief of muscle spasms.
Nonbenzodiazepines vs. placebo (3 studies)	Moderate evidence suggested that flupirtin and tolperisone are more effective than placebo for the short-term improvement of chronic LBP but not for muscle spasms or pain relief.
Exercise vs. usual conservative therapy (14 studies)	Exercise is at least as or more effective than other conservative therapies. Group aerobics and strengthening exercises resulted in less improvement in pain and functional status than behavioral therapy.
Back schools vs. control vs. placebo (6 studies)	Better short-term recovery and return-to-work data were obtained for back schools vs. control or placebo groups.
Back schools vs. other treatments (8 studies)	Moderate evidence suggested back school is more effective than exercises, spinal or joint manipulation, myofascial therapy, and counseling for short- and intermediate-term relief of pain and functional status. No differences were found in long-term pain and functional status.
Cognitive-behavioral therapy vs. control group (13 studies)	Moderate evidence suggested relaxation exercises have a large positive effect on pain and behavioral outcomes. There is little evidence to suggest it has a positive effect on short-term specific and nonspecific functional status. No significant difference was found with EMG biofeedback. There was conflicting evidence on the effect of operant conditioning therapy on short-term pain intensity and moderate evidence showing differences between operant conditioning and control group behavior outcomes in the short term.
Multidisciplinary treatment programs for subacute LBP vs. usual other interventions (12 studies)	Strong evidence suggested that intensive multidisciplinary treatment using a functional restoration approach improves function when compared with other treatments. There was moderate evidence to suggest a multidisciplinary approach reduces pain compared to outpatient, nonmultidisciplinary rehabilitation, or usual care. Intensive multidisciplinary treatment with a functional restoration approach produces significant improvements in pain and function of patients with disabling chronic LBP than non–multidisciplinary rehabilitation or usual care.
Spinal manipulation vs. sham therapy (3 studies)	Spinal manipulation was significantly more effective than sham therapy on short- and long-term pain relief and functional improvement.
Spinal manipulation vs. traditional care (11 studies)	There were no differences between spinal manipulation and other traditionally advocated therapies such as physical or exercise therapy, back school, and general practice care.
Traction vs. placebo (2 studies)	Continuous traction was no more effective on pain, functional abilities, overall improvement, or work absenteeism than placebo.
TENS vs. placebo (5 studies)	Results of one study showed significant reduction in pain intensity with active TENS intervention compared with placebo. Another study showed no significant difference between TENS therapy and placebo on pain, functional status, range of motion, and use of medical services.

Conclusions

Traditional use of NSAIDs and muscle relaxants (benzodiazepines and nonbenzodiazepines) is efficacious for short-term pain relief for patients with acute LBP. Advice from the health care provider to remain active is efficacious for long-term functional improvement.

Various interventions are effective for short-term chronic pain relief and functional improvement, including use of antidepressants, COX-2 inhibitors, back schools, progressive relaxation, cognitive-behavioral therapies, exercise, and intensive multidisciplinary care. No evidence was found to support the notion that these interventions are beneficial over the long-term in terms of pain relief and functional status.

Because the studies reviewed in this macro–meta-analysis have been used in 12 different countries for the development of clinical guidelines, one would expect that each country's guidelines are similar—and indeed they are. The decision to use a particular intervention remains with the health care provider, who should weigh the pros and cons to determine whether or not a specific patient is a suitable candidate for a course of therapy.

■ **Implications for Practice**

Many of the studies reviewed in this macro–meta-analysis had methodologic weaknesses, small effect sizes, and effects that were compared to placebo, and no treatment or waiting list controls. Large, high-quality, randomized, controlled, double-blind clinical trials with sufficient power and effect size are needed to inform health care providers of the efficacy of specific interventions used for management of acute and chronic nonspecific low back pain. Future studies should focus on reducing the incidence and severity of adverse effects.

COX-2, Cyclooxygenase 2; *EMG,* electromylogram; *IM,* intramuscular (route); *IV,* intravenous (route); *NSAIDs,* nonsteroidal antiinflammatory drugs; *PO,* by mouth; *RR,* relative risk; *TENS,* transcutaneous electrical nerve stimulation.

No one skeletal muscle relaxant is any more effective than any other for acute disorders. However, available data are more likely to support the use of cyclobenzaprine or carisoprodol. In many cases, spasms are self-limiting and can be well managed with rest, physical therapy, and/or assistive devices. Most centrally acting skeletal muscle relaxants produce sedative effects and mild pain relief by reducing muscle tone and the discomfort of the spasm. The ability of skeletal muscle relaxants to relieve discomfort appears equal to that of salicylates and other NSAIDs.

For acute muscle spasm and pain, a parenteral drug is usually preferred. Parenteral drugs are preferred for patients with pain of orthopedic etiology, because they have greater sedative and pain-relieving characteristics. Cyclobenzaprine is less likely to produce alterations in muscle function than carisoprodol, although it does have anticholinergic properties that may be bothersome.

In general, gradually increase the dosage of skeletal muscle relaxants to reduce the likelihood of adverse effects.

SPASTICITY. The management of spasticity includes careful consideration of the advantages and disadvantages of spasticity in given muscle groups and the potential consequences of treatment. The choice of drug depends on the condition being treated, its initial or presenting status, associated illness, the drug's pharmacologic actions, and the preference of the patient and the health care provider. For example, baclofen and dantrolene should not be used in patients for whom spasticity is used to maintain posture and balance.

The benefit of reducing spasticity versus the disadvantage of reducing muscle strength must be weighed individually. Although drugs such as baclofen and dantrolene provide variable relief of spasticity, their overall usefulness is limited by the annoying muscle weakness, the alterations in gait, and a variety of other adverse effects they produce. Baclofen seems to be most effective for spasticity of spinal origin. It produces no direct relaxation on peripheral muscles and hence does not decrease muscle strength. Baclofen is preferred over dantrolene in patients with borderline strength.

Spasticity caused by spinal lesions is much more responsive to oral baclofen than spasticity caused by cerebral lesions. Baclofen is particularly useful in reducing the frequency and severity of flexor and extensor spasms, and in reducing flexor tone. Although the responses are clinically relevant, results may be limited. The benefits of baclofen, on the other hand, include less sleep disruption, improved comfort, maintenance of an independent state of self-care, and an ability to participate in a rehabilitation program.

Hepatotoxicity is most likely to occur in people over 35 years who have taken baclofen for 60 days or longer. Women over 35 years who are also taking estrogen are at the highest risk. Hepatotoxicity can be prevented or minimized by administering the lowest effective dose, monitoring liver enzymes during therapy, and discontinuing the drug if beneficial effects do not occur within 45 days.

Diazepam, a benzodiazepine sometimes used for its skeletal muscle relaxant properties, was discussed in Chapter 19. Although diazepam may modulate spasticity, effective doses often cause intolerable drowsiness.

When withdrawing a patient from therapy, a gradual reduction in dosage over 2 weeks is recommended. Abrupt withdrawal (from baclofen in particular) may cause hallucinations, paranoia, nightmares, confusion, and rebound spasticity.

Despite their different chemical structures, all skeletal muscle relaxants are sedating and are abused primarily for this effect. At high doses, they have been described as producing a buzz (baclofen), euphoria (carisoprodol), and mood enhancement and pleasant misperceptions (orphenadrine). Carisoprodol has been abused more often than other drugs in this class, presumably because of its close similarity to meprobamate. Abusers of either of these drugs demonstrate signs of tolerance and also experience withdrawal symptoms.

The extent to which these drugs are abused is unclear, since they are often used in conjunction with other CNS depressants (e.g., alcohol, benzodiazepines, opioids). In such combinations, skeletal muscle relaxants can be abused to prolong the effects of alcohol or an opioid, to increase the effect of the primary drug of abuse, or to achieve the same effect of alcohol or opioid with a smaller dosage. In comparison to opioids, prescriptions for skeletal muscle relaxants are more easily acquired and are less costly. Substance abusers occasionally substitute a skeletal muscle relaxant when an opioid is not available.

The addictive potential of opioids and benzodiazepines has been well documented, requiring health care providers today to remain conscious of patients' requests for these drugs. In contrast, few health care providers have noted the potential for dependency in prescribing skeletal muscle relaxants. Because skeletal muscle relaxants are not controlled, health care providers may become complacent about their use. Carisoprodol, among other drugs, is also available through veterinary mail-order services. Health care providers and pharmacists should be watchful for patients requesting repeated refills for skeletal muscle relaxants or refills before the conclusion of their current prescription.

Patient Education

Encourage the patient to comply with adjunct therapies for muscle spasm (e.g., rest, application of heat and/or cold, physical therapy). Teach correct posture and lifting techniques. Stress the importance of stooping rather than bending to lift objects, carrying heavy objects close to the body, and not lifting excessive amounts of weight. Regular exercise and the use of warm-up exercises minimize the potential for injury. Strenuous exercise performed infrequently is more likely to cause acute muscle spasm.

Educate the patient and family about the drug prescribed, including the name, the purpose, the dose, administration times and frequency, and potential adverse effects. Warn the patient not to take double doses. If the drug is to be discontinued, instruct the patient to taper the dosage as instructed rather than suddenly stopping the drug.

Advise the patient to avoid activities requiring mental alertness, judgment, and physical coordination, such as operating a motor vehicle, if drowsiness occurs. Alcohol and other CNS depressants increase the CNS depression caused by these drugs, placing the patient at increased risk for injury. Further, because many patients have postural hypotension when taking these drugs, instruct patients to change positions slowly.

Advise the patient not to take other drugs without your or another health care provider's knowledge, including over-the-counter (OTC) products. The major risks occur with concurrent use of alcohol, antihistamines, sleeping aids, or other drugs that cause drowsiness.

Teach the patient taking baclofen that maximum benefit may not be reached for 4 to 8 weeks. The sedative effects are generally transient and usually disappear with continued therapy. Baclofen has been shown to elevate blood sugar. Instruct patients with diabetes mellitus to monitor their blood sugar levels more frequently.

Evaluation

Criteria used to evaluate the therapeutic outcome of therapy for spasms include decreased pain and tenderness, increased mobility, and the ability to participate in the activities of daily living. When a skeletal muscle relaxant is used for the spasticity of chronic neurologic disorders, therapeutic effects include increased ability to maintain posture and balance, increased ability for self-care, improvement in strength and muscle tone, improved coordination, and ease of movement. However, reduction in spasticity does not necessarily correlate with overall functional improvement.

KEY POINTS

- *Spasms* occur as a result of injury to peripheral muscle system structures such as muscles, joints, tendons, or ligaments. Specific causes of spasms include whiplash injuries, cervical root syndrome, herniated discs, and lower back pain syndrome.
- *Spasticity* occurs as a result of damage to upper motor neurons of the brain and spinal cord. Specific disorders associated with spasticity include multiple sclerosis, cerebral palsy, stroke, and closed head injuries.
- Impulses from the injured muscle are transmitted to the spinal cord and back, causing a reflex contraction. The reflex contraction stimulates the muscle, increasing the stimulation of the spinal cord, and thus increasing the contractions.
- The core feature of a spastic state is the exaggeration of stretch reflexes, which manifests as hypertonus. It results from either an increase in excitatory influences or a decrease in inhibitory influences.
- Treatment objectives include the relief of signs and symptoms of muscle spasm. Primary objectives for the management of spasticity are to control symptoms, reduce spasticity, prevent joint and muscle contractures, and improve the quality of life.

- As a general rule, drugs that are used to treat spasticity do not relieve acute muscle spasm, and vice versa. The cornerstone of any treatment of patients with spasticity is the management of underlying disease and physiotherapy.
- Educate the patient and the family about the drug prescribed, including the name, the purpose for use, the dose, administration times and frequency, and potential adverse effects.
- Advise the patient to avoid activities that require mental alertness, judgment, and physical coordination, such as operating a motor vehicle, if drowsy from the drug.
- Criteria used to evaluate the therapeutic outcome of therapy for spasms include decreased pain and tenderness, increased mobility, and the ability to participate in the activities of daily living.
- Therapeutic effects of treatment for spasticity are evidenced as increased ability to maintain posture and balance, increased ability for self-care, improvement in strength and muscle tone, improved coordination, and ease of movement.

Bibliography

Bhakta, B. (2000). Management of spasticity in stroke. *British Medical Bulletin, 56*(2), 476–485.

Brunton, L., Lazo, J., and Parker, K. (Eds.). (2006). *Goodman and Gilman's the pharmacological basis of therapeutics*. (11th ed.). New York: McGraw Hill.

DiPiro, J., Talbert, R., Yee, G., et al. (2005). *Pharmacotherapy: A pathophysiologic approach*. (6th ed.). New York: McGraw-Hill.

Freitag, F. (2003). Preventative treatment for migraine and tension-type headaches: Do drugs having effects on muscle spasm and tone have a role? *CNS Drugs, 17*(6), 373–381.

Granfors, M., Backman, J., Neuvonen, M., et al. (2004). Ciprofloxacin greatly increases concentrations and hypotensive effect of tizanidine by inhibiting its cytochrome P450 1A2-mediated presystemic metabolism. *Clinical Pharmacology and Therapeutics, 76*(6), 598–606.

Gutierrez, K., Queener, S. (2003). *Pharmacology for nursing practice*. St. Louis: Mosby.

Jackson, J., Browning, R. (2005). Impact of national low back pain guidelines on clinical practice. *Southern Medical Journal, 98*(2), 139–143.

Koes, B., van Tulder, M., Ostelo, R., et al. (2001). Clinical guidelines for the management of low back pain in primary care: An

international comparison. *Spine, 26*(22), 2504–2513, discussion 2513–2514.

Leo, R., and Baer, D. (2005). Delirium associated with baclofen withdrawal: A review of common presentations and management strategies. *Psychosomatics, 46*(6), 503–507.

Lofland, J., Szarley, D., Buttaro, T., et al. (2001). *Clinical Journal of Pain, 17*(1), 103–104.

Manniche, C., and Jordon, A. (2003). Re: Tulder, M., Touray, T., Furlan, A., et al. Muscle relaxants for non-specific low back pain: A systematic review within the framework of the Cochrane collaboration. *Spine, 29*(21), 1978–1992.

Materson, R. (1996). The AHCPR practice guidelines for low back pain. *Bulletin on the Rheumatic Diseases, 45*(2), 6–8.

National Institute of Neurologic Disorders and Stroke. Spasticity information. (2006). Available online: www.ninds.nih.gov/disorders/spasticity/spasticity.htm. Accessed April 9, 2007.

Reeves, R., Carter, O., Pinkofsky, H., et al. (1999). Carisoprodol (soma): Abuse potential and physician unawareness. *Journal of Addictive Diseases, 18*(2), 51–56.

Roosth, H. (1997). False assumptions about back pain produced flaws in the AHCPR guideline. *Journal of the Southern Orthopedic Association, 6*(1), 78–79.

CENTRAL NERVOUS

Spasticity Information Center. (2006). Exploring spasticity. Available online: www.medtronic.com/exploringspasticity/explore.html. Accessed April 9, 2007.

van Tulder, M., Touray, T., Furlan, A., et al. (2003). Muscle relaxants for non-specific low-back pain. *The Cochrane Database of Systematic Reviews*. 2003, Issue 4. Art. No. CD004252. DOI: 10.1002/14651858.CD004252.

Waldman, H. (1994). Centrally-acting skeletal muscle relaxants and associated drugs. *Journal of Pain Symptom Management, 9*(7), 434–441.

Drugs Used for Migraines

24

People have suffered from headaches for centuries. Evidence from the seventh century BC shows that one method of treatment involved creating a hole in the skull (a procedure known as trepanation), presumably to relieve the pressure and release the "evil spirits or demons" inside the head that might be causing such pain. Over the next several 1000 years, continued descriptions of headache and its various treatments are found throughout art, literature, and primitive medical texts. Aretaeus of Cappadocia (second century AD) is often credited as the "founder" of migraine science because of his classic descriptions of the condition. Migraine triggers were discovered during this era. For example, Celsus (215–300 AD) correctly described what are now recognized as typical triggers: "drinking wine, or crudity (dyspepsia), or cold, or heat of fire, or the sun." The most common trigger today is stress, followed by hormone fluctuations if the patient is female.

HEADACHES

EPIDEMIOLOGY AND ETIOLOGY

Migraine headache afflicts 10% to 20% of the population, producing a morbidity estimated to be approximately 64 million lost workdays per year in the United States. The National Headache Foundation reports that over 45 million people in the United States have chronic, recurring headaches, and 28 million have migraines. Incidence favors females, with a female-to-male ratio of 2.5:1 at puberty and 3:5.1 at age 40 years, after which the disproportion declines. The incidence declines in persons over 40 years of age, except for women in menopause, when the majority (60%) will have a decrease in headaches but 40% will stay the same or worsen.

The risk of migraine increases fourfold in first-degree relatives of patients who have migraine with aura. Although it generally demonstrates a maternal inheritance pattern, no genetic basis has yet been identified for common migraine. Why some patients experience headaches whereas others do not is unknown, but it is clear that headaches, particularly migraines, tend to cluster in families.

Migraine occurs with increased frequency in patients with mitochondrial disorders such as mitochondrial myopathy, encephalopathy, lactic acidosis, and stroke-like events. It also increases the risk of a variety of diseases such as ischemic stroke (migraine with aura is a risk factor), depression and anxiety, familial cholesterol disorders, hereditary hemorrhagic telangiectasia, hereditary essential tremor, Tourette's syndrome, and patent foramen ovale. Comorbidities also include irritable bowel syndrome (IBS) and mitral valve prolapse (MVP).

More than 99% of headaches are primary and include the tension type of headaches and migraine, cluster, and analgesic rebound headaches (Box 24-1). These headache syndromes are chronic and recurring, but are not typically associated with structural abnormalities or systemic disease. Secondary headaches account for less than 1% of all headaches, occurring as a result of other conditions such as increased intracranial pressure or infection. The prevalence of analgesic rebound headache is small but appears to be on the increase.

PATHOPHYSIOLOGY

Until the 1980s, investigators believed that migraines were linked to the dilation and constriction of blood vessels in the head. Current theory states that headache, and migraine in particular, is caused by innate abnormalities in genes that control the activities of certain cell populations in the brain. A vague and inconsistent pathophysiologic characteristic of migraine is the spreading depression of neural impulses in the cortex from a focal point of vasoconstriction followed by vasodilation. However, it is unlikely that vasoconstriction alone accounts for the local edema and focal tenderness often observed in patients with migraine. The general phases of a migraine are as follows:

- A trigger phase precipitated by external factors
- A prodromal phase (e.g., hunger, fatigue, tingling)
- An aura (visual disturbances that appear such as flashing lights, zigzag lines, or a temporary loss of vision), with inhibition of cortical activity and a reduction in blood flow leading to scotomas and paresthesias (auras occur in about 15% of patients)
- The release of vasoactive neuropeptides (calcitonin gene–related peptide [CGRP], substance P, and neurokinin A), ionic alterations, platelet release of serotonin, and degranulation of mast cells
- Activation of the locus ceruleus, excitation of 5-hydroxytryptamine (5-HT) receptors, and trigeminal nuclei resulting in vasodilation of arteries in the dura mater
- The resulting perivascular inflammation leads to the headache, which is often accompanied by extreme sensitivity to light and sound. The presence of smells, nausea, and vomiting are the criteria for diagnosis of migraine.
- Disturbances in the blood-brain barrier in the area of inflammation cause nausea and vomiting.

The aura in a migraine with aura (previously known as a common migraine) is thought to be caused by neuroelectrical events (Box 24-2). The patient may see flashing lights and colors, or have a loss of peripheral vision lasting 15 to 30 minutes. Pain usually follows the aura, but sometimes the pain and the aura happen at the same time; it is rare for pain not to develop. The pain of classic migraines may be on one side of the head or on both sides and last up to 72 hours; there may be a strange prickly or burning feeling, and a sense of weakness on one side of the body. The patient may have

---

BOX 24-1

Headache Classification

Primary Headaches
1. Migraine
   1.1 Migraine without aura (common migraine)
   1.2 Migraine with aura (classic migraine)
      1.2.1 Typical aura with migraine
      1.2.2 Typical aura with non-migraine headache
      1.2.3 Typical aura without headache
      1.2.4 Familial hemiplegic migraine
      1.2.5 Sporadic hemiplegic migraine
      1.2.6 Basilar-type migraine
   1.3 Childhood periodic syndromes that are commonly precursors to migraine
   1.4 Retinal migraine
   1.5 Complications of migraine
   1.6 Probable migraine
   1.7 Migrainous disorder not fulfilling above criteria
2. Tension type of headache
   2.1 Episodic tension type headache
   2.2 Chronic tension-type headache

   2.3. Headache of the tension-type not fulfilling above criteria
3. Cluster type of headaches and chronic paroxysmal hemicrania
   3.1. Cluster headache
   3.2. Paroxysmal hemicrania
   3.3. Cluster headache not fulfilling above criteria
4. Medication overuse headache (MOH)

Secondary Headaches
1. Miscellaneous primary headaches unassociated with structural lesion
2. Headache attributed to trauma
3. Headache attributed to cranial or cervical vascular disorder
4. Headache attributed to nonvascular intracranial disorder
5. Headache attributed to substances or its withdrawal
6. Headache attributed to noncephalic infection
7. Headache attributed to metabolic disorder or disorder of homeostasis
8. Headache or facial pain not associated with cranium, neck, eyes, ears, sinuses, teeth, mouth, or other facial or cranial structures
9. Cranial neuralgias, nerve trunk pain, and deafferentation pain
10. Headache not classifiable

Partial listing adapted from the World Headache Alliance. (2003). International Headache Society Classification of Headache Disorders. Available online: www.w-h-a.org/wha2/index.asp. Accessed April 9, 2007; and the Headache Classification Committee of the International Headache Society. (2004). The International Classification of Headache Disorders (2nd ed.). *Cephalalgia, 24*(Suppl), 1–150.

---

trouble talking, and feel depressed, grouchy, or restless (see Case Study). *Common migraines* don't start with an aura. Reductions in blood flow have not been observed in patients who have common migraine

In contrast, *tension headaches* start slowly, usually in the middle of the day, and are stress-related with a dull, achy feeling on both sides of the head. There is tightness of head or neck muscles. Tension headaches can be mild or severe. Sometimes, tension headaches are more painful than migraine. Patients with tension headaches and headaches in general frequently self-medicate and may first seek treatment for analgesic rebound headache.

Analgesic rebound headache, also known as *medication overuse headache (MOH)*, is associated with the overuse of simple analgesics, combination agents, opioids, ergot alkaloids, or triptans. An MOH occurs about 15 days a month, appearing with the overuse of drugs for headache relief and going away after withdrawal of the drugs. Although most patients report improvement shortly after withdrawal, 30% to 45% of patients relapse during the first year. Caffeine and butalbital formulations are notorious for causing MOH. Frequent, regular use (i.e., 2 or 3 times/week) is much more likely to cause MOH than taking a drug(s) frequently for several treatment days in a row separated by prolonged treatment-free periods. The initial treatment for MOH consists of withholding all analgesics for 1 to 2 weeks.

Cluster headache is diagnosed when a patient has 5 or more severe, unilateral headaches that are located in the orbital, supraorbital, or temporal regions of the head and can last 15 minutes to 3 hours. These headaches occur most often during the night in males between the ages of 20 and 40 years, although they may be seen in females. The headaches are intermittent in 80% to 90% of patients and may reappear every 2 weeks in some

patients, with each episode lasting 7 days or more. Headaches that are continually present for over 1 year or without sporadic relief are referred to as chronic cluster headaches.

Cluster headaches are often triggered by alcohol intake. Some health care providers feel that the headaches tend to be inherited (i.e., autosomal dominant). Regardless of the trigger, the ganglion of the trigeminal nerve may be partially responsible for the pain on the affected side. Dysfunction of the cranial parasympathetic nerves on the opposite side of the head has also been implicated as a trigger. In addition, it has been noted that testosterone levels decrease during a cluster headache, and the production of melatonin declines. The suprachiasmatic nucleus in the hypothalamus may also be connected to the occurrence of the headaches since this structure has a role in circadian rhythms.

The typical symptoms of a cluster headache usually include, on the affected side, the following: a red, watery eye; photophobia; unilateral sweating of the face or forehead; a stuffy or runny nose; a swollen but drooping eyelid, and pupillary dilation. Patients often describe eye pain as searing or boring inward, or as the worst headache they have ever had.

PHARMACOTHERAPEUTIC OPTIONS

Serotonin Agonists
◆ almotriptan (Axert); ♣ Almogran, Axert
◆ eletriptan (Relpax); ♣ Relert, Relpax
◆ frovatripan (Frova)
◆ naratriptan (Amerge); ♣ Amerge, Naramig
◆ rizatriptan (Maxalt); ♣ Maxalt, Rizalt
◆ sumatriptan (Imitrex); ♣ Imigran, Imitrex
◆ zolmitriptan (Zomig); ♣ Rapimelt

BOX 24-2

Diagnostic Criteria for Headaches

Episodic Tension Headache

At least 10 previous headaches that fulfill the criteria below, with fewer than 180/year or fewer than 15 headaches/month

- Headaches last from 30 minutes to 7 days
- At least two of the following pain characteristics:
  - Bilateral
  - Pressing or tightening quality
  - Mild or moderate intensity that may inhibit but not prevent activity
  - No aggravation with routine physical activities
- No photophobia, nausea, or vomiting

Migraine with Aura

At least two attacks that fulfill the criteria below

- At least three of the following characteristics:
  - One or more fully reversible aura symptoms, including focal cerebral cortex or brainstem dysfunction
  - At least one aura symptom develops gradually over more than 4 minutes, or two or more symptoms occur in succession
  - No aura symptom lasts longer than 60 minutes*
  - Headache follows aura, with a free interval of less than 60 minutes†
- At least one of the following is present:
  - History and physical and neurologic exam do not suggest an organic disorder
  - History and physical and neurologic exam do suggest an organic disorder, but one which is then ruled out through appropriate investigation
  - An organic disorder is present, but migraine attacks do not occur for the first time in close proximity to the disorder

Migraine without Aura

At least five attacks fulfilling the criteria below

- Attacks last 4 to 72 hours (untreated or unsuccessfully treated)
- At least two of the following criteria are present:

- Unilateral location
- Pulsating quality
- Moderate to severe intensity that inhibits or prohibits activities of daily living
- Aggravated by walking stairs or similar routine physical activity
- At least one of the following is present during the headache:
  - Photophobia or phonophobia
  - Nausea or vomiting
- At least one of the following is present:
  - History and physical and neurologic exam do not suggest an organic disorder
  - History and physical and neurologic exam do suggest an organic disorder, but one which is then ruled out through appropriate investigation
  - An organic disorder is present, but migraine attacks do not occur for the first time in close proximity to the disorder

Analgesic Rebound Headache

At least 15 attacks/month fulfilling the criteria below

- At least one of the following is present:
  - History and physical and neurologic exam do not suggest an organic disorder
  - History and physical and neurologic exam suggest an organic disorder, but one which is then ruled out through appropriate investigation
  - Attacks appear with the overuse of drugs for headache relief and go away after withdrawal of the drugs
- At least one of the following is present before the headache:
  - Simple analgesics used more than 5 days for over 3 months
  - Combination drugs used for more than 10 days for over 3 months
  - Opioids used more than 10 days for over 3 months
  - Ergotamine and triptans used more than 10 days/month, for over 3 months

*If migraine lasts over 60 minutes, diagnosis is migraine with prolonged aura. If more than one aura symptom is present, accepted duration is increased proportionally.
†Headache may also begin before or simultaneously with the aura.
Adapted from the Headache Classification Committee of the International Headache Society. (1988). Classification and diagnostic criteria for headache disorders, cranial neuralgias, and facial pain. *Cephalalgia*. 8(Suppl 4), 1–96; and the World Headache Alliance. (2003). International Headache Society Classification of Headache Disorders. Available online: www.w-h-a.org/wha2/index.asp. Accessed April 9, 2007.

Indications

Serotonin agonists, also known as "triptans," are used in adults for the acute treatment of migraine with or without aura. Sumatriptan, the original drug in this class, is also approved for treatment of acute cluster headache. Triptans are used for migraine prophylaxis and are contraindicated for hemiplegic or basilar migraine.

Pharmacodynamics

Serotonin is thought to act as a mediator in the development of migraine headache. As such, the triptans block serotonin (5-HT) receptors, thereby preventing the release of CGRP; they prevent vasodilation and cause a reduction in intracranial pressure; or they block the release of proinflammatory neuropeptides such as brain-derived neurotrophic factor (BDNF) and nerve growth factor (NGF) from presynaptic nerve terminals.

Pharmacokinetics

Triptans are variably absorbed following oral administration. Bioavailability ranges from 14% for oral tablets of sumatriptan to 97% for subcutaneous (subQ) injection. The other triptans average 24% to 74% bioavailability (Table 24-1). The most striking pharmacokinetic characteristic of frovatriptan is its extremely long half-life, which is the longest of the triptan class by a factor of four. This is balanced by a peak of 2 to 3 hours, a low degree of lipophilicity, and a low oral bioavailability of 24% to 30% for frovatriptan. Fifty percent of the drug is renally excreted, and the rest is partially biotransformed by CYP 1A2 enzymes. Naratriptan is eliminated in the urine. Sixty percent of sumatriptan is eliminated in the urine, and 40% in the feces.

Adverse Effects and Contraindications

The adverse effects of triptans are less common following oral than parenteral administration but include dizziness and vertigo,

CASE STUDY   Drugs Used for Migraines

ASSESSMENT

History of Present Illness	SS, a 22-year-old female college student, comes to the clinic for treatment with a severe, throbbing headache she has had for the last 12 hours. She has a lifelong history of left-sided pulsatile head pain recurring on a weekly basis but has been unable to identify headache triggers. The onset of her headache was preceded by bilateral flashes of light and a sensation of lightheadedness that lasted about 15 minutes. The ensuing pain is unilateral and accompanied by two episodes of nausea, vomiting, and photophobia. Her headache was not relieved by two tablets of either aspirin, 325 mg, or ibuprofen, 200 mg, every 4 hours. She reports the headache usually lasts all day unless she is able to lie in a quiet, dark room and sleep. The headaches interfere with her ability to continue work. Current medications include only the OTC analgesics she uses for the headache, albuterol inhaler, and Ortho-Novum 1/35. SS recalls being told by her gynecologist 2 years ago that headaches are a possible adverse effect of oral contraceptives but did not associate the drug with the recent onset of migraine attacks. No known drug allergies.
Past Health History	Past health history is unremarkable except for exercise-induced asthma. SS denies any other medical problems. Her mother and grandmother also suffer from migraine headaches on a regular basis.
Life-Span Considerations	As a senior, SS lives on the university campus in a noisy coed dormitory. She is of child-bearing age and has been taking oral contraceptives since she was 17 years of age. Her parents live three states away. She flies home once or twice a semester for a weekend visit.
Psychosocial Considerations	SS is a nonsmoker and nondrinker. She enjoys all types of sports but excels in lacrosse and is the team captain. Her lacrosse games sometimes interfere with her ability to study. She hopes to graduate next spring (with honors) with a bachelor's degree in sports medicine.
Physical Exam	VS stable. *Height:* 5'3''. *Weight:* 184 pounds. EOMI, PERRLA. No papilledema. Photophobic. CN-II-XII intact. There is an absence of sweating on the ipsilateral face and neck. No nuchal rigidity. Rapid alternative movement's intact upper and lower extremities. DTRs 2+ with equal strength and tone upper and lower extremities. Rhomberg negative.
Lab Testing	ESR and CBC within normal limits. No diagnostic imaging done.

DIAGNOSIS: Migraine with aura

MANAGEMENT

Treatment Objectives	Decrease headache frequency, duration, disability, and symptoms, time between attacks, and intensity of care using appropriate therapies.
Treatment Plan	**Pharmacotherapy** • Promethazine, 25 mg suppository per rectum now • Rizatriptan ODT (Maxalt-MLT), 10 mg now. May repeat dose every 2 hours if needed for 2 doses. Not to exceed 30 mg/24 hours. To use as rescue drug only. • Stop oral contraceptive; use alternative, nonhormonal method **Patient Education** 1. Provide list of migraine triggers and review with patient. 2. Stop aspirin and ibuprofen to avoid MOH. 3. Advise patient to take rizatriptan ODT with the onset of a headache rather than waiting for the headache to be fully involved. 4. Explain the purpose for an angiotensin receptor–blocker in headache prophylaxis. 5. Encourage the use of stress-reduction strategies. 6. Encourage patient to explore the use of nonhormonal contraceptive methods. 7. Continue albuterol inhaler, 2 puffs 20 minutes before exercise. 8. Follow-up in office in 1 month to further discuss the use of topiramate as prophylaxis. **Evaluation** Headache symptoms have decreased in terms of character, frequency, duration, disability, time between attacks, and intensity.

Continued

CASE STUDY   Drugs Used for Migraines—Cont'd

CLINICAL REASONING ANALYSIS

Q1. I thought that promethazine was a nonselective antihistamine. Why are we using it for nausea and vomiting and giving it rectally?

A. Promethazine is a nonselective H_1 blocker. By antagonizing central and peripheral H_1 receptors, the nausea and vomiting should be relieved. The drug is formulated as a tablet, syrup, IM solution, and suppository. We are using the suppository just now because she can't keep anything down.

Q2. Why did you choose rizatriptan for her acute headache rather than one of the other triptans?

A. Compared with 100 mg of sumatriptan, rizatriptan has been shown effective in relieving headache pain within 2 hours, provides long-lasting pain relief, is generally well tolerated, and has been found to consistently relieve migraine headaches. In comparison, the other triptans are less efficacious overall, and sumatriptan has too many adverse effects to be used comfortably. Eletriptan, 80 mg may be helpful, but it is not approved for use in the United States at this dose.

Q3. I read in my textbook that other drugs such as propranolol can be used as migraine prophylaxis. Why can't she take a beta blocker?

A. Since SS is a lacrosse star, she needs to be able to raise her heart rate when playing. A beta blocker such as propranolol is nonselective, thus blocking β_1 and β_2 receptors. It would keep her heart rate down and potentially narrow her airways, which will aggravate her exercise-induced asthma.

Q4. Assuming SS improves with the headache medicine you ordered for her, why do we still need to stop her birth control?

A. Oral contraceptives either worsen or precipitate migraine attacks in some women without a previous history of this problem. Although headaches usually arise within the first few months of contraceptive use, headaches can develop several years later. Also, women who have migraine symptoms while on oral contraceptives may be at increased risk for stroke.

as well as a warm, tingling sensation. For some patients, there is a feeling of chest heaviness or tightness, drowsiness, anxiety, malaise, fatigue, and weakness. There may be throat and sinus discomfort, as well as alterations in vision. Patients may note abdominal discomfort and dysphagia. **The most life-threatening adverse effects of triptans include myocardial infarction in patients with known coronary artery disease.**

Triptans are contraindicated for use in patients with hypersensitivity, ischemic heart disease, or signs and symptoms of ischemic heart disease, Prinzmetal's angina, or uncontrolled hypertension. They should be used with caution in patients with any history of cardiovascular disease, in patients of childbearing age, and during pregnancy (triptans are pregnancy category C) and lactation, as well as in children under 18 years of age.

PHARMACOKINETICS

TABLE 24-1 Drugs Used for Migraines

Drug	Route	Onset	Peak	Duration	PB (%)	$t_{1/2}$
SEROTONIN AGONISTS						
almotriptan	PO	30–60 min	1–3 hr	>12 hr	35	3–4 hr
eletriptan	PO	30–60 min	1.5 hr	>20 hr	85	4.4 hr
frovatripan	PO	1–2 hr	2–4 hr	>24 hr	15	26 hr
naratriptan	PO	30–60 min	2–3 hr	>24 hr	28–31	6 hr
rizatriptan	PO	30–60 min	1–1.5 hr	14–16 hr	14	2–3 hr
sumatriptan	PO	30–60 min	1–2 hr	10 hr	10–21	1–2 hr
	SubQ	10 min	12 min	Short	10–21	1–2 hr
	Nasal	15 min	1–1.5 hr	Short	14–21	1–2 hr
zolmitriptan	PO	45 min	1.5–2 hr	Short	Low	2–3 hr
	Nasal	2 min	5 min	Short	Low	2–3 hr
ERGOT ALKALOIDS						
dihydroergotamine	IV	15–30 min	15 min-2 hr	3–4 hr	93	9 hr
	SubQ	10 min	15 min	3–4 hr	93	18–32 hr*
	IM	10 min	15 min	3–4 hr	93	9 hr
ergotamine	SL	Rapid	30 min-3 hr	UA	90	3 hr; 21 hr*
MISCELLANEOUS DRUGS						
topiramate	PO	Rapid	2 hr; 4 days to steady state	UA	15–41	21 hr

*Half life includes metabolites.
IV, intravenous; *IM*, intramuscular; *PB*, protein binding; *PO*, by mouth; *SL*, sublingual; *subQ*, subcutaneous; $t_{1/2}$, serum half-life; *UA*, unavailable.

🔍 EVIDENCE-BASED PHARMACOTHERAPEUTICS

Neutrophins and Migraines

■ Background

Brain-derived neurotrophic factor (BDNF) is one of four neutrophins expressed throughout the central nervous system (CNS) as well as in the periphery. Although known primarily for their role in neuronal development, nerve growth factor (NGF) is one of the other neutrophins found in many cells and tissues including the brain, the meninges, and cerebral spinal fluid. BDNF and NGF protect nerve cells from programmed cell death and thus promote the survival of neuronal populations located in the CNS. BDNF and NGF have been implicated in the creation and modulation of pain. Whether or not these substances are involved in subjects suffering from nociceptive disorders, such as primary headaches, is uncertain.

Platelets are the cellular elements with the highest content of 5-hydroxytryptamine (5-HT), which is taken up from plasma and stored in dense bodies and which, upon release, exerts a pronounced vasomotor activity. Consequently, platelets have long been implicated as important contributors to the peripheral 5-HT pathogenic component of migraine headache.

■ Research Article

Blandini, F., Rinaldi, L., Tassorelli, C., et al. (2006). Peripheral levels of BDNF and NGF in primary headaches. *Cephalalgia, 26*(2), 136–142.

Purpose

To investigate whether alterations in BDNF and NGF levels can be detected in subjects affected by migraine with aura, or migraine without aura, and cluster headaches, and to verify platelet levels of 5-HT and its primary metabolite 5-HIAA in the same clinical setting.

Design

This Italian study used a control-group design to determine if peripheral (platelet and plasma) levels of BDNF and NGF were detected in subjects suffering from migraine with or without aura, or cluster headache, and in healthy volunteers. The sample group was comprised of 60 subjects suffering from migraine (27 with aura; 33 without aura) and 14 subjects affected by cluster headaches. Women participating in the study were in the follicular phase of their menstrual cycle. All subjects were initially evaluated during a headache-free period and asked to keep a daily headache diary. BDNF and NGF levels were evaluated during the interictal phase of subjects' headaches.

Methods

The control group included 57 age-and sex-matched healthy subjects, none of whom suffered from migraine or cluster headaches, or had more than two episodes per year of the tension type of headache. Subjects and the control group had not taken analgesics, nonsteroidal antiinflammatory drugs (NSAIDs), or 5-HT-related drugs for at least 7 days before the study. For subjects with cluster headaches, only symptomatic treatment with oxygen was permitted in the 7 days preceding the examination.

BDNF and NGF assays were carried out using standard laboratory procedures. Ordinary ANOVA using nonparametric methods was done for all comparisons. NGF, BDNF, 5-HT, and 5-HIAA levels were compared for all four groups using the Kruskal-Wallis test followed by the Dunn multiple comparison posthoc test, with a level of $\alpha = 0.05$ (significant difference, $p = 0.05$).

Findings

All subjects with primary headaches showed significantly decreased platelet levels of BDNF (migraine vs. controls $p < 0.001$; cluster headache vs. controls $p < 0.01$), whereas a selective reduction of platelet NGF was observed in migraine sufferers and not in cluster headache subjects, compared with control subjects (migraine vs. control; $p < 0.001$). These changes did not coincide with significant modifications in neurotrophin plasma levels.

Conclusions

These findings show for the first time that changes in peripheral levels of neurotrophins are elevated in subjects suffering from different types of primary headaches, suggesting a potential involvement in BDNF and NGG in the pathophysiology of these disorders.

■ Implications for Practice

These findings raise the possibility that differences in peripheral neurotrophins may help distinguish migraine biologically from cluster headaches. Further studies are needed to define the specificity of these findings with regard to primary headache vs. other pain disorders.

▦ *Drug Interactions*

Many drugs interact with triptans; the primary concern is sustained vasoconstriction and vasospasm leading to ischemia. These drugs include macrolide antibiotics, azole antifungal drugs, and ergotamine, caffeine, nefazodone, nelfinavir, ritonavir, and CYP 3A4 inhibitors. Naratriptan and frovatriptan interact with many drugs, with a small risk of serotonin syndrome (Table 24-2). Serotonin syndrome is caused by too much serotonin in the brain. It is manifest by headaches, dizziness, anxiety, agitation, restlessness, confusion, tremors, hyperreflexia, elevated blood pressure, and diaphoresis.

▦ *Dosage Regimen*

The dosage regimen of the triptans varies with the individual drug. Table 24-3 identifies the dosages. Most of the drug doses may be repeated in 2 hours if needed; the naratriptan dose may be repeated in 4 hours. Each of the triptans has a maximum dosage regardless of the route of administration. Sumatriptan and zolmitriptan have nasal spray formulations.

▦ *Lab Considerations*

Triptans are not known to interfere with commonly used clinical laboratory tests.

Ergot Alkaloids

◆ dihydroergotamine (DHE, Migranal); ♣ Dihydroergotamine
◆ ergotamine (Cafergot); ♣ Ergomar

▦ *Indications*

The use of moldy rye in the Middle Ages was responsible for a disease known as St. Anthony's fire (ergotism), which was characterized by hallucinations and gangrene of the limbs. The cause of the disease was actually the lack of blood flow in the extremities caused by the powerful alpha-agonist effects of the ergot alkaloids, and their associated CNS stimulatory effects.

Ergot alkaloids (i.e., alpha blockers) are used to improve cerebral circulation. Ergotamine and dihydroergotamine (DHE) are used in the management of migraine and cluster headaches. For acute moderate to severe migraines, DHE nasal spray has been found to be safe and effective. Oral or rectal ergotamine (and caffeine combinations) may also be considered for patients under age 40 years who have been unresponsive to previous therapies. SubQ, intravenous (IV), intramuscular (IM), and the nasal formulations of DHE can be used for patients with nausea and vomiting.

DRUG INTERACTIONS
TABLE 24-2 Drugs Used for Migraines

Drug	Interacting Drug	Interaction
SEROTONIN AGONISTS		
Triptans in general	ergotamine, caffeine	Prolongs vasospastic reactions
almotriptan	lithium, MAO inhibitors, SSRIs	Reduces almotriptan clearance
	erythromycin, fluoxetine, itraconazole, propranolol, ritonavir, verapamil	Increases plasma concentration of almotriptan
eletriptan	clarithromycin, ketoconazole, itraconazole, nefazodone, nelfinavir, ritonavir, CYP 3A4 inhibitors	Increases plasma concentration of eletriptan
frovatriptan, naratriptan	sibutramine	Increases risk of serotonin syndrome (additive effect)
	St. John's wort	Increases or decreases triptan levels; increases risk of serotonin syndrome
	acetaminophen, tramadol, buspirone, topical cocaine, duloxetine, mirtazapine, nefazodone, olanzapine, pentazocine, all SSRIs, trazodone, venlafaxine	Increases risk of serotonin syndrome
	butorphanol nasal	Increases risk of transient rise in BP
	propranolol	Increases levels of triptan
rizatriptan, sumatriptan, zolmitriptan	MAO-A inhibitors, propranolol, cimetidine	Increases plasma levels of triptan
	linezolid	Increases rizatriptan levels
zolmitriptan	Oral contraceptives	Delays onset of zolmitriptan
ERGOT ALKALOIDS		
dihydroergotamine	Triptans, azole antifungals	Increased risk of severe, prolonged vasospasm
	bromocriptine, clarithromycin, conivaptin, delaviridine, diltiazem, efavirenz, erythromycin, fluoxetine, grapefruit juice, metronidazole, nefazodone, olanzapine, imatinib, protease inhibitors, all SSRIs, telithromycin	Increases risk of ergot toxicity; severe vasospasm and ischemia
	Nitrates	Decreases nitrate efficacy, increases DHE levels, risk of vasoconstriction, angina, ischemia
ergotamine	Beta blockers, erythromycin	Increases risk of vasospasm
	Nitrates	Decreases nitrate efficacy
	Systemic vasoconstrictors	Increases pressor effects
MISCELLANEOUS DRUGS		
topiramate	digoxin	Decreases AUC. Clinical significance uncertain
	CNS depressants, alcohol, ethosuximide	Increases risk of CNS depression, psychomotor impairment
	Oral contraceptives	Reduces oral contraceptive efficacy and increases risk for breakthrough bleeding
	hydrochlorothiazide	Decreases potassium levels
	lithium	Decreases serum levels of lithium
	amitriptyline	Increases amitriptyline concentration
	risperidone	Decreases serum levels of risperidone
	Carbonic anhydrase inhibitors	Increases risk for renal stones, hyperthermia
	valproic acid and derivatives	Elevates serum ammonia levels; increases risk of encephalitis
	Antiepileptic drugs in general	Decreases topiramate concentration
	metformin, phenytoin,	Increases metformin levels
	pioglitazone	Decreases pioglitazone and active metabolite levels

AUC, Area under the curve; *BP,* blood pressure; *CNS,* central nervous system; *DHE,* dihydroergotamine; *MAO,* monoamine oxidase; *SSRIs,* selective serotonin reuptake inhibitors.

Pharmacodynamics

The ergot alkaloids are a group of indole-containing alkaloids produced by the mold *Claviceps purpurea*, a common mold that grows on grains, especially rye, under damp growing or storage conditions. This fungus synthesizes histamine, acetylcholine, tyramine, and other biologically active products, in addition to a score of unique ergot alkaloids.

Ergotamine and similar drugs have agonist and antagonist actions with adrenergic (α_1, α_2), serotonergic (5-HT$_{1B}$, 5-HT$_{1D}$, 5-HT$_{2A}$, 5-HT$_{2B}$), and dopaminergic (D$_2$) receptors. They may also inhibit the reuptake of norepinephrine. These drugs directly stimulate vascular smooth muscle, thus constricting veins and arteries. The spectrum of effect depends on the drug, the dosage, the species, the tissue, and the physiologic and neuroendocrine states.

Pharmacokinetics

The ergot alkaloids are variably absorbed from the gastrointestinal (GI) tract (see Table 24-1). Absorption after IM injection is slow but usually reliable. The bioavailability of oral and sublingual ergotamine is poor compared with that

CENTRAL NERVOUS

DOSAGE
TABLE 24-3 Drugs Used For Headaches

Drug	Indication(s)	Dosage Regimen	Implications
SEROTONIN AGONISTS			
almotriptan	Acute migraine with or without aura	*Adult:* 6.25–12.5 mg PO as single dose; may repeat in 2 hr to max of 2 doses/24 hr	Reduce dosage in patients with mild to moderate renal or hepatic dysfunction.
eletriptan	Acute migraine with or without aura	*Adult:* 20–40 mg PO as single dose; may repeat at 2-hr intervals to max of 80 mg/24 hr	Do not crush or break film-coated tablets. May decrease possibility of ovulation.
frovatriptan	Acute migraine with or without aura	*Adult:* 2.5 mg PO as single dose; may repeat at 2-hr intervals to max of 7.5 mg/24 hr	Do not crush or break film-coated tablets.
naratriptan	Acute migraine with or without aura	*Adult:* 1–2.5 mg PO as single dose; may repeat in 4 hr to max of 5 mg/24 hr	Reduce dosage in patients with mild to moderate renal or hepatic dysfunction.
rizatriptan	Acute migraine with or without aura	*Adult:* 5–10 mg PO or in orally disintegrating dose as single dose; may repeat in 2 hr to max of 30 mg/24 hr	Oral disintegrating tablets are packed in aluminum pouches. Place tablet on tongue, allow to dissolve, and swallow along with saliva. Administration of water is not necessary.
sumatriptan	Acute migraine with or without aura	*Adult:* 25–100 mg PO as single dose; may repeat after 2 hr to max of 200 mg/24 hr –or– 6 mg subQ to max of 2 injections/24 hr –or– 5–20 mg nasal spray; may repeat after 2 hr to max of 40 mg/24 hr	Injectable formulation should be given in presence of health care provider. Do not confuse sumatriptan with somatropin, a growth hormone.
zolmitriptan	Acute migraine with or without aura	*Adult:* 2.5 mg PO as single dose; may repeat in 2 hr to max of 10 mg/24 hr –or– 5 mg nasal spray as single dose; may repeat in 2 hr	May take without regard to food.
ERGOT ALKALOIDS			
dihydroergotamine	Acute migraine with or without aura	*Adult:* 1 mg single dose IM, subQ; may repeat hourly to max of 3 mg/day or 6 mg/wk –or– 1 mg IV to max of 2 mg/day or 6 mg/wk –or– 1 spray (0.5 mg) into each nostril; may repeat in 15 min to max of 4 sprays/24 hr or 8 sprays/wk	Initiate therapy at first sign of headache. **Prolonged administration or excessive dosage may produce ergot toxicity**. Monitor closely for evidence of overdosage as a result of unrelieved headache.
ergotamine	Acute migraine with or without aura	*Adult:* 2 mg PO at onset of headache, then 1–2 mg every 30 min PRN to max of 6 mg/episode or mg/wk –or– 1 SL tablet at onset of headache, then 1 tablet every 30 min to max of 3 tablets/day or 5 tablets/wk *Child:* 1 mg PO, SL at onset of headache, then 1 mg every 30 min to max of 3 mg/episode	Initiate therapy at first sign of headache. Prolonged administration or excessive dosage may produce ergot toxicity. Monitor closely for evidence of overdosage as a result of unrelieved headache.
MISCELLANEOUS DRUGS			
topiramate	Migraine prophylaxis	*Adult:* 25 mg daily to 50 mg twice daily. Max 600 mg/day *Child 2–16 yr:* 1–3 mg/kg/day initially to max of 25 mg/day. May increase dosage at weekly intervals.	Dosage adjustment may be needed for patients with renal disease, those on dialysis, and those >age 65 yr. Pregnancy category C.

CAD, Coronary artery disease; *IM,* intramuscular (route); *PO,* by mouth; *PRN,* as needed; *SL,* sublingual (route); *subQ,* subcutaneous (route).

of inhalation formulations. The ergot alkaloids have an extensive first-pass effect and are extensively biotransformed in the liver by largely undefined pathways. Ninety percent of ergotamine metabolites are eliminated in the bile in a biphasic process.

▥ Adverse Effects and Contraindications

The common adverse effects of ergot alkaloids include numbness, tingling of fingers and toes, extremity muscle

pain, nausea and vomiting (these drugs stimulate the chemoreceptor trigger zone), precordial distress and pain, transient tachycardia, transient changes in heart rate (e.g., bradycardia), and localized edema. Approximately 10% of patients experience nausea and vomiting after receiving therapeutic dosages of ergotamine.

Ergotism can occur with prolonged use of ergot alkaloids. Symptoms of ergotism include nausea, vomiting, diarrhea, severe thirst, hypoperfusion, chest pain, blood pressure changes, and confusion. Drug dependence and abuse may develop with extended use. Ergot alkaloids are pregnancy category X.

Drug Interactions

Most drugs that interact with ergot alkaloids have the potential to cause prolonged vasoconstriction and vasospasm with the risk of ischemia (see Table 24-2). Macrolide antibiotics increase the risk of ergot toxicity.

Dosage Regimen

Ergot alkaloids are taken by mouth during an acute attack, or the drugs may be given by subQ , IM, or IV routes (see Table 24-3). The oral dose of ergotamine is about 10 times larger than the IM dose, but the speed of absorption and peak blood levels after oral administration can be improved by administration of caffeine.

Lab Considerations

There are no significant laboratory considerations for ergotamine and DHE.

Migraine Prophylaxis Drugs

◆ topiramate (Topamax); ◆ Topamax

Indications

Topiramate is approved by the Food and Drug Administration (FDA) for migraine prophylaxis but is ineffective for treatment of acute migraine. Topiramate is also indicated in the treatment of partial seizures (see Chapter 25).

Pharmacodynamics

Gamma-aminobutyric acid (GABA) is the principal inhibitory neurotransmitter in the brain. Without adequate inhibition from GABA, the brain may be more predisposed to migraines. Topiramate is thought to block the repetitive firing of CNS neurons by enhancing the ability of GABA to cause an influx of chloride ions into CNS neurons. Topiramate also blocks sodium channels, reduces the activity of calcium channels, and inhibits the enzyme carbonic anhydrase. Through these mechanisms, there is a reduction in headache pain, frequency, and duration.

Glutamate is the principal excitatory neurotransmitter in the brain. Excessive glutamate activity may contribute to a hyperexcitable state, and blocking the effect of glutamate thus increases the efficacy of topiramate.

Pharmacokinetics

Topiramate is rapidly absorbed after oral administration (see Table 24-1). The sprinkle formulation of topiramate is both bioequivalent and therapeutically equivalent to the immediate release form. Topiramate is minimally biotransformed, and although six metabolites have been identified, they make up less than 5% of an orally administered dose of the drug. Approximately 70% of an oral dose of topiramate is eliminated unchanged in the urine.

Adverse Effects and Contraindications

Most adverse effects of topiramate are dose dependent. They occur more often during upward titration of dosage (rather than with maintenance dosages) and vary in severity from mild to moderate, although some can be severe enough to require withdrawal of the drug from therapy. The adverse effects include nervousness, somnolence, fatigue, ataxia, paresthesias, tremors, nystagmus, diplopia, and nausea. Psychomotor retardation, altered ability to concentrate, word-finding difficulties, and memory disturbances occasionally occur. Although rare, confusion, breast pain, dysmenorrhea, depression, asthenia, pharyngitis, anorexia, rash, musculoskeletal pain, sinusitis, agitation, and flulike symptoms have occurred.

Drug Interactions

Drug interactions with topiramate are identified in Table 24-2. Cautious use is warranted in patients who have diabetes because concurrent use of topiramate with metformin increases metformin levels, thus increasing the risk for hypoglycemia and lactic acidosis. Used in combination with topiramate, pioglitazone and phenytoin levels may be decreased.

Dosage Regimen

Dose and titration rates of topiramate are guided by patient response. Longer dosing intervals can be used when necessary to reduce adverse effects. Topiramate dosages range from 25 mg/day to a maximum of 500 to 600 mg/day based on patient response (see Table 24-3). Overdoses of topiramate have been reported. **Signs and symptoms of topiramate** ⚠ **overdosage include blurry vision, diplopia, difficulty speaking, drowsiness, dizziness, agitation, altered mental status and coordination, lethargy, depression, seizures, hypotension, abdominal pain, and possible seizures.** In most cases, the outcomes of topiramate overdose are not severe; however, metabolic acidosis and deaths have been reported.

Lab Considerations

Topiramate does not alter the results of commonly used laboratory tests.

Divalproex Sodium

Of all antiepileptic drugs (AEDs) used for migraine, divalproex sodium (Depakote) has undergone the most study (see Chapter 25 for further discussion of divalproex sodium). Currently, divalproex sodium is the only AED that has received FDA approval for the management of migraine. AEDs are known to be effective for neuropathic pain, so it is reasonable to conclude that divalproex sodium may also be effective for migraine prophylaxis as well as provide an alternative to conventional migraine prophylaxis. About half of the patients who use divalproex sodium for migraine have a 50% reduction in the number of attacks or days with the headache. The adverse effects of divalproex sodium are not insignificant, though, and include nausea, dizziness, and drowsiness.

CLINICAL REASONING

Treatment Objectives

Headaches vary in intensity, duration and frequency, their effects on functional abilities, and the interval between attacks. The severity of the headache is evaluated according to symptoms and functional impairments. It is inappropriate to prolong use of ineffective or poorly tolerated drugs.

CENTRAL NERVOUS

Consider ongoing headache prophylaxis (whether or not an attack is currently underway) for patients who have one to two disabling headaches per month, or two to three headaches per week, and who have not responded to acute interventions. Prophylaxis is also indicated when reliance on acute care drugs increases the potential for MOH. The short-term objectives of headache management include the following:

- Timely, consistent intervention for headache attacks
- Restoring the patient's functional abilities
- Reducing reliance on rescue drugs (see also Chapter 16)
- Optimizing self-care and reducing inappropriate use of health care resources (i.e., emergency rooms)
- Reducing the risk for adverse effects
- Maintaining a cost-effective management plan

The long-term objectives of headache management include the following:

- Reducing the frequency of, the severity of, and disability caused by the headache while avoiding adverse effects
- Reducing reliance on poorly tolerated, ineffective, or unwanted acute drug therapy
- Improving the patient's quality of life
- Avoiding escalation in the use of acute headache remedies, headache-related distress, and psychologic symptoms
- Helping patients manage and gain personal control of their headache

To meet these objectives, the health care provider must accurately diagnose and manage the headache. In patients with a long history of near-daily or daily headaches, a more realistic goal may be reducing the intensity of pain and restoring the patient's functional ability, while providing an effective strategy for acute management of severe headaches. The goals of withdrawal for patients who have MOH include the following:

- Stopping daily or near-daily drug use of analgesics and its associated symptoms
- Restoring an episodic headache pattern
- Establishing an effective management strategy that includes both preventive and acute drugs

Treatment Options

Primary prevention is the most effective modality for headaches and migraine and includes identifying migraine triggers and using non–drug therapies such as progressive muscle relaxation strategies, stress management, biofeedback, and cognitive-behavioral strategies. Failure to initiate therapy in a timely fashion increases pain, disability, and the impact of the headache (see Table 24-4).

▮ *Patient Variables*

Headaches are often underdiagnosed and undertreated even in the face of substantial disability, often because of patients' inability to recognize their headache as migraine, cluster, tension, or (MOH), or to adequately self-report symptoms. Before starting drug therapy, it is important to determine the type and frequency of the headache and identify any over-the-counter (OTC) drugs used. Uncontrolled hypertension, heart disease, and pregnancy should be identified before initiating therapy, since they may restrict treatment options.

A full neurologic exam should be done at the first visit, although ordinarily the findings will all be normal. Neuroimaging is usually not recommended in a typical presentation of headache. Simple assessment tools like the Migraine Assessment of Current Therapy (Migraine-ACT) can be used to quantify the extent of the disability on the first visit and at follow-up visits (see Box 24-3).

LIFE-SPAN CONSIDERATIONS

Pregnant and Nursing Women. Migraines occur more often in women than men, likely because of estrogen, although most headaches improve with pregnancy. Pregnancy is of primary concern, if drug therapy for migraines is to be initiated. Migraines often diminish in number and intensity during the second and third trimesters.

Drugs selected for migraine treatment or prophylaxis should be safe for use during pregnancy. Acetaminophen is the safest analgesic during pregnancy but may be ineffective for migraines. Ibuprofen may be used in the first and second trimesters only. If a stronger drug is needed, acetaminophen with codeine may be used sparingly. If prophylaxis is needed, fluoxetine (pregnancy category B) can be used. Although pregnancy category C drugs, triptans, amitriptyline, propranolol, gabapentin, or topiramate may also be used in patients with severe migraine during pregnancy, these drugs should be prescribed by a neurologist. Labetolol has been efficacious in some patients during pregnancy (Dey et al., 2002). Use of ergotamine derivatives, valproic acid and its derivatives, high dosages of vitamin B_2, angiotensin-converting enzyme inhibitors (ACEIs), and angiotensin receptor blockers (ARBs) are contraindicated during pregnancy. (Fluoxetine is further discussed under Antidepressants, Vitamin B_2 under Riboflavin, and ACEIs and the ARBs in an eponymous section under Other Prophylaxis Drugs.)

Children and Adolescents. The most common headache in children is migraine, although it presents differently than in adults. Pediatric headaches are usually shorter than those in adults, lasting 1 to 2 hours; the pain is throbbing and pulsating but tends to be frontal or temporal in location. Pediatric migraines are best managed by simple analgesics such as acetaminophen or ibuprofen along with an antiemetic drug if needed, if the child is not of adult height and weight. For adolescents who are of adult weight, recent studies have shown that triptan nasal sprays are effective, although orally administered triptans are still not acceptable for use before adulthood. Prophylaxis is the same as for an adult, either a low-dose tricyclic antidepressant (TCA; see later discussion under Antidepressants) or topiramate. Propranolol, a beta blocker, may be used for prophylaxis in some children (Victor and Ryan, 2003).

Older Adults. New-onset migraines are unusual in adults over age 50 years. However, when present, the normal changes in renal and hepatic function with advancing age may require adjustment in drug dosages or frequency. A new headache pattern in an older adult should make the health care provider suspicious of organic disease or an adverse effect of other drugs. Consider in particular a diagnosis of temporal arteritis. Temporal arteritis involves inflammation and damage to blood vessels, particularly the large or medium arteries branching from the external carotid artery of the neck. The disorder should not be overlooked as a differential diagnosis, because it may cause obstruction of the arteries of the eye, leading to blindness or ophthalmoplegia; other complications include transient ischemic attacks and stroke. The treatment goal for temporal arteritis is to

TABLE 24-4 Overview of Common Headaches

Characteristic	Migraine without Aura (Common Migraine)	Migraine with Aura (Classic Migraine)	Cluster Headache, Pericranial Headache	Tension Headache	Medication Overuse Headache (MOH)
Age of onset	Childhood, adolescence, or young adulthood	Childhood, adolescence, or young adulthood	Young adulthood, middle age	Young adulthood, middle age	Young adulthood, middle age
Sex	Female	Female	Male	Not sex-specific	Not sex-specific
Family history of headaches	Yes	Yes	No	Yes	Sometimes
Evolution	Slow to rapid	Slow to rapid	Rapid	Slow to rapid	Predictably after last dose of drug
Time course	Episodic	Episodic	Clusters in time	Episodic, but may be constant	Episodic; ~15 days/month
Quality	Usually throbbing	Usually throbbing	Steady	Steady tightness or pressure not related to activity	Steady
Location	Variable, often unilateral	Variable, often unilateral	Orbit, temple, cheek	Variable	Variable
Associated symptoms	Prodrome, vomiting	Prodrome, vomiting	Lacrimation, rhinorrhea, Horner's syndrome	Nausea (no vomiting), photophobia, tenderness pericranial and neck muscles	Early morning headache
Acute treatment*	*Specific:* naratriptan PO; rizatriptan PO; sumatriptan IN, subQ, PO; zolmitriptan PO; DHE all routes; DHE IV + antiemetic *Nonspecific:* acetaminophen, aspirin, + caffeine PO; aspirin PO, butorphanol IN, ibuprofen PO, naproxen sodium PO, prochlorperazine IV		Oxygen 8 L/mask for 10 min; subQ sumatriptan, ergotamine, DHE	Cognitive-behavioral therapy, biofeedback; stress-reduction strategies	Withdrawal therapy; clonidine patch
Prophylaxis†	Avoid triggers. Antiepileptics (divalproex sodium, sodium valproate, topiramate), TCAs (amitriptyline), SSRIs (fluoxetine), BB (timolol, propranolol), CCB (nimodipine, verapamil)		Avoid triggers. CCB verapamil), prednisone, DHE, ergotamine, lithium, valproic acid, occipital nerve steroid injection	Avoid triggers. Cognitive-behavioral therapy, biofeedback; stress-reduction strategies	Avoid triggers. BB (timolol, propranolol), antiepileptics (valproic acid); TCAs (amitriptyline), CCBs (nimodipine, verapamil)

*†Proven statistical and clinical benefit based on at least two double-blind, placebo-controlled studies and scientific and clinical impression of effect.
ACEI, Angiotensin-converting enzyme inhibitor; *ARB,* angiotensin receptor blocker; *BB,* beta blocker; *CCB,* calcium channel blocker; *DHE,* dihydroergotamine; *IM,* intramuscular (route); *IN,* intranasal (route); *PO,* by mouth; *IV,* intravenous (route); *subQ,* subcutaneous (route); *SSRI,* selective serotonin reuptake inhibitor; *TCA,* tricyclic antidepressant.
Adapted from McCance, K., and Huether, S. (2002). *Pathophysiology: The biologic basis for disease in adults and children.* (4th ed.). St. Louis: Mosby; and Srivastava, S., and Cowan, R. (2006). Pathophysiology and treatment of migraine and related headache. *eMedicine.* August 4. Available online: www.emedcine.com/neuro/topic517.htm. Accessed April 9, 2007.

minimize the irreversible tissue damage that occurs because of lack of blood flow. Most people make a full recovery, but 1 to 2 years of treatment may be necessary. Recurrence is possible for several years.

Hypnic headache is an exclusively nocturnal headache in older adults. They often occur 4 or more nights per week and usually last less than 2 hours. These headaches are worsened by lying down and typically lack autonomic or migrainous qualities. Treatment for hypnic headaches usually includes indomethacin, lithium, and caffeine.

The worsening of a migraine just before menopause may be related to hormone fluctuations. Women using hormone replacement therapy (HRT) are 40% more likely to have migraines than those not on HRT. If the woman must stay on HRT, she may be switched to pure estradiol or synthetic ethinyl estradiol, or the HRT dosage may be reduced. Continuous dosing rather than cyclical HRT therapy often reduces migraine frequency.

As menopause progresses, plasma levels of sex steroids decline and migraine headaches frequently abate. This suggests that factors other than sex hormones may contribute to the predominance of migraine in women. The reasons for this are not well understood.

Drug Variables

Most drugs cause a reduction in the severity and number of headaches. Their efficacy varies with the absence or presence of aura, the duration of the headache, its severity and intensity, and as yet undefined environmental and genetic factors. Patients with occasional, mild headache symptoms can be adequately treated with acetaminophen, nonsteroidal antiinflammatory drugs (NSAIDs; see Chapter 17), propoxyphene (see Chapter 16), or a combination of these drugs. Abortive therapy or symptomatic management interrupts acute attacks in 70% to 80% of patients given a triptan and in 60% to 70% of patients given an ergot formulation.

Patients with moderate disability may require oral migraine-specific drugs such as triptans or ergot alkaloids. Patients with severe headache need subQ, IV, or oral formulations of these drugs. Be sure these patients are well hydrated. Because nausea is one of the most disabling symptoms of a migraine, antiemetics should be used as appropriate. Do not

---

BOX 24-3

Migraine Assessment of Current Therapy

The four-item *Migraine Assessment of Current Therapy* (Migraine-ACT) is a brief assessment tool designed to be used in initial assessments and follow-up to help the health care provider quickly and easily determine whether a change in the acute therapy of their migraine patients is required. It is intended for use by the health care provider in everyday clinical practice.

The Migraine-ACT scale was shown to be highly reliable (Spearman's rho and Pearson's r measures $r = 0.82$). Four of the original 27 screening questions on the Migraine Disability Assessment Scale (MIDAS) were found to be most discriminating in terms of consistency of response, global assessment of relief, impact, and emotional response. There are four yes-no questions on the Migraine-ACT:

- Does your migraine medication work consistently, in the majority of your attacks?
- Does the headache pain disappear within 2 hours?
- Are you able to function normally within 2 hours?
- Are you comfortable enough with your medication to be able to plan your daily activities?

One or more "no" answers to these four questions may indicate a need to change treatment. An increasing number of "no" responses indicate increasing treatment needs.

Other questionnaires that help assess efficacy of migraine therapies include the following:

- Impact tools such as the Migraine Disability Assessment (MIDAS) Questionnaire and the Headache Impact Test (HIT)*
- Quality of life (QOL) questionnaires, which can be generic or migraine-specific†
- Disease management tools such as the Migraine Therapy Assessment Questionnaire (MTAQ)‡

*Stewart, W., Lipton, R., Kolodner, K., et al. (1999). Reliability of the migraine disability assessment score in a population-based sample of headache sufferers. *Cephalalgia, 19*(2), 107–114.
†Kosinski, M., Bayliss, M., Bjorner, J., et al. (2003). A six-item short-form survey for measuring headache impact: The HIT-6. *Quality of Life Research, 12*(8), 963–974.
‡Osterhaus, J., Townsend, R., Gandek, B., et al. (1994). Measuring the functional status and well-being of patients with migraine headache. *Headache, 34*(6), 337–343.

prescribe triptans or ergot alkaloids to patients with known complicated migraines; instead, use one of the other available drugs, such as an NSAID or prochlorperazine.

Approximately 40% of patients with migraine do not respond to a triptan or other drug. Patients with intractable migraine (status migrainous, a severe headache lasting over 72 hours) should be managed in an urgent care or emergency room. In some cases, hospitalization may be needed for a short time. The only effective treatment for MOH is withdrawal therapy.

Patients with MOHs are ordinarily managed in headache clinics by withdrawal of the overused drugs; treatment of withdrawal symptoms (on an inpatient or outpatient basis); headache prophylaxis therapies; and limited use of acute rescue drugs. Although the prognosis is not always what is desired, most patients respond to this therapy. Over 50% of patients may relapse during the initial 5-year follow-up period. The best and most practical strategy to prevent the overuse of drugs in the first place is thorough patient education and use of formal management strategies for treating the primary headache before it changes to an analgesic rebound headache.

About 60% of women with migraine have an increased number of headaches around the time of menses but at no other time. The term "menstrual migraine" is frequently used to depict this type of migraine, but the term is used inconsistently and lacks an accepted definition. Many headache authorities believe the term should be restricted to migraines occurring in women who experience 90% of all their attacks 2 days before and on the last day of their menstrual cycle. Menstrual migraine typically responds to a triptan or a combination drug such as Midrin, which is composed of acetaminophen, an analgesic; dichloralphenazone, a sedative; and isometheptene, a sympathomimetic agent. Triptans with a longer half-life come into consideration here to prevent recurrences.

Prophylaxis is indicated when the patient has more than two disabling migraines per month; when there are single attacks lasting longer than 24 hours; when the headache causes major disruptions in the patient's lifestyle; when abortive therapy fails or is overused; and when the patient has complicated migraine. However, up to 25% of patients with recurrent headaches do not tolerate prophylactic drugs. A 90-day trial of prophylaxis at appropriate dosages should be undertaken before abandoning therapy.

Acute Therapy

Triptans. Consistent with the premise that serotonin is a key mediator in the pathogenesis of migraine; triptans have become the mainstay for acute treatment of migraine headaches. At all FDA-approved doses, oral triptans are effective and well tolerated for the treatment of acute migraine (with or without aura), but they are not intended for migraine prophylaxis.

Clinical response to triptans varies considerably among individual patients and cannot be predicted. A 53-study meta-analysis (Ferrari et al., 2001) compared pain relief at 2 hours, sustained pain relief, the reliability of effects, and tolerability of the different oral triptans across published and unpublished studies (Table 24-5). Triptans work well when taken at the onset of the headache, and once a headache begins the drug should be taken as soon as possible; unlike many other drugs, triptans may also be effective when taken late in the course of the migraine. If one triptan fails on two separate occasions, another triptan should be tried. However, the safety of treating more than three or four headaches over a 30-day period with triptans has not been established.

SubQ formulations and nasal sprays are useful in patients with severe nausea related to migraine who cannot tolerate an oral agent. Injectable sumatriptan has the most rapid onset of action but a relatively short half-life.

Because triptans can cause an acute, although usually small, elevation in blood pressure, they should not be used by patients with uncontrolled hypertension. Triptans should not be used concurrently with or within 24 hours of administration of an ergot alkaloid; the same applies to the use of more than one triptan concurrently or within the same 24-hour period.

Ergot Alkaloids. DHE is as effective, is better tolerated (i.e., less nausea), and has only modest arterial effects compared with ergotamine. The parenteral form is particularly helpful for patients with concomitant nausea and vomiting. DHE can be used at home by patients who find other drug therapy ineffective, if the patient is taught how to safely administer the drug. A nasal spray formulation of DHE has become available and appears to offer benefit in headache relief.

TABLE 24-5 Comparison of Oral Triptans with 100 mg of Sumatriptan

Drug	2-hr Pain Relief	Long-Lasting Pain Relief	Reliability of Effect	Tolerability
almotriptan 12.5 mg	=	+	+	++
eletriptan 20 mg	−	−	−	=
eletriptan 40 mg	=/+	=/+	=	=
eletriptan 80 mg*	+(+)	+	=	−
naratriptan 2.5 mg	−	−	−	++
rizatriptan 5 mg	=	=	=	=
rizatriptan 10 mg	+	+	+(+)†	=
sumatriptan 25 mg	−	=/−	=	+
sumatriptan 50 mg	=	=	=/−	=
zolmitriptan 2.5 mg	=	=	=	=
zolmitriptan 5 mg	=	=	=	=

−, inferior; =/−, possibly inferior; =, no difference; + better; +(+) possibly much better; ++ much better compared with 100 mg of sumatriptan.
*Not an approved single dosage in the United States.
†The unusual design of the rizatriptan study makes it difficult to compare the consistency of effect with those of the other triptans.
Adapted from Ferrari, M., Roon, K., Lipton, R., et al. (2001). Oral triptans (serotonin 5-HT$_{1B/1D}$ agonists) in acute migraine treatment: A meta-analysis of 53 trials. Lancet, 22(8), 633–58.

Ergot formulations are not as effective if therapy is delayed and the pain well established. Ergotamine use can be risky in patients who have prolonged prodromal symptoms (i.e., complicated migraine), and the drug may lead to irreversible sequelae in these circumstances. Ergotamine is no longer preferred over dihydroergotamine because of its adverse effects and cardiovascular impact and thus is rarely used today. In some cases, prochlorperazine, an antiemetic drug, should be given before an ergot alkaloid administered to reduce the occurrence of nausea associated with the ergot alkaloids. Repeated dosing over an extended period may become less efficacious.

MIGRAINE PROPHYLAXIS

Topiramate. Several research studies suggest that topiramate (Topamax) is effective for migraine prophylaxis. In many of the studies it is considered the first-line drug. Three of the studies (Brandes et al., 2004; Gray et al., 1999; Silberstein et al., 2004) found that at least half of the subjects noted a 50% or greater reduction in migraines per month at dosages of 50 to 200 mg/day compared with a placebo. In the studies, subjects noted improvement within the first month of treatment. Anorexia, nausea, fatigue, and paresthesias were reported, although these adverse effects occurred more often with the 200 mg/day dosage than with lower dosages. Studies comparing other prophylactic drugs for migraine use have not been conducted.

Triptans, DHE, lidocaine, and oxygen are used to treat acute cluster headaches; however, once symptoms have improved, prophylaxis is often more helpful. The drugs that may be used for transition from acute care to prophylaxis include a 10-day course of a steroid such as prednisone, or 7 days of an ergot formulation, or of naratriptan.

OTHER PROPHYLAXIS DRUGS

Antidepressants. Amitriptyline is a tricyclic antidepressant (TCA) with consistent evidence reinforcing its use as the first line for migraine prophylaxis (Gray, 1999; Snow, 2002). One study compared dosages of 50 mg to 100 mg of amitriptyline daily, although many of the subjects also responded to dosages of 5 mg to 20 mg daily. There was a 50% improvement with amitriptyline in relation to frequency and duration of the migraine. Amitriptyline has also been compared with propranolol for migraine prophylaxis. Findings suggest that this nonselective beta blocker is efficacious for those patients who have a single type of migraine, whereas amitriptyline is helpful for patients with mixed characteristics of migraine and tension headaches.

Amitriptyline is not tolerated as well as other TCAs. In patients with intolerance to the drug, a different TCA such as nortriptyline or doxepin may be considered. There is little evidence to support the use of other TCAs for migraine prevention.

Although one study supports the use of fluoxetine (10 to 40 mg/day) for migraine prophylaxis, another study does not (Snow et al., 2002; Gray et al., 1999; respectively). Further, there is little evidence to support the use of other antidepressant drug classes, including other TCAs, and the selective serotonin reuptake inhibitors (SSRIs) for migraine prophylaxis (also see Chapter 20 for further discussion of the antidepressant drugs.)

Beta Blockers. The nonspecific beta blockers propranolol and timolol have been shown effective for migraine prophylaxis. Clinically, however, beta blockers are not as effective as TCAs or antiepileptic drugs. For migraine prophylaxis, propranolol is the most commonly used of the beta blockers, although timolol, metoprolol, and nadolol are also used. Although few trials have examined the use of propranolol for migraine prophylaxis, there is clear evidence that it is more effective than placebo in the short-term interval treatment of migraine (Rossnagel, 2004). Evidence on long-term effects is lacking. Propranolol appears to be as effective and safe as a variety of other drugs used for migraine prophylaxis.

In general, the adverse effects of beta blockers—dizziness, fatigue, insomnia, depression, reduced exercise tolerance, nausea, and depression—are generally well tolerated and rarely make it necessary to discontinue the drugs. Asthma, chronic obstructive pulmonary disease (COPD), hypotension, heart block, and hypoglycemia secondary to treatment for diabetes contraindicate the use of beta blockers for migraine, although they may be particularly helpful for patients with comorbid heart disease (see also Chapters 15 and 37).

NSAIDs. Evidence supports the use of the NSAIDs for prophylaxis, specifically naproxen sodium and naproxen (Gray et al., 1999; Snow et al., 2002). However, this statement implies daily use, which leads to NSAID abuse and MOH. Reasonable use of an orally administered NSAID, combination drugs containing caffeine, or nonopioid analgesics for mild to moderate migraine attacks have been used with some success. Although clinical effectiveness of IM ketorolac has not yet been studied, it remains a treatment option providing it is administered in a health care provider–supervised setting. In most cases, acetaminophen is not recommended, nor is it efficacious, for migraine (except in children, as noted).

Although there is little evidence to support the use of high-dose aspirin for migraine, an NSAID taken several days before menses and continuing as needed may help prevent menstrual migraines and can be particularly helpful for patients with comorbid connective tissue disorders such as osteoarthritis.

However, NSAIDs must be used cautiously because of the potential for GI distress and altered renal function (see also Chapter 17).

Antiepileptic Drugs. Evidence supports the use of divalproex and valproic acid for migraine prevention (Chronicle and Mulleners, 2004). The extended-release formulations have fewer adverse effects than previous formulations. Even so, serum drug levels of divalproex and valproic acid should be monitored if there are concerns about toxicity and when adherence is in question. However, with continued use, the adverse effects of these two drugs generally diminish. Valproic acid and its derivatives should be avoided during pregnancy and in patients with a history of pancreatitis, cirrhosis, or chronic hepatitis (see also Chapter 25).

Two studies found gabapentin effective at dosages of 1200 to 2400 mg/day (Chronicle and Mulleners, 2004; Matthew et al., 2001). The frequency of headaches was reduced by 50% or more with gabapentin at dosages of 2400 mg/day. There are concerns about the study's methodologic limitations, and further research is warranted before this drug can be recommended for first-line migraine prophylaxis. Somnolence and dizziness are the most common adverse effects of gabapentin.

ACE Inhibitors and ARBs. The ACEI lisinopril is thought to be efficacious in migraine prophylaxis. Of the patients taking lisinopril, over 50% noted a reduction in the number of days with a migraine. A randomized, double-blinded, crossover study with 55 subjects noted that 20 mg of lisinopril, taken daily for 12 weeks, reduced the average number of headache days in general and when compared with placebo (20.7 versus 24.7 days, respectively, with headache; 14.6 versus 18.7 days, respectively, with migraine) (Schrader et al., 2001). ACEIs are associated with a higher incidence of cough than placebo.

The angiotensin II receptor–blocking drug (ARB) candesartan reduced the number of migraine days by more than half in 40% of patients when compared with placebo (Tronvik et al., 2003). The severity and level of disability, and the number of sick leave days taken due to headache was also reduced with candesartan. The adverse effects of candesartan—dizziness, upper respiratory tract infection symptoms, diarrhea, and dyspepsia—are common with the drug but are similar to those of a placebo (see also Chapter 37).

Calcium Channel Blockers. Clinical experience suggests that verapamil is the best calcium channel blocker drug for migraine prophylaxis; however, dosages of over 800 mg may be necessary before patients respond. There is weak evidence to support verapamil as a first-line drug except for use in patients with cluster headaches (Gray et al., 1999). In contrast, there is no evidence to support the use of diltiazem in migraine prevention. Nifedipine is only modestly effective for migraine prophylaxis.

Botulinum Toxin Type A. Botulinum toxin type A (Botox) as migraine prophylaxis has been studied in several clinical trials (Chronicle and Mulleners, 2004; Evers et al., 2004; Gray et al., 1999; Silberstein, 2000; Snow et al., 2002). The toxin is injected into muscles around the eyes, the forehead, and sometimes the jaw, which are partially paralyzed for about 3 months. Patients whose headaches involve all of these areas may receive additional injections in the occiput region of the neck and shoulders. In one randomized, double-blind study, subjects who had chronic migraines received 25 units or 75 units of botulinum toxin type A, or a placebo (Silberstein, 2002). The group receiving 25 units of the toxin demonstrated a significant decrease in migraine frequency and severity at 3 months. Studies remain underway to identify patients who would most likely benefit from use of the toxin, the best injection sites to use, optimal dosing and dosing frequency, and the cost-effectiveness relationship.

Other Remedies.

Feverfew. Since the time of Dioscorides (78 AD), feverfew has been used for the treatment of headache and other ailments. Feverfew is a known spasmolytic, rendering the smooth muscles in the walls of cerebral blood vessels less sensitive. Furthermore, the active ingredients in feverfew are sesquiterpene lactones, which have antiinflammatory properties that block the transcription of inflammatory proteins (the transcription factor NF-κB is a key regulator of the cellular inflammatory and immune response). The adverse effects of feverfew include nausea, flatulence, diarrhea, indigestion, and, rarely, aphthous ulcerations. Withdrawal symptoms when stopping long-term use can include muscle stiffness, anxiety, and rebound headaches. Feverfew also has anticoagulant properties, so prothrombin time (PT) and international normalized ratio (INR) levels should be checked periodically. The herb should be stopped 2 weeks before surgical procedures. Fifty to 82 mg of feverfew per day was found to be more efficacious than placebo, although differences in formulations make dosage recommendations difficult (Pittler and Ernst, 2004).

Butterbur. Butterbur has been used as an herbal remedy at least since the Middle Ages and possibly much earlier. Recent scientific studies suggest that the herb extract contains petasin and isopetasin, which have vasodilation properties and inhibit leukotriene synthesis, thereby reducing inflammation. Fifty mg of butterbur daily is thought to be effective in reducing the occurrence and severity of attacks in long-term migraine sufferers. Butterbur naturally contains components called pyrrolizidine alkaloids, which are toxic to the liver and may cause cancers. No significant adverse effects have been reported in scientific studies, but more evidence of the safety of the product would be required by many health care providers before recommending widespread use.

For more information, see the Evolve Resources Bonus Content "Drug-Herb Interactions," found at http://evolve.elsevier.com/Gutierrez/pharmacotherapeutics.

Coenzyme Q_{10}. Coenzyme Q_{10} (ubiquinone, ubiquinol; CoQ_{10}) has a structure similar to that of vitamin K and is fat-soluble. It is found in mitochondrial membranes, and is also abundant in the heart, the lungs, the liver, the kidneys, the spleen, the pancreas, and the adrenal glands. The enzyme is vital in the production of adenosine triphosphate (ATP). It appears to relax veins and arteries and is a powerful antioxidant, both in its own right and in combination with vitamin E. The synthesis of an intermediary precursor of CoQ_{10}, mevalonate, is inhibited by beta blockers, antihypertensive drugs, and "statins" (statin drugs reduce serum levels of CoQ_{10} by up to 40%). In studies, 100 mg of CoQ_{10} taken 3 times/day showed a 50% or greater reduction in migraine frequency compared to placebo (Sandor et al., 2005).

Riboflavin. Research using this vitamin for migraine prophylaxis is limited, although compared with placebo, 400 mg of riboflavin (vitamin B_2) taken daily for 2 to 3 months showed some benefit in migraine prophylaxis (Ramadan et al., 2005;

Schoenen et al., 1998). Even so, the studies noted a 50% or more decrease in the number of days with headache.

Magnesium. Magnesium (trimagnesium dicitrate) is effective for migraine prophylaxis; however, diarrhea is associated with the dosages required for relief (400 to 600 mg/day). In a 12-week study done in Germany, the patients taking 600 mg of magnesium daily had the frequency of migraine attacks reduced by 41%, whereas the placebo group noted a reduction of only 16% compared to baseline (Silberstein and Goadsby, 2002). The number of days with migraine, the duration and intensity of attacks, and the use of other drugs for symptomatic patients also decreased significantly in the magnesium group.

Patient Teaching
Patients with headache or migraine should be taught about their headaches and what they can realistically expect from drug therapy. Examine the importance of holding realistic expectations for treatment and prophylaxis. Discuss the rationale for the treatment plan and how and when to contact the health care provider for assistance.

Advise the patient to take the drug with the onset of the headache rather than waiting for the headache to become established. Explain how frequently the patient can use an abortive therapy, what the maximum daily dose is, and what adverse effects the patient can expect.

Encourage patients to track their progress through the use of a headache diary. The diary should include information as to when the headache started, any precipitating or alleviating events, the duration, the severity, and any attempts at self-treatment and the results. Include in the diary identifiable triggers for the migraines such as menses, drugs, foods, alcohol intake, and environmental factors such as those identified in Box 24-4. One third of patients identify a food that triggers their migraine.

Evaluation
Careful monitoring of drug therapy is important. Patients should return to the office after a few attempts with a specific therapy to assess its effectiveness. The health care provider should monitor how frequently patients are using abortive therapies to ensure they are using the drugs correctly.

BOX 24-4

Migraine Triggers

Hormonal Factors
- Menstruation
- Pregnancy
- Menopause

Dietary Factors
- Aged, canned, cured, or processed meats (e.g., bologna, ham, herring, hot dogs, pepperoni)
- Alcohol, particularly red wines
- Aspartame
- Avocados
- Beans, including pole, broad, lima, Italian, navy, pinto, and garbanzo
- Caffeine and caffeine withdrawal
- Canned soup or bouillon cubes
- Cultured dairy products, such as buttermilk and sour cream
- Cocoa, carob, and chocolate, particularly dark chocolate
- Figs
- Lentils
- Meat tenderizer
- Monosodium glutamate (MSG; e.g., Chinese food, seasoned salts, instant foods)
- Nitrate-containing foods (processed meats)
- Nuts and peanut butter
- Onions, except small amounts for flavoring
- Papaya
- Passion fruit
- Pea pods
- Pickled, preserved, or marinated foods (e.g., olives, pickles, snack foods)
- Raisins
- Saccharin, aspartame (diet drinks and foods)
- Sauerkraut
- Snow peas
- Soy sauce
- Sulfites in shrimp
- Tyramine-containing foods (e.g., aged cheeses)

- Yeast (including fresh yeasted coffee cake, doughnuts, and sourdough bread)

Lifestyle Factors
- Too little or too much sleep
- Dieting or skipping meals
- Strenuous exercise (prolonged overexertion)
- Stress, particularly at the end of a stressful period
- Anxiety
- Depression
- Fatigue

Environmental Factors
- Weather changes
- Tobacco smoke
- Strong odors
- Loud noises
- Bright, flashing lights or glare
- High altitudes
- Strong smells and fumes

Drugs
- Analgesic overuse
- Benzodiazepine withdrawal
- Cimetidine
- Cocaine
- Decongestant overuse
- Ergotamine overuse
- Hormones (contraceptives, hormone replacement therapies)
- Indomethacin
- Mestranol
- Nicotine
- Nifedipine
- Nitrates
- Reserpine
- Theophylline

Headache frequency, duration, disability, and symptoms, time between attacks, and intensity of care should decrease with appropriate therapy. Switching to another drug is appropriate, if therapy has been unsuccessful. Be sure to document efficacy, adverse effects, and treatment failure to avoid repeating ineffective therapies in the future. Over the long term, the objective is to return patients to their activities of daily living and to improve their quality of life.

KEY POINTS

- More than 90% of headaches are primary and include the tension of type headache and migraine, cluster, and medication overdose headaches.
- Secondary headaches account for less than 10% of all headaches, occurring as a result of other conditions such as increased intracranial pressure or infection.
- A vague and inconsistent pathophysiologic characteristic of migraine is the spreading depression of neural impulses from a focal point of vasoconstriction followed by vasodilation.
- Tension headaches start slowly, usually in the middle of the day, with a dull, achy feeling on both sides of the head.
- Treating more than two headaches per week for more than a few consecutive weeks can lead to a chronic daily headache, a situation in which the patient gets a rebound headache (MOH) as each drug wears off. An analgesic rebound headache or MOH is defined as occurring about 15 days a month, appearing with the overuse of drugs for headache relief and going away after withdrawal of the drugs.
- Be sure to adequately assess the patient's headache before starting headache therapy.
- Primary prevention is the most effective modality for headaches and migraine and primarily includes identifying migraine triggers and using non–drug therapies such as progressive muscle relaxation strategies, stress management, biofeedback, and cognitive-behavioral strategies.
- The objective of drug therapy is to decrease headache frequency, duration, disability, and symptoms, time between attacks, and intensity of care using appropriate therapies.

- Triptans either cause constriction of large intracranial blood vessels, which leads to reduction in intracranial pressure, or they block the release of proinflammatory neuropeptides.
- Ergot alkaloids have agonist and antagonist actions with adrenergic, serotonergic, and dopaminergic receptors; they also inhibit the reuptake of norepinephrine. These drugs directly stimulate vascular smooth muscle, thus constricting veins and arteries.
- Topiramate, an antiepileptic drug, blocks voltage-dependent sodium channels, augments the activity of GABA, influences calcium channels, antagonizes the glutamate receptor, and inhibits the carbonic anhydrase enzyme.
- Drugs used for prophylaxis include topiramate and divalproex sodium, as well as antiepileptic drugs, antidepressants, beta blockers, ACE inhibitors, angiotensin II–receptor blockers, and calcium channel blockers.
- Feverfew, butterbur, CoQ$_{10}$, magnesium, riboflavin, and botulinum toxin type A have been evaluated for migraine prophylaxis but have limited evidence of efficacy or have adverse-effect limitations.
- Monitor how frequently patients are using abortive therapies to ensure they are using the drugs correctly. Headache frequency, duration, disability, and symptoms, time bettween attacks, and intensity of care should decrease with appropriate therapy. Switching to another drug is appropriate, if therapy has been unsuccessful.

Bibliography

Brandes, J., Saper, J., Diamond, M., et al. (2004). Topiramate for migraine prevention: A randomized controlled trial. *Journal of the American Medical Association, 291*(8), 965–973.

Chronicle, E., and Mulleners, W. (2004). Anticonvulsant drugs for migraine prophylaxis. *Cochrane Database of Systematic Reviews.* 2004, Issue 3. Art. No. CD003226. DOI: 10.1002/14651858.CD003226.pub2.

Dey, R., Khan, S., Akhouri, V., et al. (2002). Labetalol for prophylactic treatment of intractable migraine during pregnancy. *Headache, 42*(7), 642–645.

Dowson, A., Dodick, D., and Limmroth, V. (2005). Medication overuse headache in patients with primary headache disorders: Epidemiology, management and pathogenesis. *CNS Drugs, 19*(6), 483–497.

Dowson, A., Dowson, S., Tepper, V., et al. (2004). Identifying patients who require a change in their current acute migraine treatment: The migraine assessment of current therapy (Migraine-ACT) questionnaire. *Current Medical Research Opinion, 20*(7), 1125–1135.

Evers, S., Rahmann, A., Vollmer-Haase, J., et al. (2002). Treatment of headache with botulinum toxin A: A review according to evidence-based medicine criteria. *Cephalalgia, 22*(9), 699–710.

Ferrari, M., Roon, K., Lipton, R., et al. (2001). Oral triptans (serotonin 5-HT$_{1B/1D}$ agonists) in acute migraine treatment: A meta-analysis of 53 trials. *Cephalalgia, 22*(8), 633–658.

Gray, R., Goslin, R., McCrory, D., et al. (1999). *Drug treatments for the prevention of migraine.* Technical Review. 2.3. Prepared for the Agency for Health Care Policy and Research under Contract No. 290-94-2025.

Grossman, W., and Schmidramsl, H. (2001). An extract of *Petasites hybridus* is effective in prophylaxis of migraines. *Alternative Medicine Review, 6*(3), 303–310.

Headache Classification Committee of the International Headache Society. (2004). The international classification of headache disorders (2nd ed.). *Cephalalgia, 24*(Suppl.), 1–150.

Headache Classification Committee of the International Headache Society. (1988). Classification and diagnostic criteria for headache disorders, cranial neuralgias, and facial pain. *Cephalalgia, 8*(Suppl. 4), 1–96.

Katsarava, Z., Muessig, M., Dzagnidze, A., et al. (2004). Medication overuse headache: Rates and predictors for relapse in a 4-year prospective study. *Cephalalgia, 25*(1), 12–15.

Katsarava, Z., Muessig, M., Dzagnidze, A., et al. (2003). Rate and predictors for relapse in medication overuse headache: A one year prospective study. *Neurology, 60*(10), 1682–1683.

Lewis, D., Ashwal, S., Hershey, A., et al. (2004). Practice parameter: Pharmacological treatment of migraine headache in children and adolescents. *Neurology, 63*(12), 2215–2224.

Linton-Dahlöf, P., et al. (2000). Withdrawal therapy improves chronic daily headache associated with long-term misuse of headache medication: A retrospective study. *Cephalalgia*, *20*(7), 658–662.

Matthew, N., Rapoport, A., Saper, J., et al. (2001). Efficacy of gabapentin in migraine prophylaxis. *Headache*, *41*(2), 119–128.

Misakian, A. (2003). Postmenopausal hormone therapy and migraine headache. *Journal of Women's Health*, *12*(10), 1027–1036.

Modi, S., and Lowder, D. (2006). Medications for migraine prophylaxis. *American Family Physician*, *73*(1), 72–80.

Morantz, C. (2005). Practice guideline briefs: Migraines. *American Family Physician*, *71*(5), 1019–1099.

Peikert, A., Wilimzig, C., and Kohne-Volland, R. (1996). Prophylaxis of migraine with oral magnesium: Results from a prospective, multi-center, placebo-controlled and double-blind randomized study. *Cephalalgia*, *16*(4), 257–263.

Pittler, M., and Ernst, E. (2004). Feverfew for preventing migraine. *Cochrane Database of Systematic Reviews*. 2004, Issue 1. Art. No. CD002286. DOI: 10.1002/14651858.CD002286.pub2.

Ramadan, N., Silberstein, S., Freitag, F., et al. (2005). Evidence-based guidelines for migraine headache in the primary care setting: pharmacological management for prevention of migraine. Available online: www.aan.com/professionals/practice/guideline. Accessed April 10, 2007.

Rossnagel, L. (2004). Propranolol for migraine prophylaxis. *Cochrane Database of Systematic Reviews*, 2004, Issue 2. Art. No. CD003225. DOI: 10.1002/14651858.CD003225.pub2.

Sandor, P., Di Clemente, L., Coppola, G., et al. (2005). Efficacy of coenzyme Q10 in migraine prophylaxis: A randomized controlled trial. *Neurology*, *64*(4), 713–715.

Schoenen, J., Jacquy, J., and Lenaerts, M. (1998). Effectiveness of high-dose riboflavin in migraine prophylaxis: A randomized controlled trial. *Neurology*, *50*(2), 466–470.

Schrader, H., Stovner, L., Helde, G., et al. (2001). Prophylactic treatment of migraine with angiotensin converting enzyme inhibitor (lisinopril): Randomized, placebo controlled crossover study. *British Medical Journal*, *322*(7277), 19–22.

Schroeder, B. (2003). AAFP/ACP-ASIM release guidelines on the management and prevention of migraines. *American Family Physician*, *67*(6), 1392, 1395–1397.

Silberstein, S. (2000). Practice parameter: Evidence-based guidelines for migraine headache, an evidence-based review: Report of the Quality Standards Subcommittee of the American Academy of Neurology. *Neurology*, *55*(6), 754–762.

Silberstein, S., and Goadsby, P. (2002). Migraine: Preventive treatment. *Cephalalgia*, *22*(7), 491–512.

Silberstein, S., Matthew, N., Saper, J., et al. (2000). Botulinum toxin type A as a migraine preventive treatment. *Headache*, *40*(6), 445–450.

Silberstein, S., Neto, W, Schmitt, J., et al. (2004). Topiramate in migraine prevention: Results of a large controlled trial. *Archives of Neurology*, *61*(4), 490–495.

Snow, V., Weiss, K., Wall, E., et al. (2002). Pharmacologic management of acute attacks of migraine and prevention of migraine headache. *Annals of Internal Medicine*, *137*(10), 840–849.

The Medical Letter. (2001). Drugs for migraine. *The Medical Letter on Drugs and Therapeutics*. 14th ed. *2*, 131–137. Available online: medlet-best.securesites.com/restricted/articles/w943a.pdf. Accessed April 11, 2007.

The National Headache Foundation. Case studies in the differential diagnosis of headache: Migraine, sinus headache, and episodic tension-type headache. Available online: www.headaches.org/professional/educationindex.html. Accessed April 9, 2007.

Tronvik, E., Stovner, L., Helde, G., et al. (2003). Prophylactic treatment of migraine with an angiotensin II receptor blocker: A randomized controlled trial. *Journal of the American Medical Association*, *289*(1), 65–69.

Victor, S., and Ryan, S. (2003). Drugs for preventing migraine headaches in children. *Cochrane Database of Systematic Reviews*. 2003, Issue 4. Art. No. CD002761. DOI: 10.1002/14651858.CD002761

Villalon, C., Centurion, D., Valdivia, L., et al. (2002). An introduction to migraine: From ancient treatment to functional pharmacology and antimigraine therapy. *Proceedings of the Western Pharmacology Society*, *45*, 199–210.

Wasiewski, W. (2001). Preventive therapy in pediatric migraine. *Journal of Children's Neurology*, *16*(2), 71–78.

World Headache Alliance. (2003). International Headache Society classification of headache disorders. Available online: www.w-h-a.org/wha2/index.aspAccessed April 9, 2007.

Young, W., Silberstein, S., Dayno, J., et al. (1997). Migraine treatment. *Seminars in Neurology*, *17*(4), 325–333.

CENTRAL NERVOUS

25

Antiepileptic Drugs

pilepsy is a state in which a person has recurring seizures. A seizure is an abnormal, disorderly discharge of the brain's nerve cells, resulting in a temporary disturbance of motor, sensory, or mental function. In the past decade, eight antiepileptic drugs (AEDs) have been approved for use in the United States. With wider use of these new drugs, health care providers are challenged to grasp the roles that each one plays in the treatment of epilepsy. Each drug has a distinctive pharmacokinetics and pharmacodynamic profile, as well as adverse effects, making it even more difficult to arrive at an understanding of how these drugs are best utilized. Despite quality research evaluating the safety and efficacy of specific AEDs, the lack of head-to-head studies makes it difficult to recommend a single therapeutic regimen.

EPILEPSY

EPIDEMIOLOGY AND ETIOLOGY

Seizures result when electrical discharges from a *focus* (i.e., abnormally hyperexcitable neurons) spread to other areas of the brain. The manifestations of a particular seizure depend on the location of the neuronal connections to the focus.

Epilepsy is most frequently diagnosed during infancy, childhood, adolescence, and old age. The diagnosis of epilepsy applies to persons who have recurring seizures; however, around 50 million people will have a single seizure in their lifetime. Epilepsy ranks second in incidence to cerebrovascular accident (CVA) as a neurologic disorder.

Patients with biochemical and/or neurotransmitter disorders of the brain have an increased risk for epilepsy. Seizures also result from trauma sustained at birth, perinatal injuries, congenital malformations, an inherent balance in central nervous system (CNS) activity, accidents or injuries, head injury, encephalitis, brain tumors, abscesses or infections, nutritional disorders (e.g., hypoglycemia, phenylketonuria, vitamin B_6 deficiency), alcohol withdrawal, metabolic derangements, circulatory disturbances, and drug interactions. The appearance of epilepsy in older adults may suggest a CNS tumor or other organic brain disease.

Relapse of previously controlled epilepsy occurs more often in (1) patients who developed epilepsy during childhood; (2) those with an identifiable abnormality on an electroencephalogram (EEG) done in the last 12 months; (3) patients taking one or more AEDs to control seizure activity; (4) patients who experienced seizures during treatment with an AED; (5) patients with comorbid encephalopathy; and (6) patients diagnosed with myoclonic or partial seizures.

PATHOPHYSIOLOGY

The movement of sodium ions across cell membranes forms the action potential. Sodium channels become inactive once the action potential has been generated (the effective refractory period). Axons that continually fire, as with epilepsy, render the sodium channels inactive, making the generation of an action potential unlikely.

According to the concept of *seizure threshold*, every person maintains a certain balance, most likely genetically determined, between excitatory and inhibitory forces in the brain. The proportions of each person's individual balance determine his or her threshold for seizures. A low threshold would indicate a balance point that is more excitatory, whereas a high threshold would indicate a more inhibitory balance point. People with a low seizure threshold are more likely to develop epilepsy and, in general, to experience a seizure.

Epilepsy is classified by seizure type or by cause. Seizure activity where there is no known cerebral lesion is referred to as *primary idiopathic epilepsy*. More than 50% of epilepsy is idiopathic. However, in some forms of primary epilepsy, a genetic basis is apparent. If the first seizure a patient experiences occurs after age 20 years, the likelihood of this seizure being secondary to an organic or metabolic cause goes up significantly.

Partial seizures occur when the neuronal firing is confined to a very limited portion of the brain (Table 25-1). If the activity is more diffuse, a generalized seizure occurs. However, a partial seizure that becomes generalized is still primarily a partial seizure. This distinction has significant diagnostic implications since a fixed anatomic lesion (i.e., tumor, infection, or scar) serves as a local irritant or focus and generates a focal seizure, but has the capability to progress to a generalized, tonic-clonic seizure. The history of a focal seizure spreading to a generalized seizure requires a more careful search for an anatomic explanation for the event.

Focal motor symptoms that begin in the hand and progress up the arm are known as *jacksonian seizures*, although some seizures that are characterized this way appear in the face first and then spread down the arm or leg. Some proceed on to become generalized seizures.

Generalized seizures involve both hemispheres of the brain. Each seizure is a single occurrence. Single-episode seizures can be caused by such events as fever, hypoglycemia, or hyponatremia and their occurrence does not mean the patient has epilepsy. The seizure type is diagnostically significant because it is the key determinant of the treatment approach and may provide clues to the etiology.

Status epilepticus occurs when a patient has seizures in rapid succession or continuous seizures lasting 30 minutes or more. Status epilepticus has many causes, and patients who develop

TABLE 25-1 Seizure Types

Seizure Type	Manifestations
PARTIAL SEIZURES	
Simple partial seizures	Consciousness usually not impaired. Functional disturbance in motor, sensory, and/or autonomic nerves and regions of the brain. "Jacksonian march" and sensory symptoms (i.e., odor, taste) most common. Psychic symptoms (fearful feeling, sense of déjà vu). *Duration:* 1–2 min. *Age:* Older children and adults.
Complex partial seizures	Starts as simple partial seizure. Consciousness impaired at onset. Characterized by automatisms (e.g., staring; chewing; lip smacking; bizarre, purposeless motor or psychic activity; mumbled speech; unintelligible sounds). Motor, somatosensory, autonomic, or psychic symptoms. *Duration:* 1–2 min with confusion lasting 1–2 min after attack. *Age:* Any age.
GENERALIZED SEIZURES	
Absence seizures (petit mal)	Brief LOC, amnesia, or unawareness. Characterized by mild clonic movements (e.g., eye blinking, jerking movement), automatisms, and changes in postural tone. No postictal state. 50% supplanted by tonic-clonic seizures. May occur 50–100 times per day in some persons. *Duration:* 10–30 sec. *Age:* Usually at 4–8 years of age; rare before age 3 or after age 15; 40% of seizures end in adolescence.
Atypical absence seizures	Characterized by staring (as they would in any absence seizure) but often patient is somewhat responsive. Eye blinking or lip smacking may occur. Unlike other absence seizures, these seizures usually cannot be induced by rapid breathing. *Duration:* 5–30 seconds. *Age:* Usually begin before age 6. Often occur in children with below-average intelligence who experience other types of seizures that are difficult to control. Many have Lennox-Gastaut syndrome.
Myoclonic seizures	Single or multiple, short, abrupt muscular contractions of arms, legs, and/or torso and brief LOC. May be confined to face and trunk, or to one or more extremities. May not be classified as a seizure in some cases. *Duration:* 1–5 sec. *Age:* Late childhood, adolescence.
Tonic-clonic seizures	Vague aura, LOC, sudden tonic contraction with stridor if respiratory muscles involved, rigidity. May begin with shrill cry due to abrupt closure of epiglottis and secondary expulsion of air from the lungs. Muscle relaxation interrupts tonic contraction, with tone returning as rhythmic flexor spasms that become less frequent as seizure subsides. Urinary and fecal incontinence may occur during clonic phase. Amnesia after seizure. *Duration:* 10–30 sec after falling to ground. Tonic phase gives way to clonic phase, which lasts 30–50 sec. *Age:* Any age.
Status epilepticus	Two or more seizures in adults or children without full recovery of consciousness or continuous seizure activity. Can lead to brain damage and death. *Duration:* 30–60 min of continuous seizure activity or two or more seizures without full recovery of consciousness. *Age:* Any age.
OTHER SEIZURE TYPES	
Atonic seizures	Characterized by abrupt, selective loss of muscle tone or of all muscle tone. Referred to as "drop attacks" if attacks are brief and patient slumps to ground; injury possible. May be followed by postictal confusion. *Duration:* 10–30 sec. *Age:* Infants and children.
Clonic seizures	Rare. Repetitive clonic jerks that lack tonic component. Movements may be symmetric or asymmetric, synchronous or asynchronous, rhythmic or dysrhythmic. *Duration:* seconds. *Age:* Early childhood.
Tonic seizures	Altered consciousness, tonic contraction of muscle groups with no progression to clonic movement. Ocular phenomena common (e.g., fixed gaze, eyelid retraction, superior ocular deviation, nystagmus, mydriasis). Autonomia (e.g., tachycardia, hypertension, respiratory distress, capillary restriction with cyanosis). Usually activated by sleep. *Duration:* 30 seconds to several minutes. *Age:* Any age.
Unclassified seizures	Seizures cannot be classified because of inadequate or incomplete data. "Neonatal seizures" (e.g., rhythmic eye movements, chewing or swimming movements). *Duration:* 10–30 sec. *Age:* Neonates.

LOC, Loss of consciousness.

it may have no previous history of epilepsy. In these cases, the cause is often related to acute brain infections, injury to the head and brain, cerebrovascular disease, and toxic or metabolic disorders. The most severe form of status epilepticus is the tonic-clonic form. The patient experiences an unrelenting series of tonic-clonic attacks. Loss of consciousness extends throughout the entire attack.

With the sudden withdrawal of an AED or nonadherence with therapy, falling drug levels cause the seizure threshold to fall as well, which explains not only seizure occurrence but also the precipitation of status epilepticus. Status epilepticus necessitates immediate intervention and aggressive treatment to prevent damage to the CNS.

PHARMACOTHERAPEUTIC OPTIONS

AEDs are designed to modify neurons, ion channels, receptors, glia, and inhibitor and excitatory synapses. These processes favor inhibition over excitation in order to stop or prevent seizure activity. The AEDs are organized according to their primary mechanism of action, although many of them have several actions and others have unknown mechanisms of action.

The categories from which AEDs are commonly chosen for therapy include the hydantoins, the succinimides, the benzodiazepines, the oxazolidinediones, the barbiturates, and a variety of miscellaneous drugs. Barbiturates and benzodiazepines are discussed in Chapter 19 in relation to their uses as antianxiety or sedative-hypnotic drugs. They are briefly discussed here in relation to epilepsy. Magnesium sulfate, used to prevent or control preeclamptic seizures and eclamptic seizures, is discussed in Chapter 59.

Hydantoins
- fosphenytoin (Cerebryx)
- phenytoin (Dilantin); ♣ Dilantin, Epanutin

▥ *Indications*

Phenytoin, the oldest hydantoin, is the most commonly used drug in this group. Phenytoin is used for treatment of generalized tonic-clonic seizures and refractory simple and complex partial seizures; it is a second-line drug in treating status epilepticus.

Fosphenytoin, the prodrug of phenytoin, is used for the acute treatment of status epilepticus and for the treatment of seizures occurring during neurosurgery. It is a short-term parenteral substitute for oral phenytoin.

▥ Pharmacodynamics

Hydantoins keep neuronal firing in an inactive state by stabilizing sodium channels. In so doing they may also raise the seizure threshold in the motor cortex, stop or limit the neuronal discharge, or reduce the spread of excitation from the seizure focus. Phenytoin is chemically related to the barbiturates.

▥ Pharmacokinetics

Phenytoin is rapidly distributed to all tissues, with the highest concentrations occurring in the brain, the liver, and the salivary glands, and taking up to 5 days to be released from body tissues (Table 25-2). Biotransformation of phenytoin occurs in the liver, with the drug primarily eliminated in the bile. It is then reabsorbed from the gastrointestinal (GI) tract, and 5% is eliminated unchanged in the urine. Hydantoins cross the placenta and enter breast milk.

Fosphenytoin, the prodrug of phenytoin, is rapidly converted to phenytoin after parenteral administration. When administered by intravenous (IV) route, fosphenytoin reaches maximum concentrations at the end of the infusion. The pharmacologic and toxicologic effects of fosphenytoin are those of phenytoin.

Alterations in plasma protein binding may alter patient response to hydantoins. Such alterations appear to be more significant with highly bound drugs such as phenytoin (87% to 95%). Traditionally, most drug assays monitor total drug concentrations and do not quantify free drug, although only free drug (i.e., non–protein bound) is considered pharmacologically active. When alterations in plasma protein binding are present, total drug concentrations may be misleading to health care providers who are evaluating patient response.

▥ Adverse Effects and Contraindications

Patients under 23 years of age and those taking phenytoin in dosages exceeding 500 mg/day are at increased risk for gingival hyperplasia. Hypertrichosis and exfoliative dermatitis, coarsened facial features, impaired cognition, dyskinesias, urinary incontinence, and thyroid disorders occur in some patients. The most serious adverse effects of phenytoin include agranulocytosis, encephalopathy, and coma.

Exercise caution when using phenytoin in patients who have severe liver or cardiorespiratory disease or who are obese. Phenytoin hypersensitivity (fever, skin rash, lymphadenopathy) usually occurs within the first 3 to 8 weeks of therapy but may occur up to 12 weeks later. When severe, the hypersensitivity reaction can result in hepatic necrosis, rhabdomyolysis, renal failure, or death. Parenteral administration of phenytoin is limited by its poor solubility or the presence of high pH, hypotension, or arrhythmias, and the risk of soft tissue injury with extravasation of the drug into tissues.

Safe use of hydantoins during pregnancy has not been established (pregnancy category D). Both phenytoin and fosphenytoin (pregnancy category D) increase the risk of seizures because of the physiologic changes taking place during pregnancy (e.g., relative decline in plasma protein levels); careful monitoring of patients could allay this risk. Drug levels of phenytoin are reduced by about 56% in the mother during pregnancy; unbound serum levels are reduced by 31%. Because protein binding is decreased, monitoring of unbound plasma concentrations is recommended through the eighth postpartum week.

Fetal hydantoin syndrome is possible with phenytoin, producing a wide variety of teratogenic effects. The clinical features of this syndrome include craniofacial abnormalities (e.g., cleft lip, cleft palate), hypoplasia of the digits, dislocated

---

Controversy

Drug Errors from Confusing Orders and New Drugs

Jonathan J. Wolfe

Drug errors have emerged as a serious public health concern. Health care professionals have become acutely aware of the real harm and monetary cost associated with such errors. Increasingly, health care providers involved in errors find themselves subject to professional censure and discipline.

Patients as well as insurance companies are also interested in reducing drug errors. One manifestation of their participation has been the creation of the National Coordinating Council for Medication Error Reporting and Prevention (NCCMERP). This group includes founding members as diverse as the American Association of Retired Persons (AARP), the American Medical Association (AMA), the United States Pharmacopeia (USP), and the Joint Commission on Accreditation of Healthcare Organizations (JCAHO). The council uses a method that emphasizes finding problems in the medication handling system rather than assigning blame to individuals.

One illustration involves the introduction of fosphenytoin, a parenteral antiseizure drug. Numerous errors in practice have occurred because of confusion about dosage for this new product. First, phenytoin (PE), a long-established generic product, remains widely available and is in many situations entirely adequate for patient needs. Second, fosphenytoin is dosed in terms of mg-PE. This means that rather than writing a prescription for a milligram dose of fosphenytoin, the prescriber is to order fosphenytoin dosed as equivalent to a milligram dose of phenytoin. The system has proved difficult to adopt smoothly in practice. Error reports have appeared from health care providers intending one dose but inadvertently ordering another. In addition, pharmacists and nurses have prepared and administered incorrect doses when orders or prescriptions were not understood accurately.

CLINICAL REASONING

- What person in the health care system has the most immediate interest in accurate dose preparation and administration?
- What is your first concern when confronted with the possibility that an error has occurred?
- What sort of system can you imagine for classifying errors by severity or harm?
- What duty do you have to report errors or elements of your drug handling system that make errors more likely?
- What steps should drug marketers take when introducing drugs whose names or doses may be confused with similar products long established in practice?

PHARMACOKINETICS
TABLE 25-2 Antiepileptic Drugs

Agent	Route	Onset	Peak	Duration	PB (%)	t1/2	BioA (%)
ANTIEPILEPTIC DRUGS							
carbamazepine	PO	2–4 days	2–4 hr	UA	75–90	25–29 hr	85
clonazepam	PO	20–60 min	1–4 hr	6–12 hr	50–85	18–50 hr	80–98
clorazepate	PO	15 min-2 hr	1–2 hr	4–6 hr	85–98	30–100 hr	UA
divalproex sodium	PO	Slow	4–17 hr	40 hr	10–18.5	9–16 hr	89
diazepam	PO	30–60 min	0.5–2 hr	2–3 hr	96–99	20–100 min	UA
	IV	Immed	15–30 min	20–60 min	85–99	20–100 hr	100
ethosuximide	PO	Hours	1–4 hr; 3–7 hr*	>24 hr	0–10	40–60 hr; 30 hr*	UA
fosphenytoin	IM	Rapid	30 min	UA	95–99	8–15 min	100
	IV	Rapid	10 min	UA	95–99	8–15 min	100
gabapentin	PO	Rapid	2–4 hr	8 hr	0–3	5–7 hr	50–60
lamotrigine	PO	UA	1–4.8 hr	UA	55	24–30 hr	98–100
levetiracetam	PO	Rapid	1 hr	UA	<10	6–8 hr	100
lorazepam	IV	1–5 min	1–6 hr	6–8 hr	85	14–16 hr	83–100
mephobarbital	PO	20–60 min	6–12 hr	10–16 hr	40–60	34–52 hr	UA
oxcarbazepine	PO	Rapid	4.5–6 hr	UA	40–60	2; 8–10 hr†	UA
phenobarbital	PO	20–60 min	6–12 hr	6–12 hr	40–60	37–140 hr	UA
	subQ, IM	10–30 min	UA	4–6 hr	40–60	Varies	UA
	IV	5 min	15–30 min	4–10 hr	40–60	11–67 hr	100
phenytoin	PO	2–24 hr	1.5–3 hr; 4–12 hr	6–12 hr; 12–36 hr‡	87–95	7–42 hr‡	70–100
	IV	1–2 hr	End of inf	UA	90	24–30 hr	20–24
pregabalin	PO	Rapid	1 hr	UA	0	6.3 hr	>90
primidone	PO	4–7 days	7–10 days	8–12 hr	19–25	5–15 hr; 10–18 hr§	60–80
tiagabine	PO	Rapid	1 hr; 12 hr	5–8 hr	96	4–8 hr	96
topiramate	PO	Rapid	2 hr; 4 days to steady state	UA	9–15	20–30 hr	80
valproic acid	PO	Rapid	1–4 hr	40 hr	10–18.5	9–16 hr	90–95
zonisamide	PO	Rapid	2–6 hr	UA	40	63 hr; 105 hr‖	UA

BioA, Bioavailability; *ER*, Extended-release formulation; *IM*, intramuscular; *Inf*, infusion; *IV*, intravenous; *PB*, protein binding; *PO*, by mouth; *RBCs*, red blood cells; *subQ*, subcutaneous; *t1/2* half-life; *UA*, unavailable.
*Peak effects and elimination half-life of ethosuximide for adults and children, respectively.
†This is the half-life of the monohydroxymetabolite; oxcarbazepine itself has a half-life of approximately 2 hr.
‡The peak and duration of phenytoin are based on tablet and extended-release formulations, respectively. The half-life averages 22 hr but is dose dependent. Its half-life is shorter in children.
§Half-life of primidone and phenylethylmalonamide, respectively.
‖Elimination half-life of zonisamide from plasma and RBCs, respectively.

hips, congenital heart defects, microcephaly, and prenatal growth deficiencies.

At therapeutic doses, **phenytoin** produces horizontal gaze nystagmus. **View nystagmus as a sign of phenytoin toxicity until proven otherwise.** Nystagmus findings relate to elevated phenytoin concentrations as follows: far lateral nystagmus is found at serum levels of about 20 mcg/mL; a 45-degree lateral-gaze nystagmus and ataxia is found between 20 to 40 mcg/mL, decreased mentation over 40 mcg/mL, and death at levels exceeding 100 mcg/mL. The therapeutic range for phenytoin is 10 to 20 mcg/mL. Concentration-related adverse effects include not only nystagmus, but also blurry vision, diplopia, ataxia, slurred speech, dizziness, drowsiness, confusion, mood changes, lethargy, coma, rash, fever, nausea, vomiting, gingival tenderness, folic acid depletion, osteomalacia, and hyperglycemia.

Nystagmus, tinnitus, dizziness, ataxia, somnolence, hypotension, and pruritus are common adverse effects of fosphenytoin. Groin pain has been reported in up to 64% of patients who receive the drug intravenously; the discomfort ordinarily resolves within 1 hour. Fosphenytoin should not be used in patients with hypersensitivity to phenytoin and in those with sinoatrial block, second- and third-degree heart block, and Stokes'-Adams syndrome. Cautious use of fosphenytoin is advised for patients with hypotension, severe myocardial

disease, kidney or liver disease, hypoalbuminemia, and porphyria. Porphyria is a disorder caused by changes in the quantity of nitrogen-containing substances found in the blood. Porphyria can cause abdominal pain, skin lesions, light sensitivity, anemia, and neurologic changes.

Drug Interactions
Phenytoin and fosphenytoin interact with a variety of drugs including rifampin, beta blockers, calcium channel blockers, tricyclic antidepressants, estrogens, antidiabetic drugs, and a host of other drugs. Table 25-3 provides an overview of the interactions.

Dosage Regimen
The dosage for phenytoin is dependent on the patient's age and size, and on the purpose for use. Phenytoin is initially dosed at one fourth to one half the total maintenance dosages (Table 25-4). Upward titration is done slowly and is determined by serum drug levels. Phenytoin suspension must be well shaken. If this is not done, a subtherapeutic dose will be obtained from the top of the bottle and a supertherapeutic dose from the bottom.

Fosphenytoin's dosing is expressed as "phenytoin equivalents" (PE) to avoid the need to perform molecular weight–based

DRUG INTERACTIONS
TABLE 25-3 Antiepileptic Drugs

Drug	Interacting Drug	Interaction
ANTIEPILEPTIC DRUGS		
carbamazepine	cimetidine, diltiazem, erythromycin, fluoxetine, influenza virus vaccine, isoniazid, nicotinamide, propoxyphene, verapamil	Increases serum levels of carbamazepine
	Antipsychotics, corticosteroids, OCs	Decreases serum levels of carbamazepine; decreases effectiveness of interacting drug
	Acetaminophen, calcium channel blockers, doxycycline, haloperidol, quinidine, thyroid hormones, oral anticoagulants, TCAs, theophylline	Decreases level and effectiveness of interacting drug
	lithium	Increases risk of neurotoxicity
	MAOIs	Hypertensive and hyperpyretic crisis, severe seizures, death
	Phenothiazines, TCAs	Increases CNS depression; reduces antiepileptic effects of carbamazepine
	vasopressin	Increases antidiuretic effects
clonazepam, clorazepate	CNS depressants, antihistamines, alcohol	Increases CNS depression
clonazepam	valproic acid	Absence status epilepticus
	Other antiepileptic drugs	Additive sedation
	clozapine	Increases CNS and respiratory depression
ethosuximide	Hydantoins	Increases hydantoin levels
	primidone, phenobarbital	Reduces serum level of interactive drugs
diazepam	levodopa	Decreases effects of levodopa
	rifampin	Reduces effects of BZDs
	cimetidine, disulfiram, isoniazid, ketoconazole, metoprolol, OCs, opioids, propranolol, propoxyphene, valproate	Increases effects of BZDs
	Antidepressants	Increases CNS depression
	clozapine	Respiratory depression
	erythromycin, paroxetine, sertraline	Increases serum levels of diazepam
	Antacids	Delays absorption of diazepam
divalproex sodium, valproic acid	amitriptyline, diazepam, lamotrigine, lorazepam, phenobarbital, phenytoin, warfarin	Increases serum level of interactive drugs
	carbamazepine, phenobarbital, phenytoin, primidone	Increases clearance of valproic acid
	clonazepam	Absence status epilepticus develops
	Alcohol, BZDs, CNS depressants, haloperidol, phenothiazines	Increases CNS depression
	chlorpromazine, cimetidine, ranitidine, salicylates	Increases half-life of valproate
	Salicylates	Increases anticoagulation effects
	Oral anticoagulants, thrombolytic drugs, heparin, platelet aggregation inhibitors	Increases risk of bleeding or hemorrhage
fosphenytoin	phenobarbital, valproic acid	Decreases fosphenytoin binding
gabapentin	Antacids	Reduces bioavailability of gabapentin
	cimetidine	Reduces elimination of gabapentin; increases risk of gabapentin toxicity
	Oral contraceptives	Increases norethindrone levels
lamotrigine	acetaminophen	Reduces half-life of lamotrigine
	carbamazepine, phenobarbital, phenytoin	Biotransformation significantly induced
	valproic acid	Biotransformation significantly inhibited
lorazepam	loxapine, MAOIs, TCAs, scopolamine	Increases risk of sedation, irrational behaviors, toxicity
mephobarbital	isoniazid, salicylates	Changes in serum concentrations of both interactive drug and hydantoins
oxcarbazepine	phenytoin	Increases serum levels of phenytoin
phenytoin	propranolol	Additive cardiac depression with IV phenytoin
	Influenza virus vaccine	Increases, decreases, or no change in serum levels of phenytoin
	Estrogens, TCAs	Increases effects of hydantoins; decreases effects of interactive drugs
	Oral anticoagulants	Greater anticoagulant effects initially, then reduced with chronic use
	Antidiabetic drugs, acute ethanol ingestion, ranitidine, ibuprofen, sulfonamides	Increases serum glucose levels
	Antacids, antineoplastics, calcium gluconate, chronic alcohol use, continuous enteral feeding solutions	Decreases effects of hydantoin
	acetaminophen, Calcium channel blockers, Cardiac glycosides, dopamine, haloperidol, methadone, nondepolarizing muscle relaxants	Decreases effects of interacting drug
phenobarbital	metronidazole, trazodone	Increases effects of hydantoins
	meperidine, sedatives-hypnotics, primidone	Increases CNS depression
	Calcium channel blockers	Reduces blood pressure
primidone	Carbonic anhydrase inhibitors	Osteopenia
	Beta blockers, corticosteroids, ACTH, neuroleptics	Decreases effects of interactive drug
	prednisone	Exacerbates symptoms in asthmatics
	methylphenidate, nicotinamide, isoniazid	Increases serum levels of primidone
	Antihistamines, primidone, sedative-hypnotics	Increases CNS depression

DRUG INTERACTIONS
TABLE 25-3 Antiepileptic Drugs—Cont'd

Drug	Interacting Drug	Interaction
pregabalin	Gingko biloba	Decreases antiepileptic efficacy
	Acetaminophen, alpha$_2$ agonists, Antihistamine/decongestant combinations, antipsychotic drugs, barbiturates, BZDs, caffeine, dronabinol, droperidol, opiates, sedating antihistamines, tramadol, muscle relaxants, fluoxetine, olanzapine, TCAs	Increases risk of CNS depression, psychomotor impairment
topiramate	carbamazepine, phenytoin, valproic acid	Decreases serum levels of topiramate; increases serum levels of interacting drugs
zonisamide	carbamazepine, phenytoin, valproic acid	Decreases half-life of zonisamide

ACTH, Adrenocorticotropic hormone; *BZDs*, benzodiazepines; *CNS*, central nervous system; *IV*, intravenous; *MAOIs*, monoamine oxidase inhibitors; *OCs*, oral contraceptives; *TCAs*, tricyclic antidepressants.

DOSAGE
TABLE 25-4 SELECTED Antiepileptic Drugs

Drug	Use(s)	Dosage	Implications
ANTIEPILEPTICS			
carbamazepine	Tonic-clonic, complex partial, and mixed seizures	*Adult:* 200 mg PO twice daily. Increase by 200 mg/day every 7 days until therapeutic levels reached. Not to exceed 1.2 grams/day *Child 6–12 yr:* 100 mg PO twice daily. Increase dose by 100 mg/day at weekly intervals until therapeutic levels reached. Not to exceed 1 gram/day	ER formulations given once to twice daily. Dosage not to exceed 1 gram/day in 12–15-year-olds. *Therapeutic level:* 4–12 mcg/mL.
clonazepam	Absence seizures, myoclonic seizures	*Adult:* Initial daily dose not to exceed 0.5 mg PO 3 times daily. Increase by 0.5–1 mg every third day. Maintenance: Not to exceed 20 mg daily *Child <10 yr or 30 kg:* Initial daily dose 0.01–0.03 mg/kg/daily PO. Not to exceed 0.05 mg/kg/day in 2–3 divided doses. Increase by 0.25–0.5 mg PO every third day until therapeutic blood levels are reached. Not to exceed 0.2 mg/kg/day	Time to steady state: 3–7 days. Do not abruptly stop drug. *Therapeutic level:* 20–80 mcg/mL
clorazepate	Adjunctive treatment for simple partial seizures	*Adult:* 7.5 mg PO 3 times daily. May increase by 7.5 mg/day weekly. Max: 90 mg daily *Child age 9–12 yr:* 3.75–7.5 mg twice daily initially. Increase by 7.5 mg/wk. Not to exceed 60 mg/day	Time to steady state: 5 days-2 wk. *Therapeutic level:* 0.5–1.9 mcg/mL
diazepam	Status epilepticus	*Adult:* 5–10 mg IV. May repeat dose every 10–15 min to total of 30 mg. May repeat in 2–4 hr. *Child >age 5 yr:* 1 mg every 2 to 5 min IV for total of 10 mg. May repeat dose every 2–4 hr *Child <age 5 yr:* 0.2–0.5 mg/kg IV every 2–5 min to max of 5 mg. May repeat every 2–4 hr	Administer where supportive and resuscitative treatment can begin immediately. IM route may be used if IV route unavailable. Max rate of administration 5 mg/min. *Therapeutic level:* 0.1–1.5 mcg/mL
divalproex sodium	Tonic-clonic, myoclonic, absence, and complex partial seizures	*Adult:* ER formulation: 10–15 mg/kg/day. May increase by 5–10 mg/kg/wk to max of 60 mg/kg/day. If smaller dosage adjustments required, use immediate-release tablets instead.	ER formulation not studied for initial therapy. To convert to monotherapy: reduce dosage of concomitant drug by 25% every 2 wk.
ethosuximide	Absence seizures; myoclonic and complex partial seizures (rare)	*Adult and Child >6 yr:* 250 mg PO twice daily. Increase by 250 mg every 4–7 days PRN up to 1.5 g/day in 2 divided doses *Child 3–6 yr:* Titrate from 250 mg daily in 2 divided doses to effect (up to 20 mg/kg/day in divided doses). Do not exceed 1 gram/day	Time to steady state: 4–10 days. Do not abruptly discontinue. Administer with food to decrease GI effects. *Therapeutic levels:* 40–100 mcg/mL.
fosphenytoin	Generalized seizures, status epilepticus; prevention and treatment of seizures occurring during neurosurgery	*Adult: Status epilepticus:* 15–20 PE/kg IV loading dose infused at 100–150 mg PE/min. *Nonemergent seizures:* 10–20 mg PE/kg as single loading dose IM or less than 150 mg PE/min. Maintenance: 4–6 mg PE/kg/day at less than 150 mg PE/min	**Dose, concentration solution, infusion rate expressed in terms of phenytoin equivalents (PE).** A 1.5-mg dose of fosphenytoin is equivalent to 1 mg of phenytoin. *Therapeutic level:* 10–20 mcg/mL.
gabapentin	Adjunct for partial seizures with or without secondary generalized seizure activity	*Adult and Child >12 yr:* 300 mg PO at HS on first day, 300 mg PO twice daily on second day, 300 mg PO 3 times daily on third day. Maintenance: 900–1800 mg/day in 3 divided doses.	Rapid titration may be continued until desired effects obtained. Doses should not be more than 12 hr apart. *Therapeutic level:* 2–3 mcg/mL.
lamotrigine	Adjunct therapy for partial, tonic-clonic, and absence seizures; Lennox-Gastaut syndrome	*Adult and Child >16 yr presently on carbamazepine, phenytoin, phenobarbital, or primidone:* 50 mg/day as single dose for first 2 wk, then 50 mg twice daily for next 2 wk; then increase by 100 mg/day weekly to maintenance dose of 300–500 mg/day in 2 divided doses *Adult and Child >16 yr presently on valproic acid:* 25 mg every other day; increase to 300–500 mg daily given every 12 hr	Do not abruptly stop; discontinue gradually over a period of 2 wk unless safety concerns require a more rapid withdrawal. Concurrent use with valproic acid results in twofold increase in lamotrigine levels and a decrease in valproic acid levels. *Therapeutic levels:* 1–4 mcg/mL.

Continued

DOSAGE

TABLE 25-4 SELECTED Antiepileptic Drugs—Cont'd

Drug	Use(s)	Dosage	Implications
lamotrigine—cont'd		*Child 2–16 yr:* 2 mg/kg/day twice daily for 2 wk, then 5 mg/kg/day PO twice daily for 2 wk, then 10 mg/kg/day PO twice daily for 2 wk	
levetiracetam	Partial-onset seizures	*Adult:* 500 mg PO twice daily. Increase weekly in 500–1000 mg increments to max of 3 grams/day *Child 4–16 yr:* 10 mg/kg twice daily. Increase every 2 wk by 20–30 mg/kg twice daily.	Dosages greater than 3 grams/day confer additional benefit.
lorazepam	Status epilepticus	*Adult:* 15–20 mg/kg IV. Rate not to exceed 25–50 mg/min, followed by 100 mg every 6–8 hr. Give slowly—rate not to exceed 2 mg/min. *Child:* 15–20 mg/kg at 1–3 mg/kg/min	Give where supportive and resuscitative treatment can begin immediately. IM route not recommended; crystallization at injection site. *Therapeutic level:* 50–240 mcg/mL.
mephobarbital	Partial and generalized tonic-clonic and cortical focal seizures	*Adult:* 400–600 mg PO 2–4 times daily *Child <5 yr:* 16–32 mg PO 3–4 times daily *Child >5 yr:* 32–64 mg PO 3–4 times daily	Timing of administration dependent on when patient's seizures usually occur.
oxcarbazepine	Monotherapy or adjunctive therapy with partial seizures	*Adult and Child >16 yr:* 300–600 mg PO daily. Slowly titrate to 900–2400 mg/day in 2–3 divided doses. *Child 4–16 yr:* 8–10 mg/kg/day in 2 divided doses. Max: 600 mg/day	Increased effectiveness with dosages above 1200 mg/day, but most patients cannot tolerate higher dosages because of CNS effects.
phenytoin	Tonic-clonic, simple and complex partial seizures	*Adult:* 1 gram or 20 mg/kg loading dose as ER capsules in 3–4 divided doses at 2-hr intervals –or– as 400 mg capsule, then 300 mg every 2 hr for 2 doses. Maintenance: 300–400 mg daily *Older Adult:* 3 mg/kg/day PO in divided doses *Child:* 5 mg/kg/day PO in 2–3 divided doses. Maintenance: 4–8 mg/kg/day in 2–3 divided doses. Max: 300 mg/day	Give loading dose in setting where serum phenytoin levels can be rapidly monitored. Avoid loading doses in patients with hepatic or renal disease. Maintenance doses usually started 24 hr later. *Therapeutic level:* 10–20 mcg/mL.
phenobarbital	Tonic-clonic, partial and febrile seizures, status epilepticus	*Adult:* 60–250 mg PO as single dose or 2–3 divided doses –or– 100–320 mg IV as needed initially to a total of 600 mg/day. *Status epilepticus:* 10–20 mg/kg IV *Child:* 1–6 mg/kg/day PO as single dose or divided doses –or– 10–20 mg/kg IV initially followed by 1–6 mg/kg/day. *Status epilepticus:* 15–20 mg/kg IV	Give where supportive and resuscitative treatment can begin immediately. IV doses require 15–30 min to reach peak concentrations in the brain. Administer minimal dose and evaluate effectiveness before giving second dose to prevent barbiturate-induced CNS depression
primidone	Generalized tonic-clonic, complex partial seizures	*Adult and Child >8 yr:* Titrate slowly from 100 mg at HS to usual maintenance 125–250 mg 3–4 times daily. Not to exceed 2 grams/day. *Child <8 yr:* Titrate slowly 50 mg at HS to usual maintenance 125–250 mg 3 times daily –or– 10–25 mg/kg/day in divided doses. Not to exceed 1 gram/day in divided doses	Time to steady state: 1–7 days. To switch from alternative AED to primidone or when adding primidone to another regimen, increase primidone dose gradually while decreasing or continuing other drug dosages to maintain seizure control. Switch should take at least 2 wk. *Therapeutic level:* 5–12 mcg/mL.
pregabalin	Adjunct partial seizures; tonic extensor seizure; generalized tonic-clonic seizure induced by sound	*Adult:* 50 mg 3 times daily initially –or– 75 mg twice daily to max 600 mg/day	Taper dosage over 7 days if need to discontinue drug. Check dosages in patients with renal impairment.
tiagabine	Simple and complex partial and tonic-clonic seizures	*Adult and Child >12 yr:* 4 mg per wk initially, with increases of 4–8 mg/wk, to 32–64 mg/day, 4 times daily.	Dosing guidelines assume concurrent use of adjuncts such as carbamazepine, phenytoin, or primidone.
topiramate	Adjunctive therapy for partial-onset seizures	*Adult:* 50 mg daily initially; increase to 50–400 mg daily every 12 hr *Child 2–16 yr:* 5–9 mg/kg/day in 2 divided doses. Begin titration at 25 mg (or less, based on a range of 1–3 mg/kg/day) nightly for first wk. Increase dosage at 1–2-wk intervals by increments of 1–3 mg/kg/day in 2 divided doses.	Age-related renal impairment may require dosage adjustment.
valproate	Tonic-clonic, myoclonic, absence, and complex partial seizures	*Adult and Child >20 kg:* Multidrug therapy: 15 mg/kg/day PO. Monotherapy: 5–15 mg/kg/day PO. Increase by 5–10 mg/kg/day PO at weekly intervals. Maintenance: 30–60 mg/kg/day PO in 2–3 divided doses	Time to steady state: 2–7 days. Divide doses if daily dose is greater than 250 mg. *Therapeutic level:* 50–100 mcg/mL
zonisamide	Adjunctive therapy in treatment of partial seizures	*Adult and Child >16 yr:* 100 mg PO daily. After 2 wk, increase dose to 200 mg/day for 2 wk; then to 300 or 400 mg/day.	Consider stopping drug in patients who develop an otherwise unexplained rash.

AED, Antiepileptic drug; *CNS,* central nervous system; *ER,* extended release; *GI,* gastrointestinal; *HS,* bedtime; *IM,* intramuscular (route); *IV,* intravenous (route); *PE,* phenytoin equivalent; *PO,* by mouth; *PRN,* as needed.

adjustments when converting between fosphenytoin and phenytoin sodium doses. **Always prescribe fosphenytoin in PE units (150 mg PE yields 100 mg of phenytoin sodium).**

Lab Considerations
Both phenytoin and fosphenytoin increase alkaline phosphatase, gamma-glutamyltransferase (GGT), and glucose levels. Periodically obtain a serum folate level, complete blood count (CBC), platelet count, serum calcium, albumin and creatinine levels, urinalysis, and liver and thyroid function tests throughout the course of therapy.

Measure serum phenytoin levels routinely throughout therapy. Therapeutic blood level values are derived from patients who have normal serum albumin levels and renal function. Patients with reduced serum albumin levels or renal disease are at risk for phenytoin toxicity. Serum levels of the drug are measured to monitor for toxicity or subtherapeutic levels.

Valproates
* divalproex sodium (Depakote, Depakene); ✦ Depakote
* valproic acid; ✦ valproic acid
* valproate sodium (Depacon)

Indications
Valproates are indicated as monotherapy or adjunctive therapy in the treatment of patients with complex partial seizures that occur either in isolation or in association with other seizure types. They are also indicated for use as sole or adjunctive therapy in the treatment of simple and complex absence seizures, and adjunctively in patients with multiple seizure types. Divalproex is also used in the treatment of manic episodes associated with bipolar disorder (see Chapter 21) and for migraine prophylaxis (see Chapter 24). There is no evidence to suggest valproates are helpful in the acute treatment of migraine headaches.

Pharmacodynamics
The mechanism by which valproates exert therapeutic effects has not been clearly established, although it has been suggested that they act as a gamma-aminobutyric acid (GABA) agonist. Divalproex is a prodrug of valproate, dissociating to the valproate ion in the GI tract.

Pharmacokinetics
The absorption rate of valproates from the GI tract and serum drug levels vary with the dosing regimen and the formulation. Valproates are 90% to 95% protein bound at serum concentrations of 50 mcg/mL; protein binding above 50 mcg/mL is 80% to 85%. Further, as the free fraction of drug in the circulation increases, the concentration gradient of the drug to the brain increases. Divalproex is enteric-coated, so absorption is delayed by 1 to 4 hours (see Table 25-2). Valproate is primarily biotransformed in the liver, with minimal amounts eliminated unchanged in the urine.

Adverse Effects and Contraindications
The common adverse effects of valproates include blurry vision, headache, alopecia, altered appetite, tinnitus, asthenia, amnesia, somnolence, emotional lability, insomnia, nervousness, dizziness, tremor, depression, dyspnea, dyspepsia, nausea and vomiting, diarrhea, abdominal pain, altered appetite, constipation, weight changes, peripheral edema, petechiae or ecchymosis, rash, thrombocytopenia, tremor, and abnormal gait.

Serious adverse effects of valproates include hepatotoxicity (although rare), including fatal reactions, pancreatitis, syndrome of inappropriate antidiuretic hormone secretion (SIADH), hyponatremia, pancytopenia, thrombocytopenia, myelosuppression, erythema multiform, Stevens-Johnson syndrome, toxic epidermal necrolysis, hyperammonemia, and anaphylaxis. The drug is contraindicated during pregnancy (category D) because of the risk of congenital anomalies, including neural tube defects; safe use during lactation has not been established.

Exercise caution when using valproates in patients with bleeding disorders, hypoalbuminemia or a history of liver or renal disease, and organic brain disease. Valproates are contraindicated in patients with hypersensitivity to the drug or its ingredients and in those with impaired liver function. Some valproate formulations contain tartrazine; avoid using these drugs in patients with known hypersensitivity.

Drug Interactions
Drug interactions are identified in Table 25-3.

Dosage Regimen
The dosage regimen for valproates depends on the type of seizure to be treated and whether monotherapy or multidrug therapy is used (see Table 25-4).

Lab Considerations
Dose-related elevations in lactate dehydrogenase (LDH), alanine transaminase (AST), and aspartate transaminase (ALT) values may occur with the valproates. Valproates also interfere with the accuracy of thyroid function tests and produce false-positive results in urine ketone tests. Occasionally, liver function tests and serum ammonia concentrations, including serum bilirubin levels, may be elevated, and serum calcium levels decreased. Monitor CBCs, platelet counts, and bleeding times before and throughout therapy.

Other Antiepileptic Drugs
* carbamazepine (Tegretol, Carbatrol, Epirol, Equetro); ✦ Apo-Carbamazepine

Indications
Carbamazepine is one of the drugs of choice in the management of tonic-clonic and partial seizures. It is also used to manage complex partial and mixed seizures. It is ineffective for absence (petit mal) and myoclonic seizures in adults.

Pharmacodynamics
Carbamazepine decreases synaptic transmission in the CNS by affecting sodium and calcium channels in neurons.

Pharmacokinetics
Carbamazepine is erratically absorbed after oral administration, although it is rapidly absorbed when taken with food. There is wide distribution to body tissues including the brain, cerebrospinal fluid, bile, and saliva. Biotransformation occurs

in the liver, and approximately 72% of elimination occurs in the urine and 28% in the feces (see Table 25-2). Carbamazepine crosses placental membranes and accumulates in the fetal liver and kidneys. The drug is found in breast milk.

Adverse Effects and Contraindications

Restlessness, aggression, irritability, and agitation may occur with carbamazepine administration. When children take carbamazepine, they may be unable to attend to tasks. Carbamazepine causes many adverse renal effects including renal failure, glycosuria, and urinary frequency and water retention (due to stimulation of antidiuretic hormone). Depression and mood disturbances are also possible in adults and children taking the drug. Dystonias may be seen, particularly when carbamazepine is combined with phenytoin. CNS adverse effects include syncope, dizziness, confusion, ataxia, and most seriously, encephalopathy. Additional visual effects include photosensitivity, nystagmus, and visual changes.

Serious conditions associated with carbamazepine use include aplastic anemia, agranulocytosis, systemic lupus erythematosus, thrombophlebitis, arrhythmias, and heart failure. Carbamazepine should not be used in patients with hypersensitivity, bone marrow depression, blood dyscrasias, or atrioventricular heart block. It may be used cautiously in patients who are recovering from alcohol abuse, and in those with behavioral problems, heart disease (other than those conditions previously mentioned), metabolic disorders such as osteoporosis, renal and hepatic impairments, diabetes, increased intraocular pressure, and during pregnancy (category D).

Drug Interactions

Carbamazepine interacts with numerous drugs that either increase its serum levels or decrease those of the interactive drug. The interacting drugs are identified in Table 25-3.

Dosage Regimen

The extended-release formulations of carbamazepine are given once to twice daily (Table 25-4).

Lab Considerations

Carbamazepine may increase the blood, urea, nitrogen (BUN), serum glucose, protein, AST, ALT, alkaline phosphatase, bilirubin, total cholesterol, triglycerides, and low-density lipoprotein (LDL) levels. For this reason, baseline and periodic testing of these parameters is recommended. Carbamazepine decreases serum sodium and calcium levels, and thyroid function tests (triiodothyronine [T_3], T_4, and T_4 index) as well.

A baseline CBC including platelets and reticulocytes, as well as serum iron levels, should be obtained before the start of therapy. Monitor patients closely should they develop decreased platelet or white blood cell counts while taking carbamazepine. Stop the drug should bone marrow suppression occur.

Routine eye examinations, including tonometry, should also be done. Patients taking carbamazepine may have lower thyroid function test values, and hyponatremia has been reported.

Monitoring of carbamazepine serum drug levels has increased the efficacy and safety of the drug. Monitoring is especially helpful when there is a question regarding adherence to therapy and when there has been an increase in the number of seizures. Serum drug level values are also helpful if there is a question of toxicity to the drug.

Ethosuximide (Zarontin); ◆ Emeside, Zarontin

Indications

Ethosuximide is used to manage absence seizures. Ethosuximide is the drug of choice for these seizures and for absence seizures that occur during pregnancy. Ethosuximide has been used for myoclonic and complex partial seizures, although less commonly.

Pharmacodynamics

How ethosuximide acts is unclear, although it is thought to suppress the paroxysmal spike-and-wave activity related to the lapses of consciousness seen in absence seizures. The frequency of attacks is reduced, apparently by depressing the motor cortex, which subsequently elevates the seizure threshold.

Pharmacokinetics

Ethosuximide is readily and rapidly absorbed from the GI tract and distributed to the tissues and body water and across placental membranes (see Table 25-2). A steady state is reached in 4 to 6 days in children and over a longer period in adults. Biotransformation occurs in the liver. Ethosuximide is eliminated unchanged (25% to 50%) in the urine. Small amounts are eliminated via the bile and feces. Ethosuximide is found in breast milk.

Adverse Effects and Contraindications

The adverse effects of ethosuximide are many, but in general affect the CNS, the GI tract, the skin, and the hematologic system. Drowsiness, ataxia, and dizziness are common adverse CNS effects. Adverse GI effects include tongue swelling, nausea, vomiting, diarrhea, gingivitis, and vague gastric upset. Eosinophilia, thrombocytopenia, bone marrow depression, leukopenia, agranulocytosis, monocytosis, and pancytopenia can be life threatening. Systemic lupus erythematosus and renal damage are also possible. Ethosuximide may also cause vaginal bleeding.

Stevens-Johnson syndrome is seen as a serious adverse effect of ethosuximide. It is an occasionally fatal inflammatory disease of children and young adults. It is characterized by fever, bullae of the skin, and ulcers of the mucous membranes of the oral cavity, the nose, the eyes, and the genitalia. Acute toxic effects include bradycardia, confusion, apnea, laryngospasm, ataxia, extreme weakness, and visual disturbances.

Ethosuximide-related aplastic anemia has been reported; in this instance ethosuximide was used as monotherapy. This rare, but potentially fatal, complication of ethosuximide raises the question as to whether routine monitoring of blood counts during therapy is useful and should be undertaken.

Drug Interactions

As with all other drug groups, there are drug interactions to be considered. Ethosuximide interacts with phenytoin to increase serum phenytoin concentrations. Reduced primidone and phenobarbital levels have been noted with concurrent use of ethosuximide (see Table 25-3).

Dosage Regimen

The dosage regimen for ethosuximide is based on patient needs (see Table 25-4). Dosages are titrated upward at weekly intervals according to the patient's serum drug levels. The drug should be taken at regularly spaced intervals.

Lab Considerations

There are few drug–laboratory test interactions with ethosuximide. Ethosuximide increases the likelihood for a positive Coombs' test. For all patients taking ethosuximide, obtain a baseline CBC with differential and liver function testing, initially and then on a regular basis throughout therapy.

Oxazolidinedione (Trileptal); ◆ Tripletal

Indications

Oxcarbazepine is indicated for use as monotherapy in adults or as adjunctive therapy in patients with partial seizures who are older than 4 years of age.

Pharmacodynamics

Oxcarbazepine is a prodrug designed to be structurally similar to carbamazepine; it acts by regulating neuronal ion flux and inhibiting the voltage-dependent sodium channel. The majority of drug effect is the result of the metabolite, mono-hydroxycarbamazepine (MHD).

Pharmacokinetics

Oxcarbazepine, as a prodrug, is rapidly absorbed and converted to its active metabolite MHD. More than 90% of the drug is eliminated in the urine, with 4% in feces (see Table 25-2). Its elimination is catalyzed by noninducible reductases, although it induces the CYP450 system for biotransformation following first-order kinetics.

Adverse Effects and Contraindications

Somnolence, headache, diplopia, nausea, and rash are common adverse effects of oxcarbazepine. Approximately 25% to 30% of patients sensitive to carbamazepine will have a cross-sensitivity to oxcarbazepine. Aplastic anemia and agranulocytosis are possible but unusual. The risk for hyponatremia is greater with carbamazepine than with oxcarbazepine. Older adults are particularly prone to this adverse effect. Oxcarbazepine is a pregnancy category C drug.

Drug Interactions

Drug interactions are fewer with oxcarbazepine than with carbamazepine but include the oral contraceptives, whose efficacy is reduced when taken with oxcarbazepine (see Table 25-3). Oxcarbazepine does not interact with warfarin, cimetidine, erythromycin, verapamil, or dextropropoxyphene.

Dosage Regimen

Greater efficacy is noted with oxcarbazepine dosages above 1200 mg/day. However, most patients are unable to tolerate higher dosages (e.g., 2400 mg/day) because of the adverse CNS effects (see Table 25-4).

Lab Considerations

For the prodrug oxcarbazepine, therapeutic drug monitoring is useful since the active metabolite is measured. Regularly monitor serum sodium levels because of the risk of hyponatremia. Oxcarbazepine has also been associated with a drop in T_4 levels, but there are no changes in thyroid-stimulating hormone (TSH) or T_3 values.

Gabapentin (Neurontin); ◆ Neurontin

Indications

Gabapentin is an adjunct for patients with or without secondary generalization of partial seizures, and has been shown effective in decreasing neuropathic pain. It is ineffective for absence seizures.

Pharmacodynamics

The mechanism of action of gabapentin is unknown. It appears to affect the movement of amino acids across neuronal membranes.

Pharmacokinetics

Taken orally, gabapentin is well absorbed and, as a general rule, circulates unbound in the plasma. It is almost entirely eliminated (76% to 81%) through the kidneys as unchanged drug, with the remainder in the feces (see Table 25-2). Elimination is reduced in patients with impaired cardiac or renal function, and in older adults.

Adverse Effects and Contraindications

The most common adverse effects of gabapentin are somnolence and ataxia, although weakness, malaise, vertigo, depression, and anxiety have occurred. Nystagmus, abnormal vision, hypertension or hypotension, dyskinesias, respiratory symptoms, hematuria, urinary frequency, pruritus, angioedema, eczema, anorexia, flatulence, gingivitis, and muscle pain are possible.

Gabapentin is used with caution in patients with renal insufficiency and in older adults, in whom sedation is a concern. Safe use during pregnancy (category C) and lactation has not been established. Hypersensitivity to the drug or its ingredients contraindicates the use of gabapentin.

Drug Interactions

There are no known drug interactions with gabapentin and other AEDs or with oral contraceptives. When taken with antacids, the bioavailability of gabapentin is decreased 20% (Table 25-3).

Dosage Regimen

Rapid titration of gabapentin may be used until desired effects are obtained. Doses should not be more than 12 hours apart (see Table 25-4).

Lab Considerations

Gabapentin therapy can cause anemia, thrombocytopenia, leukopenia, and an increase in bleeding time. Thus laboratory monitoring of CBC, differential, and platelet count is warranted before and throughout therapy. Gabapentin may cause a false-positive reading when the Ames N-Multistix SG dipstick test for urinary protein is used. Use the sulfosalicylic acid precipitation procedure instead.

Lamotrigine (Lamictal); ◆ Lamictal

Indications

Lamotrigine may be used in adults who have partial seizures with or without secondary generation as monotherapy, or it may be used as an adjunct with other drugs. The drug has been effective for patients under 16 years of age who have Lennox-Gastaut syndrome. *Lennox-Gastaut syndrome* is a complex form of epilepsy marked by early-childhood onset, poorly controlled multiple seizure types, slow-spike EEG waves, and a high incidence of mental retardation.

Pharmacodynamics

Lamotrigine soothes sensitive neuronal membranes by inhibiting the release of neurotransmitters. Its site of action is the voltage-gated sodium channels.

Pharmacokinetics

Lamotrigine is well absorbed orally and is not affected by food (see Table 25-2). Its time to onset and duration of action are unknown. Fifty-five percent of lamotrigine is protein bound. The drug is biotransformed in the liver and eliminated in the urine. Clearance is significantly increased (i.e., half-life is reduced 50%) in the presence of other hepatic enzyme–inducing AEDs, such as carbamazepine, phenobarbital, phenytoin, and primidone. The elimination of lamotrigine is decreased in the presence of valproic acid; however, the half-life may double.

Adverse Effects and Contraindications

The most common adverse effects of lamotrigine include ataxia, dizziness, headache, somnolence, nausea, vomiting, rash, arthralgias, and photosensitivity. Complaints of rhinitis, pharyngitis, cough, infections, hematuria, anxiety, depression, and allergic reactions have also occurred with lamotrigine use. Use lamotrigine cautiously in patients with impaired cardiac or renal function. Up to 10% of patients stop the drug because of its adverse effects.

A macular, papular, or erythematous rash or systemic symptoms such as fever or lymphadenopathy develop in 10% of patients during the first 4 to 6 weeks of therapy. These symptoms require prompt discontinuation of the drug and reevaluation of the patient's condition. Angioedema, lymphadenopathy, Stevens-Johnson syndrome, and toxic epidermal necrolysis are possible though rare. The risk for these severe responses increases even more (threefold, in fact) when the lamotrigine is coadministered with a valproate. Use caution in patients who have comorbid conditions that alter kidney or liver function. Hypersensitivity to lamotrigine or its ingredients contraindicates its use.

There is a 1 in 50 chance that lamotrigine will cause rash in children; therefore the drug is not recommended for children under 16 years of age.

Use in pregnant patients is appropriate only when the benefits outweigh potential risks (category C). Withdrawal seizures may appear if lamotrigine is abruptly discontinued; thus a gradual taper over 2 weeks is recommended. Nursing is not recommended since lamotrigine is found in breast milk.

Drug Interactions

CYP-inducing AEDs that are taken concurrently (e.g., carbamazepine, phenytoin, phenobarbital, primidone) increase elimination of the drug, and valproates double the elimination half-life (see Table 25-3). Accordingly, the lamotrigine dosage must be reduced by at least 50% in patients who are also taking a valproate.

Dosage Regimen

The dosage of lamotrigine is based on its relationship with other AEDs. The dosage is adjusted downward when lamotrigine is taken concurrently with carbamazepine, phenobarbital, phenytoin, or primidone, and is especially different when it is taken with these drugs *and* valproate (see Table 25-4). Renal dosing considerations are important in patients with significant kidney impairment.

Lab Considerations

Serum drug level of lamotrigine has not been established, although such monitoring may be warranted if patients are taking lamotrigine and concomitant AEDs. This is particularly true during periods of dosage adjustment.

Pregabalin (Lyrica); ◆ Lyrica

Indications

Pregabalin (Lyrica), the newest antiepileptic drug, prevents tonic extensor seizures, which are a generalized tonic-clonic type of seizure induced by sound, but does not reduce the incidence of spontaneous absence seizures in susceptible patients. It is also approved for neuropathic pain and is used as prophylaxis for migraine headaches.

Pharmacodynamics

Although structurally related to GABA, pregabalin is not functionally related and does not directly affect GABA. It is inactive at GABA receptors and does not affect GABA uptake or degradation.

Much like with gabapentin, the potent binding of pregabalin and its structural analogues to the alpha-2-delta site reduce depolarization-induced calcium influx at nerve terminals. There is a subsequent reduction in the release of several excitatory neurotransmitters including glutamate, noradrenalin, substance P, and calcitonin gene–related peptide (CGRP), but pregabalin does not completely block calcium channel function or transmitter release even at high concentrations.

Pharmacokinetics

Pregabalin is rapidly and extensively absorbed after oral dosing and is not significantly affected by the presence of food. Pregabalin does not bind to plasma proteins and does not induce or inhibit CYP450 enzymes. The drug is eliminated entirely unchanged by the kidneys.

Adverse Effects and Contraindications

The most commonly reported adverse effects are CNS-related. Dizziness is the most common adverse effect and leads about 5% of patients to discontinue the drug. Other adverse effects include somnolence, ataxia, and asthenia. Weight gain (over 7% from baseline) is also common. No significant, serious toxicity is known. Dosages exceeding

300 mg/day are associated with a higher rate of adverse effects; the drug is considered pregnancy category C.

Drug Interactions

In vitro studies, conducted at concentrations generally 10 times those achieved in clinical trials, have shown that pregabalin does not inhibit CYP450 enzyme systems (Tassone et al., 2007). Studies have not been conducted to determine the potential of pregabalin to induce these enzymes. Steady-state trough plasma concentrations of phenytoin, carbamazepine, valproate, and lamotrigine are not affected by the concomitant administration of pregabalin at 200 mg, 3 times daily.

Dosage Regimen

The maximum recommended dose of pregabalin is 100 mg, 3 times daily, in patients with a creatinine clearance of at least 60 mL/min. Dosing should begin at 50 mg, 3 times a day, and may be increased to 300 mg/day within 1 week based on efficacy and tolerability. Because pregabalin is eliminated primarily by renal excretion, the dosage should be adjusted for patients with reduced renal function.

Lab Considerations

Pregabalin may elevate creatinine kinase (CK) levels, decrease platelet counts, and increase the PR interval on electrocardiogram (ECG).

Topiramate (Topamax); ✦ Topamax
Indications

Topiramate has been approved as initial monotherapy in patients 10 years of age and older with partial-onset or primary generalized tonic-clonic seizures. It has also been approved for migraine prophylaxis (see Chapter 24).

Pharmacodynamics

Topiramate blocks the repetitive firing of CNS neurons by enhancing the ability of GABA to cause an influx of chloride ions into CNS neurons. Topiramate also blocks the action of glutamate (an excitatory neurotransmitter), blocks sodium channels, reduces the activity of calcium channels, and inhibits the enzyme carbonic anhydrase.

Pharmacokinetics

Topiramate is rapidly absorbed after oral administration (Table 25-2). It is less than 20% bound to plasma proteins. Compared with the immediate release form, the sprinkle formulation of topiramate is both bioequivalent and therapeutically equivalent. Topiramate is minimally biotransformed, and although 6 metabolites have been identified, they make up less than 5% of an orally administered dose of the drug. With concurrent use of other AEDs, 50% of the drug is biotransformed. Approximately 70% of an oral dose of topiramate is eliminated unchanged in the urine.

Adverse Effects and Contraindications

Most adverse effects of topiramate are dose dependent, occur more often during upward titration of dosage (rather than with maintenance dosages), and vary in severity from mild to moderate. The adverse effects include nervousness, somnolence, fatigue, ataxia, paresthesias, tremors, nystagmus, diplopia, and nausea. Psychomotor retardation, altered ability to concentrate, word-finding difficulties, and memory disturbances occasionally occur. These adverse effects are generally mild to moderate but can be severe enough to require withdrawal of the drug from therapy. Although rare, confusion, breast pain, dysmenorrhea, depression, asthenia, pharyngitis, anorexia, rash, musculoskeletal pain, sinusitis, agitation, and flulike symptoms have occurred. Because of the inhibition of carbonic anhydrase the patient is at increased risk for kidney stones. Hypersensitivity to topiramate or its ingredients contraindicates use of the drug. During pregnancy, topiramate is classified as a category C drug; whether or not the drug is transmitted to breast milk is unknown.

Drug Interactions

Drug interactions with topiramate are identified in Table 25-3. Cautious use is warranted in patients who have comorbid disorders such as diabetes because concurrent use of topiramate with metformin increases metformin levels, thus increasing the risk for hypoglycemia and lactic acidosis. The levels of pioglitazone and phenytoin, when they are used in combination with topiramate, may be decreased. Avoid the concomitant use of topiramate with carbonic anhydrase inhibitors such as acetazolamide.

Dosage Regimen

Dose and titration rates of topiramate are guided by patient response. Longer dosing intervals can be used when necessary to reduce adverse effects. Dosage adjustments may be needed for patients with impaired renal function (see Table 25-4).

Lab Considerations

Measurement of baseline and serum bicarbonate levels during topiramate treatment is recommended. Monitoring drug levels of topiramate is not necessary.

Tiagabine (Gabitril)
Indications

Tiagabine is used in the treatment of simple and complex partial and tonic-clonic seizures and as monotherapy or an adjunct in patients with refractory partial-onset seizures.

Pharmacodynamics

Tiagabine is a derivative of a GABA uptake inhibitor and acts by reversibly inhibiting GABA transporter-1. It functions as an agonist to chloride conductance by blocking the reuptake of GABA and increasing synaptic levels of GABA.

Pharmacokinetics

The oral bioavailability, absorption, and protein binding of tiagabine are over 90% when the drug is taken without food (see Table 25-2). Because the drug is lipid-soluble it crosses the blood-brain barrier. A bimodal peak in plasma drug levels occurs approximately 12 hours after it is taken, likely because of enterohepatic recirculation. Linear biotransformation to inactive metabolites is accomplished by the CYP450 enzymes. Less than 3% is eliminated unchanged in the urine. The half-life of the drug is reduced to 2 to 3 hours in the presence of other enzyme-inducing AEDs.

CENTRAL NERVOUS

ⅢⅢ Adverse Effects and Contraindications

Dizziness, asthenia, nervousness, somnolence, and nausea are common adverse effects of tiagabine. Postmarketing reports have shown that tiagabine is associated with new-onset seizures and status epilepticus in patients without epilepsy (Jette et al., 2006). Patients taking concomitant drugs such as antidepressants, antipsychotics, CNS stimulants, or opioids may require dosage reduction, since these drugs are thought to lower the seizure threshold. It is a pregnancy category C drug.

ⅢⅢ Drug Interactions

Tiagabine may alter the effects of valproates. Carbamazepine, phenytoin, and phenobarbital may increase the clearance of tiagabine (see Table 25-3).

ⅢⅢ Dosage Regimen

Tiagabine is dosed orally once daily to a maximum dosage of 56 mg/day. The maximum dosage for children from 12 to 18 years of age is 32 mg/day (see Table 25-4).

ⅢⅢ Lab Considerations

Tiagabine plasma concentrations do not have an established therapeutic range. Obtaining plasma levels of tiagibine before and after adjusting the course of therapy may be useful because of the possibility for pharmacokinetic interactions between tiagabine and drugs that affect hepatic metabolizing enzymes. Tiagabine does not affect the serum concentrations of other drugs, though the effect on oral contraceptives is unestablished at higher doses.

Levetiracetam (Keppra); ✦ Keppra

ⅢⅢ Indications

Although levetiracetam (Keppra) is a potent AED, its novel design, lack of appreciable biotransformation and AED interactions, and efficacy make it an attractive choice for adult patients with persistent partial-onset seizures.

ⅢⅢ Pharmacodynamics

How levetiracetam exerts its antiepileptic action is unknown. It appears that the drug provides seizure protection against secondarily generalized activity.

ⅢⅢ Pharmacokinetics

The most attractive quality of this drug is the pharmacokinetics (see Table 25-2). Levetiracetam is rapidly and almost completely absorbed after oral administration. Biotransformation is linear, although not through the liver's CYP450 enzymes. The metabolites have no known pharmacologic activity, and more than 60% of the drug is eliminated in the urine. Levetiracetam crosses placental membranes, with concentrations similar to those of the mother (pregnancy category C).

ⅢⅢ Adverse Effects and Contraindications

Levetiracetam is generally well tolerated, with adverse effects reported in about 10% of patients. CNS-related ataxia, abnormal gait, and incoordination are most bothersome. Somnolence, asthenia, and the coordination difficulties ordinarily occur within the first 4 weeks of treatment. Behavioral abnormalities such as aggression, agitation, anger, anxiety, apathy, depersonalization, depression, emotional lability, hostility, irritability, psychotic symptoms, and psychotic depression have been reported.

The half-life of levetiracetam is increased to 24 hours in patients with renal dysfunction. No serious acute idiopathic reactions have been reported, and there is no evidence of visual field disturbances. Levetiracetam does not appear to exacerbate seizures, unlike this paradoxical effect seen in some patients taking other AEDs.

ⅢⅢ Drug Interactions

There are no significant drug interactions with levetiracetam.

ⅢⅢ Dosage Regimen

Levetiracetam is given in divided doses twice daily. The dosage is titrated upward, based on patient response, to a maximum of 3 grams/day (see Table 25-4).

ⅢⅢ Lab Considerations

Although most laboratory tests are unaltered with levetiracetam, there have been infrequent reports of abnormalities in hematologic parameters and liver function tests.

Zonisamide (Zonegran)

ⅢⅢ Indications

Zonisamide is a broad-spectrum AED that significantly reduces the frequency of complex partial seizures and generalized seizures in patients with refractory epilepsy involving one or more distinct parts of the brain. Moreover, zonisamide has demonstrated high efficacy in managing progressive myoclonic epilepsy syndromes. The properties of zonisamide highlight its potential: broad-spectrum efficacy, once-daily dosing, long half-life, and a unique mechanism of action.

ⅢⅢ Pharmacodynamics

Zonisamide's mechanisms of action include blockade of the T type of calcium channels, blockade of voltage-dependent sodium channels, and inhibition of the carbonic anhydrase enzyme.

ⅢⅢ Pharmacokinetics

Zonisamide is fully and rapidly absorbed, binding extensively to erythrocytes and resulting in 8 times the concentration of zonisamide in red blood cells (RBCs) compared to plasma. Zonisamide is biotransformed through the CYP450 system, with excretion of the drug and its metabolites primarily through the kidneys.

ⅢⅢ Adverse Effects and Contraindications

The most common adverse effects include somnolence, ataxia, loss of appetite, confusion, fatigue, and dizziness. Nephrolithiasis occurs in less than 3% of patients. **Because ⚠ of the risk for Stevens-Johnson syndrome and toxic epidermal necrolysis, discontinue zonisamide if patients develop an otherwise unexplained rash.** Seven deaths from Stevens-Johnson syndrome and toxic epidermal necrolysis were reported in the first 11 years of marketing (Sills and Brodie, 2007). **If patients taking zonisamide develop severe muscle ⚠ pain and/or weakness, either in the presence or the absence of a fever, creatinine phosphokinase (CK) and aldolase levels, markers of muscle damage, should be assessed.**

If the values are elevated, zonisamide should be discontinued, particularly in the absence of another obvious cause such as trauma or tonic-clonic seizures.

Similarly, patients taking zonisamide who manifest clinical signs and symptoms of pancreatitis should have pancreatic lipase and amylase levels monitored. If pancreatitis is evident, in the absence of another obvious cause, the drug dosage should be tapered and/or zonisamide discontinued. Zonisamide is a pregnancy category C drug.

A In addition, **oligohydrosis, sometimes resulting in heat stroke and hospitalization, is seen in children taking zonisamide. No deaths have been reported.**

Drug Interactions

Drug interactions are minimal; however, as a sulfonamide, derivative allergy to zonisamide is a concern.

Dosage Regimen

Children and adults are started on a once-daily regimen. After 2 weeks, the dosage may then be titrated upward based on patient response (see Table 25-4).

Lab Considerations

Zonisamide is associated with an elevation of serum creatinine and BUN values of approximately 8% over the baseline measurement. Consideration should be given to periodically monitoring renal function.

Barbiturates

◆ mephobarbital (Mebaral)
◆ phenobarbital (Luminal)
◆ primidone (Mysoline); ◆ Primidone

Indications

Although barbiturates all possess antiepileptic effects, even at subhypnotic dosages for many of them, the long-acting barbiturates (phenobarbital, mephobarbital) are the only ones used in an oral formulation. Barbiturates were discussed in relation to their sedative-hypnotic effects briefly in Chapter 19.

Phenobarbital is used in the prevention and treatment of tonic-clonic, simple, and complex partial seizures. It is also used for fever-induced seizures and status epilepticus. Long-term use for febrile seizures is controversial, and it is ineffective for absence seizures.

Mephobarbital is used for generalized tonic-clonic seizures and for partial seizures. It is often used as a replacement drug for phenobarbital when there is paradoxical excitement in children or there is ongoing sedation or behavioral changes in adults. It can be used as monotherapy or with other AEDs.

Primidone, used either alone or concomitantly with other AEDS, is indicated in the control of tonic-clonic seizures and focal seizures. It is use as prophylaxis for partial seizures and in combination with phenytoin or carbamazepine to control tonic-clonic seizures refractory to other AED therapy.

Pharmacodynamics

Like the benzodiazepines (BZDs) discussed in Chapter 19, barbiturates act at $GABA_A$ receptors to enhance the effects of GABA. By depressing impulse transmission from the thalamus to the cortex, barbiturates reduce the excitability of neurons and raise the seizure threshold. However, unlike BZDs, barbiturates act even in the absence of GABA to allow the movement of chloride through the channels. For this reason and because of the fact that there is no ceiling effect to the depression, barbiturates have the potential to cause greater and more widespread CNS depression than BZDs. As dosages increase, the patient's level of consciousness progresses from sedation to sleep, to general anesthesia, and to death. Primidone is the metabolite of phenobarbital.

Pharmacokinetics

Barbiturates are rapidly absorbed and distributed to all body tissues and fluids, with high concentrations in the brain, the cerebrospinal fluid, the liver, and the kidneys (see Table 25-2). Barbiturates stimulate biotransformation by promoting the synthesis of porphyrin. Porphyrin, a nitrogen-containing organic compound that is present in the protoplasm of cells, is then converted to heme, which in turn is converted to CYP450. Because many other drugs are also biotransformed by the same hepatic enzymes, barbiturates induce tolerance of other drugs (see Drug Interactions section that follows).

The lipid-solubility of barbiturates determines the speed of distribution throughout the body. Barbiturates with high lipid-solubility will be distributed more rapidly. The degree to which barbiturates bind to plasma and tissue proteins is also dependent upon lipid-solubility, with binding increasing as lipid-solubility increases. Barbiturates with the highest degree of lipid-solubility have the longest duration of action; those with the lowest degree of lipid-solubility have the shortest duration of action. The more slowly a barbiturate is altered or eliminated, the more prolonged its action. Barbiturates readily cross the placental membranes and are found in breast milk.

Adverse Effects and Contraindications

Barbiturates produce CNS depression, including drowsiness, dizziness, lethargy, and behavioral changes, which limits their use. Adverse GI effects include constipation. Rashes and urticaria have been noted. Angioedema and serum sickness are the most life-threatening adverse effects. Erythema multiforme and coma may occur with phenobarbital use. (Coma may be an intentionally induced effect in treating status epilepticus.)

The more serious adverse effects of barbiturates include hypersensitivity reactions (i.e., skin rash, exfoliative dermatitis, urticaria), sore throat, fever, edema, serum sickness, apnea, bronchospasms, and Stevens-Johnson syndrome.

Phenobarbital is contraindicated for use in patients with hypersensitivity to this drug or to primidone, and in patients with porphyria. Phenobarbital and primidone must also be used with caution in patients with nephritis or pulmonary insufficiency. Those with respiratory depression or obstruction, asthma, heart failure, severe anemia, hepatic dysfunction, hypoadrenalism, hypothyroidism, or depression, or those with acute or chronic pain, must use phenobarbital with caution. Impaired memory occurs in some children taking phenobarbital. A hydantoin-like syndrome has occurred when phenobarbital is taken during pregnancy (pregnancy category D); the newborn may manifest withdrawal symptoms as well.

Mephobarbital is reported to cause less sedation than phenobarbital. Adverse effects of mephobarbital include all of those just mentioned plus agranulocytosis, thrombocytopenia, and megaloblastic anemia (with long-term therapy). Respiratory depression, apnea, laryngospasm, and bronchospasm have been noted.

The most common adverse effects of primidone are drowsiness, ataxia, vertigo, lethargy, and anorexia. Systemic lupus erythematosus, blood dyscrasias, megaloblastic anemia, and hypersensitivity reactions are possible. Primidone must be used with caution in patients with renal impairments, hepatic dysfunction, and pulmonary insufficiency. It is contraindicated for use in patients with porphyria.

▥ Drug Interactions

Table 25-3 provides an overview of the interactions. Although barbiturates do not impair normal hepatic function, they have been found to induce CYP450 enzymes, consequently increasing and/or altering the biotransformation of themselves and other drugs. Barbiturates also interact with other CNS-depressant drugs to increase the CNS depression. The effects of certain drugs, such as acetaminophen, oral anticoagulants, some antibiotics, tricyclic antidepressants, oral contraceptives, and xanthines, are reduced. Orthostatic hypotension can occur with concurrent use of furosemide.

▥ Dosage Regimen

The dosages of barbiturates are individualized (see Table 25-4). Administer a minimal dose and evaluate effectiveness before giving a second dose, to prevent barbiturate-induced CNS depression. Administered in subanesthetic doses, phenobarbital has little analgesic effect and may intensify the response to painful stimuli. The timing of mephobarbital administration is dependent on when the patient's seizures usually occur.

▥ Lab Considerations

Periodically monitor patients on prolonged barbiturate therapy for hepatic and renal function, as well as assessing CBC and concentrations of serum folate (these drugs increase folate requirements). Phenobarbital may cause decreased serum bilirubin concentrations in neonates, in patients with congenital nonhemolytic unconjugated hyperbilirubinemia, and in patients with epilepsy. Serum phenobarbital levels should be monitored.

Benzodiazepines

Clonazepam (Klonopin) and clorazepate (Tranxene) have been approved for the treatment of absence and myoclonic seizures. Clorazepate is used concurrently with other AEDs in the treatment of partial-onset simple seizures. Diazepam (Valium) and lorazepam (Ativan) are used to treat status epilepticus (see also Chapter 19).

As discussed in Chapter 19, BZDs act at many levels to depress the CNS. Binding of GABA to GABA_A receptors in the CNS moves negatively charged chloride ions into the cell through chloride channels. The result is a more negative resting membrane potential, which is incapable of generating an action potential.

The BZDs are rapidly and well absorbed from the GI tract, although little is known about their distribution. They are thought to cross the blood-brain barrier and are known to cross the placenta. Biotransformation occurs in the liver, with elimination by the kidneys; less than 1% is eliminated as unchanged drug. BZDs are eliminated extensively into breast milk. The dosages for these drugs are listed in Table 25-4.

Sedation, restlessness, aggression, irritability, hallucinations, and agitation may occur with clonazepam and diazepam administration. Dysuria may be noted. Extrapyramidal symptoms have been noted. Impaired memory may also be seen.

Use BZDs cautiously in patients with chronic respiratory conditions and in children, older adults, debilitated patients, those with acute angle–closure glaucoma, and anyone who has a tendency toward physical or psychologic dependency. BZDs are contraindicated in patients with hypersensitivity to clonazepam and other BZDs and in patients with severe liver disease or with optic nerve or retinal disorders.

CLINICAL REASONING

Treatment Objectives

The treatment objectives for epilepsy are to prevent, or at least reduce to the greatest extent possible, the number and/or severity of seizures, while assisting the patient to maintain the highest level of independent functioning achievable.

Treatment Options

▥ Patient Variables

It is important to diagnose the etiology of seizures as early as possible, because this information influences the choice of drug and duration of therapy. Because altered consciousness often accompanies seizures, find out from family or friends what the patient's activities were before, during, and after the seizure. Also obtain specific information about the course and duration of the seizure activity, including the following:
- Where in the body did the seizures begin? Did the seizures travel through the body?
- Does the muscle tone seem tense or limp? Were color changes noted in the face or the lips?
- Was there a loss of consciousness, or loss of bladder or bowel control?
- Did the patient experience an aura before the seizure? Were there precipitating events?
- After the seizure, did the patient sleep or have any confusion, weakness, headache, or muscle ache?
- How have the seizures affected the patient's life?

Life-Span Considerations

Pregnant and Nursing Women. Women with epilepsy also have higher rates of congenital anomalies and malformations in their children; this appears to be caused by exposure of the developing fetus to AEDs taken by the mother. When AEDs must be used during pregnancy, monotherapy is preferable. Monitoring of blood levels, with as-needed dosage adjustments and stabilization, is mandatory. For absence seizures, ethosuximide is the drug of choice. Carbamazepine, although linked to malformations (e.g., spina bifida, retarded growth, congenital heart defects), is erroneously thought by some not to be recommended for use in pregnancy; in fact, it is considered one of the safest drugs for seizures during pregnancy.

Children and Adolescents. Epilepsy in infancy, childhood, and adolescence is complex to diagnose and treat because of the varying causes and concerns at these different ages and the need for family involvement. The majority of children with epilepsy lead normal, active lives. However, for some, their seizure disorder can be disabling and leads to social, emotional, and academic problems. When this occurs, children need additional resources from family, school, and community.

Seizures in newborns do not conform to the international classification of epileptic seizures. Seizures in newborns are caused by identifiable metabolic or infectious conditions. They may also be associated with perinatal complications such as electrolyte disorders, cerebral infarction, meningitis, septicemia, brain malfunctions, or hypoxic-ischemic disease.

The epilepsies in infancy range from benign to severe, with those beginning during the first year of life having the poorest prognosis. Infants may also have seizures due to transient causes, have normal clinical and EEG findings despite having seizures, and do not develop epilepsy.

Febrile seizures may result from any cause other than CNS infection. Seventy-five percent of the children who experience them have rectal temperatures above 102.2° F (39° C), although seizures may occur at lower temperature levels. These seizures are seen in children ages 3 months to 6 years, with a peak incidence at 18 months. Of children who have had a single febrile seizure, 30% to 40% will have another seizure and 3% will go on to have epilepsy by age 7 years. Although febrile convulsions are generally benign, they are extremely frightening for the child's family. Most children who have febrile seizures are otherwise completely normal. Brain damage is a possible outcome of febrile seizures, but it occurs rarely, and then only if the seizure is prolonged.

Encephalopathic epilepsies in infants and young children are associated with a cerebral disorder and mental retardation. They are referred to as West's syndrome (infantile spasms) and Lennox-Gastaut syndrome (myoclonic-astatic epilepsy of early childhood). The most common epilepsies affecting older children and adolescents are partial-onset seizures. However, they may experience generalized epilepsies with absence seizures. Benign partial epilepsies account for more than one third of all cases of epilepsy that begin in childhood.

Older Adults. Anyone with new-onset seizures after their 20s is most likely having seizures from an organic or anatomic source; it is one of those situations where "until proven otherwise," the patient has a secondary form of epilepsy. These individuals may have diseases and conditions that increase their vulnerability to seizures. They are susceptible to organ failure, metabolic disturbances, infection, CNS lesions, falls, trauma, alcohol withdrawal, and the adverse effects of polypharmacy. Epilepsy in the older adult is sometimes complicated by the normal changes of aging, as well, and other consequences of aging such as benign and malignant tumors (both primary brain and metastatic). Management with AEDs takes special assessment, intervention, and evaluation skills, as well as an understanding of the health needs of the older adult.

Factors contributing to the adverse cognitive effects of AEDs in older adults include other comorbid disorders, the patient's cognitive dysfunction before starting the drug, and polypharmacy. Gabapentin, lamotrigine, and levetiracetam cause significantly fewer cognitive adverse effects compared with carbamazepine, and are generally well tolerated.

▥ *Drug Variables*

Although AEDs may control seizures, they do not cure the underlying disorder. In cases where epilepsy is found not to be the cause of seizures, the condition that lowers the seizure threshold and/or precipitates a seizure (e.g., hypoglycemia, electrolyte imbalances, fever, exposure to toxins, and drug overdoses or withdrawal) must be controlled in addition to treating the seizures themselves. The treatment choice of an AED is dependent on accurate diagnosis of seizure type (i.e., partial, generalized, or unclassified); the pattern of seizures; age of the patient; family history; response to any previously used AED; and adverse effects of the drug.

It is usually not necessary to start an AED with the first seizure unless computed tomography (CT) or magnetic resonance imaging (MRI) scans detect a lesion, or there is an epileptic focus seen on the EEG. Begin therapy when there is a history of recurrent seizures (more than one) that cannot be explained by drug or alcohol use, arrhythmias, metabolic disorders, or other causes.

Treatment options for seizures are summarized in Table 25-5. Choose a treatment based on the importance of controlling the seizures using the fewest number of AEDs and one with the fewest adverse effects. Drug therapy for epilepsy reduces the risk of trauma arising from seizures (e.g., headbanging, falling, and prolonged periods of anoxia with status epilepticus and/or aspiration and its complications).

Development of an effective regimen that either prevents or arrests the seizures usually requires weeks of drug trial, error, and adjustment. Use seizure frequency as a guide to determine when to increase the dosage or change therapy. If seizures are infrequent, therapy is usually continued until steady-state drug levels within the therapeutic range are achieved. Once the seizure disorder is controlled, the major risk factors are nonadherence, lack of medical follow-up, and discontinuing the drug. These actions increase the risk and incidence of status epilepticus. Approximately 80% of all patients with epilepsy gain control of their disease with AEDs or show a significant reduction in the severity of the seizures (Box 25-1).

TABLE 25-5 Treatment Options for Seizures

Seizure Type	First-Line Drugs	Alternative Drugs
PARTIAL SEIZURES		
Absence seizures	ethosuximide, valproate, clorazepate	clonazepam, lamotrigine
Simple partial-onset seizures	phenytoin, carbamazepine, valproate	gabapentin, lamotrigine, phenobarbital, primidone, topiramate, tiagabine, oxcarbazepine
Complex partial-onset seizures	carbamazepine, phenytoin, phenobarbital, valproate	gabapentin, lamotrigine, primidone, topiramate, tiagabine, oxcarbazepine
GENERALIZED SEIZURES		
Myoclonic seizures	valproate, clonazepate	clonazepam
Tonic-clonic seizures	valproate, phenytoin, phenobarbital	carbamazepine
Status epilepticus	lorazepam, diazepam	phenytoin, phenobarbital

---

BOX 25-1

Principles of Prescribing AEDs

Drug Selection

a. Be sure the diagnosis is correct.

b. All things being equal, use the least expensive AED.

c. Choose an AED that can be taken once daily since this improves adherence. AEDs almost never need dosing 2, 3, or 4 times a day.

d. Use valproate for absence plus myoclonic, clonic, tonic, and/or atonic seizures.

e. Treat complex partial seizures with carbamazepine, phenytoin, primidone, and/or phenobarbital. Partial seizures may be treated using second-line drugs such as valproate or clorazepate.

f. Newer drugs are not necessarily better and are almost certainly more expensive (e.g., Topamax, Gabitril).

g. There have been no quality studies done to suggest that therapy with more than one AED used concurrently is beneficial.

h. The complexity of treating a patient with epilepsy that is refractory to treatment is compounded by the cost of the drugs and their adverse effects. Start with one AED, increasing the dosage as needed to control seizures or until clinical toxicity becomes apparent.

i. Withdraw AEDs that are ineffective.

j. Never maintain a patient arbitrarily on a regimen of more than three AEDs.

k. Use single-ingredient drugs rather than combined drug formulations (e.g., phenytoin + phenobarbital).

Evaluation

a. Readings of AED levels never replace clinical judgment; treat the patient, not the lab value.

b. Use AED levels to assess the following: poor clinical control (adherence, biotransformation); dose-related adverse effects; and drug or disease interactions. Routinely assessing levels on patients whose condition is well controlled and who are not suffering toxicity reactions is not indicated.

AED, Antiepileptic drug.

Drug treatment typically begins with one AED, with the dosage gradually increased until seizures are controlled, clinical manifestations of toxicity are noted, or serum drug levels reach the high end of the therapeutic range without controlling the seizures. In many cases, seizures can be controlled by a single drug. However, in a patient who has two or more types of seizures simultaneously, try another AED, each alone, before resorting to multidrug therapy. The efficacies of the drugs vary according to the age at onset, the type and severity of the disease, and serum drug levels.

In treatment of partial and secondary generalized tonic-clonic seizures, the success rate is higher with carbamazepine, phenytoin, or valproic acid than with phenobarbital or primidone. Gabapentin, topiramate, lamotrigine, oxcarbazepine, levetiracetam, and zonisamide are effective for partial or secondarily generalized seizures.

The pharmacokinetics and safety profiles of second-generation AEDs are much improved over those of first-generation AEDs. The fewest biotransformation and drug interactions are seen with gabapentin and levetiracetam. Reduced serum levels of second-generation AEDs (i.e., lamotrigine, tiagabine, zonisamide) occur with concurrent use of other CYP enzyme–inducing drugs.

Arriving at an appropriate dosage of an AED involves trial and error, because drug absorption and elimination vary widely from one patient to another. In the course of determining what dosage is appropriate, therapy is started at low levels (often one fourth to one third of the recommended therapeutic dosage) of a single drug and slowly increased or decreased to achieve the desired effect. Most minor adverse effects diminish after a few weeks; however, if CNS depression or other intolerable effects persist, dosages should be reduced or another drug substituted. Refer patients to a neurologist if they do not respond to monotherapy or there is a question about the organic nature of seizures.

Patients with the potential for alcohol withdrawal syndrome should receive prophylactic AED therapy to reduce the signs and symptoms of withdrawal, to prevent withdrawal seizures, and to reduce the likelihood of life-threatening events. Some experts recommend not treating this population, because frequently the discontinuation of AEDs results in more seizures than in patients not taking an AED.

Second-generation AEDs have different pharmacologic properties, and therefore, the utility of serum drug monitoring for these drugs is assessed individually. In general, the second-generation drugs have more predictable pharmacokinetics than older AEDs (i.e., phenytoin, carbamazepine, valproates).

The patient's quality of life and use of health care resources should be balanced against the cost of therapy (e.g., drug and laboratory monitoring). Second-generation AEDs are expensive; the first-generation drugs considerably less so. However, the higher cost of second-generation drugs may well be compensated for by fewer patient visits to urgent care centers, emergency departments, or the health care provider. In addition, there may be fewer hospitalizations, which are often for management of adverse effects, additional lab testing to monitor drug levels, EEGs to monitor seizure activity/control, and titrating drugs to effective dosage levels.

ABSENCE SEIZURES. Valproate is more often used in the management of absence seizures than other drugs, if there is a contraindication to use of ethosuximide, or if ethosuximide has been ineffective. It is preferred over valproic acid because of the risk of serious hepatotoxicity and pancreatitis, although the risk of hepatotoxicity with valproic acid is much lower for adults than for children. Many patients are successfully managed with ethosuximide, although GI distress is dose related, and most patients better tolerate a twice-daily regimen. Clonazepam and lamotrigine are effective alternatives for absence seizures in patients who do not tolerate or respond to first-line drugs. Clonazepam is a second-line drug because of its CNS and behavioral adverse effects.

GENERALIZED SEIZURES. Valproic acid is effective and better tolerated than phenytoin or carbamazepine for the treatment of generalized seizures. Phenytoin and carbamazepine have been associated with a greater incidence of CNS adverse effects than the valproates. Valproate is also useful if the patient has generalized tonic-clonic and absence seizures because the drug is effective for both types.

Many health care providers prefer carbamazepine over phenytoin as initial therapy. Fewer adverse effects, easier dose titration, and fewer adverse effects have been documented. On the other hand, carbamazepine is generally more expensive than phenytoin and must be dosed twice daily, compared with once-daily dosing for phenytoin.

Phenytoin is the drug of choice if an IV route is required. Phenytoin causes more cosmetic effects than carbamazepine

EVIDENCE-BASED PHARMACOTHERAPEUTICS

Rapid Versus Slow Withdrawal of Antiepileptic Drugs

■ Background

The treatment goals for a patient with epilepsy are to induce seizure remission by using antiepileptic drugs (AEDs) and to withdraw the AEDs without causing a recurrence of the seizures. AEDs produce long-term adverse effects with extended use, and therefore, when a patient who has epilepsy is in remission, it is reasonable to stop drug therapy. There is no reliable evidence available suggesting the optimal rate of taper of AEDs, and yet the question of the timing and mode of withdrawal always arises.

■ Research Article

Ranganathan, L., Ramaratnam, S. (2006). Rapid versus slow withdrawal of antiepileptic drugs. *The Cochrane Database of Systematic Reviews.* 2006, Issue 2. Art. No. CD005003. DOI: 10.1002/14651858.CD005003.pub2.

Purpose

The primary purposes of this review were to examine the evidence for the risk of seizure recurrence after a rapid or slow discontinuance of an AED in adults and children with epilepsy who are in remission, and to assess which variables modify the risk of seizure recurrence.

Design

A single, randomized, controlled clinical trial involving 149 children was examined. The trial ($N = 149$) included subjects who had a mean onset of seizure activity at 4 years and a mean age of 11 years at the time the AED taper was started. The 6-week rapid-taper group (RTG) recruited 81 subjects, with 11 subjects lost to follow-up ($N = 70$), whereas the 9-month slow-taper group (STG) had 68 subjects, with 5 lost to follow-up before the taper began ($N = 63$).

The study also examined the effect of variables such as age of seizure onset, seizure types, presence of neurologic deficits, mental subnormality, etiology of epilepsy, type of AED used, electroencephalogram (EEG) findings, or duration of seizure freedom on the risk of recurrence of seizures using the two tapering strategies.

Methods

Two independent investigators searched the Cochrane Epilepsy Group's specialized register, the Cochrane Central Register of Controlled Trials, Medline, and cross-references from the identified studies.

The outcomes examined included the percentage of subjects who had recurrence of seizure after withdrawal of an AED; time to recurrence of seizure following withdrawal; occurrence of status epilepticus; mortality; and morbidity due to seizure such as injuries, fractures, aspiration pneumonia, and quality of life.

Findings

The number of subjects who were seizure-free at the end of 1, 2, 3, 4, and 5 years is displayed in the table.

Seizure-Free Period (years)	Number of Subjects Remaining Seizure-Free		Odds Ratios (OR) and Confidence Intervals (CI)
	RTG $N = 70$	STG $N = 63$	
1	40	44	OR 0.53; 95% CI 0.27–1.03
2	30	29	OR 0.79; 95% CI 0.41–1.53
3	24	14	OR 1.62; 95% CI 0.76–3.46
4	18	8	OR 2.14; 95% CI 0.87–5.3
5	10	6	OR 1.46; 95% CI 0.5–4.23

RTG, Rapid-taper group: *STG,* slow-taper group.

Conclusions

The small sample size of this single study limits interpretation of the data; thus reliable conclusions regarding the optimal rate for AED taper cannot be determined.

■ Implications for Practice

Additional research is needed in adults and children to examine the rate of withdrawal of AEDs and to study the effects on the rate of taper of variables such as seizure types, etiology, presence of neurologic deficits, EEG abnormalities, and other comorbid conditions.

(e.g., hirsutism, coarsening of facial features, gingival hypertrophy). Phenytoin may also cause a greater incidence of adverse cognitive effects than carbamazepine.

Use phenobarbital only if valproate, phenytoin, and carbamazepine have been ineffective. Maximum drug effects of phenobarbital may not be seen for up to 30 minutes after administration. To avoid overdose, give the drug time to work before administering a second dose. Although an efficacious drug, phenobarbital has a greater potential for causing sedation and behavioral disturbances than other drugs.

PARTIAL-ONSET SEIZURES. Carbamazepine and phenytoin are equally efficacious, and the decision to choose one of these drugs is similar to that in generalized seizures. Carbamazepine has fewer adverse effects and an easier dosing regimen. Gabapentin is an effective adjunct to carbamazepine and phenytoin. Valproic acid is not as effective as carbamazepine and phenytoin, although it is an alternative for patients who do not respond to or cannot tolerate these two drugs. Phenobarbital should also be used if the other drugs are ineffective.

MYOCLONIC SEIZURES. Valproic acid is the drug of choice for myoclonic seizures. It is also the most effective drug for juvenile myoclonic epilepsy. Patients with juvenile myoclonic epilepsy generally require lower doses than adults. Clonazepam has also been used with success for myoclonic seizures.

STATUS EPILEPTICUS. Lorazepam, a BZD, is the drug of first choice of many health care providers, although diazepam is as effective and less expensive. However, diazepam administered intravenously causes more irritation than lorazepam, and it is absorbed erratically when administered by IM injection. Diazepam continues to be effective 1 to 2 days after stopping drug therapy. On the other hand, lorazepam is slow to leave the body and has a longer duration of action than diazepam (even with its shorter half-life). A longer-acting AED (e.g., phenytoin or other) is usually added after the BZD.

Patient Education

No AED is without adverse effects, and therefore patients may be nonadherent with treatment. Patients taking AEDs over an extended period need to know the adverse effects of the drug, including neurologic symptoms, GI disturbances, visual disturbances, blood dyscrasias, and hepatic and renal impairment. Reinforcement of the risk-benefit ratio is essential to ensure that

CENTRAL NERVOUS

CASE STUDY — Antiepileptic Drugs

ASSESSMENT

History of Present Illness	PS is a 29-year-old woman admitted to the surgical unit after undergoing emergency surgery for a ruptured appendix. She did well for the first 24 hours, after which she had a marked sudden change in neurologic functioning and experienced seizures. She was treated acutely with lorazepam and IV phenytoin, with resolution of status epilepticus. She was subsequently found to have a basal ganglion infarct with hematoma.
Past Health History	Past medical history is significant for an episode of Stevens-Johnson syndrome 2 years ago after being given a sulfonamide antibiotic for an upper respiratory infection. Her history is negative for both febrile and idiopathic seizures in childhood. No history of head trauma. She is a $G_1P_1Ab_0$. Her pregnancy, labor, and delivery were uneventful. No history of diabetes, hypertension, renal, or liver disease. Family history is negative for seizures. Parents and siblings are alive and well. Review of systems is as per history of present illness and the feeling that the past few years have been physically and emotionally stressful.
Life-Span Considerations	As a single parent, PS has special concerns associated with childrearing. Her 3-year-old child is being cared for by the grandmother at this time. PS notes a fear of recurrent seizures will affect her confidence and her ability to safely parent. Social history is negative for alcoholism or illicit drug use. She does not smoke cigarettes or use tobacco products.
Physical Exam Findings	Vital signs within normal limits. PS was observed while in the PACU to be having tonic-clonic seizures. The physical exam, and EEG showed signs of localized brain abnormalities, which were confirmed by the neurologist and neurosurgeon.
Diagnostic Testing	MRI 24 hours postop: basal ganglion infarct with hematoma. EEG: altered electrophysiologic activity of the brain and abnormal waveforms

DIAGNOSIS: Epilepsy

MANAGEMENT

Treatment Objective	1. Provide maximum control of seizures with minimal adverse effects.
Treatment Plan	**Pharmacotherapy** • phenytoin 400 mg loading dose then 300 mg daily. Titrate based on response. • Daily OTC multiple vitamin and vitamin C supplement **Patient Teaching** 1. Disease 2. Make and keep regular appointments with dentist. 3. Take drug as directed. Do not stop without contacting health care provider. 4. Avoid sleep deprivation and excessive alcohol use, which can lower seizure threshold and make recurrent seizure activity more likely. 5. Avoid jobs that require working at heights or near heavy machinery, flames, burners, or molten materials, and avoid swimming alone. 6. Discuss potential for pregnancy with health care provider; use contraceptives as directed when prescribed. 7. Keep follow-up appointments with health care provider. **Evaluation** PS was discharged 7 days after admission and surgery for ruptured appendix. She has had no seizure activity since 24 hours after surgery but has an appointment with the neurologist of record in follow-up.

CLINICAL REASONING ANALYSIS

Q1. Why did you choose phenytoin rather than carbamazepine or phenobarbital for PS?

A. The drugs have different mechanisms of action but are used in tonic-clonic seizures. Carbamazepine has fewer adverse effects, easier dosage titration, and fewer cosmetic adverse effects such as hirsutism, coarsening of facial features, and gingival hypertrophy that we find with phenytoin. On the other hand, carbamazepine is more expensive than phenytoin and must be dosed twice daily compared with once-daily dosing for phenytoin. Expert opinion is that phenobarbital should only be used if treatment failure occurs with the initial AED.

Q2. PS desires a simple dosing regimen to enhance her adherence. Will the phenytoin accomplish this?

A. Yes, once-daily dosing with phenytoin will foster her adherence. Phenytoin can be given as a loading dose, and the time to steady state is approximately half that for phenobarbital. Phenobarbital has the longest half-life of all the standard AEDs, and carbamazepine falls in between.

Q3. Does PS need to be a blood test to check her hydantoin level?

A. Yes, the "therapeutic" range for AEDs is a compromise between toxicity and efficacy. We will order a set of serum drug levels, considering them a target range when we first start treatment, but they should never replace thorough patient assessment and clinical judgment. Serum drug levels should be used primarily to determine clinical control (or the lack of it) and to help assess dose-related adverse effects.

Q4. Shouldn't PS be using birth control while on phenytoin?

A. Good catch. A number of AEDs, including phenytoin, are enzyme-inducing drugs that act to increase the clearance of the oral contraceptive. However, she is also taking vitamin C, which increases serum concentrations of ethinyl estradiol by competing for sulphation. We will discuss a contraceptive method, but we need to know the date of her last menstrual period and do a pregnancy test and Pap smear before starting phenytoin and the contraceptive.

the patient understands and accepts the importance of adherence with the treatment plan. Patients also need to be aware of how epilepsy affects their daily lives and of the importance of following certain principles when on drug therapy. These principles include acquiring knowledge about the following:

- Epilepsy and how it affects the patient's life and the lives of family members and friends
- Care required during a seizure and the importance of keeping a journal of all seizure activity
- The need for an adequate diet, fluid intake, and sleep, and for moderate recreation and exercise
- The importance of abstaining from alcoholic beverages and other substances
- Wearing a medical identification bracelet or tag containing pertinent medical information
- Legal protection under the law regarding employment and driving
- The availability of patient resources such as the Epilepsy Foundation of America

Evaluation

The expected course and prognosis of a patient with a seizure disorder is dependent on the seizure type. The duration of treatment with AEDs is influenced by several factors, including the probability of the patient remaining seizure-free without drugs; the adverse consequences of recurrent seizures; and the adverse effects of long-term AED therapy. In selected cases, patients may be able to discontinue the AED, although there are a number of factors to consider regarding this possibility.

It is recommended that the patient be seizure-free for at least 2 to 4 years before considering AED withdrawal, since about 33% of patients will relapse. Recurrence of seizures usually occurs within the first 6 months after withdrawal. Patients at low risk for recurrence include those with primary epilepsy, seizure onset between the ages of 2 and 35 years, and a normal EEG. The longer the patient remains seizure-free, the less likely seizures are to recur.

Patients at high risk for relapse are those who have partial complex seizures or seizures from an identifiable lesion; these patients have a 50% chance of recurrence. Patients with a history of frequent seizures or status epilepticus, multiple seizure types, persistently abnormal EEG results, and the development of altered cognition are poor candidates for drug withdrawal.

Before discontinuing drug therapy, also consider the patient's desire and motivation, along with the likelihood of success and the risks associated with recurrence of a seizure (including the possible loss of the driver's license). Advise patients not to drive during the withdrawal period and for 3 to 4 months thereafter. This restriction makes it difficult for some patients to try withdrawal.

Explain to the patient on multidrug therapy that the drugs will be withdrawn one at a time, with the least effective or the most toxic drug being stopped first. Decrease the dosage slowly over 3 to 6 months until the drug is completely withdrawn. Allow time for a new steady state to be reached before continuing with dosage reductions. If the patient remains seizure-free for 1 month, the second drug can be discontinued in the same manner, and so on. If seizures recur, restart therapy using the last drug that was withdrawn.

There are several factors to consider when an AED change is required. Second-generation AEDs have fewer drug interactions and should be added to the existing AED regimen with the objective of achieving a dosage that will be efficacious before beginning dosage reduction of the original baseline drugs. Advise patients that changing from one drug to another takes time, and help them to accept the time necessary to accomplish the task.

There are no standardized guidelines for how rapidly to taper and withdraw baseline AEDs. A safe and reasonable strategy is to reduce the dosage by 25% per step. The time between dosage reductions should be at least 5 half-lives, or a minimum of 1 week, to allow for new steady states to be reached. Further, the enzyme-inducing and -inhibiting nature of first-generation AEDs may require changes in drugs the patient is taking for other comorbid conditions during the withdrawal period.

Surgical intervention is an increasingly available option for about 5% of patients with recalcitrant seizures. Surgery is most beneficial for people whose seizures originate from clearly delineated, unilateral, anterior temporal lobe foci. The criteria for surgical intervention include failure of AED therapy and the focus of abnormal discharge being surgically accessible.

CENTRAL NERVOUS

KEY POINTS

- Epilepsy is a recurrent, paroxysmal neurologic disorder characterized by seizures that occur when the brain is subjected to abnormal, excessive discharges by localized and/or generalized neurons.
- Seizures classified as primary are of unknown origin. Seizures classified as secondary have a diagnosed cause.
- Partial seizures, particularly when associated with a cerebral disease, are more difficult to control than generalized seizures.
- Secondary seizures related to an acute, short-lasting brain disease are usually self-limiting. However, a significant proportion of those affected will go on to develop established epilepsy.
- Status epilepticus is a medical emergency that occurs when a patient has seizures in rapid succession or continuous seizures lasting at least 30 minutes.
- The diagnosis of epilepsy is made on the basis of clinical data, historical information, and observation.

- The treatment objective is to prevent or at least reduce to the greatest extent possible the number and/or severity of seizures, while assisting the patient in maintaining the highest level of individual functioning achievable.
- An effort to eliminate factor(s) that may cause or precipitate seizures should be made.
- The treatment choice of AED is dependent on accurate diagnosis of seizure type, the type or pattern of seizures, age of the patient, family history, response to any previously used AED, and any adverse effects of the drug.
- Development of an AED treatment plan that prevents or arrests the seizures usually requires weeks of trial, error, and adjustment. Seizure frequency is used as a guide in determining when to increase the dosage or change drug therapy.
- Effectiveness of therapy is demonstrated by absence of seizures and improved quality of life.

Bibliography

Antiepileptic Drug Pregnancy Registry. Available online: www.aedpregnancyregistry.org/. Accessed April 11, 2007.

Beyenburg, S., Bauer, J., and Rueber, M. (2004). New drugs for the treatment of epilepsy: A practical approach. *Postgraduate Medical Journal*, 80(948), 581–587.

Cloyd, J., and Remmel, R. (2000). Antiepileptic drug pharmacokinetics and interactions: Impact on the treatment of epilepsy. *Pharmacotherapy*, 20(8 part 2), 139S–151S.

Davenport, R., and Patel, N. (2007). Zonisamide as treatment for seizures. *Nurse Practitioner*, 32(4), 15–17.

Flomin, O., Nield, L., and Kamat, D. (2005). Seizure medications: A review for the primary care pediatrician. *Clinical Pediatrics*, 44(5), 383–391.

French, J., Kanner, A., and Mautista, J., et al. (2004a). Efficacy and tolerability of the new antiepileptic drugs, I: Treatment of new onset epilepsy. *Neurology*, 62(8), 1252–1260.

French, J., Kanner, A., and Mautista, J., et al. (2004b). Efficacy and tolerability of the new antiepileptic drugs, I: Treatment of refractory epilepsy. *Neurology*, 62(8), 1261–1273.

Jette, N., Cappell, J., and VanPassel, L., et al. (2006). Tiagabine-induced nonconvulsive status epilepticus in an adolescent without epilepsy. *Neurology*, 67(8), 1514–1518.

Johannessen, S., and Tomson, T. (2006). Pharmacokinetic variability of newer antiepileptic drugs: When is monitoring needed? *Clinical Pharmacokinetics*, 45(11), 1061–1075.

Kocak, S., Girisgin, S., and Gul, M., et al. (2007). Stevens-Johnson syndrome due to concomitant use of lamotrigine and valproic acid. *American Journal of Clinical Dermatology*, 8(2), 107–111.

Kaplan, P. (2004). Reproductive health effects and teratogenicity of antiepileptic drugs. *Neurology*, 62(6), S13–S23.

Kwan, P., and Sander, J. (2004). The natural history of epilepsy: An epidemiological view. *Journal of Neurology, Neurosurgery, and Psychiatry*, 75(10), 1376–1381.

Morrell, M., McLean, M., and Willmore, L., et al. (2000). Efficacy of gabapentin as adjunctive therapy in a large, multicenter study. The Steps Study Group. *Seizure*, 9(4), 241–248.

Ochoa, J., and Riche, W. (2005). Antiepileptic drugs: An overview. *eMedicine*. Available online: www.emedicine.com/neuro/topic692.htm. Accessed April 11, 2007.

Ramsay, R., and DeToledo, J. (1995). Intravenous administration of fosphenytoin: options for the management of seizures. *Neurology*, 46(Suppl 1), S17–SA19.

Salinsky, M., Storzbach, D., and Spencer, D., et al. (2005). Effects of topiramate and gabapentin on cognitive abilities in healthy volunteers. *Neurology*, 6(5), 792–798.

Sills, G., and Brodie, M. (2007). Pharmacokinetics and drug interactions with zonisamide. *Epilepsia*, 48(3), 435–441.

Smith, M., Wilcox, C., and White, S. (2007). Discovery of antiepileptic drugs. *Neurotherapeutics*, 4(1), 12–17.

Stoner, S., Lea, J., and Wolf, A., et al. (2005). Levetiracetam for mood stabilization and maintenance of seizure control following multiple treatment failures. *Annals of Pharmacotherapy*, 39(11), 1928–1931.

Tassone, D., Boyce, E., and Guyer, J., et al. (2007). Pregabalin: A novel gamma-aminobutyric acid analogue in the treatment of neuropathic pain, partial-onset seizures, and anxiety disorders. *Clinical Therapeutics*, 29(1), 26–48.

Zupanc, M. (2006). Antiepileptic drugs and hormonal contraceptives in adolescent women with epilepsy. *Neurology*, 66(Suppl 3), S37–S45.

26

Drugs for Parkinson's Disease and Myasthenia Gravis

Movement disorders are the broad category of neurologic diseases that include Parkinson's disease, essential tremor and other types of tremor, dyskinesias, and dystonias; all are progressive, degenerative neurologic diseases. This chapter discusses Parkinson's disease and myasthenia gravis.

PARKINSON'S DISEASE

EPIDEMIOLOGY AND ETIOLOGY

Parkinson's disease (PD) is a common movement disorder characterized by bradykinesia (slowed movement), muscle rigidity, resting tremors, and postural instability (poor balance). Originally known as *paralysis agitans*, this degenerative neurologic disease plagues people of all races and occurs around the world, affecting 1 in every 100 people over the age of 60 years. It may also been seen in people under 40 years of age. The lifetime risk of developing PD is thought to be 1% to 2%, with a variable progression rate.

Five percent to 10% of patients have a family history of PD, with persons affected in the same generation, such as a brother and sister, or across two generations, such as father and son. There are several environmental toxins that cause disorders resembling PD, including carbon monoxide, manganese, and, although rarely, certain pesticides. Gene mutations are also thought to cause PD. There was no increase in the incidence of PD in studies of identical twins in which one twin was known to have PD compared with the general population over age 60 years (Tanner, 2003). On the other hand, there is an increased risk for PD among identical twins under age 50 if one twin has been diagnosed with PD. These findings suggest that in early-onset cases of PD, heredity may play a role. To date, investigators feel that the etiology of PD involves a combination of genetics and environmental toxins.

Primary PD results from deterioration of neurons in the basal ganglia of the substantia nigra. *Secondary parkinsonism* is caused by disorders such as infection, tumor, trauma, and drug intoxication. Drug-induced PD is the most common secondary type and is often reversible. Table 26-1 provides

TABLE 26-1 Drugs Contraindicated in Parkinson's Disease

Antiemetics	metoclopramide (Reglan), prochlorperazine (Compazine), trimethobenzamide (Tigan)
Antihypertensives	diazoxide (Hyperstat), methyldopa (Aldomet), reserpine
Antipsychotics	fluphenazine (Prolixin), haloperidol (Haldol), lithium, molindone (Moban), perphenazine (Trilafon), perphenazine with amitriptyline (Triavil), trifluoperazine (Stelazine), thiothixine (Navane), thioridazine (Mellaril)

an overview of drugs associated with secondary parkinsonism and which should be avoided in these patients. Acute parkinsonism has developed in drug abusers exposed to the synthetic opioid "designer drug" N-methyl-4-phenyl-1,2,3,6-tetrahydropyridine (MPTP). Poisoning with manganese, carbon monoxide, mercury, methanol, or cyanide produces clinical abnormalities similar to those of PD. Parkinson's symptoms have also been seen in patients recovering from attempted suicide by drug overdose, during which there is a presumed central nervous system (CNS) hypoxic or ischemic injury from respiratory depression and hypotension. In addition, repeated head trauma may result in parkinsonian symptoms. Some boxers have developed pugilistic PD.

PHYSIOLOGY AND PATHOPHYSIOLOGY

Although the cause of PD is unknown, its pathology is well characterized by its extensive deterioration of neurons within the basal ganglia of the brain (Fig. 26-1). These neurons are normally needed to synthesize the neurotransmitter dopamine, which inhibits the excitatory signals produced by acetylcholine (ACh). Degeneration of neurons in the substantia nigra results in loss of dopamine, causing neurons of the striatum to fire excessively. Symptoms of Parkinson's appear when 80% of the dopamine-producing neurons are depleted. Depletion of dopamine, and thus an excess of cholinergic activity in the basal ganglia, is associated with tremor, rigidity, and akinesia.

Investigators have detected some common cellular characteristics that are thought to be a factor in neuronal degeneration and death. The existence of dense aggregates of protein, called Lewy bodies, in the neurons of the substantia nigra, the brainstem, and other parts of the brain is the leading characteristic identified thus far. Lewy bodies contain α-synuclein and other proteins that accumulate within the protein disposal system in nerve fibers. The accumulation interferes with transmission of nerve impulses. Further, dopamine neurons have a higher level of cyclooxygenase-2 (COX-2) enzyme compared to patients who are not affected by PD.

Studies of the effects of MPTP suggest that the enzyme monoamine oxidase B (MAO-B), found in the brain, and free radicals in the form of superoxide or peroxide may be involved in neuronal destruction and dopamine depletion. The two molecular MAO types, A and B, are found in the mitochondrial membranes of nerve terminals, the brain, the liver, and the intestinal mucosa. MAO regulates the metabolic degradation of catecholamines and serotonin in the CNS and peripheral tissues. MAO-B is found in the brain, regulating the concentration of dopamine by causing its breakdown. MAO-A, found in the gut, regulates entry into the body of the naturally occurring precursors of dopamine and norepinephrine that are present in the diet.

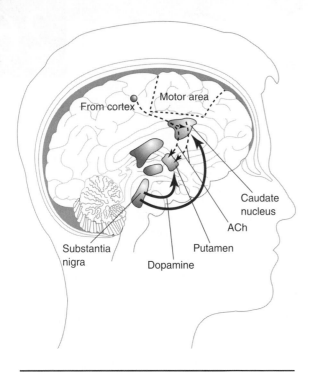

FIGURE 26-1 Neural pathways secrete dopamine and acetylcholine (ACh) in the basal ganglia, which constitute the motor axis of the central nervous system.

Of patients with PD, 100% have rigidity, a very common initial symptom that is frequently missed. *Rigidity,* a state of involuntary contraction of all skeletal muscles, seems to take over as PD worsens, impeding active and passive movement. The rigidity is present during the entire arc of movement of a joint. *Cogwheel rigidity* is a jerky, ratcheting movement demonstrated on passive motion, usually at the wrist or elbow.

Seventy-five percent of patients with PD have an asymmetric, regular, rhythmic tremor. Tremor is an asymmetric, regular, rhythmic tremor. The 8- to 10-cycles/second *resting tremor* appears when the limb is at rest and disappears with voluntary movement. The tremor produces a pronation-supination motion of the forearm. With voluntary movement, the tremor is temporarily blocked, because other motor signals arriving in the thalamus override the abnormal signals from the basal ganglia. Although they are most prominent in the hands, the tremors may also involve the tongue, the jaw, the eyelids, and the feet. A parkinsonian tremor is quite different from the tremor seen with cerebellar disease, for the former occurs during all waking hours.

A movement of the thumb against the fingers is also seen. This *pill-rolling tremor* occurs at 4 to 6 cycles/second and may begin asymmetrically. It becomes bilateral as the disease progresses.

Bradykinesia, one of the cardinal symptoms of PD, is the most crippling of all symptoms. It is a general slowness characterized by difficulty initiating movement and an inability to perform rapid, repetitive movements. The severity of bradykinesia may fluctuate markedly throughout the day.

Hypokinesia is an abnormally diminished motor response to a stimulus. It is seen when patients sit or lie for long periods

without an accompanying shift in weight. The tendency to cross the legs when sitting, to gesture with the hands when talking, or to swing the arms when walking, is lost.

The combination of rigidity and bradykinesia results in a number of other signs. There is a loss of facial expression *(masked facies),* decreased frequency of blinking, fixed flexion of the trunk, the neck, and the extremities, a slow and hesitant gait, and *postural instability,* a cardinal sign of PD. *Micrographia* (handwriting that gets progressively smaller), dysarthria, dysphagia, and general poverty of movement also are noted. Other common features of the disease include constipation, depression, intellectual impairment, orthostatic hypotension, bladder instability, eczema, and peripheral neuropathy. The symptoms and symptom intensity experienced will differ between patients. None of these secondary symptoms are fatal in and of themselves, but they may lead to other complications.

Severity Scales

Many scales have been developed to rate the severity of PD. These weighted numerical scales are based on an evaluation of the signs and symptoms. The particular symptoms assessed and the value designated for each symptom account for the differences between scales. A simple scale comes from Hoehn and Yahr, the staging of Parkinson's disease as delineated in Box 26-1; however, the more frequently used scale is the Unified Parkinson's Disease Rating Scale (UPDRS) (Box 26-2).

BOX 26-1

Hoehn and Yahr Staging of Parkinson's Disease

Stage One
- Mild signs and symptoms appear on one side only
- Symptoms inconvenient but not disabling
- Usually present with tremor of one limb
- Friends and family notice changes in posture, locomotion, and facial expression

Stage Two
- Symptoms bilateral
- Minimal disability
- Posture and gait affected

Stage Three
- Significant slowing of body movements
- Early impairment of equilibrium on walking or standing
- Generalized dysfunction that is moderately severe

Stage Four
- Severe symptoms
- Can still walk to a limited extent
- Rigidity and bradykinesia
- No longer able to live alone
- Tremor may be less than earlier stages

Stage Five
- Cachectic stage
- Invalidism complete
- Cannot stand or walk
- Requires constant nursing care

Hoen, M., and Yahr, M. (1967). Parkinsonism: Onset, progression, and mortality. *Neurology, 17,* 427–442.

BOX 26-2

Components of the Unified Parkinson's Disease Rating Scale (UPDRS)*

Mentation, Behavior, Mood
- Intellectual impairment
- Thought disorder
- Depression
- Motivation, initiative

Activities of Daily Living
- Speech
- Salivation
- Swallowing
- Handwriting
- Cutting food, handling utensils
- Dressing
- Hygiene
- Turning in bed, adjusting bed clothes
- Falling, unrelated to freezing
- Walking
- Tremor
- Sensory complaints related to parkinsonism

Motor Exam
- Speech
- Facial expression
- Tremor at rest (each extremity is measured individually)[†]
- Action or postural tremor of right and left upper extremities[†]
- Rigidity of neck and each extremity
- Finger taps (right and left)[†]
- Hand movements (open and close hands in rapid succession); right and left[†]
- Rapid alternating movements (pronate and supinate hands)
- Leg agility (tap heel on ground, amp should be 3 inches)
- Arising from chair (patient arises with arms folded across chest)
- Posture
- Gait
- Postural stability (retropulsion test)
- Body bradykinesia, hypokinesia

*The UPDRS rating tool, which is more complicated, has largely replaced the Hoehn and Yahr functional rating scale developed in 1967. The UPDRS is a tool for following the longitudinal course of PD. Each of the items is evaluated by patient and family interview.
[†]Some sections require multiple grades assigned to each extremity. A total of 199 points are possible, with 0 meaning no disability and 199 the worst (total) disability.

PHARMACOTHERAPEUTIC OPTIONS

No single drug alleviates the signs, symptoms, and disabilities of PD. Most drugs either enhance the transmission of dopamine or impede ACh transmission. Sadly, delivery of the right drug and the right dosage to counteract the disease and its symptoms is not always possible. In many cases, drugs are used in a trial-and-error fashion until the most effective drug with the fewest adverse effects is found. Drug classes commonly used to treat PD include dopaminergic drugs, dopamine agonists, anticholinergics, an MAO-B inhibitor, and/or catechol-*O*-methyltransferase (COMT) inhibitors.

Dopaminergic Drugs
- carbidopa-levodopa-entacapone (Stalevo)
- levodopa-carbidopa (Sinemet, Sinemet CR)
- levodopa (L-dopa); ✦ (Dopar, Larodopa)

Indications

Levodopa remains the most effective therapy for the tremors and rigidity of PD, including bradykinesia. Carbidopa is added to the standard oral formulation to enhance the effectiveness of levodopa and to minimize adverse effects. These drugs are also used in the management of idiopathic, postencephalitic, and symptomatic parkinsonism associated with cerebral arteriosclerosis.

Pharmacodynamics

Dopamine does not cross the blood-brain barrier. Levodopa, however, an amino acid, crosses the blood-brain barrier, where it is converted to dopamine. The dopamine then restores the normal balance between excitation and inhibition of neurons in the caudate nucleus and the putamen.

Carbidopa, a decarboxylase inhibitor, allows a greater concentration of levodopa to reach the brain and helps minimize adverse effects. Carbidopa, when combined with levodopa, permits a reduction in levodopa dosage by as a much as 70%.

Pharmacokinetics

Levodopa, taken orally, is well absorbed in the duodenum and the proximal region of the small intestine; however, the presence of food proteins competes with the levodopa for absorption, delaying achievement of peak plasma levels (Table 26-2). The absorption rate depends on the rate of gastric emptying, gastric pH, and the length of time the drug is exposed to degradative enzymes. Use of the controlled-release formulation further reduces the bioavailability of levodopa (20% to 30%); thus, higher dosages of the drug must be used to produce a satisfactory clinical response. Ninety-five percent of levodopa is biotransformed in the liver and the periphery. Its short half-life requires the patient to take multiple daily doses to maintain even intermittently effective plasma levels. Levodopa is eliminated primarily in the urine as well as through breast milk.

Adverse Effects and Contraindications

An accumulation of dopamine in the circulation contributes to the most common adverse effects of levodopa, nausea and vomiting. Syncopal episodes, dry mouth, difficulty swallowing, worsening hand tremors, and numbness have been reported. Drowsiness is also common with levodopa and other dopaminergic therapies, and sudden sleep onset is possible. Patients may not experience the warning signs of the onset of sudden sleep, particularly when starting levodopa therapy. The signs of sudden onset sleep may also occur with dosage increase or when changing drug therapies. Orthostasis

PHARMACOKINETICS
TABLE 26-2 Antiparkinsonian Drugs

Drug	Route	Onset	Peak	Duration	PB (%)	t½	BioA (%)
DOPAMINERGICS							
levodopa-carbidopa CR	PO	2–3 wk	0.5–2 hr	5–24 hr	30	1–3 hr	20–30
levodopa-carbidopa IR	PO	20–40 min	UA	2–4 hr	36	1–4 hr	UA
DOPAMINE AGONISTS							
bromocriptine	PO	30–90 min	1–3 hr	6–24 hr	90	3–7 hr*	UA
pergolide	PO	UA	1–2 hr	5–9 hr	90	24–72 hr	UA
pramipexole	PO	UA	2 hr	UA	15	7–17 hr	>90
ropinirole	PO	UA	1–2 hr	UA	40	6 hr	55
ANTICHOLINERGICS							
benztropine	PO	1–2 hr	Days	24 hr	UA	UA	UA
trihexyphenidyl	PO	60 min	2–3 hr	6–12 hr	UA	5–10 hr	100
MAO-B INHIBITORS							
selegiline	PO	2–3 days	UA	Weeks	UA	Varies†	45
rasagiline	PO	UA	1 hr	UA	88–94	3 hr	36
COMT INHIBITORS							
entacapone	PO	First dose	1 hr	UA	98	0.4–0.7; 2.4 hr‡	35
tolcapone	PO	First dose	2 hr	UA	>99.9	2–3 hr	65

*Initial phase t½ of bromocriptine is 3–7 hr, with a terminal phase of 50 hr.
†Half-lives of each of the three metabolites of selegiline range from 2 to 20.5 hr.
‡Half-life of entacapone is biphasic with an elimination half-life of 0.4 to 0.7 hr in the β-phase and 2.4 hr in the γ-phase.
BioA, Bioavailability; *COMT,* catechol-*O*-methyltransferase; *CR,* controlled-release; *IR,* immediate-release; *MAO-B,* monoamine oxidase B; *PB,* protein binding; *PO,* by mouth; *t½,* half-life; *UA,* unavailable.

is not uncommon. There is a risk that increases over time for hallucinations, paranoia, and compulsive behaviors (e.g., gambling, hypersexuality). Irregular heart rhythms may develop in patients with preexisting rhythm disturbances. The adverse effects of dopaminergic drugs are reversible and can generally be controlled by a reduction in dosage.

The most troubling adverse effect of long-term levodopa use is impaired control over ordinary muscle movement (dyskinesias). The impaired muscle control results in spasmodic movements or tics and can include writhing, twitching, and shaking. The dyskinesias typically develop in milder forms after 3 to 5 years, but may become more severe after 5 to 10 years of treatment. Dyskinesias result from the combination of continued degeneration of neurons in the substantia nigra and long-term levodopa therapy.

An *"on-off" phenomenon* appears in patients receiving long-term levodopa therapy. This phenomenon is characterized by a sudden decline in response after a period of therapeutic improvement. The decline manifests as an abrupt onset of *akinesia,* a loss or reduction of the usual power of movement. The on-off phenomenon affects 90% of patients treated with levodopa for 10 years or more, but usually appears after 2 to 3 years of treatment. The episodes become more frequent after 5 years of treatment.

Contraindications to the use of levodopa-carbidopa include hypersensitivity to the drugs or their ingredients, concurrent use of MAO-inhibitor drugs, narrow-angle glaucoma, blood dyscrasias, and uncontrolled hypertension. Avoid the use of levodopa in patients with a history of malignant melanoma, because the drug may activate this form of skin cancer.

Cautious use of levodopa-carbidopa is warranted in patients with a history of myocardial infarction, arrhythmias, psychosis, neurosis, seizures, or peptic ulcer disease; in patients with renal, hepatic, or endocrine diseases; and in patients with bronchial asthma or emphysema who are taking adrenergic drugs.

Safe use of dopaminergics during pregnancy and lactation and in children under 12 years of age has not been established (pregnancy category D).

Drug Interactions

Table 26-3 lists drug interactions of dopaminergics. Bioavailability is increased when antacids and metoclopramide are given concurrently with levodopa. Phenytoin may reduce the effectiveness of levodopa. Hypertension may be seen when MAO inhibitors or tricyclic antidepressants (TCAs) are taken concurrently with levodopa.

Dosage Regimen

Individual needs and responses to levodopa vary widely, although a therapeutic response is most often noted within days. The combination levodopa-carbidopa drugs are used most often. About 75 mg of carbidopa is needed to achieve full peripheral decarboxylation. Levodopa-carbidopa is dosed 2 to 3 times daily at evenly spaced intervals. The dosage is gradually increased, depending on the patient's history, mental impairment, and individual response. The optimal dosage is reached when the smallest dosage necessary to control symptoms and decrease disability is reached (Table 26-4). The onset of drug action may be "jump-started" by dissolving immediate-release levodopa-carbidopa tablets in orange juice; however, the duration of benefit is usually shorter as well (Box 26-3).

Lab Considerations

Baseline and periodic monitoring of the complete blood count (CBC) and liver and kidney function tests is required

DRUG INTERACTIONS

TABLE 26-3 Antiparkinsonian Drugs

Drug	Interactive Drugs	Interaction(s)
DOPAMINERGICS		
levodopa-carbidopa	Anticholinergics	Postural hypotension
	Antihypertensives, benzodiazepines, haloperidol, metoclopramide, phenothiazines, reserpine	Decreases effectiveness of interactive drugs
	MAO inhibitors, TCAs	Hypertensive reactions
	pyridoxine (large doses), phenytoin, methionine	Decreases effects of levodopa-carbidopa\
	Sympathomimetics	Increases risk of arrhythmias
DOPAMINE AGONISTS		
bromocriptine	Antihypertensive drugs	Increases drop in blood pressure
	Antihistamines, phenothiazines, haloperidol, methyldopa, reserpine, TCAs	Decreases effects of bromocriptine
	Antihistamines, alcohol, opioids, sedative-hypnotics	Increases CNS depression
	levodopa	Increases neurologic deficits
pergolide	haloperidol, metoclopramide, phenothiazines	Decreases effects of interactive drugs
ropinirole	ciprofloxacin	Increases ropinirole's AUC by 84%
	ethinyl estradiol	Decreases clearance of ropinirole
	Phenothiazines, butyrophenones, thioxanthenes, metoclopramide	Decreases effects of ropinirole
pramipexole	cimetidine, ranitidine, diltiazem, triamterene, verapamil, quinidine, quinine	Decreases clearance of pramipexole
	carbidopa, levodopa	Increases plasma levels of interacting drugs
ANTICHOLINERGICS		
trihexyphenidyl and centrally acting antimuscarinic drugs	Antacids, antidiarrheals	Decreases absorption of anticholinergic
	Antimuscarinic drugs	Increases risk, severity of CNS, peripheral atropine-like effects; possible muscarinic poisoning syndrome
	Antipsychotic drugs	Increases antimuscarinic effects; decreases effectiveness of interacting drug; worsening of psychoses
	CNS depressants in general	Increases CNS depression
MAO-B INHIBITOR		
selegiline	SSRIs, meperidine	Excitation, sweating, rigidity, hypertension, or hypotension; fatalities are also possible
	levodopa-carbidopa, opioids	Increases effectiveness of interacting drug initially
	Alcohol	Increases hypotension and sedative effects of selegiline
	chlorprothixene, haloperidol, metoclopramide, phenothiazines, reserpine (high doses), thiothixene	Decreases effects of selegiline
	Antihypertensive drugs	Increases risk of hypotension
rasagiline	levodopa	Some increase in rasagiline serum levels of rasagiline
	dextromethorphan	CNS symptoms in patients taking MAO inhibitor
	ciprofloxacin and other inhibitors of CYP 1A2	Increases AUC of rasagiline by 83%; no change in elimination half life
	SSRIs, SNRIs, TCAs, nonselective MAO-B inhibitors, meperidine	Severe CNS toxicity, hypertension, hyperthermia, death
	cyclobenzaprine, methadone, propoxyphene, mirtazapine, St. John's wort, tramadol	May cause adverse CNS and autonomic symptoms
	Vasoconstrictors (e.g., pseudoephedrine)	May cause hypertensive reactions
COMT INHIBITORS		
entacapone	selegiline	Increases risk for dyskinesias
	Dopamine agonists	Increases risk for dyskinesias, hallucinations, dystonia
	Nonselective MAO inhibitors	Inhibits majority of the pathways of normal catecholamine biotransformation
	probenecid, cholestyramine, erythromycin, rifampin, ampicillin, chloramphenicol	Interferes with elimination of entacapone through the bile
	isoproterenol, epinephrine, norepinephrine, dopamine, dobutamine, alpha-methyldopa, apomorphine, isoetherine, bitolterol	Increases heart rate, risk of arrhythmias, and excessive changes in blood pressure
tolcapone	tolbutamide, warfarin	May reduce clearance of interactive drugs
	desipramine, levodopa-carbidopa	May increase blood pressure, pulse rate, and desipramine levels

AUC, Area under the curve; *CNS,* central nervous system; *MAO,* monoamine oxidase; *SNRI,* selective norepinephrine reuptake inhibitor; *SSRI,* selective serotonin reuptake inhibitor; *TCA,* tricyclic antidepressant.

during long-term levodopa or levodopa-carbidopa therapy. Blood urea nitrogen (BUN), creatinine, and uric acid levels are lower during concomitant administration of levodopa-carbidopa than with levodopa alone. Levodopa can cause increases in serum levels of alanine transaminase (ALT), aspartate transaminase (AST), alkaline phosphatase, lactate dehydrogenase (LDH), protein-bound iodine (PBI), bilirubin, and uric acid. The Coombs' test is occasionally positive with extended levodopa therapy.

Levodopa also interferes with results of urine glucose and urine ketone testing and may produce false-positive results using the Clinitest and Ketostix methods. Although rarely used today, the Tes-Tape method for urine glucose testing may produce false-negative results.

DOSAGE
TABLE 26-4 Antiparkinsonian Drugs

Drug	Use(s)	Dosage	Implications
DOPAMINERGICS			
levodopa-carbidopa IR (IR formulation: 100 mg levodopa– 25 mg carbidopa and others)	Idiopathic PD; postencephalitic parkinsonism; symptomatic parkinsonism related to CNS injury by carbon monoxide and manganese intoxication	*Adult:* 100 mg levodopa–25 mg carbidopa 3 times a day –or– 10/100 mg PO 3–4 times daily. Increase by 1 tablet every 24 to 48 hr. Max 200/2000 mg/day	Levodopa must be discontinued at least 12 hr before starting this combination therapy.
levodopa-carbidopa CR (CR formulation: 200 mg levodopa– 50 mg carbidopa and others)	Idiopathic PD; postencephalitic parkinsonism; parkinsonism related to CO and manganese intoxication	*Adult:* 200 mg levodopa–50 mg carbidopa PO twice daily at intervals of not less than 6 hr. Increase by 0.5–1 tablet/day every 3 days. Max frequency: every 4 hr or 600/2400 mg/day	To switch from IR to CR formulation, start 10% higher than levodopa dose. Doses and dosing intervals may be altered based on response.
carbidopa-levodopa-entacapone	Idiopathic PD; adjunct to levodopa-carbidopa	*Adult:* 12.5–50–200 mg tablet PO twice daily to max of 8 tablets daily	Individual tablets should not be fractionated.
DOPAMINE AGONISTS			
bromocriptine	Idiopathic PD, postencephalitic parkinsonism, adjunct to levodopa	*Adult:* 1.25–2.5 mg PO daily. May increase by 2.5–5 mg on alternate days. Maintenance: 2.5–100 mg PO daily in divided doses. Usual dosage range: 10–40 mg daily. Not to exceed 300 mg daily.	Take with food. Patients unresponsive to levodopa are poor candidates for bromocriptine mesylate therapy.
pergolide	Parkinson's disease	*Adult:* 0.05 mg PO daily initially. May increase by 0.1–0.15 mg PO every third day over 2 wk; then increase by 0.25 mg every third day until response obtained. Total dosage in 3 equal doses at 6–8 hr intervals. Maintenance: 3 mg/24 hr. Not to exceed 5 mg/24 hr	During dosage titration, the dosage of concurrent levodopa-carbidopa may be cautiously decreased.
pramipexole	Idiopathic PD, restless legs syndrome	*Adult:* 0.125 mg 3 times daily. Increase weekly by 1.5 mg 3 times daily.	Titrate gradually in all patients to avoid dry mouth, dyskinesia, hallucinations, and somnolence.
ropinirole	Idiopathic PD, restless legs syndrome	*Adult:* 0.25 mg PO 3 times daily. Increase weekly to 1 mg 3 times daily.	Retitration of drug may be warranted if a significant interruption in therapy occurs.
ANTICHOLINERGICS			
benztropine	Adjunct for all forms of parkinsonism; control of EPS (except tardive dyskinesia) secondary to neuroleptic drugs	*Adult:* 1–2 mg PO daily. Range: 0.5–6 mg daily. Give 1–2 mg IM or IV in emergency situations.	Oral route preferred. Has cumulative action.
trihexyphenidyl	All forms of parkinsonism; adjunct to levodopa; drug-induced EPS	*Adult:* 1–2 mg first day. May increase by 2 mg every 3–5 days. Maintenance: 5 to 15 mg PO daily in divided doses. ER formulation: every 12–24 hr	Dosage may be increased or changed if tolerance develops with long-term therapy. When stopping, dosage should be tapered over 1 wk.
MAO-B INHIBITOR			
selegiline	Sometimes used as first-line adjunct with levodopa-carbidopa in PD	*Adult:* 5 mg PO daily at breakfast and lunch. Maintenance: 5 mg PO after breakfast and lunch –or– 10 mg PO daily of ODT –or– 1.25–2.5 mg/day of TBT	Dosage of levodopa-carbidopa may be reduced after starting selegiline. Safe use in adolescents and children has not been established.
rasagiline	Monotherapy or adjunct for PD across life span of the disease	*Adult:* 0.5–1 mg PO daily	**Orthostasis is most common during the first 2 mo of treatment.** ▲
COMT INHIBITORS			
entacapone	Adjunct to levodopa for idiopathic PD	*Adult:* 200 mg PO to a max of 8 tablets daily. Max: 1200 mg/day. Give with levodopa-carbidopa	Entacapone has no antiparkinsonian effect of its own.
tolcapone	Adjunct to levodopa for idiopathic PD	*Adult:* Initiate therapy at 100 mg 3 times daily. Always give as adjunct to levodopa-carbidopa therapy.	**If a patient fails to show the expected incremental benefit on the 200-mg dose after a total of 3 weeks of treatment (regardless of dose), drug should be discontinued.** ▲

CO, Carbon monoxide; *CR*, controlled-release; *DOC*, drug of choice; *EPS*, extrapyramidal symptoms; *ER*, extended-release; *IM*, intramuscular (route); *IR*, immediate-release; *IV*, intravenous (route); *ODT*, orally disintegrating tablet; *PD*, Parkinson's disease; *TBT*, transbuccal tablet.

Dopamine Agonists

◆ bromocriptine (Parlodel); ✦ Parlodel
◆ pergolide (Permax); ✦ Celance, Permax
◆ pramipexole (Mirapex)
◆ ropinirole (Requip CR); ✦ Requip CR

▌▌▌ *Indications*

Dopamine agonists produce an acute antiparkinsonian effect equal to or less than that of levodopa. Pramipexole and ropinirole are currently the most popular and most prescribed dopamine agonist drugs. Both drugs are used for idiopathic and postencephalitic PD and for the management of restless legs syndrome (RLS; also known as Ekbom syndrome). Pramipexole has also been used for bipolar disorder.

Pergolide can be used as monotherapy or as an adjunct to levodopa-carbidopa in the treatment of patients who experience intolerable dyskinesia and/or increasing "on-off" episodes when taking levodopa alone.

BOX 26-3

"Jump-Start" Dosing Using Liquid Levodopa-Carbidopa

Step 1: Mix ingredients in a 1-liter (1-quart) glass or plastic container (do NOT use metal)
- 10 tablets of 10–100 mg –or– 25–100 mg tablets of levodopa-carbidopa (equals 1000 mg of levodopa)
- One half of a teaspoon ascorbic acid crystals (approximately 2 grams)
- One liter of tap water or distilled water (1000 mL)

Rotate container or shake gently until tablets dissolve. (There is no need to crush the tablets.)

Step 2: Morning "jump-start" dose
- 60 mL of recipe, or may use amount comparable to usual tablet dose
- Adjust dose by 5 to 10 mL up or down every 3 to 5 days, until best "on" state is achieved with the least dyskinesias.

Step 3: Hourly dosing
- 30 mL of recipe on the hour while awake, or hourly proportion of usual tablet dose (e.g., patient taking 100–25 mg levodopa-carbidopa tablet every 2 hours may try 50 mL/hour of the liquid recipe)
- Adjust dose by 5 to 10 mL up or down every 3 to 5 days until "on" periods are smoother.

    NOTE: It is important that liquid levodopa-carbidopa be used under the guidance of the health care provider; optimal dosing varies greatly from one patient to another. Formula will maintain full strength and purity for 24 to 48 hours in refrigerator. Final mixture contains 1 mg of levodopa/mL, 0.1 or 0.25 mg/mL of carbidopa (depending on strength of tablet used), and 2 mg/mL of ascorbic acid.

Adapted from Marjama-Lyons, J. (2006). *Parkinson disease: Medications.* (3rd ed.). Miami, FL: National Parkinson Foundation.

Bromocriptine has also been used to prevent lactation following childbirth and to correct infertility and amenorrhea in women with high prolactin levels (see Chapter 60).

Pharmacodynamics

Pramipexole and ropinirole have a particularly strong attraction to D_3 receptors. Direct stimulation of dopamine receptors in the striatum restores the dopamine needed for correct functioning of the basal ganglia.

Pergolide and bromocriptine serve as substitutes for dopamine by directly stimulating dopamine receptor cells in the corpus striatum. The deficiency of dopamine is thus offset, which in turn diminishes rigidity, tremor, and sluggish movements.

The pathogenesis of RLS is largely unknown, although evidence suggests a fault in the striatal presynaptic dopaminergic system. Likewise, how ropinirole exerts its action in RLS is unknown, but it is thought to stimulate dopamine receptors in the presynaptic dopaminergic system.

Pharmacokinetics

Pramipexole is rapidly absorbed following oral administration with a bioavailability of 90% (see Table 26-2). Absorption is not affected by the presence of food, although time to peak plasma levels is increased by 1 hour when the drug is taken with food. There is no hepatic biotransformation. Ninety percent of pramipexole is eliminated in the urine, almost all as unchanged drug.

Pergolide is well absorbed following oral administration. Distribution is unknown. In vitro, pergolide is 10 to 1000 times more potent than bromocriptine on a milligram-to-milligram basis. Biotransformation occurs in the liver, with metabolites eliminated primarily in the urine.

Ropinirole is rapidly absorbed following oral administration, with an absolute bioavailability of 55% indicating that the drug undergoes a first-pass effect. Peak serum levels are decreased by 25%, and the time to peak effect is increased by 2.5 hours when the drug is taken with a high-fat meal. Ropinirole's pharmacokinetics profile is similar in patients with PD and patients with RLS.

Bromocriptine is poorly absorbed from the gastrointestinal (GI) tract and is completely biotransformed in the liver and eliminated in the feces.

Adverse Effects and Contraindications

The adverse drug effects of dopamine agonists are similar to those of levodopa-carbidopa, but are usually additive and more prominent. Orthostatic hypotension and GI disturbances result from peripheral and central dopaminergic effects. Dyskinesia occurs less frequently with dopamine agonists compared with the dopaminergic levodopa-carbidopa.

The confusion, hallucinations, and dyskinesia seen with dopamine agonists tends to worsen if the dose of the agonist or the levodopa (or the combination of levodopa-carbidopa) is not reduced. Although the cause is uncertain, dyspnea is thought to be the result of a combination of dopaminergic and idiosyncratic mechanisms. Angina, arrhythmias, and bilateral vasodilation of the extremities, with burning pain, increased skin temperature, and redness (erythromelalgia), are associated with dopamine agonists. Hot environments may cause orthostasis.

Bromocriptine's most common adverse effects are nausea, vomiting, dyspepsia, hypotension, hallucinations, psychosis, and dyskinesia. Leg cramps often occur in patients on long-term therapy. Use bromocriptine cautiously in patients with liver disease because of the drug's poor biotransformation in the liver and elimination via the biliary tract. It should also be used cautiously in patients with a history of cardiac disorders. The neurologic and psychiatric disturbances caused by bromocriptine may last 2 to 6 weeks after therapy is discontinued. Although rare, thickening of the pleura and pleural effusion have been noted in patients on long-term bromocriptine therapy.

The adverse reactions to pergolide are similar to those to bromocriptine and include nausea, hallucinations, dyskinesia, sedation, and postural hypotension. Use pergolide cautiously in patients with coronary artery disease, angina, arrhythmias, Raynaud's syndrome, or seizure disorders. Long-term use of pergolide may produce dyskinesias. Sudden withdrawal of pergolide can cause confusion, paranoid thinking, and severe hallucinations.

The most frequent adverse effects of pramipexole are nausea, dizziness, drowsiness, and insomnia. **"Dopamine agonists, in** ▲

clinical studies and clinical experience, appear to impair the systemic regulation of blood pressure, with resulting orthostatic hypotension, especially during dose escalation. Parkinson's disease patients, in addition, appear to have an impaired capacity to respond to an orthostatic challenge" (Pramipexole package insert). Hallucinations may occur at any time during the course of treatment. Rhabdomyolysis was reported in a single patient with advanced PD; symptoms resolved with discontinuation of the drug.

The common adverse effects of ropinirole occur in 40% to 60% of patients taking the drug and include nausea, dizziness and excessive drowsiness. **"Patients treated with ropinirole have reported falling asleep while engaged in activities of daily living, including the operation of motor vehicles, which sometimes resulted in accidents. Although many of these patients reported somnolence while on the drug, some felt that they had no warning signs such as excessive drowsiness, and believed that they were alert immediately before the event. Some of these events have been reported as late as 1 year after initiation of treatment"** (Ropinirole package insert). Somnolence has been reported more often in patients taking ropinirole for PD than when it is used for RLS.

Fewer than 12% of patients taking ropinirole experience syncope, vomiting, fatigue, viral infections, dyspepsia, diaphoresis, weakness, orthostatic hypotension, abdominal discomfort, pharyngitis, abnormal vision, dry mouth, hypertension, or confusion with hallucinations. Although rare, anorexia, peripheral edema, memory loss, rhinitis, sinusitis, palpitations, and impotence have been reported with ropinirole. There are no known contraindications to ropinirole use, although the drug should be used with caution in patients with a history of orthostatic hypotension, syncope, or hallucinations (particularly in older adults).

Safe use of dopamine agonists in children and during pregnancy has not been established (pregnancy category C).

⠿ *Drug Interactions*

Anticholinergic effects (dry mouth, blurred vision) are increased with the concurrent use of pergolide with antihistamines, phenothiazines, quinidine, TCAs, and bromocriptine. Other drug interactions are noted in Table 26-3. There are no known drug interactions with pramipexole and ropinirole.

⠿ *Dosage Regimen*

Table 26-4 identifies the dose and the administration schedule based on the patient's renal function. Retitration of pramipexole and ropinirole is needed if a significant interruption in therapy occurs.

⠿ *Lab Considerations*

Bromocriptine can cause elevations in BUN, ALT, AST, creatine kinase, alkaline phosphatase, and uric acid levels; however, the elevations hold no clinical significance. Reductions in serum levels of prolactin and growth hormone have been noted.

Pergolide can cause a marked reduction in serum prolactin levels. This appears to be its only physiologic effect that alters laboratory values. No systematic abnormalities on routine laboratory testing were noted with pramipexole or with ropinirole.

Anticholinergics

◆ benztropine (Cogentin); ✦ Apo-Benztropine, PMS-Benztropine
◆ trihexyphenidyl (Artane); ✦ Apo-Trihex

⠿ *Indications*

Anticholinergics are useful early in younger patients with PD, more to control tremor by relaxing smooth muscle than for treatment of the other manifestations of the disease. Anticholinergics are also a reasonable treatment option for middle-aged patients who have tremor but little rigidity or bradykinesia. Although this class of drugs is useful in controlling salivation and drooling, they cause dry mouth. These drugs are also the drugs of choice for treating *akathisia* (extrapyramidal symptoms [EPS]) arising from use of antipsychotic drugs (see Chapter 21).

⠿ *Pharmacodynamics*

As PD progresses, dopaminergic activity decreases and cholinergic activity becomes dominant, resulting in motor dysfunction. Anticholinergic drugs competitively inhibit ACh at postsynaptic muscarinic receptors. The muscarinic receptors are found in smooth muscle, cardiac muscle, and parasympathetic-innervated glands, as well as in the brain. This mechanism restores the cholinergic-dopaminergic balance in the striatum.

⠿ *Pharmacokinetics*

Few pharmacokinetics data are available for anticholinergic drugs. Known pharmacokinetic data is noted in Table 26-2. Anticholinergics are well absorbed when taken by mouth. The extent of distribution, biotransformation, and elimination is unknown.

⠿ *Adverse Effects and Contraindications*

The adverse effects of anticholinergic drugs are more common in older adults and are generally more disabling. The adverse CNS effects of anticholinergic drugs include headache, nervousness, disorientation, dizziness, weakness, insomnia, and cognitive impairment, and, in children, fever. Cardiovascular effects include tachycardia and palpitations. Nausea, vomiting, dry mouth, constipation, heartburn, dysphagia, paralytic ileus, and urinary retention or hesitancy in men with prostatic hypertrophy and impotence have been noted. Suppression of glandular secretions including lactation, flushed skin, and decreased perspiration with heat prostration can be troublesome in some patients. Dilated pupils, blurry vision, photophobia, and exacerbation of acute-angle glaucoma have also been documented with anticholinergic drugs.

Excessive dosages of anticholinergics may cause dry mouth, burning sensation of the mouth, difficulty in swallowing, restlessness, tachycardia, increased respirations, muscle incoordination, dilated pupils, paralysis, tremors, seizures, hallucinations, and death. If overdosage is suspected, gastric lavage or induction of emesis followed by use of activated charcoal is the treatment of choice. Anticholinergic effects can also be reversed by administering one of the cholinesterase inhibitor drugs, physostigmine or neostigmine. Artificial ventilation for paralysis of respiratory muscles may be required.

Anticholinergic drugs are contraindicated for use in patients with hypersensitivity, acute glaucoma, acute hemorrhage, tachycardia secondary to cardiac insufficiency or thyrotoxicosis, Down syndrome, asthma, or chronic lung disease. Anticholinergic drugs are also contraindicated for use in patients with bronchial asthma or emphysema who are currently taking sympathomimetic drugs.

Anticholinergic drugs should be used with caution in patients with acute or chronic kidney, cardiac, lung, or liver disease. Also use caution in prescribing anticholinergics for patients who have prostatic hypertrophy and intestinal obstruction because of the drugs' spasmolytic action on smooth muscle. Safe use of anticholinergics during childhood, pregnancy, and lactation has not been established (pregnancy category C).

▥ Drug Interactions

Anticholinergic drugs exhibit additive or antagonistic effects with other antiparkinsonian drugs and other anticholinergics (Table 26-3). The adverse effects occur most often when taken anticholinergics are taken with other CNS-active drugs such as antipsychotics, antihistamines, and antidepressants.

▥ Dosage Regimen

The dosages of anticholinergics vary with the specific drug, the severity of symptoms, the age of the patient, whether the drug is used in conjunction with another agent, and how long the patient has been using anticholinergics. Acquired tolerance is not a problem, but progression of the disease leads to an apparent loss of efficacy in many patients. Table 26-4 provides an overview of the anticholinergic drugs and their recommended dosages.

Monoamine Oxidase B Inhibitors
◆ selegiline (Eldepryl); ◆ selegiline
◆ rasagiline (Agilect, Zelapar); ◆ Agilect

▥ Indications

Selegiline is used as an adjunct to levodopa-carbidopa in all stages of PD, although it is more effective when used early in the disease and for patients with young-onset PD who have moderate to severe limitations and/or disabilities. Its use may help patients avoid the complications associated with long-term, high-dose levodopa therapy.

Rasagiline is indicated as monotherapy in early PD and as an adjunct to levodopa-carbidopa in later stages of PD. It is efficacious for end-of-dose fluctuations in motor function. There is tentative evidence that rasagiline slows the progression of PD itself as well as offers symptom relief (Guay, 2006). This has been shown in vitro and in animal studies but not in humans to date. Rasagiline and its analogues are also under investigation for use in Alzheimer's disease to enhance memory and learning (Youdim, 2006; Youdim and Weinstock, 2002).

▥ Pharmacodynamics

The mechanism of action for selegiline is not completely understood, but the drug appears to irreversibly inhibit MAO-B activity. By blocking MAO-B, selegiline prevents the breakdown of dopamine and increases dopaminergic activity by interfering with dopamine reuptake at the synapses. Selegiline indirectly raises norepinephrine levels, because dopamine can be catabolized within the brain to norepinephrine, although the extent of this is variable. Selegiline is biotransformed to amphetamine derivatives.

Rasagiline is an irreversible MAO-B inhibitor in platelets, with a potency 5 to 10 times greater than that of selegiline. By prolonging survival of dopamine neurons, normal locomotion, gait, and coordination are improved and the physical decline delayed. Unlike selegiline, rasagiline is biotransformed to a non–amphetamine compound with no adrenergic activity. In addition, at inhibitory dosages it does not provoke a "cheese reaction." However, the selectivity of rasagiline and the sensitivity to tyramine during treatment has not been adequately studied so as to eliminate the dietary restrictions on tyramine.

▥ Pharmacokinetics

Selegiline is well absorbed following oral administration, has a wide distribution, and is rapidly biotransformed to three metabolites: N-desmethydeprenyl, amphetamine, and methamphetamine. The half-lives of these metabolites differ, ranging from 2 hours to 20.5 hours (see Table 26-2). Because new MAO-B enzyme synthesis must take place for a patient to regain activity, it takes several weeks for the clinical effects of selegiline to fully disappear.

Rasagiline is well absorbed and well distributed, with rapid peak serum levels reached in 30 minutes. It is almost totally biotransformed by the CYP 1A2 isoenzyme before elimination through the kidneys.

▥ Adverse Effects and Contraindications

Selegiline has no known life-threatening or irreversible adverse effects, although it does exert numerous troublesome effects on every body system. Nausea, dizziness, lightheadedness, faintness, and abdominal discomfort appear in 4% to 10% of patients taking selegiline. Occasionally confusion, hallucinations, dry mouth, vivid dreams, and dyskinesia appear. Headaches, myalgia, anxiety, diarrhea, and insomnia occur in less than 1% of patients. Symptoms of overdosage vary from CNS depression (i.e., sedation, apnea, cardiovascular collapse, death) to severe paradoxical reactions. Impaired motor coordination (i.e., loss of balance, blepharospasm, facial grimacing, and a sense of heaviness in lower extremities, stiff neck, involuntary movements), hallucinations, confusion, depression, nightmares, delusions, overstimulation, sleep disturbance, and anger occur in some patients. Once the dosage of selegiline is reduced or the drug stopped, adverse effects resolve.

Selegiline is contraindicated for use in patients with hypersensitivity to the drug or its ingredients. Cautious use of selegiline in dosages exceeding 10 mg/day is warranted because of the higher risk of hypersensitivity reactions with tyramine-containing foods. Caution is important when the drug is used in patients with a history of peptic ulcer disease, dementia, psychosis, tardive dyskinesia, profound tremor, and arrhythmias. Safe use of selegiline during pregnancy or lactation or in children has not been established (pregnancy category C).

The adverse effects of rasagiline vary depending on whether it is used as monotherapy or in combination with levodopa. When used as monotherapy, the common adverse effects include headache, arthralgia, dyspepsia, depression, and falls. When used concurrently with levodopa, the most common adverse effects include dyskinesias, GI symptoms, headaches, weight loss, joint pain, and orthostasis.

Epidemiologic studies have shown that patients with PD may have 2 to 4 times the risk for developing melanoma than the general population, although it is unclear whether the increased risk was due to PD itself or to drugs used to treat PD (Olsen et al, 2005; Olsen, Friss, and Frederickson, 2007; Zanetti and Rosso, 2007). The increased incidence of melanoma with rasagiline was comparable to the increased risk observed in the PD populations examined in the epidemiologic studies.

Rasagiline may potentiate dopaminergic adverse effects and exacerbate preexisting dyskinesia when used as an adjunct to levodopa. Eighteen percent of patients experienced treatment-related dyskinesia when treated with rasagiline as an adjunct to levodopa compared with 10% of patients treated with placebo. Orthostasis is likely to occur during the first 60 days of therapy with rasagiline, but it generally improves over time.

Other adverse events with rasagiline include behavioral and mental status changes, syncope, dose-dependent postural hypotension, hypertension, diaphoresis, and muscular rigidity. Dose-dependent hallucinations have been reported in 3% to 5% of patients taking rasagiline as an adjunct to levodopa.

▥ Drug Interactions

Selegiline is contraindicated for use in conjunction with meperidine and other opiates (see Table 26-3). Interestingly, MAO-B isozymes lack the notable interaction that occurs with the ingestion of foods containing tyramine. Rasagiline, when used in combination with TCAs or selegiline, has been associated with CNS toxicity, including hyperpyrexia and death. Patients receiving rasagiline should not take amine-containing drugs concurrently. Adrenergic amines found in over-the-counter (OTC) drugs to be avoided include pseudoephedrine and phenylephrine.

▥ Dosage Regimen

The initial dose of selegiline is 5 mg once or twice a day (see Table 26-4). The usual maintenance dose is 10 mg/day in two divided doses, one taken after breakfast and one after lunch.

Rasagiline can be taken orally, with or without food, and is
A typically well tolerated. **"Rasagiline at any dose may be associated with a hypertensive crisis or 'cheese reaction' if the patient ingests tyramine-rich foods, beverages, or dietary supplements or amines (from OTC drugs). Hypertensive crisis, which in some cases may be fatal, consists of marked systemic blood pressure elevation and requires immediate treatment and/or hospitalization"** (Rasagiline package insert).

Catechol-*O*-Methyltransferase (COMT) Inhibitor

◆ entacapone (Comtan); ♣ Comtan, Comtess
◆ tolcapone (Tasmar)

▥ Indications

Entacapone and tolcapone are FDA-approved as adjuncts to levodopa-carbidopa for patients with idiopathic PD who experience end-of-dose "wearing off." Patients using COMT inhibitors along with levodopa-carbidopa showed a significant improvement in UPDRS motor and activities of daily living (ADLs) scores.

Because of the risk of potentially fatal, acute fulminant **A** **liver failure, tolcapone should only be used in patients with PD who are presently taking levodopa-carbidopa but who are experiencing significant fluctuations in symptoms that are unresponsive to other therapies or who are not candidates for other treatments.**

▥ Pharmacodynamics

Entacapone and tolcapone are reversible inhibitors of COMT activity in erythrocytes, thereby altering the plasma pharmacokinetics of levodopa. When given with levodopa and a decarboxylase inhibitor, such as carbidopa, plasma levels of levodopa are higher and more sustained than after administration of levodopa-carbidopa alone. Steadier dopaminergic stimulation in the brain, resulting from the higher sustained plasma levels of levadopa, can lead to great improvement in the signs and symptoms of PD. However, higher levodopa levels also contribute to a higher incidence of levodopa's adverse effects.

▥ Pharmacokinetics

Entacapone is rapidly absorbed but is poorly distributed to tissues because of its extensive binding to plasma proteins, albumin in particular. The oral bioavailability of entacapone suggests the drug has an extensive first-pass effect. Food does not affect the pharmacokinetics of entacapone. Entacapone interacts with levodopa to increase its area under the curve, and extends the half-life of levodopa without raising therapeutic levels above those that are safe. Entacapone is almost completely biotransformed before excretion, with less than 0.5% of one dose found unchanged in the urine. The pharmacokinetics of entacapone are linear over the dosing range and are independent of levodopa-carbidopa coadministration.

Given along with levodopa-carbidopa, tolcapone increases the bioavailability of levodopa twofold by reducing levodopa clearance. Therapeutic effects are evident over the long term.

▥ Adverse Effects and Contraindications

Adverse effects associated with the use of COMT inhibitors are most frequently the result of elevated levodopa availability in the brain. These dopaminergic effects, such as dyskinesias, abdominal pain, nausea, vomiting, diarrhea, discoloration of the urine, dizziness, postural hypotenstion, amnesia, agitation, confusion, and hallucinations, have been previously seen in patients undergoing levodopa therapy without using a COMT inhibitor.

Several cases of rhabdomyolysis have been reported. The complicated nature of PD and PD treatment make it difficult to establish what role, if any, entacapone has in the pathogenesis of rhabdomyolysis, although severe prolonged motor activity, including dyskinesias, may account for some of the symptoms. It is also thought that a series of signs and symptoms that appear with entacapone use may reflect neuroleptic malignant syndrome (see Chapter 21).

▥ Drug Interactions

Entacapone binds to the benzodiazepine (BZD) site on albumin but does not bind to the warfarin site. Although albumin binds certain other drugs (e.g., salicylic acid, phenylbutazone, diazepam), it is not thought that entacapone will displace these drugs, nor will it be significantly displaced.

Isoproterenol, epinephrine, norepinephrine, dopamine, dobutamine, α-methyldopa, apomorphine, isoetharine, and bitolterol are all biotransformed by COMT, and consequently, health care providers should use caution in administering these drugs to patients receiving entacapone, regardless of the route of administration. The interaction may result in tachyarrhythmias and extreme changes in blood pressure (see Table 26-3).

Dosage Regimen

Entacapone does not have an antiparkinsonian effect when taken alone; therefore the drug must be given with levodopa-carbidopa (see Table 26-4). When withdrawal from entacapone is necessary, proceed slowly. Monitor the patient closely, and adjust other dopaminergic treatments as needed. Patients who develop a high fever or severe rigidity during withdrawal from entacapone should be considered as having neuroleptic malignant syndrome until known otherwise.

Because of the risk for liver failure, and because tolcapone provides an obvious therapeutic benefit, patients who do not demonstrate significant clinical improvement within 3 weeks of starting therapy should be withdrawn from the drug.

Lab Considerations

Even though entacapone chelates iron, the effect on the body's iron supply has not been identified. The tendency of patients with PD to have lower serum iron concentrations necessitates close monitoring of ferritin levels to minimize the risk for comorbid iron deficiency. There have been no observed entacapone-related abnormalities in chemistry or liver function tests.

CLINICAL REASONING

Treatment Objectives

There are no currently available drugs that modify the disease process or affect its natural progression. Most drugs either lessen or reverse the symptoms by replacing the chemicals needed for neural transmission and movement. Until there is a prophylaxis strategy or a cure for PD, management of the patient with PD is aimed at maintaining function and independence, and reducing the symptoms and disabilities caused by the disease as much and for as long as possible. This can be accomplished by maintaining a balance between dopaminergic and cholinergic activity in the basal ganglia. In general, 85% of patients with early, mild PD achieve at least 50% improvement in function with appropriate drug therapy.

Treatment Options

Because symptoms of PD are attributable to the lack of dopamine within the striatum of the brain, the majority of anti-Parkinson's drugs are aimed at temporarily replenishing or enhancing dopamine concentration while preventing further neuronal damage. Numerous strategies can be chosen for the management of PD based on the etiology (Table 26-5).

Patient Variables

PD is defined solely by clinical signs and symptoms, especially physical signs. To evaluate the severity of the disease, the health care provider must perform an exam. However, the exam may not reveal a patient's ability to perform outside the office and to carry out ADLs. Nonetheless, a thorough assessment is required so that proper intervention can be undertaken. Key information to be obtained includes why the patient came to the hospital or clinic and when the symptoms started. What does the patient think caused the symptoms? Has the patient experienced these symptoms in the past? When? Complaints of interference with ADLs often precede recognition of PD by months or years.

CENTRAL NERVOUS

TABLE 26-5 Drugs for Parkinson's Disease and Parkinsonism

Drug	Idiopathic Disease	Drug-Induced EPS	Chemical- or Drug-Induced Disease	Arteriosclerotic Disease	Postencephalitic Disease
DOPAMINERGICS					
levodopa-carbidopa	X		X		X
carbidopa-levodopa-entacapone	Adjunct				
DOPAMINE AGONISTS					
bromocriptine	X				X
pergolide	X			Adjunct	
pramipexole	X				
ropinirole	X				
ANTICHOLINERGICS					
benztropine	X	X	X	X	X
trihexyphenidyl	X	X	X	X	X
MAO-B INHIBITORS					
selegiline	X, Adjunct			X	
rasagiline	X, Adjunct				
COMT INHIBITOR					
entacapone	Adjunct				
tolcapone	Adjunct				

EPS, Extrapyramidal symptoms.

A health history elicits information about drugs, exposure to environmental toxins, past or present alcohol or drug use, and drugs currently being taken. In addition, note information related to history of renal, hepatic, cardiovascular, or GI disorders.

Observation of the patient during the interview may reveal changes in speech and facial expression, arm swing, and gait. An exam can reveal valuable clues as to the extent of interference with ADLs. Assessment of the neurologic system may be the greatest diagnostic aid. Other systems of importance are the musculoskeletal system, the head and neck, and the skin.

Postural abnormalities appear early in PD. There may be involuntary flexion of the head and neck and a flexed, "stooped" posture. Moving as a unit, the body may be unable to correct position when changing from one position to another or merely when turning over. The patient may be slow to initiate a walk but spontaneously break into a run. When pushed forward or backward, the patient may actually have difficulty stopping.

Typically, the arms are flexed at the elbows, with the wrists slightly dorsiflexed and the fingers adducted and flexed at the metacarpophalangeal joint. During walking, arm swing is decreased or absent. There may be difficulties with handwriting (micrographia), using kitchen utensils, grooming, and fastening buttons. Rapid repetitive movements, such as tapping of the fingers or pronation and supination of the hand, are common.

There is a masklike facial expression owing to limited muscle movements. Be cautious not to mistake a "masked facies" for depression. A blank expression, decreased blinking, and characteristic stare are all common. Unfortunately, these effects are associated with other head and neck symptoms, such as difficulties in swallowing and chewing. Drooling may be noted as the disease progresses. The patient's speech may become softer and less distinct.

Commonly, the patient with PD is emotionally labile, has a flat affect, is easily upset, and shows signs of paranoia. When questioned, the patient may respond slowly owing to cognitive impairments. The same impairments may be evident as delayed reaction times in the completion of requested tasks. Evidence of dementia and acute confusion are common in the older adult with this disease.

Autonomic symptoms include diaphoresis, orthostatic hypotension, and constipation. Neuroendocrine dysfunction accounts for the excessively oily skin, especially on the face.

There are no lab tests to confirm or refute the clinical diagnosis of PD. Chemistry tests are most commonly used to seek treatable causes of dementia with parkinsonism, especially hypothyroidism. Although unreliable in diagnosing idiopathic parkinsonism, magnetic resonance imaging (MRI) has proven to be the single most useful means to look for other etiologies. Computed tomography (CT scan) is also useful. If a CT scan shows calcification of the basal ganglia, investigate for hyperparathyroidism and hypoparathyroidism by measuring serum calcium, phosphorus, and parathormone levels.

LIFE-SPAN CONSIDERATIONS

Pregnant and Nursing Women. Pregnancy in patients with PD is a rare occurrence. It is not known whether antiparkinsonian drugs cause fetal harm or affect reproductive capacity. Do not use antiparkinsonian drugs during pregnancy unless the anticipated benefits outweigh the risks arising from failure to treat PD.

Children and Adolescents. Antiparkinsonian drugs are usually not needed in children. Further, the safety and efficacy of antiparkinsonian drugs have not been established for this age group. Juvenile parkinsonism may occur but is usually associated with Wilson's disease, progressive lenticular degeneration, or Huntington's chorea.

Older Adults. Normal changes of aging alter the biotransformation and elimination of antiparkinsonian drugs, thereby increasing the risk for adverse effects. Note any existing dementia as well as occasional confusion before beginning drug therapy for PD.

CASE STUDY | Drugs for Parkinson's Disease

ASSESSMENT

History of Present Illness	DD is a 75-year-old male with complaints of a general feeling of stiffness, mild to moderate tremors in both arms, and increasing difficulty dressing and eating. His family noticed that his handwriting has changed and his speech is slower than normal. He does not exercise but has started to lose weight.
Past Health History	DD denies allergies to food or medications. His last physical exam 6 years ago was unremarkable. He has mild arthritis and takes ASA for discomfort. He denies a history of hospitalizations, illnesses, smoking, or alcohol use. Current meds: ASA 650 mg PRN for shoulder and knee discomfort (requires about 4 tablets/week).
Life-Span Considerations	Age-related physiologic changes to body systems.
Psychosocial Considerations	DD retired from working in a grocery store at the age of 55. Currently living in a retirement community with wife, who is in fair health. He has an attentive daughter and two grandchildren who live within 5 miles and visit often. Sister lives out of town. DD has access to both a medical facility and a pharmacy. Wife provides transportation as needed. Through Medicare, his supplemental insurance, and retirement benefits, the majority of medical bills and prescriptions are paid.

Continued

CASE STUDY	**Drugs for Parkinson's Disease—Cont'd**
Physical Exam Findings	*Height:* 5'11". *Weight:* 170 lb (5 lb below usual). *VSS:* Afebrile. Slight pill-rolling movements of the thumb against fingers of the left hand. Mild to moderate resting tremors bilaterally, rigidity, and bradykinesia noted. Postural instability. Low-pitched, poorly articulated speech lacks modulation. Short-term memory loss apparent.
Diagnostic Testing	Chest x-ray, ECG, CT and MRI brain, CBC, and electrolytes within normal limits.

DIAGNOSIS: Parkinson's Disease

MANAGEMENT

Treatment Objectives	1. Reduce symptoms and enhance the quality of life. 2. Maintain function and independence for as long as possible. 3. Provide patient with lowest possible treatment regimen that is effective in controlling symptoms.
Treatment Options	**Pharmacotherapy** • Low-dose immediate-release levodopa-carbidopa: ½ of scored 100-mg levodopa–25-mg carbidopa tablet initially. Increase dosage by ½ tablet at weekly intervals until improvement or toxicities are noted. • Switch to controlled-release formulation once total daily dose of 200 mg levodopa is reached. Start CR dosage 10% higher than levodopa dose to switch from IR to CR. **Patient Teaching** 1. Encourage DD to pursue as many of his pre–disease activities as possible. 2. Teach about the drug regimen, why it is taken, the correct dosages, warning signs of adverse effects, and the importance of not abruptly discontinuing the drug. 3. Restrict total dietary protein to the recommended daily allowance of 0.8 grams/kg (61 grams/day). Dietary protein may be divided into portions eaten throughout the day or may be consumed in the evening meal. 4. Avoid alcohol and OTC multiple vitamins containing pyridoxine (vitamin B_6), which interferes with levodopa activity. 5. Advise DD's wife that he is to make position changes slowly so as to minimize orthostatic hypotension. 6. Warn that perspiration may decrease, so that overheating may occur during hot weather. **Evaluation** 1. Symptoms decreased after 2 to 3 weeks of levodopa-carbidopa therapy. 2. Functional and cognitive abilities have improved or are stable.

CLINICAL REASONING ANALYSIS

Q1. When do you decide to start an anti-Parkinson's drug?
A. It depends on patient age and symptoms, but in DD's case, functional and cognitive symptoms have starting interfering with the patient's activities of daily living.

Q2. How do you know which drugs to use?
A. Dopamine agonists such as the combination of levodopa-carbidopa are the mainstay of treatment for PD and are more effective than the other drugs currently available. The combination concentrates levodopa in the brain and minimizes the adverse effects of dopamine, as well as reducing nausea and other peripheral adverse effects. The other drug options such as anticholinergics, the MAO-B inhibitors, and COMT inhibitors, which are new, are used most often as adjuncts to levodopa-carbidopa therapy. Doing so helps us to reduce the dosage of levodopa the patient gets and reduces adverse effects.

Q3. We just finished studying anticholinergic drugs. Couldn't we just use something like benztropine?
A. Well, yes, we could consider an anticholinergic drug like benztropine. However, anticholinergic drugs seem to work better in middle-aged patients with little rigidity or bradykinesia. DD isn't middle-aged any longer and already has significant rigidity and bradykinesia. Anticholinergics also have more adverse effects in older adults.

▦ Drug Variables

New evidence-based recommendations clarify which drugs are beneficial in slowing the progression of PD and which effectively treat motor fluctuations and the mental status changes associated with the disease. Left untreated, PD progresses from minimal dysfunction to severe disability in 3 to 10 years. There is no way to predict which patients will develop which symptoms, and the severity of the symptoms varies from one person to another. Treatment generally retards but does not completely halt progression of the disease. It may, however, prolong independent functioning and longevity by 5 to 15 years. Treatment is not warranted for patients with early, mild symptoms and no disability. Drug therapy is started when disability interferes with the patient's social, emotional, or work life (see Box 26-4).

There is strong evidence to suggest that aggregation of proteins in the substantia nigra starts the cascade of events that results in neural degeneration. If is this true, then inhibiting the aggregation of proteins may be an effective approach to preventing and treating PD. Current treatment strategies involve drugs that control symptoms rather than treating the underlying cause of PD (see Box 26-3). Although efficacious in the early stages of PD, they progressively fail as more and more neurons die.

Dopaminergic Drugs. Levodopa-carbidopa is probably the single most effective combination drug for PD. The addition of carbidopa allows a reduction in the oral dose of levodopa. For patients who cannot tolerate multidose regimens, the controlled-release formulation of levodopa-carbidopa may be an alternative. More stable blood levels of the drugs help to prevent the sudden and unpredictable on-off phenomenon. It has been reported that some patients show more improvement while taking fewer daily doses of the controlled-release formulation; however, some do worse. **A rule of thumb when prescribing levodopa-carbidopa and dopamine agonists is to start with one drug at a time and observe for a clinical benefit or intolerable adverse effect before changing therapy.** Abrupt cessation of levodopa-carbidopa therapy may precipitate a serious hyperpyretic state similar to neuroleptic malignant syndrome. The use of "drug holidays" from levodopa is dangerous and no longer recommended.

Loss of control in a previously levodopa-responsive symptom should not be interpreted as loss of levodopa effect or evidence of disease progression. If previously controlled symptoms recur, search for other treatable etiologies, such as drug interactions, difficulties with drug absorption, and other conditions associated with PD (e.g., dehydration). As PD progresses, the increasing dosage of levodopa required for symptom control approaches the dosage at which intolerable dyskinesias occur, which limits the continuing usefulness of levodopa. For this reason, the standard of practice today is to start a younger patient on a dopamine agonist instead of levodopa, which delays the onset of dyskinesias.

Patients who develop nausea from levodopa-carbidopa may benefit from additional carbidopa (Lodosyn) added to each dose of levodopa-carbidopa. One of the advantages of using carbidopa in combination with levodopa includes allowing patients to take vitamin B_6 (which would otherwise decrease the effectiveness of levodopa).

Excessive gastric acidity can cause erratic gastric emptying and decrease the absorption of levodopa. Gastric emptying, and consequently the absorption of levodopa, can be accelerated by taking the drug with antacids or warm liquids, by chewing the tablets before swallowing, or using the "quick-start" strategy previously identified. Food has less of an effect on the absorption of the controlled-release formulations than on the absorption of the immediate-release levodopa-carbidopa formulations and is a benefit to patients with erratic absorption.

Dopamine Agonists. Recognize the differences in potency among dopamine agonists. For example, 0.5 mg of pergolide is roughly equivalent to 0.5 mg of pramipexole or to 5 mg of bromocriptine. Ropinirole is less potent but equally effective with higher dosages; individual doses of 8 to 12 mg may be needed before clinical benefit is reached. There is no maximal dosage for dopamine agonists. Choose the lowest dose that achieves the desired clinical benefit while avoiding unacceptable adverse effects.

Before initiating treatment with ropinirole, inquire about factors that may increase the risk for drowsiness, such as

---

BOX 26-4

Treatment Guidelines for Parkinson's Disease

MOTOR STATE	CONSIDERATIONS*
No functional deficit (i.e., normal ADLs, QOL)	Drug therapy not needed
Dyskinesias	Decrease levodopa-carbidopa dosage or dosing intervals
	Add dopamine agonist†
	Substitute controlled-release formulation for levodopa-carbidopa
Dystonias	Adjust dosage of levodopa-carbidopa upward or downward
	Add baclofen (Lioresal)
	Add anticholinergic
Wearing off	Switch from levodopa-carbidopa to controlled-release formulation
	Increase dosage of controlled-release levodopa-carbidopa and/or dosing frequency
	Add dopamine agonist (to permit reduction of levodopa-carbidopa dosage)
	Add COMT inhibitor
Unpredictable on-off	Add dopamine agonist
	Evaluate as candidate for investigational drug trial or surgical procedure
Young-onset PD with cognitive changes and functional disability	Consider selegiline
	Consider dopamine agonists (delays onset of dyskinesias)

*Titrate levodopa-carbidopa by increasing by one half of a tablet with each dose every 2 wk. For example, levodopa-carbidopa 100–25 mg, one tablet 3 times daily for 2 weeks, then 1½ tablets 3 times daily for 2 weeks, then 2 tablets 3 times daily.

†Titrate dopamine agonists slowly. The lowest dose may be doubled every 1–2 wk. For example, titrate pramipexole, 0.125 mg 3 times daily for 1–2 wk, then increase to 0.25 mg 3 times daily for 1–2 wk before considering increasing to 0.375 mg. Titrate at slower rate if patient experiences intolerable adverse effects.

NOTE: Considerations are not listed in order of preference. Drug needs vary significantly from patient to patient.

ADLs, Activities of daily living; *COMT,* catechol-*O*-methyltransferase; *PD,* Parkinson's disease; *QOL,* quality of life.

concomitant use of sedative-hypnotics, the presence of sleep disorders (other than RLS), and use of drugs known to increase ropinirole serum levels. If a decision is made to stay with ropinirole, patients should be advised to not drive, to avoid alcohol-containing beverages, and other potentially harmful activities. At this time, there are insufficient data to conclude that dosage reduction eliminates episodes of falling asleep during activities.

Pergolide can be used in combination with levodopa-carbidopa for patients with advanced PD; however, the adverse effects of pergolide limit its use to administration by health care providers with experience treating PD. When a patient is taking both levodopa and pergolide, reduce the daily dosage of levodopa and note any additional relief of parkinsonian symptoms. A significant reduction in the long-term adverse effects of levodopa has also been observed with concurrent therapy. Close observation is needed because of a greater susceptibility to adverse effects that include confusion, agitation, hallucinations, and postural hypotension.

Bromocriptine does not produce early, serious fluctuations or the on-off phenomenon, as long as patients have not previously received levodopa. Dyskinesia is seen much less commonly and is less severe in patients taking bromocriptine alone. Bromocriptine may be added to a treatment regimen for a patient with unstable, fluctuating response patterns. It can also be used when additional intervention (e.g., alterations in dosage intervals or dosage reduction, or use of sustained-release levodopa formulations) is ineffective in minimizing the fluctuations.

ANTICHOLINERGICS. Anticholinergics have historically been used as first-line treatment for mild PD in which tremor was the predominant symptom and the patient had good cognitive functioning. Today, with the introduction of carbidopa and levodopa, anticholinergics have been classified as second-line drugs. However, there appears to be no difference between trihexyphenidyl and benztropine with respect to efficacy. Even so, benztropine has greater sedative properties than other anticholinergics.

MONOAMINE OXIDASE B INHIBITORS. Selegiline monotherapy can be initiated early in the course of the disease in patients without functional impairment. In early disease, it delays the progression of symptoms and the need for levodopa-carbidopa. Selegiline also slows symptom progression when added to levodopa-carbidopa therapy. Combination therapy also has a dose-sparing effect. These effects are related to selegiline's inhibition of dopamine breakdown through inhibition of MAO-B, rather than a neuroprotective effect. It is thought that the neurotoxic amphetamine metabolites of selegiline negate any possible protection conferred by the drug.

⚠ **Attention to the dose-dependent nature of selegiline's selectivity is critical if it is to be used without elaborate restrictions being placed on diet and concomitant drug use,** although as noted above, hypertensive reactions have been reported at the recommended dose.

The primary benefit for using rasagiline over selegiline is that rasagiline, once biotransformed, does not have the toxic amphetamine metabolites. Selegiline is biotransformed to R(−)-methamphetamine and R(−)-amphetamine, whereas rasagiline is biotransformed to R(+)-1-aminoindan, a non–amphetamine metabolite. The S isomer of rasagiline is 1000 times less potent as an MAO inhibitor, but it is still protective against neurotoxic insults. There is no evidence to suggest that the trace amphetamine metabolites of selegiline contribute to its neuroprotective action.

COMT INHIBITORS. When entacapone or tolcapone are given in combination with standard levodopa formulations, single doses prolong the plasma half-life of levodopa, thus increasing its bioavailability without altering the peak concentration. Patients with on-off fluctuations and those without fluctuations benefit from the addition of a COMT inhibitor to their levodopa therapy. However, the beneficial effects of levodopa are rapidly lost upon withdrawal of the COMT inhibitor.

AMANTADINE. Amantadine is used as a second-line drug to treat motor fluctuations (see Chapter 28). Amantadine increases neuronal dopamine release and inhibits its reuptake. Amantadine appears to make it easier for dopamine-producing nerve cells to release their stored dopamine into the synapse. This approach is helpful in mild cases of PD, in which amantadine works to reduce disease symptoms. Amantadine is available in liquid formulations, which can be helpful in patients with swallowing problems or for someone who requires smaller doses. As with all liquid formulations, each dose must be accurately measured; this is sometimes difficult for patients with visual problems or tremors.

SURGERY. In some cases, deep brain stimulation (DBS) may be an appropriate intervention if the disease hasn't responded to drug therapy. In DBS, which is approved by the FDA, electrodes are set into the brain and connected to an externally programmable pulse generator. When using DBS, the need for antiparkinson drugs is decreased; in turn, the adverse effects associated with dopaminergic drug therapy, such as dyskinesias, are decreased as well. DBS also helps alleviate symptom fluctuation and reduces the incidence of tremors, bradykinesia, and gait problems.

Patient Education

Advise the patient who is prescribed antiparkinsonian drugs to take them as ordered to achieve maximal therapeutic effects while minimizing adverse effects. Teach the patient and family what the treatment regimen involves, why each drug is taken, the correct dosages, the warning signs of adverse effects, and the importance of strict adherence to the dosing schedule. Adherence to the dosing schedule lowers the risk of motor fluctuations, thereby permitting better control of PD motor symptoms. Sudden withdrawal of the drug can cause a dramatic increase in parkinsonian symptoms and deterioration of control.

Abrupt withdrawal of antiparkinsonian drugs can render ⚠ **the patient totally immobile and cause significant problems with breathing and swallowing. Tapering is required when any antiparkinsonian drug discontinued.**

Teach the patient and family that antiparkinsonian drugs may cause drowsiness or dizziness and to avoid driving or other activities that require alertness until the response to the drug is known. Caution the patient to make position changes slowly to minimize orthostatic hypotension. Also, warn that perspiration may decrease, and thus that overheating can occur during hot weather. Patients should remain indoors in an air-conditioned environment during hot weather. Nonetheless, encourage patients to pursue as many of their pre–disease activities as possible. Support groups and psychotherapy for patients with PD and their families have proven beneficial.

Dietary factors may alter the effects of levodopa action in the brain and, subsequently, affect motor performance. High-protein diets interfere with the absorption of immediate-release levodopa-carbidopa. This phenomenon is most common in persons who have significant on-off motor fluctuations: those requiring four or more doses of levodopa-carbidopa per day. Patients known to be "protein-sensitive" may choose to consume the majority of their daily protein requirement (45 to 60 mg/day for adults) in the evening when activity levels are ordinarily decreased. Other patients may choose several small meals throughout the day, avoiding high-protein foods near dosing times of levodopa-carbidopa to minimize motor fluctuations. The effects of protein and timing of meals on the absorption of the controlled-release formulation of levodopa-carbidopa are less clear.

Gastroparesis is seen in many patients with PD and can be aggravated by foods high in fat or fiber. If these are taken with levodopa-carbidopa, gastroparesis can cause levodopa to remain in the stomach for extended periods. For this reason it is wise to take levodopa-carbidopa on an empty stomach with 6 to 8 ounces of water whenever possible, so as to maximize absorption and obtain better relief of motor symptoms.

Advise patients to increase their level of activity and fluids in the diet as much as possible to minimize the constipating effects of the drugs. Also instruct patients to avoid alcohol while taking antiparkinsonian drugs. The combined effects of the drugs and alcohol may exaggerate the blood pressure–lowering and sedative effects of the drugs. Tell patients that frequent rinsing of the mouth, good oral hygiene, and use of sugarless gum or candy may decrease the dry mouth associated with antiparkinsonian drugs; but patients should also report persistent dryness, since saliva substitutes may be required. A dentist should be consulted if mouth dryness interferes with denture use. Also, patients should notify the dentist of their drug regimens before undergoing oral surgery or dental work.

Teach patients with diabetes who are taking levodopa-carbidopa to perform fingerstick glucose monitoring. Ketone monitoring may be done using urine dipsticks.

Evaluation

The management of PD is guided by the impact of the patient's symptoms on ADLs. Therapeutic effects, usually noted as a decrease in symptoms, become evident after 2 to 3 weeks of therapy but may require up to 6 months to be seen in some patients. The patient should be seen at regular intervals, every 2 to 6 months, to monitor response to therapy and assess for adverse effects.

Hot Topics

▓ Estrogen

The observation that PD occurs more often in men than in women has led investigators to question whether female hormones may help delay or prevent the development of PD. A recent study compared women who were diagnosed with PD to women of the same age who did not have PD. Study results suggested that women diagnosed with PD had a threefold rate of hysterectomy, a higher rate of early menopause, and a lower rate of using hormone replacement therapy after menopause. These findings suggest that estrogen or other female hormones may help protect dopamine neurons and in turn prevent or delay the onset of PD.

▓ Nicotine

For some time now it has been observed that people who smoke have a lower rate of PD. Some believe that the nicotine protects dopamine neurons from injury. Animal studies found that nicotine was protective against MPTP-induced dopamine cell death. Others have proposed that nicotine may regulate the release of dopamine in the brain and improve memory and cognition. In contrast, however, a double-blind study demonstrated that patients with PD who used a nicotine patch showed no improvement in motor symptoms compared to those using a placebo patch. The relationship between PD and nicotine use is poorly understood and warrants further investigation.

In an effort to develop drugs that provide a more continuous stimulation of dopamine receptors, investigators have developed a dopamine agonist formulated as a patch. Rotigotine is a transdermal dopamine agonist that is well tolerated and effective in patients with early idiopathic Parkinson's disease. It may reduce "wearing off" and lessen the risk of dyskinesia. Study reports indicate that patients who use the dopamine patch had significant improvement in mobility compared to those using a placebo (Guldenpfennig, et al., 2005; Watts, et al., 2007). Potential advantages of transdermal delivery are similar to other transdermal drug formulations and include ease of administration for patients unable to swallow, the lack of effect on food intake or gastric emptying, convenient once-daily dosing, and maintenance of constant serum levels. Another benefit of the drug is that a patient could potentially take less or, possibly, no oral drug while using the patch. The most common adverse effects include application site reactions, dizziness, somnolence, and nausea.

Swarz Pharma, the developer of the ritogotine patch, filed a new drug application with the FDA in February 2006. That same month, the company received approval authorizing the European Medicines Agency marketing authority for the ritogotine patch as monotherapy for PD. It has not yet been approved in the United States.

▓ Caffeine

Caffeine consumption has been associated with a lower incidence of PD. One study suggests that caffeine may have neuroprotective effects. This finding came from a longitudinal study of Japanese-American men (see the Evidence-Based Pharmacotherapeutics box).

MYASTHENIA GRAVIS

EPIDEMIOLOGY AND ETIOLOGY

Myasthenia gravis (MG) is a degenerative neurologic disease characterized, as its name implies, by "grave muscle weakness" (without atrophy). It presents as muscular weakness and fatigue that worsens with exercise and improves with

EVIDENCE-BASED PHARMACOTHERAPEUTICS

Coffee and Caffeine Intake and Risk for Parkinson's Disease

■ Background

Parkinson's disease (PD) affects 3% of the U.S. population of persons over 65 years of age and is a significant source of morbidity and use of health services. No treatment has been definitively shown to prevent or slow the progression of PD. Coffee intake has been inversely associated with PD in some studies, but findings have been equivocal.

■ Research Article

Ross, G., Abbott, R., Petrovitch, H., et al. (2000). Association of coffee and caffeine intake with the risk of Parkinson disease. *Journal of the American Medical Association, 283*(20), 2674–2679.

Purpose

The purpose of this study was to explore the relationship between dietary caffeine intake and the risk of Parkinson's disease.

Design

This prospective, longitudinal study began between 1965 and 1968 and continues today. In this study, 30 years of follow-up data were used. Data sources before 1991 included (1) reviews of cohort members [$N = 8006$] medical records for all diagnoses of PD; (2) ongoing review of all Hawaiian death certificates; and (3) medical record review from local neurologist offices cross-checked with the cohort member list. After 1991, the diagnosis of PD was based on complete record reviews and interviews of the cohort from 1991 to 1993 and 1994 to 1996. The Unified Parkinson's Disease Rating Scale was used.

Methods

Nutrient intake of Japanese-American men ages 45 to 68 years was determined by a dietitian based on 24-hour dietary recall records. Caffeinated coffee intake was measured as the number of 120-mL cups consumed per 24 hours. Total dietary caffeine and caffeine from non–coffee sources were calculated from the baseline dietary recall. Other variables measured included saturated fat intake, energy level, alcohol consumption, total serum cholesterol levels, and physical activity. Coffee and caffeine intake was reported at 6-year intervals using 24-hour recall methods.

Incident rates in person-years were estimated within the categories of caffeine consumption (i.e., none; 4–8 oz/day; 12–16 oz/day; 20–24 oz/day; and over 28 oz/day). Proportional hazard regression models were used to test the effect of coffee and caffeine intake on PD change over time. Relative hazards for PD were estimated by comparing the risk of PD disease with amount of coffee. All reported p values for covariants were based on two-sided tests of significance.

Findings

The age-adjusted occurrence of PD steadily declined when the intake of coffee increased from 10.4 in men who drank no coffee, to 1.9 per 10,000 person-years in men who consumed over 28 oz/day ($p < 0.001$ for trend). During the study period, 102 men were identified as having PD.

Similar findings were noted for total caffeine intake ($p < 0.001$ for trend) and caffeine from non–coffee sources ($p = 0.03$ for trend). There was no relationship between caffeine in which milk and sugar had been added and PD, or to other ingredients in the coffee. The increased consumption of coffee was also related to a lower risk for PD in males who were never smokers, were past smokers, or who were current smokers at baseline ($p = 0.049$, $p = 0.22$, and $p = 0.02$, respectively, for trend).

Conclusions

Independent of smoking, this study's findings suggest that caffeine intake is linked with a significantly lower incidence of PD. According to data collected, the mechanism for such findings is associated with the intake of caffeine itself and not the other components contained in coffee. Although the protective value of dietary caffeine showed a similar dose-response pattern for drinkers and nondrinkers of coffee, it was significant only in coffee drinkers. Among other nutrients contained in coffee (i.e., niacin), no associations with risk for PD were identified. Adjustments for alcohol consumption, hypertension, cholesterol level, energy level, and saturated fat level had no effect on the model.

Other possible explanations for the study findings must be considered. If coffee consumption was associated with increased mortality, then selective survival of non–coffee drinkers may help explain the inverse relationship between PD and coffee intake. A previous article from the Hawaiian Heart study (from which the cohort was selected) found that coffee drinking is associated with elevated cholesterol levels. If this effect was enough to cause cardiovascular mortality, then heavy coffee drinkers were more likely to die before developing PD. Since coffee intake was not associated with mortality in nondrinkers, it is unlikely that inadequate data gathering from members of the cohort played a part in the results of the study. One other possibility is that cohort members destined to develop PD used caffeine-containing analgesics and other drugs more commonly than other members and reduced their caffeine intake to avoid excess.

Potential limitations to the study include the population of men (older age at time of diagnosis). A recent concordance study of twins suggests that older-onset PD may be more likely related to environmental conditions compared with younger-onset cases, with a strong genetic component. Generalizations cannot be made to younger-onset cases, women, and other ethnic groups with any certainty.

■ Implications for Practice

The observational nature of this study design prevents concluding that coffee and caffeine intake from non–coffee sources directly protect against the development of PD. The strengths of the study were the prospective design and unbiased case-finding methodologies. Any differences that were found with PD and coffee and caffeine intake are related to case-finding and case-definition methods. The possibility that coffee and caffeine have a protective effect should be investigated further with future epidemiologic, clinical, and basic science research.

---

rest. Although weakness and easily fatigued extremities were identified in the 1600s, drug therapies were not discovered until the 1930s. The cause of MG is unknown, but 80% to 90% of people with the generalized form have elevated ACh antibody titers.

MG may appear at any age, with two peaks of onset. Between the ages of 20 and 30 years, women are most often affected; and after the age of 50 years, men are more often affected. MG associated with a tumor of the thymus gland usually appears at a later age and is rare in patients younger than 30. The overall incidence of MG is 0.4 persons/100,000. The prevalence is 0.5 to 5/100,000.

PATHOPHYSIOLOGY

The functional defect of MG appears to be a lack of ACh or an excess of cholinesterase at the neuromuscular junction. Thus nerve impulses fail to produce normal muscle contraction. Normal neuromuscular transmission is mediated by ACh stored within nerve terminals. In the presence of a nerve impulse, a large amount of ACh is released, resulting in depolarization and production of an action potential. The action potential travels along the muscle to cause contraction. In MG, the same amount of ACh is released, but receptor sites are blocked, either directly or indirectly, by immunoglobulin G (IgG) antibodies (Fig. 26-2). The antibodies fix to receptor sites, blocking the binding of ACh. The electrical impulse to the muscle is diminished, thus causing a weak contraction.

The life of the ACh receptor is also diminished in MG, from a normal life span of 7 days to an average of 1 day. The body attempts to compensate by increasing the number of ACh receptors.

Types of Myasthenia Gravis

Five distinct types of MG have been identified: neonatal, congenital, juvenile, adult, and drug-induced. The *neonatal* form appears in 15% of children born to women with MG. It is usually transient but is secondary to the passive transfer of MG-specific IgG from the mother. Interestingly, it is thought that neonates develop antibodies to their own ACh-activated ion channels, supporting the notion that MG is an autoimmune disorder. Neonates have been observed to carry myasthenic symptoms for 7 to 14 days after birth. However, once antibodies are gone, symptoms also disappear.

Congenital MG may be evident at birth as generalized weakness with poor muscle tone, sucking ability, and cry as well as with dysphagia and respiratory distress. Respiratory depression and arrest may occur. MG can be life threatening during the first 2 weeks after birth. More commonly, the disease manifests during the first 2 years of life and is characterized by ptosis or ophthalmoplegia. *Juvenile MG* is rare but closely resembles adult and drug-induced MG.

Drug-induced MG can be caused by a number of different drugs (Table 26-6). The drugs are thought to trigger antibody production to ACh receptors. In approximately 70% of patients who develop MG while taking the disease-modifying

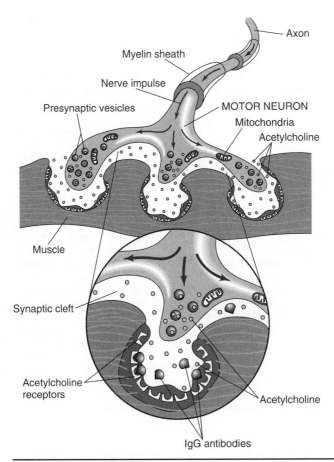

FIGURE 26-2 Myasthenia Gravis. Acetylcholine (ACh) is released, accumulates within the synaptic cleft, and stimulates postsynaptic neurons. The result is depolarization and production of an action potential. In myasthenia gravis, the same amount of ACh is present but not available to the membrane receiving the impulse. Immunoglobulin G (IgG) antibodies fix to receptor sites in postsynaptic membranes and block the binding of ACh. More ACh is exposed to cholinesterase breakdown. The electrical impulse from the nerve to the muscle is diminished, the muscle contraction is weak, and muscle weakness results.

TABLE 26-6 Drugs that Exacerbate Myasthenia Gravis

Anesthetics	chloroprocaine, fluothane, tetracaine, trichloroethylene, tubocurarine
Antibiotics	Aminoglycosides, clindamycin, chloroquine, ciprofloxacin, colistin, erythromycin, imipenem, interferon-alpha, lincomycin, oxytetracycline, polymyxin B, prednisone, pyrantel, streptomycin, tetracyclines, trimethoprim-sulfamethoxazole
Anticonvulsants	magnesium sulfate, phenytoin, trimethadione
Cardiovascular drugs	Beta blockers, calcium channel blockers, disopyramide, lidocaine, oxyprenolol, phenytoin, procainamide, quinine, quinidine
DMARDs	chloroquine, D-penicillamine
Hormonal drugs	ACTH, corticosteroids, oral contraceptives, thyroid hormones
Psychoactive drugs	chlorpromazine, lithium, phenothiazines, gabapentin
Neuromuscular blockers	Botulinum toxin
Sedatives	Antihistamines, barbiturates, opioids
Ocular drugs	Mydriatics

ACTH, Adrenocorticotropic hormone; *DMARDs*, disease-modifying antirheumatic drugs.

antirheumatic drug (DMARD) D-penicillamine, remission occurs within a year of stopping the drug.

Stages of Myasthenia Gravis

Stage 1 MG comprises the first 5 to 7 years of the disease. Visual symptoms are found in approximately 50% to 70% of persons affected with MG and include *ptosis* (drooping eyelids), blurry vision, and/or *diplopia* (double vision). Ptosis is caused by paresis of the levator palpebrae superioris muscle in one or both eyes. Bright sunlight can precipitate ptosis and blurry vision. The symptoms may subside for months or years, with relapses following remissions.

Stage 2 MG is divided into A and B substages, but both are characterized by ocular manifestations. It lasts about 15 years or to a point in the disease at which respiratory reserve diminishes. Stage 2 is more prevalent among men and responds best to corticosteroid drugs. Temporary improvement may be achieved with immunosuppressive drugs.

Stage 2A is mild and generalized, with slow progression, and is responsive to drug therapy. There is a weakness of the facial and levator palpebrae muscles, giving the patient a masklike, expressionless appearance. The patient has droopy eyelids and full lips, with the lower slightly everted. When the patient attempts to smile, a snarl appears instead. The jaw sags when muscles of mastication are involved. Further, the patient may hold a hand under the chin to support the head if flexor muscles of the neck are affected. Laryngeal muscle involvement results in a nasal sound to the voice or difficulty in articulation. *Aphonia*, an inability to produce vocal sounds, may develop with severe involvement.

Weakness of arm, hand, and leg muscles is seen in 20% of newly diagnosed patients. The upper extremities are affected before the lower, and the proximal muscles before the distal. When muscles of respiration are affected, there is an impaired ability to cough and swallow, which predisposes the patient to aspiration and pneumonia.

Stage 2B is seen most often in the juvenile patient and is moderately generalized, with severe skeletal and bulbar involvement. Its response to drug therapy is less satisfactory.

Stage 3 of MG is referred to as the "burnout" stage. It appears 14 to 20 years after the onset of the disease. This stage includes patients who initially manifested ocular symptoms but who rapidly progressed to severe disability and respiratory problems. There is a higher incidence of muscular atrophy and reduced response to cholinesterase inhibitor drugs in this stage.

Clinical symptoms vary from patient to patient, and the onset of symptoms in MG is usually insidious but may be sudden in some cases. Variability in the strength of voluntary muscles throughout the day is characteristic of MG. Muscle weakness may be worse in the morning or evening, with symptoms fluctuating in severity from day to day. Symptoms can be exacerbated by febrile illness, heat, stress, or repetitive tasks and may worsen during periods of menstruation and infection. Simple tasks such as brushing the teeth or combing the hair may trigger muscle weakness, requiring the patient to stop and rest. Pregnancy and postpartum states are typical times when a woman first experiences symptoms or when there is an abnormal response to muscle relaxants used during general anesthesia.

Recovery after rest is often incomplete. Once the muscles are involved, the patient cannot perform sustained or repeated muscle contractions such as walking or keeping the eyelids open.

PHARMACOTHERAPEUTIC OPTIONS

Cholinesterase Inhibitors

◆ edrophonium (Enlon, Reversol, Tensilon); ✦ Enlon
◆ neostigmine (Prostigmin); ✦ Prostigmin
◆ pyridostigmine (Mestinon, Regonol); ✦ Mestinon

▓ Indications

Cholinesterase inhibitors (i.e., anticholinesterase drugs) are used in the diagnosis and treatment of MG. They effectively and rapidly restore muscle strength in the majority of patients. Pyridostigmine is used as the first-line treatment for MG. Neostigmine is used to reverse the effects of tubocurarine (see Chapter 18). Neostigmine and edrophonium are useful in determining whether a patient with confirmed MG is in cholinergic or myasthenic crisis (see discussion that follows under management).

▓ Pharmacodynamics

Cholinesterase inhibitors act by decreasing the amount of the enzyme acetylcholinesterase at sites of cholinergic transmission, thereby halting destruction of available ACh. More ACh is available for a longer time. Because the drugs do not increase ACh production, they are effective only as long as ACh is released at motor nerve endings and ACh receptors are intact. In stage 3 MG, this may not be so. Cholinesterase inhibitors also take direct cholinergic action on skeletal muscle, and there is a possibility that the drugs have a cholinergic effect on autonomic ganglion cells and CNS neurons as well.

▓ Pharmacokinetics

The pharmacokinetics of cholinesterase inhibitors vary from drug to drug (Table 26-7). The drugs are lipid-soluble and do not enter the CNS to affect central cholinergic function.

PHARMACOKINETICS
TABLE 26-7 Myasthenia Gravis Drugs

Drug	Route	Onset	Peak	Duration	PB (%)	t½	BioA (%)
CHOLINESTERASE INHIBITORS							
edrophonium	IM	2–10 min	Rapid	5–30 min	UA	UA	UA
	IV	30–60 sec	Rapid	5–10 min	UA	UA	100
neostigmine	PO	45–75 min	1–2 hr	2–4 hr	15–25	40–60 min	1–2
	IM	10–30 min	20–30 min	2–4 hr	15–25	50–90 min	100
	IV	10–30 min	20–30 min	2–4 hr	15–25	40–60 min	100
pyridostigmine	PO	30–45 min	UA	3–6 hr	UA	3–7 hr	11–17
	ER	30–60 min	Rapid	6–12 hr	UA	3–7 hr	UA
	IM	15 min	UA	2–4 hr	UA	3–7 hr	100
	IV	2–5 min	UA	2–3 hr	UA	1–9 hr	100
CORTICOSTEROID							
prednisone	PO	60 min	1–2 hr	1–2 days	70–75	3–4 hr	80–90
IMMUNOSUPPRESSANTS							
azathioprine	PO	3–6 mo	2–3 yr	Days-weeks	30	3–5 hr	80–90
cyclophosphamide	IV	Immed	1 hr	UA	60*	4–10 hr	>75%
cyclosporine	PO	UA	3.5 hr	UA	90	19 hr; 7 hr†	10–60
mycophenolate mofetil	PO	UA	6–12 hr	UA	97	11–24 hr	94

*Plasma protein binding of unchanged cyclophosphamide is low but some metabolites are bound to an extent greater than 60%.
†The half-life of cyclosporine in adults and children, respectively.
BioA, Bioavailability; *ER*, extended-release; *IM*, intramuscular; *IV*, intravenous; *PB*, protein binding; *PO*, by mouth; *t½*, half-life; *UA*, unavailable.

Although pyridostigmine is an analogue of neostigmine, it varies in several clinically significant aspects. For example, pyridostigmine is characterized by a longer duration of action and fewer GI adverse effects. Neostigmine is lipid-soluble but is poorly absorbed from the GI tract. It is biotransformed in the liver and eliminated in the urine.

▦ Adverse Effects and Contraindications

Adverse effects are usually attributed to overdosage, when pharmacologic effects of the drugs are amplified. The most common adverse effects with use of cholinesterase inhibitors are gastrointestinal or respiratory in nature. Salivation and fasciculation occur most often, but dysphagia, nausea and vomiting, abdominal cramps, diarrhea, and flatulence have also been documented. Respiratory adverse effects may be potentially serious and include excessive oral, pharyngeal, and bronchial secretions. Bronchospasm, laryngospasm, dyspnea, and respiratory depression are most serious.

Cardiovascular adverse effects of cholinesterase inhibitors include bradycardia, tachycardia, hypotension, ECG changes, atrioventricular block, nodal rhythms, and cardiac arrest in susceptible patients. Miosis, lacrimation, hyperemia of the conjunctiva, double vision, and visual changes have also been noted. The musculoskeletal, CNS, genitourinary, and dermatologic systems are also affected by cholinesterase inhibitors in a variety of ways.

The cholinesterase inhibitors are contraindicated for use in patients with mechanical obstruction of the GI or genitourinary tract or peritonitis, and those having a history of bromide sensitivity, urinary bladder outlet obstruction, or hypersensitivity. Do not use cholinesterase inhibitors in patients with a previous history of reaction to bromides, because these drugs contain bromide ions.

Use these drugs cautiously in patients with a history of peptic ulcer disease, bronchial asthma, PD, epilepsy, cardiac disease, hypotension, bradycardia, and hyperthyroidism, and during lactation. These drugs can cause uterine irritability when administered by IV route during the third trimester of pregnancy and to induce premature labor (pregnancy category C). It is not known if the drugs are present in breast milk.

▦ Drug Interactions

Table 26-8 summarizes the drug interactions of cholinesterase inhibitors. The drugs with the most significant interactions are atropine, guanethidine, procainamide, quinidine, and quinine. These drugs, when used concurrently, decrease the effect of the cholinesterase inhibitors. The actions of neostigmine are antagonized by any drug with anticholinergic properties (e.g., antihistamines, antidepressants). With concomitant alcohol use, weakness and unsteadiness are exacerbated.

▦ Dosage Regimen

Dosage regimens for the cholinesterase inhibitors vary with the drug (Table 26-9). Pyridostigmine is formulated as a syrup, as tablets, and as prolonged-action tablets. Neostigmine is available in both tablet and injection formulations. Frequently, administration is required day and night. Larger doses of the total daily dosage may be administered at times when the patient is more likely to become fatigued (e.g., afternoon, mealtimes).

Corticosteroids

▦ Indications

Corticosteroids are useful for use in the patient with MG who is over 50 years of age and who cannot be managed with cholinesterase inhibitors, those with severe generalized MG, those who have had the thymus gland removed, and those with pure ocular MG. In many cases, the disease goes into remission and the possibility of relapse is minimized. It has been suggested that corticosteroids are more beneficial in adolescents and young females with MG. Chapter 56 contains a thorough discussion of the corticosteroids.

DRUG INTERACTIONS
TABLE 26-8 Myasthenia Gravis Drugs

Drug	Interactive Drugs	Interaction(s)
CHOLINESTERASE INHIBITORS		
neostigmine	Antihistamines, antiarrhythmics, local and general anesthetics	Antagonizes neostigmine action
	neomycin, streptomycin, kanamycin	Accentuates neuromuscular blockade
pyridostigmine	Anticholinergic drugs, antidepressants, haloperidol, other cholinesterase inhibitors, phenothiazines, succinylcholine	May precipitate cholinergic crisis
	atropine, clozapine, corticosteroids, cyclobenzaprine, glycopyrrolate, magnesium sulfate, nondepolarizing neuromuscular blockers, scopolamine, procainamide, tolteradine, trihexyphenidyl	Decreases efficacy of pyridostigmine
	Beta blockers, decongestant-opioid combinations, dicyclomine, dipyridamole, flavoxate, hydrocodone-ibuprofen combination, hyoscyamine, mefloquine, meperidine-promethazine combination, opioids and opioid antagonists, orphenadrine, oxybutynin, quinidine	Increases risk for AV blockade and risk of bronchospasm and hypotension
	bupropion, tiagabine, tramadol	Increases risk of seizures
CORTICOSTEROID		
prednisone	warfarin	Increases effects of anticoagulant and results in hypoprothrombinemia and possible bleeding
	Barbiturates, colestipol, ephedrine, phenytoin, rifampin, theophylline	Decreases action of prednisone
	Anticonvulsants, antidiabetic drugs, cholinesterase inhibitors, salicylates, somatrem	Decreases effects of interacting drug
	Alcohol, amphotericin B, cyclosporin, digoxin, diuretics, indomethacin, ketoconazole, macrolides, salicylates	Increases action of prednisone and the risk for adverse effects
	Estrogens	Increases the antiinflammatory effect of corticosteroids by reducing breakdown in the liver
	Oral contraceptives	Reduces effectiveness of oral contraceptives
IMMUNOSUPPRESSIVE DRUGS		
azathioprine	allopurinol	Inhibits biotransformation of azathioprine
	Antineoplastics, myelosuppressive drugs	Additive myelosuppression
	tubocurarine	Decreases effects of interactive drug
	warfarin	Decreases in efficacy of warfarin
	Corticosteroids	Muscle wasting with prolonged therapy
	benazepril, captopril, lisinopril	Increases risk of leukopenia
	erythromycin	Increases absorption of azathioprine
cyclosporine	amphotericin B, aminoglycosides, erythromycin, fluoroquinolones, ketoconazole, NSAIDs, melphalan, sulfonamides	Increases risk for nephrotoxicity
	Anabolic steroids, calcium channel blockers, cimetidine, danazol, erythromycin, fluconazole, ketoconazole, miconazole	Blood levels and risk of toxicity of cyclosporine are increased
	azathioprine, cyclophosphamide, glucocorticoids, verapamil	Additive immunosuppression and increases risk for lymphoma
	Barbiturates, carbamazepine, phenytoin, rifampin, sulfonamides	Decreases effects of cyclosporine
	ACE inhibitors, potassium-sparing diuretics, potassium supplements	Increases risk for hyperkalemia
	digoxin	Increases risk for digoxin toxicity
	Neuromuscular blocking drugs	Prolongs action interactive drugs
	imipenem-cilastatin	Increases risk for seizures
	Live virus vaccines	Decreases Ab response to vaccine
	lovastatin	Increases risk for rhabdomyolysis
cyclophosphamide	phenobarbital	Biotransformation and leukopenic activity of cyclophosphamide increases with chronic, high doses of phenobarbital
	succinylcholine	Marked and persistent inhibition of cholinesterase activity; potentiates effect of succinylcholine
mycophenolate mofetil	acyclovir, valacyclovir, ganciclovir	Increases plasma levels of acyclovir
	Magnesium and aluminum antacids, cholestyramine	Decreases absorption of mycophenolate mofetil
	Levonorgestrel-containing OCs	Reduces levonorgestrel serum level
	Antibiotics and other drugs that act on intestinal flora	Antibiotics disrupt enterohepatic recirculation, making less mycophenolate mofetil available.
	Live attenuated vaccines	Reduces effectiveness of vaccine

Ab, Antibody; *ACE,* angiotensin-converting enzyme; *AV,* atrioventricular; *NSAIDs,* nonsteroidal antiinflammatory drugs; *OCs,* oral contraceptives.

❚❙ *Pharmacodynamics*

Corticosteroids are thought to protect ACh receptor sites from attack by IgG, thus increasing the amount of ACh available at the site. Further, it is thought that the drugs reduce the total number of circulating antibodies and the degradation of the receptor sites, thereby increasing the effectiveness of ACh. Overall, corticosteroids suppress the patient's immune response.

❚❙ *Pharmacokinetics*

Corticosteroids are well absorbed when taken orally. Prednisone is biotransformed in the liver to prednisolone, with a half-life of about 3.4 hours. Prednisone is about 3 to 5 times more potent than cortisone or hydrocortisone. In contrast, when prednisone is given by IM route, it is absorbed very slowly from the injection site with a duration of action of up to 4 weeks.

CENTRAL NERVOUS

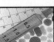

DOSAGE
TABLE 26-9 Myasthenia Gravis Drugs

Drug	Use(s)	Dosage	Implications
CHOLINESTERASE INHIBITORS			
edrophonium	Diagnosis of myasthenia gravis; differentiation of myasthenic crisis from cholinergic crisis	*Adult:* 2 mg IV initially. If no response, give 8 mg more. May repeat in 30 min. *Child <34 kg:* 1 mg IV. If no response, give 1 mg every 30–45 min to total of 10 mg. *Child >34 kg:* 2 mg IV. If no response, give 1 mg every 30–45 min to a total of 10 mg.	Patient may feel flushed, dizzy, hypotensive immediately after injection. If cholinergic response occurs, give atropine.
neostigmine (bromide or methylsulfate)	Improvement of muscle strength in myasthenia gravis; reversal of neuromuscular nondepolarizing neuromuscular blockers	*Adult:* 15–30 mg PO initially in divided doses *–or–* 0.5–2 mg every 1–3 hr IM or IV. Maintenance: 75–150 mg/day. May go as high as 375 grams/day *Child:* 2 mg/kg/day in divided doses	15 mg of PO neostigmine bromide is equivalent to 1 mg of parenteral neostigmine methylsulfate owing to poor bioavailability. Larger doses of the total daily dosage may be administered at times when the patient is more likely to become fatigued (e.g., afternoon, mealtimes).
pyridostigmine	Improvement of muscle strength in myasthenia gravis; reversal of nondepolarizing neuromuscular blockers	*Adult:* 60–120 mg PO initially 6–8 times/day *–or–* 2 mg IM or IV. May repeat every 2 hr. Maintenance doses to 1500 mg daily *Child:* 7 mg/kg/day in 5–6 divided doses	Dose may be increased daily until desired response achieved. Large doses should be avoided in situations where there may be an increased absorption rate from the intestinal tract.
CORTICOSTEROID			
prednisone	Adjunct in treatment of myasthenia gravis	*Adult:* 20–25 mg PO daily	ADT or single daily dose may be used for maintenance. Dosage should be tapered when drug is being discontinued.
IMMUNOSUPPRESSIVE DRUGS			
azathioprine	Myasthenia gravis	*Adult:* 1 mg/kg/day. Max of 2.5 mg/kg/day	Contraceptive use is recommended up to 12 wk after drug is discontinued.
cyclosporine	Myasthenia gravis	*Adult:* 14–18 mg/kg/day PO *–or–* 5–6 mg/kg/day IV. Maintenance: 5–10 mg/kg/day	Check serum drug levels regularly. **Microemulsion products (Neoral) and other formulations (Sandimmune) are not interchangeable.**
cyclophosphamide	Myasthenia gravis	*Adult:* 25 mg PO daily to max of 2–5 mg/kg daily.	Dosages based on patient response.
mycophenolate mofetil	Myasthenia gravis	*Adult:* 250 mg PO twice daily. Titrate upward as needed to 1–2 grams/day.	CBC weekly for the first month; every 2 wk for 6–8 wk; and monthly thereafter.

ADT, Alternate-day therapy; *CBC,* complete blood count.

⚈ *Adverse Effects and Contraindications*

The adverse effects of corticosteroids are many and varied, and some may be life threatening. Chapter 56 contains a thorough discussion of the corticosteroids. Corticosteroids are contraindicated for use in the presence of active, untreated infections, because these drugs mask infection. Their use is also contraindicated in patients who are lactating or those who have psychoses, Cushing's syndrome, active tuberculosis, heart failure, varicella, or peptic ulcer disease. Exercise caution when using corticosteroids in patients with diabetes, hypertension, chronic nephritis, seizure disorders, hepatic or renal disorders, or thrombophlebitis. Safe use during pregnancy and in children has not been established (pregnancy category C).

⚈ *Drug Interactions*

Table 26-8 lists the drug interactions of corticosteroids. These drugs have additive or antagonistic effects when combined with many other drugs.

⚈ *Dosage Regimen*

The dosage of corticosteroids is highly individualized. The usual course of treatment for MG extends over 2 years with initial high dosages, and then, when improvement is seen, the regimen is changed to alternate-day therapy. The dosage is gradually reduced to the smallest effective maintenance level so as to have the fewest possible adverse effects. Never withdraw corticosteroids abruptly; gradually taper the dosage

downward when discontinuing the drug. Long-term use may cause serious adverse effects.

⚈ *Lab Considerations*

Corticosteroids play havoc with lab test results. They decrease white blood cell counts, as well as serum potassium, calcium, uric acid, protein-bound iodine, and thyroxine concentrations. On the other hand, they increase serum glucose (especially in patients with diabetes), amylase, and sodium, cholesterol, and lipid values. Males may have a decrease in sperm production and count when taking corticosteroids.

Immunosuppressants

- azathioprine (Imuran, Azasan); ♣ Imuran
- cyclophosphamide (Cytoxan)
- cyclosporine (Sandimmune, Neoral, Gengraf); ♣ Neoral
- mycophenolate mofetil (CellCept)

⚈ *Indications*

Although approved by the FDA for use in treating MG, immunosuppressive therapy with azathioprine is aimed at reducing antireceptor antibody production. Azathioprine is useful for patients with MG who have not responded to corticosteroids or who have a flare-up during a corticosteroid taper. Remission of MG symptoms is possible in 30% to 50% of patients treated with azathioprine, although the benefits may take 3 months to appear and a year to be fully achieved.

Cyclosporine is useful in patients in whom corticosteroid drug therapy and azathioprine treatment are limited by the adverse effects and/or the lack of improvement.

Cyclophosphamide has been used successfully in patients whose disease is refractory to other treatments. Clinical trials demonstrate a response in 75% to 80% of patients with steroid-refractory MG, with improvement demonstrated within 4 weeks (Ciafaloni et al., 2000).

There have been reports of successful treatment for MG using mycophenolate mofetil (Geevasinga, Wallman, and Katelaris, 2005). About two thirds of patients with MG gained strength or were able to reduce their need for prednisone after taking mycophenolate mofetil for several months. Mycophenolate mofetil appears to be effective as adjunctive therapy in the treatment of refractory and steroid-dependent MG.

Pharmacodynamics

Azathioprine is an analogue of the antineoplastic drug mercaptopurine (see Chapter 33). It suppresses the immune system, thus reducing the production of ACh receptor antibodies, which allows the receptors to regenerate and function normally. A return in muscle strength results. The patient will notice a gradual improvement in muscle strength over 3 to 12 months, and the improvement may then decrease the need for other drug therapies.

Cyclosporine is a fungal peptide with potent immunosuppressive activity. It inhibits normal immune responses by inhibiting interleukin-2, a factor necessary for initiation of cytotoxic T-cell activity. It inhibits both T-helper-cell and T-suppressor-cell activity.

Mycophenolate mofetil inhibits guanosine synthesis, thus reducing the quantity of monophosphate dehydrogenase in activated T and B lymphocytes. In doing so, it selectively inhibits the production of T and B cells while leaving other cell lines intact.

Pharmacokinetics

Azathioprine is readily absorbed from the GI tract. The therapeutic response to azathioprine is much slower than that to corticosteroids, usually occurring between 3 and 6 months (see Table 26-7). It is biotransformed to 6-mercaptopurine, which inhibits T-cell development. Azathioprine is eliminated through the kidneys, with minimal elimination of unchanged drug.

Cyclosporine is erratically absorbed after oral administration, but is widely distributed to extracellular fluid and blood cells. Cyclosporine is biotransformed by the liver to inactive metabolites, which are then eliminated primarily through the bile. This drug crosses the placenta and enters breast milk.

Cyclophosphamide in its unchanged form has a relatively low plasma protein binding, although its metabolites are more than 60% bound. Several cytotoxic and noncytotoxic metabolites of cyclophosphamide have been identified in plasma and in urine. There is no evidence that any single metabolite is responsible for either the therapeutic or the toxic effects of cyclophosphamide. Forty percent or more is eliminated through the stool following oral administration.

Following oral and intravenous administration, mycophenolate mofetil is rapidly biotransformed to mycophenolic acid (MPA), an active metabolite. MPA is then further biotransformed to the inactive metabolite (MPAG).

Adverse Effects and Contraindications

Azathioprine therapy is limited by its adverse effects, the most serious and limiting of which is bone marrow suppression. Symptoms common to bone marrow suppression include macrocytic anemia, thrombocytopenia, pancytopenia, and leukocytopenia. Bruising and bleeding may also occur as a result. Allergic reactions to azathioprine include rashes and serum sickness. Azathioprine can cause mild taste alterations when given by IV route. Allergic reactions to azathioprine include rashes and serum sickness. It is a pregnancy category D drug.

Cyclosporine's most common adverse effects are tremor, gingival hyperplasia, diarrhea, hypertension, renal dysfunction, hirsutism, and acne. Hepatotoxicity can be life threatening. Cyclosporin is contraindicated for use in patients who have a hypersensitivity to cyclosporine or polyoxyethylated castor oil, in patients during lactation, and in patients taking potassium-sparing diuretics. Use caution in administering cyclosporine to patients with liver and kidney disorders, untreated infections, and malabsorption disorders, as well as during pregnancy (pregnancy category C).

Three fourths of patients treated with cyclophosphamide develop alopecia, which is often complete but occasionally reversible. Leukopenia, nausea, and vomiting are also common. Cyclophosphamide sometimes causes a (sterile) hemorrhagic cystitis. The delayed consequences include acute leukemia and bladder cancer. The drug is contraindicated for use in patients with known leukopenia, thrombocytopenia, or systemic infections, as well as during pregnancy (pregnancy category D).

The principal adverse effects of mycophenolate mofetil include diarrhea, leukopenia, sepsis, and vomiting, and there is evidence of a higher frequency of certain types of opportunistic infections, for example, cytomegalovirus. GI hemorrhage and pulmonary edema are also possible. It is a pregnancy category C drug.

Use of immunosuppressant drugs is contraindicated in pregnancy unless the potential benefits outweigh the risks. Long-term use of immunosuppressants in children decreases growth and development. Further, the drugs mask signs of infection (fever, inflammation). With long-term use of such drugs, the patient's adrenal function becomes suppressed, leading to hypotension, weight loss, weakness, nausea and vomiting, anorexia, lethargy, confusion, and restlessness.

Drug Interactions

Azathioprine is partially biotransformed by xanthine oxidase. Allopurinol, an inhibitor of this enzyme, increases the potential for toxicity by decreasing the biotransformation of azathioprine in the liver. Reduce the dosage of azathioprine by 75% when using it concurrently with allopurinol. Decreases in the efficacy of warfarin with concomitant azathioprine administration may be due to reduced bioavailability, enhanced warfarin biotransformation, or increased prothrombin and factor II activity. Table 26-8 identifies drug interactions with azathioprine.

Cyclosporine interacts with many drugs. The risk of lymphoma and immunosuppression rises when cyclosporine

CENTRAL NERVOUS

is taken with other immunosuppressants. Corticosteroids increase immunosuppression through the suppression of lymphocytes. Infection and malignancy may also occur with the concurrent use of the corticosteroids. Nephrotoxicity may occur when this drug is given concurrently with other nephrotoxic drugs, such as the systemic antifungal drug amphotericin B or any of the NSAIDs.

Acyclovir, probenecid, cholestyramine and antacids, and drugs that undergo tubular renal excretion interact with mycophenolate mofetil. Interaction studies have not been conducted with other drugs that are commonly administered for renal or cardiac problems or liver transplant. Avoid the use of live or attenuated vaccines during treatment with mycophenolate mofetil, and advise patients that vaccinations may be less effective.

▥ Dosage Regimen

The actual dosages of immunosuppressants are primarily based on patient response, although it is common to administer these drugs to a patient with advanced MG for 12 to 36 months. This duration of therapy helps prevent a relapse of symptoms in an otherwise stable patient. Dosages of some immunosuppressant drugs may be reduced in patients with renal dysfunction.

▥ Lab Considerations

Azathioprine specifically affects renal, hepatic, and hematologic functions. Urine uric acid and serum uric acid and plasma albumin levels may fall. Increases in serum alkaline phosphatase, bilirubin, ALT, AST, and amylase values may suggest hepatotoxicity. Bone marrow depression is suspect with a decrease in hemoglobin values. A leukocyte count less than 3000/mm^3 or a platelet count less than 100,000/mm^3 may indicate the need to decrease dosage.

Lab values that may be increased when the patient is taking cyclosporine are the BUN, total bilirubin, serum creatinine, uric acid, alkaline phosphatase, serum potassium, cholesterol, LDL, and apolipoprotein B. Further, cyclosporine use requires frequent serum drug levels to be obtained. Adverse effects can be lessened by keeping serum trough levels between 250 and 800 mcg/mL or plasma levels between 50 and 300 mcg/mL per 24 hours.

The development of neutropenia may be related to mycophenolate mofetil itself or to concomitant drugs, viral infections, or some combination of these causes. Interrupt or reduce dosing of mycophenolate mofetil, perform appropriate diagnostic tests, and manage the patient appropriately if neutropenia develops.

CLINICAL REASONING

Treatment Objectives

The primary treatment objective does not include a cure for MG; rather, the objective is to achieve the maximum muscle strength and endurance possible with the fewest adverse effects (i.e., excessive salivation, sweating, nausea, diarrhea, abdominal cramps, or tachycardia).

Treatment Options

The stage of myasthenia and the extent of disability determine the treatment regimen, with each regimen individualized and developed for the most part on a trial-and-error basis. The optimal dose and administration schedule will fluctuate during periods of stress.

Like therapy for parkinsonism, drug therapy for MG is lifelong. Plan the treatment regimen giving consideration to the patient's lifestyle and disability. Persons with preexisting neuromuscular disorders are especially susceptible to the adverse effects of drugs used for MG. Even the most perfect drug regimen is ineffective if the patient is unable or unwilling to comply with the therapy because of its impact on lifestyle.

CASE STUDY	Drugs for Myasthenia Gravis
ASSESSMENT	
History of Present Illness	JJ is a 56-year-old white male in moderate distress with complaints of blurry vision and an inability to open his left eyelid over the last 2 days. It was first noticed while sailing his yacht 2 days ago. He reports bright sunlight worsens the "droopy eyelid," and he has noticed more fatigue recently than in the past. He jogs 2 miles/day now, down from 5 miles/day 3 months ago, and follows a low-cholesterol diet. He states, "I'm just getting older."
Past Health History	JJ is allergic to aspirin and penicillin. He has no food allergies. His last physical exam was 6 months ago. He denies hospitalizations and injuries, but has been told he has borderline-high cholesterol. He denies using alcohol, smoking, or drugs. He takes no routine or OTC medications.
Life-Span Considerations	At 56 years old, JJ has age-related physiologic changes to body systems. He has had no disabilities until recent symptoms developed.
Psychosocial Considerations	JJ is the owner of a local chain discount store. He is married, and his wife is in excellent health. He is very health-conscious and visits his physician semiannually for a complete physical. JJ has access to both a medical facility and pharmacy. JJ has a late-model sports car and yacht; wife reports he is able to drive both without difficulty until his recent symptoms arose.
Physical Exam Findings	*Height:* 5'11". *Weight:* 165 lb (no recent weight loss or gain). VSS. Lg. Snellen: 20/200 corrected left eye; ptosis of left eyelid noted. Neuromuscular: Weakness noted in lifting and movement of the left shoulder only. Remainder of exam unremarkable.

Continued

CASE STUDY Drugs for Myasthenia Gravis—Cont'd

Diagnostic Testing	Edrophonium test positive–shoulder felt much better with improved strength and less ptosis and diplopia. CT of chest and chest x-ray negative for thymoma. ECG: sinus bradycardia at 56 bpm. Anti-ACh–receptor antibody titer elevated. All of chemistry panels WNL.

DIAGNOSIS: Myasthenia gravis

MANAGEMENT

Treatment Objectives	1. Alleviate current ocular problems and muscular weakness and worsening fatigue. 2. Achieve maximal muscle strength and endurance with least adverse effects.
Treatment Options	**Pharmacotherapy** • Pyridostigmine, 600 mg PO in divided doses spaced to provide maximum relief. Optimal control may require supplementation with the more rapidly acting syrup. • Low-dose prednisone based on patient response to pyridostigmine. **Patient Teaching** 1. Teach the names of the drugs prescribed along with the dose, the reason for use, and possible adverse effects. The importance of taking drugs on time–not too late or too early–and how to intervene in a crisis situation should also be explained. 2. Teach the patient and family to recognize signs and symptoms of cholinergic and MG crises. 3. Wear a form of medical alert identification and carry written information regarding prescribed drugs and dosages. Also carry a list of drugs contraindicated for persons with MG. **Evaluation** JJ has increased muscle strength, decreased fatigue, and improved vision.

CLINICAL REASONING ANALYSIS

Q1. I always thought patients with myasthenia gravis were placed on a ventilator. When do you start drug therapy?
A. The stage of JJ's myasthenia and the extent of disability determine the treatment regimen. Treatment will be individualized, on a trial-and-error basis for the most part, to meet JJ's needs for muscle strength and endurance.

Q2. We learned in pharmacology that there are several drugs that are used to treat myasthenia gravis. What drugs will you be using for JJ?
A. There is no distinct protocol for the treatment of patients who have MG. Cholinesterase inhibitors stop destruction of available ACh. Corticosteroids protect receptors from destruction by immunoglobulin G. Immunosuppressants depress immune response. We will choose an appropriate drug from one of these categories.

Q3. Okay, so which drug are we going to use?
A. We will start with pyridostigmine since it is the initial drug of choice for JJ's nonprogressive eye-muscle weakness and mild limb-muscle weakness, and it has few serious adverse effects. We will also add prednisone to his regimen to reduce serum levels of ACh-receptor antibodies and increase the possibility of remission. We must monitor his therapy regardless, but we will also be watching for complaints that may suggest avascular necrosis, an adverse effect of the prednisone, even at a low dosage.

Q4. I cared for a transplant patient the other day who was on CellCept and doing well. Why not use CellCept for JJ?
A. Oh, do you mean mycophenolate mofetil? Mycophenolate mofetil has a shorter onset of action, a low risk for late malignancies, and no major organ toxicities. It may be particularly useful when prednisone cannot be used or is ineffective. Its high cost is a disadvantage, however. Also, the onset of action may not occur for 6 to 12 months, and at the current time there is limited experience in using the drug for MG. We may need to consider its use at a later date, but for now we will stick with the prednisone and pyridostigmine regimen.

▥ Patient Variables

In most cases, the diagnosis of MG is obvious to a neurologist from the history and physical exam findings. However, edrophonium testing confirms a diagnosis of MG and helps monitor worsening of symptoms. A test dose is given and muscle strength assessed. If there is no improvement, a second dose is given. Improvement in muscle strength suggests the diagnosis of MG. Further, edrophonium and neostigmine are useful in determining whether a patient with confirmed MG is in cholinergic or myasthenic crisis.

Immediately following the edrophonium dose, the patient may complain of feeling dizzy, flushed, or faint and may experience a drop in blood pressure. However, because the drug action is short-lived, these effects rarely last longer than

5 minutes. The patient in cholinergic crisis becomes temporarily worse (a negative test), whereas the patient in myasthenic crisis has a temporary improvement in muscle strength, which signifies a positive test (see discussion that follows).

Of patients with MG, 10% to 15% have a tumor of the thymus gland. Routine anteroposterior and lateral chest x-ray studies, chest CT, and possibly MRI have been useful in identifying a thymoma.

Pulmonary function tests, nerve conduction tests, and electromyography (EMG) are helpful in determining patients' baseline status. EMG is helpful in demonstrating the fatigability of affected muscles. A 10% or more decrease in amplitude during progressive stimulation generally indicates defective neuromuscular transmission.

Other lab testing includes a lupus screen (to rule out lupus erythematosus); tests for antinuclear antibodies, rheumatoid factor, and antithyroglobulin antibodies; a tuberculin test; and a fasting blood glucose measurement. Approximately 5% of patients with MG have thyrotoxicosis. Serum anti–ACh receptor antibody titers may be elevated.

LIFE-SPAN CONSIDERATIONS

Pregnant and Nursing Women. The pregnant woman with MG should be in the care of a neurologist specializing in neuromuscular diseases. No specific effects of pregnancy on MG have been documented; however, either significant improvement in symptoms or drastic worsening may occur. Labor proceeds as in the nonmyasthenic patient except that sedatives and opioid analgesics should be used sparingly and with careful measurement of vital capacities. Injectable cholinesterase inhibitors should be available in the event of a myasthenic crisis and for use during labor, when nausea may preclude oral administration.

The second stage of labor is associated with muscle fatigue and increased risk of myasthenic crisis. The vaginal route is the preferred method of delivery because a Cesarean section is thought to be too stressful and it has the potential to precipitate a myasthenic crisis. Epidural anesthesia is recommended to decrease fatigue and provide adequate analgesia.

The postpartum period may also be associated with exacerbations of MG. Drug dosages must be adjusted as the mother returns to her prepregnant state. Breastfeeding is not advised for patients with a myasthenic exacerbation, for those receiving high doses of cholinesterase inhibitors, and for those with high circulating antibody titers.

Children and Adolescents. It is very rare for a mother with MG to have more than one child affected with the disease. Neonatal MG develops in 10% to 12% of neonates born of myasthenic mothers. No prenatal prognostic factors or test has yet identified neonates at risk for this problem. Full resuscitation equipment should be available and the child closely monitored for 12 to 72 hours after birth. The neonate may have poor muscle tone and a weak cry and may be unable to take a bottle because of a decrease in muscle tone. However, breastfeeding is not advised because the antibodies of MG cross into the breast milk, and thus breastfeeding prolongs the myasthenic state for the neonate.

Older Adults. The older adult is not immune to MG, although the disease is more likely to have been diagnosed earlier in life. However, older adults are more prone to complications and have more frequent crises than younger patients. Stress factors that tend to precipitate crises in the older adult include the complications of immobility, fractures secondary to falls, urosepsis, pneumonia, and a generalized poor state of health. The natural decline of kidney function in the aging adult warrants the administration of smaller drug dosages to prevent drug accumulation. Further, some patients may not have the mental capacity and/or proper vision to take the drug as scheduled and in the proper dosage.

▥ *Drug Variables*

There is no distinct protocol for the treatment of patients who have MG. Health care providers must decide when aggressive management must be undertaken. In general, the rate of disease progression and the distribution of weakness as well as severity are the most important considerations when developing a treatment plan.

CHOLINESTERASE INHIBITORS. Pyridostigmine is the initial drug of choice for nonprogressive eye muscle weakness and mild limb muscle weakness. Because cholinesterase inhibitors provide only transient, symptomatic relief of MG, they are of limited use in most cases of moderate to severe MG. Pyridostigmine used in conjunction with prednisone increases the possibility of remission and is likely the most effective treatment regimen.

CORTICOSTEROIDS. The corticosteroid drug prednisone reduces serum ACh receptor antibodies levels; however, clinical improvement can occur even when there is no significant decrease in antibody levels. Corticosteroids may temporarily worsen symptoms; such a response is ordinarily followed by gradual improvement in muscle strength. Once peak improvement is reached and maintained for several weeks, the dosage of both prednisone and the cholinesterase inhibitor may be gradually decreased over 3 to 6 months to the smallest effective maintenance level. A low maintenance dose of prednisone on alternate days may be effective for many months or years. If prednisone is discontinued in the absence of any other immunosuppressive therapy, MG will recur in almost all patients.

IMMUNOSUPPRESSANTS. When used alone, immunosuppressant drugs are useful in reducing prednisone requirements and lead to improvement or remission. They are believed overall to be slightly less toxic than corticosteroids used long-term. Use of an immunosuppressant prevents prolonged use of cholinesterase inhibitors, promotes remission, and minimizes the possibility of relapse. When azathioprine is used in combination with prednisone, a lower prednisone dose may be used, thus reducing the adverse effects of the corticosteroid.

Cyclosporine is used for patients in whom prednisone and immunosuppressant therapy are limited by adverse effects and/or lack of optimal response. Its benefit is similar to that of azathioprine, but cyclosporine acts more promptly, usually within 1 to 3 months.

More than half the patients treated with cyclophosphamide become asymptomatic after 1 year. Life-threatening infections are a significant risk, but this risk is limited to patients with invasive thymoma. The long-term risk of malignancy has not been established, but there are no reports of an increased incidence of malignancy in patients with MG undergoing immunosuppression.

Mycophenolate mofetil may be an effective alternative to azathioprine with fewer adverse effects, a more rapid onset of action, low risk for late malignancies, and no major organ toxicity. It may be especially useful in patients who cannot take prednisone or in whom prednisone use is ineffective. Its high cost is a disadvantage. Furthermore, the onset of action may not occur for 6 to 12 months, and at the current time there is limited experience in using the drug for MG.

Patient Education

A patient's adjustment to MG depends on the extent of the loss of independence, the resultant body changes, and merely the nature of the disease. The generalized weakness and fatigue, the neck and shoulder muscle weakness, and the loss of fine motor control associated with MG contributes to social isolation and changes in body image. The patient may become frustrated with the changes.

Impaired verbal communication is often an area of frustration. It may be necessary to identify effective communication strategies before impairment becomes severe. The patient may be taught to use sign language, or the patient can write on an erasable board.

Teach patients with MG and their families' strategies that facilitate chewing and swallowing and thus help prevent weight loss and aspiration. Remaining upright while eating, using foods that are the consistency of thick liquid, and eating a soft diet all reduce the risk of aspiration. Small, frequent meals with high-calorie snacks may help minimize weight loss. Encourage patients to take small bites and eat slowly. As the disease worsens, patients may require tube feedings.

Visual difficulties compound the other problems. Ptosis and ocular palsy lead to an inability to close the eyes, increasing the risk of corneal abrasions. Teach the patient to use a patch and a shield to protect the eyes. The eyes also have a tendency for excessive dryness. Artificial tears can be used to keep the eyes moist. Alternating eye patches may help to relieve diplopia.

Teach the patient and family to identify measures that help prevent or modify fatigue and to incorporate those measures into daily activities. Assist the patient in planning to alternate activities with periods of rest. Activities that can be completed in short periods of time or divided into several segments are desirable; for example, read one chapter of a book at a time, or avoid scheduling two energy-draining activities for the same day. Conserving energy through rest, planning, and priority-setting helps prevent or alleviate fatigue.

Instruct the patient and family on the names of the drugs prescribed along with the dosage, the reason for use, and possible adverse effects. Stress the proper administration technique for the dosage form. Additionally, teach them to recognize the symptoms of cholinergic and MG crises. And finally, explain the importance of taking drugs on time—not too late or too early—and how to intervene in a crisis situation.

Both patients and families should be aware that it may take weeks or months before the full benefits of a particular drug are seen. Advise patients to avoid immunizations while taking immunosuppressants, which decrease the effectiveness of any therapy that enhances immunity.

Patients should wear a form of medical alert identification and carry written information regarding their prescribed drugs and dosages and a list of drugs contraindicated for persons with MG (see Table 26-6). Refer patients and families to local, state, and/or national MG support groups for additional information.

The importance of taking an antimyasthenic drug as prescribed cannot be overstated. The risk of a myasthenic or a cholinergic crisis increases with improper dosing or with improper administration. All drugs used in the management of MG should be taken with food or milk. Space doses evenly to minimize gastric distress and adverse effects. In older adults, it is often helpful to have a family member oversee the treatment regimen.

Always implement precautions against the adverse effects of corticosteroids. These include a low-sodium diet, supplemental potassium and calcium, and the use of antacids or proton pump inhibitors to prevent GI problems (see Chapter 45). All MG patients started on prednisolone fulfilled current guidelines for osteoporosis prophylaxis, indicating that most patients in this situation should be started on osteoporosis prophylaxis at onset. For patients facing medium- to long-term steroid therapy, perform a bone mineral density scan; and for most patients, begin bisphosphonates, such as alendronate.

Advise women of childbearing age to use contraception before starting mycophenolate mofetil therapy. Contraception should continue throughout treatment and for 6 weeks following treatment.

Evaluation

Drug therapy for MG is thought successful if the patient experiences improved muscle strength and endurance with few troublesome adverse effects. The highest possible level of functioning should be achieved. The patient and family should be able to identify community resources, such as the Myasthenia Gravis Foundation of America, which will help them maintain an effective level of functioning. The patient should also be able to identify measures that will help prevent or modify fatigue.

Differentiate between myasthenic crisis and cholinergic crisis. With early recognition, effective therapy, and modern intensive care units, death from such crises is now a rare occurrence (Table 26-10). *Myasthenic crisis* is the sudden onset of muscular weakness usually caused by a late dose or inadequate dosing with a cholinesterase-inhibiting drug. Symptoms are noted about 3

TABLE 26-10 Comparison of Cholinergic and Myasthenic Crises

	Cholinergic Crisis	Myasthenic Crisis
Cause	Excessive dosage of cholinesterase inhibitor drug	Insufficient dosage of cholinesterase inhibitor drug; late dose
Signs and symptoms*	Nausea, vomiting, diarrhea, abdominal cramps, blurred vision, pallor, facial muscle twitching, pupillary miosis, respiratory failure, hypotension, muscle weakness	Inability to speak or swallow; loss of gag reflex and ability to cough; tachycardia, tachypnea, elevated blood pressure, anoxia, cyanosis, bladder and bowel incontinence, decreased urinary output, muscle weakness
Management	Prompt withdrawal of all cholinesterase inhibitor drugs	Intensive cholinesterase inhibitor therapy, atropine (may lead to inadvertent cholinergic crisis; use cautiously)

*Testing with edrophonium may determine whether the patient is in myasthenic or cholinergic crisis.

hours after the dose was due. Myasthenic crisis manifests as an inability to swallow or speak; weakness of respiratory, laryngeal, pharyngeal, and bulbar muscles; and sudden respiratory distress. The patient in myasthenic crisis is in danger of respiratory arrest. Extreme quadriparesis or quadriplegia may also be noted.

Symptoms of *cholinergic crisis* arise within 1 hour of an excessive dose of a cholinesterase inhibitor. The clinical picture is much like that of myasthenic crisis but includes other symptoms (see Table 26-10). As in myasthenic crisis, the patient is at risk for respiratory arrest.

KEY POINTS

- Epidemiologic data suggest vascular, viral, genetics, and metabolic factors as possible causes of Parkinson's disease. The possibility of an environmental contributor, such as toxins found in the workplace or used in industry, is also being explored.
- PD is characterized by a large deterioration of neurons within the basal ganglia. These neurons are normally needed to synthesize the neurotransmitter dopamine.
- Diagnosis of PD is based on the history and physical exam. There are no lab tests to confirm or refute the clinical diagnosis.
- Treatment is aimed at abolishing, as far as possible, the symptoms and disabilities caused by the disease. There is no universal antiparkinsonian drug; thus there is no single drug to alleviate all symptoms and disabilities.
- Dopaminergic drugs such as combination levodopa-carbidopa are generally the drugs of choice for initial therapy. COMT-inhibitor use is becoming more frequent.
- Dopamine agonists are considered first-line treatment for PD. Anticholinergic drugs are used for patients with minimal symptoms.
- Therapeutic effectiveness of antiparkinsonian drug therapy is noted as a decrease in signs and symptoms, with the effects usually becoming evident after 2 to 3 weeks of therapy.
- Myasthenia gravis (MG) is a disorder of voluntary muscles characterized by muscle weakness and fatigability.
- MG is an autoimmune disease resulting from a defect in nerve impulse transmission at the neuromuscular junction. IgG antibody is secreted against ACh receptors, blocking the binding of the neurotransmitter.

- Early clinical manifestations include weakness of the muscles of the face and throat, but the weakness may involve muscles of the diaphragm and chest wall.
- The diagnosis of MG is confirmed using the cholinesterase inhibitor edrophonium. Improved muscle strength indicates a positive test and the diagnosis of MG.
- Treatment options for MG include cholinesterase inhibitors, corticosteroid drugs, and immunosuppressants.
- Cholinesterase inhibitors decrease the breakdown of ACh. They provide transient symptomatic relief and are most useful for nonprogressive eye muscle weakness and mild limb muscle weakness.
- Corticosteroids such as prednisone protect ACh receptor sites and are given early in large doses until improvement is seen.
- Immunosuppressants reduce corticosteroid requirements and produce improvement and remission when used alone.
- The patient in either myasthenic or cholinergic crisis is in danger of respiratory arrest.
- The patient and family should be taught strategies that will facilitate chewing and swallowing and thus help prevent weight loss and aspiration.
- Drug therapy for MG is considered successful if the patient experiences improved muscle strength and endurance with few troublesome adverse effects.

Bibliography

Barichella, M. (2006). The use of low-protein food in Parkinson's disease patients on levodopa therapy. 1st World Parkinson Congress. Feb. 22–26. Washington, DC.

Boehringer Ingelheim. (2006). Mirapex (pramipexole dihydrochloride). Package insert. Available online:www.fda.gov/MEDWATCH/safety/2006/Nov_PIs/Mirapex_PI.pdf. Accessed April 14, 2007.

Cahoon, W., and Kockler, D. (2006). Mycophenolate mofetil treatment of myasthenia gravis. *Annals of Pharmacotherapy, 40*(2), 295–298.

Chen, J., and Ly, A. (2006). Rasagiline: A second-generation monoamine oxidase type-B inhibitor for the treatment of Parkinson's disease. *American Journal of Health System Pharmacy, 63*(10), 915–928.

Ciafaloni, E, Nikhar, N., Massey, J., et al. (2000). Retrospective analysis of the use of cyclosporine in myasthenia gravis. *Neurology, 55*(3), 448–450.

Ferrero, S., Pretta, S., Nicoletti, A., et al. (2005). Myasthenia gravis: Management issues during pregnancy. *European Journal of Obstetrics, Gynecology, & Reproductive Biology, 121*(2), 129–138.

Geevasinga, N., Wallman, L., and Katelaris, C. (2005). Mycophenolate mofetil: A review of indications and use in a large tertiary hospital. *Iranian Journal of Asthma, Allergy, and Immunology, 4*(4), 159–166.

Gladstone, D., Brannagan, T., Schwartzman, R., et al. (2004). High dose cyclophosphamide for severe refractory myasthenia gravis. *Journal of Neurology Neurosurgery and Psychiatry, 75*(5), 789–791.

Goetz, C., Poewe, W., Rascol, O., et al. (2005). Evidence-based medical review update: Pharmacological and surgical treatments of Parkinson's disease: 2001 to 2004. *Movement Disorders, 20*(5), 523–539.

Guay, D. (2006). Rasagiline (TVP-1012): A new selective monoamine oxidase inhibitor for Parkinson's disease. *American Journal of Geriatric Pharmacotherapy, 4*(4), 330–346.

Guldenpfennig, W., Poole, K., Sommerville, K., et al. (2005). Safety, tolerability, and efficacy of continuous transdermal dopaminergic stimulation with rotigotine patch in early-stage idiopathic Parkinson disease. *Clinical Neuropharmacology, 28*(3), 106–110.

Hughes, B., Moro De Casillas, M., and Kaminski, H. (2004). Pathophysiology of myasthenia gravis. *Seminars in Neurology, 24*(1), 21–30.

Kothari, M. (2004). Myasthenia gravis. *Journal of the American Osteopathic Association, 104*(9), 377–384.

Lacomis, D. (2005). Myasthenic crisis. *Neurocritical Care, 3*(3), 189–194.

Lyytinen, J., Kaakkola, S., Ahtila, S., et al. (1997). Simultaneous MAO-B and COMT inhibition in L-dopa-treated patients with Parkinson's disease. *Movement Disorders, 12*(4), 497–505.

McCance, K., and Huether, S. (2005). *Pathophysiology: The biologic basis for disease in adults and children.* (6th ed.). St. Louis: Mosby.

National Institute for Neurologic Disorders and Stroke. National Institutes of Health. (2004). Parkinson's disease: Challenges, progress, and promise. NIH Publication: N0. 05–5595. Available online: www.ninds.nih.gov/disorders/parkinsons_disease/parkinsons_research.htm. Accessed April 14, 2007.

Novartis Pharmaceuticals. (2000). Comtan (entacapone). Package insert. Available online:www.pharma.us.novartis.com/product/pi/pdf/comtan.pdf. Accessed April 14, 2007.

Olsen, J., Friss, S., and Frederickson, K. (2007). Malignant melanoma and other types of cancer preceding Parkinson disease. *Epidemiology, 17*(5), 582–587.

Olsen, J., Friss, S., Frederickson, K., et al. (2005). Atypical cancer pattern in patients with Parkinson's disease. *British Journal of Cancer, 92*(1), 201–205.

Reider, C., Halter, C., Castelluccio, P., et al. (2003). Reliability of reported age at onset for Parkinson's disease. *Movement Disorders, 18*(3), 275–279.

Ross, G., Abbott, R., Petrovitch, H., et al. (2000). Association of coffee and caffeine intake with the risk of Parkinson's disease. *Journal of the American Medical Association, 283*(20), 2674–2679.

Rostedt, A., Padua, L., and Stalberg, E. (2006). Correlation between regional myasthenic weakness and mental aspects of quality of life. *European Journal of Neurology, 13*(2), 191.

Rotenberg, M., Levy, Y., Shoenfeld, Y., et al. (2000). Effect of azathioprine on the anticoagulant activity of warfarin. *Annals of Pharmacotherapy, 34*(1), 120–122.

Ruottinen, H., and Rinne, U. (1996). Effect of one month's treatment with peripherally acting catechol-*O*-methyltransferase inhibitor, entacapone, on pharmacokinetics and motor response to levodopa in advanced parkinsonian patients. *Clinical Neuropharmacology, 19*(3), 222–233.

Seppa, N. (2000). An alternate approach to Parkinson's. *Science News, 157*(June 10), 381.

Siep, J. (2005). Myasthenia gravis: Emerging new therapy options. *Current Opinion in Pharmacology, 5*(3), 303–307.

Tanner, C. (2003). Is the cause of Parkinson's disease environmental or hereditary? Evidence from twin studies. *Advances in Neurology, 91*, 133–142.

Teva Pharmaceutical Industries. (2003). Rasagiline. Package insert. Available online: www.rasagiline.com. Accessed April 14, 2007.

Valeant Pharmaceuticals. (2006). Tasmar (tolcapone). Package insert. Available online: www.tasmar.com/HTML-INF/index.shtml. Accessed April 14, 2007.

Watts, R., Jankovic, J., Water, C., et al. (2007). Randomized, blind, controlled trial of transdermal rotigotine in early Parkinson disease. *Neurology, 68*(4), 272–276.

Youdim, M. (2006). The path from anti-Parkinson drug selegiline and rasagiline to multifunctional neuroprotective anti Alzheimer drugs ladostigil and m30. *Current Alzheimer Research, 3*(5), 541–550.

Youdim, M., and Weinstock, M. (2002). Novel neuroprotective anti-Alzheimer drugs with anti-depressant activity derived from the anti-Parkinson drug, rasagiline. *Mechanisms of Aging and Development, 123*(8), 1081–1086.

Zanetti, R., and Rosso, S. (2007). Levodopa and the risk of melanoma. *Lancet, 369*(9558), 257–258.

Zanetti, R., Loria, D., and Rosso, S. (2006). Melanoma, Parkinson's disease and levodopa: Causal or spurious link? A review of the literature. *Melanoma Research, 16*(3), 201–206.

CENTRAL NERVOUS

Antibiotics

An *antibiotic* is a compound that has the ability to kill or inhibit the growth of bacteria. Antibiotics sufficiently nontoxic to the host are used in the treatment of infectious disease caused by bacterial pathogens. Generally, one antibiotic is sufficient. However, in some instances, multidrug antibiotic therapy is needed to eradicate an infectious process.

Infections have been of great concern throughout world history. During the first half of this century, infections were among the most common causes of death. The discovery and use of sulfonamides and penicillins offered the first real pharmaceutical armamentarium against infectious disease, specifically, bacterial infections; and for many years progress was steady. That has changed somewhat. Many factors have contributed to today's global resurgence of infectious disease. Among them are the development of strains of bacteria resistant to antibiotics; larger populations of immunocompromised individuals; increases in the number and complexity of invasive medical procedures; and the prolonged survival of patients who have chronic, debilitating diseases. Indeed, the issue of drug resistance has provoked an ongoing reexamination of the use of antibiotics. Widespread misuse of these drugs has led to the development of drug resistance, to which the existence and further development of other pathogenic bacteria also contributes. This inappropriate use of antibiotics arises from a lack of knowledge regarding the treatment regimens suitable for specific infections, together with a lack of understanding of how bacteria mutate. As microbiochemistry continues to evolve, health care providers can acquire a clearer understanding of the complex interactions of microorganisms as well as of new drugs designed to target specific diseases.

Antibiotics effective in the laboratory do not necessarily work in an infected patient. The effectiveness of treatment depends on the drug's activity against the bacteria, or how well it is absorbed into the blood stream, how much of the drug reaches the sites of infection in the body, and how quickly the body eliminates the drug. In selecting which antibiotic to use, the health care provider also considers the nature and seriousness of the infection, the drug's possible adverse effects, the possibility of allergies or other serious reactions to the drug, and the cost of the drug.

BACTERIAL INFECTIONS

EPIDEMIOLOGY AND ETIOLOGY

Almost 2 million patients in the United States contract a hospital-acquired infection every year; 90,000 of these patients die as a result of their infection. Furthermore, hospital-acquired infections are increasingly hard to treat, given

that more than 70% of the bacteria that produce these infections are resistant to at least one of the antibiotics most commonly used. Extended hospital stays and treatment with second- or third-line drugs that may be less effective, more toxic, and more costly are often the result of infections caused by antibiotic-resistant organisms. Overall, antimicrobial resistance pushes up health care costs and increases both the severity of disease and death rates from certain infections.

In ambulatory care settings, infections account for about 20% of all acute and chronic illnesses, with about 70% of these being acute upper respiratory tract illnesses (URI). The vast majority of infections are preventable and curable. The specific illnesses that hold the attention of health care providers—and, occasionally, the public—shift from time to time, but the challenges of dealing with infections endure.

The vast majority of bacteria commonly residing in or on the body do so without causing disease, and many are actually beneficial. By and large, these bacteria, often referred to as normal flora, compete with and prevent infection by pathogenic bacteria. Unfortunately, in many cases, the organisms function as parasites, living at the expense of their human host when host defense mechanisms are down. *Subclinical infections* cause no apparent response in the patient and are accompanied by no signs and symptoms. On the other hand, *clinical infections* cause overt injury and are marked by a variety of signs and symptoms.

PATHOPHYSIOLOGY

The human body is not, under normal conditions, devoid of bacteria. The skin for example, is loaded with bacteria, much of which does not cause illness. However, in relation to numbers of bacteria, the gastrointestinal (GI) tract has the most, more than 10 trillion bacteria/mL.

The transport of pathogens to or into the body is an essential characteristic of infection. However, the mere presence of a pathogen does not mean that infection will necessarily occur. For an infection to develop there must be an interaction of six elements including (1) a susceptible host; (2) a pathogen; (3) a reservoir or source for pathogen growth; (4) a portal of exit from the reservoir; (5) a mode of transmission; and (6) a port of entry into the body. If any one of these elements is absent, there can be no infection.

Bacteria

Bacteria are prokaryotes—that is, single cells that do not contain a nucleus (Fig. 27-1). The Gram stain is a way of identifying the bacteria so that they can be classified into groups. About 75% of known bacteria are *gram-negative*: spherical (coccus), rodlike (bacillus), or spiral or corkscrew (spirochete

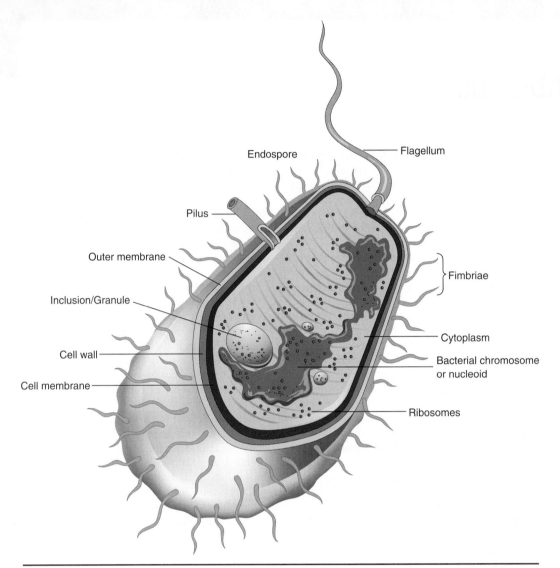

Endospore

Flagellum

Pilus

Outer membrane

Fimbriae

Inclusion/Granule

Cytoplasm

Cell wall

Bacterial chromosome or nucleoid

Cell membrane

Ribosomes

FIGURE 27-1 Structure of Typical Rod-Shaped Bacterium. The external structures of bacteria consist of flagella (whiplike organelles), pili (minute filamentous appendages), and a capsule (a layer of gelatinous material around the cell). The capsule protects the organism from phagocytosis. Various types of pili are involved in conjugation and the adherence of bacteria to mucosal surfaces. The rotary action of flagella, like that of a propeller, permits the organism to travel through a liquid environment. Note that there is no nucleus.

or spirilla) in appearance. Some bacteria also have a shape like that of a comma and are known as *vibrio*. *Gram-positive* bacteria are not as varied as the gram-negative bacteria but include gram-positive cocci and rods, and actinomycetes (Fig. 27-2).

The physical arrangements of the cell walls of gram-negative and gram-positive bacteria are different. In gram-positive cells, the peptidoglycan, a multilayered, cross-linked polysaccharide and peptide chain, makes up 90% of the weight of the cell wall. In contrast, in gram-negative bacteria the peptidoglycan is thinner and irregularly cross-linked and makes up only 15% to 20% of the cell wall.

Bacteria cause disease by producing toxins, causing inflammation, or provoking a hypersensitivity reaction. *Exotoxins* are exceedingly powerful poisons produced by some gram-positive (and some gram-negative) bacteria; *endotoxins* are components

of the outer membrane of gram-negative cell walls and are released by cell lysis.

Infections caused by bacteria can occur in almost any organ. The infections can range from a simple invasion of intact skin to localized visceral infection involving the lungs, the kidneys, the spleen, or the heart. Sepsis occurs when there is widespread invasion of the blood stream. The bacteria spread through lymphatic channels if phagocytic mechanisms are overcome. Given the right circumstances, septicemia can lead to death.

Chlamydiae

Falling between viruses and bacteria in complexity, chlamydiae are obligate intracellular parasites. These organisms contain both DNA and RNA, have a cell wall, and contain ribosomes. Chlamydiae organisms are unable to synthesize

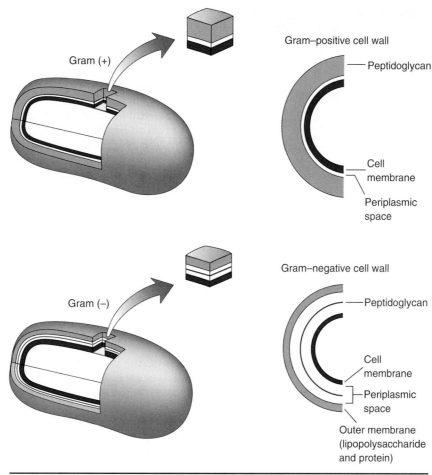

Gram (+)

Gram–positive cell wall
— Peptidoglycan
— Cell membrane
— Periplasmic space

Gram (−)

Gram–negative cell wall
— Peptidoglycan
— Cell membrane
— Periplasmic space
— Outer membrane (lipopolysaccharide and protein)

FIGURE 27-2 Differences Between Gram-Positive and Gram-Negative Bacteria. Gram-negative bacteria have a cell membrane; gram-positive bacteria have a cell wall. Drugs interfering with the production of bacterial cell walls are toxic to bacteria but harmless to the host. Further, the bacterial ribosome is sufficiently different from human ribosomes, making bacterial ribosomes good targets for antibacterial drug action. NOTE: teicoplanin is not available in the United States.

compounds such as adenosine triphosphate (ATP) and so depend on energy from the host cell to survive. These organisms are easily engulfed by phagocytes; however, they have an unusual ability to proliferate within the phagosome. Chlamydial antigens prevent phagosome-lysosome fusion, and the organism is thus protected from normal host defenses. Through a long developmental cycle, chlamydiae develop inclusion bodies, which nearly fill entire host cells. Reproduction occurs in the inclusion bodies, with the new organisms continually infecting susceptible host cells. This group of organisms includes those that cause *Chlamydia* vaginitis, pelvic inflammatory disease, and conjunctivitis of the newborn.

Mycoplasmas

Mycoplasmas are intracellular parasites that have a cell membrane but no cell walls and contain just enough DNA to code a functioning cell. Because they have no cell wall, antibiotics that act on cell walls have no effect on mycoplasmas. Pharyngitis, pneumonia, pyelonephritis, and pelvic inflammatory disease are often caused by mycoplasmas.

Rickettsiae

Rickettsiae are small, gram-negative coccobacilli that structurally resemble bacteria, but are on the average only one tenth to one half as large. They are obligate intracellular pathogens that produce disease in humans through the bite of an insect vector such as a tick, flea, or mite. Culture of these bacteria is virtually impossible except in specialized laboratories. Rickettsiae, most commonly known for causing Rocky Mountain spotted fever, produce a group of illnesses characterized by fever, headache, and rash. Because most of these illnesses are transmitted by an insect vector, they are frequently limited by climate and, to a lesser extent, by geographic location.

Protozoa

More than 65,000 species of protozoa have been identified, although only a few are pathogenic in humans. Protozoal organisms cause localized gastrointestinal (GI) illness such as amebiasis and giardiasis, genitourinary tract infection such as trichomoniasis, or widespread infection of the blood stream and the hematopoietic system.

IMMUNE

PRINCIPLES OF ANTIBIOTIC THERAPY

A number of factors are taken into consideration when considering which drug to use for an infection: (1) the status of the host patient's defenses; (2) the site of the infection; (3) the infecting organism, either suspected or confirmed; (4) the specific drug; (5) the susceptibility and sensitivity of the particular bacteria to the antibiotic, and (6) the drug's mechanism of action.

SITE AND HOST DEFENSES

No antibiotic will cure an infection if the patient's defense mechanisms are inadequate. Many infections do not require antibiotics and are adequately eradicated by the patient's defense mechanisms, which include antibody production, phagocytosis, interferon production, fibrosis, or GI rejection. However, patient defense mechanisms may be diminished, necessitating supportive therapy of various types to ensure adequate oxygenation, fluid and electrolyte balance, and optimal nutrition for antibiotics to be effective. In some cases, surgical intervention may be required in addition to the antibiotic.

It is also important to consider the location of the infection when determining selection and dosage of an antibiotic. A particular antibiotic may not reach the necessary body compartment, such as the cerebrospinal fluid, in sufficient concentrations to be effective. Thus, it is important to select a drug that penetrates the appropriate tissues in concentrations sufficient to inhibit or destroy the pathogens.

THE INFECTING ORGANISM

Most of the available antibiotics have a specific effect on a limited range of bacteria. The drug to be used for a given infection is best chosen after the infecting bacteria have been identified. It is desirable to have culture and sensitivity reports available before starting antibiotics. In some cases, though, it is impractical to wait for these reports. In acute, life-threatening situations, therapy must be started without delay. In these situations, the antibiotic chosen for initial therapy is based on the suspected bacterium. Treatment that is started before establishing a definitive diagnosis is known as empiric therapy. When positive identification is difficult, *broad-spectrum* antibiotic drugs, or several different drugs, can be prescribed. However, widespread use of broad-spectrum antibiotics almost invariably leads to emergence of resistant strains of the pathogen. On the other hand, the sicker the patient and the less certainty there is regarding the responsible pathogen, the more important initial empiric broad-spectrum coverage becomes. Once the culture results are available, the antibiotic can be changed if necessary to one that is more specific for the identified bacterium.

DRUG ACTION

Antibiotics exert their bactericidal or bacteriostatic effects in one of four ways. Unlike host cells, bacteria are not isotonic with body fluids; their contents are under high osmotic pressure, and their viability depends on the integrity of cell walls.

Further, drugs that inhibit any step in the synthesis of the cell wall cause it to weaken and the cell to lyse. These antibiotics are known as *bactericidal*, that, is capable of killing the bacteria. In contrast, some drugs disrupt or alter the permeability of the cell membrane resulting in leakage of essential bacterial components. These drugs may be either bactericidal or *bacteriostatic* (e.g., tetracyclines, sulfonamides). Bacteriostatic antibiotics inhibit or retard bacterial growth, allowing the body's defense mechanisms to handle the infection. Bactericidal activity of these drugs is possible if concentrations of the antibiotic are high enough for a long enough period. Whether effects are bacteriostatic or bacteriocidal depends on many variables such as dosage and the bacterium treated. The speed with which antibiotics act is often concentration-dependent, and the extent of their action is concentration-dependent, concentration- and time-dependent, or time-dependent.

For some antibiotics, the ratio of effective to toxic concentrations is narrow (i.e., narrow therapeutic index). Serum levels of these drugs must be monitored to ensure appropriate dosing and to avoid toxicity (e.g., aminoglycosides, vancomycin).

SUSCEPTIBILITY AND SENSITIVITY

Sensitivity is the ability of a particular antibiotic to exert bacteriostatic or bacteriocidal effects on a given type of bacteria. A *susceptible* bacterium is one whose growth is inhibited by antibiotics taken in usual dosages. A bacterium that is *moderately susceptible* is one whose activity is inhibited with maximum dosages of antibiotic. A *resistant* bacteria is one likely to be unaffected by the antibiotic. Health care providers often rely more on published reports of the drug's effectiveness against the isolated pathogen than on sensitivity reports, because sensitivity is an in vitro test (in the test tube), and the antibiotic will be used in vivo (in the body).

ANTIBIOTIC RESISTANCE

Antibiotic resistance is the ability of bacteria (or other organisms) to quickly adapt to new environmental conditions and thus resist the action of the antibiotic. There are several mechanisms by which drug resistance develops, including (1) physical alterations in receptors; (2) enzyme interactions with the drug; (3) a decrease in the amount of drug reaching receptors; (4) synthesis of resistant metabolic pathways; and (5) failure of biotransformation (of the drug).

Since bacterial reproduction occurs every few hours, the bacterial population can grow rapidly. A mutation that promotes pathogen survival against an antibiotic will quickly become dominant. Bacteria have small numbers of genes, so even a single random mutation can greatly improve the bacteria's capacity to survive and cause disease.

Antibiotic resistance can be gradual or sudden. Resistance is suspected when an infection does not respond to antibacterial treatment or when the patient's condition worsens. Resistance is usually related to antibiotic therapy whose duration is too short.

Genetic Modification

Genetic modifications of the organism can be responsible for drug resistance when it brings about an alteration in proteins that are the specific target for a drug. If the drug cannot interact with the altered protein, organisms containing the genetic modification will survive at the expense of the others, a "survival of the fittest." For example, sulfonamide antibiotics inhibit the growth of sensitive bacteria by competing with para-aminobenzoic acid (PABA) for binding sites on an enzyme; thus they inhibit the first step in the synthesis of folic acid, a vitamin essential to the growth of bacteria. In resistant bacteria, the sulfonamide no longer interacts effectively with the enzyme and consequently does not inhibit the incorporation of PABA into folic acid.

Genetic material can be transferred between bacteria by transduction, conjugation, or transformation. The most common mechanism of resistance is *transduction.* Fundamentally, transduction occurs when a virus containing DNA (i.e., a *bacteriophage*) inadvertently incorporates bacterial DNA into surrounding bacteria. The bacteria thus invaded die, and new bacteriophages with their newly repackaged DNA move on to infect other bacteria.

DNA is released into the environment when cells die. *Transformation* is the incorporation of this free-floating DNA into the DNA of surrounding bacteria. The scavenged DNA may contain antibiotic-resistant genes that benefit the recipient organism.

Conjugation, the transfer of DNA from one organism to another during mating, is accomplished through a *plasmid,* a circular form of DNA that reproduces without aid of the chromosome. When two cells abut each other, a pilus is formed between them (Fig. 27-3). This bridge-like structure allows for duplication and transfer of plasmids from one bacterium to another, thereby enabling them to become resistant to a particular antibiotic. For example, Enterobacteriaceae and *Shigella flexneri* are transferred by conjugation.

Efflux

Bacterial resistance can also come about through *efflux.* An efflux pump removes the antibiotic from the organism

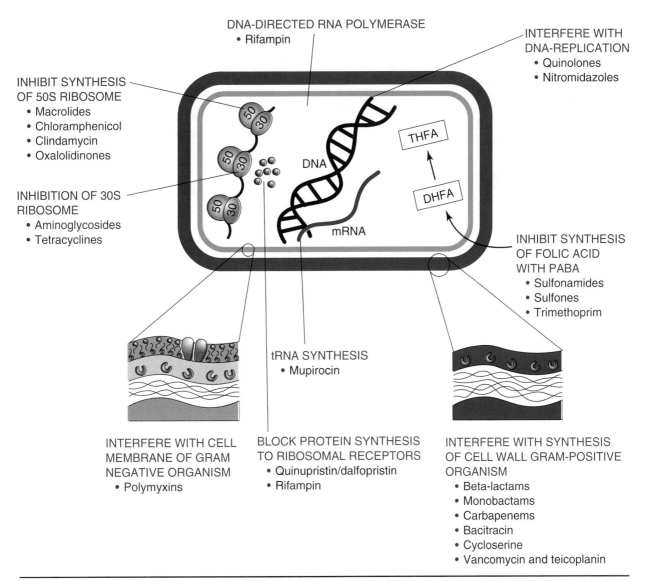

FIGURE 27-3 Sites and Mechanisms of Antibiotic Action. Antibiotics act at various sites within the bacterial organism; some act on the bacterial cell wall, and others alter replication of DNA or RNA synthesis or folic acid synthesis, or act by inhibiting ribosomes.

through a channel known as a *porin*, thus preventing accumulation of the antibiotic and the death of the organism that would otherwise ensue. Malarial parasites have become resistant to antimalarial drugs through this mechanism, just as some organisms have become resistant to tetracyclines (see Chapter 30).

Strategies to Reduce Resistance

It is estimated that 95% of antibiotic use is unnecessary and inappropriate. The more antibiotics are used, the faster drug-resistant organisms emerge. Moreover, not only do antibiotics promote emergence of drug-resistant organisms, but they also promote overgrowth of normal flora. Box 27-1 identifies strategies that help delay antibiotic resistance, three of which are vital to effective therapy:

⚠ 1. **Use narrow-spectrum drugs whenever possible**. Most importantly, use antibiotics only when truly indicated. Conventional use of broad-spectrum drugs is discouraged.

⚠ 2. **Reserve newer antibiotics for situations in which older drugs are ineffective or too dangerous.** Extensive use of the newer antibiotics will only expedite their obsolescence.

⚠ 3. **Prescribe the drug for the appropriate length of time**. The duration of use may vary from a single dose to weeks, months, or even years, in some cases. For most acute infections, the average duration of treatment is 7 to 10 days, or until the patient has been afebrile and symptomatic for 48 to 72 hours, but this varies based on the type of infection and the antibiotic used.

PHARMACOTHERAPEUTIC OPTIONS

The primary tool to manage infection is pharmacotherapy. Several classifications of antibiotics have been developed over the past decades. The antibiotic selected for treatment of an infection should be the one that is most effective in eradicating the causative organisms and yet creates the least harmful adverse effects.

Beta-lactam antibiotics, which owe their effectiveness to the beta-lactam ring that is part of their chemical structure, are commonly used. This broad group of drugs includes penicillins, cephalosporins, carbapenems, and monobactams. Some bacterial strains produce beta-lactamase, an enzyme that provides a mechanism for bacterial resistance. The enzyme breaks the chemical bonds between carbon and nitrogen atoms within the beta-lactam ring. Breaking the bond causes beta-lactam drugs to lose their antibacterial effectiveness. For this reason, a second drug known as a beta-lactam inhibitor is added to several different beta-lactam penicillins.

Penicillins

PENICILLINASE-SENSITIVE PENICILLINS (FIRST-GENERATION)
◆ penicillin G benzathine (Bicillin LA); ✦ penicillin G benzathine
◆ penicillin G potassium aqueous; ✦ Megacillin, Novopen-G, Pfizer-pen
◆ penicillin G procaine (Wycillin, others)
◆ penicillin VK (Veetids); ✦ Apo-Pen-VK, Novo-Pen-VK

PENICILLINASE-RESISTANT PENICILLINS (SECOND-GENERATION)
◆ dicloxacillin sodium (Dycill, Dynapen, Pathocil)
◆ methicillin (Staphcillin)
◆ nafcillin
◆ oxacillin (Bactocill, Prostaphlin)

AMINOPENICILLINS (THIRD-GENERATION)
◆ amoxicillin (Amoxil, others); ✦ Amoxil
◆ ampicillin (Omnipen, others); ✦ ampicillin

ANTIPSEUDOMONAL PENICILLINS (FOURTH-GENERATION)
◆ carbenicillin (Geopen, Geocillin)
◆ mezlocillin (Mezlin)
◆ piperacillin (Pipracil)

PENICILLIN–BETA-LACTAMASE INHIBITOR COMBINATIONS
◆ amoxicillin + clavulanate (Augmentin); ✦ Augmentin
◆ ampicillin + sulbactam (Unasyn)
◆ piperacillin + tazobactam (Zosyn)
◆ ticarcillin + clavulanate (Timentin)

BOX 27-1

Recommendations for Controlling Antibiotic Resistance

Appropriate Antibiotic Prescribing
- Use guidelines for antibiotic use.
- Use narrow-spectrum antibiotics whenever possible.
- Reserve newer antibiotics for situations in which older drugs are ineffective or too dangerous.
- Prescribe the drug's use for the appropriate length of time.
- Use combination therapy when appropriate.
- Rotate antibiotics.
- Restrict use of selected antibiotics (e.g., vancomycin).

Surveillance Programs
- Detect new resistance patterns.
- Detect resistant pathogens promptly.

Infection Control
- Isolate patients; use barrier precautions for patients infected or colonized with resistant organisms.
- Follow proper handwashing protocol.

Education
- Carry out education of physicians and staff.
- Place emphasis on multidisciplinary team approach to infection control.
- Use computer-based monitoring; get feedback on antibiotic prescribing using benchmark data.
- Review hospital infection control procedures according to The Joint Commission.*

*Formerly the Joint Commission on Accreditation of Healthcare Organizations (JCAHO).

Indications

Penicillins are derived from a mold fungus often seen on bread or fruit. Penicillins are used for respiratory and genitourinary (GU) tract, skin, soft tissue, bone, joint, and intraabdominal infections. Other diagnoses for which penicillins are considered the drug of choice include tetanus, meningitis, pneumonia, Lyme disease, anthrax, botulism, gas gangrene, gonorrhea, syphilis, and bacterial septicemia. Penicillins are also used as prophylaxis for patients with bacterial endocarditis or valvular heart disease who are undergoing dental procedures or minor upper respiratory tract surgery.

Pharmacodynamics

Penicillins are classified according to their spectrum of activity. The classifications include those that are penicillinase-sensitive (natural penicillins); penicillinase-resistant penicillins (narrow-spectrum penicillins); aminopenicillins (broad-spectrum penicillins); and antipseudomonal penicillins (extended-spectrum penicillins). Regardless of the spectrum of activity, they all act by inhibiting bacterial cell wall synthesis.

PENICILLINASE-SENSITIVE PENICILLINS. Penicillinase-sensitive penicillins, the natural penicillins, were first introduced in the early 1940s, during World War II, and to date have remained very effective and safe antibiotics. These bactericidal antibiotics are active against aerobic, gram-positive organisms, including various species of streptococci, enterococci, and non–penicillinase-producing staphylococci. They are also active against certain gram-negative organisms such as non–penicillinase-producing strains of *Neisseria gonorrhoeae* and *Neisseria meningitides,* and certain anaerobic oral flora. Further, penicillinase-sensitive penicillins are highly effective against *Actinomyces israelii, Pasteurella multocida, Listeria monocytogenes,* and *Treponema pallidum.*

PENICILLINASE-RESISTANT PENICILLINS. Penicillinase-resistant penicillins are narrow-spectrum drugs effective against *Staphylococcus aureus* and *Staphylococcus epidermidis.* These second-generation drugs were developed to preserve the beta-lactam ring by attaching a protective chain around it, thus preventing penicillinase from destroying or inactivating the antibiotic. However, *S. aureus* and *S. epidermidis* are becoming increasingly resistant and are able to survive the activity of penicillinase-resistant penicillins (and cephalosporins; see following discussion) and a few other drugs. The resistant bacteria are referred to as methicillin-resistant *S. aureus* (MRSA) or methicillin-resistant *S. epidermidis* (MRSE). Both organisms are becoming increasingly resistant to this class of penicillins (whether or not they receive MRSA or MRSE classification).

AMINOPENICILLINS. Aminopenicillins are broad-spectrum drugs effective against many of the same organisms as penicillin G, but they are also active against certain gram-negative bacilli. This group of antibiotics has enhanced activity with gram-negative urinary tract pathogens (see Chapter 41) and *Enterococcus faecalis.* Non–penicillinase-producing strains of *Haemophilus influenzae* type B are also sensitive to aminopenicillins.

ANTIPSEUDOMONAL PENICILLINS. These fourth-generation antibiotics are antipseudomonal, extended-spectrum penicillins with enhanced effectiveness against gram-negative bacilli, especially *Pseudomonas aeruginosa;* they retain activity similar to that of the aminopenicillin antibiotics. Mezlocillin and piperacillin are effective against *P. aeruginosa* and other enteric gram-negative rods. Mezlocillin also is effective against the *Klebsiella* species. Antpseudomonal penicillins are often used as monotherapy or in combination with an aminoglycoside (see discussion later in chapter) to treat nosocomial gram-negative infections.

PENICILLIN–BETA-LACTAMASE INHIBITOR COMBINATIONS. The addition of beta-lactamase inhibitors such as clavulanate, sulbactam, and tazobactam to aminopenicillins and certain antipseudomonal penicillins has broadened the spectrum of penicillins.

Pharmacokinetics

Penicillins are well absorbed following oral administration; however, penicillin G is unstable in acid, and the majority of an oral dose is destroyed in the stomach. Food slows gastric emptying, thus prolonging exposure of the penicillin to gastric acid. Accordingly, in order to achieve serum levels comparable to those of parenteral formulations, the oral dose must be 4 to 5 times greater and the drug taken on an empty stomach. All forms of penicillin may be given by intramuscular (IM) route. However, the various penicillin salts (i.e., sodium, potassium, procaine, benzathine) are absorbed at different rates. The procaine and benzathine formulations are preferred as depot agents (Table 27-1).

Penicillins are distributed well to most tissues and body fluids; however, in the absence of inflammation, penetration into the cerebrospinal fluid (CSF), joints, and eye fluids is poor. However, in the presence of inflammation, the distribution of penicillins into CSF, joints, and the eyes is enhanced.

The penicillins are biotransformed in the liver. Antipseudomonal penicillins are eliminated through the bile, and the others through the urine. As with many other drugs, renal insufficiency prolongs the half-life and increases the risk of penicillin toxicity.

Adverse Effects and Contraindications

Fewer than 10% of patients receiving penicillins are allergic to penicillins, although as many as 30% report a penicillin allergy. Ten percent of allergic reactions are life threatening, and of those, 10% are fatal. A wide variety of idiosyncratic (unpredictable) reactions can occur including maculopapular eruptions (2% with penicillin; 5.2% to 9.5% with ampicillin), eosinophilia, Stevens-Johnson syndrome, and exfoliative dermatitis. The most severe reactions are most likely to occur with parenteral use.

Anaphylaxis can occur 2 to 30 minutes after drug administration and is generally manifested by nausea, vomiting, pruritus, tachycardia, severe dyspnea, diaphoresis, stridor, vertigo, loss of consciousness, and peripheral circulatory failure. Because of cross-sensitivity, patients allergic to one penicillin are generally considered allergic to all penicillins. Additionally, 5% to 10% of penicillin-allergic patients display a cross-sensitivity to cephalosporins and carbapenems because of the close structural similarity (i.e., all have a beta-lactam ring) between the three classes of drugs.

Other adverse effects of penicillins include heartburn, anorexia, abdominal pain, and mild to severe diarrhea. Taste alterations, sore mouth, and discolored or sore tongue (black, furry tongue) have also been noted.

Penicillins may cause neurologic, nephrologic, or hematologic toxicities. Neurotoxic reactions are manifested as

IMMUNE

PHARMACOKINETICS

TABLE **27-1** Selected Penicillins

Drug	Route	Onset	Peak	Duration	PB (%)	t½	BioA (%)
PENICILLINASE-SENSITIVE PENICILLINS (FIRST-GENERATION)							
penicillin G benzathine	IM, IV	Delayed	12–24 hr	1–4 wk	UA	30–60 min	100
penicillin G procaine	IM, IV	Delayed	1–4 hr	1.5 hr	UA	30–60 min	100
penicillin G potassium	IM, IV	Rapid	15–30 min	4–6 hr	UA	30–60 min	100
penicillin VK	PO	Rapid	0.5–1 hr	4–6 hr	80	0.5 hr	60
PENICILLINASE-RESISTANT PENICILLINS (SECOND-GENERATION)							
dicloxacillin	PO	30 min	1–2 hr	UA	96	0.8 hr	UA
methicillin	IM, IV	Rapid	0.5–1 hr	6 hr	40	0.4 hr	100
nafcillin	IM, IV	Rapid	0.5–1 hr	UA	80	0.5–1.5 hr	100
oxacillin	PO	Rapid	30–60 min	UA	90	20–50 min	33
	IM, IV	Rapid	30 min	UA	90	20–50 min	100
AMINOPENICILLINS (THIRD-GENERATION)							
amoxicillin	PO	30 min	1–2 hr	6–8 hr	20	1–1.3 hr	80
ampicillin	PO	Variable	1.5–2 hr	4–6 hr	20	0.7–1.4 hr	50
	IM	Rapid	1 hr	UA	20	1–1.3 hr	100
	IV	Immed	End of inf	UA	20	1–1.3 hr	100
ANTIPSEUDOMONAL PENICILLINS (FOURTH-GENERATION)							
carbenicillin	PO	30 min	30 min–2 hr	6 hr	UA	0.8–1 hr	UA
	IV	Immed	30 min–2 hr	UA	UA	0.8–1 hr	100
mezlocillin	IM	Rapid	5 min	Variable	30	0.7–1.3 hr	100
	IV	Immed	End of inf	Variable	30	0.7–1.3 hr	100
piperacillin	IM	Rapid	0.5–1 hr	UA	19	0.5–1.2 hr	100
	IV	Immed	End of inf	UA	19	0.5–1.2 hr	100
PENICILLIN–BETA-LACTAMASE INHIBITOR COMBINATIONS							
ampicillin-sulbactam	IM	Rapid	1–2 hr	UA	20	1–1.3 hr	50
	IV	Immed	End of inf	UA	20	1–1.3 hr	100
amoxicillin-clavulanate	PO	30 min	1–2 hr	UA	20	1–1.3 hr	80
piperacillin-tazobactam	IM	Rapid	30–50 min	4–6 hr	16; 30	0.7–1.2 hr	80
	IV	Rapid	End of inf	4–6 hr	16; 30	0.7–1.2 hr	100
ticarcillin-clavulanate	IV	Variable	15 min	4 hr	50	1–1.3 hr	100

BioA, Bioavailability; *immed,* immediate; inf, infection; *IM,* intramuscular; *IV,* intravenous; *PB,* protein binding; *PO,* by mouth; *t½,* half-life; *UA,* unavailable.

lethargy, twitching, confusion, dysphasia, hyperreflexia, agitation, depression, hallucinations, seizures, and coma. Signs of nephropathy, which can progress to renal failure, include fever, macular rash, eosinophilia, proteinuria, hematuria, leukocyturia, and eosinophiluria. Hematologic toxicity is reflected as neutropenia, thrombocytopenia, and prolonged bleeding time.

Penicillins are contraindicated for use in patients with a history of allergy to penicillins. In addition, cautious use is warranted in patients with an allergy to cephalosporins, and in patients with anemia, thrombocytopenia, or bone marrow depression. Penicillins are pregnancy category B drugs.

▥ *Drug Interactions*

Table 27-2 lists drug interactions of selected penicillin drugs. The majority of interactions are with antigout drugs (e.g., probenecid, sulfinpyrazone), potassium-sparing diuretics, aminoglycosides, anticoagulants, rifampin, oral contraceptives, and colestipol.

▥ *Dosage Regimen*

Dosage regimens of penicillins vary based on the type and the severity of infection and the desired route of administration (Table 27-3). Note that dosages of penicillin G formulations are prescribed in units (1 unit = 0.6 mcg). Other penicillin formulations are prescribed in milligrams or grams.

▥ *Lab Considerations*

Penicillins cause elevated serum uric acid concentrations and an elevated value for urine specific gravity.

Cephalosporins

FIRST-GENERATION CEPHALOSPORINS

- ◆ cephalexin (Keflex); ✦ Keflex, Apo-Cephalex
- ◆ cefazolin (Ancef); ✦ cephazoline
- ◆ cefadroxil (Duricef); ✦ Duracef
- ◆ cephradine (Velosef)

SECOND-GENERATION CEPHALOSPORINS

- ◆ cefaclor; ✦ Ceclor
- ◆ cefotetan disodium (Cefotan); ✦ Cefotan
- ◆ cefoxitin sodium (Mefoxin)
- ◆ cefuroxime axetil (Ceftin); ✦ Ceftin
- ◆ cefuroxime sodium (Kefurox, Zinacef)
- ◆ cefprozil (Cefzil); ✦ Cefzil
- ◆ loracarbef (Lorabid)

THIRD-GENERATION CEPHALOSPORINS

- ◆ cefdinir (Omnicef)
- ◆ ceftibuten (Cedax)
- ◆ cefixime (Suprax); ✦ Suprax
- ◆ cefoperazone (Cefobid); ✦ Cefobid
- ◆ cefotaxime (Claforan); ✦ Claforan
- ◆ cefpodoxime sodium (Vantin); ✦ Vantin

DRUG INTERACTIONS
TABLE **27-2** Antibiotics

Drug	Interactive Drugs	Interaction
ANTIBIOTIC CLASSES		
Penicillins	Aminoglycosides, clavulanate, warfarin	Enhances bactericidal effects of interactive drug
	probenecid, sulfinpyrazone	Delays renal elimination of penicillin
	Oral contraceptives, rifampin	Decreases activity of interactive drug
	NSAIDs	Increases penicillin action and half-life
	Potassium-sparing diuretics	Increases risk of hyperkalemia
	colestipol	Decreases serum levels of penicillin
Cephalosporins	Alcohol	Disulfiram-like reaction
	probenecid	Increases cephalosporin absorption
	Nephrotoxic drugs	Increases nephrotoxicity
	Antacids, H$_2$ antagonists	Decreases absorption of cephalosporin
Sulfonamides	Alcohol	Increases serum urate levels
	Oral anticoagulants	Increases risk of hypoprothrombinemia
	Oral antidiabetic drugs	Increases risk of hypoglycemia
	nitrofurantoin, phenytoin	Increases toxicity risk to interactive drug
	Cephalosporins, penicillin G	Prolongs serum antibiotic levels
	Salicylates	Decreases uricosuric activity
	methotrexate, sulfonylureas	Increases action of interactive drug
Tetracyclines	Aminoglycosides, antacids, antidiarrheal drugs, barbiturates, cimetidine, iron salts, penicillins	Decreases antibacterial action of tetracycline
	carbamazepine, phenytoin	Decreases half-life of doxycycline
	Oral anticoagulants	Decreases activity of interactive drug
Aminoglycosides	ethacrynic acid, furosemide	Increases nephrotoxicity and ototoxicity of aminoglycoside
	Penicillins	Inactivates aminoglycosides (in vitro)
	General anesthetics, neuromuscular blockers	Increases neuromuscular blockade
	Nephrotoxic drugs, neurotoxic drugs, oral anticoagulants, ototoxic drugs	Increases activity of interactive drug
Quinolones	Caffeine, theophylline, warfarin	Increases risk of toxicity to interactive drug
	Class IA and III antiarrhythmics (e.g., amiodarone, bepridil, disopyramide, quinidine, sotalol)	Increases risk for dangerous arrhythmias
	Antacids, bismuth subsalicylate, sucralfate, iron salts, zinc salts	Decreases absorption of quinolone
	Antineoplastic drugs	Decreases serum levels of quinolone
	cimetidine	Interferes with elimination of quinolone
	Glucocorticoids	Increases risk of tendon rupture
	nitrofurantoin, probenecid	Interactive drug antagonizes ciprofloxacin
	foscarnet	Increases risk of seizures if taken with ciprofloxacin
Macrolides	carbamazepine, cyclosporine, digoxin, midazolam, triazolam, theophylline, warfarin	Enhances effect and increases risk for toxicity of interactive drug
	ergotamine	Increases ischemia, dysesthesia, peripheral vasospasm
MISCELLANEOUS ANTIBIOTICS		
imipenem-cilastatin	Penicillins, cephalosporins	Antagonizes action of interactive drug
	probenecid	Increases serum levels of imipenem-cilastatin
	ganciclovir	Increases risk of seizures
clindamycin	chloramphenicol, erythromycin	Decreases action of interactive drugs
chloramphenicol	Oral hypoglycemics, oral anticoagulants, phenytoin	Increases effects of interactive drugs
	phenobarbital, rifampin	Decreases chloramphenicol levels
	folic acid, vitamin B$_{12}$	Delays response to interactive drug
	Antineoplastics	Additive bone marrow depression
	acetaminophen	Increases risk of toxicity
ertapenem	probenecid	Reduces renal elimination of ertapenem
linezolid	pseudoephedrine	Increases blood pressure
quinupristin-dalfopristin	Antihistamines, carbamazepine, cyclosporine, delavirdine, diazepam, diltiazem, disopyramide, docetaxel, HMG-CoA reductase inhibitors, indinavir, lidocaine, methylprednisolone, midazolam, nifedipine, nevirapine, paclitaxel, quinidine, ritonavir, tacrolimus, verapamil, vinblastine	Increases concentrations of interactive drugs
telithromycin	itraconazole, ketoconazole	Increases concentration of telithromycin
	rifampin, phenytoin, carbamazepine, phenobarbital	Decreases telithromycin concentration
	digoxin, simvastatin, atorvastatin, lovastatin, metoprolol, theophylline, pimozide	Increases concentration toxicity of interactive drugs
	sotalol	Decreases sotalol concentrations
vancomycin	Aminoglycosides, aspirin, cisplatin, cyclosporine, loop diuretics	Additive ototoxicity and nephrotoxicity
	Nondepolarizing neuromuscular blockers	Enhances neuromuscular blockade
	Anesthetics	Increases risk of histamine flush in children

HMG-CoA, 3-Hydroxy-3-methylglutaryl coenzyme-A; *NSAIDs,* nonsteroidal antiinflammatory drugs.

IMMUNE

DOSAGE
TABLE **27-3** Penicillins

Drug	Dosage	Implications	
PENICILLINASE-SENSITIVE PENICILLINS (FIRST-GENERATION)			
penicillin G sodium	*Adult:* 4 million units IM or IV every 4 hr. Max: 24 million units/day. *Infant and Child:* 250,000–400,000 units/kg/day in divided doses every 4–6 hr. Max: 24 million units/day	**Dosages are identified in units rather than mg or grams.**	⚠
penicillin G potassium	*Adult:* 4 million units IM or IV every 4 hr *Child:* 50,000–250,000 units/kg/day IM or IV in divided doses every 4 hr	**Dosages are identified in units rather than mg or grams.**	⚠
penicillin G benzathine	*Adult:* 1.2–2.4 million units IM as a single dose *–or–* 400,000–600,000 units IM every 4–6 hr *Child:* 25,000–90,000 units/kg/day PO in 3–6 divided doses *–or–* 0.9 million units IM as single dose	**Dosages are identified in units rather than mg or gram. 1 mg = 1600 units. Never give by IV—may cause embolism or toxic reactions.**	⚠
penicillin G procaine	*Adult:* 600,000–1.2 million units/day IM as single dose or divided doses every 6–12 hr *Child:* 0.05 million units IM daily	**Dosages are identified in units rather than mg or gram. 1 mg = 1600 units.**	⚠
penicillin VK	*Adult:* 250–500 mg PO 3–4 times daily *Child:* 25–50 mg/kg/day PO every 6–8 hr. Max: 3 grams/day	Dosage depends on reason for use. **250 mg = 400,000 units.** Take on empty stomach.	
PENICILLINASE-RESISTANT PENICILLINS (SECOND-GENERATION)			
dicloxacillin	*Adult and Child >40 kg:* 125–500 mg PO every 6 hr to 4 grams/day *Child <40 kg:* 12.5–25 mg/kg/day in divided doses every 6 hr. Max: 4 grams/day	Acidic juices decrease absorption.	
methicillin	*Adult:* 1 gram IM every 4–6 hr *–or–* 1–2 grams IV over 5–10 min every 4 hr *Child:* 100–200 mg/kg/day IM in 4 divided doses every 6 hr	FDA-approved for infection due to penicillinase-producing *Staphylococcus aureus.*	
nafcillin	*Adult:* 500–2000 mg IM every 4–6 hr. Max: 12 grams *Child:* 50–100 mg/kg/day PO in 4 divided doses	Past history of hypersensitivity to corn or corn products may precipitate an allergic reaction.	
oxacillin	*Adult and Child >40 kg:* 500–2000 mg PO, IM, or IV every 4–6 hr Max: 12 grams/day *Child <40 kg:* 50–100 mg/kg/day PO, IM, or IV in 4 divided doses every 6 hr	Long-term treatment (500 mg PO 4 times daily for approximately 5 years) may result in congestive cardiomyopathy.	
AMINOPENICILLINS (THIRD-GENERATION)			
amoxicillin	*Adult and Child >20 kg:* 250–500 mg PO every 8 hr *Child <20 kg:* 20–40 mg/kg/day in divided doses every 8 hr	Obtain baseline creatinine and monitor periodically if therapy is prolonged.	
ampicillin	*Adult and Child >20 kg:* 250–500 mg PO, IM, or IV every 6 hr *Child <20 kg:* 25–100 mg/kg/day in divided doses every 6 hr	Dosage depends on reason for use	
ANTIPSEUDOMONAL PENICILLINS (FOURTH-GENERATION)			
carbenicillin	*Adult:* 382–764 mg PO every 6 hr	Take on empty stomach	
mezlocillin	*Adult:* 150–200 mg/kg/day IM or IV in 4–6 divided doses. Max: 24 grams/day *Child 1 mo-12 yr:* 50–75 mg/kg IM or IV in 6 divided doses every 4 hr	Manufacturer recommends 200–300 mg/kg/day by IV for serious infections. For life-threatening infections, doses up to 350 mg/kg/day IV may be used.	
piperacillin	*Adult:* 3–4 grams IM or IV in divided doses every 4–6 hr. Max daily dose: 24 grams	Safe use in children <12 not established	
ticarcillin	*Adult:* 1–2 grams IM or IV every 6 hr *Child <40 kg:* 50–200 mg/kg/day IM or IV every 6–8 hr	Injections should not exceed 2 grams.	
PENICILLIN–BETA-LACTAMASE INHIBITOR COMBINATIONS			
ampicillin-sulbactam	*Adult:* 1.5–3 grams IM or IV every 6 hr. Max: 12 grams/day *Child >40 kg:* 300 mg/kg/day divided every 6 hr. Max: 12 grams/day	Age-related renal impairment may require dosage adjustment.	
amoxicillin-clavulanate	*Adult:* 250–500 mg amoxicillin and 125 mg clavulanic acid PO every 8 hr *–or–* 500 mg amoxicillin and 125 mg clavulanic acid to 875 mg amoxicillin and 125 mg clavulanic acid PO twice daily *Child <40 kg:* 20–40 mg/kg/day PO every 8 hr *–or–* 200–400 mg PO twice daily	**Dosage is expressed in terms of amoxicillin.**	⚠
piperacillin-tazobactam	*Adult:* 3.375 grams IV every 6 hr	Safe dosage not established for children	
ticarcillin-clavulanate	*Adult:* 3.1 grams IV every 4–6 hr *Child <60 kg:* 200–300 mg/kg/day IV in divided doses every 4–6 hr	Safe dosage not established for children <3 months of age	

FDA, U.S. Food and Drug Administration; *IM,* intramuscular (route); *IV,* intravenous (route); *PO,* by mouth.

- ceftazidime (Fortaz); ✦ Ceptaz
- ceftidoren (Spectracef)
- ceftizoxime (Cefizox); ✦ Cefizox
- ceftriaxone (Rocephin); ✦ Rocephin

FOURTH-GENERATION CEPHALOSPORINS
- cefepime (Maxipime)

▌ Indications
Cephalosporins are indicated for infections caused by susceptible organisms that have invaded the respiratory, urinary, and biliary tracts or the skin, soft tissue, or bone.

Cephalosporins are also used in serious conditions such as septicemia, meningitis, endocarditis, peritonitis, acute pelvic-inflammatory disease, and gonorrhea.

Prophylactic use of cephalosporins is indicated in perioperative patients who are undergoing surgical procedures associated with a high risk of infection. Examples of such procedures include biliary, cardiovascular, obstetric, gynecologic, orthopedic, or potentially contaminated surgery.

▌ Pharmacodynamics
These broad-spectrum, chemically altered derivatives of a fungus are categorized into four generations based on their

order of development. They are structurally and pharmacologically related to penicillins. Although the exact mechanisms of action have not been fully explained, cephalosporins are thought to interfere with mucopeptide synthesis. This interference results in the formation of defective cell walls and bacterial cell death.

Each generation differs significantly with respect to its spectra. There is increasing activity against gram-negative organisms and anaerobes as the generations increase, increasing stability against beta-lactamase, and increasing ability of the drug to enter cerebrospinal fluid (CSF).

FIRST-GENERATION CEPHALOSPORINS. First-generation cephalosporins have the best gram-positive coverage and are most active against *S. aureus* (except MRSA), *S. epidermidis*, *Streptococcus agalactiae*, and *Streptococcus pneumoniae*. First-generation cephalosporins have limited action against gram-negative bacteria and do not reach effective concentrations in CSF.

SECOND-GENERATION CEPHALOSPORINS. Second-generation cephalosporins are active against organisms susceptible to first-generation drugs and gram-negative organisms, including most strains of *H. influenzae*, *Enterobacter*, *Klebsiella*, *Escherichia coli*, and some strains of *Proteus*. Each of the drugs has a somewhat different antimicrobial spectrum; therefore susceptibility tests must be performed for each drug rather than for the entire group. None of the second-generation drugs are active against *P. aeruginosa*, and they do not reach effective concentrations in CSF. The exception is cefuroxime, which penetrates into the CSF. Cefotetan has anaerobic activity also.

THIRD-GENERATION CEPHALOSPORINS. Third-generation cephalosporins are active against organisms susceptible to the first- and second-generation cephalosporins and further extend the spectrum of activity against gram-negative organisms. These drugs are also active against unusual strains of enteric organisms such as *Citrobacter*, *Enterobacter*, *Morganella*, *Providencia*, and *Serratia*. Some third-generation cephalosporins are effective against *P. aeruginosa*, although drug-resistant strains can emerge when a cephalosporin is used alone for treatment of a pseudomonal infection. The third-generation drugs reach clinically effective concentrations in the CSF.

FOURTH-GENERATION CEPHALOSPORINS. Although there is only one fourth-generation drug, cefepime, this drug has a greater spectrum of antibiotic activity and greater stability against beta-lactamase enzymes compared with third-generation drugs. Cefepime is active against both gram-positive and gram-negative organisms and is considered a broad-spectrum antibiotic.

Pharmacokinetics
Most cephalosporins are poorly absorbed from the GI tract and must be administered parenterally. Cephalosporins are variously bound to plasma proteins, with half-lives ranging from less than 1 hour to over 10 hours (Table 27-4).

Only third-generation cephalosporins are distributed to the CSF in sufficient quantities to produce bactericidal effects, but even these depend on the presence of meningeal inflammation. For example, ceftriaxone passes easily through the blood-brain barrier and can be used to treat meningitis. Notably, only one third-generation cephalosporin, cefoperazone, is unable to produce therapeutic concentrations in the CSF.

Most of the cephalosporins are eliminated through the kidneys. Only two drugs, cefoperazone and ceftriaxone, are eliminated by nonrenal routes; therefore they can be used with relative safety in patients with significant renal impairment.

Adverse Effects and Contraindications
Like penicillins, cephalosporins are usually tolerated well and are one of the safest groups of antimicrobial drugs. The most common systemic adverse effects involve mild diarrhea, abdominal cramping or distress, rash, pruritus, redness, and edema. Other adverse effects include vertigo, hallucinations, malaise, fatigue, nightmares, headache, hepatic dysfunction, menstrual irregularities, vaginitis, genital pruritus, and vaginal moniliasis. Nephrotoxicity is associated with cephalothin. In rare situations, cephalosporins have caused drug-induced pseudomembranous colitis due to overgrowth with *Clostridium difficile*. In this case, stop the cephalosporin and, if necessary, treat the patient with oral vancomycin or metronidazole.

Cefoperazone and cefotetan have been associated with bleeding tendencies, because they interfere with the metabolism of vitamin K. The hematologic reactions are particularly dangerous in older adults, in debilitated and malnourished patients, and in those with severe renal insufficiency.

Because cephalosporins eliminate the inhibitory influence of normal flora, they can cause an overgrowth of nonsusceptible organisms, leading to superinfection. *Superinfection* is defined as a secondary infection that appears during the course of treatment for a primary infection. Broad-spectrum antibiotics are more likely than narrow-spectrum antibiotics to cause superinfection. Clinically significant superinfections due to *Pseudomonas*, *Candida*, and enterococci are more often associated with third-generation drugs. Superinfections can be difficult to treat because they are, by definition, caused by organisms that are drug-resistant.

Research has shown that the incidence of cross-sensitivity with penicillins is between 1% and 18%. However, only those patients who have had an anaphylactic reaction to penicillin should avoid cephalosporins.

Drug Interactions
Table 27-2 lists drug interactions of cephalosporins. As with penicillins, probenecid delays the renal excretion of some cephalosporins and therefore prolongs their effects. Cefoperazone and cefotetan produce a disulfiram-like reaction when taken with alcohol. The disulfiram effect is brought about by accumulation of acetaldehyde and can be dangerous. Further, drugs that promote bleeding (i.e., anticoagulants, nonsteroidal antiinflammatory drugs, and thrombolytics) place the patient at risk if they are used concurrently with cephalosporins.

Dosage Regimen
The dosage regimens of cephalosporins are noted in Table 27-5. Reduce the dosages of cephalosporins (excepting cefoperazone and ceftriaxone) in patients with renal impairment. Generally, treatment is continued for a minimum of 48 to 72 hours after the patient achieves an asymptomatic state. Perioperative prophylaxis is usually discontinued 24 to 48 hours after surgery.

PHARMACOKINETICS

TABLE 27-4 Cephalosporins

Drug	Route	Onset	Peak	Duration	PB (%)	t½	BioA (%)
FIRST-GENERATION CEPHALOSPORINS							
cephalexin	PO	15–30 min	1 hr	6–12 hr	6–15	0.5–1.2 hr	UA
cefazolin	IM	Variable	1–2 hr	Variable	74–86	1.5–2.5 hr	0
	IV	10 min	End of inf	Variable	74–86	1.5–2.5 hr	100
cefadroxil	PO	Rapid	1.5–2 hr	UA	15–20	1.5–2 hr	90
cephradine	PO	Rapid	1 hr	UA	6–20	0.7–2 hr	>90
	IM	Rapid	1 hr	UA	6–20	0.7–2 hr	>90
	IV	Immed	End of inf	UA	6–20	0.7–2 hr	100
SECOND-GENERATION CEPHALOSPORINS							
cefaclor	PO	15 min	30–60 min	UA	25	0.6–0.9 hr	High
cefotetan	IM	Rapid	1–3 hr	UA	88	3–5 hr	0
	IV	Immed	End of inf	UA	88	3–5 hr	100
cefoxitin	IM	Variable	20–30 min	Variable	73	0.7–1.1 hr	0
	IV	Immed	End of inf	Variable	73	0.7–1.1 hr	100
cefuroxime	PO	Variable	2–2.3 hr	6–8 hr	UA	1.3 hr	UA
	IM	Rapid	15–60 min	UA	UA	1.3 hr	0
	IV	Immed	End of inf	UA	UA	1.3 hr	100
cefprozil	PO	UA	1.5 hr	UA	36	1.3 hr	95
loracarbef	PO	Rapid	1 hr	8–12 hr	25	0.8–1.1 hr	79
THIRD-GENERATION CEPHALOSPORINS							
cefdinir	PO	Slow	2–4 hr	UA	UA	1.7 hr	20–25
cefditoren*	PO	Slow	1.5–3 hr	UA	88	1.6 hr	13–19
ceftibuten	PO	Rapid	2–3 hr	24 hr	65	2–2.4 hr	UA
cefixime	PO	15–30 min	3–4.4 hr	12–24 hr	65–70	3–4 hr	30–50
cefoperazone	IM	Rapid	1–2 hr	UA	82–93	1.6–2.6 hr	0
	IV	5 min	End of inf	UA	82–93	1.6–2.6 hr	100
cefotaxime	IM	Rapid	0.5 hr	UA	13–38	0.9–1.7 hr	0
	IV	Rapid	End of inf	UA	13–38	0.9–1.7 hr	100
cefpodoxime	PO	Rapid	UA	UA	22–40	2.09–2.84 hr	UA
ceftazidime	IM	Rapid	1 hr	8–12 hr	5–24	2 hr	0
	IV	Immed	End of inf	UA	5–24	2 hr	100
ceftizoxime	IM	Rapid	0.5–1.5 hr	UA	30	1.5–2 hr	0
	IV	Immed	End of inf	UA	30	1.5–2 hr	100
ceftriaxone	IM	Rapid	1–2 hr	6–8 hr	58–95	5.4–10.9 hr	0
	IV	Immed	End of inf	6–8 hr	58–95	5.4–10.9 hr	100
FOURTH-GENERATION CEPHALOSPORIN							
cefepime	IM	30 min	1.5–2 hr	8–12 hr	20	1.7–2.3 hr	UA
	IV	Immed	End of inf	8–12 hr	20	1.7–2.3 hr	100

*Cefditoren is given with a low-fat meal.
BioA, Bioavailability; *immed*, immediate; *inf*, infection; *IM*, intramuscular; *IV*, intravenous; *PB*, protein binding; *PO*, by mouth; *t½*, half-life; *UA*, unavailable; *UK*, unknown.

▥ Lab Considerations

Monitor the prothrombin time and international normalized ratio (PT, INR) for appropriate dosage adjustment when administering oral anticoagulants with cephalosporins. Cephalosporins can cause transient increases in blood urea nitrogen (BUN), alanine transaminase (ALT), aspartate transaminase (AST), alkaline phosphatase, lactate dehydrogenase (LDH), and bilirubin levels. Cefotetan causes falsely elevated serum and urine creatinine concentrations. Do not draw blood for these tests within 2 hours of drug administration.

Sulfonamides

- sulfadiazine (Microsulfon)
- sulfamethoxazole (Gantanol, Urobak); ♣ Apo-Sulfamethoxazole
- sulfisoxazole
- trimethoprim-sulfamethoxazole (TMP-SMX; Bactrim, co-trimoxazole, Septra); ♣ Apo-Sulfatrim

▥ Indications

Sulfonamides are a chemically related group of drugs that are all synthetic derivatives of sulfanilamide. They were once a major treatment modality for infection and originally were active against a wide range of gram-positive and gram-negative bacteria. Sulfonamides are used in the treatment of urinary tract infections, otitis media, and bronchitis. Sulfonamides are also used in the treatment of malaria, ulcerative colitis, dermatitis herpetiformis, chlamydia, nocardiosis, gonorrhea, and protozoal infections (e.g., toxoplasmosis, *Pneumocystis jirovecii* [previously known as *Pneumocystis carinii*] pneumonia). Sulfonamides are also used prophylactically in patients with a history of rheumatic fever, penicillin-allergic patients, adults and children infected with human immunodeficiency virus (HIV), granulocytopenic patients, and patients with traveler's diarrhea. Sulfasalazine is used for ulcerative colitis and rheumatoid arthritis and not as an antibiotic. The more commonly used sulfonamides are sulfadiazine, sulfamethoxazole, and sulfisoxazole.

▥ Pharmacodynamics

Sulfonamides are bacteriostatic against a wide range of bacteria, including pneumococci, *E. coli*, *Streptococcus pyogenes*,

DOSAGE
TABLE **27-5** Selected Cephalosporins

Drug	Dosage	Implications
FIRST-GENERATION CEPHALOSPORINS		
cephalexin	*Adult:* 250–500 mg PO every 6 hr. Max: 4 grams/day *Child:* 25–50 mg/kg/day PO in 2 divided doses every 12 hr	Somewhat less active against penicillinase-producing staphylococci than cephalothin
cephapirin	*Adult:* 500–1000 mg IM or IV every 4–6 hr *Child:* 40–80 mg/kg/day IM or IV in 3–4 divided doses	More active against *Escherichia coli* and *Klebsiella* than cephalothin
cefazolin	*Adult:* 500–2000 mg IM or IV every 6–8 hr. Max: 12 grams/day *Child >1 mo:* 25–50 mg/kg/day in divided doses every 6–8 hr. Max: 100 mg/kg/day	Do not use if solution is cloudy or contains precipitate.
cefadroxil	*Adult:* 1–2 grams PO twice daily *Child:* 30 mg/kg/day PO in 2 divided doses every 12 hr	A derivative of cephalexin but with longer half-life and reduced dosing frequency
cephradine	*Adult:* 250–500 mg PO every 6 hr –or– 500–1000 mg every 12 hr –or– 2–4 grams/day IM or IV in 2 divided doses *Child >9 mo:* 25–50 mg/kg/day PO in divided doses every 6–12 hr –or– 50–100 mg/kg/day IM or IV in divided doses every 6 hr	Reconstituted parenteral doses may vary in color from light straw to yellow. Color changes do not alter potency.
SECOND-GENERATION CEPHALOSPORINS		
cefaclor	*Adult:* 250–500 mg PO every 8 hr *Child >1 mo:* 20–40 mg/kg/day PO in divided doses every 8–12 hr	Suspension is stable for 14 days if refrigerated.
cefotetan	*Adult:* 1–2 grams IM or IV every 12 hr for 5–10 days. Max: 3 grams every 12 hr for life-threatening infections	Highly resistant to beta-lactamase enzymes. Effective against most organisms except *Pseudomonas*
cefoxitin	*Adult:* 1–2 grams IM or IV every 6–8 hr *Child:* 80–160 mg/kg/day IM or IV in divided doses every 4–6 hr. Max: 12 grams/day	More active against gram-negative organisms; less active against gram-positive organisms
cefuroxime	*Adult:* 125–500 mg PO twice daily depending on the infection –or– 750–1500 mg IM or IV every 8 hr *Child 3 mo-12 yr:* IM and PO dosage based on weight and type of infection every 6–12 hr	**Do not confuse with cefotaxime, cefzil, or deferoxamine.**
cefprozil	*Adult:* 250–500 mg PO every 12–24 hr *Child:* 15 mg/kg PO every 12 hr	Similar to cefaclor and cefuroxime
loracarbef	*Adult and Child >13 yr:* 200–400 mg PO every 12 hr *Child 6 mo-12 yr:* 15–30 mg/kg/day PO in divided doses every 12 hr	No significant drug interactions
THIRD-GENERATION CEPHALOSPORINS		
cefdinir	*Adult:* 300 mg PO every 12 hr –or– 600 mg PO every 24 hr *Child 6 mo-12 yr:* 7 mg/kg PO every 12 hr –or– 14 mg/kg PO every 24 hr	Renal dosing adjustment required.
cefditoren	*Adult and Child >12 yr:* 200–400 mg PO twice daily	Renal dosing adjustment required.
ceftibuten	*Adult and Child >40 kg:* 400 mg PO daily for 10 days *Child >6 mo:* 9 mg/kg PO once daily	Renal dosing adjustment required.
cefixime	*Adult and Child >12 yr or >50 kg:* 400 mg PO as single dose –or– 200 mg PO every 12 hr *Child:* 8 mg/kg/day as single dose or in 2 divided doses every 12 hr	Use suspension only when treating otitis media.
cefoperazone	*Adult:* 1–2 grams/day IM or IV in divided doses every 12 hr	Active against gram-negative organisms resistant to previous cephalosporins.
cefotaxime	*Adult:* 1–2 grams IM or IV every 6–12 hr. Max: 12 grams/day *Child >1 mo:* 50–180 mg/kg/day IM or IV in divided doses every 4–6 hr	**Do not confuse with cefoxitin, ceftizoxime, or cefuroxime.**
cefpodoxime	*Adult:* 200 mg PO twice daily	Renal dosing adjustment required.
ceftazidime	*Adult and Child >50 kg:* 1–2 grams IM or IV every 8–12 hr. Max: 6 grams/day *Child >1 mo:* 30–50 mg/kg/day IM or IV in divided doses every 8 hr	Active against most gram-negative and gram-positive bacteria. Some activity against *Pseudomonas* resistant to second-generation cephalosporins
ceftizoxime	*Adult:* 1–2 grams IM or IV every 8–12 hr *Child >6 mo:* 50 mg/kg IM or IV every 6–8 hr. If needed, increase to total daily dose of 200 mg/kg.	Renal dosing adjustment required. Broader gram-negative and anaerobic activity. Active against *Bacteroides fragilis*
ceftriaxone	*Adult:* 1–2 grams/day IM or IV *Child:* 50–75 mg/kg/day IM or IV. Max: 2 grams daily in divided doses every 12 hr	Reconstituted parenteral doses vary in color from light straw to yellow. Color changes do not alter potency.
FOURTH-GENERATION CEPHALOSPORIN		
cefepime	*Adult:* 0.5–2 grams IM or IV every 12 hr for 7–10 days. Can be given every 8 hr for serious infections *Child:* 50 mg/kg every 12 hr	Renal dosing adjustment required.

IM, Intramuscular (route); *IV,* intravenous (route); *PO,* by mouth.

S. pneumoniae, H. influenzae, Haemophilus ducreyi, Nocardia and *Actinomyces* organisms, *Klebsiella granulomatis, and Chlamydia trachomatis.* Protozoa susceptible to sulfonamides include *Toxoplasma gondii* and *P. jirovecii.*

As mentioned earlier, sulfonamides inhibit bacterial growth by preventing the synthesis of bacteria of folic acid, a B-complex vitamin required for the proper synthesis of purines and nucleic acid. Specifically, the sulfonamide enters the reaction instead of PABA, competing for the enzyme involved, and causing the formation of nonfunctional derivatives of folic acid. Thus sulfonamides stop growth, development, and multiplication of new bacteria but do not kill mature, fully formed bacteria. Only organisms that synthesize their own folic acid are inhibited by sulfonamides.

Some bacteria alter their metabolic pathways to use precursors or other forms of folic acid, thereby developing resistance to the antibacterial action of sulfonamides. Once resistance to one sulfonamide develops, cross-resistance to others is common.

▥ Pharmacokinetics

The pharmacokinetics of sulfonamides are identified in Table 27-6. Most sulfonamides are well absorbed following oral administration and are distributed throughout all body tissues with good penetration of pleural, peritoneal, synovial, and ocular fluids. They cross placental membranes and the blood-brain barrier, diffusing into CSF. The largest percentages of sulfonamides are eliminated by the kidneys; therefore dosage adjustments are necessary in patients with renal insufficiency.

▥ Adverse Effects and Contraindications

Sulfonamides are a common cause of allergic reactions. The sulfa moiety is found in several other drug classes including diuretics, oral hypoglycemics, and carbonic anhydrase inhibitors. Although immediate allergic responses are possible, sulfonamides typically cause delayed cutaneous reactions. These begin with fever and are followed by a rash (e.g., morbilliform eruptions, erythema multiforme, or toxic epidermal necrolysis).

The most common adverse effects of sulfonamides include headache, anorexia, nausea, vomiting, diarrhea, and rash. Other adverse effects include urticaria, weakness, flushing, vertigo, stomatitis, glossitis, abdominal pain, photosensitivity, peripheral neuritis, oliguria, anuria, crystalluria, uric acid kidney stones, and exacerbations of gout.

The more serious adverse effects of sulfonamides involve hemolytic anemia, thrombocytopenia, convulsions, hepatic necrosis, and renal failure. Stevens-Johnson syndrome is the most serious form of cutaneous sensitivity and has been noted with all sulfonamides. It manifests as erythema and ulceration of mucous membranes (eyes, mouth, and urethra). Serum sickness and drug fever are also noted. Patients with acquired immunodeficiency syndrome (AIDS) are more likely to develop rashes secondary to sulfonamide therapy than patients without AIDS.

Acute hemolytic anemia results from increased destruction of red blood cells. Hemolytic anemia is most likely to occur in patients whose red blood cells have been sensitized because of a glucose-6-phosphate dehydrogenase (G6PD) deficiency. When red blood cells are challenged by one of several sulfonamides, glutathione is depleted, Heinz bodies form, and glucose use is inhibited.

Agranulocytosis or aplastic anemia can occur in patients taking a sulfonamide because of the direct toxic effects of the drug on the bone marrow. Also rare but serious is focal or diffuse necrosis of the liver secondary to direct toxicity or hypersensitivity. These reactions are rare; however, should they develop, prompt discontinuation of the offending drug is essential.

Sulfonamides are contraindicated for use in patients who have blood dyscrasias, porphyria, uric acid kidney stones, or excessive elimination of uric acid (over 1000 mg/day); in patients who are having or are within 2 or 3 weeks of having had an acute gout attack; and in patients who have a creatinine clearance below 50 mL/min. Sulfonamides are also contraindicated for use during pregnancy and lactation, and in infants younger than 2 months of age (unless the infant is being treated for congenital toxoplasmosis). The primary danger of using sulfonamides during pregnancy occurs when these drugs are given close to delivery. The sulfonamides compete with bilirubin for binding to plasma albumin. In utero, the fetus clears free bilirubin through the placental circulation. However, after birth this mechanism is no longer available, and unbound bilirubin is free to cross the blood-brain barrier, resulting in kernicterus.

▥ Drug Interactions

Sulfonamides have clinically significant interactions with a number of other drugs. Table 27-2 lists drug interactions of selected sulfonamide drugs. The most common drug interactions involve anticoagulants, oral hypoglycemic drugs, and phenytoin.

▥ Dosage Regimen

Sulfonamides fall into two major categories: systemic sulfonamides and sulfonamides used for local effects (e.g., burns). The systemic sulfonamides are more widely used and are identified in Table 27-7.

▥ Lab Considerations

Sulfonamides increase serum levels of alkaline phosphatase, AST, and creatinine, and the bilirubin value may be elevated.

PHARMACOKINETICS
TABLE 27-6 Sulfonamides

Drug	Route	BioA (%)	Onset	Peak	Duration	PB (%)	t½
sulfadiazine	PO	70–100	Varies	3–6 hr	UA	32–56	13 hr
sulfamethoxazole	PO	70–100	1 hr	3–4 hr	UA	65	7–12 hr
sulfisoxazole	PO	70–100	UA	2–4 hr	UA	90	5–8 hr
	IV	100	Rapid	End of inf	UA	<10	2–3 hr
trimethoprim- sulfamethoxazole	PO	UA	Rapid	1–4 hr	UA	65; 50*	10–13 hr; 8–10 hr†

*Protein binding of sulfamethoxazole and trimethoprim, respectively.
†Half-life of trimethoprim and sulfamethoxazole, respectively.
BioA, Bioavailability; *inf,* infection; *IV,* intravenous; *PB,* protein binding; *PO,* by mouth; *t½,* half-life; *UA,* unavailable.

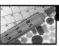

DOSAGE
TABLE 27-7 Selected Sulfonamides

Drug	Dosages	Implications
sulfadiazine	*Adult:* 2–4 grams PO initially, then 2–4 grams daily in 3–6 divided doses *Child >2 mo:* 75 mg/kg PO initially, then 150 mg/kg/day in 4–6 divided doses. Max: 6 grams/day	Low solubility, short-acting, rapidly eliminated
sulfamethoxazole	*Adult:* 2 grams PO initially, then 1–2 grams 2–3 times daily *Child >2 mo:* 50–60 mg/kg PO initially, then 25–30 mg/kg every 12 hr. Max: 75 mg/kg/day	Absorbed and eliminated more slowly than sulfisoxazole. More likely to cause high blood levels and crystalluria than sulfisoxazole
sulfisoxazole	*Adult:* 2–4 grams PO, IV, or subQ in divided doses every 4–6 hr, then 4–8 grams/day PO in 4–6 divided doses *Child >2 mo:* 75 mg/kg, then 150 mg/kg/day in 4–6 divided doses. Not to exceed 6 grams/day	Fluid intake should be at least 1200–1500 mL/day if drug is taken orally, to minimize crystalluria.
trimethoprim-sulfamethoxazole (TMP-SMZ)	*Adult:* 160 mg TMP + 800 mg SMZ PO every 12 hr –*or*– 8–10 mg/kg TMP + 50 mg/kg SMZ every 6–12 hr IV in divided doses *Child >2 mo:* 4–6 mg/kg TMP + 20–30 mg/kg SMZ PO every 12 hr –*or*– 8–10 mg/kg TMP + 50 mg/kg SMZ every 6–12 hr IV in divided doses PCP: 15–20 mg/kg/day TMP PO in divided doses every 6 hr	**Dosages are based on trimethoprim.** Phlebitis possible with IV route. Fluid intake should be at least 1200–1500 mL/day to minimize crystalluria.

IM, Intramuscular (route); *IV,* Intravenous (route); *PCP, Pneumocystitis jirovecii* pneumonia (previously known as *Pneumocystitis carinii pneumonia*); *PO,* by mouth; *subQ,* subcutaneous (route).

Tetracyclines

- doxycycline (Doryx, Doxy, Monodox, Vibramycin, Vibra-Tabs); ♣ Doxycin, Novo-Doxylin, Vibramycin
- minocycline (Minocin); ♣ Minocin, Soladyn
- tetracycline (Achromycin V, Panmycin, Sumycin, Tetracyn); ♣ Novo-Tetra
- tigecycline (Tygacil)

Indications

The extensive use of these broad-spectrum drugs has resulted in increased bacterial resistance. As a result, they are now rarely the drug of first choice for common bacterial infections. Disorders for which tetracyclines are considered first-line drugs include Rocky Mountain spotted fever, typhus fever, Q fever (rickettsial infections), trachoma, lymphogranuloma venereum, urethritis, cervicitis *(C. trachomatis),* pneumonia *(Mycoplasma pneumoniae),* peptic ulcer disease *(Helicobacter pylori),* brucellosis *(Brucella* species), and cholera *(Vibrio cholera).*

Other diseases in which tetracyclines render effective treatment include sinusitis, tularemia, anthrax, yaws and plague *(Treponema pertenue),* tetanus, rat-bite fever, tropical sprue, and cystitis. Tetracycline has also been used to treat Lyme disease *(Borrelia burgdorferi),* but it is not approved by the U.S. Food and Drug Administration (FDA) for such use. Tetracycline is also effective for acne. Doxycycline appears to be effective and inexpensive prophylaxis for patients traveling to most countries where malaria is prevalent.

Tigecycline, a derivative of minocycline, is approved for the treatment of complicated intraabdominal and skin and skin-structure infections. It is the first of a new class of antibiotics called *glycylcyclines.* It has activity against many gram-positive organisms including MRSA, glycopeptide intermediate-resistant *S. aureus* (GISA), penicillin-resistant *S. pneumoniae,* and vancomycin-resistant *Enterococcus faecium* (VREF). Tigecycline is also active against many gram-negative organisms including *Acinetobacter baumanii, Stenotrophomonas maltophilia,* and most *Enterobacteriaceae,* including strains producing extended-spectrum beta-lactamases, and against atypical bacteria and anaerobes such as *Bacteroides fragilis, Clostridium perfringens, and C.*

difficile. The drug does not have clinically significant activity against *P. aeruginosa* or *Proteus* species. Tigecycline is not affected by the two major mechanisms of tetracycline resistance: ribosomal protection proteins and efflux pumps.

Pharmacodynamics

Tetracyclines are derivatives of *Streptomyces* organisms. They are bacteriostatic, entering microbial cells by passive diffusion and an active transport system to interfere with the synthesis of bacterial proteins. They do so by competing for the binding of the 30S subunit site of the RNA ribosome. Tetracyclines are bactericidal in high concentrations.

The exact action of tetracycline on acne has not been fully clarified. Tetracyclines appear to inhibit the growth of *Propionibacterium acnes* on skin surfaces and reduce the concentration of free fatty acids in sebum. Sebum is believed to cause the inflammatory acne lesions (e.g., papules, pustules, nodules, and cysts).

Pharmacokinetics

The absorption of orally administered tetracyclines is incomplete but can be enhanced by taking the drugs on an empty stomach. Food is less likely to interfere with the absorption of doxycycline and minocycline. Alterations in gastric pH (e.g., after antacid administration) also decrease the absorption of tetracyclines. The presence of milk and dairy products, aluminum- or magnesium-containing antacids, or iron and zinc salts causes a considerable reduction in absorption.

Doxycycline and minocycline are the most lipid-soluble forms and thus are distributed to various tissues, crossing the blood-brain barrier and placental membranes. Fetal plasma concentrations reach 60% of the level in the maternal circulation. The drugs are also found in breast milk. As a class, tetracyclines undergo enterohepatic recirculation and are eliminated in the urine and the feces (Table 27-8).

Adverse Effects and Contraindications

GI effects appear more often after oral administration of tetracyclines but may also appear after IM and intravenous

PHARMACOKINETICS
TABLE 27-8 Tetracyclines

Drug	Route	Onset	Peak	Duration	PB (%)	t½	BioA (%)
doxycycline	PO	1–4 hr	1.5–4 hr	To 12 hr	25–93	14–24 hr	93
	IV	Immed	End of inf	To 12 hr	25–93	14–24 hr	100
minocycline	PO	Rapid	2–3 hr	UA	55–88	15–20 hr	90
	IV	Immed	End of inf	UA	55–80	15–20 hr	100
tetracycline	PO	1–2 hr	2–4 hr	UA	20–67	6–12 hr	60–80
tigecycline	IV	Immed	End of inf	UA	71–89	27–42 hr	100

BioA, Bioavailability; *immed*, immediate; *inf*, infection; *IV*, intravenous; *PB*, protein binding; *PO*, by mouth; *t½*, half-life; *UA*, unavailable.

(IV) administration. The most common adverse effects are nausea, vomiting, diarrhea, and photosensitivity. Lightheadedness, dizziness, vertigo, and vestibular reactions are common with minocycline. The drugs bind to calcium in bones and teeth, resulting in yellow or brown discolorations. The intensity of tooth discoloration is related to the total cumulative dose. The staining becomes darker with prolonged and repeated treatment. The risk of discoloration is less with doxycycline than with other tetracyclines. Hypoplasia of tooth enamel may also occur.

Photosensitivity reactions (i.e., sunburn and tingling and burning of the nose, hands, and feet) occur most often with doxycycline. The onset of photosensitivity occurs a few minutes to several hours after sun exposure and may last 1 or 2 days after the drug has been discontinued. Minocycline appears to be the least likely to cause the sunburn reaction, although a blue-gray or muddy brown pigmentation, accentuated in sun-exposed areas of the skin, has been noted.

The most important characteristic of tetracyclines is their ability to bind to divalent (calcium, magnesium) and trivalent metallic (aluminum) ions to form insoluble complexes. For this reason, coadministration with milk and dairy products, antacids, or iron salts causes a considerable reduction in absorption. Their strong affinity for calcium usually precludes their use in children under the age of 8 years because they can cause significant tooth discoloration. Tetracyclines taken after the fourth month of pregnancy causes staining of deciduous teeth in offspring. In premature infants, tetracyclines also suppress long-bone growth. Bone growth can be depressed up to 40% after prolonged exposure to tetracyclines.

Sometimes, the effects are reversible on discontinuation of treatment.

Tetracyclines lead to superinfection because of alterations in the normal flora of the respiratory tract, the GI tract, and the vagina. *Candida* superinfections are more likely to occur with prolonged therapy and in debilitated patients.

All tetracyclines have the potential to cause fatty infiltration of the liver. It appears that dosages over 2 grams/day, tetracyclines given by IV infusion, and use during pregnancy have been associated with hepatotoxicity.

▮ Drug Interactions

The primary drug interactions associated with tetracyclines include antacids (magnesium, calcium, aluminum, iron), and dairy products (see Table 27-2), which decrease the absorption of tetracycline if they are taken concurrently. The net effect is a decrease in the antibacterial efficacy of tetracycline. Tetracyclines have also been reported to decrease the efficacy of oral contraceptives because these undergo the same enterohepatic recirculation as tetracyclines. There appears to be interference with the hydrolytic process, thus reducing or abolishing the reabsorption of the oral contraceptive drug, and the risk of pregnancy increases.

Tigecycline is not a substrate of, an inhibitor of, or induced by CYP450 enzymes; thus few interactions have been noted. However, serum levels of warfarin may be elevated, but PT and INR were not affected in clinical studies (Kasbekar, 2006).

▮ Dosage Regimen

The dosage regimen of tetracyclines varies according to the reason for use (Table 27-9). Tetracyclines may be administered

DOSAGE
TABLE 27-9 Tetracyclines

Drug	Dosage	Implications
doxycycline	*Adult:* 100–200 mg/day PO, IV daily or in divided doses every 12 hr *Child >8 yr:* 2.2–4.4 mg/kg/day PO or IV daily or in divided doses every 12 hr	**Avoid dairy products, antacids, iron supplements, sodium bicarbonate, calcium supplements, and antidiarrheal drugs within 1–3 hr of oral tetracyclines.** Prevent extravasation if given by IV.
minocycline	*Adult:* 100–200 mg PO initially, then 100 mg every 12 hr *Child >8 yr:* 4 mg/kg PO initially, then 2 mg/kg every 12 hr *–or–* 4 mg/kg IV initially, then 2 mg/kg every 12 hr	
tetracycline	*Adult:* 1–2 grams/day in divided doses every 6–12 hr *Chronic acne treatment:* 500–1000 mg/day for 3 wk, then decrease to 125–1000 mg/day *Child >8 yr:* 25–50 mg/kg/day in divided doses every 6–12 hr	
GLYCYLCYCLINES		
tigecycline	*Adult:* 100 mg IVPB initially, followed by 50 mg every 12 hr	Decrease dosage in patients with liver disorders.

IV, Intravenous (route); *IVPB*, intravenous piggy-back; *PO*, by mouth.

by mouth or parenterally. The IV route is used only when oral therapy cannot be tolerated or has proven inadequate. IM injections are painful, and the route is rarely used.

Lab Considerations

Tetracyclines may cause a false elevation in fluorometric determinations of urine catecholamines. Depending on the dose, tetracyclines can cause elevated BUN levels. Increased serum amylase concentrations, hyperbilirubinemia, and increases in BUN have occurred with tigecycline.

Aminoglycosides

- ◆ amikacin sulfate (Amikin); ♣ Amikin
- ◆ gentamicin sulfate (Garamycin, Gentamicin); ♣ Alcomicin; Cidomycin
- ◆ kanamycin sulfate (Kantrex)
- ◆ neomycin sulfate (Mycifradin, Myciguent)
- ◆ netilmicin (Netromycin); ♣ Netromycin
- ◆ streptomycin sulfate
- ◆ tobramycin sulfate (Nebcin, Tobrex); ♣ Tobrex

Indications

Aminoglycosides are narrow-spectrum antibiotics. They are used for serious, systemic infections, caused by susceptible aerobic, gram-negative organisms, of the blood stream, the respiratory tract, the bones and joints, the skin and soft tissue, and the intraabdominal area. Aminoglycosides are reserved for situations in which less toxic drugs have proved ineffective, as well as for very serious, life-threatening infections. Gentamicin, tobramycin, and amikacin are the most commonly used drugs in this class.

Oral neomycin is used to suppress the normal flora of the bowel in preparation for intestinal surgery. A few aminoglycosides are administered topically to the eye or to the skin. These are discussed in Chapters 61 and 63, respectively.

Pharmacodynamics

Aminoglycosides are bactericidal, primarily targeting *P. aeruginosa, E. coli, Klebsiella, Serratia,* and *Proteus mirabilis.* They are similar to the tetracyclines in that they are derived from *Streptomyces* organisms. They act by penetrating the bacterial cell to bind to the 30S ribosome, a structure that must be functioning for protein synthesis to occur. By disrupting this process, the synthesis of proteins necessary for bacterial function and replication is inhibited, and the bacteria eventually die.

Pharmacokinetics

The pharmacokinetics of aminoglycosides is identified in Table 27-10. All aminoglycosides carry multiple positive charges. As a result, these drugs are not absorbed from the GI tract and therefore must be administered parenterally and distributed largely in extracellular fluids. Distribution to amniotic fluid and fetal plasma occurs; thus, use aminoglycosides only if their potential benefit outweighs the risk. Sufficient concentrations occur in peritoneal fluids, making them useful for treating peritonitis. Similarly, periocular injections may be used for serious eye infections. The low CSF concentrations that result following parenteral administration make it necessary to inject these antibiotics directly into the CSF. They are eliminated via glomerular filtration. There is little tubular secretion and no hepatic biotransformation.

Adverse Effects and Contraindications

The adverse effects most commonly associated with aminoglycosides include nausea, vomiting, and diarrhea. Other undesirable adverse effects consist of syncope, vertigo, skin rash, fever, headache, neuromuscular blockade, paresthesia, and superinfection. Hypersensitivity symptoms manifest as a rash, urticaria, stomatitis, pruritus, generalized burning, fever, and eosinophilia.

The most serious adverse effects associated with aminoglycosides are neurotoxicity, nephrotoxicity, and ototoxicity. Neurotoxicity manifests as neuromuscular blockade, respiratory depression, and paralysis. The risk for paralysis is more likely to occur with concurrent use of neuromuscular blocking drugs, aminoglycosides, or general anesthetics. Most episodes of neuromuscular blockade occur following intrapleural or intraperitoneal instillation of aminoglycosides. Exercise caution when administering these drugs to patients with myasthenia gravis and other neuromuscular disorders, because muscle weakness may be escalated. Nephrotoxicity usually manifests as acute tubular necrosis with proteinuria, oliguria, or white blood cells (WBCs) or casts in the urine; hematuria; elevated BUN; and serum creatinine. Patients at risk for nephrotoxicity

PHARMACOKINETICS
TABLE 27-10 Aminoglycosides

Drug	Route	Onset	Peak	Duration	PB (%)	t½
amikacin	IM	Rapid	0.75–1.5 hr	8–12 hr	4	2–3 hr
	IV	Immed	End of inf	8–12 hr	4	2–3 hr
gentamicin	IM	Rapid	0.5–2 hr	8–12 hr	<10	2–3 hr
	IV	Immed	End of inf	8–12 hr	<10	2–3 hr
kanamycin	IM	Rapid	1–2 hr	UA	<10	2–3 hr
	IV	Rapid	End of inf	UA	<10	2–3 hr
neomycin	PO	Varies	1–4 hr	6–8 hr	UA	2–3 hr
	IM	Rapid	1–2 hr	6–8 hr	UA	2–3 hr
netilmicin	IM	Rapid	1–2 hr	UA	10	2–3 hr
	IV	Immed	1–2 hr	UA	10	2–3 hr
streptomycin	IM	Rapid	1–2 hr	UA	30	2–3 hr
tobramycin	IM	Rapid	1 hr	UA	<10	2–3 hr
	IV	Immed	End of inf	UA	<10	2–3 hr

BioA, Bioavailability; *immed,* immediate; *inf,* infection; *IM,* intramuscular; *IV,* intravenous; *PB,* protein binding; *PO,* by mouth; *t½,* half-life; *UA,* unavailable.

are those with trough levels of the drug above 2 mg/dL. The incidence ranges from 7% to 16% depending on the specific aminoglycoside.

Ototoxicity is caused by damage to the eighth cranial nerve and is manifested by vestibular symptoms (e.g., vertigo, ataxia, nystagmus) and auditory symptoms (e.g., tinnitus and varying degrees of hearing impairment). Factors increasing the risk of ototoxicity include renal dysfunction, concurrent use of other drugs with ototoxic properties of their own, and the use of excessive doses of aminoglycosides for longer than 10 days.

Owing to their potential nephrotoxic effects, aminoglycosides are contraindicated for use in infants and in patients with known renal impairment. Aminoglycosides are also contraindicated in patients with allergy to bisulfites, because most parenteral formulations contain this allergen. Cross-sensitivity among aminoglycosides may occur.

Drug Interactions

Table 27-2 lists drug interactions of selected aminoglycoside drugs. There is increased nephrotoxicity and ototoxicity when the drugs are taken with diuretics such as ethacrynic acid or furosemide. The activity of oral anticoagulants is increased.

Dosage Regimen

Aminoglycosides are usually given by parenteral means because of their poor GI absorption (Table 27-11). Further, because of the multiple toxicities associated with aminoglycosides, dosages are calculated based on milligrams per kilograms of body weight rather than using a fixed dosage. If the patient is obese, base the calculation on lean or ideal body weight, because these drugs have no significant distribution to body fat. Serum drug levels can be used to determine dosage adjustments needed in patients with impaired renal failure, or the time interval between doses can be adjusted based on creatinine clearance levels.

Ordinarily, an initial loading dose is given to rapidly achieve therapeutic serum levels. For gentamicin and tobramycin, peak levels above 10 to 12 mcg/mL and trough levels above 2 mcg/mL for prolonged periods are associated with nephrotoxicity.

Greater interest has been shown in once-daily or extended-interval aminoglycoside dosing. Two factors allow for and even suggest the merits of once-daily dosing with aminoglycosides: concentration-dependent bactericidal effects and postantibiotic effects. Concentration-dependent effects mean the drugs are most effective in killing organisms when given in large doses and high peak serum concentrations are obtained. Postantibiotic effects mean that aminoglycosides continue killing organisms even at low serum concentrations. The combination of these two factors allows regimens to achieve optimal killing of organisms as long as dosages are sufficiently high to produce high peak serum levels. The 24-hour period between doses permits serum levels to fall to very low levels as the drug is eliminated. During this period with low serum drug levels, the postantibiotic effect is active and there is minimal drug accumulation in the body. There are several reported advantages to this regimen: antibacterial effects are enhanced, and there is less nephrotoxicity, reduced need to draw and calculate peak and trough drug levels, and reduced time for administration.

Lab Considerations

Aminoglycosides can elevate BUN, AST, and ALT, serum alkaline phosphatase, bilirubin, creatinine, and LDH

DOSAGE
TABLE 27-11 Aminoglycosides

Drug	Dosage	Implications
amikacin	*Adult and Older Child:* Loading dose: 5–7.5 mg/kg, then 7.5 mg IM or IV every 12 hr *Neonate:* 10 mg/kg IV initially, then 7.5 mg/kg IV every 12 hr.	*Peak:* 20–30 mcg/mL. *Trough:* <10 mcg/mL. Peak and trough levels checked with third dose. Used primarily for infections resistant to other aminoglycosides. Broader spectrum than other aminoglycosides For obese patients, use adjusted weight = IBW + 0.4(ABW−IBW)
gentamicin	*Adult:* Loading dose: 1.5–2 mg/kg, then 3–5 mg/kg/day IM or IV in divided doses every 8 hr *Child:* 6–7.5 mg/kg/day IM or IV in divided doses every 8 hr	*Peak:* 5–8 mcg/mL. *Trough:* <2 mcg/mL. Peak and trough levels checked with third dose.
kanamycin	*Adult and Child:* 15 mg/kg/day IM or IV in 2–3 divided doses *Suppression of GI bacteria:* 1 gram PO every hr for 4 doses, then 1 gram PO every 6 hr for 36–72 hr	*Peak:* 25–35 mcg/mL. *Trough:* 4–8 mcg/mL. Peak and trough levels checked with third dose.
neomycin	*Adult: Suppression of GI bacteria:* 1 gram PO every hr for 4 doses, then 1 gram every 4 hr for 5 doses. Max: 4–12 grams/day	**Most toxic aminoglycoside. Poorly absorbed from GI tract. Toxic levels possible in presence of renal failure.**
netilmicin	*Adult:* Initial loading dose: 1.5–2 mg/kg, then 2–3.3 mg/kg/day IM or IV in 2–3 divided doses every 12 hr *Child 6 wk–12 yr:* 1.8–2 mg/kg/day in 2–3 divided doses every 8–12 hr	*Peak:* 4–12 mcg/mL. *Trough:* <4 mcg/mL. Similar in spectrum to gentamicin. Less active against *Pseudomonas*. Peak and trough levels checked with third dose.
streptomycin	*Adult:* 15 mg/kg/day IM to max of 1 gram *–or–* 25–30 mg/kg 2–3 times weekly. Max: 1.5 grams/dose *Child:* 20–40 mg/kg/day IM in 2 divided doses every 12 hr to max of 1 gram/day	The first aminoglycoside. Less favored today because of nerve damage (CN VIII) and emergence of resistant organisms.
tobramycin	*Adult and Child:* Initial loading dose: 1.5–2 mg/kg, then 3–5 mg/kg/day IM or IV every 24 hr *–or–* 1.5–2.5 mg/kg IM or IV every 12 hr *–or–* 1–1.7 mg/kg IM or IV every 8 hr *Neonates <1 wk:* Up to 4 mg/kg/day IM or IV in 2 divided doses every 12 hr	*Peak:* 5–12 mcg/mL. *Trough:* <2 mcg/mL. Similar in spectrum to gentamicin. Used when penicillins or less toxic drugs are contraindicated. Peak and trough levels checked with third dose.

ABW, Adjusted body weight; *CN*, cranial nerve; *GI*, gastrointestinal; *IBW*, ideal body weight; *IM*, intramuscular; *IV*, intravenous; *PO*, by mouth.

concentrations. They may decrease serum calcium, magnesium, potassium, and sodium concentrations.

Quinolones

- ciprofloxacin (Cipro); ◆ Cipro
- gemifloxacin (Factive)
- levofloxacin (Levaquin); ◆ Levaquin
- lomefloxacin (Maxaquin)
- moxifloxacin (Avelox, Vigamox); ◆ Avelox, Vigamox
- norfloxacin (Chibroxin, Noroxin); ◆ Noroxin
- ofloxacin (Floxin); ◆ Floxin
- sparfloxacin (Zagam)

▓ Indications

Quinolones are the newest and a very potent classification of broad-spectrum antibiotics. They are chemically related to nalidixic acid, a narrow-spectrum antibiotic used only for urinary tract infections. Quinolones used for urinary tract infections are discussed in Chapter 41.

Quinolones are used for a variety of infections caused by gram-negative and other organisms. They can be used to treat bacterial infections of the respiratory, the GU, and the GI tracts, as well as infections of bones and joints and skin and soft tissues. They are also used to treat multi–drug-resistant tuberculosis (see Chapter 29), infections caused by atypical mycobacteria (e.g., *Mycobacterium avium*) in patients with AIDS, and fever in neutropenic patients with cancer.

▓ Pharmacodynamics

Quinolones act by interfering with DNA gyrase. DNA gyrase is the enzyme responsible for the stranding of bacterial DNA synthesis, as well as bacterial growth and replication. Without the ability to strand for DNA synthesis, the ability of the organism to grow and reproduce is halted.

Ciprofloxacin, norfloxacin, ofloxacin, and levofloxacin are active against an extensive spectrum of gram-negative bacteria including *Enterobacteriaceae* and *P. aeruginosa*. Lomefloxacin is effective against slightly fewer gram-negative bacteria and, among the gram-positive bacteria, only against *Staphylococcus* species. Sparfloxacin and levofloxacin are somewhat more active than older quinolones against gram-positive organisms such as *Enterococcus* and *S. aureus*. Moxifloxacin is 4 to 8 times more active than levofloxacin again *S. pneumoniae*, including

strains highly resistant to penicillins. MRSA and VREF are generally resistant to moxifloxacin.

▓ Pharmacokinetics

Quinolones are well absorbed when taken orally, with the exception of norfloxacin, and are widely distributed to tissues and fluids such as saliva, nasal and bronchial secretions, sputum, bile, lymph, and peritoneal fluid (Table 27-12). The majority of quinolones is biotransformed in the liver and eliminated unchanged by the kidneys. A small percentage of lomefloxacin is eliminated unchanged in the feces.

▓ Adverse Effects and Contraindications

Common adverse effects of quinolones include nausea, vomiting, diarrhea, abdominal pain, and restlessness. An unpleasant taste, decreased appetite, dry mouth, and photophobia have been reported. The most serious adverse effects include seizures and bone and cartilage toxicities (e.g., tendon rupture), but these are rarely noted. However, until further studies are conducted, it seems prudent to avoid this drug in children whose skeletal growth is incomplete. Hypersensitivity is uncommon, but anaphylaxis has occurred. Superinfections such as vaginitis have developed from *Candida* overgrowth with long-term use of quinolones. Crystalluria has been reported with large doses.

Quinolones are contraindicated for use in patients with hypersensitivity. Cross-allergenicity among quinolone drugs may occur. Do not use these drugs during pregnancy or lactation, or in persons under the age of 18 years. Use caution when using quinolones in patients with underlying CNS pathology (seizures have been reported in patients with a history of seizures) and renal impairment (quinolones are substantially eliminated by the kidneys). Older adults and dialysis patients are at greater risk for tendon rupture.

▓ Drug Interactions

There are several drugs that interact with quinolones, some with significant consequences. Dangerous arrhythmias have appeared when quinolones are administered concurrently with class IA and III antiarrhythmic drugs such as disopyramide and amiodarone. Quinolones interfere with the biotransformation of caffeine, warfarin, and theophylline because of effects on CYP450 enzymes. The serum

PHARMACOKINETICS
TABLE 27-12 Quinolones

Drug	Route	Onset	Peak	Duration	PB (%)	t½	BioA (%)
ciprofloxacin	IV	Immed	End of inf	12 hr	UA	3–4.8 hr	100
	PO	1 hr	1–2.3 hr	12 hr	UA	3–4.8 hr	UA
gemifloxacin	PO	UA	30 min–2 hr	UA	60–70	4–12 hr	71
lomefloxacin	PO	Rapid	UA	UA	10	8 hr	95–98
levofloxacin	PO	Rapid	1–2 hr	UA	24–38	6–8 hr	99
moxifloxacin	PO	Rapid	72 hr	UA	30–50	10–13 hr	90
	IV	Immed	End of inf	UA	30–50	12.2–17 hr	100
norfloxacin	PO	Rapid	2–3 hr	12 hr	10–15	6.5 hr	30–40
ofloxacin	PO	Rapid	1–2 hr	12 hr	20–25	5–7 hr	89
	IV	Immed	End of inf	12 hr	20–25	5–7 hr	100
sparfloxacin	PO	Rapid	3–6 hr	24 hr	45	20 hr	92

BioA, Bioavailability; *immed*, immediate; *inf*, infection; *IV*, intravenous; *PB*, protein binding; *PO*, by mouth; *t½*, half-life; *UA*, unavailable.

IMMUNE

concentration of these drugs is thus increased, resulting in possible toxicity (see Table 27-2).

Dosage Regimens

Adjust dosages in patients with creatinine clearance values below 30 mL/min. Dosage recommendations are identified in Table 27-13.

Lab Considerations

Quinolone use leads infrequently to some lab abnormalities. Eosinophilia, leukopenia, and elevated ALT, AST, BUN, and serum creatinine concentrations may occur after use, but are all reversible with discontinuation of the drug.

Macrolides

◆ azithromycin (Zithromax); ◆ Zithromax
◆ clarithromycin (Biaxin, Biaxin XL); ◆ Biaxin, Biaxin XL
◆ dirithromycin (Dynabec)
◆ erythromycin base (E-Base, E-Mycin, EryC, Ery-Tab); ◆ Erybid, Erythromid
◆ erythromycin ethylsuccinate (E.E.S., Ery-Ped); ◆ Eryc
◆ erythromycin lactobionate (Erythrocin)
◆ erythromycin stearate (Erythrocin Stearate); ◆ Apo-Erythro-S, Novo-Rythro

Indications

The macrolides are a large class of antibiotics that first became available in the 1950s with the introduction of erythromycin. There are four primary macrolide antibiotics in the United States: azithromycin, clarithromycin, dirithromycin, and erythromycin. Macrolides are indicated for susceptible infections located in the upper and lower respiratory tract, the skin, and soft tissue; pertussis; diphtheria; intestinal amebiasis; pelvic inflammatory disease; nongonococcal urethritis; syphilis; legionnaires' disease; and rheumatic fever. Clarithromycin, used in combination with the proton pump inhibitor omeprazole, has been approved for treatment of active ulcers associated with *H. pylori.*

Macrolides are often used as alternatives for patients with allergies to beta-lactam antibiotics and are commonly used for dental prophylaxis. Erythromycin formulations are used less often today because of microbial resistance and the development of newer macrolides. Ophthalmic and topical formulations of macrolides are discussed in Chapters 61 and 63, respectively.

Pharmacodynamics

Macrolides are bacteriostatic; however, in high enough concentrations they may be bactericidal to some bacteria.

Macrolides are thought to inhibit protein synthesis by penetrating the wall of sensitive bacteria. They reversibly bind to the 50S ribosomal subunit to inhibit polypeptide chain formation. The ribosomal binding fails to occur in resistant bacteria. Bacteria become more and more resistant to azithromycin because of its long half-life and misuse by health care providers and patients alike.

Macrolides are effective against *S. pyogenes* (group A beta hemolytic streptococci) and *H. influenzae.* They are unique in that they are particularly effective against several bacteria that reproduce inside host cells instead of in the blood stream or interstitial spaces. Examples of such bacteria include *N. gonorrhea* (gonorrhea), *Legionella pneumophila* (legionnaires' disease); and *Campylobacter jejuni. T. pallidum* (syphilis) and Lyme disease are also susceptible to macrolides, as are *M. pneumoniae* and *C. trachomatis* (chlamydia) organisms.

Azithromycin and clarithromycin are also active against the atypical mycobacteria that cause *M. avium* complex disease. This disease is an opportunistic infection that occurs primarily in people with HIV infection.

Outside of its antibiotic actions, erythromycin stimulates smooth muscle and GI motility. This action is beneficial in increasing GI motility in conditions such as the gastroparesis of diabetes. It has also been used with some success to facilitate the passage of feeding tubes from the stomach into the small bowel.

Pharmacokinetics

Erythromycin base and stearate formulations are susceptible to inactivation by gastric acid. To avoid this problem, enteric coating has been added and alterations made to the chemical structure of the estolate and ethylsuccinate formulations. Macrolides are widely distributed to most body tissues and fluids, except the brain and CSF. Penetration into the prostate gland is approximately 40% of the simultaneous serum concentration. Drug levels in bronchial secretions and middle ear and sinus fluids reach in excess of the inhibitory concentrations of several pathogens causing community-acquired pneumonias, otitis media, or acute sinusitis. The drugs cross the placental membranes, attaining fetal plasma concentrations 20% of that of maternal circulation. Erythromycin concentrates in the liver and is eliminated mainly via the bile. Some of the drug is also eliminated in urine.

Clarithromycin and azithromycin are well absorbed from the GI tract and are not inactivated by gastric acids, although food decreases the absorption of azithromycin by as much as 40% to 50%; therefore the drug is usually administered at least

DOSAGE
TABLE 27-13 Quinolones

Drug	Dosage*	Implications
ciprofloxacin	*Adult:* 250–750 mg PO every 12 hr –or– 200–400 mg IV every 12 hr	Fluid intake should be at least 2000–3000 mL/day to minimize crystalluria.
gemifloxacin	*Adult:* 320 mg PO once daily	No renal or hepatic dosing considerations required.
levofloxacin	*Adult:* 250–500 mg PO or IV once daily	Much like sparfloxacin
lomefloxacin	*Adult:* 400 mg PO once daily.	Much like ciprofloxacin
moxifloxacin	*Adult:* 400 mg PO or IV once daily	Use IV formulation for complicated abdominal infections.
norfloxacin	*Adult:* 400 mg PO twice daily	Used only for UTI and uncomplicated GC.
ofloxacin	*Adult:* 200–400 mg PO or IV every 12 hr	Much like ciprofloxacin. Used for UTI and uncomplicated GC.
sparfloxacin	*Adult:* 400 mg PO initially, then 200 mg PO daily	Fluid intake should be at least 1500–2000 mL/day to prevent crystalluria.

*Quinolones not usually recommended for children because of risk of tendon damage.
GC, Gonorrhea; *IV,* intravenous (route); *PO,* by mouth; *UTI,* urinary tract infection.

1 hour before or 2 hours after a meal. Clarithromycin is widely distributed, with high concentrations being deposited in the nasal mucosa, the tonsils, and the lungs. Serum concentrations are relatively low for azithromycin, but both drugs penetrate polymorphonuclear leukocytes and macrophages. Tissue concentrations last for days. The half-life of azithromycin is much longer than that of erythromycin or clarithromycin. About 20% of clarithromycin is eliminated unchanged in the urine. Azithromycin is hepatically biotransformed, with only 6% of the dose recovered unchanged in the urine (Table 27-14). Dirithromycin is eliminated primarily in bile.

Adverse Effects and Contraindications

The most common adverse effects of macrolides include dose-related abdominal pain and cramping, nausea, vomiting, diarrhea, stomatitis, flatulence, anorexia, heartburn, and pruritus ani. A reversible, mild acute pancreatitis has been noted. Other adverse effects of erythromycin include palpitations, chest pain, headache, vertigo, somnolence, tinnitus, and bilateral hearing loss. Hearing loss in a susceptible patient develops 36 hours to 1 week following IV administration, but it is reversible in 24 hours to 2 weeks after the drug is discontinued. Recovery time is not dose related.

Most GI adverse effects seem less of a problem with azithromycin or clarithromycin, but they can still occur. Adverse effects unrelated to dosage include hypersensitivity reactions (e.g., skin rash, drug fever, eosinophilia) and hepatotoxicity (e.g., cholestatic jaundice). Hepatotoxicity occurs with the estolate and ethylsuccinate forms of erythromycin, and thus these formulations are used less often.

The only usual contraindication to macrolide use is hypersensitivity. Use them cautiously in patients with impaired liver function.

Drug Interactions

Table 27-2 lists drug interactions of selected macrolide drugs. Two properties of macrolides are the source of drug interactions: they are highly protein bound and biotransformed in the liver. Competition for albumin-binding sites results in additional active, free drug in the circulation. Macrolides inhibit the biotransformation of other drugs by CYP450 enzymes. Concomitant use of other ototoxic drugs increases the potential for ototoxicity. Relatively few studies examining other macrolide-drug interactions are available.

Dosage Regimen

The dosage regimen for macrolides depends on the type of infection (Table 27-15). Erythromycin is available in oral and parenteral formulations. Parenteral formulations of erythromycin are reserved for severe infections but are rarely used.

PHARMACOKINETICS
TABLE 27-14 Macrolides

Drug	Route	Onset	Peak	Duration	PB (%)	t½	BioA (%)
azithromycin	PO	Variable	2.5 hr	24 hr	7–50	25–68 hr	37
clarithromycin	PO	Variable	2–4 hr	6–8 hr	65–75	3–7 hr; 5–7 hr*	55
dirithromycin	PO	Variable	2–4 hr	6–8 hr	15–30	16–65 hr	10
erythromycin	PO	1 hr	1–4 hr	UA	70–90	1.4–2 hr	60

*Clarithromycin's half-life and that of its metabolites, respectively.
BioA, Bioavailability; *PB*, protein binding; *PO*, by mouth; *t½*, half-life; *UA*, unavailable.

DOSAGE
TABLE 27–15 Macrolides

Drug	Dosage	Implications
azithromycin	*Adult: Respiratory and skin infections:* 500 mg PO first day, then 250 mg PO daily for 4 more days *Nongonococcal urethritis or cervicitis:* *Adult:* 1 gram PO single dose *Child >6 mo to 2 yr: Acute otitis media:* 10 mg/kg PO as single dose on first day, then 5 mg/kg PO once daily for 4 days *Child >2 yr: Pharyngitis, Tonsillitis:* 12 mg/kg PO once daily for 5 days –or– 7.5 mg/kg every 12 hr. Not to exceed 500 mg PO every 12 hr	Food decreases absorption by 43%. Take on empty stomach. Increasing reports of bacterial resistance. Consider other options when possible. Also available in IV formulation
clarithromycin	*Adult:* 250–500 mg PO every 12 hr for 7–14 days *Child:* 7.5 mg/kg every12 hr. Not to exceed 500 mg every12 hr	May be used in combination with omeprazole (PPI) in the treatment of *Helicobacter pylori* infections
dirithromycin	*Adult:* 500 mg PO daily for 7, 10, or 14 days based on purpose for its use	Safe dosage in children has not been established.
erythromycin base	*Adult:* 250–500 mg PO every 6–12 hr. Max: 4 grams daily in divided doses *Child:* 30–50 mg/kg/day in divided doses every 6–12 hr. For severe infections, may increase to 100 mg/kg/day in divided doses.	Renal dosing regimen required. Available as delayed-release capsules and tablets, and film-coated tablets
erythromycin ethylsuccinate	*Adult:* 400 mg PO every 6 hr. Max: 4 grams/day *Child:* Depends on reason for use	Seldom used because of risk of hepatotoxicity. Renal dosing regimen required.
erythromycin lactobionate	*Adult and Child:* 15–20 mg/kg/day IV in divided doses. For severe infections, up to 4 grams PO daily	Renal dosing regimen required.
erythromycin stearate	*Adult:* 250 mg PO every 6 hr –or– 500 mg PO every 12 hr. For severe infections, up to 4 grams PO daily	Renal dosing regimen required.

IV, Intravenous (route); *PO*, by mouth.

▒ Lab Considerations

Macrolides may cause several altered test results. Elevations of AST, ALT, and alkaline phosphatase concentrations may be seen. Readings of catecholamines, 17-hydroxycorticosteroids, and 17-ketosteroids can be falsely elevated. Clarithromycin also alters liver function tests but rarely causes elevated PT or INR, BUN, or serum creatinine levels. It may occasionally cause a decrease in the number of WBCs. In addition, azithromycin may cause a decreased platelet count. Serum albumin, chloride, hematocrit, hemoglobin, neutrophils, platelet counts, and total protein levels may be decreased in the presence of dirithromycin. Dirithromycin can cause elevation of alkaline phosphatase, ALT, AST, bands, basophils, total bilirubin, creatinine, leukocytes, monocytes, and uric acid levels.

Carbepenems

- ◆ ertapenem (Invanz)
- ◆ imipenem-cilastatin (Primaxin); ♣ Primaxin
- ◆ meropenem (Merrem)

▒ Indications

Ertapenem is used to treat moderate to severe intraabdominal infections, community-acquired pneumonia, complicated urinary tract infections, acute pelvic infections, and complicated skin and soft tissue infections for patients with diabetes ("the diabetic foot").

The primary use of imipenem-cilastatin is the treatment of infections caused by organisms that are resistant to other drugs.

Meropenem has a broad spectrum of activity and may be used as empirical monotherapy before culture results are available. It is used most often in the treatment of intraabdominal infections and bacterial meningitis in children older than 3 years of age. It has been used for hospital-acquired pneumonia and febrile neutropenia, although the drug is not approved by the FDA for these uses.

▒ Pharmacodynamics

Ertapenem penetrates bacterial organisms to inhibit cell wall synthesis. It is efficacious against methicillin-susceptible isolates of *S. aureus, S. agalactiae,* penicillin-susceptible isolates of *S. pneumoniae, S. pyogenes, E. coli,* beta-lactamase–negative isolates of *H. influenzae, K. pneumoniae, Moraxella catarrhalis, P. mirabilis, B. fragilis, Bacteroides* species, *Clostridium clostridioforme* and others.

Imipenem-cilastatin has the broadest antibacterial action of any beta-lactam antibiotic and is extremely effective against staphylococci and streptococci, with variable activity against *enterococci,* and *Proteus, Enterobacter, Klebsiella, Serratia,* and *Pseudomonas* species. In addition, it maintains activity against *H. influenzae, N. meningitides, N. gonorrhoeae, B. fragilis, Peptostreptococcus,* and *Fusobacterium.* It is not effective against MRSA.

Imipenem has an unusual problem: after imipenem is removed from the circulation by glomerular filtration and secreted, it is biotransformed by a renal peptidase that is found on the brush border of the proximal renal tubules. The metabolites are toxic. To overcome this problem, a specific peptidase inhibitor, cilastin, was synthesized. Cilastin totally blocks the biotransformation of imipenem in the kidney, thus blocking toxicity. Cilastin has virtually no antibacterial activity of its own, but by inhibiting the enzyme

activity; the amount of bacterially active imipenem eliminated in the urine is markedly increased, enabling imipenem to be used in urinary tract infections. The compounded drug became the combination imipenem-cilastatin.

Meropenem is reported to be effective against penicillin-susceptible staphylococci and *S. pneumoniae,* most gram-negative aerobes *(E. coli, H. influenzae, Klebsiella pneumoniae, Pseudomonas),* and some anaerobes including *B. fragilis.*

▒ Pharmacokinetics

Ertapenem is almost completely absorbed following IM administration but can also be given intravenously. The drug is widely distributed to body tissues and is ordinarily eliminated in the urine, with smaller amounts eliminated in feces.

Imipenem-cilastatin is not absorbed by mouth and thus is only available for IV or IM use. The drug is well distributed to most tissues and body fluids, and penetrates inflamed meninges. Approximately 50% of a dose is eliminated by the kidneys via glomerular filtration, 25% by tubular secretion, and 25% by nonrenal routes. The pharmacokinetics, drug interactions, and dosage regimens are noted in Tables 27-2, 27-16, and 27-17, respectively.

Meropenem is widely distributed to body tissues and fluids, entering the CSF in bactericidal levels when the meninges are inflamed. Three fourths of the drug is eliminated unchanged through the kidneys, with the remaining drug eliminated as an inactive metabolite. Pharmacokinetics, drug interactions, and dosage regimens are noted in Tables 27-2, 27-16, and 27-17, respectively.

▒ Adverse Effects and Contraindications

Nausea, vomiting, and diarrhea are the most common adverse effects of ertapenem. A small percentage of patients note abdominal pain, vomiting, constipation, peripheral edema, and fever. Dizziness, cough, oral candidiasis, anxiety, tachycardia, and IV-site phlebitis are rare. Pseudomembranous colitis ranging in severity from mild to serious has been reported. Superinfections are possible.

Patients should have a neurologic evaluation and be started on another antiepileptic drug if focal tremors, myoclonus, or seizures occur. Reexamine the dosage of ertapenem to determine whether it should be decreased or discontinued. Serious and occasionally fatal anaphylactic reactions may occur in patients taking ertapenem who also have a history of sensitivity to multiple allergens, particularly the beta-lactam antibiotics.

Ertapenem is contraindicated for use in patients with known hypersensitivity to any component of this product or to other drugs in the same class or in patients who have demonstrated anaphylactic reactions to beta-lactams. Patients with an allergy to lidocaine should avoid ertapenem; lidocaine is used as the diluent for the IM formulation. It is a pregnancy category B drug.

Adverse effects of imipenem-cilastatin are the same as those occurring with other beta-lactam antibiotics. Patients allergic to penicillins should be considered to be allergic to imipenem-cilastatin. Infrequent reactions have included drug fever, urticaria, pruritus, and other rashes. Seizures have been noted in 1.5% of patients and appear to be more common in older adults with renal insufficiency and in patients with head injury, intracranial neoplasm, or a history of seizures or alcohol abuse. The most common adverse effects include nausea,

PHARMACOKINETICS
TABLE 27-16 Miscellaneous Antibiotics

Drug	Route	Onset	Peak	Duration	PB (%)	t½	BioA (%)
aztreonam	IM	Rapid	60 min	6–12 hr	56–60	1.5–2.2 hr	UA
	IV	Immed	End of inf	6–12 hr	56–60	1.5–2.2 hr	100
clindamycin	PO	Rapid	1.5–2 hr	UA	93	2–3 hr	>90
	IM	Rapid	90 min	UA	93	2–3 hr	0
	IV	Immed	End of inf	UA	93	2–3 hr	100
chloramphenicol	PO	15 min	1–3 hr	UA	60	1.5–3.5 hr	UA
	IV	Immed	End of inf	UA	60	1.5–3.5 hr	100
ertapenem	IM, IV	Rapid	2.3 hr	UA	85–95	2.5–4 hr	90
imipenem-cilastatin	IM	Rapid	UA	UA	20	1–1.3 hr	UA
	IV	Immed	30–60 min	UA	20	1–1.3 hr	100
linezolid	PO, IV	Rapid	1–2 hr	UA	31	11.6 hr	100
meropenem	IV	Immed	End of inf	8 hr	2	1 hr	100
quinupristin-dalfopristin	IV	Immed	End of inf	9–10 hr	50	0.85 hr; 0.7 hr*	100
telithromycin	PO	Rapid	1 hr	UA	60–70	10 hr	57
vancomycin	PO	UA	1 hr	To 12 hr	52–56	4–6 hr	< 1
	IV	Immed	End of inf	To 12 hr	52–56	4–6 hr	100

*Terminal half-life of quinupristin and dalfopristin, respectively.
BioA, Bioavailability; *immed*, immediate; *inf*, infection; *IM*, intramuscular; *IV*, intravenous; *PB*, protein binding; *PO*, by mouth; *t½*, half-life; *UA*, unavailable.

DOSAGE
TABLE 27-17 Miscellaneous Antibiotics

Drug	Dosage	Implications
aztreonam	*Adult:* 0.5–2 grams IM or IV every 8–12 hr. *Serious infections:* 2 grams IM or IV every 6–8 hr	Monobactam. Warn patient that drug may cause taste alteration or superinfection.
clindamycin	*Adult:* 150–450 mg PO every 6–8 hr *–or–* 300–900 mg IM or IV in 2–4 divided doses. Max: 4.8 gram/day IV. *Child >10 kg:* 8–25 mg/kg/day PO in divided doses every 6–8 hr	Single IM doses over 600 mg are not recommended.
chloramphenicol	*Adult:* 50–100 mg/kg PO or IV in 4 divided doses every 6 hr. *Child and Full-Term Infants >2 wk:* 50 mg/kg/day PO in 3–4 divided doses every 6–8 hr	Therapeutic level: 10–25 mcg/mL. Concentrations over 25 mcg/mL increase risk of reversible BMD and gray baby syndrome. Monitor serum drug levels weekly for toxicity.
ertapenem	*Adult:* 1 gram IM daily. *Child 3 mo–12 yr:* 15–20 mg/kg twice daily IM or IV	Carbapenem. Do not use diluents containing dextrose.
imipenem-cilastatin	*Adult:* 2–4 grams IV daily in divided doses every 6 hr *–or–* 500–750 mg IM every 12 hr (max dose 4 grams/day)	Carbapenem. Renal dosing considerations required. Cross-sensitivity with cephalosporins
linezolid	*Adult:* 400–600 mg PO every 12 hr *–or–* 600 mg IV every 12 hr	Newest in oxazolidinone class. Dosage depends on reason for use.
meropenem	*Adult:* 1 gram IV every 8 hr as bolus or infusion. *Child >3 mo:* 20–40 mg/kg IV every 8 hr. Max: 2 grams every 8 hr	Renal dosing considerations required.
quinupristin-dalfopristin	*Adults: VREF:* 7.5 mg/kg IV every 8 hr. *Skin:* 7.5 mg/kg IV every 12 hr	PICC line and infusion pump recommended.
telithromycin	*Adult:* 800 mg PO daily	Renal dosing considerations required.
vancomycin	*Adult:* 500 mg–1 gram IV every 12 hr over 60–90 min. *Child:* 40 mg/kg/day in divided doses every 6–12 hr	IV bolus or rapid IV administration increases risk for thrombophlebitis, hypotension, and *red-neck syndrome.*

BMD, Bone marrow depression; *IM*, intramuscular; *IV*, intravenous; *PICC*, peripherally-inserted central catheters; *VREF*, vancomycin-resistant *Enterococcus faecalis*.

vomiting, and diarrhea. Hypotension may or may not occur; it is unpredictable and may occur inconsistently in the same patient. If it does occur, slowing the infusion may be the only intervention necessary. It is a pregnancy category C drug.

The most common adverse effects of meropenem have not yet been identified, although there is evidence that the drug may cause nausea, constipation, diarrhea, glossitis (children only), rash, pruritus, dizziness, and headache. Pseudomembranous colitis, apnea, and seizures are the most serious adverse effects to be identified to date.

◗ Drug Interactions
Probenecid reduces renal elimination of ertapenem and meropenem, and therefore they should not be used concurrently. There are no known drug interactions with imipenem-cilastatin.

◗ Dosage Considerations
Although the dosage recommendations for ertapenem are similar, the duration of therapy varies from 5 to 14 days. Dosages of imipenem-cilastatin and meropenem vary depending on the reason for use, the patient's age, and the presence of renal impairment.

◗ Lab Considerations
Ertapenem can reduce the hemoglobin, hematocrit, platelet count, and serum potassium values and may increase AST, ALT, and alkaline phosphatase.

Imipenem-cilastatin increases the AST, ALT, alkaline phosphatase, LDH, bilirubin, BUN, and creatinine values, and decreases hemoglobin and hematocrit values.

Meropenem increases the AST, ALT, alkaline phosphatase, LDH, bilirubin, BUN, and creatinine values, and may

IMMUNE

decrease hemoglobin, hematocrit, and serum potassium levels. Meropenem may cause positive results on a direct or indirect Coombs' test.

Miscellaneous Antibiotics

Aztreonam

Aztreonam (Azactam) is a monobactam, the only drug in its class, with activity against aerobic gram-negative rods (e.g., *E. coli, K. pneumoniae, Proteus* species, *Enterobacter* species, *P. aeruginosa*). It is effective against *N. gonorrhoeae* and *H. influenzae* but has no activity against anaerobic or gram-positive organisms. Aztreonam is used to eliminate urinary tract infections, lower respiratory tract infections, septicemia, and abdominal and gynecologic infections caused by susceptible organisms. Its ability to preserve normal gram-positive and anaerobic flora may be an advantage over most other antibiotic drugs.

Aztreonam has the same adverse effects profile as that of penicillins and cephalosporins. Cross-allergenicity with other beta-lactam drugs is minimal to nonexistent. Seizures are the most serious adverse effect.

Aztreonam is rapidly distributed following administration, with penetration to CSF in patients with inflammation of the blood-brain barrier (e.g., meningitis). Small amounts of the drug are biotransformed in the liver, with 70% to 80% of the drug eliminated unchanged in the urine. The pharmacokinetics, drug interactions, and dosage regimens of aztreonam are noted in Tables 27-16 and 27-17.

Clindamycin

Clindamycin (Cleocin; ✦ Cleocin) has limited uses because of its potential to cause severe antibiotic-associated colitis. It is indicated only for gram-positive anaerobic infections located outside the CNS. Clindamycin is indicated for the treatment of serious respiratory infections (e.g., empyema, pneumonia, lung abscess), bacterial endocarditis, toxoplasmosis, acne, serious skin and soft tissue infections, septicemia, intraabdominal infections, and infections of the female pelvis and genital tract (e.g., endometritis, pelvic cellulitis, nongonococcal tuboovarian abscess, pelvic inflammatory disease, bacterial vaginosis). Clindamycin is also used as prophylaxis against bacterial endocarditis or in patients who are allergic to penicillin or do not tolerate erythromycin. Clindamycin is also used in patients who are having dental procedures or minor respiratory tract surgery.

Susceptible organisms include *B. fragilis, Fusobacterium, C. perfringens,* and anaerobic streptococci. Its actions are usually bacteriostatic, but it may produce bactericidal effects if the target organism is particularly sensitive. Drug resistance is significant with *B. fragilis.*

The most notable adverse effect of clindamycin is antibiotic-associated diarrhea and pseudomembranous colitis. These adverse effects are not unique to clindamycin and are noted with other broad-spectrum antibiotics (e.g., ampicillin, cephalosporins). It alters the normal colonic flora to allow overgrowth of *C. difficile,* which produces a powerful toxin that causes the diarrhea. If a patient receiving clindamycin develops persistent diarrhea, the drug is usually stopped; it may be continued, but only with frequent observation of the patient. A metallic taste may develop from high IV doses of clindamycin. Sensitivity reactions of skin rash, urticaria, pruritus, fever,

hypotension, and contact dermatitis have been reported. A few anaphylactoid reactions have been reported. Superinfection (e.g., *Candida*) is common with clindamycin. Use caution in patients with a history of colitis or renal or hepatic impairment.

Much like erythromycin, clindamycin inhibits bacterial protein synthesis by binding to the 50S ribosomal subunit. Oral administration results in complete absorption, with significant concentrations of the drug found in bile and pleural and peritoneal fluids. However, in the absence of inflammation, penetration of the CSF is poor, and in the presence of common bile duct obstruction, no drug is detected. Clindamycin readily crosses placental membranes. Both the parent drug and its metabolites are eliminated in the bile and the urine. The pharmacokinetics, drug interactions, and dosage regimens are noted in Tables 27-2, 27-16, and 27-17, respectively.

Clindamycin increases bilirubin, alkaline phosphatase, and AST levels, as well as the incidence of transient leukopenia, neutropenia, eosinophilia, thrombocytopenia, and agranulocytosis. Perform periodic liver and renal function tests and blood cell counts.

Chloramphenicol

Chloramphenicol (Chloromycetin) use is limited to treatment of meningitis, bacteremia, and skin, intraabdominal, CNS, and soft tissue infections when less toxic drugs cannot be used. It is a broad-spectrum drug with activity against meningococcal and pneumococcal infections; in addition, it is used to treat *H. influenzae* meningitis in penicillin-allergic patients, anaerobic brain abscess, *B. fragilis* infections, rickettsial infections, brucellosis when tetracyclines are contraindicated, and *Klebsiella* and *Haemophilus* infections that are resistant to other drugs. It is the drug of choice only in typhoid fever. It is ineffective against *Pseudomonas* species. Chloramphenicol is rarely used in infections caused by gram-positive organs because of the effectiveness and the low toxicity of penicillins, cephalosporins, and macrolides. Chloramphenicol acts by interfering with microbial protein synthesis.

Chloramphenicol has two major adverse effects: there is an irreversible, idiosyncratic hypersensitivity reaction, and a fatal aplastic anemia reported to occur in 1 of 40,000 courses of therapy. These effects are unpredictable, independent of serum drug levels, and unrelated to dosage, and may occur more often during prolonged therapy or in patients with previous chloramphenicol exposure.

Anemia may appear even with a normal-appearing bone marrow. The anemia is predictable and reversible, correlates with serum drug concentrations, and is a dose-related effect. It can be minimized by maintaining serum drug levels below 25 mcg/mL. Patients with anemia, leukopenia, or thrombocytopenia during therapy are suspected to have a drug-related toxicity. Consider dosage reduction.

Chloramphenicol is well absorbed when taken by mouth, with peak serum concentrations similar to those found after IV administration. It is well distributed to most body tissues and fluids, penetrating ocular fluid and CSF (over 50% of the simultaneous serum concentration) in the presence of inflammation. Chloramphenicol crosses placental membranes and enters breast milk. Repeated administration of high doses of chloramphenicol to neonates leads to accumulation of large amounts of drug and interference with tissue respiration. This effect is known as "gray baby syndrome" and is characterized by abdominal distention, cyanosis, and circulatory collapse. The pharmacokinetics, drug interactions, and dosage regimens are noted in Tables 27-2, 27-16, and 27-17, respectively.

Linezolid

Linezolid (Zyvox; ◆ Zyvox) is the first antibacterial drug in a new class, the oxazolidinones. Approved by the FDA in 2000, it became the first drug to be introduced to the U.S. market in over 40 years for treatment of MRSA; it was also approved to treat infections associated with VREF, including cases with blood stream infection. Hospital- and community-acquired pneumonia, and complicated and uncomplicated skin infections, including cases of MRSA, have been effectively treated with linezolid; it is thought to be as effective as vancomycin for these infections.

Linezolid binds to the 70S subunit site of the RNA ribosome, thus preventing formation of functional ribosomes. It is active against gram-positive infections caused by MRSA, MRSE (in particular, penicillin- and cephalosporin-resistant S. pneumoniae), and vancomycin-susceptible and vancomycin-resistant E. faecium and E. faecalis. Linezolid is bacteriostatic against enterococci and staphylococci. For streptococci, linezolid is bactericidal for the majority of strains. The susceptibility of gram-positive organisms to linezolid is attributed to a lack of gram-positive transmembrane pumps with oxazolidinone specificity. It is thought that linezolid penetrates the E. coli outer membrane but is rapidly excreted from the cell via the family of efflux pumps.

Linezolid is 100% bioavailable after oral or IV dosing and achieves blood levels well in excess of the mean inhibitory concentration-90 (MIC$_{90}$; see later section on Drug Variables) for staphylococci, enterococci, and streptococci. The drug is not cross-resistant with other antibiotic classes. Elimination of most linezolid is primarily nonrenal, with minimal amounts through the feces. Linezolid is not acted upon by CYP450 enzymes, and it does not inhibit the activities of clinically significant CYP isoforms (i.e., 1A2, 2C9, 2C19, 2D6, 2E1, 3A4).

Headache, nausea, vomiting, and diarrhea are the most commonly reported adverse effects of linezolid. Anemia, leukopenia, pancytopenia, and thrombocytopenia have been reported. Affected hematologic parameters return to pretreatment levels once the drug is stopped. Antibiotic-associated colitis may result from the altered bacterial balance in the GI tract. Excessive amounts of tyramine-containing foods (e.g., red wine, aged cheese) may cause severe headache, neck stiffness, diaphoresis, and palpitations in patients receiving linezolid.

Over-the-counter (OTC) cold remedies containing pseudoephedrine, which elevates blood pressure, interact with linezolid. This is particularly a problem in patients with uncontrolled blood pressure. Linezolid tends to lower the platelet count.

Quinupristin-dalfopristin

Quinupristin-dalfopristin (Synercid) is used to treat infections caused by staphylococci and by VREF. It is the first injectable member of a class of antibiotics known as *streptogramins*. The first streptogramin, called pristinamycin, was isolated from an Argentine soil sample. It was difficult to manufacture and for years was outranked by vancomycin. It is not effective against E. faecalis infections.

Use of quinupristin-dalfopristin for VREF-caused life-threatening infections is based upon the drug's ability to clear VREF from the circulation. The two antibiotic components act synergistically to keep bacteria from multiplying, and together they are bactericidal. Dalfopristin inhibits early-phase protein synthesis and quinupristin the later phase of protein synthesis within the bacterial ribosome. The two components are more efficacious than either component used alone.

Elevated drug plasma levels result when quinupristin-dalfopristin is taken concurrently with other drugs biotransformed by the CYP 3A4 enzyme system. The elevated drug level prolongs therapeutic effects but also increases the risk for adverse reactions. A prolonged QTc interval may result when other drugs that interfere with the biotransformation of quinupristin-dalfopristin are taken; the drug itself does not induce QTc prolongation. The pharmacokinetics, drug interactions, and dosage regimens of vancomycin are noted in Tables 27-2, 27-16, and 27-17.

Telithromycin

Telithromycin (Ketek; ◆ Ketek) is the first drug in its class of ketolides. It has been approved for use in mild to moderate acute community-acquired pneumonia caused by S. pneumoniae (including multi–drug-resistant isolates), H. influenzae, M. catarrhalis, Chlamydophila pneumoniae, or M. pneumoniae. Multi–drug-resistant S. pneumoniae includes isolates known as penicillin-resistant S. pneumoniae (PRSP), which are resistant to two or more of the following antibiotics: penicillin, second-generation cephalosporins (e.g., cefuroxime), macrolides, tetracyclines, and trimethoprim-sulfamethoxazole. It acts by blocking protein synthesis to ribosomal receptor sites of bacterial cell walls, causing lysis and death of the bacterial cell.

It is estimated that approximately 50% of the biotransformation of telithromycin is mediated by CYP 3A4, and the remaining 50% is CYP450-independent. It concentrates in WBCs, exceeding plasma concentrations, and is eliminated more slowly from the WBCs than from plasma. It is minimally eliminated in the feces and the urine.

The adverse effects of telithromycin limit its use. These include hepatotoxicity and severe hypersensitivity reactions; atrial arrhythmias are rare. Superinfections, particularly pseudomembranous colitis, may result from altered bacterial balance. It is contraindicated for use in patients with allergy to its ingredients or to macrolide antibiotics. It is a pregnancy category C drug. It is unknown if the drug is distributed to breast milk. The pharmacokinetics, drug interactions, and dosage regimens are noted in Tables 27-2, 27-16, and 27-17, respectively.

Vancomycin

Vancomycin (Vancocin, Vancoled; ◆ Vancocin) is a narrow-spectrum bactericidal drug; its use has increased because of the development of MRSA and MRSE, and endocarditis caused by Streptococcus viridans (in patients allergic to, or with infections resistant to, penicillins or cephalosporins), or E. faecalis (with an aminoglycoside). Vancomycin is also indicated in the treatment of rickettsial, chlamydial, mycoplasmal, gonorrheal, and spirochetal infections. It is also active against gram-positive bacteria such as streptococci, staphylococci, pneumococci, enterococci, and clostridia.

IMMUNE

Vancomycin acts in both a bactericidal and bacteriostatic manner, depending on dosage. It enters the CSF only in the presence of inflammation. Approximately 90% of an IV dose is eliminated by the kidneys. Eosinophilia and leukopenia appear in transient fashion with use of vancomycin.

Treatment options for infections caused by such organisms as vancomycin is often used for (i.e., MRSA, MRSE, and VREF) are very limited. Because of vancomycin's widespread use, VREF is encountered more often, particularly in critical care units. Patients colonized with VREF remain so for prolonged periods. **To reduce the spread of VREF, the Centers for Disease Control (CDC) recommend limiting the use of vancomycin** to the following:

- Serious infections caused by beta-lactam–resistant gram-positive microorganisms
- Infections caused by gram-positive microorganisms in patients who have serious allergies to beta-lactam antibiotics
- Antibiotic-associated colitis that is unresponsive to metronidazole therapy or that is potentially life-threatening
- Prophylaxis following certain procedures in patients at high risk for endocarditis
- Prophylaxis for major surgical procedures involving implantation of prosthetic materials or devices (e.g., cardiac and vascular procedures, total hip replacement) where there is a high rate of MRSA or methicillin-resistant *S. epidermidis* infections. A single dose of vancomycin administered immediately before surgery is sufficient unless the procedure lasts over 6 hours, in which case the dose should be repeated. Prophylaxis should be discontinued after a maximum of two doses.

Vancomycin can cause serious adverse effects such as ototoxicity, nephrotoxicity, hypersensitivity reactions, anaphylaxis, and superinfections. Red-neck or red-man syndrome is unique to vancomycin and is related to rapid infusion of large doses. It is characterized by fever, chills, paresthesias, and erythema at the base of the neck and the upper back. It may be followed by hypotension. It usually begins 10 minutes after the start of the infusion and resolves 15 to 20 minutes after the infusion is stopped. Patients receiving IV vancomycin may also develop thrombophlebitis, neutropenia, and thrombocytopenia. The pharmacokinetics, drug interactions, and dosage regimens of vancomycin are noted in Tables 27-2, 27-16, and 27-17.

CLINICAL REASONING

Treatmenat Objectives

The objectives of antibiotic therapy are to ameliorate the signs and symptoms of infection, prevent sepsis and death, and prevent complications associated with therapy. Achievement of the treatment objectives is promoted by accurate diagnosis, accurate administration of drug therapy, and close monitoring for toxicities.

Treatment Options

When and what to prescribe, and when not to, are decisions based on clinical evidence of infection. The evidence may be, for example, cellulitis or pus for soft tissue infections; frequency and dysuria for cystitis; or fever, rigors, tachycardia, or hypotension. Isolation of an organism without signs and symptoms of an infection usually represents colonization rather than infection and does not necessitate treatment—in other words: no symptoms, no treatment.

The first rule of antibiotic therapy is to buy time; that is, keep the patient stable and/or alive until the etiology and antibacterial susceptibility of the invading bacteria is known, thereby permitting precisely targeted treatment. Until that point, there is an important distinction to be made, and the decision whether or not to begin empiric therapy depends on its outcome: (1) Can the patient be considered a "diagnostic dilemma"? In this case, the health care provider awaits culture results before prescribing antibiotics. (2) Alternatively, does the patient have a "therapeutic emergency" whereby antibiotics would be administered empirically? Does the patient have an abnormality that increases the risk from an inadequately treated bacteremia—for example, an abnormal heart valve, prosthetic joint, or prosthetic vascular graft? If the answer is yes, the health care provider will begin antibiotics, wait for culture results to return, and then reevaluate the patient and adjust treatment accordingly.

However, whenever possible and before antibiotic therapy is begun, obtain a culture and sensitivity of the target area of infection to identify the specific bacteria. Sensitivity testing indicates which antibiotic will be most effective in killing the specific pathogen. Because 48 to 72 hours are required to obtain results from culture and sensitivity testing, knowledge of additional factors is needed to guide antibiotic selection, including a drug's ability to penetrate infected tissue, toxicity, and cost (see Controversy box).

Because certain pathogens are associated with a specific site of infection, empiric therapy guided by a well-informed guess can often be directed against these organisms. Although a number of antibiotics can be considered, clinical efficacy, adverse effects profile, pharmacokinetic disposition, and cost considerations ultimately guide the choice of therapy. Once a drug has been selected, the dosage must be based on patient size, site of infection, route of elimination, and other factors such as the likelihood of drug resistance.

▥ Patient Variables

The basic question always is, or should be, this: what is the best antibiotic for this patient? To answer the question, the health care provider must have information about patient allergies; any abnormal organ function (e.g., renal, hepatic, bone marrow) and the effects of various antibiotics on those organ systems; the need for bactericidal as opposed to bacteriostatic drugs; what drugs the patient is receiving concurrently and potential drug interactions; and, of course, the severity of the patient's illness.

Adverse effects such as hypersensitivity to prior administration of a specific antibiotic should be foremost in the consideration of available treatment options. Some antibiotics may be administered with more ease if the patient is in the hospital setting, because the patient is accessible for close monitoring (this also applies to drugs that are only available for intravenous administration).

A dosage reduction may be needed for patients with renal insufficiency or failure and must be undertaken with caution. Dosage calculations are usually based on creatinine clearance rates. In general, antibiotic use in patients with renal dysfunction falls into one of the following four categories:

Controversy

Should Health Care Providers Perform Diagnostic Tests on Patients Before Prescribing Antibiotics?

Jonathan J. Wolfe

The availability of antibiotics probably enhanced the reputation of traditional medicine among patients as much as any advance after the introduction of anesthesia. Health care providers who had previously been powerless in the face of infectious disease found a new power. No longer limited to comforting the patient and offering supportive care, they were able to apply remedies that through understandable scientific processes struck at the root cause of illness. The lay public was quick to applaud the accomplishments of antibiotic therapy.

Decades have passed since sulfonamides, penicillins, and other classic antibiotics appeared. Patients and health care providers alike have come to accept antibiotics as commonplace. One result has been unthinking and even irrational use of this class of drugs. Patients frequently demand an antibiotic prescription, even if the underlying cause of discomfort and fever is a viral disease. Health care providers frequently choose to cover the possibility of a bacterial infection by ordering broad-spectrum antibiotics. This may reduce opportunistic infections and return clinic visits.

The hazard is that inappropriate use of antibiotics promotes drug resistance. Bacteria exhibit resistance in several ways. The classic scenario is that susceptible organisms die out, beneficial commensal organisms also die out, and resistant organisms overgrow in the absence of these two classes of bacteria. More threatening is that organisms may, through plasmid transfer, share the genetic basis for drug resistance. When this occurs, bacteria exhibit drug resistance even before exposure to a particular antibiotic. When such strains become established in a health care facility, they exacerbate all the hazards of nosocomial infections.

CLINICAL REASONING

- What is the most common setting in which your patients receive prescriptions for antibiotics?
- When antibiotics are prescribed for prophylaxis, what steps should be taken afterward to ensure that appropriate drug therapy has been used?
- Failure of patients to complete courses of antibiotic therapy may lead to drug resistance. What counseling and follow-up are appropriate to ensure that patients use antibiotics as directed?

- Antibiotics that should not be given unless the infecting organism is sensitive only to a particular drug (e.g., tetracyclines except doxycycline)
- Antibiotics that are not used unless the infection is caused by organisms resistant to safer drugs (e.g., aminoglycosides, carbenicillin, cephalexin)
- Antibiotics requiring dosage reduction (e.g., penicillin G, ampicillin, methicillin, oxacillin, most cephalosporins, trimethoprim-sulfamethoxazole)
- Antibiotics that require little or no dosage adjustment (e.g., cloxacillin, dicloxacillin, nafcillin, erythromycin, doxycycline, clindamycin, chloramphenicol)

Monitoring of toxicities is very important. Many antibiotics increase the risk for hepatotoxicity, nephrotoxicity, and ototoxicity. Therefore, once drug therapy is started, close monitoring is necessary to prevent toxicity from reaching the irreversible stage. Monitoring for nephrotoxicity includes measurement of BUN, serum creatinine levels, evidence of proteinuria and azotemia, and intake and output. Ototoxicity is monitored with audiometric tests. The dosage of antibiotics biotransformed by the liver must be reduced for patients with severe liver disease. Drugs specifically affected include erythromycin, clindamycin, and chloramphenicol.

The cost of antibiotics has risen sharply and presents a hardship to many patients, especially older adults and those who are disadvantaged. In addition, many antibiotics require expensive follow-up testing. Peak and trough testing is necessary with most aminoglycosides to ensure a dosage adequate for therapeutic effectiveness and to avoid drug toxicity. Health care insurance systems are in flux; many payment systems are inadequate or nonexistent, and many patients have a high deductible. The high cost of antibiotics is of major concern (see Case Study).

LIFE-SPAN CONSIDERATIONS

Pregnant and Nursing Women. Antibiotic therapy in perinatal patients should be undertaken carefully owing to the potential for teratogenicity. The general principles of perinatal antibiotic therapy are as follows.

Because of the danger of kernicterus to the neonate, sulfonamides are contraindicated for use during the last 3 months of pregnancy, especially if premature delivery is expected. Sulfonamides also reach levels in breast milk sufficient to cause kernicterus and should not be administered during lactation. Sulfonamides may be prescribed for use during the first two trimesters to treat urinary tract infections.

Penicillins, first- and second-generation cephalosporins, and erythromycins are safe to use during pregnancy in patients who are not allergic. However, there is a paucity of clinical experience with the newer drugs; therefore consider these drugs only when another, better-studied antibiotic cannot be used. Tetracyclines cross placental membranes and are deposited in fetal teeth and bones. An increased incidence of toxicity from tetracycline use during pregnancy is characterized by hepatic necrosis, pancreatitis, renal damage, and in extreme cases, death.

Aminoglycosides are used during pregnancy only when serious gram-negative infections are present. Gentamicin is preferable to tobramycin, amikacin, or netilmicin, because it has been more extensively studied.

As a general guideline, avoid administering antibiotics and all other drugs to women who are breastfeeding.

Children and Adolescents. General principles of antibiotic therapy for children include the following. Penicillins, cephalosporins, and erythromycins are generally considered safe for most age groups but should be used cautiously in neonates because of immature renal function. The safety of some drugs (e.g., imipenem-cilastatin, aztreonam, clarithromycin, azithromycin, ciprofloxacin) has not been established in children younger than 12 years of age.

Aminoglycosides may cause nephrotoxicity and ototoxicity in any patient population, but neonates are at higher risk

IMMUNE

CASE STUDY | Antibiotics—Soft Tissue Infection

ASSESSMENT

History of Present Illness	LM, an 82-year-old white male, comes to ER triage today with a puncture wound on the bottom of his right foot. He was working inside the barn when he stepped on a rusty nail, which penetrated his work boot and the bottom of his foot. The wound did not bleed at the time of injury. The wound is now red, swollen, warm, and painful, and he has had a fever and fatigue. He has been unable to ambulate for 2 days because of the pain. He reports his blood sugars, which are normally in good control, have been elevated since the injury. He is accompanied by a daughter-in-law, who reports he self-treated by soaking his foot in hydrogen peroxide and water twice a day. However, it doesn't appear to be improving, and now he has some "stinky" drainage from the hole where the nail was.
Past Health History	LM has an allergy to penicillin and cephalosporins (anaphylaxis for both). Does not remember when he had a tetanus shot. Diagnosed with type 2 diabetes mellitus 25 years ago and takes Lantus insulin, 25 units twice daily; lisinopril, 20 mg; and lovastatin, 20 mg daily. LM also had an aortic valve replacement 1 month ago and is receiving warfarin therapy. Daughter-in-law reports that LM has consumed large quantities of water his whole life, which makes it difficult to monitor for excessive thirst. He has been urinating more than usual and can't seem to get enough to eat. His degree of adherence with medical therapies is unknown.
Life-Span Considerations	LM may have impaired renal function due to aging process as well as his diabetes. He lives alone on his small ranch, with occasional assistance from two aging sons. One son wants LM to move into his home until his foot heals; the other thinks he should stay and work the farm. LM has limited income, surviving on Social Security and the little money he earns from selling a calf now and then. LM no longer drives and needs assistance for grocery shopping, errands, and medical appointments.
Physical Exam Findings	*Height:* 5′8″. *Weight:* 176 lbs. *BP* 138/88. 100.2°F-92-24. HRRR. BSCTA. Abd soft, round, NT. 4-cm area of induration around puncture wound, distal plantar surface right foot. Area warm, minimal pain with palpation. Small amount of cloudy, yellow, foul-smelling exudate expressed and on dressing. Noticeable pedal edema.
Diagnostic Testing	*WBC:* 20,000. *BUN:* 20 mg/dL. *Creatinine:* 1.3 mg/dL. *CrCl:* 45 mL/min. *FSBS 2 hr after lunch:* 326 mg/dL. *UA:* 2^+ glucose; small amount protein. *HbA1c:* 12%. *ECG:* Sinus rhythm. Wound culture results pending; preliminary report: likely polymicrobial with risk for *Pseudomonas aeruginosa.*

DIAGNOSIS: Diabetes Mellitus with Wound Infection (Foot)

MANAGEMENT

Treatment Objectives	1. Ameliorate signs and symptoms of infection. 2. Prevent complications such as tissue necrosis, local extension of infection, bone destruction, loss of limb, thrombophlebitis. 3. Reduce risk for worsening sepsis. 4. Regain control of diabetes.
Treatment Plan	**Pharmacotherapy** • Stop warfarin. • Begin subcutaneous enoxaparin, 30 mg subcutaneously twice daily. • Continue other currently prescribed medications. • Tetanus immune globulin 0.5 mL IM now • Tetanus and diphtheria toxoid 0.5 mL IM now • Gentamicin sulfate, 80 mg (4 mg/kg) IVPB every 12 hr. Infuse over 60 min using infusion pump. Check peak and trough level with third dose. • Metronidazole, 600 mg (30 mg/kg) day IVPB every 6 hr **Patient Education** 1. Teach purpose for prescribed drugs, adverse effects (e.g., muscle and bone pain), and when to contact health care provider. 2. Importance of wearing medical alert bracelet identifying penicillin-cephalosporin allergy 3. Signs and symptoms of superinfection 4. Importance of adequate fluid intake to minimize risk of crystalluria

Evaluation
1. Monitor peak and trough levels with third dose of gentamicin sulfate.
2. Evaluate for signs and symptoms of worsening infection as well as signs of improvement.
3. Monitor for complications such as tissue necrosis, local extension of infection, bone destruction, and thrombophlebitis.
4. Observe for signs of worsening sepsis or nephrotoxicity, ototoxicity, or neurotoxicity.
5. Evaluate blood sugars as prescribed so as to adjust insulin dosage if needed.

CLINICAL REASONING ANALYSIS

Q1. Why can't he just soak his foot in peroxide or Betadine like he was doing at home? Why does he need IV antibiotics?
A. Think about the organisms he was exposed to in the barn area. He is febrile and has an elevated WBC count, his foot looks awful, and his underlying health problems such as the aortic valve replacement and insulin-dependent diabetes indicates need for hospitalization, IV antibiotics, and an improvement in his diabetes control.

Q2. Tell me again what drug you ordered? It was a combination of something, right?
A. No, I ordered gentamicin sulfate at 4 mg/kg IVPB every 12 hr. Gentamicin sulfate is bactericidal and should cover *P. aeruginosa*, which is often associated with puncture wounds.

Q3. Are you sure you want to order the gentamicin every 12 hours? Why not give it every 8 hours like I have seen with other patients?
A. Did you check the chart for his renal function test results? His creatinine clearance is 45 mL/min. A creatinine clearance of 41 to 60 mL/min makes every 12-hr dosing necessary. If it was between 20 and 40 mL/min, we would administer the drug every 12 hrs. I have also ordered peak and trough levels with the third dose so we can check for therapeutic levels as well as the risk for nephrotoxicity.

Q4. Are there any other antibiotic choices that could be considered? According to my copy of the Sanford Guide, he could have several other drugs. Why didn't you order one of those?
A. For several reasons: traumatic polymicrobic wound infections like his are typically sensitive to ampicillin-sulbactam, ticarcillin-clavulanate, piperacillin-tazobactam, imipenem-cilastatin, or meropenem as first-line drugs. He is allergic to penicillins and cephalosporins, so that eliminates these drugs. Imipenem-cilastatin is a beta-lactam with the possibility of cross-sensitivity, and meropenem is given by IM. The metronidazole I also ordered covers the anaerobic bacteria.

Q5. Will the gentamicin and metronidazole interfere with his warfarin?
A. Yes, they both will. They can raise the PT and INR levels, but we are somewhat limited in what drugs we can use. It seems better to stop the warfarin and perhaps we can use enoxaparin, a low–molecular weight heparin, for anticoagulation while he is on these antibiotics; but we will clarify this change with his cardiologist. We will still watch his PT and INR values closely for the next 3 to 4 days to be sure his levels remain in a safe range.

because of immature renal function. Tetracyclines are contraindicated for use in children younger than 8 years of age because of the adverse effects on bones and teeth.

Older Adults. Many antibiotics are contraindicated for use in older adults, or at least they should be administered with caution; unfortunately, the data in older adults are limited. General principles of antibiotic therapy in the older adult include the following. Penicillins, cephalosporins, and erythromycins are generally considered safe. However, hyperkalemia can develop with large IV doses of penicillin and is more likely to occur in patients with impaired renal function. Although rare, cephalosporins may aggravate existing renal dysfunction, especially when given with other nephrotoxic drugs. Clarithromycin and azithromycin have not been used extensively in older adults but appear to be relatively safe. Dosages of certain antibiotics may have to be reduced in the older adult with declining renal function. Aminoglycosides and tetracyclines are contraindicated for use in the presence of renal dysfunction if less toxic drugs are available. Older adults are at high risk of nephrotoxicity and ototoxicity from aminoglycosides.

▌ Drug Variables
Remember, not all positive cultures necessitate treatment with antibiotics. Consider whether culture results are the result of colonization, contamination, a self-limiting infection, or a true infection. Because there are many classifications of antibiotics, the selection process centers on several variables. Appropriate therapy is based on one of the following:

- *Positive identification of the organism.* Once an antibiotic has been started, cultures are unlikely to contain bacteria in sufficient numbers; even though viable pathogens remain. Avoid contaminating specimens when collecting cultures.
- *Empiric therapy.* In many situations the exact organism causing the infection is unknown. Before culture results are available, the health care provider uses "bacteriologic statistics" (i.e., an awareness of which organism most likely to cause the infection of a particular site) together with knowledge of the local antibiotic resistance patterns.
- *Change of drug therapy.* A change of drug therapy results from knowing culture results. Because bacteria vary in their

susceptibility to antibiotics, it is important that there is a process available for identifying antibiotic susceptibility.

- *The risk for drug toxicity.* Use drug assays with narrow therapeutic indices to estimate the risk for drug toxicity. Antibiotics with narrow therapeutic indices, such as the aminoglycosides and vancomycin, are more likely to cause toxicity than drugs with a wide therapeutic index. Serum drug levels are useful in reducing the risk for toxicity and yet allowing therapeutic levels to be achieved.

There are four important principles that must come into play for an antibiotic to be effective:

- The antibiotic must interact with a specific binding site in order to exert bacteriocidal or bacteriostatic action.
- The greater the drug concentration, the greater the binding on the bacterial organism.
- To be effective, the antibiotic must adhere to the binding site for a long enough period.
- The minimum inhibitory concentration (MIC) must be the lowest concentration of the antibiotic with which the bacteria have come into contact.

OPTIMIZING PHARMACOKINETIC AND PHARMACODYNAMIC PRINCIPLES. The optimizing of antibiotic regimens on the basis of pharmacokinetic and pharmacodynamic principles plays a role in reducing antibiotic resistance and maximizing efficacy (Table 27-18). A greater length of time (T) during which the serum drug concentration remains above the MIC *(time-dependent killing)* of the antibiotic (i.e., higher T/MIC) enhances bacterial eradication with beta-lactams (i.e., penicillins, cephalosporins), carbapenems (i.e., ertapenem, imipenem-cilastatin, meropenem), monobactams (i.e., aztreonam), glycopeptides (e.g., vancomycin), and the oxazolidinone linezolid (Table 27-19). Frequent dosing, prolonged infusion times, or

continuous infusions increase the T/MIC ratio and improve cure rates. In addition, to maximize the bactericidal effects of aminoglycosides, optimize the ratio of maximum drug concentration (C_{max}) to MIC. A C_{max}/MIC ratio above 10:1 using once-daily aminoglycoside dosing (5 to 7 mg/kg) prevents the emergence of resistant bacteria, improves clinical outcomes, and reduces the risk for toxicity. As a general rule, bacteria resistant to a drug in a particular class tend to be equally insensitive to chemically related drugs (i.e., those drugs in the same class). However, they remain sensitive to chemically dissimilar drugs.

DOSING CONSIDERATIONS. An optimum dosing interval for a given antibiotic is calculated as the time needed for most bacteria to be killed plus the length of time the antibiotic effects exist *(postantibiotic effects),* plus the time required for bacterial lag. It must be pointed out that there is no way, in clinical settings, to compute the best possible dosing interval. Nonetheless, it is an important consideration when making decisions among treatment options.

In general, dosage recommendations found in medical and pharmaceutical references are reasonably effective for most infections. Pharmacologic and patient factors are used to modify dosing and dosing intervals, and to evaluate current therapy. Postantibiotic effects continue for several hours after some drugs have been discontinued. With sufficient serum concentrations, bacterial growth does not take place for some time after drug concentrations fall below the MIC.

Peak serum concentrations (C_{max}) are most crucial for bacteriocidal antibiotics. The mean steady-state concentration of antibiotic needed to eradicate an organism regarded as susceptible varies according to the drug and the organism; but in general, the steady-state mean concentration must be at least twice the MIC.

TABLE 27-18 Bacteria Kill

Pharmacodynamic Characteristics	Representative Antibiotics	Goal of Drug Regimen	Parameters Correlating with Clinical Efficacy
Concentration-dependent killing	Aminoglycosides, quinolones, metronidazole	Maximize concentration	Ratio of maximum peak concentration to MIC; ratio of AUC to MIC
Time-dependent killing	Penicillins, cephalosporins, aztreonam	Maximize exposure time	Time above MIC

AUC, Area under the curve; *MIC,* mean inhibitory concentration.

TABLE 27-19 Resistance Mechanisms for Selected Antibiotics

Drug	Class	Target	Mutant, Plasmid	Efflux	Porin	Inactive	Target Alteration
ampicillin	PCN	E	+ / +	√	√	√	√
ceftriaxone	Ceph	E	+ / +	√	√	√	√
chloramphenicol	Misc	R	+ / +	√		√	√
ciprofloxacin	Quin	D	+ / +	√			√
clindamycin	Misc	R	+ / +			√	√
erythromycin	Mac	R	+ / +	√		√	√
gentamicin	Amin	R	+ / +	√		√	√
imipenem	Carb	E	+ / +	√	√	√	
linezolid	Oxaz	R	+ / −				√
quinupristin-dalfopristin	Strept	R	+ / +	√		√	√
telithromycin	Keto	R	+ / +	√		√	√
tetracycline	Tetra	R	+ / +	√		?	√
vancomycin	Misc	E	+ / +				√

Amin, Aminoglycoside; *Carb,* carbapenem; *Ceph,* cephalosporin; *D,* replication; *E,* envelope, *Keto,* ketolide; *Mac,* macrolide; *Misc,* miscellaneous; *Oxaz,* oxazolidinone; *PCN,* penicillin; *Quin,* quinolone; *R,* ribosome; *Strept,* streptogramin; *Tetra,* tetracycline.

Measuring the steady-state trough concentration helps reduce the risk for nephrotoxicity and ototoxicity, for in theory, the antibiotic is more efficacious if the bacteria are allowed to grow at the end of each dosing interval (i.e., during the trough period). However, trough values are only crucial when aminoglycosides and vancomycin are used. Despite the variable pharmacokinetics of antibiotics, most are safe enough in recommended dosages, which achieve serum concentrations that exceed the MIC.

Other considerations to include when choosing an antibiotic are the location of the infection and the offending organism, the spectrum of activity against the organisms, potential drug resistance, potential for hypersensitivity and harm to the patient in light of age or physical state (e.g., health, pregnancy, lactation), and the speed with which the drug's action is needed. The more compromised the patient's immune system, or the more rapid a cure is needed, the greater the serum and tissue concentrations of the antibiotic have to be.

PROPHYLAXIS. The probability of infection without the use of antibiotics, the morbidity, and the cost of complications caused by infection must all be contemplated before establishing a "prophylaxis indicated" status for a procedure. Appropriate timing of antibiotic prophylaxis provides for effective tissue concentrations during a procedure should contamination occur. Give the antibiotic no later than 30 minutes and no longer than 2 hours before surgery. Antibiotic administration should occur approximately 30 minutes before skin incision and should be repeated at 1 to 2 half-lives (e.g., for cefazolin, every 3 to 4 hours).

The drug of choice depends on the organisms most likely to enter the site. The microbiology of the wound is also influenced by the type of contamination, the degree of contamination, and the specific nature of the wound. A first-generation cephalosporin (e.g., cefazolin) is warranted for all procedures in the categories of clean-contaminated, contaminated, or dirty (Table 27-20). Patients with a known allergy to cephalosporins

TABLE 27-20 Classification of Operative Wounds and Risk for Infection

Classification	Criteria	Risk
Clean	Elective, not emergency, nontraumatic, primarily closed; no acute inflammation; no break in technique; respiratory, gastrointestinal, biliary and genitourinary tracts not entered	<2%
Clean-contaminated	Urgent or emergency case that is otherwise clean; elective opening of respiratory, gastrointestinal, biliary, or genitourinary tract with minimal spillage (e.g., appendectomy) not encountering infected urine or bile; minor technique break	<10%
Contaminated	Nonpurulent inflammation; gross spillage from gastrointestinal tract; entry into biliary or genitourinary tract in the presence of infected bile or urine; major break in technique; penetrating trauma <4 hr old; chronic open wounds to be grafted or covered	~20%
Dirty	Purulent inflammation (e.g., abscess); preoperative perforation of respiratory, gastrointestinal, biliary, or genitourinary tract; penetrating trauma >4 hr old	~40%

Data from Cruse, P., and Foord, R. (1980). The epidemiology of wound infection. A 10-year prospective study of 62,939 wounds. *Surgical Clinics of North America, 60,* 27–40.

can be given vancomycin for coverage of *Staphylococcus*, and metronidazole or clindamycin and an aminoglycoside for coverage of anaerobic and gram-negative organisms, respectively. Aztreonam can be used in conjunction with clindamycin but not with metronidazole in the same setting. Quinolones, such as ciprofloxacin, may also be effective for coverage of gram-negative organisms, although there are no data available within the context of prophylaxis (Woods and Dellinger, 1998). In most cases, antibiotic prophylaxis is not given beyond the intraoperative period; however, it is warranted with dirty, traumatic wounds or ruptured viscera.

Patients with a history of congenital or valvular heart disease and those with prosthetic valves are especially susceptible to bacterial endocarditis. Bacterial endocarditis can develop following surgery, dental procedures, or other interventions that may cause bacteria to enter the blood stream. Hence these patients should receive prophylactic antibiotic treatment before undergoing such procedures.

There is evidence that antibiotic prophylaxis reduces the risk of infection in patients with severe neutropenia. However, antibiotic therapy also escalates the risk of infection caused by fungi. By killing off normal flora, whose presence restrains fungal growth, antibiotics encourage fungal invasion. An infectious disease consultation is appropriate for these patients.

MULTIDRUG THERAPY. Failure of initial IV antibiotic therapy in hospital patients with complicated skin and skin structure infections may cost the U.S. health care system more than $800 million each year and results in increased mortality. Patients with an initial antibiotic treatment failure are 3 times more likely to die in the hospital than are patients whose therapy did not fail. In many cases, treatment failure was due to the presence of multiple organisms.

There are four basic situations in which multidrug antibiotic therapy is recommended: (1) an infection that is typically caused by multiple organisms; (2) a serious infection in which a combination of drugs would be synergistic; (3) the likely emergence of drug-resistant organisms; and (4) the presence of a fever or other evidence that the patient is immunosuppressed. However, there are also disadvantages to multidrug therapy. There is an increased risk of allergic and toxic reactions, as well as possible antagonism of antibiotic effects. There is also an increased risk of superinfection; and, not insignificantly, the costs are increased. For these reasons, use multidrug therapy only when clearly warranted.

Patient Education

Teach patients about the drugs they are receiving and the purpose for the drugs. Knowledge is helpful in improving the patient's adherence with the treatment regimen. It is important that patients understand that antibiotics are to be taken as prescribed in regard to doses and frequency, and for the specified time, even though symptoms may abate before the full course of therapy is completed. For example, if an oral antibiotic is prescribed every 12 hours, it should be taken as much as possible every 12 hours, or the drug level of the antibiotic will not be maintained adequately to fight the pathogens. Likewise, if the antibiotic is to be taken every 6 hours, each dose should be taken 6 hours apart, not at the usual 4-hour intervals between breakfast, lunch, dinner, and bedtime. If the serum drug level drops below the MIC because of late dosing or stopping the drug too soon, pathogens have

IMMUNE

an opportunity to increase in virulence or become resistant to the drug.

Advise patients to report any signs or symptoms of allergic response. Some antibiotics initially cause dizziness; thus caution is warranted when driving or operating machinery until response to the drug is known. Advise patients with allergies to antibiotics to wear some form of identification (e.g., MedicAlert). Carrying the identification in a wallet or purse is usually not of help if emergency care is needed.

In addition to common adverse effects, teach patients to report these signs and symptoms: drug-specific adverse effects and toxicities such as blood dyscrasias (e.g., bruising, bleeding), nephrotoxicity (e.g., oliguria, hematuria), and ototoxicity (e.g., tinnitus, dizziness). Advise patients to report severe or persistent GI upset. Evidence of superinfection (e.g., diarrhea, vaginal or anal itching, black and furry appearance of the tongue) should be reported. Superinfection by *Candida* can usually be managed by stopping the antibiotic or by administering an antifungal drug.

Because the effects of hormonally based contraceptives are reduced in combination with many of the antibiotics, advise patients that a second form of birth control is needed during treatment and for up to 2 weeks after completing the antibiotic regimen.

Evaluation

In general, therapeutic response to antibiotic therapy can be checked using clinical criteria alone. Thus the subsidence of

fever, the return of WBC counts to normal limits, the return of the patient's vital signs to normal ranges, and the disappearance of local and systemic signs of infection all reflect an appropriate response. Other variables that help identify treatment effectiveness are an increase in appetite and energy level, a general sense of well-being, and negative culture and sensitivity testing for the offending organism. No further monitoring or interventions are needed in most cases.

Treatment failure may be caused by a number of variables, all of which should be examined before proceeding with additional interventions. Such variables include the following:

- The drug may be unable to reach or concentrate at the site of infection (i.e., poor absorption or distribution to the site of infection; rapid drug elimination; or inactivation of the drug at the infection site)
- The patient may be immunocompromised (e.g., patients with granulocytopenia or AIDS)
- There may be a need for surgical intervention (e.g., an abscess or the presence of necrotic tissue)
- There is bacterial resistance before starting therapy or one that emerges during therapy
- A wrong diagnosis has been made (e.g., the patient may not have an infectious process taking place)
- An error has been made in microbial susceptibility testing

KEY POINTS

- Factors contributing to susceptibility for infection include an individual's general health, age, immune status, nutritional status, hormonal balance, concurrent diseases, living conditions, drug use, hygiene, and sexual practices.
- A culture and sensitivity test determines the specific causative pathogen and drug sensitivities and should be done *before* initiation of antibiotic therapy.
- The objectives of antibiotic therapy include amelioration of signs and symptoms of infection, prevention of sepsis, and prevention of complications.
- Treatment options include several different antibiotic classifications: penicillins, cephalosporins, sulfonamides, tetracyclines, macrolides, aminoglycosides, quinolones, and several miscellaneous drugs.
- When and what to prescribe and when not to are decisions based on clinical evidence of infection. The drug of choice for a particular infection is based on culture and sensitivity reports, severity of the infection, patient allergies, presence of renal or hepatic disease, and life-span considerations.

- Isolation of an organism without signs and symptoms of an infection usually represents colonization rather than infection and does not necessitate treatment—in other words: no symptoms, no treatment.
- Drug resistance develops when bacterial growth resumes and is unaffected by the same concentration of a drug that was originally inhibitory or lethal.
- Prophylaxis is appropriate for patients with a history of congenital or valvular heart disease and those with prosthetic valves or artificial joints.
- Multidrug therapy is warranted when the infection is known to be caused by multiple organisms, when the combination would be synergistic, if emergence of drug-resistant organisms is expected, and when there is fever or other evidence the patient is immunosuppressed.
- Patient teaching and adherence to therapy are vital for successful resolution of infection.
- Evidence of successful antibiotic therapy includes subsidence of fever, normalization of the WBC count, and return of the patient's vital signs to normal; disappearance of local and systemic signs of infection; and an increase in appetite and energy level and a general sense of well-being. Culture and sensitivity testing is negative for the offending organism.

Bibliography

Allington, D., and Rivey, M. (2001). Quinupristin/dalfopristin: A therapeutic review. *Clinical Therapeutics, 23*(1), 24–44.

Bernstein, J., and Meller, M. (2006). Antimicrobial prophylaxis to prevent surgical site infection. *Journal of Bone and Joint Surgery, American Volume, 88*(5), 1149–1150.

Carattoli, A., Miriagou, V., Bertini, A., et al. (2006). Replicon typing of plasmids encoding resistance to newer beta-lactams. *Emerging Infectious Disease, 12*(7), 1145–1148.

Collignon, P., Frederick, J., and Angulo, F. (2006). Fluoroquinolone-resistant *Escherichia coli:* Food for thought–Editorial commentary. *The Journal of Infectious Diseases, 194*(1), 8–10.

Cruse, P., and Foord, R. (1980). The epidemiology of wound infection. A 10-year prospective study of 62,939 wounds. *Surgical Clinics of North America, 60*, 27–40.

Furuno, J., McGregor, J., Harris, A., et al. (2006). Identifying groups at high risk for carriage of antibiotic-resistant bacteria. *Archives of Internal Medicine, 166*(5), 580–585.

Gilbert, D., Moellering, R., Eliopoulos, G., et al. (2007). *The Sanford guide to antimicrobial therapy.* Hyde Park, VT: Antimicrobial Therapy.

Kasbekar, N. (2006). Tigecycline: A new glycylcycline antimicrobial agent. *American Journal of Health-System Pharmacy, 63*(13), 1235–1243.

Kowalski, T., Berbari, E., and Osman, D. (2005). Epidemiology, treatment, and prevention of community-acquired methicillin-resistant *Staphylococcus aureus* infections. *Mayo Clinic Proceedings, 80*(9), 1201–1207.

Manzella, J. (2001). Quinupristin-dalfopristin: A new antibiotic for severe gram-positive infections. *American Family Physician, 64*(11), 1863–1866.

Sherman, M. (2006). An overview of antibiotic resistance. *U.S. Pharmacist, 31*(01), HS24–HS28.

Sivapalasingam, S., Nelson, J., Joyce, K., et al. (2006). High prevalence of antimicrobial resistance among *Shigella* isolates in the United States tested by the National Antimicrobial Resistance Monitoring System from 1999 to 2002. *Antimicrobial Agents and Chemotherapy, 50*(1), 49–54.

The Hospital Infection Control Practices Advisory Committee, Hospital Infections Program, National Center for Infectious Diseases, U.S. Department of Health and Human Services, Public Health Service, Centers for Disease Control and Prevention. (1995). Recommendations for preventing the spread of vancomycin resistance: Recommendations of the hospital infection control practices advisory committee. *American Journal of Infection Control, 239*(2), 87–92.

The Medical Letter. (2006). Treatment of community-associated MRSA infections. *The Medical Letter, 48*(1228), 13–14.

The Medical Letter. (2005). Tigecycline. *The Medical Letter, 47*(1217), 73–74.

The Medical Letter. (2004). Telithromycin (Ketek) for respiratory infections. *The Medical Letter, 46*(1189), 66.

National Institute of Allergy and Infectious Diseases. National Institutes of Health. (2006). The problem of antimicrobial resistance. Available online: www.niaid.nih.gov/factsheets/antimicro.htm. Accessed April 19, 2007.

National Institute of General Medical Sciences. (2006). New strategies take on antibiotic resistance. Available online: www.nigms.nih.gov/News/Results/brief_20050427.htm. Accessed April 19, 2007.

Rubenstein, E., and Vaughan, D. (2005). Tigecycline: A novel new glycylcycline. *Drugs, 65*(10), 1317.

Warters, R., Szmuk, P., Pivalizza, E., et al. (2006). The role of anesthesiologists in the selection and administration of perioperative antibiotics: A survey of the American Association of Clinical Directors. *Anesthesia and Analgesia, 102*(4), 1177–1182.

Wilcox, M., Nathwani, D., and Dryden, M. (2004). Linezolid compared with teicoplanin or the treatment of suspected or proven gram-positive infections. *Journal of Antimicrobial Chemotherapy, 53*(2), 335–344.

Woods, R., and Dellinger, E. (1998). Current guidelines for antibiotic prophylaxis of surgical wounds. *American Family Physician, 57*(11), 2731–2740.

Zirakzadeh, A., and Patel, R. (2006). Vancomycin-resistant enterococci: Colonization, infection, detection, and treatment. *Mayo Clinic Proceedings, 81*(4), 529–536.

IMMUNE

28

Antiviral and Antifungal Drugs

The number of viral and fungal infections occurring worldwide is nearly impossible to accurately measure. Indeed, viruses are the most common cause of acute infections in the United States that do not result in hospitalization (e.g., common cold, influenza, chicken pox, warts, hepatitis). If one takes into account the prominent viral infections found only in other regions of the world (e.g., hemorrhagic fever), the total easily exceeds several billion cases each year. Some infections have very high mortality rates (e.g., acquired immunodeficiency syndrome [AIDS], Ebola), whereas others lead to long-term disability (e.g., neonatal rubella, polio). Current research is focusing on the possible connection of viruses to chronic diseases of unknown cause such as multiple sclerosis, various cancers, and diabetes.

Viruses are infectious particles (i.e., virions) that invade every known cell type. They are not alive, yet they are able to redirect the metabolism of living cells to reproduce viral particles. Viral replication inside a cell usually causes death or loss of function of that cell. Until recently, viruses were thought to be the simplest pathogens producing infection in humans. They are submicroscopic, filterable organisms that rely entirely on host cells for protein synthesis and replication; they are, therefore, obligate intracellular parasites. Their size relegates them to the realm of ultramicroscopic organisms (i.e., an electron microscope is necessary to detect them). For example, more than 2000 bacterial viruses fit into an average bacteria cell, and more than 50 million polioviruses could be accommodated by an average human cell.

Viral illnesses range in severity from upper respiratory infections produced by relatively benign adenoviruses, to the progressive AIDS associated with the human immunodeficiency virus (HIV). While viruses differ greatly in size and shape, infectious outcomes, and specific mechanisms of action, they all rely on susceptible host cells to reproduce. Therefore the formulation of antiviral drugs has proven more complex than the development of antibiotics and antifungals, both of which work by disrupting the pathogen's cell membrane, nuclear division, or nuclear acid synthesis. Instead, antiviral drugs target one of the steps between host cell reception and virion reproduction.

Of the more than 50,000 species of fungi, approximately 50 are generally recognized as being pathogenic in humans. Fungi are organisms that live in soil enriched by decaying nitrogenous matter. Humans become accidental hosts through the inhalation of spores or by introduction into the tissues through trauma. Yet, inhalation alone is not sufficient to produce invasive fungal infection in most hosts—the majority of patients who develop invasive disease are immunocompromised by underlying disease and/or drug therapy. Most fungi exist in a yeast form, round to ovoid cells that may reproduce by budding, or a mold form, a complex of tubular structures that grow by branching or extension. The cell walls of fungi are primarily composed of polysaccharide, which permits cell synthesis even in the presence of antifungal drugs.

The incidence of both mucosal and invasive fungal infections (*Candida* species, *Cryptococcus neoformans*, *Aspergillus* species, and other emerging molds such as *Fusarium, Scedosporium,* and *Rhizopus* species) in immunocompromised patients has increased steadily over the past 2 decades. Several reasons have been proposed for the increase in invasive fungal infections, including the use of broad-spectrum antibiotics, antineoplastic and immunosuppressive drugs, prosthetic devices and grafts, and more aggressive surgery. Apart from organ transplant recipients, individuals with AIDS, and patients hospitalized with severe illnesses, major increases in invasive fungal infections have also been observed in patients with hematologic malignancies who receive antineoplastic therapy and those who undergo bone marrow transplantation. Patients with burns, neutropenia, HIV infection, and pancreatitis are also predisposed to fungal infection.

INTRODUCTION TO VIRUSES

Viruses contain only those parts needed to invade and control a host cell: a core of one or more single- or double-stranded RNA or DNA (but not both), and an external coating. The sum total of the genetic information carried by the virus is known as its *genome*. The external protein coating, also known as a *capsid*, surrounds and protects strands of nucleic acid. The capsid also plays a role in the fusion process between the virions and the host cells. The envelope is the outmost layer of the virion and occurs in some, but not all, viruses. The envelope is made up of lipoproteins containing viral antigens specific for various proteins on the surface of the host cell membranes. Enveloped viruses are more susceptible to harsh environmental conditions compared to nonenveloped viruses. This biochemical specificity, when present, facilitates the virus's attachment process so it can multiply and take control of the host cell's genetic material and regulate the synthesis and assembly of new viruses. HIV operates in this fashion.

In addition to the protein of the capsid, the lipoproteins of envelopes, and the nucleic acids of the core, some viruses also contain enzymes needed for viral replication within the host cell. Examples of these enzymes include the *polymerases* that synthesize DNA and RNA, and the *replicases* that copy RNA. The HIV virus comes equipped with *reverse transcriptase* for synthesizing DNA from RNA. Other viruses completely lack the genes necessary for synthesis of enzymes. However, this deficiency has little consequence, since viruses have adapted to completely take over their host's metabolic resources.

The general phases in the life cycle of a virus are (1) absorption, (2) penetration, (3) uncoating, (4) synthesis, (5) assembly, and (6) release. These events turn the cell into a factory with the sole purpose of making and shedding new viruses, which ultimately results in destruction of the cell. The length of the entire viral replication cycle varies from 8 hours in polioviruses to 36 hours in herpes viruses.

Absorption begins when the virus encounters a susceptible host and enters the body through inhalation, ingestion, or inoculation via the skin or mucous membranes, or passes across the placenta from mother to infant. The mode of transmission can be sexual contact, blood transfusions, sharing of syringes or needles, and animal bites (human, animal, insect, spiders, others).

What follows is *penetration* of the flexible cell membrane of the host by a whole virus or its nucleic acid by endocytosis. The entire virus is engulfed by the cell and enclosed in a vacuole or vesicle. *Uncoating* occurs when the intracellular enzymes in the vacuole dissolve the viral envelope, a process that releases viral nucleic acid into the cytoplasm of the host cell. The uncoating frees viral nucleic acid for replication and *synthesis* of new virions. *Assembly* occurs when the DNA virus enter the host cell's nucleus and replicates. With few exceptions, the retrovirus of HIV being one, RNA viruses are replicated and assembled in the cytoplasm of the host cell.

Release of the mature virus occurs in two ways. Nonenveloped, complex viruses are released with cell lysis or rupture. Enveloped viruses are released by budding from the membranes of the cytoplasm, nucleus, endoplasmic reticulum, or vesicles and go on to infect other host cells, where the replication process continues.

The effects of viral infections are well documented. The cytopathic effects (i.e., viral-induced cell damage) change individual cells so that they become unstable and undergo changes in their shape or size, or develop intracellular changes. Accumulated damage from a viral infection kills most host cells, although in some cases, the cells and the virus maintain a carrier relationship, the cell harboring virus that is not immediately lysed. Persistent infections can last from a few weeks to the remainder of the host's life, periodically becoming activated. Examples include the herpes simplex viruses that most often cause cold sores (HSV-1) and genital herpes (HSV-2), and the varicella zoster virus (VZV) that is responsible for chickenpox and shingles. In another example, a dormant HIV infection, in which the virions remain inside host cells but do not actively replicate to any significant degree, may have a lengthy dormant phase of 10 years or more before giving rise to AIDS.

Host-cell DNA or RNA may also be transformed as a result of the viral invasion, resulting in mutation of host-cell DNA or RNA and the development of cancerous host cells (see also Chapter 33). Viruses that introduce cancer in this fashion are known as *oncogenic* viruses. In most cases, the host's immune system acts to eradicate viral infections, but it can become overwhelmed depending on the strength, or virulence, of the virus, how rapidly it replicates inside host cells, and the health of host cells.

INFLUENZA

EPIDEMIOLOGY AND ETIOLOGY

The term influenza, also known as the "flu," has its origins in fifteenth-century Italy, where the cause of the disease was attributed to unfavorable astrologic influences. Evolution in medical thought led to its modification to "*influenza di freddo,*" meaning "influence of the cold," which by the eighteenth-century became the prevalent terminology in the English-speaking world as well. Many different illnesses cause flulike systemic and respiratory symptoms such as fever, chills, aches and pains, cough, and sore throat. To be accurate, the term influenza refers to illness caused by influenza virus. In addition, influenza itself has many different illness patterns, ranging from mild common-cold symptoms of typical flu to life-threatening pneumonia and other complications, including secondary bacterial infections.

Each year the impact of influenza is felt globally when the disease develops in approximately 20% of the world's population. In the United States, influenza outbreaks occur each winter, generally between late December and early March. On average, 5% to 20% of the population becomes infected with influenza, with more than 200,000 people hospitalized annually from complications; about 36,000 people die from flu each year. Pandemics have occurred approximately every 10 to 15 years since the 1918–1919 pandemic. Persons at risk for influenza and its subsequent complications include young children, older adults, and persons with health conditions such as heart disease, diabetes, and chronic obstructive pulmonary disease (COPD). Human cases of avian influenza ("bird flu") have heightened awareness of the threat of a pandemic and have spurred efforts to develop plans for its control.

PATHOPHYSIOLOGY

Influenza viruses, with single-stranded RNA, are members of the orthomyxoviruses group of RNA viruses. This group of viruses is known by their ability to mutate and to rearrange the antigens on the viral surface. The viruses are contained within an outer lipoprotein envelope with two viral glycoprotein spikes. The antigenic nature of the glycoprotein spikes (i.e., neuramidase and haemagglutinin) on the viral surface can change dramatically in some instances. These glycoproteins are needed for viral entry into the host cell.

The first spike is a box-shaped protein called *neuraminidase* (NA), of which there are nine major antigenic types; it has enzymatic properties, as the name implies. NA functions at the end of the life cycle of the virus to facilitate the release of virus particles from infected cell surfaces during the budding process and prevents self-aggregation of virions. It is also thought that NA crosses the mucoid layer of the lungs to reach epithelial cells, the intended cells for viral activity.

The other envelope spike is called *haemagglutinin* (HA), of which there are 13 major antigenic types. An antigenic protein called the matrix protein lines the inside of the envelope and is chemically bound to ribonucleic protein. The HA protein binds virus particles to susceptible cells and can combine with specific receptors on a number of different types of cells, including red blood cells.

Influenza viruses are classified into categories (i.e., A, B, C) based on the antigenic differences in their lipoproteins and matrix proteins. The differences involve factors including the type of virus, the host, geographic origins, whether the virus was isolated, and the number of isolates. Viral subtypes are identified using NA and HA antigenic variants. An example is provided in Table 28-1.

TABLE 28-1 Examples of Viral Classification System

Virus Type	Host of Origin	Geographic Origin	Number of Isolates	Year of Isolation	HA and NA Type
A		Singapore	6	1986	H1N1
A		Hong Kong	3	1968	H3N2
A	Swine	Iowa	15	1930	H1N1

HA, Haemagglutinin; *NA*, neuraminidase.

Influenza is transmitted from person to person by droplets (e.g., coughing and sneezing), although sometimes people become infected by touching inanimate objects contaminated with the virus and then touching their mouth or nose. This viral infection is transmissible to others from the onset of symptoms up to 5 days after contact.

Every 10 to 15 years, a major new pandemic strain of influenza, with a completely new HA and sometimes a new NA as well (antigenic shift), emerges in the human population. The result is a pandemic. Over the subsequent period of 2 to 3 years, the strain undergoes slight changes, also known as antigenic drift, most likely driven by selective antibody pressure in the populations of humans infected.

PHARMACOTHERAPEUTIC OPTIONS

Influenza vaccine is the principal means of preventing and controlling this viral illness; antiviral drugs are not a substitute for vaccine and should be used only as an adjunct to vaccine in control of influenza. Four antiviral drugs active against influenza are commercially available in the United States. The four drugs are classified into two categories, the adamantine derivatives and the neuramidase inhibitors, on the basis of their chemical properties and activity against influenza virus. However, all four of the drugs may not always be effective against different influenza virus strains because of viral resistance to one or more of the drugs. Amantadine and rimantadine, the adamantine derivatives, have activity limited to the type A virus, whereas oseltamivir and zanamivir, the neuramidase inhibitors, have activity against both type A and type B viruses (Table 28-2).

Neuramidase Inhibitors

◆ oseltamivir (Tamiflu); ♣ Tamiflu
◆ zanamivir (Relenza); ♣ Relenza

▥ Indications

Both of the neuramidase inhibitors are effective as prophylaxis and are used in the treatment of types A and B influenza virus. However, recent data indicate there may be reduced activity against the B strain of the virus.

▥ Pharmacodynamics

Neuraminidase inhibitors break the bond holding influenza virus particles to the outside of a host cell. In so doing, the drugs prevent the new virion from being released, which in turn limits the spread of the virus. The efficacy of neuramidase inhibitors diminishes substantially when administered 60 hours after symptoms develop; efficacy is suboptimal when started later in the course of illness.

▥ Pharmacokinetics

Oseltamivir is readily absorbed following oral administration and extensively converted by hepatic esterases to oseltamivir carboxylate, its active form. The binding of oseltamivir to human plasma proteins is ordinarily insufficient to cause significant displacement-based drug interactions. At least 75% of an oral dose reaches the systemic circulation as oseltamivir carboxylate. Oseltamivir is excreted through the kidneys.

Of an inhaled dose of zanamivir, 17% is systemically absorbed. Distribution sites are unknown. The drug is primarily excreted by the kidneys as unchanged drug; any unabsorbed drug is eliminated in the feces. Table 28-3 provides an overview of the pharmacokinetics of these non-HIV antiviral drugs.

▥ Adverse Effects and Contraindications

Common adverse drug effects of oseltamivir include headache, and mild nausea and vomiting the first day or two of therapy. Rare adverse effects include hepatitis and elevated liver enzymes, rash, and allergic reactions including anaphylaxis and Stevens-Johnson syndrome. Although rare, there have been reports of changes in level of consciousness, confusion, abnormal behaviors, hallucinations, seizures, arrhythmias, toxic epidermal necrolysis, aggravation of diabetes, and hemorrhagic colitis.

Because zanamivir is administered as an inhaled powder, patients may develop cough or throat irritation. In patients with preexisting lung disorders (e.g., COPD), zanamivir may cause severe bronchospasm and respiratory decline. Zanamivir treatment of acute influenza in patients with asthma and COPD does not change airway resistance. There are

TABLE 28-2 Treating Viral Infections Other Than HIV/AIDS

Influenza A*	Influenza B†	HSV-1 and HSV-2‡	Varicella Zoster‡	Cytomegalovirus‡
amantadine	oseltamivir	acyclovir	acyclovir	cidofovir
rimantadine	zanamivir	famciclovir	cidofovir	ganciclovir
oseltamivir		foscarnet	famciclovir	fomivirsen§
zanamivir		penciclovir	penciclovir	foscarnet
		valacyclovir	valacyclovir	

*Drugs for influenza A act in the uncoating step of viral replication.
†Drugs for influenza B act in the release and budding step of viral replication.
‡Most drugs for HSV-1, HSV-2, VZV, and CMV act in the RNA or DNA replication step of viral reproduction.
§Fomivirsen acts in the translation step of viral replication.
AIDS, Acquired immunodeficiency syndrome; *HIV*, human immunodeficiency virus.

PHARMACOKINETICS
TABLE 28-3 Non-HIV Antiviral Drugs

Drug	Route	Onset	Peak	Duration	PB (%)	t½	BioA (%)
NEURAMIDASE INHIBITORS							
oseltamivir	PO	Rapid	UA	UA	42	6–10 hr	75
zanamivir	NS	Rapid	1–2 hr	12 hr	<10	2.5–5.1	14–17
ADAMANTANE DERIVATIVES							
amantadine	PO	48 hr	1–4 hr	UA	67	9–37	62–93; 53–100*
rimantadine	PO	Rapid	5–7 hr	UA	40	19–37	75–93
NUCLEOSIDE ANALOGUES AND OTHERS							
acyclovir	PO	UA	1.5–2.5 hr	UA	9–33	2.5–3.3 hr	15–20
	IV	Immed	End of inf	UA	9–33	2.5–3.3 hr	100
cidofovir	IV	Immed	End of inf	UA	6	17–65 hr	100
famciclovir	PO	Rapid	1 hr	8–12 hr	20	2.1–3 hr	77
fomivirsen	IO	Rapid	Hours	7–10 days	40	UA	UA
foscarnet	IV	Immed	End of inf	NA	14–17	3 hr; 90 hr†	100
ganciclovir	PO	UA	UA	UA	1–2	2.5–3.6 hr	3–9
	IV	Immed	1 hr	UA	1–2	3–7.3 hr	100
ribavarin	INH	Rapid	60–90 min	UA	INS	24 hr; 9.5 hr; 40 days‡	NA
valacyclovir	IV	Immed	1 hr	UA	1–2	3–7.3 hr; 14 hr§	100
valganciclovir	PO	Rapid	2 hr	UA	1–2	4 hr	60

*Bioavailability of amantadine in the young and older adults, respectively.
†The long elimination half-life of foscarnet may reflect release of the drug from bone.
‡The elimination half-life of ribavirin and red blood cells (RBCs), respectively.
§Elimination half-life of valacyclovir is 2.5–3.3 hr. The half-life may extend (as acyclovir) to as much as 14 hr in patients with renal impairment.
BioA, Bioavailability; *Immed*, immediate; *inf*, infection; *INH*, inhaled; *INS*, insignificant; *IO*, intraocular; *IV*, intravenous; *NA*, not applicable; *NS*, nasal spray; *PB*, protein binding; *PO*, by mouth; *subQ*, subcutaneously; *t½*, half-life; *UA*, unavailable.

limited data about the use of neuramidase inhibitors during pregnancy (category C), lactation, and in children under age 7 years.

Drug Interactions

There are no known drug interactions with oseltamivir or zanamivir. However, advise patients using an inhaled bronchodilator such as albuterol to administer the bronchodilator before inhaling zanamivir.

Dosage Regimen

For prophylaxis, these drugs are generally given for the duration of the influenza season; for treatment, a 5-day course is recommended (Table 28-4). In more severe cases, treatment with higher doses and a longer course of therapy may be recommended.

Lab Considerations

Zanamivir may increase liver function test and creatine phosphokinase (CPK) values. There are no known lab considerations for oseltamivir.

Adamantane Derivatives

◆ amantadine (Symmetrel); ♣ Symmetrel
◆ rimantadine (Flumadine)

Indications

Both amantadine and rimantadine are effective when used as prophylaxis during outbreaks of influenza A. Prophylaxis is used to control influenza outbreaks and to protect high-risk patients immunized after an epidemic has begun. They can also be used as prophylaxis for patients who are immunodeficient; for those who may respond poorly to the vaccine; and in patients for whom the vaccine is contraindicated

because of egg allergy. Either drug may be given alone or along with influenza vaccine. Amantadine is also used to treat active influenza A, although neither drug is active against type B influenza, colds, or other viral illnesses.

Pharmacodynamics

Amantadine and rimantadine are thought to act in a similar fashion. Both drugs bind inside the ion channel formed by the M2 transmembrane protein in the envelope of the virion. Binding creates a steric block preventing activation of the H^+ ion-transport function of the channel, which normally acidifies the interior of the virion. The latter is essential for the release of the RNA genome from the cell.

The mechanism of resistance is the same for both adamantane derivatives; viruses resistant to one drug are also resistant to the other. The mutations prevent drug binding to the target site, confer shared drug resistance on the virion, and result in clinical treatment failure. There is no evidence indicating that adamantane-resistant viruses are any more transmissible or virulent than adamantane-sensitive viruses. Cross-resistance between adamantane derivatives and neuramidase inhibitors does not occur.

Pharmacokinetics

Amantadine and rimantadine are available only as oral formulations. Their pharmacokinetics are related to their high pKa and lipophilicity, with almost complete ionization in the low pH of the stomach and slow but relatively complete absorption from the intestine (see Table 28-3). They are widely distributed, rimantadine 3 times more than amantadine. Amantadine is primarily eliminated through the kidneys in urine. Renal clearance can be enhanced by urinary acidification.

Compared with amantadine, rimantadine is extensively biotransformed in the liver, with less than 25% of the dose

IMMUNE

DOSAGE
TABLE 28-4 Non-HIV Antivirals

Drug	Use(s)	Dosage	Implications
NEURAMIDASE INHIBITORS			
oseltamivir	Treatment influenza A and B	*Adult and Child >age 13 yr:* 75 mg PO twice daily for 5 days. Not recommended for children under 12 mo of age*	The dose should be reduced by 50% in patients whose CrCl is <30 mL/min.
	Prophylaxis influenza A and B	*Adult:* 75 mg PO once daily for 5 days	
zanamivir	Treatment influenza A and B	*Adult and Child >12 yr:* 10 mg (2 inhalations) twice daily for 5 days	Must have 2 hr between initial doses; and then give 12 hr apart on subsequent days.
	Prophylaxis influenza A and B	*Adult and Child >5 yr:* 10 mg (2 inhalations) once daily	
ADAMANTANE DERIVATIVES			
amantadine	Treatment influenza A	*Adult and Child >age 10 yr:* 100 mg PO twice daily *Child <age 10 or <40 kg:* 5 mg/kg/day up to 150 mg in 2 divided doses	Renal dosing considerations required. Duration of treatment usually 10 days for treatment; prophylaxis is continued until the epidemic abates (usually in 5–6 wk. Prophylaxis may be discontinued 2 wk after vaccination received.
	Prophylaxis influenza A	*Adult:* 100 mg PO twice daily *Child <age 10 or <40 kg:* 5 mg/kg/day up to 150 mg in 2 divided doses	
rimantadine	Treatment influenza A	*Adult:* 100 mg PO twice daily *Child:* Not approved	Renal dosing considerations required. Duration of treatment usually 5 days; prophylaxis is continued until the epidemic abates (usually in 5–6 wk)
	Prophylaxis influenza A	*Adult and Child >age 13 yr:* 100 mg PO twice daily *Child >10 kg or <40 kg:* 5 mg/kg/day up to 150 mg in 2 divided doses	
HERPES, VARICELLA, AND CMV			
cidofovir	CMV retinitis	*Adult:* 5 mg/kg IV. Probenecid must be administered PO with each cidofovir dose; 2 grams is given 3 hr before cidofovir dose, and 1 gram given 2 and 8 hr after the completion of cidofovir infusion, for a total of 4 grams	IV infusion weekly for 2 consecutive wk. To minimize potential nephrotoxicity, probenecid and IV saline rehydration must be given along with cidofovir infusion.
foscarnet	CMV retinitis	*Adult:* 90 mg/kg IV every 12 hr *—or—* 60 mg/kg IV every 8 hr. Maintenance: 90–120 mg/kg/day IV	Renal dosing considerations required. Adequate hydration minimizes renal toxicity. Regular ophthalmologic exams needed.
	HSV in patient with AIDS	*Adult:* 40–60 mg/kg IV every 8 hr for 2–3 wk. May be followed by 50 mg/kg/day for 5–7 days/wk, up to 15 wk	Dilute to 12 mg/mL if peripheral line; standard 24 mg/mL may be given via central line.
	Acyclovir-resistant HSV infection in immunocompromised patients	*Adult:* 40 mg/kg IV every 8–12 hr for up to 3 wk	
ganciclovir	CMV retinitis in patients with AIDS	*Adult:* 10 mg/kg/day IV in divided doses every 12 hr for 14–21 days, then 5 mg/kg/day.	Renal dosing considerations required. Intravitreal implant is an effective longer term alternative.
valacyclovir	Herpes zoster	*Adult:* 1 gram PO 3 times daily for 7 days	Renal dosing considerations required. Avoid intercourse during course of therapy to minimize risk of passing HSV-2 to partner.
	Initial outbreak genital herpes	*Adult:* 1 gram PO twice daily for 10 days	
	Recurrent genital herpes	*Adult:* 500 mg PO twice daily for 3 days	
	Prevention genital herpes	*Adult:* 500–1000 mg PO daily	
	Herpes simplex orolabial	*Adult:* 1 gram twice daily for 1 day	
valganciclovir	CMV retinitis	*Adult:* 900 mg PO twice daily for 21 days. Maintenance: 900 mg PO daily with food	Prodrug of ganciclovir. Take with food. Steady state AUC increases 30% with high-fat meal.

*The dosage recommendation of oseltamivir for children <15 kg is 30 mg PO twice daily; for children 15–23 kg, dosage is 30 mg PO twice daily; for 23–40 kg child, the dosage is 60 mg PO twice daily, and for children >40 kg, the dosage is 75 mg PO twice daily.
AIDS, Acquired immunodeficiency syndrome; *AUC,* area under the curve; *CrCl,* creatinine clearance; *HSV,* herpes simplex virus; *IV,* intravenous (route); *CMV,* cytomegalovirus; *PO,* by mouth.

excreted unchanged in the urine. A dosage reduction of rimantadine is recommended in patients with severe liver disease.

▥ Adverse Effects and Contraindications

Both amantadine and rimantadine cause dose-related adverse effects including insomnia, dizziness, headache, nervousness, or an inability to concentrate. These adverse effects occur less often with rimantadine than amantadine, and they

are more common in patients also taking antihistamines. Anorexia, nausea, and vomiting have been reported in 1% to 3% of patients. More serious, but less frequent, adverse effects (i.e., seizures, confusion) have been reported in older adults and, most commonly, in adults who have seizure disorders. Lowering the dose (to 100 mg once daily for 7 days rather than twice daily) reduces these adverse effects without reducing the effectiveness of the drug. Adverse effects decrease after 1 week of use and reverse as soon as treatment stops. The safe use of amantadine and rimantadine during pregnancy (category C) has not been established.

Both drugs have been associated with rapid development of drug-resistant strains, because a single point mutation at certain amino acid positions confers cross-resistance to both amantadine and rimantadine. The influenza viruses resistant to one drug are also resistant to the other. The drug-resistant viruses spread to contacts of treated patients, including persons receiving prophylaxis therapy.

Drug Interactions

Drugs that interact with amantadine and rimantadine are identified in Table 28-5.

Dosage Regimen

Treatment is generally based on time to clinical response, which generally ranges from 3 to 5 days (see Table 28-4). Prophylaxis of influenza A or B is continued for the duration of the outbreak. Dosage reductions for amantadine are essential for safe use of the drug in patients with kidney disease.

Lab Considerations

There are no known lab considerations with amantadine or rimantadine.

CLINICAL REASONING

Treatment Objectives

Annual influenza vaccination remains the primary means for preventing morbidity and mortality associated with influenza. Treatment of influenza is aimed at reducing morbidity and mortality.

Treatment Options

Patient Variables

Patients at high risk for contracting influenza should receive annual influenza vaccinations. These individuals are identified in Box 28-1.

Drug Variables

Oseltamivir and zanamivir are over 70% effective in reducing the risk of both influenza A and influenza B when taken before and after exposure to the illness. The efficacy of these drugs in preventing the complications of influenza A is unknown, but they have relatively few adverse effects. Oseltamivir is generally better tolerated by patients with nausea and may be easier to use in persons who have trouble using the inhaled formulation of zanamivir, and in frail or confused persons.

DRUG INTERACTIONS

TABLE 28-5 Antiviral Drugs

Drug	Interactive Drug	Interaction
NON-HIV ANTIVIRAL DRUGS		
amantadine	Antihistamines, disopyramide, phenothiazines, quinidine, tricyclic antidepressants	Increases anticholinergic effects of amantadine
	hydrochlorothiazide, triamterene, quinine, quinidine	Increases concentration and risk for amantadine toxicity
rimantadine	Acetaminophen, aspirin, cimetidine	Decreases plasma levels of rimantadine
	Alcohol	Increases risk of CNS depression
	CNS stimulants	Increase risk of CNS stimulation
PROTEASE INHIBITORS		
darunavir	clarithromycin, tenofovir, rifabutin	Increases serum levels interactive drug
	warfarin	Reduces serum warfarin levels
indinavir	midazolam, triazolam	Causes arrhythmias and excessive sedation
	didanosine	Reduces absorption of indinavir
	fluconazole, rifampin	Reduces serum levels of indinavir
	ketoconazole, isoniazid, oral contraceptives, rifabutin, saquinavir	Increases plasma levels of interactive drug
nelfinavir	rifabutin	Decreases biotransformation and may increase effects of interactive drug
	carbamazepine, oral contraceptives, phenobarbital, phenytoin, theophylline, zidovudine	Reduces plasma concentration and effectiveness of interactive drug
	erythromycin, midazolam, indinavir, ritonavir, saquinavir, triazolam, warfarin	Increases plasma concentration and effectiveness of interactive drug
	ketoconazole	Increases plasma concentration of nelfinavir
ritonavir	amiodarone, bepridil, bupropion, clozapine, encainide, flecainide, meperidine, piroxicam, propafenone, propoxyphene, quinidine, rifabutin	Produces large increases in serum levels and effects of interactive drug
	disulfiram	Causes disulfiram-like reaction
	alprazolam, clorazepate, diazepam, estazolam, flurazepam, midazolam, triazolam, zolpidem	Increases serum levels and risk for excessive sedation and respiratory depression
	Selected opioids and NSAIDs, antiarrhythmics, antimicrobials, antidepressants, antiemetics, beta blockers, calcium channel blockers, antineoplastic drugs, glucocorticoids, antilipidemics, immunosuppressants, antipsychotics, methamphetamine, saquinavir, warfarin	Increases plasma levels and effects of interactive drugs
	Protease inhibitors in general	Synergistic effects if used concurrently
	Oral contraceptives, zidovudine, sulfamethoxazole, theophylline	Decreases plasma levels of interactive drugs
	Ergotamine, dihydroergotamine	Possible ergot toxicity
saquinavir	Calcium channel blockers, clindamycin, dapsone, quinidine, triazolam, ketoconazole, ritonavir	Increase plasma concentration of saquinavir
	carbamazepine, dexamethasone, phenobarbital, phenytoin, rifampin	Decreases plasma concentration of saquinavir

Continued

IMMUNE

DRUG INTERACTIONS
TABLE 28-5 Antiviral Drugs—Cont'd

Drug	Interactive Drug	Interaction
NUCLEOSIDE REVERSE TRANSCRIPTASE INHIBITORS		
didanosine	dapsone, fluoroquinolones, itraconazole, ketoconazole, tetracycline	Decreases gastric absorption of interactive drug
	Antacids	Increases bioavailability of didanosine
	tenofovir	Increases serum levels of didanosine
	zalcitabine	Reoccurrence or exacerbation of neuropathy
	Alcohol, clotrimazole, diuretics, pentamidine	Increases risk for pancreatic toxicity
lamivudine	trimethoprim-sulfamethoxazole	Increases serum levels of lamivudine
	zidovudine	Increases serum levels of zidovudine
stavudine, zalcitabine	chloramphenicol, cisplatin, dapsone, didanosine, disulfiram, ethionamide, ethambutol, glutethimide, gold, hydralazine, isoniazid, lithium, metronidazole, nitrofurantoin, phenytoin, vincristine, zalcitabine	Increases risk of peripheral neuropathy
	zidovudine	Possible viral antagonism
zalcitabine	Antacids	Decreases bioavailability of zalcitabine
	Alcohol, asparaginase, azathioprine, estrogens, furosemide, methyldopa, nitrofurantoin, pentamidine, sulfonamides, tetracyclines, thiazide diuretics, valproic acid	Increases risk for pancreatitis
	pentamidine	Increases risk for pancreatic toxicity
	Aminoglycosides, amphotericin B, foscarnet	Decreases renal clearance of zalcitabine and increases risk of peripheral neuropathy
	ribavirin	Antagonizes antiviral activity of zalcitabine
	zidovudine	Synergistic antiviral activity
	probenecid	Increases blood levels of zalcitabine
zidovudine	acyclovir, didanosine, foscarnet, ganciclovir, GM-CSFs, interferon alfa, zalcitabine, zidovudine	Synergistic antiviral activity
	ganciclovir, ribavirin	Antagonizes antiviral activity; increases risk of hematologic toxicity
	acyclovir	Additive neurotoxicity
	fluconazole, phenytoin, probenecid, trimethoprim	Increases risk of zidovudine toxicity
	acetaminophen, clarithromycin	Decreases levels of zidovudine
	phenytoin, trimethoprim	Increases levels of zidovudine
	Myelosuppressive drugs, nephrotoxic, or directly toxic to circulating blood cells	Increases risk of hematologic toxicity
NON-NUCLEOSIDE REVERSE TRANSCRIPTASE INHIBITORS		
nevirapine	rifampin, rifabutin	Decreases bioavailability of nevirapine
	Protease inhibitors, oral contraceptives	Reduces plasma levels of interactive drug
efavirenz	Ergot derivatives, midazolam, triazolam	Severe life-threatening arrhythmias, prolonged sedation, respiratory depression
	Alcohol, psychoactive drugs	Additive CNS depression
	phenobarbital, rifampin, rifabutin	Decreases efavirenz plasma concentration
delavirdine	Alprazolam, antiarrhythmics, dihydropyridine CCBs, clarithromycin, dapsone, ergot alkaloids, midazolam, quinidine, warfarin	Increases plasma levels of interactive drug
	Antacids, didanosine	Decreases absorption of delavirdine
NUCLEOSIDE ANALOGS AND OTHERS		
acyclovir	amphotericin B	Synergistic effects
	probenecid	Increases serum levels of acyclovir
	Nephrotoxic drugs	Increases risk of nephrotoxicity
	methotrexate (intrathecal), zidovudine	Increases risk of CNS adverse effects
cidofovir	Aminoglycosides, amphotericin B, foscarnet, pentamidine	Increase risk of nephrotoxicity with concurrent use
	acetaminophen, acyclovir, ACE inhibitors, barbiturates, benzodiazepines, bumetanide, methotrexate, famotidine, furosemide, NSAIDs, theophylline, zidovudine	Interacts with probenecid that is required for concurrent use
famciclovir	cimetidine, probenecid	Increases serum levels of famciclovir
	digoxin	Increases plasma levels of digoxin and risk of toxicity
	theophylline	Decreases renal clearance of famciclovir
foscarnet	Parenteral pentamidine	Severe life-threatening hypocalcemia
	imipenem	Increases risk of seizures
	didanosine	Decreases elimination of foscarnet
	amphotericin B, aminoglycosides	Increases risk of nephrotoxicity
ganciclovir	amphotericin B, antineoplastics, dapsone, flucytosine, immunosuppressives, other nucleoside analogs, pentamidine, pyrimethamine, radiation therapy	Increases risk of bone marrow depression
	didanosine, zidovudine	Antagonizes antiretroviral activity of interactive drug
	foscarnet	Additive or synergistic activity
	probenecid	Increases risk of toxicity to ganciclovir
	imipenem-cilastatin	Increases risk of seizures
	amphotericin B, cyclosporine, nephrotoxic drugs	Increases risk of nephrotoxicity
ribavirin	zalcitabine, zidovudine	Antagonizes antiviral activity of ribavirin and potentiates hematologic toxicity
	didanosine	Potentiates action of interactive drug
valacyclovir	cimetidine, probenecid	Increases levels of acyclovir component of valacyclovir
	zidovudine	Increases drowsiness and lethargy

ACE, Angiotensin converting enzyme; *CCBs,* calcium channel blockers; *CNS,* central nervous system; *GM-CSFs,* granulocyte-macrophage colony stimulating factors; *HIV,* human immunodeficiency virus; *NSAIDs,* nonsteroidal antiinflammatory drugs.

BOX 28-1

Who Should Get Vaccinated?

People Who Should be Vaccinated Each Year for Influenza

1. **People at high risk for complications from influenza, including the following:**
   - Persons 65 years of age and older
   - All children between 6 and 23 months of age
   - People residing in nursing homes and other long-term care facilities that house those with long-term illnesses
   - Adults and children 23 months of age and older who have chronic heart or lung conditions, including asthma
   - Adults and children 23 months of age and older who needed regular medical care or were in a hospital during the previous year because of a metabolic disease (e.g., diabetes), chronic kidney disease, or weakened immune system (including immune system problems caused by drugs or by infection with the human immuno-deficiency virus [HIV/AIDS])
   - Children 23 months to 18 years of age who are on long-term aspirin therapy **(Children given aspirin for a viral illness such as influenza are at risk for Reye's syndrome)**
   - Women who will be pregnant during the influenza season
   - People with any condition that compromises respiratory function or the handling of respiratory secretions (e.g., brain injury or disease, spinal cord injuries, seizure disorders, or other nerve or muscle disorders)

2. **People between 50 and 64 years of age**
   Nearly one third of persons between 50 and 64 years of age in the United States have one or more medical conditions that place them at increased risk for serious complications of influenza; thus vaccination is recommended for all persons aged 50 to 64

3. **Persons who may transmit influenza to others at high risk for complications**
   Any person in close contact with another in a high-risk group (see above) should be vaccinated. This includes all health-care workers, household contacts, and out-of-home caregivers of children 6 to 23 months of age, and close contacts of people 65 years of age and older

People Who Should *Not* be Vaccinated
People who should not be vaccinated without first consulting with their health care provider, include the following:
- Persons who have a severe allergy to chicken eggs
- **Persons who have had a severe reaction to an influenza vaccination in the past**
- Persons who developed Guillain-Barré syndrome (GBS) within 6 weeks of receiving a previous influenza vaccination
- Children under 6 months of age (influenza vaccine is not approved for this age group)
- Persons who have a moderate or severe illness with a fever should wait to be vaccinated until symptoms lessen and fever is gone.

Both oseltamivir and zanamivir reduce viral shedding when they are taken within 48 hours of the onset of symptoms. One study of oseltamivir found a sizeable reduction in complications of influenza such as pneumonia and bronchitis associated with antibiotic use, and a significant reduction in hospitalizations. The one critical variable was that patients had to start taking the drug within 2 days of the onset of symptoms; when that condition was met, patients were less contagious, symptoms reduced, and the length of illness shortened by 1 or 2 days (Kaiser et al., 2003). Genetic mutation of neuraminidase, which is required for viral resistance, may also make the virus less likely to cause an infection. In contrast to amantadine-resistant viral strains, there are no documented cases of influenza caused by a resistant virus.

The adverse effects of amantadine may limit its use in the treatment of influenza. Five percent to 15% of patients taking amantadine prophylaxis report adverse effects. The major adverse effects of amantadine are the result of CNS stimulation but usually resolve once the drug is stopped.

Another disadvantage of amantadine is that within 5 days of starting therapy, one third of patients begin to shed resistant virus as a result of genetic mutation of the M2 protein. In these cases, family members of the person treated with amantadine can be infected. The spectrum of amantadine covers only influenza A, whose strains cause most epidemics.

A report on the global prevalence of adamantane-resistant influenza viruses showed a significant increase (from 1.9% to 12.3%) in drug resistance over the past 3 years (Ward et al., 2005). In the United States, the frequency of adamantane-resistant influenza virus increased from 1.8% during the 2001-2002 season to 14.5% during the first 6 months of the 2004 and 2005 influenza seasons (*Morbidity and Mortality Weekly Report*, 2006). **The Centers for Disease Control and Prevention (CDC) recommended during the 2005-2006** **influenza season to avoid the use of adamantane derivatives because of drug resistance.**

Patient Education

Advise patients that antiviral drugs are not a substitute for an annual influenza vaccination. Patients should receive the vaccination according to immunization guidelines (see also Chapter 31). Teach them to take their antiviral drug as prescribed for the time prescribed, and to contact the health care provider if they have questions or develop an infection.

Instruct patients about the importance of preventive self-care and what to do should they get influenza. The best way to limit the spread of viruses is to exercise good personal hygiene. The following are examples. Handwashing etiquette includes using soap and tissues and disposing of them correctly. Cough etiquette involves covering the mouth and nose or coughing into the upper sleeve, avoiding the hands; put used tissues in a waste basket, put on a mask if appropriate, and clean your hands with soap and water, or alcohol-based hand cleaner. Avoid touching contaminated surfaces. Make sure food preparation areas are clean and sanitary. It is unwise for a patient with a genuine case of influenza to go to work, especially anyone working in retail and food service, or health care. Patient responsibilities and where they work determines where to draw the stay-at-home line. If working in direct patient care, ensure that Occupational Safety and Health Administration (OSHA) regulations are being followed.

Some patients ask about the usefulness of nasal tissues treated with virucidal compounds. Although there have been no conclusive studies supporting their use, in theory, these tissues interrupt transmission of viral infections by blocking hand contamination and/or small particle aerosols from nose-blowing, sneezing, and coughing (see Evidence-Based Practice box). According to the manufacturer, the three-ply paper tissue contains a middle layer

IMMUNE

EVIDENCE-BASED PHARMACOTHERAPEUTICS

Virucidal Nasal Tissues

■ Background
Although this study was carried out several years ago, in some respects it is still relevant since the incidence and prevalence of viral illnesses has not declined and, in fact, may be worsening as the result of viral mutations.

■ Research Article
Farr, B., Hendley, J., Kaiser, D., et al. (1988). Two randomized controlled trials of virucidal nasal tissues in the prevention of upper respiratory infections. *American Journal of Epidemiology, 128*(5),1162–1172.

Purpose
The purpose of this study was to evaluate the results from two studies evaluating the effectiveness of virucidal nasal tissues in the prevention of natural upper respiratory infections.

Design
This was a mini meta-analysis of two 6-month, randomized, placebo-controlled, double-blind studies carried out between 1983 and 1986 by the faculty of the University of Virginia School of Medicine in Charlottesville, Virginia.

Methods
The two studies analyzed a total of 186 families in the first study and 98 families in the second study. Families in the first placebo-controlled study group used nasal tissues containing saccharin. The treatment group used virucidal nasal tissues impregnated with malic and citric acids and sodium lauryl sulfate. The second placebo-controlled study group used nasal tissues containing a mixture of saccharine and succinic acid. The treatment group also used virucidal nasal tissues impregnated with malic and citric acids and sodium lauryl sulfate.

Findings
The antiviral tissues were associated with 14% and 5% relative reductions in the overall rate of colds in the first and second trials, respectively. In the first study, this appeared to be due to an appropriate fall in secondary illnesses, with a relative reduction in the ratio of secondary to primary illnesses of 32%. However, in the second trial, the small and statistically insignificant reduction was primarily due to a drop in the rate of primary illness (which cannot be attributed to tissue efficacy), but the ratio of secondary to primary illness was actually 5% higher in the group with active tissues than in the placebo group.

Conclusions
The study investigators conclude that when used in a rigorous study protocol, virucidal tissues may offer a modest reduction of secondary colds in the home, but for reasons currently unknown, do not have a major effect on the overall rate of colds.

■ Implications for Practice
It is well known that standard statistical procedures become invalidated when applied to cluster randomized trials in which the unit of inference is the individual. One consequence is that researchers conducting such trials are faced with a multitude of design choices, including selection of the primary unit of inference, the degree to which clusters should be matched or stratified by prognostic factors at baseline, and decisions related to cluster subsampling. Future research studies should be done using randomized, placebo-controlled, double-blind studies with larger, more well-defined sample groups, and a study design that includes power analyses. Perhaps other combinations of virucidal compounds could be used on the tissues, or different brands of virucidal nasal tissues tested.

---

impregnated with citric acid, a common additive in detergents, and sodium lauryl sulfate, which is found in many shampoos. Sodium lauryl sulfate disrupts the lipid envelope of many viruses. Although rhinoviruses, which are responsible for a high percentage of upper respiratory illnesses, do not have a lipid envelope, they are sensitive to acids and are disrupted by citric acid. The active ingredients in the tissues are reported to inactivate 99% of types 1A and 2 rhinoviruses, influenza A and B, and the respiratory syncytial virus present in the tissue after 15 minutes. Teach patients to use the tissues only on the face since they are not effective as hand wipes or surface disinfectants. In fact, a used tissue with active virus remains a potential means of transmission of the virus to hands or inanimate objects. Handwashing does more to lessen viral transmission than use of virucidal tissues.

Evaluation
Clinical response to therapy is evaluated by noting a decrease in the signs and symptoms of influenza (i.e., malaise, fever, headache, myalgia, cough, sore throat). If the antiviral drugs were used as prophylaxis and influenza infection was prevented, treatment was successful.

HIV AND AIDS

EPIDEMIOLOGY AND ETIOLOGY

Globally, there are approximately 40 million individuals infected with HIV (CDC, 2005) with another 950,000 persons who are estimated to be infected but are not yet diagnosed.

Nearly 2.5 million of HIV-infected persons are under the age of 15 years. The numbers are highest among minority populations, with HIV the leading killer of black males' ages 25 to 44 years of age. Since 2003, two thirds of those affected by AIDS were black women and children.

HIV-1 and HIV-2 both cause AIDS, but HIV-2 is primarily confined to western Africa. HIV-1 causes much of the HIV pandemic in the rest of the world. A number of variables contribute to the risk for HIV-related illness including the patient's susceptibility to infection, the size and virulence of the viral inoculum, and the route of exposure. The average length of time from initial HIV infection to the development of opportunistic infections is about 10 years; however, more than 95% of patients exposed to HIV seroconvert within 6 months.

A diagnosis of AIDS cannot be made until the HIV-infected patient meets the definitive criteria that were established by the CDC in 1993: (1) a cluster designation 4 cell (CD4) count less than 200 cells/mm^3 (the median CD4 count at the time of an AIDS-defining illness is 67cells/mm^3); and (2) at least one condition indicative of severe immunosuppression, especially of defective cell-mediated immunity (*Pneumocystis jirovecii* pneumonia [PCP], cytomegalovirus [CMV] retinitis, tuberculosis [TB], or Kaposi's sarcoma). Remember, HIV infection is not synonymous with AIDS, which usually develops years after HIV infection is acquired.

HIV Transmission

▥ *Sexual Contact*
Sexual contact with an infected partner is the most common mode of HIV transmission. The highest risk for

transmission is through unprotected anal intercourse. Inflammation of the anal mucosa enhances the risk for infection, particularly in the presence of ulceration. The risk for infection is greatest for the receptive partner because of prolonged contact with semen. HIV may also be transmitted via vaginal and oral mucosa. Heterosexual intercourse is responsible for 75% of all adult HIV infections.

Contaminated Needles

HIV transmission by sharing contaminated needles is the next most common mode of transmission. Any previously used syringes and needles are potential sources of HIV infection.

Blood and Blood Products

Parenteral exposure to HIV-infected blood carries a significant risk for infection; in fact, the risk is almost 100%. Today, with better screening procedures in place, the risk of receiving a unit of blood infected with HIV is 2 in 1 million.

In 1992, screening for both HIV-1 and HIV-2 started; and in 1995 screening for the p24 antigen began as well. Because p24 levels rise and fall with HIV levels, the test may also be used to monitor anti-HIV therapy and to evaluate disease progression. The advantage of the p24 test is that it can detect HIV infection days before antibodies develop. The p24 quantitative test helps to identify the intensity of HIV expression in the body; the more p24 protein present, the higher the quantity of HIV in the blood. Its utility is limited, however, since p24 is only detectable for a short time. Nonetheless, this test can still be used when other tests are unavailable.

Mother-to-Child

Vertical transmission from mother to child accounts for over 90% of all HIV infections worldwide in infants and children. Perinatal transmission from an HIV-infected mother to an infant can occur during pregnancy, at the time of delivery, or after birth through breastfeeding. The risk of mother-to-infant transmission is greatest in women whose plasma HIV RNA levels are high; among patients with advanced HIV disease and low antibody titers to gp120; and when there is extended time from rupture of membranes, invasive fetal monitoring, or a prolonged, complicated labor. Other risk factors include the route of delivery (i.e., vaginal vs. cesarean section), gestational age of the infant at time of delivery, clinical presence of chorioamnionitis, and persistent illicit drug use. Infants at risk include the first born of twins, premature infants, and infants with neonatal bacterial infections.

Occupational Exposure

HIV can be transmitted to health care providers as a result of exposure to HIV-infected body fluids. The average risk of occupational HIV infection from all types of percutaneous exposures to HIV-infected blood is 0.3% (i.e., 1 in 300). The risk is even higher if the exposure is caused by a blood-filled, large-bore needle with blood from a person whose HIV status is unknown. Infected patients near death from AIDS, or patients with symptoms of acute HIV infection, usually have higher quantities of HIV in their blood and may pose increased risk. Percutaneous exposures involving larger blood volumes and high HIV titers may increase the risk above 0.3%. The risk of occupational HIV exposure by HIV-infected blood to mucous membranes of the eye, the nose, or the mouth and nonintact skin is 0.1% or 1 in 1000. Seroconversion to an HIV-positive state occurs 6 to 12 weeks after a needlestick injury.

PATHOPHYSIOLOGY

HIV infection is caused by a retrovirus, a group of RNA viruses that are so named because they carry the enzyme reverse transcriptase. Like all other viruses, HIV lacks the machinery needed for self-replication. In order to replicate, retroviruses must first transcribe their RNA into DNA (Fig. 28-1). The enzyme used for this process is reverse transcriptase (also known as RNA-dependent DNA polymerase).

Functional CD4 cells (i.e., T helper cells) of the host are required for the production of antibodies by B cells and for activation of T killer cells. For that reason, as HIV kills the CD4 cells, the immune system undergoes a downward decline and the infectious person becomes increasingly vulnerable to opportunistic infections, the major cause of death in persons with HIV. Reverse transcriptase selectively destroys the CD4 antigens found on T helper cells.

The HIV attacks CD4 cells because they are the major attachment points for the retrovirus; without the attachment points, HIV would be unable to connect with and penetrate host cells. Once the HIV infects the host cell, it dies in about 1.25 days. However, a small percentage of CD4 cells circulate in the blood; the vast majority is found in lymph nodes and other lymphoid tissues. Macrophage and microglial cells (the central nervous system [CNS] counterparts of macrophages) also have CD4 surface receptor sites that provide targets for the HIV. Macrophages and microglial cells are more resistant to the cytopathic consequences of HIV infection than CD4; they survive despite being infected. It is thought that macrophages and microglial cells play critical roles in the persistence of an HIV infection by providing reservoirs of chronically infected cells. Skin, lungs, bone marrow, and CNS tissues are directly infected.

Lymph nodes serve as a major reservoir for the virus. The network of dendritic cells with lymphoid tissue acts as a filter, trapping free virus and infected CD4 cells. This reservoir of free virus infects large numbers of previously uninfected CD4 lymphocytes as they flow through the lymph nodes. The architecture of the lymph nodes break down and the entrapped HIV escapes, resulting in even more free virus in the blood. The thymus, also an early target of HIV infection and damage, limits effective T cell production in younger patients.

The outer envelope of the HIV contains glycoproteins needed for attachment to host cells. Each glycoprotein consists of two subunits. The smaller of the two, gp41 is embedded in the lipid layer of the viral envelope; gp120 is firmly connected to gp41. Once attached, the virus sheds its protein coat, gaining entry into the cytoplasm of the cell. As soon as the viral particle gains entrance, reverse transcriptase enables the virus to reproduce its genetic material.

Another important enzyme is protease, which serves to chemically separate new viral RNA from virion protein molecules. These components are initially synthesized as a large

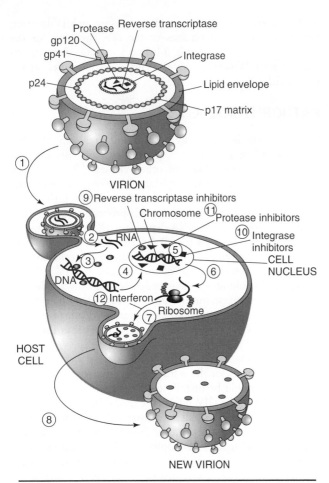

FIGURE 28-1 Life Cycle of a HIV Virion.

1. Attachment and injection of virion into core of susceptible host cell.
2. Uncoating of viral RNA
3. Reverse transcriptase converts single-stranded RNA to double-stranded DNA.
4. Entrance of DNA into host cell's nucleus
5. Viral DNA is integrated into host's own DNA. Integrase enzyme splices DNA into the host cell's chromosomes.
6. New viral RNA is translated into viral protein precursors at ribosomes.
7. Newly made proteins fold together to form new virion.
8. Budding and release of new virion.
9. Nucleoside reverse transcriptase inhibitors (NRTIs) prevent transcription of viral RNA to DNA. Non-nucleoside reverse transcriptase inhibitors (NNRTIs) bind directly to HIV viral reverse transcriptase to disrupt the active center of the enzyme.
10. Integrase inhibitors
11. Protease inhibitors (PIs) inhibit viral protease and prevent processing of PR 160, the precursor to all structural proteins and viral enzymes.
12. Interferon keeps virus from reassembling itself and budding out of the cell.

macromolecular strand, and the protease enzyme carefully breaks up this strand into its key components.

Clinical Course of HIV Infection

Without clinical intervention, HIV follows a distinct clinical course. Viral replication occurs during all stages of HIV infection, although it heightens during the initial infection. The enormous viral replication occurs because the population of CD4 cells is still large (thereby providing a large viral breeding ground), and the host has not yet mounted an immune response against the virus. Plasma levels of HIV can exceed 10 million virions/mL. At this point, patients usually have acute retroviral syndrome.

Primary HIV infection occurs in the first few weeks or months after initial HIV exposure and seroconversion, and disappears within a week to a month. The symptoms are nonspecific and are often mistaken for those of another viral infection (e.g., mononucleosis). The symptoms include headache; fever; pharyngitis; lymphadenopathy; mucocutaneous ulcerations involving the mouth, the esophagus, or the genitals; maculopapular erythematous rash, which may involve the palms and the soles of the feet; myalgias; and nausea, vomiting, and diarrhea. During this period, the patient is highly infectious, with HIV present in sizeable amounts in genital secretions. The viremia is associated with the spread of the virus to the CNS and lymphatics. Lymph nodes, spleen, tonsils, and adenoids are the major reservoir of HIV burden and replication.

Symptoms may not appear in an adult for 10 years or more after the first exposure to HIV, or within 2 years in children born with HIV infection. During the *asymptomatic infection* period, the virus actively multiplies, infects, and kills cells of the immune system. Except for a persistent generalized lymphadenopathy, enlarged lymph nodes involving at least two noncontiguous sites other than inguinal lymph nodes, the patient may have no clinical findings on physical exam. Vague symptoms include fatigue, headaches, low-grade fevers, and night sweats. Demyelinating peripheral neuropathies resembling Guillain-Barré syndrome may occur. The viral burden in peripheral blood is low. As the disease progresses, the lymph node architecture is disrupted and more HIV is released. The rate of CD4 decline correlates with viral burden. The patient may be unaware of the infection during this asymptomatic phase, posing a tremendous risk to public health.

Toward the end of this asymptomatic phase but before a diagnosis of AIDS is made, the CD4 count drops below 500 to 600 cells/mL and *early symptomatic disease* develops. Early symptoms include persistent fatigue, headache, fevers, weight loss, recurrent night sweats, and chronic diarrhea. The patient may experience persistent or frequent oral or vaginal yeast infections, persistent skin rashes or flaky skin, pelvic inflammatory disease in women that does not respond to treatment, and short-term memory loss. Frequent, severe herpes simplex outbreaks causing painful lesions of the mouth, the genitals, or the anus or herpes zoster (i.e., shingles) may be noted. Failure to thrive and recurrent illnesses arise in children.

In the advanced stages of HIV infection, the presence of certain opportunistic infections signals the transition to AIDS (Box 28-2). The median survival time for a patient with AIDS who is not taking highly active antiretroviral therapy

---

BOX 28-2

AIDS-Defining Opportunistic Illnesses*

Protozoal Infections
- Cryptosporidiosis with diarrhea
- Isopsoriasis with diarrhea
- Toxoplasmosis of the brain

Fungal Infections
- Candidiasis of the gastrointestinal tract and lungs
- Cryptococcosis
- Coccidioidomycosis (disseminated)
- Histoplasmosis (disseminated)

Viral Infections
- Cytomegalovirus disease (CMV)
- Herpes simplex virus (persistent or disseminated)
- Hairy leukoplakia (caused by Epstein-Barr virus)

Bacterial Infections
- Any "atypical" mycobacterial disease
- Extrapulmonary tuberculosis
- *Mycobacterium avium* complex (disseminated)
- Pyogenic bacterial infections (multiple or recurrent)
- *Salmonella* septicemia (recurrent)

Opportunistic Neoplasms
- Kaposi's sarcoma
- Non-Hodgkin's lymphoma
- Primary lymphoma of the brain

Other
- HIV encephalopathy
- HIV wasting syndrome
- Lymphoid interstitial pneumonia

*Based on Centers for Disease Control and Prevention (CDC) criteria.

(HAART) is 12 to 18 months. Patients who die of AIDS-related complications typically have a CD4 count under 50/mm^3.

Dramatic advances continue to evolve in clinical research and treatment of HIV and AIDS. The availability of more efficacious, potent drugs that inhibit HIV replication has led to multidrug therapies that offer nearly complete suppression of detectable HIV replication.

PHARMACOTHERAPEUTIC OPTIONS

To date, there are five types of antiretroviral drugs: reverse transcriptase inhibitors (RTIs): (1) nucleoside (NOTE the *s*) reverse transcriptase inhibitors (NRTIs); (2) structural analogues of nucleosides known as nucleotide (NOTE the *t*) reverse transcriptase inhibitors (NtRTIs); (3) nonnucleoside reverse transcriptase inhibitors (NNRTIs); (4) protease inhibitors (PIs); and (5) a single drug known as a fusion inhibitor. In addition, a variety of other drug classifications are used to treat opportunistic and secondary infections.

Nucleoside and Nucleotide Reverse Transcriptase Inhibitors

- Abacavir; ♣ Ziagen
- didanosine (Videx, dideoxyinosine, ddl); ♣ Videx
- emtricitabine (Emtriva); ♣ Emtriva
- lamivudine (Epivir, 3TC); ♣ Epivir, Heptovir, Epivir HBV

- stavudine (Zerit, d4T); ♣ Zerit
- zalcitabine (Hivid, ddC)
- zidovudine (Retrovir); ♣ Retrovir

Nucleotide Reverse Transcriptase Inhibitor (NtRTI)
- tenofovir (Viread, TDF); ♣ Viread

▌ Indications

NRTIs were the first drugs used against HIV infections, and they remain a vital component of HIV treatment. They can also be used as prophylaxis for occupational health exposure to HIV. When RTIs are used in combination with other anti-HIV drugs, usually a total of three drugs, the combination therapy blocks replication of HIV. All of the drugs listed above are currently approved by the U.S. Food and Drug Administration (FDA) for use in combination therapies; **the NRTIs should not be used as monotherapy for HIV** ⚠ **disease.**

▌ Pharmacodynamics

NRTIs block the replication cycle of HIV at the point where reverse transcriptase is used to convert RNA to DNA. As an HIV-specific enzyme, reverse transcriptase draws from the infected cell's pool of deoxynucleosides (e.g., thymidine, guanosine, adenosine, and cytidine) to synthesize the DNA chain. NRTIs lack a second hydroxyl group needed for the addition of subsequent bases to the growing DNA strand. By incorporating reverse transcriptase, elongation of the DNA strand is halted (NRTIs are chain-terminating drugs). They also have a competitive, inhibitory effect on reverse transcriptase itself. These drugs prevent the spread of HIV to new cells but do not interfere with viral replication in cells that are already infected. All NRTIs are considered prodrugs.

NtRTIs (tenofovir is the only nucleotide approved at this time) are technically different than nucleoside analogues, although they act very much the same way. In order for nucleoside analogues to work, they must undergo chemical changes (phosphorylation) to become active in the body. NtRTIs bypass this step, given that they are already chemically activated.

Neither NRTIs nor NtRTIs are selective for HIV reverse transcriptase, so their actions cause damage to other cells (especially the mitochondria) of the body. For this reason, it is common to see serious adverse effects such as lactic acidosis, hepatic steatosis, pancreatitis, neuropathy, and lipodystrophy syndrome with use of these drugs.

VIRAL RESISTANCE. Viral resistance is a function of both the duration of therapy and the severity of the HIV infection. Although viral resistance is discussed here under NRTI drugs, the risk of resistance exists for the other HIV drug classes as well. There are several commercially available HIV drug–resistance tests, but none are yet approved by the FDA.

HIV drug–resistant genetic mutations (HIV variants) can occur. Variants developing before the start of treatment are often the result of natural selection or the result of an error made during replication of the virus. Variants may be sufficiently robust to replicate but may not be capable of competing with the wild-type virus. Some variants are associated with the development of anti-HIV–drug resistance. Cross-resistance is also possible. Avoiding the development of drug resistance is the primary purpose for using multidrug therapy; variants that resist one anti-HIV drug almost always respond to multidrug therapy.

Pharmacokinetics

NRTIs are well absorbed when taken by mouth and widely distributed. The absorption of NRTIs is variable and depends on dose, gastric pH, and the presence of food in the gastrointestinal (GI) tract. NRTIs and NtRTIs are rapidly eliminated, with half-lives that vary from less than 1 hour for zidovudine to about 17 hours for tenofovir (Table 28-6). All RTIs, except abacavir, are eliminated through the kidneys in urine. Urinary elimination of zidovudine occurs after phase 1 biotransformation (glucuronidation) in the liver, whereas other RTIs are eliminated unchanged. NRTI biotransformation does not depend on the CYP450 enzyme system, the drugs are not highly protein bound, and they penetrate the CNS in significant, though varying, concentrations.

Adverse Effects and Contraindications

Hypersensitivity reactions to NRTIs are common in patients with HIV. No factors have been identified that assist the health care provider to identify which patients are likely to experience the adverse effects of these drugs. There is no evidence to support the conclusion that hypersensitivity reactions are related to the prescribed dosage. Symptoms of hypersensitivity (e.g.,

rash) usually subside within a few days of stopping treatment. However, if the patient is once again given the drug, cardiovascular collapse and death may result.

Lactic acidosis is rare but has been reported in patients taking NRTIs. The signs and symptoms of lactic acidosis include a patient history of NRTI use, unexplained GI complaints (e.g., nausea, vomiting, abdominal pain, loose stools); tachycardia, tachypnea; and myopathy and neuropathy. Hepatomegaly with steatosis (i.e., fatty liver) is associated with monotherapy as well as multidrug therapy. The myopathy and neuropathy are usually reversible once the drug is stopped.

The risk of hematologic toxicity is increased with high-dose therapy, advanced HIV infection, folic acid and B$_{12}$ deficiencies, and concurrent use of myelosuppressive, nephrotoxic drugs, or drugs that are directly toxic to circulating blood cells. A macrocytic anemia (i.e., a hemoglobin value below 5 mg/dL or 25% of baseline) commonly develops 4 to 6 weeks after treatment with zidovudine and appears to be related to impaired erythrocyte maturation. Granulocytopenia (i.e., a neutrophil count below 750 cells/mL or 50% of baseline) usually occurs after 6 to 8 weeks of therapy.

There is a 2.3% dose-related risk for pancreatitis in patients taking didanosine for 1 to 6 months. Alcohol ingestion, advanced HIV disease with CD4 counts less than 50 cells/mm^3, and a history of pancreatitis increase the risk that pancreatitis will develop. Concomitant use of didanosine with drugs

PHARMACOKINETICS
TABLE 28-6 Anti-HIV Drugs

Drug	Route	Onset	Peak	Duration	PB (%)	t½	BioA (%)
NUCLEOSIDE REVERSE TRANSCRIPTASE INHIBITORS							
abacavir	PO	Rapid	UA	UA	50	1.5 hr	83
emtricitabine	PO	Rapid	1–2 hr	UA	<4	10	75; 90*
didanosine tablets	PO	Rapid	0.5–1.0 hr	UA	<5	1.6 hr; 0.8 hr†	20–25
lamivudine	PO	Rapid	0.9 hr	12 hr	<36	3–6 hr; 2 hr†	86; 66†
stavudine	PO	Rapid	0.5–1.0 hr	3–5 hr	<5	3.0 hr	82; 78‡
zalcitabine	PO	Rapid	1–2 hr	8 hr; 3 hr‖	<4	2.6–10 hr	85
zidovudine	PO	UA	0.4–1.5 hr	3–5 hr	34–38	0.8–1.8 hr	52–75
NUCLEOTIDE REVERSE TRANSCRIPTASE INHIBITORS (NtRTIs)							
tenofovir§	PO	UA	1 hr	UA	<7.2	17 hr	25
NON-NUCLEOSIDE REVERSE TRANSCRIPTASE INHIBITORS (NNRTIs)							
delavirdine	PO	Rapid	1 hr	UA	98	5.8 hr	85
efavirenz	PO	Rapid	5 hr	UA	99	40–55 hr	UA
nevirapine	PO	2 hr	2–4 hr	24 hr	60	25–30 hr	>90
PROTEASE INHIBITORS							
amprenavir	PO	Rapid	1–2 hr	UA	90	7.1–10.6 hr	UA
atazanavir	PO	Rapid	2–2.5 hr	UA	86	5–8 hr	UA
darunavir	PO	Rapid	UA	UA	UA	UA	UA
fosamprenavir¶	PO	Rapid	2.5 hr	UA	90	7.7 hr	UA
indinavir	PO	2 wk	0.5–1 hr	6 mo	60	1.5–2 hr	30
nelfinavir	PO	Rapid	2–4 hr	8 hr	98	3.5–5 hr	20–80
ritonavir	PO	Rapid	4 hr	12 hr	98–99	3–5 hr	60–70
saquinavir	PO	Rapid	2 hr	7 hr	90	1–2 hr	4
tipranavir	PO	Rapid	UA	UA	99.9	6 hr	Low
FUSION INHIBITOR							
enfuvirtide	SubQ	UA	3–12 hr	UA	92	3.8 hr	84

*Absolute bioavailability of emtricitabine capsules and oral solution, respectively.
†Half-life of the active metabolites of didanosine, lamivudine, and stavudine for adult and child, respectively.
‡Half-life and bioavailability of stavudine for adult and child, respectively.
§Tenofovir is always combined with other anti-HIV drugs, or in the combination capsules tenovir + emtricitabine (Truvada), or tenofovir DF + emtricitabine + efavirenz (Atripla).
‖Duration of action of zalcitabine and its metabolites for adult and child, respectively.
¶Fosamprenavir is the prodrug of amprenavir.
BioA, Bioavailability; *INS*, insignificant; *NA*, not applicable; *PB*, protein binding; *PO*, by mouth; *subQ*, subcutaneously; *t½*, half-life; *UA*, unavailable.

that are likely to cause pancreatitis (e.g., stavudine and hydroxy-urea) also increases the chances that patients will manifest the signs and symptoms of pancreatitis. Although didanosine-induced pancreatitis can be fatal, the disorder usually resolves within a few weeks of stopping the drug. Patients with pancreatitis complain initially of vague abdominal pain, nausea, and vomiting. Elevations in serum triglycerides or glucose concentrations may appear before the onset of symptoms. Obtain baseline amylase and lipase concentrations for all patients who will be taking a didanosine-containing regimen; these values should also be checked periodically

Most NRTIs cause mild to moderately severe GI distress, including didanosine, zidovudine, and tenofovir. There is a transient nausea in 46% of patients, particularly with zidovudine, that ordinarily subsides within the first month of treatment. The nausea can usually be minimized by taking the drug with food and eating smaller but more frequent meals. However, in some cases the drug may have to be stopped owing to severe nausea. Because of the magnesium-hydroxide buffer that is added to the tablet formulation of didanosine, diarrhea can develop.

Peripheral neuropathy has been noted with didanosine (14% to 34%), zalcitabine (17% to 31%), and stavudine (15% to 21%). The neuropathy appears to be dose related and is generally described by patients as having a stocking-like distribution in the feet. Patients may also complain of an aching sensation or bilateral tingling and burning of their hands. The paresthesias and peripheral neuropathy are more likely to occur in children taking lamivudine than in adults.

⚠ **Safe use of NRTIs and NtRTIs during pregnancy and lactation and in children has not been established. Breastfeeding should be avoided by HIV-infected mothers because of the risk for transmitting the virus in breast milk.**

▥ Drug Interactions

Table 28-5 identifies key drug interactions with the NRTIs and NtRTIs.

▥ Dosage Regimen

The dosage regimens of NRTIs and NtRTIs are identified in Table 28-7. As mentioned, these drugs must be used in combination to reduce drug resistance. It is recommended that tenofovir be taken with a meal to increase absorption.

▥ Lab Considerations

NRTI therapy makes it necessary to obtain complete blood counts with differentials, at the start of treatment and regularly thereafter. Patients may require multiple blood transfusions if the CBC drops below a safe level.

Given the risk for liver and pancreatic adverse with RTIs, it is also important to check CD4 values, electrolytes, alkaline phosphatase, aspartate transaminase (AST) and alanine transaminase (ALT), amylase, lipase, bilirubin, triglycerides, and uric acid levels. In addition, patients taking stavudine should have a prothrombin time (PT) and international normalized ratio (INR) assessed and kidney function tests done.

Nonnucleoside Reverse Transcriptase Inhibitors (NNRTIs)

◆ delavirdine (Rescriptor); ♣ Rescriptor
◆ efavirenz (Sustiva); ♣ Sustiva
◆ nevirapine (Viramune); ♣ Viramune

▥ Indications

NNRTIs are also used for the treatment of HIV infection. These drugs are often used in combination with NRTIs such as zidovudine. Single-dose nevirapine reduces transmission of HIV by 50%, which makes it the drug of choice in developing countries.

▥ Pharmacodynamics

NNRTIs differ from NRTIs and NtRTIs in structure and mechanism of action. In contrast with these latter drug types, NNRTIs are not incorporated into viral DNA; rather, they directly inhibit HIV replication by binding noncompetitively to reverse transcriptase at sites separate from the RTI binding sites. NNRTIs are selective for the HIV-1 reverse transcriptase, allowing for fewer adverse effects.

RESISTANCE. Resistance and cross-resistance may develop rapidly with each NNRTI and, as a result, could eliminate this entire class from future treatment regimens. Therefore these drugs should only be used in potent combination regimens that maximally suppress viral replication. Do not use NNRTIs as monotherapy. Higher viral loads associated with NNRTI resistance may contribute to the high frequency of transmitted NNRTI resistance. There is no cross-resistance between the NNRTIs and NRTIs or protease inhibitors.

▥ Pharmacokinetics

NNRTIs are generally well absorbed following oral administration. The bioavailability of nevirapine is over 90% and is not food dependent (see Table 28-6). It is highly lipophilic; approximately 60% is protein bound, and cerebrospinal fluid (CSF) levels are 45% of those in plasma. Nevirapine is extensively biotransformed by the CYP 3A4 enzyme to metabolites and then eliminated through the kidneys.

Delavirdine is about 85% orally bioavailable but is reduced in the presence of antacids. It is extensively bound to plasma proteins. CSF levels are much less compared with nevirapine (0.4%) of the corresponding plasma levels, representing about 20% of the unbound fraction.

Efavirenz is moderately well absorbed following oral administration, with bioavailability increased to about 65% following a high-fat meal. Peak plasma levels are seen 3 to 5 hours after administration, with steady-state levels reached in 6 to 10 days. CSF levels range from 0.3% to 1.2% of plasma levels or approximately 3 times the free fraction of drug in the plasma. Efavirenz is principally biotransformed by CYP 3A4 and CYP 2B6 to inactive metabolites, with the remainder of the drug eliminated unchanged in the feces.

▥ Adverse Effects and Contraindications

Hypersensitivity reactions are particularly common during the induction phase of antiretroviral therapies that include an NNRTI. One third of patients treated with nevirapine develop a rash within 4 to 6 weeks of starting therapy; less than one fourth of patients taking delavirdine develop the rash, which is characterized by maculopapular, erythematous lesions that appear on the face, the trunk, and the extremities. It may or may not itch. Serious rashes have been reported in children taking efavirenz.

Unlike therapy with delavirdine or efavirenz, the cautious, upward dosage titration of nevirapine is unlikely to produce a

DOSAGE
TABLE 28-7 Anti-HIV Drugs

Drug	Dosage	Implications
NUCLEOSIDE REVERSE TRANSCRIPTASE INHIBITORS*		
abacavir	*Adult:* 300 mg PO twice daily†	Do not challenge after "hypersensitivity reaction." Take with or without food; alcohol increases serum levels by 41%.
emtricitabine	*Adult:* 200 mg PO once daily	May take without regard to meals.
didanosine	*Adult and Child >60 kg:* 200 mg PO enteric-coated tablets twice daily *–or–* 400 mg PO daily *Adult or Child <60 kg:* 125 mg PO twice daily *–or–* 250 mg PO once daily	Renal dosing considerations required. Take 30 min before meals or 2 hr after. Also available in delayed-release capsules and oral solutions.
lamivudine	*Adult:* 150 mg PO twice daily *–or–* 300 mg daily *Child:* 4 mg/kg PO twice daily. Maximum: 150 mg PO twice daily	Renal dosing considerations required. May take without regard to meals. Also used to treat patients with HBV, but at a different dose. If patient has both HIV and HBV, use dosage indicated for HIV therapy.
stavudine	*Adult:* 40 mg PO every 12 hr *Adult <60 kg:* 30 mg PO every 12 hr *Child:* Check package literature for pediatric dosing.	Renal dosing considerations required. May take without regard to meals.
zalcitabine	*Adult:* 0.75 mg PO every 8 hr	Renal dosing considerations required. May take without regard to meals.
zidovudine	*Adult:* 200 mg PO 3 times daily *–or–* 300 mg PO twice daily *Symptomatic Child 3 mo to 12 yr:* 180 mg/m² PO every 6 hr. Not to exceed 200 mg PO every 6 hr.	May take without regard to meals. Monitor CBC every 2–4 wk during initial therapy. Anemia may develop 2–4 wk after starting treatment. Granulocytopenia usually occurs after 6–8 wk of therapy.
NUCLEOTIDE REVERSE TRANSCRIPTASE INHIBITOR (NtRTI)		
tenofovir	*Adult:* 300 mg PO once daily	Take with a meal to enhance absorption.
NONNUCLEOSIDE REVERSE TRANSCRIPTASE INHIBITORS		
efavirenz	*Adult:* 600 mg PO daily	Preferred drug for treating HIV. Take before HS.
delavirdine	*Adult:* 400 mg PO 3 times daily	Used in combination therapy. Disperse tablets in 3 oz of water and stir.
nevirapine	*Adult:* 200 mg PO daily for 14 days, then 200 mg PO twice daily	Lead-in therapy; helps reduce incidence of rash. If therapy is interrupted for longer than 7 days, restart at 200 mg PO daily. May take without regard to meals.
PROTEASE INHIBITORS		
amprenavir	*Adult:* 1.2 grams PO every 12 hr if used as monotherapy. With ritonavir: 1.2 grams PO every 12 hr + 200 mg ritonavir. *Child:* Based on mg/kg body weight	Drug is available in 150-mg capsules.
atazanavir	*Adult:* 400 mg PO once daily for ARV-naïve patients. For experienced patients: 300 mg PO with retonavir 100 mg once daily	Take with food.
darunavir	*Adult:* 600 mg PO darunavir + 100 mg ritonavir twice daily	Take with food.
fosamprenavir	*Adult:* 1.4 grams PO twice daily or once daily with ritonavir 200 mg	Combination therapy
indinavir	*Adult:* 800 mg PO every 8 hr with ritonavir	Seldom used. Take 1 hr before or after low-fat meals.
nelfinavir	*Adult:* 1250 mg PO every 12 hr *Child:* 20–30 mg/kg/dose	Take with food.
ritonavir	*Adult:* 600 mg PO every 12 hr	Rarely used for its ARV activity, rather for its ability to boost concentrations of other PIs; given at much smaller dosage.
saquinavir	*Adult:* 600 mg PO 3 times daily. Fortovase tablets: 1.2 grams PO 3 times daily. Invirase capsules: 1 gram twice daily	Rarely given without ritonavir. Take within 2 hr of high-fat meal.
tipranavir	*Adult:* 500 mg PO twice daily with 200 mg of ritonavir twice daily	Genotypic or phenotypic testing and/or treatment history should guide use of tipranavir or ritonavir.
FUSION INHIBITOR		
enfuvirtide	*Adult:* 90 mg subQ twice daily *Child 6–16 yr:* 2 mg/kg subQ twice daily, to max of 90 mg twice daily	May take without regard to meals but must avoid high-fat meals, which increase absorption by 50%.

*Lactic acidosis rare but potentially fatal with *all* NRTIs.
†Special warnings are reviewed in the "Black-Box Warnings" that the U.S. Food and Drug Administration (FDA) has required manufacturers to list in the package inserts for some HIV drugs. These are the most dangerous adverse effects of which health care providers and people living with HIV should be aware. However, drugs without black-box warnings can still have serious adverse effects.
ARV, Antiretroviral; *HBV*, hepatitis B virus; *HIV*, human immunodeficiency virus; *HS*, bedtime; *PO*, by mouth, *subQ*, subcutaneous (route).

rash. Patients whose rash is erythematous, macular, or maculopapular do not necessarily need to have therapy stopped. On the other hand, patients whose reactions are more serious (e.g., desquamation, edema, fever, malaise, myalgias) may require hospitalization. In these cases, the NNRTI drug is permanently discontinued.

NNRTIs can cause drug-induced hepatitis. The risk of hepatitis is even higher in patients with high CD4 counts who are taking nevirapine. If liver function tests are moderately or severely elevated, the drug should be discontinued.

Headache, fatigue, nausea, vomiting, and diarrhea may be found in 2% of patients taking delavirdine. Cardiovascular adverse effects are rare but include syncope, bradycardia, tachycardia, and vasodilation. Anemia, bruising, neutropenia, and prolonged PT and INR values may be seen.

Approximately 52% of patients taking efavirenz have mild to severe adverse effects including dizziness, vivid dreams, insomnia, confusion, impaired concentration, amnesia, agitation, depersonalization, hallucinations, and euphoria. Occasionally patients report a mild to moderate maculopapular rash (27%), fatigue, headache, diarrhea, fever, and cough (less than 26%). There are no known toxic effects.

Safe use of NNRTIs during pregnancy (category C) and lactation and in children under age 16 has not been established.

Drug Interactions

Drug interactions are of concern with this class, since each NNRTI is a substrate of the CYP450 enzyme system. Nevirapine tends to induce biotransformation; delavirdine inhibits biotransformation; and efavirenz is both an enzyme inducer and inhibitor. Specific drug interactions are identified in Table 28-5.

Dosage Regimen

The dosage regimen for NNRTIs is identified in Table 28-7. As discussed previously, the drugs are used in combination with other antiretroviral drugs. Avoid high-fat meals since they may increase absorption of efavirenz.

Lab Considerations

Lab abnormalities noted with delavirdine therapy include neutropenia, anemia, thrombocytopenia, and increased ALT, AST, amylase, and bilirubin levels. Hyperkalemia, hypocalcemia, hyponatremia, and hypophosphatemia may also occur. Patient evaluation before initiation of therapy includes CBC, PT and INR, partial thromboplastin time (PTT), electrolytes, and renal and liver function studies. In addition, the glutamyltransferase (GGT) level may be increased after nevirapine administration. Efavirenz may produce false-positive urine test results for cannabinoids. It also increases total cholesterol and triglyceride levels along with ALT and AST values.

Protease Inhibitors

◆ amprenavir (Agenerase)
◆ atazanavir (Reyataz)
◆ darunavir (Prezista)
◆ fosamprenavir (Lexiva)
◆ indinavir (Crixivan); ♣ Crixivan
◆ nelfinavir (Viracept); ♣ Viracept
◆ ritonavir (Norvir, RTV); ♣ Norvirsec
◆ saquinavir (Invirase, Fortovase)
◆ tipranavir (Aptivus)

Indications

Protease inhibitors (PIs) are the most effective antiretroviral drugs, but they are not to be used as monotherapy. When used in combination, viral loads can be reduced to an undetectable level. The first protease inhibitor approved for HIV was saquinavir, but its efficacy was limited by poor bioavailability. The development of ritonavir and indinavir launched the era of HAART. Their use improves survival and reduces hospitalizations for patients with HIV. Suppression rates of viremia are as high as 80% or better for up to 3 years.

Pharmacodynamics

PIs, in combination with NRTIs and NtRTIs (and with NNRTIs), are potent inhibitors of HIV-1 and HIV-2 replication. Once HIV RNA is inside the DNA of a CD4 cell, a long strand of genetic material is produced that must be disassembled and put back together correctly to form new copies of the virus. To cut the strand, a scissor-like enzyme called protease is required. PIs block this enzyme to prevent the breakdown of viral proteins into the components needed for viral assembly and budding. Their actions do not require intracellular activation to be effective.

PIs are active in both acutely and chronically infected cells, and show activity with chronically infected monocytes and macrophages unaffected by reverse transcriptase inhibitors. Early stages of the HIV replication cycle are not affected.

RESISTANCE. Resistance is a problem with PIs and is, as with the other anti-HIV drugs, the major obstacle to the long-term efficacy of antiretroviral therapy. There are two primary tests used to assess viral susceptibility, genotype and phenotype. In genotype resistance, the viral genetic material mutates. In phenotype resistance, the virus becomes less sensitive to the drug. Cross-resistance with PIs is also possible when viral strains resistant to one PI become resistant to the others as well. Nelfinavir has less of a problem with cross-resistance than other PIs.

Pharmacokinetics

The oral bioavailability of PIs ranges between 4% to as much as 80% (see Table 28-6). PIs are protein bound at 89% to 99% except for indinavir, which is 60% protein bound. CSF penetration is limited, although data suggest that indinavir may achieve clinically significant concentrations in the CNS. This fact provides justification for the use of CNS-penetrating NRTI drugs with PIs. The PIs are biotransformed through the CYP450 enzyme system and eliminated in the urine.

Adverse Effects and Contraindications

The primary adverse effects of PIs are on the GI tract, with nausea predominating in 3% to 30% of patients. Ritonavir and amprenavir have the highest incidence of nausea. Other typical GI adverse effects include vomiting, acid reflux, flatulence, abdominal cramps, constipation, and diarrhea (5% to 30%). Ritonavir is more likely than nelfinavir to cause severe diarrhea.

Ritonavir-induced pancreatitis has been reported (Chapman et al., 2007). The serum triglyceride value in one patient, after 5 months of treatment with ritonavir, was 1563 mg/dL. In another patient, the triglyceride value was 5957 mg/dL after 2 months of treatment with ritonavir. In another patient, whose triglyceride levels were normal, nelfinavir-induced pancreatitis was reported shortly after treatment was started. The elevated triglyceride levels and subsequent pancreatitis appear to resolve once the PI is discontinued.

An accumulation of body fat is associated with all PIs except amprenavir. There is increased fat in the breasts, in the abdomen ("protease paunch"), and over the dorsocervical vertebrae ("buffalo hump"). The cause for the fat redistribution is unclear, and whether it accounts, at least in part, for the adverse effects of HAART is still not understood. Researchers regard the symptoms as different aspects of a complex syndrome or syndromes. It should also be noted that the body fat changes have also been seen in a number of patients with HIV who are not taking PIs.

Dyslipidemia associated with the use of PIs is a risk factor for premature atherosclerosis. Patients treated with PIs also show significantly greater degrees of thickening of the intima media, compared with either PI-naive or HIV-negative control subjects.

The risk for adverse liver effects is greater in patients who have chronic hepatitis B or C, or who have existing liver disease from other causes. These patients are nearly 4 times as likely to develop drug-induced hepatitis and liver failure, particularly patients taking indinavir and ritonavir. Some 10% of patients experience liver damage severe enough to warrant stopping anti-HIV therapy.

PIs can increase blood glucose levels, increase insulin resistance, alter insulin metabolism, and worsen existing diabetes. It appears that the insulin resistance contributes to the body fat changes.

Increased risk for bleeding and hematomas in patients with hemophilia may occur with PIs, although the cause is unknown. Patients should be advised of the possibility of bleeding, although it is rare to stop a PI regimen for this reason.

Nephrolithiasis has been reported in almost half of the patients taking over 2.4 grams of indinavir daily and appears to be dose related. The symptoms of nephrolithiasis include costovertebral angle tenderness, flank or groin pain, and hematuria.

In one study, osteopenia developed in approximately 50% of patients taking PIs, and 21% experienced osteoporosis compared to 6% of those not taking the drugs (Annapoorna et al., 2004). Why osteopenia and osteoporosis develop is unclear, as is the best way to manage the problem. Men were twice as likely to develop osteoporosis as women.

Loss of libido and erectile dysfunction is 3 times more common in men taking PIs. Acute myeloblastic leukemia, hemolytic anemia, and Stevens-Johnson syndrome have been reported with saquinavir, although they are rare.

▥ Drug Interactions

All PIs are substrates of the CYP 3A4 enzyme (see Table 28-5). Saquinavir is subject to extensive first-pass effect and functions as a CYP 3A4 inhibitor as well as the substrate. Drugs that induce this enzyme reduce plasma concentrations of the drug. Conversely, concomitant administrations of drugs that inhibit the CYP 3A4 enzyme result in decreased biotransformation, causing drug levels to rise. Ritonavir increases the amount of other drugs within the body since it prevents the liver from eliminating drugs.

Administration of indinavir with grapefruit juice results in a decrease in indinavir plasma levels. In contrast, the bioavailability of saquinavir is increased when it is taken with grapefruit juice.

Both the PIs and HMG CoA reductase inhibitors ("statins") are biotransformed in the liver, thus contributing to the risk for elevated liver function test values. For this reason, many health care providers avoid using statin drugs in people taking HAART. Atorvastatin is the only statin reported to reduce serum concentrations of saquinavir.

▥ Dosage Regimen

The dosages of protease inhibitor drugs vary with the specific drug (see Table 28-7). Indinavir is taken 1 hour before or after a low-fat meal. In contrast, saquinavir is taken within 2 hours of a high-fat meal.

▥ Lab Considerations

The ALT, AST, lactate dehydrogenase (LDH), alkaline phosphatase, amylase, bilirubin, creatine phosphokinase, cholesterol, glucose, and uric acid levels should be obtained before initiating therapy and then on a regular basis. A CBC

and comprehensive metabolic panel usually are sufficient to monitor these parameters.

HIV Fusion Inhibitor

◆ enfuvirtide (Fuzeon, T-20)

▥ Indications

Patients with HIV who become resistant to NRTIs, NtRTIs, NNRTIs, and PIs will likely benefit from the fusion inhibitor enfuvirtide. As the only drug in this class, enfuvirtide treats HIV infection resistant to other antiretroviral drugs; it is not used for monotherapy. It may be used in patients who are treatment-experienced and who have evidence of viral replication despite ongoing antiretroviral therapy. Enfuvirtide, when combined with other anti-HIV drugs, is thought to have strong activity against HIV in patients who are treatment-naïve. Enfuvirtide, taken alone, reduces the viral load as much as 60% in treatment-naïve patients.

▥ Pharmacodynamics

Enfuvirtide binds to the gp41 subunit of the viral envelope, thus preventing the changes required for the virus to fuse to cellular membranes, and consequently viral entry and replication is prevented.

RESISTANCE. Resistance to enfuvirtide is possible; the mechanism thought responsible is a structural change in gp41. When other drugs in the patient's regimen are still effective, resistance to enfuvirtide develops somewhat slowly. If there is significant resistance to other drugs, resistance to enfuvirtide will rapidly develop. However, it is known that enfuvirtide completely lacks cross-resistance to other currently approved anti-HIV drugs.

▥ Pharmacokinetics

The bioavailability of enfuvirtide given subcutaneously is about 84%, regardless of the injection site (see Table 28-6). High-fat meals increase absorption by 50%. It is highly protein bound to albumin. Biotransformation does not involve the CYP450 enzymes but rather is carried out by proteolytic hydrolysis.

▥ Adverse Effects and Contraindication

Injection site reactions occur in 98% of patients, usually within the first week of use. Although generally mild to moderate, injection site reactions can also be severe. A local reaction usually resolves in less than a week but may persist longer. Injection site reactions may be worse if the drug is administered intramuscularly rather than subcutaneously.

In clinical trials, patients taking enfuvirtide with other anti-HIV drugs developed bacterial pneumonia more often than patients not receiving enfuvirtide (Jamjian and McNicholl, 2004). The development of pneumonia has not definitively been tied to use of enfuvirtide. Eosinophilia has been noted. Although rare, hypersensitivity reactions may occur; if they do, they are of varying severity and may reappear on rechallenge.

Respiratory distress, glomerulonephritis, Guillain-Barré syndrome, and primary immune complex reactions have been reported with enfuvirtide. Peripheral neuropathy, insomnia, depression, decreased appetite, fatigue, muscle pain, constipation, and pancreatitis have also been noted. It is unknown if enfuvirtide passes into breast milk and what effect it may have on a nursing infant. To prevent transmission of the virus, it is recommended that mothers with HIV not breastfeed.

RESISTANCE. Resistance to enfuvirtide develops rapidly when the drug is used as monotherapy. With combination therapy, HIV mutates much more slowly. Enfuvirtide does not have cross-resistance with any other antiviral drugs.

▥ Drug Interactions

No drug interactions with enfuvirtide have been identified.

▥ Dosage Regimen

Because of its fragile structure, enfuvirtide must be given subcutaneously (see Table 28-7). The manufacturers of enfuvirtide are experimenting with needle-free injection devices and are also looking at the possibility of administering the drug once daily.

▥ Lab Considerations

Enfuvirtide may elevate serum lipase, amylase, triglycerides, ALT, AST, creatine kinase, and blood glucose levels. The hemoglobin value and WBC counts may decrease.

CLINICAL REASONING

Treatment Objectives

The goal of early therapy is to suppress viral loads to undetectable levels, suppress viral replication, preserve immune function, prolong health and life, and decrease the risk of drug resistance due to early suppression of viral replication.

Treatment Options

Viral load testing measures the amounts of viral RNA in the plasma and is critical in determining the effectiveness of HIV treatment. The results are reported as the number of HIV RNA copies/mL of serum. The goal is to make all viral loads undetectable, because high loads drive CD4 loss and, ultimately, immune suppression. The Department of Health and Human Services guidelines recommend deferring antiretroviral therapy for patients with a CD4 count over 350 cells/mm³ and a viral load less than 100,000 copies/mL. On the other hand, asymptomatic patients with CD4 counts between 201 and 350 cells/mm³ and patients with a CD4 count over 350 cells/mm³ and a viral load over 100,000 copies/mL

▲ should be offered antiretroviral therapy. **Antiretroviral drugs are not a cure for HIV infection, nor do they reduce the risk of transmission to others.**

▥ Patient Variables

Recent social history and current prejudices constitute a large portion of what preoccupies HIV-infected people. Health care providers should focus vital information on issues that relate to housing, family and community support, family dynamics, employment, and health insurance. It may be necessary to remove system barriers to treatment in order to stabilize patients' lives before the initiation of drug therapy. Recommendations regarding the use of antiviral drugs in HIV are in flux. When and what to initiate, when to change regimens, and how to minimize the development of resistance and cross-resistance are continually being reevaluated. Clearly, monotherapy results

in resistance and loss of efficacy as a result of the huge viral load, short viral half-life, and tendency for mutations.

Antiretroviral drugs used in the treatment of HIV are effective as long as patients adhere to the prescribed treatment regimen. However, each of the drugs can cause a variety of unpleasant, adverse effects that range from bothersome to fatal. Weigh the risk-benefit ratio for each drug in the multidrug combination. Since all antiretroviral drugs have the potential for toxicity, particular attention is needed to teach patients about the potential effects and at what point they are to contact their health care provider.

All patients on HAART should have liver function tests ▲ done once monthly for the first 3 months of therapy and then every 3 to 6 months thereafter. Increased liver function test values may indicate hepatotoxicity. Increased serum creatinine levels, proteinuria, or glucosuria are warning signs of renal toxicity.

LIFE-SPAN CONSIDERATIONS. Diagnosis of HIV infection is often missed at initial encounters with the health care provider. Although most patients seek medical attention during their acute illness, only 25% are diagnosed at that time. Early diagnosis of acute primary HIV infection is important for explaining a patient's often undiagnosed complaints. Early diagnosis is also important in counseling, preventing further transmission, determining the natural history of the infection, and starting early treatment with drug therapy. Consider the possibility of HIV infection in all patients who have symptoms consistent with acute viral syndrome.

The complexities of HIV and AIDS make care of these patients challenging and sometimes frustrating for both patient and health care provider. Nonadherence seems to be a major obstacle in maximizing benefit from drug therapy. Even minimal nonadherence contributes to drug resistance and loss of efficacy. To help resolve the problem of too many pills, the pharmaceutical industry often formulates two or three of the drugs into one tablet (see Case Study—Antiviral Drugs).

Pregnant and Nursing Women. Women should receive optimal antiretroviral therapy regardless of pregnancy status (Kourtis, Lee, and Abrams, 2006). Treatment is based on the health of the mother as well as preventing transmission to the fetus and ensuring the health of the child after birth. To date the only drugs with a demonstrable ability to reduce the risk of perinatal HIV transmission are zidovudine and nevirapine. Zidovudine is effective in reducing perinatal HIV transmission regardless of maternal viral load. Oral zidovudine is started at 14 weeks' gestation and continued throughout pregnancy. Zidovudine is then administered intravenously during the intrapartum period and to the newborn for the first 6 weeks of life.

Women receiving antiretroviral drugs at the time pregnancy is diagnosed should continue therapy. All drugs in a multidrug treatment regimen should be discontinued at the same time if antiretroviral drug therapy is discontinued. When the antiretroviral regimen is restarted, all drugs should be started simultaneously.

The choice of which antiretroviral drug to administer requires consideration of pharmacokinetics and the safety of antiretroviral drugs in pregnancy. It is important to note the potential effects of drugs on the fetus and newborn. Only the pharmacokinetics of zidovudine and lamivudine have been evaluated in infected women.

CASE STUDY · Antiviral Drugs

ASSESSMENT

History of Present Illness	JD is a 43-year-old man diagnosed HIV infection within the last year. Until the last few weeks he was feeling fine. Today he comes in to be seen with fatigue, weakness, fever, chills, dyspnea on exertion, and a dry cough. This "bad cold" has been creeping up on him over the last 3 weeks. He suspects his HIV infection may have been the result of a single same-sex encounter he had on a business trip 3 years ago and may be responsible for his current illness. He refused antiretroviral therapy at the initial visit when the diagnosis of HIV was made.
Past Health History	JD has no known allergies. Follows vegetarian diet. Nonsmoker, nondrinker. Denies recent or past IV drug use. He reports no other sexual partners in the 20 years he was married.
Life-Span Considerations	JD lives alone and is currently on leave from his employment as a horticulturist. His support system includes a twin sister who lives nearby and several colleagues from work. Without work, his health insurance plan (COBRA) will lapse in another 12 months. He has no pharmacy plan.
Physical Exam Findings	*Height:* 72 inches. *Weight:* 148. *BP:* 124/82. 102.2° F. 128. 32. *SpO₂ room air:* 68%. Weight down 40 lb since last visit 6 months ago. Skin dusky, no skin lesions or masses. Lymphadenopathy. Breath sounds with crackles, wheezing, and rhonchi all lobes. No E>A changes noted. HRRR. Abdomen soft, flat, no HSM, masses, or bruits. EOMI, PERRLA, CN II-XII intact. Rhomberg negative.
Diagnostic Testing	*CXR:* diffuse bilateral interstitial infiltrates. Viral load pending. *CD4 count:* 128/mm³. *WBC:* 5.8/mm³; *RBC:* 3.35/mm³; *Hgb:* 10.6 mg/dL; *Hct:* 30 mg/dL; *Lymph:* 15%; *K:* 3.9 mEq/L; *BUN:* 10 mg/dL; *Creatinine:* 1.5 mg/dL. ABGs reveal hypoxemia. PPD negative at previous visit.

DIAGNOSIS: HIV⁺ with *Pneumocystitis jirovecii* pneumonia

MANAGEMENT

Treatment Objectives	1. Maintain and improve oxygenation. 2. Maintain immune function as near a normal state as possible. 3. Slow disease progression and prolong survival. 4. Preserve quality of life by effectively suppressing HIV replication.
Treatment Plan	**Pharmacotherapy** • trimethoprim-sulfamethoxazole 15 mg/kg/day IV in divided doses every 6 hr for 21 days • prednisone 40 mg PO twice daily for 5 days; then 40 mg daily for 5 days; and then 20 mg daily • tenofovir DF 300 mg PO once daily • efavirenz 600 mg PO once daily • atazanavir 400 mg PO once daily • Home O₂ @ 3L/NC continuously **Patient Education** 1. Follow-up in office tomorrow morning for repeat blood gases and to make arrangements for home care IV therapy until patient is able to manage antibiotic therapy himself 2. How to manage home O₂ therapy and IV antibiotic therapy 3. The implications of a PCP infection and a relatively new diagnosis of HIV-positive status 4. Importance of taking efavirenz 30 minutes before a meal and the remainder of the drugs with a meal to reduce gastric upset and enhance absorption of the drugs 5. Pharmacodynamics of each anti-HIV drug and the importance of combination therapy 6. Complete a patient drug list identifying what to take, when to take it, the adverse effects of each drug, and when to contact the health care provider for assistance. 7. Purpose of taking prednisone along with trimethoprim-sulfamethoxazole 8. Importance of avoiding others who are ill; remove plants from the home 9. Provide list of HIV resources for financial assistance and support. **Evaluation** 1. Follow-up visit: SpO₂ on 3L O₂NC 89% at rest; with exertion, SpO₂ 85% 2. Too early in treatment to determine drug effectiveness on CD4 count and viral load 3. Fever down to 100° F, pulse down to 88, and respirations down to 24; skin color improved 4. JD is asking more questions about his therapy, which suggests he is beginning to understand the purpose for antiretroviral drug therapy and the implications of his disease.

CLINICAL REASONING ANALYSIS

Q1. **What criteria did you use to determine when to start his HIV drugs?**

A. Therapy should be initiated in any patient who is symptomatic, or when the CD4 count is less than 500 cells/mm^3, or the viral load is greater than 5000 copies/mL. JD is symptomatic with his PCP, and even though we don't have his viral load back yet, his CD4 count is only 128/mm^3.

Q2. **Why combination therapy? Wouldn't he do just as well with monotherapy for his HIV?**

A. Combination therapy during early-stage disease produces significant and sustained reduction of viral load, as well as an increase in CD4 counts. The same combination in late-stage disease with CD4 cell counts of less than 50 cells/mm^3 usually lowers death rates. Triple therapy demonstrates a benefit over double nucleoside therapy in both viral load and clinical benefit.

Q3. **Some HIV drugs are taken 2 to 3 times a day and one even every 4 hours. Why is he only taking his once a day?**

A. Well, first of all, efavirenz is a preferred NNRTI for HIV and it is formulated as a once-daily tablet. Secondly, treatment for HIV, and now his PCP, is hard enough without having to take any more drugs than are absolutely necessary. At least with this regimen, he will take one tablet before breakfast, and then the rest of the morning tablets after he eats. If he would like, he can take the other drugs with his evening meal. It really doesn't make all that much difference, as long as he takes them at about the same time each day.

Q4. **I heard the other health care providers talking in the hallway about a rule for changing his treatment regimen once he is over the PCP. What rule were they talking about?**

A. A very basic rule: when changing drug therapy, never change a single drug but at least two at a time. We also choose drugs that have not been taken before. By following this rule, the likelihood of viral resistance is reduced. We now have enough anti-HIV drugs that the rule is easier to follow than in the past.

Q5. **How will you know when it is time to change his HIV treatment regimen?**

A. Therapy should be changed when toxicity or intolerance occurs, or there is evidence of drug failure, as in a fall in his CD4 count.

Q6. **I understand why the anti-HIV drugs and the IV drug were started, but why the prednisone? Isn't it going to reduce his immune status even more?**

A. Mortality is reduced in patients with moderate to severe PCP whose SpO$_2$ is less than 70 mm Hg when prednisone is started within 72 hours of his PCP diagnosis. JD's SpO$_2$ is 68% today with activity, and 82% at rest.

Q7. **Everyone says these HIV drugs are so expensive. They can't be that expensive, can they?**

A. Oh, they are expensive all right. That's why we need to get him connected with the social worker and other HIV resources for financial assistance. For example, for 30 tablets that are a month's supply of efavirenz, the cost is $400; the tenofovir tablets are $430/month; and the atazanavir capsules, since they are the newer drugs, are $1600/month—that comes to a total of almost $2500/month.

All NRTIs except didanosine are classified as FDA pregnancy category C; didanosine is classified as category B. However, only nevirapine has been evaluated during pregnancy. Nevirapine crosses the placenta, reaching neonatal serum concentrations equivalent to those in the mother. Studies on the use of other NNRTIs in pregnancy have not been conducted.

Children and Adolescents. **Antiretroviral therapy is recommended for infants infected with HIV (soon after delivery), children, and adolescents, regardless of age, clinical status, or viral load.** As a result, a growing number of adolescents are long-term survivors of perinatal or blood-product HIV infection as children. However, some health care providers defer therapy and closely monitor the clinical, immunologic, and virologic status of the patient. The viral load indicative of increased risk for disease progression is not well defined in children, so any child with a viral load greater than 100,000 copies/mL should be started on antiretroviral therapy. Combination therapy is recommended for all infants, children, and adolescents.

Children are dependent on caregivers for the administration of drug therapy. The environment, as well as the willingness of the parents or caregiver to adhere to a complex multidrug regimen, should be evaluated. Because absorption of some antiretroviral drugs is affected by food, it can be difficult to juggle drug administration times around feedings. Adolescents do not want to be different from their peers; it is difficult to obtain adherence to a treatment regimen when the adolescent generally feels well.

Older Adults. HIV infection in the older adult has been called the great imitator because it can masquerade as dementia and be mistaken for Alzheimer's or other chronic illness. Subtle differences between Alzheimer's disease and related dementias and HIV dementia also make patient assessment difficult. In addition, other symptoms such as fatigue, weakness, anorexia, and weight loss occur in many conditions other than HIV infection. Risk factors most often associated with HIV transmission in the older adult include sexual contact, blood transfusions earlier than 1985, and illicit drug use.

Currently the only way to slow the progression of HIV infection is with antiretroviral drug therapy; however, older adults are generally more prone to adverse effects than their younger counterparts. Older adults are also more prone to adverse effects of drugs because of polypharmacy. Nephron mass and renal blood flow decreases with age, which may affect the dosing of drugs eliminated by the kidneys. Lean muscle mass decreases, whereas the proportion of body fat increases. This lengthens the effects of fat-soluble drugs. It is important to note if older adults' cognitive status, hearing, and visual acuity enable them to hear, understand, read, and follow directions with regard to drug therapy.

▥ Drug Variables

Multidrug therapy exerts constant maximal suppression of HIV replication and is the best approach in reducing the risk of drug-resistant variants. HAART can be used by patients newly infected with HIV, as well as those with established AIDS. HAART should be started with all drugs started simultaneously. Triple combinations containing a PI are considered the most potent of all regimens (Tables 28-8 and 28-9). Consultation with experts in HIV/AIDs therapy is recommended (Table 28-10).

A   **Viral resistance emerges in weeks to months with monotherapy, and therefore antiretroviral drugs should not be used as monotherapy or added sequentially.** Sequential introduction of antiretroviral drugs increases the likelihood of incomplete suppression of HIV replication. Indeed, there is a transient decrease in plasma viral load with monotherapy, but future therapies are compromised by viral variants resistant to one or more antiretroviral drugs. The one

exception is the use of zidovudine specifically for the purpose of reducing the risk of perinatal HIV transmission in pregnant women with high CD4 counts and low viral loads, and who have decided not to initiate antiretroviral therapy. This time-limited use of zidovudine has important benefits to infants and is not likely to compromise the mother's ability to benefit from combination antiretroviral therapy in the future.

TREATMENT FAILURE. It is important not to abandon specific therapeutic regimens too soon, since each decision to alter therapy limits future alternative options. Factors that may contribute to treatment failure include the following: (1) poor health before starting the treatment regimen; (2) poor adherence to the treatment regimen; (3) previous anti-HIV treatment and/or drug resistance; (4) alcohol or drug abuse; (5) adverse effects of the drugs, including toxicities, or drug interactions; (6) poor absorption of the drugs; and (7) any comorbid conditions or illnesses other than HIV infection.

TABLE 28-8 Combination Anti-HIV Formulations

Brand Name	Combination	Abbreviation
Atripla	tenofovir DF + emtricitabine + efavirenz	TDF + FTC + EFV
Combivir	zidovudine + lamivudine	AZT + 3TC
Epzicom	abacavir + lamivudine	ABC + 3TC
Kaletra	lopinavir + ritonavir	LPV
Trizivir	abacavir + zidovudine* + lamivudine	ABC + AZT + 3TC
Truvada	tenofovir DF + emtricitabine	TDF + FTC

*Consider possibility of lactic acidosis whenever a patient receiving zidovudine develops unexplained tachypnea or dyspnea, or there is a fall in serum bicarbonate level. Zidovudine therapy should be suspended under these circumstances.

TABLE 28-9 Constructing an Anti-HIV Treatment Regimen*

DRUG	Column A				Column B
	NNRTI	OR	Protease Inhibitor	+	Dual-NRTI Options
Preferred	efavirenz[†]	–OR–	atazanavir + ritonavir	+	tenofovir-emtricitabine[§] –or– zidovudine-lamivudine[§]
Alternatives	nevirapine[‖]	–OR–	atazanavir[¶] fosamprenavir fosamprenavir + ritonavir (once/day) lopinavir-ritonavir[‡] (once/day)	+	abacavir-lamivudine didanosine + emtricitabine –or– lamivudine

	OTHER OPTIONS	
Option	Reasons for Not Recommending as Initial Therapy	Special Circumstances Whereby Drug May Be Used
trizivir	Inferior virologic activity	When NNRTI or PI regimens cannot be used because of toxicities or concerns about significant drug-drug interactions
nelfinavir	Inferior virologic activity	Has had most experience in pregnancy, with good tolerability and adequate pharmacokinetic data
saquinavir (boosted with ritonavir)	Inferior to lopinavir-ritonavir. Minimal efficacy data in treatment-naive patients	When preferred or alternative regimen cannot be used based on toxicities or concerns about significant drug-drug interactions
stavudine + lamivudine	Significant toxicities including neuropathy, lipoatrophy, hyperlactatemia (including symptomatic lactic acidosis, hepatic steatosis, and pancreatitis)	When preferred or alternative regimen cannot be used

*To construct an antiretroviral regimen, select one drug from column A and one from column B.
[†]Efavirenz is not recommended during first trimester of pregnancy or in sexually active women of child-bearing age who are not using contraception.
[‡]Lopinavir-ritonavir as a preferred PI was based on twice-daily dosing. There is similar efficacy with once-daily dosing but a higher incidence of moderate to severe diarrhea.
[§]Emtricitabine may be used in place of lamivudine and vice versa.
[‖]Nevirapine should not be used in women with CD4 cell counts >250 cells/mm^3 or in men with cell counts >400 cells/mm^3 because of increased risk for symptomatic hepatic events.
[¶]Atazanavir must be boosted with ritonavir if used in combination with tenofovir.
NNRTI, Non-nucleoside reverse transcriptase inhibitor; *PI*, protease inhibitor.

TABLE 28-10 Situations Warranting Expert Consultation*

Situation	Reasoning
Delayed exposure report (>24–36 hr)	Interval after which lack of benefits from PEP undefined
Unknown source of exposure	Use of PEP decided on case-by-case basis Consider severity of exposure and epidemiologic likelihood of HIV exposure. Do not test needles or other devices for HIV.
Known or suspected pregnancy of exposed person; exposed person is breastfeeding	Use of optimal PEP regimens not excluded PEP not denied solely on basis of pregnancy or breast-feeding
Resistance of source virus to antiretroviral drugs	Influence of drug resistance on transmission risk unknown If source person's virus is known or suspected to be resistant to one or more of the drugs considered for PEP, selection of drugs to which the source person's virus is unlikely to be resistant is recommended Resistance testing of the source person's virus at the time of exposure not recommended Initiation of PEP not to be delayed while awaiting results of any resistance testing
Toxicity of the initial PEP regimen	Adverse symptoms (e.g., nausea, diarrhea) common with PEP Symptoms often manageable without changing PEP by using antiemetics and antidiarrheal drugs In other situations, modifying the dose interval (e.g., taking drugs after a meal, or administering a lower dose more frequently throughout the day as recommended by the manufacturer) may help alleviate symptoms.

*Either with local experts or by calling the National Clinicians' Postexposure Prophylaxis Helpline (PEP-line) number 888–448–4911.
HIV, Human immunodeficiency virus; *PEP,* postexposure prophylaxis.
From Panlilio, A., Cardo, D., Grohskopf, L., et al. (2005). Updated U.S. Public Health Service guidelines for the management of occupational exposures to HIV and recommendations for postexposure prophylaxis. *Morbidity and Mortality Weekly Report Recommendation, 54*(RR-9), 1–17.

Before a decision is made to change antiretroviral therapy based on viral loads, the test should be repeated using the same type of test. There are three types of treatment failure. *Virologic failure* is when viral loads fail to drop by 10-fold (1 log) within the first 4 weeks of treatment, or if the virus is found again after treatment had previously lowered the viral load to undetectable levels. Virologic failure is the most common failure type.

An *immunologic failure* occurs when CD4 counts continue to drop despite antiretroviral therapy, or do not rise above baseline within the first year of treatment. A *clinical failure* occurs if the patient develops an opportunistic infection or a decline in physical health despite at least 3 months of anti-HIV drug therapy. Because there are small numbers of antiretroviral drugs available, options for changing therapeutic regimens are clearly limited.

Patients who experience toxic reactions to a specific drug in the treatment regimen should have that drug discontinued. The toxic drug should be replaced with one of equal efficacy

from the same class. For example, if a patient were to experience toxicity from zidovudine therapy, that drug should be discontinued and replaced with another NRTI such as lamivudine. Changing one drug is considered correct procedure when toxicity is the reason for altering the treatment regimen. When resistance or suboptimal treatment is the reason, all drugs should be changed.

Do not discontinue antiretroviral therapy for patients with advanced AIDS and an acute opportunistic infection or malignancy unless the patient becomes intolerant or develops drug toxicity, or there are concerns about drug interactions.

Long, slow recovery of the immune system with continued viral shutdown is reported with highly active HAART. It appears that slow recovery of the immune function is possible as long as the virus is kept in check.

OCCUPATIONAL EXPOSURE. The current recommendations for prophylaxis after occupational exposure to HIV are determined by type of exposure and the source material. The potential toxicity of antiretroviral drugs must be carefully considered when prescribing postexposure prophylaxis (PEP) since most occupational exposures do not result in transmission of the virus. Health care providers with exposures to patients with an unknown HIV status should be considered for the initiation of PEP on a case-by-case basis. Tables 28-11 and 28-12 identify the prophylaxis recommendations for persons with occupational HIV exposure. Again, consultation with experts in HIV/AIDs therapy is wise (Box 28-3; see also Table 28-10).

Patient Education

HIV/AIDS treatment is lifelong. Therefore, before starting antiretroviral therapy, a detailed discussion between the patient and his or her primary caregiver is necessary to assess the patient's ability and willingness to commit to a complex, costly, and potentially toxic drug regimen. This is very important in asymptomatic patients whose illness is at an early stage and for whom the ability to maintain a long-term adherence to the regimen is a major challenge.

Psychologists believe that the biggest predictor of adherence with prescribed drug protocols is the amount of chaos in the patient's life. For many, the circumstances are such that the patient has neither the capacity, nor the will, to adhere to drug therapy. Patients may discontinue treatment for varying reasons. It is difficult for some patients to adhere to a treatment regimen when they are symptom-free, particularly if the drugs adverse effects are interfering with their activities of daily living. Schedules that require fewer daily doses make life easier for patients. The cost of drugs for many patients is significant.

Once the decision has been made to start therapy, specific information concerning drug administration, dosing frequencies, adverse effects, and expected outcomes must be discussed with the patient and his or her family. Inform the patient that antiretroviral drug therapy is not a cure for HIV infection, nor does it reduce the risk of transmission of HIV to others through sexual contact, contaminated blood, or contact with body fluids.

Instruct the patient to take the drugs exactly as prescribed. In the past, HIV treatment required dosing around the clock, even if sleep was interrupted. Now that the effects of most PIs are boosted with ritonavir, this is not necessary. Many drugs in the treatment regimen can be given once daily, and others twice daily. The importance of adherence with therapy, not taking more than the prescribed dosage, and not discontinuing a drug without first consulting with the health care provider must be strongly emphasized.

The health care provider must be clear when teaching patients about their drug regimen. Some drugs must be taken on an empty stomach and others with a high-fat meal; some are taken with water, and others are mixed with juice, milk, or formulas. For example, patients with achlorhydria require an acidic beverage when taking the drug delavirdine for maximum benefit. In contrast, patients using the powdered formulation of didanosine should be advised to mix the powder with water (not fruit juice or acid-containing beverages). Some drugs, such as retonavir, may be mixed with chocolate milk, Ensure, or formulas to improve the taste.

The impact of drug therapy on the overall monthly costs of HIV care is significant, adding significantly to the cost of illness. Inform patients that there are compassionate-use drug programs, available through pharmaceutical manufacturers, that offer assistance with the economic realities of care (see Box 28-3).

The patient should be instructed on the proper storage of the drugs. Some drugs are sensitive to moisture, others need to be stored in the refrigerator, and some may be kept at room temperature.

Instruct the patient to call promptly if adverse effects appear. Some drugs may cause drowsiness and blurred vision (e.g., didanosine); therefore the patient should be cautioned to avoid driving or other activities that require alertness until the response to the drugs is known. Frequent oral rinses, sugarless gum or candy, and good oral hygiene may help relieve the dry mouth associated with some of the drugs. Advise the patient to contact the health care provider if dry mouth persists longer than 2 weeks; saliva substitutes may be prescribed. Adequate fluid intake, at least 1 to 2 liters of water daily, should be taken to reduce the risk of adverse effects (e.g., kidney stones with indinavir). Similarly, the health care provider should be sure the patient understands which drugs are to be taken with meals and which should be taken on an empty stomach. It is often necessary to use a "drug box" that conveniently organizes the day's or week's drugs according to administration time. Also tell the patient to discuss a nonhormonal method for birth control.

TABLE 28-11 Recommended Postexposure Prophylaxis for Percutaneous Injuries

	Exposure Type	
	Less severe exposure*	More severe exposure†
HIV-positive class 1‡	Basic two-drug PEP recommended	Expanded three-drug PEP recommended
HIV-positive class 2§	Expanded three-drug (or more) PEP recommended	Expanded three-drug (or more) PEP recommended
HIV status of source unknown	Generally no PEP warranted; consider‖ two-drug PEP for source with HIV risk factors¶	Generally no PEP warranted; consider‖ two-drug PEP for source with HIV risk factors¶
Unknown source**	Generally, no PEP warranted; consider‖ two-drug PEP in settings where exposure to HIV is likely	Generally, no PEP warranted; consider‖ two-drug PEP in settings where exposure to HIV is likely
HIV-negative	No PEP warranted	No PEP warranted

*Less severe: e.g., a needle from a container for sharps disposal.
†More severe: e.g., large-bore needle, deep puncture, blood present on device, or needle used in patient artery or vein.
‡HIV-positive class 1: Asymptomatic HIV infection or known low viral load (<1500 RNA copies/mL).
§HIV-positive class 2: Symptomatic HIV infection, AIDS, acute seroconversion, or known high viral load. If drug resistance is a concern, obtain expert consultation. Initiation of PEP should not be delayed pending consultation. Because expert consultation alone cannot substitute for face-to-face counseling, arrangements should be made for immediate evaluation, counseling, and follow-up care for all exposures.
‖The phrase "consider using PEP" implies treatment is optional. The benefits and risks of initiating PEP should be discussed between the person exposed and the health care provider.
¶If PEP is offered and administered and later the source is found, to be HIV-negative, PEP should be discontinued
**For example, source person is deceased, with no samples available for HIV testing.

TABLE 28-12 Recommended Postexposure Prophylaxis for Mucous Membrane and Nonintact* Skin Exposures

Status of Source	Small-Volume Exposure†	Large-Volume Exposure‡
HIV-positive class 1§	Consider‖ basic two-drug PEP	Recommend basic two-drug PEP
HIV-positive class 2¶	Recommend basic two-drug PEP	Recommend expanded three-drug (or more) PEP
HIV status of source unknown**	Generally, no PEP warranted††	Generally, no PEP warranted; consider‖ basic two-drug PEP for source with HIV risk factors††
Unknown source‡‡	Generally, no PEP warranted	Generally, no PEP warranted; consider‖ basic two-drug PEP in settings in which exposure to HIV is likely
HIV-negative	No PEP warranted	No PEP warranted

For nonintact skin exposure, follow-up recommended if evidence of compromised skin integrity (e.g., dermatitis, abrasion, or open wound).
†Small volume: e.g., a few drops.
‡Large volume: e.g., a major skin splash.
§HIV-positive class 1: Asymptomatic HIV infection or known low viral load (<1500 RNA copies/mL).
‖The phrase "consider" implies treatment is optional. The benefits and risks of initiating PEP should be discussed between the person exposed and the health care provider.
¶Symptomatic HIV infection, AIDS, acute seroconversion, or known high viral load. If drug resistance is a concern, obtain expert consultation. Initiation of PEP should not be delayed pending consultation. Because expert consultation alone cannot substitute for face-to-face counseling, arrangements should be made for immediate evaluation, counseling, and follow-up care for all exposures.
**For example, source person is deceased with no samples available for HIV testing.
††If PEP is offered and administered and later source is found to be HIV-negative, PEP should be discontinued.
‡‡For example, splash from inappropriately disposed-of blood.
AIDS, Acquired immunodeficiency syndrome; *HIV*, human immunodeficiency virus; *PEP*, postexposure prophylaxis.

BOX 28-3

HIV Information Resources

- HIV Telephone Consultation Service, 800–933–3413
- AIDS Clinical Trials Information Service (ACTIS), 800-TRIALS-A (874–2572) (English and Spanish)
- The American Foundation for AIDS Research, 800–39AMFAR (392–6327)
- AIDS Treatment Data Network, 212–268–4196
- AIDS Treatment News, 800-TREAT1–2 (893–2812)
- National AIDS Hotline, 800–342-AIDS (342–2437) (English), 800–344-SIDA (344–7432) (Spanish), 800-AIDS-TTY (243–7889) (hearing-impaired)

- National Association of People with AIDS, 202–898–0414
- Hemophilia and AIDS/HIV Network for Dissemination of Information (HANDI), 800–42-HANDI (424–2634)
- National Pediatric HIV Resource Center, 800–362–0071
- Antiretroviral Pregnancy Registry, Post Office Box 13398, Research Triangle Park, NC 27709–3398; 919–483–9437, 800–722–9292, ext 39437; FAX 929–315–8981
- HIV Postexposure Prophylaxis (PEP) Registry, 888–737–4448

Avoidance of temperature extremes is necessary when taking certain anti-HIV drugs. Teach the patient to slowly change positions so as to minimize the orthostatic hypotension associated with some antiretroviral drugs. Additionally, if diarrhea develops, it can usually be controlled with over-the-counter (OTC) drugs (e.g., loperamide), but advise the patient to first contact the health care provider before self-treating.

Caution patients to avoid crowds and people with known infections. Have them use a soft toothbrush, exercise caution when using toothpicks or dental floss, and have dental work performed before therapy and regularly thereafter, when possible. The importance of regular follow-up examinations and lab testing to determine progress and to monitor for adverse effects should be emphasized (Controversy: Ethical Challenges in HIV Treatment of the Homeless).

Evaluation

The goal of therapy in treating HIV infection is to control viral replication. This preserves the immunocompetence of the patient and prevents emergence of viral resistance. It also sustains the effectiveness of the combination regimen, which is demonstrated by decreasing viral load values, increasing CD4 counts, and general improvement of health status. Benefits of therapy for specific populations of patients and in various settings can be measured by population-based morbidity and mortality data. HIV/AIDS research is a dynamic field, and information about care and treatment advances may be obtained from a variety of resources (see Box 28-3). Guidelines for the use of antiretroviral drugs in HIV were updated in October 2006 and are available online from the Department of Health and Human Services. New information on HIV pathogenesis, viral load monitoring, and the impact of potent antiretroviral drug regimens continues at a rapid pace. Recommendations for treatment should be continuously reevaluated in order to integrate the latest developments in basic science, drug development, and clinical investigation. Evidence suggests that prevention education and early treatment of HIV infection slows disease progression and, according to mathematical models, may eradicate HIV.

Controversy

Ethical Challenges in HIV Treatment of the Homeless

The standard of care for patients infected with human immunodeficiency virus (HIV) has become combination antiretroviral therapy. The cost of these three drugs often exceeds $25,000 per year. New therapeutic advances raise many ethical challenges, including questions related to equal access to medical care, limits of patient autonomy, medical paternalism, and threats to public health caused by poor drug-regimen adherence.

Controversy exists over whether the new drugs should be made available to homeless patients, who make up a substantial subset of the urban poor. There are reasons for caution in prescribing protease inhibitors for the homeless. These drugs require specific regimens for storage and administration. Combination therapy with protease inhibitors must be timed around meals. Some drugs are taken with meals and others on an empty stomach. Ritonavir must be refrigerated. Also, patients must continually be monitored for adverse effects as well as undergo frequent blood testing. Adherence to treatment is thought to be poor enough in this patient group to disrupt the effectiveness of therapy. Nonadherence leads to the development of drug resistance in viruses. Furthermore, the cost of protease inhibitors may well be spent in other interventions that have the potential for greater success.

The homeless population has an HIV infection rate of 8% to 20%. The prevalence of mental illness, alcoholism, and drug abuse also is high in this group of patients. Before the initiation of combination drug therapy for HIV infection, patients should be stabilized with respect to housing, contact with the health care system, chemical dependency, and mental illness. Patients can then be informed of the risks and benefits of treatments. Health care providers, social workers, dietitians, and others involved with these patients should work as a team to facilitate holistic treatment.

Access to therapy should never be based on broad social characteristics such as mental illness, homelessness, or drug use. However, these conditions should trigger a careful, individualized assessment of the ability of individual patients to comply with treatment regimens. Remediation of social conditions that undermine a patient's capacity for compliance should be the initial step in treatment. Provision of housing may do more to increase life expectancy than initiation of drug therapy.

CLINICAL REASONING ANALYSIS

- What issues of social justice exist concerning the availability of combination antiretroviral drug therapy?
- Should there be requirements for supervised administration of HIV treatment regimens for populations of patients that may be noncompliant?
- Can our society choose to restrict successful therapies to select groups of patients? On an economic basis? On a public health basis?

IMMUNE

Antiviral drugs are also used to treat infections other than HIV/AIDS. The other viral infections include herpes simplex virus 1 and 2 (HSV), varicella zoster virus (VZV), cytomegalovirus (CMV) retinitis, and hepatitis A, B, and C. Hepatitis treatment is discussed in Chapter 32.

HERPESVIRUS INFECTIONS

Herpes simplex virus (HSV), when it attacks the skin and neurons of the dorsal root ganglia, causes a lifelong latent infection. Once the virus reactivates, it spreads down the axons of spinal or trigeminal nerves and is either shed asymptomatically in saliva (HSV-1) or in genital secretions (HSV-2). However, be aware that HSV-1 may also appear on the genitals and HSV-2 as orolabial lesions. The herpesvirus can also cause disease of the skin, the mucosa, and occasionally, major organs.

Exposure to HSV-2 ordinarily occurs with sexual contact during adolescence or early adulthood, often in people who have had a previous HSV-1 outbreak. Women are generally infected at an earlier age than men. The number of lifetime sexual partners is the one factor increasing the risk for contracting the virus. An outbreak of HSV-2 is often an *initial* rather than a primary infection. A primary infection occurs when HSV-2 is acquired in the absence of HSV-1 antibodies.

Children with a primary HSV infection are often asymptomatic; most HSV-1 seroconversions occur in the first 5 years of life. By adolescence and adulthood, 80% of persons have antibodies to HSV. The lesions of HSV-1 are ordinarily localized to the oral mucosa and lips, but can cause much discomfort. In some cases, severe stomatitis results in hospitalization.

Varicella zoster virus (VZV) is the same herpesvirus that causes chicken pox. The virus is commonly associated with varicella zoster (also known as shingles), a painful disorder characterized by a unilateral vesicular rash. The reactivated virus follows sensory nerve fibers (a dermatome) to the skin area innervated by the affected nerve. Before the vesicular rash develops there is tingling, itching, and pain in the area. The vesicles crust over in 3 to 5 days, and the lesions resolve in 2 to 4 weeks.

Pharmacotherapy for Herpes Simplex and Varicella Zoster

Three systemic antiviral drugs are used for the treatment of HSV and VZV infections: acyclovir, famciclovir, and valacyclovir. These drugs act by opposing the activity of a thymidine kinase–dependent polymerase enzyme that normally catalyzes the synthesis of new viral genomes; the result is impaired viral replication.

Acyclovir

Acyclovir (Zovirax; ◆ Zovirax, acyclovir) has multiple uses. The oral formulation of acyclovir is most commonly used for infections caused by HSV and VZV. Of these two viruses, the HSV variants are most sensitive. When used to treat primary genital herpes, oral acyclovir shortens the duration of symptoms, the time of viral shedding, and the time to resolution of lesions by about 5 days; with recurrent genital herpes, the outbreak is shortened by 1 to 2 days. Chronic suppressive

therapy of genital herpes decreases the frequency of symptomatic recurrences and of asymptomatic viral shedding, thus reducing sexual transmission of the virus. Outbreaks may resume when the drug is stopped. There are two topical antiviral drugs for the treatment of oral HSV symptoms: acyclovir ointment and penciclovir cream, however, efficacy of topical use has not been proven.

IV acyclovir is the treatment of choice for HSV encephalitis, serious HSV and VZV infections, and neonatal HSV infection. For patients who are immunocompromised and have VZV, IV acyclovir reduces the incidence of cutaneous and visceral dissemination.

Acyclovir is virustatic. It is converted to acyclovir triphosphate before becoming part of the DNA chain, thereby interfering with DNA synthesis and viral replication.

▥ *Resistance*

Clinical resistance to acyclovir has been reported in immunocompromised patients. Most viral isolates are resistant to acyclovir on the basis of deficient thymidine kinase activity and are therefore cross-resistant to famciclovir and valacyclovir.

Acyclovir is poorly absorbed when taken by mouth but is widely distributed in body tissues and fluids including the brain, the kidneys, saliva, uterine and vaginal mucosa, semen, CSF, and the fluids within herpetic lesions. Acyclovir crosses placental membranes (pregnancy category B) and is distributed in breast milk. Acyclovir is partially biotransformed by cellular enzymes and is eliminated in the urine (see Table 28-3).

Although acyclovir is generally well tolerated, nausea, diarrhea, and headache have been reported. Rapid IV infusion of acyclovir is associated with reversible crystalline nephropathy and neurotoxicity. However, these effects are uncommon, providing the patient is adequately hydrated. No adverse effects have been reported with long-term (>10 years) suppressive therapy. Drug interactions and dosages are identified in Tables 28-4 and 28-5.

Valacyclovir

Valacyclovir (Valtrex; ◆ Valtrex) is a prodrug of acyclovir. This drug delivers acyclovir more efficiently so the body absorbs more of the drug, which means it can be taken fewer times during the day. As with acyclovir, valacyclovir can be used for the treatment of initial attacks or recurrences of HSV-2, suppression of recurrent outbreaks, or treatment of VZV, and recently it has been introduced as a 1-day treatment for orolabial herpes. Valacyclovir has also shown to be efficacious in preventing CMV after organ transplantation.

Valacyclovir inhibits the synthesis of viral DNA and therefore suppresses HSV and VZV replication. It is rapidly absorbed from the GI tract when taken by mouth and is widely distributed to body tissues including CSF, saliva, and major body organs. Fifty-four percent of valacyclovir reaches systemic circulation as acyclovir and L-valine by first-pass biotransformation (see Table 28-3). Valacyclovir crosses placental membranes and is excreted in breast milk.

Valacyclovir is contraindicated for use in patients with known hypersensitivity or intolerance to valacyclovir or acyclovir and in patients who are immunocompromised. Death has resulted from valacyclovir therapy in patients with bone and renal transplants. The cause of death was thrombocytopenic purpura–hemolytic uremic syndrome. This disorder is not seen in immunocompetent patients receiving valacyclovir. Exercise caution when using valacyclovir in patients with acute renal failure (creatinine clearance [CrCl] <50 mL/min), and in patients with glomerulonephritis. Safe use of valacyclovir during pregnancy (category B) and lactation and in children has not been established. Drug interactions and dosages are identified in Tables 28-4 and 28-5.

Famciclovir

Famciclovir (Famvir; ◆ Famvir) is used for HSV infections, including treatment of genital herpes, and also in the treatment of localized VZV. Famciclovir prevents the appearance of new VZV lesions, decreases viral shedding, reduces pain, and promotes healing.

Famciclovir is a diacetyl ester prodrug of 5-deoxypenciclovir, an acyclic guanosine analogue. Its active metabolite, penciclovir (Denavir), stops HSV from replicating. Penciclovir is active against HSV-1, HSV-2, VZV, Epstein-Barr virus, and hepatitis B virus. Its action is much like that of acyclovir or valacyclovir. Penciclovir triphosphate has a lower affinity for viral DNA polymerase than acyclovir triphosphate, but it achieves higher intracellular concentrations and has more prolonged intracellular effects. Variants of HSV are commonly encountered with famciclovir that are cross-resistant to acyclovir and famciclovir.

Famciclovir is well absorbed (although distribution sites of the drug are unknown), persists for a longer time in the body, and can be taken less frequently than acyclovir. Food does not alter the absorption of famciclovir (see Table 28-3). It is rapidly converted in the intestinal wall and the liver to penciclovir, the active compound, and eliminated in the urine.

The most frequent adverse effects of famciclovir are headache and nausea. Dizziness, insomnia, somnolence, and paresthesia may be seen occasionally. Diarrhea, abdominal pain, dyspepsia, flatulence, constipation, and vomiting have been reported. Fatigue, pain, fever, rigors, pharyngitis, and sinusitis have also been reported. Confusion, delirium, disorientation, and confusional states are sometimes reported in older adults but are rare.

Famciclovir is contraindicated for use in patients with hypersensitivity to the drug or its ingredients. Use it with caution in patients with impaired renal function (CrCl <60 mL/min in those with herpes zoster; or <40 mL/min in patients who have HSV-2). Safe use during pregnancy (category B) and lactation and in children under the age of 18 has not been established. Monitor BUN and creatinine levels before and throughout therapy. Drug interactions and dosages are identified in Tables 28-4 and 28-5.

INVASIVE CMV RETINITIS

CMV antibodies are found in the majority of adults by age 40 years. Of women who become infected with CMV for the first time during pregnancy, 33% pass the virus to their fetus. Congenital CMV is a common cause of serious disabilities such as Down syndrome, fetal alcohol syndrome, and neural tube defects. Approximately 1 in 150 children is born with congenital CMV infection; 1 in 750 children suffer permanent disabilities as a result of either congenital CMV or later exposure. Each year, 8000 children have permanent disabilities as a result of acquired CMV infection.

CMV is found in body fluids including urine, saliva, breast milk, blood, tears, semen, and vaginal fluids. Once a person is exposed, CMV remains in the body for life. Most CMV infections are silent, meaning they cause no signs or symptoms in an infected person. Patients receiving antineoplastic therapy, those taking immunosuppressive drugs for bone marrow or organ transplants, and those with AIDS can develop serious CMV infections.

CMV retinitis develops in 25% of persons with AIDS. The disorder usually begins in one eye but often involves the other eye. Symptoms of CMV retinitis include blurry vision, eye pain, photophobia, redness, floaters, decreased visual acuity, decreased peripheral vision, and blind spots. Without treatment, CMV retinitis and the subsequent destruction of the retina create the risk for retinal detachment (25% to 40% of patients) with blindness occurring in 4 to 6 months. Patients with AIDS who have a CD4 count less than 100 cells/mm^3 must have periodic eye exams for retinitis, even if they are symptom-free.

Pharmacotherapy for CMV Retinitis

Antiviral drugs are commonly used to treat invasive CMV retinitis. The drugs may be administered orally or intravenously, or the drug may be injected directly into the eye (intravitreal) or via an intravitreal implant. The latter procedures require the skills of a retinal specialist.

Some patients with CMV develop a relatively new condition known as immune recovery uveitis (IRU) (Thorne et al., 2006). IRU occurs when the poor immune response of an immunocompromised individual is suddenly increased as the patients restored immune system recognizes and reacts to viral antigens in the retina. This reaction can lead to several complications, including uveitis, which leads to hypotony, cataract, and glaucoma; epiretinal membrane (ERM); and cystoid macular edema (CME).

Valganciclovir, ganciclovir, foscarnet, and cidofovir given by IV route have all been shown to improve CMV retinitis; however, valganciclovir is the first-line drug. To prevent the progression of CMV retinitis, treatment must be sustained indefinitely, or until blindness occurs. Ganciclovir and foscarnet are also formulated as intravitreal implants, small capsules of drugs surgically implanted in the eye. The implant delivers a particularly high dosage of drug to the eye and is changed every 8 months. These implants, when used along with oral valganciclovir, are beneficial in reducing the progression of CMV retinitis.

Fomivirsen (Vitravene), is an intravitreal administered drug used to treat CMV retinitis in patients with AIDs who are unresponsive or intolerant to other treatments. The benefit of acyclovir for prevention of CMV infection in patients with transplants remains controversial.

Valganciclovir

Valganciclovir (Valcyte) is a valine ester prodrug of ganciclovir and is used to treat CMV retinitis in patients with AIDS. It has good bioavailability and may be used in place of IV ganciclovir for maintenance therapy and for the prevention of CMV retinitis recurrences. It is rapidly hydrolyzed to the active compound ganciclovir by intestinal and hepatic esterases when taken orally. As with ganciclovir, the major route of elimination is renal.

IMMUNE

Valganciclovir is contraindicated for use in patients with hypersensitivity to the drug or its ingredients, who have severe renal dysfunction or are undergoing hemodialysis, who are pregnant or lactating, or who have an absolute neutrophil count (ANC) less than 500 cells/mm^3, a platelet count less than 25,000/mm^3, or a hemoglobin level below 8 grams/dL. Strict adherence to dosage guidelines is essential to avoid overdose. Valganciclovir tablets may not be substituted for ganciclovir capsules on a one-to-one basis; adjust dosage according to CrCl values in patients with impaired renal function.

Ganciclovir

Ganciclovir (Cytovene; ✦ Cytovene) is approved for the treatment of CMV retinitis and CMV infections of the GI tract, and for the treatment of CMV pneumonitis, hepatitis, and viremia; it is better tolerated than foscarnet (see following discussion), although ganciclovir has been largely replaced by valganciclovir, one of its esters (see discussion that follows). It is 10 to 100 times more potent than acyclovir against CMV in vitro. Although ganciclovir prophylaxis reduces the incidence of CMV end-organ disease by up to 50%, its use usually is not recommended, because most patients would be using it unnecessarily and the incidence of adverse effects is high.

Ganciclovir competes with viral DNA polymerases for incorporation into the growing viral DNA chains, thus interfering with viral replication. Oral ganciclovir is poorly absorbed (3% to 9%) from the GI tract (see Table 28-3). It is widely distributed in tissues, crossing the blood-brain barrier and demonstrating good ocular distribution following IV administration. Ganciclovir may be distributed in human milk and crosses the placenta, and is eliminated unchanged in the urine.

The most common adverse effect of ganciclovir, confusion, occurs in 1% to 3% of patients, although adverse CNS effects of ganciclovir range in severity from headache to coma. Anorexia, nausea, vomiting, diarrhea, GI bleeding, and abnormal liver function tests have been reported. Impaired renal function is common in patients receiving ganciclovir for prevention of CMV infection following transplant. Localized inflammation, phlebitis, and pain at the site of IV infusion may occur and are related to the high pH of the infusion solution. Fever, rash, malaise, arrhythmias, decreased blood glucose, dyspnea, alopecia, hyponatremia, and syndrome of inappropriate secretion of antidiuretic hormone (SIADH) are rare.

Neutropenia, defined as an ANC less than 1000/mm^3, occurs in 25% to 50% of patients and can be fatal. Neutropenia usually occurs within the first 2 weeks of treatment but may develop at any time. Thrombocytopenia occurs frequently in patients receiving ganciclovir.

Retinal detachment is a consequence of ganciclovir-induced resolution of retinitis and has been reported in 30% of patients. The detachment is thought to result from the hastening of the involutional stage of the disease, in which the retina thins as necrotic tissue is mobilized and edema disappears. These changes predispose the retina to tears and detachment. Discontinuing the drug leads to relapse at a rate of 100% within 4 weeks.

Ganciclovir adversely affects spermatogenesis and fertility. Advise patients to use barrier contraceptive methods during therapy and for at least 90 days after therapy has been discontinued. Ganciclovir is teratogenic. Safe use during pregnancy and lactation and in children has not been established. Drug interactions with ganciclovir are identified in Table 28-5.

Evaluate the CBC and electrolytes values and hepatic and renal function before starting therapy with ganciclovir. Obtain neutrophil and platelet counts at least every other day during twice-weekly ganciclovir therapy, and weekly thereafter. Do not administer ganciclovir if the ANC is less than 500/mm^3 or if the platelet count is less than 25,000/mm^3. Neutrophil recovery begins 3 to 7 days after discontinuation of therapy. Granulocytopenia usually occurs within the first 2 weeks of therapy but may occur at any time.

Monitor renal function frequently, checking serum creatinine or CrCl every 2 weeks throughout therapy. Closely monitor the renal function of older adults. Periodic monitoring of AST, ALT, and serum bilirubin levels is indicated. The drug may also cause a decrease in blood glucose levels.

Foscarnet

Foscarnet (Foscavir) is used in the treatment of CMV retinitis in patients with HIV and in the management of acyclovir-resistant mucocutaneous HSV infections. Foscarnet has also been used in a limited number of patients with AIDS for the management of acyclovir-resistant varicella viral infections.

Foscarnet is an organic analogue of inorganic pyrophosphate. Its antiviral activity occurs through the selective inhibition of virus-specific DNA polymerases at pyrophosphate binding sites. It does so at concentrations that do not affect cellular DNA polymerases. It also prevents viral replication by inhibiting reverse transcriptase. In patients who do not respond to oral or parenteral acyclovir, foscarnet reduces the time of viral shedding, the time required for crusting and healing of lesions, and the number of positive cultures in AIDS patients with HSV infections who did not respond to oral or parenteral acyclovir therapy.

The absorption of foscarnet is essentially complete with IV administration, but it has variable penetration (15% to 70%) into CSF (see Table 28-3). It concentrates in and is slowly released from bone. Some 80% to 90% of foscarnet is eliminated unchanged in the urine.

Adverse effects to foscarnet occur frequently and can be serious. Patients receiving foscarnet usually have serious comorbid illnesses that are being treated concomitantly with other drugs. Renal impairment, the most common adverse effect, is most likely to become clinically evident during the second week of induction therapy but may occur at any time. Dosage adjustments of foscarnet may be required. Elevations in serum creatinine are usually reversible following discontinuation or dosage adjustments of foscarnet.

Headache, seizures, fatigue, malaise, paresthesia, dizziness, confusion, and anxiety have been reported with foscarnet. Anemia has been noted in one third of patients but is manageable with transfusions. Leukopenia and thrombocytopenia are seen less frequently. Adverse GI effects include nausea, vomiting, diarrhea, and esophageal ulceration, although ulceration is rare.

Foscarnet chelates divalent metal ions and alters serum concentrations of calcium and magnesium, potassium, and phosphate, which contributes to the risk of arrhythmias and seizures. The drug is also associated with hypocalcemia, hypophosphatemia, hyperphosphatemia, hypomagnesemia, and hypokalemia. The dose-related decrease in ionized serum calcium may not be reflected in total serum calcium levels. The seizures that may occur are often associated with renal failure and hypocalcemia. Safe use during pregnancy (category C) and lactation and in children under the age of 18 years has not been established. Dosages and drug interactions of foscarnet are identified in Tables 28-4 and 28-5, respectively.

Check serum calcium level and electrolytes periodically, particularly if the patient complains of perioral tingling, numbness, and paresthesia. Increases may be seen in AST, ALT, alkaline phosphatase, bilirubin, and creatinine levels. Monitor serum creatinine before and 2 to 3 times weekly during induction therapy and at least once weekly during maintenance therapy. Obtain a 24-hour urine collection for CrCl measurement before and periodically throughout therapy. If the CrCl rate drops below 0.4 mL/min/kg, foscarnet may be discontinued.

Cidofovir

Cidofovir (Vistide) is also used in the treatment of CMV retinitis for patients with HIV infection. The safety and efficacy of cidofovir have not been established for treatment of other CMV infections or in non-HIV infected individuals.

Cidofovir suppresses CMV replication by selective inhibition of viral DNA synthesis. By incorporating cidofovir into growing viral DNA chains, there is a reduction in the rate of viral DNA synthesis. CMV variants with reduced susceptibility to cidofovir have been identified. Table 28-3 identifies the pharmacokinetics of cidofovir.

The most common adverse effects of cidofovir include headache, weakness, dyspnea, anorexia, nausea, vomiting, diarrhea, abdominal pain, fever, chills, alopecia, rash, infection, and proteinuria. Anemia, neutropenia, granulocytopenia, and thrombocytopenia, asthma, bronchitis, coughing and dyspnea, amblyopia, conjunctivitis, and ocular hypotony have been noted.

Dose-dependent proteinuria may be an early indicator of cidofovir-related nephrotoxicity. Continued administration of cidofovir leads to additional proximal tubular cell injury resulting in glycosuria, decreases in serum phosphate, uric acid, and bicarbonate levels, and elevations in serum creatinine levels. To reduce the risk for kidney injury, all patients must receive IV hydration with each infusion. Renal function may not return to baseline after discontinuation of cidofovir.

Cidofovir is contraindicated for use in patients with hypersensitivity to cidofovir or its ingredients, probenecid, or sulfonamides. It is also contraindicated in patients whose serum creatinine values exceed 1.5 mg/dL, CrCl rates are less than 55 mL/min, or urine protein levels exceed 100 mg/dL (>2+ proteinuria). Use caution when prescribing cidofovir during pregnancy (category C), and in children. Breastfeeding is not recommended. Any condition that increases the risk of dehydration warrants extreme caution with the use of cidofovir. Dosages of cidofovir are identified in Table 28-4, and drug interactions in Table 28-5.

Fomivirsen

Fomivirsen (Vitravene), a drug recently approved by the FDA, is an oligonucleotide that inhibits CMV activity via an "antisense" mechanism. Binding of the drug to viral mRNA inhibits protein synthesis, thus inhibiting viral replication. Although resistant isolates have been identified, clinical resistance has not been observed to date. To date, cross-resistance between fomivirsen and other anti-CMV drugs has not been documented.

Fomivirsen is injected into and slowly cleared from the vitreous humor (see Table 28-3). No measurable systemic drug levels have been identified following intraocular injection. Concurrent systemic anti-CMV therapy is recommended to protect against extraocular and contralateral retinal CMV disease.

There are no known systemic adverse effects of fomivirsen, although the drug has been associated with inflammation of the anterior chamber and increased intraocular pressure in less than 20% of patients. In most cases, beta blocker or corticosteroid eye drops relieved these adverse effects.

FUNGAL INFECTIONS

EPIDEMIOLOGY AND ETIOLOGY

Few fungi are capable of causing disease in humans, but when present, the disorders they cause can range from mild, superficial infections to life-threatening systemic infections. Systemic, opportunistic mycoses have become more common, largely because of AIDS, the use of immunosuppressant drugs to treat cancer patients and organ transplant recipients, the use of indwelling catheters for prolonged IV therapy or parenteral nutrition, more frequent use of implantable prosthetic devices, burns, and widespread use of broad-spectrum antibiotics.

Mycoses are fungal infections whereby the fungi bypass the body's first lines of defense to establish infection. Dermatophytes are fungi that live only in nonviable tissues of the skin, hair, and nails (i.e., keratinized tissues). These are generally acquired infections commonly referred to as "tinea" infections. The source of acquisition may be other individuals, animals, or less often, the soil. The common dermatophytes include *Microsporum*, *Trichophyton*, and *Pityrosporum* species. The ubiquitous *Candida* species cause the most common fungal pathogens that affect humans.

Systemic mycoses originate primarily in the lungs but may spread to other organ systems. Fungi that cause systemic mycoses are inherently virulent; however, host factors such as an immunocompromised state determine whether a particular fungal infection leads to invasive disease. In general, primary systemic mycoses are caused by opportunistic fungi that invade patients who would not be affected if it were not for their immunosuppressed condition. Systemic fungal infections, such as coccidioidomycosis, aspergillosis, and histoplasmosis are difficult to treat. Of these, aspergillosis presents the greatest diagnostic and treatment challenge (primarily because of lack of specific diagnostic tests), although they all require more intensive therapy compared to superficial fungal infections. Systemic fungal infections occur much less often than superficial infections but are significantly more dangerous.

PATHOPHYSIOLOGY

Fungi are self-contained, highly organized cells containing a nucleus bounded by a nuclear membrane. Fungi have a rigid cell wall and feature a spore stage somewhere in their life cycle. They occur naturally in soil, water, and air and on plants. Fungi are separated into two groups, yeasts and molds. Dimorphic fungi are capable of growing as yeasts at one temperature and as molds at another temperature.

As dimorphic organisms, fungi exhibit two different growth phases, forming typical mycelial colonies on laboratory culture media but forming small, yeast-like structures in the tissues. The oval, single-celled yeast organism reproduces by *budding*. The buds separate from the parent cell and mature into identical daughter cells. Mold reproduction, on the other hand, involves a three-step process. In the first stage, a *spore* produces branches called *hyphae*. As the hyphae grow and mass together, they are called a *mycelium*. Mycelia break away from the parent structure to become a free-standing mold. The spore form most readily spreads infection and is commonly associated with asymptomatic colonization of tissues. The mycelium form is associated with symptomatic infections.

PHARMACOTHERAPEUTIC OPTIONS

There are several classes of antifungal drugs: polyene antifungals, triazole antifungals, imidazoles, allylamines, glucan synthesis inhibitors (used for invasive fungal infections), and the proverbial "miscellaneous" category, which includes griseofulvin and flucytosine (Box 28-4). Topical formulations are the most commonly used drugs in this class and are most often available over the counter for the treatment of cutaneous or subcutaneous mycoses. A few are available by prescription in special formulations for the eye (Chapter 61).

Indications for the various antifungal drugs are specific to both the drug and the type of infection. In general, the adverse effects of the newer antifungal drugs are fewer and less serious than those of the older drugs.

Polyene Antifungals
Amphotericin B
Amphotericin B deoxycholate (Fungizone) is a broad-spectrum polyene antifungal available for systemic and topical use. Amphotericin B is a broad-spectrum drug and was long considered the drug of choice for nearly all invasive fungal infections. Topical formulations are available for treatment of cutaneous candidiasis.

⚠ **This drug should be used primarily for treatment of patients with progressive and potentially life-threatening fungal infections; it should not be used to treat noninvasive forms of fungal disease such as oral thrush, vaginal candidiasis, and esophageal candidiasis in patients with normal neutrophil counts.**

The mechanism of action is the same for all formulations of amphotericin B. As a lipophilic polyene antifungal, amphotericin B binds preferentially to ergosterol in the fungal cell–membrane to disrupt its osmotic integrity, making the membrane more permeable (Fig. 28-2). The increased permeability results in leakage of intracellular cations such as potassium, magnesium, sugars, and metabolites, which is followed by cellular death. Depending on concentration and the susceptibility of the fungus, the drug may be fungistatic or fungicidal.

Amphotericin B formulations are active against a broad spectrum of fungi. They are effective against the clinically significant yeasts including all species of *Candida* (with the

exception of *Candida lusitaniae*) and *C. neoformans*; endemic fungal pathogens such as *Histoplasma capsulatum, Blastomyces dermatitidis,* and *Coccidioides immitis*; and pathogenic molds such as *Aspergillus fumigatus*. Some protozoa (e.g., *Leishmania braziliensis*) are also susceptible.

Resistance to amphotericin B is extremely rare; however, fungi that are resistant have membranes whose ergosterol content is reduced or absent. Amphotericin B resistance develops when the fungus alters the amount of ergosterol on its membrane, or modifies its structure so that the drug binds less strongly.

Amphotericin B is poorly absorbed from the GI tract; thus oral formulations are only effective on fungi within the lumen of the GI tract and cannot be used for treatment of systemic disease (Table 28-13). For systemic disease, conventional amphotericin B is administered by IV route as a colloidal suspension. Amphotericin B formulations are widely distributed to most tissues, but less than 3% reaches CSF. Occasionally, intrathecal therapy for certain types of fungal meningitis is required. While most amphotericin B is biotransformed, some is slowly eliminated in the urine over a period of several days. Liver disease has little impact on drug concentrations, and therefore no dosage adjustment is needed.

Adverse effects of amphotericin B, particularly renal insufficiency, are dosage-limiting factors. AmBisome is the only true liposomal formulation; Abelcet is a ribbon-like formulation; and Amphotec has a disc-like formulation. These newer formulations were developed, in part, because of the concerns about renal function, and because of their improved safety profile compared with the original formulation. The three formulations differ in regard to shape, size, reticuloendothelial clearance, maximum drug concentration (C_{max}), area under the curve (AUC), and visceral diffusion. All formulations are less toxic to the kidneys than conventional amphotericin B.

BOX 28-4

Antifungal Classes

Polyene Antifungals
- amphotericin B lipid complex
- amphotericin B colloidal dispersion
- amphotericin B (conventional formulation)
- liposomal amphotericin B
- nystatin

Triazole Antifungals
- ketoconazole
- itraconazole
- fluconazole
- posoconazole
- voriconazole

Imidazole Antifungals
- butoconazole
- clotrimazole
- econazole
- miconazole

- oxiconazole
- sulfonazole
- terconazole
- tioconazole

Allylamine Antifungals
- butenafine
- naftifine
- terbinafine

Glucan Synthesis Inhibitors
- anidulafungin
- caspofungin
- micafungin

Miscellaneous Antifungals
- cyclopirox
- flucytosine
- griseofulvin
- tolnaftate

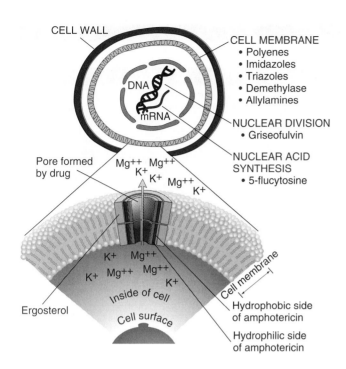

FIGURE 28-2 Sites and Mechanism of Antifungal Drug Action. Polyene antifungals (e.g., amphotericin) bind to membrane ergosterol; imidazoles (e.g., ketoconazole) and triazoles (e.g., fluconazole) inhibit the CYP450 enzyme system; and allylamines (e.g., naftifine, terbinafine) prevent ergosterol synthesis. Demethylase blocks the synthesis of ergosterol. Ergosterol binding damages the fungal cell membrane, with subsequent leakage of ions.

Up to 20% of patients have minimal to no immediate, infusion-related adverse reactions. Reactions that do occur are ordinarily seen within 90 minutes of the infusion and usually remit in 3 to 4 hours. Tolerance to the immediate reactions usually develops over time. Stimulation of the host immune cells causes the release of inflammatory cytokines by circulating monocytes, resulting in nearly universal adverse effects that include fever, chills, rigor, nausea, vomiting, myalgias, arthralgias, and headache. The adverse effects can be considerably reduced by slowing the infusion rate, decreasing the total daily dosage, and by pretreating with diphenhydramine and/or acetaminophen, antihistamines, meperidine, or corticosteroids. Since the majority of patients now receive the lipid formulations, administration of test doses of the drug is no longer standard practice. If pretreatment is used, it is done early in the treatment course, and the need for it is reevaluated weekly. Consider withholding pretreatment drugs after several days if the infusion-related adverse effects have resolved.

Nephrotoxicity is the major adverse effect limiting the use of amphotericin B. Infusions of the drug cause constriction of afferent arterioles, which in turn leads to a drop in renal blood flow (RBF) and glomerular filtration rate (GFR). Clinically, these effects on the kidney are evidenced by an increase in serum creatinine and increasing BUN (i.e., azotemia) levels. Serum creatinine levels ordinarily stabilize at 2 to 3 mg/dL and fall once the drug is discontinued.

Amphotericin B is also directly toxic to cellular membranes of the distal tubules, resulting in wasting of Na^+,

K^+, and Mg^{++}, impaired urinary acidification and concentration, and eventual renal tubular acidosis, a reversible component of nephrotoxicity. Hypokalemia is typically the first sign of distal tubular toxicity and may necessitate the administration of supplemental potassium to maintain normal serum levels. Hypokalemia and hypomagnesemia frequently precede changes in serum creatinine, especially in patients who are well-hydrated or receiving lipid formulations of amphotericin B. However, continued tubular damage eventually decreases the GFR through compensatory tubular-glomerular feedback mechanisms that further constrict the afferent arterioles. Renal tubular acidosis is most often associated with prolonged administration of the drug (>4 grams cumulative dose). Renal injury also reduces erythropoietin production and leads to a normochromic normocytic anemia.

Thrombocytopenia is possible but rarely observed. Amphotericin B formulations are contraindicated for use in patients with hypersensitivity to the drug or its ingredients. Safe use during pregnancy (category B) and lactation has not been established.

Nystatin

Nystatin (nystatin) is a polyene antifungal that is too toxic for parenteral administration, and therefore its clinical use is limited to topical applications for the skin and mucus membranes (buccal and vaginal), and oral administration to suppress *Candida* in the lumen of the gut in infants and those with impaired immunity. Like amphotericin, it acts by binding to sterols in the cell membrane of susceptible *Candida* species; the resultant increase in membrane permeability permits loss of potassium and other intracellular components. Nystatin is both fungistatic and fungicidal in vitro against a wide variety of yeasts and yeastlike fungi. There is no significant resistance of *Candida albicans* to nystatin in vitro; other *Candida* species become quite resistant. Nystatin exhibits no appreciable activity against bacteria, protozoa, or viruses.

Oral formulations of nystatin are generally well tolerated. Nystatin is not absorbed from the skin, the mucous membranes, or the GI tract; orally administered nystatin is eliminated unchanged in the feces. Significant plasma concentrations of nystatin occasionally occur in patients with renal insufficiency who are receiving conventional dosages of oral nystatin. High dosages may cause nausea, vomiting, diarrhea, and GI distress. Skin and vaginal irritation may develop.

Nystatin is dispensed as a suspension and in tablets, troches, creams, ointments, and powders. Suspensions are dosed from 100,000 to 1 million units 3 to 4 times daily. Cream and ointment formulations are applied twice daily, the powder 3 times daily. Vaginal applicators are contraindicated for use during pregnancy; thus manual insertions of the tablets are used; vaginal tablets are also dosed in units.

There are no known drug interactions with nystatin since the majority of formulations are used for topical purposes. Perform cultures to establish accurate diagnosis before prescribing nystatin.

Triazole Antifungals

All of the antifungal drugs in the triazole class have the same mechanism of action; they inhibit lanosterol 14-alpha demethylase activity. By inhibiting this critical enzyme in

PHARMACOKINETICS
TABLE 28-13 Selected Antifungal Drugs

Drug	Route	Onset	Peak	Duration	PB (%)	t½	BioA (%)
POLYENE ANTIFUNGALS							
amphotericin B	IV	Rapid	End of inf	20–24 hr	90–95	24–48 hr; 15 days*	100
liposomal amphotericin B (AmBisome)	IV	Rapid	End of inf	UA	UA	100–1153 hr	100
amphotericin B (Abelcet)	IV	Rapid	5–7 days	UA	UA	7.2 days	100
TRIAZOLE ANTIFUNGALS							
fluconazole	IV	Immed	1–2 hr	2–4 days	11–12	22–31 hr	90–100
itraconazole	PO	Rapid	1.5–5 hr	12–24 hr	99	24–42 hr	55
	IV	Immed	UA	UA	99	21 hr; 12 hr†	100
ketoconazole	PO	Rapid	1–4 hr	24 hr	99	7–10 hr	75
posoconazole	PO	Rapid	UA	UA	98	UA	UA
voriconazole	IV	Rapid	2 hr	UA	98	6hr	98
	PO	Rapid	UA	UA	UA	6–24 hr	98
IMIDAZOLE ANTIFUNGALS							
butoconazole	Vag	Rapid	UA	24 hr	NA	21–24 hr	NA
clotrimazole	Vag	Rapid	UA	24 hr	NA	NA	NA
econazole	Top	Slow	UA	UA	NA	UA	NA
miconazole	IV	Rapid	End of inf	8 hr	90	0.4, 2.1; 24 hr‡	50
	Vag	Slow	6 days	8 hr	NA	21–24 hr	NA
oxiconazole	Top	Slow	UA	UA	NA	UA	NA
sulconazole	Top	Slow	UA	UA	NA	UA	NA
terconazole	Vag	3 days	6.6 hr	24 hr	NA	6.9 hr	NA
tioconazole	Vag	Rapid	NA	NA	NA	UA	NA
ALLYLAMINE ANTIFUNGALS							
amorolfine	NL	Slow	NA	NA	NA	NA	NA
butenafine	Top	Slow	7–23 hr	UA	NA	UA	NA
naftifine	Top	7 days	UA	UA	UA	2–3 days	NA
terbinafine	PO	Slow	2 hr	UA	99	22–26 hr§	40
GLUCAN SYNTHESIS INHIBITORS							
anidulafulgin	IV	Immed	UA	UA	84	40–50 hr	100
caspofungin	IV	Immed	UA	24–48 hr	97	9–11 hr; 40–50 hr‖	100
micafulgin	IV	Immed	14–21 days	~70 hr	99	14–15 hr	100
MISCELLANEOUS ANTIFUNGALS							
flucytosine	PO	Rapid	2 hr	UA	2–4	2.5–6 hr	78–90
griseofulvin	PO	4 hr	4–8 hr	2 days	UA	9–22 hr	100

*The half-life of amphotericin B is biphasic, with the initial phase lasting 24–48 hr and the terminal phase 15 days.
†Half-lives of itraconazole and its metabolite, respectively.
‡Plasma concentrations of miconazole decline triphasically with sequential biologic half-lives.
§A terminal half-life of 200–400 hr for terbinafine may represent the slow elimination of terbinafine from tissues such as skin and adipose tissue.
‖Caspofungin has a biphasic half-life

BioA, Bioavailability; *Immed*, immediate; *inf*, infection; *IV*, intravenous;, *NA*, not available; *NL*, nail lacquer; *PB*, protein binding; *t½*, elimination half-life; *NA*, not available; *Top*, topical; *UA*, unavailable; *Vag*, vaginal.

the ergosterol synthesis pathway, ergosterol within cell membranes is depleted and there is an accumulation of toxic intermediate sterols, which causes increased membrane permeability and inhibition of fungal growth.

Ketoconazole

Ketoconazole (Nizoral; ✦ Nizoral) was the first orally active triazole antifungal. It is less toxic, but also less effective, than amphotericin B; however, it is an alternative to amphotericin B for the treatment of disseminated and mucocutaneous candidiasis, chromomycosis (a chronic fungal infection of the skin, producing wart-like nodules or papillomas that may ulcerate), coccidioidomycosis, and histoplasmosis. It is distinguished from other azoles by its greater propensity to inhibit CYP450 enzymes, and it is less selective for fungal CYP450 enzymes than newer azoles. In general, systemic use of ketoconazole has fallen out of clinical favor in the United States, but will be briefly discussed here for comparative purposes.

Ketoconazole is well absorbed and distributed when taken orally, although CSF concentrations are low and unpredictable. The absorption of ketoconazole from the GI tract is pH dependent. Increasing the pH of the stomach decreases absorption. Ketoconazole is highly protein bound and partially biotransformed by the liver; it is eliminated in the feces. The drug crosses placental membranes and is found in breast milk. Resistance to azole drugs is rare, but resistant strains of *Candida* have been recovered from AIDS patients who have chronic mucocutaneous candidiasis.

The most common adverse effects of ketoconazole are nausea and vomiting. Other adverse effects are relatively mild and include headache, rash, itching, dizziness, fever, chills, constipation, diarrhea, and photophobia. Gynecomastia has been reported. Hepatotoxicity is rare, but potentially fatal; therefore do not use the drug for superficial fungal infections.

Adverse effects reported in patients receiving topical ketoconazole as a shampoo include increased hair loss, skin irritation, abnormal hair texture, scalp pustules, dry skin, pruritus, and oiliness or dryness of hair and scalp. In some patients with permed hair, loss of curl occurred.

Ketoconazole is contraindicated for use in patients with hypersensitivity to the drug or its ingredients. Use it cautiously in patients with a history of liver disease, achlorhydria, or hypochlorhydria, and in patients who abuse alcohol. Ketoconazole may increase AST, ALT, alkaline phosphatase, and bilirubin concentrations. Discontinue the drug if even minor abnormalities occur.

Itraconazole

Itraconazole (Sporanox; ♣ Sporanox), also a member of the azole family, is a potent antifungal active against a broad spectrum of fungal pathogens. It has been approved for the treatment of blastomycosis, histoplasmosis, onycomycosis, and oral and esophageal candidiasis, and for the second-line pulmonary and extrapulmonary aspergillosis. Because it is a broad-spectrum drug, it has been used for other systemic fungal infections such as coccidioidomycosis and crytococcosis, and for superficial fungal infections.

Absorption of itraconazole capsules is sporadic but can be much improved by use of the suspension formulation rather than the capsule. On the other hand, food decreases the absorption of the oral suspension formulation. Use of the suspension is also limited by poor taste and the incidence of diarrhea (it is formulated with sorbitol). Once absorbed, the drug is widely distributed to lipophilic tissues. Although itraconazole displays potent antifungal activity, effectiveness can be limited by reduced bioavailability. Itraconazole is biotransformed by the liver and eliminated in the feces. Hydroxyitraconazole, the major metabolite, has antifungal activity. Concentrations in the CSF and saliva are negligible. The drug undergoes significant biotransformation in the liver, with elimination in the urine.

The most common adverse effect of itraconazole is nausea, although many other adverse effects have been reported such as fatigue, malaise, headache, somnolence, dizziness, tinnitus, and fever. Hypertension, edema, anorexia, flatulence, diarrhea, abdominal pain, a decreased libido, and impotence have been noted. Rhabdomyolysis, hypokalemia, hepatotoxicity, adrenal insufficiency, toxic epidermal necrolysis, and albuminuria are reported. The IV formulation may cause local venous irritation, swelling, and discomfort. The IV formulation of itraconazole is made with cyclo-beta dextrin, which accumulates in patients with renal failure, and therefore its use is contraindicated.

Itraconazole carries a black box warning because it produces negative inotropic action that may cause transient decreases in cardiac output; however, there is a return to normal about 12 hours after administration. As such, the drug is contraindicated for use in patients with ventricular dysfunction and a history of heart failure. Although a causal link has not been established at this time, itraconazole has been associated with liver failure and death in patients taking the drug. Much like other azole antifungal drugs, itraconazole inhibits CYP450 enzymes and therefore has many drug interactions (Table 28-14). Dosage regimens are identified in Table 28-15.

Itraconazole is contraindicated for use in patients with hypersensitivity to the drug or its ingredients and in patients who are lactating. Cross-sensitivity with other azole antifungals (i.e., miconazole, ketoconazole) may occur. Exercise caution when using the drug in patients with hepatic impairment and in patients with achlorhydria or hypochlorhydria. Safe use during pregnancy (category C) and lactation has not been established.

Fluconazole

Fluconazole (Diflucan; ♣ Diflucan) is the drug of choice for the treatment and secondary prophylaxis of cryptococcal meningitis in certain patient populations (not in HIV-positive patients with cryptococcal meningitis). In many cases, it is preferred over amphotericin B. IV fluconazole is equivalent to amphotericin B in treatment of candidemia. Fluconazole is also commonly used for the treatment of mucocutaneous and vaginal candidiasis. It provides excellent coverage against many fungi.

Although there are concerns about fluconazole-resistance in persons with AIDS and recipients of bone marrow transplant, it has also been used as prophylaxis to reduce fungal disease in these patients. Activity against dimorphic fungi is limited to coccimeningitis.

Unlike ketoconazole and itraconazole, the oral bioavailability of fluconazole is high, and it is highly water-soluble with good penetration to CSF. There are fewer CYP450 enzyme interactions and better GI tolerance compared with other azole antifungals. The oral and parenteral formulations are identical. Because of its wide therapeutic index, more aggressive dosing regimens are possible. Fluconazole is contraindicated for use in patients with hypersensitivity.

Fluconazole has a much better adverse effects profile than conventional amphotericin B and is better tolerated than ketoconazole and itraconazole. Common adverse effects of fluconazole include nausea, headache, rash, vomiting, abdominal pain, and diarrhea. Although rare, fluconazole has been associated with hepatic necrosis, Stevens-Johnson syndrome, and anaphylaxis. Fluconazole is thought to be teratogenic.

Drug interactions with fluconazole are identified in Table 28-14 but in general include warfarin, phenytoin, cyclosporin, zidovudine, rifabutin, and the oral hypoglycemic sulfonylurea drugs. Dosages are identified in Table 28-15.

Posaconazole

Posaconazole (Noxafil) is relatively new to the azole antifungal drug class. It is indicated for prophylaxis of invasive *Aspergillus* and *Candida* infections in immunocompromised patients who are at high risk for infections; for example, stem cell transplant recipients with graft-versus-host disease and cancer patients with protracted neutropenia. Like other drugs in the class, it acts by inhibiting the lanosterol 14a-demethylase enzyme. It is significantly more potent than itraconazole, particularly for the *Aspergillus* species.

Posaconazole is generally well tolerated when taken by mouth and widely distributed throughout the body. Steady state serum concentrations are reached in 1 to 2 weeks with repeated dosing. There is limited biotransformation of the drug with no major active metabolites. Posaconazole has a lengthy elimination half-life and is primarily eliminated unchanged in the feces.

The most common adverse effects of posaconazole are nausea and headache. Dizziness, taste disturbances, flushing,

DRUG INTERACTIONS
TABLE 28-14 Drug Interactions

Drug	Interactive Drug	Interaction
amphotericin B	Aminoglycosides, capreomycin, colistin, cisplatin, cyclosporine, furosemide, methoxyflurane, pentamidine, polymyxin B, vancomycin	Increases risk of renal toxicity
	Corticosteroids	Sodium retention, potassium depletion
	tubocurarine	Enhances effects of muscle relaxants
	digoxin	Increases risk of digoxin toxicity with hypokalemia
	flucytosine	Synergistic effect; greater risk of toxicity to flucytosine
	Antineoplastic drugs	Increases renal toxicity, bronchospasm, hypotension
	Corticosteroids, diuretics, mezlocillin, piperacillin, ticarcillin	Potentiates hypokalemia and risk for arrhythmias
	norfloxacin	Possible enhancement of antifungal activity
fluconazole	warfarin	Increases prothrombin times
	cyclosporine	Increases cyclosporine concentrations in renal transplant recipients
	phenytoin	Increases phenytoin levels
	rifampin	Decreases plasma levels of fluconazole
	glyburide, glipizide, tolbutamide	Increases plasma concentrations of antidiabetic drugs; hypoglycemia
	Thiazide diuretics	Increases plasma concentrations of fluconazole
flucytosine	amphotericin B	Increases toxicity of flucytosine; synergistic
	norfloxacin	Enhances antifungal activity of antifungal
	cytarabine	Antagonizes antifungal activity of flucytosine
	Antineoplastic drugs, radiation therapy	Additive bone marrow depression
griseofulvin	Alcohol	Flushing and tachycardia
	Barbiturates	Decreases activity of griseofulvin
	Oral anticoagulants	Decreases hypoprothrombinemic effects of oral anticoagulants
	Oral contraceptives	Decreases efficacy of oral contraceptives
ketoconazole	Alcohol	Increases risk for hepatotoxicity. Sunburnlike reaction may occur.
	triazolam	Increases peak and prolongs half-life of triazolam
	Sulfonylureas	Severe hypoglycemia
	Antacids, antimuscarinics, didanosine, histamine$_2$ antagonists, lansoprazole, omeprazole	Increases gastric pH; decreases absorption of ketoconazole
	Alcohol, hepatotoxic drugs	Concurrent use may cause severe liver disease
	isoniazid, rifampin	Decreases serum levels of ketoconazole
	warfarin	Enhances activity of interactive drug
	cyclosporin, glucocorticoids	Increases serum levels and toxicity of interactive drug
	phenytoin	Alters the biotransformation of interactive drug
	theophylline	Decreases serum levels and effectiveness of interactive drug
itraconazole	midazolam, triazolam	Prolongs sedation
	Antacids, histamine$_2$ antagonists, drugs that increase gastric pH	Decreases absorption of itraconazole
	Cardiac glycosides	Increases risk of glycoside toxicity in presence of hypokalemia
	carbamazepine, isoniazid, phenytoin, phenobarbital, rifampin	Increase biotransformation of itraconazole
	cyclosporine, phenytoin, tacrolimus, oral hypoglycemic drugs, warfarin	Decrease biotransformation of and increase effects of interactive drug
miconazole	warfarin	Enhances anticoagulation effects
	isoniazid, rifampin	Decreases serum levels and effectiveness of miconazole

a mild rash, dry skin, and abdominal pain have been reported. Some patients have trouble sleeping. Posaconazole can cause abnormalities in liver function test results and serious liver disease in some patients, although death is rare. No dosage adjustment is needed for patients with hepatic dysfunction or renal insufficiency.

Voriconazole

Voriconazole (Vfend) is one of the newer IV antifungals to be licensed in the United States for the treatment of life-threatening fungal infections. It is less toxic than amphotericin B and is approved only for the treatment of invasive aspergillosis infections caused by *Scedosporium apiospermum* or *Fusarium* species in patients unresponsive to other drugs, for the treatment of candidemia and invasive candidiasis in nonneutropenic patients, and in those with esophageal candidiasis. The rate of cross-resistance between voriconazole and fluconazole is variable.

Compared with amphotericin B, voriconazole is equally efficacious and incurs a much lower risk of kidney damage. However, voriconazole has its own adverse effects, including hepatotoxicity (i.e., hepatitis, cholestasis, fulminant hepatic failure). Fortunately, these disorders are uncommon and, for the most part, reversible. Dose-related reversible visual disturbances occur in 30% of patients. They usually start within 30 minutes after dosing and include decreased visual acuity, photophobia, altered color perception, and increased brightness; the effects tend to diminish over the next 30 minutes. Voriconazole may cause skin reactions ranging from a simple rash to Stevens-Johnson syndrome and photosensitivity. Anaphylaxis has occurred during infusion of the drug, which is manifested by tachycardia, tight chest, dyspnea, syncope, flushing, fever, and diaphoresis. Voriconazole is teratogenic; avoid it during pregnancy (category D) unless the benefits outweigh the risks to the fetus.

DOSAGE

TABLE 28-15 Selected Antifungal Drugs

Drug	Use(s)	Dosage	Implications
POLYENE ANTIFUNGALS			
conventional amphotericin B (Fungizone)	Systemic mycoses	*Adult:* 0.5 mg/kg/day IV. Can give up to 1 mg/kg/day or 1.5 g/kg/every other day. *Child:* 0.25 mg/kg. Increase by 0.25 mg/kg every other day to max of 1 mg/kg/day.	Usually fungistatic but may be fungicidal with very high dosage or very susceptible organisms. Give test dose before administering drug. Hydration minimizes risk for nephrotoxicity
liposomal amphotericin B (AmBisome)	Empiric therapy in febrile neutropenia; *Aspergillus, Candida, Cryptococcus* infections	*Adult and Child:* 3 mg/kg/day IV over 2 hr	Renal dosing considerations required. 1:1 drug-to-lipid molar ratio. Individualize dosing and rate of infusion to patient needs to ensure maximum efficacy while minimizing systemic toxicities or adverse events.
	Systemic infections with *Aspergillus, Candida, Cryptococcus*	*Adult:* 3–5 mg/kg/day IV over 2 hr	
	Cryptococcal meningitis in patient with HIV	*Adult:* 6 mg/kg/day IV over 2 hr	
amphotericin B (Abelcet)	Invasive fungal infections refractory or intolerant to conventional amphotericin B	*Adult:* 5 mg/kg/day IV at rate of 2.5 mg/kg/hr	Fever and chills may occur 1–2 hr after starting drug; reactions are more common with first few doses; generally diminish with subsequent doses. Infusion has been rarely associated with hypotension, bronchospasm, arrhythmias, and shock.
nystatin	Oropharyngeal candidiasis	200,000–400,000 units 4 times daily as swish and swallow. Max: 14 days	100,000 units/mL. Retain suspension in the mouth for as long as possible before swallowing.
	Intestinal candidiasis	1–2 tablets (500,000 units/tab) PO 3 times daily	Continue treatment for 48 hr after clinical cure.
	Vulvovaginal candidiasis	1–2 tablets inserted high into vagina once or twice daily	Continue treatment during menstruation
TRIAZOLE ANTIFUNGALS			
ketoconazole	Mucocutaneous and disseminated candidiasis, histoplasmosis	200–400 mg PO as single daily dose *Child >2 yr:* 3.3–6.6 mg/kg as single dose	Do not take H_2 antagonists within 2 hr of ketoconazole.
itraconazole	Blastomycoses, histoplasmosis	200 mg PO daily. Increase by 100 mg/day to 200 mg PO twice daily	Administer with meal or snack to increase absorption. Do not give with antacids or other drugs that increase gastric pH.
	Aspergillosis	200 mg PO once-twice daily for minimum of 3 mo	
	Onychomycosis	200 mg/day for 3–6 mo	
fluconazole	Oropharyngeal candidiasis	200 mg PO initially, then 100 mg daily for at least 2 wk	Because bioavailability of oral and IV formulations is similar, doses are equal.
	Esophageal candidiasis	50–400 mg/day IV for 2 wk following symptom improvement	
	Vulvovaginal candidiasis	150 mg PO as a single dose *–or–* if recurrent, 150 mg PO every 7 days for 6 mo	Hepatotoxic. Monitor LFTs.
	Cryptococcal meningitis	200 mg PO or IV every 24 hr. Start PO at 400 mg for one dose, then increase to 400 mg PO or IV	Continue 10–12 wk after cultures negative, and then begin suppression regimen if AIDS.
	Tinea corporis, tinea cruris, tinea versicolor, tinea pedis, cutaneous candidiasis	Apply to affected areas and surrounding skin once *–or–* twice daily for 2 wk	4–8 wk are necessary if cream formulation used.
posaconazole	*Aspergillus*	600–800 mg PO daily in 2–4 divided doses	Optimal efficacy when taken with food or a nutritional supplement.
voriconazole	Aspergillosis, esophageal and systemic candidiasis	6 mg/kg PO loading dose every 12 hr for first 24 hr. Maintenance: 4 mg/kg every 12 hr for a minimum of 7 days	Switch after 7 days to oral drug at 200 mg every 12 hr. Take oral formulation on empty stomach.
IMIDAZOLE ANTIFUNGALS			
butoconazole	Vulvovaginal candidiasis	*Nonpregnant adult:* One applicator vaginally at HS for 3 days *Pregnant patient:* One applicator vaginally at HS for 6 days	Continue treatment during menstruation. Insert applicator gently if pregnant.
clotrimazole	Vulvovaginal infections	One applicator vaginally at HS for 7–14 days *–or–* 2 vaginal tablets nightly for 3 nights *–or–* 1,500-mg vaginal tablet as a single HS dose	Advise patient that sexual partner may experience burning and irritation of penis or urethritis. Advise partner to use condoms.
	Oropharyngeal candidiasis	One lozenge (10 mg) 5 times daily (every 3 hr while awake) for 14 days	Patient condition must permit him or her to dissolve lozenge in mouth.
econazole	Tinea cruris, tinea corporis, tinea pedis, tinea versicolor; cutaneous candidiasis	Apply sufficient cream to cover the affected area once daily. Use for the full time prescribed.	If no improvement is noted after recommended treatment, notify primary care provider.
miconazole	Disseminated pulmonary fungal infections	200 mg–3.6 grams/day IV in divided doses every 8 hr *Child 1–12 yr:* 20–40 mg/kg/day in divided doses every 8 hr. Not to exceed 15 mg/kg/dose.	Reduce nausea and vomiting by slowing rate, avoiding meal times, or administering antiemetic or antihistamine before infusion.

IMMUNE

Continued

DOSAGE
TABLE 28-15 Selected Antifungal Drugs—Cont'd

Drug	Use(s)	Dosage	Implications
miconazole—cont'd	Bladder mycoses	200 mg every 6–12 hr by continuous bladder irrigation	
	Tinea pedis, tinea cruris, tinea corporis	Apply to affected area twice daily.	Treat for 1 month to prevent recurrence.
	Vulvovaginal candidiasis	One 200-mg vaginal suppository at HS for 3 days –or– 100-mg suppository vaginally at HS for 7 days	Consult with primary health care provider if symptoms persist longer than 7 days.
oxiconazole	Tinea pedis, tinea cruris, tinea corporis	Apply to affected area once daily in the evening for 2–4 wk.	Treat for 1 month to reduce the possibility of recurrence.
sulconazole	Tinea pedis, tinea cruris, tinea corporis	Apply cream to affected areas once or twice daily for 3–4 wk.	If improvement not seen, an alternate diagnosis should be considered.
terconazole	Vulvovaginal candidiasis	One applicator vaginally at HS for 3 days –or– 1 supp vaginally at HS for 3 days –or– 1 applicator cream vaginally at HS for 7 days	Terconazole interacts with diaphragms and latex condoms. Not recommended for children.
tioconazole	Vulvovaginal candidiasis	One applicator as single dose at HS	Systemic absorption negligible
ALLYLAMINE ANTIFUNGALS			
butenafine	Tinea versicolor, tinea corporis, tinea cruris	Apply cream to affected areas once daily for 2 wk	Avoid contact with eyes or mucous membranes.
	Tinea pedis	Apply twice daily for 7 days or once daily for 4 wk	
naftifine	Tinea pedis, tinea cruris, tinea corporis	Apply cream to affected area once daily or the gel twice daily. May use up to 4 wk.	Avoid contact with eyes or mucous membranes.
terbinafine	Onychomycosis	250 mg PO daily for 6 wk for fingernail disease; 12 wk for toenail disease	Hepatotoxicity possible. ALT and AST levels needed before starting therapy. Improvement may continue for 2–6 wk after completion of therapy.
	Tinea pedis	Apply twice daily for 2 wk.	
	Tinea cruris, tinea corporis	Apply once-twice daily for 1–4 wk.	
GLUCAN SYNTHESIS INHIBITORS			
anidulafungin	Candidemia; esophageal candidiasis	200 mg loading dose PO, then 100 mg PO for 14 days after last positive culture. Safety and efficacy in children has not been established.	Dosage adjustment unnecessary in patients with renal disease.
caspofungin	Esophageal candidiasis	50 mg IV daily	Treat 14 days after last positive culture to prevent recurrence.
	Fungal infections in febrile, neutropenic patients; invasive aspergillosis refractory to other therapies	Single 70-mg loading dose on day 1, followed by 50 mg daily thereafter based on clinical response	Reduce dosage to 35 mg in patients with moderate hepatic insufficiency.
micafungin	Esophageal candidiasis	150 mg PO daily for 15 days (range 10–30 days)	Not currently approved for use in children. Efficacy against infections caused by fungi other than *Candida* has not been established.
	Hematopoietic stem cell transplant (HSCT) recipient prophylaxis	50 mg PO daily for 19 days (range 6–51 days)	
MISCELLANEOUS ANTIFUNGALS			
ciclopirox	Onychomycosis	Apply 8% solution over entire nail plate once daily or 8 hr after bathing. Make daily applications over previous coats, and remove with alcohol every 7 days.	This cycle should be repeated throughout the duration of therapy.
flucytosine	Mycoses caused by *Candida* species and *Cryptococcus neoformans*	12.5–37.5 mg/kg PO every 6 hr in conjunction with amphotericin B, until patient is afebrile and culture is negative.	Dosage requires 10 or more capsules/dose. Nausea and vomiting can be reduced by taking drug over 15 min.
griseofulvin	Tinea capitus, tinea pedis, tinea cruris, tinea corporis, tinea unguium, tinea barbae; onychomycosis	500-mg microsize tabs PO every 12 hr –or– 330–375 mg of ultramicrosize tabs in single or divided doses	Determine whether microsize or ultramicrosize formulations are used; they require different dosages. Take with high-fat meals to increase absorption..
tolnaftate	Tinea pedis, tinea cruris, tinea corporis	Apply to affected areas of skin twice daily.	Available without a prescription.

AIDS, Acquired immunodeficiency syndrome; *ALT,* alanine transaminase; *AST,* aspartate transaminase; *HS,* bedtime; *IV,* intravenous (route); *LFTs,* liver function tests; *PO,* by mouth; *supp,* suppository.

Voriconazole is both a substrate for, and an inhibitor of, CYP450 enzymes, and has the most significant drug interactions among the listed azole antifungal drugs (see Table 28-12). As a consequence, drugs inhibiting CYP450 can lower voriconazole serum levels as well as raising serum levels of other drugs.

Imidazole Antifungals
Butoconazole, Terconazole, and Tioconazole
Like the triazoles, imidazole antifungals are a subclass of azole antifungals and have the same mechanism of action. Butoconazole, terconazole, and tioconazole are approved only for vulvovaginal candidiasis. All three drugs are fungicidal, and systemic adverse effects are rare. There is a small risk of fetal harm with these drugs, and thus they are not recommended for use during the first trimester of pregnancy.

Butoconazole (Femstat-3, Mycelex-3, Gynazole-1) is absorbed (5%) from vaginal mucosa with a plasma half-life of 21 to 24 hours. It is formulated as a vaginal cream that causes itching and burning in 2% to 6% of patients. The drug is eliminated in both urine and feces in small amounts.

Terconazole (Terazol-3, Terazol-7; ✦ Terazol) is systemically absorbed (approximately 5% to 15%), with a half-life of 6.9 hours for the parent drug and 52.2 hours for its metabolite. The drug is eliminated equally in urine and feces. It is available as vaginal suppositories and cream that cause a headache in over 10% of patients; some patients complain of vulvovaginal burning. Dysmenorrhea, pain in the genitals, abdominal pain, fever, and itching are possible. Chills are rare.

Tioconazole (Monistat-1, Vagistat-1; ✦ Monostat 3 Duo Pak) is a broad-spectrum antifungal drug formulated as an ointment and supplied in a ready-to-use, prefilled, single-dose vaginal applicator. It is not systemically absorbed, and its half-life and elimination routes are unknown. Adverse effects include burning, pruritus, soreness, swelling, pelvic pain or cramps, and abdominal pain. The ointment base of tioconazole interacts with rubber or latex products such as condoms or contraceptive diaphragms; therefore use of such products within 72 hours following treatment is not recommended. It is a pregnancy category C drug. It is not known whether this drug is eliminated in breast milk.

Clotrimazole
Clotrimazole (Mycelex, Lotrimin; ✦ Canesten) troches are indicated for the treatment of oropharyngeal candidiasis, and the cream and lotion for multiple forms of tinea and for cutaneous candidiasis. Clotrimazole is also indicated prophylactically to reduce the incidence of oropharyngeal candidiasis in patients immunocompromised by conditions that include antineoplastic therapy, radiation or steroid therapies used in the treatment of leukemia, solid tumors, or renal transplantation.

Clotrimazole is minimally absorbed (3% to 13%). It is fungistatic at serum drug concentrations up to 20 mcg/mL and may be fungicidal in vitro against *C. albicans* and other species of the genus *Candida* at higher concentrations. It is primarily eliminated in the feces but also, to some extent, in the urine. There are no known serious adverse effects to orally administered clotrimazole, although nausea, vomiting, cramps, and elevated liver function test values have been reported.

Econazole
Econazole (Spectazole) is another antifungal drug with the same mechanism of action as the other imidazoles. As a broad-spectrum antifungal it is effective against *Epidermophyton floccosum*, *Microsporum audouinii*, *Microsporum canis*, *Microsporum gypseum*, *Trichophyton mentagrophytes*, *Trichophyton rubrum*, and *Trichophyton tonsurans*, as well as the yeasts *C. albicans* and *Malassezia furfur*.

Absorption of topically applied econazole is extremely low. Most of the applied drug remains on the skin surface. Inhibitory concentrations are achieved in the epidermis and the middle region of the dermis. Less than 1% of the applied dose is recovered in the urine and feces.

Early symptom relief is reported by the majority of patients with clinical improvement seen soon after treatment is begun; however, candidal infections, tinea cruris, and tinea corporis should be treated for 2 weeks and tinea pedis for 1 month to reduce the possibility of recurrence. Patients with tinea versicolor usually show clinical improvement after 2 weeks of treatment.

Econazole should be avoided during pregnancy. It is not known whether econazole is passed into breast milk. The drug is contraindicated for use in patients hypersensitive to the drug or its ingredients.

Miconazole
Miconazole (Monistat, Monistat-Derm, Micatin, Lotrimin, and Fungoid Tincture; ✦ Monostat 3 Duo Pak) is similar to ketoconazole but is primarily used for the treatment of vaginal candidiasis. The topical form of miconazole is also used for cutaneous candidiasis and the multiple forms of tinea. Because of its toxicity, the drug is rarely used for systemic fungal infections, although it has been used in some cases of severe, disseminated pulmonary infections. IV use is associated with a high incidence of adverse effects including fever, rash, nausea, vomiting, phlebitis, and thrombocytosis.

Miconazole is minimally absorbed following oral administration. It is widely distributed following IV administration, although penetration of CSF is poor. Intrathecal administration would be needed in the treatment of meningitis. Miconazole is mostly biotransformed by the liver and is a CYP 2C9 and 3A4 inhibitor. The half-life is 24 hours, with elimination in the urine.

The common adverse effects of miconazole used vaginally include burning, itching, soreness, and swelling of tissues; pelvic and abdominal pain has been reported. The most common adverse effects of IV miconazole are phlebitis and pruritus. Other adverse effects include drowsiness, dizziness, anxiety, headache, blurred vision, dry eyes, nausea, vomiting, diarrhea, a bitter taste in the mouth, anemia, and hyponatremia. The drug is contraindicated for use in patients with hypersensitivity to the drug or hypersensitivity to castor oil or parabens.

Women taking warfarin should not use intravaginal miconazole, since it intensifies the anticoagulant action of warfarin. If miconazole is absolutely required, PT and INR values and the warfarin dosage must be closely monitored, and the latter adjusted downward as appropriate.

IMMUNE

Oxiconazole

Oxiconazole (Oxistat) is indicated for the topical treatment of the following dermal infections: tinea pedis, tinea cruris, and tinea corporis due to *T. rubrum*, *T. mentagrophytes*, or *E. floccosum*. Oxiconazole cream is indicated for the topical treatment of tinea versicolor due to *M. furfur*.

Tinea versicolor gives rise to hyperpigmented or hypopigmented patches on the trunk that may extend to the neck, the arms, and the upper thighs. Treatment of the infection may not immediately result in restoration of pigment in the affected sites. Normalization of pigmentation following successful therapy is variable and may take months, depending on the person's skin type and incidental sun exposure. Although tinea versicolor is not contagious, it may recur because the organism that causes the disease is part of the normal skin flora. Drug interactions between oxiconazole and other drugs have not been systematically evaluated.

Sulconazole

Sulconazole (Exelderm) is a broad-spectrum azole antifungal that inhibits in vitro growth of common pathogenic dermatophytes including *T. rubrum*, *T. mentagrophytes*, *E. floccosum*, and *M. canis*. It also inhibits the organism responsible for tinea versicolor, *M. furfur*. Sulconazole is active against *C. albicans* and certain gram-positive bacteria, although clinical efficacy has not been established. The drug has been approved for tinea pedis, tinea cruris, and tinea corporis.

Sulconazole is contraindicated for use in patients who have a history of hypersensitivity to any of its ingredients. It is a pregnancy category C drug; it is not known whether sulconazole is present in breast milk.

Allylamines

Allylamines work much like azole antifungals by inhibiting the synthesis of ergosterol. However, allylamines act by inhibiting squalene epoxidase, an earlier step in the ergosterol synthesis pathway. There are now three allylamines on the market: butenafine, naftifine, and terbinafine.

Butenafine

Butenafine (Mentex) is used for the topical treatment of tinea versicolor due to *M. furfur*, interdigital tinea pedis, tinea corporis, and tinea cruris due to *E. floccosum*, *T. mentagrophytes*, *T. rubrum*, and *T. tonsurans*. Use of butenafine cream has not been studied in immunocompromised patients.

The amount of butenafine absorbed through the skin into the systemic circulation has not been quantified, although low levels of butenafine are thought to remain in the plasma 7 days after the last application. Marginal benefit from the drug was noted 6 weeks after therapy started.

Naftifine

Naftifine (Naftin) has shown fungicidal activity in vitro against a broad spectrum of organisms including *T. rubrum*, *T. mentagrophytes*, *T. tonsurans*, *E. floccosum*, *M. canis*, *M. audouini*, and *M. gypseum*; and fungistatic activity against *C. albicans*. Naftifine is indicated for the topical treatment of tinea pedis, tinea cruris, and tinea corporis.

Naftifine penetrates the stratum corneum in sufficient concentrations to inhibit growth of dermatophytes. Occlusive dressings or wrappings should be avoided unless otherwise directed. Naftifine is a pregnancy category B drug. It is not known whether the drug passes into breast milk.

Terbinafine

Terbinafine (Lamisil, ♣ Apo-Terbinafine, Novo-Terbinafine) is in the same class as naftifine and has the same mechanism of action. It is highly active against dermatophytes, but less so for *Candida* species, and has activity against most strains of *T. mentagrophytes* and *T. rubrum*. It is used in the treatment of tinea pedis, tinea corporis, and tinea cruris. Oral therapy is used for onychomycosis.

Terbinafine is well absorbed when taken orally, and well distributed. It is lipophilic, with high concentrations found in adipose tissue, the stratum corneum, the dermis, the epidermis, and the nails after oral administration. It is biotransformed in the liver to two metabolites, 80% of which are eliminated primarily through the kidneys, with 20% in the feces.

The adverse effects of orally administered terbinafine are many, affecting most body systems to one degree or another. Dermatologic reactions include acute generalized exanthematous pustulosis, alopecia, bullous pemphigoid, erythema multiforme, lupus erythematosus, psoriasiform drug eruption, Stevens-Johnson syndrome, and toxic epidermal necrolysis. GI adverse effects include an altered appetite, diarrhea, taste disorders, nausea, and parotid swelling. Other GI adverse effects include cholestasis, jaundice, elevated liver enzymes, and liver failure. Hematologic adverse effects include agranulocytosis, neutropenia, and thrombocytopenia. Malaise, dizziness, fatigue, and vertigo have been reported, as well as arthralgias, and anaphylaxis. Terbinafine is a pregnancy category B drug, but it is unknown whether the drug passes into breast milk. Check package literature for information regarding other adverse effects.

Results of the first toenail study at week 48 (12 weeks of treatment with follow-up 36 weeks after completing therapy), demonstrated "mycologic cure," defined as simultaneous occurrence of negative potassium hydroxide (KOH) test plus negative culture, in 70% of patients (Jennings et al., 2006). Fifty-nine percent of patients experienced mycologic cure with no nail involvement or over 5 mm of new, unaffected nail growth; 38% of patients experienced mycologic and clinical cure (0% nail involvement). Fingernails evaluated at week 24 (6 weeks of treatment with follow-up at 18 weeks after completing therapy) demonstrated mycologic cure in 79% of patients, effective treatment in 75% of the patients, and mycologic cure plus clinical cure in 59% of the patients.

Like the azoles, terbinafine has the potential for interactions with other drugs biotransformed through the CYP450 pathway.

Glucan Synthesis Inhibitors
Caspofungin

Caspofungin (Cancidas) is used as salvage therapy in patients with invasive aspergillosis, candidemia, intraabdominal abscess, peritonitis, and esophageal candidiasis who did not respond to amphotericin B. Caspofungin is also used empirically for invasive fungal infections in febrile patients with neutropenia. Caspofungin has shown activity in regions of active cell growth of the hyphae of *A. fumigatus* and against *Candida* species. Mutants of *Candida* with reduced susceptibility to caspofungin have been identified in some patients during treatment.

Caspofungin, as a glucan synthesis inhibitor, blocks fungal cell wall synthesis by inhibiting 1,3-beta-D-glucan synthase. Inhibition of this enzyme causes the fungal cell wall to be depleted of glucan polymers (as glycogen or cellulose), and the result is a weak cell wall that is unable to withstand osmotic stressors.

Caspofungin is water-soluble and highly protein bound (see Table 28-13). The active metabolites of the drug are eliminated through the urine and the feces. It is well tolerated, with minor adverse GI effects and flushing reported infrequently. Other adverse effects of caspofungin include fever, headaches, nausea, and phlebitis at the IV site. Although rare, paresthesia, vomiting, diarrhea, abdominal pain, muscle aches, chills, tremor, and insomnia have been reported. Hypersensitivity reactions are characterized by rash, facial swelling, pruritus, and a sensation of warmth. Caspofungin may be embryotoxic (pregnancy category C) and is distributed in breast milk.

Micafungin

Micafungin (Mycamine) is approved for candidal prophylaxis in patients with stem cell transplant and for the treatment of esophageal candidiasis. It acts much like the other two drugs in this category, inhibiting the synthesis of 1,3-beta-D-glucan, an essential component of the cell wall of filamentous fungi.

Isolated cases of serious anaphylaxis and anaphylactoid reactions have been reported in patients receiving micafungin. Significant hepatic dysfunction, hepatitis, and liver failure have been reported. In addition, elevations in BUN and creatinine values, and occasional cases of significant renal dysfunction or acute renal failure have been reported in patients who received the drug. Isolated cases of significant hemolysis and hemolytic anemia have also been reported. Closely monitor patients who develop clinical or laboratory evidence of hemolysis or hemolytic anemia during therapy for evidence of worsening of these conditions. Micafungin is a pregnancy category C drug; it is unknown whether the drug passes into breast milk.

Anidulafungin

Anidulafungin (Eraxis) inhibits the synthesis of 1,3-beta-D-glucan. It is approved for patients with candidemia, esophageal candidiasis, and disseminated candidiasis (intraabdominal and peritonitis). Anidulafungin is effective against *Candida* and *Aspergillus* species and *P. jirovecii*, and is also used for immunocompromised patients who have superficial or disseminated candidiasis (primarily in azole or amphotericin B resistance). It may be especially useful in azole-refractory patients who have renal impairment or failure. Anidulafungin is not uniformly fungicidal; the growth medium influences activity. Resistance patterns have not been studied.

Anidulafungin does not undergo hepatic biotransformation, but rather has a slow chemical degradation at physiologic temperature and pH. It does not act as a substrate, inducer, or inhibitor of CYP450 enzymes.

There are few adverse effects of anidulafungin, but they include hypokalemia and diarrhea in about 3% of patients. Deep vein thrombosis, hypotension, and abnormal liver function test results are rare. Liver dysfunction, significant and worsening liver failure, and hepatitis have occurred. Contraindications include hypersensitivity to anidulafungin, or any component of the solution or other echinocandins. Anidulafungin is a pregnancy category C drug.

Miscellaneous Antifungals
Ciclopirox

Ciclopirox (Pen-Lac) is a topical antifungal drug used for the treatment of mild to moderate onychomycosis of fingernails and toenails without involvement of the white area at the base of the nail (the lunula).

Ciclopirox acts by chelating polyvalent cations (Fe^{+3} or Al^{+3}). The chelation process results in the inhibition of enzymes responsible for the breakdown of peroxides within fungal cells. Nail plate concentrations of the drug are reduced as a function of nail depth. Treatment may necessitate monthly removal of the infected nails.

Adverse effects of ciclopirox include redness, irritation, and itching at the application site. Treatment should be discontinued if a hypersensitivity reaction develops. The drug should be used cautiously in patients with diabetes mellitus or diabetic neuropathy. No studies have been conducted to determine whether ciclopirox might reduce the effectiveness of systemic antifungals for onychomycosis. The concomitant use of the topical and oral formulations of antifungal drugs is not recommended.

Flucytosine

Flucytosine (Ancobon) is used as an adjunct for susceptible fungal infections. It is taken up by susceptible fungal cells and converted to 5-fluorouracil (5-FU), a pyrimidine antimetabolite, in the cytoplasm (see also Chapter 33). A phosphate group is added to 5-FU and incorporated into RNA, where it stops protein synthesis. In addition, phosphorylated 5-FU inhibits DNA synthesis by hindering the activities of an enzyme required for DNA replication. As a result, DNA synthesis within the fungal cell is disrupted.

Flucytosine is well absorbed from the GI tract following oral administration (see Table 28-13). It is widely distributed, crossing the blood-brain barrier and the placental membranes. The majority of the drug (80% to 90%) is eliminated unchanged in the urine.

The most common adverse effects of flucytosine are similar to but less severe than those of the antineoplastic drug 5-FU; they include nausea, vomiting, diarrhea, and bone

IMMUNE

marrow suppression. Adverse effects are commonly seen when serum drug levels exceed 100 mcg/mL. Other reported adverse effects of flucytosine include dizziness, drowsiness, confusion, photosensitivity, anemia, and thrombocytopenia. Measure serum drug levels, CBC, and renal function values regularly.

Griseofulvin

Griseofulvin (Grifulvin V, Fulvicin U/F, Fulvicin P/G; ✦ Grifulin Forte) is derived from species of *Penicillium griseofulvum*. It is used in the treatment of tinea capitus, tinea pedis, tinea cruris, tinea corporis, tinea unguium, and tinea barbae. Use of oral griseofulvin is not warranted for minor infections that ordinarily respond to topical antifungal drugs.

Griseofulvin acts by inhibiting mitosis; thus spindle formation, a critical step in cellular division, is disrupted. The drug acts systemically to inhibit the growth of *Trichophyton, Microsporum,* and *Epidermophyton* genera of fungi. Fungistatic amounts are deposited in the keratin, which gradually exfoliates and is replaced by noninfected tissue.

Griseofulvin absorption varies considerably among individuals, primarily because of the insolubility of the drug in the aqueous media of the GI tract. Note that some patients are consistently poor acetylators and tend to have lower serum levels at all times. This may explain the unsatisfactory therapeutic results seen in some patients. Better serum levels are achieved when griseofulvin tablets are taken after a high-fat meal.

Because griseofulvin is derived from species of *P. griseofulvum*, the possibility of cross-sensitivity with penicillin exists; however, known penicillin-sensitive patients have been treated without difficulty. Since a photosensitivity reaction is occasionally associated with griseofulvin therapy, warn patients to avoid exposure to intense natural or artificial sunlight. Lupus erythematosus may be aggravated in persons hypersensitive to griseofulvin. Perform periodic monitoring of renal, liver, and bone marrow function. The safety and efficacy of griseofulvin for prophylaxis of fungal infections has not been established.

Tolnaftate

Tolnaftate (Tinactin) is available OTC and is also used topically to treat tinea pedis, tinea cruris, and tinea corporis. The most common adverse effect is skin irritation. Improvement is ordinarily seen within 1 month. The dose of tolnaftate will be different for different patients. To help prevent reinfection after treatment, the powder or the spray powder formulation may be used each day, after bathing and carefully drying the affected area.

CLINICAL REASONING

Treatment Objectives

Treatment objectives for the patient with a fungal infection include controlling symptoms (e.g., local pain, altered taste, dysphagia, itching, visible lesions, vaginal irritation), avoiding preventable adverse effects secondary to the use of systemic drugs, preventing reinfection, and reducing morbidity and mortality associated with invasive fungal infections.

Treatment Options

▥ Patient Variables

Skin diseases are visible and therefore may have profound psychologic effects on patients. Visually and physically disabling chronic skin disorders have been associated with chronic unemployment, poor mental health, and even suicide. There are a variety of cultural attitudes toward illness. In light of this, it is best not to assume that a certain idea or belief is held about the illness. Stereotyping inhibits an effective patient–health care provider relationship. It is better to ask patients how they feel about the condition and to individualize care.

Adherence with a treatment plan and return for follow-up care are influenced by social expectations or the financial ability to pay for desired drugs and treatments. Many topical therapies are expensive, and cost is a factor that influences patient adherence to the treatment plan.

Intermittent or long-term prophylaxis may be considered for patients who have frequent or severe recurrences of fungal infections. However, several factors should be considered when initiating therapy, such as the impact of recurrences on the patient's well-being and quality of life, the need for prophylaxis against other fungal infections, the cost of prophylaxis, drug toxicities, and drug interactions.

LIFE-SPAN CONSIDERATIONS

Pregnant and Nursing Women. Except for vaginal infections secondary to *Candida*, fungal infections in healthy pregnant women are uncommon. Pregnancy, however, predisposes the woman to dissemination of an otherwise acute, self-limited infection. Vulvovaginal candidiasis is common during pregnancy and is evidenced by the characteristic curdy, white, itchy discharge. In contrast, however, coccidioidomycosis can be very severe in pregnancy, and disseminated infections are usually fatal if left untreated.

Children and Adolescents. Oral candidiasis is common in infants who pass through a birth canal affected with *Candida*. Fetal loss may be as high as 50% in instances where the fungus invades the placenta. Infants of mothers with certain fungal diseases (e.g., cryptococcosis) may be born without infection, indicating the absence of placental transfer of the fungus.

Children are at increased risk for systemic toxicity from topically applied drugs for two reasons. First, because of their greater surface area–to–weight ratio, a given amount of applied drug represents a greater dose (in mg/kg) compared with adults. Second, at least in preterm neonates, the permeability of the skin is increased (see Chapter 7).

Older Adults. Physiologic changes of aging affect the skin. Progressive impairment of the peripheral vascular circulation alters the older adult's cutaneous response to physical trauma, cold, or infection. In contrast to children, the skin of older adults is less permeable to drugs, perhaps because of the altered lipid content and loss of subcutaneous tissue (see Chapter 8). Changes in the CNS modify the perception of itching and pain, and atrophy of the reticuloendothelial system may impair the immune response. Emotional factors are certainly important and may prolong or exacerbate a skin disorder.

Controversy

Using Topical Antifungal and Antiviral Drugs

Jonathan J. Wolfe

A central problem to the use of both antifungal and antiviral drugs relates to the nature of infections caused by the pathogens. In both cases, patients may be slow to commence therapy, and then prove reluctant to treat the infections for as long as needed. This problem is particularly true when topical preparations of such drugs are needed.

Fungi are notoriously slow-growing. Therefore they usually prove difficult to kill, since the most susceptible microorganism is typically one in the process of cell division. This means that the patient must treat fungi for weeks or even months in order to eradicate the problem. Many fungi represent cosmetic defects in the eye of the sufferer. The patient may easily become discouraged and stop treatment in the face of continued disfigurement. It is difficult to promote best drug therapy under such circumstances.

Various topical antifungals have been available for years. Some, such as gentian violet and silver nitrate, are of ancient origin. Topical drugs to treat viral infections, however, are of more recent origin. HSV-1 lesions of the nose, the lip, and the buccal mucosa are both disfiguring and painful. Patients may try inappropriate treatment for a time, like products containing camphor, but usually request more effective drugs to deal with viral infec-

tions. It is difficult to refuse such requests. It also proves difficult to prevent patients from sharing topical antivirals with friends who exhibit similar lesions.

CLINICAL REASONING

- Is drug resistance a serious matter when considering the use of topical antiviral drugs? Justify your answer, based on the history of viruses to exhibit drug resistance.
- One feature of viruses is their incredible variance from one year to the next. Based on the frequent changes encountered in viruses, do they offer a greater or lesser hazard for developing resistance if the patient is frequently treated with antiviral drugs?
- What supportive instruction can you offer to the patient discouraged by the persistence of a prominent HSV-1 infection on the upper lip?
- One problem with systemic antifungal drugs is liver toxicity. What methods would you employ to encourage a patient suffering from alcoholism who has become discouraged over a persistent and unsightly fungal infection of her toenails?

Drug Variables

Treatment of fungal infections is based on the type and the location of fungi and includes both topical and systemic antifungal drugs. Each antifungal drug has a distinct spectrum of antifungal activity and specific therapeutic uses. Because of the vast number of drugs available, it would be impossible to discuss them all. Further, not all generic topical drugs are equivalent to their brand-name counterparts, either in potency or in the presence of ingredients that may cause further irritation or allergy.

The basis for deciding which drugs to use includes (1) whether the lesion is dry or moist, pruritic, or inflammatory; (2) whether there is an infectious pathogen involved; and (3) the location and spread of the lesions. In general, it is best for the health care provider to be thoroughly familiar with a few dermatologic diseases, drugs, and treatment methods, rather than attempting to use a great many. As one might expect, the course of some endogenous skin diseases cannot be altered, but steps can be taken to prevent their occurrence and to minimize their effects.

The response rate to topical therapy usually decreases with repeated episodes, as evidenced by the increased time needed to achieve symptomatic relief with each new episode, as well as a shortening of the symptom-free interval between episodes. In such cases, it is helpful to change to systemic antifungal drugs. The increased expense, potential adverse effects, and risk of interactions of the drugs used for systemic therapy are warranted if persistent symptoms are severe enough. A combination of topical and systemic therapy is generally not recommended; it does not usually increase the effectiveness of treatment.

Management of the patient with a fungal infection may also require monitoring of systemic parameters (e.g., CBC,

kidney function and renal function values), as well as monitoring of the skin. Because the primary effect of most antifungal drugs is to prevent colonization of new fungi, any drug should be used a minimum of 4 weeks to eradicate the infection. Fungal infections of the nails begin in the matrix, and cure thus consists of eradication of fungi from that protected site. Treatment can take 6 to 12 months for fingernails and 12 to 24 months for toenails. However, the success rate is probably less than 60%.

Patient Education

Inform the patient and family that **systemic fungal infections are not contagious; however, superficial fungal infections are highly contagious.** A likely source of infection can be identified if the species of fungus is known.

The risk of cryptococcosis can be reduced by wearing masks when working in and around pigeon nests and droppings. Rodent burrows are the reservoir for coccidioidomycosis. The fungus can be transmitted to humans, cattle, cats, dogs, horses, burros, sheep, swine, coyotes, chinchillas, llamas, and other animal species given the appropriate temperature, moisture, and soil requirements. Advise the patient to avoid dusty occupations, such as road building. The risk of histoplasmosis can be reduced by teaching the patient to avoid old chicken houses, caves harboring bats, and the roosts of starlings and blackbirds.

Tinea infections can be prevented by educating the patient, especially parents, about the danger of acquiring the infection from infected children as well as from dogs, cats, and other animals. In some cases, the child may need to stay home from school or other activities until the treatment regimen is established and a response is noted. The fungus is transmitted by direct skin-to-skin contact or

IMMUNE

indirect contact, especially from the backs of theater seats, barber clippers, toilet articles such as combs and hairbrushes, or clothing and hats contaminated with hair from infected persons or animals. Fungal infections can also be spread by sharing towels and hairbrushes. Careful attention to drying and ventilation of intertriginous areas help prevent candidiasis. Emphasize the importance of good handwashing. Teach parents of children with a fungal infection how to care for the child.

Tinea cruris and tinea corporis infections can be prevented with fungicidal drugs and thorough laundering of towels and clothing with hot water and detergents. Remind patients that fungus can be transmitted by direct or indirect contact with the skin lesions of infected persons or inanimate objects. General cleanliness in showers and dressing rooms of gymnasiums and frequent hosing and rapid draining of shower rooms may help.

Onychomycosis is transmitted presumably by direct contact with skin or nail lesions of infected persons, and possibly from contaminated floors and shower stalls. Even so, patients should be told that there is a low rate of transmission, even to close family associates. Advise the patient and family members that organism growth can be reduced with general cleanliness, the use of a fungicidal drug to disinfect floors in common use, and with frequent hosing and rapid draining of showers.

Advise women who are pregnant that treatment is required if they develop vulvovaginal candidiasis during their pregnancy. Timely treatment helps prevent neonatal candidiasis.

Instruct patients who are immunocompromised to contact their health care provider as soon as possible for early detection and treatment of candidiasis to prevent systemic spread. In addition, advise patients who are neutropenic or otherwise immunocompromised to decrease their exposure to environmental fungi. For example, soil that is used to hold plants should be disposed of or removed from the patient's immediate environment. Regular inspection of air conditioning systems should also be performed.

Evaluation

The effectiveness of antifungal treatment is demonstrated by a decrease in skin irritation and resolution of infection. Early symptom relief may be seen in 2 or 3 days; however, systemic fungal infections may take several weeks or months to clear. Recurrent topical fungal infections may be a sign of systemic illness.

KEY POINTS

ANTIVIRAL DRUGS

- The mechanism of action for viral infections allows either DNA or RNA viruses to take over a susceptible host cell and use it to replicate new virions, which then systemically spread disease.
- The success of antiviral therapy is based on the integrity of the patient's immune system.
- HIV infection presents clinically in stages: primary infection or HIV-positive but asymptomatic patients, those who are HIV-positive and symptomatic, and those whose disease has progressed to AIDS.
- The pathogenicity of HIV appears to be a function of the destruction and disruption of CD4 cells, which are central to the maintenance of immunocompetency.
- Non–AIDS-defining opportunistic infections begin to appear as the CD4 count drops below 500/mm^3. AIDS-defining opportunistic infections develop as the CD4 count falls below 300/mm^3.
- The primary objectives of therapy are to decrease symptoms, slow the progression of the disease, and improve and prolong the quality of life.
- Protease inhibitors (PIs) are the most effective antiretroviral drugs. They act by binding HIV protease, thereby preventing the enzyme from cleaving HIV polyproteins. The enzymes and structural proteins of HIV remain nonfunctional, and therefore the virus remains immature and noninfectious.
- All protease inhibitors inhibit CYP450 and therefore suppress biotransformation of other drugs, causing their serum levels to rise.
- Reverse transcriptase inhibitors (RTIs) suppress HIV replication by incorporating into the growing strand of viral DNA by reverse transcriptase to prevent strand growth and by competing with natural nucleoside triphosphates for binding to reverse transcriptase, thereby competitively inhibiting the enzyme.
- Non-nucleoside reverse transcriptase inhibitors (NNRTIs) act by causing direct noncompetitive inhibition of reverse transcriptase by binding to its active center.
- All patients with primary HIV disease or advanced, symptomatic HIV disease should receive multidrug therapy. Multidrug therapy with a PI, or an NNRTI-based regimen with an NRTI, is recommended. Monotherapy is contraindicated because of the high risk of developing resistance.
- Changing antiretroviral drug regimens is appropriate when there is (1) failure of the viral load to drop to an undetectable level, (2) a rebound in viral load after it had previously fallen to an undetectable level, (3) continued decline of CD4 counts, and/or (4) continued progression of clinical disease.
- If treatment failure is caused by drug resistance, the preferred response is to change all drugs in the regimen. The drugs used should be ones the patient has not previously taken and that have no cross-resistance.
- CMV retinitis develops in 25% of persons with AIDS. The disorder usually begins in one eye but often involves the other eye as well. Without treatment, CMV retinitis and the subsequent destruction of the retina create the risk for retinal detachment (25% to 40% of patients) with blindness occurring in 4 to 6 months.
- Acyclovir, famciclovir, and valacyclovir are used to treat herpesvirus infections. These drugs act by opposing the enzyme that normally catalyzes the synthesis of new viral genomes; the result is impaired viral replication.

ANTIFUNGAL DRUGS

■ Infections caused by fungi are called mycotic infections or mycoses. They can be superficial or systemic.

■ Broad-spectrum antibiotics such as the penicillins, the tetracyclines, and the cephalosporins eliminate the normal protective vaginal flora, thereby permitting an overgrowth of *Candida* and other fungi.

■ Immunosuppressed states (as in newborns, malignancies, leukemia, and HIV infection), pregnancy, and diabetes mellitus may also predispose the patient to a fungal infection.

■ Management objectives for patients with fungal infections include controlling symptoms, eradicating the infection, avoiding preventable adverse effects secondary to the use of systemic drugs, and preventing reinfection.

■ The duration of antifungal therapy depends on the formulation and dosage employed, the dosage schedule, the severity of the infection, and the degree of patient compliance.

Bibliography

Annapoorna, N., Rao, G., Reddy, N., et al. (2004). An increased risk of osteoporosis during acquired immunodeficiency syndrome. *International Journal of Medical Sciences, 1*(3):152–164.

Bright, R., Shay, D., Shu, B., et al. (2006). Adamantane resistance among influenza A viruses isolated early during the 2005-2006 influenza season in the United States. *Journal of the American Medical Association, 295*(8), 891–894.

Burney, W., Liesnard, C., Donner, C., et al. (2004). Epidemiology, pathogenesis, and prevention of congenital cytomegalovirus infection. *Expert Review of Anti-infective Therapy, 2*(6), 881–894.

Cagnoni, P., Walsh, T., Prendergast, M., et al. (2000). Pharmacoeconomic analysis of liposomal amphotericin B versus conventional amphotericin B in the empirical treatment of persistently febrile neutropenic patients. *Journal of Clinical Oncology, 18*(16), 2476–2483.

Centers for Disease Control and Prevention. (2005). Control of influenza: Recommendations of the Advisory Committee on Immunizations Practices (ACIP). *MMWR Morbidity and Mortality Weekly Report, 52*(RR-8), 1–34.

Chapman, S., Woolley, I., Visvanathan, K., et al. (2007). Acute pancreatitis caused by tipranavir/ritonavir-induced hypertriglyceridemia. *AIDS, 21*(4), 532–533.

Collazos, J., Martinez, E., Mayo, J., et al. (2002). Sexual dysfunction in HIV-infected patients treated with highly active antiretroviral therapy. *Journal of Acquired Immune Deficiency Syndromes, 31*(3), 322–326.

Cooper, N., Sutton, A., Abrams, K., et al. (2003). Effectiveness of neuramidase inhibitors in treatment and prevention of influenza A and B: Systematic review and meta-analysis of randomized controlled studies. *British Medical Journal, 326*(1), 1–7.

Cowan, K., and Talaro, I. (2006). *Microbiology: A systems approach.* Boston: McGraw-Hill Higher Education.

Demicheli, V., Jefferson, T., Rivetti, D., et al. (2000). Prevention and early treatment of influenza in healthy adults. *Vaccine, 18*(11–12), 957–1030.

DHHS Panel on Antiretroviral Guidelines for Adults and Adolescents. (2006). Guidelines for the use of antiretroviral agents in the treatment of HIV-1 infected adults and adolescents. Available online: http://AIDSinfo.nih.gov. Accessed April 24, 2007.

Dupont, B. (2002). Overview of the lipid formulations of amphotericin B. *Journal of Antimicrobial Chemotherapy, 49*(Suppl S1), 31–36.

Enoch, D., Ludlam, H., and Brown, N. (2006). Invasive fungal infections: A review of epidemiology and management options. *Journal of Medical Microbiology, 55*(Part 7), 809–818.

Fluckiger, U., Marchetti, O., Bille, J., et al. (2006). Treatment options of invasive fungal infections in adults. *Swiss Medical Weekly, 136* (29–30), 447–463.

Graybill, J. (2001). The echinocandins, first novel class of antifungals in two decades: Will they live up to their promise? *International Journal of Clinical Practice, 55*(9), 633–638.

High levels of adamantane resistance among influenza A (H3N2) viruses and interim guidelines for use of antiviral agents–United States, 2005–2006 influenza season. (January 20, 2006). *MMWR Mortality and Morbidity Weekly Report, 55*(2), 44–48.

Hodge, W., Boivin, J., Shapiro, S., et al. (2005). Iatrogenic risk factors for cytomegalovirus retinitis. *Canadian Journal of Ophthalmology, 40*(6), 701–710.

Jamjian, M., and McNicholl, I. (2004). Enfuvirtide: First fusion inhibitor for treatment of HIV infection. *American Journal of Health System Pharmacy, 61*(12), 1242–1247.

Jefferson, T., Deeks, J., Demicheli, V., et al. (2004). Amantadine and rimantadine for preventing and treating influenza A in adults. *The Cochrane Database of Systematic Reviews* 2004, Issue 3. Art. No. CD001169. DOI: 10.1002/14651858.CD001169.pub2.

Jefferson T., Demicheli V., Rivetti D., (2006). Antivirals for influenza in healthy adults: Systematic review. *Lancet, 367*(9507), 303–313.

Jennings, M., Pollack, R., Harkless, L., et al. (2006). Treatment of toenail onychomycosis with oral terbinafine plus aggressive debridement: IRON-CLAD, a large, randomized, open-label, multicenter trial. *Journal of the American Podiatric Medical Association, 96*(6), 465–473.

Kaiser, L., Wat, C., Mills, T., et al. (2003). Impact of oseltamivir treatment on influenza-related lower respiratory tract complications and hospitalizations. *Archives of Internal Medicine, 163*(14), 1667–1672.

Kourtis, A., Lee, F., and Abrams, E. (2006). Mother-to-child transmission of HIV-1: Timing and implications for prevention. *Lancet, 6*(11), 726–732.

Moscona, A. (2005). Neuramidase inhibitors for influenza. *Drug Therapy, 353*(13), 1363–1373.

Panlilio, A., Cardo, D., Grohskopf, L., et al. (2005). Updated U.S. Public Health Service guidelines for the management of occupational exposures to HIV and recommendations for postexposure prophylaxis. *MMWR Morbidity and Mortality Weekly Report Recommendation, 54*(RR-9), 1–17.

Pfaller, M., Messer, S., Boyken, L., et al. (2004). Cross-resistance between fluconazole and ravuconazole and the use of fluconazole as a surrogate marker to predict susceptibility and resistance to ravuconazole among 12,796 clinical isolates of *Candida* spp. *Journal of Clinical Microbiology, 42*(7), 3137–3141.

Product Information. (2006): Eraxis (™) IV injection: Anidulafungin IV injection. New York: Pfizer.

Product Information. (2006). Mycamine ® IV injection: Micafungin sodium IV injection. Deerfield, IL: Astellas Pharm US.

IMMUNE

Ross, D., Dollard, S., Victor, M., et al. (2005). The epidemiology and prevention of congenital cytomegalovirus infection and disease: Activities of the Centers for Disease Control and Prevention Workgroup. *Journal of Women's Health, 15*(3), 224–229.

Steiver, D. (2003). Treatment of influenza with antiviral drugs. *Canadian Medical Association Journal, 168*(1), 49–56.

Thorne, J., Jabs, D., Kempen, J., et al. (2006). Incidence of and risk factors for visual acuity loss among patients with AIDS and cytomegalovirus retinitis in the era of highly active antiretroviral therapy. *Ophthalmology, 113*(8), 1432–1440.

U.S. Preventive Services Task Force. (2005). Screening for HIV: Recommendation statement. *Clinical Guidelines, 143*(1), 43–47.

Volmink, J., Siegfried, N., van der Merwe, L., et al. (2007) Antiretrovirals for reducing the risk of mother-to-child transmission of HIV infection. *Cochrane Database of Systematic Reviews.* 2007, Issue 1. Art. No. CD003510. DOI: 10.1002/14651858.CD003510.pub2.

Ward, P., Small, I., Smith, J., et al. (2005). Oseltamivir (Tamiflu) and its potential for use in the event of an influenza pandemic. *Journal of Antimicrobial Chemotherapy, 55*(Suppl 1), i5-i21.

29

Antitubercular and Antileprotic Drugs

Tuberculosis (TB) and leprosy (Hansen's disease) remain a major concern to public health officials throughout the world. The mycobacterial organisms that cause TB, *Mycobacterium tuberculosis*, and leprosy, *Mycobacterium leprae*, are slow-growing microbes. The infections they cause create the need for multiple drug regimens and prolonged therapy. TB is a disease with social and medical implications. It generally occurs disproportionately among disadvantaged populations such as the homeless, the malnourished, and the overcrowded. Although few primary care providers are called upon to treat TB or leprosy, the development of effective treatment regimens permits most patients to be managed within the community rather than in acute care settings.

TUBERCULOSIS

EPIDEMIOLOGY AND ETIOLOGY

Robert Koch, a German physician and scientist, reported his discovery of *M. tuberculosis*, the bacterium that causes TB, on the evening of March 24, 1882. Koch became known as "The Father of Bacteriology" and received the Nobel Prize in Physiology or Medicine in 1905 for his investigations and discoveries. As significant as his work on TB are *Koch's postulates*, which state that to establish that an organism as the cause of a disease, the following must hold: (1) the organism must be found in all cases of the disease examined; (2) the organism must be prepared and maintained in a pure culture; (3) the organism must be capable of producing the original infection, even after several generations in culture; and (4) it must be possible to retrieve the organism from an inoculated animal and to culture it again.

In the 1940s, and as a result of Koch's work, the first of several drugs used in the treatment of TB were discovered. The prevalence of TB slowly began to decrease in the United States. However, as the acquired immunodeficiency syndrome (AIDS) epidemic captured the attention of the nation, and efforts to combat this public health crisis dominated the health care field in the 1970s and early 1980s, the number of cases of TB jumped. Between 1985 and 1992, they increased by 18%. After this increase there was a recorded 50% decline in cases of TB from 1992 through 2002, with roughly 15,000 new U.S. cases reported in 2002 alone. This was presumably due in part to improved public health education, surveillance, and treatment programs. However, the prevalence of TB is much greater and continues to grow in the larger global community, with millions affected worldwide with some form of TB; in the United States, an estimated 15 million people are infected with *M. tuberculosis*. According to the Foundation for Better Health Care, a number of interrelated and interdependent factors are behind the reappearance of TB.

The human immunodeficiency virus (HIV) and AIDS epidemic: According to the Centers for Disease Control and Prevention (CDC), an estimated 100,000 HIV-infected people in the United States also carry *M. tuberculosis*. The presence of TB may indicate an immunocompromised state and be diagnosed at the same time as HIV infection. Because of the overlap of risk groups, the index of suspicion for TB should be high in HIV-infected persons. Similarly, the index of suspicion for HIV infection should be high in persons diagnosed with TB. The risk for transmission is highest in crowded environments such as shelters, hospitals, long-term care facilities, and prisons

Increased numbers of immigrants: Approximately 66% of the cases of TB in the United States today occur among ethnic minorities (e.g., Native Americans, Alaskan Natives, Hispanics, Blacks, Asians, and Pacific Islanders) who come from countries where TB is endemic. Because of psychosocial obstacles and language barriers, many of the immigrants do not receive even basic health care services. The largest increase is in males 25 to 44 years old and, to a lesser extent, children under age 15 years.

The culture of poverty: Exposures to M. tuberculosis often go unnoticed and unchecked in those who abuse alcohol or other substances, IV drug abusers, and the homeless. They are more vulnerable to exposure to *M. tuberculosis*.

Poor adherence with treatment: Some disadvantaged groups remain contagious, and other people go on to develop and spread resistant strains of *M. tuberculosis* to others.

Increasing numbers of residents in long-term care facilities, prisons, and mental institutions: As people age, the body's normal immune system function declines, placing them at risk for TB. Most of these individuals likely acquired the latent infection during early adulthood.

Drug-resistant strains of TB bacilli: TB is also on the rise because of greater numbers of drug-resistant strains of the tuberculosis bacillus. Drug therapy that is too short contributes to the development of resistant strains.

PATHOPHYSIOLOGY

There are five closely related strains in the *Mycobacterium tuberculosis* complex: *M. tuberculosis, M. bovis, M. africanum, M. microti,* and *M. canetti*. Transmission of *M. tuberculosis* is through respiratory drops; there are no known animal reservoirs for the mycobacterium. Mycobacteria have fatty cell walls whose structure and function are unknown, but which allow the organism to survive inside macrophages. Ordinarily, pathogens are degraded by enzymes within the cell. The waxy coat of *M. tuberculosis* makes it impervious to antitubercular drugs. Mycobacteria are referred to as "acid-fast," because their waxy coat repels the acid solutions used during diagnostic testing.

M. bovis can invade the respiratory tract, the lymph system, and the gastrointestinal (GI) tract when unpasteurized milk is consumed. The risk of infection from *M. bovis* has dropped appreciably as a result of the pasteurization of milk and effective TB control programs for cattle. Airborne transmission of *M. africanum* can also occur.

Bacille Calmette-Guérin (BCG) vaccine is a live-attenuated strain of *M. bovis* routinely given in foreign countries to increase resistance to TB. Vaccination of uninfected persons is thought to induce sensitivity in more than 90% of those vaccinated. Recipients of the BCG vaccine will have a positive tuberculin skin test and should be evaluated for the disease by means of a chest x-ray exam. Protection given by BCG may persist for as long as 20 years. BCG may also be used as an agent to enhance immunity against transitional-cell carcinoma of the bladder. When used in this manner, adverse reactions such as dissemination may be encountered, and in such cases *M. bovis* BCG may be cultured from specimens of systems other than the urinary tract (e.g., blood, sputum, bone marrow).

M. tuberculosis multiply only once every 24 hours and take a month to form a colony. In contrast, other bacteria such as *Escherichia coli* form colonies within 8 hours. TB bacilli tend to form in clumps, making them difficult to separate and count.

Incubation Period

TB is usually transmitted after prolonged exposure to a person infected with active TB because most infected people expel a relatively small amount of bacilli. It has been estimated that most people have a 50% chance of infection if they spend 8 hours a day for 6 months, or 24 hours a day for 2 months working or living with someone infected with active TB. Coughing, sneezing, laughing, talking, and singing aerosolize the 1 to 5 micron mycobacteria which are carried by air currents over large areas and for long periods. Once inhaled, the bacilli deposit in alveoli, infection develops and spreads to other organs and tissues. Certain areas of the body favor replication of the bacillus, including the upper lobes of the lungs, the bones, the kidneys, and the brain.

The incubation period from infection to discernible primary lesions or significant tuberculin reaction is 4 to 12 weeks. The subsequent risk of pulmonary or extrapulmonary TB is greatest during the first 1 to 2 years after infection, but may exist for a lifetime as a latent infection. The disease remains communicable as long as there are viable bacilli in the sputum. Communicability depends on the number and the virulence of the bacilli, the adequacy of ventilation, exposure of the bacilli to the sun or ultraviolet light, and opportunities for aerosolization.

Forms of TB

TB occurs in three forms: primary, reactivation, and miliary. The appearance of a lung infection with no known prior exposure to the organism is referred to as *primary* TB. Activation of cell-mediated immunity leads to resolution of primary infections in most persons, but they remain at risk for reactivation for life. Children with primary TB are generally not infectious.

Reactivation (secondary) TB results when dormant bacilli become endogenously active or the person is again exposed to TB. Reactivation TB occurs anytime, even years after the primary event, at sites seeded with bacilli at the time of primary infection. Seeded areas are most commonly found in the upper lobes of the lungs, perhaps because of the relatively high oxygen tension.

Miliary TB (disseminated disease), more common in older adults, occurs when bacilli are dispersed throughout other organs and tissues of the body. The bacilli produce lesions resembling tiny seeds.

TB and HIV Infection

TB may develop in patients with HIV months or years before other opportunistic infections. In fact, a diagnosis of TB may be the initial sign of a comorbid HIV infection. In late stages of HIV, it often occurs in areas outside the lungs. Each year, 8% of people in the United States who have latent TB and HIV develop active TB. In contrast, the lifetime risk of developing active TB for healthy individuals infected with *M. tuberculosis* is 10%. A multi–drug-resistant TB (MDR-TB) develops more rapidly and is more deadly in patients who also have HIV compared with MDR-TB patients who are otherwise healthy. MDR-TB is sometimes resistant to two or more of the most important antitubercular drugs: isoniazid (INH) and rifampin (RIF).

Stages of TB

Progression of TB occurs in two stages. The first is a primary infection, or active disease. The patient has a positive tuberculin skin test, a normal chest x-ray exam, and sputum cultures negative for acid-fast bacilli. Of those infected with TB, 90% never develop active disease, because they have an intact immune system. The American Thoracic Society (ATS) has assigned a grading system for TB to aid in evaluation and determination of appropriate drug therapy; the grading system is summarized in Table 29-1.

▥ *Primary Infection*

Once bacilli are inhaled and multiply, they cause nonspecific, exudative pneumonitis and necrosis. The inflammatory response brings neutrophils and alveolar macrophages to the area. Bacilli are taken up and killed by the neutrophils and the macrophages. However, in certain situations, the bacilli multiply within the phagocytes; they are resistant to the cell's destructive action. Monocytes from the blood are attracted to the infected area but are unable to kill the bacilli. The multiplying bacilli disperse from the original pulmonary site with extensive hilar lymph node involvement. In addition, the spillover from lymphatic vessels to the blood stream causes infection in lung apices and in other organs and tissues. The process ordinarily resolves within a few weeks as a result of cell-mediated immunity. Coincidental to the resolution, a marked increase develops in the ability of macrophages to inhibit multiplication of the bacilli.

▥ *Reactivation of Tuberculosis*

Endogenous reactivation of dormant bacilli may occur as the result of poor nutritional status, diabetes mellitus, long-term steroid therapy, and other debilitating circumstances or diseases. Necrosis, a conspicuous feature of reactivation of the bacilli, is due to tissue destruction following the inflammatory

TABLE 29-1 Grading of Tuberculosis (TB)

Grade	Classification	Associated Findings
0	No tuberculosis, no exposure, no infection	No history of exposure; negative tuberculin test
1	Exposure to TB, no infection	History of exposure; negative tuberculin test
2	Latent TB infection, no active disease	Significant reaction to tuberculin skin test; negative bacteriologic studies (if done); no x-ray, bacteriologic, or clinical evidence compatible with TB
3	TB, clinically active disease	Clinical and x-ray exam findings of current TB.* Definitive isolation of *M. tuberculosis* organism.
4	TB, not clinically active	History of previous episode of TB *or* abnormal, stable x-ray exam findings in person with significant reaction (in mm) to tuberculin skin test; negative bacteriologic studies (if done); no clinical or x-ray exam evidence of active disease
5	TB suspected but diagnosis not yet definitive or unsubstantiated	Diagnosis pending; independent of whether treatment has started†

*Grade 3 TB is also characterized by location of disease: pulmonary, pleural, lymphatic, in bone and/or joint, genitourinary tract, disseminated (miliary), meningeal, peritoneal, and other. Chest x-ray exam findings: normal, abnormal, cavitary or noncavitary, and stable or worsening or improving. Positive skin test with area of induration identified.
†Patients should not remain in this grade longer than 3 months. Move to other class once testing has been completed.
Data from the American Thoracic Society. (2000). Diagnostic standards and classifications of TB in adults and children. *American Journal of Respiratory Critical Care Medicine, 161*(4), 1376–1395.

reaction. The resultant granulomatous area is surrounded by collagen, fibroblasts, and lymphocytes, thus sealing off colonies of bacilli. The lesion, referred to as *Ghon's tubercle,* prevents the spread of organisms. The necrotic areas calcify, and the organisms remain dormant for life. If, however, the bacilli reactivate, *caseation necrosis* (liquefaction) may occur. Caseation necrosis occurs as infected tissues within the tubercle die, forming a cheese-like material. The liquid material enters the bronchus, whereby the evacuated area becomes a cavity *(cavitation)* (Fig. 29-1).

▥ *Miliary Tuberculosis*

If the immune system is compromised or if there is an erosion of Ghon's tubercles, bronchogenic spread may occur. When a blood vessel is affected, the bacilli spread through the circulation. These changes are referred to as *miliary* TB. Active disease develops because macrophages and lymphocytes do not function or survive in necrotic areas, and therefore the value of cell-mediated immunity is lost. The acute systemic manifestations of miliary TB include fever, dyspnea, and cyanosis, or, in the case of a chronically ill patient, with manifestations such as weight loss, fever, and GI disturbances. In addition, generalized lymphadenopathy, hepatomegaly, and splenomegaly may be present.

Pleural effusions form with the release of caseous material into the pleural cavity. Pleuritis develops from a superficial lesion that involves the pleura. Acute pneumonia can also be found when large numbers of bacilli are discharged from a liquefied lesion into the lung or lymph node. The meninges, the bones and joint tissues, the kidneys, and the genital tract may also be involved.

In open cavities, oxygen tension is fairly high, the medium neutral or slightly alkaline, and the multiplication of bacilli active. In closed caseous lesions, the oxygen tension is low and the medium neutral, so the replication of bacilli is slow and intermittent. In addition, the intracellular environment of macrophages is acidic and multiplication of bacilli relatively slow.

PHARMACOTHERAPEUTIC OPTIONS

Primary treatment for TB consists of first-line and second-line antitubercular drugs. First-line therapy includes isoniazid, rifampin, ethambutol, and pyrazinamide. These drugs provide the most effective antitubercular activity, with an acceptable

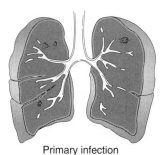

Primary infection

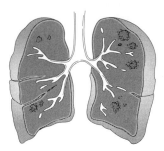

Cavitation of a caseous tubercle

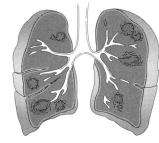

Progression of cavitations

FIGURE 29-1 Tubercular lesions may occur in any lobe of the lung. Lesions in various stages of development and resolution are noted: primary infection, cavitation of a caseous tubercle, and progression of the cavitations with erosion into bronchi. Cavitations are illustrated as empty areas.

degree of toxicity. Second-line drugs such as cycloserine, capreomycin, ethionamide, and kanamycin provide acceptable antimicrobial activity but with excessive toxicity; thus these drugs are reserved for second-line therapy. With the reemergence of MDR-TB, the use of second-line drugs has gained even greater importance. However, because of the toxicity associated with these agents, clinical trials of newer drugs for the treatment of MDR-TB are underway.

First-Line Drugs

- ethambutol (EMB, Myambutol); ♣ Myambutol, Etibi
- isoniazid (INH, Laniazid); Isotamine, ♣ PMS-Isonizaid
- isoniazid + rifampin (Rifamate)
- isoniazid + pyrazinamide + rifampin (Rifater)
- pyrazinamide (PZA); ♣ PMS-Pyrazinamide, Tebrazid
- rifabutin (Mycobutin)
- rifampin (RIF, Rifadin, Rimactane); ♣ Rifadin, Rimactane

- rifapentine (RPT, Priftin)
- streptomycin

Indications

Patients diagnosed with both pulmonary and extrapulmonary TB should receive first-line therapy. The daily use of first-line antitubercular drugs helps eliminate actively multiplying extracellular bacilli, rendering the sputum noninfectious. Treatment thereafter is designed to eliminate intracellular bacilli. Persons exposed to TB (close contacts, HIV-infected persons with significant reactions to a tuberculin test, and newly infected persons) but who have not developed active disease are candidates for prophylaxis with isoniazid (Box 29-1). The benefits of prophylaxis are prevention of active disease and minimization of the spread of infection. Isoniazid is usually combined with other drugs to enhance adherence to therapy and promote destruction of *M. tuberculosis.*

🔍 EVIDENCE-BASED PHARMACOTHERAPEUTICS

Levofloxacin for Active Tuberculosis?

■ Background
Tuberculosis (TB) treatment necessitates the use of traditional first-line drugs, often for 6 months or longer. For some patients, drug resistant bacilli or intolerance to the drugs necessitated the use of an alternative regimen; often the alternative regimen included levofloxacin, a quinolone antibiotic. Clinical research using fluoroquinolones as first- or second-line drugs for the treatment of TB or multiple–drug-resistant *Mycobacterium tuberculosis* is limited. Even with the increasing use of fluoroquinolones, there is little data on patient tolerance to the drugs outside of clinical research settings.

Research Article
Marra, F., Marra, C., Moadebi, S., et al. (2005). Levofloxacin treatment of active tuberculosis and the risk of adverse events. *Chest, 128*(3), 1406–1413.

Purpose
The purpose of this study was to compare the overall incidence of adverse effects associated with levofloxacin-containing regimens with that of standard anti-TB therapy.

Design
A case-controlled, retrospective design was used for this 3-year study. Subjects taking levofloxacin (*N* = 102) were matched by age and sex to control subjects (*N* = 358) taking traditional first-line antitubercular drugs in a 1:4 ratio. Residents of British Columbia diagnosed with active TB were eligible for the study. Both the attending physician and the nurse practitioner had to agree that the drug was responsible for an observed adverse effect for it to be considered as such. Operational definitions of the severity of adverse effects were categorized by body system affected or by laboratory value as mild, moderate, or severe. Using five criteria, the chance for a relationship between adverse effects to levofloxacin was categorized as probable, possible, or unlikely.

Methods
A diagnosis of active TB was established in all subjects by isolating *M. tuberculosis* from a sputum culture. Subjects were included in the study if they had taken levofloxacin for 7 days or more (with no additional antitubercular drugs taken), or traditional first-line drugs (i.e., INH, RIF, EMB, and PZA). Data collected from subject medical records included country of birth, age, sex, weight, comorbid conditions, the dosage, duration of treatment, and any intolerances or adverse effects to other antitubercular drugs, previous hospitalizations, and reasons for discontinuing therapy.

Data analysis was done using the *t* test. Cross-tabulations and x^2 tests for homogeneity were calculated for sex and other descriptors. A Poisson regression model determined the overall rate of occurrence of any major adverse effects in the two groups. Because most of the adverse effects appeared during the first 3 months of treatment, post hoc analysis was done that looked at the rate of major adverse effects in the first 100 days of treatment.

Findings
No significant differences in adverse effects were found between the two groups with one exception: 82% of subjects taking levofloxacin had an antecedent adverse event to first-line drugs, whereas 18% took the drug because of resistance to another.

The rate of major adverse events in subjects taking levofloxacin was almost half that of subjects taking first-line drugs (relative risk [RR] 0.6; 95% confidence interval [CI], 0.44–0.82). After adjusting for variations in the use of concomitant drugs, the rate of major adverse effects was found comparable between the levofloxacin group and the control group (adjusted RR [ARR], 0.83; 95% CI, 0.66–1.03). In addition, no differences were found between the two groups in relation to central nervous system (ARR 0.94%; 95% CI, 0.61–1.43), gastrointestinal (ARR, 0.81; 95% CI, 0.58–1.13), skin (ARR, 0.65; 95% CI, 0.38–1.10), or musculoskeletal adverse effects (ARR, 0.87; 95% CI, 0.48–1.6) within the first 100 days of treatment. Time to the first major adverse effect was also similar between the two groups (adjusted hazard ratio, 1.01; 95% CI, 0.76–1.34).

Conclusions
Subjects treated with levofloxacin were treated with fewer drugs, and thus they could be expected to have fewer adverse effects. Despite a history of adverse effects, use of a treatment regimen that included levofloxacin resulted in a rate of adverse effects that was similar to the rate when using traditional first-line drugs. Major confounding variables were controlled for in the study design or were dispersed equally between the two study groups.

■ Implications for Practice
The results of this study, although not conclusive in recommending TB treatment regimens that contain levofloxacin, do suggest that such regimens may result in fewer adverse effect and thus greater adherence to the treatment regimen. Additional research is needed to evaluate a potential protective effect of levofloxacin and other quinolones (e.g., ofloxacin, ciprofloxacin, moxifloxacin) against the major adverse effects of traditional first-line treatment.

EMB, Ethambutol; *INH*, isoniazid; *PZA*, pyrazinamide; *RIF*, rifampin.

BOX 29-1

Recommendations for Isoniazid Prophylaxis

The Following Persons Should Receive Isoniazid Prophylaxis
1. HIV-infected persons with significant reactions to a tuberculin test
2. Household members and other close contacts of patients with active pulmonary TB
3. Newly infected persons (i.e., those with a tuberculin skin test conversion during the previous 2 years)
4. People with a history of TB and inadequate treatment
5. People with a tuberculin skin test and an abnormal chest x-ray film consistent with previous (nonprogressive) disease
6. People who demonstrate significant reactions to a tuberculin test and who are at special risk of developing active disease because of factors such as

- Silicosis
- Diabetes mellitus
- Certain hematologic and reticuloendothelial diseases (e.g., leukemia, Hodgkin's disease)
- End-stage renal disease
- Conditions associated with substantial weight loss or chronic undernutrition, including postgastrectomy states, intestinal bypass surgery, chronic peptic ulcer disease, chronic malabsorption syndromes, and carcinomas of the oropharynx and upper GI tract that inhibit adequate nutritional intake
- Long-term therapy with adrenal corticosteroids or immunosuppressive therapy
- Age less than 35 years

GI, Gastrointestinal; *TB,* tuberculosis, tuberculin.

Rifabutin is indicated for the prevention of disseminated *Mycobacterium avium* complex (MAC) disease in patients with advanced HIV infection. The Advisory Council for the Elimination of Tuberculosis, the ATS, and the CDC also recommend that either streptomycin or ethambutol be added to the rifabutin regimen unless the likelihood of isoniazid resistance is very low.

Pharmacodynamics

Ethambutol inhibits the synthesis of mycolic acids, important constituents of the mycobacterial cell wall. Because mycolic acids are unique to mycobacteria, this action explains the high selectivity of ethambutol. Bacterial resistance develops when ethambutol is given as monotherapy.

Isoniazid is a potent bactericidal drug. The precise mechanism of action is unknown, although several hypotheses have been proposed. The hypotheses include effects of the organism on lipids, nucleic acid biosynthesis, and glycolysis. Like ethambutol, it is also believed that isoniazid inhibits synthesis of mycolic acids.

Pyrazinamide is an analogue of nicotinamide and has bacteriostatic or bactericidal effects, depending on the susceptibility of the particular bacilli and the concentration of drug at the site of infection. Its mechanism of action is unknown; however, pyrazinamide requires an acidic environment to be active.

Rifabutin is a semisynthetic derivative of the bactericidal rifamycins. It is effective against gram-positive and some gram-negative organisms. It is not known whether rifabutin inhibits DNA-dependent RNA polymerase in *M. avium* or in *Mycobacterium intracellulare,* which comprise MAC.

Rifampin inhibits DNA-dependent RNA polymerase, leading to suppression of RNA synthesis, and it may also inhibit DNA synthesis. Bactericidal action results in destruction of both multiplying and inactive *M. tuberculosis* bacilli. Human cells are not as sensitive as mycobacterial cells and therefore are not affected by rifampin except at high dosages.

Rifapentine is fairly well absorbed and distributed following oral administration and carries a similar microbiologic profile to that of rifampin. At therapeutic levels, rifapentine exhibits bactericidal activity against both intracellular and extracellular *M. tuberculosis* organisms. The drug is primarily bound to albumin and hydrolyzed by an esterase enzyme to form an active metabolite. Most of the drug and its metabolite are eliminated in the feces, with a small portion in the urine. Rifapentine resistance to *M. tuberculosis* strains is principally the result of one of several single-point mutations that occur in the gene coding for the beta submit of DNA-dependent RNA polymerase.

Streptomycin is bactericidal in the extracellular, alkaline environment. The longer therapy is continued, the higher the incidence of bacterial resistance. Approximately 80% of patients treated with streptomycin alone harbor resistant bacilli after 4 months of treatment.

Pharmacokinetics

Ethambutol is rapidly absorbed when taken orally and widely distributed (Table 29-2). The main path of biotransformation appears to be an initial oxidation of the alcohol to an aldehydic intermediate, followed by conversion to dicarboxylic acid. Approximately 50% of ethambutol is eliminated via the urine, and another 20% via the feces.

Isoniazid is rapidly absorbed after oral administration. It is readily distributed into all body tissues and fluids, including cerebrospinal fluid (CSF) and breast milk. It penetrates well into caseous material. Drug concentration is initially higher in plasma and muscle than infected tissue. However, muscle retains the drug for a longer time in quantities above those required for bacteriostasis. Biotransformation of isoniazid occurs in the liver, with elimination in the urine.

Rifabutin, owing to its high lipophilicity, has a high propensity for distribution and intracellular tissue uptake. Rifabutin is a synthetic drug derived from rifamycin. The metabolite of rifabutin has an activity equal to the parent drug and contributes up to 10% to the total antimicrobial activity. Approximately 60% of the oral dose is excreted in the urine as both metabolites and unchanged drug, and the remainder is excreted in the feces.

Rifampin is rapidly absorbed from the GI tract on an empty stomach and distributed to most body tissues and fluids, including breast milk and CSF. Most rifampin is protein bound (80%) and therefore is not ionized to diffuse freely into tissues. Up to 60% of the drug is eliminated in the feces, with 30% in the urine.

Pyrazinamide is rapidly absorbed from the GI tract, with distribution throughout most body tissues and fluids,

IMMUNE

PHARMACOKINETICS
TABLE 29-2 Antitubercular and Antileprotic Drugs

Drug	Route	Onset	Peak	Duration	PB (%)	t½	BioA (%)
FIRST-LINE DRUGS							
ethambutol	PO	Variable	2–4 hr	24 hr	20–30	3–4 hr	69–85
isoniazid	PO	Variable	1–2 hr	24 hr	10–15	1–4 hr	90–95
pyrazinamide	PO	Variable	2 hr	24 hr	50	9–10 hr	UA
rifabutin	PO, IV	Rapid	2.1–4.3 hr	UA	85	16–68 hr	85*
rifampin	PO	Variable	2–4 hr	24 hr	88–90	1.5–5 hr	90–95
rifapentine	PO	UA	5–6 hr	UA	98	14–17 hr	70
streptomycin	IM	Variable	1–2 hr	24 hr	34–62	2–3 hr	Poor
SECOND-LINE DRUGS							
capreomycin	IM	Rapid	1–2 hr	UA	UA	4–6 hr	UA
cycloserine	PO	Rapid	3–4 hr	12 hr	0	10 hr	70–90
ethionamide	PO	Rapid	1 hr	UA	30	2–3 hr	80
ANTILEPROTIC DRUGS							
clofazimine	PO	Variable	1–6 hr	5 days	UA	10 days	42–62
dapsone	PO	Variable	4–8 hr	8–12 days	70–90	10–58 hr	70–80

*Bioavailability depends on formulation of rifabutin: capsules, IV, or solution.
BioA, Bioavailability; *IM,* intramuscular; *IV,* intravenous; *PB,* protein binding; *PO,* by mouth; *t½,* half-life.

including CSF, lungs, and liver. Pyrazinamide is hydrolyzed in the liver to its major active metabolite, pyrazinoic acid, and eliminated in the urine.

Streptomycin is rapidly absorbed after IM injection but not from the GI tract. Appreciable concentrations are found in all organ tissues except the brain, with significant amounts in pleural fluid and tuberculous cavities. Streptomycin is eliminated almost entirely by the kidneys.

▮ Adverse Effects and Contraindications

Generally, first-line antitubercular drugs are less toxic than their second-line counterparts, with the occurrence of adverse effects related to patient age, dose, and length of therapy.

The most significant adverse effect associated with ethambutol is dose-related optic neuritis with signs and symptoms such as decreased visual acuity, loss of red-green color detection, diminished visual fields, or loss of vision. Other adverse reactions are acute episodes of gout, peripheral neuritis, and skin rash. Contraindications to the use of ethambutol include hypersensitivity and optic neuritis, as well as age under 13 years. Optic neuritis is generally reversible, but the drug should be stopped immediately should symptoms develop. Although considered pregnancy category C drug, ethambutol has been used safely in pregnancy. Use ethambutol cautiously in the presence of impaired renal function.

The major adverse effects of isoniazid are peripheral neuritis and hepatitis. Peripheral neuritis occurs in about 2% of patients receiving 5mg/kg/day who are not concurrently taking pyridoxine (vitamin B$_6$). Pyridoxine prevents the development of peripheral neuritis, especially in patients with diabetes mellitus, alcoholism, and malnutrition, even if therapy lasts as long as 2 years. The risk of hepatitis is greater in patients who are older than 35 years and/or consume alcohol on a daily basis. Prodromal symptoms of hepatitis are anorexia, nausea and vomiting, malaise, fatigue, and weakness. When isoniazid and rifampin are given concurrently, the incidence of hepatotoxicity is 4 times that seen with isoniazid therapy alone. In addition, severe hepatic injury leading to death has occurred in some patients. Isoniazid is contraindicated for use in patients with hypersensitivity to the drug or

to its ingredients and in patients with acute liver disease. Isoniazid is considered pregnancy category C, and although it does cross the placenta, because of the risk of tuberculosis to the fetus, treatment is started and therapy with pyridoxine recommended. Its cautious use is warranted in the presence of renal dysfunction and during lactation.

Dose-related hepatotoxicity is the most serious adverse effect associated with pyrazinamide. Arthralgia is a common reaction, occurring in about 40% of patients taking the drug. Contraindications to the use of pyrazinamide are patient hypersensitivity, acute liver disease, and acute gout. Pyrazinamide is considered pregnancy category C, so weigh the risks versus the benefits of the drug before using it. Cautious use of this drug is warranted in the presence of renal failure, chronic gout, diabetes mellitus, and acute intermittent porphyria, and in women who are lactating.

Although adverse effects are uncommon with rifabutin, it can cause pressure in the chest. Other uncommon adverse effects of rifabutin include hepatitis and thrombocytopenia. It is a pregnancy category B drug.

The most common adverse effects associated with rifampin are nausea, vomiting, diarrhea, flatulence, and abdominal pain. A red-orange discoloration of urine, feces, saliva, sputum, sweat, and tears also occurs. Other less common reactions include a flulike syndrome, hypersensitivity with pruritus and rash, and thrombocytopenia. Rifampin use is contraindicated in the presence of allergy to any rifamycin, acute liver disease, and concurrent use of protease inhibitors for HIV treatment. Cautious use is warranted during pregnancy (category C) because teratogenic effects have been reported.

The most common adverse effects of rifapentine occur in less than 4% of patients. They include a red-orange or red-brown discoloration to urine, feces, saliva, skin, sputum, sweat and tears; arthralgia, pain, nausea, vomiting, headache, dyspepsia, hypertension, dizziness, and diarrhea. The more serious adverse effects are also rare; they include hyperuricemia, neutropenia, proteinuria, hematuria, and hepatitis. It is a pregnancy category C drug.

The most significant adverse effect associated with streptomycin is ototoxicity. Damage to the eighth cranial nerve

(CN VIII) results in vertigo, loss of hearing, and nausea and vomiting. High dosages and a lengthy treatment regimen increase the risk for ototoxicity. The risk of nephrotoxicity increases in patients with renal failure. Contraindications to streptomycin use include allergy to aminoglycosides; herpes, vaccinia, varicella, and fungal infections; and pregnancy (category D) or lactation. Cautious use is warranted in older adults or patients with diminished hearing, decreased renal function, dehydration, or neuromuscular disorders.

▓ Drug Interactions

Table 29-3 lists drug interactions of antitubercular drugs. A large number of other drugs interact with antitubercular drugs. In addition, patients on isoniazid therapy should avoid consuming cheese (e.g., Swiss or Cheshire cheese), fish (e.g., tuna, skipjack) and, possibly, tyramine-containing foods. When such foods are taken concurrently with isoniazid, redness or itching of the skin, warmth, palpitations, diaphoresis, chills, cold clammy sensations, headache, or lightheadedness

may result. There are no known drug-food interactions with the other antitubercular drugs.

▓ Dosage Regimen

The ATS and CDC recommend that initial treatment for active TB be given as the standard "short-course" treatment of isoniazid, rifampin, pyrazinamide, and ethambutol, although there are four different regimens that may be considered (Tables 29–4 and 29–5). Standard treatment for latent TB is identified in Table 29-6.

▓ Lab Considerations

Isoniazid, rifampin, pyrazinamide, and streptomycin cause elevations in the levels of liver enzymes, alanine transaminase (ALT), aspartate transaminase (AST), and bilirubin in approximately 10% to 20% of patients; thus liver enzymes should be closely monitored.

Treatment with rifampin also necessitates a complete blood count (CBC), B_{12} and folate levels, and prothrombin

DRUG INTERACTIONS
TABLE **29-3** Antitubercular and Antileprotic Drugs

Drug	Interactive Drug(s)	Interaction
FIRST-LINE DRUGS		
isoniazid	rifampin	Increases risk for hepatotoxicity
	alfentanil	Prolongs duration of alfentanil
	carbamazepine	Increases serum level and toxicity of carbamazepine; increases risk of isoniazid hepatotoxicity
	cycloserine, disulfiram	Increases CNS effects
	phenytoin	Increases phenytoin serum levels
	Aluminum antacids	Decreases isoniazid absorption
	Corticosteroids	Decreases isoniazid effectiveness
pyrazinamide	Antigout drugs, ethambutol	Increases serum levels of ethambutol and uric acid
	Neurotoxic drugs, streptomycin	Increases risk of optic neuritis
	Other ototoxic drugs	Increases risk of ototoxicity
	Other nephrotoxic drugs	Increases risk of nephrotoxicity
	Neuromuscular blockers	Increases neuromuscular blocking effect
rifabutin	clarithromycin, delavirdine, fluconazole, indinavir, nelfinavir, ritonavir	Increases the AUC of rifabutin
	clarithromycin, delavirdine, indinavir, itraconazole, nelfinavir, oral contraceptives, trimethoprim-sulfamethoxazole, saquinavir	Decreases concentration of interactive drugs
rifampin	Oral anticoagulants	Decreases effectiveness of anticoagulants
	digoxin	Decreases serum levels of digoxin
	quinidine	Decreases serum levels of quinidine
	verapamil	Decreases serum level of verapamil
	Estrogen-based oral contraceptives	Decreases effectiveness of contraceptive
	cyclosporine	Increases metabolism of cyclosporine
	phenytoin	Increases elimination of phenytoin
rifapentin	indinavir	Increases indinavir biotransformation
SECOND-LINE DRUGS		
capreomycin	cycloserine, other ototoxic and nephrotoxic drugs	Additive ototoxicity and nephrotoxicity
	isoniazid, ethionamide	Additive adverse CNS effects
	phenytoin	Inhibition of phenytoin biotransformation
	ethionamide, other neurotoxic drugs	Increased risk of neurotoxicity
ANTILEPROTIC DRUGS		
dapsone	rifampin	Decreases blood levels of dapsone
	clofazimine	Increases urinary elimination of dapsone
	Hemolytics	Increases risk for agranulocytosis, aplastic anemia, and blood dyscrasias
	dideoxyinosine	Decreases absorption of dapsone
	trimethoprim	Increases serum levels of dapsone
clofazimine	rifampin	Decreases rate of rifampin absorption and delays time to reach peak serum concentrations of rifampin
	isoniazid	Increases serum and urinary concentrations of clofazimine

AUC, Area under the curve; *CNS,* central nervous system.

DOSAGE
TABLE 29-4 Antitubercular Drugs

Drug	Use*	Dosage	Implications
ATS AND CDC GUIDELINES FOR 6-MONTH REGIMEN*			
ethambutol	Active disease	*Adult and Child:* 15–25 mg/kg PO daily for initial 2 months of therapy. Max: 2.5 grams daily	Either EMB or streptomycin initially used when INH resistance occurs. Not for very young children
isoniazid	Active disease	*Adult:* 5 mg/kg PO or IM daily for initial 2 months of therapy. Max: 300 mg daily *Child:* 10 to20 mg/kg PO or IM daily	Initial treatment of TB except in cases of drug resistance or toxicity
pyrazinamide	Active disease	*Adult and Child:* 15–30 mg/kg PO daily for initial 2 months of therapy. Max: 2 grams daily (per CDC)	Taken along with INH and RIF for first 2 months, then INH and RIF for 4 additional months
rifabutin	Active disease	*Adult:* 150 mg PO twice daily *–or–* 300 mg PO once daily	High-fat meals slow the rate without influencing extent of absorption from the capsule formulation. Do not confuse with rifamate, rifapentin, or ritalin.
rifampin	Active disease	*Adult:* 10 mg/kg PO daily *Child:* 10–20 mg/kg daily Max: 600 mg daily	Usually taken along with isoniazid. May cause orange discoloration of urine, feces, sputum, sweat, or tears.
rifapentine	Active disease	*Adult:* 600 mg (four 150 mg tablets) initially given twice weekly with an interval of not less than 72 hours between doses for 2 months; then once weekly for 4 months	Food increases drug concentration. Do not confuse with rifampin.
streptomycin	Active disease	*Adult:* 15 mg/kg IM daily *Child:* 20–40 mg/kg IM daily for 2 months. Max: 1 gram daily	ACET, ATS, and CDC suggest either streptomycin or ethambutol be added as fourth drug in regimen (INH, RIF, and PZA) for initial treatment unless likelihood of INH or RIF resistance is very low.
SECOND-LINE ANTITUBERCULAR DRUGS†			
cycloserine	Failure of first-line drugs	*Adult and Child:* 15–20 mg/kg PO daily *–or–* 500 mg PO twice daily	Give equal doses twice a day.
capreomycin	MDR-TB	*Adult and Child:* 15–30 mg/kg IM daily or up to 1 gram for 60–120 days	Should not be used together with streptomycin or kanamycin.
ethionamide	Failure of first-line drugs	*Adult and Child:* 15–20 mg/kg PO daily	Concomitant use of pyridoxine (B₆) is recommended.

*Joint statement by ATS and CDC. These drugs are used in combination with other antitubercular drugs.
†The fluoroquinolones ciprofloxacin, levofloxacin, and ofloxacin are discussed in Chapter 27, as are the aminoglycosides amikacin and kanamycin.
ACET, Advisory Council for the Elimination of Tuberculosis; *ATS,* American Thoracic Society; *EMB,* ethambutol; *CDC,* Centers for Disease Control and Prevention; *IM,* intramuscular; *INH,* isoniazid; *MDR-TB,* multidrug-resistant tuberculosis; *PO,* by mouth; *PZA,* pyrazinamide; *RIF,* rifampin.

time (PT) and international normalized ratio (INR) to be obtained before and during therapy. Rifampin and isoniazid interfere with the determination of vitamin B₁₂ and folate levels. Further, PT and INR monitoring should be done more frequently since rifampin decreases the effectiveness of anticoagulants. Carefully monitor phenytoin levels of patients taking phenytoin and rifampin concurrently. Serum uric acid levels may be increased in the presence of pyrazinamide and ethambutol. Obtain blood urea nitrogen (BUN), creatinine, and urine specific gravity measurements as well as a urinalysis, especially for patients with impaired renal function.

Second-Line Drugs
◆ amikacin (Amikin)
◆ capreomycin (Capastat)
◆ ciprofloxacin (Cipro), levofloxacin (Levaquin); ◆ ofloxacin (Floxacin)
◆ cycloserine (Seromycin)
◆ ethionamide (Trecator)
◆ kanamycin (Kantrex)
◆ para-aminosalicylic acid (PAS)

▌▌▌ Indications
Second-line drugs are especially useful in the treatment of MDR-TB. However, they are less effective than first-line drugs, and they have greater toxicity. Ciprofloxacin, levofloxacin, and ofloxacin are fluoroquinolones that have demonstrated effectiveness against a number of gram-negative organisms, as have the aminoglycosides amikacin and

kanamycin. Neither of these classes is FDA-approved for TB, but both have been used for MDR-TB. They are discussed further in Chapter 27. Cycloserine is an antibiotic-antimycobacterial drug effective in the treatment of TB, but it is rarely prescribed. PAS has been used in the past in the treatment of TB but has lost favor among health care providers in recent years because of its marked GI toxicities. For this reason it will not be discussed further.

▌▌▌ Pharmacodynamics
Capreomycin is an antimycobacterial cyclic peptide derived from *Streptomyces capreolus*. It inhibits RNA synthesis, thereby decreasing the replication of bacilli. Bacterial resistance to capreomycin develops when it is given alone, and the resistant organisms show cross-resistance to kanamycin.

Ciprofloxacin, levofloxacin, and ofloxacin exert their effects by disrupting the action of DNA gyrase and topoisomerase IV, enzymes that are the major catalysts in the transcription, duplication, and repair of DNA in bacterial cells.

Cycloserine, as an analog of D-alanine (a nonessential amino acid occurring in proteins and found at high levels in plasma), inhibits mycobacterial cell wall synthesis. There is no cross-resistance between cycloserine and other antitubercular drugs.

Depending on the concentration of ethionamide at the infection site and the susceptibility of infecting bacilli, the drug is bacteriostatic or bactericidal. The exact mechanism of action is unclear, but it is thought to inhibit peptide synthesis in susceptible bacilli. Resistance can develop when the

TABLE 29-5 Examples of First-Line Treatment Regimens for TB*

Regimen	Drug Combinations
1	INH, RIF, PZA, and EMB daily for 2 months. After INH and RIF sensitivities are established, INH and RIF or RPT alone daily or 2–3 times weekly for 4 months
2	INH, RIF, PZA, and EMB daily for 2 weeks; then DOT twice weekly for 6 weeks, then DOT of INH and RIF or RPT weekly for 4 months
3	INH, RIF, PZA, and EMB for 2 months of DOT; then DOT with INH and RIF for 18 weeks
4	INH, RIF, PZA, and EMB for 2 months, then INH and RIF daily or twice weekly for 8 months

*Treatment regimens in order of preference. All regimens are continued for a minimum of 6 months, and should continue for 3 months after cultures become negative. If cultures remain positive after that 3-month period, referral to specialist is warranted. Patients with HIV require a minimum of 9 months of treatment and should continue therapy for 6 months after cultures are negative.
DOT, Directly-observed therapy; *EMB*, ethambutol; *INH*, isoniazid; *PZA*, pyrazinamide; *RIF*, rifampin; *RPT*, rifapentin.

TABLE 29-6 Recommended Treatment for Latent TB*

Regimen	Drugs and Dosage	Comments
First-line	INH 300 mg PO daily for 6–9 months; then twice weekly dosing using DOT	9–12 months in HIV patients. Add pyridoxine (B$_6$) supplement 50 mg/day to patients with diabetes, CRF, alcohol abuse, and those who are taking antiepileptic drugs or are malnourished or pregnant.
Second-line	RIF 10 mg/kg + PZA 15–30 mg/kg PO daily for 2 months; then twice weekly for 3–4 months using DOT	For patients with known INH resistance, RIF-susceptible contacts
Third-line	RIF 10 mg/kg PO daily for 4 months (with/without DOT)	For patients intolerant to PZA, with INH-resistant, RIF-susceptible contacts

*Treatment regimens in order of preference. Note comments.
CRF, Chronic renal failure; *DOT*, directly-observed therapy; *INH*, isoniazid; *PO*, by mouth; *PZA*, pyrazinamide; *RIF*, rifampin.

drug is used as monotherapy. Acquired resistance to both isoniazid and ethionamide are possible with MDR-TB. The majority of isolates resistant to one are usually susceptible to the other. There is no evidence of cross-resistance.

Pharmacokinetics

Cycloserine and ethionamide are rapidly absorbed from the GI tract following oral administration. Both are distributed throughout most body tissues and fluids. Both drugs readily cross the blood-brain barrier, with CSF concentrations in all patients approximately the same as plasma concentrations (see Table 29-2). The majority of both drugs is eliminated in the urine as inactive metabolites.

Capreomycin is poorly absorbed from the GI tract and must be given by intramuscular (IM) injection. Elimination of capreomycin occurs primarily through the urine.

Adverse Effects and Contraindications

Capreomycin's most common adverse effects are ototoxicity and nephrotoxicity, although hepatic dysfunction has also been evident in some patients. Leukocytosis, leukopenia, eosinophilia, and hypokalemia have also been demonstrated in patients taking capreomycin. Avoid the concomitant use of capreomycin with other ototoxic and nephrotoxic drugs, including streptomycin and kanamycin. The risk-benefit ratio for capreomycin use during pregnancy (category C) should be based on available data. Its safe use in children has not been established.

The most common adverse effects of cycloserine involve the CNS. Seizures have been known to occur when cycloserine is used concomitantly with isoniazid or ethionamide. Ingestion of alcohol further increases the likelihood of seizures. Some neurologic effects may be prevented by using pyridoxine (vitamin B$_6$) with cycloserine. Because limited information is available to date on the use of cycloserine during pregnancy (category C), a specific indication is necessary for it to be considered.

The most common adverse effects of ethionamide are GI disturbances, including anorexia, nausea, and vomiting. Some patients develop a metallic taste in the mouth. Less common effects are hepatitis and optic and peripheral neuritis. Ethionamide may increase the risk for neurotoxicity when used with other neurotoxic drugs. Ethionamide is contraindicated in patients with hypersensitivity and severe hepatic impairment. Ethionamide is considered pregnancy category C, and caution should be used during lactation.

Dosage Regimen

Because second-line antitubercular drugs are potentially ototoxic and nephrotoxic, do not give any drugs from this group concurrently (Table 29-7). Further, do not use these drugs in combination with streptomycin.

Lab Considerations

Increased AST levels have been reported in patients with liver disease who are taking cycloserine. Dosage adjustments may be required on the basis of renal function tests and serum drug levels.

Renal impairment associated with capreomycin use results in increased blood urea nitrogen and decreased creatinine clearance levels as well as electrolyte disturbances. Eosinophilia occurs often during therapy with capreomycin but usually subsides when the dosage is reduced.

Ethionamide therapy results in increased ALT and AST levels. Measure these levels before and during therapy.

CLINICAL REASONING

Treatment Objectives

Treatment objectives for the patient with TB are to eliminate the infectious state as quickly as possible and to maintain consistently negative sputum cultures thereafter. Preventing

IMMUNE

DOSAGE
TABLE 29-7 Antileprotic Drugs

Drug	Use	Dosage	Comments
clofazimine*		**WHO Recommendations**	
	Multibacillary forms	*Adult:* 50 mg PO daily and 300 mg monthly	DOT in children. Self-administered in adult.
		Child: 50 mg PO given on alternate days, supplemented by 200 mg monthly	Given for 2 yr or until skin tests are negative
		NHDC Recommendations	
	Sulfone-resistant strains of paucibacillary forms	*Adult:* 50–100 mg PO daily for 2 yr	DOT. In place of dapsone, given in the same regimen.
	Sulfone-resistant strains multibacillary forms	*Adult:* 50–100 mg PO daily indefinitely	In combination with rifampin
dapsone		**WHO Recommendations**	
	Paucibacillary form	*Adult:* 100 mg PO daily for 6 months	Self-administered in adults, in combination with rifampin
		Child: 1–2 mg/kg PO daily for 6 months	
	Multibacillary form	*Adult:* 100 mg PO daily for a minimum of 2 yr or until skin tests are negative	Self-administered in adults, combined with rifampin
		Child: 1–2 mg/kg PO daily for a minimum of 2 yr	
		NHDC Recommendations†	
	Sulfone resistant strains of paucibacillary form	*Adult:* 100 mg PO daily for 6 months, given with rifampin	For indeterminate and tuberculoid forms, continue drug for 3 yr after skin tests negative
	Sulfone-sensitive strains of multibacillary form	*Adults:* 100 mg PO daily for 3 yr	For midborderline form, drug is continued for 10 yr after skin tests negative. For borderline and lepromatous forms, drug is continued indefinitely
rifampin		**WHO Recommendations**	
	Paucibacillary form	*Adult:* 600 mg PO monthly for 6 months	DOT. Used in combination with dapsone
	Multibacillary form	*Adults >35 kg:* 600 mg PO monthly for 2 yr	DOT. Used in combination with dapsone and clofazimine.
		Adults <35 kg: 450 mg PO monthly for 2 yr	
		Child: 10 mg/kg PO monthly	
		NHDC Recommendations	
	Sulfone-sensitive strains of paucibacillary form	*Adult:* 600 mg PO monthly for 6 months	In combination with dapsone
	Multibacillary form due to sulfone-sensitive strains	*Adult:* 600 mg PO monthly for 3 yr	In combination with dapsone
	For sulfone-resistant strains	*Adult:* 600 mg PO monthly for 3 yr	In combination with clofazimine

*For WHO regimens when clofazimine is unacceptable to patients, ethionamide, 250–375 mg PO daily may be self-administered in adults. For NHDC regimens, when clofazimine is unacceptable to patients, ethionamide, 250 mg PO daily, along with rifampin, 600 mg PO daily may be given to adults.
†The NHDC regimens have no recommendations for pediatric dosages of dapsone.
DOT, Directly-observed therapy; *NHDC,* National Hansen's Disease Centers; *PO,* by mouth; *WHO,* World Health Organization.

drug-resistant strains of TB from forming and avoiding a reactivation of the TB are equally important. To accomplish these objectives, treatment is designed to eradicate three replicating populations of bacilli: those in cavitary lesions, those in closed caseous lesions, and those existing within macrophages.

Treatment Options

▥ *Patient Variables*

A tuberculin skin test (Mantoux test) is useful for screening groups at high risk for TB. A small amount (0.1 mL) of intermediate-strength purified protein derivative (PPD) containing 5 tuberculin units is administered intradermally in the forearm, and the site is evaluated 48 to 72 hours after injection. An area of induration measuring 10 mm or more in diameter is considered a positive reaction. A positive reaction does not suggest active disease, but rather indicates exposure to the bacilli or dormant disease and the development of antibodies. Information on the interpretation of tuberculin skin test results is found in Boxes 29–2 and 29–3. When sputum is required for culture, in most instances, three samples are obtained for acid-fast smear. A positive sputum culture confirms the diagnosis of TB. Once drug therapy is started, sputum samples are again obtained to monitor the effectiveness of therapy.

Once a skin test is positive, a chest x-ray study is essential to rule out clinically active TB or to detect old, healed lesions. Nodules, calcifications, and cavities may be seen in the upper lobes, as can hilar enlargement or mediastinal lymphadenopathy. Routine skin tests and chest x-ray exams are no longer recommended in these patients. Advise these patients to seek medical attention if they develop symptoms suggestive of TB. It is difficult to identify *M. avium* TB in patients with HIV, because the skin test may be negative. The negative finding is due to the patient's weak immune response (i.e., anergy). In addition, sputum cultures may remain negative for acid-fast bacilli.

LIFE-SPAN CONSIDERATIONS

Pregnant and Nursing Women. A diagnosis of TB in a pregnant woman is not an indication for an abortion. Pregnancy itself has no impact on the progression of latent TB to active TB. However, treatment is mandated to protect the fetus, the mother, family members, and others. In most cases, treatment of latent TB in women who have an intact immune system may be delayed in most cases until the postpartum period. If, however, the pregnant woman has risk factors for disease progression, begin treatment with INH immediately.

Discuss the risks and benefits of antitubercular therapy with the pregnant patient. She should understand that problems associated with not treating the TB far outweigh the possible risks to her and her unborn child. Isoniazid,

CASE STUDY   Antitubercular Drugs

ASSESSMENT

History of Present Illness	SE, a homeless, 45-year-old male, arrives at the infectious disease clinic with complaints of increasing fatigue ("I can hardly stand on my corner anymore"), fatigue, and productive cough with blood-streaked sputum. He reports weight loss, lethargy, and periodic chills. SE does not know when his symptoms started but some of the people he lives with also "have the same shit."
Past Health History	Poor historian. Unknown family history. Denies drug or food known allergies.
Psychosocial History	He admits to a daily consumption of 16 ounces of alcohol ("if my pan-handling gets me coin, else I share with my friends"). SE has a 25-py smoking history.
Life-Span Considerations	No permanent address; lives with other homeless people under the bridge at Bannock Street and 8th Avenue, just across from the clinic. He has been "down on his luck" for years. SE retrieves his social security disability income check from a nearby post office box.
Physical Exam Findings	*Height:* 72 inches. *Weight:* 155 pounds. TPR: 99.6° F-100–28 and labored with hemoptysis when coughing. SpO$_2$: 90%. Physically unkempt with sour body odor and alcohol on breath. Skin dry. ENT negative. Teeth poor repair. Barrel chest. Breath sounds diminished all lobes, no E>A changes or fremitus. HRRR. Scaphoid abdomen, NT, mild hepatomegaly, no splenomegaly. BS×4. DP and PT 2+ but extremities cool to touch.
Diagnostic Findings	BUN and creatinine within normal limits. AST, ALT, bilirubin mild elevations. GGT within normal limits Chest x-ray: Hilar enlargement, suspicious area in the right middle lobe. Sputum culture × 3 positive for acid-fast *Mycobacterium tuberculosis* bacilli. Mantoux positive with 12 cm of induration. Liver function tests within normal limits.

DIAGNOSIS: Active TB of unknown duration

MANAGEMENT

Treatment Objectives	1. Render patient noninfectious. 2. Prevent bacilli replication and resistance. 3. Minimize risk for drug-induced adverse effects (i.e., hepatitis, peripheral neuritis).
Treatment Plan	**Pharmacotherapy** • Rifater (pyrazinamide 300 mg + isoniazid 150 mg + rifampin 150 mg) daily for 2 months • Ethambutol 1050 mg PO daily for 2 months • Pyridoxine 20 mg PO daily for 3 weeks; then 5 mg daily thereafter **Patient Education** 1. Significance of taking drugs regularly and for regular follow-up during clinic hours 9–2 PM 2. Advise him that infectious disease case workers will go to his living site if he does not appear daily for DOT. 3. Take Rifater on empty stomach. 4. Avoid alcohol; if not possible, at least reduce intake. 5. Return to clinic if he notices vision difficulties, nausea and vomiting, red-orange or red-brown urine, yellowing of skin or eyes, worsening fatigue, or numbness of extremities. 6. Avoid foods such as tuna, sauerkraut, aged cheese, smoked fish (tyramine-containing foods) to avoid tyramine reaction. **Evaluation** 1. Infectious disease case workers have contacted those he lives with for evaluation of disease status and treatment if needed. 2. Liver function tests remain within normal limits; no evidence of drug-induced hepatitis or peripheral neuritis. 3. Sputum no longer contains *M. tuberculosis* bacilli.

IMMUNE

Continued

Q1. Why does SE need to take all three drugs, even if they are in one pill, for such a long time? Isn't there a single drug of choice for TB?

A. No, there isn't a single drug of choice. Multidrug therapy is used to reduce the risk of mycobacterial resistance. TB requires long-term therapy because mycobacteria are slow-growing organisms. Even without symptoms, ES can harbor tubercle bacilli lifelong unless the drugs are given to eliminate the inactive bacilli.

Q2. These drugs are considered first-line for TB, but what does that mean and how are first-line drugs different from second-line drugs?

A. Second-line drugs are less effective and more toxic than first-line drugs. They are used when first-line drugs are not effective in killing the bacilli of TB.

Q3. How long will SE have to take these drugs? Do you think he will really come to the clinic every day?

A. I hope so, but we will do what we can to encourage him to come every day. The Volunteers of America provide lunch at 12 PM for those coming to the clinic for DOT. Perhaps a nice hot meal daily will entice him to come and help put a few pounds on him. He will need to be here every day for at least 2 months. After that he will take Rifamate, a combination of isoniazid 150 mg and rifampin 300 mg daily for another 4 months.

Q4. Why is it essential to treat SE's contacts prophylactically for TB?

A. Preventive therapy is required for persons in close contact with SE or others with TB to prevent spread of primary infection.

Q5. What do you think about prophylaxis for the other homeless people he lives with under the bridge? Shouldn't they also be tested and take drugs?

A. The infectious disease case workers will aid us in finding his contacts so they can be evaluated, treated if necessary, and followed. Prophylaxis would be with isoniazid, but people with liver disease and those with serious adverse reactions to isoniazid in the past should not take the drug.

rifampin, and ethambutol have not been shown to be teratogenic. PZA may be used in pregnant women in whom drug resistance is suspected, but it is not a first-line drug. Streptomycin, capreomycin, and kanamycin should not be used during pregnancy because of documented fetal ototoxicity. The safe use of pyrazinamide and cycloserine during pregnancy has not been established. Do not discourage pregnant women receiving antitubercular therapy from breastfeeding. Toxicity among breastfed infants is rare.

Children and Adolescents. The incidence of TB has risen significantly in children, with a 36.1% increase noted in children up to 4 years old and a 34.1% rise in children ages 5 to 14 years. The increases have been attributed in part to the immigration of many TB-positive persons to the United States.

Children are susceptible to both types of TB, *M. tuberculosis* and *M. bovis*. The bovine type is a common source of infection in children in parts of the world where TB in cattle is not controlled or pasteurization of milk is not practiced. The morbidity and mortality of TB are higher in girls than in boys, particularly in later childhood and adolescence.

Older Adults. At the opposite end of the spectrum is the older adult. The physical changes of aging affect biotransformation and elimination of drugs by the kidneys that can lead to toxicity. Further, distribution of drugs that are highly protein bound is influenced by the level of albumin in the serum. Rifampin, for example, is 88% to 90% protein bound, so its time in the body may be extended. On the other hand, isoniazid has little to no protein binding, so more free drug is available to act on the mycobacterium.

The incidence of TB is higher among older adults (65 years of age and older) than in any other group, except for persons in developing countries who have HIV. Some of the older adult populations were infected and became hosts of the dormant bacilli many years before antitubercular drugs were available.

TB among older adults is reactivated by several factors, including diabetes mellitus, poor nutrition, long-term corticosteroid therapy, smoking, alcohol, and immunosuppression. Older adult residents of long-term care facilities are at greater risk than older adults in the general population. Careful screening for TB is required in all long-term care facilities.

▮ Drug Variables

There are two main principles of antitubercular therapy. First, the therapy must consist of two or more drugs to which the bacilli are sensitive. Second, treatment must continue for at least 3 to 6 months after the sputum becomes negative. This practice sterilizes the lesions and prevents relapse. Because there are three different populations of bacilli, antitubercular drugs differ in their bacteriostatic and/or bactericidal activity. Further, because *M. tuberculosis* is slow-growing and the disease often chronic, patient compliance, drug toxicity, and the development of bacterial resistance present special therapeutic problems. The adverse effects of antitubercular therapy usually occur within the first 100 days of treatment.

ACTIVE DISEASE. In the United States, initial intensive therapy is accomplished using a combination of isoniazid, rifampin, pyrazinamide, and ethambutol. Streptomycin is

BOX 29-2

Factors Contributing to False-Negative Tuberculin Skin Test

Factors Related to the Person Being Tested
- Current viral infection (e.g., measles, mumps, chicken pox, HIV)
- Current bacterial infection (e.g., typhoid fever, typhus, leprosy, pertussis, overwhelming TB)
- Current fungal infection (e.g., South American blastomycosis)
- Recent receipt of live virus vaccination (e.g., measles, mumps, polio, varicella)
- Metabolic derangements (e.g., chronic renal failure)
- Low-protein states (e.g., severe protein depletion, afibrinogenemia)
- Lymphoid diseases (e.g., Hodgkin's disease, lymphoma, chronic leukemia, sarcoidosis)
- Drugs taken (e.g., corticosteroids and other immunosuppressive drugs)
- Age (e.g., newborns, older adults with "waned" sensitivity)
- Stress (e.g., surgery, burns, mental illness, graft-versus-host reactions)

Factors Related to the Method of Administration
- Injection of too little antigen
- Subcutaneous injection (i.e., rather than intradermal)
- Delayed administration after drawing into syringe (drug adheres to plastic of syringe)
- Injection too close to other skin test sites

Factors Related to Reading the Test and Recording Results
- Inexperienced reader
- Conscious or unconscious bias
- Error in recording results

Factors Related to the Tuberculin Used
- Improper storage (i.e., exposure to light and heat)
- Improper dilutions; adsorption (partially controlled by formulation)
- Chemical denaturation or contamination

HIV, Human immunodeficiency virus; *TB*, tuberculosis, tuberculin.
Data from the American Thoracic Society. (2000). Diagnostic standards and classifications of tuberculosis in adults and children. *American Journal of Respiratory Critical Care Medicine, 161*(4), 1376–1395.

BOX 29-3

Interpretation of Tuberculin Skin Test Results*

- A *15-mm or larger area of induration* is considered positive in all persons.
- A *10-mm or larger area of induration* is considered positive in persons with one or more of the following characteristics:
  - Work in a health care environment
  - Were born in high-prevalence areas in countries in Asia, Africa, Latin America, Oceania
  - Are intravenous drug abusers
  - Are members of any medically underserved, low-income populations, including high-risk racial or ethnic minorities (blacks, Hispanic Americans, Native Americans, Eskimo Americans) and the homeless
  - Reside in long-term care facilities (e.g., nursing homes, prisons, mental institutions) or congregate living settings

- Have medical conditions that are thought to increase the risk of TB: silicosis, gastrectomy, jejunoileal bypass, 10% or greater loss of body weight, chronic renal failure, diabetes, high-dose corticosteroid use, immunosuppressive therapies, hematologic disorders (e.g., leukemia, lymphoma), and other malignancies
- A *5-mm or greater area of induration* is considered positive in patients with one or more of the following characteristics:
  - Are known HIV-positive or have an unknown HIV status and high-risk factors for TB
  - Have, or have had, close or recent contact with patients with confirmed active TB
  - Have chest x-ray results consistent with old, healed TB

*In adults older than 50 years, a two-step testing procedure is recommended. The patient is retested in 1–2 weeks if the first test was negative. A positive second test indicates that the patient was previously infected.

added to the regimen if resistance is suspected. A large proportion of organisms from Latin American, African, and Asian immigrants are found resistant to isoniazid. Two or more drugs are used to treat active disease, because the combination provides additive antitubercular activity, and because one drug minimizes or delays the development of resistance to the other.

Second-line antitubercular drugs are similar in several respects. They are all used only for treatment of disease caused by resistant organisms or by nontuberculous mycobacteria. The second-line drugs are given either parenterally or by mouth and have similar pharmacokinetics and toxicities. Ototoxicity and nephrotoxicity are possible; therefore no two drugs from this group should be used together, nor should any of these drugs be used in combination with streptomycin.

PROPHYLAXIS. In general, the benefits of prophylaxis outweigh the risks of hepatotoxicity associated with isoniazid. However, prophylaxis is contraindicated in persons who have liver disease or have had serious adverse reactions to isoniazid in the past. Persons older than 35 years should not be routinely treated, because the risk of isoniazid-induced liver damage increases significantly with age. Reserve prophylaxis for persons who have other factors placing them at increased risk for TB (e.g., diabetes, leukemia, drug-induced immunosuppression). Postpone prophylaxis for a pregnant woman until after delivery where possible.

Directly observed therapy (DOT) is recommended in areas where patients do not complete at least 90% of the recommended therapy. DOT requires that another person actually watch the patient as the prescribed drugs are taken. This approach is feasible for patients taking their drugs on daily, twice-weekly, or thrice-weekly regimens. It improves adherence in both rural and urban settings and is cost-effective even though it requires additional resources. Further, DOT is the standard of care for newborns, infants, children, and adolescents, as well as for their contacts (see Controversy box).

IMMUNE

Directly Observed Therapy for Tuberculosis

Sandra Franklin

The incidence of tuberculosis (TB) declined for 30 years with the introduction of antitubercular drugs. Unfortunately, TB has now reemerged as a serious threat to public health. The significant rise in TB can be attributed in part to the increased prevalence of human immunodeficiency virus (HIV) infections, but resurgence of TB has been documented in a variety of health care settings.

Standard treatment regimens for TB involve self-administration of specific drugs for a period of several months. However, approximately one third of patients with active disease do not follow the prescribed treatment regimen, and their disease then relapses.

Current protocols promote directly observed therapy (DOT) as an effective alternative to the standard self-administration strategy. DOT requires that patients receive and swallow their drugs under supervision. DOT significantly decreases the frequency of primary drug resistance, and reduces the rates of acquired drug resistance and relapse.

Management costs for DOT and standard antitubercular therapy are comparable. The costs for one patient who fails standard treatment regimens and develops multi–drug-resistant TB far outweigh the cost of implementing DOT for several hundred patients.

CLINICAL REASONING

- What factors make self-administration of a drug difficult for the patient?
- What is primary drug resistance? How is it different from acquired drug resistance? In what way is/are the difference(s) significant in determining treatment regimens?
- What constitutes a relapse of TB? Why is relapse considered a public health menace as well as a problem for the patient?

Patient Education

In the United States, it is mandatory for health care providers to report newly diagnosed cases of TB, as well as patients who discontinue treatment prematurely, to state public health officials. Detailed records of treatment must be kept, including changes in the drug regimen, all bacteriologic reports, and the results of sensitivity testing. Advise patients of this regulation and answer their questions in a straightforward manner. As recently as the 1960s, patients with TB were often confined for months or years in TB sanatoriums for treatment. The patient with suspected TB may be aware of a nonspecific anxiety or nervousness in others with whom they associate. Explain each aspect of the treatment regimen to the patient. Most treatment failures occur because patients neglect to take their drugs, discontinue treatment prematurely, or take their drugs irregularly.

Teach patients to cover the mouth and nose when coughing or sneezing. Persons in close contact with those who cannot or will not cover their mouths or who are coughing should wear masks. Patients who have primary TB or whose sputum is bacteriologically negative, but who do not cough and are known to be receiving adequate drug therapy, need not be isolated. Hospitalization is necessary only for patients with severe illness and for whom medical or psychosocial circumstances make treatment at home difficult or impossible.

Most patients need careful instruction in order to manage their drug regimens properly. Adherence is a key factor in the success of treatment for TB, especially among specific high-risk populations. Question patients regularly about adherence to drug regimens.

To verify adherence, perform spot urine and serum drug level testing and maintain strict record-keeping. Advise patients to keep clinic appointments for drug dispensing, laboratory testing, and follow-up physical exams. Notify public health officials if appointments are not kept. It may be beneficial to offer incentives for improved adherence, such as taxi fare to and from the clinic, food vouchers, or free day care.

TB prophylaxis may be indicated for close contacts of patients with TB. BCG vaccination of tuberculin-negative household contacts, especially infants and children, may be warranted under special circumstances. Continuing exposure to untreated or ineffectively treated persons with sputum-positive TB necessitates additional intervention strategies.

Teach patients to recognize the signs and symptoms of hepatitis and optic neuritis. Instruct them to promptly report signs and symptoms of hepatitis (i.e., yellow eyes and skin, nausea and vomiting, anorexia, fatigue or weakness, or dark urine), optic neuritis (i.e., eye pain, blurred vision, and/or loss of vision), hearing disturbances and/or dizziness, tinnitus, or vertigo. Regular ophthalmologic examinations aid in the detection and follow-up of optic neuritis. Warn patients receiving rifampin that the drug may turn body fluids and urine a red-orange. Reassure them that this is harmless. Advise patients to wear glasses instead of contact lenses to prevent discoloration of lenses while taking rifampin.

Evaluation

Monitor for indications that the TB infection is under control. Diminished cough and sputum production, decreased fever and night sweats, amelioration of anorexia with a concomitant weight gain, and fewer bacilli in sputum specimens are all evidence of improvement. Successful therapy is further noted as an absence of observable bacilli in the sputum and in sputum cultures. Once sputum cultures are negative, continue treatment for another 3 to 6 months. Monitor the patient's liver function tests and electrolyte values regularly. As discussed previously, a baseline visual examination should be performed before the start of antitubercular therapy, and the drug stopped should symptoms of optic neuritis develop. Serum uric acid levels and coagulation studies should remain within normal limits, and patient records should indicate that the patient is keeping follow-up appointments.

LEPROSY

EPIDEMIOLOGY AND ETIOLOGY

Leprosy is also known as Hansen's disease, after Armauer Hansen, the Norwegian physician who first identified the microorganism that causes the disease. Known and dreaded since biblical times because of the severe deformities that can occur, it was considered incurable until the 1940s. The culprit is a slow-growing bacterium, *M. leprae,* which is related to *M. tuberculosis*, the microorganism that causes TB.

Ninety percent of the patients with currently active Hansen's disease are found in Brazil, Madagascar, Mozambique, Tanzania, and Nepal. This CDC information is also supported by World Health Organization (WHO) data. The CDC only reported 92 new cases in 2002. The disease also occurs in colder climates of Tibet, Nepal, Korea, and Siberia. Small numbers (300 to 500 per year) of cases currently occur in the United States. Cases have been reported in California, Hawaii, Texas, Florida, Louisiana, New York City, and Puerto Rico. The rise in leprosy incidence in the United States has been attributed to immigration from areas where it is endemic.

There is some evidence to suggest that single-lesion paucibacillary leprosy is a clinical entity. It refers to those patients with a single hypopigmented or reddish lesion with definitive loss of sensation but without nerve trunk involvement. It accounts for a significant number of newly diagnosed cases of leprosy (e.g., 20% to 30% of cases in Malawi, nearly 60% of cases in India).

Worldwide, the prevalence of leprosy has declined by 90%–from 21.1 cases per 10,000 inhabitants to less than 1 case per 10,000 inhabitants in 2000. There has also been an annual, worldwide decrease in cases of leprosy by 20% since 2001. At the start of 2005, 290,000 patients were receiving treatment for leprosy.

There has also been a dramatic decline in disease burden since 1985. According to WHO, leprosy has been eradicated in 113 of the 122 countries where it was considered a public health problem in 1985. An additional 13 countries have eliminated leprosy since 2000. The WHO criterion for elimination of the disease is less than 1 reported case per 10,000 population.

The incubation period for leprosy is unknown but is thought to be 3 to 5 years. Symptoms may take 20 years to appear. Most people exposed to infected patients do not develop leprosy. Cattle, birds, armadillos, and humans serve as the main reservoirs for these mycobacteria. Many primates, pigs, sheep, goats, rabbits, cats, dogs, and ferrets are susceptible to infection, and contribute to the spread of the disease. In the United States, armadillos are extending their range northward from Louisiana and Texas to as far north as Illinois.

In general, prolonged and/or close contact with an infected reservoir is needed for transmission of mycobacteria, although even a short period of contact may be all that is needed for susceptible individuals to contact the infection. Intrafamilial contact with multibacillary form carries greater risk than an occasional exposure outside of the family. Transmission of leprosy is determined by the infectiousness of the person, the susceptibility of the contact person, and the closeness, frequency, and duration of contact.

PATHOPHYSIOLOGY

M. leprae is a slow-growing bacillus that proliferates in the cooler parts of the body. Contact need not be "skin to skin" for the infection to be passed on since the nose, and not the skin, is the primary exit portal for the bacilli from patients with multibacillary infection. However, ulcerated, scratched, or abraded skin of a susceptible individual can be a portal of entry for the bacilli. Each day, untreated patients with leprosy may discharge as many as 100 million bacilli from their nasal secretions, which remain viable for 7 days. Damage to nasal epithelium (e.g., picking the nose, the common cold, and allergies) may facilitate transmission. Although semen, ovaries, a fetus, the umbilical cord, and the placenta are possible transmission routes, the risk for congenital leprosy is unlikely. Some instances of transmission via tattoo equipment or contaminated needles have been reported.

Although the prevalence of leprosy is high in hot, humid climates, the environment seems to have a little role in transmission. Malnutrition is known to be a part of lepromatous leprosy since these patients have been found to have severe deficiencies of magnesium, calcium, zinc, and vitamins A and E. Leprosy transmission is 7 times higher in children who sleep with their infected, but untreated, parents on mats compared with children who sleep separately.

The type of leprosy contracted appears to be related to the human lymphocyte antigen (HLA). Evidence is mounting that a predisposition to tuberculoid leprosy may be coded by HLA-DR2 and/or HLA-DR3. A significant relationship between HLA-DR3 and tuberculoid leprosy has been found in a Mexican population (Baker et al., 2003). The HLA-MT1 haplotype is more common among European, Japanese, Chinese, Burmese, Parsee, and Anglo-Indian populations who are more likely to contact lepromatous leprosy compared with their Africans or Indian counterparts.

Classifications and Forms of Leprosy
There are two classifications of leprosy: paucibacillary and multibacillary. The three forms of *paucibacillary leprosy* are indeterminate, tuberculoid, and borderline tuberculoid (Box 29-4 and Fig. 29-2). The three forms of *multibacillary* leprosy are midborderline, borderline, and lepromatous. Differences in cell-mediated immunity may account for the various forms of leprosy. Host resistance to *M. leprae* is more prominent in the indeterminate and tuberculoid forms of paucibacillary leprosy, but much less prominent in the lepromatous form.

Leprotic reactions are manifestations of delayed hypersensitivity to the *M. leprae* organism and occur in approximately 50% of patients during treatment. Type 1, or "reversal," reactions are seen in the tuberculoid and midborderline forms of leprosy. Type 1 reversal reactions often result in irreversible tissue damage and nerve destruction. Type 2 reactions ("Lucio's phenomenon"), seen in borderline lepromatous and lepromatous forms, are characterized by the appearance of raised, tender, intracutaneous nodules, severe constitutional symptoms, and high fever.

A type 2 reaction is thought to be an Arthus type of reaction related to the release of microbial antigens in patients harboring large numbers of bacilli. Most cases have been reported to have a leukocytoclastic vasculitis as the underlying pathologic abnormality. The histologic picture of an early lesion of Lucio's phenomenon shows a milky, mononuclear cell infiltration, endothelial swelling, vascular thrombosis, and ischemic necrosis. Lepra bacilli are abundant around nerves and blood vessels, and many are noted in vascular walls and endothelium.

BOX 29-4

The Ridley-Joplin Classification of Leprosy

Types of Paucibacillary Leprosy

Patients with an intact immune response who are able to self-heal or to localize the disease. Patients with a bacterial index* (BI) of 0 on skin scrapings at all sites at the time of diagnosis and only rare bacilli on biopsy specimens.

- Indeterminate (B0)
  - Occurs very early in course of infection
  - Macular lesions reflect limited cellular response on biopsy but not specific type
  - 75% heal spontaneously; the remainder progress to other forms of leprosy
- Tuberculoid (B0)
  - More benign than other types
  - Characterized by one or a few macular skin lesions
  - Lesions usually hypopigmented on dark-skinned persons and erythematous on light-skinned persons
  - There is hair loss and loss of sensation at skin lesions
  - Incubation period ranges from 9 months to 20 years, with an average of 4 years
- Borderline tuberculoid (B0)
  - Lesions appear in greater numbers
  - Lesions more symmetric and associated with a loss of sensation and hair
  - Alterations in perception of light touch, pain, and temperature

Types of Multibacillary Leprosy

Patients with the least intact immune response whose disease becomes generalized. Patients with the identified BI at time of diagnosis. Infective capacity of this type is 4 to 11 times greater than that of patients with the paucibacillary form of leprosy.

- Midborderline (BI 2–3$^+$)
  - Numerous lesions with raised plaque appearance with punched-out areas
  - Loss of sensation is variable
- Borderline lepromatous (BI 3–5$^+$)
  - Lesions occur in greater numbers; similar to midborderline form
  - Macular, papular, or nodular lesions have a shiny appearance and are bilaterally symmetric
- Lepromatous (BI 6$^+$)
  - Markedly impaired cell-mediated immunity
  - Diffuse, ill-defined localized infiltrates; skin becomes thick, glossy, corrugated
  - Skin lesions too numerous to count; smooth, shiny erythematous areas
  - Sensory loss occurs late in lepromatous leprosy
  - Large nerve trunks involved; anesthesia, atrophy of skin and muscle, absorption of small bones, ulcerations, and spontaneous amputations may occur
  - Earlobes enlarge; eyebrows and lashes disappear; *leonine facies* develops
  - Nasal stuffiness and epistaxis develop along with a saddle-nose deformity
  - Incubation period of lepromatous leprosy ranges from 18 months to 40 years.
  - More easily spread than other two types

*Bacterial Index (BI): A semilogarithmic scale ranging from 0 (indicating no bacilli in 100 oil immersion fields) to 6$^+$ (indicating more than 1000 organisms per oil immersion field); specimens are obtained from biopsy sections and skin scrapings.

PHARMACOTHERAPEUTIC OPTIONS

First-Line Drugs

- clofazimine (Lamprene)
- dapsone (DDS); ✦ Avlosulfon
- ethionamide (Trecator)
- rifampin (RIF) (Rifadin, Rimactane); ✦ Rifadin, Rimactane

⊞ Indications

According to the WHO guidelines, clofazimine, dapsone, and rifampin are used for the treatment of multibacillary leprosy. The antiinflammatory effects of clofazimine are useful in the treatment of leprotic reactions. At the National Hansen's Disease Centers (NHDC), dapsone is used in conjunction with rifampin for the treatment of paucibacillary and multibacillary forms of leprosy because of sulfone-resistant strains. Dapsone is also used to control the dermatologic symptoms of dermatitis herpetiformis.

Rifampin and ethionamide were discussed previously in relation to treatment of TB but are also useful in treating leprosy. Rifampin is used for all forms of leprosy. Ethionamide is used for multibacillary leprosy. It is only weakly bactericidal to the *M. leprae* organism.

⊞ Pharmacodynamics

Dapsone is a synthetic sulfone, a compound containing two hydrocarbon radicals attached to an SO_2 group. The action of a sulfone is similar to that of the sulfonamide antibiotics. They interfere with the bacterial synthesis of folic acid by competing with para-aminobenzoic acid (PABA). Dapsone and sulfonamide antibiotics (see Chapter 27) possess approximately the same ranges of antibacterial activity. It is essentially bacteriostatic, but weakly bactericidal. Do not use dapsone as monotherapy because of the risk of mycobacterial resistance.

The exact mechanism of action of clofazimine is unclear. The drug binds with mycobacterial DNA to inhibit the multiplication and growth of the *M. leprae* organism. Cross-resistance to dapsone and rifampin has not been demonstrated.

⊞ Pharmacokinetics

Dapsone is slowly absorbed from the acidic environment of the GI tract following oral administration (see Table 29-2). It is well distributed to skin, kidneys, liver, and muscle. Eighty-five percent of the daily dosage is recoverable from urine, mainly in the form of water-soluble metabolites. Elimination of the drug is slow, and a constant blood level can be maintained with the usual dosage.

Clofazimine is absorbed at variable rates depending on several factors, including the site of administration, the dosage, and whether or not food is present in the GI tract. The onset of action varies considerably from patient to patient, but the duration of action is measured in months, because clofazimine tends to accumulate in fatty tissues, the

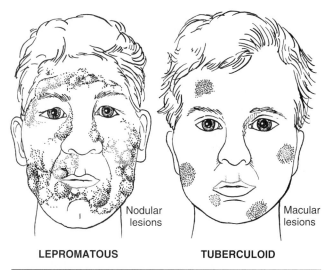

Nodular lesions

Macular lesions

LEPROMATOUS   **TUBERCULOID**

FIGURE 29-2 Comparison of Lepromatous and Tuberculoid Forms of Leprosy. Lepromatous leprosy is characterized by diffuse, ill-defined localized infiltrations of the skin. The lesions, too numerous to count, become thickened, glossy, and corrugated, with smooth, shiny erythematous areas. Tuberculoid leprosy is characterized by one or a few macular skin lesions produced by a granulomatous reaction. The lesions are usually hypopigmented on dark-skinned persons, and erythematous on light-skinned persons. There is hair loss and a loss of sensation at skin lesions. (From Cotran, R., Kumar, V., and Robbins, S. [1994]. *Pathologic basis of disease.* [5th ed.]. Philadelphia: WB Saunders. Used with permission.)

reticuloendothelial system, and the small intestines. Clofazimine is eliminated very slowly from the body, primarily through feces. The drug has an impressive half-life of nearly 70 days.

▥ *Adverse Effects and Contraindications*

The patient taking dapsone should watch for sore throat, fever, pallor, purpura, or jaundice. Deaths associated with the administration of dapsone have been reported from agranulocytosis, aplastic anemia, and other blood dyscrasias. Obtain frequent CBCs in patients receiving dapsone. The U.S. Food and Drug Administration (FDA) recommends that, when feasible, blood counts should be done weekly for the first month, monthly for 6 months, and semiannually thereafter. If a significant reduction in leucocytes, platelets, or hemolysis is noted, discontinue dapsone and follow the patient intensively. Do not use dapsone if the patient is allergic to sulfonamide preparations.

The overall incidence of adverse reactions to dapsone and rifampin treatment regimens is about 0.4%. The most common adverse effect of dapsone is a dose-dependent hemolytic anemia. Anemia develops in patients who receive more than 200 mg a day. The hematologic effects are most severe in patients with a glucose-6-phosphate dehydrogenase (G6PD) deficiency. A syndrome similar to mononucleosis has also occurred occasionally. Signs and symptoms of the syndrome are skin rashes, fever, jaundice, hepatitis, methemoglobinemia, and anemia.

Hypersensitivity reactions to dapsone are manifested by a variety of skin rashes. If the reaction is severe, it may be necessary to discontinue the drug. GI and CNS adverse effects have

also occurred. Hepatic adverse effects include jaundice and hepatitis. Blurred vision, tinnitus, and fever also may occur.

The most serious adverse effects of clofazimine are dose-related GI problems. At doses of 100 mg or less, nausea, vomiting, or diarrhea may be present. More serious effects occur with higher doses of several months' duration. The more serious adverse effects include abdominal pain, perhaps related to the accumulation of drug in the small intestines. On rare occasions, bowel obstruction, GI bleeding, and splenic infarction have been reported.

Clofazimine contains a red-hued dye that leads to discoloration of the skin and conjunctiva in 75% to 100% of patients. There are general skin color changes from red to a brown-black discoloration, with the macules, papules, patches, and plaques also affected. The skin discoloration is reversible, but it may take several months or years to disappear completely. Tears, sweat, sputum, urine, and feces are also discolored. In addition to discoloration, 8% to 38% of patients experience itching and dry skin.

Clofazimine crosses placental membranes and may cause deep pigmentation of the skin of an unborn child, although no teratogenicity has been documented. Clofazimine should be used during pregnancy only if the potential benefit justifies the fetal risk.

▥ *Drug Interactions*

Table 29-3 lists drug interactions of antileprotic drugs. Although drug interactions are fewer than those found with antitubercular drugs, it is important they be noted before these drugs are used.

▥ *Dosage Regimen*

The patient with leprosy usually takes a daily dose of dapsone of 100 mg (or 1 to 2 mg/kg of body weight). With repeated dosing, peak serum levels exceeding the MIC by a factor of about 500 are reached. The high levels inhibit the multiplication of *M. leprae* mutants that have moderate or even low levels of dapsone resistance. The full dosage should therefore be given from the start of therapy and taken without interruption. Dapsone resistance should be confirmed clinically in cases that show no response to therapy within 3 to 6 months, and when the patient's adherence with therapy can be assured. The drugs are available without charge from the U.S. Public Health Service (USPHS) in Carville, Louisiana. DOT is recommended to ensure patient adherence, regardless of the type or form of leprosy treated.

▥ *Lab Considerations*

Dapsone has been shown to decrease the platelet count and hemoglobin levels by 1 to 2 grams/dL, and to increase the reticulocyte count by 2% to 12% of RBCs (adult normal: 0.5% to 2%); therefore blood counts are recommended at regular intervals during the first few weeks of therapy and then every 3 to 6 months. The decrease in hemoglobin levels is related to altered hemoglobin synthesis and bone marrow suppression with an accompanying reduction in hematocrit. The reticulocyte elevation is a response to increased peripheral RBC destruction and increased bone narrow activity. As a result of its long half-life, dapsone may be present in the body up to 3 weeks after it is discontinued. To date, there is no correlation between serum concentrations and therapeutic effects of the drug.

IMMUNE

Dapsone has also been associated with increased serum levels of alkaline phosphatase, AST, ALT, lactate dehydrogenase, and bilirubin. Monitor these values before and during therapy. Methemoglobinemia may be present; monitor hemoglobin levels if patients develop cyanosis, headache, fatigue, and/or shortness of breath.

The erythrocyte sedimentation rate, serum albumin, AST, bilirubin, and glucose levels may be raised in the presence of clofazimine. Serum potassium level is reduced, and therefore serum chemistry panels are warranted at the start of therapy and periodically thereafter.

On The Horizon

Quinolones have shown new promise in the treatment of leprosy. As noted earlier in the discussion of TB, floxacin and ciprofloxacin are thought to be bactericidal. These drugs act by inhibiting DNA synthesis during bacterial replication, probably by interfering with DNA gyrase activity. The bactericidal activity of ofloxacin when given alone to previously untreated multibacillary patients is significantly more rapid than that of either dapsone or clofazimine, but less effective than rifampin. Its antileprosy activity is currently being explored by the WHO. Single-dose and multiple-dose regimens are being used in clinical trials.

Minocycline is the most lipid-soluble of the tetracyclines and inhibits bacterial protein synthesis. It has been shown consistently bactericidal against *M. leprae*. The clearance of viable *M. leprae* from the skin is more rapid than that of dapsone or clofazimine, similar to that for ofloxacin, and slower than that of rifampin. The safety record of minocycline has been previously established.

The efficacy of single-dose therapy using a combination known as ROM of 600 mg of rifampin (the *R*), 400 mg of ofloxacin (the *O*), and 100 mg of minocycline (the *M*) has been for the treatment of paucibacillary leprosy. A single dose of ROM was slightly less effective than standard MDT over 6 months. A single dose of ROM could be an alternative regimen for these patients. However, before recommending a single dose of ROM, examine the entire body of the patient in a good light to exclude more than one lesion and nerve trunk involvement. Follow patients receiving a single dose of ROM for at least 6 months for evidence of advancing disease. Therefore, lepromatous leprosy should be excluded as the possible cause of the lesion before recommending a single-dose ROM regimen.

CLINICAL REASONING

Treatment Objectives

The objective of treatment is to render the patient with leprosy noninfectious, thereby preventing the spread of the disease. To achieve this objective, give the patient the correct dose and combination of drugs for an appropriate duration and, if necessary, arrange supervision to ensure adherence.

Treatment Options

▮▮ *Patient Variables*

Leprosy affects the body of the patient and the mind of the public. The social stigma associated with leprosy has been noted throughout history. The Hebrew word "leper" (from Greek translations) meant someone who was an outcast from society. Dating back to biblical times, the marginalization of persons with leprosy is gradually ceding to the attitude that holds leprosy to be a disease, not a social stigma. Even today, however, the word *leprosy* has negative connotations.

The attitudes of health care providers toward patients with leprosy influence public opinion. As previously stated, infectious patients need not be hospitalized, provided (1) there is adherence with the treatment plan and adequate supervision; (2) the home environment meets specific conditions; and (3) the local health officer concurs in the disposition of the case.

LIFE-SPAN CONSIDERATIONS

Pregnant and Nursing Women. Transmission of the disease from an untreated, infected mother to an infant is not uncommon. Pregnancy and the subsequent 6 months of lactation are said to result in an exacerbation of symptoms in about one third of patients with leprosy. The fetal effects are said to include low birth weight, small placenta, and a high incidence of infant mortality.

Exercise caution when undertaking drug therapy for leprosy during pregnancy. Studies have demonstrated no adverse effects on the fetus from dapsone. However, because of the risk for tumor development in animal studies, dapsone is not recommended for nursing mothers. The patient should make an informed decision regarding whether to discontinue nursing the infant or taking the drug. Thoroughly explain the risk-benefit ratio of the use of rifampin. Rifampin is secreted in breast milk and has tumorigenic effects similar to those of dapsone. Clofazimine is not recommended during the first trimester of pregnancy, or during lactation. Ethionamide is not recommended in pregnant or lactating women with leprosy. It crosses the placenta to cause developmental anomalies.

Children and Adolescents. Leprosy can manifest at any age, but it is seldom seen in children under 3 years of age. The age-specific incidence peaks during childhood in most developing countries. Up to 20% of cases appear in children younger than 10 years. Because leprosy is most prevalent in poorer socioeconomic groups, this figure may simply reflect the age distribution of the high-risk population. Boys and girls are equally affected (1:1 ratio) during childhood, although in adulthood, manifestation in males dominates by a 2:1 ratio. The physiologic immunodeficiency of the newborn may lead to an early colonization with the bacillus.

Older Adults. The immunosuppression found in the older adult causes infections to be a significant risk factor for this age group. Thymic mass is steadily lost, so that serum activity of thymic hormones is almost undetectable. With the decline in T-cell activity and the presence of higher numbers of immature T cells in the thymus, a significant decline in cell-mediated immunity occurs. Thus T lymphocytes are less able to proliferate in response to *M. leprae*.

▮▮ *Drug Variables*

The principal treatment for leprosy is drug therapy. Treatment recommendations for leprosy, according to the WHO and the NHDC consist of dapsone, rifampin, and clofazimine. Clinical evidence suggests that in most instances, infectiousness is lost within 3 months of continuous and regular treatment with antileprotic drugs, or within 3 days of treatment with rifampin. (See Box 29-5.)

CASE STUDY   Antileprotic Drugs

ASSESSMENT

History of Present Illness	MF, a 30-year-old white female with symmetric "red spots that don't itch or hurt" on arms and face near the eyes and in nares, is referred to the infectious disease clinic. States they first appeared 7 weeks ago.
Past Health History	Denies allergies to food or drugs. She takes no current medications. Only hospitalization was at age 16 for appendectomy. FH unremarkable for skin disorders or allergies.
Psychosocial Considerations	Currently active-duty military who just returned from a 4-year assignment in Southeast Asia. MF is unmarried and shares a 2-bed room in the barracks with another soldier. Her roommate is due back from the same Southeast Asian region in another 2 weeks. Military health care system provides health care and pharmacy services without cost while on active duty. She has one to two beers/week but denies other drug use.
Life-Span Considerations	Worried about changes in self-image caused by presence of lesions and that she will not be able to get married and have children.
Physical Exam Findings	Afebrile. Macular, papular, and nodular lesions on forearms and left forehead near eyes shiny in appearance and bilaterally symmetric. Lesions within nares apparent. Loss of hair and sensation in and around all affected areas.
Diagnostic Testing	CBC, LFTs, and renal function test results all within normal limit. Pregnancy test negative. Skin smears confirm *Mycobacterium leprae*. Lepromin skin test negative. Sulfone sensitivity testing confirms sensitivity to dapsone and rifampin.

DIAGNOSIS: Borderline lepromatous leprosy

MANAGEMENT

Treatment Objectives	1. Render patient noninfectious. 2. Support and improve immune system. 3. Prevent spread of infection. 4. Minimize risk of mycobacterial resistance.
Treatment Plan	**Pharmacotherapy** • Dapsone 100 mg PO daily (unsupervised) • Rifampin 600 mg once monthly (supervised) • Contraceptive of choice (through GYN clinic) **Patient Teaching** 1. The etiology and pathophysiology of leprosy, adverse effects of drug treatment, and importance of adherence with drug therapy 2. Period of infectiousness once treatment is begun 3. Importance of clinic follow-up on regular basis. If needed, military orders can be written to that effect. 4. Take drugs on empty stomach. 5. Be sure to use contraceptive regularly to avoid pregnancy. 6. Notify clinic promptly if she experiences fever, loss of appetite, malaise, nausea and vomiting, darkened urine, yellowish discoloration of the skin and eyes, and pain or swelling of the joints. **Evaluation** 1. CBC and liver and renal function test results all within normal limits. 2. She has an appointment next month for a skin smear as part of her follow-up care. 3. She has joined a support group and reports doing well in relation to her depression. 4. She is taking an oral contraceptive to reduce the risk of pregnancy. 5. No evidence of skin changes at this time (too early in therapy).

IMMUNE

Continued

CASE STUDY Antileprotic Drugs—Cont'd

CRITICAL REASONING ANALYSIS

Q1. How long will she be infectious? Do I need to worry about being exposed to leprosy?

A. In general, prolonged and/or close contact with an infected individual is needed for transmission of mycobacteria, although intrafamilial contact with the multibacillary form carries a greater risk than an occasional exposure outside of the family. Studies suggest that in most instances, infectiousness is lost within 3 months of continuous and regular treatment with antileprotic drugs, or within 3 days of treatment with rifampin. We can arrange for you to be screened for the disease, but contact is unlikely.

Q2. We learned in class that TB is treated using several drugs at once. Is the same thing done for leprosy?

A. Yes, combinations of dapsone and rifampin are effective for leprosy but only when used together. When given together, the likelihood of mycobacterial resistance is reduced.

Q3. How long will MF have to take the dapsone and rifampin? Can this kind of leprosy be cured?

A. Yes, some types of leprosy can be cured. Because she has a more serious type, she will need to take the dapsone for at least 3 years after her skin smears are negative. There is also a likelihood that she may need to take the drug the rest of her life.

Q4. I remember hearing something specific about why 100 mg of dapsone is taken, rather than some other dosage. Do you know the reasoning?

A. The 100-mg dosage results in peak serum levels that exceed the minimum effective concentration by a factor of 500. The high levels inhibit the multiplication of *M. leprae* mutations that may have moderate or even low levels of dapsone resistance.

Q5. My clinical instructor wants me to talk with MF about the adverse effects of the drugs she will be taking, dapsone and rifampin. I know about the sore throat, fever, being pale, bruising, and getting jaundiced; but what do I tell her about the skin changes? She will be taking it an awfully long time.

A. Explain to her that the skin changes to a red-orange or a red-brown color, but these changes are reversible over time. Given that she has a light complexion and is already upset about the lesions on her face and arms, she will be at risk for depression. There have been reports of patient suicide because of the severe depression associated with the pigmentation effects. Tell the patient that there are support groups available to help with this issue.

BOX 29-5

Leprosy Take-Home Points

- Paucibacillary leprosy patients treated with MDT are cured within 6 months
- Multibacillary patients treated with MDT are cured within 12 months
- Patients are no longer infectious to others after the first dose of MDT
- There are virtually no relapses (i.e., recurrences of the disease after treatment is completed)
- No resistance of the bacillus to MDT has been identified
- Early detection and treatment with MDT has prevented about 4 million people from being disabled. This suggests great cost-effectiveness of MDT as a health intervention, considering the economic and social loss averted.
- WHO provides free MDT for all patients in the world, as it has since 1995.

MDT, Multidrug therapy; *WHO*, World Health Organization.

Because of the emergence of dapsone-resistant strains of *M. leprae*, combination drug therapy is recommended. The use of combination drug therapy rapidly decreases a patient's infectious state and reduces the likelihood that resistant strains will develop. With a long half-life (10 to 80 hours),

the serum concentration of dapsone remains high for days, thus creating a wide therapeutic margin. As a result, *M. leprae* bacilli are prevented from multiplying, even when there is moderate resistance to the drug.

Rifampin, in combination with other antileprotic drugs, is recommended for all forms of leprosy. It has a rapid effect, and a single dose has been found to kill 99% of the bacilli, thus rendering the patient noninfectious. The bactericidal effect of ethionamide appears sooner than that of dapsone but later than that of rifampin.

The bactericidal effects of clofazimine fall between that of dapsone and rifampin. However, it takes approximately 50 days for clofazimine's bactericidal activity to occur. Concurrent use of clofazimine with rifampin decreases the rate of absorption of rifampin. This factor becomes an important consideration when patient response to leprosy treatment is poor.

Patient Education

Give the patient and family written instructions about all drugs, including the name, the prescribed dose, the reason for taking the drug, its adverse effects, and when to contact the health care provider. Remind the patient of the importance of completing the entire drug regimen, which may take years.

Discuss the adverse effects of the drugs, particularly skin discoloration and serious GI problems, with the patient. Reassure the patient that skin color changes are usually reversible, although they may take several months to years to disappear. Some patients have committed suicide because of the depression associated with changes in pigmentation. Inform the patient of the support groups available to help with this issue.

Evaluation

Note symptoms indicating resolution of the leprotic infection. Evaluate adherence to therapy regularly, depending on the type of leprosy; some treatment regimens may last as long as 10 years, and others for life. Resolution of skin lesions may take 8 to 12 weeks, depending on the severity of the disease.

KEY POINTS

TUBERCULOSIS

- The highest incidences of TB are in males aged 25 to 44 years and in children younger than 15 years, as well as in the Native Americans, Alaskan Natives, Hispanics, blacks, Asians, and Pacific Islander populations.
- Nonadherence, crowded institutional settings, increasing numbers of homeless persons, substance abuse, the immigration of infected persons, and lack of access to health care have contributed to the rising incidence of TB.
- Two primary factors have been associated with the rise in TB incidence: the epidemic of HIV and AIDS, and the growing numbers of drug-resistant strains of the tubercular bacillus.
- The extent of communicability of TB depends on the number and virulence of discharged bacilli, adequacy of ventilation, exposure of the bacilli to the sun or ultraviolet light, and opportunities for aerosolization.
- The appearance of a lung infection with no known prior exposure to the organism is referred to as *primary TB*. The term r*eactivation TB* applies when dormant bacilli become endogenously reactive or the individual is exposed to TB again.
- In *miliary TB* (disseminated disease), more common in older adult patients, bacilli are dispersed throughout body organs and tissues.
- The objectives of treatment are eliminating the patient's infectious state and preventing the development of drug-resistant strains of TB.
- First-line antituberculosis therapy includes isoniazid, rifampin, ethambutol, and pyrazinamide. Streptomycin may be an option in select cases.
- Second-line antituberculosis therapies are amikacin, kanamycin, capreomycin, ciprofloxacin, levofloxacin, ofloxacin, cycloserine, ethionamide, and occasionally, para-aminosalicylic acid.
- Short-term therapy takes place over 6 to 9 months, whereas conventional therapy typically lasts 18 to 24 months.
- A positive sputum culture for acid-fast bacilli confirms the diagnosis of TB. An area of induration measuring 10 mm or more in diameter on the Mantoux test indicates exposure to TB and the production of antibodies against the bacillus.
- Because therapy for TB is complex and lengthy, drug toxicity, poor patient adherence, and the development of microbial resistance present significant problems.

- To achieve treatment objectives, the patient should be given the correct dose and combination of drugs for an appropriate period of time and, if necessary, should be supervised to ensure adherence.
- Successful antitubercular therapy is noted as an absence of observable mycobacteria in the sputum and as the failure of sputum cultures to yield colonies of bacilli.

LEPROSY

- *Mycobacterium leprae (M. leprae)*, a slow-growing bacillus, causes leprosy.
- Humans are the only reservoir of proven significance, and although the exact mode of transmission is not clearly known, household and prolonged close contacts appear to be important.
- The incubation period for leprosy ranges from 9 months to 20 years, with an average of approximately 4 years for the tuberculoid form, and twice that for lepromatous leprosy.
- Paucibacillary leprosy comprises indeterminate, tuberculoid, and borderline tuberculoid forms. Multibacillary leprosy comprises midborderline, borderline lepromatous, and lepromatous forms.
- Differences in cell-mediated immunity may account for the various forms of leprosy.
- The objectives of treatment are to render patients noninfectious and to prevent spread of the disease.
- The primary treatment options for leprosy are dapsone, rifampin, and clofazimine.
- Dapsone is the drug of choice for all forms of leprosy caused by sulfone-sensitive strains. Clofazimine is especially potent against sulfone-resistant strains of M. leprae. Ethionamide may be used as a substitute for clofazimine in the treatment of multibacillary forms of leprosy.
- Patients should understand that the key to controlling leprosy is to prevent the spread of the disease. This may require a life-long commitment by the patient to comply with therapy.
- To achieve treatment objectives, the patient should be given the correct dose and combination of drugs for an appropriate period of time and, if necessary, should be supervised to ensure compliance.
- Symptoms that indicate resolution of the infection should be monitored.

Bibliography

American Thoracic Society, Centers for Disease Control and Prevention, and Infectious Diseases Society of America. (2005). Treatment of tuberculosis. *American Journal of Respiratory Critical Care Medicine, 172*(9), 1169–1227.

American Thoracic Society. (2000). Diagnostic standards and classifications of tuberculosis in adults and children. *American Journal of Respiratory Critical Care Medicine, 161*(4), 1376–1395.

IMMUNE

Baker, B., Evans, M., DeCastro, F., et al. (2003). Leprosy in a Mexican immigrant. *Journal of the Kentucky Medical Association, 101*(7), 289–294.

Bayer, R., and Wilkinson, D. (1995). Directly observed therapy for tuberculosis: History of an idea. *Lancet, 345*(4), 1545–1548.

Burman, W., Goldberg, S., Johnson, J., et al. and the Tuberculosis Trials Consortium. (2006). Moxifloxacin versus ethambutol in the first 2 months of treatment for pulmonary tuberculosis. *American Journal of Respiratory and Critical Care Medicine* 2006, *174*(3), 331–338.

Centers for Disease Control and Prevention. (2005). Controlling tuberculosis in the United States: Recommendations from the American Thoracic Society, CDC, and the Infectious Diseases Society of America. *MMWR Morbidity and Mortality Weekly Report, 54*(No. RR-12), 1–81.

Centers for Disease Control and Prevention. (2003). Trends in tuberculosis morbidity–United States 1992–2002. *MMWR Morbidity and Mortality Weekly Report,* 52 (No. RR-11), 217–220, 222. Available online: www.cdc.gov/mmwr/preview/mmwrhtml/mm5211a2.htm. Accessed April 28, 2007.

Foundation for Better Health Care. *Tuberculosis.* Available online: www.fbhc.org/Patients/Modules/tb.cfm. Accessed April 29, 2007.

Holtz, T., Sternberg, M., Kammerer, S., et al. (2006). Time to sputum culture conversion in multidrug-resistant tuberculosis: Predictors and relationship to treatment outcome. *Annals of Internal Medicine, 144*(9), 650–660.

Ishii, N. (2003). Recent advances in the treatment of leprosy. *Dermatology Online Journal, 9*(2), 5.

Jensen, P., Lambert, L., Iademarco, M., et al. (2005). Guidelines for preventing the transmission of *Mycobacterium tuberculosis* in health-care settings. *MMWR Morbidity and Mortality Weekly Report, 54* (No. RR-17), 1–141.

Lee, L., Lobato, M., Buskin, S., et al. (2006). Low adherence to guidelines for preventing TB among persons with newly diagnosed HIV infection, United States. *International Journal of Tuberculosis and Lung Disease, 10*(2), 209–214.

Manangan, L., Moore, M., and Macaraig, M., (2006). Health department costs of managing persons with suspected and noncounted tuberculosis in New York City, three Texas counties, and Massachusetts. *Journal of Public Health Management and Practice, 12*(3), 248–253.

Miller, T., Hilsenrath, P., Lykens, K., et al. (2006). Using cost and health impacts to prioritize the targeted testing of tuberculosis in the United States. *Annals of Epidemiology, 16*(4), 305–312.

Reichman, L., Lardizabal, A., and Hayden, C. (2004). Considering the role of 4 months of rifampin in the treatment of latent tuberculosis infection. *American Journal of Respiratory Critical Care Medicine, 170*(8), 832–835.

Sterling, T., Bethel, J., Goldberg, S., et al. and the Tuberculosis Epidemiologic Studies Consortium. (2006). The scope and impact of treatment of latent tuberculosis infection in the United States and Canada. *American Journal of Respiratory and Critical Care Medicine, 173*(8), 927–931.

World Health Organization. (2001). *Leprosy status report.* Geneva, Switzerland: Author.

World Health Organization. (2000). *Guide to eliminate leprosy as a public health problem.* Geneva, Switzerland: Author.

Yawalkar, S. (2002). *Leprosy for medical practitioners and paramedical workers.* (7th ed.). Basle, Switzerland: Novartis Foundation for Sustainable Development.

Uniformed Services University. (2006). Leprosy. USU Tropical Medicine. Available online: http://tmcr.usuhs.mil/. Accessed April 29, 2007.

Anthelmintic, Antimalarial, and Antiprotozoal Drugs

30

Symbiosis is defined as any two organisms living in close association, one commonly living in or on the body of another. There are four main means for organisms of different species to come together in a symbiotic relationship: (1) phoresis, organisms traveling together; (2) mutualism, an association where both organisms benefit from the relationship with each other; (3) commensalism, an association where one organism benefits, but the host is neither helped nor harmed; and (4) parasitism, an obligatory association between two different species of organisms in which the dependence of the parasite upon the host is metabolic. Parasitic associations can provide for requirements for protection, nutrition, and both geographical and temporal dispersion of the organism. However, these relationships can give rise to extreme pathology in the host, with the possibility of injury or death.

Parasitism is carried out by many organisms; the main categories include groups of helminths, protozoa, and arthropods, as well as some higher organisms (Box 30-1). Generally, however, and partly for historical reasons, the term *parasitology* refers only to the study of infestation with invertebrate metazoan parasites (metazoa are the division of the animal kingdom that includes multicellular animals, i.e., all animals except the protozoa) and eukaryotic protozoans; not bacteria or viruses. Most of these organisms cause infestations by being ingested in the form of eggs or larvae, which most often are present on contaminated food or clothing; others gain entry through skin abrasions.

Parasitic diseases account for major health problems throughout the world, particularly in developing countries where they are endemic. Health care providers are becoming more familiar with the diseases as a group because of increased travel to and immigration from these regions. Although major infestations are more commonly associated with tropical climates, outbreaks are becoming universal in distribution. Parasitic infestations discussed in this chapter include helminthiases; protozoal infestations such as malaria, amebiasis, giardiasis, and leishmaniasis; and ectoparasitic infestations such as scabies. Emphasis is placed on diseases seen more frequently in the United States.

HELMINTHIASIS

EPIDEMIOLOGY AND ETIOLOGY

Helminths are simple, invertebrate animals, some of which are infectious parasites. They are multicellular and have differentiated tissues. *Helminthiasis* is a disease in which the body is infested with worms (e.g., roundworm, tapeworm, flukes). Because they are animals, their physiology is similar in some ways to that of humans. This makes infestations difficult to treat because drugs that kill helminths are frequently very toxic to human cells. Typically, the worms reside in the gastrointestinal (GI) tract but may also burrow into the liver and other organs. The presence of worms, most often in the GI tract, the bladder, the lungs, and the liver of a human, is called an "infestation" rather than an "infection."

The incidence of helminthic infestations is rapidly growing in the United States. This phenomenon is in part related to the greater incidence of travel and immigration. Parasitic helminths are divided into three groups: *nematodes* (roundworms), *cestodes* (flatworms or tapeworms), and *trematodes* (flukes) (Table 30-1). Relatively unchanged from the beginnings of organic life forms, these creatures live dependently by sharing body juices of plants, animals, and humans.

Nematode Infestations

Nematode, or roundworm, infestations are the most common helminthic diseases in the world, with over 500,000 different species described; over 15,000 are parasitic. Nematode infestations are more common in tropical and temperate zones, where their prevalence often exceeds 50%, but they are also found in locations as diverse as Antarctica and oceanic trenches; distribution in the United States is limited to the southeastern states. Roundworm infestations produce a number of clinical disorders, ranging from an occult infestation to a fulminating, fatal disease, depending on the number of larvae ingested. The common nematode infestations include

---

BOX 30-1

Definitions in Parasitology

Types of Parasites

Ectoparasites	Lives outside of host
Endoparasites	Lives inside of host as obligate parasites but many have free-living stages
Facultative parasites	Not normally parasitic, but won't pass up the opportunity
Accidental parasites	Attaches or enters the wrong host; may or may not survive, but can be very pathogenic
Permanent parasites	Live adult lives in, or on, the host

Types of Hosts

Definitive host	Where the parasite reaches sexual maturity (e.g., humans, domestic animals, wild animals)
Intermediate host	Required for development; but not sexual maturity (i.e., freshwater snails)
Transport host	Parasite does not develop but remains infective to another host
Reservoir host	Any organism that can harbor an infection that can be transmitted to humans

---

TABLE 30-1 Helminth Infestations

Helminth Disease/Disorder	Location	Source of Infestation	DOC, TOC, and ALT*
NEMATODES (ROUNDWORMS)			
Necator americanus (Hookworm) **Ancylostomiasis**	Africa, Far East, Southeast Asia, South Pacific	Contaminated soil; human fecal contact through skin	**DOC:** albendazole or mebendazole **ALT:** pyrantel
Ascaris lumbricoides (Intestinal roundworm) **Ascariasis**	Warm, moist climates; temperate climates	Agricultural products; human fecal-oral contact	**DOC:** albendazole or mebendazole **ALT:** pyrantel
Enterobius vermicularis (Pinworm) **Enterobiasis**	Temperate zones; United States	Human fecal-oral contact	**DOC:** albendazole or mebendazole **ALT:** pyrantel
Strongyloides stercoralis (Threadworm) **Strongyloidiasis**	Most tropics, southern United States	Human fecal-oral contact; soil	**DOC:** ivermectin **ALT:** thiabendazole
Trichinella spiralis (Pork roundworm) **Trichinosis**	Northern hemisphere	Raw or uncooked meat	**DOC:** Steroids plus albendazole†
Trichuris trichiura (Whipworm) **Trichuris**	Warm, moist climate; rare in United States	Human fecal-oral contact	**DOC:** albendazole **ALT:** mebendazole
CESTODES (TAPEWORMS)			
Echinococcus multilocularis (Lung tapeworm) **Alveolar hydatid disease**	Primarily northern hemisphere; central Europe	Dog feces; mice, rats, hamsters, gerbils, and squirrels	**TOC:** Surgical excision **DOC:** albendazole and mebendazole
Echinococcus granulosus (Tissue tapeworm) **Cystic hydatid disease**	Sheep pastures, worldwide	Feces: dogs, wolves, deer, foxes, coyotes, hyenas, cats, jackals, lynxes, black bears, reindeer, sheep, cattle, goats, horses, camels	**TOC:** Percutaneous aspiration and albendazole **ALT:** praziquantel
Cysticercus cellulosae (Tissue tapeworm) **Cysticercosis**	Mexico, Central and South America, India, Spain, Portugal, eastern Europe	Food or water contaminated with *T. solium* eggs; fecal-oral contact	**TOC:** Surgery **DOC:** praziquantel; albendazole and mebendazole
Diphyllobothrium latum (Segmented fish flatworm) **Diphyllobothriasis**	Eastern Europe, Africa, North and South America, Canada	Raw or pickled fish	**DOC:** praziquantel and B$_{12}$ injections
Hymenolepis nana **Dwarf tapeworm infestation**	Warm climates; southern United States	Human feces	**DOC:** praziquantel
Taeniasis saginata **Beef tapeworm infestation**	Middle East, Africa, South America, Mexico, Russia	Human feces	**DOC:** praziquantel **ALT:** albendazole
Taenia solium **Pork tapeworm infestation**	Central America, South America, India, Mexico	Human feces; pigs, dogs, cats, sheep	**DOC:** praziquantel **ALT** albendazole
TREMATODES (FLUKES)			
Fasciolopsis buski; Heterophyes heterophyes; Metagonimus yokogawai **Intestinal fluke infestation**	Far East, Spain, eastern Europe	Ingestion of freshwater aquatic plants infected with metacercariae	**DOC:** praziquantel
Fasciola hepatica **Liver fluke infestation**	Worldwide	Ingestion of aquatic plants, watercress infected with metacercariae	**DOC:** triclabendazole **ALT:** bithionol
Clonorchis sinensis **Liver fluke infestation**	Far East, Southwest Asia	Raw, partially cooked freshwater fish; dried, salted, or pickled fish	**DOC:** praziquantel or albendazole
Paragonimus westermani **Lung fluke infestation**	Africa, Far East, South America; rare in United States	Ingestion of snails, freshwater crabs or crayfish	**DOC:** praziquantel or bithionol‡
Schistosoma japonicum **Blood fluke infestation**	Africa, Far East, South America	Skin penetrated by cercariae	**DOC:** praziquantel
Schistosoma mansoni **Blood fluke infestation**	Africa, Latin America	Skin penetrated by cercariae	**DOC:** praziquantel **ALT:** oxamniquine§
Schistosoma haematobium **Blood fluke infestation**	Africa, Near East	Water contaminated by cercariae	**DOC:** praziquantel

*Treatment information from Gilbert, D., Moellering, R., and Eliopoulos, G. (2007). *The Sanford Guide to Antimicrobial Therapy*. (37th Ed). Hyde Park, VT: Antimicrobial Therapy.
†Corticosteroid use with trichinosis may prolong the intestinal phase of trichinosis infestation.
‡There are availability problems with bithionol (Lorothidol, Bitin).
§Oxamniquine is difficult to obtain in the United States.
ALT, Alternative; *DOC,* drug of choice; *TOC,* treatment of choice,

enterobiasis ("pinworm"), *ascariasis, hookworm, strongyloidiasis, trichinosis,* and *trichuriasis* (Fig. 30-1).

Nematodes are ever-present in freshwater, marine, and terrestrial environments. Some species of roundworm may contain more than 27 million eggs at one time and lay more than 200,000 of them in a single day. The prevalence and intensity of infestations are usually highest in children between the ages of 3 and 8 years. Most roundworm eggs or larvae are found in the soil and can be picked up on the hands and transferred to the mouth or can enter through the skin.

Nematodes range in size from 1 mm to several inches. They have no circulatory or respiratory systems so they use diffusion to breathe and to circulate substances around their body. They are thin and round in cross-section, though they are actually bilaterally symmetric. Live worms, passed in feces and occasionally vomited or coughed up, are often the first-recognized sign of infestation.

Signs and symptoms vary somewhat for each infestation but in general include malaise, anorexia, nausea, vomiting, abdominal pain, and muscle or joint aches. Serious infestations result in symptoms arising from inflammatory responses on vital organs and nutritional deficiencies. Some patients have pulmonary manifestations (i.e., sneezing, coughing, fever, eosinophilia, pulmonary infiltration). Bowel obstructions, particularly in children, or obstruction of the bile duct, the pancreatic duct, and the appendix by one or more adult worms may occur. In time, the larvae become walled-off in the tissues, remaining in the body for 10 years or longer. Strongyloidiasis may be fatal in newborns and those who are immunocompromised.

Cestode Infestations

Cestodes, more commonly called tapeworms or flatworms, are the largest of all of the parasites. These very mobile worms are made up of 3,000 to 4,000 segments with each body segment containing up to 50,000 eggs. They can release up to 1,000,000 eggs into a person's body each day. Some tapeworms live up to 25 years within the GI tract of the host, growing in length to as much as 33 feet (10 meters).

Cestodes parasitize the intestinal tract of vertebrates to absorb nutrients through their tegument. Microtriches, or minute projections covering the tegument, lie in proximity to the host's intestinal villi and greatly increase the surface area of the cestode, thus maximizing nutrient absorption. The adult consists of a head where the worms attach to the intestinal mucosa; a neck; and a segmented body that contains both male and female gonads. Segments expand in the creation of eggs, which are then passed into the stool of the host.

Since each segment of the cestode contains both male and female reproductive organs, cestodes are capable of self-fertilization. However, the eggs of the *Diphyllobothrium* must first enter an aquatic environment to finish their development

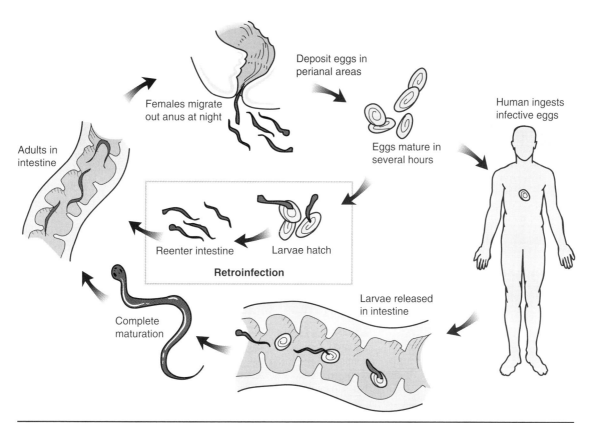

FIGURE 30-1 Life Cycle of *Enterobius vermicularis.* Pinworm infestation is caused by direct transfer of infective eggs by hand from the anus to the mouth of the same or another person. Larvae from ingested eggs hatch in the small intestine. Young worms mature in the cecum and upper portions of the colon. (From Mahon, C., and Manuselis, G., Jr. [1995]. *Textbook of diagnostic microbiology* [p. 781]. Philadelphia: WB Saunders. Used with permission.)

and become infective. Cestodes are not invasive, and mortality is rare. Infested persons are usually asymptomatic, although when present, the symptoms are most often related to vitamin deficiencies and anemia.

Trematode Infestations

Trematodes are the flukes (not to be confused with *coincidence* or *stroke of luck*) of the worm world and cause various clinical infestations. Fluke-worm infestation in the United States is extremely rare. The parasites are so named because of their conspicuous suckers, the organs of attachment (*trematos* means "pierced with holes"). They are unsegmented worms, leaf-shaped and flattened dorsoventrally. Flukes have one sucker that surrounds the mouth and another on the ventral body surface. The suckers attach the worm to the host's body. Depending on the location in the body, these worms are classified as blood flukes (e.g., *Schistosoma* species); liver flukes (*Clonorchis sinensis*); lung flukes (*Paragonimus westermani*); or intestinal flukes (*Fasciolopsis buski*). There are more than 50 different species of intestinal trematodes.

Trematodes penetrate the skin and then migrate to the hepatic portal circulation or into the duodenum. From these locations, they migrate to the bladder or the intestines, or to the bile ducts or the pancreas, respectively. Trematodes are found in the larval stage of development, but these worms also develop within sporocysts that parasitize snails or bivalve mollusks, using them as an intermediary. They emerge from the mollusk either to enter their final host directly or to encyst in an intermediate host that is eaten by the final host. For example, the larvae of *C. sinensis* are eaten by fish, which in turn are eaten by humans, in whom they invade the intestinal tract. They can live in the human liver for 20 to 50 years, continually passing eggs into the feces. These organisms even live through the pickling process used to preserve many varieties of fish.

Symptoms of trematode infestation are diverse, ranging from asymptomatic to "swimmer's itch," a benign form of schistosomiasis, to those with findings only at autopsy. Penetrating larvae cause fever, urticaria, eosinophilia, hepatosplenomegaly, and lymphadenopathy. When the adult worms reach their chosen location in the body, symptoms such as cystitis and chronic diarrhea arise. It is not uncommon to diagnose ascites of unknown etiology in a patient in whom an infestation has been overlooked.

PATHOPHYSIOLOGY

Both larval and adult helminths can cause disease. An important distinction between infestation with parasitic helminths and infection with bacterial, viral, or protozoan parasites is that the parasites generally are unable to complete their life cycle within the human host. Larval helminths or some nematodes such as *Strongyloides* species may present exceptions to this rule; that is, each larval helminth infecting the host will give rise to a single adult parasite. Therefore, infestation begins when a larval helminth enters the host from without and continues with each larva's development into a single adult parasite. In turn, since pathology produced by helminth infestation is generally dependent on the quantity of worms a host carries (i.e., only high worm burdens will cause severe

pathology), the degree of pathology is determined by the rate at which larval parasites enter the host. The significance of this characteristic of the helminth diseases lies in its potential for control or possible elimination of incidence and prevalence of the diseases.

Helminthic infestations usually do not generally cause clinical signs and symptoms, although they may be detrimental for a number of reasons. Heavy infestations produce nutritional deficits, particularly in children. Host tissues can be traumatized, thus predisposing the patient to bacterial infection, or toxic substances produced by the helminth may be absorbed by the host. In large numbers, helminths cause intestinal obstruction and blood loss, as well as obstruction of lymphatic channels with massive edema.

PHARMACOTHERAPEUTIC OPTIONS

The major drugs used in the treatment of helminth infestations are discussed in the following sections. These drugs differ from one another in spectrum; some are relatively active against several types of worms, whereas others are more selective. For this reason, the drugs are discussed separately rather than in the format usual for this text. Table 30-1 provides an overview of the infestations and the treatment options.

Some anthelmintics act directly to "starve the worm to death" or to paralyze it through destruction of its central nervous system. Others interfere with production of adenosine triphosphate (ATP) in the helminth or act on specific enzymes in the worm itself, not touching the host's structures. Other substrates affected by anthelmintic drugs are glycogen, glucose, and phosphorylase phosphatase.

Albendazole

Albendazole (Albenza) is an orally administered, broad-spectrum anthelmintic. It is used in the treatment of neurocysticercosis, a pork tapeworm infestation of *Taenia solium* that affects the cerebral parenchyma, the meninges, the spinal cord, and the eyes. Large numbers of cysts will trigger a response from the body's immune system, but smaller quantities can exist undetected in the host for many years. Live cysts may survive for as many as 5 years without detection until cyst death or symptom precipitation. The lesions caused by the infestation and considered responsive to albendazole are seen as nonenhancing cysts with no surrounding edema on contrast-enhanced computerized tomography (CT). With treatment, patients with lesions of this type demonstrate a 74% to 88% reduction in number of cysts; 40% to 70% of albendazole-treated patients showed resolution of all active cysts.

Albendazole is also approved for the treatment of cystic hydatid disease of the liver, lung, and peritoneum, produced by the larval form of the dog tapeworm, *Echinococcus granulosus*. After taking albendazole for three 28-day cycles of treatment, 80% to 90% of patients exhibit noninfectious cysts. Albendazole is also used off-label for the treatment of pinworms, roundworms, hookworms, tapeworms, and flukes.

Albendazole acts primarily by inhibiting tubulin polymerization, which results in the loss of cytoplasmic microtubules, which in turn causes blockage of the ventricular aqueducts. Albendazole also appears effective against the larval forms of *E. granulosus* and *T. solium*. To avoid the infestation-related inflammatory response in the central nervous system (CNS), the patient must also receive an antiepileptic drug and high-dose glucocorticoids.

Albendazole is slowly absorbed from the GI tract because of its solubility in water. Oral bioavailability is enhanced 4 to 5 times when taken with a fatty meal (Table 30-2). The drug is rapidly converted to its active metabolite before reaching systemic circulation. It has been suggested that the albendazole metabolite may induce its own biotransformation. Biliary elimination accounts for about 99% of the drug; 1% is eliminated in the urine.

The adverse effects of albendazole include headache, nausea, dizziness, vomiting, and abnormalities in liver functions. Increased intracranial pressure resulting from cyst death is also a possibility. Observe children for the first 24 to 48 hours for evidence of increased intracranial pressure. Rare adverse effects include alopecia, rash, fever, and pancytopenia, so obtain initial and biweekly complete blood counts (CBCs) and monitor liver function test (LFT) values throughout therapy. Albendazole may be continued if reductions in total white blood cell (WBC) counts and absolute neutrophil counts (ANC) appear modest and do not progress.

Albendazole should not be used in patients with documented hypersensitivity to the benzimidazole compounds or any components of albendazole. It is wise to avoid albendazole if possible during pregnancy (category C) and wait 1 month after use before getting pregnant. It is unknown if the drug is excreted in breast milk.

Information on drug interactions and dosages for albendazole can be found in Tables 30-3 and 30-4, respectively.

Ivermectin

Ivermectin (Strometol, ◆ Mectizan) is used for the treatment of intestinal strongyloidiasis caused by the nematode parasite *S. stercoralis*. Ivermectin is also used in the treatment of onchocerciasis, a multisystem disease also known as "river blindness" that is caused by the *Onchocerca volvulus* nematode. Transmission of onchocerciasis is through the bite of the black fly (genus *Simulium*), an intermediate host.

Ivermectin acts by binding to glutamate-chloride channels to increase cell wall permeability to chloride ions. The result is hyperpolarization of nerve and muscle cells, paralysis, and death of the nematode. Ivermectin is effective against the tissue microfilariae of *O. volvulus* but not against the adult form of the nematode. The adult form of *O. volvulus* is found in nonpalpable subcutaneous nodules, which are removed by surgical excision. Remind the patient that ivermectin does not kill the adult *Onchocerca* nematode, and therefore repeated follow-up and retreatment is usually required. Perform stool examinations to verify eradication of infestation.

Ivermectin is well absorbed when taken orally on an empty stomach. Distribution to the CNS is poor, although plasma concentrations of the drug are proportional to the dosage given. Ivermectin is biotransformed in the liver, with the parent drug and its metabolites eliminated almost entirely in the feces. Less than 1% is eliminated in the urine.

A Mazotti reaction may occur in patients treated with ivermectin for onchocerciasis and is characterized by fever, tender lymphadenopathy, alterations in vision, bone damage, a pruritic rash, and bone and joint pain. Interestingly, the reaction does not develop in patients with strongyloidiasis who are treated with ivermectin. A Mazotti reaction is an allergic and inflammatory response to the death of microfilariae. Patients with hypersensitivity onchodermatitis are more likely

PHARMACOKINETICS
TABLE **30-2** Selected Anthelmintic Antimalarial Drugs

Drug	Route	Onset	Peak	Duration	PB (%)	t½	BioA (%)
ANTHELMINTIC DRUGS							
albendazole	PO	Slow	2–5 hr	UA	70	8–4–12 hr	<5
ivermectin	PO	Slow	4 hr	UA	UA	18 hr	UA
mebendazole	PO	UA	1.5–7.5 hr	UA	95	2.5–5.5 hr	2–3
praziquantel	PO	Varies	1–2 hr	UA	80	0.8–1.5 hr; 4–5 hr*	<80
pyrantel	PO	UA	1–3 hr	UA	UA	2.5–9 hr	2–10
thiabendazole	PO	Rapid	1–2 hr	UA	UA	UA	UA
ANTIMALARIAL DRUGS							
amodiaquine	PO	Rapid	0.5–1 hr	UA	UA	3.5–6.9 hr	UA
atovaquone-proguanil	PO	UA	UA	UA	99; 75†	2–3 days; 12–21 hr‡	23
chloroquine	PO	3–3.5 hr	1–2 hr	UA	55	Dose-related; 30-60 days	89
mefloquine	PO	1–2 hr	1–2 hr	UA	98	2–3 wk	85
primaquine	PO	Rapid	3 hr	<24 hr	100	5 hr	96
quinine	PO	1–3 hr	1–3 hr	UA	90	4–5 hr	80
sulfadoxine-pyrimethamine	PO	Rapid	2.5–6 hr	UA	UA	111 hr	UA
ANTIPROTOZOAL DRUG							
paromomycin	PO	UA	UA	UA	UA	UA	UA

*Half-life is 4–5 hours for the praziquantel metabolites.
†The protein binding of atovaquone and proguanil, respectively.
‡The half-lives of atovaquone-proguanil, respectively but may be longer in slow acetylators.
BioA, Bioavailability; *PB*, protein binding; *PO*, by mouth; *t½*, half-life; *UA*, unavailable.

DRUG INTERACTIONS
TABLE 30-3 Selected Anthelmintic and Antimalarial, Drugs

Drug	Interactive Drugs	Interaction
ANTHELMINTIC DRUGS		
albendazole	dexamethasone	Increases albendazole levels by 58%
	praziquantel	Increases albendazole levels by 50%
	cimetidine, carbamazepine	Increases albendazole serum levels; may increase albendazole metabolism
ivermectin	diazepam	Enhances actions of diazepam
mebendazole	Insulins, oral hypoglycemics	Increases potential for hypoglycemia
	carbamazepine, phenytoin	Decreases plasma concentration of mebendazole
	cimetidine	Increases serum concentration of mebendazole
thiabendazole	theophylline, mirtazapine, fluvoxamine	Increases serum levels of interactive drugs
ANTIMALARIAL DRUGS		
atovaquone-proguanil	tetracycline, rifampin, rifabutin	Significant reduction in level of atovaquone
	metoclopramide	Decreases bioavailability of atovaquone
chloroquine	Highly protein-bound drugs	Decreases effects of other highly protein-bound drugs
	cimetidine	Increases effects of chloroquine
	magnesium trisilicate	Decreases absorption of both drugs
mefloquine	chloroquine	Increases risk for seizures
	quinine, quinidine	Increases risk for cardiac toxicity and seizures
primaquine	Hemolytic drugs, immunosuppressants	Increases risk of bone marrow depression
quinine	mefloquine	Increases incidence of seizures and electrocardiogram (ECG) abnormalities
	amiodarone, digoxin, verapamil	Increases levels of interacting drug
	Neuromuscular blockers, succinylcholine	Excessive muscle weakness and respiratory difficulties with concurrent use
	Oral anticoagulants	Increases anticoagulant effects
	Antacids, sodium bicarbonate	Increases cardiac depressant effects
	phenobarbital, hydantoins, rifampin	Decreases quinine levels
ANTIPROTOZOAL DRUGS		
paromomycin	digoxin	Reduces rate and extent of digoxin absorption
	succinylcholine	Potentiation of neuromuscular blockade

than others to have severe adverse effects, particularly edema and worsening of the dermatitis. Symptomatic treatment controls the related itching and does not affect treatment outcomes. Ivermectin is a category C drug and should not be taken during pregnancy. Advise the breastfeeding patient to avoid such on the day of treatment and for the following 3 days.

Information on drug interactions and dosages for ivermectin can be found in Tables 30-3 and 30-4, respectively.

Mebendazole

Mebendazole (Vermox; ◆ Nemasole) and is indicated for the treatment of *Enterobius vermicularis, Trichuris trichiura, Ascaris lumbricoides, Ancyclostoma duodenale,* and *Necator americanus infestations* and trichinosis. Because it is a broad-spectrum anthelmintic, it is particularly useful in mixed infestations. There is no evidence that mebendazole, even at high dosages, is effective for echinococcosis, also known as hydatid disease, a potentially fatal parasitic disease of the liver, lung, and peritoneum. Anyone can get echinococcosis by ingesting the eggs of the *E. granulosus* or the *Echinococcus multilocularis* tapeworm.

Echinococcal infestations among humans occur worldwide, although they are rare. E. granulosus is found in the sheep-raising regions of Arizona, California, New Mexico, and Utah. E. multilocularis has been found in the north central region from eastern Montana to central Ohio, as well as Alaska and Canada.

Mebendazole inhibits the formation of microtubules and irreversibly inhibits the uptake of glucose. Because glucose uptake into the nematode is prevented, glucose distribution

throughout the nematode is affected. Eventually the nematode's energy stores become depleted; it becomes immobilized, and dies over a period of about 3 days. Dead nematodes are eliminated in the feces within days. Efficacy varies as a function of transit time through the GI tract, the presence of preexisting diarrhea, the extent of infestation, and the helminth strain. Mean cure rates range from 95% for *E. vermicularis* to 96% for *N. americanus* and 98% for ascariasis.

When taken by mouth, 2% to 3% of mebendazole is absorbed and rapidly biotransformed (see Table 30-2). Two percent of the unabsorbed fraction of the drug is eliminated in the urine, with the remainder eliminated unchanged in the feces.

Adverse effects of mebendazole are rare, likely because the drug is so poorly absorbed. However, abdominal pain and diarrhea may occur in patients who have massive infestation. In addition, teratogenicity and fetal toxicity has been demonstrated in rodents. Mebendazole is pregnancy category C; it is unknown if the drug is excreted in breast milk.

Information on drug interactions and dosages for mebendazole can be found in Tables 30-3 and 30-4, respectively.

Praziquantel

Praziquantel (Biltricide) is the drug of choice for the treatment of schistosome infestations (including those caused by *Schistosoma mekongi, Schistosoma japonicum, Schistosoma mansoni,* and *Schistosoma haematobium*), and infestations due to liver fluke (e.g., *Fasciola hepatica*).

Praziquantel causes a rapid contraction of the schistosome, which in turn causes spastic paralysis and detachment of the worm from body tissues. The drug further causes

DOSAGE

TABLE 30-4 Selected Anthelmintic, Antimalarial, and Antiparasitic Drugs

Drug	Use(s)	Dosage	Implications
ANTHELMINTIC DRUGS			
albendazole	Neurocysticercosis; hydatid disease	*Adult >60 kg:* 400 mg PO twice daily with meals *Adult <60 kg:* 15 mg/kg in divided doses twice daily with meals. Max: 800 mg/day	A 28-day cycle is followed by a 14-day albendazole-free interval, for total of three cycles. Corticosteroids are coadministered to prevent IIOP episodes during first week of anticysticercosal therapy.
ivermectin	Strongyloidiasis Onchocerciasis	*Adult:* 200 mg/kg PO as a single dose *Adult:* 150 mg/kg PO as a single dose	In mass drug-distribution campaigns, the dosing interval is 12 months. For individuals, consider retreatment at 3-month intervals.
mebendazole	Ascariasis; ancylostomiasis; *Trichuris trichiura* enterobiasis	*Adult or Child:* 100 mg PO twice daily for 3 days *Adult or Child:* 100 mg as single dose	Repeat regimen in 2 wk if treatment unsuccessful. Safe use in children <2 yr has not been established.
pyrantel	Ascariasis; ancylostomiasis; *T. trichiura*; enterobiasis	*Adult or Child >12 yr:* 5 mg/kg PO as a single dose —or— 11 mg/kg; not to exceed 1 gram	May be mixed with juice or milk.
praziquantel	Schistosomiasis, hermaphroditic infestations Fish, beef, and pork tapeworm infestations Dwarf tapeworm *Cysticercus cellulosae*	*Adult:* 40 to 75 mg/kg 3 times daily for 1 day *Child:* 40–60 mg/kg 3 times daily for 1 day *Adult or Child:* 5–10 mg/kg as single dose *Adult:* 5–10 mg/kg as single dose *Child:* 25 mg/kg as single dose *Adult or Child:* 50 mg/kg/day divided in three doses for 15 days	**Although approved by FDA, drug is considered experimental for these purposes.** ⚠
thiabendazole	Enterobiasis	*Adult or Child <150 lb:* 50 mg/kg twice daily for 2 days —or— 2 doses/day for 2 successive days. Max: 3 grams/day	Repeat in 7 days to reduce risk of reinfestation.
ANTIMALARIAL DRUGS			
chloroquine	*Plasmodium vivax, Plasmodium ovale, Plasmodium malariae,* chloroquine-susceptible *Plasmodium falciparum*	*Adult Prophylaxis:* 500 mg PO the same day each week for up to 8 wk after leaving endemic area *Adult Treatment:* 1 gram PO followed by 500 mg after 6–8 hr and a single dose of 500 mg on each of 2 consecutive days *Child Prophylaxis:* 8.3 mg/kg salt (5 mg/kg base) orally, once/week, up to max adult dose of 300 mg base *Child Treatment:* 10 mg base/kg. Max: 600 mg base, then 5 mg base/kg 6 hr later, then 5 mg base/kg at 24 and 48 hr. Dosage should not exceed adult dose, regardless of weight.	Each 500-mg tablet = 300 mg base. Begin 1–2 weeks before travel to malarious areas. Take weekly on the same day of the week while in the malarious area and for 4 weeks after leaving such areas. May worsen existing psoriasis.
mefloquine	Multi–drug-resistant *P. falciparum*	*Adult Prophylaxis:* 228 mg base (250 mg salt) orally, once/week *Adult Treatment:* 1250 mg PO as a single dose. *Child Prophylaxis:* <9 kg: 4.6 mg/kg base (5 mg/kg salt) orally, once/week 10–19 kg: 1/4 tablet once/week 20–30 kg: 1/2 tablet once/week 31–45 kg: 3/4 tablet once/week ≥46 kg: 1 tablet once/week *Child Treatment:* 25 mg/kg base PO divided in 2 doses and taken 6–8 hr apart	**Contact CDC for current prophylaxis regimen.** ⚠ Drug has many contraindications. Begin 1 wk before departure; take on same day each wk; continue for an additional 4 wk after leaving area.
primaquine	*P. vivax, P. ovale, P. malariae, P. falciparum*	*Adult:* 26.3 mg (15 mg base) PO daily for 14 days. Start during last 2 wk of, or following a course of suppression with, chloroquine or a comparable drug. *Child:* 0.5 mg/kg/day PO (0.3 mg/kg base) PO daily for 14 days. Max: 15 mg/kg base/dose	**Effective against all stages of all species, but growing resistance is a problem. An option for prophylaxis in special circumstances.** ⚠ Call CDC Malaria Hotline (770–488–7788) for additional information. Combination therapy with chloroquine phosphate to eliminate erythrocytic forms of the parasite.
quinine sulfate	*P. vivax, P. ovale, P. malariae,* Chloroquine-resistant *P. falciparum*	*Adult:* *Chloroquine-Resistant Malaria:* 650 mg PO every 8 hr for 3–7 days. *Chloroquine-sensitive malaria:* 600 mg PO every 8 hr for 5–7 days *Child:* *Chloroquine-Resistant Malaria:* 30 mg/kg PO every 8 hr for 3–7 days. *Chloroquine-sensitive malaria:* 10 mg/kg PO every 8 hr for 5–7 days	Duration of therapy may be shortened if drug is taken concurrently with other antimalarial drugs.
sulfadoxine-pyrimethamine	Chloroquine-resistant *P. falciparum*	*Adult:* 3 tablets PO as single dose (500 mg sulfadoxine + 25 mg pyrimethamine/tab)	Presumptive treatment of travelers in remote areas who suspect infestation or infestation but will not have ready access to medical attention

Continued

IMMUNE

DOSAGE
TABLE 30-4 Selected Anthelmintic, Antimalarial, and Antiparasitic Drugs—Cont'd

Drug	Use(s)	Dosage	Implications
atovaquone-proguanil	P. falciparum	Adult Prophylaxis: 1 adult tablet/daily Adult Treatment: 2 tabs PO twice daily –or– 4 adult tabs once daily for 3 days Child Prophylaxis: 5–8 kg: ½ pediatric tablet daily 8–10 kg: ¾ pediatric tablet daily 10–20 kg: 1 pediatric tablet daily 20–30 kg: 2 pediatric tablets daily 30–40 kg: 3 pediatric tablets daily	Adult (250 mg + 100 mg) and pediatric (62.5 mg + 25) mg tablets available. Start prophylaxis 1–2 days before travel; continue daily prophylaxis during travel and for 7 days after leaving the area.
amodiaquine	Nonimmune adults with acute malarial attack	Adult: 600 mg base, followed by 200 mg after 6 hr, then 400 mg daily for 2 days Child <15 yr: 7 mg base/kg weekly for up to 6 wk after last exposure	For partially immune subjects, a single dose of 600 mg of base is often sufficient.
ANTIPROTOZOAL DRUGS			
iodoquinol	Intestinal amebiasis	Adult: 650 mg PO 3 times daily for 20 days	Tissue-acting amebicide
paromomycin	Intestinal amebiasis	Adult: 25–35 mg/kg PO 3 times daily for 7 days	Luminal amebicide
diloxanide	Intestinal amebiasis	Adult: 500 mg PO 3 times daily for 10 days	Luminal amebicide; second-line agent
metronidazole	Severe intestinal amebiasis	Adult: 750 mg PO 3 times daily for 10 days	Tissue-acting drug; use in combination with another antiprotozoal drug.
stibogluconate sodium	Cutaneous leishmaniasis Visceral or mucocutaneous leishmaniasis	Adult: 20 mg/kg IV –or– IM daily for 20 days Adult: 20 mg/kg IV –or– IM daily for 30 days	Cure rates high if treatment regimen followed.

CDC, Centers for Disease Control and Prevention; FDA, U.S. Food and Drug Administration; IM, intramuscular (route); IIOP, increased intraocular pressure; IV, intravenous (route); PO, by mouth.

vacuolization and disintegration of the schistosome tegument, rendering it vulnerable to attack by host defenses.

Praziquantel is rapidly absorbed from the GI tract (see Table 30-2). It undergoes extensive biotransformation, with the metabolites eliminated in the urine.

Praziquantel is relatively free from adverse effects. Transient headache and abdominal discomfort are the most common reactions. Drowsiness is possible. High serum drug concentrations are associated with a greater incidence of adverse effects in patients with liver disease. The drug is contraindicated for use in patients with hypersensitivity, women who are pregnant or lactating, and patients with ocular cysticercosis. Hydantoins decrease praziquantel levels, resulting in treatment failure (see Table 30-3).

Pyrantel

Like mebendazole, pyrantel (Antiminth, Ascarel, Pin-X, Reese's Pinworm Medicine; ♣ Combantrin, Helmex), is used in the treatment of E. vermicularis, T. trichiura, A. lumbricoides, A. duodenale, trichinosis, and N. americanus in single or mixed infestations. It can also be used if mebendazole is ineffective.

By stimulating the release of acetylcholine, inhibiting cholinesterase, and stimulating ganglionic neurons, the drug acts as a depolarizing neuromuscular blocker in the lumen of the intestine. These actions cause depolarization of the helminth and spastic paralysis. After their hold on the intestinal wall is released, they are cleared in the feces.

Pyrantel is poorly and incompletely absorbed when taken by mouth. The majority of the dose taken is eliminated unchanged in the feces along with the parasites.

Serious adverse effects of pyrantel are rare. The most common are nausea, vomiting, cramps, abdominal pain, and diarrhea. CNS effects have been reported and include dizziness, drowsiness, headache, and insomnia.

Information on dosages for pyrantel can be found in Table 30-4.

Thiabendazole

Thiabendazole (Mintezol) is indicated for the treatment of strongyloidiasis, cutaneous larva migrans (creeping eruption), visceral larva migrans, and trichinosis, and for symptom relief, fever reduction, and eosinophilia reduction during the invasive stage of the disease. Thiabendazole is used only for N. americanus and A. duodenale, and for Trichuris and ascariasis when more specific therapy is not available or cannot be used, or when further therapy with a second drug is desirable. Its effect on larvae of T. spiralis that have migrated to muscle is questionable.

The mechanism of action for thiabendazole is not clear; however, it appears to suppress production of eggs or larvae and their subsequent development during passage through the GI tract. It does so by inhibiting a helminth-specific enzyme, fumarate reductase.

Thiabendazole is rapidly absorbed after oral administration (see Table 30-2). The drug is almost completely biotransformed in the liver. More than 90% of the conjugates (sulfate and glucuronide) are recovered from the urine in 24 hours.

The adverse effects noted with thiabendazole include tinnitus, conjunctival injection, blurry vision, hypotension, syncope, anaphylaxis, numbness, seizures, and transient leukopenia. A few cases of erythema multiforme and Stevens-Johnson syndrome have been reported.

Thiabendazole is a powerful inhibitor of the CYP 1A2 enzyme system. Information on drug interactions and dosages for thiabendazole can be found in Tables 30-3 and 30-4, respectively.

CLINICAL REASONING

The currently available anthelmintic drugs are very specific in the worms they can destroy. For this reason, accurately identify the infesting helminth before starting treatment. Lab identification of helminths can be made by examining freshly passed stool, obtained early mornings on 3 to 5 consecutive days. The frequency of stool collection is guided by the expectations of worm load. Light infestations may not demonstrate eggs or larvae in some stool samples. Heavy infestations may demonstrate adult worms in the first stool sample.

Requests for examination of fresh stool specimens for ova and parasites must include information about the suspicion of helminths, and special instructions must be given for handling the specimen, for a correct diagnosis to be made. For example, it is not unusual to confuse hookworm larvae with *Strongyloides* larvae if the specimen is not examined within a half hour after being taken. Advise patients to collect the specimen at the lab or to make sure the fresh specimen is delivered within this time frame. Notify the lab of the specimen's arrival so it isn't left sitting in a collection box. Blood, tissue fluid, or skin snips are better scanned when they are fresh. Complement fixation tests, immunofluorescent antibody testing, and enzyme-linked immunosorbent assays are not routinely available except in special parasitology laboratories.

Treatment Objectives

The primary treatment objective for helminthic infestations is to destroy the adult helminths, thus reducing the helminth load. The life cycle of many helminths is complex, offering a formidable challenge to disease eradication and even to drug treatment. Consultation with a representative from the public health department and/or the Centers for Disease Control and Prevention (CDC) is wise, although light helminthic infestations are self-limiting and usually do not require treatment.

Treatment Options

▥ Patient Variables

Since many of those most likely to be affected are not in the social mainstream, and their behaviors and attitudes already seem odd or even suspect others, an infestation only arouses further embarrassment and discomfort. The primary psychosocial implication of an infestation is embarrassment if the condition becomes public knowledge. Patients are often reluctant to discuss the problem, and thus many use home remedies for a time before seeking help from their health care provider. The public health departments and other public resources can be invaluable for support and education of an individual with an infestation. Before treatment, the parasites must be identified using tests that look for parasites, eggs, or larvae in feces, urine, blood, sputum, or tissues.

▥ Drug Variables

A key to eradication of infestation is to use anthelmintic drugs that interfere with the life cycle of adult parasites. Antibiotics are inappropriate for the treatment of infestations. Because helminths feed on the substrates of nutrition processes in the body, the drug chosen must be effective in blocking parasitic dependence on these processes. Further, when evaluating drug treatment options, consider the substrate component. For example, pyrantel pamoate is a neuromuscular blocking drug that releases acetylcholine. Inhibiting cholinesterase produces seizures in the helminth.

Most anthelmintic drugs are only active against specific parasites; however, some are also toxic to the host. In some cases, the initial regimen using the drug of choice does not effect a cure, and alternative treatment options are hazardous. Try retreating the patient with the first drug before prescribing another anthelmintic drug. The advantage of many antihelminthic drugs is their short duration of treatment.

Many of the anthelmintic drugs are not routinely available in the United States. In some cases, the drugs may be available only through the Parasitic Disease Drug Service at the CDC in Atlanta, Georgia.

Patient Education

The compliance and dependability of the person being treated are crucial factors for successful elimination of the parasites. Careful instructions must be given for timing of return visits, for submission of specimens, and for taking of drugs.

Emphasize the importance of meticulous hygiene: namely, washing hands before eating and after toileting, and keeping hands or objects away from the mouth. Toilet facilities should be disinfected daily. Instruct the patient to take frequent showers rather than baths, and to change clothing, bed linens, and towels daily to prevent reinfestation. The importance of follow-up with the health care provider cannot be stressed enough.

Travelers to other countries must be cautioned regarding the reservoirs for helminths there. This is particularly important if their travel takes them to underdeveloped areas with primitive facilities for, eating, drinking, and toileting.

Evaluation

Depending on the specific infestation, the stool should be reexamined between 1 week and 3 to 6 months after treatment to determine whether the infestation has cleared. Stool specimens for intestinal, liver, and blood flukes are collected at 1 week, and again at 1, 6, and 12 months following treatment. A stool specimen is collected at 1 month following treatment for lung flukes; and at 1 and again at 3 months following treatment for tapeworms.

For most patients with helminthic infestation, three stool samples examined after completion of therapy should be negative. After roundworm infestation, the patient's stool samples should be free of ova, larvae, or worms 2 to 3 weeks after completion of therapy. Specimens from a patient with flukes should be negative for several months before the patient is considered cured. For pinworm infestation, perianal swabs should be negative for 7 days.

IMMUNE

MALARIA

EPIDEMIOLOGY AND ETIOLOGY

Malaria was first described by the Egyptians in the third millennium BC. The Crusades, the building of the Panama Canal, and World War II are historical examples of malaria's ability to kill more people than even combat or construction accidents. It is a devastating disease in terms of human suffering and economic cost. Malaria affects the largest number of people (between 300 and 500 million cases are reported each year) of any natural or man-made affliction, and over 2 million of its victims die, most of them young children in sub-Saharan Africa. The primary reasons for the high number of deaths are failure to take prophylaxis, inappropriate prophylaxis, delay in seeking care, and misdiagnosis.

Malaria is caused by the parasites *Plasmodium falciparum*, *Plasmodium vivax*, *Plasmodium ovale*, and/or *Plasmodium malariae*. These parasites have different biologic patterns, but all of them affect humans. The species with the highest morbidity and mortality in humans is *P. falciparum*, posing the greatest risk to immunocompromised persons and children younger than 5 years.

P. falciparum is the most pathogenic form of the organism. Common in the tropics (and formerly in temperate zones), it accounts for about 50% of malaria cases worldwide. *P. vivax* is common in temperate zones and responsible for about 43% of cases in these zones. *P. malariae* is not found in contiguous distribution but accounts for 7% of cases worldwide; and *P. ovale*, found primarily in tropical south Africa and the Western Pacific, is rare in humans (<1%).

Emigration from and travel to regions where malaria is endemic constitutes a continuing public health concern in the United States. Attempts in the 1950s to eradicate the malaria parasites failed, primarily because of the development of resistance to insecticides and antimalarial drugs. Since 1960, transmission rates of malaria and the degree of resistance to antimalarial drugs has increased. If mosquito populations themselves become infected by imported disease, they could reemerge in the future as endemic disease vectors. Additionally, the climate influences all three components of the *Plasmodium* life cycle and is thus a key determinant in the geographic distribution and seasonal pattern of malaria.

PATHOPHYSIOLOGY

Malarial parasites were named *Plasmodium* because of their affinity for red blood cells (RBCs). The sporozoite (a tissue parasite), is injected into the host by the *Anopheles* mosquito. *P. vivax*, *P. ovale*, or *P. malariae* invade RBCs traveling to the liver, where they reproduce asexually and periodically seed the body. It is unusual for more than 1% of RBCs to become infested. The exception is *P. falciparum*, in which more than 50% of the RBCs contain the parasite. Patients at this stage are largely asymptomatic (Fig. 30-2).

With time, the intracellular parasite multiplies to such an extent in each cell that it cannot be contained. Daughter cells of *Plasmodium*, known as merozoites, cause death of the hepatocytes: membranous vesicles shuttle malaria parasites from the liver to blood cells during infestation while simultaneously holding in check the cues that would ordinarily signal phagocytosis of the dying cell. This alteration allows membrane-bound extensions of the infested cells to bud off and shuttle merozoites directly into the blood stream.

Symptoms of infestation appear after an incubation period of 10 to 35 days, often with a break period of flulike symptoms. The patient's fever cycles correspond with the release of merozoites from the liver. *P. falciparum* infestation begins with a chilly sensation rather than a shaking chill, and the temperature rises and falls with lysis. The episodes may last 20 to 36 hours, with prominent headache and increasing prostration. In a patient with a fever of 104° F or higher and a severe headache with drowsiness, delirium, or confusion, cerebral malaria should be suspected.

P. vivax and *P. ovale* cause less severe, but abrupt, attacks consisting of shaking chills, fever, and sweats, as well as irregular, intermittent fevers. Headache may precede the first chill. Rigors occur at 48-hour intervals and last 1 to 8 hours, with no symptoms in between. The severity of rigors in malaria is related to the number of species present, differences in the strains, and the immunity of the host.

Chronic malaria exists in residents of hyperendemic areas of the world. Infestation with *P. malariae* begins with severe paroxysm that recurs in 72 hours. The paroxysms of chronic malaria are shorter and lighter than those seen with an acute attack.

PHARMACOTHERAPEUTIC OPTIONS

Major drugs used in the prophylaxis and treatment of malaria are discussed in the following sections. These drugs differ from one another in efficacy; some are relatively active against *Plasmodium* whereas others are more selective. For this reason, the drugs are discussed separately rather than in the format usual for the text.

Chloroquine

Chloroquine (Aralen) is classified as a blood schizonticide and is indicated for suppression and treatment of acute attacks of malaria due to *P. vivax*, *P. malariae*, *P. ovale*, and susceptible strains of *P. falciparum*. The drug is also used in the treatment of extraintestinal amebiasis.

Chloroquine does not prevent relapses in patients with *P. vivax* or *P. malariae* malaria, because it is ineffective against exoerythrocytic forms of the parasite. Nor will it prevent *P. vivax* or *P. malariae* infestation when administered as prophylaxis. However, chloroquine use plays a significant role in lengthening the interval between treatment and relapse; a second drug is used to eliminate the plasmodia. Thus relapse is preventable with initial effective treatment. In patients with *P. falciparum* malaria, chloroquine abolishes the acute attack and eliminates the hepatic form of the parasite; however, the parasite has shown resistance to the drug.

Chloroquine binds to a product of heme breakdown that is highly lytic to RBCs, thus preventing hemolysis and accumulating in the acidic lysosome compartments of the parasite. As a weak base, chloroquine neutralizes these compartments; the parasite thus cannot utilize protein substances involved in heme breakdown, an operation essential for its survival.

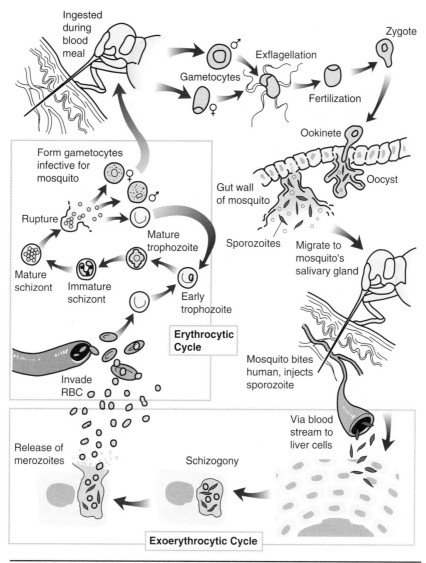

FIGURE 30-2 Life Cycle of *Plasmodium*. The organism is transmitted to the blood stream of humans by the bite of anopheline mosquitoes. The sporozoites migrate to the liver, where they develop and multiply and ultimately invade red blood cells. (From Mahon, C., Manuselis, G., Jr. [1995]. *Textbook of diagnostic microbiology* [p. 754]. Philadelphia: WB Saunders. Used with permission.)

Resistance of *P. falciparum* to chloroquine is widespread and, at present, particularly prevalent in sub-Saharan Africa, Southeast Asia, the Indian subcontinent, and over large portions of South America, including the Amazon basin. Cases of *P. vivax* resistance have also been reported.

Chloroquine is rapidly absorbed in the GI tract and well distributed to all body tissues, with concentration in erythrocytes, liver, spleen, kidneys, lung, heart, and brain, as well as melanin-containing tissues such as the retina and the epidermis. Chloroquine is a major substrate and moderately inhibits the CYP 2D6 isoenzyme. It is eliminated in the urine (70%) as a metabolite (diethylchloroquine). Any unabsorbed drug is eliminated in the feces, although it can remain in urine for years after the drug is stopped. Elimination of chloroquine is increased in acid urine. It penetrates the CNS and crosses the placenta (pregnancy category C) and enters breast milk.

Chloroquine is associated with relatively mild adverse effects including headache, nausea, and visual disturbances (blurring, diplopia). Prolonged treatment may cause a lichenoid skin eruption, toxic myopathy, cardiomyopathy, or peripheral neuropathy in a few patients. The conditions subside promptly when the drug is discontinued. When chloroquine has been used for treatment of diseases other than malaria, prolonged high doses have resulted in irreversible retinopathy. Doses over 5 grams are usually fatal.

Chloroquine is contraindicated for use in patients with psoriasis or porphyria, which may be exacerbated by the drug, and in patients with ocular disease. Psoriasis and porphyria are exacerbated by chloroquine.

Information on drug interactions and dosages for chloroquine can be found in Tables 30-3 and 30-4, respectively.

Hydroxychloroquine

Hydroxychloroquine (Plaquenil) may be used to treat malaria; however, it is more often used in the treatment of rheumatoid arthritis and systemic lupus erythematosus. The drug is used as a second-line treatment for *P. vivax*, *P. ovale*, or *P. malariae* infestations. Its mechanism of action and contraindications are similar to that of chloroquine. The basic pharmacology of hydroxychloroquine was discussed in Chapter 17.

Mefloquine

Mefloquine (Lariam, Mephaquin) is indicated for the treatment of mild to moderate acute malaria caused by those strains of *P. falciparum* that are sensitive to it (including both chloroquine-sensitive and chloroquine-resistant strains) or by *P. vivax*. Clinical data are insufficient to document the effect of mefloquine in malaria caused by *P. ovale* or *P. malariae*.

Mefloquine is a structural derivative of quinine. Like chloroquine and quinine, mefloquine concentrates in lysosomal compartments of the parasite. Although mefloquine's action is largely unclear, it is known to raise the intravascular pH in parasitic vesicles, thereby causing plasmodial death. Because resistance to this drug is already occurring, limitations on its use are prudent.

Mefloquine is rapidly absorbed when taken by mouth, with a bioavailability over 85% (see Table 30-2). Tissue concentrations remain relatively high for extended periods. Peak plasma concentrations are attained in a few hours and then slowly decline, with half-lives of the metabolites lasting 2 to 3 weeks. Mefloquine is a substrate of the CYP 3A4 enzyme and weakly inhibits 2D6 and 3A4. Elimination is primarily through the feces.

Mefloquine produces dose-related nausea, vomiting, abdominal pain, and dizziness. Rare manifestations of CNS toxicity are seen, such as disorientation, hallucinations, seizures, and depression. It is contraindicated for use in patients with known hypersensitivity and in cases of overwhelming acute *P. falciparum* infestation. Patients should initially receive the drug by intravenously, and oral administration of mefloquine should follow. The drug is also contraindicated for use in patients with seizure disorders or psychiatric disturbances. Suicidal ideation has been reported in patients taking this drug. Do not use mefloquine during pregnancy because of its teratogenic and embryotoxic effects (category X). It also enters breast milk.

Information on drug interactions and dosages for mefloquine can be found in Tables 30-3 and 30-4, respectively.

Primaquine

Primaquine (Primaquine) is classified as a tissue schizonticide. It also has prophylactic activity, but it is seldom used for this purpose because of its toxicity. Primaquine is the only tissue schizonticide available to eradicate tissue forms of plasmodia that cause relapse.

Little is known about the mechanism of action of primaquine, especially why it is more active against tissue forms and gametes than against asexual forms of plasmodia.

The bioavailability of primaquine after oral administration is 96%. The plasma concentration after a single dose peaks in 3 hours and then falls, with a half-life of 6 hours (see Table 30-2). It is rapidly biotransformed, with only a small fraction eliminated as the parent drug. Three metabolites of primaquine (i.e., 5-hydroxyprimaquine, 5-hydroxydemethylprimaquine, and 5,6-dihydroxy-8-aminoquinoline) have considerably less antimalarial activity but greater hemolytic activity than the parent compound. Primaquine crosses the placenta, but whether it is excreted into breast milk is unknown.

Primaquine, even when used in therapeutic doses, may cause dark-colored urine, anorexia, pallor, unusual fatigue or weakness, and back, leg, or abdominal pain. These symptoms suggest the development of hemolytic anemia. Bluish fingernails, lips, or skin, dizziness, breathing difficulty, or unusual fatigue or weakness may indicate methemoglobinemia. These occur most frequently with high-dosage therapy. Immediate stoppage of the drug is required if any of these adverse effects appear.

Because of its association with hematologic problems, use the drug cautiously in blacks and ethnic groups from the eastern Mediterranean region, where glucose-6-phosphate dehydrogenase (G6PD) deficiency is most prevalent. Mild to moderate cramping and occasional epigastric distress occur in some people given larger doses. Mild hemolytic anemia, methemoglobinemia, and leukocytosis have been observed. Because of cross-sensitivity, primaquine is contraindicated for use in patients with hypersensitivity to iodoquinol (Yodoxin).

Information on drug interactions and dosages for primaquine can be found in Tables 30-3 and 30-4, respectively.

Quinine sulfate

Quinine (Quinamm; ◆ Novo-Quinine) is the oldest antimalarial drug. It has been used to treat malarial fevers since 1633. Quinine sulfate and related derivatives, such as mefloquine, have been used for clinical or suppressive cure of malaria and to destroy sexual erythrocytic forms of plasmodia. The action of quinine is much like that of chloroquine.

Quinine is readily absorbed when taken orally, even in patients with diarrhea, and distributed to the liver, the lungs, the kidneys, and the spleen. The drug is poorly distributed to cerebrospinal fluid (2% to 7%). Steady state levels are achieved and maintained with regular dosing. Plasma concentrations of 8 to 15 mg/L are clinically effective and are generally nontoxic. Quinine is extensively biotransformed in the liver; only about 10% of the dose is eliminated unchanged in the urine. Renal elimination is twice as rapid when the urine is acidic.

Quinine, when given in full therapeutic dosages, produces a typical dose-related cluster of symptoms termed *cinchonism*. In mild form, cinchonism consists of tinnitus, headache, nausea, and disturbed vision. There can also be adverse reactions in patients with untreated or undertreated hypothyroidism. When the drug is continued or after large single doses, GI, cardiovascular, and dermal manifestations may appear. Hearing and vision are particularly affected.

The visual manifestations of cinchonism include blurred vision, altered color perception, photophobia, diplopia, night blindness, constricted visual fields, scotomata, and mydriasis. Functional impairment of the eighth cranial nerve results in tinnitus, decreased auditory acuity, and vertigo. GI symptoms result from the local irritant effect of quinine, but nausea and emesis also have a central origin. Vomiting, abdominal pain, and diarrhea result from the irritation. The cardiovascular adverse effects of quinine are qualitatively related to those of its isomer, quinidine. Therapeutic doses of quinine have little, if any, effect on the normal heart or blood pressure. When given as an intravenous (IV) bolus, quinine sometimes causes alarming and even fatal hypotension.

Quinine is contraindicated for use in patients with a history of G6PD deficiency (it increases the risk for hemolytic anemia), myasthenia gravis (it produces neuromuscular blockade exacerbating muscle weakness, respiratory distress, and dysphagia), and arrhythmias (prolonged QT intervals). Do not use quinine in patients with hypoglycemia, because it stimulates the release of insulin and reduces serum glucose levels. *P. falciparum* attacks can also lower serum glucose levels. Avoid quinine in patients with optic neuritis or tinnitus, because it can exacerbate these conditions. The American Academy of Pediatrics considers quinine compatible with breastfeeding; however it is considered category X during pregnancy. It should not be used in patients with a known hypersensitivity.

Information on drug interactions and dosages for quinine sulfate can be found in Tables 30-3 and 30-4, respectively.

Sulfadoxine-pyrimethamine

The combination drug sulfadoxine-pyrimethamine (Fansidar) is used for prophylaxis (even in pregnant women) against the *P. falciparum* species. In combination with quinine, it has been used in the treatment of acute malarial attacks resulting from chloroquine-resistant strains.

Sulfadoxine-pyrimethamine is a folic acid antagonist that acts selectively to inhibit plasmodial dihydrofolate reductase. This enzyme is important to the cellular biosynthesis of proteins. The *Plasmodium* enzyme is much more sensitive to sulfadoxine-pyrimethamine than its mammalian counterparts. This drug is not effective against the tissue forms of malaria, so it will not cure infestations caused by *P. ovale* or *P. vivax*. It is the drug of choice for all chloroquine-sensitive strains of malaria. However, the development of resistance to sulfadozine-pyrimethamine in *Plasmodium* parasites is a major setback in the effective treatment of malaria, especially *P. falciparum*.

Factors promoting the development and transmission of resistance to sulfadozine-pyrimethamine by *Plasmodium* parasites are unclear. It appears that the development of resistance involves three stages:

1. The falciparum parasites look for and reproduce with other parasites with mutations in the dihydrofolate reductase or dihydropteroate synthetase gene. **Typically, drugs with long half-lives tend to reduce development of resistance by maintaining higher mean inhibitory concentrations (MICs) when dosed appropriately.**

2. Parasites with allelic types of higher resistance within the host during infestation are chosen. The dosages used and the timing of treatment relative to the initiation of a specific anti-*P. falciparum* immune response are important factors during this stage.

3. Lastly, treatment failure becomes prevalent as the parasites develop enough resistant mutations to survive therapeutic dosages of the combined drug.

Therefore it is important to treat malaria properly to prevent the development of resistance. Partially immune patients tend to respond better to treatment than hosts not previously exposed to malaria.

Sulfadoxine-pyrimethamine is well absorbed in the GI tract following oral administration. Distribution is throughout the kidney, the lungs, the liver, and the spleen. Elimination half-life averages 111 hours (see Table 30-2).

The adverse effects of sulfadoxine-pyrimethamine are few when it is used in dosages employed for treatment of malaria. Excessive dosages produce a megaloblastic anemia that resembles folic acid deficiency. The anemia readily reverses upon discontinuation of the drug or administration of leucovorin (folinic acid). In rare cases, Stevens-Johnson syndrome, toxic epidermal necrosis, serum sickness types of reaction, urticaria, exfoliative dermatitis, and hepatitis have been associated with sulfadoxine-pyrimethamine. The combination drug is teratogenic in laboratory studies.

Dosage information for sulfadoxine-pyrimethamine can be found in Table 30-4.

Atovaquone-proguanil

Atovaquone-proguanil (Malarone) is highly effective for both prophylaxis and treatment of malaria caused by chloroquine-resistant *P. falciparum*. Both drugs are active against the erythrocytic and exoerythrocytic forms of *P. falciparum*, including strains that are resistant to chloroquine, mefloquine, and sulfadoxine-pyrimethamine. The drug is also used in the treatment of *Pneumocystis jirovecii* (previously called *P. carinii*) pneumonia.

Atovaquone-proguanil interferes with the biosynthesis of pyrimidines required for replication of nucleic acids. Atovaquone selectively disrupts mitochondrial electron transport to inhibit the synthesis of pyrimidines. No other antimalarial drug exhibits this action. The prodrug, proguanil, acts by inhibiting the dihydrofolate reductase inhibitor cycloguanil, thus preventing activation of folic acid. In the absence of useable folic acid, *P. falciparum* is unable to make proteins, DNA, or RNA. This combination drug may not be effective for treatment of recurrent malaria that develops after one course of the drug.

Atovaquone-proguanil is poorly soluble in water and should be taken with a meal; absorption is greatly enhanced in the presence of fatty foods. Atovaquone is highly protein bound. There is evidence that atovaquone undergoes limited biotransformation; however, a specific metabolite has not been defined. In contrast, proguanil is extensively absorbed, both in the presence and absence of food. Proguanil concentrates in RBCs and is biotransformed to the metabolite cycloguanil via CYP 2C19, and to the metabolite 4-chlorophenylbiguanide. Forty percent to 60% of proguanil is eliminated by the kidneys.

Atovaquone-proguanil is generally well tolerated. When used alone, atovaquone may cause a rash in 20% to 40% of patients. Other adverse effects of atovaquone include headache, fever, nausea, vomiting, diarrhea, and insomnia. When proguanil is used alone, the most common adverse effects include stomatitis, GI upset, and headache. In addition, the proguanil component may cause hair loss, urticaria, hematuria, thrombocytopenia, and scaling of the soles of the feet and the palms. The combined drug is a pregnancy category C agent.

Information on drug interactions and dosages for atovaquone-proguanil can be found in Tables 30-3 and 30-4, respectively.

Amodiaquine

Amodiaquine (Basoquin, Fluroquin, and Miaquin) is used for the treatment of acute malarial attacks. It is comparable to chloroquine in almost all aspects and is also effective against some chloroquine-resistant strains, although resistance to amodiaquine has been reported as well. It has also been used, with variable success, in the treatment of leprae reactions, lupus erythematosus, rheumatoid arthritis, giardiasis, hepatic amebiasis, and urticaria. Any possible prophylactic advantage that amodiaquine may afford is not justified by the risk of agranulocytosis associated with its use.

The mechanism of action of amodiaquine has not yet been determined; in general, however, the drug appears to bind to nucleoproteins to inhibit DNA an RNA polymerase. High drug concentrations of the drug are found in the malaria parasite's digestive vacuoles.

Amodiaquine is rapidly absorbed and undergoes rapid and extensive biotransformation to desethylamodiaquine, which concentrates in RBCs. It is likely that this metabolite, not amodiaquine, is responsible for most of the antimalarial activity, and that the toxic effects of amodiaquine may, in part, be due to the metabolite. It appears to be eliminated in the urine.

Oral administration of a single dose of amodiaquine may be followed by abdominal discomfort, nausea, vomiting, headache, dizziness, blurring of vision, mental and physical weakness, and fatigue. These symptoms are usually mild and transient. More severe adverse reactions include itching, cardiac muscle depression, impaired cardiac conductivity, vasodilation with resultant hypotension, dyskinesia, ocular damage, neuromuscular disorders, and hearing loss. There have been several reports of agranulocytosis, and these have limited its use in prophylaxis. Because amodiaquine concentrates in the liver, use the drug with caution in patients with liver disease or alcoholism, and in patients receiving hepatotoxic drugs. Hepatitis and peripheral neuropathy have also been reported.

Information on dosages for amodiaquine can be found in Table 30-4.

CLINICAL REASONING

Identification of plasmodia in serial blood smears is definitive for malaria. If a drug-resistant strain of *P. falciparum* is suspected, mark the lab order forms accordingly. A commercial kit is available for the diagnosis of *P. falciparum* infestation. The identification of the type of plasmodium is important for effective therapy. In some cases, the patient is infested with more than one strain of plasmodia. Before initiating drug therapy, perform baseline lab tests, including CBC, platelet count, electrolytes, renal function tests, LFTs, and G6PD measurements.

Treatment Objectives

Treatment objectives for malaria are to eradicate the parasite in both its erythrocytic and exoerythrocytic forms, to reduce or eliminate signs and symptoms of malaria, and to decrease patient discomfort. Plasmodia are killed most easily in the erythrocytic stage. Plasmodia in the exoerythrocytic stage are more difficult to eradicate, but it can be done.

Treatment Options

▥ Patient Variables

Ten percent of blacks, and 5% to 10% of Sephardic Jews, Greeks, Iranians, Chinese, Filipinos, and Indonesians have G6PD deficiency. There is evidence that G6PD is essential for metabolism in the plasmodia, so persons with this genetic deficiency are believed to have some natural immunity to malaria. Africans who carry hemoglobin C, rather than hemoglobin A, were noted to have immunity against malarial infestation.

Since malaria tends to be a chronic disease, treatment may be long-term or recurrent. Further, because antimalarial drugs cause discomfort and are not without adverse effects, patients may have difficulty complying with their treatment regimen. There are alternative drugs available for the treatment of malaria, although they are less effective, require difficult dosage schedules, cause serious adverse effects, and/or are too expensive.

Pregnant women are at higher risk for death and serious complications resulting from *P. falciparum* malaria; maternal death and fetal loss are both known complications. Pregnant women who must travel to areas where malaria is endemic should use personal protection against mosquito bites.

▥ Drug Variables

Malaria Prophylaxis. Malaria prophylaxis begins with a prescription for drugs to be used before traveling to a malaria-endemic area. Prophylaxis cannot prevent primary infestation of the liver, because the drugs have no effect on sporozoites; however, it does prevent the erythrocytic stage, which causes symptoms. Once the liver is affected, the patient can have an acute attack whenever the drug is no longer taken.

In general, in chloroquine-sensitive areas, chloroquine or sulfadoxine-pyrimethamine are the drugs of choice for prophylaxis. In chloroquine-resistant areas, mefloquine is the preferred drug. Alternative drugs include hydroxychloroquine and doxycycline (Vibramycin). Check with the CDC for the latest recommendations on prophylaxis and treatment of malaria.

Malaria Treatment. Drugs that eradicate plasmodia in the erythrocytic stage of the life cycle are used to treat an acute attack. These drugs include chloroquine, mefloquine, primaquine, sulfadoxine-pyrimethamine, and quinine. The choice of drugs depends on the specific plasmodium involved. The exoerythrocytic stage of the disease requires multi–drug therapy. Few drugs are available for the treatment of malaria, and what is available is in danger of becoming ineffective in treating the disease.

Relapse Prevention. A cure for malaria is necessary for strains of *P. vivax*, because the infestation is harbored in the liver. Treatment is ordinarily withheld until the patient is out of the endemic area, because reinfestation is almost a certainty. The drug of choice for relapse prevention is primaquine.

CASE STUDY | Antimalarial Drugs

ASSESSMENT

History of Present Illness	JD is a 26-year-old female missionary trainee who returned 3 days ago from 3-month stay with the people of Shan, Myanmar. She reports faithfully taking mefloquine for malaria prophylaxis while she was gone and still has 4 more weeks to go. She complains of general malaise, fevers ranging from subnormal to 38° C, headaches, intermittent cold sensations, nausea, vomiting, intermittent diarrhea, and myalgias. Thinks she may have the flu, because her traveling companions have also been ill. She is scheduled to return to Shan 6 weeks from now.
Past Health History	Health good, passed full physical before the church appointment 9 months ago. Denies history of diabetes, hypertension, or cancer. Family health history benign. Mother and father alive and well, as are two younger siblings. She has a history of tetracycline allergy (anaphylaxis).
Life-Span Considerations	JD voices concerns about the type of illness and chronicity, the need for continual drug therapy, and obligations to church program in Burma. Therapy and laboratory fees will probably be paid by church insurance. Infestation may be considered a job-related illness with long-term implications.
Physical Exam Findings	WNL (within normal limits) except for temp elevation of 37.8° C. Pulse and respirations WNL. Skin intact, pink, clear. Nail beds clear, no clubbing. Deep tendon reflexes WNL. Abdomen benign, bowel sounds present. Lungs clear to auscultation.
Diagnostic Testing	Cultures revealed the presence of *Plasmodium falciparum* and sensitivities.

DIAGNOSIS: Mefloquine-resistant *plasmodium falciparum* malaria

MANAGEMENT

Treatment Objective	1. Cure infestation and relieve symptoms of acute attack. 2. Prevent chronic state if *Plasmodium vivax* or *Plasmodium ovale* are also present.
Treatment Plan	**Pharmacotherapy** • Stop mefloquine now. • Start atovaquone-proguanil 250 mg/100 mg PO once daily. • IV fluids for next 24 hours per protocol **Patient Education** 1. Follow up in office 24 hours after discharge. 2. Take atovaquone-proguanil tablets at the same time each day with food or a milky drink. Repeat the dose of atovaquone-proguanil if vomiting occurs within 1 hour after dosing. 3. Protective clothing, insect repellents, and bed nets are important factors in malaria prophylaxis. 4. No drug regimen is 100% effective; seek medical attention for any febrile illness that occurs during or after return to or from a malaria-endemic area and inform her health care provider in Myanmar that she has had an outbreak of *P. falciparum* malaria. 5. *P. falciparum* malaria holds a higher risk of death and serious complications in pregnant women than in the general population. Discuss the risks and benefits of birth control at follow-up visit. **Evaluation** 1. Symptoms of acute attack (i.e., fever, chills, malaise, muscle aches, etc.) have been relieved. 2. Malaria NOT caused by *P. viva* or *P. ovale*. 3. Patient provided with supply of Malarone tablets for return trip to Shan, Myanmar. 4. Birth control has been started.

CLINICAL REASONING ANALYSIS

Q1. What made the infectious disease health care provider recommend Malarone rather than mefloquine? I thought mefloquine was standard treatment?

A. JD was in Shan, Myanmar, a remote area northeast of Thailand. It used to be called Burma. Anyway, that area of the country has a high incidence of *P. falciparum* malaria. According to the CDC website on international travel, that part of Myanmar has had reports of mefloquine and chloroquine resistance.

Continued

CASE STUDY   Antimalarial Drugs—Cont'd

Q2. I thought Malarone was a single drug. You told JD that it's two drugs in one. Don't they both do the same thing?

A. Malarone is two drugs in one, but they have different mechanisms of action. Atovaquone selectively disrupts mitochondrial electron transport. No other antimalarial drug exhibits this action. Proguanil acts by inhibiting cycloguanil, a dihydrofolate reductase inhibitor, which prevents activation of folic acid. In the absence of usable folic acid, the malaria organism can't make proteins, DNA, or RNA and can't replicate.

Q3. But don't we have to worry about drug interactions with the combination drug?

A. Yes, we always worry about drug interactions; however, although atovaquone is highly protein bound, it does not displace other highly protein-bound drugs. This means that significant drug interactions arising from displacement are unlikely. We need to watch out for the proguanil part, since it is a minor substrate of the CYP 1A1, 2C19, and 3A4 enzyme.

Q4. I heard the infectious disease specialist talking about using doxycycline on someone else going to the Middle East. Why can't she take doxycycline instead? Seems like the drug interaction issue would be prevented that way.

A. Well, doxycycline is in the tetracycline family of drugs; and JD had an anaphylactic reaction to tetracyclines a few years ago.

Q5. Oh, I remember. Even if she could take a tetracycline, I thought it was an antibiotic, not an antimalarial drug. How does it work for malaria?

A. Doxycycline has been found to be active against the asexual erythrocytic form of *P. falciparum*, which is what JD has. It is not effective against the gametocytes of *P. falciparum*. The precise mechanism of action of the drug is not known.

PLASMODIA RESISTANCE. During the past decade, the malaria parasite has become resistant to drugs used for its suppression and cure. Even chloroquine, once the drug of choice, may be unreliable in some cases. Antibiotics are not usually effective against the malarial parasites; however, sulfonamides, tetracyclines, and chloramphenicol have been used. They are most useful when administered in combination with either quinine or pyrimethamine to treat drug-resistant strains of parasites. Doxycycline is used as an alternative when mefloquine cannot be tolerated or its use is contraindicated. Antibiotics are discussed in more detail in Chapter 27.

INFORMATION SOURCES. There are a variety of sources available for information about drugs used to treat and prevent malaria:

- Centers for Disease Control and Prevention: www.cdc.gov
- Malaria Foundation International: www.malaria.org
- Food and Drug Administration (FDA) Medication Guide: www.fda.gov/cder
- World Health Organization (WHO): www.who.int/en

Within the WHO website is a link to the Roll Back Malaria website, an international partnership of the WHO, the World Bank, the United Nations Development Programme, and the United Nations Children's Fund. The partnership was formed with the goal of reducing the burden of malaria worldwide by 50% by 2010. The website is a repository of information from all countries, including information on grants and research projects and reports on the progress being made in reducing the global burden of malaria.

MALARIA VACCINE. A malaria vaccine is not available at this time, although many pharmaceutical companies are actively testing malaria vaccines. It is hoped that this goal will ultimately be achieved. Because the major parasitic stages of malaria in humans are antigenically distinct, a successful vaccine will likely need to contain at least three parasite antigens (sporozoite, merozoite, and gametocyte). A vaccine that limits the magnitude of the parasitemia could have a marked effect on survival, even if it had no effect on the incidence of infestation, because severe morbidity and mortality are associated with high parasitemias.

Patient Education

Because of growing drug resistance, greater emphasis is placed on reducing exposure to the anopheline mosquito, especially in hyperendemic areas such as Africa. Successful strategies include the application of insect repellents containing diethyltoluamide (DEET) and the use of netting impregnated with pyrethrin (insecticide) over the bed for protection during sleep. Despite resistance, dichlorodiphenyltrichloroethane (DDT) remains effective in most regions of the world. Advise exposed nonimmune persons to consider malaria prophylaxis, to use insect repellents, and otherwise to reduce their exposure to the *Anopheles* mosquito. The WHO recently endorsed the use of DDT indoors as a persistent insecticide for the control of mosquitoes.

Regardless of the drug chosen for treatment, adherence with the regimen is important. Instruct patients to take the drug exactly as prescribed. A calendar can be prepared for the patient taking the antimalarial drugs for prophylaxis, with the dosage days marked. Mefloquine, for example, should be taken on the same day each week, beginning 1 week before exposure and continuing for 4 weeks after the traveler has returned to a malaria-free area.

Persons who harbor the sexual forms of plasmodia are referred to as *carriers*. It is from the carriers that mosquitoes receive the forms of the parasite that perpetuate the disease. Advise carriers to avoid giving blood, because it is possible that the recipient of their blood will contract malaria or become a carrier. A growing number of malaria cases have been associated with transfusion of infected blood. Any person who has had malaria or has been exposed to the disease by visiting a region where it is prevalent must be disqualified as a blood donor.

Evaluation

For patients receiving malaria suppression, no therapeutic monitoring is needed. However, for patients under treatment for active disease, frequent follow-up is required. Before and throughout therapy, monitor CBC, renal function, and LFT values, blood pressure measurements, and neurologic exam findings (including muscle strength and deep tendon reflexes). Because chloroquine affects the eyes, obtain a complete baseline ophthalmologic exam (including fundoscopic and slit-lamp and visual fields). Serial laboratory and eye exams should be done twice yearly. Glucose monitoring is needed for patients receiving quinine. Patients receiving mefloquine should also have routine electrocardiogram (ECG) monitoring.

Treatment effectiveness for malaria results from killing plasmodia in erythrocytes and is evident by the absence of clinical signs and symptoms, by negative cultures, and by lack of adverse drug effects. If fever or other symptoms persist after adequate antimalarial therapy, the diagnosis must be reevaluated.

AMEBIASIS

EPIDEMIOLOGY AND ETIOLOGY

Amebiasis is an infestation of the intestine caused by the one-cell parasite *Entamoeba histolytica*. Because of its worldwide distribution and serious GI manifestations, amebiasis is one of the more important parasitic diseases. Approximately 50 million cases of invasive amebiasis occur each year, leading to 100,000 deaths. Although anyone can have this disease, it is most common in those living in developing countries that have poor sanitary conditions. In the United States, the incidence of amebiasis is estimated at 2% to 4% of the population; it is most often found in immigrants from developing countries. The highest incidence is found in institutionalized patients with mental illness, men who have sex with men, patients with acquired immunodeficiency syndrome (AIDS), the Native American population, and new immigrants from countries where it is endemic (e.g., Mexico, India, West and South Africa, and portions of Central and South America).

PATHOPHYSIOLOGY

E. histolytica must be differentiated from *Entamoeba dispar*, which is considered nonpathogenic and is associated with an asymptomatic carrier state. Although both protozoa are indistinguishable morphologically, recent research has been able to separate the two; *E. dispar* is about 10 times more common than *E. histolytica* and does not necessitate treatment. Invasive amebiasis is almost exclusively the result of *E. histolytica* infestation.

Transmission of amebiasis occurs through ingestion of cysts in fecally contaminated food or water, which is common when human feces is used as fertilizer. It can also be spread person-to-person, via oral or anal contact. Cockroaches and house flies can also spread the cysts. The cyst invades colonic epithelium, producing a classic flask-shaped ulcer in the submucosa. The trophozoite has a cytocidal effect on cells through a toxin. If the trophozoite reaches portal circulation,

it is carried to the liver, where it causes abscesses and periportal fibrosis. Amebic ulcerations can affect genitalia and the perineum, and abscesses can occur in the lungs and the brain (extraintestinal amebiasis). The most common signs and symptoms of intestinal amebiasis range from vague abdominal discomfort and malaise to severe abdominal cramping, flatulence, vomiting, odoriferous bloody diarrhea with mucus, and tenesmus. Eosinophilia is usually absent, although mild leukocytosis is not unusual. If liver involvement has occurred, the patient will have a high fever (e.g., 105° F) and significant leukocytosis, an increased number of cells and an increase in the percentage of immature cells (mainly band cells) in the blood. This change is called a "shift to the left." Other symptoms of liver involvement include elevated alkaline phosphatase, right upper quadrant pain, hepatomegaly, and palpable tenderness. Pain may be referred to the left or right shoulder because of pressure on the phrenic nerve. Signs of peritonitis will be present with erosion of liver abscesses.

PHARMACOTHERAPEUTIC OPTIONS

The goals of treatment for amebiasis are, initially, to eradicate the protozoa by use of amebicides, and then to provide supportive therapy. With the exception of metronidazole, each of these drugs is only active against *E. histolytica*. Although the following discussion is limited to drugs of choice, be aware that other antiprotozoal drugs are available. Also remember that a systemic drug may be so well absorbed that only a minimal amount is found in the intestinal lumen, and thus the drug may prove ineffective as a luminal drug. On the other hand, a luminal-acting drug may be too poorly absorbed to be effective in tissues.

Metronidazole, tetracycline, dehydroemetine, and chloroquine are tissue-acting drugs, whereas iodoquinol, paromomycin, and diloxanide are luminal amebicides. For asymptomatic patients and those with mild intestinal amebiasis, prescribe one of the following intraluminal drugs: iodoquinol, paromomycin, or diloxanide so as to prevent amebic liver abscess. These three drugs have cure rates of 84% to 96%.

For patients with severe intestinal disease or liver abscess, use metronidazole first to eliminate surviving protozoa, followed by a course of one of the intraluminal drugs noted above. Patients too ill to take oral metronidazole should receive the equivalent dosage using the IV route.

Iodoquinol

Iodoquinol (Yodoxin, Diquinol, Yodoquinol; ♣ Diodoquin) is the drug of choice for asymptomatic intestinal amebiasis. Iodoquinol is active against both the trophozoite and encysted forms of the protozoa.

Iodoquinol is poorly absorbed from the GI tract but reaches high concentrations in the intestinal lumen. It acts at the precise location of the infestation without significant systemic absorption (8%). The small amount that is absorbed is eliminated as metabolites in the urine.

The adverse effects of iodoquinol include mild GI upset (nausea, vomiting, diarrhea, cramps, and pruritus ani), acne and discoloration of the hair and nails, slight thyromegaly, fever, chills, headache, dizziness, and malaise. Taking the drug with food or milk may help reduce the GI upset. Although rare, prolonged therapy at high dosages has caused peripheral

IMMUNE

neuropathy and optic atrophy with permanent vision loss. There are no known drug significant drug interactions. Iodoquinol may alter the results of thyroid function tests for as long as 6 months after stopping therapy. Iodoquinol contains a substantial amount of organic iodine and should be used with caution in patients with thyroid disease.

Diloxanide

Diloxanide (Entamide; ◆ Furamide) is an orphan drug available from the CDC. It is used as second-line treatment for asymptomatic and very mild, but symptomatic, cases of amebiasis. If the course of treatment is ineffective, another course may be given; however, no more than three courses should be given in any 12-month period. The mechanism of action of the drug is unknown.

Diloxanide is hydrolyzed before absorption from the GI tract. The resulting diloxanide is readily absorbed and eliminated primarily in the urine as the glucuronide; less than 10% of a dose appears in the feces.

Flatulence is the most common adverse effect of diloxanide. Dry mouth, vomiting, esophagitis, persistent or recurrent diarrhea, cramping, pruritus, and urticaria occur occasionally. Adverse effects including headache, lethargy, vertigo or dizziness, disorientation, diplopia, and paresthesia have been reported occasionally. There are no significant drug interactions.

Paromomycin

Paromomycin (Humatin) is an oral aminoglycoside. It is used in the treatment of intestinal amebiasis and to treat hepatic coma; it is ineffective for extraintestinal amebiasis. It has also been used for cestodiasis, although it is not the drug of choice because it can cause release of viable eggs from the tapeworm. It is also used in the treatment of *Cryptosporidium parvum* infestation in patients with human immunodeficiency virus (HIV).

The effects of paromomycin are localized in the intestine. It is contraindicated for use in patients with intestinal obstruction or renal impairment. Patients who have an inflammatory bowel disease such as ulcerative colitis can inadvertently absorb the drug. It is completely eliminated, unchanged, in the feces.

The adverse effects of paromomycin include nephrotoxicity, ototoxicity, neuromuscular blockade, hypercholesterolemia, malabsorption, rash, headache, vertigo, eosinophilia, exanthema, and unexplained hematuria. Paromomycin is contraindicated for use in patients with a history of previous hypersensitivity reactions to it. It is also contraindicated in the presence of intestinal obstruction. It is compatible with breastfeeding since it is not absorbed systemically.

GIARDIASIS

Giardiasis, also known as "beaver fever," is caused by the flagellate protozoan *Giardia lamblia* (also *Giardia intestinalis*). The *Giardia* organism inhabits the upper intestinal tract of a number of different animals, both domestic and wild, as well as humans. It is the most frequently identified protozoan in the United States, with a prevalence of 16% in some areas. Fifty percent of infested persons remain symptom-free.

Giardiasis is transmitted via the fecal-oral route. Personal contact and contaminated water and food are the main routes of transmission. Susceptibility is increased in people who spend time in institutional or day-care settings, travelers and those who consume improperly treated water, and people hiking or backpacking in wilderness areas worldwide. It is suspected that *Giardia* is zoonotic, that is, communicable between animals and humans. Beavers, dogs, cats, horses, and cattle all serve as major reservoir hosts.

Most people infected with giardiasis will not exhibit symptoms; however, symptoms that are both unpleasant and uncomfortable may develop. Symptoms of giardiasis include profound malaise, loss of appetite, lethargy, explosive diarrhea, loose or watery stool, stomach cramps, upset stomach, malodorous belching, bloating, and flatulence. The protozoan occasionally migrates to the bile ducts and the gallbladder. The symptoms of giardiasis often mimic that of cholelithiasis, appendicitis, peptic ulcers, or hiatal hernia. Symptoms usually begin 1 to 2 weeks after infestation and may wax and wane cyclically. Symptoms are largely produced by the layer of *Giardia* protozoa coating the inside of the small intestine and blocking the absorption of nutrients.

PHARMACOTHERAPEUTIC OPTIONS

The drug of choice for patients with giardiasis is metronidazole. The alternative drug paromomycin was previously discussed.

Metronidazole is an antibacterial and antiprotozoal drug approved for the treatment of anaerobic infestations of the skin, the CNS, the lower respiratory tract, and bones and joints, as well as for intraabdominal or gynecologic infections, endocarditis, and septicemia. In addition, the drug is used in the treatment of trichomoniasis, amebiasis, and antibiotic-associated pseudomembranous colitis.

Metronidazole inhibits nucleic acid synthesis which results in antibacterial, amebicidal, and trichomonacidal effects. It is well absorbed from the GI tract and widely distributed to body tissues including the blood-brain barrier. Metronidazole is biotransformed in the liver to active metabolites and eliminated primarily in the urine, with a small amount eliminated in the feces. The drug readily crosses placental membranes (pregnancy category B) and is distributed in breast milk. Age-related liver impairment may require dosage adjustment.

Common adverse effects of metronidazole include anorexia, nausea, dry mouth, metallic taste, abdominal pain and discomfort, and uterine pain. Occasionally, the patient develops diarrhea or constipation, vomiting, dizziness, urticaria, an erythematous rash, and dark, reddish-brown urine. The drug is contraindicated in patients with hypersensitivity to metronidazole or other nitroimidazole derivatives and should be used with caution in patients with blood dyscrasias or a predisposition to edema, and those who are on concurrent corticosteroid therapy. Avoid the concurrent use of alcohol to reduce the risk of a disulfiram-like adverse reaction.

LEISHMANIASIS

Leishmaniasis is an infestation by selected protozoal species. Worldwide, the incidence of leishmaniasis is estimated at 10 million. The highest incidence occurs during the summer months, especially in persons working near forested areas. The forms of leishmaniasis vary significantly in severity from mild to potentially fatal.

The cutaneous form of leishmaniasis ("oriental sore") seen in the United States is caused by *Leishmania braziliensis* or by *Leishmania mexicana*, endemic to south Mexico and Central Mexico. Nodular formations are seen at exposure sites, which then evolve into slow-healing ulcers. The mucocutaneous leishmaniasis is characterized by mucosal ulcerations in the nose, the mouth, and the pharynx.

Visceral leishmaniasis (kala-azar, "black fever," or Assam fever) is transmitted to humans most often by the bites of infected female phlebotomine sandflies. These flagellated extracellular organisms live in the GI tract and the saliva of the insect vector, which passes the infestation on to humans during a blood meal. Once in the host, the organisms multiply in macrophages and in cells of the reticuloendothelial system. With visceral leishmaniasis, all internal organs may be affected, but the liver, the spleen, and the bone marrow are most involved. It is characterized by fever, hepatosplenomegaly, liver dysfunction, hypoalbuminemia, pancytopenia, lymphadenopathy, and hemorrhage. Left untreated, the disease is fatal. No effective prophylaxis against leishmaniasis is available at this time.

Visceral leishmaniasis may also be acquired from transfusion of contaminated blood and accidental needlestick injuries. Patients with advanced AIDS are highly susceptible to leishmaniasis. Military veterans of Desert Storm, the Sudan campaigns, African assignments, Iraq or Afghanistan service, or Central American service must be considered suspect for having leishmaniasis if symptoms dictate.

PHARMACOTHERAPEUTIC OPTIONS

Liposomal amphotericin B

Two antifungal drugs, fluconazole (taken by mouth), and liposomal amphotericin B (administered by IV route) are highly effective alternative drugs (see Chapter 28). Several factors explain the suitability of lipid formulations of amphotericin B for the treatment of visceral leishmaniasis. *Leishmania* resides in the macrophages, and liposomes are rapidly taken up by the macrophages. Amphotericin B, known to be an effective antileishmanial drug, can be formulated as a liposomal preparation. For these reasons, delivery of liposomal amphotericin B can be targeted to the desired site for antiparasitic action, reducing the risk for drug toxicities. In addition, liposomes offer an amplification effect, through concentrated encapsulation of numerous molecules in each liposome particle that are delivered at the desired site of action. Liposomal amphotericin B has been used extensively throughout the world as the best option for treatment of visceral leishmaniasis, even in cases resistant to standard drugs (see also Chapter 28).

Stibogluconate sodium

All three forms of leishmaniasis may be treated with stibogluconate sodium, which is available only from the CDC. There is some suggestion that it interferes with the parasite's production of energy and genetic material (DNA). The drug is poorly absorbed from the GI tract and therefore must be given parenterally. It undergoes little biotransformation and is eliminated rapidly in the urine.

Because stibogluconate sodium is a heavy metal (an antimonial compound), it is considered a toxic drug. Its adverse effects include pain at the injection site, joint pain, and GI upset. In some cases, liver failure and renal failure have occurred. Changes in the ECG are common and occasionally precede serious arrhythmias. Renal and liver dysfunction, shock, and sudden death are possible, but rare.

ECTOPARASITES

Ectoparasites are insects living on the outer surface of the body. Strictly speaking, the term encompasses fungal infections of the skin as well as infestations by mites and lice. In practice, it refers only to mites and lice. Treatment of ectoparasitic infestations includes the use of scabicides and pediculicides. As a rule, ectoparasitic infestations are treated with topical agents available in the form of shampoos, creams, lotions, and gels. Only one ectoparasitic drug is administered orally, ivermectin.

PEDICULOSIS

Pediculosis is a general term referring to any infestation with lice. The incidence of infestation has been increasing in North America and Western Europe. It was once thought that overcrowding, poor hygiene, lack of laundry and bathing facilities, and general uncleanliness promoted the infestation. However, this assumption has proven to be untrue. The infestation is transmitted from one person to another by close contact or through sharing of combs, clothing, or towels. Since humans are the only hosts for these obligate parasites, infestation cannot be acquired from pets or other animals. Transmission via toilet seats is unlikely.

Pediculosis capitus is the presence of nits or lice in the hair and scalp. The nits or lice are found most often over the postauricular and occipital regions of the head. Less commonly, lice are found on axillary hair, beards, mustaches, eyebrows, and eyelashes. Head lice may be transmitted by close personal contact and perhaps by contact with infested clothing, hairbrushes, furniture, and other objects.

Pediculosis corporis, or body lice, are not actually found directly on the body. The lice move to the body only to feed and are therefore seldom seen. Body lice are more likely to be seen on bed linens and the seams of clothing. Body lice are relatively uncommon in the United States, where regular laundering precludes infestation. Infestations are more often found among the homeless and other people whose clothes are not laundered regularly. The majority of lice can be removed from the body by simply removing the clothes.

Pediculosis pubis (commonly known as crabs) is the presence of nits or lice attached to pubic hairs. Pubic infestations are found only in postpubertal individuals. Common signs and symptoms are pruritus and, occasionally, sky-blue macules on the inner thighs or the lower abdomen. As a rule, pubic infestations are transmitted through sexual contact. Pubic lice are common among persons with multiple sexual partners. Advise patients with pubic lice that sexual partners should be treated and bedding, towels, and clothing washed or dry-cleaned. Pubic lice do not survive longer than 24 hours away from the body.

As a rule, ectoparasitic infestations are treated with topical agents available in the form of shampoos, creams, lotions, and gels. Four successive wet combings are thought to be as effective as an over-the-counter (OTC) product at eliminating lice.

SCABIES

Scabies is a highly communicable disease caused by the itch mite, *Sarcoptes scabiei.* It is transmitted from one person to another by close contact. Transmission between bed partners is common and does not require body contact. Infestation occurs most often along the sides of the fingers, in interdigital webs, and on the flexor surfaces of the wrists, the elbows, the skin around the nipples, and the penis. Other lesions including erythematous papules, lichenified patches, and pustules can occur on the abdomen, the thighs, and the buttocks. In infants and young children, the mites burrow in the palms and the soles, and papular lesions may be seen on the scalp, the face, and the neck.

Intense pruritus begins 2 to 6 weeks after the first exposure. Definitive diagnosis is often difficult because of excoriation. Itching occurs almost exclusively at night, when the pests move around. Nits (eggs) and egg cases may be seen with the naked eye. The head and neck are usually exempt from infestation. Diagnosis depends on observing the mite in skin scrapings, or by gently raising the top of the burrow with a sterile needle, obtaining a sample of *Sarcoptes* mites or parts,

and examining the specimen under high-power magnification. Typically fewer than 10 mites will be found on a human body.

PHARMACOTHERAPEUTIC OPTIONS

Permethrin

Permethrin (Nix, Elimite) is 90% effective in treating lice after a single application. In addition to nits and lice, permethrin is active against fleas and ticks. It acts on the louse's nerve cell membranes to disrupt the sodium channel, thereby delaying repolarization and paralyzing the parasite. The 1% formulation is the drug of choice for lice; the 5% formulation is used for scabies.

Permethrin fails to eradicate head lice in about 5% of patients. Drug resistance is suspected, although evidence is lacking. To manage drug-resistant head lice, some health care providers suggest prolonged treatment. Leave permethrin in the hair for 8 to 14 hours before shampooing and combing, rather than the usual 10 minutes recommended on the package instructions.

Very little of topical permethrin is absorbed. The fraction absorbed is rapidly inactivated and eliminated in the urine. The adverse effects of topical permethrin are few and occur rarely. However, the drug may cause some exacerbation of the itching, erythema, and edema that is commonly seen with pediculosis. Other adverse effects include temporary burning, stinging, and numbness. Do not use permethrin in patients with chrysanthemums sensitivities.

Malathion

The organophosphate pediculicide malathion (Ovide) has been shown to destroy lindane-resistant (see later section on lindane) lice by inhibiting cholinesterase. The drug kills the lice and their eggs. Humans are not harmed, because an enzyme in the blood of the lice converts malathion to

CASE STUDY	Antiprotozoal Drugs
ASSESSMENT	
History of Present Illness	GB, a 63-year-old debilitated male, arrives at the local urgent care center with complaints of a fine rash and bad itching on his hands, feet, and genitalia. The rash first started about 1 to 2 months ago after he moved into a boarding home; has a roommate. Unable to sleep because of itching. His roommate has the same rash and itching. He reports no other illnesses.
Past Health History	He is known to the staff of the urgent care center because of PTSD. He is seen an average 2 to 3 times a year for PTSD-related problems. He takes no routine medications and has no known allergies.
Life-Span Considerations	Unemployed. Lives on social security disability. He has no family in this area. Widower of 5 years. He has a 40-py smoking history.
Physical Exam Findings	Well developed, poorly nourished male in mild distress. Evidence of scratching on interdigital webs, flexor surfaces of wrists, ankles, genitalia, perineum, and inner thighs. Heavy perineal involvement. Burrows noted in areas of scratching.
Diagnostic Testing	Microscopic hair and skin sampling obtained from burrows in affected areas reveal mites, eggs, and cases.

DIAGNOSIS: Scabies; posttraumatic stress disorder

MANAGEMENT

Treatment Objectives	1. Clear infestation of pediculus corporis. 2. Relieve pruritus. 3. Avoid secondary infection from scratching.
Treatment Plan	Investigate and treat source(s) of infestation. **Pharmacotherapy** • permethrin 5% cream as single-dose regimen applied from neck down at bedtime and washed off in AM. Repeat same treatment in 1 week. • fexofenadine 180 mg each AM • diphenhydramine 25 mg PO at bedtime **Patient Education** 1. Remember, while you may be distressed by the thought of the bugs, scabies is not a reflection on personal hygiene. 2. It's easier said than done, but try to avoid scratching. Take fexofenadine or cetirizine and diphenhydramine regularly to help with itching. 3. Arrange to have all personal clothing and linens dry-cleaned or laundered in hottest water possible. Clean clothing hanging in a closet is okay. 4. Keep appointment with dermatology clinic in 1 week. 5. Discuss with boarding home supervisor the need for a thorough vacuuming of carpets and bedding; personal item that cannot be laundered may also be placed in a sealed plastic bag and placed in the garage for 2 weeks. Mites will die after 1 week if they have not eaten. 6. No alcohol or driving when taking diphenhydramine **Evaluation** 1. No evidence of eggs, nits, or lice 2. No evidence of secondary infection 3. Pruritus is lessening.

CLINICAL REASONING ANALYSIS

Q1. **I am new on the infectious disease service and haven't seen scabies before. How is it treated?**
A. The treatment of choice at the moment is permethrin, in view of its relative safety, ease of application, and the fact that is tends not to irritate the skin. The 5% permethrin cream is applied to the skin from the neck down, including the palms of the hands, under fingernails, the soles of the feet, and the groin and the thighs at bedtime, and washed off the next morning. It should be left on for 8 to 14 hours. A second treatment 1 week later usually takes care of the infestation.

Q2. **And then his itch will go away?**
A. The treatment kills the mites, but their bodies are still in the skin; and since it is the bodies that cause the itch, the itch will remain until his natural defense systems break down and get rid of what is left of the mites. This process takes about 2 weeks, and therefore the itch will continue for about 2 weeks after treatment.

Q3. **What about all the people he lives with? Will he give it to them when he returns to the boarding home tonight?**
A The critical issue in treating scabies is the elimination of the mites. Although not everyone in the boarding home may be experiencing itching, symptoms may not manifest for 6 to 8 weeks (the incubation time). If not everyone is treated, the infestation can continue to spread.

IMMUNE

nontoxic metabolites. The drug is approved for the treatment of head lice.

The formulation used for lead lice is typically devoid of significant adverse effects, although scalp irritation sometimes occurs. No systemic toxicity has been reported, and there are no known drug interactions. Instruct patients that hair dryers and other sources of heat should be avoided until the drug has dried, since the lotion is 78% alcohol by content, and that the head should not be covered while the drug is drying.

Crotamiton

Crotamiton (Eurax) is used in the treatment of scabies but not for pediculosis. It has scabicidal activity and may help to relieve the itching through an independent mechanism. Mild adverse effects include dermatitis and conjunctivitis, although these are uncommon.

Lindane

At one time, lindane (Kwell) was the drug of choice for pediculosis and scabies. However, owing to the risk of seizures, the FDA now recommends that lindane be reserved for patients who do not respond to safer drugs such as permethrin or malathion. Avoid repeated dosing of lindane. Do not use during pregnancy, in women who are breastfeeding, for infants, or for anyone who falls under the any of the following categories:

- Has atopic dermatitis or psoriasis
- Has open or crusted lesions or extensive areas of broken skin in the treatment area
- Has not tried a safer drug for lice and scabies eradication
- Has used lindane in the past few months
- Has a seizure disorder or a history of seizures
- Had an adverse effect to lindane in the past

KEY POINTS

HELMINTHIASIS

- Helminthiasis, an infestation of parasitic worms, is a major health problem in many parts of the world.
- The presence of worms is called an "infestation" rather than an "infection."
- Roundworms, hookworms, tapeworms, threadworms, and pinworms make up the bulk of helminth infestations. Trematodes are the so-called flukes of the worm world.
- A variety of drugs are used in the treatment of infestation and act directly or indirectly to interfere with the life cycle of the adult parasite.
- The primary treatment objective is to kill or destroy the adult worm, thus reducing the worm load.
- Adherence and dependability of the patient being treated are crucial factors for successful elimination of the parasites.

MALARIA

- Malaria remains a devastating human infestation in parts of the world where the *Anopheles* mosquito continues to flourish.
- The pharmacodynamics of antimalarial drugs are unclear, but they appear to bind to a product of heme breakdown that is highly lytic to RBCs and to accumulate in the acidic lysosome compartments of the parasite.

- Treatment objectives for malaria include a reduction in or elimination of signs and symptoms, and decreasing patient discomfort.
- Prophylaxis and treatment regimens should be followed closely to prevent adverse drug effects as well as to promote efficacy.

PROTOZOAL INFESTATIONS

- Leishmaniasis is a spectrum of diseases caused by a variety of protozoal species. The disease is transmitted to humans by the bites of infected female sandflies.
- The two principal *Leishmania* species cause distinct diseases and differ in geographic distribution and species of vector.
- Treatment for leishmaniasis relies most often on antimonial compounds (heavy metals).

ECTOPARASITIC INFESTATIONS

- Ectoparasites live on the outer surfaces of the body as infestations by mites and lice. The two most common infestations are scabies and pediculosis.
- Scabies and pediculosis are highly communicable.
- The drug of choice for the treatment of scabies is permethrin, but crotamiton is also effective.
- For pediculosis, the drug of choice is permethrin, although malathion is also useful.

Bibliography

Abramowicz, M. (Ed.). (2004). Drugs for parasitic infections. *The Medical Letter, 46*(1198), 1–12.

Aksoy, D., Kerimoglu, U., Oto., A., et al. (2005). Infection with *Fasciola hepatica. Clinical Microbiology and Infections, 11*(11), 859–861.

Berg, R. (Ed.) (1993). *APIC curriculum for infection control practice.* Dubuque, Iowa: Kendall Hunt.

Centers for Disease Control and Prevention. *Malaria.* Available online: www2.ncid.cdc.gov/travel/yb/utils/ybGet.asp?section =dis&obj=index.htm&cssNav=browsecyb. Accessed May 2, 2007.

Crompton, D., Crompton C., and Crompton, D. (2006). *Handbook of human helminthiasis for public health.* Boca Raton, FL: CRC Press.

Del Brutto, O., Roos, K., Coffey, C., et al. (2006). Meta-analysis: Cysticidal drugs for neurocysticercosis: Albendazole and praziquantel. *Annals of Internal Medicine, 145*(1), 43–51.

Enk. C. (2006). Onchocerciasis–river blindness. *Clinics in Dermatology, 24*(3), 176–180.

Garcia, H., Evans, C., Nash, T., et al. (2003). Consesus: Current guidelines for the treatment of neurocysticercosis. *Clinical Microbiology Reviews, 15*(4), 747–756.

Gatton, M., Martin, L., and Cheng, Q. (2004). Evolution of resistance to sulfadoxine-pyrimethamine in *Plasmodium falciparum. Antimicrobial Agents and Chemotherapy*, June, 2116–2123.

Gilbert, D., Moellering, R., and Eliopoulos, G. (2007). *The Sanford guide to antimicrobial therapy.* (37th ed.). Hyde Park, VT: Antimicrobial Therapy.

Martin, M., and Humphreys, M. (2006). Social consequence of disease in the American South: 1900-World War II. *Southern Medical Journal, 99*(8), 862–864.

Minodier, P., and Parola, P. (2007). Cutaneous leishmaniasis treatment. *Travel Medicine and Infectious Disease, 5*(3), 150–158.

Rose, S., and Keystone, J. (2006). International Travel Health Guide: 2006–2007. Philadelphia: Mosby.

Shoff, W., Chen, E., and Shepherd. S. (2005). Shistosomiasis (Parts I and II). *Infectious Disease Practice, 29,* 419–436.

Zaccome, P., Fehervari, Z., Phillips, J., et al. (2006). Parasitic worms and inflammatory disease. *Parasite Immunology, 28*(10), 515–523.

IMMUNE

31

Sera, Vaccines, and Other Immunizing Drugs

Many infectious diseases can be prevented through active or passive immunization, which offers an opportunity not only to prevent disease but also to improve clinical outcomes for those at high risk, and realize significant savings to the person in terms of cost, time, and resources. Vaccines are one of the most effective disease prevention tools available in the world. Widespread immunization of children in the United States led to a reduction of over 90% of all childhood diseases. Although there is a propensity to focus on the immunizations of infants and children, prophylaxis is essential for all age groups, including adults.

Immunizations are considered the most basic of all preventive health care strategies. The effectiveness of immunization campaigns has been demonstrated through a measurable reduction in the *incidence* of vaccine-preventable infectious disease in this country. The *prevalence* rate of vaccine-preventable diseases is one of the traditional measures of the quality and effectiveness of a nation's overall health care delivery system.

IMMUNITY

Immunity is a state in which the host is resistant to a specific disease. Immunity can be innate or acquired. The terms *vaccination* and *immunization* are often used interchangeably to refer to active immunization, although they are not synonymous (Box 31-1). The administration of a vaccination cannot be equated with the development of immunity.

TYPES OF IMMUNITY

Innate Immunity
Innate immunity is nonspecific and derived from all of the elements with which a person is born. It is always available on short notice to protect the body from challenges by foreign agents. Innate immunity is conferred via physical, cellular, and chemical barriers. Physical barriers include skin, mucous membranes, and the cough reflex. Phagocytic cells make up the cellular barrier. Biologically active substances including degradative enzymes, toxic free radicals, and lipids, together with low pH, are barriers to invasion by foreign agents. These nonspecific defense mechanisms work against all foreign agents; no recognition of a specific agent is required. The innate system does not confer long-lasting immunity to the host.

▮▮ Antigens
Antigens (Ags) are defined as a live or inactivated substance (i.e., protein or polysaccharide) capable of producing an immune response. Two types of lymphocytes originate from stem cells in the bone marrow: T lymphocytes (T cells) and B lymphocytes (B cells). When an Ag is first introduced into the body, it is phagocytized by a macrophage, which then transfers the Ag to T cells. The T cells contain a receptor for that specific Ag and become activated. Both the macrophage and the activated T cells secrete substances that stimulate replication of the activated T cells. Some activated T cells (i.e., killer cells [TK]) destroy cells containing the Ag. The T cells that provide long-term acquired immunity are called memory T cells (TM). These cells recognize a specific Ag, thereby stimulating a faster and more intense response if the same Ag is encountered again.

▮▮ Antibodies
Antibodies (Abs) are specific proteins released from B cells. B cells are responsible for *humoral immunity*. Like T cells, each B cell responds to only one Ag. Unlike T cells, B cells do not act directly on the Ag but instead are responsible for the production of antibodies that react with the Ag or substances produced by the Ag. Abs are found in body fluids. Ab-mediated immunity is most effective against bacteria, viruses that are outside body cells, and toxins.

In general, all antibodies have a similar amino acid structure, but one portion of the molecule is different. That component allows each Ab the ability to react with a specific Ag. They belong to a class of proteins known as globulins. Because they are involved in the immune response they are known as *immunoglobulins.*

An Ab is an immunoglobulin (Ig) with a specific amino acid sequence that gives it the ability to adhere to and interact only with a specific Ag. This initial action is the primary response (Fig. 31-1). When Ags are destroyed, macrophages clean up the debris, and T suppressor cells reduce the immune response. Memory B cells remain dormant in lymphatic tissue until the same Ag again enters the body. The TM cells recognize the Ag and launch a rapid and intense response. This is called a secondary response. The purpose of vaccinations is to provide an initial exposure so TM cells are available for a rapid and intense response against subsequent exposure to the Ag.

There are five classes of antibodies (i.e., immunoglobulins): IgM, IgG, IgA, IgE, and IgD. They differ not only in their specific physiologic roles in immunity but also in their structures. IgM is the first Ab produced during a primary immune response and is distributed primarily in intravascular spaces. IgM reflects an early response of the immune system; it eliminates pathogens in the early stages of B cell–mediated immunity (i.e., before there is sufficient IgG to do the job). IgM activates complement and is efficient in agglutinating Ab. The serum half-life of IgM ranges from 8 to 23 hours.

IgG reflects immunity of longer standing and is found after infection. Immunoglobulins of the IgG class are called *gamma globulins.* IgG is most abundant in the serum but is also found in the intravascular and extravascular spaces. IgG is responsible for most responses to Ags, including activation of complement, sensitization of target cells for destruction by TK cells,

BOX 31-1

Terminology of Immunizations

Active immunity—Protection that is produced by a person's own immune system

Acquired immunity—Develops after a person has contracted an illness or has been injected with a vaccine or a toxoid

Antisera—A serum containing antibodies. Usually obtained from an animal that received the antigen, either by injection into the tissues or blood, or by infection

Antitoxins—A specific antibody manufactured in the body in response to the presence of a toxin

Attenuated vaccine—The result of changing the virulence of a disease-causing virus by repeated culturing in a laboratory

Incidence—The number of new cases of a specific disease occurring during a certain period

Immunity—A state in which a person is resistant to a specific disease

Live virus—A virus that replicates in the body and creates enough virus to stimulate an immune response

Innate immunity – A natural, nonspecific immunity that is provided through receptors encoded in a person's germline

Immunization— Term used when referring to active immunization

Passive immunity—Achieved by introducing antibodies into a human that are produced by an animal or another human

Prevalence—The total number of cases of a specific disease in existence in a given population at a given time

Sera—The blood serum from persons or animals whose bodies have built antibodies, called antisera or immune serum. Used when person has already been exposed or contracted the disease. Plural for *serum*

Seroconversion—The change of a serologic test from negative to positive, indicating the development of antibodies in response to immunization or infection

Trivalent—An antibody with three antigen binding sites

Toxoid—A toxin treated by heat or a chemical agent to destroy its deleterious properties. The toxin's pathogenic quality is destroyed, but its antigenic properties remain.

Vaccine—A suspension of live or attenuated organisms administered for the purpose of establishing active immunity to an infectious disease

Vaccination—Term used when referring to active immunization

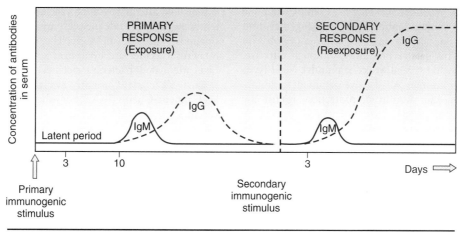

FIGURE 31-1 Time course of antibody release on first exposure vs. subsequent exposure.

neutralization of toxins and viruses, and immobilization of bacteria. IgG crosses the placenta and is present in colostrum. The serum half-life of IgG is approximately 5 hours.

IgA is part of the first-line immune barriers in mucosa but is also found in intravascular spaces and breast milk. IgA recognizes the Ag and immobilizes it through agglutination, and its effector functions eliminate the Ag. IgA's external function is that of protection against various forms of bacterial and viral aggression. Its general mechanism is "the immune exclusion of antigens" (i.e., prevention of the penetration of Ags into the organism by confining them to external secretions followed by elimination). The serum half-life of IgA is 6 hours.

IgE mediates hypersensitivity and allergic reactions. It is found in parasitic infections as an allergic response and is located on basophils and mast cells and in saliva and nasal secretions. The serum half-life of IgE is 2.5 hours.

IgD is located on the surface of B lymphocytes, with a trace found in the serum. IgD functions primarily as an Ag-specific receptor on B cells and is thought to be involved with differentiation of B cells. The half-life of IgD is 2.5 to 3 hours.

Natural Immunity

Natural Passive Immunity

The most common type of passive immunity comes into being when antibodies are transferred from a pregnant woman across the placenta to the infant before birth. These antibodies, IgG developed by the mother in response to the pathogens she encountered throughout her lifetime, are often called "maternal antibodies." They protect the infant, for the first 6 months of life, against illnesses to which the mother is immune. Breast milk contains IgA, which may extend the length of protection. Natural passive immunity provides protection as long as the Ab remains in the blood and is active. This is unlike natural active immunity, which lasts a lifetime.

Natural Active Immunity

A person can achieve natural active immunity by having the disease. For example, a child with chicken pox responds to the virus by developing Ab. After initial exposure the child does not get chicken pox again because the immune system has a ready supply of Ab and T$_M$ cells that respond quickly to the second exposure to chicken pox. Because the body produced the Ab with no stimulation by deliberate, artificial means such as a vaccination, this type of immunity is called *natural active immunity*.

Acquired Immunity

The body also has an ability to develop specific immunity against Ag such as lethal bacteria, viruses, toxins, and even foreign tissues from other animals, without actually developing the disease state. This is called *acquired immunity* and, unlike innate immunity, is not present at birth but develops as the infant grows and matures. Acquired immunity is not fully exhibited until the person has had two sequential exposures to the same Ag. Each Ag contains one or more specific components that make it different from all others. In general these are proteins, large polysaccharides, or lipids found on cell surfaces. The Ag initiates the acquired immune response when attacked by lymphocytes.

Acquired Passive Immunity

Ab from another person or animal can be injected or transfused to provide *acquired passive immunity*. For example, immune globulin (Ig), which contains antibodies pooled together from the blood of many donors, can be injected into a person who needs antibodies. This passive immunity, although effective, usually disappears within several weeks or months. Most types of transfused blood contain Ab. Passive acquired immunity provides immediate, but short-lived, protection against the injurious Ag.

Acquired Active Immunity

Acquired active immunity, which can also be termed *artificial immunity* to help distinguish it from natural active immunity, is achieved by deliberately administering a specific vaccine or toxoid. A vaccine is an Ag-containing substance injected into a person in an attempt to stimulate Ab production. The vaccine usually consists of attenuated, inactivated, or killed pathogens or their toxins. The Ags still stimulate the immune system, but they are altered so they do not produce symptoms of the disease. Because a vaccine stimulates the body to produce its own Ab, active immunity is induced.

A vaccine can be prepared from the toxin secreted by a pathogen. The toxin is altered to reduce its harmfulness, but still acts as an Ag to induce an immune response. The altered toxin is known as a *toxoid*. Because a toxoid incites Ab production, it also produces active immunity.

DRUGS FOR ACTIVE IMMUNITY

Natural immunity is the basis for development of most immunizations and vaccines, but the results are not completely equivalent. With the injection of an Ag, the immune system responds by producing Ab. It is often assumed that active immunization provides lifelong protection the way natural active immunity does, but in reality, it does not. Periodic boosters are needed with many vaccinations to further stimulate Ab production to maintain acquired, active immunity (Table 31-1).

Vaccines

There are two general classes of vaccines, viral and bacterial. Viral vaccines include live attenuated viruses (e.g., measles, mumps, rubella, varicella, influenza [intranasal]); inactivated whole virus (e.g., influenza, rabies, inactivated poliovirus, hepatitis A); and antigenic components of the virus particle (e.g., influenza "split-virus" vaccine, hepatitis B vaccine, acellular pertussis). Because the microorganisms found in these formulations cannot replicate in the host, inactivated viral vaccines must contain sufficient amounts of Ag to induce the desired immune response. Repeated dosing is usually necessary to provoke long-term immunity.

Live Attenuated Vaccines

Live attenuated viruses (LAVs) generate an immune response when they replicate within the vaccinated person. LAVs usually do not cause disease and are usually effective with one dose. Disease resulting from an LAV is generally moderate compared to the "wild-type" disease-causing organism, and is labeled as an adverse effect. Severe adverse effects caused by LAVs are usually seen in persons who are immune-suppressed (e.g., those with human immunodeficiency virus [HIV], patients on antineoplastic therapies).

The live attenuated viral vaccines (LAVVs) that are currently available include measles, mumps, rubella, yellow fever, smallpox, varicella, and varicella zoster. Live oral polio and rotavirus vaccines are no longer used in the United States. Live attenuated bacterial vaccines (LABV) are made from weakened bacteria. Currently available LABVs include bacillus Calmette-Guérin (BCG), for tuberculosis, and oral typhoid vaccines.

Inactivated Vaccines

Inactivated vaccines can be made from whole viruses or bacteria, or fractions of either. Inactivated virus cannot cause disease. The inactivated vaccines include (1) *fractionated vaccines* that are protein-based such as hepatitis B, influenza, and acellular pertussis; (2) polysaccharide-based vaccines such as pneumococcal, meningococcal, and *Salmonella typhi* (with virulence [Vi] antigen); (3) *whole-cell vaccines* composed of a polysaccharide such as polio, rabies, and hepatitis A; (4) *conjugate vaccines*, which are chemically altered proteins combined with polysaccharides, such as *Haemophilus* influenza, type b, and pneumococcal vaccines; and (5) *toxoids*, which are protein-based, inactivated bacterial toxins and subvirion products such as diphtheria and tetanus. There are no whole-cell bacterial vaccines in use in the United States.

In conjugate vaccines, the chemical bond between a protein and a polysaccharide increases the potency of the polysaccharide vaccine; however, the Ab titer diminishes over time. The predominant Ab produced by polysaccharide vaccines is IgM; little IgG is produced. Multiple doses of inactivated protein vaccines cause the antibody level to increase; this is not seen with polysaccharide vaccines.

Recombinant vaccines are produced by placing a segment of an organism's gene, such as hepatitis B, into the gene of a yeast cell. In this example, the altered yeast cell produces pure hepatitis B surface Ag during growth. There are two other recombinant vaccines, typhoid and influenza. Live typhoid vaccine (i.e., Ty21a) is genetically modified from *Salmonella typhi* and does not cause illness. Another example is that of

TABLE 31-1 Drugs for Active Immunity

Drug	FRM	Indications	Efficacy and Duration	Implications
Bacille Calmette-Guérin (TICE BCG)	LA/L	TB in adults and children with negative skin tests who reside in high risk households; for HCW exposed to resistant TB; travelers to areas with endemic disease	Protection variable Duration variable	Avoid persons with active TB for 6–12 wk after immunization. Conduct postvaccination TB test in 2–3 mo. Repeat dose in 2–3 mo if still TB-negative.
Hepatitis A vaccine (Havrix)	IVV	Prophylaxis for high-risk persons including military personnel and travelers to areas with endemic disease	Efficacy: 80%–98% Duration: 10 yr Booster: after 6–12 mL	May give concurrently with other travel vaccines without interfering with immune responses. Contraindications: bleeding disorders or febrile illness
Hepatitis B vaccine (Energix B, Heptavax B, Recombivax B)	IVV	Prophylaxis for infants, young children, and persons with environmental or lifestyle risk, including those with hemophilia or who are on dialysis	Efficacy: 96% children; 88% adults Duration: Unknown	Dialysis patients should receive special formulation of 40 mcg surface antigen/mL
Influenza vaccine (Fluogen, Fluzone, FluShield, Fluvirin, Flu-Immune, Influenza Virus, Vaccine)	IVV	Prophylaxis for adults over age 65, persons with asthma or COPD, and health care providers	Efficacy: 60%–75% Maximum Ab protection in 2 wk Duration: 1 mo	Children <9 yr not previously immunized need two doses 1 mo apart. Contraindications: egg allergy, history of Guillain-Barré syndrome
Japanese encephalitis vaccine (JE-VAX)	IVV	Prophylaxis for adults and children traveling to or residing in areas with endemic disease	Effectiveness: 78% after second dose, 99% after third dose Duration: 3–6 mo	Do not travel within 10 days of vaccination. Booster in 1–3 years depending on exposure
Lyme vaccine (LYMErix)	RLP	Prophylaxis for persons age 15–70 yr residing in high-risk areas	Unknown at this time	Safety and efficacy dependent on administration of second and third doses several weeks before onset of *Borrelia* transmission season
Measles-mumps-rubella vaccine (MMR II)	LAVV	Children to age 12 yr	Efficacy: 95% Duration: Years to life Second dose on entry to grade school, middle school, or high school	Contraindications: allergy to eggs or neomycin Combination drug preferred over single formulations
Measles vaccine (Attenuvax; rubeola)	LAVV	Children and adults born after 1956 without a history of measles or LVV on or after their first birthday	Efficacy: 95% Duration: Years to life	Usually given with mumps and rubella vaccines. May invalidate TB test if given within 6 wk of immunization
Measles-rubella vaccine (MR-vax II)	LAVV	Susceptible persons >12 yrs who have immunity to mumps	Duration: 8 yr	A mixture of live attenuated rubeola virus and rubella virus
Meningococcal vaccine (Menomune-A/C/Y/W-135)	IBV	Military personnel, persons without a spleen or who are immunosuppressed, and those with household, institutional, or travel contact with the disease	Efficacy: 90% in adults; variable in young children Duration: 3 yr Effectiveness drops to 67% after 3 yr.	Not for routine immunization
Mumps vaccine (Mumpsvax)	LAVV	Adults born after 1956 without history of mumps or LVV on or after their first birthday	Efficacy: Permanent immunity in 75%–90% of patients Duration: 10 yr	Not for routine immunization
Mumps-rubella vaccine (Biavax II)	LVV	Susceptible persons >12 yr old; except pregnant women	Permanent immunity	Used less often than MMR
Pneumococcal vaccine (Pneumovax 23, Pnu-Imune 23)	IBV	Adults >65 yr and persons at risk, including those with weakened immune systems, cancers, organ transplants, or chronic diseases	Duration: Years	Available as heptavalant conjugate or polysaccharide; check formulation before using. Contraindication: hypersensitivity to phenol
Pneumococcal 7-valent (Prevnar)	IBV	Universal immunization of children 2–23 mo and high-risk children 24–59 mo	Efficacy: 92%–100% Duration: Unknown	Requires a series of four injections
Poliovirus vaccine [Salk] (IPV, IPOL)	IVV	Children 6 wk to adulthood and adults at high risk	Efficacy: 90% Booster required	Although protective immune response cannot be assured in compromised individual, IPV is still recommended because the vaccine is safe and some protection may result from its administration.
Rabies human diploid cell vaccine (HDCV, Imovax)	KVV	Preexposure prophylaxis for persons at risk through animal handling; postexposure prophylaxis	Boosters recommended	For postexposure prophylaxis, administer rabies immunoglobulin (RHIg) at same time as initial dose of HDCV
Rabies vaccine (Absorbed, RVA)	IV	Postexposure prophylaxis in adults	Duration: 2 yr	Check Ab levels after 2 years; give booster if needed.
Rubella (Meruvax II)	LAV	Persons >12 yr old, nonpregnant women, postpartum women with no history of immunization, and persons traveling to areas with endemic disease	Efficacy: 95% Duration: 6–15 yr Booster not recommended	Contraindications: pregnancy, immunosuppression, allergy to neomycin
Smallpox (calf lymph, DryVax)	LVV	Preexposure and postexposure prophylaxis	Efficacy: Unknown Duration: Unknown	Vaccine take rate is >90% for current stockpile of drug.
Typhoid vaccine (Ty2 *S. typhi*)	IBV	Military personnel and persons in or traveling to areas with endemic disease	Efficacy: 70%–90% Duration: 3 yr Booster: 5 yr later	Avoid concurrent use with antibiotics or within 7 days of antibiotic use.

IMMUNE

Continued

TABLE 31-1 Drugs for Active Immunity—Cont'd

Drug	FRM	Indications	Efficacy and Duration	Implications
Typhoid oral TY21a (Vivotif Berna)	LAVV	Persons in or traveling to areas with endemic disease	Duration: 6 yr Booster required	Avoid concurrent use with antibiotics or within 7 days of antibiotic use.
Varicella vaccine (Varivax)	LAVV	Healthy adults and children with no history of chicken pox	Efficacy: 96%–97% ages 1–12 yr; 79% ages 13–17 yr	Can be given along with MMR, using separate syringes and injection sites.
Yellow-fever (YF-Vax)	LAVV	Persons >9 yr who are living in or traveling to areas of So. America or Africa where yellow fever is endemic	Efficacy: 100% after 7–10 days Duration: 10 yr	Caution advised in patients with allergy to chicken or egg products. Contraindications: children <6 mo, during pregnancy, immunosuppression
TOXOIDS				
Diphtheria-tetanus-acellular pertussis (DTaP, Acel-Immune, Tripedia, Infanrix)	T	Children 2 mo–7 yr	Efficacy: High, 10 yr Boosters required for tetanus toxoid component	Decreases serious adverse effects associated with whole-cell vaccine
Tetanus-diphtheria vaccine (Adult absorbed type, Td)	T	Adults and susceptible children >7 yr	Duration: 10 yr Booster required every 6–10 yr	Reactions are usually mild.
Tetanus-diphtheria (Pediatric, DT)	T	Adults and routine administration for children up to 6 yr in whom pertussis vaccine is contraindicated	Duration: 10 yr	Do not administer to child with a fever or to someone with history of neurologic or severe hypersensitivity reaction to previous dose.
Tetanus toxoid	T	All children and adults	Efficacy: High Duration: 10 yr Booster required	Available as fluid and absorbed formulations containing different concentrations of tetanus toxoid

Ab, Antibody; *COPD*, chronic obstructive pulmonary disease; *FRM*, formulation; *HCW*, health care worker; *IBV*, inactivated bacterial vaccine; *IWV*, inactivated whole cell virus; *KVV*, killed viral vaccine; *LAVV*, live attenuated viral vaccine; *LA/L*, live attenuated/live; *RLP*, recombinant lipoprotein; *T*, toxoid.

the live attenuated influenza vaccine; it has as been genetically modified to effectively replicate in the nasopharynx but not the lungs.

DISEASES AND DRUGS OF ACTIVE IMMUNITY

Diphtheria, Tetanus, and Pertussis

Diphtheria results from infection by *Corynebacterium diphtheriae*. The endotoxin leaves patches of an adherent grayish membrane with surrounding inflammation on the tonsils, the pharynx, the larynx, the anterior nose, and, occasionally, other mucous membranes. The skin and sometimes the conjunctivae or the genitalia are affected. Late effects appear 2 to 6 weeks after absorption of the toxin and include neuritis, most often affecting motor nerves with paralysis of the soft palate, the eye muscles, the limbs, and the diaphragm, and myocarditis.

Formerly a prevalent disease, diphtheria has largely disappeared in areas with effective immunization programs. Immunity is often acquired through asymptomatic infection. Recovery from a clinical attack of diphtheria is not always followed by lasting immunity. Prolonged active immunity can be induced by toxoid. Diphtheria vaccine provides active immunity and is most often administered in combination with tetanus (DT, Td), or with tetanus and acellular pertussis (DTaP, TdaP).

Tetanus is a bacterial infection resulting from the *Clostridium tetani* exotoxin tetanospasmin. *C. tetani* is a large, grampositive, nonencapsulated bacillus with terminal spores that lives in the soil. The organisms require strict anaerobic conditions for growth and toxin elaboration and are very resistant to destruction. The exotoxin invades devitalized tissue. Fifty to 90 cases of tetanus and 20 to 30 deaths are reported annually in the United States. Approximately 60% of the cases occur in

persons older than 60 years. Tetanus is more common in areas where contact with animal feces is likely and immunization inadequate. The disease is characterized by painful muscular contractions, primarily of the masseter and neck muscles. Trunk muscles may be involved secondarily.

Td is routinely administered to adults to provide immunity against both tetanus and diphtheria. Ab levels wane 10 years after administration. The Td vaccine is formulated with a lower "adult" dose of diphtheria toxoid than in the DT vaccine, because adverse reactions to that component increase with age. Td has 2 units of diphtheria per dose, in contrast to pediatric formulations that contain 6.7 to 12.5 units per dose.

Childhood immunization with DTaP, adolescent immunization with TdaP (with the lower dose of diphtheria toxoid), adult immunization with Td, and careful wound management has reduced the incidence of tetanus. Susceptibility to the disease is directly related to immunization status. The primary immunization series is given in infancy; booster doses are needed every 10 years.

Human tetanus Ig is a solution of globulins derived from the plasma of people hyperimmunized with tetanus toxoid. Human tetanus Ig is used to prevent tetanus in patients with wounds possibly contaminated with *C. tetani*. It is also recommended for patients whose immunization history is uncertain, or that includes less than two immunizing doses of tetanus toxoid. It is used in the treatment of tetanus. Give tetanus toxoid at the same time as the Ig formulation to initiate active immunization.

Pertussis (commonly known as whooping cough) is an acute bacterial infection of the respiratory tract. It is caused by the gram-negative bacillus *Bordetella pertussis*. The initial catarrhal stage (inflammation of mucous membranes with free discharge) has an insidious onset with an irritating cough that gradually becomes paroxysmal. This stage usually develops within 1 to 2 weeks of exposure and lasts 1 to 2 months or longer. Paroxysmal coughing episodes commonly end with the expulsion of clear, tenacious mucus, followed by vomiting. Adults and infants under 6 months of age often do not have the cough with the typical "whoop" sound.

Acellular pertussis vaccines contain inactivated pertussis toxin and may contain one or more other bacterial components. There is considerably less endotoxin found in acellular pertussis vaccines than whole-cell pertussis vaccines. Mild local and systemic adverse events occur less frequently among infants vaccinated with acellular pertussis vaccines for the first three or four doses than among those vaccinated with whole-cell DTP. Infants who receive acellular pertussis vaccines generally experience the more serious adverse events (e.g., fever greater than or equal to 105° F, crying lasting more than 3 hours, hypotonic hyporesponsive episodes, and seizures) less frequently than infants vaccinated with whole-cell DTP.

Complications of pertussis include pneumonia, seizures, and encephalitis. Approximately 90% of deaths are children under 1 year of age, with 75% in those younger than 6 months. Morbidity and mortality is higher in females. In nonimmunized populations, particularly patients with underlying malnutrition and multiple enteric and respiratory infections, pertussis is the most lethal disease of infants and young children. Pneumonia is the most common cause of death.

Standard pertussis vaccines were introduced in the 1950s, resulting in a marked decline in the incidence of pertussis. The disease is on the rise again, however, largely owing to waning of the immunity in adolescent and adult populations. The acellular vaccines DTaP and TdaP are currently used.

Pediarix, the first five-component vaccine licensed in the United States, was approved by the FDA in 2002. Pediarix is composed of DTaP, hepatitis B, and inactivated polio vaccine (IPV). Pediarix can be administered at 2 months of age, with two additional doses administered at 6- to 8-week intervals. Pediarix is not approved for the fourth and fifth doses of DTaP and IPV.

▥ Adverse Effects and Contraindications

Both local and systemic effects can occur with administration of DT, DTaP, TdaP, or Td vaccines. Most reactions occur within 48 hours of vaccine administration and include redness, swelling, and pain at the injection site. A nodule may be palpable at the injection site. Local reactions occur most commonly; mild systemic reactions are less common, and neurologic reactions are the least common. Systemic effects include fever, drowsiness, persistent and inconsolable crying in infants, anorexia, vomiting, collapse, and seizures. Severe systemic reactions (generalized urticaria, anaphylaxis, or neurologic complications) have rarely been reported following administration of DT, DTaP, TdaP, or Td.

The Advisory Committee on Immunization Practices (ACIP) states that DTaP or TdaP vaccination is contraindicated in patients who have had an immediate anaphylactic reaction, encephalopathy occurring within 7 days after vaccination that is not related to another cause, or any acute, severe, central nervous system disorder occurring within 7 days following vaccination. Contraindications also include

major alterations in consciousness, unresponsiveness, and generalized or focal seizures persisting longer than a few hours with failure to recover within 24 hours.

Haemophilus Influenza, Type B

Before the introduction of the vaccine, *Haemophilus* influenza, type B (*H. influenza* B, or Hib, which generally signifies the vaccine rather than the organism), was the leading cause of bacterial infection in preschool children, with an estimated 12,000 cases of meningitis occurring annually as a result of infection. As many as 6% of meningitis patients died, and up to 30% of survivors suffered permanent damage, which ranged from mild hearing loss to profound mental retardation. *H. influenza* infection is seen most often in children between the ages of 3 months and 3 years.

H. influenza B are gram-negative coccobacilli consisting of both encapsulated and nonencapsulated strains. The virulence of the bacterium is attributed to its outer capsule, which triggers an unusual immune response difficult for infants to handle. Nonencapsulated strains are common constituents of upper respiratory flora and can cause otitis media, sinusitis, and bronchitis.

The first Hib vaccines licensed for use in the United States contained polyribosyl ribitol phosphate (PRP) and were effective against type B strains in children at 18 months of age. Because most Hib invasive disease occurs in infants and children younger than 18 months, a vaccine using the PRP polysaccharide attached to protein carriers was developed and licensed for use in infants. Four conjugate vaccines are now available for use in infants. All have similar efficacy. The carrier proteins used in three of these are derived from the toxoids used in the DTP vaccine.

The major component of the Hib vaccine is a capsular polysaccharide. The polysaccharide is T cell–independent, because it does not stimulate a T_M response. It is attached to a protein to enhance its immunogenicity in infants, who have more immature immune systems. Infants less than 7 months old require multiple doses of Hib conjugate to reach protective levels of anticapsular Ab. Hib conjugate vaccines may be administered simultaneously with DTaP, IPV, measles-mumps-rubella (MMR), influenza, and hepatitis B vaccines.

▥ Adverse Effects and Contraindications

Adverse reactions to polysaccharide conjugate vaccines are rare. These vaccines are considered the safest of all vaccine products. Swelling, redness, and pain at the injection site have been reported but usually resolve in 12 to 24 hours. Systemic reactions such as fever and irritability are uncommon. Vaccination with Hib conjugate vaccine is contraindicated in persons known to have had anaphylaxis following a prior dose of the vaccine.

Hepatitis A

Hepatitis A virus (HAV) occurs worldwide. It is caused by an RNA virus, a member of the picornavirus group (a positive-stranded RNA virus) and spread by the fecal-oral route to replicate in the liver. HAV is characterized by fever, malaise, anorexia, nausea, and abdominal discomfort. Jaundice follows these symptoms within a few days. The disease can range in severity from a mild illness that lasts 1 to 2 weeks to an incapacitating manifestation of several months. The mortality rate is low (0.6%). When death occurs, it is usually in an older adult with fulminant disease. Most infections in infants and preschool children are either asymptomatic or cause mild, nonspecific symptoms without jaundice. The highest rates of hepatitis A are among children 5 to 14 years of age.

HAV vaccine is licensed for use in persons 1 year of age and older, travelers going to areas with endemic disease, and other high-risk groups. High-risk groups include international travelers, men who have sex with men, IV drug users, immunocompromised persons with occupational risk, and persons with chronic liver diseases, including hepatitis C. Continue to routinely vaccinate persons at increased risk for hepatitis A or those who are at increased risk for complications from HAV infection. This two-dose series (or three doses if combined with hepatitis B) can be administered simultaneously with other vaccines and toxoids.

▌▌ *Adverse Effects and Contraindications*

Mild injection site soreness, erythema, or swelling occurs in 20% to 50% of patients. Transient headache, fatigue, fever, malaise, anorexia, and nausea have been reported but are uncommon. Safe use of the HAV vaccine in pregnancy has not been established.

Hepatitis A immune globulin (HAIg) is recommended for those who are exposed to or who have close household contact with a patient who has hepatitis A, measles, or varicella. Ig provides immediate Ab to the recipient. When there is an outbreak of hepatitis A in childcare facilities, administration of Ig is recommended for employees in contact with the child and for children in the same room as the index case. Household contacts of persons with hepatitis A should also receive HAIg, and it is recommended for prophylaxis for all susceptible travelers to developing countries.

Hepatitis B

Hepatitis B virus (HBV) is a double-stranded DNA virus that causes a wide spectrum of infections, ranging from asymptomatic seroconversion to clinical hepatitis with jaundice, arthralgias, arthritis, or macular rashes. Complications of hepatitis B infection include fulminant hepatitis, cirrhosis, and hepatocellular carcinoma.

Transmission of the virus occurs via parenteral or mucosal exposure to HBV-infected body fluids from persons who are carriers or who have the acute HBV infection. Sexual contact with an infected person is the most important route of transmission in the United States. Groups at risk for HBV infection include the following:

- Users of illicit parenteral drugs; direct exposure through needle sharing
- Heterosexual persons with multiple partners
- Men having sex with men
- People with occupational exposure to blood and blood products
- Staff of institutions and residential child care programs for the developmentally disabled
- Patients receiving hemodialysis
- Sexual or household contacts of persons with acute or chronic infections
- International travelers who plan to spend more than 6 months in areas with high rates of HBV infection

Mucosal surfaces may become contaminated through direct contact with infective serum or plasma—eye splashes, mouth pipetting, or hand-to-eye or hand-to-mouth contact when hands are contaminated with infective blood or serum.

Chronic HBV infection, which is seen in the carrier state, occurs in as many as 90% of infants who become infected through perinatal transmission and in 6% to 10% of others who acquire HBV infection. Most HBV-related morbidity and mortality can be attributed to chronic infection. Chronic carriers are at increased risk for liver disease or primary hepatocellular carcinoma in later life.

Preexposure immunization of susceptible persons is the most effective means of preventing HBV transmission. HBV vaccination is recommended for all infants as part of the routine childhood immunization schedule. For persons not immunized in infancy, immunization before adolescence is recommended. The American Academy of Pediatrics (AAP) recommends that adolescents and all infants be vaccinated shortly after birth or before hospital discharge.

Hepatitis B immune globulin (HBIg) is a solution of Ig containing Abs to hepatitis B surface Ag (HBsAg). It is used in specific situations in which nonimmunized patients have been exposed to HBV. HBIg is used in the prevention of perinatal HBV infection in infants born to HBsAg-positive mothers, and is given concurrently with HBV vaccination within 12 hours of birth. Other candidates for HBIg are susceptible sexual partners of persons with acute HBV infection, household contacts having identifiable blood exposure to persons with acute HBV infection, susceptible infants (younger than 12 months) who were exposed to a caregiver with acute HBV infection, and an individual exposed through percutaneous or permucosal contact. All of these persons should receive the series of three HBV vaccinations

▌▌ *Adverse Effects and Contraindications*

Pain at the injection site and a temperature higher than 37.7° C are the most commonly reported adverse effects of hepatitis B vaccine. Allergic reactions have been reported but are rare. Pregnancy is not a contraindication for immunization against hepatitis B. HBV vaccine is considered equivalent to a thimerosal-free product. HBV vaccine may contain trace amounts (less than 3 mcg) of mercury left after post-production thimerosal removal, but these amounts have no biologic effect.

Influenza

Influenza is an acute viral disease of the respiratory tract that manifests with an abrupt onset of fever, prostration, cough, headache, myalgia, and sore throat. It is spread by way of airborne droplets and direct contact. Influenza derives its significance from the speed with which epidemics evolve, the widespread morbidity, and the seriousness of complications; viral and bacterial pneumonias are most notable. During major epidemics, severe disease and deaths occur predominantly among older adults and persons debilitated by chronic disease (e.g., cardiac, pulmonary, renal, or metabolic), anemia, or immunosuppression.

Three types of influenza virus are identified, A, B, and C. Influenza A causes moderate to severe illness in all age groups and affects humans and other animals. Influenza B primarily affects children and causes milder disease than type A. Influenza C cases are subclinical and rarely reported as a cause of human illness. Clinical attack rates during epidemics range from 10% to

30% of the general population, to more than 50% in closed populations (e.g., nursing homes, boarding schools).

The most frequent complication of influenza is pneumonia. Other complications include myocarditis and worsening of chronic bronchitis and other chronic pulmonary disease. Older adults, younger children, and persons of any age with underlying medical conditions are at greatest risk for complications and hospitalizations. Older adults (65 years and older) account for more than 90% of deaths attributed to pneumonia and influenza.

The influenza vaccine is reformulated every year to try to match the strains that specialists predict are most likely to strike the following winter. Because influenza is caused by a changeable virus, and vaccine-induced immunity wanes within a few months, an annual vaccination is required. New vaccine is produced each year containing the inactivated particles of viral strains expected to cause disease that year. Each year's vaccine is inactivated and made trivalent (i.e., it contains two strains of type A and one strain of type B). In 2003, the United States approved the use of the live attenuated influenza vaccine (LAIV). LAIV is administered by the intranasal route and contains the same three influenza viruses as the trivalent formulation.

The optimal time for vaccination is mid-October to mid-November. The incidence of influenza ordinarily peaks between late December and early March. The vaccine is recommended for persons susceptible to influenza-related complications. These target groups include the following:

- All adults 65 years or older and children aged 6 to 23 months
- Residents of nursing homes and other institutional facilities
- Adults and children with chronic disorders of the pulmonary or cardiovascular system
- Adults and children who required regular medical follow-up or hospitalization during the preceding year because of chronic metabolic diseases, renal dysfunction, hemoglobinopathies, or immunosuppression
- Pregnant women—specifically those who will be in at least the fourteenth week or later of gestation during influenza season
- Children and adolescents receiving long-term aspirin therapy and who may be at risk for developing Reye's syndrome
- Any person at least 6 months of age who is considered at high risk for influenza complications
- People in contact with high-risk groups, such as health care providers, employees of nursing homes and chronic care facilities, providers of home care, and household members of persons in high-risk groups

▌ Adverse Effects and Contraindications

The most common adverse effects of influenza immunization are localized reactions at the injection site lasting up to 2 days. Fever, malaise, myalgia, and other symptoms are uncommon but, if present, usually start 6 to 12 hours after vaccination. Anaphylaxis can occur in persons with hypersensitivity to some vaccine component.

The influenza vaccine is contraindicated for use in persons known to have a hypersensitivity to eggs, because the vaccine is grown in chick embryos. Do not vaccinate adults with acute febrile illnesses until symptoms have disappeared. Minor acute illnesses in children do not contraindicate use of the influenza vaccine.

Measles, Mumps, and Rubella

Measles (rubeola, "hard measles," "14-day measles") is an acute, highly communicable viral disease characterized by a prodromal fever, cough, coryza, conjunctivitis, and pathognomonic enanthema (Koplik's spots) on the buccal mucosa. An erythematous maculopapular rash appears 2 to 4 days after the prodrome. The rash begins at the hairline and spreads to the face and upper neck, and gradually proceeds downward and outward. The rash fades in the same order as it appeared, lasting 4 to 7 days. The disease is more severe in children under the age of 5 years and adults over the age of 20 years. Complications of the disease may result from viral replication or bacterial superinfection and include diarrhea, otitis media, bronchopneumonia, and encephalitis.

Persons in the United States who received killed measles vaccine before 1968 and who were subsequently exposed to a wild-type measles virus may develop atypical measles manifestations, including pneumonitis, pleural effusion, and peripheral edema. There is a predilection for an atypical rash on extremities that resembles the rash of Rocky Mountain spotted fever.

Measles is transmitted person-to-person through large respiratory droplets. Measles was extremely contagious before widespread immunization programs for preschool and young school-age children. Since 1963, when measles vaccine was licensed, the incidence has decreased dramatically in all age groups. In the late 1980s, the incidence of measles began to increase, especially in preschool children. Low vaccination coverage was determined to be the most important cause of this measles resurgence. Measles outbreaks in school settings are now uncommon as a result of requiring a second dose of measles vaccine for school-age children.

Mumps is also an acute viral illness spread by respiratory droplets or direct contact with infected droplets or saliva. Mumps most often occurs during the winter and spring seasons and is characterized by low-grade fever, malaise, and parotitis. Complications of mumps include aseptic meningitis, orchitis (most common complication in postpubertal males), oophoritis, and sensorineural deafness. Oophoritis occurs in about 5% of females after puberty. Sterility is extremely rare. Central nervous system (CNS) involvement is common and can occur early or late in the disease. CNS involvement usually results in aseptic meningitis, almost always without sequelae. The mortality rate for mumps averages 1.4%. Mumps infection during the first trimester of pregnancy may cause spontaneous abortion, but there is no firm evidence that mumps during pregnancy causes congenital malformations.

Rubella (German measles, "3-day measles") is a mild, febrile viral illness caused by an enveloped RNA virus. Rubella is characterized by a diffuse, punctate, and maculopapular rash, generalized lymphadenopathy, and a slight fever. The rash of rubella usually begins on the face and progresses from head to foot. The rash sometimes resembles that of measles or scarlet fever, although up to 50% of infections occur without evident rash. Children usually show few or no constitutional symptoms at the outset. Adults may have a prodromal period of low-grade fever, headache, malaise, mild coryza, and conjunctivitis before rubella develops 1 to 5 days later. Postauricular,

IMMUNE

occipital, and posterior cervical adenopathy usually precedes the rash by 5 to 10 days.

The primary objective for rubella vaccinations in the United States is the prevention of congenital rubella syndrome (CRS). Congenital rubella syndrome occurs in more than 25% of infants born to women who acquired rubella during the first trimester of pregnancy. The rubella virus can affect virtually all organs and lead to deafness, eye defects, cardiac defects, and neurologic abnormalities. Rubella can lead to fetal death, spontaneous abortion, or premature delivery. Defects are rare when maternal infection develops after the twentieth week of gestation.

The measles-mumps-rubella (MMR) vaccine is a trivalent live virus vaccine first licensed in 1968. It produces serum Ab levels in approximately 95% of patients. The incidence of the three diseases declined dramatically until 1986, when the incidence of measles and mumps began to rise. Through the remainder of the 1980s and into the early 1990s, the incidence of measles remained high. More than half of the cases occurred in individuals older than 5 years, many of whom had already been immunized. Before this, it was recommended that children receive one dose of MMR at 15 months of age. Following the outbreaks in the late 1980s, immunization recommendations were changed to include a second dose of MMR when the child starts school (age 4 to 6 years). For those children who have not received the second dose by age 11 to 12 years, the second dose is recommended at that time.

Children whose mothers received MMR vaccine as children were found to have a lower level of passive Ab to measles, which waned by the time the child was 1 year of age. As a result, the recommended age for the initial MMR immunization has been changed from 15 months to 12 to 15 months, with a second immunization given between 4 and 6 years of age.

Adverse Effects and Contraindications

Five percent to 15% of recipients susceptible to the measles component of MMR develop a fever 7 to 12 days after vaccination. The fever generally lasts 1 to 2 days. Five percent of recipients report a transient rash. Less common adverse effects are encephalitis and transient thrombocytopenia.

MMR vaccine is contraindicated for use in patients with a previous anaphylactic reaction to rubeola vaccine or to a component of the vaccine (e.g., gelatin, neomycin), and in patients with altered immune status (not including HIV). Because blood products may interfere with the replication of live parenteral viral vaccines, wait 3 months following administration of Ig, plasma, or whole blood products before administering the MMR vaccine. Both the MMR vaccine and tuberculin skin testing using purified protein derivative (PPD) can be administered at the same visit. If MMR has been administered recently, delay PPD screening at least 4 weeks. This delay removes the concern of transient suppression of PPD reactivity from the MMR vaccine.

Meningococcal Disease

Meningococcal meningitis is an acute bacterial disease caused by *Neisseria meningitidis*. It is the leading cause of bacterial meningitis and sepsis in the United States. Meningitis is characterized by sudden onset of fever, intense headache, stiff neck, and other symptoms such as nausea, vomiting, photophobia, and altered mental status. Substantial

morbidity results for survivors of meningococcal disease, including neurologic disabilities, limb loss, and hearing loss. The mortality rate exceeds 50%, but with early diagnosis, modern therapy, and supportive measures, the rate drops below 10%. The Centers for Disease Control and Prevention (CDC) noted that higher rates of disease were seen among students living in college dormitories than among students living off campus.

There are two meningococcal vaccines available in the United States: meningococcal polysaccharide vaccine (MPSV4), available since the 1970s, and meningococcal conjugate vaccine (MCV4), available since 2005. According to the National Immunization Program (2007), MCV4 is preferable to the polysaccharide formulation because it provokes a longer-lasting immune response. Then again, the polysaccharide vaccine (MPSV4) is highly effective against meningitis caused by serogroups A, C, Y, and W-135, and may be used instead of MCV4. The polysaccharide vaccine is a good alternative in persons who have brief elevations in disease risk, such as college freshmen living in dorms.

The ACIP recommends routine MCV4 vaccination of people from 11 to 55 years of age in high-risk groups. MPSV4 can be used if MCV4 is not available. MCV4 induces immunity against serogroups A, C, Y, and W-135. The ACIP recommends vaccinations for adolescents entering high school (at approximately age 15 years) who have not previously received the vaccine. Meningococcal vaccine is also recommended for the following:

- Military personnel and travelers to areas where disease is recognized to be endemic, especially the parts of sub-Saharan Africa known as the "meningitis belt" (Ethiopia in the east to Senegal in the west). The government of Saudi Arabia requires vaccination for all travelers to Mecca during the annual Hajj.
- Persons who have terminal complement component deficiencies
- Person with functional or anatomic asplenia
- Persons who are exposed routinely to *N. meningitides* in solutions that may be aerosolized such as research, industrial, and clinical laboratory personnel

Adverse Effects and Contraindications

About half of the people who receive meningococcal vaccines have mild adverse effects such as redness or pain at the injection site. They are more common after MCV4 than after MPSV4, the older version of the vaccine. When present, the reaction usually resolves in 1 to 2 days. A small percentage of persons develop a fever.

Serious allergic reactions to meningococcal vaccine are rare but, when they occur, they do so within a few minutes of the injection. A few cases of Guillain-Barré syndrome, a serious nervous system disorder, has been reported among persons who received MCV4. There is not yet enough evidence to tell whether they were caused by the vaccine. This is still under investigation by health officials.

Meningitis vaccination is contraindicated for use in persons with a documented severe allergic reaction to any component of the vaccine, such as diphtheria toxoid or dry natural rubber latex. Minor acute illness (e.g., diarrhea or mild upper respiratory infection with or without fever) is not a contraindication to vaccination.

Pneumococcal Disease

The most common clinical presentation of pneumococcal disease in adults is pneumonia. Pneumococcal pneumonia is an acute bacterial infection characterized by a sudden onset of shaking chills, fever, pleuritic chest pain, and dyspnea, a productive cough with "rusty" sputum, malaise, and weakness. Pneumonococcal infection is a common bacterial complication of influenza. The case/fatality rate may be greater than 7% in elderly persons. Pneumococcal pneumonia is responsible for 13% to 19% of all cases of bacterial meningitis, with the mortality rate in older adults as high as 80%.

In children under 2 years of age, pneumococcal disease may first appear as bacteremia without a known site of infection. Before the routine immunizations for pneumococcal disease, the majority of the children affected were under 5 years of age. Children (under 59 months) attending day care have 2 to 3 times the risk for invasive pneumococcal disease.

There are two types of pneumococcal vaccines: polysaccharide pneumococcal vaccine and conjugate pneumococcal vaccine. The current pneumococcal polysaccharide vaccine formulation (Pneumovax-23) is composed of purified, capsular polysaccharide Ag of 23 pneumococcal serotypes (PPV23). These 23 strains of *Pneumococcus* cause approximately 85% to 90% of serious pneumococcal infections in the United States. Prophylactic administration is effective in older children and adults. PPV23 is specifically recommended for all adults 65 years of age or older and persons older than 2 years with a normal immune system who have a chronic illness. Like other polysaccharide Ags, some pneumococcal serotypes have limited immunogenicity in children younger than 2 years.

The current 23-valent vaccine (PPV23) can be administered to patients who previously received the 14-valent formulation. Only one dose should be administered, except in persons with certain medical problems. Protection begins at about the third week after vaccination and is thought to last up to 9 years. Long-term follow-up data concerning Ab levels in persons who have been revaccinated are not available; however, the overall increase in Ab levels among older adults has been determined to be lower after revaccination than following primary vaccination.

A one-time revaccination with PPV23 is recommended for persons over 2 years of age who are at highest risk for serious infection and those who are likely to have a rapid decline in pneumococcal antibody levels. At least 5 years must have elapsed since the first dose of PPV23. Children at highest risk who would be under 10 years of age at the time of revaccination should be revaccinated in 3 years. Children with a rapid antibody decline secondary to nephrotic syndrome, kidney failure, or kidney transplant, and those with sickle cell disease or who have had their spleen removed are candidates for the 3-year revaccination cycle. The vaccine is contraindicated for use in persons who have had an anaphylactic reaction or a localized Arthus type of reaction to the initial dose of PPV23.

The pneumococcal conjugate vaccine is a purified capsular polysaccharide of seven serotypes of *Streptococcus pneumoniae* (PCV7). After the four recommended doses of PCV7 vaccine, over 90% of healthy infants develop Ab to all seven serotypes. Routinely administer PCV7 to all children less than 24 months of age and to children ages 24 to 59 months who have a high-risk medical condition. Do not revaccinate children who were vaccinated with age-appropriate primary series of PCV7.

▥ Adverse Effects and Contraindications

Injection site tenderness occurs with the administration of pneumococcal vaccine. Local reactions are more common with the fourth dose of PCV7 than with the first three doses. Fever, myalgia, and severe local reactions are very uncommon. Anaphylaxis is rare. Hypersensitivity to phenol contraindicates the use of pneumococcal vaccine.

Poliomyelitis

Poliomyelitis is an acute viral illness that ranges from asymptomatic infection through nonspecific febrile illness, aseptic meningitis, and paralytic disease to death. The incidence of asymptomatic infections and minor illness is usually 100 times that of paralytic cases, especially when infection occurs in early life. Highly infectious poliomyelitis is more common in infants and young children, but the diseases causes paralysis more often in older individuals.

Poliomyelitis is caused by serotypes P_1, P_2, and P_3 of the poliovirus. It is transmitted by the fecal-oral route in areas where sanitation is poor and during epidemics. The virus is detectable more easily and for longer periods in feces than in pharyngeal secretions. The ingested virus multiplies first in the gastrointestinal (GI) tract, with viremia following. Invasion of the CNS and selective involvement of motor neurons results in flaccid paralysis, most commonly of the lower extremities.

The mortality rate for paralytic polio varies from 2% to 10% in different epidemics, with mortality increasing markedly with age. Before 1955, more than 20,000 cases of paralytic poliomyelitis occurred every year, leaving half its victims with neurologic complications. Paralytic polio was virtually eliminated in the United States with the introduction of the Salk (inactivated) poliovirus vaccine (IPV) in 1955. The Sabin vaccine (oral poliovirus vaccine, OPV), a superior strain of live virus, became available in 1960.

In 2000, IPV was exclusively recommended for infants and children. IPV is highly effective in producing immunity (90% after two doses) to all three serotypes of poliovirus. From 1980 to 1999, one case of vaccine-associated paralytic polio (VAPP) occurred for every 2 to 3 million doses of OPV (trivalent oral polio vaccine) administered. VAPP accounted for 95% of all cases of paralytic poliomyelitis in the United States from 1980 to 1999. The exclusive use of IPV has eliminated the shedding of the live vaccine virus in the stool and thus eliminated the risk of vaccine-associated poliomyelitis.

Poliomyelitis is rare in the United States at this time but is still prevalent in developing countries, where it is a potential threat to travelers. It is recommended that adults who are at a greater risk of exposure to wild-type poliovirus than the general population be immunized. Those at greater risk include the following:

- Travelers to areas where poliomyelitis is epidemic or endemic (Indian subcontinent, the eastern Mediterranean, and Africa)
- Members of communities experiencing disease caused by wild-type poliovirus

IMMUNE

- Laboratory workers who handle specimens containing poliovirus
- Health care workers in close contact with patients who have poliovirus

A pentavalent (five-component) combination vaccine, Pediarix, was approved in the United States in 2002. Pediarix is a combination of DTaP, a pediatric dose of hepatitis B, and IPV and is approved only for the first three doses of the DTaP and IPV series. Pediarix is not approved for the booster doses of DTaP and IPV.

▥ Adverse Effects and Contraindications

No serious adverse effects of the currently available IPV have been documented. Trace amounts of streptomycin and neomycin are found in IPV, so its use in patients with sensitivity to those antibiotics is contraindicated.

Rabies

Rabies results in an almost universally fatal acute viral encephalomyelitis. Rabies' onset is often heralded by a sense of apprehension, headache, fever, and malaise. The RNA virus is found in the saliva of wild animals such as skunks, bats, raccoons, foxes, and coyotes. These wild animals in turn may infect domestic animals (in the United States, most often dogs) by bites. Most infections in humans are from contact with these domestic animals. Annually, there are an estimated 30,000 deaths worldwide, almost all in developing countries. In developed countries, rabies infection in humans is uncommon. At present, the only locales free of rabies are Australia, New Zealand, New Guinea, Japan, Hawaii, Taiwan and the Pacific Islands, the United Kingdom, Ireland, mainland Norway, Sweden, Portugal, and some of the West Indies and Atlantic islands. Preexposure immunization is recommended for persons in high-risk groups such as the following:

- Veterinarians and animal handlers
- Certain laboratory workers
- People living in areas where canine rabies is endemic

Postexposure immunization is used prophylactically for people who have been bitten by a potentially rabid animal or who have scratches or abrasions exposed to animal saliva (such as when an animal licks a wound on a human being), urine, or blood. Active immunization after exposure involves vaccination with one of three approved rabies vaccines. These vaccines are human diploid cell vaccine (HDCV), rabies vaccine absorbed (RVA), and purified chicken embryo cell (PCEC). Any of these vaccines may be administered as a five-dose series. Administer human rabies immune globulin (HRIg) concurrently with the first dose of rabies vaccine.

Immunity to rabies develops 7 to 10 days after immunization. Serum Ab titers decline 2 years after the primary series. Boosters are not routinely recommended except for persons whose risk of exposure is likely to be continuous or frequent. In such individuals, draw rabies serum Ab titers at 6-month intervals, and use boosters to maintain antibody concentrations. HRIg is not useful in the treatment of clinical rabies.

▥ Adverse Effects and Contraindications

Systemic reactions such as headache, nausea, abdominal pain, muscle aches, and dizziness have been reported in adults receiving rabies vaccinations. Local reactions such as pain, erythema and swelling or itching at the vaccine injection site have been reported. It is uncommon for children to have reactions to the rabies vaccine. Immune complex–like reactions have been noted in persons receiving booster doses of human diploid cell vaccine. These manifest as generalized urticaria, arthralgia, arthritis, angioedema, nausea, vomiting, fever, and malaise. Pregnancy is not a contraindication to the use of postexposure vaccine.

Tuberculosis

Tuberculosis is caused by *Mycobacterium tuberculosis*, an acid-fast bacillus (see Chapter 29). Exposure in high-prevalence regions (e.g., Asia, Middle East, Africa, and Latin America) usually occurs as a result of prolonged contact with respiratory droplets from infected persons. For travelers, the best approach to tuberculosis prevention is pretravel and posttravel tuberculin testing rather than immunization.

BCG vaccine is widely used outside North America for immunization against tuberculosis. The World Health Organization (WHO) recommends a single dose at birth, and most of the world's children receive BCG vaccine according to varying schedules. The BCG vaccine is approved by the AAP for children who will be living in areas where tuberculosis is prevalent. The United States has not endorsed the use of BCG vaccine for prevention of tuberculosis.

BCG vaccine may be considered for uninfected children who are at unavoidable risk of exposure and for whom other methods of prevention and control are not feasible. BCG can be given to infants from birth to 2 months of age without tuberculin testing. Thereafter, BCG is given only to children who have a negative tuberculin skin test.

▥ Adverse Effects and Contraindications

The adverse effects of BCG include redness and mild swelling where the injection was given. These symptoms will improve over time. Swollen glands, aching bones, aching muscles, and fever have also been reported. Abscess formation with a discharging ulcer, nausea, vomiting, conjunctivitis, and anaphylaxis have also been reported.

BCG is contraindicated for use in persons who have an impaired immune response from the following: HIV; congenital immunodeficiency; leukemia; lymphoma; generalized malignancy; high-dose steroid therapy; therapy with alkylating and antimetabolite drugs; or radiation therapy. It is also prudent to avoid giving BCG vaccination to pregnant women, although no harmful effects of BCG on the fetus have been observed.

Varicella

Varicella (chickenpox) is an acute, generalized viral illness characterized by a sudden onset of slight fever, mild constitutional symptoms, and skin eruptions that are usually pruritic. The maculopapular rash lasts a few hours and then changes to vesicles for 3 to 4 days, leaving a granular scab over the lesions. The lesions occur in crops, with several stages of maturity present at the same time. Lesions first appear on the scalp and then on the trunk and then progress to the extremities. Lesions tend to be more abundant on the trunk. Mild, atypical, and asymptomatic infections occur.

Varicella in children is a self-limiting but highly contagious disease spread by direct contact, droplet nuclei, and aerosols from vesicles or respiratory tract secretions. In adults, the fever and constitutional symptoms may be severe. Lifetime immunity usually develops after recovering from primary varicella infection.

Varicella develops primarily in children younger than 8 years of age. By age 12, only 10% of children are still at risk for this disease. In the United States, the number of adults contracting varicella appears to be increasing as a result of recent immigrations from tropical countries. Although adults account for only 2% of varicella cases, they have a 50% mortality rate, with 25% of deaths occurring in patients who are immunocompromised.

Herpes zoster (shingles) is caused by the reactivation of a latent varicella-zoster virus. About 15% of people who had varicella in their younger years develop zoster. The incidence of herpes zoster in immunocompromised patients and older adults is related to a decline in cellular immunity. Histologically, the two disorders are identical. Severe pain and paresthesias are common with the disorder. Herpes zoster occurs primarily in adults, although there is evidence to suggest that approximately 10% of children treated for malignancy are likely to develop the viral infection. Persons who have HIV or are immunosuppressed are also at increased risk.

Varicella vaccine, a live attenuated viral vaccine, is 95% effective in preventing chickenpox, but not as protective as live virus vaccines; however, the risk of zoster is considerably reduced in patients receiving the vaccine. Seroconversion occurs in 97% of susceptible children aged 1 to 12 years, but in only 79% of recipients aged 13 to 17 years. The ACIP strongly recommends that varicella vaccine be administered in the following manner:

- At 12 to 18 months of age; if varicella and MMR vaccines are not administered at the same visit, they should be administered 28 days apart.
- To healthy adults and adolescents with no history of the disease and/or who are at high risk of exposure to varicella
- To those who will have close contact with persons at high risk for serious complications of varicella
- The ACIP recommends that all health care workers be immune to varicella, either from evidence of vaccination or from a reliable history of varicella disease.

Varicella vaccine can be given simultaneously with MMR at separate injection sites. In 2005, a new formulation of measles, mumps, rubella, and varicella (MMRV) was approved for administration in children from 12 months to 12 years of age. It must be noted that MMRV is not to be used in children less than 1 year of age. The ACIP noted that MMRV should not be given as the second dose of MMR except when a dose of varicella is also indicated, or if no MMR vaccine is available at the time the second dose of MMR is indicated.

Varicella zoster vaccine (Zostavax) is a live, attenuated vaccine approved by the FDA for persons over 60 years old to reduce the risk for varicella zoster and postherpetic neuralgia. It is not approved to treat varicella zoster. It is thought to act by increasing immunity to VZV. The vaccine's effectiveness has been documented in older adults from 60 to 69 years of age but then declines with increasing age.

Varicella-zoster immune globulin (VZIg) is used to prevent or decrease the severity of varicella infections in children younger than 15 years who are immunosuppressed because of illness (e.g., lymphoma, leukemia) or drug therapy (e.g.,

antineoplastic or corticosteroid drugs), and who have had significant exposure to varicella or herpes zoster. The Ab provides only temporary protection.

▥ *Adverse Affects and Contraindications*

Pain and redness at the site of injection are the common adverse effects of the varicella vaccine and ZVZ, although a generalized varicella-like rash may occur in immunocompromised individuals. Although the virus can be transmitted from recently immunized individuals to others, it does not become more virulent.

Varicella vaccine is contraindicated for use in patients with a history of allergic reactions (i.e., anaphylaxis) to neomycin or gelatin, or to ingredients in the vaccine; patients with a history of HIV or AIDS; patients with any type of lymphoma or other malignancies involving bones or the lymphatic system; patients on high-dose corticosteroids; those with untreated active tuberculosis, and women of childbearing age who may become pregnant (category C). It is not known if ZVZ is transmitted to breast milk. Salicylates are not recommended for the 6 weeks after immunization because of the association among varicella, salicylates, and Reye's syndrome.

DRUGS FOR PASSIVE IMMUNITY

Antitoxins

An *antitoxin* is an Ab with the ability to neutralize a specific *toxin* (Table 31-2). Antitoxins are used therapeutically when a person has been exposed to a toxin-secreting organism, but are also used for prophylaxis. Antitoxins are obtained by injecting a purified toxin into an animal such as a horse. Once Abs have time to develop, blood is withdrawn from the animal and the antitoxin prepared from it. Examples of antitoxins are those for tetanus, botulism, diphtheria, and rabies. The disadvantage of antitoxins is related to the hypersensitivity (serum sickness) that many people have to horse serum. To reduce the risk of serum sickness, the antitoxin used is generated from the same species (i.e., use human antitoxin to treat humans). The symptoms of serum sickness include fever, urticaria, maculopapular rash, arthritis or arthralgia, and lymphadenopathy.

Antisera

Animal *antisera* (Ab of animal origin) are derived from serum of horses. Antisera are used for illnesses in which specific Ig of human origin are unavailable (i.e., diphtheria and botulism). Each patient is tested for sensitivity to that animal by means of a scratch or intradermal test before administration of the serum. If sensitivity is evident, begin desensitization, because anaphylaxis reaction is probable. Other reactions that may occur to antisera are acute febrile reactions and serum sickness occurring 1 to 3 weeks after administration.

Sera

Sera, or gamma globulins, are used as postexposure prophylaxis to prevent infectious diseases after exposure or to relieve symptoms of the disease. Sera provide passive immunity. Human serum Ig is used, a sterile, concentrated protein solution (15% to 18%) composed primarily of the Ig fraction with trace amounts of IgA or IgM in proportion to the infection and immunization experience of the population from which it is derived. Peak serum levels of Ab are achieved 48 to 72 hours

TABLE 31-2 Drugs for Passive Immunity

Drug	FRM	Indications	Efficacy and Duration	Implications
ANTITOXINS				
Diphtheria antitoxin	KAT	Diphtheria	———	Used in conjunction with antibiotics to eliminate bacteria but does not eliminate bacterial toxins
Tetanus antitoxin	AT	Tetanus	———	Rarely used; tetanus immune globulin is used if available
SERA				
Cytomegalovirus human immunoglobulin (CMV-IGIV, CytoGam)	AS	CMV infection	Weeks to months	May interfere with immune response to LVV; wait 3 mo before administering
Hepatitis B immune globulin (Human, H-BIG, Hyper-Hep, Hep-B-Gammagee)	AS	Postexposure prophylaxis	Efficacy: 70%-80% after second dose; 94%-98% after third dose Duration: 2 mo	Not for fulminant acute or chronic active hepatitis B
Immune serum globulin (gamma globulin, ISG, Gammar, Gamastan)	IgG with trace amount IgA and IgM	Primary immunodeficiency states, ITP, bone marrow transplant, pediatric HIV	Produces adequate serum levels of IgG in 2–5 days	Routine use in early pregnancy is not recommended.
Immune serum globulin (IGIV, Gamimune, Sandoglobulin)	IgG with trace amount IgA and IgM	Primary immunodeficiency states, ITP, bone marrow transplant, pediatric HIV	May be given more often or dosage increased if clinical response or serum level of IgG insufficient	May interfere with immune response to LVV; wait 3 mo before administering
Rabies immune serum globulin (RIG, Hyperab, Imogam)	AS	Postexposure prophylaxis with rabies exposure who lack a history of preexposure or postexposure prophylaxis with rabies vaccine	Duration: 21 days	Preferable to give with first dose of vaccine but can be given up to 8 days after vaccination. One half dose may be infiltrated around the wound.
Rh₀ human immune globulin (Gamulin Rh, HypRho-D, RhoGam)	IgG-antiD (Rh1)	Obstetric use; transfusion mishap	Duration: 12 weeks	Consult package insert for blood typing and drug administration procedures.
Tetanus immune globulin (human, TIG, Hyper-Tet)	IgG	Prophylaxis in patients whose immunization status is incomplete or uncertain	Duration: 21 days	Preferred to antitoxin; less likely to cause allergic reactions and has longer duration of action; toxoid should be given at same time to initiate active immune response.
Varicella-zoster immune globulin (human, VZIG)	AS	Varicella zoster in children <15 yr and adults with significant risk factors on an individual basis	Duration: 21 days	Not for immunocompromised individuals; most effective given within 72 hr of exposure; no evidence that drug modifies established infection

AS, antiserum; *AT*, antitoxin; *CDC*, Centers for Disease Control and Prevention; *CMV*, cytomegalovirus; *FRM*, formulation; *HIV*, human immunodeficiency virus; *IgA*, immunoglobulin A; *IgG*, immunoglobulin G; *IgM*, immunoglobulin M; *ITP*, idiopathic thrombocytopenic purpura; *KAT*, killed antitoxin; *LVV*, live virus vaccine.

after inoculation. The dosage of Ig is based on body weight. Ig is indicated as replacement therapy for Ab deficiency disorders, hepatitis A, and measles prophylaxis. Adverse effects include discomfort and pain at the site of administration.

TRAVEL IMMUNIZATIONS

The increased risk of contracting infectious diseases during international travel results from two primary factors: the close proximity of individuals during travel and exposure to exotic infectious agents through contact with foreign populations and natural environments. The number and kind of immunizations needed are determined by the person's itinerary. The health care provider must consider the geographic location, the style of accommodation, and planned activities when determining which immunizations are needed. The patient's age, prior immunization history, allergies, and general health must also be taken into account. The efficacy and adverse effects of vaccines are important considerations.

Before international travel, children and adolescents should be up to date on routinely recommended immunizations for their age (see *Epidemiology and Prevention of Vaccine-Preventable Diseases: The "Pink Book"* at www.cdc.gov/nip/publications/pink/). Consider additional vaccines to prevent hepatitis A, yellow fever, meningococcal disease, typhoid fever, rabies, and Japanese encephalitis for all persons. *Health Information for International Travel: The "Yellow Book"* (online at www.cdc.gov/travel/yb/), updated and reissued every 2 years by the CDC, is an excellent reference for people regarding health risks for international travel.

Cholera

Cholera is an acute bacterial disease caused by *Vibrio cholerae*. It is acquired by ingesting large numbers of organisms from contaminated food such as shellfish or water; boiling or other disinfection of water prevents transmission. Cholera is transmitted by uncooked seafood and by the fecal-oral route in environments where hygienic preparation of food and sanitary disposal of human wastes are lacking. Asymptomatic infection is more common than clinical illness. Cholera is characterized by its sudden onset; profuse, painless, and watery stools; and occasional vomiting, rapid dehydration, acidosis, and circulatory collapse. When untreated, severe cases can result in death within a few hours. The mortality rate may exceed 50%, but with proper treatment, the rate falls below 1%.

At present, the manufacture and sale of the only licensed cholera vaccine in the United States has been discontinued. It has not been recommended for travelers because of the brief and incomplete immunity it offers. Two recently developed vaccines for cholera are licensed and available in other countries (Dukoral and Mutacol). Both vaccines appear to provide somewhat better immunity and fewer adverse effects than the previously available vaccine. There are no cholera vaccination requirements for entry or exit in any country, although cholera presents a continuing health risk in Asia, Africa, and Latin America.

Japanese Encephalitis

Japanese encephalitis is a mosquito-transmitted, inflammatory viral disease of short duration that involves the brain, the spinal cord, and the meninges. Japanese encephalitis is prevalent in many areas of subcontinental India, Southeast Asia, China, and eastern Russia. It appears from June to September in temperate zones and throughout the year in tropical zones of the Far East. The disease primarily affects young children and adults over 65 years. Japanese encephalitis carries high mortality and morbidity rates, and therefore vaccination is considered for travelers, although the risk is low for those traveling to urban areas and staying for a brief period.

The Japanese encephalitis vaccine is an inactivated vaccine derived from the brain of an infected mouse. The recommended immunization series consists of three doses. The onset of drug action begins with the second dose. Vaccination is about 78% effective after the second dose and 99% effective after the third dose.

Typhoid

Typhoid is a systemic bacterial disease caused by *S. typhi* characterized by an insidious onset of sustained fever, headache, malaise, anorexia, bradycardia, splenomegaly, rose-colored spots on the trunk, nonproductive cough, constipation (more often than diarrhea), and lymphadenopathy. The disease rarely occurs in the United States; the typhoid that does occur is contracted through international travel. The risk of transmission is particularly high in the Indian subcontinent, Latin America, Asia, and Africa. Typhoid vaccine is not routinely recommended for residents in the United States or for foreign travelers. Typhoid vaccine is recommended for persons who expect to consume food and water at nontourist facilities in areas where it is endemic.

Two typhoid vaccines are available for travelers: an oral vaccine containing live attenuated *S. typhi* (Oral Ty21a) and an injectable Vi capsular polysaccharide vaccine (ViCPS). Immunization with ViCPS is recommended for persons over 2 years of age and consists of one dose. If continued or renewed exposure is expected, the manufacturer of ViCPS vaccine recommends a booster dose every 2 years.

The primary series of oral Ty21a vaccine consists of four capsules; one of the capsules, which must be refrigerated, is taken with cool liquids every other day, approximately 1 hour before a meal. A booster is required 5 years later, which means taking the entire four-dose series again. The vaccine is approved for children over 6 years of age and in adults.

▥ Adverse Effects and Contraindications

Adverse effects of oral Ty21a vaccine are fewer than from the injectable vaccine. Common adverse effects include fever, headache, and, with ViCPS, local reactions at the site of injection. Ty21a is contraindicated for in persons who are immunocompromised (e.g., HIV). The injectable typhoid vaccine is thought to be safer in these patients. Because information is not available on the safety of these vaccines when used during pregnancy, it is prudent on practical grounds to avoid vaccinating pregnant women. Do not administer oral Ty21a vaccine to patients currently taking antibiotics, or within 7 days of a patient's concluding a course of an antibiotic.

Contraindications to vaccination with ViCPS vaccine are a history of severe local or systemic reactions after a previous dose. Do not give either of the typhoid vaccines to persons with a fever. Typhoid vaccinations may be administered together with viral vaccines. Simultaneous administration of Ty21a and Ig does not appear to pose a problem.

Yellow Fever

Yellow fever is a serious and potentially fatal viral infection of short duration and varying severity. It is characterized by a sudden onset of fever, chills, headache, backache, generalized muscle pain, nausea, and vomiting. After a brief period of remission the disease progresses to hemorrhagic fever, with GI bleeding, hemorrhage, jaundice, and cardiovascular instability.

Yellow fever is transmitted by the *Aedes aegypti* mosquito in tropical and subtropical regions of the world. The mortality rate among indigenous populations of endemic regions is less than 5%. The mortality rate can exceed 50% among nonindigenous groups and during epidemics. Although the disease is now rare, many countries have retained an entrance requirement for yellow fever immunization despite years of having had no reported cases.

Yellow fever vaccine is a live attenuated vaccine. Yellow fever vaccine is given only at approved vaccination centers. The onset of immunity after a single dose of vaccine is 10 days. Boosters are required at 10-year intervals.

▥ Adverse Effects and Contraindications

Reactions to yellow fever vaccine are less likely to occur after a booster dose of the vaccine than after the first dose. The mild adverse effects include soreness, redness, or swelling at the injection site, fever, and muscle aches. If these problems occur, they usually begin soon after the injection and last 5 to 10 days. In studies, they occurred in as many as 25% of vaccine recipients. Severe reactions include life-threatening allergic reactions, severe nervous system reactions, and major organ system failure (particularly in people over age 60). More than half of the patients who develop severe adverse effects to yellow fever vaccine die.

Contraindications to use of the vaccine are an allergy to eggs and immunosuppression. It is not recommended for use in children younger than 6 months because of a higher incidence of adverse effects. It is also contraindicated for use in pregnancy, except when travel cannot be avoided to an area where endemic disease is highly prevalent.

IMMUNE

CLINICAL REASONING

Treatment Objectives

The immediate goal is to prevent disease in individuals and groups. The long-term goal of immunization programs is eradication of disease. To achieve these goals, participation in immunization programs must be a high priority for people of all ages–children, adolescents, and adults. *Healthy People 2010* objectives include achieving a 90% primary immunization rate for children aged 19 to 35 months and adolescents. Factors that interfere with these goals must be addressed. Cultural barriers, adverse effects, and contraindications must be considered in the design of an effective immunization campaign.

Treatment Options

Health care providers play an active role in immunization programs when they understand immunity and the types of vaccines used, as well as the indications and current recommendations for these vaccines. Knowledge of administration guidelines and potential vaccine reactions are also required. In addition, stay familiar with the legislative rules and societal concerns associated with this important component of health promotion and disease prevention.

▥ *Patient Variables*

Recommendations for infant, child, and adult immunizations are influenced by the age-specific risks for disease and for complications, by the ability of persons of a given age to respond to the vaccine, and by potential interference with the immune response by passively transferred maternal antibodies. Consider the benefits and risks associated with the use of all immunobiologics, because no vaccine is completely safe or completely effective (see Controversy box).

Ask patients if they have food or drug allergies and to bring their immunization record to the appointment. If they do not have an immunization record, start one. Determine what previous immunizations or allergic reactions the patient has had. Because some immunizations may not be given in close proximity to others, pay attention to the dates of previous immunizations.

Certain constituents of vaccines (e.g., egg protein, gelatin, neomycin, latex) may cause allergic reactions, and individuals known to have severe allergies should not receive vaccines containing them. The ACIP removed egg allergy as a contraindication to measles and mumps vaccines. Both of the vaccines are now developed in the fibroblasts of chick embryos rather than whole eggs. Before administering influenza or yellow fever vaccines, screen for allergy risk.

The Immunization Action Coalition developed the set of screening questions shown in Box 31-2. Effective screening is crucial in preventing serious adverse reactions.

In the patient for whom pregnancy status is questionable, perform a pregnancy test before giving immunizations. For pregnant women not known to be immunized against rubella, measure serum Ab titers to determine resistance or susceptibility to the disease.

Individualize immunization for adults, considering age, physical health, chronic health problems, immunocompromised conditions, and possible allergic reactions. Also, many parents have questions or misconceptions about the safety and efficacy of immunizations for their child. Health care providers have a responsibility to listen to and try and understand the parents' fears and apprehensions. The CDC has numerous publications both for health care providers and parents that address misconceptions and answers questions frequently posed by parents.

Economic and ethnic disparities exist that still may hinder children and adults from receiving recommended

---

Controversy

Immunization Policy Issues

Jonathan J. Wolfe

Immunization is the primary response to communicable disease, because it is proactive. Successful immunization prevents disease and all its sequelae. However, immunization is not a perfectly benign process. Although patients rarely suffer harm from vaccines, there are adverse reactions including neurologic sequelae and anaphylaxis. Occasionally, a patient may contract the disease that the vaccine seeks to prevent. Also, people who are immunocompromised are at some risk for reactions if the vaccine is made with live attenuated virus. The benefits to health must be weighed against the risks.

The acceptance of an immunization by parents, guardians, and adults is important. However, many parents and guardians refuse to subject their children to risks associated with immunization. Sometimes a person's religious convictions prohibit receiving vaccines. At other times, the person's fear of even the slightest risk of harm prevents participation. Indeed, the media may exacerbate the problem by reporting rare adverse events without adequately presenting the countervailing benefit. Stories of people harmed by vaccines make gripping headlines and television sound bites. The long-term benefits of disease-free health are less obvious to readers and listeners.

Health care reform, with its suggestions of rationing care, adds urgency to the discussion of immunization. Public and private payers alike want to know where the right of individuals to refuse immunization infringes on the right of the majority to lower health care costs resulting from responsible preventive care.

CLINICAL REASONING

- The discovery and preparation of vaccines was watched and welcomed as a sign of progress in the late nineteenth century and on through the advent of the Salk poliomyelitis vaccines in the 1950s. How have public perceptions of vaccines changed since that time?
- To what extent do you think concerns about legal liability for the harmful effects of vaccines inhibit wider immunization?
- What particular issues of individual autonomy must be respected in any debate about immunization?
- Health care providers are no longer the sole source for vaccinations. Describe the role health care providers play in the immunization programs.
- What harm do you foresee to our society if immunization coverage were to fall to low levels?
- What geographic areas of the United States are at greatest risk from low levels of immunization?
- What one vaccine is most important to discover and make available in the next 10 years?
- Given the above issues, to what extent should we immunize against potential bioterrorism agents?

BOX 31-2

Immunization Screening Questions*

- Are you sick today?
- Do you have allergies to drugs, foods, or any vaccine?
- Have you had a serious reaction to a vaccine in the past?
- Do you have a seizure or a brain problem?
- Do you have cancer, leukemia, AIDS, or other immune system problem?
- Have you taken cortisone, prednisone or other steroids, or anticancer drugs or had radiation treatments in the past 3 months?
- Have you received a transfusion of blood or blood products, or been given a drug called immune (gamma) globulin in the past year?
- For women: Are you pregnant, or is there a chance you could become pregnant during the next month?
- Have you received any vaccinations in the past 4 weeks?
- For patients exposed to infectious disease or illness: What exposure(s) have you had, and when did it occur? Was the exposure to household contacts or to a brief, casual contact?
- For patients with wounds: How and when the wound was sustained, and what was done for treatment?

*Questions may be directed to the parents of a child but apply to both adults and children.

AIDS, Acquired immunodeficiency syndrome.

From the Immunization Action Coalition. Available online: www.immunize.org. Accessed April 29, 2007.

---

immunizations in a timely manner. There is a greater risk for underimmunization of children and adults in lower income brackets and in certain ethnic groups. These disparities may exist because of a lack of understanding of the importance of up-to-date immunizations, lack of access to immunization clinics, and lack of insurance or economic assistance in paying for the immunizations.

▥ Drug Variables

In the United States, the Committee on Infectious Diseases appointed by the AAP and the Public Health Service's ACIP, in collaboration with the CDC, review immunization data, provide recommendations, and publish updated information (Box 31-3). The AAP and its publications address pediatric and general practice in conjunction with public health. In

Canada, The *Canadian Immunization Guide* from the National Advisory Council on Immunization is used to determine immunization schedules. Thus there may be some differences between its recommendations and those of the ACIP in its journal, *Morbidity and Mortality Weekly Report (MMWR).* Read each vaccine's package insert to become familiar with its components. Seek consultation if there is ANY doubt about administering a vaccine.

The benefits of immunization range from partial to complete protection against the consequences of the infection. The risks vary from common, minor, and inconvenient effects to rare, severe, and life-threatening conditions. Benefits, costs, and risks must be considered in achieving optimal protection against infectious diseases. Recommendations attempt to minimize the risk by providing specific advice on dose, route, and timing of vaccines, and by delineating circumstances that warrant precaution in, or abstention from, administration of a particular vaccine.

TIMING OF ADMINISTRATION. The recommended childhood and adolescent immunization schedules are noted in Table 31-3. Some vaccines require more than one dose for adequate Ab response. Others require (booster doses) to maintain protection. The ACIP recommends the interval between administration of doses and vaccines. Box 31-4 provides safety tips for vaccine administration. Many common vaccines and immunizations can be used concurrently and still maintain safety and efficacy, and other vaccines can be administered on the same day but at a different anatomic site.

Administration of Ig can inhibit the immune response to live vaccines for 3 months or more. Therefore MMR and its individual components should be given 3 months after administration of Ig. Ig formulations are less likely to interact with toxoids and inactivated vaccines and as such can be given concurrently or at any interval. They should be administered at different anatomic sites.

STORAGE. Vaccines and immunizations are stored according to manufacturer's directions to maintain efficacy of vaccines and other biologic preparations. Most are stored in the body of the refrigerator (not in the door) at temperatures ranging from 35.6° to 46.4° F (2° to 8° C). Some vaccines (e.g., MMR and IPV) require protection from light. If immunizing

---

BOX 31-3

Immunization Information Resources

Advisory Committee for Immunization Practices (ACIP)	http://immunize.org/acip/index.htm
American Academy of Pediatrics	www.cispimmunize.org/
Health and Human Services National Vaccine Program Office	www.hhs.gov/nvpo/
Immunization Action Coalition	www.immunize.org/
Morbidity and Mortality Weekly Report (MMWR)	www.cdc.gov/mmwr/
National Network for Immunization Information	www.immunizationinfo.org/
The Children's Hospital of Philadelphia Vaccine Education Center	www.chop.edu/consumer/jsp/microsite/microsite.jsp?id=75918
The National Immunization Program (NIP) at the Centers for Disease Control and Prevention	www.cdc.gov/nip
Tips for Evaluating Immunization Information on the Internet	www.metrokc.gov/health/immunization/immweb.htm
Report of the Committee on Infectious Diseases (Redbook)	www.aap.org
The Pink Book from The National Immunization Program	www.cdc.gov/nip/publications/pink
University of Alabama School of Medicine (bioterrorism education)	www.bioterrorism.uab.edu
Vaccine Adverse Event Reporting System	http://vaers.hhs.gov/
Vaccine Information Statements (VIS)	www.immunize.org/vis

IMMUNE

TABLE 31-3 Immunization Schedules

Age or Time	HBV	DTaP or DTP	OPV or IPV	Hib	MMR	Td	PPD
RECOMMENDED IMMUNIZATION SCHEDULE FOR HEALTHY INFANTS AND CHILDREN							
Birth–12 hr	✓						
1–2 mo	✓						
2 mo		✓	✓	✓			
4 mo		✓	✓	✓			
6 mo		✓					
6–18 mo	✓		✓				
12–15 mo				✓*	✓		✓
15–18 mo		✓					
4–6 yr		✓	✓		✓†		
11–12 yr					✓		
14–16 yr						✓	
RECOMMENDED IMMUNIZATION SCHEDULES FOR INFANTS AND CHILDREN NOT IMMUNIZED AS ABOVE							
First visit	✓	✓	✓				✓
1 mo later	✓				✓‡		
2 mo after first visit		✓	✓	✓			
4 mo after first visit	✓	✓	✓				
10–16 mo after last dose		✓	✓	✓			
4–6 yr		✓	✓				
14–16 yr		✓					✓

*Hib #3 may be needed at 12–15 mo if not received at age 6 mo.
†MMR #2 is given at age 11–12 yr if not given at age 4–6 yr (entry to school).
‡MMR is not given before age 15 mo. Hib is used for children between the ages of 18 and 60 mo.
DTaP, Diphtheria-tetanus–acellular pertussis; DTP, diphtheria-tetanus-pertussis; Hib, Haemophilus influenza, type b; HBV, hepatitis B; IPV, inactivated polio vaccine; MMR, measles-mumps-rubella; MMRV, measles-mumps-rubella-varicella; OPV, oral polio vaccine; PPD, purified protein derivative; Td, tetanus-diphtheria.

drugs are to be transported, use ice packs and polystyrene foam containers. Keep varicella vaccines frozen until ready to reconstitute before administration. Those immunizations requiring reconstitution (MMR and varicella) are mixed just before use.

Patient Education

Many people think that certain diseases have been eradicated and are no longer a threat, so it is not unusual for patients or parents to resist immunization. Others fear serious adverse effects, are deterred by the cost of the vaccine, or say they do not have the time for successive vaccinations or boosters. Public education is vital so that people understand the need for prevention, the reasons for seeking health care in the event of injury, animal bite, or exposure to contagious diseases, and the role of vaccination in both.

Advise the vaccine recipient that adverse reactions have been reported for all vaccines. The reactions are usually local and transient, but they can be systemic, and either immediate or delayed. Local inflammatory reactions at the injection site are the most common. Fever, rash, and hypersensitivity occur uncommonly. Most reactions resolve within 48 hours and can usually be effectively managed with symptomatic treatment. This information is transmitted through vaccine information statements (VIS) available through the CDC website (www.cdc.gov/nip/publications/vis/).

Information about travel immunizations is an important part of travel preparation. Instruct individuals traveling to high-risk areas to contact you, the health department, and/or a travel clinic for guidance about required immunizations. Information about vaccinations is also available from the CDC.

Evaluation

The benefit of immunization is difficult to ascertain directly. However, when universal immunization of infants is successful, there will be a dramatic decline in the transmission and incidence of infectious diseases. Greater attention to the vaccination of high-risk individuals would accelerate the decline.

It is not unusual for a health care provider to encounter people without adequate documentation of immunizations. Do not postpone immunizations because of a lack of records.

LEGAL IMPLICATIONS OF IMMUNIZING

Vaccine Information Statements

The National Childhood Vaccine Injury Act (NCVIA) of 1986 mandates that a VIS be provided to either the adult vaccinee or to the child's parent or legal representative before administering any vaccine. Be sure that the most recent version of the VIS is given to the recipient of the vaccine and that enough time is given to read the VIS before administering the drug (Box 31-5).

Vaccine information statements are developed by the staff of the CDC and undergo intense scrutiny for accuracy by panels of experts. Each VIS provides information to properly inform the adult or the minor child's parent or legal representative about the risks and benefits of each vaccine. A VIS is not meant to replace interactions with health care providers. Answer questions and address concerns that the vaccinee or the parent or legal representative may have.

Foreign-language versions of VISs are not officially available from the CDC. However, several state health departments have arranged for their translations. These versions do not require CDC approval. There are more than 30 languages available through the Immunization Action Coalition's website (www.immunize.org/) or from individual state health departments.

Immunization Records

The International Certificate of Vaccination (document number PHS-731), available from the Superintendent of

BOX 31-4

Tips for Vaccine Immunizations

1. *The more similar a vaccine is to the natural disease, the better the immune response to the vaccine.* Inactivated vaccines are not usually affected by circulating Ab to the Ag. Live attenuated vaccines may be affected by circulating Ab to the Ag.
2. ***Killed vaccines can be administered simultaneously at separate sites.*** **Live and inactivated vaccines may be administered at the same time. Whenever possible, live virus vaccines should be administered at least 30 days apart.**
3. Live attenuated vaccines generally produce long-lasting immunity with a *single dose.* Inactivated vaccines require *multiple doses* and may require periodic boosting to maintain immunity.
4. *Separate administration of live vaccines by at least 4 weeks if they are not given simultaneously.* The live vaccine given first interferes with the second vaccine, and the person may not develop active immunity to the second vaccine. There are no concerns if one or both of the drugs are inactivated vaccines.
5. *If two live vaccines are given less than 4 weeks apart, the second vaccine should be repeated in 4 weeks.* The efficacy of the second vaccine can be determined by serologic testing.
6. *Decreasing the interval between doses of a multidose vaccine interferes with Ab response and production.* It is not necessary to restart the vaccination series or add doses of any vaccine because of an extended interval between doses.
7. *For routine immunizations, combined formulations of vaccine are preferred (e.g., DTaP, TdaP, MMR, MMRV, DTaP-Hib-HepB, HepB-Hib).* Single antigenic formulations are recommended when other components in the formulation are contraindicated.
8. *Adverse reactions following administration of live attenuated vaccines are similar to a mild form of the natural disease.* Adverse reactions following administration of inactivated vaccines are mostly local and may occur with or without fever. The type of adverse reaction depends on the type of vaccine given.
9. *Do not give live attenuated injectable vaccines or intranasal influenza vaccine to immunosuppressed persons.* Use inactivated vaccines, because they do not replicate. However, immunosuppression can cause a poor immune response, therefore vaccination may not result in immunity.
10. *Know your workplace's policies about administering vaccines to immunosuppressed persons.* If there are questions about whether a vaccine can be given to a person who has a condition that suppresses the immune system, consult the person's health care provider.
11. *Recent receipt of Ab-containing products necessitates a temporary precautionary hold on administration of live attenuated vaccines.* Because circulating Ab interfere with development of active immunity, do not give live vaccines until after the person's Ab level goes back down. If there are questions about whether to administer a vaccine, ask for help.
12. *Always consult the person's health care provider before giving any vaccine to a person who has had a stem cell or bone marrow transplant.* Certain vaccines are currently not recommended (varicella and pneumococcal conjugate), and other vaccines must be given at specific intervals after a transplant.
13. There are only two permanent contraindications to vaccination:
    A. *Anaphylaxis* in response to prior exposure to a vaccine component or occurring *after a prior dose of vaccine is a contraindication to vaccination.* Patients who have had only mild allergic reactions can be vaccinated. If a patient has had a severe allergic reaction to a vaccine or vaccine component, do not give additional doses of that vaccine.
    B. *Encephalopathy without a known cause* that occurs within 7 days of a dose of pertussis vaccine is a contraindication to administering more doses of pertussis-containing vaccine. If encephalopathy occurs after pertussis vaccination, you may give other vaccines, but do not give pertussis-containing vaccine again.

Data from the Centers for Disease Control and Prevention. *General Recommendations on Immunization.* Available online: www.cdc.gov/Nip/publications/pink/genrec.rtf. Accessed May 4, 2007.

Ab, Antibody; *Ag,* antigen; *DTaP,* diphtheria-tetanus–acellular pertussis; *HepB,* hepatitis B; *Hib, Haemophilus* influenza, type b; *MMR,* measles-mumps-rubella; *MMRV,* measles-mumps-rubella-varicella; *TdaP,* tetanus, diphtheria,–acellular pertussis.

BOX 31-5

Vaccines Requiring a VIS

A vaccine complication case in Florida highlights the importance of distributing the most recent VIS to patients. In 1997, a 3-month-old boy developed vaccine-associated paralytic poliomyelitis following his first dose of live polio vaccine (OPV). The boy's parents reported that their physician furnished them with the 1994 polio VIS at the time of vaccination. However, the polio VIS had been revised in 1997 to reflect the ACIP preference for sequential use of inactivated polio vaccine (IPV) followed by OPV; in other words, the 1994 polio statement that was given to the parent was outdated.

- Anthrax*
- Diphtheria, tetanus, pertussis (DTP, DTaP)
- Hepatitis A (HepA)
- Hepatitis B (Hep B)
- Influenza
- *Haemophilus* influenza, type b (Hib)
- Measles, mumps, rubella (MMR)
- Meningococcal
- Pneumococcal conjugate vaccine
- Polio
- Rabies
- Typhoid vaccines*
- Varicella
- Yellow fever*

*VIS use is recommended but not required by federal law at this time.

ACIP, Advisory Committee on Immunization Practices; *VIS,* vaccine information statement.

IMMUNE

Documents at the United States Government Printing Office, may be used as validation of immunization status of locally required vaccinations and of those received for the purpose of international travel.

Health care providers who administer vaccines must ensure that the patient's permanent medical records include the date the vaccine was given (or the prescription written), the vaccine's manufacturer, the lot number, and the name, address, and title of the person administering the vaccine. The ACIP recommends that this information be kept for all vaccinations. In addition, it is recommended that parents establish a permanent immunization record for each newborn child and that it be continuously updated.

Vaccine Adverse Event Report (VAER)

Under the NCVIA, provisions are made for a one-time payment to families of children who have significant adverse reactions following the administration of vaccines. The legislation acts as an alternative to civil litigation under the traditional tort system. A report of the adverse reaction must be submitted and an agreement made not to pursue litigation, before payment is made. The filing process is outlined in the VIS for the individual vaccine or immunization. Separate from the claims process is the legally mandated filing of a vaccine adverse event report (VAER) (42 USC 300aa-25) to the Vaccine Adverse Event Reporting System (VAERS) whenever an immunization recipient experiences an adverse reaction to any vaccine (Fig. 31-2 and Table 31-4). Information about this process can be obtained on the website of this national vaccine safety surveillance program (http://vaers.hhs.gov/), which is jointly administered by the CDC and the U.S. Food and Drug Administration (FDA) (http://vaers.hhs.gov/).

BIOTERRORISM

Bioterrorism is the use of biologic, nuclear, or chemical agents to bring harm to peoples in large geographic areas. Terrorists may use genetically engineered agents that resist current therapies and circumvent vaccine-induced immunity. Individuals and communities may develop symptoms but fail to recognize that they have been exposed to weapons of mass destruction (WMDs). For some, symptoms may not appear for days or weeks; given our mobile society, people who are thus unaware of their condition may unknowingly infect others, including health care providers. The impact of bioterrorism may be exacerbated if emergency medical personnel and procedures are inadequate to respond to WMD events in an effective and timely manner.

DISEASES AND DRUGS OF BIOTERRORISM

Although vaccines can offer protection when administered after exposure to certain biologic agents, none are available against many of the potential threats of biologic warfare. The primary benefit of passively acquired immunity against biologic illness is that it grants an immediate state of immunity that extends for weeks and possibly months. Some of the vaccines have half-lives of 30 days or more.

Vaccination reduces a community's vulnerability to specific threats, assuming a safe and effective vaccine is available that will provoke an immune response in the populace. Unfortunately, provoking an immune response through vaccination often takes longer than the period between threat exposure and onset of illness. Further, many of the vaccines require repeated injections to achieve adequate immunity, thus limiting their ability in an emergency vaccination program to provide rapid prophylaxis after exposure.

Viral Hemorrhagic Fevers

The viral hemorrhagic fevers (VHF) include Argentine, Ebola, Marburg, Junin, and Lassa viruses. The two greatest threats to the United States as well as other countries are Ebola and Marburg, category A biologic weapons. The VHFs are a group of febrile illnesses with a tendency to cause significant bleeding. They are caused by a group of RNA viruses that belong to four distinct viral families. These viruses are characteristically associated with high mortality and morbidity, are spread person-to-person, are highly infectious at a low dose delivered by the aerosol route, and are stable in the environment; furthermore, large-scale production is possible.

Prodromal symptoms are typical, with several days of fever, myalgias, headache, malaise, arthralgias, nausea, diarrhea, and abdominal pain. With some VHFs, abdominal pain may be pronounced, mimicking an acute condition in the abdomen. After the prodrome period, patients may develop conjunctivitis and pharyngitis, and most VHF patients have a rash, with the dermal manifestations varying by etiology. As the disease progresses, patients may show evidence of a progressively worsening bleeding diathesis, with petechiae, conjunctival and mucosal hemorrhage, hematuria, hematemesis, and melena, followed by disseminated intravascular coagulation (DIC) and hypotension. As the patient's condition worsens, CNS signs appear, including delirium, seizures, and coma. Shock and multiple organ system failure precede death.

Passive immunization has been used for the treatment of Ebola, Argentine, and Lassa hemorrhagic fevers, with promising results. However, there are two caveats in the use of passive Ab therapy against VHF: (1) disease-enhancing antibodies must exist and, (2) high-titer sera are needed to achieve protection. Two vaccines are currently available for VHF, yellow fever virus and Argentine hemorrhagic fever vaccines. Treatment is primarily supportive.

Anthrax

Anthrax is an acute infectious disease caused by the spore-forming bacterium *Bacillus anthracis*. Anthrax most commonly occurs in wild and domestic lower vertebrates (cattle, sheep, goats, camels, antelopes, and other herbivores), but it can also occur in humans who are exposed to infected animals or to tissue from infected animals, or when anthrax spores are used as a bioterrorist weapon. Anthrax infection is not contagious and cannot be transmitted by human-to-human contact.

Inhalational anthrax develops once spore-bearing particles reach the alveolar spaces. The spores are ingested by macrophages, some of which are lysed and destroyed. Any remaining spores germinate into vegetative cells and are transported to mediastinal lymph nodes, where they multiply. Illness follows soon after multiplication has begun.

Cutaneous anthrax results from the deposition of anthrax spores in the skin through lacerations or abrasions. Once the spores germinate in the tissues, toxin production leads to localized edema.

VAERS

VACCINE ADVERSE EVENT REPORTING SYSTEM
24 Hour Toll-free information line 1-800-822-7967
P.O. Box 1100, Rockville, MD 20849-1100
PATIENT IDENTITY KEPT CONFIDENTIAL

For CDC/FDA Use Only

VAERS Number _____

Date Received _____

Patient Name:	Vaccine administered by (Name):	Form completed by (Name):
Last　　　First　　　M.I.	Responsible Physician _____	Relation ☐ Vaccine Provider ☐ Patient/Parent
Address	Facility Name/Address	to Patient ☐ Manufacturer ☐ Other
		Address (if different from patient or provider)
City　　State　　Zip	City　　State　　Zip	City　　State　　Zip
Telephone no. (_____)_____	Telephone no. (_____)_____	Telephone no. (_____)_____

1. State	2. County where administered	3. Date of birth ___/___/___ mm dd yy	4. Patient age	5. Sex ☐ M ☐ F	6. Date form completed ___/___/___ mm dd yy

7. Describe adverse event(s) (symptoms, signs, time course) and treatment, if any	8. Check all appropriate:
	☐ Patient died　(date ___/___/___)
	☐ Life-threatening illness mm dd yy
	☐ Required emergency room/doctor visit
	☐ Required hospitalization (_____days)
	☐ Resulted in prolongation of hospitalization
	☐ Resulted in permanent disability
	☐ None of the above

9. Patient recovered ☐ YES ☐ NO ☐ UNKNOWN	10. Date of vaccination	11. Adverse event onset
12. Relevant diagnostic tests/laboratory data	___/___/___ mm dd yy Time_____ AM PM	___/___/___ mm dd yy Time_____ AM PM

13. Enter all vaccines given on date listed in no. 10

	Vaccine (type)	Manufacturer	Lot number	Route/site	No. previous doses
a.					
b.					
c.					
d.					

14. Any other vaccinations within 4 weeks prior to the date listed in no. 10

	Vaccine (type)	Manufacturer	Lot number	Route/site	No. previous doses	Date given
a.						
b.						

15. Vaccinated at: ☐ Private doctor's office/hospital ☐ Military clinic/hospital ☐ Public health clinic/hospital ☐ Other/unknown	16. Vaccine purchased with: ☐ Private funds ☐ Military funds ☐ Public funds ☐ Other /unknown	17. Other medications

18. Illness at time of vaccination (specify)	19. Pre-existing physician-diagnosed allergies, birth defects, medical conditions (specify)

20. Have you reported this adverse event previously? ☐ No ☐ To health department ☐ To doctor ☐ To manufacturer	**Only for children 5 and under**
	22. Birth weight _____ lb. _____ oz.
	23. No. of brothers and sisters

21. Adverse event following prior vaccination (check all applicable, specify)

Only for reports submitted by manufacturer/immunization project

	Adverse event	Onset age	Type vaccine	Dose no. in series	24. Mfr. / imm. proj. report no.	25. Date received by mfr. / imm. proj.
☐ In patient	_____	_____	_____	_____		
☐ In brother	_____	_____	_____	_____	26. 15 day report?	27. Report type
or sister	_____	_____	_____	_____	☐ Yes ☐ No	☐ Initial ☐ Follow-Up

Health care providers and manufacturers are required by law (42 USC 300aa-25) to report reactions to vaccines listed in the Table of Reportable Events Following Immunization. Reports for reactions to other vaccines are voluntary except when required as a condition of immunization grant awards.

Form VAERS -1

IMMUNE

FIGURE 31-2 Vaccine Adverse Event Report. The Food and Drug Administration (Law 42 USC 300aa-25) requires that a report be filed whenever a recipient of an immunization has an adverse reaction to vaccines listed in Table 31-4. (From Vaccine Adverse Event Reporting System. (2002). *The reportable events table.* Rockville, MD: Author.)

TABLE 31-4 Table of Reportable Events Following Vaccination

Event	Interval from Vaccination
TETANUS AND PERTUSSIS IN ANY COMBINATION; DTAP, DTP, DTP-HIB, P	
Anaphylaxis or anaphylactic shock	7 days
Brachial neuritis	28 days
Any sequelae of above events (including death)*	No limit
Events as described in manufacturer's package insert are contraindications to additional doses of vaccine.	See package insert
PERTUSSIS IN ANY COMBINATION; DTAP, DTP, DTP-HIB, P	
Anaphylaxis or anaphylactic shock	7 days
Encephalopathy or encephalitis	7 days
Any sequelae of above events (including death)	No limit
Events as described in manufacturer's package insert are contraindications to additional doses of vaccine.	See package insert
MEASLES, MUMPS, AND RUBELLA IN ANY COMBINATION; MMR, MR, M, OR R	
Anaphylaxis or anaphylactic shock	7 days
Encephalopathy or encephalitis	15 days
Any sequelae of above events (including death)	No limit
Events as described in manufacturer's package insert are contraindications to additional doses of vaccine.	See package insert
RUBELLA IN ANY COMBINATION; MMR, MR, R	
Chronic arthritis	42 days
Any sequelae of above events (including death)	No limit
Events as described in manufacturer's package insert are contraindications to additional doses of vaccine.	See package insert
MEASLES IN ANY COMBINATION; MMR, MR, M	
Thrombocytopenic purpura	7–30 days
Vaccine-strain measles viral infection in an immunodeficient recipient	6 months
Any sequelae of above events (including death)	No limit
Events as described in manufacturer's package insert are contraindications to additional doses of vaccine.	See package insert
ORAL POLIO VACCINE (OPV)	
Paralytic polio	30 days, 6 months
Vaccine-strain polio viral infection	30 days, 6 months
Any sequelae of above events (including death)	No limit
Events as described in manufacturer's package insert are contraindications to additional doses of vaccine.	See package insert
INACTIVATED POLIO VACCINE (IPV)	
Anaphylaxis or anaphylactic shock	24 hours
Any sequelae of above events (including death)	No limit
Events as described in manufacturer's package insert are contraindications to additional doses of vaccine.	See package insert
HEPATITIS B (HBV)	
Anaphylaxis or anaphylactic shock	24 hours
Any sequelae of above events (including death)	No limit
Events as described in manufacturer's package insert are contraindications to additional doses of vaccine.	See package insert
***HAEMOPHILUS* INFLUENZA, TYPE B, (CONJUGATE) (HIB)**	
Events as described in manufacturer's package insert are contraindications to additional doses of vaccine.	See package insert
VARICELLA	
Events as described in manufacturer's package insert are contraindications to additional doses of vaccine.	See package insert
ROTOVIRUS	
Intussusception	30 days
Any sequelae of above events (including death)	No limit
Events as described in manufacturer's package insert are contraindications to additional doses of vaccine.	See package insert
PNEUMOCOCCAL CONJUGATE	
Events as described in manufacturer's package insert are contraindications to additional doses of vaccine.	See package insert

*The term *sequela* means a condition or event that was actually caused by a condition listed in the Reportable Events Table (RET).
Effective date: August 26, 2002. The RET reflects what is reportable by law (42 USC 300aa-25) to the Vaccine Adverse Event Reporting System (VAERS) including conditions found in the manufacturers package insert. In addition, individuals are encouraged to report any clinically significant or unexpected events (even if not certain the vaccine caused the event) for any vaccine, whether or not it is listed on the RET. Manufacturers are also required by regulation (21CFR 600.80) to report to the VAERS program all adverse events made known to them for any vaccine.
DTaP, Diphtheria-tetanus–acellular pertussis; *DTP*, diphtheria-tetanus-pertussis; *Hib*, *Haemophilus* influenza, type b; *HBV*, hepatitis B; *IPV*, inactivated polio vaccine; *M*, measles; *MMR*, measles-mumps-rubella; *MMRV*, measles-mumps-rubella-varicella; *MR*, measles-rubella; *OPV*, oral polio vaccine; *P*, pertussis; *PPD*, purified protein derivative; *Td*, tetanus-diphtheria. Data from Centers for Disease Control. (2006). Vaccine Adverse Event Reporting System. Rockville, MD: The Centers. Available online: http://wonder.cdc.gov/wonder/help/vaers/reportable. htm. Accessed April 27, 2007.

TABLE 31-5 Vaccines Relevant To Bioterrorism

Drug	FRM	Indications	Efficacy and Duration	Implications
Anthrax vaccine, absorbed	KBV	Anthrax	Efficacy: Unknown Duration: Unknown	Effective against inhalational anthrax and may help prevent onset of disease postexposure, if given with appropriate antibiotics
Botulism antitoxin (Bivalent anti-AB equine antitoxin, Anti-AB human antitoxin for infant botulism)	KAT	Botulism	Efficacy: 100% with three doses Duration: Unavailable	Test for hypersensitivity to horse serum before administering antitoxin. Available from the CDC
Smallpox (calf lymph, DryVax)	LVV	Preexposure and postexposure prophylaxis	Efficacy: Unknown Duration: Unknown	Vaccine take rate is >90% for current stockpile of drug. Vaccination administered within 4 days of first exposure has been shown to offer some protection against acquiring infection and significant protection against a fatal outcome.

CDC, Centers for Disease Control and Prevention; KAT, killed antitoxin; KBV, killed bacterial vaccine; LVV, live virus vaccine.

Germination of anthrax spores in the oropharyngeal area results in edema, esophageal ulceration, regional lymphadenopathy, and sepsis. Once deposited in the ileocecal area, necrosis of the intestines causes an acute condition in the abdomen, ascites, blood diarrhea, and sepsis.

An FDA-licensed vaccine derived from an attenuated, non-encapsulated *B. anthracis* strain of anthrax is available and has been used in military troops and at-risk civilians (Table 31-5). The vaccine, designated as "anthrax vaccine absorbed," is nonliving. The vaccination series consists of six IM doses, administered at 0, 2, and 4 weeks, and again at 6, 12, and 18 months, followed by annual boosters.

The U.S. Army has also developed a second-generation vaccine for anthrax based on the same Ag. There are no grounds to believe the new vaccine will be more protective; however, it is more easily manufactured, may be less likely to cause adverse reactions, and is possibly less expensive if made in large quantities. The CDC has recommended the manufacture of Ab formulations from the serum of persons previously vaccinated for anthrax.

A small percentage of persons receiving the anthrax vaccine experience local reactions. A headache is the vaccine's most common adverse effect. In addition, other adverse effects may include fever and chills, sore throat, blurry vision, dizziness, anorexia, nausea, vomiting, diarrhea, malaise, muscle and joint pains, and urticaria. No long-term adverse effects have been reported.

Botulism

Botulinum toxins are some of the most potent toxins known. Botulism is caused by a group of neurotoxins produced by the bacterium *Clostridium botulinum*. The toxins do not penetrate intact skin but rather are absorbed into the circulation through the pulmonary or GI mucosa or a wound.

Botulinum toxins bind to neuromuscular junctions preventing the release of acetylcholine (ACh), which in turn causes muscular paralysis. Although it may take weeks or months for an improvement to be seen, damage to the neuromuscular junctions is potentially reversible with the growth of new axons.

Symptoms of botulism are related to the ingestion of foods containing botulinum. The symptoms begin with symmetrical flaccid paralysis with cranial nerve palsies that manifest first as dysphagia, dysphonia, or blurry or double vision, followed by dilated pupils, dysconjugate gaze, dry mouth, loss of gag reflex, extremity weakness and paresthesias, and sometimes ataxia. In some patients, the neurologic manifestations may be preceded by nausea, vomiting, diarrhea or constipation, and abdominal cramps. Sensation is not affected, and mentation is preserved. The severity of symptoms varies with the amount of toxin consumed as well as individual patient variables.

Treatment should be started with the appearance of the signs and symptoms of botulism. There are two antitoxins available: bivalent anti-AB equine antitoxin, anti-AB human antitoxin for infant botulism. The trivalent formulation of equine antitoxin, available through the CDC, contains Ab against three of the seven causes of human botulism, toxin types A, B, and E. Administration of a botulinum antitoxin effectively slows or may halt progression of paralysis to respiratory failure by binding the remaining circulation toxins, provided the antitoxin is given within 24 hours of disease onset. Once respiratory failure requiring artificial ventilation is present, the antitoxin is unlikely to be useful.

Plague

Plague (bubonic plague, also called pneumonic plague) is a bacterial disease caused by *Yersinia pestis*, a gram-negative bacillus. It is transmitted from rodents and their fleas to animals and people. Plague occurs most commonly in the western United States, in parts of South America, and in Africa and Asia. Those at risk for exposure include field biologists and people who reside or work in rural or mountainous areas.

Plague is characterized by lymphadenitis in nodes receiving drainage from the site of the fleabite. Lymphadenitis occurs more often in the inguinal area and less commonly in axillary and cervical nodes. The nodes become edematous, inflamed, tender, and suppurative. Fever, chills, headache, and weakness are characteristic symptoms. Secondary pulmonary involvement results in pneumonia, mediastinitis, or pleural effusion.

No plague vaccine is currently available for use in the United States, although a killed vaccine was previously licensed. Animal and preliminary human studies have indicated that a killed plague vaccine is not effective for preventing bubonic plague. A recombinant vaccine for the prevention of bubonic plague after an inhalational exposure is under investigation.

Smallpox

Smallpox is a potentially fatal disease caused by the variola virus invading the pharynx and airways, and traveling to regional lymph nodes. In general, lengthy periods of face-to-

IMMUNE

face contact are required for the virus to be disseminated, although variola can be transmitted via body fluids and contaminated objects. Once replication begins, the disease progresses rapidly to viremia. Viremia is characterized by headache, malaise, a fever of 101° F to 104° F, chills, pharyngitis, lymphadenopathy, vomiting, backache, and, in some patients, delirium.

Red lesions develop on the tongue and in the mouth 48 to 72 hours after the development of viremia. The patient becomes contagious once the lesions in the oral cavity break open, spreading large amounts of virus into the mouth and throat. The rash spreads next to the face and then to the arms and the legs. The hands and feet are the last areas to be affected. By the third day, the rash becomes firm, pustular, raised lesions, followed in another week by the formation of scabs with depigmented, pitting scars. The patient remains contagious until all of the scabs have fallen off, approximately 2 to 3 weeks after the onset of the infection.

Variola major, the most common form of smallpox, accounts for over 90% of the cases. A less severe form may occur in persons who have previously received smallpox vaccination. Overall, variola major has a 30% fatality rate. Variola minor appears as often as the major form of smallpox but is much less severe. The incubation period is 7 to 17 days.

Except for stockpiles of the virus in specialized infectious disease laboratories, variola virus has been eliminated worldwide. The last known case of smallpox was in 1997 in Somalia; the last known case in the United States was in 1949. Since then, routine vaccination against smallpox has not been done in the United States. Nonetheless, the bioterrorism events of September 11, 2001, in the United States have increased concerns that variola may be released into the populace to cause widespread illness and subsequent death.

Smallpox vaccine (vaccinia; calf lymph, DryVax) is a live virus vaccine currently used in persons in special-risk categories, including laboratory workers directly involved with smallpox or closely related orthopoxviruses. Since 2002, U.S. Department of Defense announced that certain military personnel, half a million first responders, and other health care providers have received smallpox vaccinations. Vaccinia immune globulin (VIG) is reserved for persons who would be in close contact with patients with smallpox. The use of VIG significantly reduces the incidence of disease compared with persons who have not received passive smallpox immunization.

Patients in whom smallpox vaccination is contraindicated, because of the risk for complications, include (1) persons who are immunosuppressed or have HIV; (2) those with a history or evidence of eczema, (3) those in current close contact with persons characterized by the foregoing conditions, and (4) pregnant women. The benefits of administering the vaccine to these groups must be weighed against the greater risk to others should they contract the disease. When available, VIG can be given simultaneously with the smallpox vaccination, although the risk of reducing the immune response must be taken into account

Adverse effects are usually self-limiting but include fever, headache, fatigue, myalgia, chills, local skin reactions, nonspecific rashes, erythema multiforme, lymphadenopathy, and pain at the vaccination site. Smallpox can be transmitted from a vaccinee's unhealed vaccination site to other persons by close contact. Adverse effects that require further evaluation are generalized vaccinia (manifested by skin lesions and organ involvement), eczema vaccinatum, progressive vaccinia, postvaccinial encephalopathy, and fetal vaccinia (which often results in fetal or neonatal death).

Tularemia

Francisella tularensis, a nonmobile gram-negative coccobacillus, is a facultative intracellular parasite that is found naturally in the United States in animals (e.g., rodents, rabbits). The bacillus is transmitted via the bite of an infected deerfly or other insect; by eating or drinking contaminated water or food; and through the handling of infected animal carcasses. Tularemic meningitis, gastrointestinal disease, and bacterial endocarditis may result from an aerosolized formulation of the bacilli.

The incubation period for tularemia is 2 to 5 days. The signs and symptoms of pneumonic tularemia include fever, headache, muscle pain, difficulty breathing, shortness of breath, cough, and pleural pains. An x-ray study will reveal spotty infiltrates in lungs, lobular consolidation, and pleural exudate. The signs and symptoms of typhoidal tularemia include fever, but no lymphadenopathy or visible skin lesions.

The live vaccine for tularemia is derived from strain 15 of *F. tularensis*. This avirulent strain was acquired by the United States from the Soviet Union, otherwise known as the United Soviet Socialists Republic or USSR, in trade for strain Schu SD4. The Soviet Union used their newly acquired strain to enlarge their cache of WMD, whereas the United States used the Soviet strain to develop a vaccine. Despite incomplete efficacy in preventing tularemia, the vaccine can minimize its severity. Although the vaccine is recommended for those at significantly high risk for exposure to tularemia, it is currently undergoing a safety review by the FDA.

KEY POINTS

- Sera, vaccines, and other immunizing agents are used to produce active and passive immunity.
- Active acquired immunity develops when the host forms antibodies after exposure to modified pathogens or toxins.
- Passive immunity develops when the host is given antibodies from another individual or animal.
- The specific drug to be used for active immunity depends on how prevalent the disease is, the degree of exposure, the season, and the duration of exposure.
- The patient history should include a thorough immunization history and documentation of screening questions for precautions and contraindications, medical history, and history of chronic illness or immunosuppression.

■ The immediate goal in the use of vaccines and other immunizing agents is to prevent disease in individuals and groups. The long-term goal of immunization programs is eradication of disease.

■ Universal immunization of infants and other at-risk individuals produces a dramatic decline in the transmission of infectious diseases.

■ The CDC develops immunization schedules under the guidance of the Advisory Committee for Immunization Practices (ACIP).

■ Patient education includes information about the recommended immunization schedule and addressing parents' and patients' fears about vaccinations.

■ The federal government accepts responsibility for adverse reactions under the National Childhood Vaccine Injury Act (NCVIA) of 1986.

■ The FDA requires a vaccine adverse event report (VAER) to be completed whenever an immunization recipient experiences an adverse reaction to a specific vaccine.

■ The ACIP recommends that the following information be kept for all vaccinations: the date each vaccine was administered, the vaccine manufacturer, the vaccine lot number, and the name, address, and title of the person administering the vaccine.

■ It is not unusual for a health care provider to encounter persons without adequate documentation of immunizations. Immunizations should not be postponed for lack of records.

■ The NCVIA mandates that a vaccine information statement (VIS) be provided to either the adult vaccinee or to the child's parent or legal representative before administration of any vaccine.

■ Pathogens that have been identified as potential biologic warfare agents include those that cause anthrax, botulism, plague, smallpox, tularemia, and viral hemorrhagic fevers. Although there are vaccines for anthrax, botulism, and smallpox, their use is restricted.

Bibliography

Advisory Committee on Immunization Practices. (2004). Prevention and control of influenza. *MMWR Morbidity and Mortality Weekly Report, 53*(RR 6), 1–40.

American Academy of Pediatrics. *2006 Immunization schedule.* Available online: www.cispimmunize.org. Accessed April 29, 2007.

Centers for Disease Control and Prevention. *Bioterrorism overview.* Available online: www.bt.cdc.gov/bioterrorism/. Accessed April 29, 2007.

Centers for Disease Control and Prevention. (2000). Guidelines for preventing opportunistic infections among hematopoietic stem cell transplant recipients: Recommendations of the CDC, the Infectious Disease Society of America, and the American Society of Blood and Marrow Transplantation. *MMWR Morbidity and Mortality Weekly Report, 49*(RR-10), 1–128.

Centers for Disease Control and Prevention. (2000). Poliomyelitis prevention in the United States: Updated recommendations of the Advisory Committee on Immunization Practices (ACIP). *MMWR Morbidity and Mortality Weekly Report, 49*(RR-5), 1–22.

Centers for Disease Control and Prevention. (2000). Prevention and control of meningococcal disease: Recommendations of the Advisory Committee on Immunizations Practices (ACIP). *MMWR Morbidity and Mortality Weekly Report, 49*(RR-7), 1–10.

Centers for Disease Control and Prevention. (2002). Progress toward elimination of *Haemophilus* influenza type B disease among infants and children–United States, 1998–2000. *MMWR Morbidity and Mortality Weekly Report, 51*(11), 234–237.

Centers for Disease Control and Prevention. *Summary of October (2002) ACIP Smallpox Vaccination Recommendations.* Available online: www.bt.cdc.gov/agent/smallpox/vaccination/acip-recs-oct2002. asp. Accessed April 29, 2007.

Centers for Disease Control and Prevention. (2005). Prevention and control of influenza: Recommendations of the Advisory Committee on Immunization Practices (ACIP). *MMWR Morbidity and Mortality Weekly Report, 54*(RR-8), 1–40.

Centers for Disease Control and Prevention. (2005). Recommended adult immunization schedule–United States 2005. *MMWR Morbidity and Mortality Weekly Report, 54*(40), Q1-Q4.

Centers for Disease Control and Prevention. (2005). Recommended childhood and adolescent immunization schedule–United States 2006. *MMWR Morbidity and Mortality Weekly Report, 54*(51, 52), Q1-Q4.

Centers for Disease Control and Prevention. (2005). *Recommended adult immunization schedule, by vaccine and age group. United States, October 2005–September 2006.* Available online: www.cdc.gov/nip/recs/adult-schedule.pdf. Accessed July 16, 2007.

Centers for Disease Control and Prevention and Kozarsky, P., Arguin, P., and Navin, A. (2005). *Health information for international travel 2005–2006–CDC Yellow Book.* St Louis: Mosby. Available online: www2.ncid.cdc.gov/travel/yb/utils/ybBrowseO.asp. Accessed March 5, 2007.

Centers for Disease Control and Prevention. (2006). *Childhood immunization schedule.* Available online: www.cdc.gov/nip/recs/child-schedule.htm. Accessed July 16, 2007.

Centers for Disease Control and Prevention and Atkinson, W., Hamborsky, J., Wolfe, S., eds. (2007). *Epidemiology and prevention of vaccine-preventable diseases.* (10th ed.). Washington, DC: Public Health Foundation. Available online: www.cdc.gov/nip/publications/pink/. Accessed April 29, 2007.

Centers for Disease Control and Prevention. (2005). *Six common misconceptions about vaccinations and how to respond to them.* Available online: www.cdc.gov/nip/publications/6mishome.htm. Accessed April 29, 2007.

Colorado Training Center. (2004). Biological, nuclear, incendiary, chemical, explosive (BNICE) WMD clinical care course. Denver, Colorado: Denver Health Medical Center.

Diekema, D. (2005). Responding to parental refusals of immunization of children. *Pediatrics, 115*(5), 1428–1431.

Hoard, M., Williams, J., Helmkamp, J., et al. (2002). Preparing at the local level for events involving weapons of mass destruction. *Emerging Infectious Diseases, 8*(9), 1006–1007. Available online: www.cdc.gov/ncidod/EID/vol8no9/01-0520.htm. Accessed March 1, 2007.

Kimberlin, D., and Whitley, R. (2007). Varicella-zoster vaccine for the prevention of herpes zoster. *New England Journal of Medicine, 356*(13), 1338–1343.

Macintyre, A., Christopher, G., Eitzen, E., et al. (2000). Weapons of mass destruction events with contaminated casualties: effective planning for health care facilities. *Journal of the American Medical Association, 283*(2), 242–249.

National Foundation for Infectious Diseases (NFID). (2004). *The changing epidemiology of meningococcal disease among U.S. children, adolescents, and young adults.* Available online: www.nfid.org/publications/meningococcalepid.pdf. Accessed April 29, 2007.

National Immunization Program. (2006). *Vaccines for Children Program.* Available online: www.cdc.gov/nip/vfc. Accessed April 29, 2007.

Offit, P., and Jew, R. Addressing parents' concerns: Do vaccines contain harmful preservations, adjuvants, additives, or residuals? Available online: http://pediatrics.aappublications.org/cgi/content/full/112/6/1394. Accessed April 29, 2007.

IMMUNE

Oxman, M., Levin, M., Johnson, G., et al. (2005). A vaccine to prevent herpes zoster and postherpetic neuralgia in older adults. *New England Journal of Medicine, 352*(22), 2271–2284.

Pickering, L. (2003). *The 2003 Red Book: Report of the Committee on Infectious Diseases*. (26th ed.). Elk Grove Village, IL: American Academy of Pediatrics.

Plotkin, S., and Orenstein, W. (2003). *Vaccines*. (4th ed.). Philadelphia: WB Saunders.

Rose, S., and Keystone, J. (2006). International Travel Health Guide 2006–2007. Philadelphia: Mosby.

Schleiss, M. (2005). Cytomegalovirus infection. *eMedicine*. Available online: www.emedicine.com/PED/topic544.htm. Accessed April 29, 2007.

The Group on Immunization Education of the Society of Teachers of Family Medicine (website). Available online: www.immunizationed.org. Accessed April 29, 2007.

United States Agency for Healthcare Research and Quality, University of Alabama School of Medicine. *CDC Category A high-priority biological diseases*. Available online: www.bioterrorism.uab.edu/eipba.html. Accessed April 29, 2007.

United States Department of Health and Human Services. (2000). *Healthy people 2010: National health promotion and disease prevention objectives*. Washington, DC: U.S. Government Printing Office.

University of Alabama. *Bioterrorism and emerging infections*. Available online: www.bioterrorism.uab.edu/. Accessed May 2, 2007.

Zimmerman, R. (2001). Pneumococcal conjugate vaccine for young children. *American Family Physician, 63*(10), 1991–1998.

32

Biologic Response Modifiers

Two scientific developments in the mid-to-late 1970s fostered the development of biologic response modifiers (BRM), substances that boost the body's immune system against diseases: hybridoma and recombinant DNA technology. Hybridoma technology allows the production of monoclonal antibodies by using the antigen-antibody (Ag-Ab) reaction when targeting cancers and other diseases. Each hybridoma produces large quantities of identical Abs (Fig. 32-1). By allowing the hybridoma to multiply in culture, it is possible to produce a population of cells, each of which produces identical Ab molecules. *Monoclonal antibodies (MoAbs)* are produced by the identical progeny of a single, cloned antibody-producing cell, the hybridoma cell. Abs produced by traditional methods, on the other hand, are derived from preparations containing many kinds of cells, and for this reason are called *polyclonal antibodies*. Today's generation of MoAbs allow for newer and more precise therapeutic and diagnostic possibilities, particularly for the treatment of cancer and autoimmune conditions, and early detection of viral infections.

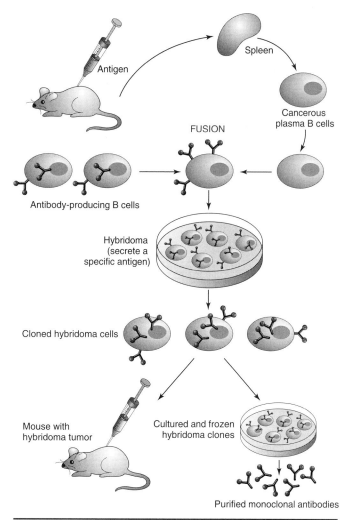

FIGURE 32-1 Hybridoma Technology. Monoclonal antibodies are produced by hybridizing B cells from the spleens of mice that have been injected with a specific Ag and B cells from a plasma cell tumor. The result is a hybridoma that is both Ag-specific and capable of indefinite proliferation.

The second major scientific development was recombinant DNA technology. The fundamental components of recombinant DNA technology are *bacterial plasmids,* small, circular sections of self-replicating DNA. Plasmids can be removed from or inserted into bacteria without severely disrupting bacterial growth or reproduction. The plasmid is withdrawn from the bacterial host and exposed to restrictive enzymes that cut the plasmid's DNA at a precise site in the nucleotide sequence (Fig. 32-2). For example, the common enzyme *EcoRI* (named for the bacteria that produce it, *Escherichia coli*) cuts a strand of the plasmid's DNA where the nucleotide sequence G-A-A-T-T-C is found. Human DNA can also be exposed to *EcoRI* and cut at the same site. The pieces of human DNA and bacterial DNA can then be recombined. The plasmid, which now contains human genes in addition to its own, is then reintroduced into the bacterium, where it divides and replicates, copying itself and the recombinant DNA. This product of cell fusion now combines the desired qualities of the two different types of cells: the ability to grow continually, and the ability to produce large amounts of pure Ab. Through cell division, millions of bacterial clones are formed, all containing the same human gene. The human gene directs protein synthesis in the bacteria, resulting in the production of human proteins by the bacteria. Because protein enzymes are responsible for most chemical reactions within cells, the ability to replicate specific proteins becomes extremely important to the understanding and manipulation of cell activity and the most basic elements of body function.

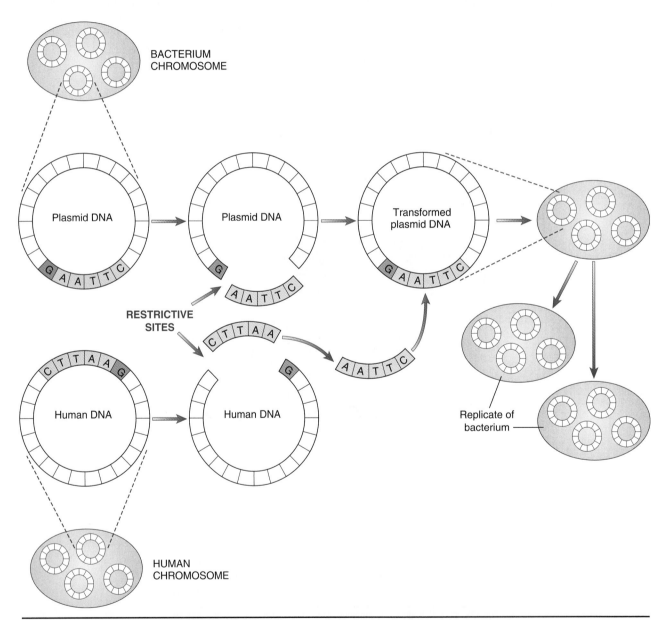

FIGURE 32-2 Recombinant DNA Technology. Human DNA and plasmid DNA from a bacterium (e.g., *Escherichia coli*) are cleaved by a restrictive enzyme. The enzymes cut both DNA fragments at a precise site in the nucleotide sequence, for example, where the nucleotide sequence G-A-A-T-T-C is found. The human DNA is then recombined with bacterial DNA. The plasmids, which now also contain human genes, are introduced back into the bacterium, which divide and replicate, copying its original and the recombinant DNA. (**G,** Guanine; **A,** adenine; **T,** thymine; **C,** cytosine.)

CATEGORIES OF BRMS

BRMs are organized into two primary categories: immunostimulants and immunosuppressants. *Immunostimulants* augment the immune response by stimulating reticuloendothelial cells (i.e., monocytes, macrophages) to initiate action against foreign invaders. The best example of immunostimulation is the practice of administering vaccines (see also Chapter 31). Patients who receive vaccines acquire either active or passive immunity to specific foreign proteins or Ags (see also Chapter 31). The major *immunosuppressant* drugs inhibit or suppress the immune response and are employed in the control of organ transplant rejection and to reduce the inflammatory process associated with autoimmune diseases.

PATHOGENESIS

The ability of multicellular organisms to coordinate cellular proliferation, survival, and differentiation and other cell functions is dependent on the ability of different cell types to communicate with each other. Nature has a well-designed solution for cell-to-cell communication that does not require cell-to-cell contact: cytokines and colony stimulating factors. A *cytokine* is a cell-derived factor that mediates communication between cells. The cytokines are not required for maintenance of a steady-state but instead are important in the accelerated production of these cells in the presence of inflammation and infection. The maturation of each cell is depicted in the hematopoietic cascade (Fig. 32-3). The efficacy of the immune response relies on the interactions between the humoral and cell-mediated immune systems.

The primary cell of the immune response is the lymphocyte. Lymphocytes originate in the liver and the spleen of the fetus and the bone marrow of the child or adult as lymphocyte precursors or stem cells. To become immunocompetent, they must migrate through the lymphatic system, the blood vessels, and then through lymphoid tissues in various parts of the body. While passing through these tissues, they mature and undergo changes that entrust them to one of two cell lines: B and T cells.

Lymphocytes that migrate through lymphoid tissues (i.e., *lymphokines*) are referred to as *B cells* and are responsible for humoral immunity. When B cells encounter Ags, they mature into plasma cells that produce antibodies (i.e., IgG, IgM, IgA, and IgE). Lymphocytes migrating through the thymus gland become *T cells*. The T cells then become sensitive to and recognize specific Ags, which they attack directly to destroy cells bearing foreign Ags (e.g., virus-infected cells, tumors, or foreign grafts). T helper cells produce lymphokines that trigger macrophage activity, but do not appear to mediate any other function.

Whereas T helper cells and T suppressor cells control both humoral and cell-mediated immune processes, T memory cells induce a secondary immune response. When the body first meets an Ag, it destroys the Ag. T memory cells remember the Ag throughout the patient's lifetime.

Natural killer (NK) cells are a major part of the innate immune system, and are distinctive in that they attack cells infected by microorganisms, but not the organisms themselves. NK cells contain perforin and proteases, proteins that lyse target cells upon contact. Perforin creates pores in the membranes of target cells through which other molecules can enter to cause cell death (i.e., apoptosis). The distinction between cell lysis and apoptosis is important in immunology: lysing a virus-infected cell only releases the virions, whereas apoptosis leads to intracellular destruction of the virus.

Lymphocytes produced by monocyte-macrophage cells are called *monokines*. Some of the monokines are referred to as *interleukins* (ILs), which are polypeptide molecules secreted by lymphocytes. ILs help regulate the production of white blood cells (WBCs) by serving as chemical communicators between various WBCs. Healthy adults produce about 2 million new WBCs every hour, mostly in the bone marrow. These cells survive, proliferate, and differentiate only if they are provided with colony-stimulating factors (CSFs). CSFs are glycoproteins that regulate the differentiation of specific types of blood cells (one "colony" has at least 50 cells). Because infection is the most common cause of death among patients undergoing antineoplastic therapy, CSFs are administered after antineoplastic therapy to increase the speed at which WBC counts return to normal. This also allows higher dosages of antineoplastic drugs to be administered because the risk for immunosuppression is lessened and infection improved.

Interferons (IFNs) are small, low–molecular weight proteins produced and released by host cells that have been invaded by a virus. They are naturally occurring antiviral proteins that are host-specific but not virus-specific. Neutrophils and macrophages release IFN-alpha (IFN-α) and IFN-beta (IFN-β); T cells release IFN-gamma (IFN-γ). IFN-α and IFN-β possess antiinflammatory, antiproliferative, and antitumor effects, whereas IFN-γ is proinflammatory and enhances cell-mediated immunity (see Fig. 32-4).

IFNs confer resistance against most viruses, hinder multiplication of intracellular parasites, and inhibit the proliferation of normal as well as cancer cells. They also enhance granulocyte and macrophage phagocytosis and augment T-cell activity (specifically NK cell activity) and several other activities.

MoAbs are high–molecular weight proteins designed to attack one specific Ag. They are laboratory-grown clones of either a hybridoma or a virus-transformed lymphocyte that is more abundant and uniform than naturally existing Ab. That is, they are derived from a single Ab-producing cell. Hybrid cells are cloned to establish cell lines that produce a specific Ab that is chemically and immunologically homogeneous. MoAbs are able to bind specifically to almost any chosen Ag, or to reveal previously unknown Ab sites.

The early MoAbs were 100% murine (derived from mice), and the incidence of an adverse reaction, most notably anaphylaxis, was common. The use of recombinant drugs containing human DNA has reduced the incidence of hypersensitivity reactions.

This chapter will review the immunopharmacotherapeutic options in the management or treatment of cancers, autoimmunity disorders, patients with transplants, and those with other immune system–related disease. The common classes of BRMs include interferons, interleukins, colony-stimulating factors, and MoAbs. In addition, there are a variety of miscellaneous BRM drugs.

IMMUNE

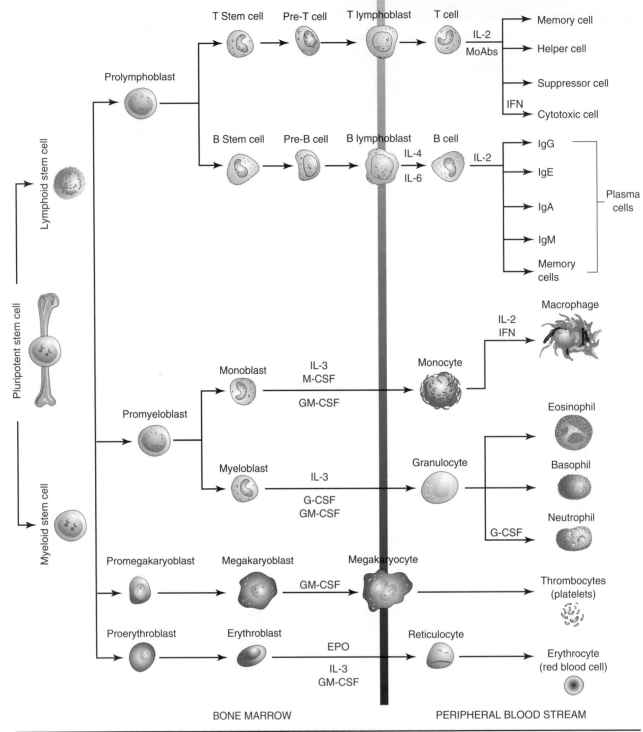

FIGURE 32-3 **Hematopoietic Cascade.** Blood cell production occurs in the liver and spleen of the fetus; however, it occurs in the bone marrow in an adult. The process involves proliferation and differentiation. Each cell type is derived from a stem cell undergoing mitosis in response to specific biochemical signals. The pathway by which natural killer (NK) cells develop is unknown. Biologic response modifiers work at various stages of the hematopoietic cascade. (**GM-CSF,** Granulocyte-macrophage colony–stimulating factor; **G-CSF,** granulocyte colony–stimulating factor; **M-CSF,** macrophage colony–stimulating factor; **IFN,** interferon; **IL,** interleukin.)

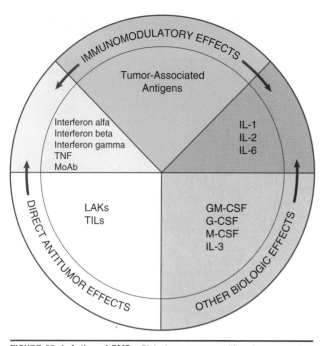

FIGURE 32-4 Action of BMRs. Biologic response modifiers have more than one drug action, including immunomodulatory, direct antitumor, and other biologic effects. (**GM-CSF,** Granulocyte-macrophage colony–stimulating factor; **G-CSF,** granulocyte colony–stimulating factor; **M-CSF,** macrophage colony–stimulating factor; **TNF,** tumor necrosis factor; **MoAb,** monoclonal antibody; **LAKs,** lymphocyte activated killer cells; **IL,** interleukin.)

PHARMACOTHERAPEUTIC OPTIONS

Interferons

- interferon alfa-2a, recombinant (Roferon-A); ✦ Roferon-A
- interferon alfa-2b, recombinant (Intron-A); ✦ Intron B
- interferon alfacon-1 (Imagent; Infergen); ✦ Infergen
- interferon alfa-3n (Alferon-A, Alferon-N); ✦ Avonex
- interferon beta-1a (Avonex); ✦ Rebif
- interferon beta-1b, recombinant (Betaseron); ✦ Betaferon
- interferon gamma-1b, recombinant (Actimmune)
- peginterferon alfa-2a (Pegasys)
- peginterferon alfa-2b (Peg-Intron)

▓ Indications

There are different synthetic formulations of IFNs, all designed to augment the body's immune system in targeting disease. IFNs are used to manage hepatitis B, chronic hepatitis C, renal cell carcinoma, hairy cell leukemia, chronic myelogenous leukemia (CML), malignant melanoma, non-Hodgkin's lymphoma, and cutaneous T-cell lymphomas, and Kaposi's sarcoma related to acquired immunodeficiency syndrome (AIDS). Other uses include the treatment of laryngeal papillomatosis in children, and for selected cases of condylomata acuminata involving external surfaces of the genital and the perianal areas. The response to IFN treatment with each of these diseases is evaluated in terms of individual patient outcomes.

Interferon beta is used to reduce the frequency of exacerbations of relapsing, remitting multiple sclerosis, Kaposi's sarcoma, renal cell carcinoma, malignant melanoma, and acute hepatitis C. In addition, interferon beta-1 has been used in the treatment of cutaneous T-cell lymphoma (off-label use).

Interferon gamma is distinct from interferon alfa and interferon beta. It functions not so much as an antiviral drug, but as a signal between T helper cells and mononuclear phagocytes. Interferon gamma reduces the frequency and severity of infections from chronic granulomatous disease and delays the effects of osteopetrosis in patients with severe malignant disease.

Peginterferon alfa-2a and peginterferon alfa-2b, alone or in combination with ribavirin, are used in the treatment of adults with chronic hepatitis C with compensated liver disease who have not been previously treated with interferon alfa.

▓ Pharmacodynamics

IFNs bind to specific receptors on the cell surface, initiating intracellular signaling through a complex cascade of protein-protein interactions and leading to rapid activation of gene transcription. IFN-mediated genes modulate many biologic effects including the inhibition of viral replication in infected cells, inhibition of cell proliferation, and immunomodulation.

When cancer cells are exposed to IFNs, they begin to look and behave more like normal cells. Although the exact mechanisms remain unclear, IFN inhibits DNA and protein synthesis in tumor cells (antiproliferative effects), and stimulates human lymphocyte antigen (HLA) and tumor-associated Ag expression on tumor cell surfaces (antitumor effects). Research is ongoing as to whether IFN has an inhibiting effect on cell growth by prolonging the phases of the cell cycle.

▓ Pharmacokinetics

The serum concentrations of IFNs following subcutaneous (subQ), intravenous (IV), or intramuscular (IM) administration of IFNs are comparable, thus demonstrating consistent absorption. IFN serum half-lives range from 2 to 8.5 hours. Undetectable levels of IFN occur approximately 4 hours after administration, representing a rapid elimination from the body (Table 32-1).

▓ Adverse Effects and Contraindications

There are a variety of well-defined adverse effects associated with IFNs, all of which are dose-dependent. The most common is a flulike syndrome with fever, chills, malaise, headache, mild anorexia, myalgias, arthralgias, xerostomia, taste alterations, weight loss, pervasive fatigue, and conjunctivitis. Hematuria and proteinuria are possible, but rare. Neurologic alterations may occur over time, including slowed thinking, poor concentration, and decreased short-term memory and attention span. Myelosuppression, neutropenia, mild anemia, paranoia, and psychoses are also possible. With high dosage, IFNs can cause hypotension, tachycardia, somnolence, confusion, and peripheral neuropathies. Although rare, acute hypersensitivity reactions have been reported with urticaria, angioedema, bronchoconstriction, and anaphylaxis.

▓ Drug Interactions

The interaction of IFNs with other drugs is not fully understood. Exercise caution when administering IFNs with other myelosuppressive drugs; the combination may result in profound neutropenia and increased risk of infection (Table 32-2). IFN increases theophylline levels by inhibiting its biotransformation. ◆

IMMUNE

PHARMACOKINETICS

TABLE 32-1 Biologic Response Modifiers (Cytokines)

Drug	Route	Onset	Peak	Duration	PB (%)	t½	BioA (%)
INTERFERONS							
interferon alfa-2a	IM	Rapid	3–4 hr*	Weeks	UA	3.7–8.5 hr	UA
	SubQ	Slow	7.3 hr	UA	UA	3.7–8.5 hr	UA
	IV	Rapid	30 min	Minutes	UA	2 hr	100
interferon alfa-2b	IM, subQ	Varies†	6–8 hr; 3–5 days to 4–8 wk‡	UA	UA	2–7 hr	UA
interferon alfa-n3	IL	Varies	UA	UA	UA	6–8 hr	UA
interferon beta-1a	IM	Varies	3–15 hr	4 days	UA	10 hr	UA
interferon beta-1b	SubQ	Rapid	1–8 hr	UA	UA	8 min–4.3 hr	50
interferon gamma-1b	SubQ	Slow	4–7 hr	UA	UA	2.9–5.9 hr	89
INTERLEUKINS							
interleukin-2	IV	5 min	13 min	3–4 hr	UA	85 min	100
COLONY STIMULATING FACTORS							
epoetin alfa	IM, IV	7–14 days	5–24 hr	24 hr	UA	4–13 hr	100
filgrastim	IV, subQ	UA	2–8 hr	4 days§	UA	3.5 hr	100
pegfilgramstim	SubQ	UA	UA	Varies	UA	15–80 hr	100
sargramostim	IV	UA	2 hr	6 hr	UA	2 hr	100
MONOCLONAL ANTIBODIES							
adalimumab	SubQ	UA	3.1–4.6 hr	UA	UA	2 wk	64
alemtuzumab	IV	Rapid	UA	UA	UA	12 days	100
bevacizumab	IV	Rapid	100 days	UA	UA	20 days	100
cetuximab	IV	Rapid	UA	UA	UA	114 hr	100
dacliximab	IV	Rapid	UA	UA	UA	480 hr	100
etanercept	SubQ	UA	UA	UA	UA	170–230 hr	UA
infliximab	IV	Rapid	UA	UA	UA	8–9.5 days	100
muromonab-CD3	IV	Rapid	3 days	3–14 days	UA	18 hr	100
natalizumab	IV	Rapid	UA	UA	UA	7–15 days	100
omalizumab	SubQ	Slow	7–8 days	UA	UA	26 days	62
rituximab	IV	Rapid	UA	3–6 mo	UA	76.3 hr	100
trastuzumab	IV	Rapid	UA	UA	UA	5.8 days	100
MISCELLANEOUS BMRS							
azathioprine	PO	UA	1–2 hr	5 hr	30	UA	UA
	IV	Rapid	UA	UA	UA	UA	100
cyclosporine	PO	UA	3–4 hr	UA	90	19–27 hr	20–50
	IV	UA	End of inf	UA	90	19–27 hr	100
etanercept	SubQ	UA	34–103 hr	UA	UA	115 hr	UA
levamisole	PO	UA	1.5–2 hr	UA	UA	3–4 hr	UA
lymphocyte IG	IV	Rapid	UA	UA	UA	3–9 days	100
mycophenolate	PO	Rapid	0.8–1.3 hr	NA	UA	17.9 hr‖	UA
RhoGam	IM	Rapid	5 days	UA	UA	24.2 days	100
tacrolimus	IV	Rapid	UA	UA	99	10–11 hr	100

*Interferon alfa-2a effect on blood count. Onset of clinical response may take 1–3 months.
†Interferon alfa-2b onset of clinical response is 1 to 3 months; onset of effects on platelet counts unknown; onset of changes in liver function tests seen in approximately 2 wk.
‡Interferon alfa-2b peak effect on platelet count seen in 3 to 5 days; 4 to 8 wk.
§Filgrastim (G-CSF) return of neutrophil count to baseline.
‖The half-life of mycophenolate's metabolite, mycophenolic acid (MPA).
IG, Immunoglobulin; IM, intramuscular; inf, infection; IV, intravenous; PB, protein binding; PO, by mouth; SubQ, subcutaneous; t½, half-life; UA, unavailable.

Dosage Regimen

Because IFNs are proteins, they would be destroyed by digestive enzymes if taken by mouth (Table 32-3). Each FDA-approved interferon has a different route and dosage regimen.

Interferon alfa-2a (human lymphoblastoid interferon) and interferon alfa-2b (human fibroblast interferon) are not interchangeable. Interferon alfa and beta share a multicomponent cell surface receptor and elicit a similar range of biologic responses including antiviral, antiproliferative, and immunomodulatory activities. They are different in several very complex biologic properties that are beyond the scope of this text. For more information, check references on biochemistry.

Lab Considerations

There are several lab values to monitor when IFNs are used. IFNs may increase aspartate transaminase (AST), alanine transaminase (ALT), and triglyceride values. Hemoglobin, hematocrit, white blood cell count, and platelet counts may decrease in the presence of IFNs. Prothrombin time and international normalized ratio (INR) values may be falsely elevated in patients taking interferon alfa-3n. Blood urea nitrogen (BUN), and creatinine values may be falsely elevated in the presence of interferon beta-1a and interferon beta-1b.

Interleukins

Indications

The only FDA-approved drug in this category is interleukin-2, recombinant (aldesleukin, Proleukin; ◆ Proleukin). Although others have been approved, some for rheumatoid arthritis, they remain in clinical trials and may be ready for use in the future. IL-2 is indicated for use in patients with metastatic renal cell

DRUG INTERACTIONS

TABLE **32-2 Biologic Response Modifiers (Cytokines)**

Drug	Interactive Drugs	Interaction
INTERFERONS		
interferon alfa-2a, interferon alfa-2b, interferon alfa-3, interferon gamma	Myelosuppressive drugs Radiation therapy	Profound neutropenia Increases risk of infection
interferon alfa-2a	theophylline, aminophylline	Decreases biotransformation and increases serum levels of interactive drug; toxicity
interferon alfa-2b	zidovudine	Increases risk of neutropenia
interferon alfa-3n	Alcohol, CNS depressants	Enhances CNS-depressant effects of either drug
INTERLEUKINS		
interleukin-2	Antianxiety drugs, Antiemetics, Opioids, Sedatives Aminoglycosides, Antineoplastics, indomethacin Corticosteroids, NSAIDs Antihypertensives, Beta blockers	Additive CNS effects Increases risk for organ toxicity Reduces antitumor effectiveness of IL-2 Increased potential for hypotension
COLONY-STIMULATING FACTORS		
filgrastim	Antineoplastic drugs	Increases risk of neutropenia
sargramostim	Corticosteroids, lithium	Potentiates myeloproliferative effects of sargramostim
MONOCLONAL ANTIBODIES		
adalimumab	methotrexate	Reduces clearance of adalimumab
adalimumab, infliximab, etanercept	abatacept, Imunosuppressants anikinra, TNF-blocking drugs imatinib natalizumab Live virus vaccines Vaccines (toxoids)	Increases risk of infection Increases risk of serious infection and neutropenia Increases risk of immunosuppression Increases risk of infection, including progressive multifocal leukoencephalopathy (PML) Inadequate immunologic response to vaccine; increases risk of disseminated infection Inadequate immunologic response to vaccine or toxoid
muromonab-CD$_3$	Immunosuppressant drugs Live virus vaccines	Increases risk of infection, lymphoproliferative disorders Increases adverse effects of interactive drug; decreases Ab response
rituximab	cisplatin natalizumab Live virus vaccines	Increases risk of nephrotoxicity Increases risk of infection, including PML Inadequate immunologic response to vaccine; increases risk for disseminated infection
trastuzumab	alefacept, allopurinol, methotrexate Anthracyclines, mitoxantrone natalizumab paclitaxel warfarin Live virus vaccines; Bacterial vaccines; Toxoids	Increases risk of infection, immunosuppression Concurrent or past use of either drug may increase risk of cardiotoxicity Increases risk of infection, including PML Increases trastuzumab levels Increases INR values and risk of bleeding Inadequate immunologic response to vaccine, increase risk of disseminated infection
MISCELLANEOUS BIOLOGIC RESPONSE MODIFIERS		
cyclosporine A	amphotericin B, Aminoglycosides, erythromycin, Fluoroquinolones, ketoconazole, NSAIDs, melphalan, Sulfonamides Anabolic steroids, Calcium channel blockers, cimetidine, danazol, erythromycin, fluconazole, ketoconazole, miconazole, Oral contraceptives azathioprine, Corticosteroids, cyclophosphamide, verapamil Barbiturates, carbamazepine, phenytoin, rifampin, Sulfonamides ACE inhibitors, Potassium-sparing diuretics, Potassium supplements digoxin Neuromuscular blockers imipenem-cilastin Live virus vaccines lovastatin	Increases risk of nephrotoxicity Increases blood levels and risk of cyclosporine toxicity Additive immunosuppression Decreases effects of cyclosporine Additive hyperkalemia Increases risk of toxicity to digoxin Prolonged action of interactive drug Increases risk for seizures Decreases Ab response; increases risk of adverse reactions Increases risk of rhabdomyolysis
levamisole	Antineoplastic drugs, radiation therapy Alcohol phenytoin warfarin	Increases bone marrow suppression Disulfiram-like reaction Increases blood levels and risk of toxicity to interacting drug Increases effects of interactive drug

Continued

IMMUNE

DRUG INTRACTIONS

TABLE 32-2 Biologic Response Modifiers (Cytokines)—Cont'd

Drug	Interactive Drugs	Interaction
mycophenolate	acyclovir, ganciclovir	Competes with metabolite for renal excretion; increases risk of toxicity to mycophenolate
	Aluminum antacids, cholestyramine, colestipol, Magnesium antacids	Decreases absorption of mycophenolic acid
tacrolimus	Aminoglycosides, cisplatin, cyclosporin	Increases risk for toxicity
	Antifungal drugs, Calcium channel blockers, cimetidine, danazol, erythromycin	Increases blood levels of tacrolimus
	carbamazepine, phenobarbital, phenytoin, rifampin	Decreases blood levels of tacrolimus

CNS, Central nervous system; *INR,* international normalized ratio; *NSAIDs,* nonsteroidal antiinflammatory drugs; *ACE,* angiotensin-converting enzyme.

DOSAGE

TABLE 32-3 Selected Biologic Response Modifiers (Cytokines)*

Drug	Use(s)	Dosage	Implications
INTERFERONS (IFN)			
interferon alfa-2a	Kaposi's sarcoma	*Adult:* Give 3 MIU on day 1; 9 MIU on day 2; 18 MIU on day 3; then begin 36 MIU/day for remainder of 10–12 wk. Maintenance: 36 MIU 3 times/wk	Approx cost: $29,348 for 70-day supply
	Hairy cell leukemia	*Adult:* 3 MIU subQ or IM daily for 16–24 wk. Maintenance: 3 MIU 3 times weekly.	Approx cost: 3-MIU vial = $8400/wk
	CML	*Adult:* 9 MIU subQ or IM daily	Approx cost: $40,698/yr
interferon alfa-2b	Hairy cell leukemia	*Adult:* 2 MIU/m² subQ or IM 3 times weekly	**Interferon alfa-2b is not interchangeable with interferon alfa-2a.** Approx cost: 12 3-MIU vials = $500/mo
	Condylomata acuminata	*Adult:* 10 MIU/mL IL 3 times weekly for 3 wk	Approx cost: $2100/3 wk
	Chronic hepatitis B	*Adult:* 30–35 MIU/wk subQ or IM -or- 10 MIU 3 times wk for 16 wks	Approx cost: $6500-$8200 for 112-day supply
	Hepatitis C	*Adult:* 3 MIU subQ or IM 3 times wk for up to 6 months	Approx cost: Unavailable
peginterferon alfa-2b	Chronic hepatitis C in patients not previously treated with IFN	*Adult:* Once weekly for 1 year on same day each week. Dosage based on weight and purpose for use.	Modify dosage or temporarily discontinue drug if adverse reactions occur. Approx cost: $6500-$8200 for 112-day supply
interferon alfa-N3	Condylomata acuminata	*Adult:* 250,000 international units/0.05 mL IL twice weekly up to 8 wk. Max: 2.5 international units/session	Do not repeat for 3 months after initial 8 wk of treatment unless warts enlarge or new warts appear. Approx cost: $132 for 56-day supply
interferon beta-1alfa	Relapsing-remitting multiple sclerosis	*Adult:* 30 mcg IM once weekly	Approx cost: 4, 30-mcg vials = $1500/mo
interferon beta-1beta	Relapsing-remitting multiple sclerosis	*Adult:* 8 MIU (0.25 mg) subQ every other day	Approx cost: 15, 30-mcg vials = $1400/mo
interferon gamma-1beta	Chronic granulomatous disease	*Adult and Child with BSA >0.5 m²:* 50 mcg/m² (1.5 million units/m²) subQ 3 times weekly	Approx cost: 1.5 million–unit vial = $2309/mo
COLONY-STIMULATING FACTORS			
epoetin alfa	Antineoplastic drug-induced anemia	*Adult:* 150 units/kg subQ 3 times weekly. May increase after 2 mos to 300 units/kg 3 times weekly.	Patients taking AZT with serum erythropoietin levels over 500 milliunits likely will not respond to therapy. Approx cost: $1700–1800/mo
	Anemia in ZVD-treated patients with HIV	*Adult:* 100 units/kg subQ or IV 3 times weekly for 2 months. May increase by 50–100 units/kg every 1–2 months up to 300 units/kg 3 times weekly.	Therapeutic response in reticulocyte count should appear in 1–2 wk. Approx cost: $1500 for 10 days
filgrastim	Neutropenia related to nonmyeloid malignancy; bone marrow transplant	*Adult:* 5 mcg/kg/day subQ as single dose. May increase by 5 mcg/kg in each treatment cycle. Give daily for up to 2 wk until the ANC is 10,000/m³.	Response is much greater with subQ than IV therapy. Approx cost: $10,780 for 21-day supply
pegfilgrastim	Nonmyeloid malignancies in patients on myelosuppressive therapy	*Adult:* 6 mg subQ injection once per antineoplastic therapy cycle	**Do not give 14 days before or 24 hr after a cytotoxic antineoplastic drug.** Approx cost: $3190/treatment cycle
sargramostim	Autologous bone marrow transplant; non-Hodgkin's lymphoma, ALL, bone marrow transplantation failure or engraftment delay	*Adult:* 250 mcg/m²/day IV. For 21 days as a 2-hr infusion. Begin 2–4 hr after autologous bone marrow infusion and not less than 24 hr after last dose of antineoplastic drug or not less than 12 hr after last dose of radiation treatment.	When used for myeloid recovery purposes, may be repeated in 7 days with dosage increased to 500 mcg/m²/day for 14 days. Approx cost: $3000–$6000/day for up to 21 days depending on purpose.

INTERLEUKIN			
interleukin-2	Metastatic renal cell cancer	*Adult:* 600,000 international units/kg every 8 hr for 14 doses; rest 9 days, repeat 14 doses. Total of 28 doses.	A 9-day rest period should separate treatment cycles. Approx cost: $48,615/29-day supply
MISCELLANEOUS BMRS			
azathioprine	Kidney transplant rejection	*Adult:* 3–5 mg/kg PO daily beginning at time of transplant	Chronic immunosuppression increases risk of neoplasia. Approx cost: $157–$333/mo
levamisole	Adjunct colorectal cancer; advanced malignant melanoma (unlabeled use)	*Adult:* 50 mg PO every 8 hr for 3 days every 2 wk. Repeat every 14 days for 1 yr.	Start treatment no sooner than 7 days and no later than 30 days after surgery. Approx cost: Unavailable
cyclosporine-A	Solid organ transplantations	*Adult and Child:* 12–15 mg/kg/day PO for 1–2 wk. Maintenance: 5 to10 mg/kg/day	**The microemulsion formulation (Neoral) and other formulations (Sandimmune) are not interchangeable.** Approx cost: 30 100-mg capsules = $135.
lymphocyte immune globulin	Acute graft rejection; aplastic anemia	*Adult:* 10–30 mg/kg/day IV for 14 days	Approx cost: $30, 274 for 14 days of therapy
mycophenolate	Allogenic renal transplantation	*Adult:* 1gram PO twice daily	Start within 72 hours of transplant. Approx cost: 100 500-mg tabs = $550
Rh$_o$(D) immune globulin	Prevent during L&D, abortions, miscarriages, or amniocentesis	*Adult before delivery:* 300 mcg IM at 28 wk *Adult following delivery:* 300 mcg IM within 72 hr of delivery *Termination of pregnancy <13 wk gestation:* 50 mcg IM within 72 hr of termination *Termination of pregnancy >13 wk gestation:* 300 mcg IM within 72 hr of termination	**Check formulation carefully. Rh$_o$(D) *immune globulin* is for IM use only. Rh$_o$(D) *immune globulin* IV is for IM *or* IV use.** Approx cost: $46–$350/dose based on reason for use
	Idiopathic thrombocytopenic purpura (ITP)	*Adult:* 50 mcg/kg IV initially. If Hgb less than 10 grams/dL, reduce dose to 25–40 mcg/kg.	Further dosing and frequency determined by clinical response. Approx cost: $2500 for single dose
tacrolimus	Solid organ transplantations	*Adult and Child:* Dosage varies with organ transplanted.	Approx cost: = $1200/mo

*Approximate costs courtesy of *2007 Mosby's Drug Consult* software.
ALL, Acute lymphocytic leukemia; *ANC,* absolute neutrophil count; *AZT,* zidovudine; *BSA,* body surface area; *ESRD,* end-stage renal disease; *G-CSF,* granulocyte colony–stimulating factor; *GI,* gastrointestinal; *Hgb,* hemoglobin; *IL,* intralesion; *IM,* intramuscular (route); *IV,* intravenous (route); *L&D,* labor and delivery; *MIU,* million international units; *PO,* by mouth; *subQ,* subcutaneous (route); *ZVD,* zidovudine.

carcinoma, Kaposi's sarcoma (along with zidovudine), metastatic melanoma (along with cyclophosphamide), and non-Hodgkin's lymphoma (along with lymphokine-activated killer cells), and in the treatment of human immunodeficiency virus (HIV). IL-2 has recently been used in the management of multiple sclerosis.

Pharmacodynamics

The secretion of one IL produces a cascade of other ILs and cytokines. The action of each IL is unique, but many have actions shared by other ILs as well. IL-1 is produced by many cell types but is only secreted from monocytes, macrophages, and dendritic cells. IL-1 is an important part of the inflammatory response of the body against infection. It increases the expression of adhesion factors on endothelial cells to enable movement of leukocytes to sites of infection. It also resets the thermoregulatory center in the hypothalamus, leading to an increased body temperature that expresses itself as fever. It is therefore an endogenous pyrogen. The increased temperature helps the body's immune system to fight infection. Excessive, persistent IL-1 release has been implicated in the pathogenesis of rheumatoid arthritis, cachexia, and atherosclerosis. The IL-1 inhibitor anakinra was discussed in Chapter 17.

Many of the immunosuppressive drugs used in the treatment of autoimmune diseases (e.g., corticosteroids, cyclosporine-A, tacrolimus) work by inhibiting the production of IL-2 indirectly by Ag-activated T cells.

IL-2 is well known from its first identification as a T-cell growth factor. It acts as a growth and differentiation factor for cytotoxic T cells, T helper cells, T suppressor cells, and NK cells. It induces lymphokine production by T cells and monocytes and enhances NK cell activity. IL-2 also stimulates lymphokine-activated killer (LAK) cells and induces IFN-γ. The exact mechanism of how IL-2 affects tumor cells is unknown.

Pharmacokinetics

High plasma concentrations of IL-2 are reached after IV infusion with rapid distribution to extravascular and extracellular spaces. IL-2 is quickly biotransformed to amino acids in the cells lining the proximal convoluted tubules, with its metabolites eliminated in urine. The half-life of IL-2 is 85 minutes (see Table 32-1).

Adverse Effects and Contraindications

Most adverse effects of IL-2, although quite significant, are dose-dependent and self-limiting, and usually reverse 2 to 3 days after the drug is stopped. The adverse effects are less severe when IL-2 is used in smaller doses and when administered by subQ instead of IV route.

Flulike symptoms are among the most common adverse effects of IL-2. However, sinus congestion, low blood pressure, liver toxicity, and changes in mental status, as well as increased levels of albumin, potassium, and magnesium can also occur. Dry skin, sensory disorders, dermatitis, arthralgia, myalgia, weight loss, conjunctivitis, hematuria, and proteinuria are possible but rare.

There can also be temporary stimulation of viral replication, since IL-2 stimulates the immune system, particularly

IMMUNE

the CD4 cells where a virus may harbor. Unfortunately, IL-2 cannot replace cell types that are destroyed as a result of viral infections. Instead, it can only increase what is left. For example, the very low numbers of cells left to fight *Pneumocystis jirovecii* pneumonia (previously known as *Pneumocystis carinii* pneumonia) may very well increase in number with IL-2 therapy, preserving and enhancing what remains of the ability to cope with this specific infection.

Capillary leak syndrome is a serious complication of IL-2 therapy. Plasma proteins and fluid leak into extravascular spaces, resulting in a loss of vascular tone that 2 to 12 hours after administration. Patients with significant cardiac, pulmonary, renal, hepatic, or central nervous system (CNS) impairment related to use of IL-2 require very close monitoring.

▥ Drug Interactions

IL-2 affects CNS functioning. Therefore interactions can appear with concomitant use of IL-2 and opioids, antiemetics, sedatives, or antianxiety drugs. Beta blockers and other antihypertensive drugs may cause additive hypotension. The risk for organ toxicity may be increased with the use of nephrotoxic drugs such as aminoglycosides or indomethacin, or antineoplastic drugs that are myelotoxic, cardiotoxic, or hepatotoxic. Corticosteroids are generally contraindicated because they reduce the antitumor effectiveness of IL-2.

▥ Dosage Regimen

A course of IL-2 therapy generally consists of two 5-day treatment cycles separated by a 9-day rest period; however, a minimum rest period of 7 weeks between further courses of therapy is required (see Table 32-3). If there is a positive response, the patient continues on with the next course. Patient response is evaluated 4 weeks after treatment, and then immediately before the next course of therapy. The short half-life of IL-2 necessitates frequent, short-dosing schedules.

▥ Lab Considerations

IL-2 increases bilirubin, BUN, serum creatinine, transaminase, and alkaline phosphatase values. Monitoring of magnesium, calcium, phosphorous, potassium, and sodium levels is required, as these electrolytes commonly decrease with therapy.

Colony-Stimulating Factors

◆ epoetin alfa (EPO, Epogen)
◆ filgrastim (rG-CSF, Neupogen)
◆ pegfilgrastim (rG-CSF, Neulasta)
◆ sargramostim (rHuGM-CSF, Leukine, Prokine)

▥ Indications

To date, CSFs have been used to treat iatrogenic bone marrow dysfunction, AIDS myelodysplasia, myelosuppression related to antineoplastic therapy, and bone marrow transplantation. They also have been used in the management of intrinsic bone marrow dysfunction states such as myelodysplasia, congenital cyclic neutropenia, and aplastic anemia, and other states of bone marrow infiltration such as hairy cell leukemia. Although sargramostim, filgrastim, and pegfilgrastim are used clinically to prevent febrile neutropenia after administration of standard dosages of antineoplastic drugs, only the latter two drugs are FDA-approved for this indication.

Epoetin alfa was the first approved CSF for patients with end-stage renal diseases who are on dialysis and are transfusion-dependent, and for patients with HIV infection who are receiving myelosuppressive therapy such as zidovudine. Epoetin alfa decreases the need for transfusion support (see Chapter 44). It is also used for patients with chronic anemia resulting from cancer or cancer therapy.

▥ Pharmacodynamics

CSFs, a group of polypeptide hormones named for their parent cell, are secreted by macrophages. CSFs stimulate stem cells to produce neutrophils, eosinophils, basophils, and additional macrophages. Some CSFs have multilineage effects; that is, they are influenced by several cell lines. CSFs increase the production of granulocytes and monocytes by stimulating stem and precursor cell replication and maturation. The precise location where the drugs exert their action is unclear.

Also known as sargramostim when the CSF protein is expressed in yeast cells (i.e., *Saccharomyces cerevisiae*), this CSF is used to stimulate the production of WBCs, especially granulocytes and macrophages, following antineoplastic therapy.

Do not confuse granulocyte-stimulating factor (G-CSF) ▲ with granulocyte-macrophage stimulating factor (GM-CSF), a different hematopoietic growth factor. G-CSF is a lineage restricted glycoprotein, meaning it stimulates cell division and maturation in only one cell line (see Fig. 32-3). G-CSF is produced by the endothelium, macrophages, and a number of other immune cells to stimulate the bone marrow to produce granulocytes. GM-CSF, on the other hand, is a potent, species-specific stimulator of bone marrow cells. M-CSF stimulates only macrophage activity by interacting with specific cell surface receptors.

▥ Pharmacokinetics

Knowledge of the pharmacokinetics of CSFs is limited. Filgrastim and pegfilgrastim are well absorbed after subQ administration (see Table 32-1). The polyethylene glycol formulation (peg), pegfilgrastim, has a much longer half-life than filgrastim, reducing the necessity of daily injections.

▥ Adverse Effects and Contraindications

CSFs are well tolerated in the recommended dosages. Alopecia, nausea, vomiting, diarrhea, fever, and fatigue are common; anorexia, dyspnea, cough, headache, and skin rash are rare. Although atypical, exacerbations of preexisting inflammatory conditions have been noted, such as have psoriasis, hematuria, proteinuria, thrombocytopenia, arrhythmias, myocardial infarction, and osteoporosis. Adults with sepsis may go on to develop adult respiratory distress syndrome (ARDS).

The adverse effects of CSFs are more commonly seen with sargramostim than with filgrastim and pegfilgrastim, and are thought to be related to the drug's ability to enhance the binding of neutrophils to endothelial cells, or to the activation of monocytes and macrophages, which may stimulate the release of cytokines such as IL-1 and tumor necrosis factor. Bone pain occurs most often in patients receiving high IV doses and appears to be related to extensive bone marrow regeneration, but it is transient and usually managed easily with acetaminophen. Bone pain is seen less frequently with a low-dose, subQ route of administration. Other adverse effects of sargramostim include rash, pruritus, myalgia, fatigue, anorexia, diarrhea, malaise, phlebitis, and thrombosis. Peripheral edema, weight gain, dyspnea, fever, and leukocytosis occur occasionally. At high dosages, capillary leak syndromes with pericardial and pleural effusions and edema have been seen. The development of eosinophilia may signal toxicity; therefore, lab monitoring should include a baseline and then twice-weekly complete blood count (CBC) with differential, platelets, and reticulocyte count.

Drug Interactions

There are no known drug interactions with filgrastim. Lithium and corticosteroids increase the effects of sargramostim and pegfilgrastim.

Dosage Regimen

Sargramostim is given for 21 days, or until the bone marrow has recovered (see Table 32-3). Recovery is defined as an absolute neutrophil count (ANC) over 20,000/mm^3, or a platelet count that exceeds 500,000/mm^3. Begin the IV infusion of sargramostim 2 to 4 hours after autologous bone marrow infusion; not less than 24 hours after the last dose of antineoplastic therapy; and not less than 12 hours after the last radiotherapy treatment, bone narrow transplant failure, or engraftment delay. Discontinue sargramostim if blast cells appear or the underlying disease progresses. Filgrastim is given daily for 2 weeks or until the ANC is 10,000/m^3.

Lab Considerations

Lab values for alkaline phosphatase, lactate dehydrogenase (LDH), uric acid, and leukocytes may be elevated in the presence of G-CSF. Albumin levels may decrease in the presence of GM-CSF, with elevations noted in bilirubin, creatinine, and liver enzyme values.

Monoclonal Antibodies
- adalimumab (Humira)
- alemtuzumab (Campath)
- bevacizumab (Avastin)
- cetuximab (Erbitux)
- dacliximab (Zenapax)
- etanercept (Embrel)
- infliximab (Remicade); ♣ Remicade
- muromonab-CD3 (Orthoclone OKT3); ♣ Orthoclone OKT3
- natalizumab (Tysabri)
- omalizumab (Xolair)
- rituximab (Rituxan); ♣ Rituxan
- trastuzumab (Herceptin); ♣ Herceptin

Indications

MoAbs are used in diagnosing or screening cancers, and monitoring disease progression; as therapeutic agents in the treatment of cancer to stop tumor growth; and in the treatment of inflammatory disorders. MoAbs have also been effective in the treatment of autoimmune diseases such as rheumatoid arthritis, Crohn's disease, ankylosing spondylitis, systemic lupus erythematosus (SLE), Takayasu's arteritis (an inflammation of the aorta and its major branches), multiple sclerosis, and asthma. By virtue of their specific actions, MoAbs are treatment options for various other medical conditions.

There are two classifications of MoAbs: unconjugated and conjugated. Unconjugated MoAbs are used alone in therapies, whereas conjugated MoAbs are combined with another drug such as antineoplastics, toxins, or radioisotopes.

Pharmacodynamics

The basis for cancer treatment using an Ag-Ab response is the knowledge that all cells, including tumor cells, have Ags unique to that cell. This unique characteristic is referred to as *specificity*. Ab therapy utilizes this characteristic to target certain cells for destruction. The "bullets" are MoAbs programmed to destroy the target cells. The MoAbs can be used for tumor detection; to deliver drugs, toxins, or radioactive material directly to a tumor; in the treatment of inflammatory and autoimmune conditions such as asthma and rheumatoid arthritis; in the treatment of cardiovascular diseases; and in infectious disease management.

MoAbs block graft rejection by binding to CD3 receptors on mature circulating T cells and medullary lymphocytes. This action blocks the ability of cells to recognize foreign Ags, thereby inhibiting the generation and function of cytotoxic T cells responsible for graft rejection. Further, the Ag may incite an inflammatory response through recognition of a specific portion of an Ab.

Pharmacokinetics

MoAbs are well absorbed following subQ and IV administration. The distribution of most MoAbs is similar to that of albumin. Serum levels and half-life are proportional to dosage. The wide range of half-lives may reflect the variable tumor burden among cancer patients. Rituximab is usually detectable in the serum of patients 3 to 6 months after completion of treatment, which is the foundation for treatment every 12 weeks in rheumatoid arthritis.

Adverse Effects and Contraindications

Many possible adverse effects can occur with MoAb therapies, although they often are uncommon (occur in less than 1% of patients). Some reactions that occur more frequently include flulike symptoms such as fever, chills, and headache, nausea, vomiting, diarrhea, and general malaise, which generally decrease with additional treatments. Less frequent adverse effects include reversible thrombocytopenia, marked hypotension, chest pain, and pulmonary edema in fluid-overloaded patients, aseptic meningitis, and an acute decline in the glomerular filtration rate. Hair loss had been noted for a small percentage of patients receiving rituximab. Trastuzumab use has resulted in ventricular dysfunction and heart failure.

Patients can develop human antimurine Abs after treatment with any murine MoAb. This concept forms the basis for why many therapies lose their effectiveness. The lack of effectiveness is commonly seen in patients with autoimmune diseases. In these situations, where repeated treatments are indicated, an immune suppressant such as methotrexate (MTX) is used to decrease the opportunity for the body to again develop an Ab against the treatment drug and to enhance therapeutic response.

Drug Interactions

Drug interactions with MoAbs include increased risks of infection and lymphoproliferative disorders, particularly in the presence of corticosteroids. Vaccines formulated with live viruses may increase the adverse effects, and patients taking

IMMUNE

these drugs may have a decreased Ab response to the vaccine. Table 32-2 identifies the drug interactions associated with MoAbs.

▥ *Dosage Regimen*

MoAbs are administered by IV route in most cases, based on body weight. Dosage and duration of treatments vary depending on the condition treated (Table 32-4). It is recommended that purified protein derivative (PPD) tuberculosis testing or an anergy panel be done before use of MoAb therapy because of the risk for activating latent tuberculosis.

▥ *Lab Considerations*

Standard lab testing, usually performed with each infusion, includes a CBC, reticulocyte count, C-reactive protein, complete metabolic panel, and sedimentation rate. These lab values, combined with patient assessment, are the baseline measures used to determine dosage and frequency of drug administration, or both.

Miscellaneous BRMs

TRANSPLANT THERAPEUTICS
◆ azathioprine (Imuran); ✦ Imuran
◆ cyclosporine A (cyclosporine, cyclosporine A, Sandimmune, Neoral); cyclosporin, Neoral
◆ mycophenolate (CellCept); ✦ CellCept
◆ tacrolimus (Prograf); ✦ Prograf, Procytox
GLOBULINS AND OTHERS
◆ cyclophosphamide (Cytoxan, Neosar); ✦ Cytoxan
◆ etanercept (Enbrel); ✦ Enbrel
◆ levamisole (Ergamisole)
◆ lymphocyte immune globulin (Atgam, Thymoglobulin)
◆ Rho(D) immune globulin (RhIG, RhoGam, Gamulin RH)
◆ tumor necrosis factor

Azathioprine

Azathioprine is an immunosuppressive antimetabolite (also see Chapters 17 and 33). Azathioprine (combined with prednisone) has been the mainstay of attempts to suppress rejection of transplanted organs for the last 20 years; it made renal transplants possible. Prophylactic antirejection therapy using azathioprine is usually initiated 1 to 2 days before transplantation.

Rejection can usually be controlled by suppressing the body's immune response and the ability to recognize foreign substances. Azathioprine is a prodrug that acts to inhibit the synthesis of purine, needed for the proliferation of cells, particularly lymphocytes and leukocytes. It is subsequently converted to mercaptopurine-containing nucleotides that then act on the synthesis and utilization of the precursors of

DOSAGE
TABLE **32-4 Monoclonal Antibodies***

Drug	Use	Dosage	Comments
adalimumab	Rheumatoid arthritis; psoriatic arthritis	*Adult:* 40 mg subQ every 2 wk	PPD required before starting therapy. Approx cost: $1440 for 28-day supply
alemtuzumab	CLL with failure on fludarabine	*Adult:* 3 mg IV daily to maximum of 30 mg/day 3 days/week for 12 wk	High dosages associated with greater risk for pancytopenia. Approx cost: $66,452 for 84-day supply
bevacizumab	Advanced metastatic colon cancer	*Adult:* 5 mg/kg IV every 14 days	Approx cost: $2406/mo
cetuximab	Metastatic colorectal cancer, squamous cell head and neck cancer	*Adult:* 250 mg/m² IV weekly	90% of severe infusion reactions are seen with first dose. Approx cost: $5100 for 2-wk supply
dacliximab	Acute renal transplant rejection	*Adult:* 1 mg/kg IV every 14 days for 5 doses	Treatment associated with 3-yr post-transplant survival. Approx cost: Unavailable
etanercept	Rheumatoid arthritis; psoriatic arthritis; ankylosing spondylitis; plaque psoriasis	*Adult:* 50 mg subQ once weekly. Duration depends on disorder treated.	PPD required before starting therapy. Approx cost: 4 50-mg units = $5000
infliximab	Rheumatoid arthritis; Crohn's disease; enterocutaneous and rectovaginal fistulas; ankylosing spondylitis, psoriatic arthritis; ulcerative colitis	*Adult:* 5 mg/ kg IV every 6–8 wk depending on disorder treated	**PPD required before starting therapy. Tuberculosis and invasive fungal infections have been noted.** Some of these infections have been fatal. Approx cost: $1450–$2120/dose based on reason for use
muromonab-CD₃	Acute allograft rejection in renal, heart and liver transplants.	*Adult:* 5 mg IV daily for 10–14 days	Common first-dose reaction fever, chills, dyspnea, malaise. Approx cost: $8583 for 10 days of therapy
natalizumab	Relapsing multiple sclerosis	*Adult:* 300 mg IV every 4 wk	Restricted access in United States. Approx cost: Unavailable
omalizumab	Moderate to severe persistent asthma	*Adult:* 150–375 mg subQ every 2–4 wk to max of 150 mg/site	Approx cost: $1082 for 28-day supply
rituximab	Refractory rheumatoid arthritis; non-Hodgkin's lymphoma; breast cancer	*Adult:* 375–1000 mg IV every 1–4 wk depending on disorder treated	**Approximately 80% of fatal infusion reactions occur within 24 hr of first infusion.** Approx cost: $14,264/mo.
trastuzumab	Metastatic breast cancer	*Adult:* 2 mg/kg IV weekly	Compared to antineoplastic therapy alone, MoAb and antineoplastic drugs have significantly longer time to disease progression, higher overall response rate, longer median duration of response, and higher 1-yr survival rate. Approx cost: $3328 per 4 wk

*Approximate costs courtesy of *2007 Mosby's Drug Consult* software.
CLL, Chronic lymphocytic leukemia; *IV,* intravenous (route); *MoAb,* monoclonal antibody; *PPD,* purified protein derivative.

RNA and DNA. However, by reducing the immune response, azathioprine also reduces the body's ability to ward off infections.

Hematologic toxicity to azathioprine appears as thrombocytopenia and leukopenia. Nausea and vomiting are common but ordinarily do not restrict therapy. Although hepatic toxicity is rare, a severe hepatic venoocclusive disease has been seen in some patients with transplants.

Cyclophosphamide

Cyclophosphamide is an alkylating drug with extremely potent humoral immunosuppressive properties. It is used to treat a variety of disorders including Hodgkin's disease, malignant melanoma, leukemia, mycosis fungoides, neuroblastoma, ovarian and breast cancers, glomerulonephritis, autoimmune blood dyscrasias, and systemic lupus erythematosus. Additional information about cyclophosphamide can be found in Chapters 17 and 33, where its uses as a disease-modifying antirheumatic drug (DMARD) and antineoplastic, respectively, are discussed.

Cyclosporine A

Cyclosporine is a fungus-derived peptide. It is used most often to prevent rejection of solid organ transplants. It is a potent immunosuppressor of T helper cells and acts by blocking the synthesis and secretion of IL-2 (IL-2 is required for the proliferation and growth of Ag-stimulated cells). It impairs cell-mediated responses without destroying the effector lymphocytes. It has minimal to no effect on T suppressor cells, B cells, granulocytes, or macrophages. Further, it does not prevent immune cells already present and activated by an Ag from maturing and differentiating.

Cyclosporine A is erratically absorbed after oral administration, with a significant first-pass effect by the liver. The oral bioavailability of cyclosporine A varies from 20% to 50%. The microemulsion products (Neoral) have greater bioavailability. Cyclosporine A is widely distributed, primarily into extracellular fluid and blood cells. It crosses placental membranes and enters breast milk. About 60% to 70% of the drug in whole blood is contained in red blood cells (RBCs). Despite their small contribution to blood volume, leukocytes contain 10% to 20% of circulating cyclosporine A. It is primarily eliminated in the bile, with small amounts eliminated unchanged in the urine. There are many drug interactions to cyclosporine (see Table 32-2).

The most common adverse effects of cyclosporine A include oral candidiasis, hyperplasia of the gums, headache, hirsutism, tremors, and headache. Hirsutism and gingival hyperplasia are seen in 10% to 30% of patients who receive cyclosporine A, but these reactions rarely require discontinuation of therapy. Life-threatening adverse effects include hepatotoxicity, albuminuria, hematuria, proteinuria, and renal failure. Treatment with cyclosporine is also associated with an increased risk for infections, but this problem is generally less prominent than with other immunosuppressive drugs. There is a relatively low incidence of cancers appearing in patients treated with cyclosporine alone. However, when cyclosporine A is used in combination with other drugs, the drug causes lymphomas and an unusually high incidence of brain metastases.

Cyclosporine A is contraindicated for use in patients with a known hypersensitivity to the drug and in patients on disulfiram therapy or who have known alcohol intolerance (IV and oral liquid dosage formulations contain alcohol). Cautious use is warranted in patients with severe liver or kidney disease, in those with active infection, and in children.

The microemulsion formulation (Neoral) and other ⚠ **formulations of cyclosporine A (Sandimmune) are not interchangeable.** Table 32-4 identifies the most common dosages.

About 50% of patients taking cyclosporine A will have elevated liver function test results or concentrations of bilirubin in the plasma. These abnormalities generally disappear if the dosage is reduced or the drug discontinued. Cyclosporine A may elevate serum potassium, uric acid, and serum lipid levels. Monitor serum cyclosporine levels periodically during therapy, and adjust dosages in response to serum concentrations. The guidelines for desired serum levels vary among institutions.

Etanercept

Etanercept is used to reduce the signs and symptoms of moderate to severe rheumatoid arthritis in adults and children. Elevated levels of tumor necrosis factor (TNF) are found in patients with ankylosing spondylitis, psoriatic arthritis, and chronic moderate to severe plaque psoriasis. Etanercept helps reduce the signs and symptoms of these diseases. It has been used off-label in the treatment of Crohn's disease.

There are two distinct receptors for TNF (i.e., TNF-α, TNF-β). Etanercept binds to TNF, blocking its interaction with cell surface receptors and thus rendering it inactive. The drug also modifies cellular activities that are induced or regulated by the TNF (e.g., expression of the adhesion molecules necessary for leukocyte migration, serum levels of cytokines). Tables 32-1 and 32-4 identify the pharmacokinetics of etanercept and its dosage, respectively. (See the discussion of TNF later in this chapter.)

Adverse effects are frequent with etanercept and include injection-site reactions (i.e., redness, itching, pain, edema). The incidence of abdominal pain and vomiting is greater in children than adults. Occasionally, headache, rhinitis, pharyngitis, cough, dizziness, dyspepsia, abdominal pain, and asthenia occur. The more serious adverse effects of etanercept include pyelonephritis, cellulitis, osteomyelitis, wound infection, leg ulcers, septic arthritis, and diarrhea. Upper respiratory tract infections such as bronchitis and pneumonia occur frequently. Although rare, pancytopenia, heart failure, hypertension or hypotension, pancreatitis, reactivation of hepatitis B, and GI hemorrhage have been reported. A threefold increase in the incidence of lymphomas has been reported with etanercept use. Allergic reactions occur in fewer than 2% of patients.

Although the causal relationship remains unclear, etanercept has been associated with rare instances of new onset or exacerbation of demyelinating disorders of the CNS. Some patients were noted to have mental status changes. Other patients presented with transverse myelitis, optic neuritis, multiple sclerosis, and new onset or exacerbation of seizure disorders. Because animal studies are not always predictive of human response, this drug should only be used during

IMMUNE

pregnancy with caution (category B). It is not known if etanercept is transferred to breast milk.

There are no known drug or herbal interactions with etanercept and no interferences in lab testing.

Levamisole

Levamisole is an antineoplastic, immunomodulating drug (see Chapter 33). It is used as adjunct therapy after surgery for colorectal cancer (along with 5-fluorouracil) and for treatment of advanced malignant melanoma. Levamisole returns leukocyte function to normal levels after antineoplastic therapy or surgery; its effects include fostering the formation of antibodies, T-cell response, phagocytosis, and chemotaxis.

Levamisole is rapidly absorbed after oral administration, although its distribution is unknown. It is extensively biotransformed in the liver.

The most common adverse effects of levamisole include fatigue, stomatitis, nausea, vomiting, diarrhea, dermatitis and alopecia, anemia, leukopenia, and thrombocytopenia. CNS impairment is rare but when present includes ataxia, blurred vision, confusion, mental status changes, paresthesias, seizures, tardive dyskinesia, and tremors. Agranulocytosis is the most life-threatening adverse effect. Use levamisole cautiously in patients with bone marrow depression and other chronic debilitating diseases, and in patients of child-bearing age. Safe use during lactation and in children has not been established.

Lymphocyte Immune Globulin

Lymphocyte immune globulin is an immunosuppressive, lymphocyte-selective, polyclonal Ab. It is utilized primarily to treat allograft rejection related to renal transplantation, but also for the management of aplastic anemia.

Lymphocyte immune globulin reduces the number of circulating thymus-dependent lymphocytes. It also acts by altering the function of T cells that are responsible for cell-mediated and humoral immunity and stimulates the growth of hematopoietic growth factors.

Lymphocyte immune globulin's adverse effects include fever, chills, itching, erythema, and hemolysis in about 5% of patients. Anaphylaxis is possible. Because patients who receive this drug are also being treated with other immunosuppressive drugs, allergic reactions to its equine protein are not as frequent or as severe as would otherwise be expected. To minimize the risk of anaphylaxis, intradermal skin testing is done before the first dose and the patient is monitored for 30 minutes to 1 hour. A positive skin test is distinguished by the presence of erythema or an area of induration that exceeds 10 mm in diameter at the site of administration.

The usual adult dose, when used for transplantation rejection, is given once daily for 14 days, then every other day for 14 days or 21 total doses, if needed. When used in the management of aplastic anemia, the drug is administered daily for 8 to 14 days. Infuse the drug through a central line, vascular shunt, or arterial venous fistula, using an in-line filter; drug-induced phlebitis can occur if the drug is infused through peripheral veins. Administer lymphocyte immune globulin over 4 to 12 hours, monitoring the patient continually for adverse effects.

Mycophenolate

Mycophenolate is an immunosuppressant used to prevent rejection in patients who have undergone allogenic renal transplantation. It is ordinarily used in conjunction with cyclosporine and corticosteroids.

Mycophenolate inhibits inosine monophosphate dehydrogenase, an enzyme required for synthesis of guanine nucleotides that are necessary for DNA synthesis. The inhibition results in suppression of both T- and B-cell proliferation and in impairment of immune responses that promote rejection of transplanted organs. Begin therapy within 72 hours after transplantation.

Mycophenolate is rapidly hydrolyzed to mycophenolic acid (MPA), its active metabolite, after oral administration. Its distribution is unknown. MPA is extensively biotransformed, with less than 1% eliminated unchanged in the urine. Some enterohepatic recirculation of MPA occurs. Peak drug levels of MPA are significantly decreased when the drug is taken with food.

The most common adverse effects of mycophenolate include diarrhea, vomiting, leukopenia, and sepsis. Gastrointestinal (GI) bleeding is the most life-threatening adverse effect. There is an increased risk of malignancy because of the patient's reduced immune response. Use mycophenolate with caution in patients with active, serious pathologic conditions of the GI tract, severe chronic renal impairment, delayed graft function following transplant, and in women of child-bearing age. Safe use in children has not been established.

Mycophenolate elevates serum alkaline phosphatase and other liver function test values. It may also cause hypercalcemia or hypocalcemia, hyperuricemia, hyperlipidemia, hypoglycemia, and hypoproteinemia. Monitor the patient's hepatic, hematopoietic, and renal status periodically during therapy. Neutropenia occurs most frequently 31 to 180 days after transplantation. If the ANC is less than $1000/mm^3$, reduce the dosage or discontinue the drug.

Rho(D) Immune Globulin

Rho(D) immune globulin (RhIG) is a human Ab directed at the D Ag of the Rh system. It is used to prevent isoimmunization (sensitization) in Rh-negative women who are exposed to Rh-positive blood in the process of labor and delivery, abortion, ectopic pregnancy, version, trauma, fetomaternal hemorrhage, chorionic villi sampling, or amniocentesis.

When the mother with an Rh-positive fetus is Rh-negative, the mother's immune system responds by producing anti-Rho(D) antibodies. During subsequent pregnancies these antibodies cross placental membranes to enter fetal circulation. The anti-Rho(D) antibodies attack the RBCs of the Rh-positive fetus to cause hemolysis. RhIG grants passive immunity by coating fetal Rh-positive cells as they enter maternal circulation. The coating prevents the maternal immune system from identifying the cells as foreign, thereby preventing Ab formation. Administration of RhIG has decreased the incidence of hemolytic disease of the newborn (i.e., erythroblastosis fetalis) by 70%.

Note that many other blood Ags also trigger the development of antibodies. For example, idiopathic thrombocytopenic purpura (ITP) is a disorder that results in a reduced number of platelets. The cause is unknown. RhIG has been used for the management of this disorder because it helps to increase platelet counts and decrease the episodes of bleeding.

Little is understood about the pharmacokinetics of RhIG. The drug is well absorbed from IM and IV administrations, but its distribution, biotransformation, and elimination are unknown. The half-life of RhIG is approximately 30 days when given intramuscularly and 24 days when given intravenously. Keep in mind that the drug is given to the mother, not the infant, within 72 hours of delivery.

The most common adverse effects of RhIG are irritation at the injection site, fever, lethargy, and myalgias. Anemia is possible when the drug is used in the management of ITP. RhIG is contraindicated for use in patients with previous immunization with this drug and in Rho(O)-positive–D^u-positive patients. Exercise caution when using RhIG in patients with previous hypersensitivity to immune globulins or thimerosal and in patients with ITP who have a preexisting anemia. Thimerosal, one of the most widely used preservatives in vaccines, is almost 50% mercury by weight. It is metabolized or degraded to ethylmercury and thiosalicylate. Thimerosal-free formulations are available.

Identify the blood type of the mother and newborn to identify the need for the drug. The mother must be Rho(D)-negative and D^u-negative. The infant must be Rho(D)-positive. Administer the drug if there is any doubt regarding the infant's blood type, or if the father is Rho(D)-positive. An infant born to a woman previously treated with RhIG during the antepartum period may have a weakly positive direct Coombs' test on cord or infant blood.

The Kleihauer-Betke test, which quantifies the amount of fetal blood entering maternal circulation, is used as the basis for RhIG dosage after delivery. One unit of RhIG (i.e., 300 mcg) neutralizes 30 mL of fetal whole blood or 15 mL of fetal RBCs. For most vaginal deliveries, this is more than enough RhIG. However, if the quantity of fetal blood entering maternal circulation exceeds this amount, a larger dose of RhIG may be necessary to prevent an Ab response. Situations that may require a larger dose include cesarean birth, manual removal of the placenta, breech birth, stillbirth, placenta previa, or abruptio placentae.

Monitor platelet counts, RBC counts, hemoglobin levels, and reticulocyte levels to determine the effectiveness of RhIG for ITP.

Tacrolimus

Tacrolimus is a macrolide immunosuppressant used in organ transplantation to prevent rejection. It has been used as a primary immunosuppressant to suppress T-cell activity after kidney, heart, heart-lung, pancreas, lung, small intestine, liver, and islet-cell transplantation.

Tacrolimus is 100 times more potent than cyclosporine and acts by inhibiting T-cell activity, which in turn inhibits cell-mediated immune response by blocking the production of IL-2 and other lymphokines. It has a powerful hepatotrophic effect; that is, it fosters regeneration and repair of the liver. Even though it is more potent than cyclosporine, it has fewer adverse effects. The effects are most pronounced when it is administered in conjunction with a high-fat meal.

The most common adverse effects of tacrolimus include headache and tremors. Nausea, vomiting, diarrhea, constipation, hypertension, insomnia, paresthesia, fever and chills, a rash, and flushing also may be noted. The metabolic adverse effects include hirsutism, hyperglycemia, hyperkalemia, hyperuricemia, hypokalemia, and hypomagnesemia. Life-threatening adverse effects of tacrolimus include anemia, leukocytosis, thrombocytopenia, albuminuria, hematuria, proteinuria, and renal failure. Pleural effusion and atelectasis have also been noted. Tacrolimus is contraindicated for use in patients with hypersensitivity to this drug or to some kinds of castor oil. Use it with caution in patients with renal disease, diabetes, hyperkalemia, hyperuricemia or gout, or lymphomas, and during pregnancy or lactation. Safe use in children under 12 years of age has not been established.

Known drug interactions of tacrolimus include an increased risk of renal toxicity with concurrent use of aminoglycosides, cisplatin, or cyclosporine A. There may be increased serum levels of antifungal drugs, calcium-channel blockers, cimetidine, danazol, and erythromycin. Carbamazepine, phenobarbital, phenytoin, and rifampin blood levels are decreased in the presence of tacrolimus. The effects of live virus vaccines are diminished.

Tumor Necrosis Factor

Tumor necrosis factor (TNF) is a naturally occurring intracellular mediator protein produced by monocytes and macrophages. TNF is used for the management of metastatic adenocarcinoma of the colon and rectum, the liver, and the bladder. It is also being used experimentally for non–small cell lung cancer, renal cell cancer, and malignant melanoma. Clinical trials are still underway to determine tumor response, extent of immunomodulation, therapeutic dosage, route of administration, and expected adverse effects of TNF for these cancers and other disorders. Studies also continue as to TNFs effectiveness with regional therapy such as isolated limb perfusion for melanoma and IV administration for a variety of tumors. In combination with antineoplastic drugs, the TNF is believed to produce the highest possible cell kill of malignant cells.

TNF is thought to exert a direct effect on tumor cells by binding with receptors on the cell surface. Drug action occurs at the G_2 phase of the cell cycle (see Chapter 33), producing immediate cell death and cytostasis (arrest of growth). Some tumor cells are resistant to the effects of TNF. Although the exact mechanism is unclear, it is thought that TNF may cause capillary endothelial damage by supplying the tumor and causing hemorrhage. Another possible mechanism of action is that the TNF may augment and increase NK cell cytolytic activity, and increase the number of B cells and polymorphonucleocytes. Perhaps TNF incites an inflammatory response by stimulating macrophage cytotoxicity or by inducing the release of IL-1 by monocytes.

Receptors for TNF are found on several mononuclear cells, in the synovial membrane as well as in the peripheral blood and synovial fluid. There are also soluble receptors: receptors that are free in solution after being shed from mononuclear cells. Increased soluble receptors are seen in rheumatoid arthritis and to a certain degree in osteoarthritis, SLE, and systemic sclerosis. The soluble TNF receptors block the action

IMMUNE

of TNF by binding it so that less free TNF is available to activate the mononuclear cells.

The therapeutic use of this soluble receptor is restricted because the half-life of TNF is short; to increase the half-life and thus enable therapeutic applications, the strategy of combining TNF with an immunoglobulin or other molecule has been attempted. It is the combination of the recombinant soluble form of human p75 TNF receptor to the Fc fragment of immune gamma globulin that is known as etanercept (see earlier discussion).

The adverse effects of TNF are similar to those of IFN and are dose-dependent, resolving quickly after discontinuance of the TNF. An acute flulike syndrome is most common. Hypotension, fatigue, and malaise are possible. There may be local skin reactions if the TNF is administered by IM or SC route. TNF enhances coagulation, thereby increasing the risk for a thrombus.

Different routes of administration are being studied, including intraperitoneal and arterial. No specific dosage has been identified at this time. TNF causes an elevation in liver function tests and a transient increase in blood counts. Coagulation studies should be monitored as they are commonly elevated.

CLINICAL REASONING

Treatment Objectives

Treatment objectives for the patient receiving BRMs depend somewhat on the reason for use of the drug. In general, the major objective is to decrease the risk of organ toxicities and constitutional adverse effects of the BRMs. For example, for patients receiving G-CSFs, the objective is to abate the risk of infection by accelerating the recovery of neutrophils after high-dose antineoplastic therapy. With GM-CSFs, the therapeutic objective is to hasten myeloid recovery in patients who have received autologous bone marrow transplantation subsequent to high-dose antineoplastic therapy. The treatment objective for the patient receiving ILs may be to reduce the size of the tumor. The objective for patients receiving epoetin alfa is the restoration and maintenance of erythrocyte counts. If infection does occur, some therapies are discontinued until the infection resolves. For all patients receiving BRMs, early detection and treatment of infection is paramount.

Treatment Options

▥ Patient Variables

Many of the BRMs are administered as self-injections. This method is generally not covered by insurance, as it assumes the patient can be taught to give the drug. However, not all patients are able and/or willing to administer the drug to themselves, or have another person who can assist. In addition, many patients are too ill to reliably take the drug but are not sick enough to be hospitalized.

BRM drugs are expensive. Prices are established to offset the high cost of years of research and development. The technology used to produce the products (hybridoma and recombinant DNA) is expensive as well. For example, one hospitalization for 14 doses of IL-2 therapy can easily exceed $30,000.00; one course of an antineoplastic drug with the

additional support of a TNF can increase the cost of treatment by $2500. The cost of one regimen of sargramostim to the pharmacist is more than $4000.

Life-Span Considerations

Pregnant and Nursing Women. BRMs are generally not recommended for use during pregnancy or lactation. To prevent undesirable complications to the fetus or newborn child, determine whether the patient is pregnant or nursing before administering BRMs.

Children and Adolescents. BRMs are ordinarily not used in persons under the age of 18. However, if the drug is required and the patient is an infant, determine if the child is breastfed or bottle-fed. Breastfeeding introduces Ab to the infant's GI tract, conferring some immunity. For all children, determine which immunizations they have received (e.g., measles, mumps, and pertussis). Epoetin alfa was recently approved for use in children with oncologic disorders, and many of the TNF inhibitors now have indications in children.

Older Adults. There is an increased risk of adverse effects in older adults. With increasing age, the patient may experience alterations in hepatic and renal function, decreasing cardiovascular function, altered neurosensory function, and decreased integrity of tissue, skin, and mucous membranes. All of these changes place the older person at more risk for the adverse effects of BRM therapy. Every patient must be assessed individually for the appropriateness of BRM therapy.

Increasing age is identified as a risk factor for the constitutional, cardiovascular, and neurologic adverse effects of BRMs. Older patients are more likely to have preexisting cardiovascular dysfunction as well. The headache, fever, chills, fatigue, malaise, and weakness common with many of the BRMs are more pronounced in older patients. Increased monitoring is needed in older adult patients using BRMs because of the increased risk of adverse effects.

▥ Drug Variables

Because of the unique nature of BRMs, concurrent biotherapy is being used more often and for a wider range of disorders. Combined with antineoplastic drugs, BRMs provide immunomodulatory, direct antitumor, and other biologic effects (Fig. 32-4). Certain drugs, such as IFN or IL-2, are used as conventional treatment for cancer, with the expected response of tumor shrinkage. BRMs have made it possible to successfully control rejection of transplanted tissues without compromising all the patient's immune functions. The branch of the immune system that must be controlled is cell-mediated immunity.

The advantage of using MoAbs over conventional antisera (Ab-containing sera) is that a single Ab of known antigenic specificity is generated rather than a mixture of different antibodies; monoclonal antibodies have a single, constant binding affinity. Further, a MoAb can be diluted to a uniform titer because the actual concentration of Ab is known. The MoAb can also be refined easily to homogeneity. MoAbs can be chosen for a specific antigenic determinant of a virus and manufactured in large amounts. As a result of hybridoma technology, the health care provider can order tests for viral Ag that are specific and diagnostic, and can detect disease early in its course.

CSFs reduce inpatient hospital stays, antibiotic use, febrile days, and transfusion requirements. These benefits are reflected in reduction in the cost of treatment and improvement in the quality of life.

The use of BRMs has raised many economic issues because the ways these drugs are used goes beyond current criteria for reimbursement. The first economic consideration in the use of BRMs is the investigational status of most of the drugs. FDA indications are usually narrow, whereas clinical applications are quite broad. Reimbursement is frequently refused when use is outside the approved FDA indications (see Controversy).

BRM therapy often includes the use of other drugs to reduce or minimize the adverse effects of the biologic drug. Strategies that may be recommended to minimize or prevent the flulike symptoms include acetaminophen to reduce fever. Meperidine may be used to reduce shaking chills (rigors). Proton pump inhibitors (e.g., omeprazole, esomeprazole) may be used for prophylaxis of GI irritation and bleeding. Antiemetics and antidiarrheal drugs may also be needed. Patients with indwelling catheters should receive prophylactic antibiotic therapy for *Staphylococcus aureus*. Have epinephrine readily available in the event of anaphylaxis.

Be sure to check the results of lab testing before administering a BRM. Assess patients who are at high risk for organ or drug toxicities.

Patient Education

Patients receiving BRMs have the same educational needs with regard to drug therapy as other patients. Information and the ability to participate in self-care activities increase self-esteem and enhance coping ability. The basic function of the immune system, the drug's mechanism of action, and therapeutic results that are expected from treatment should

be taught. The expected adverse effects, of both the specific BRM and of combination therapy (BRM plus antineoplastic drug, or more than one BRM), and administration techniques should also be covered. The importance of lab testing and follow-up with the health care provider cannot be overemphasized. Also advise patients to avoid driving or operating hazardous machinery if blurry vision or drowsiness occurs. Teach female patients that contraceptive measures are required during and up to 12 weeks after BRM therapy stops.

Consider the patient's family a resource as they coach each other during the physical and emotional strain of BRM therapy. It is important to teach the family to identify and report adverse effects that the patient may be unable to recognize (e.g., neurologic changes). Be sure the patient and the family know when and how to contact the health care provider.

Because the patient is at risk for infection while taking immunosuppressing BRMs, conscientious handwashing is required of all who come in contact with the patient. Teach the patient and the family to monitor specifically for signs and symptoms of infection. Teach patients how to take their temperature. Advise them to avoid persons who have just received immunizations containing live vaccine. Some patients need to avoid exposure to house plants and animals. In some cases, the immunocompromised patient may require reverse isolation so as to reduce the risk of contracting an infection.

Patient and family knowledge about what constitutes adequate nutrition is vital. Encourage the patient to consume high-quality dietary nutrients and to avoid as much as possible "empty" calories. Use of supplemental vitamins and

---

Controversy

Tumor Necrosis Factor-α Antagonists: Helpful or Harmful?

The biologic response modifiers (BMRs) are a division of the disease-modifying antirheumatic drugs (DMARDs), but unlike the DMARDs, the drugs essentially stop progression of the disease. In some cases, use of a BRM drug launches a long-lasting remission for the patient. Furthermore, the BRM drugs are often efficacious in patients for whom other interventions have been unsuccessful.

Even though the mechanisms of action for BRMs are sometimes different for each drug within the larger class, all of them act to inhibit cytokines, the proteins that contribute to inflammation. Because BRMs improve disease in patients unresponsive to traditional therapies and retard radiographic progression of their disease, the BRMs have redefined therapy for rheumatoid arthritis (RA).

Adalimumab (Humira) is approved for RA; etanercept (Enbrel) for RA, psoriatic arthritis, ankylosing spondylitis, and adult and juvenile RA; and infliximab (Remicade) for RA and Crohn's disease. These BRMs block the cytokine receptor known as tumor necrosis factor-alpha (TNF-α), and anakinra (Kineret) blocks a cytokine known as interleukin-1 (IL-1). Pegfilgrastim (Neulasta) and infliximab (Remicade) took the fourth and fifth positions, while adalimumab took the hundred and fifty-sixth position on the list of the top 200 drugs used in hospitals (*Drug Topics.* [2007]. *151* [8], 19) during the year 2006. For 2006, the wholesale acquisition cost of pegfilgrastim totaled $860,663,090; for infliximab, $749,934,062; and for adalimumab, $54,658,622—all significant figures in the health care

arena. Yet, what are the costs of these drugs to the individual patient? Refer back to Tables 32-3 and 32-4 for approximate costs.

CLINICAL REASONING ANALYSIS

Your 65-year-old patient's activities of daily living continue to be limited by her rheumatoid arthritis. At today's visit she tells you that she has just come from the rheumatologist, who recommended etanercept (Enbrel) to help control her debilitating disease. The patient expresses worry over the possible adverse effects she has seen in direct-to-consumer advertising, yet she is anxious to start therapy.

- Could monoclonal antibodies such as etanercept really hold the promise your patient hopes for?
- Your patient is normally reluctant to take new drugs until the adverse effects are well known. How will you go about discussing with her the benefits and risks of monoclonal antibody therapy?
- Would a breakthrough in monoclonal antibody research change the nature of your discussion?
- Will allowing limited federal funding for patients in need reignite a fierce battle over the use of the new drugs?
- Is there an ethical difference between creating human embryos specifically for the development of monoclonal antibody drugs versus extraction from embryos left over from fertility treatments or abortion?

IMMUNE

minerals may have to be considered for some patients. Protein supplements also may be required.

Evaluation

The effectiveness of BRM therapy is specific to the disorder under treatment. For example, therapeutic effectiveness may be demonstrated by immunosuppression of an autoimmune disorder or the absence of graft rejection for patients who have undergone transplantation. In some cases, tumor regression and decreased spread of malignant cells can be noted as early as 4 weeks after completion of the first course of IL therapy. Patients taking ILs for relapsing-remitting multiple sclerosis may see a decrease in the frequency of relapse, further providing evidence of drug effectiveness. Normalized blood chemistry and CBC parameters also provide evidence of therapeutic response. The time to hematopoietic response is related to the interval required for the maturation of immature cells to become fully mature and to be released into the peripheral circulation. The rate and extent of a hematopoietic response are influenced by available iron stores, baseline hematocrit, and presence of concurrent medical problems.

KEY POINTS

- Biologic response modifiers are produced through hybridoma and recombinant gene technologies.
- BRMs act in conjunction with the immune system to destroy tumor cells, influence chronic granulomatous disease and multiple sclerosis, and in the treatment of the hematologic adverse effects of autologous bone marrow transplantation.
- There may be one or more treatment objectives for the use of BRMs, depending on the disease or condition for which it is used.
- The development of all biotherapy drugs is based on the prototype drug interferon. Colony-stimulating factors, interleukins, monoclonal antibodies, and tumor necrosis factor were developed later.
- Other FDA-approved CSFs include granulocyte colony-stimulating factor (filgrastim and pegfilgramstim), and granulocyte-macrophage colony-stimulating factor (sargramostim).
- Monoclonal antibodies are highly specific to lymphocyte membrane Ags. These antibodies impair cell-mediated immune responses, specifically, T-cell activity.

- BRMs tend to be more effective when the disease entity or tumor mass is quantitatively small. For this reason, they are used in combination with other drugs or treatment modalities.
- BRMs affect every organ system in the body. Adverse effects can be acute (anaphylaxis) or chronic (fatigue), constitutional (fever, chills), or system specific (hypotension).
- Administration and patient education must be tailored according to the individual BRM being given.
- Quality of life is a great issue with the use of BRMs. There is a significant incidence of adverse effects because BRM therapy often continues for months to years.
- Remember, tumor response and survival does not directly correlate with enhanced quality of life.

Bibliography

Abbas, A., and Lichtman, A. (2003). *Cellular and Molecular Immunology*. Philadelphia: WB Saunders.

Armitage, J. (1998). Emerging applications of recombinant of human granulocyte-macrophage colony stimulating factors. *Blood, 92*(12), 4491–4508.

Bagot, M., Nikolova, M., and Schirm-Chabanette, F., et al. (2001). Crosstalk between tumor T lymphocytes and reactive T lymphocytes in cutaneous T cell lymphomas. *Annals of the New York Academy of Science, 941*, 31–38.

Breedveld, F. (2000). Therapeutic monoclonal antibodies. *Lancet, 355* (9205), 735–740.

Cunnane, G., Doran, M., and Bresnihan, B. (2003). Infections and biological therapy in RA. *Best Practices and Research in Clinical Rheumatology, 17*, 345–363.

Ellerin, T., Rubin, R., and Weinblatt, M. (2003). Infections and anti-tumor necrosis factor alpha therapy. *Arthritis and Rheumatism, 48* (11), 3013–3022.

Feldman, M. (2002). Development of anti-TNF therapy for rheumatoid arthritis. *Nature Reviews: Immunology, 2*(5), 364–371.

Gardam, M., Keystone, E., and Menzies, R., et al. (2004). Anti-tumor necrosis factor agents and tuberculosis risk: Mechanisms of action and clinical management. *Lancet Infectious Disease, 3*, 148–155.

Guyton, A., and Hall, J. (Eds.). (2000). *Textbook of Medical Physiology*. (10th ed). Philadelphia: WB Saunders.

Hainsworth, J., Burris, H., and Morrissey, L., et al. (2000). Rituximab monoclonal antibody as initial systemic therapy for patients with low-grade non-Hodgkin lymphoma. *Blood, 95*(10), 3052–3056.

Hainsworth, J. (2000). Monoclonal antibody therapy in lymphoid malignancies. *Oncologist, 5*(5), 376–384.

Hanauer, S., Feagan, B., and Lichtenstein, G., et al. (2002). Maintenance infliximab for Crohn's disease: The ACCENT I randomized trial. *Lancet, 359*(9317), 1541–1549.

Imperato, A., Smiles, S., and Abramson, S. (2004). Long-term risks associated with biologic response modifiers used in rheumatic diseases. *Current Opinions in Rheumatology, 16*(3), 199–205.

Janeway, C., Travers, P., and Walport, M., et al. (2005). *Immunobiology: The Immune System in Health and Disease*. New York: Churchill Livingston.

Kalofonos, H., and Grivas, P. (2006). Monoclonal antibodies in the management of solid tumors. *Current Topics in Medicinal Chemistry, 6*(16), 687–705.

Mousa, S., Goncharuk, O., and Miller, D. (2007). Recent advances of TNF-alpha antagonists in rheumatoid arthritis and chronic heart failure. *Expert Opinion on Biological Therapy, 7*(5), 617–625.

Press, O. (2003). Radioimmunotherapy for non-Hodgkin's lymphomas: A historical perspective. *Seminars in Oncology, 30*(2 Suppl 4), 10–21.

Rader, C., Sinha, S., and Popkov, M., et al. (2003). Chemically programmed monoclonal antibodies for cancer therapy: Adaptor immunotherapy based on a covalent antibody catalyst. *Proceedings of the National Academy of Sciences of the United States of America*, *100*(9), 5390–5400.

Runkel, L., Lawrence, P., and Lewerenz, M., et al. (1998). Differences in activity between alpha and beta type I interferons explored by mutational analysis. *Journal of Biological Chemistry*, *273*(14), 8003–8008.

Slamon, D., Leyland-Jones, B., and Shak, S., et al. (2001). Use of chemotherapy plus a monoclonal antibody against HER-2 for metastatic breast cancer that overexpresses HER-2. *New England Journal of Medicine*, *344*(11), 783–792.

Solal-Celigny, P. (2001). Rituximab as first-line monotherapy in low-grade follicular lymphoma with a low tumor burden. *Anticancer Drugs*, *12*(Suppl 2), S11–S14.

Sompayrac, L. (2003). *How the Immune System Works* (2nd ed.). Ames, IA: Blackwell.

ten Hove, T., van Montfrans, C., and Peppelenbosch, M., et al. (2002). Infliximab treatment induces apoptosis of lamina propria T lymphocytes in Crohn's disease. *Gut*, *50*(2), 206–211.

Tremblay, F., Fernandes, M., and Habbab, F., et al. (2007). Malignancy after renal transplantation: Incidence and role of type of immunosuppression. *Annals of Surgical Oncology*, *9*(8), 758–788.

Vogel, C., Cobleigh, M., and Tripathy, D., et al. (2002). Efficacy and safety of trastuzumab as a single agent in first-line treatment of HER-2-overexpressing metastatic breast cancer. *Journal of Clinical Oncology*, *20*(3), 719–726.

Vose, J., Link, B., and Grossbard, M., et al. (2005). Long-term update of a phase II study of rituximab in combination with CHOP chemotherapy in patients with previously untreated, aggressive non-Hodgkin's lymphoma. *Journal of Clinical Oncology*, *46*(11), 1569–1573.

IMMUNE

33

Antineoplastic Drugs

ancer is no longer considered an immediate death sentence because of modern treatment options. Today, malignant diseases that were previously considered incurable can be cured. Paired with increased public awareness of the importance of cancer screening for common malignancies, major advances have also been made in basic and translational research relating to prevention and early intervention as well as adjuvant therapies. However, cancer remains the second leading cause of death in the United States, preceded only by cardiovascular disease. The rate of occurrence for certain types of neoplastic disease, including breast, lung, and skin cancer, continues to increase. Antineoplastic therapy is the treatment of choice for hematolymphatic malignancies and solid tumors that have undergone regional or distant metastasis. The ultimate goals of antineoplastic therapy are to provide cure, control, or palliation of disease. Future advances in individualizing cancer treatment and patient surveillance are promised by newer gene-based diagnostic technology. In addition to gene technology, research in DNA microarrays has the potential to enhance the effectiveness of drug therapies by helping us to target the specific populations who will derive the greatest benefit.

CANCER

EPIDEMIOLOGY AND ETIOLOGY

The occurrence, distribution, and outcomes of malignant diseases reflect varying patterns, depending upon sex, age, geographic location, and socioeconomic status. Cancers of the lung are equally likely to occur in men and women and account for the highest rates of mortality in both sexes. In women, the leading sites of fatal cancers are the lung, the breast, the colon, and the rectum, while the lung, the prostate, the colon, and the rectum are the leading sites in men. Age-adjusted death rates over the last few decades show a steady increase in cancer death rates for both sexes, which may be due, at least in part, to improved detection and diagnosis of the disease.

The exact cause of cancer remains unknown. There is evidence to suggest that cellular genes, normally responsible for cellular metabolism, division, and growth, change to malignant *oncogenes* (genes found in chromosomes of tumor cells) that cause uncontrolled cell growth and replication. Data support the commonly held belief that environmental agents are the major causes of human cancers. Various substances have been identified as *carcinogenic* (cancer-causing) or able to promote the development of cancer.

Environmental Agents
The earliest chemical carcinogens to be identified were tobacco snuff in 1759 and soot in 1775. Today, cigarette

smoking is responsible for one fourth of all cancers in the United States. These days, it is well known that tars and other carcinogens emitted by a cigarette increase the risk for cancer tenfold over nonsmokers. The risk increases with the number of cigarettes and length of time smoked. Secondhand smoke, or passive smoking, has been implicated as a cause of lung cancer in those indirectly exposed to tobacco smoke, including children, spouses, and fellow workers. To date, smoking is known to be a causative factor in the development of cancer of the lung, the larynx, the oral cavity, the bladder, the kidney, the colon, and the cervix, and has been implicated in leukemia. Heavy alcohol consumption is related to cancers of the oral cavity, the esophagus, and the liver, and may be synergistic or additive to the effects of tobacco use.

Physical carcinogens alter DNA structure and create chromosomal alterations and translocations. Ionizing radiation (x-ray therapy, radon gas, and nuclear power), ultraviolet radiation, and radon are well-known carcinogens. Ionizing radiation is associated with cancers of the lung, the bone, the liver, the thyroid, the thymus, and the breast. Leukemia has been reported following exposure to radioactive gas from the atomic bomb blasts in Nagasaki and Hiroshima during World War II and at nuclear reactors at Three Mile Island and in Chernobyl, Russia. Arsenic, beryllium, cadmium, nickel, and uranium are among numerous other carcinogens primarily seen with occupational exposures. Asbestos has been linked to lung cancer and mesothelioma. Mesothelioma is a malignant tumor composed of cells that line the pleura, pericardium, and peritoneum. A smaller number of leukemias and various solid tumors have been attributed to high-dose radiation therapy.

Lifestyle and Diet
A relationship appears to exist between excessive alcohol intake and cancers of the oropharynx, the esophagus, and the liver. Evidence from laboratory, animal, and epidemiologic studies suggest vitamin D may be protective against some types of cancers. Epidemiologic studies have related higher dietary intake of calcium and vitamin D with a lower incidence of cancer. Crude petroleum, coal tar, and polycyclic aromatic hydrocarbons are formed by cooking noncarcinogenic hydrocarbons in food and oil to high temperatures. Cancers of the larynx and the scrotum, and chromosomal aberrations in cord blood and in adults have been linked to aromatic hydrocarbons.

High dietary fat intake has been associated with increased incidence of many solid tumors. Cancers of the breast, the prostate, the colon, and the rectum are more common in the Western world and higher economic groups, where dietary fat intake is higher. Studies have shown a rise in the incidence of cancer in females from Asian countries after migration to the United States and increases in dietary fat intake. The role of fat in colon cancer is supported by both the increased incidence with dietary change and the potential relationship of fat consumption to bile acids, which are known to be mutagenic. Cancer of the breast, the ovaries, the endometrium, the pancreas, and the prostate and colorectal cancer are also related to high fat intake, but the evidence is not conclusive. However, obesity is a documented risk factor for endometrial cancer and breast cancer, and for an increased severity and progression of ovarian cancer.

Genetics

Neoplasia has been attributed to abnormalities in one or more of the genes that regulate growth and differentiation, with chromosomal disorders often preceding some neoplasms. Some genes contain instructions for controlling cell growth, division, and death. Genes that promote cell division are referred to as *oncogenes*. Tumor suppressor genes slow cell division, or cause cells to die at the right time. Cancers are caused by mutations in DNA that turn oncogenes on, or turn tumor suppressor genes off.

The BRCA genes (i.e., *BRCA1* and *BRCA2*), for example, are tumor suppressor genes. When mutated, they no longer suppress abnormal growth and cancer is more likely to develop. Certain inherited DNA changes can cause an increased risk for developing breast cancer in women who carry these genes and are responsible for the breast cancers that run in some families. However, DNA mutations in patients with breast cancer usually occur in individual breast cells during the woman's lifetime rather than being inherited. These acquired mutations may be the result of radiation or cancer-causing chemicals. To date, the cause of most acquired mutations remains unknown.

Infections

Certain types of cancers can have an infectious component. Primary liver cancer has been linked with hepatitis B viral infections, and the Epstein-Barr virus (EBV) has been associated with Burkitt's lymphoma, a form of undifferentiated malignant lymphoma. In addition to EBV, a member of the *Herpes* group associated with nasopharyngeal cancer, herpes simplex virus II, and human papilloma virus (HPV) have both been linked to cancer of the cervix. Human T-cell leukemia-lymphoma virus is associated with leukemias and lymphomas.

Drugs

Some drugs, including antineoplastics, are associated with increased risk for certain cancers. Alkylating drugs interact with DNA directly or indirectly and may cause secondary leukemias years later. Unopposed estrogen therapy use or oral contraceptives containing only estrogen do not cause cancer, but may allow potentially neoplastic changes to take place, increasing the risk for endometrial cancer. For example, tamoxifen use has been linked to endometrial and uterine cancer, which is significant because patients take tamoxifen to prevent breast cancer.

PATHOPHYSIOLOGY

Cancer is characterized by both uncontrolled cell proliferation and impaired differentiation. *Tumors* are neoplastic or new growths of cells. Benign tumors do not *metastasize* or

spread from their original location. Malignant tumors spread by direct extension into surrounding tissues, via the lymphatic system, and hematogenously via blood circulation. Most cancers are clonal in origin, which means they emerge from a single progenitor cell versus a group of cells. This finding supports a genetic link to cancer, but it is also now understood that the formation of cancer in a specific cell type or tissue is caused by a series of mutations.

Cancer cells proliferate only when the normal capacity to identify and repair mutations in the genome is lost. A *genome* is a complete set of hereditary factors contained in the haploid set (one half) of chromosomes. Except for the germ cells of the gonads, each body cell is programmed for a limited number of cell divisions. The program involves telomeres located at the ends of the chromosome and produced and maintained by telomerase, an enzyme in both germ and embryonic cells. Telomeres pair and align at mitosis. They normally lose function during development because a portion of the telomere is lost with each cell division. Telomeric loss serves as a cellular clock. In contrast, cancer cells reexpress telomerase, which allows continued proliferation. Loss of normal cell cycle controls causes ongoing expression of the enzyme. Ninety-five percent of cancer cells express the telomerase enzyme, making it a potential target for drug intervention.

Tumor Suppressor Genes

Tumor suppressor genes regulate mitosis and cell division. These genes act as gatekeepers for passage from the S (synthesis) phase of the cell cycle to G_2 and mitosis (see following discussion). Activation of these genes, which may occur if DNA replication cannot be successfully completed, triggers apoptosis, or programmed cell death. When the activation of tumor suppressor genes is faulty, the result is uncontrolled cell growth. There are two primary ways for a cell to lose the function of its tumor suppressor genes: (1) hereditary gene mutations and (2) acquired gene mutations.

Hereditary Gene Mutations

Hereditary gene mutations, also known as germline mutations, initially occur in the sperm cells of males or egg cells of females but are integrated into cells throughout the body. In these cases, almost all the cells of the body will inherit the same mutation, which is then passed on from generation to generation. These mutations are a major contributing factor in 5% to 10% of cancers. However, a single faulty tumor suppressor gene is usually not sufficient to cause cancer since individual cells contain two copies of each gene, one from each parent.

Acquired Gene Mutations

Most cancers are caused by acquired mutations that develop as cellular DNA changes over time. Acquired gene mutations, also known as sporadic or somatic mutations, can be caused by environmental influences such as exposure to radiation or toxins. Acquired mutations start in one cell and are found only in the progeny of that cell. Unlike hereditary mutations, these mutations are found only in cancer cells.

For example, chromosomal aberrations can occur in which two different chromosomes swap locations. The most common aberration is in the translocation of chromosomes 11 and 22. Occurring in 10 to 15 of every 10,000 newborns, this translocation is the most common cause of childhood leukemia. In another example, chronic myelogenous leukemia (CML) is the result of translocation of chromosomes 9 and 22, which gives rise to the Philadelphia chromosome.

DNA Repair Genes

As a major defense against environmental damage to cells, DNA repair is present in all organisms including bacteria, yeast, fish, amphibians, rodents, and humans. DNA repair involves processes that minimize apoptosis, mutations, replication errors, persistence of DNA damage, and genetic instability.

Toxic and mutagenic gene consequences are minimized by distinct pathways of repair, and 150 known human DNA repair genes have been profiled. Some noteworthy characteristics include four enzymes that can remove uracil from DNA, seven recombination genes related to *RAD51* (a homologous pairing gene), DNA polymerases that bypass damage, and one system to remove the main DNA lesions provoked by ultraviolet light (Wood et al., 2005). A listing of the DNA repair genes can be found online at the National Center for Biotechnology Information on Science.

Tumor Growth

Understanding the basic processes of cellular proliferation is essential to understanding the mechanisms of antineoplastic drugs. *Cell cycle time* involves a series of events during which both neoplastic and normal cells grow and reproduce. Rapidly growing cancers are more susceptible to antineoplastic drugs than slower-growing cancers. The term *growth fraction* refers to the percentage of cells that are actively dividing at any given time. During the early stages of tumor expansion, the growth fraction is high and the tumor doubling time rapid.

Tumor growth is best described using Gompertzian kinetics (Table 33-1). The *log kill hypothesis* assumes that drugs kill a constant fraction of tumor cells (relative to the log number of cells) and not a constant number of cells. Log kill varies with cell growth rate; thus, there is a gradual decrease in log kill in the late stages of tumor growth, when cells stop cycling. Early return of slow-growing tumors occurs because the log kill is small. Late return of rapid-growing tumors may occur despite effective treatment if too few courses of treatment are given.

Doubling time is the time required for a tumor mass to increase twofold. When tumor volume is low and the cells

TABLE 33-1 Gompertzian Growth Kinetics

Cell Burden	Number of Cells Present	Clinical Response
10^0	1	Clinical disease undetectable by physical exam or by cell burden
10^5	100,000	Clinical disease undetectable by physical exam or by cell burden
10^9	1,000,000,000	Clinical symptoms begin to appear*
10^{10}	10,000,000,000	Regional spread of cancer cells
10^{11}	100,000,000,000	Metastasis of cancer cells
10^{13}	10,000,000,000,000	Cancerous process likely to be lethal

*A cell burden of 10^9 is typically the smallest tumor physically detectable. The patient has approximately 1 billion cancer cells at this point, equivalent to a tumor the size of a small grape and weighing 1 gram. Clinical symptoms usually begin to appear.

are rapidly dividing, a high proportion of cells undergo division. As a result, these tumor cells are more sensitive to antineoplastic drugs. Similarly, a tumor with a relatively vigorous doubling time (e.g., testicular cancer–21 days, Ewing's sarcoma–22 days) is more sensitive to antineoplastic drugs than tumors with a slow doubling time (e.g., colon cancer–96 days, breast cancer–129 days, adenocarcinoma of the lung–134 days).

The larger the tumor cell population, the longer the tumor doubling time. Large tumors have a less efficient blood supply than smaller tumors, divide more slowly, and respond more favorably to drugs effective in any phase of the cell cycle. For this reason, cell cycle–nonspecific drugs are likely to be more effective against slow-growing cancers. In contrast, cell cycle–specific drugs tend to be effective against rapid-growing cancers. Unfortunately, as the tumor burden increases, the patient becomes more and more debilitated and less able to withstand antineoplastic therapy. The patient's ability to withstand therapy is related to the fact that normal cells also have a high growth fraction. This is why the gastrointestinal (GI) tract, hair follicles, and bone marrow display the most toxicity when exposed to antineoplastic drugs.

▓ *Cell Cycle Concepts*

At any given time, tissue cells are actively dividing and differentiating, and some are dormant. The term *cell cycle* describes the series of events during which both neoplastic and normal cells grow and reproduce. Cell cycles vary depending on the type of tissue, which accounts for differences in response by specific cell types to antineoplastic drugs.

PHASES OF THE CELL CYCLE. Four distinct phases of the cell cycle are recognized. During the first phase known as gap 1 (G_1), proteins, RNA, and enzymes required for the synthesis of DNA are formed (Fig. 33-1). The G_1 phase may be virtually absent, as in embryonic cells, or so prolonged that it becomes dormant (G_0).

In the synthesis (S) phase, DNA is formed and chromosomes double within the cell in preparation for mitosis. The activity of replicative enzymes such as thymidine kinase, DNA polymerase, dihydrofolate reductase, ribonucleotide reductase, RNA polymerase II, and topoisomerases I and II is increased. The S phase can last 12 to 18 hours depending on cell type. Many antineoplastic drugs cause direct damage to the DNA code during this phase, thereby decreasing the cell's ability to replicate.

In the gap 2 (G_2) phase, the second period of RNA and protein synthesis, the mitotic spindle forms. This phase lasts 1 to 8 hours, with the DNA complement becoming twice the normal number of chromosomes.

During mitosis (M), the parent cell divides into two new daughter cells. Each daughter cell contains the same number and kind of chromosomes as the parent cell. This phase lasts about 1 to 2 hours. After mitosis, cells will either return to the G_1 phase or go into the resting stage (G_0).

Antineoplastic drugs that target the cell cycle are classified according to their mechanism of action and how they act within a specific phase of the cell cycle. Drugs characterized as *cell cycle–specific* (CCS) act on cells undergoing specific phases in cell production (Box 33-1). These drugs include most subcategories of antimetabolites that act specifically in the S phase of the cell cycle, and topoisomerase inhibitors,

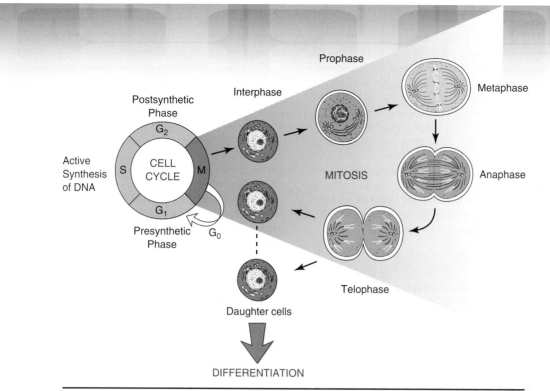

FIGURE 33-1 The Cell Cycle. The cell cycle represents the interval from the midpoint of mitosis to the ensuing end point of mitosis, where a daughter cell is produced. The phases include synthesis (S), in which DNA is synthesized in the cell's nucleus; gap 2 (G_2), in which RNA and protein synthesis occurs (construction of mitotic apparatus); mitosis (M), where both nuclear and cytoplasmic division take place; and gap 1 (G_1), the postmitotic period between the M phase and the start of DNA synthesis, when RNA and protein synthesis is increased and cell growth occurs.

BOX 33-1

Summary of Cell Cycle Active Drugs

Cell Cycle–Specific Drugs	Cell Cycle–Nonspecific Drugs
Phase S	• carboplatin
• busulfan	• carmustine
• cytarabine	• chlorambucil
• fluorouracil	• cisplatin
• hydroxyurea	• cyclophosphamide
• methotrexate	• daunorubicin
• thioguanine	• doxorubicin
	• idarubicin
Phase G_2	• lomustine
• dactinomycin	• mechlorethamine
• bleomycin	• melphalan
• etoposide	• mitomycin
• teniposide	• plicamycin
Phase M	
• ifosfamide	
• vinblastine	
• vincristine	
• vindesine	
• paclitaxel	
Phase G_1	
• mitoxantrone	
• ʟ-asparaginase	
• prednisone	

specific to the late G_2 and M phases. For example, the antimetabolite drug methotrexate is most effective in the S phase of the cell cycle. It binds with folic acid reductase, thus inhibiting synthesis of DNA and RNA. *Cell cycle–nonspecific* (CCNS) drugs act on the cell, whether it is dividing or in a resting state. CCNS drugs include alkylating drugs (e.g., cyclophosphamide, chlorambucil) and antitumor antibiotics (e.g., mitomycin, doxorubicin, and daunorubicin) as well as the other drugs.

Combination drug regimens act in different phases of the cell cycle to yield greater tumor cell kill compared to single drug regimens. In addition, multidrug treatment regimens decrease the risk for developing a drug-resistant tumor cell line. It is important to consider the potential for toxicity when combining antineoplastic drugs, particularly when moderate to high doses are used, and when the drugs are given for extended periods of time.

Concept of Cell Kill

The effects of antineoplastic drugs on cancer cells follow the concept of first-order kinetics. This concept refers to the destruction of a constant percentage of cancer cells, rather than a constant number, regardless of the number of cells present. To eradicate all viable cancer cells, the antineoplastic drug or drug combination must be administered at repeated intervals over time until the drug, along with the patient's immune system, destroys all cancer cells. According to the *cell kill hypothesis,* if the cancer contains 1 million cells and the treatment regimen has a 90% kill rate, the first course of therapy would theoretically destroy 90% of tumor cells, leaving 10% unaffected. The second dose would kill 90% of the remaining cells, leaving 10%, and so on until one cell remains. The body's immune response would then destroy the final remaining cell. This hypothesis explains why most antineoplastic regimens use multidrug therapy administered at regular intervals over a period of months or years.

The degree of cell kill is directly proportional to the dosage administered. Ideally, with each additional course of therapy, the dosage remains the same, even though the cancer may be getting progressively smaller. The patient must be able to tolerate the same level of drug toxicity if therapy is to continue. This theory provides useful insight into applications and antineoplastic treatment strategies but fails to account for variations in the tumor's responsiveness to treatment.

Tumor Cell Resistance

Tumor cell heterogeneity is important because it is linked to the emergence of antineoplastic-resistant tumor cells. The origin of the resistance is thought to be predictable and due to random mutational events. A tumor contains subsets of cells whose characteristics vary greatly, including their responsiveness to antineoplastic therapy.

Tumor cell resistance is intrinsic or acquired. *Intrinsic resistance* is resistance to a specific drug without any prior exposure to that drug. *Acquired resistance* develops after the start of therapy and represents a change in the tumor cells themselves.

Tumor cell resistance may be temporary or permanent. Factors related to *temporary resistance* include alterations in the bioavailability, biotransformation, or elimination of the drug; the presence of tumor in sanctuary sites; limited drug diffusion; alteration in cell kinetics; host toxicity; and the blood supply of the tumor. A *sanctuary site* is defined as an area in the body that is not readily perfused by antineoplastic drugs.

Permanent resistance to antineoplastic drugs is genetically based. The probability of having at least one drug-resistant cell is based on the mutation rate and the size of the tumor. The mechanisms associated with permanent drug resistance include defective drug transport or biotransformation, transformed nucleotide pools, increased drug activation, altered repair of DNA, gene amplification, altered target proteins, and multidrug resistance. In some cases, cancer cells repair DNA damage caused by the antineoplastic drug or decrease permeability to prevent drug activation. Tumor cell resistance also occurs because of the inability of a tumor to change a drug to its active form and/or its ability to inactivate a drug. The larger the tumor mass (i.e., the greater the heterogeneity), the greater the likelihood of drug-resistant and multi–drug-resistant clones. Fortunately, tumor cell mutation that results in resistance to one drug does not usually result in resistance to drugs in other different classes. This provides a rationale for combination drug therapy.

ANTINEOPLASTIC DOSING REGIMENS

There is no exact way to predict which drug will be most effective (i.e., killing the largest number of cancer cells). Thus, dosage recommendations and schedules must be followed as closely as possible for maximal effectiveness. Dosage regimens of antineoplastic drugs vary significantly from drug to drug but in general are based on body weight (mg/kg) or body surface area (mg/m²). Dosage modifications of antineoplastic regimens may be required based on patient age, organ impairment, and patient response.

Plasma concentrations of the various antineoplastic drugs have no clear relationships with efficacy and/or safety. Additionally there is often a delay of days to weeks between measurement of drug concentrations and the clinical effects of many antineoplastics. It is often difficult to observe patients' daily antineoplastic therapy, thus valuable information about a drug's efficacy and toxicity may not be observed or understood. For example, after four cycles of antineoplastic therapy, a patient with lung cancer may have a repeat computed tomography (CT) scan. **Monitoring for drug efficacy is not a surrogate for monitoring drug toxicity. Dosing strategies generally prioritize safety over efficacy at the expense of maximum tumor suppression or reduction in tumor volume.** ▲

Monitoring Therapeutic and Adverse Effects

Most antineoplastic drugs cause bone marrow suppression; therefore, monitoring blood cell counts is particularly important. **Neutrophils are important in protecting the body from infection; a patient receiving an antineoplastic drug must be alert to the possible signs of a low neutrophil count and take protective measures against infection.** ▲

The degree of neutropenia is reflected in the absolute neutrophil count (ANC) (Box 33-2). Platelet counts less than 50,000/mm³ and hemoglobin values lower than 11 mg/dL

BOX 33-2

Calculating the Absolute Neutrophil Count (ANC)

When a patient's immune system is compromised and the patient is at increased risk for infection, look at more than the white blood cell (WBC) counts to determine if the patient is neutropenic. Look at the differential and calculate the absolute neutrophil count (ANC). By using ANC values, the precursors of the WBCs (i.e., the immature WBCs), a more accurate prediction of a patient's risk for infection can be made and used to guide therapy.

Measuring the ANC:
Example
WBC 4000 cells/mm³
Neutrophils* 50% of WBCs
Bands 8% of WBC

1. Add percentages of neutrophils and bands together:	50% + 8% = 58%
2. Then, convert to a decimal by dividing the figure obtained by 100:	58/100 = 0.58
3. Multiply the decimal figure by the total WBC to get the ANC:	0.58 × 4000 = 2320

Risk of Infection:

Neutropenia	ANC <2000	Slight risk of infection; antineoplastic therapy given
Mild neutropenia	ANC >1000 but <2000	Minimal risk of infection; antineoplastic therapy given
Moderate neutropenia	ANC >500 but <1000	Moderate risk of infection; antineoplastic therapy held
Severe neutropenia	ANC <500	Severe risk of infection

*Neutrophils are sometimes also called ''segs'' (segmented neutrophils) or ''polys'' (polymorphonucleocytes).

require attention and will likely cause antineoplastic therapy to be withheld. Additionally, liver function tests and blood urea nitrogen (BUN) and creatinine levels must be carefully monitored because most of these drugs are biotransformed and eliminated through the liver and kidneys. Any compromise in liver or kidney function alters antineoplastic drug action and increases the toxicity of antineoplastic drugs.

Monitor serum alanine aminotransferase (ALT), aspartate aminotransferase (AST), bilirubin, alkaline phosphatase, lactate dehydrogenase (LDH), uric acid, BUN, and creatinine levels and electrolyte values before and periodically throughout antineoplastic drug therapy. How frequently the monitoring takes place depends on the drugs used and the patient's tolerance for therapy.

PHARMACOTHERAPEUTIC OPTIONS

Antineoplastic drugs are divided into several categories based on how they act within specific cancer cells, which cellular activities or processes the drug interferes with, and which specific phases of the cell cycle the drug affects. Knowing this helps oncologists decide which drugs are likely to work well together and, if more than one drug will be used, plan exactly when each of the drugs should be given (i.e., in which order and how often).

Drugs Interacting with DNA Synthesis: Alkylating Drugs

- altretamine (Hexalen, Nexistat, HMM); ◆ Hexalen
- busulfan (Mielucin, Myleran, Sulfabutin); ◆ Myleran
- carmustine (BCNU, BiCNU, Gliadel); ◆ BiCNU
- carboplatin (Paraplatin); ◆ Paraplatin-AQ
- chlorambucil (Leukeran); ◆ Leukeran
- cisplatin (CDDP, Platinol, Platinol AQ, CIS); ◆ Platinol-AQ
- cyclophosphamide (Cytoxan, Neosar); ◆ Cytoxan, Procytox
- dacarbazine (DTIC-Dome); ◆ DTIC
- ifosfamide (Ifex); ◆ Ifex
- lomustine (CeeNu, Gliadel); ◆ CeeNU
- mechlorethamine (Mustargen, nitrogen mustard); ◆ Mustargen
- melphalan (Alkeran); ◆ Alkeran
- oxaliplatin (Eloxatin)
- polifeprosan 20 with carmustine implant
- procarbazine (Matulane)
- temozolomide (Temodar); ◆ Temodal
- thiotepa (ThioTEPA, triethylenethiophosphoramide, Thioplex, Tespa)

Indications

Alkylating drugs are the oldest and largest group and the most useful of the antineoplastic drugs used in the United States. They are a potent group of drugs but also have a large number of adverse effects and drug interactions. The uses for these drugs are identified in Table 33-2.

Pharmacodynamics

All of the alkylating drugs act through covalent bonding of highly reactive alkyl groups or substituted alkyl groups with nucleophilic proteins and nucleic acids. Some of the drugs act directly with biologic molecules, whereas others form an intermediate compound that reacts with target receptors. The sites for alkylation are widespread and include proteins (i.e., enzymes and cell membranes) and nucleotides, accounting for adverse as well as therapeutic effects.

The most common binding site for alkylating drugs is the 7-nitrogen group of guanine. Binding to this site leads to miscoding and cross-linking between two DNA strands or between two bases in the same strand of DNA. Reactions between DNA and RNA and between the alkylating drug and proteins may also occur, although the main insult that results in cell death is inhibition of DNA replication (the DNA strands do not separate as required for replication).

Alkylating drugs are CCNS, with their effects seen in rapidly dividing cells. As a whole, these drugs are cytotoxic, mutagenic, teratogenic, carcinogenic, and myelosuppressive. Nevertheless, some are cytocidal to cells in particular phases of the cell cycle (e.g., lomustine in G_1 or G_2; mechlorethamine, which is most active in phases M and G_1).

Tumor resistance to these drugs is often multifactorial. Resistance may be the result of decreased membrane transport (e.g., for melphalan and cisplatin) or it may be bound by glutathione in the cytoplasm and inactivated. The alkylating drug can also be transformed to an inactive metabolite (e.g., by enzymes such as aldehyde dehydrogenase).

Pharmacokinetics

The pharmacokinetics of alkylating drugs is found in Table 33-3. Alkylating drugs react with water and are inactivated by hydrolysis, making spontaneous degradation an important component of their elimination from the body.

Adverse Effects and Contraindications

Alkylating drugs differ in their patterns of antitumor activity and in the sites and severity of adverse effects. Most of the drugs cause a dose-limiting toxicity to bone marrow and to a lesser degree to intestinal mucosa. Chlorambucil, cyclophosphamide, ifosfamide, melphalan, and mechlorethamine produce an acute myelosuppression, with a nadir (see Myelosuppression section later in chapter) of the peripheral neutrophil count of 6 to 10 days and recovery in 14 to 21 days. Cyclophosphamide has lesser adverse effects on neutrophil counts than the other alkylating drugs.

Busulfan suppresses all cellular components, particularly stem cells, and may produce prolonged and cumulative myelosuppression that closely simulates the hematologic effects of whole-body radiation therapy. For this reason, busulfan is used as a preparative regimen in allogenic bone marrow transplantations. Carmustine and other chloroethylnitrosureas cause delayed and prolonged suppression of both neutrophils and platelets, reaching a nadir 4 to 6 weeks after administration.

Alkylating drugs, in addition to the effects on the hematopoietic system, are highly toxic to dividing mucosal cells, leading to stomatitis and intestinal denudation. The stomatitis is particularly a problem with high-dosage protocols associated with bone marrow reconstitution, since they predispose to bacterial sepsis arising from the GI tract. Melphalan and thiotepa have advantages over some of the other drugs in that they cause less mucosal damage. In high-dosage protocols, a number of toxicities become apparent compared with conventional dosages.

Nausea and vomiting are most often associated with carmustine and mechlorethamine and are presumably the result

IMMUNE

```
┌─────────────────────────────────────────────────────────────────────┐
│ TABLE 33-2 Uses of Selected Antineoplastic Drugs                     │
└─────────────────────────────────────────────────────────────────────┘
```

Drug	Use(s)
ALKYLATING DRUGS	
altretamine	Persistent or recurrent ovarian cancer, germ cell testicular cancer
busulfan	CML, ANLL
carboplatin	Ovarian, head and neck, testicular, and lung cancers
carmustine	CNS cancers; colorectal, stomach, liver cancers; multiple myeloma, Hodgkin's disease, non-Hodgkin's lymphoma, melanoma, small lymphocytic lymphoma, nongastric MALT lymphoma
chlorambucil	Ovarian, testicular cancers; CLL, malignant lymphomas, breast cancer, hairy cell leukemia, small cell lymphocytic lymphoma, multiple myeloma, trophoblastic neoplasms, follicular lymphoma, nongastric MALT lymphoma
cisplatin	Testicular, ovarian, bladder, brain, breast, adrenal cortex, endometrium, cervical, uterine, head and neck, esophagus, lung, prostate, stomach cancers; trophoblastic neoplasms, melanoma, non-Hodgkin's lymphoma, osteosarcoma
cyclophosphamide	Breast, bladder, cervical, endometrium testicular, prostate, head and neck, lung cancers; AIDS-related B cell lymphoma, diffuse large B cell lymphoma, non-Hodgkin's lymphoma, NLPHD, Hodgkin's disease, melanoma, myeloma, cutaneous T-cell lymphoma, lymphoblastic lymphoma, neuroblastoma, ALL, ANLL, cervical, CML, Ewing's sarcoma, Burkitt's lymphoma, small lymphocytic lymphoma, small cell lung cancer, osteosarcoma, Wilm's tumor, sarcomas, rhabdomyosarcoma, retinoblastoma, trophoblastic neoplasms, nongastric MALT lymphoma, germ cell tumors, mantle cell lymphoma, Waldenström's macroglobulinemia, splenic zone lymphoma
dacarbazine	Malignant melanoma, Hodgkin's disease, islet cell carcinoma, neuroblastoma, soft tissue sarcomas
ifosfamide	Ovarian, cervical, germ cell testicular cancers; AIDS-related B cell lymphoma, Burkitt's lymphoma, diffuse large B cell lymphoma, mesenchymal chondrosarcoma, intra-abdominal soft tissue sarcomas other than GIST, nongastric MALT lymphoma, NSCLC, splenic zone lymphoma
lomustine	Breast, lung, colorectal, kidney, CNS tumors, Hodgkin's disease, melanoma, myeloma, non-Hodgkin's lymphoma
mechlorethamine	Hodgkin's disease, lymphosarcoma, CML, CLL, polycythemia vera, mycosis fungoides, bronchogenic cancer, metastatic cancers resulting in effusion, CNS tumors, NLPHD
melphalan	Breast, thyroid, ovarian, testicular cancers; amyloidosis, multiple myeloma, melanoma, diffuse large B cell lymphoma, Waldenström's macroglobulinemia, nongastric MALT lymphoma
oxaliplatin	Metastatic colorectal cancer in patients whose disease has recurred or progressed
polifeprosan 20	CNS tumors (with carmustine implant)
procarbazine	Advanced Hodgkin's disease, nodular lymphocyte-predominant Hodgkin disease (NLPHD), primary and metastatic CNS tumors, SCLC, classic Hodgkin's
temozolomide	Refractory anaplastic astrocytoma, melanoma
thiotepa	Breast, bladder, lung, ovarian cancers; intracavitary effusions, lymphoma, Hodgkin's disease
ANTIMETABOLITES	
5-azacitidine	Myelodysplastic syndromes
cladribine	Hairy cell leukemia, advanced cutaneous T-cell lymphoma, CLL, non-Hodgkin's lymphoma, AML, mycosis fungoides or Sézary syndrome, autoimmune hemolytic anemia
capecitabine	Colorectal, breast, kidney, pancreas, gastric cancers
cladribine	Hairy cell leukemia (leukemic reticuloendotheliosis)
cytarabine	ANLL, ALL, CML, meningeal leukemia, Hodgkin's and non-Hodgkin's lymphoma
decitabine	Myelodysplastic syndromes
fludarabine	B-cell CLL, non-Hodgkin's lymphoma
5-fluorouracil	Solid tumors of stomach, gallbladder, colon, rectum, breast, pancreas, bladder, cervical, endometrium, esophagus, head and neck, islet cell, liver, lung, ovarian, prostate; premalignant actinic keratoses and superficial skin cancers, occult primary cancers
floxuridine	Brain, breast, bladder, cervical, gallbladder, head and neck, kidney, ovarian, prostate cancers: GI adenocarcinoma metastatic to liver, ANLL, ALL
gemcitabine	Head and neck, breast, liver, bladder, kidney, testicular, cervical, uterine, ovarian cancers; locally advanced metastatic cancer of pancreas in patients who have previously received 5-FU, Hodgkin's lymphoma, soft tissue cancers other than GIST, NSCLC
hydroxyurea	CML, malignant melanoma, metastatic or inoperable ovarian cancer, head and neck cancer, occult primary cancers, lymphoblastic lymphoma
6-mercaptopurine	ALL, ANLL, CML, APL non-Hodgkin's lymphoma
methotrexate	Breast, head and neck, lung, bladder, brain, cervical, esophagus, kidney, ovarian, prostate, stomach, testicular cancers; choriocarcinoma, hydatidiform mole, prophylaxis and treatment of meningeal lymphocytic lymphoma, Burkitt's lymphoma, non-Hodgkin's lymphoma, osteosarcoma, psoriasis (severe, recalcitrant, disabling), rheumatoid arthritis (second- or third-line treatment), ANLL, cutaneous T-cell lymphoma, myeloma, rhabdomyosarcoma, APL, AML, AIDS-related B-cell lymphoma, desmoid tumors, mantle cell lymphoma
pemetrexed	NSCLC; currently being evaluated for use in the treatment of bladder and breast cancer, non-Hodgkin's lymphoma, and pancreatic cancer
pentostatin	Hairy cell leukemia, chronic lymphocytic leukemia or small lymphocytic lymphoma, mantle cell lymphoma
thioguanine	ALL, CML, remission induction, consolidation, and maintenance therapy for ANLL
MITOTIC INHIBITORS	
docetaxel	Breast, prostate, ovarian, cervical, uterine, esophageal, gastric, head cancers; NSCLC, SCLC, melanoma, and soft tissue sarcomas, germ cell tumors, intraabdominal soft tissue sarcomas other than GIST, NSCLC
etoposide	Refractory testicular tumors, SCLC, Kaposi's sarcoma
estramustine	Prostate cancer
irinotecan	Colon and breast cancer, SCLC, leukemia
paclitaxel	Ovarian, cervical, breast, bladder, testicular, prostate cancers; advanced NSCLC, esophageal and gastric cancers, germ cell cancers, occult primary cancers, NSCLC
teniposide	Refractory ALL in children
topotecan	Colorectal, head and neck cancers; malignant glioma
vinblastine	Testicular, breast, upper GI cancers; classic Hodgkin's disease, neuroblastomas, histiocytosis X, Kaposi's sarcoma, lymphomas, choriocarcinomas, desmoid tumors, germ cell tumors, NLPHD, melanoma, NSCLC
vincristine	Breast, bladder, lung, cervical cancers; AIDS-related B-cell lymphoma, ALL, primary amyloidosis, CLL, classic Hodgkin's disease, Burkitt's lymphoma, Ewing's sarcoma, rhabdomyosarcoma, germ cell tumors, neuroblastoma, Wilm's tumor, diffuse large B-cell lymphoma, sarcomas, follicular lymphoma, gastric MALT lymphoma, nongastric MALT lymphoma, NLPHD, lymphoblastic lymphoma, mantle cell lymphoma, myeloma, SCLC, splenic zone lymphoma

vindesin	Melanoma and lung cancers and with other drugs, to treat uterine cancers
vinorelbine	Breast, cervical, ovarian cancers; soft tissue sarcomas, NSCLC
ANTITUMOR ANTIBIOTICS	
bleomycin	Head and neck, skin, testicular, penis, cervical, vulva, ovarian cancers; classic Hodgkin's disease, NLPHD
dactinomycin	Testicular cancer; Wilms' tumor, rhabdomyosarcoma, Ewing's sarcoma, osteosarcoma, Kaposi's sarcoma, choriocarcinoma, germ cell tumors
daunorubicin	ALL, AML, APL, CML, lymphoblastic lymphoma
doxorubicin	Thyroid, ovarian, uterine, prostate, breast, stomach, lung, pancreas, kidney, bladder cancers; AIDS-related B-cell lymphoma, Burkitt's lymphoma, classical Hodgkin's disease, non-Hodgkin's lymphoma, NLPHD, ALL, AML, osteogenic sarcoma, Ewing's sarcoma, rhabdomyosarcoma, neuroblastomas, Wilm's tumor, desmoid tumors, diffuse large B-cell lymphoma, mesenchymal chondrosarcoma, osteosarcoma, follicular lymphoma, gastric MALT lymphoma, nongastric MALT lymphoma, sarcoma other than GIST, islet cell tumors, mantle cell lymphoma, multiple myeloma, primary amyloidosis, soft tissue sarcomas, SCLC, splenic zone lymphoma
epirubicin	Solid tumors of breast cancer; cervical, gastric cancer; uterine sarcoma
idarubicin	AML, APL, CML
mitomycin	Anus, stomach, pancreas, bladder, cervical cancers; NSCLC
mitoxantrone	Prostate cancer; AML, ANLL, CML, diffuse large B-cell lymphoma, follicular lymphoma, gastric MALT lymphoma, lymphoblastic lymphoma, mantle cell lymphoma, nongastric MALT lymphoma, splenic zone lymphoma
plicamycin	Hypercalcemia, hypercalciuria
MISCELLANEOUS	
L-asparaginase	Pediatric ALL, lymphoblastic lymphoma
mitotane	Palliation of inoperable cancer of adrenal cortex
pegaspargase	ALL patients sensitive to L-asparaginase

AIDS, Acquired immunodeficiency syndrome; *ALL,* acute lymphocytic leukemia; *AML,* acute myelocytic leukemia; *ANLL,* acute nonlymphocytic leukemia; *APL,* acute promyelocytic leukemia; *CML,* chronic myelocytic leukemia; *CNS,* central nervous system; *GI,* gastrointestinal; *GIST,* gastrointestinal stromal tumor; *MALT,* mucosa-associated lymphoid tissues; *NLPHD,* nodular lymphocyte-predominant Hodgkin's disease; *NSCLC,* non–small cell lung cancer; *SCLC,* small cell lung cancer.

of CNS stimulation. They occur with all drugs that interfere with DNA, but they can be particularly severe with cisplatin and mechlorethamine. Cisplatin may cause both acute and delayed nausea and vomiting since it is biphasic; use it with antiemetic drugs. Ifosfamide is the most neurotoxic drug of this class.

Neurotoxicity is more common and is a dose-limiting toxicity of cisplatin. Carboplatin, on the other hand, carries a greater risk of neurotoxicity but with cumulative dosages. Neurotoxicity is worse when the drugs are given by intravenous (IV) route because of higher peak levels. Neurotoxicity is manifested as somnolence, confusion, mood changes, and paresthesias.

In any acute treatment cycle, 30% of patients treated with oxaliplatin noted acute neurotoxicity. Oxaliplatin causes an acute, reversible, primarily peripheral sensory neuropathy that is of early onset and occurring within hours or 1 to 2 days of dosing. The neuropathy ordinarily resolves within 14 days. The symptoms are precipitated or exacerbated by exposure to cold or cold objects and usually appear as transient paresthesias, dysesthesia, and hypoesthesia in the hands, feet, perioral area, or throat. For some patients, these symptoms can be triggered by anything cold, such as iced drinks and cold air. Jaw spasm, abnormal tongue sensation, dysarthria, eye pain, and a feeling of chest pressure have been reported.

Additionally, pulmonary fibrosis is noted in approximately 43% of patients using oxaliplatin. In the event of unexplained respiratory symptoms (i.e., dyspnea, nonproductive cough, crackles, or radiologically identified infiltrates), the drug should be discontinued until further examination excludes pulmonary fibrosis and interstitial lung disease.

Both cellular and humoral immunity are suppressed by alkylating drugs. Immunosuppression is reversible at dosages used in most antineoplastic regimens. Although bone marrow toxicity is predictable with standard dosages of alkylating drugs, other organ toxicities are less common. For example, all alkylating drugs can cause pulmonary fibrosis; interstitial pneumonitis is seen with the nitrosureas busulfan, carmustine, and lomustine. In high dosages, endothelial damage may give rise to occlusive venous disease of the liver; the nitrosureas can lead to renal failure after multiple treatment cycles; and ifosfamide frequently causes a central neurotoxicity with seizures, coma, and, at times, death. Busulfan at high dosages can precipitate seizures.

Cyclophosphamide and ifosfamide are associated with renal and bladder toxicities. Cyclophosphamide-related bladder irritation is associated with dosages over 2 grams/m^2. Hemorrhagic cystitis is a major concern with ifosfamide but of less concern with cyclophosphamide. Giving the drug during the day reduces the risk of a dehydration-related bladder irritation and cystitis. In addition, cyclophosphamide may cause syndrome of inappropriate secretion of antidiuretic hormone (SIADH).

Teratogenesis and gonadal atrophy are common but variable depending on the specific drug, its administration schedule, and its route of administration. In women, amenorrhea of several months' duration sometimes follows a course of therapy with alkylating drugs. Impairment of spermatogenesis (i.e., azoospermia) is noted in men. Damage to hair follicles is much more pronounced with cyclophosphamide than with other nitrogen mustards, frequently resulting in alopecia. This effect is usually reversible, even with continued therapy.

As a class, alkylating drugs carry a major risk for the **A** **induction of or secondary development of acute nonlymphocytic leukemia,** which is associated with partial or total deletion of chromosomes 5 or 7. The incidence peaks about 4 years after therapy was started and affects up to 5% of patients treated with alkylating drugs. Melphalan, the nitrosureas, and procarbazine carry the greatest risk for leukemia. Cyclophosphamide is the least potent in this regard.

PHARMACOKINETICS

TABLE 33-3 Selected Antineoplastic Drugs

Drug	Route	Onset	Peak	Duration	PB (%)	t½
ALKYLATING DRUGS						
altretamine	PO	UA	3–4 wk	6 wk	6; 25; 50*	4.7–10.2 hr
busulfan	PO	10–15 days	Weeks	1 mo†	30–32	2.5 hr
carboplatin	IV	UA	21 day	28 days	High	2.6–5.9 hr
carmustine	IV	Days	4–5 wk	96 hr	UA	UA
chlorambucil	PO	7–14 days	7–14 days	14–28 days	99	1.5 hr
cisplatin	IV	UA	18–23 days	39 days	90	30–100 hr
cyclophosphamide	PO	7 days	7–15 days	21 days	>60	4–6.5 hr
dacarbazine‡	IV	16–20 days	16 days	3–5 days	Low	5 hr
ifosfamide	IV	UA	7–14 days	21 days	UA	15 hr
lomustine	PO	UA	4–7 wk	1–2 wk	50	1–2 days
mechlorethamine	IV	Immed	Min	Min	UA	Min
melphalan	PO	5 days	2–3 wk	5–6 wk	<30	1.5 hr
oxaliplatin	IV	Immed	UA	UA	>90	0.43 hr; 16.8 hr
temozolomide	PO	Rapid	1 hr	UA	14	1.8 hr
thiotepa	IV	10–30 days	14 days	21 days	UA	2.4–17.6 hr
ANTIMETABOLITES						
5-azacitidine	IV	Immed	30 min	UA	UA	33–49 min
capecitabine	PO	UA	1.5 hr	UA	<60	45 min
cladribine	IV	UA	UA	5 wk§	20	5.4–7 hr
cytarabine	IV	24 hr; 15–24 hr‖	24 days	12 days; 25–34 days	15	1–3 hr
fludarabine	IV	Immed	13–16 days	UA	19–29	20 hr
5-fluorouracil	IV	1–9 days	9–21 days	30 days	UA	20 hr
gemcitabine	IV	Immed	30 min	UA	UA	1–19 hr
hydroxyurea	PO	7 days	10 days	21 days	UA	3–4 hr
6-mercaptopurine	PO	7–10 days	14 days	21 days	20	45 min; 2.5 hr; 10 hr¶
methotrexate	PO, IV	4–7 days	7–14 days	21 days	35	8 hr
pentostatin	IV	4–7 mo	UA	7.7–35 mo**	4	6 hr
pemetrexed	IV	Immed	UA	UA	81	3.5 hr
6-thioguanine	PO	7–10 days	14 days	21 days	UA	11 hr
MITOTIC INHIBITORS						
docetaxel	IV	Immed	8 days	7 days	94–97	11.1 hr
estramustine	PO	UA	UA	UA	UA	20 hr
paclitaxel	IV	UA	11 days	3 wk	89–98	5.3–17.4 hr
vinblastine	IV	5–7 days	10 days	7–14 days	75	24 hr
vincristine	IV	UA	4 days	7 days	75	85 hr
vindesin	IV	Immed	UA	UA	UA	24 hr
vinorelbine	IV	UA	7–10 days	7–14 days	UA	28–44 hr
TOPOISOMERASE INHIBITORS						
etoposide	PO, IV	7–14 days	9–16 days	20 days	97	3–12 hr
irinotecan	IV	Immed	1.5 hr	UA	30–68	6 hr
teniposide	IV	UA	16–18 days	15 days	99	5 hr
topotecan	IV	Days	11 days	7 days	35	2–3 hr
ANTITUMOR ANTIBIOTICS						
bleomycin	IV	Immed	10–20 min	UA	UA	2 hr
dactinomycin	IV	7 days	14 days	21–28 days	UA	36 hr
daunorubicin	IV	7–10 days	10–14 days	21 days	UA	18.5 hr; 26.7 hr††
doxorubicin	IV	10 days	14 days	21–24 days	UA	16.7 hr
epirubicin	IV	Immed	UA	UA	77	3 min; 2.5 hr; 33 hr‡‡
idarubicin	IV	UA	10–14 days	21 days	97; 94§§	4–46 hr
mitomycin	IV	3–8 wk	4–8 wk	3 months	UA	50 min
mitoxantrone	IV	10 days	10 days	21 days	78	5.8 days
plicamycin	IV	UA	7–10 days	3–4 wk	UA	UA
MISCELLANEOUS						
L-asparaginase	IV	Immed	UA	23–33 days	UA	8–30 hr
mitotane	PO	2–4 wk	6 wk	UA	UA	18–159 hr
pegaspargase	IV	Immed	UA	14 days	UA	5.7 days
procarbazine	PO	14 days	2–8 wk	28–42 days	UA	10 min

*Protein binding of the 3 altretamine metabolites.
†Recovery from busulfan may take up to 20 months.
‡Onset, peak, and duration of dacarbazine effects on white blood cells and platelets, respectively.
§Cladribine's time to normalization of blood counts.
‖Onset and duration of cytarabine's phase 1 and 2 effects on WBC count.
¶6-Mercaptopurine has a triphasic half-life.
**The duration of inhibition of metabolite lasts over 1 week following administration of pentostatin.
††Half-life of daunorubicin and its metabolite, respectively.
‡‡The plasma concentration of epirubicin declines in a triphasic manner with mean half-lives for the alpha, beta, and gamma phases, respectively.
§§Protein binding of idarubicin and its metabolite, respectively.
BioA, Bioavailability; *Immed,* immediate; *IV,* intravenous; *NA,* not applicable; *PB,* protein binding; *PO,* by mouth; *t½,* half-life; *UA,* unavailable.

Drug Interactions

Drug interactions with alkylating drugs are many (Table 33-4). All alkylating drugs interact with other antineoplastic drugs and total body radiation therapy to increase the risk of bone marrow suppression.

Lab Considerations

Alkylating drugs cause bone marrow suppression; therefore, careful attention must be paid to monitoring the ANC, hemoglobin, and platelet counts. Serum ALT, AST, bilirubin, alkaline phosphatase, LDH, uric acid, BUN, and creatinine levels and electrolyte values should be monitored before and periodically throughout alkylating drug therapy. Any alterations in liver or kidney functions alter the action and toxicity of the alkylating drug.

Busulfan may cause elevated uric acid levels and produce false-positive cytology results of breast, bladder, cervix, and lung tissues. Cisplatin may cause decreased serum sodium,

DRUG INTERACTIONS
TABLE 33-4 Selected Antineoplastic Drugs

Drug	Interactive Drug	Interaction
ALKYLATING DRUGS		
Alkylating drugs in general	Antineoplastics, radiation	Additive bone marrow suppression
	Live virus vaccines	Decreases antibody response and risk for adverse effects of interactive drug
carboplatin, cisplatin	Aminoglycosides, amphotericin B, vancomycin	Increases risk for nephrotoxicity of cisplatin and carboplatin
	Aminoglycosides, furosemide	Increases risk for ototoxicity
carmustine	Smoking	Increases risk for pulmonary toxicity
cyclophosphamide	phenobarbital, rifampin	Increases toxicity of cyclophosphamide
	allopurinol	Exaggerates bone marrow depression
	succinylcholine	Prolongs neuromuscular blockade
	Diuretics	Increases risk for leukopenia
	Insulin	Increases risk for hypoglycemia
	cytarabine, daunorubicin, doxorubicin	Additive cardiotoxicity
	warfarin	Potentiates effects of interactive drug
	Adrenocorticosteroids, azathioprine, chlorambucil, cyclosporine, mercaptopurine	Increases risk for infection and development of other neoplasms
	probenecid, sulfinpyrazone	Hyperuricemia and gout may develop
	cocaine	Prolongs effects of cocaine
dacarbazine	phenobarbital, phenytoin	Increases biotransformation of dacarbazine and decreases effectiveness
melphalan	carmustine	Increases risk for pulmonary toxicity
	cyclosporine	Increases risk for renal failure
	nalidixic acid	Increases risk for enterocolitis
thiotepa	succinylcholine	Prolongs neuromuscular blockade
ANTIMETABOLITES		
methotrexate	Aspirin, NSAIDs	Decreases elimination of MTX and increases risk for toxicity
	leucovorin	Decreases MTX toxicity
	probenecid	Increases MTX displacement and increases toxicity
	sulfonamides	Additive enzyme inhibition and increased toxicity
floxuridine	dexamethasone	Decreases floxuridine hepatotoxicity
5-fluorouracil	allopurinol	Decreases fluorouracil toxicity
	cimetidine	Increases serum concentration of fluorouracil
	interferon-alfa, leucovorin, MTX	Increases toxicity to fluorouracil
cytarabine	digoxin	Decreases serum levels of interactive drug
6-mercaptopurine	allopurinol	Inhibits biotransformation of mercaptopurine and increases risk for toxicity
	Nondepolarizing muscle relaxants	Decreases neuromuscular blockade
	warfarin	Potentiates or antagonizes activity
6-thioguanine	Myelosuppressants	Increases risk for toxicity, bleeding, hepatotoxicity
ANTITUMOR ANTIBIOTICS		
Antitumor antibiotics in general	Antineoplastic drugs, radiation	Increases risk for pulmonary and hematologic toxicity
	Live virus vaccines	Decreases antibody response and increases risk for adverse effects
bleomycin	cisplatin	Decreases elimination of bleomycin; increases risk of toxicity
dactinomycin	doxorubicin	Increases risk for cardiotoxicity
daunorubicin	cyclophosphamide	Increases risk for cardiotoxicity
doxorubicin	cyclophosphamide	Increases risk for hemorrhagic cystitis from cyclophosphamide
	6-mercaptopurine	Increases risk for hepatitis from 6-mercaptopurine
	cyclophosphamide, radiation	Increases risk for cardiotoxicity

Continued

IMMUNE

DRUG INTERACTIONS
TABLE 33-4 Selected Antineoplastic Drugs—Cont'd

Drug	Interactive Drug	Interaction
mitomycin	vinblastine, vincristine, vindesine, vinorelbine	Increases risk for respiratory toxicity
plicamycin	aspirin, Cephalosporins (some) dextran, heparin, NSAIDs, sulfinpyrazone, Thrombolytic drugs, valproic acid, warfarin	Increases risk for bleeding
	Aminoglycosides, amphotericin B, vancomycin	Increases risk for hepatotoxicity
	Nephrotoxic drugs	Increases risk for nephrotoxicity
MITOTIC INHIBITORS		
Mitotic inhibitors in general	Antineoplastics, radiation	Additive bone marrow depression
	Live virus vaccines	Decreases antibody response and increases risk of adverse effects
docetaxel	cyclosporine, ketoconazole, erythromycin, troleandomycin	Significantly alters effects of docetaxel
mitoxantrone	dactinomycin, doxorubicin, idarubicin	Increases risk for cardiomyopathy with previous use of interactive drugs
paclitaxel	ketoconazole	Inhibits biotransformation of paclitaxel and increases risk for serious toxicity
vinblastine	mitomycin	Bronchospasm in patients previously treated with mitomycin
vincristine	L-asparaginase	Decreases biotransformation of vincristine
vinorelbine	cisplatin	Increases risk and severity of myelosuppression
	mitomycin, radiation to chest	Increases risk of acute pulmonary reactions
TOPOISOMERASE INHIBITORS		
irinotecan	Laxatives	Exacerbates diarrhea
	Diuretics	Increases risk of dehydration if diarrhea occurs
	dexamethasone	Increases risk of hyperglycemia and lymphocytopenia
	prochlorperazine	Increases risk for akathisia if given the same day
teniposide	Antineoplastic drugs, radiation, sodium salicylate, sulfamethizole, tolbutamide	Increases myelosuppression
topotecan	G-CSF	Prolongs neutropenia
MISCELLANEOUS		
hydroxyurea	Antineoplastics, radiation	Additive bone marrow suppression
	Live virus vaccines	Decreases Ab response and increases risk for adverse effects
L-asparaginase	vincristine	Decreases hepatic clearance of vincristine
	MTX	Diminishes effects of MTX
	prednisone	Increases toxicity to L-asparaginase
mitotane	phenytoin	Decreases effectiveness of mitotane
	Alcohol, Antihistamines, Antidepressants, Opioids, Sedative-hypnotics, warfarin	Additive CNS depression
	spironolactone	Blocks effects of mitotane in Cushing's disease
pegaspargase	Anticoagulants, Antiplatelet drugs	Alters response to interactive drug
procarbazine	Alcohol, Antidepressants, Antihistamines, Opioids, Sedative-hypnotics	Additive CNS depression
	Alcohol	Disulfiram-like reaction
	Antidepressants. Levodopa, Local anesthetics, guanadrel, guanethidine, reserpine, Sympathomimetics	Increases risk for hypertensive episodes since procarbazine contains MAO inhibitory properties
	meperidine, Opioids	Severe paradoxical reactions
	carbamazepine, fluoxetine, MAO inhibitors, Tricyclic antidepressants	Increases risk for seizure and hyperpyrexia
	Antineoplastics, radiation	Additive bone marrow suppression
	Insulin, Oral hypoglycemic drugs	Potentiates hypoglycemia

Ab, Antibody; *CNS*, central nervous system; *G-CSF*, granulocyte colony stimulating factor; *MAO*, monoamine oxidase; *MTX*, methotrexate; *NSAIDs*, nonsteroidal antiinflammatory drugs.

potassium, calcium, and magnesium concentrations. Cyclophosphamide may suppress positive reactions to skin tests for *Candida*, mumps, *Trichophyton*, and purified protein derivative (PPD) tuberculin tests. It may also produce false-positive results on Papanicolaou (PAP) smears. Melphalan may elevate 5-hydroxyindoleacetic acid (5-HIAA) concentrations as a result of tumor breakdown.

Drugs Damaging DNA: Antimetabolites

- 5-azacitidine (azacytidine, 5-AC, Ara C, Vidaza)
- cladribine (Leustatin); ◆ Leustatin
- clofrabine (Clofarabine)
- capecitabine (Xeloda); ◆ Xeloda
- cytarabine (Ara-C, Cytosar-U, Tarabine); ◆ Cytosar
- fludarabine (Fludara); ◆ Fludara
- 5-fluorouracil (5-FU, Adrucil, Efudex); ◆ Adrucil, Efudex, Fluoroplex
- gemcitabine (Gemzar); ◆ Gemzar
- hydroxyurea (Hydrea); ◆ Hydab
- 6-mercaptopurine (6-MTP, Purinethol); ◆ Purinethol
- methotrexate (MTX, Folex, Mexate, Mexate AQ, Rheumatrex); ◆ Folex, Mexate
- permetrexed (Alimeta); ◆ Alimeta
- pentostatin (Nipent); ◆ Nipent
- 6-thioguanine (Lanvis); ◆ Lanvis

▮ Indications

Antimetabolites are divided into four categories: folic acid analogues, purine analogues, pyrimidine analogues, and cytosine analogues. Antimetabolites structurally resemble naturally occurring metabolites within a cell; the names of these subclasses are derived from the metabolite affected: (1) The folate analogues include MTX and pemetrexed; (2) the purines and purine antimetabolites include 6-mercaptopurine, 6-thioguanine, fludarabine, cladribine, and pentostatin; (3) the pyrimidines include 5-fluorouracil and capecitabine; and (4) the cytosine analogues include cytarabine, gemcitabine, and azacitidine.

Antimetabolites have been used to treat the entire spectrum of cancers. The effectiveness of the individual drugs varies with the different types of cancer (see Table 33-2).

Pharmacodynamics

Anticancer antimetabolites take advantage of the need for dividing cells to have a constant supply of the deoxynucleic acids required for DNA synthesis. Cells get their supply of nucleic acids by salvaging them from within the body or by synthesizing them de novo. Growing cells synthesize deoxythymidine monophosphate, required for DNA synthesis, from deoxyuridine monophosphate. They are all CCS within the S phase of the cell cycle; however, to be effective the drugs must be present for an extended period.

The cells incorporate folic acid, pyrimidines (e.g., cytosine, thymine, uracil), or purines (e.g., adenine, guanine, hypoxanthine) into themselves during cellular metabolism, disrupting critical metabolic processes. Thus the neoplastic cells are unable to continue dividing, and die.

Folic acid analogues inhibit DNA and/or RNA synthesis; therefore, their mode of action means that their toxic effects are most marked in rapidly proliferating tissues. Folic acid is a cofactor in purine and pyrimidine synthesis and includes pteridine, para-aminobenzoic acid (PABA), and glutamate complexes. Polyglutamates are the more efficient cofactors because they are retained longer in the cells.

The best understood folic acid analogue is MTX, which is transported into cancer cells via active transport. The drug enters the cells by passive diffusion. However, this strategy also subjects normal cells to extremely high levels of MTX. In order to save normal cells, a "leucovorin rescue" (Jaffee regimen) is given to rescue the lining of the GI tract and the bone marrow cells from MTX toxicity. Most of the complications and adverse effects of MTX can be either prevented or treated by using leucovorin, which is usually given 24 hours after MTX. Leucovorin bypasses the metabolic impedance caused by MTX, thus permitting normal cells to synthesize thymidylate and other compounds. Cancer cells are not affected by the leucovorin because uptake requires the same transport system as MTX.

Tumor resistance occurs as a result of decreased uptake of the drug, or an increased synthesis of dihydrofolate reductase. Dihydrofolate reductase reduces dihydrofolic acid to tetrahydrofolic acid, using nicotinamide adenine dinucleotide phosphate (NADPH) as an electron donor, which can be converted to the kinds of tetrahydrofolate cofactors used in 1-carbon transfer chemistry. Because tetrahydrofolate, the product of this reaction, is the active form of folic acid, inhibiting dihydrofolate reductase causes functional folic acid deficiency. Because folic acid is needed by rapidly dividing cells to make thymine, this effect may be therapeutic.

Resistance may also occur as a result of the synthesis of a modified form of dihydrofolate reductase that has a reduced affinity for the drug. Pemetrexed, a multitargeted antifolate, inhibits dihydrofolate reductase as well as thymidine synthase and glycinamide ribonucleotide formyltransferase, therefore decreasing the risk of drug resistance.

Purine analogues (i.e., adenine, guanine, and hypoxanthine) are bases used in the synthesis of nucleic acids. The major site of purine synthesis is in the liver. Purine analogues act to reduce purine levels in tumor cells. For example, 6-mercaptopurine inhibits purine synthesis, the first step in purine synthesis. It does so by mimicking the purine nucleoside, glutamine 5-phosphoribosylpyrophosphate aminotransferase. Azathioprine, a widely used immunosuppressant, is a prodrug of 6-mercaptopurine (see also Chapter 17).

Pyrimidine analogues are structurally similar to the naturally occurring pyrimidines (i.e., cytosine, thymine, and uracil). All pyrimidines are prodrugs that must be converted to active metabolites for drug action to take place. They inhibit the synthesis of pyrimidines and of DNA and RNA, and they are incorporated into DNA and RNA. Cytarabine is a nucleoside analogue of cytosine; it requires phosphorylation to produce the active monophosphate product and subsequently a triphosphate.

5-Fluorouracil (5-FU) is a fluorinated analogue of the naturally occurring pyrimidine uracil. In order to be active, it must be transformed to its nucleotide form. 5-FU binds tightly to, and interferes with, thymidylate synthase, one of the four essential building blocks of DNA. RNA incorporation of 5-fluoro-deoxyuracil monophosphate corresponds to the cytotoxicity in many cell lines. Another metabolite of 5-FU (triphosphate nucleotide) is incorporated into RNA as a false base, thus interfering with its function. Although 5-FU nucleotides can also be incorporated directly into DNA and affect its stability, the contribution to cell damage remains blurred. Further, the route of administration influences the mechanism of action. Inhibition of thymidylate synthesis plays a greater role in continuous-infusion regimens, with incorporation of RNA being more important in intermittent-bolus regimens.

Capecitabine is a prodrug of 5-FU. Because of its conversion it shares the same mechanism of action, selectively generating higher levels of 5-FU within some tumors. Twice-daily oral dosing of capecitabine produces sustained 5-FU levels and a risk for toxicities similar to that found with continuous IV infusions.

Gemcitabine, as a cytidine analogue, is related to cytarabine and is CCNS. It is incorporated into DNA, inhibits DNA synthesis, inhibits ribonucleotide reductase, and interferes with DNA chain elongation. It is 5 to 8 times more active against solid tumors than cytarabine. The triphosphate form of gemcitabine is retained within cells much longer than cytarabine.

Cytidine analogues, such as 5-azacitadine, are believed to exert their antineoplastic effects by causing hypomethylation of DNA and direct cytotoxicity on abnormal hematopoietic cells of the bone marrow. The concentration of the drug required for maximum inhibition of DNA methylation does not cause major suppression of DNA synthesis. Hypomethylation may restore normal function to genes that are critical to differentiation and proliferation. The cytotoxic effects of 5-azacitidine cause the death of rapidly dividing cells, including cancer cells that have lost their normal response to growth control mechanisms.

Hydroxyurea was synthesized over 100 years ago. It inhibits ribonucleotide reductase, and the result of its cellular mechanism is inhibition of S-phase cells and synchronization of cells at the G_1-S interphase of the cell cycle. The effects of hydroxyurea are reversed by deoxyribonucleotides; in the absence of the nucleotides, DNA cannot be made.

Adverse Effects and Contraindications

The primary adverse effects of MTX and other antineoplastic folate antagonists are exerted against rapidly dividing cells of the bone marrow, epithelial lining of the GI tract, and hair follicles. Mucositis, myelosuppression, and thrombocytopenia reach their maximum 5 to 10 days after administration and reverse shortly thereafter.

MTX, fludarabine, and pentostatin can cause pneumonitis and pulmonary fibrosis, which is characterized by patchy inflammatory infiltrates that rapidly regress upon discontinuation of the drug. In some patients, a rechallenge may be attempted without toxicity. Pentostatin has also been linked to anaphylaxis and myocardial infarction.

Nausea, vomiting, and stomatitis also occur with many of the drugs in the antimetabolite class. Other toxicities of MTX include spontaneous hemorrhage or life-threatening infection that may require prophylactic transfusion of platelets and broad-spectrum antibiotics if a fever is present. Adverse effects usually disappear in 2 weeks, but prolonged suppression of bone marrow may occur in patients with renal dysfunction. Reduce the dosage of MTX in proportion to any reduction in creatinine clearance. It is important to alkalinize the urine after using high-dose MTX because the precipitates in the renal tubules can cause severe and irreversible renal failure. There are dosing modification guidelines required for patients with renal impairment. Approximately 30% to 40% of patients have decreased renal function after receiving pentostatin.

In general, antimetabolites should be used with caution in patients with peptic ulcer disease, ulcerative colitis, impaired renal or hepatic function, aplasia, leukopenia, thrombocytopenia, bone marrow suppression, or anemia. 5-FU should be used with caution in patients who have undergone high-dose pelvic radiation, or therapy with alkylating drugs. Irinotecan causes much more significant diarrhea than 5-FU or MTX. The administration of live virus vaccines (i.e., measles, mumps, and rubella [MMR]) during treatment with 5-FU should be avoided since it suppresses normal defense mechanisms and may increase replication of the virus, causing adverse effects.

Drug Interactions

Drug interactions with antimetabolite drugs are identified in Table 33-4. In many cases, antimetabolite drugs increase the risks of myelosuppression when used with other antineoplastic drugs.

Lab Considerations

Antimetabolites produce myelosuppression; thus routine monitoring of CBC, ANC, and platelet counts is important before and periodically throughout therapy. Serum ALT, AST, bilirubin, alkaline phosphatase, LDH, uric acid, BUN, creatinine levels, and electrolyte values should be monitored before and periodically throughout antimetabolite drug therapy. Urinary

pH should be monitored for patients taking high-dose MTX therapy and every 6 hours during leucovorin rescue. Urine pH should be kept above 7 to prevent renal damage.

Bone marrow aspiration and biopsy may be required every 2 to 3 months for patients receiving pentostatin to assess response to therapy. Renal dosage modifications for pentostatin are based on creatinine clearance values. Patients with high tumor burdens who are receiving antineoplastic drugs may also have elevated uric acid levels.

Drugs Damaging DNA: Antimitotic Drugs

◆ docetaxel (Taxotere); ◆ Taxotere
◆ estramustine (Emcyst); ◆ Emcyst
◆ albumin-bound nab-paclitaxel (Abraxane)
◆ paclitaxel (Taxol); ◆ Taxol
◆ vinblastine (Velban, Velsar); ◆ Velbe
◆ vincristine (Oncovin, Vincasar PFS, VCR); ◆ Oncovin
◆ vindesin (Eldisine, Fildesin)
◆ vinorelbine (Navelbine); ◆ Navelbine

Indications

Vinblastine, vincristine, vinorelbine, and vindesin are vinca alkaloids derived from the periwinkle plant and are widely used today in the treatment of testicular cancer, Hodgkin's disease, breast cancer, neuroblastomas, lymphomas refractory to alkylating drugs, and a host of other cancers, including ovarian cancer (see Table 33-2).

Taxanes (i.e., docetaxel and paclitaxel) are plant alkaloids with antimitotic activity; they are derivatives from the bark and the needles of yew trees. They are used in the treatment of advanced breast cancer, non–small cell lung cancer (NSCLC), prostate cancer, ovarian cancer, small cell lung cancer (SCLC), bladder cancer, gastric cancer, head and neck cancers, melanoma, and soft tissue sarcomas.

Estramustine is an unusual drug in that it structurally combines the hormone estradiol with the alkylating drug normechlorethamine. It is used in the treatment of prostate cancer.

Pharmacodynamics

Microtubules are filaments that move chromosomes during cell division. In the absence of the microtubules, the distribution of chromosomes to daughter cells becomes random, leading to cell death.

Vinca alkaloids are CCS drugs and, in common with other drugs such as colchicine, podophyllotoxin, and taxanes, block cells in mitosis. They enter cells by nonsaturable, energy-dependent membrane transport and bind to tubulin, thereby inhibiting the formation and assembly of the microtubular components of the mitotic spindle. The inhibition leads to arrest of mitosis in the metaphase portion of the cell cycle. Although the vinca alkaloids act throughout the cell cycle, they are particularly effective in the last phase or G_2-M phase of the cell cycle. Tumor resistance to vinca alkaloids involves mutations in tubulin-binding sites.

Taxanes promote the assembly of microtubules and inhibit the disassembly of these structures by stabilizing the tubulin polymers. By inhibiting disassembly of the microtubules, the division in the tumor cells in the M and G_2 phases of the cell cycle is effectively stopped. Although both drugs have similar mechanisms of action, cross-resistance between them is incomplete.

Despite falling into the category of alkylating drugs, estramustine does not function as such. Estramustine phosphate is a combination of estradiol with nitrogen mustard. The precise mechanism of action of estramustine is unknown. It is thought that estramustine acts by covalently binding to microtubule-associated proteins that are part of the structural support for microtubules. The binding causes separation of microtubule-associated proteins from the microtubules, which in turn inhibits microtubule assembly and eventually causes the organism to disassemble.

▥ Adverse Effects and Contraindications

In terms of adverse effects of vinca alkaloids, vinblastine and vinorelbine are more likely to cause bone marrow suppression, and vincristine is more likely to cause peripheral neuropathy. Neutropenia develops in about half of patients treated with vinca alkaloids. Other adverse effects of vinca alkaloids include alopecia, constipation, nausea, and vomiting. Like vinblastine and vincristine, vinorelbine can cause local tissue necrosis if extravasation occurs.

Myelosuppression and peripheral neuropathy is the major dose-limiting toxicities for the taxanes. Peripheral neuropathy may be more problematic if these drugs are administered in combination with other neurotoxic agents, such as cisplatin.

Allergic reactions may occur with any naturally derived substance but are most frequently seen with the taxanes, paclitaxel and docetaxel. There is a black box warning for paclitaxel indicating that patients are to be pretreated with corticosteroids, diphenhydramine, and H_2 antagonists to reduce the risk for hypersensitivity responses. The reason for pretreatment is cremaphor, a solvent contained in paclitaxel. Paclitaxel needs a solvent because it is too water-insoluble. Nab-paclitaxel, a newer formulation of the drug, lacks the solvent and therefore the need for pretreatment.

Similarly, with docetaxel, all patients should be pretreated with oral corticosteroids such as dexamethasone for 3 days starting 1 day before docetaxel administration in order to reduce the incidence and severity of fluid retention as well as the severity of hypersensitivity reactions. For hormone-refractory metastatic prostate cancer, given the concurrent use of prednisone, the recommended premedication regimen is oral dexamethasone at 12 hours, 3 hours, and 1 hour before the docetaxel infusion.

▥ Drug Interactions

Drugs that interact with the mitotic inhibitors are identified in Table 33-4. Mitotic inhibitors interact with other antineoplastic drugs or radiation therapy to increase myelosuppression. Live virus vaccines (e.g., MMR) given to patients taking a mitotic inhibitor may not produce the desired response, and the risk of adverse effects of the vaccine is increased.

Drugs Damaging DNA: Topoisomerase Inhibitors

* etoposide (VP-16, VePesid); ◆ Vepesid
* irinotecan (Camptosar); ◆ Camptosar
* teniposide (VM-26, Vumon); ◆ Vumon
* topotecan (Hycamtin)

▥ Indications

Topoisomerase inhibitors are derived from the mandrake plant. This was used as a folk remedy by the American Indians

and early colonists for its emetic, cathartic, and anthelmintic properties. The two synthetic glycosides (e.g., etoposide and teniposide) of the active principle, podophyllotoxin, show significant therapeutic effects in several neoplasms including pediatric leukemia, SCLC, testicular tumors, Hodgkin's disease, and large cell lymphomas.

Irinotecan and topotecan are currently the most widely used camptothecin analogues in the clinical setting, with established activity in colorectal, ovarian, and SCLC.

▥ Pharmacodynamics

Two classes of topoisomerase inhibitors (I and II) are known to mediate DNA strand breakage and resealing, and both have become the target of antineoplastic therapies. Structurally, etoposide and teniposide are semisynthetic topoisomerase inhibitors with similar actions and spectrum of tumors affected. They do not arrest cells in mitosis but rather act by inhibiting topoisomerase II, a DNA enzyme responsible for initiating the separation of daughter DNA strands before mitosis. This activity results in permanent cross-linking of DNA strands and eventual cell death. The enzyme remains bound to the free end of the strand breaks and cell death ensues.

In contrast, irinotecan and topotecan are topoisomerase I inhibitors that create reversible single-strand breaks in DNA. The drugs bind to the DNA-topoisomerase I complex, thereby preventing repair of strand breaks caused by topoisomerase. Cytotoxicity is believed to result from impaired DNA replication. Thus the drug effects are manifest during the S phase of the cell cycle. However, clinical trials failed to show antitumor activity, and the drugs produced severe and unpredictable toxicities.

▥ Adverse Effects and Contraindications

The dose-limiting toxicity of the topoisomerase inhibitor ▲ **II topotecan is neutropenia, with or without thrombocytopenia.** The incidence of severe neutropenia at the recommended dosages may be as high as 81%, with a 26% incidence of febrile neutropenia.

In patients with hematologic cancers, GI adverse effects such as mucositis and diarrhea become dose-limiting. Other adverse effects of topotecan are generally mild but include nausea and vomiting, elevated liver function tests, fever, fatigue, and rash. In addition, topotecan can cause alopecia, stomatitis, abdominal pain, and headache.

Irinotecan, a topoisomerase II inhibitor drug, has a dose-limiting toxicity of early and delayed diarrhea (up to 35% of patients treated), with or without neutropenia. Early diarrhea occurs in half of the patients treated with irinotecan, manifesting within 24 hours of the onset of the infusion. Late diarrhea occurs in about 88% of the patients, developing 24 hours or more after the infusion. Late diarrhea can be prolonged, causing severe dehydration and electrolyte imbalance. Loperamide, an antidiarrheal drug, started at the appearance of loose stools, has reduced the incidence of severe diarrhea by more than 50% (see Chapter 46). However, once the severe diarrhea is established, standard dosages of antidiarrheal drugs tend to be ineffective. The diarrhea episode generally resolves within a week unless accompanied by fever and neutropenia, and is rarely fatal.

Irinotecan can also cause asthenia, alopecia, abdominal discomfort, anorexia, fever, and weight loss. Less common adverse effects include stomatitis, dyspepsia, headache, cough, rhinitis, insomnia, and rash. Serious thrombocytopenia is uncommon in patients treated with irinotecan, although neutropenia occurs 54% of the time and anemia 61% of the time. Sepsis secondary to neutropenia has resulted in death.

The adverse effects of irinotecan and topotecan include myelosuppression, especially a dose-limiting neutropenia, thrombocytopenia, and anemia. Myelosuppression and toxicity are not cumulative.

⚠ **The dose-limiting adverse effect of etoposide is leukopenia, with a nadir of 10 to 14 days and recovery in 3 weeks.** Thrombocytopenia occurs less often and is usually mild. Nausea, vomiting, stomatitis, and diarrhea are reported in about 15% of patients treated with IV etoposide and in 55% of patients treated with the oral formulation. Alopecia is common but reversible.

Other reported adverse effects of etoposide include fever, phlebitis, dermatitis, and allergic reactions (including anaphylaxis). Liver toxicity is particularly apparent after high-dose therapy with etoposide. The risk of toxicity is increased in patients with reduced serum albumin levels, an effect related to decreased protein binding of the drug. Acute problems, such as arrhythmia and pericarditis, do not appear to be dose related. Chronic myocardial damage, however, is correlated to cumulative dose.

Nausea, vomiting, diarrhea, alopecia, and myelosuppression are the primary toxic effects of teniposide. However, severe hypersensitivity reactions (urticaria, angioedema, bronchospasm, and hypotension) have occurred in patients receiving teniposide. Secondary leukemias have developed within 8 years of initial drug exposure.

Drugs Damaging DNA: Antitumor Antibiotics

- bleomycin (Blenoxane); ♣ Blenoxane
- dactinomycin (Cosmegen); ♣ Cosmegen
- daunorubicin (Cerubidine); ♣ Cerubidine
- doxorubicin (Adriamycin, Rubex, Myocet); ♣ Adriamycin PFS, Adriamycin RDF
- epirubicin (Ellence); ♣ Pharmorubicin, Pharmorubicin RDS
- idarubicin (Idamycin); ♣ Idamycin
- mitoxantrone (Novantrone); ♣ Novantrone
- mitomycin C (Mutamycin); ♣ Mutamycin
- plicamycin (Mithracin)

▥ *Indications*

Antitumor antibiotics are derivatives of soil fungus and have some antiinfective activity; however, they are too toxic for this use. The four categories of antitumor antibiotics include the anthracyclines, anthracenediones, chromomycins, and miscellaneous drugs. The anthracycline antibiotics and their derivatives are among the most important antitumor drugs. Today, the most widely used and best understood antitumor antibiotic is doxorubicin. Although they differ slightly in chemical structure, daunorubicin and idarubicin have been used in the treatment of acute leukemias, whereas doxorubicin displays broader activity against neoplasms, including a variety of solid tumors. Other members of this antitumor antibiotic group include epirubicin and mitoxantrone.

▥ *Pharmacodynamics*

The antitumor antibiotics produce antineoplastic effects by forming complexes with DNA, thereby inhibiting DNA activity, a process known as intercalation (i.e., the insertion or introduction of a thing among others).

Bleomycin is phase-specific to the G_2-S phases of the cell cycle. All active bleomycin compounds bind reduced iron (Fe^{2+}) so their molecular action is not directed at tissues. It produces breaks in single- and double-stranded DNA. These breaks are reflected as DNA chromosomal gaps, deletions, and fragments. These result from a secondary action in which free radical formation from Fe^{2+}-bleomycin-oxygen forms an intercalated complex between DNA strands. The complex catalyzes the reduction of molecular oxygen to superoxide or hydroxyl radicals. This reduction causes breaks in the DNA strands and inhibition of DNA synthesis. There appears to be inhibition of RNA and protein synthesis as well.

The anthracyclines are CCNS drugs. Daunorubicin and doxorubicin are produced by the fungus *Streptomyces peucetius*, differing only slightly in their chemical structure. These drugs interact with DNA, affecting DNA and RNA synthesis. Single- and double-strand breaks occur, as does sister chromatid exchange. The dividing of DNA is thought to be mediated either by the action of topoisomerase II, or by the generation of free radicals. As would be expected of drugs that inhibit DNA function, maximal toxicity occurs during the S phase of the cell cycle. At low concentrations of drug, tumor cells will proceed through the S phase and die in phase G_2.

Free radical formation via electron reduction is a second cytotoxic mechanism. All anthracyclines are quinones capable of producing free radicals, which in turn damage membranes, proteins, and lipids. Enzymatic defenses (e.g., superoxide dismutase, catalase) are believed to play an important role in protecting cells against the toxicity of daunorubicin and doxorubicin. Glutathione and catalase detoxify the free radical quinones; the lack of catalase in cardiac tissue is the basis for anthracycline cardiotoxicity. Further, it appears that enzymatic defenses can be enhanced with the exogenous intake of antioxidants (e.g., alpha tocopherol).

Although dactinomycin is a CCNS drug, its activity seems to be greatest in phase G_1 of the cell cycle. It intercalates between adjacent base pairs in DNA and becomes bound to DNA. The intercalation process distorts DNA structure, which in turn prohibits RNA polymerase from using DNA as a template. The result is inhibition of RNA synthesis.

Mitoxantrone interacts with topoisomerase II and DNA, resulting in breaks in DNA strands. It does not produce free radicals like some of the other drugs.

Mitomycin activity is dependent on bioreductive alkylation under anaerobic reducing conditions. It has to be reduced at quinone sites to form unstable intermediates that react monofunctionally at a position on guanine. It is therefore a prodrug. Free radical formation under aerobic conditions may lead to single-strand breaks in DNA, or these may result from unsuccessful alkylation repair.

▥ *Adverse Effects and Contraindications*

The adverse effects of bleomycin are confined to the lungs and skin. Pulmonary toxicity is the major problem and is manifested as subacute or chronic interstitial pneumonitis and, later, pulmonary fibrosis. Risk factors for pulmonary fibrosis include decreased renal function and cumulative dosing. The most common adverse effect of bleomycin is fever; the recommendation is to pretreat the patient with acetaminophen before treatment.

The clinical value of anthracyclines is limited by an unusual, and often irreversible, dose-related cardiomyopathy. Mitoxantrone, an anthracenedione, has significantly less cardiotoxicity than the anthracyclines.

▲ Although conventional doxorubicin has shown excellent antitumor activity, its use in the clinical setting is limited by acute and chronic toxicities, specifically cardiotoxicity, myelosuppression, nausea, and vomiting; and although often underestimated, alopecia is obviously a very important issue for patients. Irreversible cardiac damage is the most critical toxicity induced by conventional doxorubicin use. Damage to the heart can significantly limit the cumulative lifetime dose. In a patient with no cardiac risk factors, the cumulative lifetime dose receiving a weekly regimen of doxorubicin is 750 mg/m^2. For the patient with known cardiac risk factors, the cumulative lifetime dose when receiving weekly regimens of doxorubicin is 550 mg/m^2.

Cardiac toxicity is cumulative across members of the anthracycline (doxorubicin, epirubicin, daunorubicin, idarubicin) and anthracenedione (mitoxantrone) classes of drugs. Carefully monitor patients who have taken these drugs, since they have a heightened risk of cardiac toxicity. In patients who have undergone radiation to the mediastinal area combined with other cardiotoxic drug therapy (i.e., cyclophosphamide), smaller cumulative dosages suffice to produce cardiotoxicity. Increased toxicity has also been noted when conventional doxorubicin is used concurrently with other biologic therapy. Young patients with comorbid heart disease, and those with hypertension or mediastinal radiation therapy, are at high risk for cardiotoxicity, which can lead to irreversible heart failure.

However, there are methods to reduce the heart damage associated with use of anthracyclines. Cardiac toxicity may be prevented by reducing the cumulative anthracycline dose; by using a 48- or 96-hour continuous infusion schedule; by using a cardioprotectant (e.g., dexrazoxane); or by choosing an anthracycline formulation with a lower potential for cardiac toxicity, such as a liposomal anthracycline. Further, liposomal anthracyclines have shown similar effects to conventionally formulated doxorubicin, while also having favorable toxicity profiles, including less cardiac toxicity. There have been phases 2 and 3 clinical trials that support the use of liposomal doxorubicin (Myocet) alone or in combination with other biologic agents (Yamaguchi et al., 2007).

The use of doxorubicin before, during, and after radiation therapy can result in increased radiation injury to tissues. So-called "radiation recall reactions" advance radiation injury most commonly to the skin, but internal organs can also be affected. Doxorubicin use typically produces skin reactions (i.e., erythema followed by dry desquamation) only if drug administration is within 7 days of radiation. Although atypical, reactions occurring after 30 days have been observed. Skin reactions can cause discomfort, but the enhanced radiation injury to internal organs can be serious. Concurrent drug and radiation therapy results in the most severe enhancement of radiation injury to the esophagus and the GI tract. Injury to a previously irradiated site may be repeated weeks to months after radiation.

Other adverse effects of doxorubicin and daunorubicin include myelosuppression, mucositis, and stomatitis. Stomatitis is especially likely with a continuous infusion of doxorubicin rather than with bolus dosing. The adverse effects of dactinomycin include nausea, vomiting, stomatitis, dose-limiting myelosuppression, and dermatologic manifestations.

Mitoxantrone lacks the ability to produce free radicals and therefore has far less inherent cardiotoxicity than doxorubicin. Other adverse effects include extravasation injuries, alopecia, nausea, and a dose-limiting myelosuppression. Overall, the adverse effects profile is much more favorable than that for anthracyclines, especially as it relates to cardiotoxicity.

Anaphylaxis can occur with any of the antitumor antibiotics, particularly if the drug is a derivative of a naturally occurring substance. Most of the antitumor antibiotics are also vesicants. Vesicants are drugs with the potential to cause severe tissue damage if they extravasate from the vein. For this reason it is recommended that they be administered through a central-line IV.

▥ Drug Interactions

As with the other antineoplastic drugs, interactions with antitumor antibiotics can be significant if the drugs are used concurrently with other antineoplastic drugs or in patients who are receiving radiation therapy (see Table 33-4). Receipt of live virus vaccines (e.g., MMR) may increase the risk of adverse effects owing to inadequate antibody response.

Miscellaneous Antineoplastic Drugs

Not all antineoplastic drugs can be neatly categorized into a major classification group, either because the exact mechanism of action is unknown or the chemical structure poorly understood.

L-Asparaginase

L-Asparaginase ([Elspar]; ◆ Kidrolase) is an enzyme derived from culture of either *Escherichia coli* or *Erwinia carotovora* (a plant parasite). Most normal tissues synthesize what asparagine they need for protein synthesis. However, the lymphoblasts in patients with acute lymphocytic leukemia appear to lack the enzyme asparagine synthetase. L-Asparaginase, by catalyzing the hydrolysis of circulating asparagine to aspartic acid and ammonia, deprives the lymphoblasts of the asparagine necessary for tumor protein synthesis in patients with acute lymphocytic leukemia. The drug is probably CCS for the G$_1$ phase of the cell cycle, but its usefulness is limited by acute hypersensitivity reactions, which are more likely to occur with repeated treatments. L-Asparaginase is used along with vincristine and prednisone to induce remission of acute lymphocytic leukemia.

Because normal tissues as well as leukemic cells are sensitive to L-asparaginase, a variety of adverse effects may occur. L-Asparaginase does not cause alopecia or stomatitis and is rarely associated with bone marrow suppression. However, 40% of patients experience hypersensitivity reactions ranging from urticaria to anaphylactic shock. Have emergency life support equipment readily available before this drug is administered. The incidence of anaphylaxis is greater with IV administration than with intramuscular (IM) routes. Neurotoxic reactions are caused by inhibition of protein synthesis in the brain. Reverse encephalopathy, with manifestations ranging from confusion to coma, occurs in 25% of patients.

Thrombosis and hemorrhage have been reported with L-asparaginase because of the drug's effects on clotting factors. Pancreatitis may occur and progress to severe, even fatal, hemorrhagic pancreatitis. Liver function tests are elevated but return to normal when the drug is discontinued. Acute renal insufficiency can be fatal.

L-Asparaginase may negate the antineoplastic activity of MTX and enhance the hepatotoxicity of other hepatotoxic drugs (see Table 33-4). Additive hypoglycemia has been reported when L-asparaginase is used with glucocorticoids. The concurrent IV use of L-asparaginase with or immediately preceding vincristine may result in increased neurotoxicity and hyperglycemia. As with other antineoplastic drugs, L-asparaginase may alter the patient's response to live vaccines by decreasing antibody response and increasing the risk of adverse reactions.

Mitotane

Mitotane (Lysodren; ✦ Lysodren) is a structural analogue of two insecticides, dichlorodiphenyldichloroethane (DDD) and dichlorodiphenyltrichloroethane (DDT). It is used in the palliation of inoperative carcinoma of the adrenal cortex. The drug is selectively toxic to tumor cells, but normal cells are also damaged. This isomer of the pesticide DDT acts to inhibit corticosteroid biosynthesis.

Adverse reactions and toxicities of this drug include anorexia, nausea, vomiting, diarrhea, skin rash, and gynecomastia in males. Patients receiving this drug should be well hydrated to prevent nephrotoxicity and should undergo periodic monitoring of renal function and CBCs.

Other adverse effects of mitotane include depression, sedation, lethargy, vertigo, and dizziness. Anorexia, nausea, vomiting, diarrhea, and rash also occur. Adrenal insufficiency develops because of the action of mitotane on the adrenal cortex with corticosteroid replacement therapy needed. Mitotane does not cause inflammation of the GI tract or bone marrow depression.

Pegaspargase

Pegaspargase (Oncaspar, Peg-L-asparaginase) is used along with other drugs in the treatment of acute lymphoblastic leukemia in patients who have had a previous hypersensitivity reaction to L-asparaginase. Pegaspargase consists of L-asparaginase bound to polyethylene glycol (PEG). The two drugs are essentially very similar. They have the same mechanism of drug action and produce the same spectrum of adverse effects, including liver and kidney dysfunction, pancreatitis, coagulopathy, and hypersensitivity reactions.

Normal cells are able to produce their own asparagine and thus are unlikely to be affected by asparaginase. The polyethylene glycol-pegaspargase compound depletes asparagine, which leukemic cells cannot synthesize. Binding to polyethylene glycol renders asparaginase less antigenic, and therefore the drug is less likely to induce hypersensitivity reactions.

As with other antineoplastic drugs, hematologic adverse effects are possible, including leukopenia, pancytopenia, and thrombocytopenia, decreased fibrinogen levels, and increased thromboplastin levels. Paresthesia, myalgia, arthralgia, and extremity pain are also common. Seizures and pancreatitis are the most life-threatening adverse effects. Pegaspargase used concurrently with anticoagulants or antiplatelet drugs increases the risk of bleeding, and the response to other drugs that are biotransformed by the liver may be altered.

Hormones and Hormone Antagonists

Hormones used in antineoplastic therapy include androgens, antiandrogens, estrogens, antiestrogens, adrenocorticosteroids, adrenocorticosteroid inhibitors, gonadotropin-releasing hormone analogues, progestins, and luteinizing hormone–releasing (LHRH) analogues (Box 33-3). Hormones and hormone antagonists exert beneficial effects by altering the hormonal environment that promotes cancer growth. The primary indications for these drugs are cancers of the breast, the endometrium, and the prostate. In addition, the corticosteroids are used against lymphomas and certain leukemias.

BOX 33-3

Drugs with Emetogenic Potential

Almost Certainly Emetogenic (90%)
Alkylating Drugs
- cisplatin
- cyclophosphamide
- dacarbazine
- mechlorethamine

Antimetabolites
- cytarabine

High Emetogenic Potential (60%-90%)
Alkylating Drugs
- carboplatin
- carmustine
- lomustine

Antitumor Antibiotics
- dactinomycin
- daunorubicin
- doxorubicin

Moderate Emetogenic Potential (30%-60%)
Alkylating Drugs
- altretamine
- ifosfamide

Antimetabolites
- pentostatin

Antitumor Antibiotics
- idarubicin
- mitomycin
- plicamycin

Mitotic Inhibitors
- etoposide
- mitoxantrone
- topotecan

Miscellaneous Antineoplastics
- L-asparaginase
- procarbazine

Low Emetogenic Potential (0%-30%)
Alkylating Drugs
- busulfan
- chlorambucil
- melphalan
- thiotepa

Antimetabolites
- cytarabine
- fludarabine
- fluorouracil
- floxuridine
- methotrexate
- mercaptopurine
- thioguanine

Antitumor Antibiotics
- bleomycin

Mitotic Inhibitors
- paclitaxel
- vinblastine
- vincristine
- vindesine
- vinorelbine

Miscellaneous Antineoplastics
- hydroxyurea

The sex hormones such as estrogens (e.g., diethylstilbestrol, ethinyl estradiol), progestins (e.g., medroxyprogesterone, megestrol), and androgens (e.g., fluoxymesterone, testosterone) are useful in cancers of the breast and the prostate gland.

Estrogens

Estrogens and other hormones are second-line drugs for treating prostate cancer. Their benefits stem from suppressing androgen production, which prostate cells need to survive. Estrogens change the hormonal environment of the tumor and suppress androgen production, acting in the pituitary to suppress the release of interstitial cell–stimulating hormone. In the absence of this hormone, production of androgens by the testes declines.

Progestins

Progestins, such as megestrol acetate, are used in the treatment of metastatic endometrial carcinoma. Megestrol acetate is also often used in patients with cancer to increase their appetite. The progestins promote palliation and tumor regression; their exact mechanism in suppressing tumor growth is unknown. The basic pharmacology of estrogens and progestins is discussed in Chapter 58.

Antiestrogenic Drugs

Antiestrogenic drugs (e.g., bicalutamide, flutamide, tamoxifen) compete with estrogen for binding sites in breast tissues. Tamoxifen is a competitive inhibitor of estradiol, binding to the estrogen receptor. When bound to the receptor, tamoxifen induces a change in the three-dimensional shape of the receptor, inhibiting its binding to the estrogen-responsive element on DNA. Under normal conditions, estrogen stimulation increases tumor cell production by transforming growth factor β, an autocrine inhibitor of tumor cell growth. By blocking these pathways, the net effect of tamoxifen is to decrease the autocrine stimulation of breast cancer growth. It appears that estrogen receptor–positive tumors treated with tamoxifen are arrested in the G_0 and G_1 phases of the cell cycle, immediately after mitosis.

Tamoxifen is also thought to inhibit the production of several growth factors that stimulate tumor cell growth, including growth factor A, epidermal growth factor, and insulin-like growth factor. Insulin-like growth factor is a paracrine growth factor for the breast cancer cell. Tamoxifen also enhances the production of transforming growth factor B, an inhibitor of breast tumor cell growth. In addition, estrogen agonist effects are thought to offer some protection against osteoporosis in postmenopausal women.

The most frequent adverse effects of tamoxifen include hot flashes, nausea, and vomiting. The severity of these adverse effects is such that it is rare to require discontinuation of therapy. Menstrual irregularities, vaginal bleeding and discharge, pruritus vulvae, and dermatitis are frequent occurrences, depending on the menopausal status of the patient.

In addition, there is growing concern about the potential for tamoxifen to cause endometrial cancer; the incidence is at least twofold in women who received the drug for 2 years or longer compared to untreated patients. Regular pelvic examines and PAP smears are to be done and any symptoms of pelvic discomfort or vaginal bleeding investigated.

Tamoxifen increases the risk of thromboembolic events. The drug also causes retinal deposits, decreased visual acuity, and cataracts in susceptible patients, although the frequency of these changes is unclear. Tamoxifen also lowers total serum cholesterol and low-density lipoproteins while raising apolipoprotein A_1 levels, potentially decreasing the risk for myocardial infarction.

Aromatase Inhibitors

Aromatase inhibitors include exemestane, letrozole, and anastrazole, which prevent the peripheral conversion of estrogen in adipose tissue in postmenopausal women. These drugs have been used in the treatment of advanced breast cancer in postmenopausal women whose disease has progressed despite tamoxifen therapy. Aromatase inhibitors act just as the name implies: they inhibit the enzyme aromatase, which is partially responsible for conversion of precursors to estrogen. By lowering levels of circulating estrogen, the progression of estrogen-sensitive breast cancer may be halted.

Letrozole is another selective, nonsteroidal aromatase inhibitor that inhibits the conversion of estrogen. One of the problems with aromatase inhibitors is the risk of osteopenia and osteoporosis.

▥ Exemestane

Additional drugs function as antiestrogens. Exemestane is an irreversible steroidal aromatase "inactivator" that prevents the conversion of androgens to estrogen. Fulvestrant is a pure antiestrogen approved for use in postmenopausal women after tamoxifen has failed to control their breast cancer. It is a receptor antagonist that down-regulates estrogen receptor protein binding in breast cancer cells.

Antiandrogenic Drugs

Antiandrogenic drugs such as flutamide act either to inhibit the uptake of androgens or to inhibit the nuclear binding of androgen in target tissues. Bicalutamide competitively inhibits the action of androgens by binding to androgen receptors in target tissue. Accordingly, the effects of androgen on androgen-sensitive tissues are reduced.

Gonadotropin-Releasing Hormone

Gonadotropin-releasing hormone (GnRH) analogues such as goserelin and leuprolide are alternative therapies (e.g., to orchiectomy, estrogen) for men with advanced prostate cancer. They are synthetic analogues of LHRH. They increase the production of luteinizing hormone (LH) and follicle-stimulating hormone (FSH) in the pituitary gland, resulting in transient increases in testosterone and dihydrotestosterone in males. With prolonged administration, LH and FSH receptors are down-regulated in the pituitary gland. Eventually, gonadotropin secretion is reduced, which in time decreases testosterone to castration levels. The drug's effects persist for up to 3 years. Goserelin and leuprolide are as effective as an orchiectomy (surgical removal of the testicles) in lowering testosterone levels (see also Chapter 57).

IMMUNE

The gonadotropin-releasing hormone antagonist abarelix (Plenaxis) directly competes with GnRH receptors in the pituitary gland. This action leads to suppression of LH and FSH production, and reduces testosterone secretion from the testes. A major challenge with this drug is the potential for an immediate, life-threatening hypersensitivity reaction.

Adrenocorticosteroids

Adrenocorticosteroids interfere with the mitosis of lymphocytes and lymphoid proliferation, resulting in cell death. This may result in glucose deprivation. Adrenocorticosteroids are CCS drugs active in phase G_1 of the cell cycle. They are used to induce remission in children with acute lymphocytic leukemia and to relieve the complications of cancer and cancer treatment, such as nausea, vomiting, hypercalcemia, hemorrhagic thrombocytopenia, and intracranial metastasis; and they are components of various antineoplastic regimens. They are used for palliation and symptom relief because they reduce pain and fever and increase appetite, strength, and sense of well-being. They are used at times in radiation therapy to reduce edema in the mediastinum, the brain, and the spinal cord.

Adrenocorticosteroid Inhibitors

The *adrencocorticosteroid-inhibitor* drug aminoglutethimide is useful in patients with advanced prostatic cancer and produces a state that mimics an adrenalectomy. Chapter 57 discusses this adrenocorticosteroid inhibitor drug in more depth.

Other Types of Cancer Drug Therapies

Other drugs and biologic treatments are used to treat cancer but are not antineoplastics. These other drugs target different characteristics that separate cancer cells from normal cells. They often have less serious adverse effects than those commonly caused by standard antineoplastic drugs; some are even used in combination with antineoplastics.

Angiogenesis Inhibitors

Angiogenesis inhibitors (e.g., angiostatin, endostatin) are also used to treat cancers. When cancer cells are still very small (1 to 2 mm diameter) they do not need blood vessels to survive. However, in order to grow to any size at all, they need a sufficient blood supply to provide the needed nutrients. To do so, tumor cells convince nearby capillaries to extend outward, thus carrying the required nutrients to the tumor cells.

Angiogenesis inhibitors are thought to block the construction of the new capillaries, thereby preventing the tumor cells from receiving nutrients. As a result, the tumor may stop growing, shrink, or in some cases regress to a microscopic dormant lesion (Fig. 33-2). Angiogenesis inhibitors have the potential to treat cancer as well as a variety of other angiogenic diseases such as blindness and arthritis that depend on new blood-vessel growth.

Angiostatin, a potent naturally occurring inhibitor of angiogenesis and tumor metastasis, is generated by proteolysis of plasminogen. To date, it is known that in a defined cell-free system, plasminogen activators (e.g., tissue plasminogen

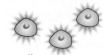

• Isolated cancer cells

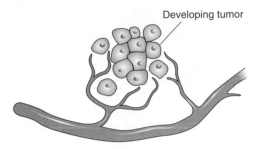

• Capillary network forms

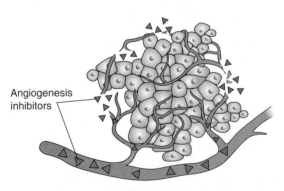

• Angiogenesis feeds tumor's growth

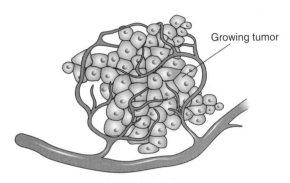

Angiogenesis inhibitors

• Angiogenesis inhibitors destroy capillary network

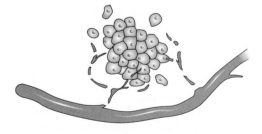

• Without the blood supply, the tumor shrinks

FIGURE 33-2 Angiogenesis-Inhibiting Drugs. Currently under investigation, angiogenesis-inhibiting drugs such as angiostatin and endostatin act by preventing the formation of the capillary network that nourishes the malignant tumor and provides access to the circulatory system.

activator [tPA], streptokinase) in combination with *N*-acetyl-L-cysteine, D-penicillamine, captopril, L-cysteine, or reduced glutathione, generate angiostatin from plasminogen. It is also known that prostate carcinoma cells possess enzymes that convert plasminogen to angiostatin.

Endostatin is a natural antiangiogenic protein shown to inhibit the growth of blood vessels, thereby starving cancerous tumors. Endostatin is produced by hemangioendothelioma. Hemangioendothelioma is used to describe a group of vascular neoplasms that can be considered benign or malignant. They have been described as masses that fall between a hemangioma and angiosarcoma. Endostatin specifically inhibits endothelial proliferation and potently inhibits angiogenesis and tumor growth. Using a sustained release method, *E. coli*–derived endostatin is thought to cause regression of primary tumors.

In addition to angiostatin and endostatin, a number of other drugs are being investigated for their effects on blood vessels. Marimastat, a matrix metalloproteinase enzyme synthesized in the laboratory, may stop the growth of lung cancer by stopping blood flow to the tumor. It is not yet known if marimastat is an effective treatment for SCLC. Marimastat is currently in phase 3 clinical trials.

Cartilage is an avascular tissue that is thought to inhibit angiogenesis. Neovastat, an extract of spiny-dogfish shark cartilage, remains in phase 1 clinical trials. The cartilage is also thought to inhibit tumor progression by acting directly on the transformed cells to lower their proliferation rate. None of the factors responsible for these biologic activities has yet been purified to homogeneity.

Combretastatin, from the African bush willow, has shown promise in drastically reducing the hypervascular nature of solid tumors. This ability sets it apart from angiogenesis inhibitors that act by inhibiting the growth of new blood vessels. The drug affects the microtubules that form the cytoskeleton of the endothelial cells lining the tumor vasculature. When microtubule function is disrupted, the shape of endothelial cells changes from flat to round, causing flow through the capillary to stop, which in turn starves the tumor of nutrients; death ensues.

Combretastatin acts primarily on tumors with newly formed blood vessels. The protein actin, present in endothelial cells, protects tubulin, which is responsible for maintaining cell shape as the cell matures. Tubulin appears days after the creation of the new endothelial cells.

Targeted Therapies

As researchers learn about the workings of cancer cells, they are developing biologic response modifying (BRM) drugs that attack cancer cells more specifically than standard antineoplastic drugs (see Chapter 32). Most BRMs attack cells containing certain gene mutations, or cells expressing too many copies of these genes. Only a handful of these drugs are available at this time. Examples include imatinib (Gleevec), gefitinib (Iressa), erlotinib (Tarceva), rituximab (Rituxan), and bevacizumab (Avastin). There will likely be many more in the future.

CLINICAL REASONING

Treatment Objectives

Choices of antineoplastic therapies are guided by the most realistic and achievable treatment objectives. The three major goals of antineoplastic therapy are cure, control, and palliation. An increasing number of cancers are curable, particularly if they are identified and treated before metastasis has occurred.

Cure is defined as eradication of all clinically detectable cancer, giving the patient the same life expectancy as a person who does not have cancer. Highly proliferative tumors (e.g., pediatric acute lymphocytic leukemia, Hodgkin's disease, neuroblastoma, testicular carcinoma, choriocarcinoma) are often curable. However, cure must not be achieved at the cost of a poor quality of life or disabling treatment-related symptoms. The common reference points used in predicting the likelihood of cure and to judge the results of therapy are 5- and 10-year survival rates without evidence of disease. Advanced solid tumors are not generally curable using antineoplastic therapies.

Control of the disease is the next goal of antineoplastic therapy. When the disease is found to be incurable, prolonging life is the purpose for treating the cancer. Given the variety of drugs and treatment options available, it is often possible to control metastatic disease for many months or years while providing an optimal quality of life for the patient.

Palliation is defined as providing relief of distressing symptoms (e.g., pain, shortness of breath) and maintaining function as near normal as possible when it is no longer possible to achieve a remission. When cure or control is no longer possible, relief of symptoms may still be achieved by antineoplastic therapy, particularly if doses are adjusted to minimize toxicities.

Treatment Options

▌▌ *Patient Variables*

Factors influencing the treatment outcome include the status of the patient's immune system, presence of comorbid medical illnesses, nutritional status, psychologic state, availability of supportive care, social support, and of course, personal preference. Patients who are relatively asymptomatic and able to carry out normal activities of daily living are more likely to have positive outcomes from therapy compared to the patient who is bedridden, cachectic, and dependent on others for care.

LIFE-SPAN CONSIDERATIONS. Patients faced with a potentially fatal illness exhibit a wide array of coping behaviors. It is the responsibility of the health care provider to determine which patients exhibit ineffective or harmful coping mechanisms requiring psychologic intervention and counseling and to determine the social support available to the patient. Social support, as well as coping skills, have been well documented as important factors in the successful completion of treatment regimens.

A diagnosis of cancer may have devastating economic effects on the patient and the family members. Inability to work may lead to loss of insurance coverage, which then jeopardizes the patient's access to life-saving medical care. Basic insurance coverage may be insufficient to cover the cost of cancer therapy, placing the patient's home, savings, and financial earnings at risk. Most patients with a diagnosis of cancer benefit from a referral to social services for assistance with their financial affairs.

Pregnant and Nursing Women. Malignant diseases occurring in pregnancy include, in order of decreasing frequency, breast cancer, hematopoietic malignancy, melanoma, gynecologic

IMMUNE

cancer, and bone tumors. The glandular hyperplasia of the breast that accompanies pregnancy makes recognition of suspicious breast masses difficult. However, when matched for age and stage of cancer, survival rates for breast cancer found during pregnancy are no different from the nonpregnant state. Survival is generally not improved by terminating the pregnancy. However, it may be appropriate to avoid the risk of fetal exposure to either antineoplastic drugs or radiation therapy. Treatment recommendations for pregnant women with cancer vary depending on the type and location of the cancer, stage of the disease, gestational age of the fetus, and maternal health in general.

Administration of antineoplastic drugs during the first trimester of pregnancy increases the risk of spontaneous abortion and fetal malformations. Second and third trimester exposure to antineoplastic drugs may result in low birth weight or prematurity. Contraceptives should be used for birth control during therapy and for up to 2 years following completion of antineoplastic therapy.

Children and Adolescents. Having a child diagnosed with cancer may be an extraordinary stressor for the family. The health care provider must be prepared to give the extra time needed to provide patient and family teaching and emotional support. Give the parents and child detailed information on the implications of the diagnosis, adverse effects and toxicities associated with antineoplastic therapy, and desired therapeutic effects. It is particularly important that parents understand the potential for late effects of antineoplastic drugs, including sterility, hypogonadism, growth retardation, cognitive impairment, and secondary cancers such as leukemia. These late effects may be worsened by brain surgery or radiation therapy. Psychologic evaluation should be considered for all children following cancer treatment if development is slowed or disturbed. It is also important to note that toxicity and pharmacokinetic patterns may be significantly different between children and adolescents and adult patients. Individualize therapy based on parameters specific for these patients, rather than considering children or adolescents as small adults.

Older Adults. Older adults may have impaired communication ability, sensory deficits, and decreased cognitive function. There is an increased incidence of organ damage due to changes associated with age and chronic disease. Physiologic changes associated with aging and pathophysiologic alterations associated with various chronic diseases may influence the safety and efficacy of antineoplastic therapies.

▥ Drug Variables

When planning antineoplastic treatment regimens, the variables to be considered include the type of tumor and cell types involved, and the degree of cellular differentiation, the growth rate, and the heterogeneity of the tumor (Box 33-4). *Neoadjuvant therapy* (primary antineoplastic therapy, induction therapy) is used before other local therapies (e.g., surgery, radiation therapy) in an attempt to reduce tumor size and bulk and increase surgical resectability of the tumor. **Many solid tumors have micrometastatic disease, becoming systemic diseases incurable by surgery alone.** This fact justifies the use of antineoplastic therapy in combination with surgery or radiation therapy. Administration of adjuvant antineoplastic therapy is therefore based on the biologic behavior of the

---

> **BOX 33-4**
>
> ### Take Away Points About Antineoplastic Therapy
>
> **Cell-cycle–Specific Drugs (CCS)**
> - Most effective against rapidly growing cancer cells
> - Antimetabolites
>
> **Cell-cycle–Nonspecific Drugs (CCNS)**
> - Most effective against large, slow-growing tumors
> - Most alkylating drugs
> - Antitumor antibiotics
> - Hormones
>
> **Combination Therapy**
> - Most commonly used type of regimen today
> - Provides best chance of "cure"
> - Attacks multiple facets of cancer cell growth
> - Allows for lower dosages of drugs
>
> **Risk Factors for Antineoplastic Toxicity**
> - Drug dose, route, and method of administration
> - Extent of cancer and overall condition
> - Concomitant organ dysfunction or illness
> - Age
> - Nutritional status
> - Self-care behaviors
> - Combination versus monotherapy
>
> **Principles of Antineoplastic Drug Administration**
> - Allow for full recovery of myelosuppression before resuming therapy, although this principle may not apply for aggressive leukemias and lymphomas
> - Avoid drug interactions involving CYP450 enzyme system
> - Avoid concomitant administration of platelet-inhibiting drugs
> - Dosage adjustment is warranted if there is hepatic or renal impairment.

---

cancer that metastasizes early in the course of the disease. The goal of *adjuvant therapy* is to eradicate any micrometastatic deposits when they are most susceptible.

Administering multiple drugs that have different mechanisms of action and different toxicities produces greater cell kill than monotherapy. This concept is based on the Goldie-Coldman hypothesis, which describes the heterogenicity of tumor cells and the likelihood of drug resistance. **The dose of an individual antineoplastic drug is limited by the toxicity the patient can tolerate.** Choosing drugs with minimal or no overlapping toxicities allows the maximum tolerated dose of each drug to be administered. Cell kill is additionally produced because the combination of drugs assaults the cancer cells by a variety of mechanisms rather than one action produced by a single drug.

Tumors that microscopically display the fewest number of normal cellular characteristics tend to grow more rapidly, spread more readily, and impose more lethal consequences on the host. Because of their cellular characteristics, poorly differentiated tumors tend to be more responsive to drug therapy in the short term than slow-growing, well-differentiated cancers. The growth fraction of the tumor, or the number of cells that are cycling at any given time, also affects how the tumor responds to therapy.

The stage of the tumor must also be considered when evaluating treatment options. Patients with extensive metastatic disease may not be candidates for antineoplastic therapy, because dosages required to eradicate the disease may have toxicities that decrease the quality of life and therefore may not be appropriate.

▲ **Remember, antineoplastic drugs damage cancer cells as well as healthy cells.** The ultimate goal of antineoplastic therapy is to limit damage to healthy cells while yielding a 100% kill rate for cancer cells. An intermittent schedule of drug therapy allows normal cells to repair themselves and grow between doses of antineoplastic therapy. During the break from therapy, however, the cancer cells also have time to repair damage caused by the drugs. For intermittent therapy to be successful, healthy cells must be able to repair damage and repopulate faster than the cancer cells. If the cancer cells repopulate faster than normal cells, intermittent therapy will fail.

▲ **Treatment regimens that use multiple drugs are generally more successful than regimens that employ a single drug.** Choose drugs for combination therapy that are individually effective against the targeted neoplasm, minimize toxicity to normal cells, produce minimally overlapping toxicities, and have different mechanisms of actions.

Experience has shown that cancer cells are capable of
▲ developing temporary and permanent drug resistance. **The degree and type of drug resistance depends on the blood supply and the nutrients available to the tumor, the bioavailability of the drug, and the presence of tumor in sanctuary sites.** Permanent drug resistance is genetically based and is the result of random cell mutations. The more rapid the mutation rate, the less likely it is that cure or control of the disease will occur. Tumor cells can possess innate resistance to a specific drug without having had previous exposure to the drug. Tumor cells may also acquire drug resistance after exposure to the drug and may develop cross-resistance to other antineoplastic drugs.

Toxicities associated with antineoplastic therapy adversely affect almost any body organ, but in general are a reflection of damage to rapidly dividing cells. Normal tissues with a high growth fraction, such as the GI mucosa, bone marrow, hair follicles, and reproductive system tissues, are most likely to be damaged. The damage varies in severity depending upon the drugs administered, drug dosages, treatment protocol, and the patient's health status before the start of treatment.

MYELOSUPPRESSION. Myelosuppression is a general term used to describe the suppressive effects of cytotoxic drugs on the bone marrow. As a consequence of disease or therapy, many patients experience neutropenia, thrombocytopenia, and anemia to varying degrees. Neutropenia occurs frequently because the life span of leukocytes is very brief (12 hours). The time after antineoplastic drug administration when the white blood cell (WBC) or platelet count is at the lowest point is referred to as the *nadir*. For most myelosuppressive drugs, the WBC nadir occurs within 7 to 14 days after drug administration (Table 33-5). Knowledge of the blood count nadirs helps the health care provider predict when the patient is at greatest risk for infection and bleeding. A normal leukocyte count is 4000 to 10,000 cells/mm^3. A patient is neutropenic if his or her ANC is 1000 cells/mm^3. The frequency of infection increases as the ANC falls below 500 cells/mm^3 and the longer the patient remains neutropenic.

A normal platelet count is 140,000 to 440,000 cells/mm^3. Thrombocytopenia increases the risk of bleeding when platelet counts fall below 50,000 cells/mm^3. Most health care providers will order a transfusion for the patient to keep the platelet count above 20,000 cells/mm^3. Fatal CNS hemorrhage or massive GI bleeding can occur when platelet counts fall below 10,000 cells/mm^3. Some controversy exists as to whether patients should receive prophylactic transfusions when platelet count falls below a certain level, or when the patient is actively bleeding.

Anemia is a reduction in the concentration of hemoglobin and circulating red blood cells (RBCs). Anemia leads to tissue hypoxia because of impaired oxygen-carrying capacity. Anemia is manifested as a drop in hemoglobin, hematocrit, or RBC count. Dehydration may raise the hematocrit, thus masking an anemia. A normal hemoglobin is 12 to 15 grams/dL in females and 13 to 16 grams/dL in males. The patient is anemic if values fall below 12 grams/dL. Anemia that falls below this lower value can result in hypotension and myocardial infarction. One unit of blood ordinarily raises the hemoglobin by 1 gram/dL.

Many patients tolerate varying degrees of anemia and may be reluctant to accept transfusions. However, packed RBCs may be required to relieve anemia that is symptomatic. Erythropoietin may be ordered to maintain or elevate the RBC level and decrease the need for transfusions (see Chapter 44).

GASTROINTESTINAL EFFECTS. In general, most nausea and vomiting can be successfully controlled with careful administration of antiemetic therapy in conjunction with the drug treatments. Antiemetics are ordinarily administered 30 minutes before therapy and, depending on the treatment regimen, may be continued for up to 5 days after treatment.

Antineoplastic therapy can also cause nausea, stomatitis, oral mucositis, an aversion to food, changes in taste and smell, nausea, vomiting, and diarrhea. The emetic potential of a particular antineoplastic regimen depends on the drugs given, the dosage and route of administration, and the patient's susceptibility to emesis (Box 33-3). **Uncontrolled** ▲ **nausea and vomiting contributes to anorexia, malnutrition, dehydration, metabolic imbalances, psychologic depression, and reduced immunity.**

Three patterns of nausea and vomiting are often seen in patients receiving antineoplastic therapy:
1. Anticipatory nausea and vomiting may occur before the next treatment, once the patient has experienced nausea and vomiting related to antineoplastic therapy
2. Acute posttherapy nausea and vomiting that occurs within the first 24 hours after drug administration
3. Delayed nausea and vomiting that persists or develops 24 hours after drug administration

The health care provider responsible for drug administration must be thoroughly familiar with antiemetic drugs and adjunct measures that can be used to control nausea and vomiting (see also Chapter 47).

Stomatitis or oral mucositis is a consequence of delayed cell renewal caused by antineoplastic drugs. Lesions seen in the mouth are present throughout the GI tract. **The drug** ▲ **classes commonly associated with stomatitis include the antimetabolites (i.e., MTX and 5-FU) and the antitumor antibiotics (i.e., doxorubicin).** The oral lesions may be so severe that patients are unable to eat, drink, speak, or swallow

IMMUNE

TABLE 33-5 Nadir and Recovery of Selected Antineoplastics

Drug	WBC Nadir (Days)	WBC Recovery (Days)	Platelet Nadir (Days)	Comments
ALKYLATING DRUGS				
busulfan	7–10	24–54	10–30	—
carmustine	28–42	42–56	28–35	Myelosuppressive effects cumulative, delayed, and prolonged
chlorambucil	6–10	14–21	14–21	—
cisplatin	18–23	29	14	—
cyclophosphamide	6–10	14–21	14–21	Somewhat platelet-sparing
dacarbazine	10–14	24	14–28	—
ifosfamide	8–14	14–21	Platelet-sparing	—
lomustine	42	60	28	Myelosuppressive effects are cumulative, delayed, and prolonged; thrombocytopenia more common than leukopenia
mechlorethamine	6–10	14–21	14–21	—
melphalan	8–14	14–21	14–21	Thrombocytopenia more common than neutropenia
thiotepa	10–14	28	14–28	—
ANTIMETABOLITES				
cytarabine	12–14	22–24	12–15	Somewhat platelet-sparing
fludarabine	3–25	UA	2–32	—
fluorouracil	9–14	20–30	7–17	—
mercaptopurine	7–14	14–21	10–14	—
methotrexate	7–14	14–21	5–12	—
thioguanine	14–28	28–35	14	—
ANTITUMOR ANTIBIOTICS				
dactinomycin	14–21	21–25	10–14	—
daunorubicin	8–10	21	10–14	Profound myelosuppression is dose-limiting
doxorubicin	10–14	22	14	—
idarubicin	10–15	21	10–14	—
mitomycin	21–28	28–42	30	Effects cumulative and prolonged
mitoxantrone	10–14	21	8–16	Profound myelosuppression is dose-limiting
MITOTIC INHIBITORS				
docetaxel	8	7	UA	—
paclitaxel	8–11	15–21	UA	Platelet-sparing
vinblastine	5–9	14–21	4–10	—
vincristine	4–10	7–14	UA	Platelet-sparing
vindesine	7	14	7	—
vinorelbine	7–10	7–14	UA	Platelet-sparing
TOPOISOMERASE INHIBITORS				
etoposide	7–14	21	9–16	Thrombocytopenia occurs less often and is usually not severe.
irinotecan	7	14–21	UA	Mild thrombocytopenia
teniposide	16–18	15	16–18	—
topotecan	11	18	15	—
MISCELLANEOUS ANTINEOPLASTIC DRUGS				
hydroxyurea	7	14–21	UA	Somewhat platelet-sparing
L-asparaginase	4–7	10–14	5–10	Somewhat platelet-sparing; myelosuppression is seldom a problem
procarbazine	25–36	35–50	21	Myelosuppression is prolonged and delayed

UA, Unavailable; *WBC*, white blood cell.

their own oral secretions. Severe stomatitis is a dose-limiting toxicity for the patient taking certain antineoplastic drugs.

Diarrhea is most often associated with antimetabolites. Constipation is frequently the effect of vinca alkaloids because it causes neuropathy of the GI tract. Other causes of constipation include the use of opioid analgesics, immobility, decreased fluid and fiber intake, tumor invasion of the GI tract, and depression.

DERMATOLOGIC EFFECTS. Dermatologic toxicities include alopecia, skin and nail hyperpigmentation, and onycholysis of the nails. Toxicities and adverse effects gradually resolve with cessation of treatment. The extent of hair loss depends on the specific drug, the dosage, and the mode of administration. Alopecia is temporary; hair regrowth ordinarily begins before antineoplastic therapy ends, although the hair color and texture may change. Scalp hypothermia (i.e., ice packs) decreases blood flow to the hair follicles, thereby reducing contact between the drug and epithelial cells. It is rarely used today owing to the risk of creating a sanctuary site for metastatic disease. Scalp hypothermia is contraindicated or use in patients with brain tumors or metastatic disease to this area.

Hyperpigmentation of the nail bed, the mouth, the gums, or the teeth, and along veins used for IV therapy is not uncommon. The hyperpigmentation usually occurs 2 to 3 weeks after therapy and continues for 10 to 12 weeks after stopping. Photosensitivity may result in acute sunburn after short sun exposure. The skin effects range from redness, shedding, or peeling to blisters and oozing. Once the skin heals, it is permanently darkened. Radiation recall may occur in patients who received radiation therapy weeks or months before the administration of antineoplastic drugs.

REPRODUCTIVE EFFECTS. The effects of antineoplastic drugs on gonadal function and reproduction capacity can be temporary or permanent. The effect varies with respect to the patient's age, the drug administered, and total dosage. Azoospermia, oligospermia, and sterility have been documented in males. Amenorrhea, manifestations of menopause, and sterility has been noted in females.

PREPARATION AND ADMINISTRATION. For the most part, all antineoplastic drugs are carcinogenic, teratogenic, and mutagenic. Primary exposure routes include absorption through the skin, inhalation, ingestion through contaminated food, or from contact with contaminated surfaces. Preparation and administration of antineoplastic drugs should be done only by specially trained health care providers. Personnel should be familiar with the Occupational Safety and Health Administration (OSHA) guidelines, Oncology Nursing Society (ONS) guidelines, and individual agency policies regarding antineoplastic drug administration.

Selection of the administration site is an important consideration when using antineoplastic drugs. Large veins in the forearm are the preferred sites. If a drug does extravasate, there is maximum soft tissue coverage to prevent functional impairment. Vesicants should not be administered through veins in the hands, in the antecubital fossa, or over bony prominences (Box 33-5). Extravasation in these areas leads to destruction of nerves and tendons, resulting in loss of function. Veins that are damaged or sclerosed and sites that have been damaged by burns, grafts, surgery, amputation, and mastectomy should be avoided. An extravasation kit containing agency-approved antidotes should be kept at the patient's side whenever a vesicant is being administered. Blood return and infusion site should be monitored before, during, and after drug administration.

Central venous access devices (e.g., Hickman or Groshong single-lumen catheters, Port-A-Cath Dual-Lumen Venous Access System, OmegaPort, Infusaid Microport) are recommended for continuous infusion of vesicants. Because the termination site of the catheter is in a large central vein, hyperosmolar solutions can be safely administered, and rapid dilution and distribution of irritating drugs will be improved.

Regional administration of antineoplastic drugs includes topical, intrathecal, intracavitary, and intraarterial routes. Although intraarterial routes pose some risk, major organs or tumor sites receive maximal exposure with limited serum drug levels. As a result, systemic adverse effects are minimal.

Almost all antineoplastic drugs are given in relatively high doses, on an intermittent or a cyclic schedule. This appears to be more efficacious than low doses given continuously or massive doses given only once. It also causes less immunosuppression and provides for drug holidays, during which normal tissues can repair themselves from antineoplastic drug-induced damage. Fortunately, normal cells repair more quickly than neoplastic cells. Subsequent dosages are usually administered as soon as tissue repair becomes evident, usually when neutrophil and platelet counts return to acceptable levels.

Multidrug therapies follow a precise schedule because safety and efficacy of the drugs are usually schedule-dependent. When used as an adjunct to surgery, the drug is started as soon as possible and given in maximal doses (as tolerated), just as if advanced disease were present. Therapy is continued for several months to a year. Examples of multidrug therapies are identified in Table 33-6.

Patient Education

Provide patients with a complete explanation of their treatment regimen, including adverse effects, before informed consent is obtained for antineoplastic drug therapy. Care should be taken to discuss not only the life-threatening and

TABLE 33-6 Examples of Antineoplastic Regimens

Regimen	Drug Combinations
ABVD	**A**driamycin (doxorubicin) + **b**leomycin + **v**inblastine + **d**acarbazine
MOPP	**m**echlorethamine + **O**ncovin (vincristine) + **p**rocarbazine + **p**rednisone
BACOP	**b**leomycin + **A**driamycin (doxorubicin) + **c**yclophosphamide + **O**ncovin (vincristine) + **p**rednisone
BEP	**b**leomycin + **e**toposide + **p**latinum
CAF	**c**yclophosphamide + **A**driamycin (doxorubicin) + **f**luorouracil
CMF(P)	**c**yclophosphamide + **m**ethotrexate + **f**luorouracil + **p**rednisone
CDOP	**c**yclophosphamide + **d**oxorubicin + **O**ncovin (vincristine) + **p**rednisone
CDOP + R	**c**yclophosphamide, **d**oxorubicin, **O**ncovin (vincristine) + **p**rednisone + **r**ituximab
COP	**c**yclophosphamide + **O**ncovin (vincristine) + **p**rednisone
COPP	**c**yclophosphamide, **O**ncovin (vincristine) + **p**rednisone + **p**rocarbazine
ECF	**E**pirubicin + **c**isplatin + **f**luorouracil
FAM-BCNU	**F**luorouracil + **A**driamycin (doxorubicin) + **m**itomycin + **BCNU** (carmustine)
FOLFOX	**f**luorouracil + **l**eucovorin + **ox**aliplatin
PCV	**p**rocarbazine, **l**omustine, **v**incristine
Thaldex	**thal**idomide + **dex**amethasone
VAD	**v**incristine + **a**driamycin + **d**examethasone

BOX 33-5

Vesicants

- dacarbazine
- dactinomycin
- daunorubicin
- doxorubicin
- idarubicin
- mechlorethamine
- mitomycin
- paclitaxel
- platinol
- vinblastine
- vincristine

pathologic condition–producing adverse effects, but also the adverse effects that produce discomfort and embarrassment. In the past, patients with cancer could rely on health care professionals to monitor their health status. However, drug administration is quickly becoming the domain of outpatient and home settings, and it is imperative for patients to know how to monitor their own health status. Instruction sheets for most antineoplastic drugs are available in English, Spanish, and other languages from the National Cancer Institute.

Because antineoplastic drugs typically induce periods of low neutrophil and platelet counts, patients should become familiar with what desirable cell counts are. The risk for infection is reduced by teaching patients to avoid potential sources of infection. These sources include individuals with a cold or flu and live plants and flowers (sources of microscopic fungus, bacteria, and insects). Advise patients against receiving live virus vaccines (e.g., MMR) for several months after antineoplastic therapy has been discontinued. In addition, persons in close contact with the patient should not receive nasal influenza vaccine, because the live virus is excreted by the person receiving it and can be transmitted to the patient. Additionally, help patients to understand the importance of early reporting of early signs and symptoms of infection (i.e., low-grade fever, sore throat, or cough). The single most important practice to prevent infection is for all health care workers, patients, families and friends to know about, and follow, strict handwashing regimens.

⚠ **Low platelet counts create additional risk factors for patients receiving antineoplastic drugs**. The potential for hemorrhage can be minimized by teaching patients to avoid aspirin and other over-the-counter drugs that prolong clotting times, substitute electric shavers for razors (to reduce the risk of nicks and cuts), refrain from using suppositories (since they may cause tears to rectal tissue), hold pressure over cuts and venipuncture sites for 5 to 10 minutes, and avoid IM injections as much as possible. Most importantly, help patients understand the signs and symptoms of internal bleeding and to promptly report these symptoms to their health care provider or oncologist.

Teach patients who have thrombocytopenia to avoid aspirin-containing products or drugs that inhibit platelet activity without first checking with their health care provider. Some patients may require activity restrictions or bed rest to decrease the risk of injury. Blood counts must be scrutinized closely before a patient undergoes surgery or any invasive procedure.

The patient with stomatitis requires education about how to perform oral hygiene. This includes frequent gentle mouth care using a soft toothbrush, the importance and cautions of flossing, and measures to relieve pain, maintain comfort, and promote hygiene.

Evaluation

Decision-making guidelines for potentially active new drugs, as well as routine practice in cancer treatment, are based on evaluation of tumor response. In 1981, the World Health Organization (WHO) established guidelines in an attempt to standardize criteria for assessment of tumor response. Since then, the criteria were simplified in a version known as RECIST (response evaluation criteria in solid tumors); it uses one-dimensional (a line) instead of bidimensional measurements (a plane) for evaluation; a reduced number of lesions are measured; the disease progression criteria are withdrawn based on an isolated size increase in a single lesion; and different thresholds are used when defining tumor response and progression. However, the rules are not easily applicable and often not strictly followed in day-to-day oncology practice or even in the clinical research settings. Table 33-7 provides a comparison of the 1981 WHO criteria and the response evaluation criteria in solid tumors (RECIST). Assuming that an adequate trial of antineoplastic therapy has been conducted, disease progression indicates a treatment failure.

There are many possible explanations for the failure of antineoplastic drug therapy:

1. *Antagonism between antineoplastic drugs;* for example, if one drug prevents cancer cells from entering the S phase of the cell cycle, using another S phase–specific drug in concurrent combination would not be helpful.
2. *The sanctuary sites* for the cancer cells (e.g., the CNS or the center of large poorly vascular zed tumors) may not be reached by the antineoplastic drug.
3. *Toxicity to normal cells* may prevent the use of effective dosages that have steep dose-response curves.
4. *Tumors with low growth fraction and long doubling times* are less responsive.
5. *The numbers of tumor cells* may be too great and contain resistant cells.
6. *Active drugs fail* to enter the cell, are biotransformed to inactive metabolites, or are eliminated too quickly.
7. *The drug dosage, schedule, or route of administration* was badly chosen. The highest dose with acceptable risk of toxicity should be used.
8. *Previous therapy* may have given resistant cells a growth advantage.
9. *Comorbid diseases, intolerance to drug therapy or the patient's physical state* limits treatment options.

TABLE 33-7 Comparison of Who and Recist Tumor Evaluation Criteria

Parameter	1981 WHO Criteria	2000 RECIST Criteria
Measurement methodology	Bidimensional	Unidimensional
Number of measured lesions	Not specified	Maximum of 5/organ; 10 in total
Definition of partial response	Over 50% decrease in tumor area	Over 30% decrease in tumors longest diameter
Definition of disease progression	Over 25% increase in tumor area or appearance of a new lesion or over 25% increase in size of 1 lesion	Over 20% increase in tumor's longest diameter or the appearance of a new lesion

RECIST, Response evaluation criteria in solid tumors; *WHO*, World Health Organization.
Adapted from Miller, A., Hoogstraten, B., Staquet, M., et al. (1981). Reporting results of cancer treatment. *Cancer, 47*(1), 207–214; and Therasse, P., Arbuck, S., Eisenhauer, E., et al. (2000). New guidelines to evaluate the response to treatment in solid tumours. *Journal of the National Cancer Institute, 92*(3), 205–216.

The ultimate goal of antineoplastic therapy is to achieve a cure, without unreasonable toxicities and adverse reactions. When cure is impossible, antineoplastic drugs are valuable tools in prolonging life and minimizing suffering. The health care provider must be knowledgeable about the antineoplastic drugs and their toxicities so as to ensure patient's safety, minimize adverse effects, and assist the patient and the family to cope with a life-threatening illness.

KEY POINTS

- Cell cycle–specific drugs are effective only during a specific phase of the cell cycle (i.e., S, G_2, M, G_1).
- Cell cycle–nonspecific drugs are effective throughout the cell cycle, including G_0.
- Alkylating drugs act by causing interstrand and intrastrand cross-linkages in DNA, thus blocking replication. They are CCNS drugs, although in some cases cells appear to be more sensitive in one phase than another.
- Antimetabolites are CCS, acting in phase S to interfere with DNA synthesis.
- The antitumor antibiotics act by forming complexes with DNA, thereby inhibiting DNA activity through the process of intercalation.
- Mitotic inhibitors act by interfering with assembly of the microtubular components of the mitotic spindle.
- Hormones used in antineoplastic therapy include androgens, antiandrogens, estrogens, antiestrogens, adrencocorticosteroids, adrenocorticosteroid inhibitors, gonadotropin-releasing hormone analogues, and progestins.
- The three major goals of antineoplastic therapy are cure, control, and palliation. *Cure* is defined as eradication of all cancer, giving the patient treated the same life expectancy as an individual who does not have cancer. *Control* of the disease and prolonging life are necessary when cancer is found to be incurable. *Palliation* provides relief of symptoms and maintenance of function as near normal as possible when it is no longer possible to achieve a remission.
- Primary antineoplastic therapy (i.e., neoadjuvant therapy or induction therapy) is used before other treatments in an attempt to reduce tumor size and bulk and increase surgical resectability of the tumor.

- The goal of adjuvant therapy is to eradicate possible micrometastatic deposits when they are most susceptible.
- Selecting an antineoplastic regimen is based on the type of tumor and cell types involved, and the degree of cellular differentiation, the growth rate, and the heterogeneity of the tumor. Selection of an antineoplastic regimen involves a complex series of decisions that includes considerations as to the type of tumor, the cell types involved, and the degree of cellular differentiation.
- The toxicities of antineoplastic drug therapy are a reflection of damage to rapidly dividing cells. Normal tissue with high growth fractions, such as the GI mucosa, bone marrow, hair follicles, and reproductive system tissue, are most likely to be damaged.
- Host factors that influence treatment outcome include immune function, nutritional status, psychologic status, availability of supportive care, and social support.
- The nadir is the period after antineoplastic drug administration when the WBC or platelet count is at the lowest point. For most myelosuppressive drugs, the nadir occurs 7 to 14 days after drug administration.
- Assuming that an adequate trial of antineoplastic therapy has been conducted, disease progression indicates treatment failure.
- *Complete response* is defined as the disappearance of all non–target lesions and normalization of tumor marker level.
- *Incomplete response–stable disease* is the persistence of one or more non–target lesion(s) and/or maintenance of tumor marker level above the normal limits.
- *Progressive disease* is the appearance of one or more new lesions and/ or unequivocal progression of existing non–target lesions.

Bibliography

Abeloff, A., Armitage, J., Niederhuber, J., et al. (2004). *Clinical oncology* (3rd ed.). Philadelphia: Churchill Livingstone.

Ambati, B., Joussen, A., Ambati, J., et al. (2002). Angiostatin inhibits and regresses corneal neovascularization. *Archives of Ophthalmology*, 120(8), 1063–1068.

American Cancer Society (website). Available online: www.acs.org. Accessed May 5, 2007.

Balmer, C., Valley, A., Iannucci, A., et al. (2005). Cancer treatment and chemotherapy. In: DiPiro, J., Talbert, R., & Yee, G., et al. *Pharmacotherapy: A pathophysiologic approach* (6th ed). NY: McGraw Hill.

Burnham, B., Hall, I., and Gringauz, A. (2007). *Introduction to medicinal chemistry: How drugs act and why* (3rd ed). Indianapolis: Wiley.

Calabresi, P., and Chabner, B. (2001). Chemotherapy of neoplastic diseases. In Hardman, J., Limbird, L., and Gilman A. (Eds.). *Goodman and Gilman's the pharmacologic basis of therapeutics* (10th ed). NY: McGraw-Hill.

Glinghammar, B., Venturi, M., Rowland, I., et al. (1997). Shift from a dairy product-rich to a dairy product-free diet: Influence on cytotoxicity and genotoxicity of fecal water–potential risk factors

for colon cancer. *American Journal of Clinical Nutrition*, 66(5), 1277–1282.

Kufe, D., Pollock, R., Weichselbaum, R., et al. (2003). *Cancer medicine* (6th ed). Hamilton, Ontario: BC Decker.

Langman, M., and Boyle, P. (1998). Chemoprevention of colorectal cancer. *Gut*, 43(4), 578–585.

La Vecchia, C., Braga, C., Negri, E., et al. (1997). Intake of selected micronutrients and risk of colorectal cancer. *International Journal of Cancer*, 73(4), 525–530.

Miller, A., Hoogstraten, B., Staquet, M., et al. (1981). Reporting results of cancer treatment. *Cancer*, 47(1), 207–214.

National Comprehensive Cancer Care Network. (2006). Drugs and biologics compendium. Available online:www.nccn.org/default.asp. Accessed May 5, 2007.

Rostom, A., Dube, C., Lewin, G., et al. (2007). Nonsteroidal anti-inflammatory drugs and cyclooxygenase-2 inhibitors for primary prevention of colorectal cancer: A systematic review prepared for the U.S. Preventive Services Task Force. *Annals of Internal Medicine*, 146(5), 376–389.

IMMUNE

Therasse, P., Arbuck, S., Eisenhauer, E., et al. (2000). New guidelines to evaluate the response to treatment in solid tumours. *Journal of the National Cancer Institute, 92*(3), 205–216.

Wood, R. D., Mitchell, M., and Lindahl, T. (2005). Human DNA repair genes. *Mutation Research/Fundamental and Molecular Mechanisms of Mutagenesis, 577*(1–2), 275–283.

Yamaguchi, M., Tsutsumi, K., Abe, M., et al. (2007). Release of drugs from liposomes varies with particle size. *Biological and Pharmaceutical Bulletin, 30*(5), 963–966.

34

Inotropic Drugs

Heart failure (HF) is a syndrome rather than a primary diagnosis. It has many possible causes, assorted clinical features, and numerous clinical subsets. Patients may have a variety of primary cardiovascular diseases and never develop cardiac dysfunction, and those in whom cardiac dysfunction is identified may never develop clinical HF. In addition to cardiac dysfunction, other factors, such as vascular stiffness and how the body manages sodium (Na$^+$), play major roles in the signs and symptoms of the syndrome of HF.

Patients at risk for cardiovascular diseases are at risk for HF. Early identification and treatment of risk factors is perhaps the most significant step in limiting the public health impact of HF. Emphasis on primary and secondary prevention is particularly critical because of the difficulty of successfully treating left ventricular (LV) dysfunction, especially when severe. Current therapeutic advances in the treatment of HF do not make prevention any less important.

Although HF is progressive, current therapy provides stability and even reversibility. The relentless progression from LV remodeling and dysfunction to HF is no longer inevitable. Prolonged survival with mild to moderate LV dysfunction is now possible. Treatment with angiotensin-converting enzyme inhibitors (ACEIs), or angiotensin II–receptor blockers (ARBs) and beta blockers lead to slowing or to partial reversal of remodeling. Because of prolonged survival, comorbid conditions such as coronary artery disease or renal failure can progress, complicating treatment. Reducing the risk of sudden death, predominantly from ventricular tachyarrhythmia, has been a major new focus of clinical research. The purpose of this chapter is to address treatment for heart failure.

HEART FAILURE

Heart failure (HF) is defined as a state in which the heart is unable to pump an adequate amount of blood to meet the metabolic needs of the body at rest or during exercise. Impaired cardiac function is responsible for failure of the heart to pump blood at a volume commensurate with venous return, hence, the term failure. The term congestive heart failure (CHF) refers to circulatory overload secondary to HF. Pump failure results in hypoperfused tissues followed by pulmonary and vascular congestion. In addition, fluid overload secondary to activation of the body's compensatory mechanisms compounds the difficulty. As cardiac performance deteriorates, blood backs up behind the failing ventricles, causing venous distention and edema, hence the descriptive term congestive. Other terms used to denote HF include cardiac decompensation, cardiac insufficiency, and ventricular failure.

EPIDEMIOLOGY AND ETIOLOGY

Cardiovascular disorders are a leading cause of morbidity and mortality in all industrialized nations. HF affects approximately 5 million Americans; more than 2% of the population. Approximately 500,000 to 900,000 new cases of HF are diagnosed each year. In 2005, the direct cost of HF in the United States was estimated to exceed $25 billion.

HF is the most common cause of in-hospital mortality in patients with cardiovascular disease. It is responsible for one third of all deaths in patients who have had a myocardial infarction (MI). Both the incidence and prevalence of HF increase dramatically with advancing age. It is projected that the number of Americans over age 65 will double in the next 30 years; so too will the number of persons at risk for HF. Statistics like these have given impetus to clinical research in HF, which in turn has revealed promising new strategies for preventing and managing this costly and debilitating disease.

When the heart is overloaded with blood, there is excessive preload (i.e., the degree of stretch of ventricular myocardial muscle fibers at the onset of contraction). The increased preload lessens the force and efficiency of ventricular contraction. Conditions that contribute to increased preload include valvular regurgitation, hypervolemia, congenital defects (i.e., septal defects), patent ductus arteriosus, and HF.

Afterload is the systemic pressure that opposes LV ejection, that is, the tension the heart must overcome for sufficient ventricular emptying to occur–how hard the heart must pump to force blood into the circulation. Afterload, a measure of vascular resistance, is determined by the vascular tone of the arterioles, the elasticity of the aorta and the large arteries, the thickness and size of the ventricle, the condition of the aortic valve, and the viscosity of the blood. Elevated peripheral vascular resistance and high blood pressure require the ventricles to work harder. With prolonged high pressure, the ventricles eventually fail. Conditions contributing to increased afterload include aortic and mitral valve stenoses, pulmonary valve stenosis, pulmonary hypertension, high peripheral vascular resistance, and systemic hypertension. In 75% of the cases, hypertension preceded the HF.

Intrinsic conditions that contribute to abnormal myocardial function include an MI, myocarditis, cardiomyopathy, and ventricular aneurysm. These disorders impair function of myocardial muscle fibers and reduce ventricular emptying and stroke volume (SV). Extrinsic conditions can also cause abnormal function of the heart muscle. Constrictive pericarditis (an inflammatory, fibrotic process of the pericardial sac) and cardiac tamponade (accumulation of fluid or blood in the pericardial sac) hamper ventricular filling and contractility. Because the pericardium encompasses the entire heart, compression decreases ventricular relaxation, thereby increasing diastolic pressure and hampering forward blood flow through the heart.

HF can also be precipitated or exacerbated by hypervolemia. Expanded circulatory volume increases venous returnto the heart and in turn increases preload. Possible causes of hypervolemia include poor renal function, underlying cardiac disease, corticosteroid therapy, and excessive intake of Na^+.

There is no conclusive evidence that caffeine or alcohol intake increases the risk of heart disease. Nevertheless, caffeine increases the heart rate and the blood pressure, each of which raises the myocardial workload and can precipitate HF. As failure worsens, patients find that activities of daily living and social activities are restricted because of dyspnea, chest pain, or peripheral edema. Furthermore, the social isolation that results may significantly affect the patient's ability to cope with his or her disease.

Emotional or physical stress increases the workload of the heart by increasing sympathetic nervous system (SNS) activity. Fever and infection increase the oxygen demands of body tissues. Thyrotoxicosis increases the body's metabolic rate, thus accelerating heart rate and myocardial workload. Anemia reduces the oxygen-carrying capacity of the blood, necessitating increased cardiac output to meet the body's needs for oxygen. Pregnancy, like thyrotoxicosis and anemia, increases the metabolic needs of the body and increases the workload. Thiamine (vitamin B_1) deficiency, often associated with excessive use of alcohol, interferes with cardiac function by decreasing contractility, increasing the heart rate, and causing ventricular dilation. Pulmonary diseases such as chronic airway limitation (previously known as chronic obstructive pulmonary disease or COPD), severe pulmonary embolism, and primary pulmonary hypertension produce sizable resistance to right ventricular emptying. The resistance can lead to right ventricular hypertrophy and HF.

PATHOPHYSIOLOGY

Normally, the pumping action of the left and the right sides of the heart complement each other, producing a continuous blood flow. However, as a result of pathologic conditions, one side may fail while the other side continues to function normally for a period of time. With prolonged strain, the functional side of the heart also eventually fails, resulting in biventricular failure. Biventricular failure may be unresponsive to treatment because myocardial disease renders the myocardium unable to contract more forcefully no matter what the stimulus.

When the heart fails as a pump and cardiac output (i.e., the volume of blood ejected from the ventricle/minute) decreases, three primary compensatory mechanisms arise to maintain the cardiac output: SNS stimulation; ventricular dilation; and ventricular hypertrophy (Table 34-1). As a result of decreased cardiac output and the SNS stimulation of baroreceptors, epinephrine and norepinephrine are released. Arterial vasoconstriction increases blood pressure and decreases blood flow to the periphery to maintain blood flow to vital organs. However, arterial vasoconstriction has a downside in that it increases afterload and myocardial oxygen requirements. Venous vasoconstriction increases preload.

To monitor preload, the index of *left ventricular end diastolic (LVED) pressure* is used. When preload decreases, the amount of blood in the ventricles at the end of diastole decreases, and

TABLE 34-1 Etiology of Heart Failure Symptoms

Mechanism	Signs	Symptoms
Decreased cardiac output	Decreased blood pressure, pulse pressure	Anxiety and fear
	Pulsus alternans	Dizziness
	Tachycardia	Syncope
	Supraventricular rhythms	Decreased exercise tolerance, fatigue
	S_3 and S_4 present	Chest pain
Pulmonary congestion (left ventricular failure)	Dyspnea	Cough with frothy sputum
	Orthopnea	Tachypnea
	Paroxysmal nocturnal dyspnea	Bibasilar crackles
	Nocturia	Increased PADP, PAWP
Systemic congestion (right ventricular failure)	Nausea	Vomiting
	Indigestion	Jugular vein distention
	Weakness	Peripheral and sacral edema
		Hepatosplenomegaly, ascites
		Abdominal distention
		Increased RAP

PADP, Pulmonary artery diastolic pressure; *PAWP*, pulmonary artery wedge pressure; *RAP*, right atrial pressure.

therefore SV is decreased. When other factors are held constant (i.e., heart rate, contractility, and afterload), the force of muscle contraction is directly proportional to the preload. Knowledge of pressure changes is important because excessive LV filling pressures cause blood to back up into pulmonary circulation, where it forces plasma out through vessel walls. The fluid accumulation in lung tissues is *pulmonary edema.*

In addition to SNS stimulation of heart rate and SV, the failing heart attempts to compensate, via Starling's law, to increase cardiac output either by ventricular dilation or hypertrophy. Ventricular dilation and increased contractility create greater wall tension, but also increase myocardial oxygen consumption.

Hypertrophy of the heart muscle increases contractile powers of the working muscle mass. There are trade-offs, however. Eventually, ventricular hypertrophy becomes inadequate as the elasticity of muscle fibers is strained. The overstretched muscle fibers increase contractile forces and the dilation and hypertrophy result in a decrease in coronary blood flow. Hypertrophied ventricles become stiff, requiring greater left LVED pressures to achieve adequate filling. According to Starling's law, the force of a contraction is determined primarily by the length of muscle fibers and is proportional to the amount of blood remaining in the ventricle at the end of diastole. The situation is somewhat like stretching a rubber band; the more it is stretched, the harder it contracts. The larger the preload, the greater the SV, until a point is reached when the ventricle is so stretched that it can no longer contract.

The mechanism of fluid retention and subsequent elevation of LVED pressure in patients with HF is multifactorial. As cardiac output falls, blood flow to the kidneys also falls. The juxtaglomerular apparatus interprets this as decreased volume. The kidneys release renin, which interacts with angiotensinogen to form angiotensin I, which is converted by ACE to

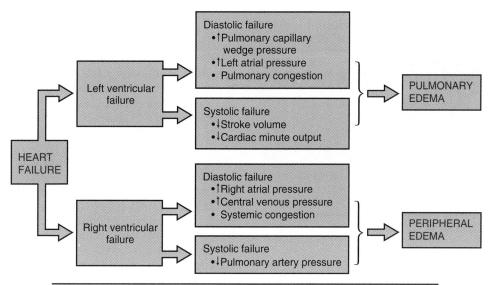

FIGURE 34-1 Compensatory Mechanisms Associated with Right and Left Ventricular Failure.

angiotensin II, a potent vasoconstrictor. Angiotensin II causes the adrenal cortex to release aldosterone, which in turn causes Na^+ retention that increases blood volume and further increases arterial pressure. The posterior pituitary senses the increased osmotic pressure (due to Na^+ and water retention) and subsequently secretes antidiuretic hormone (ADH). ADH increases water reabsorption in the distal convoluted tubules and collecting ducts of the nephron. The process is cyclical, creating a downward spiral in the patient's condition (Fig. 34-1).

When compensatory mechanisms function properly to provide adequate cardiac output, the patient has compensated HF. When the compensatory mechanisms can no longer assist in maintaining cardiac output, and therefore adequate tissue perfusion, the patient has decompensated HF. Even with treatment, the prognosis for decompensated HF is poor and is often fatal.

Classifications of Heart Failure

There are three primary classifications of HF: systolic vs. diastolic failure; left ventricular vs. right ventricular failure; and acute vs. chronic failure.

▮ Systolic vs. Diastolic Failure

Although both types of dysfunction are often present in HF, systolic HF reflects impaired contractile function whereas diastolic HF results from reduced ventricular compliance.

▮ Left Ventricular vs. Right Ventricular Failure

Both left and right ventricular dysfunction are present in HF. Blood accumulates within the chamber that first fails. Because contractility is altered, there is an accumulation of blood in the left ventricle, the left atrium, and the pulmonary circulation; hence, left ventricular failure occurs. Left ventricular failure is responsible for the signs and symptoms of pulmonary edema and reduced systemic cardiac output. However, because the cardiovascular structures are a closed system, failure of one ventricle frequently progresses to failure of the other.

Right ventricular failure produces elevated jugular venous pressure and peripheral edema. It is common for right-sided HF to follow left-sided failure; however, the reverse is rare. Right ventricular HF is most often caused by pulmonary vasoconstriction due to hypoxia from COPD. Right-sided failure due to pulmonary disease is referred to as *cor pulmonale.*

▮ Acute vs. Chronic Failure

Acute and chronic failure are sometimes referred to as *high-output* (acute) *and low-output* (chronic) HF. Acute failure occurs when the heart is unable to meet the accelerated needs of the body. Causes of acute HF include sepsis, Paget's disease, anemia, thyrotoxicosis, arteriovenous fistula, pregnancy, and an acute MI.

Chronic HF occurs in most forms of heart disease, with the underlying symptoms developing slowly because of the various compensatory mechanisms in operation. The underlying problem is related to ineffective ventricular pumping and low cardiac output, which in turn is related to the increased metabolic needs of the body. Patients may have a superimposed acute HF caused by an aggravating factor such as uncontrolled atrial fibrillation.

The New York Heart Association (NYHA) classifies the functional capacity of patients with HF into four levels depending on the degree of effort needed to elicit symptoms (Table 34-2).

PHARMACOTHERAPEUTIC OPTIONS

In 1785, William Withering published his famous book, *An Account of the Foxglove and Some of Its Medical Uses: With Practical Remarks on Dropsy and Other Diseases.* Indeed, the most current drugs used in the treatment of HF include the cardiac glycosides, but also comprise phosphodiesterase inhibitors, ACEIs, ARBs, diuretics, and vasodilators; and soon a newer class of inotropic drugs will join them, the calcium sensitizers. This chapter focuses on the cardiac glycosides and the phosphodiesterase inhibitors. Chapter 35 provides further discussion of beta blockers, Chapter 37 discusses vasodilators,

TABLE 34-2 New York Heart Association Functional Classification of Heart Failure

Class	Definition
I	IA. No limitation of physical activity. Ordinary physical activity does not cause undue fatigue or dyspnea.
	IB. Patients may have symptoms of HF only at levels that would produce symptoms in healthy individuals.
II	Slight limitation of physical activity. Comfortable at rest, but ordinary physical activity results in fatigue or dyspnea.
III	Marked limitation of physical activity. Comfortable at rest, but less than ordinary activity causes fatigue and dyspnea
IV	Unable to carry out any physical activity without symptoms. Symptoms are present even at rest. If any physical activity is undertaken, symptoms are increased.

Heart Failure Society of America. (2006). 2006 HFSA Comprehensive Heart Failure Practice Guideline. *Journal of Cardiac Failure, 12*(1). Available online: www.heartfailureguideline.com/. Accessed May 7, 2007.

ACEIs, and ARBs, and Chapter 42 discusses the diuretics. Box 34-1 identifies key terminology necessary to appreciate the action and effects of cardiovascular drugs.

Angiotensin-Converting Enzyme Inhibitors

Recognition that patients with HF often have elevated peripheral vascular resistance led to the introduction of vasodilator therapy. Of the vasodilators, the ACEIs appear to be the most efficacious because they counteract the major adverse hormonal and vasoconstrictor mechanisms, relieve symptoms, diminish ventricular dilation after myocardial infarction, and improve exercise capacity and ejection fraction (EF).

BOX 34-1

Terminology

Inotropic Actions
- *Positive inotropic* actions increase the contractile forces of the heart, causing the ventricles to empty more completely, thus improving cardiac output. Positive inotropic drugs include digoxin, a cardiac glycoside, and adrenergic drugs such as dobutamine, dopamine, epinephrine, and isoproterenol (see also Chapters 14 and 36).
- *Negative inotropic* actions weaken or decrease the force of myocardial contraction. Negative inotropic drugs include lidocaine, quinidine, and propranolol (see Chapter 36).

Chronotropic Actions
- *Positive chronotropic* actions accelerate the heart rate by increasing the rate of impulse formation at the sinoatrial (SA) node. An example of a positive chronotropic drug is norepinephrine.
- *Negative chronotropic* actions slow the heart rate by decreasing the rate of impulse formation. An example of a negative chronotropic drug is propranolol.

Dromotropic Actions
- *Positive dromotropic* action increases the speed with which impulses from the SA node pass through conduction pathways (i.e., the conduction velocity). An example of a positive dromotropic drug is phenytoin.
- *Negative dromotropic* action decreases conduction velocity. Example of drugs with a negative dromotropic action is verapamil, a calcium channel blocker.

The clinical and mortality benefits of ACEI have been shown in numerous uncontrolled and controlled, randomized clinical trials (e.g., SOLVD [The SOLVD Investigators, 1991], RESOLVD [The RESOLVD Investigators, 1999]). ACEIs are now recommended for patients with asymptomatic HF who have an LVEF of less than 40%. In patients with evidence for or a prior history of fluid overload, ACEIs are usually used in combination with diuretics.

Angiotensin Receptor Blockers

The ARBs were developed to offer the advantages of increased selectivity and specificity and to maintain blockade of the circulating and tissue renin-angiotensin-aldosterone system (RAAS) at the angiotensin-1 receptor, without the adverse effects associated with ACEIs (Table 34-3). When ARBs were first introduced to the marketplace, it was thought that reducing the production of angiotensin II with an ACEI and opposing the remaining angiotensin II with an ARB would be more efficacious than either drug alone; however, the VAL-Heft trial showed that adding an ARB to ACEI regimen is not beneficial.

Two ARBs are approved for use in HF: valsartan (Diovan) and candesartan (Atacand). However, of the seven ARBs currently on the market, losartan (Cozaar) has been the most extensively studied in patients with HF. Losartan lowers blood pressure, peripheral vascular resistance, pulmonary capillary wedge pressure (PCWP), and heart rate, and raises cardiac output. Losartan also decreases dyspnea on exertion and exacerbation of HF. Compared with the ACEI enalapril (Vasotec), losartan demonstrates no significant difference in terms of clinical status, the incidence of adverse effects, neurohumoral activation, altered exercise capacity, or laboratory evaluation. Losartan was also associated with fewer hospital admissions for any reason and less all-cause mortality than captopril (Capoten), another ACEI.

ARBs act by blocking angiotensin II at the receptor sites. ARBs do not block the degradation of vasoactive substances such as bradykinin, enkephalins, and substance P, and may not cause the adverse effects such as cough related to ACEI-induced accumulation of bradykinin.

The adverse effects of ARBs include first-dose hypotension, which may also occur with upward titration of the drug or when the patient's clinical status worsens. Hypotension is most likely to be a problem in patients with hyponatremia, hypovolemia, low baseline blood pressure, renal impairment, and high baseline levels of renin or aldosterone. Potentiation of bradykinin and prostaglandins by these states appear to contribute to the hypotension.

Beta Blockers

In the past, use of beta blockers has been contraindicated in HF. The negative inotropic and chronotropic actions and the peripheral vasoconstriction of beta blockers can all worsen HF. With HF, the nervous system is overstimulated, which raises norepinephrine levels. The increased levels of circulating norepinephrine cause myocardial remodeling and are directly toxic to myocardial cells, increasing the risk of hospitalization and death. On the other hand, prolonged activation of the SNS accelerates progression of HF. Research has now determined that the risk of HF progression can be considerably decreased by using drugs that interfere

TABLE 34-3 Recommended Therapy by Stage of Heart Failure

Stage	Patients With:	Goals	Therapy
A	Hypertension Atherosclerosis Diabetes Obesity Metabolic syndrome Cardiotoxic drugs Family history of cardiomyopathy	Treat hypertension Encourage smoking cessation Treat lipid disorders Encourage regular exercise Discourage alcohol intake, illicit drugs Control metabolic syndrome	**DRUG(S):** ACEIs • captopril • enalapril • fosinopril • lisinopril • quinapril • ramipril (post-MI*) • trandolapril (post-MI*) ARBs • candesartan • valsartan (post-MI*)
B	Previous MI LV remodeling including LVH and EF <40%	Same as above	**DRUG(S):** ACEIs or ARBs Beta blockers • bisoprolol • carvedilol (post-MI*) • metoprolol succinate **DEVICES:** • Implantable defibrillators
C	Known structural heart disease *and* shortness of breath and fatigue; reduced exercise tolerance	Same as above *plus* Dietary salt restriction	**DRUGS FOR ROUTINE USE:** Diuretics • Thiazides† • Loops‡ • Potassium-sparing§ • Sequential nephron blockade‖ ACEIs Beta blockers **DRUGS FOR SELECTED PATIENTS:** Aldosterone antagonists • eplerenone¶ (post-MI*) • spironolactone ARBs digoxin hydralazine, nitrates **DEVICES:** Biventricular pacing Implantable defibrillators
D	Marked symptoms at rest despite maximal medical therapy (e.g., those recurrently hospitalized or cannot be safely discharged without specialized interventions)	Same as for A, B, and C above *plus* Decisions regarding appropriate level of care	End-of-life care; hospice **EXTRAORDINARY MEASURES:** • Heart transplant • Chronic inotropes • Permanent mechanical support • Experimental surgery or drugs

Stage A: At risk for HF but without structural heart disease or symptoms of HF. ACEIs are the cornerstones of therapy for HF. They should be prescribed for all patients with EF less than 40%, even those who are asymptomatic.
Stage B: Structural heart disease but without signs or symptoms of HF.
Stage C: Structural heart disease with prior or current symptoms of HF. Used for patients with volume overload. Decreased K$^+$ levels (less than 4.0 mEq/L) may precipitate potentially dangerous arrhythmias, even in patients without a history of arrhythmias. K$^+$ should be used to correct hypokalemia for patients who are treated with non–K$^+$-sparing diuretics. Use of digoxin or spironolactone should be considered in patients with NYHA class III/IV HF. In a patient with mild HF, use a K$^+$-sparing diuretic when serum K$^+$ level is less than 4.0 mEq/L.
Stage D: Refractory HF requiring specialized interventions.
*Reduction in HF or other cardiac events following MI.
†Thiazide diuretics: chlorothiazide, chlorthalidone, hydrochlorothiazide, indapamide, metolazone.
‡Loop diuretics: bumetanide, furosemide, torsemide.
§Potassium-sparing: amiloride, spironolactone, triamterene.
‖Sequential nephron blockade: metolazone plus loop diuretic; hydrochlorothiazide plus loop diuretic; chlorothiazide IV plus loop diuretic.
¶Eplerenone, although also a diuretic, is primarily used in chronic HF as a suppressor of the RAAS.
ACE, Angiotensin-converting enzyme; *ACEI,* angiotensin-converting enzyme inhibitor; *ARB,* angiotensin II–receptor blocker; *EF,* ejection fraction; *HF,* heart failure; *LV,* left ventricular; *LVH,* left ventricular hypertrophy; *MI,* myocardial infarction; *RAAS,* renin-angiotensin-aldosterone system.
Adapted from the ACC/AHA 2005 Guideline Update for the diagnosis and management of chronic heart failure in the adult. *Journal of the American College of Cardiology, 46*(6), e1–82 and *Circulation 112*(12), e154-e235. The classification is meant to complement but not replace the New York Heart Association (NYHA) functional classification, which primarily gauges the severity of symptoms in patients in stages C or D heart failure.

CARDIOVASCULAR

TABLE 34-4 Large Beta Blocker Trials in Heart Failure

Studies	Patient HF Class			Relative Risk Reduction with Beta Blocker			
	2	3	4	All-Cause Mortality	Heart-Related Mortality	All-Cause Hospitalization	Heart-Related Hospitalization
US Carvedilol HF Study*	582 53%	480 44%	32 3%	65%	63%	NA	27%
MERIT-HF†	1636 41%	2210 55%	145 4%	34%	38%	12.6%	19.8%
CIBIS-II‡	0 0%	2202 83%	445 17%	33%	29%	20%	36%
BEST§	0 0%	2491 92%	217 8%	8.5%	12.5%	NA	16.7%
COPERNICUS‖	0	0	2289	11.4%	35%	27%	40%
A-HeFT¶	—	1050		43%	43%	NA	33%

*Target dose: 25–50 mg carvedilol twice daily, based on patient weight. Trial stopped early: carvedilol patients' 65% lower risk of death than placebo patients and a reduced risk for hospitalization for heart causes.

†Target dose: 190 mg metoprolol ER daily. Trial stopped early: metoprolol patients had 34% lower risk of death than placebo patients. Metoprolol reduced mortality and all-cause hospitalization by 19%. All-cause mortality plus hospitalization went down 31%. All-cause hospitalization alone was lowered by 13%, hospitalization for all heart-related causes by 20%, and hospitalization for worsening HF by 32%.

‡Target dose: bisoprolol 10 mg daily. Trial stopped early: risk of death in the bisoprolol group was 33% lower than in placebo group. Bisoprolol patients had fewer heart-related deaths and were hospitalized less.

§Target dose: 50–100 mg bucindolol twice daily, based on patient weight. Study stopped early: no difference in all-cause mortality between bucindolol and placebo groups. However, there were fewer heart-related deaths with bucindolol. The EF was increased with bucindolol. Fewer bucindolol patients were hospitalized for HF. Black patients did not have any survival benefit with bucindolol.

‖Target dose: 3.125 mg carvedilol twice daily, titrated upward every 2 weeks to 25 mg twice daily. Study stopped early: highly significant survival benefit in group treated with carvedilol compared with placebo.

¶Target dose: total daily dose of 225 mg hydralazine and 120 mg isosorbide dinitrate. Study stopped early: significantly higher mortality in the placebo group. Mean composite score significantly better in the group treated with both drugs. Improved quality of life scores in active treatment arm.

A-HeFT, African-American heart failure trial; *CIBIS*, cardiac insufficiency bisoprolol study; *COPERNICUS*, carvedilol prospective randomized cumulative survival; *EF*, ejection fraction; *ER*, extended release; *MERIT-HF*, metoprolol CR/XL randomized intervention trial in congestive heart failure; *NA*, not applicable.

with SNS activity on the heart and periphery (Table 34-4). Thus beta blockers are now used to improve symptoms and clinical status and decrease the risk of hospitalization and death in patients with class II HF (NYHA class II), or moderate to severe failure in patients with an EF of less than 35% to 40%.

Vasodilators

HF affects about 5 million Americans, including about 750,000 blacks, and this number is expected to grow to 900,000 by the year 2010. Further, blacks with HF are more likely to die from HF at an earlier age than whites. Given this information, in 2005, the Food and Drug Administration approved hydralazine with isosorbide dinitrate (BiDil), specifically for black patients. This drug significantly reduces the number of hospitalizations and the risk for death in the black population. The approval of this combination drug is especially noteworthy because **blacks between ages 45 and 64 years are 2.5 times more likely to die from HF than whites in the same age range**. There is no cure for HF, and more than half of patients die within 5 years of diagnosis.

The hydralazine component of BiDil relaxes coronary arteries so there is less difficulty perfusing the heart muscle. The isosorbide dinitrate component relaxes both veins and arteries equally. Isosorbide dinitrate acts by releasing nitric oxide at vessel walls; the hydralazine may avert the loss of this effect. Exactly how the drugs work in combination to improve HF remains unclear. The pharmacokinetics of this combination of drugs is similar to those of each of the drugs used alone.

The common adverse effects of BiDil include amblyopia, headache, dizziness, asthenia, rhinitis and sinusitis, low blood pressure, tachycardia, bronchitis, hyperglycemia, and nausea. The serious adverse effects include angioedema, a lupuslike syndrome, severe hypotension, blood dyscrasias, peripheral neuritis, and methemoglobinemia.

BiDil is taken orally at a starting dosage of 37.5 hydralazine/20 mg of isosorbide dinitrate 3 times daily. The dosage may be adjusted based on patient response. Adverse effects include headaches and dizziness.

Cardiac Glycoside

Indications

Digoxin (Lanoxin, Lanoxicaps; ◆ Lanoxin, Lanoxicaps) used alone, or in combination with diuretics and vasodilators, has traditionally been used in the management of HF. In addition, digoxin is occasionally used to control the ventricular rate of patients with atrial fibrillation, atrial flutter, and paroxysmal atrial tachycardia (PAT). In a sense, digoxin is palliative in that it improves cardiac functioning without treating the underlying cause. It is most useful for patients with a dilated heart, a low EF, and an S_3 gallop.

Pharmacodynamics

Digoxin produces a mild inotropic effect by inhibiting the sodium-potassium–adenosine triphosphatase (Na^+-K^+-ATPase) enzyme. This enzyme normally hydrolyzes adenosine triphosphate (ATP) to provide the energy needed for the Na^+ pump to release Na^+ and transport K^+ into the cardiac cell during repolarization. By binding specifically to the Na^+-K^+-ATPase complex, digoxin inhibits active transport of Na^+ and K^+ across cell membranes. With the complex inhibited, more calcium is allowed to enter the cell, rendering it irritable and providing for a greater force and velocity of myocardial contraction. The mild positive inotropic action thus increases cardiac output, which in turn reduces preload

PHARMACOKINETICS
TABLE 34-5 Inotropic Drugs

Drug	Route	Onset	Peak	Duration	PB (%)	t½	BioA (%)
CARDIAC GLYCOSIDE							
digoxin	PO	0.5–2 hr	6–8 hr	2–4 days	20–30	26–52 hr	57–83
	IV	5–30 min	1–5 hr			32–48 hr	100
PHOSPHODIASTERASE INHIBITORS							
inamrinone	IV	2–5 min	10 min	2 hr	35–49	3.6–5.8 hr	100
milrinone	IV	Immed	UA	Varies	70	2.3 hr	100

BioA, Bioavaliability; *Immed*, immediate; IV, intravenous; *PB*, protein binding; *PO*, by mouth; *t½*, half-life.

and, secondarily, the LVED pressure, while at the same time there is no overall increase in oxygen consumption. However, ATPase is further inhibited when serum K^+ or serum magnesium levels are too low, leading to arrhythmias.

Pharmacokinetics

Digoxin is completely absorbed from the gastrointestinal (GI) tract, primarily the jejunum. Digoxin tablets are 60% to 85% absorbed, whereas liquid-filled capsules are 90% to 100% absorbed and elixirs approximately 75% to 80% (Table 34-5).

Digoxin is slowly, but widely, distributed to the heart, the kidneys, the liver, the intestine, the stomach, and skeletal muscle. Serum levels are not significantly altered by body fat concentration. At equilibrium, serum concentrations in the myocardial tissues are 15 to 30 times that of plasma. Fourteen percent of digoxin is biotransformed by hepatic enzymes, with the drug almost entirely eliminated by the kidneys. The half-life of orally administered digoxin is dependent on adequate renal function and the oral formulation used. Digoxin crosses the blood-brain barrier and placental membranes and is found in breast milk.

Adverse Effects and Contraindications

Central nervous system (CNS) adverse effects of digoxin include headache, drowsiness, fatigue, and confusion. CNS adverse effects are most common in older adults. Visual disturbances appear as blurred vision or double vision. White borders or halos may appear on dark objects (hence the term "*white vision*"), and the objects may appear frosted. Color vision may be disturbed, with the colors green and yellow most commonly affected (chromatopsia). In some cases red, brown, and blue colors are also affected.

Noncardiac symptoms are related to the CNS and the GI tract. Diarrhea may also be noted and, in rare cases, it is the only GI sign of digoxin toxicity. Abdominal discomfort often accompanies other symptoms. Because adverse effects are caused, at least in part, by stimulation of the chemoreceptor trigger zone in the medulla, nausea occurs with parenteral as well as oral forms of the drug.

Gynecomastia, although rare, can be seen in both sexes and is related to the steroid component of digoxin. Generalized muscle weakness and fatigue are particularly prominent. Other less common adverse effects include pruritus, mental depression, and respiratory depression. The noncardiac symptoms do not always precede cardiac symptoms.

Signs of digoxin toxicity develop in approximately 20% ▲ of patients with HF, and up to 18% of patients with digoxin toxicity die from the subsequent arrhythmias. The earliest sign of chronic digoxin toxicity is anorexia, but this is often overlooked.

High serum levels of digoxin are typically associated ▲ with rhythm disturbances. The therapeutic effect of slowing conduction through the atrioventricular (AV) node, although beneficial and desirable in most cases of HF, can also produce varying degrees of arrhythmias and heart block. Cardiac toxicity manifested by arrhythmias can take the form of almost any known rhythm disturbance. For example, premature ventricular contractions (PVCs) are among the most common digoxin-induced arrhythmias and are usually described by the patient as "skipped beats." PVCs can arise from several causes, however, and are not specific to digoxin toxicity. Bradycardia, a slowing of the pulse rate to 60 beats/min (bpm) or less, is an extension of the drug's therapeutic action of slowing AV nodal conduction and of sinoatrial (SA) nodal suppression.

DIGOXIN TOXICITY. Toxicity to digoxin is relatively common, occurring in 10% to 20% of patients, and can be life threatening. The overall incidence of toxicity is uncertain, but it has been estimated that approximately 25% of hospitalized patients taking digoxin show some signs and symptoms. It is important, therefore, to understand the signs and symptoms that point to toxicity.

There are two primary causes of digoxin toxicity: ▲ improper dosing, and hypokalemia secondary to the concurrent administration of diuretics. The most obvious cause of toxicity is the administration of too large a dose of digoxin. However, the overdosage may result from a health care provider's decision, the patient independently increasing the dosage, or increased absorption of the drug. For example, increased absorption may occur as the result of changing to a formulation with greater bioavailability. Rapid intravenous (IV) administration produces toxicity. Decreased renal elimination increases serum concentrations of the drug to a toxic level. Hypothyroidism increases the likelihood of digoxin toxicity because elimination of the digoxin is reduced and because the heart is more sensitive to the drug.

K^+ loss can occur with non–K^+-sparing diuretics as a result of vomiting or diarrhea, steroid or laxative use, concurrent use of certain extended-spectrum penicillins (e.g., carbenicillin, ticarcillin, piperacillin, mezlocillin), or amphotericin B, an antifungal drug. Poor dietary intake of K^+, the continuous use of K⁺-free IV solutions, and dialysis may also contribute to low serum K⁺ levels.

In addition, abnormally large concentrations of serum Ca^{++} may also contribute to toxicity. A hypercalcemic state can result from sustained bed rest, multiple myeloma, parathyroid disease, or iatrogenic Ca^{++} supplements. A low serum magnesium level, commonly found in persons who abuse alcohol, produces effects similar to those of hypercalcemia.

⚠ Heart rates below 60 bpm in adults or below 90 bpm in children are considered undesirable and generally contraindicate further dosing until the patient's heart rate improves. Likewise, prolongation of the PR interval (indicating depressed AV conduction rate), a shortened QT interval, and an altered P wave also necessitate evaluation before giving another dose.

It is important to note, however, that not all rhythm disturbances are associated with high serum or tissue concentrations of digoxin and are not necessarily manifestations of toxicity. Moreover, low plasma concentrations of digoxin do not preclude the possibility of drug-induced arrhythmias. Serum concentrations provide a crude, although useful, guide to the likelihood of efficacy and toxicity. **A good rule of thumb ⚠ when evaluating a new rhythm disturbance in a patient receiving digoxin is to assume it is drug-induced until proven otherwise.**

When toxicity is diagnosed, the drug is discontinued. **Timely administration of antigen-binding fragments of ⚠ digoxin-specific antibody (Digibind) is appropriate if the toxicity is severe** (Table 34-6). The antibody, produced in sheep, acts antigenically to bind the cardiac glycoside, decreasing the concentration of free drug available to interact with myocardial membranes. Total plasma concentration of the cardiac glycoside rises markedly because of binding to the antibody, but the fraction of free drug in the plasma is reduced to extremely low levels. Digibind is readily eliminated in the urine.

Contraindications to digoxin include hypersensitivity, uncontrolled ventricular arrhythmias, AV block, idiopathic hypertrophic subaortic stenosis (IHSS), constrictive pericarditis, and known alcohol intolerance. Exercise caution when using digoxin in patients with electrolyte abnormalities or a recent MI, and in older adults because of a particular sensitivity to toxic effects.

TABLE **34-6** Digibind for Overdose

Indications	Management of serious life-threatening overdose of digoxin
Pharmacodynamics	Binds to free digoxin in the serum
Pharmacokinetics	Absorption and distribution: 100%; widely distributed Onset: variable Biotransformation: liver; elimination: kidneys Duration of action: 2 to 6 hours
Adverse effects, contraindications	Hypokalemia, reemergence of atrial fibrillation, heart failure
Dosage	*When digoxin dosage is unknown*: 800 mg (20 vials) *When the dosage of digoxin is known:* Digibind dose (mg) = ingested glycoside dose (mg) × 0.8 × 40 *When dosage is known for digoxin capsules, or IV digoxin:* Digibind dose (mg) = ingested glycoside dose (mg) × 40

Single ingestion of digoxin overdose in adults and children:		
Quantity Ingested*	**Digibind (mg)**	**No. Digibind Units**
25	340	8.5
50	680	17
75	1000	25
100	1360	34
150	2000	50
200	2680	67

When adult serum digoxin concentration and weight in kg is known:						
Wt (kg)	**Serum Digoxin Concentration (mcg/mL)**					
	1	2	4	8	12	16	20
40	0.5	1	2	3	5	6	8
60	0.5	1	2	5	7	9	11
70	1	2	3	5	8	11	13
80	1	2	3	6	9	12	15
100	1	2	4	8	11	15	18

- Obtain serum digoxin levels prior to administration of Digibind.
- Continuously monitor ECG and VS before and during treatment.
- Patients with atrial fibrillation may develop a rapid ventricular response.
- Monitor serum K⁺ levels since they may rapidly drop, especially during the first few hours of administration.
- Treat hypokalemia promptly.
- Skin test patients who have a history of allergy to Digibind or sheep proteins.

*Number of 0.25 mg digoxin tablets or 0.2 mg capsules ingested.
ECG, Electrocardiogram; *IV,* intravenous; *K⁺,* potassium; *VS,* vital signs.

DRUG INTERACTIONS
TABLE 34-7 Inotropic Drugs

Drug	Interactive Drug	Interaction
CARDIAC GLYCOSIDE		
digoxin	Adrenocorticosteroids, amphotericin B, Loop and thiazide diuretics, mezlocillin, piperacillin, ticarcillin	Increases risk for hypokalemia that can lead to digoxin toxicity
	amiodarone, Anticholinergics, cyclosporine, diltiazem, diflunisal, hydroxychloroquine, propafenone, quinidine, spironolactone, verapamil	Increases serum levels leading to increased risk of toxicity
	Beta blockers, diltiazem, quinidine, verapamil, disopyramide	Additive bradycardia
	Antacids, Antidiarrheals, cholestyramine, colestipol, Laxatives, Oral aminoglycosides	Decreases absorption and effectiveness of cardiac glycoside
	magnesium sulfate, succinylcholine, Thyroid preparations	Increases risk for arrhythmias and cardiac toxicity
	indomethacin	Decreases excretion of glycoside
PHOSPHODIESTERASE INHIBITORS		
inamrinone	furosemide, Glucose-containing IV solutions, sodium bicarbonate	Precipitates in IV line
	disopyramide	Hypotension
milrinone	digoxin	Additive effects

Drug Interactions

Drug interactions with digoxin are many (Table 34-7). Additive, synergistic, and even antagonistic effects can occur. Biotransformation of digoxin is enhanced with the concurrent administration of hepatic enzyme–inducing drugs such as phenobarbital, rifampin, and phenytoin.

Concurrent ingestion of a high-fiber meal may decrease the absorption of digoxin. Advise patients to avoid milk, cheeses, yogurt, and ice cream for at least 2 hours before and after taking digoxin.

Dosage Regimens

At any given maintenance dose, there is a close correlation between creatinine clearance and the concentration of digoxin in the plasma. Before administering an initial loading dose of digoxin, determine if the patient has taken any other formulations in the previous 2 to 3 weeks.

DIGITALIZING DOSAGES. For rapid effects, a larger initial loading dose (*digitalizing dose*) may be given several times (e.g., every 4 to 8 hours by IV route, or every 6 hours by mouth) over 12 to 24 hours. Digitalization allows saturation of plasma proteins and other body tissues before therapeutic serum concentrations are achieved. Nomograms and formulas are available to estimate digoxin dosage. However, most calculations are based on the patient's body weight (Table 34-8). In any given situation, loading doses are somewhat relative depending on age, body size, and the medical condition of the patient, the formulation, and the route of administration.

MAINTENANCE DOSES. Maintenance doses are based on the patient's renal function and individual response and on the proportion of daily losses. However, dosages of digoxin that achieve a concentration of drug in plasma in the range of 0.5 to 1 ng/mL are suggested given the limited evidence currently available. There have been no randomized clinical trials of the relative efficacy or safety of different plasma concentrations of digoxin. Some health care providers have voiced concerns that serum digoxin levels that are consistently in the therapeutic range (0.8 to 2 ng/mL) over the short term may cause harmful effects in the long run.

Dosages required for atrial arrhythmias are higher than those for inotropic effects. In patients taking digoxin who have normal renal function, this is about 35% of total body stores. Whether the desired effect has been achieved is evaluated through careful and frequent observation of the patient. Electrocardiograms (ECGs) and plasma drug levels are helpful in adjusting the dosage. Evaluation of therapeutic response includes noting changes in the signs and symptoms of HF, such as weight loss, reduced venous pressure, and improved exercise tolerance.

Lab Considerations

Evaluate digoxin levels, serum electrolytes, and hepatic function periodically throughout therapy. Hypokalemia, hypomagnesemia, and hypercalcemia make the patient more susceptible to toxicity. There are no known drug-laboratory test alterations with digoxin.

Phosphodiesterase Inhibitors

◆ inamrinone (Inocor); ◆ Inocor
◆ milrinone (Primacor); ◆ Primacor

Inamrinone

Inamrinone is the only phosphodiesterase inhibitor approved for use in the United States for the short-term management (2 to 3 days) of heart failure in patients who have not responded to diuretics, digoxin, or vasodilators. The official name of amrinone was changed to inamrinone by the United States Pharmacopeia nomenclature committee and the United States Adopted Name council effective July 1, 2000. The drug was discovered in a search for positive inotropic drugs that had a better therapeutic/toxic ratio than digoxin. When given to digitalized patients, inamrinone increases stroke volume and cardiac output, decreases left ventricular end diastolic pressure and pulmonary artery wedge pressure, promotes vasodilation, and increases exercise tolerance.

DOSAGE
TABLE **34-8 Inotropic Drugs**

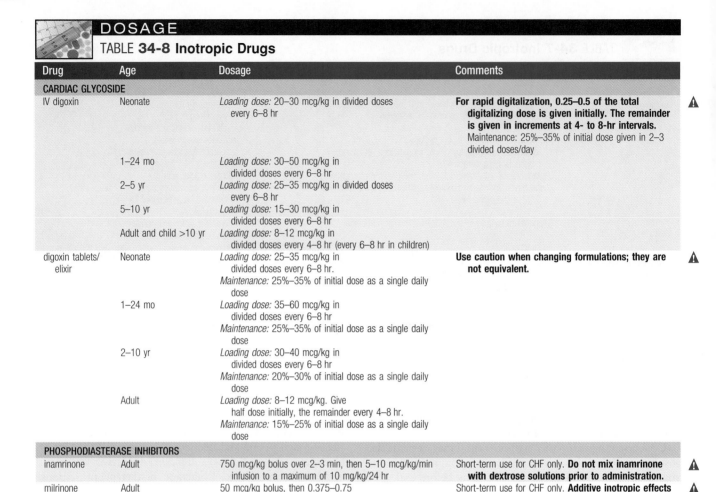

Drug	Age	Dosage	Comments
CARDIAC GLYCOSIDE			
IV digoxin	Neonate	*Loading dose:* 20–30 mcg/kg in divided doses every 6–8 hr	**For rapid digitalization, 0.25–0.5 of the total digitalizing dose is given initially. The remainder is given in increments at 4- to 8-hr intervals.** Maintenance: 25%–35% of initial dose given in 2–3 divided doses/day ⚠
	1–24 mo	*Loading dose:* 30–50 mcg/kg in divided doses every 6–8 hr	
	2–5 yr	*Loading dose:* 25–35 mcg/kg in divided doses every 6–8 hr	
	5–10 yr	*Loading dose:* 15–30 mcg/kg in divided doses every 6–8 hr	
	Adult and child >10 yr	*Loading dose:* 8–12 mcg/kg in divided doses every 4–8 hr (every 6–8 hr in children)	
digoxin tablets/ elixir	Neonate	*Loading dose:* 25–35 mcg/kg in divided doses every 6–8 hr. *Maintenance:* 25%–35% of initial dose as a single daily dose	**Use caution when changing formulations; they are not equivalent.** ⚠
	1–24 mo	*Loading dose:* 35–60 mcg/kg in divided doses every 6–8 hr *Maintenance:* 25%–35% of initial dose as a single daily dose	
	2–10 yr	*Loading dose:* 30–40 mcg/kg in divided doses every 6–8 hr *Maintenance:* 20%–30% of initial dose as a single daily dose	
	Adult	*Loading dose:* 8–12 mcg/kg. Give half dose initially, the remainder every 4–8 hr. *Maintenance:* 15%–25% of initial dose as a single daily dose	
PHOSPHODIASTERASE INHIBITORS			
inamrinone	Adult	750 mcg/kg bolus over 2–3 min, then 5–10 mcg/kg/min infusion to a maximum of 10 mg/kg/24 hr	Short-term use for CHF only. **Do not mix inamrinone with dextrose solutions prior to administration.** ⚠
milrinone	Adult	50 mcg/kg bolus, then 0.375–0.75 mcg/kg/min infusion	Short-term use for CHF only. **Additive inotropic effects occur with digoxin use.** ⚠

Inamrinone does not inhibit Na⁺-K⁺-ATPase. Instead, the effects result from intracellular accumulation of cyclic adenosine monophosphate secondary to inhibition of phosphodiesterase III, the enzyme that normally degrades cyclic adenosine monophosphate. In so doing, it reduces preload and afterload by directly affecting vascular smooth muscle. The phosphodiesterase inhibitors do not stimulate α or β receptors or provoke the release of histamine or prostaglandins. They are considered nonglycoside, noncatecholamine drugs that relax vascular tone, thus decreasing peripheral and pulmonary vascular resistance and dilating coronary vessels.

Inamrinone is available only as an IV injection. Inamrinone is 100% bioavailable when given intravenously. The distribution sites of inamrinone are unknown, although it is 10% to 49% bound to plasma proteins. The effects of inamrinone can last up to 2 hours after the infusion is discontinued. One half of a dose of inamrinone is biotransformed in the liver. Sixty-three percent of the drug is eliminated in the urine as both parent compound and metabolites. Approximately 18% is eliminated in the stool.

The most common adverse effects of inamrinone include arrhythmias, thrombocytopenia, and tachyphylaxis. Dyspnea,

nausea, vomiting, diarrhea, hepatotoxicity, hypokalemia, fever, and hypersensitivity reactions are also possible adverse effects. The drug is contraindicated in patients with hypersensitivity to inamrinone or bisulfates and in patients with idiopathic hypertrophic subaortic stenosis (IHSS). It should be used with caution in patients with atrial fibrillation or flutter because it can increase ventricular response. In this case, pretreatment with digoxin may be necessary. Inamrinone should also be used with caution in patients who have had recent aggressive diuretic therapy and in pregnancy and lactation. Safe use in children younger than age 18 years has not been established.

Drug interactions with inamrinone are few, but they can be significant. There may be additive inotropic effects when inamrinone is used concurrently with digoxin. Hypotension may be exaggerated in the presence of disopyramide.

The dosage of inamrinone is adjusted based on patient response. Tachyphylaxis (rapid development of tolerance) develops within the first 72 hours.

Platelet counts, serum electrolytes, liver enzymes, and hepatic and renal function should be evaluated periodically throughout therapy. If the platelet count drops below 150,000/mm³, the health care provider should be promptly notified. Increased liver enzymes may indicate hepatotoxicity. Inamrinone may decrease serum potassium levels.

Milrinone

Milrinone is also used for the short-term management of heart failure unresponsive to conventional therapy with digoxin, diuretics, and vasodilators. It has been shown to increase myocardial contractility and to decrease preload and afterload by direct action on vascular smooth muscle. Its actions overall are similar to those of inamrinone. In general, milrinone in combination with digoxin for patients with moderately severe heart failure is no more effective than digoxin alone.

Adverse effects of milrinone include headache, tremor, hypotension, hypokalemia, thrombocytopenia, angina pectoris, and chest pain. Its life-threatening effects include supraventricular arrhythmias and ventricular arrhythmias. Milrinone has been associated with an increased mortality rate. Milrinone is contraindicated in patients with hypersensitivity, severe aortic or pulmonary valvular heart disease, and hypertrophic subaortic stenosis. It should be used cautiously in patients with a history of arrhythmias, electrolyte imbalances, and abnormal digoxin levels. Insertion of vascular catheters for patients receiving milrinone increased the risk for ventricular arrhythmias. Safety during pregnancy and lactation and in children has not been established.

Milrinone is 100% bioavailable, although its distribution is unknown. From 80% to 90% of milrinone is eliminated unchanged in the urine, with a half-life of 2.3 hours. The half-life is increased in patients with renal impairment.

Laboratory testing of electrolytes and renal function is required frequently during milrinone therapy. Hypokalemia should be corrected prior to administration to reduce the risk of arrhythmias. As with inamrinone, platelet counts are to be monitored throughout therapy.

On the Horizon

Levosimendan (Simdax), the first drug to reach clinical trials in a new class, is a Ca^{++}-sensitizing drug used in the treatment of acute and chronic HF in patients who have not improved with treatment with diuretics and vasodilators. Levosimendan use improves patient outcomes relative to the standard of care, and has the potential to reduce hospital costs associated with HF. Levosimendan also appears to be a safe alternative to dobutamine for treatment of acute, decompensated HF. Prospective clinical trials are still needed to confirm the effect of levosimendan on long-term survival and its role in HF in the setting of myocardial infarction.

Levosimendan shows signs of having a dual mechanism of action and is the most potent Ca^{++} sensitizer to date. It combines a positive inotropic action mediated by Ca^{++} and a vasodilator property via ATP-dependent K^+ channels, thus reducing the risk for myocardial necrosis. In addition, the drug also dilates coronary and peripheral vessels to improve coronary blood flow and reduce afterload. Levosimendan is a significant improvement over the classic inotropic drugs, such as digoxin, because of its ability to enhance inotropic action without a concurrent increase in cardiac events.

The short half-life of levosimendan is advantageous in that it reduces the risk for arrhythmias; however, there appears to be a small secondary increase in the QTc interval of 15 msec, but this has to be evaluated in relation to the ability of levosimendan to open ATP-sensitive K^+ channels. In addition, the drug has not been studied in patients with additional risk factors for torsades de pointes, a potentially deadly form of ventricular tachycardia.

CLINICAL REASONING

Treatment Objectives

The overall management of HF includes improving hemodynamics, identifying and correcting precipitating factors, relieving symptoms, and improving exercise tolerance and the patient's quality of life. This goal often is accomplished with the use of inotropic drugs. Symptom relief, improved exercise tolerance, and improved quality of life can be enhanced with drug therapy.

Consider drug therapy in all patients once symptomatic HF is documented and acute reversible precipitating factors are removed. Symptoms that warrant drug therapy include decreased exercise tolerance, orthopnea, shortness of breath, and nocturnal polyuria. Begin drug therapy immediately for patients with acute failure.

Treat the underlying cause of HF. If arrhythmias precipitated the failure, treat the arrhythmias accordingly. When the underlying cause is hypertension, antihypertensive drugs are helpful. Surgery may be required if valvular or septal defects are the contributing factors to HF.

Treatment Options

Patient Variables

Ensure that all patients with suspected or clinically evident HF have documented assessment of ventricular function (EF) before starting drug therapy. All patients with LV dysfunction (EF <40%) should be started on an ACEI.

LIFE-SPAN CONSIDERATIONS

Pregnant and Nursing Women. The incidence of heart disease in pregnant women ranges from 0.5% to 2%; however, HF still ranks high among the causes of death during pregnancy. Rheumatic fever, once responsible for 88% of cardiac disease during pregnancy, is now on the decline, and is responsible for only about 50% of cardiac disease cases in pregnancy; congenital heart disease now plays a more prominent role. However, because of increases in total body water and changes in cardiovascular, renal, and hormonal function, the woman with preexisting heart disease can develop HF. In addition, pregnancy in a woman with preexisting cardiac disease increases the risk for thromboembolism, palpitations, and fluid retention.

There is considerable controversy about how much of a drug crosses placental membranes. Because of the expansion of maternal blood volume and the increased glomerular filtration rate during pregnancy, a larger dosage of a drug may be necessary to maintain therapeutic serum levels as the pregnancy progresses. Balance the benefit of inotropic drugs with the potential for harm to the mother and the fetus.

Children and Adolescents. Drugs chosen for the treatment of pediatric HF are based on the child's symptomatology and the severity of the HF. Infants require higher dosages than adults because of increased renal clearance. The dosage regimen must be individualized according to the degree of maturity of the infant. Because drug dosages are determined in part by the child's weight, an increase in dosage will usually be necessary following a weight gain.

Older Adults. HF in older adults is a fairly common occurrence that increases with age. Resting systolic LV function appears to be preserved, but perhaps at the expense of LV enlargement. A dwindling of diastolic function has been documented in otherwise normal older adults. Exercise capacity declines with age, most likely from a combination of cardiac and peripheral vascular factors, and ventricular-vascular coupling (defined as the ratio of arterial elasticity to left ventricular systolic elasticity, and its components, at rest and during exercise). Although these cardiovascular changes tend to reduce exercise capacity, their impact on health and quality of life remains modest compared with the detrimental effects of HF. Signs and symptoms of HF in older adults include confusion, insomnia, wandering during the night, agitation, depression, anorexia, nausea, weakness, dyspnea, orthopnea, weight gain, and bilateral ankle edema. The management of HF in the older adult is basically the same as for middle-aged adults (see Case Study).

▥ Drug Variables

The revised Agency for Health Care Policy and Research (AHCPR) clinical practice guidelines changed the approach to the management of patients with HF. Routinely manage patients who have HF with a combination of three classes of drugs: a diuretic, an ACEI or an ARB, and a beta blocker (see Table 34-3). Few patients will be able to maintain "dry weight" (weight without extra fluid volume) without a diuretic. One pint (2 cups/16 ounces) of fluid equals 1 pound on the scale. The goal is to keep patients' weight within 4 pounds of their dry weight without using a diuretic. Digoxin may be started at any time to reduce symptoms, control heart rhythm, enhance exercise tolerance, and reduce the risk for hospitalizations. Health care providers today have a more complete understanding of strategies that will improve the prognosis of HF (i.e., by blocking the RAAS and SNS). Drugs noted to accomplish this goal include ACEIs, ARBs, beta blockers, diuretics, and calcium sensitizers (see Evidence-Based Pharmacotherapeutics box).

Three classes of drugs have been shown to exacerbate HF and are therefore not recommended for most patients (American College of Cardiology–American Heart Association [ACC-AHA] 2006 guidelines). (1) Antiarrhythmic drugs in general (although there are some exceptions) exert significant cardiodepressant and proarrhythmic effects. Of the available drugs, only amiodarone and dofetilide do not adversely affect survival. (2) Calcium channel blockers (CCBs) can worsen heart failure and are associated with an increased risk of cardiovascular events. Only the vasoselective CCBs have been shown not to adversely affect survival. (3) Nonsteroidal antiinflammatory

CASE STUDY   Inotropic Drugs

ASSESSMENT

History of Present Illness	MB is a 70-year-old black male admitted for evaluation of increasing fatigue and ankle edema. Until recently he was able to remain active. During the past month, the persistent dyspnea confined him to his home. He reports that the dyspnea awakens him at night, and he sits by an open window to "catch his breath." He reports he has "lost my good appetite." He feels the water pill he started 6 weeks ago is not working. Current meds: enalapril 2.5 mg PO twice daily and furosemide 20 mg PO daily. Records indicate previous non–drug therapies have failed. No known drug allergies.
Past Health History	MB had an acute MI 5 years ago with subsequent development of chronic HF. Since then, he has had occasional PVCs. Although he has a history of coronary artery disease (CAD), he attributes his otherwise healthy state to the fact that he never drank or smoked and that he always eats nutritious meals, including salads. "They are easy to fix and easy for my wife and me to eat. They are also cheaper than some other things."
Life-Span Considerations	MB reports he is "simply waiting for his turn to meet God." MB retired 3 years ago after 40 years as a railroad mechanic. On several occasions he has expressed concern that he will become a "cardiac cripple" to his wife, who is 74 years old and physically unable to assume the responsibility for his care. He feels that if he needs changes in his medicine, he wants to go to once-daily dosing so he will remember to take it. MB has one son and one daughter who live nearby. They visit their parents regularly and help with transportation to grocery store, medical appointments, and so forth. MB is covered by Medicare and a railroad supplemental insurance policy that includes pharmacy coverage. He and his wife live on his railroad retirement income.
Physical Exam Findings	*Ht:* 5'8". *Wt:* 195 lb (up 9 lb from usual weight). *VS:* 130/70, 98.6° F-120-28. Color pale, but no evidence of cyanosis. Skin warm and dry. ENT negative. No lymphadenopathy, thyromegaly, JVD, carotid bruits. Bibasilar breath sounds with crackles and rhonchi at the bases on auscultation. S_3 gallop present. Hepatomegaly. 2+ pitting edema of ankles.
Diagnostic Testing	CXR: Left ventricular enlargement with congestion of pulmonary vasculature; fluid level more prominent right side than left. ECG: Atrial fibrillation with apical rate of 124 bpm. Eight PVCs/tracing. Na^+ 131 mEq/L, K^+ 3.2 mEq/L, Cl^- 91 mEq/L, BUN 35 mg/dL, serum creatinine 1.6 mg/dL. TSH 3.25 mg/dL.

DIAGNOSIS: Worsening Heart Failure

MANAGEMENT

Treatment Objectives	Enhance cardiac performance. Relieve symptoms of heart failure. Identify and correct precipitating factors.
Treatment Options	**Pharmacotherapy** 1. Continue enalapril 2.5 mg PO twice daily. 2. Add hydralazine 37.5 mg with isosorbide dinitrate 20 mg PO 3 times daily. First dose at HS. 3. Continue furosemide 20 mg PO daily PRN for weight gain of more than 5 pounds/week. 4. Klor-Con 20 mEq PO today then PRN with each furosemide taken **Patient Education** 1. Low Na^+ diet; check with health care provider regarding the use of salt substitutes. 2. Do not restrict fluids unless advised by health care provider. 3. Obtain daily weights at the same time each day, on the same scale, and in similar clothing. Contact office if there is weight gain of more than 5 pounds in 1 week. 4. Importance of taking K^+ supplement each time furosemide is taken to minimize risk for hypokalemia and subsequent arrhythmias 5. Provide written listing of prescribed drugs, dosages, times to be taken, and the reasons for use. 6. Avoid concurrent use of other drugs without first checking with the health care provider. **Evaluation** • Breath sounds are clear of crackles and rhonchi. • Salt intake has been reduced and weight has come down by 5 pounds since last visit. • Patient understands the monitoring of heart rate, blood pressure, and weight so as to appropriately use his PRN furosemide and potassium. • Signs and symptoms of heart failure are relieved.

CLINICAL REASONING ANALYSIS

Q1. I thought you ordered two different drugs for MB. What is BiDil?

A. BiDil is an adjunct in the treatment of heart failure. It is a combination of hydralazine, a selective vasodilator of arterial smooth muscle and isosorbide dinitrate, a vasodilator that acts on both arteries and veins. Research has suggested that the combination of the two drugs improves survival, prolongs the time to hospitalization for heart failure, and improves patient-reported functional status.

Q2. Why did we need to add this drug in the first place? I thought patients with heart failure are supposed to take an ACE inhibitor?

A. And he will remain on the ACE inhibitor. We added BiDil because MB remains symptomatic despite the ACE inhibitor.

Q3. I thought we didn't need to worry about him taking K^+ if he is on an ACE inhibitor? Doesn't the ACE inhibitor cause K^+ retention?

A. ACE inhibitors conserve K^+. However, did you look at his serum K^+ level? It is at the low end of a normal range, which predisposes him to arrhythmias. He will use the loop diuretic furosemide.

Q4. Why did you tell MB to take his first dose of the combination drug at bedtime?

A. I told him that because vasodilating drugs have a first-dose phenomenon. That is, they can cause a drop in blood pressure with subsequent lightheadedness. If he goes to bed right after taking the drug, he is less likely to notice the initial dose's effects.

Q5. Why does he need to take the BiDil 3 times daily? Why not just once a day?

A. The isosorbide dinitrate component of BiDil has a half-life of about 2 hours. The half-life of hydralazine is about 4 hours. Relatively short half-lives require more frequent dosing. Also, isosorbide undergoes a rapid first-pass effect, and once steady state has been reached, isosorbide accumulates significantly in pectoral muscle and the walls of saphenous veins relative to the plasma concentration; these sites act as a storage depot of sorts.

🔍 EVIDENCE-BASED PHARMACOTHERAPEUTICS

Phosphodiesterase Inhibitors

■ Background

The introduction of phosphodiasterase inhibitors (PDEIs), such as inamrinone (previously known as amrinone) and milrinone was a major breakthrough in intravenous (IV) drug therapy for patients with HF. However, it has been suggested that PDEIs may actually do more harm.

Several possible explanations for the harmful effects of PDEIs on mortality have been proposed including the following: (1) an excessive increase of intracellular cAMP, which decreases in patients with chronic HF; (2) a proarrhythmic effect; or (3) a potentiation of the harmful effects of PDEIs with concomitant use of vasodilators. This last phenomenon may account either for the observed increase in mortality rate or for the adverse effects, such as hypotension, blurry vision, and syncope. Whether PDEIs exert direct proarrhythmic effects or hasten structural remodeling of the ventricle, thus providing a basis for ventricular tachycardia and fibrillation is unknown. The positive effects of ACEIs, of the combination of isosorbide dinitrate and hydralazine (BiDil), and of beta blockers on the incidence of sudden death appear related to the regression of ventricular remodeling and thus provide, conceivably, a link between ventricular dilation and lethal arrhythmias.

■ Research Article

Amsallem, E., Kasparian, C., Haddour, G., et al. (2005). Phosphodiesterase III inhibitors for heart failure. *Cochrane Database of Systematic Reviews* 2005, Issue 1. Art. No. CD002230. DOI: 10.1002/14651858.CD002230. pub2.

Purpose

The intent of this project was to analyze data obtained from all studies that used PDEIs (in relation to placebo) in the treatment of patients with symptomatic, chronic HF. The main outcomes were (1) total mortality; (2) HF requiring hospitalization, modification of treatment regimen, or withdrawal from the study; (3) occurrence of myocardial infarction, cardiac transplantation, or arrhythmias, as defined by the study's authors; (4) the presence of vertigo, dizziness, lipothymia, or syncopal episodes; and (5) etiology-specific mortality. The project also examined whether the therapeutic effects of treatment were constant in subgroups based on the severity of HF, the concurrent use of vasodilator drugs, and the specific PDEI used.

Design

This meta-analysis examined the use of PDEIs vs. placebo in 21 studies ($N = 8408$) having a follow-up duration of at least 3 months or more. Four PDEI drugs and eight molecules of PDEI were identified in the analyses.

Methods

Two investigators independently obtained data from the studies based on previously determined inclusion criteria. For each study that met inclusion criteria, an evaluation of methodology (i.e., allocation, concealment, and blinding) was done. PDEI studies were included if they were (1) randomized, placebo-controlled, double-blind studies of an orally administered PDEI drug; (2) had well-defined "a priori" end-points; (3) lasted a minimum of 3 months; (4) an intention-to-treat data sets were available for analyses; (5) no more than 10% of subjects were lost to follow-up on relevant clinical outcomes; and (6) subjects with NYHA classes II to IV HF were included provided subject age, range, and diagnosis criteria were present.

Findings

Compared with placebo, PDEIs were associated with a significant 17% increased mortality rate (relative risk [RR], 1.17; 95% confidence interval [CI], 1.06–1.30; $p = 0.001$). Further, PDEIs significantly increased cardiac deaths (RR 1.16; 95% CI 1.05–1.30; $p = 0.005$); sudden death (RR 1.30; CI 95% 1.11–1.152; $p = 0.001$), arrhythmias (RR 1.25; 95% CI 1.02–1.54; $p = 0.03$), and vertigo (RR 1.81; 95% CI 1.41–2.23; $p = 0.001$). There was a nonsignificant decrease for worsening of HF (RR 0.93; 95% CI 0.84–1.02; $p = 0.12$) and cardiac transplantation (RR 0.5; 95% CI 0.23–1.09; $p = 0.08$). There was also a nonsignificant increase in myocardial infarction (MI) (RR 1.41; 95% CI 0.82–2.43, $p = 0.21$). The adverse effects of PDEIs appears to be the same, given the mortality from all causes, regardless of whether vasodilators were or were not used concurrently, the severity of HF, or the PDEI used or its derivative.

Conclusions

PDEI use is associated with increased mortality rates in patients with chronic HF compared to placebo. The adverse effects were the same for all outcomes, including total mortality, mortality of cardiac origin, and sudden death. The results did not support the notion that increased mortality is the result of additional vasodilator use. The use of PDEIs, therefore, should be avoided in all HF patients.

■ Implications for Practice

A major bias innate to meta-analyses is the "iceberg phenomenon" or "file drawer" problem of unpublished trials. These trials often have nonsignificant results, whereas published trials often have significant results. Further, it is impractical to take into account the unavoidable differences in baseline characteristics of subjects, such as the cause of HF, or the duration of heart disease before joining the study. The percentage of subjects with ischemic heart disease likely differed from one trial to another, and the proportion of patients who died while taking the placebo, which is an indirect measure of the severity of heart failure, varied from 0% to 24%. The length of the actual follow-up studies varied from 3 to 52 months, but the meta-analytical approach assumes a constant therapeutic effect and a relative stability of the odds ratio over time.

Alternative strategies for patients with chronic HF must be considered. For example, studies may be conducted that use discontinuous treatment methodologies during periods of worsening HF. Replication studies could be carried out in further randomized, controlled trials that have suitable power, endpoints, and follow-up built into the study.

---

drugs (NSAIDs) should be avoided because they cause Na⁺ retention and peripheral vasoconstriction, and attenuate the efficacy and enhance the toxicity of diuretics and ACEIs.

Patient Education

One of the most common causes for exacerbation of HF is nonadherence to the low-Na⁺ diet, but control of excessive salt and water retention can be achieved by restricting salt intake. Sodium levels in the average American diet usually far exceed the recommended daily allowance of intake. Approximately 4 grams of Na⁺ are contained in the average 10 grams of table salt consumed daily. A 4-gram Na⁺ diet can be achieved by avoiding salty foods and not adding salt at the table. For people with more severe disease, a 2-gram Na⁺ diet (i.e., no added salt) may be prescribed. It is unusual to restrict fluid intake except with dilutional hyponatremia results. Advise patients to check with you or another health care provider before using salt substitutes. When treatment of HF with digoxin and diuretics necessitates concurrent use of K⁺ supplements, instruct the patient on which foods are good sources of K⁺.

Teach patients the name of the drug(s) taken, the dosages, and the reasons for use. Encourage them to carry the

Controversy

Inotropics: Expectations and Limitations

Jonathan J. Wolfe

Cardiotonic glycosides, derived from the plant genus *Digitalis,* established the classic definition of inotropic drugs. Their therapeutic use was established by William Withering in the eighteenth century. These drugs slow the pulse rate and simultaneously strengthen the force of cardiac contraction, thus providing a significant advantage in therapy that continues to have value today. As with most drugs, even these classic inotropic drugs present a mixed effect. The challenge now is to use them rationally in an era that offers the health care provider a broad choice of drugs, some of which are clearly superior for a given patient.

The advent of intravenous drugs has allowed rescue of patients once beyond the reach of treatment. Inamrinone represents an almost pure inotropic drug among injectable drugs, but dopamine and dobutamine are often considered as inotropes because of their predominant effects. The ability to resuscitate patients or help high-risk patients make a smooth transition through surgery and recovery with the aid of these drugs means that many more patients survive to require chronic therapy.

What drugs ought to be used for the long haul? The issue of this choice is clouded by cost. Digoxin is an inexpensive, elegant, and universally available product. However, it is not proper to try every patient who requires inotropic therapy on cardiac glycosides. The precision of diagnosis possible with present-day technology allows clear sorting of patients into categories whose best treatment is discoverable. The standard of practice has carried us far beyond the day of the stethoscope and monitoring of edema in the extremities. The same parallel exists in drug choice. The addition of new drugs allows increased sophistication in treatment, but requires vigilance in balancing the elements of a particular drug regimen.

CLINICAL REASONING ANALYSIS

1. Your patient has been stable on digoxin for 11 years. Her dosage has required little adjustment, except to decrease the dose around her eightieth birthday. Her general health is good, with only age-related decrease in renal function. A new calcium channel–blocking drug has come to market that may benefit her. What concerns do you have in regard to cost, compliance, and outcome for this patient?

2. The 18-month-old boy about to be discharged from your postsurgical care unit has done well since closure of his ventricular septal defect. He was smoothly digitalized after surgery and now receives oral liquid digoxin every 12 hours. What three points are most important for you to make in teaching his parents about giving this drug?

3. A 64-year-old man who has been your patient comes to the clinic today complaining of nausea, dizziness, and visual disturbance. He has been taking digoxin 250 mcg orally once daily without incident for the past 10 months. The only remarkable element of his history today is that he has decided to use vitamin and mineral supplements in order to bolster his health, as advised by a new book he bought at the Herbal Boutique in the nearby mall. What mineral would you be most concerned to find he is taking in megadose quantities?

information in written form. Patients should know how to take a radial pulse and to do so at least once daily. Advise them to take the drug at the same time each day to maintain consistent blood levels and to assist in remembering to take the drug. Also advise the patient to avoid concurrent use of other drugs without a health care consultation and to avoid taking antacids or antidiarrheal drugs within 2 hours of digoxin (if taken). Instruct patients to keep their drugs in the original containers and not to mix them in pill containers with other drugs. This helps to ensure patients do not make an error when taking their drugs and helps patients to remember which drugs still have to be taken.

Evaluation

Once therapeutic lifestyle changes and drug therapy are initiated, there should be improvement in dyspnea, orthopnea, and fatigue. The evaluation of drug therapy is based on the information obtained from the patient database. Generally the evaluation criteria include sufficient knowledge of the disease process and treatment regimen to actively participate in the plan of care; maintenance of a therapeutic blood level; reduction in symptoms; adherence with dietary modifications; and an understanding of, and adherence with, an exercise regimen.

The effectiveness of drug and non–drug therapies is demonstrated by an increase in cardiac output. Therefore there should be a decrease in the severity of the HF with fewer signs and symptoms of pulmonary congestion (dyspnea, orthopnea, cyanosis, cough, hemoptysis, crackles, anxiety, and restlessness). The pulmonary symptoms that develop with HF are the result of events initiated by insufficient cardiac output. The improved strength of myocardial contraction reverses the potentially fatal chain of events.

Fewer signs and symptoms of peripheral congestion (absence of pitting edema, decreased abdominal girth, and weight loss) are indicators of more effective right heart function. Increased activity tolerance indicates a more adequate blood supply to tissues. Diuresis and decreasing edema result from the improved circulation and renal blood flow. Therapeutic levels of drugs also alter certain aspects of the ECG. They cause a narrowing of the QRS complex, depress or invert the T waves, and slow the heart rate.

KEY POINTS

- HF develops when the pumping action of the heart is impaired and cardiac output falls below venous return.
- In left-sided failure there is an accumulation of blood in the left ventricle, the atrium, and pulmonary circulation. With right-sided failure, blood backs up in systemic circulation.
- Treatment objectives are to enhance cardiac performance, identify and correct precipitating factors, and relieve symptoms.
- Drug management of HF includes use of ACEIs, ARBs, diuretics, vasodilators, and digoxin.
- ACEIs are shown to reduce mortality rates and improve the quality of life.
- Diuretics, used alone or in combination with other drugs, decrease plasma volume and preload.

■ Venous and arterial vasodilators have recently been used to treat chronic HF. They act to decrease preload, afterload, or a combination of preload and afterload.

■ Digoxin reduces the workload of the heart, improves cardiac contractility, and increases renal blood flow. It is most useful for patients with a dilated heart, a low EF, and an S_3 gallop.

■ Digoxin produces positive inotropic effects and negative dromotropic and chronotropic effects.

■ An initial loading or digitalizing dose is used if a rapid response is desired.

■ The potential for digoxin toxicity increases in the presence of diuretics. The patient should be closely monitored for hypokalemia and signs and symptoms of toxicity.

■ Digibind may be used to manage severe digoxin toxicity.

■ Patients should be advised to continue non–drug therapies (e.g., low Na^+ diet, rest) while on drug therapies for HF.

■ The effectiveness of drug therapy is demonstrated by an increase in cardiac output and therefore a decrease in the severity of the HF, with fewer signs and symptoms of pulmonary congestion.

■ Therapeutic levels of digoxin produce a narrowing of the QRS complex, depress or invert the T wave, and slow the heart rate.

Bibliography

American College of Cardiology-American Heart Association. (2005). ACC/AHA 2005 Guideline update for the diagnosis and management of chronic heart failure in the adult. *Journal of the American College of Cardiology, 46*(6), 1116–1143.

Amsallem, E., Kasparian, C., and Haddour, G, et al. (2005). Phosphodiesterase III inhibitors for heart failure. *Cochrane Database of Systematic Reviews*, 2005, Issue 1. Art. No. CD002230. DOI: 10.1002/14651858.CD002230.pub2.

Boswell-Smith, V., Spina, D., and Page, C. (2006). Phosphodiasterase inhibitors. *British Journal of Pharmacology, 147*, S252–S257.

Camara, K., Chen, Q., and Rhodes, S., et al. (2004). Negative inotropic drugs alter indexes of cytosolic (Ca2+)-left ventricular pressure relationships after ischemia. *American Journal of Physiology and Heart Circulation Physiology, 287*(2), H667–H680.

Segev, A., and Mekori, Y. (1999). The cardiac insufficiency bisoprolol study II: A randomized trial. *Lancet, 353*(9146), 9–13.

CIBIS Investigators and Committees. (1994). A randomized trial of beta-blockade in heart failure: The cardiac insufficiency bisoprolol study (CIBIS). *Circulation, 90*(4), 1765–1773.

Crouch, M. (2006). Pharmacotherapy implications of revised chronic heart failure guidelines. *The Consultant Pharmacist, 21*(7), 576–582.

Domanski, M., Krause-Steinrauf, H., and Massie, B., et al. (2003). A comparative analysis of the results from 4 trials of beta-blocker therapy for heart failure: BEST, CIBIS-II, MERIT-HF, and COPERNICUS. *Journal of Cardiac Failure, 9*(5), 354–363.

Earl, G., and Fitzpatrick, J. (2005). Levosimendan: A novel inotropic agent for treatment of acute, decompensated heart failure. *The Annals of Pharmacotherapy, 39*(11), 1888–1896.

Ernhardt, L. (2005). An emerging role for calcium sensitization in the treatment of heart failure. *Expert Opinion on Investigational Drugs, 14*(6), 659–670.

Farrell, M., Foody, J., and Krumholz, H. (2002). Beta blockers in heart failure: Clinical applications. *Journal of the American Medical Society, 287*(7), 890–897.

Fowler, M. (2004). Carvedilol prospective randomized cumulative survival (COPERNICUS) trial: Carvedilol in severe heart failure. *American Journal of Cardiology, 93*(9A), 35B–39B.

Heart Failure Society of America. (2006). 2006 HFSA Comprehensive Heart Failure Practice Guideline. *Journal of Cardiac Failure, 12*(1). Available online:www.heartfailureguideline.com/. Accessed May 7, 2007.

Howard, P., Cheng, J., and Crouch, M., et al. (2006). Drug therapy recommendations from the 2005 ACC/AHA guidelines for treatment of chronic heart failure. *Annals of Pharmacotherapy, 40*(9), 1607–1617.

Hunt, S., Baker, D., and Chin, M., et al. (2001). ACC/AHA guidelines for the evaluation and management of chronic heart failure in the adult: Executive summary: A report of the American College of Cardiology/American Heart Association Task Force on Practice Guidelines (Committee to Revise the 1995 Guidelines for the Evaluation and Management of Heart Failure). *Circulation, 104*(24), 2996–3007.

Hurst, J., Morris, D., and Alexander, R. (1999). The use of the New York Heart Association's classification of cardiovascular disease as part of the patient's complete Problem List. *Clinical Cardiology, 22*(6), 385–390.

Lehtonen, L., Antila, S., and Pentikainen, P. (2004). Pharmacokinetics and pharmacodynamics of intravenous inotropic agents. *Clinical Pharmacokinetic, 43*(3), 187–203.

McBride, B., and White, C. (2003). Levosimendan: Implications for clinicians. *Journal of Clinical Pharmacology, 43*(10), 1071–1081.

McKee, P., Castelli, W., and McNamara, P., et al. (1971). The natural history of congestive heart failure: The Framingham study. *New England Journal of Medicine, 285*(26), 441–446.

MERIT-HF Study Group. (1999). Effect of metoprolol Cr/XL in chronic heart failure: Metoprolol CR/XL randomized intervention trial in congestive heart failure (MERIT-HF). *Lancet, 353*(9169), 2001–2007.

Persone, S., and Kaplinsky, E. (2005). Calcium sensitizer agents: A new class of inotropic agents in the treatment of decompensated heart failure. *International Journal of Cardiology, 3*(3), 248–255.

Rocci, M., and Wilson, H. (1987). The pharmacokinetics and pharmacodynamics of newer inotropic agents. *Clinical Pharmacokinetics, 13*(2), 91–109.

Swynhedauw, B., and Charlemagne, D. (2002). What's wrong with positive inotropic drugs? Lessons from basic science and clinical trials. *European Heart Journal Supplement, 4*(Suppl D), D43–D49.

Taylor, A., Ziesche, S., and Yancy, C., et al. (2004). The African-American Heart Failure Trial Investigators. Combination of isosorbide dinitrate and hydralazine in blacks with heart failure. *New England Journal of Medicine, 351*(20), 2049–2057.

The RESOLVD Investigators. (1999). Comparison of candesartan, enalapril, and their combination in congestive heart failure: Randomized evaluation of strategies for left ventricular dysfunction (RESOLVD) pilot study. *Circulation, 100*(10), 1056–1064.

The SOLVD Investigators. (1991). Effect of enalapril on survival in patients with reduced left ventricular ejection fractions and congestive heart failure. *New England Journal of Medicine, 325*(5), 293–302.

Wedel, H., Demets, D., and Deedwania, P., et al. (2001). Challenges of subgroup analyses in multinational clinical trials: Experiences from the MERIT-HF trial. *American Heart Journal, 142*(3), 502–511.

Withering, W. (1977). *An account of the foxglove and some of its medical uses: With practical remarks on dropsy and other diseases.* (Reprint of 1785 edition.) Wakefield, NH: Longwood.

Zineh, I., Schofield, R., and Johnson, J. (2003). The evolving role of nesiritide in advanced or decompensated heart failure. *Pharmacotherapy, 23*(10), 1266–1280.

Antianginal Drugs

In healthy individuals, coronary arteries supply blood to the myocardium, which adequately meets tissue metabolic demands. When sufficient oxygen extraction does not take place, coronary arteries dilate to increase the flow of oxygenated blood to the myocardium. However, a variety of pathologic mechanisms interfere with the ability of coronary arteries to dilate, thereby contributing to myocardial ischemia and anginal pain.

Angina pectoris (also known as angina) is not a disease in and of itself, but rather a symptom of coronary artery disease (CAD). Anginal pain can appear spontaneously and has a dramatic onset, usually intensifying during exercise and dissipating with rest. Drugs used in the management of angina are typically separated into three categories: nitrates, beta blockers, and calcium channel blockers. The purpose for using these groups of drugs for relief of anginal pain is to improve the balance between myocardial oxygen supply and demand.

ANGINA PECTORIS

EPIDEMIOLOGY AND ETIOLOGY

The term angina pectoris is derived from the Latin words *angere,* "to choke," and *pectoralis,* referring to the chest or breast. Although angina has many characteristics, the term is used to describe the sensation of choking or strangling in the chest area accompanied by anxiety or fear of death. The chest pain of angina is a sensory response to a transient lack of oxygen. Box 35-1 classifies the various types of angina.

Each year, there are an estimated 6.3 million people in the United States with angina. Additionally, there are 1.1 million newly diagnosed and recurrent acute coronary events, 40% of which are fatal. Angina, which is often atypical in presentation, is the most common complaint in women with CAD. Women also have a higher mortality rate from CAD compared with men, in part because women are older when diagnosed with angina and because of the lack of the classical signs of angina (Fig. 35-1).

Angina also occurs in patients with normal coronary arteries but is less common. Any condition that increases myocardial contractility or heart rate (e.g., exercise, stress, anemia, polycythemia, hyperthyroidism) raises the risk for an anginal episode. Left ventricular hypertrophy (LVH) caused by disorders that increase systemic vascular resistance (e.g., aortic stenosis, heart failure, high systolic blood pressure) also contribute to the risk for an anginal episode. Hypercholesterolemia, defined as excess cholesterol in the blood, and smoking are known risk factors for angina, hypertension, acute myocardial infarction (MI), and sudden coronary death.

BOX 35-1

Classifications of Angina

Stable Angina	Paroxysmal chest pain or discomfort provoked by physical exertion or emotional stress and relieved by correction of precipitating event, resting, and/or nitroglycerin. Predictable. Pain reaches maximal intensity before dissipating. Pain may occur in the morning (Fig. 35-3). Exists when characteristics of pain and precipitating factors have not changed for the past 30 days. An electrocardiogram (ECG) completed in early morning hours may show ST-T–wave abnormalities. Also known as classic, stable exertional, or predictable angina.
Unstable Angina	A change in the stability of a previously established pattern of pain or a new onset of severe angina. Symptoms at rest or which are triggered by minimal physical exertion. Seldom predictable. Onset and course of pain differ with each episode. Patient at high risk for myocardial infarction (MI). Symptoms may be only partially relieved by rest or vasodilating drugs. Also known as preinfarction angina, crescendo angina, or intermittent coronary syndrome.
Variant Angina	Related to vasospasm of coronary vessels. Not necessarily associated with atherosclerosis. Attacks may be cyclical, occurring at the same time of the night, and often during the rapid eye movement phase of sleep. Also known as Prinzmetal's, vasospastic, or nocturnal angina.
Angina Decubitus	Paroxysmal chest pain that occurs when patient reclines and lessens when the patient sits or stands.
Intractable Angina	Chronic, incapacitating chest pain; often unresponsive to intervention.
Postinfarction Angina	Occurs after an MI, when residual ischemia may cause anginal episodes.

PATHOPHYSIOLOGY

Oxygen Demand vs. Supply

Coronary arteries ordinarily supply the myocardium with blood during diastole, thus meeting its metabolic needs. When oxygen demand increases, vessels dilate to supply additional blood to myocardium. The hemodynamic mechanisms responsible for alterations in total and regional coronary blood flow are not clearly understood; however, it is known that relaxation of vascular smooth muscle reduces cardiac workload. However, vessels filled with atherosclerotic plaque build-up cannot dilate. Fixed atherosclerotic lesions of at least 90% almost completely abolish blood flow; patients with these lesions may have angina at rest.

As vessels become more and more occluded, the growing mass of plaque accumulates platelets, fibrin, and cellular

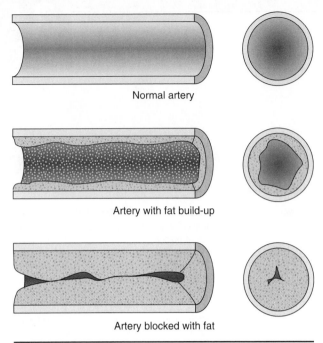

FIGURE 35-1 Stages of Atherosclerotic Plaque Formation. Cross-section of a normal artery and an artery altered by disease. The affected artery is obstructed by a mass of platelets, red blood cells, and cholesterol bodies and is indicative of coronary heart disease. With progressive disease, the artery becomes almost completely obstructed.

debris. Platelet aggregates release thromboxane A$_2$, a vasoconstrictor compound that can cause coronary artery spasms. Ironically, thromboxane A$_2$ also promotes platelet aggregation, resulting in a vicious circle of vasoconstriction and platelet build-up in vessel walls.

Nicotine promotes platelet adhesiveness and plaque build-up, although the mechanism by which it does so is uncertain. Nicotine enhances platelet adhesiveness, raising the risk for clot formation and contributing to an ischemic episode. The carbon monoxide in smoke reduces arterial oxygen content, thereby stimulating the release of epinephrine and norepinephrine, which in turn results in increased blood pressure, cardiac workload, and oxygen demand.

Other factors contributing to angina include arterial spasm, coronary arteritis, hypotension, potent antihypertensive drugs, blood loss, spinal anesthesia, and any other disorders that lessen venous return to the heart. Aortic stenosis or insufficiency lowers the filling pressure of the coronary arteries. Polycythemia increases the viscosity of the blood and slows flow through coronary arteries. Exercise, cold, and emotion increase catecholamine release and thus the heart rate. A large meal shunts blood toward the gastrointestinal tract (GI) and away from other structures. Anemia and hypoxemia reduce myocardial perfusion. Hyperthyroidism increases the production of thyroid hormones, which raises blood pressure, myocardial contractility, heart rate, and cardiac output. In addition, rhythm disturbances such as premature ventricular contractions (PVCs), atrial fibrillation, and paroxysmal atrial tachycardia (PAT) associated with hyperthyroidism also contribute to anginal pain.

Pain associated with focal coronary artery spasm and ST-segment elevation is known as *Prinzmetal's angina*. This form of angina is thought to be caused by a focal deficiency of nitric oxide production, hyperinsulinemia, low intracellular

magnesium levels, cigarette smoking, or cocaine use. Although some patients with Prinzmetal's angina have fixed atherosclerotic lesions of coronary vessels, some patients have normal coronary arteries on angiography.

Syndrome X angina is characterized by pain, ST-segment elevation, and/or myocardial perfusion defects during stress testing but angiographically normal coronary arteries. The mechanisms responsible for syndrome X are thought to include any or all of the following: (1) increased release of local vasoconstricting compounds; (2) dysfunction of endothelium; (3) abnormalities in normal adrenergic innervation within the myocardium; (4) fibrosis and hypertrophy of microcirculation; and/or (5) estrogen deficiency. A reduction in the oxygen-carrying capacity of blood, as seen with severe anemia (hemoglobin less than 8 grams/dL), also contributes to angina. The majority of patients with syndrome X are postmenopausal women.

In some patients, coronary arteries supply adequate blood when the patient is at rest. However, with exercise or in otherwise taxing situations, angina develops. Myocardial cells become ischemic within 10 seconds of a coronary artery occlusion. Within several minutes, the heart loses its ability to contract, impairing pump function and depriving the myocardium of the glucose necessary for aerobic metabolism. Anaerobic metabolism takes over with an accumulation of lactic acid. Anginal pain develops as the lactic acid accumulates.

Under ischemic conditions, myocardial cells remain viable for about 20 minutes. If blood flow is restored, aerobic metabolism resumes, contractility is restored, and cellular repair begins. Myocardial infarction occurs when coronary arteries are unable to compensate for the lack of oxygen. Afferent sympathetic fibers, entering the spinal cord from levels C3–T4, account for the variety of locations and for the radiation pattern of anginal pain (Fig. 35-2).

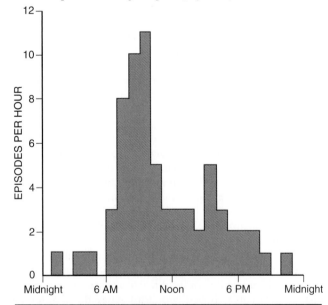

FIGURE 35-2 Distribution of Ischemic Episodes. Some patients with chronic stable angina, both silent and symptomatic episodes of angina, clearly have a peak incidence in the morning and early afternoon hours. The frequency gradually declines in the late afternoon and is lowest in the early morning. (Adapted from Nademanee, K., Intarachot, V., Josephson, M., et al. [1987]. Circadian variations in occurrence of transient overt and silent myocardial ischemia in chronic stable angina and comparison with Prinzmetal's angina in men. *American Journal of Cardiology, 60,* 498. Used with permission.)

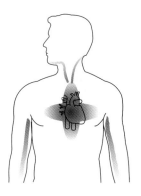
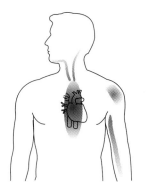
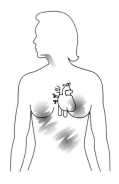

- Upper chest or epigastric radiation to neck, jaw, and arms

- Beneath sternum radiation to neck and jaw or radiation down left arm

- Nausea, shortness of breath, or vague discomfort in upper abdomen or jaw

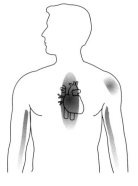
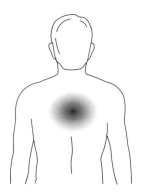
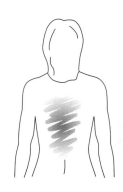

- Epigastric or left shoulder radiating down both arms

- Intrascapular

- Discomfort in back

FIGURE 35-3 Common Sites of Anginal Pain *(shaded areas).* The locations of the pain are similar in males and females.

PHARMACOTHERAPEUTIC OPTIONS

The major categories of drugs used in the management of angina pectoris include nitrates, beta blockers, calcium channel blockers, antiplatelet drugs, and opioids. Opioids were discussed in Chapter 16. Antiplatelet drugs are discussed in Chapter 39; the nitrates, the beta blockers, and the calcium channel blockers (CCBs) are discussed here as they relate to the management of angina pectoris.

Nitrates

SHORT-ACTING NITRATES
- nitroglycerin (Nitrostat, Nitrobid IV, Nitrostat IV, Nitrolingual, Nitroglyn, Nitrobid, Nitrospan, Nitrol, Nitrodisc, Transderm-Nitro, Nitrogard); ◆ Minitran, NitroBid, Nitro-Dur, Nitro-Quick, Nitrostat, Transderm-Nitro

LONG-ACTING NITRATES
- isosorbide dinitrate (Isordil, Sorbitrate, Dilatrate-SR, ISDN, Iso-Bid, Isordil, Sorbitrate SA); ◆ Apo-ISDN, Cedocard-SR, Corones
- isosorbide mononitrate (Imdur, Ismo, Monoket); ◆ Imdur, Ismo

▦ *Indications*
Nitroglycerin, the short-acting ester of nitric acid, has been the drug of choice against anginal attacks since 1867. Today,

nitrates remain the major weapon for immediate relief of acute angina, for prevention of angina when an attack is anticipated, and for the long-term prevention of chronic anginal attacks. Nitrates can be used as monotherapy, or concurrently with beta blockers and calcium channel blockers. Nitrates are also used to increase the exercise capacity of patients with CAD.

▦ *Pharmacodynamics*
Of the general mechanisms by which nitrates reduce myocardial ischemia, their ability to reduce myocardial oxygen demand by reducing preload is the most important. Low-dose nitrates preferentially cause dilation of veins over arterioles (they relax vascular smooth muscle by stimulating intracellular cyclic guanosine monophosphate [cGMP]), resulting in a pooling of blood in the periphery. In turn, there is a decrease in venous return to the heart and filling of the left ventricle. Decreasing venous return to the heart reduces left end-diastolic pressure and volume and oxygen consumption. With the reduced filling of the left ventricle, the workload of the heart is also reduced and therefore the heart requires less oxygen, blood pressure is reduced, and angina relieved. In addition, a reduction in preload generates a higher pressure gradient across the ventricular wall, which favors

subendocardial perfusion. Nitrates do not directly change the inotropic or chronotropic state of the heart.

Independent of autonomic nervous system activity, nitrates also dilate arteries by direct action on arterial smooth muscle. Most resistance to the ejection of blood from the left ventricle comes from the arterioles. The greater the arteriolar constriction, the more resistance to ejection of blood from the left ventricle. Nitrates decrease afterload by dilating arterioles. Systemic vascular resistance is usually unaffected, the heart rate is unchanged or slightly increased, and pulmonary vascular resistance and cardiac output are reduced. The apparent selectivity of some nitrates for different vascular beds may relate to differences in bioavailability and cellular biotransformation of the drugs.

▥ Pharmacokinetics

Nitrates are well absorbed following oral, buccal, sublingual, or topical administration. The onset, peak, and duration of action vary with the route of administration. Table 35-1 summarizes the pharmacokinetics of nitrates. Orally administered nitrates are rapidly biotransformed in the liver, leading to decreased bioavailability. **An extensive first-pass effect limits ▲ the usefulness of oral nitroglycerin therapy in most cases.** As a consequence of reduction hydrolysis, nitrates are transformed from lipid-soluble organic esters to more water-soluble metabolites and inorganic nitrites. Elimination is through the kidneys.

▥ Adverse Effects and Contraindications

In general, the adverse effects of nitrates are almost all secondary to their action on the cardiovascular system. The decreased afterload from arteriolar dilation causes hypotension. The reduced preload and cardiac output results in worsened hypotension, which is most noticeable when the patient assumes an upright position. Transient episodes of dizziness, weakness, and

PHARMACOKINETICS
TABLE 35-1 Antianginal Drugs

Drug	Route	Onset	Peak	Duration	PB (%)	t½	BioA (%)
SHORT-ACTING NITRATES*							
nitroglycerin	SL	1–3 min	3–5 min	30–60 min	60	1–4 min	12–64
	IV	Immed	Immed	3–5 min	60	1–4 min	100
	Buccal	2–4 min	UA	3–5 hr	60	1–4 min	UA
	Ointment	15 min	30–120 min	2–12 hr	60	1–4 min	52–92
	TD	30–60 min	1–3 hr	18–24 hr	60	1–4 min	52–92
	PO, SR	40–60 min	3–4 hr	4–8 hr	60	1–4 min	<1
	TL	2 min	UA	30–60 min	60	1–4 min	UA
LONG-ACTING NITRATES							
isosorbide dinitrate	SL or chewable	2–5 min	30–60 min	1–2 hr	UA	50 min, 5 hr†	22–38‡
isosorbide mononitrate	PO, IR	30–60 min	UA	4–6 hr	UA	4 hr	8–36‡
	PO, SR	20–45 min	1–3 hr	4–8 hr	UA	UA	UA
NONSELECTIVE BETA BLOCKERS§							
propranolol	PO	1–2 hr	60–90 min	6 hr	90	4–6 hr	16–36
	PO, ER	UA	6 hr	24 hr	90	3.4–6 hr	UA
	IV	2 min	1 min‖	4–6 hr	90	3–6 hr	100
nadolol	PO	>5 days	2–4 hr	24 hr	30	16–18 hr	29–39
SELECTIVE BETA BLOCKERS§							
atenolol	PO	60 min	2–4 hr	24 hr	<5	6–9 hr	26–86
metoprolol	PO	30–60 min	90 min	24 hr	12	3–7 hr	24–52
	IV	Immediate	20 min	5–8 hr	12	3–4 hr	100
CALCIUM CHANNEL BLOCKERS							
amlodipine	PO	50 min	12 hr	24 hr	98	30–50 hr	64–90
bepridil	PO	8 days¶	UA	24 hr	99	42 hr**	UA
diltiazem	PO	30 min	2–3 hr	4–8 hr	70–85	3–5 hr	UA
isradipine	PO	<2 hr	2–3 hr	12 hr	95	8 hr	64–90
felodipine	PO	60 min	2–4 hr	Up to 24 hr	99	11–16 hr	UA
nicardipine	PO	20 min	0.5–2 hr	8 hr	>95	2–4 hr	UA
nifedipine	PO	20 min	30 min	2.5–3 hr	92–98	2–5 hr	UA
verapamil	PO	1–2 hr	1–2 hr	6–8 hr	83–92	3–7 hr	UA
	PO, SR	UA	5–7 hr	24 hr	83–92	4–12 hr	UA
PIPERAZINE DERIVATIVE							
ranolazine	PO	UA	2–5 hr	UA	62	7 hr	76

*Cardiovascular effects of nitrates.
†Half-life values for isosorbide dinitrate and isosorbide mononitrate, respectively.
‡Bioavailability calculations from single doses, because systemic clearance may be reduced with long-term use of isosorbide formulations.
§Because beta blockers are not used for relief of acute anginal pain, their onset of action is difficult to measure.
‖Antianginal effects of propranolol are manifest at 15–90 mcg/mL to achieve a 50% decrease in exercise-induced cardioacceleration.
¶Onset of steady-state antianginal effects with long-term dosing of bepridil.
**Half-life of bepridil following cessation of multiple dosing.
ER, Extended release; *Immed,* immediate; *IR,* immediate release; *IV,* intravenous; *NA,* not applicable; *PO,* by mouth; *PB,* protein binding; *SL,* sublingual; *SR,* sustained release; *t½,* half-life; *TD,* transdermal patch; *TL,* translingual spray; *UA,* unavailable.

other symptoms of postural hypotension may occur, particularly when the patient stands immobile. Hypotension occasionally progresses to a loss of consciousness, especially when accompanied by alcohol ingestion. Even with the most severe syncopal episode, positioning and other strategies that facilitate venous return to the heart are the only therapeutic measures needed.

Approximately 50% of patients receiving nitrates for acute angina attacks experience flushing and a pounding headache after administration. The headache, caused by dilation of meningeal blood vessels, usually disappears after several days of continued treatment and often can be effectively controlled by reducing the dose of the nitrate. They occur less commonly with long-term prophylaxis therapy.

Other adverse effects include blurry vision, dry mouth, and increased peripheral edema. Methemoglobinemia (a condition in which more than 1% of hemoglobin has been oxidized to the ferric form) occurs with large, continuous doses of nitrates. The principal sign of methemoglobinemia is cyanosis, which occurs because the oxidized hemoglobin is unable to transport oxygen.

A rash caused by isosorbide mononitrate is reported less often than with isosorbide dinitrate. There is also less flushing and halitosis with the mononitrate formulation of isosorbide.

Drug Interactions

Drug interactions associated with nitrates usually result in additive hypotension. The absorption of sublingual and buccal nitroglycerine formulations is reduced when nitrates are used concurrently with drugs that have anticholinergic properties (antihistamines, antidepressants, and phenothiazines) (Table 35-2).

Dosage Regimen

Nitrates are available in a variety of formulations (Table 35-3). Nitrate dosages are determined by the frequency and intensity of anginal episodes, as well as by the patient's response to therapy. In years past, the dosage regimen was to take a sublingual tablet with the onset of chest pain, and then every 5 minutes until a total of three tablets have been taken, after which emergency service assistance is required. The current recommendation is to take one tablet and call for emergency medical assistance.

Although used less often today, nitroglycerin ointment is titrated according to the patient's response and blood

DRUG INTERACTIONS
TABLE 35-2 Antianginal Drugs

Drug	Interactive Drugs	Interaction
NITRATES		
nitroglycerin	Alcohol, Antihypertensives, Beta blockers, Calcium channel blockers, Diuretics, haloperidol, Phenothiazines	Additive hypotension
	Antihistamines, sildenafil, tadalafil, TCAs	Decreases absorption of SL and buccal nitroglycerin
BETA BLOCKERS		
atenolol	Antacids	Decreases absorption from GI tract
metoprolol, nadolol	NSAIDs	Decreases hypotensive effects
propranolol	Barbiturates	Increases biotransformation of BB
	Calcium channel blockers	Increases toxic effects of both drugs
	digoxin	Increases bradycardia and AV nodal depression
	cimetidine	Decreases biotransformation of BB; increases ability of BB to reduce pulse
	clonidine	Increases antihypertensive and bradycardia effects
	Insulins	Hypoglycemia, hyperglycemia
	Oral hypoglycemics	Masks tachycardia as a sign of hypoglycemia (other symptoms still present)
	lidocaine	Increases plasma levels of lidocaine; may potentiate toxicity and produce additive cardiac depression
	rifampin	Inhibits response to BB
	albuterol, dobutamine, dopamine, epinephrine, isoproterenol, metaproterenol, terbutaline, ritodrine	Hypertension and reflex bradycardia from unopposed alpha effects and increased vagal tone
CALCIUM CHANNEL BLOCKERS		
amlodipine, bepridil	cimetidine	Decreases hepatic clearance of CCB
diltiazem, felodipine	Calcium salts, vitamin D	Decreases response to CCB
isradipine	digoxin	Increases serum digoxin level
nicardipine, nifedipine	Beta blockers, disopyramide phosphate	Causes myocardial depression
verapamil	carbamazepine, cyclosporine, Nondepolarizing blockers	Enhances action of interacting drug
PIPERAZINE DERIVATIVE		
ranolazine	Antipsychotics, dextromethorphan, digoxin, simvastatin, TCAs, diltiazem, ketoconazole, verapamil	Increases plasma levels of interactive drugs
		Increases plasma levels of ranolazine and increases risk of QTc prolongation
	Class I and II antiarrhythmics, Certain macrolide and quinolone antibiotics, TCAs, thioridazine, ziprasidone	Increases QTc interval

AV, Atrioventricular; *BB*, beta blocker; *CCB*, calcium channel blocker; *GI*, gastrointestinal; *QTc*, QT interval on electrocardiogram; *SL*, sublingual; *TCAs*, tricyclic antidepressants.

DOSAGE

TABLE **35-3 Antianginal Drugs**

Drug	Use(s)	Dosage	Comments
NITRATES			
nitroglycerin	Acute unstable angina, acute myocardial infarction, angina prophylaxis, adjunct in heart failure	*Adult:* 0.15–0.6 mg SL *–or–* 5 mcg/min IV drip *Low-dose therapy:* Titrate by 10 to 20 mcg *High-dose therapy:* Titrate by 10 to 20 mcg *Adult:* 1–2 SL (0.4 mg) sprays PRN *Adult:* ½-inch to 5 inch ribbon (7.5 to 75 mg) of ointment every 3–4 hr *Adult:* 0.1 to 0.8 mg/hr TD patch every 24 hr	Titrate IV formulation until desired fall in systolic BP and/or chest pain relief occurs. Highly flammable. Do not inhale or swallow. Do not touch ointment with hands. Cover with plastic wrap for better absorption. Remove patch before defibrillation to avoid arcing.
isosorbide dinitrate	Angina prophylaxis, adjunct in heart failure	*Adult:* 2.5–10 mg SL PRN *–or–* IR 10–30 mg PO 2–3 times daily *–or–* SR 10–30 mg PO 2–3 times daily *–or–* 80–120 mg PO daily IR	Do not crush or chew tablets
isosorbide mononitrate	Angina prophylaxis, adjunct in heart failure	*Adult:* 10–20 mg PO 2–3 times daily SR *–or–* 30–120 mg PO daily	
NONSELECTIVE BETA BLOCKERS			
propranolol	Chronic exertional angina	*Adult:* 10–20 mg PO 3–4 times daily. Increase every 3–7 days to desired effect. Maintenance: 160 mg/day in divided doses	**Contraindicated for use in patients with respiratory disorders. Abrupt withdrawal may result in life-threatening arrhythmias.**
	Myocardial infarction	*Adult:* 180–240 mg PO daily in 3–4 divided doses.	
nadolol	Chronic exertional angina	*Adult:* 40 mg PO daily. Increase every 3–7 days to desired effect Maintenance: 80–240 mg PO daily	**Contraindicated for use in patients with respiratory disorders. Abrupt withdrawal may result in life-threatening arrhythmias.**
SELECTIVE BETA BLOCKERS			
atenolol	Angina hypertension	*Adult:* 50 mg PO daily. Increase by 50 mg/day every 3 days to desired effect *–or–* titrate until exercise-induced heart rate is reduced by 15%.	Reduce dosage to 50 mg every other day in renal failure.
	Myocardial infarction	*Adult:* 5 mg IV every 2 min for 3 doses; then 5 mg PO every 6 hr for 36–48 hr; then 100 mg every 12 hr	Withhold if apical pulse rate before administration is less then 50 bpm.
metoprolol	Exertional angina, hypertension	*Adult:* 100–450 mg PO single dose or twice daily. Increase every 7 days as needed up to 450 mg/day. ER formulation given once daily.	Hypotensive effects may persist for up to 4 wk after discontinuation.
CALCIUM CHANNEL BLOCKERS			
amlodipine	Prinzmetal's angina	*Adult:* 5–10 mg PO daily. Maintenance: 2.5–10 mg PO daily.	May take without regard to meals.
verapamil	Angina	*Adult:* 80–120 mg PO 3 times daily *–or–* 120–240 mg of SR formulation daily. Increase in daily or weekly intervals as needed. Maintenance: 240–480 mg PO daily *–or–* 5–10 mg IV. May repeat with 10 mg after 30 min.	Initial dose lower in patients with hepatic impairment or poor left ventricular function, or in older adults.
bepridil	Exercise-induced angina	*Adult:* 200 mg PO daily Increase after 10 days to 300 mg daily. Maintenance dose not to exceed 400 mg/day.	May be administered with meals if gastrointestinal distress is a problem.
diltiazem	Prinzmetal's angina, exercise-induced angina	*Adult:* 30–120 mg PO 3–4 times daily *–or–* 60–120 mg PO twice daily as SR capsules *–or–* 180–240 mg PO daily as CD or XR capsules Maintenance: Not to exceed 360 mg daily	Useful addition if BB and nitrates are not effective. Usually the best-tolerated CCB
isradipine	Angina, essential hypertension	*Adult:* 2.5 mg PO twice daily. Increase at 3–4-wk intervals to 10 mg twice daily.	Limit consumption of caffeine.
felodipine	Angina, hypertension	*Adult:* 5 mg PO daily. May increase every 2 wk. Usual daily dose 5–10 mg. Not to exceed 20 mg daily.	Start older adults at 2.5 mg PO daily.
nicardipine	Stable angina, hypertension	*Adult:* 20 mg PO 3 times daily. Increase after 3 days to max dose of 30 mg 3 times daily if needed. Maintenance: 20–40 mg PO 3 times daily *–or–* 60 mg SR PO formulation twice daily	Absorption may be increased with concurrent intake of high-fat meal.
nifedipine	Prinzmetal's angina	*Adult:* 10–30 mg PO 3 times daily *–or–* 30–90 mg daily of ER formulation *–or–* 10 mg SL. Maintenance: Not to exceed 180 mg of oral formulation or 120 mg of SR formulation.	SL formulation may be repeated in 15 min if necessary, although this route has not been approved by the FDA.
PIPERAZINE DERIVATIVE			
ranolazine	Chronic angina unresponsive to other treatments	*Adult:* 500 mg PO twice daily initially. Max: 1000 mg PO twice daily.	Serum levels increase as much as 50% in patients with renal impairment.

BP, Blood pressure; *bpm,* beats/min; *IR,* immediate release; *ER,* extended release; *IR,* immediate release; *IV,* intravenous; *PO,* by mouth; *PRN,* as needed; *SL,* sublingual; *SR,* sustained release.

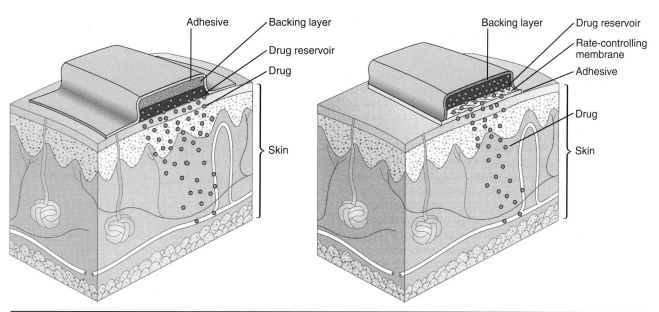

FIGURE 35-4 **Transdermal Drug Delivery Systems.** *Left*, Matrix formulation: drug is slowly dispersed through polymer matrix to absorption site. *Right*, Reservoir delivery system: drug migrates to absorption site through rate-controlled permeable membrane.

pressure. Topical formulations can be applied anywhere on the body surface, but the skin should be clean, dry, and free of hair. Transdermal, controlled-release nitrates are currently compounded one of two ways, as a matrix or a reservoir (Fig. 35-4). Transderm-Nitro uses a reservoir formulation in which the drug migrates to the absorption site through a rate-controlled permeable membrane. Nitro-Dur and Nitrodisc are matrix formulations; the nitrate is slowly dispersed through the polymer matrix to the absorption site.

▌ *Lab Considerations*

All nitrates cause falsely elevated serum cholesterol levels. Nitrates also increase urine concentrations of catecholamines and vanillylmandelic acid. Excessive doses may raise methemoglobin values.

For more information, see the Evolve Resources Bonus Content "Influence of Selected Drugs on Laboratory Values," found at http://evolve.elsevier.com/Gutierrez/pharmacotherapeutics.

Beta Blockers

NONSELECTIVE
- ◆ labetalol (Normodyne, Trandate); ✦ Trandate
- ◆ nadolol (Corgard); ✦ Syn-Nadolol
- ◆ pindolol (Visken); ✦ Novo-Pindol, Syn-Pindolol
- ◆ propranolol (Inderal, Inderal LA); ✦ Apo-Propranolol

SELECTIVE
- ◆ acebutolol (Sectral); ✦ Monitan
- ◆ atenolol (Tenormin); ✦ Apo-Atenolol, Novo-Atenol
- ◆ metoprolol (Lopressor, Toprol XL); ✦ Betaloc, Betaloc Durules, Lopresor, Lopresor SR, Novo-Metoprol

▌ *Indications*

Beta blockers constitute a major treatment modality for angina, second only to nitrates. The drugs currently approved

by the Food and Drug Administration (FDA) for use as antianginal drugs are the nonselective beta blockers propranolol and nadolol, and the cardioselective drugs atenolol and metoprolol. Beta blockers are effective in reducing the severity and frequency of exertional angina attacks. Acebutolol, labetalol, and pindolol have not been approved by the FDA for angina, but they are occasionally prescribed.

Patients using a beta blocker for angina usually note improved exercise tolerance and report a decrease in the number and severity of attacks. The beta blockers are also used for the treatment of hypertension, migraine headaches, anxiety, pheochromocytoma, arrhythmias, and open-angle glaucoma associated with hyperthyroidism. The uses of beta blockers as antiarrhythmics and antiglaucoma drugs are discussed in Chapters 36 and 61, respectively.

▌ *Pharmacodynamics*

Beta blockers reduce the oxygen requirements of the myocardium by preventing stimulation of sympathetic nervous system (SNS) receptors, inhibiting catecholamine action at these sites, and reducing contractility, sinus node rate, and atrioventricular conduction velocity (negative dromotropic action). These actions, in turn, raise the exercise tolerance of patients with reduced coronary blood flow. The competitive blocking action occurs not only at adrenergic nerve receptors, but also in the adrenal medulla. Drug action at these two sites accounts for the widespread effects of beta blockers. Certain beta blockers (e.g., propranolol, metoprolol) also produce central nervous system (CNS) activity, with effects exerted at the vasomotor center of the brainstem.

Selective beta blockers preferentially act at β_1 receptor sites. The principal effects are slowing of the heart rate (negative chronotropic effect), a reduction in the force of the contraction (negative inotropic effect), and suppression of impulse conduction through the atrioventricular node. Because of the blockade, these drugs decrease the workload of the heart, oxygen demand is brought into balance with oxygen supply, and anginal pain is prevented. In contrast, nonselective beta blockers act on both β_1 and β_2 receptors, preventing not only cardiac excitement but also bronchodilation.

▥ Pharmacokinetics

Only orally administered beta blockers are used to treat angina. These drugs have varying pharmacokinetic properties, which are listed in Table 35-1.

▥ Adverse Effects and Contraindications

The most common adverse effects of beta blockers occur when the drug is started. Hypotension, bradycardia, and bronchospasm are potentially harmful. Heart failure may be precipitated or exacerbated because of the negative inotropic effect and greater preload produced by beta blockers. **A rapid discontinuance of a beta blocker may precipitate an anginal attack, hypertension, arrhythmias (especially atrioventricular block), or an acute MI.**

Although occurring most often with propranolol, adverse CNS effects of the beta blockers include dizziness, fatigue, lethargy, confusion or depression, and decreased libido. The GI tract adverse effects of nausea, vomiting, and diarrhea are usually transient.

⚠ **Significant bronchoconstriction can result from blockade of beta receptors.** Although this reaction is more likely to occur with nonselective drugs (i.e., nadolol, propranolol), it can also occur with high doses of selective drugs such as atenolol and metoprolol. Beta blockers are contraindicated for use in variant angina. The deleterious effect of beta blockers on variant angina is probably due to an increase in coronary resistance caused by the unopposed effects of catecholamines on α receptors.

Nonselective beta blockers are contraindicated for use in patients with heart failure, acute bronchospasm, some forms of valvular heart disease, bradyarrhythmias, and heart block. In low dosages, metoprolol and atenolol induce full cardiac beta blockade without causing wheezing in patients who have pulmonary disease. At larger doses, selective beta blockers become nonselective and block both cardiac and bronchial beta receptors. Use them cautiously in pregnant and lactating females, because they may cause fetal bradycardia and hypoglycemia.

▥ Drug Interactions

Drug interactions with beta blockers are numerous and are summarized in Table 35-2. Cimetidine increases the beta blocking effects of propranolol by slowing its hepatic clearance and elimination. Adrenergic agonists, which stimulate β-receptors, can reverse the bradycardia induced by beta blockers.

▥ Dosage Regimen

Table 35-3 identifies the dosage regimens for beta blockers used in the management of angina pectoris. As with most drugs, the dosage for the individual formulations varies.

▥ Lab Considerations

Selective and nonselective beta blockers may increase blood urea nitrogen (BUN), serum lipoproteins, and potassium, triglyceride, and uric acid levels. Antinuclear antibody titers (ANA) and blood glucose levels may rise. Metoprolol can cause elevations in serum alkaline phosphatase, lactate dehydrogenase, aspartate transaminase (AST), and alanine transaminase (ALT) levels.

Calcium Channel Blockers

- amlodipine (Norvasc)
- bepridil (Vascor)
- diltiazem (Cardizem, Cardizem SR, Cardizem CD, Dilacor XR); ♣ Cardizem, Cardizem LA, Cardizem CD, Cardizem SR
- felodipine (Plendil); ♣ Plendil
- isradipine (Dynacirc); ♣ Dynacirc
- nicardipine (Cardene, Cardene SR); ♣ Cardene SR
- nifedipine (Adalat, Adalat CC, Procardia, Procardia XL); ♣ nifedical, nifedipine, Adalat CC, Adalat PA, Adalat XL, Procardia XL
- verapamil (Calan, Calan SR, Isoptin, Isoptin SR, Verelan); ♣ verapamil, Calan SR, Covera HS, Isoptin SR, Verelan PM

▥ Indications

Verapamil is considered the prototype drug and was the first calcium channel blocker (CCB) approved for use in the United States. CCBs are used alone or with other drugs in the management of angina and hypertension, as well as of arrhythmias (see Chapter 36). Although not approved by the FDA for this use, some CCBs have been used for the prevention of migraine headaches, to treat arrhythmias and heart failure, and in the management of cardiomyopathy. Bepridil, the newest CCB, is used only for the management of angina. The clinical use of these drugs varies with the manner in which each affects the heart.

▥ Pharmacodynamics

CCBs produce antianginal effects by mechanisms different from those of nitrates or beta blockers. Physiologically, cardiac tissue is rapidly depolarized by the rapid influx of Na^{++} ions. The depolarization is quickly followed by a slow inward current of Ca^{++}. By inhibiting Ca^{++} entry into cardiac and smooth muscle cells, CCBs dilate peripheral arteries and arterioles. Nifedipine and amlodipine have the greatest peripheral arterial vasodilating effect, verapamil has a moderate effect, and diltiazem has the least effect on peripheral vasculature. The pacer cells of the sinoatrial (SA) and atrioventricular (AV) nodes are depolarized primarily by Ca^{++}. Myocardial contractility is decreased, as are AV nodal conduction and heart rate.

▥ Pharmacokinetics

The absorption of CCBs varies considerably, from 64% to 90%. Isradipine, felodipine, and nifedipine are well absorbed following oral administration, but they are extensively biotransformed, decreasing their bioavailability. CCBs are significantly bound to plasma proteins. All have a relatively rapid onset of action, reaching peak serum levels in 1 to 2 hours. Specific information on pharmacokinetics can be found in Table 35-1.

▥ Adverse Effects and Contraindications

The vasodilating effect of CCBs can predictably result in dizziness, headache, flushing, and weakness, especially with nicardipine and nifedipine. Hypotension can occur as a result of the decrease in afterload and the force of ventricular contraction.

Other possible adverse effects include dry mouth, anorexia, dyspepsia, nausea (with bepridil), vomiting, constipation, diarrhea, and abnormal liver function values. Some patients complain of weight gain, muscle cramps, and joint stiffness. Long-term use of amlodipine can cause gingival hyperplasia, which may necessitate discontinuing the drug if the patient and the dentist are unable to adequately care for the teeth. It is not known if the hyperplasia is a class effect of calcium channel blockers.

CCBs decrease afterload and the force of ventricular contraction, and can cause hypotension. Arrhythmias (e.g., bradycardia, tachycardia) and chest pain can occur as the result of inhibition of SA and AV nodes, particularly with verapamil and diltiazem. The depressant action of CCBs on myocardial contractility contributes to the onset or worsening of heart failure. Peripheral edema is possible and is more likely to occur with amlodipine and nifedipine.

A rash or dermatitis, pruritus, and urticaria have been reported with CCBs, particularly nifedipine, but are less likely to occur with verapamil. **Stevens-Johnson syndrome can be life threatening.** Sexual dysfunction, urinary frequency, polyuria, dysuria, and nocturia are possible. Shortness of breath, dyspnea, congestion, cough, and epistaxis has occurred in susceptible patients.

There are a number of contraindications to the use of CCBs. Hypersensitivity, sick sinus syndrome, and second- or third-degree heart block (unless a pacemaker is in place) contraindicates use of these drugs. Avoid the use of bepridil, diltiazem, and verapamil in patients with systolic blood pressures less than 90 mm Hg. A recent MI or the presence of pulmonary congestion contraindicates use of diltiazem. Verapamil is contraindicated for use in patients with heart failure, severe ventricular dysfunction, cardiogenic shock, severe bradycardia, or hypotension.

Exercise caution when using CCBs in patients with severe hepatic or renal dysfunction, those with a history of serious ventricular arrhythmias or heart failure, and older adults. The safe use of these drugs during pregnancy and lactation has not been established.

Drug Interactions

CCBs interact with a variety of other drugs (see Table 35-2). For example, cimetidine decreases the hepatic clearance of CCBs. Disopyramide and beta blockers can produce additive myocardial depression when given in combination with CCBs.

Dosage Regimen

The dosages of other CCBs are given in Table 35-3. Use caution in administering oral as opposed to sustained-release formulations of the same drug, because the dosages are different.

Lab Considerations

Total serum Ca^{++} levels are not affected by CCBs. Hypokalemia increases the risk of arrhythmias, and thus K^+ levels should be corrected before these drugs are used, especially for patients to be given bepridil. CCBs such as nifedipine may increase creatine kinase, lactate dehydrogenase, AST, and ALT levels, and may cause a positive Coombs' test. Liver function values generally return to normal by stopping the drug. Although the AST level is always increased in acute myocardial infarction, the ALT level does not necessarily rise proportionately. Nifedipine can cause positive ANA and direct Coombs' test results. Platelet counts are occasionally decreased with nimodipine.

Angiotensin-Converting Enzyme Inhibitors

Also useful in the management of angina are the angiotensin-converting enzyme inhibitors, commonly known as ACE inhibitors (ACEIs). The primary end point of antianginal treatment is to lower the blood pressure, which in turn lessens the workload on the heart. Sadly, too many health care providers still perceive that a blood pressure of 130 to 140 mm Hg over 75 to 85 mm Hg is acceptable and does not require drug therapy.

The problem is not whether these figures are normal, but more importantly, whether the blood pressure is too high for a patient with heart disease, since patients with low blood pressures generally have fewer episodes of chest pain and a reduced incidence of myocardial infarction. For these reasons, the blood pressure is reduced and kept at the lowest reasonable level that does not interfere with the patient's activities of daily living.

Ordinarily, stress does not elevate blood pressure to an extreme, but when the patient has preexisting, uncontrolled blood pressure elevations, stress can send the values as high as 180/100 in a matter of seconds. However, if the patient's blood pressure is normally about 110/70 and is carefully controlled, stress is unlikely to elevate the reading to a dangerous high. Even when stress does cause an elevation, it is unusual for the increase to be greater than 10 to 15 mm Hg. Antihypertensive drugs are discussed further in Chapter 37.

Antianginal and Antiischemic Drug
Ranolazine

Ranolazine (Ranexa) is used, in addition to a CCB (e.g., amlodipine), beta blocker, or nitrate for the management of chronic angina unresponsive to other antianginal therapies. This new drug does not depend on reductions in heart rate or blood pressure to provide antianginal and antiischemic actions but rather reduces angina by partially inhibiting the oxidation of fatty acids, thereby increasing the oxidation of glucose and generating more ATP/molecule of oxygen consumed. The benefit of this drug on the incidence of anginal pain and of exercise tolerance is greater in men compared to women.

Ranolazine is a piperazine derivative whose absorption is highly variable but unaffected by food. Ranolazine is rapidly absorbed and extensively biotransformed by the CYP 3A and CYP 2D6 enzymes. Less than 5% of ranolazine is eliminated unchanged in urine and feces. The pharmacologic activity of the metabolites has not been well defined.

Common adverse effects of ranolazine include dizziness, headache, nausea, and constipation. Patients with severe renal impairment may note a blood pressure increase of about 15 mm Hg. The parent drug, ranolazine, and not its metabolites, is shown to prolong the QT interval, reduce the amplitude of T waves, and in some cases, dose-related, notched T waves appear. **The clinical significance of a prolonged QT interval resulting from ranolazine use is unknown; however, other drugs with this same potential are associated with torsades de pointes type of arrhythmias and sudden death.** Cautious use is warranted. The contraindications to ranolazine use include documented hypersensitivity to the drug or its ingredients, preexisting prolonged QT intervals, QT-prolonging drugs, and liver disease. Ranolazine is a moderately potent CYP 3A4 inhibitor.

Drug interactions associated with ranolazine are primarily the result of interactions with the CYP 3A enzyme (see Table 35-2). Toxicity is possible when ranolazine is coadministered with other drugs that increase QT interval.

CLINICAL REASONING

Treatment Objectives

The primary treatment objective in the management of angina is to enhance cardiac performance, thereby restoring the balance between myocardial oxygen supply and demand. This objective can be accomplished by reducing the duration and intensity of symptoms, preventing attacks, and improving exercise capacity (even though angina may still occur). The ultimate outcome is to prevent or delay the onset of MI.

Treatment Options

▥ Patient Variables

Treat diseases or conditions that predispose an individual to angina as part of a comprehensive therapeutic program. When choosing a management strategy, consider comorbid conditions and the psychosocial, cultural, economic, and religious background of the patient (Table 35-4). Adherence may be improved by using drugs that simplify the treatment

TABLE 35-4 Initial Treatment of Angina Based on Comorbidities

Comorbid Condition	Nitrate	Beta Blocker	CCB
All patients	1st	—	—
Chronic obstructive pulmonary disease	1st	NR	2nd
Diabetes mellitus	1st	NR	2nd
Heart failure	1st	NR	NR
Hypertension	2nd	1st	3rd
Hyperthyroidism	NA	1st	NA
Intermittent claudication	1st	1st	1st
Migraine	NR	1st	2nd
Raynaud's phenomenon	2nd	NR	1st

1st, First-choice drug; 2nd, alternative drug; 3rd, possible alternative drug if patient is unable to tolerate the alternative drug.
CCB, Calcium channel blocker; NA, not applicable; NR, not recommended.
NOTE: Where no drug of choice is identified, there may be no specific recommendation.

regimen, such as those requiring once-daily dosing, that come in a lingual spray, or that require little psychomotor skill for application. For example, the use of transdermal nitroglycerin rather than nitroglycerine ointment may be less bothersome, and therefore the patient may be more adherent to therapy.

Consider the patient's clinical response to therapy when prescribing any drug. Drug response may vary as a consequence of individual physiologic or psychologic compositions. If a patient is psychologically distressed by recurrent anginal episodes, or has symptoms more than 2 to 3 times a week, consider maintenance drug therapy (Case Study).

CASE STUDY | Antianginal Drugs

ASSESSMENT

History of Present Illness	JS, a 49-year-old male, comes to the clinic accompanied by his wife. He complained of chest pain after shoveling snow this morning but is in no acute distress at this time. He reports that the pain radiated to his jaw and left arm. It was relieved with rest and two nitroglycerin tablets. During the attack, he complained of being dizzy and anxious. His wife noticed he was breathing rapidly and that he looked pale. JS first experienced nonradiating chest pain 3 years ago. A stress test showed ischemic ST-T waves. He was diagnosed with exercise-induced angina and prescribed nitroglycerin tablets, 0.3 mg. SL PRN chest pain. He reports taking the nitroglycerin 2 or 3 times during the past year but did not go to the emergency room. JS has a history of exercise-induced asthma. He noticed a tightening in his chest shortly after starting atenolol for high blood pressure a few months ago. Today, he requests a refill on his albuterol inhaler since he has been using it more often lately.
Past Health History	JS has been on a low-cholesterol diet and taking fenofibrate, 145 mg daily since diagnosed with elevated lipid levels a few months ago. He was also prescribed atenolol, 50 mg daily for hypertension. He uses an albuterol inhaler PRN for reactive airway disease he has had since childhood. JS has a 20 pack/year smoking history but lately is trying to quit. Denies alcohol use. Father age 89, living, CAD, diabetes, hyperlipidemia, HTN, prostate cancer; mother age 86, living, HTN, CAD, hypothyroidism; brother age 44, HTN and CAD; sister age 41, HTN and elevated lipids
Life-Span Considerations	JS has three children under the age of 10. The 7-year-old boy is developmentally disabled and has been having behavioral difficulties at school recently. JS's wife does not work outside the home. JS is a self-employed accountant who has been spending long periods at the office owing to tax season. He remains an active coach for the local basketball team for developmentally disabled children. JS considers the family as middle-class with a "large mortgage payment each month and medical care for their son" but no other unusual financial stressors. The family has health insurance through a local PPO but doesn't have pharmacy coverage.

Physical Exam Findings	*VS:* BP 168/90, 37 °C-94(AP)-26 and irregular. SpO_2 90%. Skin warm and dry. Dyspnea observed. Breath sounds clear bilaterally. No wheezes, crackles, rhonchi, E > A changes. PMI palpable at left 5th ICS, MCL. S_1 > S_2 at the apex. No murmur, S_3, or S_4 heart sounds, gallops, rubs noted on auscultation. Peripheral pulses are strong bilaterally. No carotid, aortic, renal artery, or femoral artery bruits noted.
Diagnostic Testing	CBC: WNL. Cardiac enzymes/isoenzymes: unremarkable. Cholesterol: 220 mg/dL; HDL: 35 mg/dL; triglycerides: 320 mg/dL. LDL: 130 mg/dL. LFTs: within normal limits. ECG: Slight ST-T wave elevation; unchanged since previous tracing 2 years ago.

DIAGNOSIS: Angina

MANAGEMENT

Treatment Objectives	1. Enhance cardiac performance. 2. Decrease the duration and intensity of anginal attacks. 3. Improve exercise capacity.
Treatment Options	**Pharmacotherapy** 1. Change to nitroglycerin spray 0.4 mg 1 to 2 SL sprays PRN chest pain. If no relief in 5 minutes, contact emergency services. 2. Stop atenolol. Change to diltiazem SR 180 mg PO daily. 3. Continue fenofibrate 145 mg PO daily. Recheck LFTs and lipids in 6 weeks. 4. Start aspirin 81 mg daily. **Patient Education** 1. Educate the patient about angina pectoris, hypertension, and the drugs used in treatment. 2. Educate all patients about therapeutic lifestyle changes 3. Strongly encourage patients to quit smoking now, and take an active role in helping them to achieve this goal. 4. Maintain lipid levels within normal ranges given comorbidities; discuss diet and exercise plan. 5. Describe the importance of taking 81 mg of aspirin daily. 6. Advise patient to take the nitroglycerin as needed, but to sit or lie down to avoid hypotension and to stand up slowly. 7. Seek medical attention immediately if acute chest pain is not relieved with rest and nitroglycerin spray. 8. Do not abruptly continue either drug without contact with the health care provider first. 9. Make and keep follow-up appointments for reevaluation. **Evaluation** Documentation of enhanced cardiac performance as evidenced by a decrease in the frequency and severity of anginal attacks, improved activity tolerance, and sense of well-being

CLINICAL REASONING ANALYSIS

Q1. I am a student who will be caring for JS today. I have read his chart but don't understand why he will be taking isradipine rather than the atenolol he was originally on. Can you help me?

A. JS has a history of asthma since childhood, even though it has not been bothering him. Atenolol is a nonselective beta blocker that narrows airways. By changing JS to a calcium channel blocker, we will not only help control his angina and blood pressure, but also reduce his risk for respiratory distress caused by atenolol-induced narrowing of the airways.

Q2. I was reading about the nitroglycerin drugs. How do you know which drug would be best for JS?

A. Well, the choice of antianginal drug and route of administration is made with consideration of the desired onset of therapeutic effects, the suitability of various routes of administration for the individual patient, the need for stable drug concentration, comorbid conditions such as his asthma, and the likelihood of tolerance or toxicity. We chose to use sublingual nitroglycerine spray because he has only 2 or 3 episodes of angina per year, which are relieved by the nitroglycerine and rest. Nitroglycerin spray is more expensive per dose than the sublingual tablets. However, if nitroglycerin is used infrequently, the spray may be more cost-effective in the long run. Sublingual tablets are outdated in 6 months, but the lingual spray is good for about 3 years.

Continued

CASE STUDY   Antianginal Drugs—Cont'd

Q3. How do you know if the nitroglycerin spray is being effective?

A. JS should report a decrease in the frequency and severity of anginal attacks, improved activity tolerance, and a sense of well-being. He should be able to correctly identify his drug, proper administration technique, and dose, as well as signs and symptoms of hypotension, ways to minimize orthostatic changes, and the importance of keeping follow-up appointments.

Q4. I recently heard that instead of taking three tablets of sublingual nitroglycerin 5 minutes apart and then calling 911, that patients are being advised to take only 1 tablet before calling 911. How can I find out if this is true?

A. I would be inclined to look in the ACLS textbook or call the American Heart Association or the American College of Cardiology for guidance. You can also check the evidence-based practice materials online. The treatment recommendations for a whole variety of conditions are always changing. Find a reliable resource and use it.

LIFE-SPAN CONSIDERATIONS

Pregnant and Nursing Women. Pregnancy is normally accompanied by significant physiologic changes in the maternal cardiovascular system (i.e., blood volume, cardiac output, pulse, blood pressure, and peripheral vascular resistance) (see Chapter 6). In the majority of patients, these changes present no significant risk to maternal or fetal well-being. However, certain patients experience a sudden decompensation of heart function during pregnancy.

Both the myocardium and the myometrium of the uterus possess α and β receptors. The smooth muscle of the uterus contracts in response to α stimulation and relaxes with β stimulation. Consider secondary uterine effects in patients treated with cardiac drugs that cause either type of stimulation. Further, there is controversy regarding the safety of beta blockers in pregnancy, and it is thought that propranolol lowers umbilical blood flow. There have been reports of blunting of fetal heart rate accelerations during the intrapartum period, bradycardia, increased incidence of growth retardation, delayed neonatal respirations, and hypoglycemia described with the use of beta blockers. Whether these phenomena are dose-related or are caused by the underlying cardiac disease is unclear. There is no evidence that identifies beta blockers as being teratogenic.

Older Adults. Physiologic changes in the cardiovascular system manifest a variety of ways in the older adult. The efficiency and contractile strength of the myocardium declines, resulting in a 1% reduction per year in cardiac output. Stroke volume is thought to decrease by 0.7% yearly, and the systolic and diastolic phases of the myocardial cycle are prolonged. Ordinarily, older adults adjust to these changes without much difficulty. However, when unusual demands are placed on the heart (e.g., shoveling snow, running to catch a bus), the changes become more evident. Pulse rates may not reach the levels of younger persons, and tachycardia lasts longer. There is some disagreement among health care providers as to when the normal elevation becomes hypertension. In some older adults, the blood pressure may remain stable while tachycardia progresses to anginal episodes and eventual heart failure.

Resistance to peripheral blood flow increases by 1% each year. Decreased elasticity of the arteries is responsible for vascular changes to the heart. Because of the rigidity of vessel walls and narrowing of lumens, more force is required to move blood through the vessels, increasing the risk of angina.

These changes also lead to a higher diastolic blood pressure. Further, there is a decrease in the ability of the aorta to distend, which in turn raises systolic pressure; vagal tone increases and the heart becomes more sensitive to carotid sinus stimulation. There is also reduced sensitivity of the baroreceptors, which potentiates orthostatic hypotension.

▓ *Drug Variables*

The ideal antianginal drug establishes a balance between ▲ coronary blood flow and metabolic demands of the heart. The choice of antianginal drug and route of administration is made with consideration of the desired onset of therapeutic effects; the suitability of various routes of administration for the individual patient; the need for stable drug concentrations; any comorbid conditions; and the likelihood of tolerance or toxicity. The drug would produce local effects by acting directly on coronary vessels rather than on other organ systems, and would promote oxygen extraction by the heart from arterial circulation. It would be effective when taken orally and would have sustained action and an absence of tolerance. Currently, no drug meets this ideal. A summary of the systemic effects of nitrates, beta blockers, and CCBs is presented in Table 35-5.

All patients with suspected or proven angina should receive drug therapy in an attempt to reduce the severity and frequency of anginal symptoms, enhance the quality of life, and minimize the risk of a MI. Because nitrates, beta blockers, and CCBs are useful in the treatment of angina, and each reduces oxygen consumption through different means, concurrent therapy may be advised in some patients (Fig. 35-5).

When relief of acute anginal pain is the desired goal and a rapid onset of drug action is necessary, the duration of action is less important. Conversely, for angina prophylaxis, the duration of action and the predictability of effect are key issues. The rapidity of onset and the duration of action of any drug are directly related to the route of administration.

NITRATES. Nitroglycerin, taken orally, has a significant first-pass effect. For this reason, nitroglycerin is available in several other formulations so as to bypass the first-pass effect.

Buccal extended-release tablets are placed between the cheek and the gum and allowed to dissolve. These tablets begin working within 2 to 3 minutes. If a second anginal attack occurs while there is an extended-release buccal tablet

TABLE 35-5 Effects of Antianginals on Heart Function

Response	Nitrates	Beta Blockers*	CCBs Nifedipine	Verapamil	Diltiazem
Afterload	↓	0 or ↓	↓↓↓	↓↓	↓↓
Arterial pressure	↓↓	↓	↓	↓	↓
Collateral blood flow	↑	NC	↓	↓	↓
LVEDV (Preload)	↓↓↓	↑	↓ or 0	↓ or 0	↓ or 0
Heart rate (chronotropic effect)	0 or ↑ †	↓↓↓	↑ or 0	↓↓	↓↓
Myocardial contractility (inotropic effect)	0 †	↓↓↓	↓	↓↓↓	↓↓
Preload	↓	↑	↓ or 0	0	0 or ↓
Vasodilation of epicardial coronary arteries	↑↑	↑ or 0	↑↑↑	↑↑↑	↑↑↑

*Beta blockers that are cardioselective and do not have intrinsic sympathomimetic activity (ISA).
†Reflex increase in heart rate and contractility with nitrate.
↑, Increased; ↓, Decreased; 0, little or no effect.
LVEDV, Left ventricular end diastolic volume; *NC,* no change.

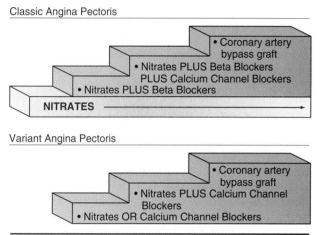

FIGURE 35-5 Progression of Antianginal Regimens for Classic and Variant Angina.

in place, a second tablet can be placed on the opposite side of the mouth.

Sublingual and buccal formulations have a similar onset time, but the effects of the buccal form last only as long as the tablet remains intact (approximately 5 hours). Nitroglycerin spray is more expensive per dose than the sublingual tablets. However, if nitroglycerin is used infrequently, the spray may be more cost-effective, because sublingual tablets are outdated in 6 months whereas the lingual spray is good for about 3 years. The onset and duration of action of the lingual spray are comparable to that of sublingual tablets, and it is equally effective.

Oral nitrates have a long history of safety and effectiveness as well as low cost. Nitrate tablets such as isosorbide dinitrate are longer-acting than sublingual forms of nitroglycerin and, when used in adequate doses, are effective for anginal prophylaxis. Because oral nitrates lack serious adverse effects, they should be used in patients in whom beta blockers are ineffective, contraindicated, or are not tolerated. The advantages of isosorbide mononitrate over the dinitrate formulation are that it does not require conversion in the body from dinitrate to mononitrate form, and it has proven efficacy in dosages that tend to circumvent tolerance. No evidence indicates that long-acting nitrates improve survival in patients with coronary artery disease.

Topical formulations may be useful for the patient with nocturnal and unstable angina because they have a longer duration of action than sublingual and lingual formulations. Paste formulations come in a tube, much like toothpaste, with a specially designed paper applicator. The drug is prescribed and measured by the inch (e.g., 1 inch) onto the paper applicator and then applied to a nonhairy skin surface.

Topical formulations have the same advantages as the sublingual and buccal formulations in that they bypass the liver and therefore the first-pass effect. The other advantage of a topical formulation over oral nitrates is that the effects can be stopped relatively quickly by simply wiping the drug off the skin. The disadvantages, however, are that some topical formulations are often messy, have a relative short duration of action, necessitating repeated application, and the dosage cannot be accurately controlled.

Both the reservoir and the matrix transdermal patch systems offer steady-state plasma levels within the therapeutic range over 24 hours, thus making only one application necessary per day. The disadvantage of the reservoir system is "dose dumping" if the seal is punctured or broken. Dose dumping does not occur with the matrix system. Both systems achieve plasma steady state levels in approximately 2 hours. However, **transdermal formulations of nitroglycerin must be removed** ▲ **for 10 to 12 hours each day to reduce the risk for nitrate tolerance.**

The greatest benefit of an IV nitrate is noted when the drug is administered within 4 to 8 hours of the onset of symptoms. Its beneficial effects include decreases in the number of anginal episodes, ventricular ectopic beats, and left ventricular failure. The dosage of IV nitroglycerin is adjusted according to patient responses. Check blood pressure and pulse every 5 to 15 minutes during dosage titration and every hour thereafter. Note, however, that IV nitroglycerin binds to the polyvinyl chloride plastic used in most IV solutions and infusion sets. In fact, so much of the drug binds to the plastic that an increase in dosage may be required to achieve treatment goals. The tubing that comes with IV nitroglycerin is made of a special plastic to which the drug does not bind.

Nitrate Tolerance. Tolerance, the loss of ability of the smooth muscles to respond to the action of the nitrates, develops with sustained, long-term use. Patients appear to develop tolerance not just to specific nitrates, but to the entire class of drugs. Tolerance is both dose- and time-dependent and can be seen after as few as 7 to 10 days of continuous administration. It may also develop with frequent sublingual administration of nitrates, if the oral tablets are taken 4 times daily in evenly spaced intervals, or if the transdermal patches are left in place for 24-hour periods.

To minimize tolerance, individualize nitrate therapy, using the lowest effective dose and an intermittent dosing schedule. One nitrate-free period per day is necessary, which means that the intervals between doses need not be equal. For example, a patient taking oral tablets can take the drug 3 times during the day only. No drug is used during the night. Transdermal formulations are applied upon arising and removed 12 hours later. Tolerance has not been reported with buccal forms of nitroglycerin, possibly because of the drug-free interval at night. Use combination antianginal drug therapy (e.g., a beta blocker plus a long-acting nitrate) for patients whose anginal symptoms are not controlled during the nitrate-free period.

⚠ *Nitrate Overdose.* **Nitrate overdose causes dose-dependent hypotension and reflex tachycardia. The simultaneous increase in oxygen demand and decrease in oxygen supply contributes to myocardial ischemia and possible MI. Severe hypotension causes cerebral ischemia and stroke.** Proper management includes temporarily stopping the nitrate, because the drug's short duration of action usually allows blood pressure to rise in a relatively short period. If an intentional overdose was taken orally, induced emesis and other measures to decrease drug absorption may be indicated. Vasopressors can be used to correct excessive hypotension; however, exercise caution to avoid coronary artery vasoconstriction that will further aggravate angina. Epinephrine use almost always increases oxygen demand by causing tachycardia and should be avoided since it may lower myocardial blood flow and oxygen supply by reducing diastolic pressure. Oxygen therapy is warranted to help overcome inadequate tissue oxygenation. Oxygen improves saturation and assists in meeting tissue oxygenation needs. It helps also to relieve the dyspnea associated with ischemic episodes.

⚠ Beta Blockers. **Beta blockers are used first-line in conjunction with sublingual nitroglycerin, for the prevention of ischemic events, and in the treatment of angina in patients with no comorbid conditions.** Beta blockers are also used as first-line drugs in patients who have hypertension, hyperthyroidism, intermittent claudication, or migraine headaches. Beta blockers may be chosen over nitrates to treat both angina and hypertension using a single drug. Their use is generally contraindicated in patients with chronic obstructive pulmonary disease (COPD), diabetes mellitus, heart failure, or Raynaud's phenomenon. However, when introduced slowly, beta blockers can improve, not worsen, heart failure.

Beta blockers (e.g., atenolol, nadolol) are effective and inexpensive, can be given once daily, and lower the likelihood of arrhythmia, reinfarction, and even sudden cardiac death after MI. Concurrent use of beta blockers and nitrates reduces coronary vascular resistance associated with beta blockade. Beta blockers can be used for patients in whom coronary vasospasm plays a role in the development of anginal pain during exercise and at rest. The additive benefit is primarily a result of one drug blocking the adverse effects of the other on myocardial oxygen consumption.

Nadolol, a nonselective beta blocker with low lipid-solubility, may be used initially because it has proven effectiveness and several advantages over propranolol. The absorption of nadolol is consistent, and can be given once daily. Nadolol also offers distinct advantages in that it blocks catecholamine-induced (β_2) arrhythmias and hypokalemia. Acebutolol, another selective beta blocker, and atenolol can be used instead of nadolol if the drugs are found to be less expensive, or if the patient has a problem with cold extremities, since this condition can be worsened by antagonizing β_2 receptors.

Calcium Channel Blockers. CCBs are useful additions to antianginal therapy if nitrates and beta blockers are ineffective. All CCBs are equally effective as antianginal drugs; however, they are relatively expensive and are often taken more than once daily. Diltiazem is usually the best tolerated, however, and should be chosen over other drugs unless there are significant price differences. Sustained-release formulations are recommended, because they are more convenient and there is often little price difference compared with the immediate-release formulations.

Long-acting CCBs reduce the heart rate in patients for whom beta blockers cannot be used, and for those in whom symptomatic relief of angina cannot be achieved with the use of nitrates, immediate-acting beta blockers, or both. Avoid short-acting dihydropyridine CCBs because they increase the risk of adverse cardiac events.

CCBs are more effective than beta blockers for patients with Prinzmetal's angina, although they are more expensive. CCBs may also be used first-line in patients with intermittent claudication or Raynaud's phenomenon. They are often second-line drugs for the patient with COPD, diabetes, or migraines. CCBs can be used for patients with angina and hypertension who are unable to take beta blockers. **Patients** ⚠ **with heart failure, particularly those with left ejection fractions less than 30%, should not use CCBs because they depress left ventricular function.**

However, variant angina is best treated with nitrates and CCBs to reduce the vasospasm of coronary arteries. The combination of a nitrate and a CCB provides greater relief of severe stable or variant angina than can be obtained with either drug alone. CCBs are as effective as nitrates and may even be preferred to beta blockers in the management of variant or unstable angina. Nitrates reduce preload, whereas CCBs reduce afterload. The net effect on reduction of oxygen demand is additive. It should be noted, however, that excessive vasodilation can occur.

Use of cardiac glycosides (i.e., digoxin) may be indicated if the patient with angina has preexisting heart failure contributing to difficulties in oxygen supply, demand, and extraction. The opioid morphine offers analgesia and lowers myocardial oxygen demand by reducing preload. Peak respiratory depression occurs 10 minutes after the dose, but if the patient is still in pain 5 minutes after the initial dose, it is highly unlikely that respiratory depression will occur at 10 minutes. Give the patient morphine (2 mg) every 5 minutes until the pain is relieved. The disadvantage of morphine, though, is that it blocks the perception of pain, an important indicator of the severity of ischemia.

The patient with angina may also receive anticoagulants or antiplatelet drugs to prevent thrombus formation. Use of fibrinolytics (see Chapter 39), antihypertensives (see Chapter 37), and cholesterol-lowering drugs (see Chapter 38) may also be indicated. Antiplatelet drugs (e.g., aspirin) interfere with platelet aggregation by inhibiting the formation of thromboxane A$_2$. When used to treat patients with unstable angina, aspirin lowers the risk of developing an acute MI and reduces mortality by 50%. Aspirin currently is the only antiplatelet drug recommended for the prevention of acute MI in patients with unstable angina. No other antiplatelet drug has been found to be as effective. All patients with angina should take 80 to 325 mg of aspirin daily. For patients in whom aspirin cannot be used because of allergy or GI complications, consider the antiplatelet drug clopidogrel (Plavix).

Patient Education

For optimal control of anginal symptoms, educate the patient on the disorder and the drugs used in treatment. Inform the patient of the seriousness of CAD and the potential consequences of untreated angina. Provide education to all patients about therapeutic lifestyle changes as often as possible. Also teach patients how to recognize worsening symptoms so that medical care can be sought in a timely manner.

Regularly inform family members about the storage location and the proper use of the drugs in case the patient needs assistance in taking them. In addition, teach the patient or family members how to recognize and report signs and symptoms of hypotension and to minimize the effects of orthostatic hypotension. Clearly explain that the dosage of these drugs is individualized to maximize therapeutic effects and minimize adverse reactions and that abrupt discontinuance of antianginal drugs is associated with increases in anginal episodes and possible MI.

Advise patients that sublingual tablets generally cause a tingling or slight burning sensation when placed under the tongue. For many years, the tingling, burning sensation was used as an indicator of the drug's "freshness." Advise patients not to use the tingling and burning as an indicator that the drug will be effective. Older patients may not have the tingling, even with new sublingual nitroglycerin tablets. Patients who doubt the potency of their drug should have their prescription refilled and then discard the old drug. Advise the patient not to eat, drink, or smoke while an undissolved tablet remains in the mouth.

Teach the patient and/or the family as to the proper storage of antianginal preparations. Sublingual formulations are effective for a period of 5 to 6 months when stored in a dark, cool location. Tablets are inactivated by light, heat, air, and moisture; they should be stored at room temperature in an amber glass container with a tight-fitting lid. Lingual sprays are viable for up to 3 years. Tell patients not to transfer the drug to other containers and to discard any unused nitroglycerin tablets in an appropriate manner.

▥ Smoking Cessation

Clearly encourage patients to stop smoking now, and take an active role in helping them to achieve this goal. Smoking cessation results in a significant reduction (37%) of acute adverse effects on the heart and may reverse, or at least slow, the progression of atherosclerosis. Smoking raises carboxyhemoglobin levels in the blood, reducing the amount of oxygen available to the myocardium and possibly precipitating anginal episodes. Patients exposed for 2 hours to smoke not only suffer elevations in carboxyhemoglobin concentrations but

also experience shortened exercise time, and increased heart rate and blood pressure. Second-hand smoke should also be avoided.

▥ Lipid Management

For patients with established CAD, reducing low-density lipoprotein (LDL) levels with a 3-hydroxy-3-methylglutaryl (HMG) coenzyme A reductase inhibitor (i.e., a "statin") is associated with significant reductions in both mortality and morbidity rates (see Chapter 38). A 10% reduction in lipid levels reduces the risk of CAD by 20%. In patients with established CAD who have a low HDL and low-risk LDL levels, drug therapy that raises HDL levels, lowers triglyceride levels, but has no effect on LDL levels (e.g., gemfibrozil) significantly reduces the risk of angina and major cardiac events.

A diet low in saturated fat and cholesterol and high in fiber is the basis for the Step I and Step II diet from the American Heart Association. Anginal episodes and CAD are less common in patients who have a high intake of dietary fiber. Encourage patients to eat small meals high in fiber, abstain from gas-forming foods, and rest for short periods after eating.

▥ Exercise and Stress Management

Advise patients who lead active, hectic lives to adjust activities to below the level that precipitates anginal episodes. Try for brief rest periods throughout the work day, an early bedtime, and longer or more frequent vacations. Help patients who are anxious or nervous to understand the importance of counseling, relaxation exercises, and other stress reduction techniques.

Strenuous exercise can precipitate an anginal attack but can be effectively managed with appropriate exercise limitations. Exercise enlarges heart volume and mass, increases capillary vascularity, raises the threshold for ischemia, and decreases the heart rate—all of which protects the myocardium from the effects of ischemic damage, and improves the patient's well-being. However, the patient with documented evidence of ischemic heart disease should be cautioned against engaging in strenuous exercise because it raises myocardial oxygen demand.

▥ OTC Drugs and Adherence to Therapy

Teach the patient the importance of avoiding concurrent use of other drugs without first checking with the health care provider. Over-the-counter decongestants, cold remedies, and diet pills stimulate the heart and constrict blood vessels, which can contribute to anginal episodes.

Also advise patients to avoid abruptly discontinuing their antianginal drug. Inform patients and their families that if it is necessary to discontinue an antianginal drug, the drug should be slowly tapered off over several days to prevent rebound angina, hypertension, arrhythmias, and acute MI.

Evaluation

With appropriate therapy, the patient with angina should report a decrease in the frequency and severity of anginal attacks, improved activity tolerance, and sense of well-being. Improvement in lifestyle should be judged not only as the ability to sustain normal activities without symptoms, but also on the basis of the inconvenience caused by treatment. The patient should be able to correctly identify his or her drug, proper administration technique, and dose, as well as signs and symptoms of hypotension, methods to minimize orthostatic changes, and the importance of keeping follow-up appointments.

KEY POINTS

- CAD secondary to atherosclerosis is the most common cause of angina pectoris.
- Risk factors for the development of angina are CAD, hypertension, hypercholesterolemia, smoking, and lack of regular exercise.
- Angina typically takes one of three forms: stable angina (classic, stable exertional, predictable), unstable angina (acute coronary insufficiency, crescendo, preinfarction), and variant angina (Prinzmetal's, vasospastic).
- Classic angina pain is located in the retrosternal region, but the pain may occur anywhere in the chest, the neck, the arms, or the back. It commonly radiates to the left arm, the mandible, or the neck. Levine's sign is often displayed when patients explain the location of their discomfort.
- Associated signs and symptoms are diaphoresis, dizziness, dyspnea, vomiting, weakness, palpitations, and pallor. In some patients with a myocardial infarction, chest pain is minimal or absent.
- The goals of antianginal therapy are to decrease the duration and the intensity of pain during an attack, reduce the frequency of attacks, and improve exercise capacity.

- Drug therapy used in the treatment of angina includes single as well as combination therapy with nitrates, beta blockers, and/or CCBs.
- Choice of antianginal drug and route of administration are made with consideration of the onset of effects, the suitability of the route for that patient, the need for stable drug concentrations, and the likelihood of tolerance or toxicity.
- Patients taking long-acting nitrates must have a supply of a short-acting nitrate on hand in case of anginal attack requiring additional nitrate.
- Intermittent treatment rather than continuous therapy minimizes the potential for tolerance to nitrates.
- Monitor the patient for toxicities associated with nitrates, beta blockers, and CCBs.
- Teach patients the name of their antianginal drug, its correct use and adverse effects, and when to seek medical attention if anginal pain is unrelieved.
- The therapeutic effects of antianginal therapy are demonstrated by patient reports of a decrease in the frequency and severity of anginal attacks along with improved exercise tolerance.

Bibliography

Alaeddini, J., Alimohammadi, B., and Shirani, J. (2006). Angina pectoris. *eMedicine*, Available online: www.emedicine.com/med/topic133.htm. Accessed May 7, 2007.

American Heart Association. (2004). *Heart and stroke facts: 2006 Update*. Dallas, TX: Author.

Beaulieu, M., Brophy, J., and Jacques, A., et al. (2004). Drug treatment of stable angina pectoris and mass dissemination of therapeutic guidelines: A randomized controlled trial. *QJM: Monthly Journal of Physicians*, 97(1), 21–31.

Belardinelli, L., Shryock, J., and Fraser, H. (2006). The mechanism of ranolazine action to reduce ischemia-induced diastolic dysfunction. *European Heart Journal Supplement*, 8(Suppl A), A10–A13.

Berger, P. (2004). Ranolazine and other antianginal therapies in the era of the drug-eluting stent. *Journal of the American Medical Association*, 291(3), 365–367.

Braunwald, E., Antman, E., and Beasley, J., et al. (2002). ACC/AHA guideline update for the management of patients with unstable angina and non-ST-segment elevation myocardial infarction–2002: Summary article: A report of the American College of Cardiology/American Heart Association Task Force on Practice Guidelines (Committee on the Management of Patients with Unstable Angina). *Circulation*, 106(14), 1893–1900.

Braunwald, E., Califf, R., and Cannon, C., et al. (2000). Redefining medical treatment in the management of unstable angina. *American Journal of Medicine*, 108(1), 41–53.

Chaitman, B., Pepine, C., and Parker, J., et al. (2004). Effects of ranolazine with atenolol, amlodipine, or diltiazem on exercise tolerance and angina frequency in patients with severe chronic angina: A randomized controlled trial. *Journal of the American Medical Association*, 291(3), 309–316.

Gibbons, R., Abrams, J., and Chatterjee, K., et al. (2003). ACC/AHA 2002 guideline update for the management of patients with chronic stable angina: A report of the American College of Cardiology/American Heart Association Task Force on Practice Guidelines (Committee to Update the 1999 Guidelines for the Management of Patients with Chronic Stable Angina). *Journal of the American College of Cardiology*, 41(1), 159–168.

Jerling, M., Huan, B., and Leung, K., et al. (2005). Studies to investigate the pharmacokinetic interactions between ranolazine and ketoconazole, diltiazem, or simvastatin during combined administration in healthy subjects. *Journal of Clinical Pharmacology*, 45(4), 422–433.

National Heart Lung and Blood Institute. (2005). What is angina? National Institutes of Health. Available online: www.nhlbi.nih.gov/index.htm. Accessed May 7, 2007.

U.S. Department of Health and Human Services, Public Health Service, Agency for Health Care Policy and Research. (2005). *Clinical practice guideline: Diagnosing and managing unstable angina*. Rockville, MD: Author.

Yusef, S., Sleight, P., and Pogue, J., et al. (2000). Effects of an angiotensin-converting enzyme inhibitor, ramipril, on cardiovascular events in high-risk patients: The Heart Outcomes Prevention Evaluation Study. *New England Journal of Medicine*, 342(3), 154–160.

36

Antiarrhythmic Drugs

Antiarrhythmic drugs are used for the prevention and treatment of cardiac arrhythmias. The use of antiarrhythmic drugs in the United States has become less popular owing to their proarrhythmic effects and evidence linking many of the drugs to increased mortality. Antiarrhythmic drugs continue to be used for emergent indications. One of these drugs in particular, namely amiodarone, has become the most commonly prescribed drug in this class. Non–drug alternatives in the management of arrhythmia have also more recently made an impact on the care of patients with arrhythmias.

An *arrhythmia*, also known as a *dysrhythmia*, is defined as an abnormal, disordered, or disturbed rhythm—any deviation from normal sinus rhythm (NSR). There are two basic rhythm disturbances: *tachyarrhythmias*, seen as rapid, and sometimes irregular, beats; and *bradyarrhythmias*, which are rhythm irregularities with a slow heart rate. This chapter primarily discusses drugs used to treat, suppress, or prevent two major mechanisms for arrhythmias—an abnormality in impulse formation (i.e., automaticity) or an abnormality in impulse conduction (i.e., reentry). In general, the goal of antiarrhythmic drug therapy is to maximize the time a patient spends in normal sinus rhythm.

ARRHYTHMIAS

EPIDEMIOLOGY AND ETIOLOGY

Arrhythmias are common in patients with cardiac disorders but also occur in people with normal hearts. Abnormalities of cardiac rhythm and conduction can cause sudden cardiac death and may be symptomatic (i.e., with syncope, dizziness, or palpitations) or asymptomatic. The irregularities may be mild or severe, acute or chronic, episodic or relatively continuous.

Although a variety of medical conditions and drugs can cause arrhythmias, the most common cause is myocardial infarction (MI) secondary to coronary artery disease (CAD). Rhythm disturbances occur in approximately 80% of all patients having an MI. Other causes of arrhythmias include electrolyte imbalance, hypoxia, and drug toxicity. Multiple factors can precipitate or contribute to the development of arrhythmias. These factors include sympathetic nervous system (SNS) stimulation (e.g., catecholamine excess), metabolic disturbances (e.g., acidosis, alkalosis, or hyperthyroidism), electrolyte disturbances (e.g., potassium imbalance), and hemodynamic abnormalities (e.g., a reduction in coronary perfusion associated with hypertension or presence of diseased myocardial tissue). Rhythm disturbances are dangerous to the extent that they reduce cardiac output and impair perfusion of the brain or myocardium, or that they deteriorate, as is their tendency, into more serious arrhythmias with the same consequences.

Cardiac Electrophysiology

The electrophysiologic characteristics of cardiac muscle include excitability, automaticity, conductivity, and refractoriness. Normally, these characteristics result in effective myocardial contraction and proper circulation. Each cardiac cycle consists of four events: (1) stimulation from an electrical impulse; (2) transmission of the impulse to conductive or contractile tissue; (3) contraction of atria and ventricles; and (4) and relaxation of atria and ventricles. During relaxation, the atria and ventricles refill with blood in preparation for the next cycle.

Excitability is the capacity of cardiac muscle cells to respond to an electrical stimulus. At rest, the inside of the myocardial cell is more negative than the outside, thus classifying the cell as polarized. This *resting membrane potential* results from differences in sodium (Na^+) and potassium (K^+) concentrations on either side of cell membranes. K^+ is primarily concentrated in the intracellular space, whereas Na^+ is more concentrated in the extracellular space.

Automaticity is the ability of the heart cell to automatically depolarize and generate an action potential. This characteristic resides in the cells of the sinoatrial (SA) node and the atrioventricular (AV) nodes and in the bundle of His. When the myocardial cell is stimulated to a certain threshold, the membrane potential changes. The movement of ions changes the membrane potential from a state of electrical neutrality to an energized state. This change in the membrane potential is known as an *action potential.* Box 36-1 describes the phases of the action potential. Depolarization, the discharge of the electrical energy, results in myocardial muscle contraction.

The initial depolarization of atrial and ventricular tissues, which occurs rapidly, is generally due to an influx of Na^+

BOX 36-1

Phases of Action Potential

Phase 0: Rapid depolarization. Results from rapid influx of Na^+.

Phase 1: Initial repolarization. Inactivation of inward Na^+ current and activation of outward K^+ current.

Phase 2: Plateau. Little change in membrane potential. Outward K^+ movement with inward Ca^{++} movement through Ca^{++} channels.

Phase 3: Rapid depolarizat ion with K^+ efflux.

Phase 4: Gradual depolarization of cell. Na^+ gradually leaks into intracellular spaces to balance decreased efflux of K^+. Increases in Na^+ permeability lead to phase 0.

ions. Not all cardiac cells, however, depend on Na^+ for this initial depolarization and may depolarize in response to the entry of calcium (Ca^{++}) ions. Ca^{++}-responsive cells are found primarily in automatic tissues such as the SA and the AV nodes. The conduction of an electrical impulse generated by Ca^{++} is slower than one produced by a change in Na^+. In general, activation of the SA and AV nodes depends on a slow depolarizing current through Ca^{++} channels. Activation of the atria and the ventricles depends on a rapid depolarizing current through Na^+ channels. These two types of conduction tissues are often called *slow* and *fast* channels, respectively.

Following myocardial muscle contraction there is a period of repolarization, that is, a period of decreased excitability during which the cell cannot respond to a new stimulus. During this refractory period, Na^+ and Ca^{++} ions return to the extracellular space, and K^+ ions return to the intracellular space. Muscle relaxation occurs, and the cell prepares for the next cycle of electrical activity and contraction.

Conductivity is the ability of the heart to convey electrical impulses along and across cell membranes. The systematic, rhythmic transmission of impulses results in effective myocardial muscle contraction. Normally, electrical impulses originate in the SA node. The impulses are transmitted to the atria where they cause atrial contraction. Impulses continue through conduction pathways to the AV node, the bundle of His, bundle branches, and Purkinje fibers, resulting in ventricular contraction.

Refractoriness is the inability of the heart to respond to new stimuli while it is still in a state of contraction from a previous stimulus. Refractoriness develops as a result of inactivation of Na^+ channels during depolarization. Thus the heart does not respond to restimulation during the action potential, reducing the likelihood of tetanic contractions. Refractoriness normally prevents uncontrolled, rapid myocardial contractions, helping to preserve heart rhythm. Damaged cardiac cells may maintain a constant state of refractoriness or may not be refractory at all.

Types and Origins of Disturbances

Arrhythmias result from disruptions in electrophysiology, including the spontaneous initiation of an impulse (automaticity), the conduction of the impulse (conductivity), or both. Arrhythmias may originate in any part of the conduction system: the SA node, atria, AV node, bundle of His, bundle branches, Purkinje fibers, or ventricles. Table 36-1 provides examples of arrhythmias according to their site of origin and mechanism.

▥ Automaticity Disturbances

A disturbance in the spontaneous initiation of an electrical impulse increases or decreases heart rate and rhythm. The SA node is the pacemaker of the heart because it holds the highest level of automaticity. It normally produces a rhythm of 60 to 100 beats/min (bpm). A decrease in the automaticity of the SA node results in sinus bradycardia (heart rate below 60 bpm). Sinus bradycardia frequently occurs in young adults and well-trained athletes and is common at night. An increase in automaticity produces sinus tachycardia (heart rate above 100 bpm).

On the other hand, an arrhythmia can be the result of an ectopic focus. An *ectopic focus* is a shift in the site of impulse

TABLE 36-1 Organization of Arrhythmias

Automaticity Disturbances	Conduction Disturbances
SUPRAVENTRICULAR ARRHYTHMIAS	
Sinus tachycardia	Paroxysmal supraventricular tachycardia (PSVT)
Sinus bradycardia	Atrial tachycardia
	Atrial flutter
	Atrial fibrillation
	Wolff-Parkinson-White syndrome
NODAL ARRHYTHMIAS	
Premature junctional contractions	First-degree AV heart block
Junctional escape rhythm (HR 40–60 bpm)	Second-degree AV heart block
Premature AV junctional tachycardias	• Mobitz type I block (Wenckebach)
Nonparoxysmal AV junctional tachycardia (HR >60 bpm)	• Mobitz type II block
	Third-degree AV heart block (complete HB)
VENTRICULAR ARRHYTHMIAS	
Premature ventricular contraction (PVC)	Right bundle branch block (RBBB)
Ventricular tachycardia	Left bundle branch block (LBBB)
Ventricular fibrillation	Ventricular asystole
Torsades de pointes*	

*Torsades de pointes is a rapid form of polymorphic ventricular tachycardia associated with a long QT interval.
AV, Atrioventricular; *bpm;* beats/min; *HR*, heart rhythm.

formation from the SA node to another site within the myocardium. For example, if the SA node fails to fire, other sites in the atria can fire. If the atria do not initiate a beat, it can begin in the AV node; and if the AV node does not initiate a beat, one can start in the ventricles. If the ectopic focus depolarizes at a rate faster than the SA node, the ectopic focus becomes the dominant pacemaker. Ectopic foci indicate myocardial irritability and potentially serious impairment of cardiac function. Ectopic foci can be activated by hypoxia, ischemia, hyperkalemia, hypocalcemia, increased catecholamine activity, digoxin toxicity, and administration of atropine.

▥ Conduction Disturbances

Altered conduction probably accounts for more arrhythmias than changes in automaticity. Conduction can be too rapid or too slow. Conduction disturbances result from a delay or block of impulse formation, or from what is referred to as the *reentry phenomenon* (Fig. 36-1). Under normal circumstances, an electrical impulse moves down the conduction pathway until it reaches recently excited tissues refractory to stimulation. This causes the impulse to be extinguished. Reentry is a phenomenon whereby an impulse continues to reenter an area of the heart rather than becoming extinguished. For a reentry phenomenon to occur, an obstacle must be present within the normal conduction pathway. The obstacle permits electrical conduction in one direction only, thus causing a circuitous movement of the impulse. The obstacle is ordinarily an area of damage. The damage can be caused by electrolyte imbalance, impaired cellular metabolism, cardiac glycoside toxicity, ischemia, beta blockers, increased atrial preload, scarring of conduction pathways, compression of the AV node by scar tissue, AV-nodal inflammation, excessive vagal stimulation of the heart, MI (particularly an inferior location),

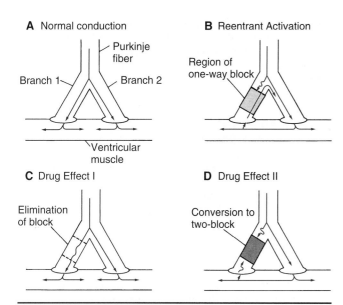

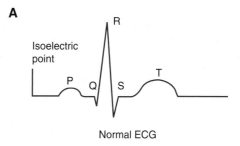

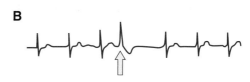

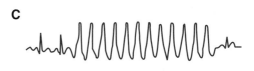

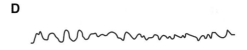

FIGURE 36-1 Reentry Phenomenon. Reentry phenomenon is the result of a barricade (e.g., myocardial muscle damage) located in the normal conduction pathway. Electrical impulses continue to reenter an area of the heart rather than being extinguished. The damaged area permits conduction in only one direction, causing a circular movement of the impulse. (From Lehne, R. [1998]. *Pharmacology for nursing care* [3rd ed., p. 500]. Philadelphia: WB Saunders. Used with permission.)

FIGURE 36-2 Electrocardiographic (ECG) Pattern. A, Normal ECG pattern recognized by impulse waves arbitrarily designated by the following letters: *P* (atrial depolarization); *PR* interval (impulse spreads from atria to ventricles); *QRS* (ventricular depolarization); *ST* interval (completion of ventricular depolarization); and *T* (ventricular repolarization); *QT* interval (represents electrical systole). **B,** Premature ventricular contraction. Represented by discrete and identifiable premature QRS complexes; usually of an abnormal shape. **C,** Ventricular tachycardia. Recognized by a rapidly occurring series of consecutive premature ventricular contractions (three or more) with no normal beats in between. P wave and PR interval absent; QRS complex widened. Ventricular tachycardia can progress to fibrillation at any time. **D,** Ventricular fibrillation. Recognized by individual deflections that vary in size and frequency. (Adapted from Page C., Curtis M., Sutter M., et al. [2002] *Integrated pharmacology* [2nd ed., p. 367]. Edinburgh: Mosby.)

and valvular surgery. If reentry is repetitive, sustained ventricular arrhythmias can occur.

Types of Arrhythmias

Most arrhythmias are classified according to site of origin and mechanism. For example, sinus tachycardia is a common arrhythmia. The term *sinus* refers to the site, and *tachycardia* refers to the mechanism of the arrhythmia.

▥ Supraventricular Arrhythmias

Supraventricular arrhythmias are viewed along a continuum of rate acceleration and a progressive reduction in atrial function: premature atrial contraction (PAC), atrial tachycardia (a rate of approximately 150 bpm), atrial flutter (a rate of about 300 bpm), and atrial fibrillation (quivering, uncoordinated activity). The AV node does not conduct atrial impulses at rates exceeding 180 bpm, which protects the ventricles from responding to extreme rates.

PACs are recognized on the electrocardiogram (ECG) by the presence of premature P waves that differ in appearance, size, or shape. Atrial tachycardia is characterized by P waves that become lost in the preceding T wave. The PR and QRS intervals may be normal. Atrial flutter is identified by inverted or bidirectional P waves that produce a saw-tooth pattern. Only every second or third impulse is conducted in atrial flutter. Atrial fibrillation is characterized by erratic or no P waves, an irregular RR interval, and a baseline that appears to be irregular and undulating (Fig. 36-2). The hemodynamic response to atrial arrhythmias depends on ventricular rate and myocardial contractility.

Supraventricular arrhythmias are usually significant only in the presence of underlying heart disease. In CAD, atrial tachycardia increases myocardial oxygen consumption and shortens diastole. As a result, anginal pain may occur. With aortic valvular disease or hypertrophic myopathies, atrial flutter or atrial fibrillation decreases ventricular filling by as much as 30%; thus cardiac output is severely impaired. Atrial fibrillation and flutter may also lead to the formation of thrombi in the atria.

Nodal Arrhythmias

Nodal arrhythmias consist of tachycardia, with increased workload for the heart, or bradycardia from heart block. Heart block involves impaired conduction of the electrical impulse through the AV node. With first-degree heart block, conduction is impaired, but not significantly. The ECG reveals a regular P wave followed by a QRS complex. The PR interval is prolonged beyond normal. With second-degree heart block, every second, third, or fourth impulse is blocked and does not reach the ventricles (a 2:1, 3:1, or 4:1 block). Atrial and ventricular rates thus differ. Second-degree heart block may interfere with cardiac output or progress to third-degree block. Third-degree block is the most serious because no atrial impulses can pass the AV node to reach the ventricles. As a result, the ventricles beat independently of the atria at a rate of 30 to 40 bpm. The slow ventricular rate severely reduces cardiac output.

Ventricular Arrhythmias

Occasional PVCs occur in everyone and are rarely significant. However, PVCs occurring after an acute MI, those that occur more than 5 times per minute, and those that are coupled, grouped, or multifocal, or that occur during the resting phase of the cardiac cycle, are considered life threatening. These arrhythmias lead to ventricular tachycardia, ventricular flutter, ventricular fibrillation, and asystole. Ventricular tachycardia increases myocardial oxygen consumption and shortens diastole. Ventricular flutter or fibrillation results in ineffective myocardial contraction. As a result, there is little to no cardiac output. Death results unless effective cardiopulmonary resuscitation or defibrillation is instituted.

PHARMACOTHERAPEUTIC OPTIONS

There are no universally effective drugs for all arrhythmias. Antiarrhythmic drugs are often classified using the Vaughan Williams classification, which organizes the drugs according to their fundamental mechanism of action. Table 36-2 provides a summary of antiarrhythmic drug classifications, their mechanisms of action, their indications, and the therapeutic ECG changes they are expected to produce. The majorities of antiarrhythmic drugs are used to treat tachyarrhythmias and as such are myocardial depressants.

There are five distinct characteristics to the ideal antiarrhythmic drug. (1) It should possess a high degree of efficacy for a well-defined group of arrhythmias; (2) it should have minimal adverse effects, including proarrhythmic effects, and no clinically significant drug interactions; (3) oral dosage forms would exhibit minimal first-pass effects and be available as an intravenous (IV) formulation; (4) it should have a half-life conducive to infrequent dosing, which in turn improves patient adherence with therapy; and (5) the drug would have a positive correlation between efficacy and plasma concentration. To date, not one antiarrhythmic drug meets all of these criteria. However, the characteristics can be used when surveying the advantages and disadvantages of the various drugs.

Class I antiarrhythmics are similar in structure and action to local anesthetics. They are divided into subclasses based on the type of Na$^+$ channel blockade produced. Class I drugs have specific receptor-binding characteristics, showing an affinity for a particular state of a channel. Because these drugs are weak bases and inhibit Na$^+$ channels in their ionized form, health care providers must consider the impact of pH when prescribing class I drugs. Generally, acidosis increases activity whereas alkalosis leads to reduced Na$^+$ channel inhibition.

Class I$_A$ Antiarrhythmics

◆ disopyramide (Norpace, Norpace CR); ✦ Rhythmodan, Rhythmodan LA
◆ procainamide (Procan SR, Promine, Pronestyl, Pronestyl-SR); ✦ Procan SR
◆ quinidine gluconate (Quinaglute Dura-Tabs, Quin G)
◆ quinidine sulfate (Quinidex Extentabs, Quinora); ✦ Apo-Quinidine, Novo-Quinidin

Indications

Class I$_A$ antiarrhythmics have powerful direct effects on most types of myocardial cells. Although there is no one overall prototypical antiarrhythmic, procainamide is considered a prototype of sorts for class I$_A$ drugs. It is the most widely used class I$_A$ antiarrhythmic, and it is effective in the management of a wide variety of atrial and ventricular arrhythmias, including PACs, premature ventricular contractions (PVCs), ventricular tachycardia, and paroxysmal atrial tachycardia. Quinidine is also used to help maintain normal sinus rhythm in patients with atrial flutter or atrial fibrillation.

With the advent of cardioversion, quinidine and procainamide are now used as prophylaxis in the management of atrial flutter and fibrillation. Of the patients scheduled for cardioversion who are treated with drug therapy 1 to 2 days before the procedure, approximately one third with atrial fibrillation and atrial flutter convert to NSR before cardioversion. However, the majority of patients still require cardioversion. Maintenance therapy with quinidine or procainamide helps prevent recurrence of the arrhythmia. However, in randomized, controlled clinical studies, maintenance therapy has been associated with a twofold to threefold increase in mortality.

Disopyramide is also used for the suppression and prevention of unifocal and multifocal PVCs and ventricular tachycardia. It has also been used for the prevention and treatment of supraventricular tachyarrhythmias, although it has not been approved by the FDA for such use.

Pharmacodynamics

Class I$_A$ drugs produce local anesthetic effects by their ability to block neuronal Na$^+$ channels, which in turn slows the rate of rise of the action potential depolarization and slows conduction velocity in Purkinje fibers. Class I$_A$ drugs tend to suppress automaticity by lowering the pacemaker potential needed to provoke spontaneous depolarization. Refractory periods are prolonged, and premature electrical stimulation is less likely to occur. The shift in the threshold is due to blockade of fast Na$^+$ channels and slowing of the reactivation rate. Indirectly, quinidine also possesses strong anticholinergic properties. There is little effect on the heart rate, but the drugs exert a direct negative inotropic effect.

Responses to class I$_A$ antiarrhythmic drugs typically include an increased pulse rate, a widening of the QRS complex, and prolongation of the PR and QT intervals. Effects

TABLE 36-2 Antiarrhythmic Drug Classifications*

Drugs	Indications	Effects on ECG
CLASS I—MEMBRANE STABILIZERS		
CLASS I$_A$		
disopyramide, procainamide, quinidine	Atrial flutter Arial fibrillation (conversion/prophylaxis) Premature atrial contractions Premature ventricular contractions Ventricular tachycardia	Widens QRS complex Prolongs QT interval Prolongs PR interval (slightly)
CLASS I$_B$		
lidocaine, mexiletine, phenytoin	Premature ventricular contractions Ventricular tachycardia Ventricular fibrillation	Widens QRS complex Prolongs QT interval Prolongs PR interval (slightly)
CLASS I$_C$—Na$^+$ CHANNEL BLOCKERS		
flecainide, propafenone	Severe ventricular arrhythmias only	Widens QRS complex Prolongs PR interval
CLASS II—BETA BLOCKERS		
acebutolol	Premature ventricular contractions	Normal or slightly prolonged PR interval
esmolol	Atrial fibrillation Atrial flutter Sinus tachycardia	Shortens QT interval (occasionally)
propranolol	Atrial flutter Atrial fibrillation Paroxysmal supraventricular tachycardia Sinus tachycardia	
CLASS III—PROLONG ACTION POTENTIAL		
amiodarone	Life-threatening supraventricular arrhythmias and ventricular arrhythmias resistant to other drugs	Widens QRS complex Prolongs QT interval† Prolongs PR interval
dofetilide	Atrial fibrillation Atrial flutter	
ibutilide	Atrial fibrillation Atrial flutter	
sotalol	Ventricular tachycardia Ventricular fibrillation	
CLASS IV— Ca^{++} CHANNEL BLOCKERS		
diltiazem	Atrial fibrillation Atrial flutter Paroxysmal supraventricular tachycardia	Decreases heart rate Increases pulse rate
verapamil	Paroxysmal supraventricular tachycardia	
COMBINED-ACTION DRUGS—SHARES ACTIVITY OF CLASSES I$_A$, I$_B$, AND I$_C$ DRUGS		
amiodarone	Life-threatening ventricular arrhythmias Ventricular fibrillation Unstable ventricular tachycardia	Widens QRS complex Prolongs QT interval Prolongs PR interval
moricizine	Life-threatening ventricular arrhythmias Supraventricular tachycardia	

*Antiarrhythmic drugs are placed in classifications based on Vaughan Williams classification system of major electrophysiologic effects. Drugs in the same class share common action and effects, but otherwise are so different that a prototype cannot be identified.
†Avoid use of class III antiarrhythmics concomitantly with other drugs that can prolong QT interval to minimize risk of torsades de pointes.
ECG, Electrocardiogram.

on the QRS complex and the QT interval are caused by slowing conduction through the bundle of His, Purkinje fibers, and ventricular fibers. Prolongation of the PR interval is caused by slowing the conduction through the AV node.

Pharmacokinetics

Table 36-3 provides an overview of the pharmacokinetics of antiarrhythmic drugs. There are three quinidine salts: quinidine sulfate, quinidine gluconate, and quinidine polygalacturonate. The active drug content is different for each formulation, as are the absorption and time to peak plasma levels.

Seventy-five percent to 90% of procainamide is absorbed from the gastrointestinal (GI) tract. Food and extremes in gastric pH hasten or delay drug absorption. Procainamide is well distributed through all body tissues. Procainamide is extensively biotransformed in the liver by the enzyme *N*-acetyltransferase to *N*-acetylprocainamide (NAPA). Acetylation of procainamide occurs primarily as a first-pass effect after oral administration. The rate of biotransformation varies widely and is determined by genetic factors. Rapid acetylators have higher plasma concentrations of the metabolite NAPA and eliminate greater quantities of NAPA in the urine than slow

PHARMACOKINETICS
TABLE 36-3 Antiarrhythmic Drugs

Drug	Route	Onset	Peak	Duration	PB (%)	t½	BioA (%)
CLASS I ANTIARRHYTHMICS							
CLASS I_A							
quinidine sulfate	PO	30 min	1–3 hr	6–8 hr	70–95	6–8 hr	70–73
quinidine gluconate	PO	UA	3–5 hr	6–8 hr	75–95	6–8 hr	70–73
procainamide	PO	30 min	30–120 min	3–4 hr	15–20	2.5–4.7 hr*	75–90
disopyramide	PO, SR	0.5–3.5 hr	2.5–4.9 hr	1.5–12 hr	35–95	4–10 hr	90
CLASS I_B ANTIARRHYTHMICS							
lidocaine	IV	Immed	Immed	10–20 min	60–80†	7–30 min; 90–120 min‡	100
mexiletine	PO	30–120 min	2–3 hr	8–12 hr	50–70	10–12 hr	90
phenytoin	IV	Immed	Immed	UA	90	DD	100
CLASS I_C ANTIARRHYTHMICS—NA+ CHANNEL BLOCKERS							
flecainide	PO	UA	2–3 hr	12 hr	32–47	11–14 hr	95
propafenone	PO	Hr	4–5 days§	Hours	97	2–17 hrs§	3–11
CLASS II ANTIARRHYTHMICS—BETA BLOCKERS							
acebutolol	PO	60 min	4–6 hr	10 hr	26	3–4 hr; 8–13 hr‖	<50
esmolol	IV	5 min	10–30 min	20–30 min	55	5–23 min	100
propranolol	PO	30 min	60–90 min	6–12 hr	93	3–5 hr	25
CLASS III ANTIARRHYTHMICS—PROLONG ACTION POTENTIAL							
amiodarone	PO	1–3 wk	UA	Weeks to months	96	13–107 days¶	35–65
	IV	2 hr	UA	UA			100
dofetilide	PO	UA	2–3 hr		60–70	10 hr	90
ibutilide	IV	Immed	UA	UA	UA	2–12 hr	100
sotalol	PO	UA	2–3 hr	UA	50	10–15 hr	100
CLASS IV ANTIARRHYTHMICS—CA++ CHANNEL BLOCKERS							
diltiazem	PO, SR	30 min	2–3 hr	6–8 hr; 12 hr**	70–80	3.5–9 hr	UA
	IV	2–5 min	UA	UA	70–80	3.5–9 hr	100
verapamil	IV	1–5 min††	3–5 min	2 hr	90	4.5–12 hr	100
	PO, SR	1–2 hr	30–90 min‡‡	3–7 hr	90	4.5–12 hr	UA
MISCELLANEOUS ANTIARRHYTHMICS							
adenosine	IV	Immed	UA	1–2 min	UA	<10 sec	100
moricizine	PO	UA	30–120 min	8–12 hr	95	1.5–3.5 hr	35

*Over 90% of patients taking procainamide are considered extensive metabolizers so half-life is 2 to 10 hr. In slow metabolizers the half-life is 10–32 hr.
†Protein binding of lidocaine depends on blood levels.
‡The half-life of lidocaine is biphasic, with the initial phase lasting 7–30 min and the terminal phase 90–120 min.
§Peak drug action with chronic dosing of propafenone. Plasma concentrations have limited usefulness because of variability between rapid (2–10 hr) and slow (10–32 hr) metabolizers.
‖Half-life of acebutolol and the metabolite, respectively.
¶The half-life of amiodarone is biphasic.
**Duration of drug action for rapid-release and sustained-release formulations of diltiazem.
††Onset of antiarrhythmic effects and hemodynamic effects of verapamil is 3–5 min following injection; these persist for up to 20 min.
‡‡Peak concentration of a single dose of verapamil. Effects of multiple doses may not be evident for 24–48 hr.
BioA, Bioavailability; DD, dose-dependent; Immed, immediately; PB, protein binding; SR, sustained-release formulation; t½, half-life; UA, unavailable.

acetylators. Both procainamide and NAPA are eliminated by active tubular secretion and glomerular filtration.

Quinidine is rapidly absorbed when taken by mouth. Quinidine is extensively biotransformed in the liver to several metabolites. Whether the metabolites possess antiarrhythmic activity remains controversial. In patients with hepatic insufficiency or cirrhosis, the unbound fraction may be significantly increased and the elimination half-life prolonged. The effect of renal dysfunction on disposition of quinidine also remains controversial. Alkaline urine retards drug elimination, whereas urinary acidification facilitates elimination of quinidine.

Disopyramide is also well absorbed from the GI tract, with variable binding to plasma proteins depending on plasma drug concentration. The hepatic biotransformation of disopyramide is not clear. About 50% is eliminated in the urine as unchanged drug and 30% as metabolites. A small percentage of the drug is eliminated in the feces.

Adverse Effects and Contraindications

The most common adverse effects of procainamide include GI upset such as abdominal pain and cramping, nausea, vomiting, and diarrhea. Occasionally dizziness, giddiness, weakness, and hypersensitivity reactions appear. One of the best characterized adverse effects of procainamide is a lupuslike syndrome. The syndrome is characterized by arthralgia, myalgia, skin rash, and the development of antinuclear antibodies (ANAs). It affects 1 in 3 patients receiving high-dose therapy for a year or longer. Treatment is usually discontinued because of the possibility of pleural effusion and potentially lethal pericardial tamponade. In some cases, a corticosteroid drug is added to the treatment regimen to permit continued use of procainamide. Rapid acetylators are less likely to develop the syndrome. Procainamide can also cause myelosuppression and agranulocytosis.

Life-threatening adverse effects of procainamide include ventricular arrhythmias, torsades de pointes, and agranulocytosis (with repeated use). Evidence of bone marrow dysfunction usually occurs during the first 3 months of therapy. Some health care providers consider the extended-release formulation of procainamide to be particularly responsible for these problems.

Procainamide is contraindicated for use in patients with hypersensitivity to the drug or its ingredients, AV block, or myasthenia gravis and in patients sensitive to tartrazine (FD&C Yellow No. 5 dye), which is present in some oral formulations. Use it with caution in patients with MI or cardiac glycoside toxicity, heart failure, or renal or hepatic insufficiency. Cautious use is also warranted in older adults. Safe use during pregnancy or lactation or in children has not been established.

The most common adverse effects of quinidine include nausea, vomiting, diarrhea, and abdominal pain. Disopyramide predisposes the individual to constipation. Disopyramide and procainamide exert anticholinergic effects that cause dry mouth and eyes, blurred vision, and urinary hesitancy. Further, procainamide is likely to cause urinary retention because of its potent antimuscarinic effects. Both quinidine and disopyramide are hepatotoxic.

Cinchonism is a constellation of adverse effects of quinidine and is characterized by tinnitus, hearing loss, headache, vertigo, dizziness, lightheadedness, disturbed vision, nausea, and vomiting. These adverse effects can occur after a single dose of quinidine. If the adverse effects are severe, diplopia, photophobia, and altered color perception may occur.

Life-threatening adverse effects of quinidine include worsening of underlying heart failure, widened QRS complex, heart block, ventricular flutter, ventricular fibrillation, hepatitis, thrombocytopenia, acute hemolytic anemia, agranulocytosis, respiratory depression, vascular collapse, and torsades de pointes (see Fig. 36-2). Torsades de pointes is an atypical rapid ventricular tachycardia with periodic waxing and waning of amplitude of the QRS complexes on the ECG. It is either self-limiting or progresses to ventricular fibrillation. Hyperkalemia enhances the effects of quinidine, whereas hypokalemia reduces the drug's effectiveness.

Quinidine is generally contraindicated for use in patients with hypersensitivity, conduction defects, and digoxin toxicity. Use it cautiously in patients with heart failure or severe liver disease. Safe use in pregnancy or lactation or in children has not been established.

The most common adverse effects of disopyramide include anticholinergic effects such as dry mouth, blurred vision, constipation, and urinary hesitancy and retention. Life-threatening adverse effects include hypotension, heart block, torsades de pointes, cardiogenic shock, and respiratory distress (e.g., laryngospasm). Other potential effects include hypoglycemia and hepatic cholestasis.

Disopyramide is contraindicated for use in patients with hypersensitivity to the drug or its ingredients, cardiogenic shock, second- and third-degree heart block, or in patients with sick sinus syndrome who do not have a pacemaker. Exercise caution when using the drug in patients with left ventricular dysfunction, decompensated heart failure, or hepatic or renal insufficiency. Cautious use is also warranted in older men with prostatic enlargement and in patients with glaucoma or myasthenia gravis, because of its anticholinergic effects. Safe use during pregnancy or lactation has not been established.

Drug Interactions

Class I$_A$ antiarrhythmic drugs exhibit additive or antagonistic effects with other antiarrhythmics as well as with anticholinergic drugs (Table 36-4). Foods that alkalinize the urine may increase serum quinidine levels and increase the risk of toxicity. These foods include cheeses, fish, meats, poultry, cranberries, breads and cereals, plums, prunes, and eggs.

Dosage Regimen

Quinidine formulations are not interchangeable without appropriate dosage adjustment (Table 36-5). The sulfate salt contains 83% quinidine base, whereas quinidine gluconate contains 62% active drug.

Lab Considerations

Because of the narrow therapeutic index and toxicity potential of class I$_A$ antiarrhythmic drugs, patients should be closely monitored. Patient surveillance may include regular assays of serum blood levels. Procainamide can increase liver transaminases and alkaline phosphatase values as well as produce a positive Coombs' test. Obtain a complete blood count (CBC) every 2 weeks during the first 3 months of therapy. Neutropenia, leukopenia, and thrombocytopenia rarely occur; however, discontinue therapy if leukopenia does occur. Monitor ANAs periodically during prolonged therapy or if symptoms of lupuslike reactions occur. Discontinue procainamide therapy if a steady increase in ANA titers occurs.

Quinidine increases creatine kinase (CK) values. Monitor serum K$^+$ levels, particularly if the patient has received digoxin in conjunction with quinidine treatment.

Disopyramide can cause increased values for aspartate aminotransferase (AST), alanine aminotransferase (ALT), bilirubin, lipids, blood urea nitrogen (BUN), and creatinine. Blood glucose values may be decreased in the presence of disopyramide.

Class I$_B$ Antiarrhythmics

◆ lidocaine (Anestacon, Baylocaine, Lidopen, Xylocaine); ✦ Zylogard
◆ mexiletine (Mexitil)
◆ phenytoin (diphenylhydantoin, Dilantin, Diphenylan); ✦ Dilantin

Indications

Class I$_B$ drugs are most effective when used in the treatment or palliation of both acute and chronic arrhythmias, including PVCs and ventricular tachycardia. Although there are fewer indications for class I$_B$ drugs, they are more effective in treating acute ventricular arrhythmias and cause fewer adverse effects. They are generally ineffective in treatment of supraventricular arrhythmias.

Lidocaine is the drug of choice for treating serious ventricular arrhythmias associated with acute MI, cardiac surgery, cardiac catheterization, cardioversion, and digoxin toxicity. There is no evidence of a teratogenic potential with lidocaine, so it can be safely administered in pregnancy as the drug of choice for acute ventricular tachycardias.

Mexiletine is an oral analogue of lidocaine, used because of its resistance to first-pass biotransformation. It is used to suppress ventricular arrhythmias, including frequent PVCs and

DRUG INTERACTIONS
TABLE 36-4 Antiarrhythmics

Drug	Interactive Drugs	Interaction
CLASS I$_A$ ANTIARRHYTHMICS		
quinidine	digoxin	Increases serum levels of digoxin
	Antiarrhythmics, pimozide	Increases cardiac effects of quinidine
	Antacids, Urinary alkalinizers	Decreases elimination of quinidine
	Oral anticoagulants, Neuromuscular blockers	Increases effects of interactive drugs
	Antimyasthenia gravis drugs	Decreases effects of interactive drug
disopyramide	Anticholinergics	Increases intensity of atropine-like adverse effects
	Antiarrhythmics, verapamil	Additive cardiac toxicity effects
	erythromycin	Increases disopyramide levels and risk of arrhythmias
	phenytoin, phenobarbital, rifampin	Decreases serum levels of disopyramide
	quinidine	Increases risk for disopyramide toxicity when high doses of disopyramide are used
	warfarin	Increases anticoagulant effect of warfarin
	cimetidine	Increases serum levels of disopyramide
procainamide	Antiarrhythmics	Additive or antagonistic effects
	lidocaine	Additive neurologic toxicity
	Antihypertensives, Nitrates	Additive hypotensive effects
	Neuromuscular blockers	Potentiates effects of interactive drug
	Anticholinesterase drugs	Antagonizes effects of interactive drug
	Antihistamines, Antidepressants, atropine, haloperidol, Phenothiazines	Additive anticholinergic effects
	cimetidine, quinidine, ranitidine, trimethoprim	Increases effects of procainamide
	Alcohol	Increases or decreases response to antiarrhythmic depending on acute or chronic use of interactive drug
	amiodarone	Increases serum levels of amiodarone
	cimetidine	Increases serum level and half-life of procainamide
CLASS I$_B$ ANTIARRHYTHMICS		
lidocaine	Beta blockers, cimetidine, phenobarbital	Decreases biotransformation of lidocaine; increases risk of toxicity
	phenytoin, procainamide, propranolol, quinidine	Additive cardiac depression and toxicity
mexiletine	Antacids, atropine, Opioids	Slows absorption of mexiletine
	metoclopramide	Speeds absorption of mexiletine
	phenytoin, phenobarbital, rifampin, smoking	Increases biotransformation and decreases effectiveness of mexiletine
	cimetidine	Slows biotransformation and increases risk of toxicity
	Antiarrhythmics	Additive cardiac effects
	Alkalinizing drugs	Increases reabsorption and serum level
	Acidifying drugs	Increases excretion and decreases serum levels
phenytoin	Barbiturates, chronic alcohol abuse, warfarin	Stimulates biotransformation and decreases effectiveness of interactive drugs
	cyclosporin, methadone, Oral contraceptives, streptozocin, theophylline	Stimulates phenytoin biotransformation and decreases serum levels
	Benzodiazepines, chloramphenicol, cimetidine, disulfiram, felbamate, fluconazole, influenza vaccine, isoniazid, ketoconazole, metronidazole, miconazole, omeprazole, Succinimides, Sulfonamides	Decreases phenytoin biotransformation and increases serum levels
	Alcohol, Antihistamines, Opioids, Sedative-hypnotics	Additive CNS depression
	warfarin	Alters effectiveness of interactive drug
	Antacids	Decreases absorption of orally administered phenytoin
	carbamazepine, valproic acid	Increases or decreases phenytoin serum levels
	felbamate	Decreases serum level interactive drug
CLASS I$_C$ ANTIARRHYTHMICS—Na$^+$ CHANNEL BLOCKERS		
flecainide	Antiarrhythmics, CCBs	Increases risk of arrhythmias
	Beta blockers, disopyramide, verapamil	Additive myocardial depressant effects
	amiodarone	Doubles serum flecainide levels
	digoxin	Increases digoxin levels by 15% to 25%
	Beta blockers	Increases levels of both flecainide and beta blocker
	Acidifying drugs	Increases renal elimination and decreases effectiveness of flecainide
	Alkalinizing drugs	Promotes reabsorption and increases risk of toxicity
propafenone	digoxin	Increases digoxin levels by 35% to 85%
	metoprolol, propranolol	Increases blood levels of interactive drugs
	quinidine	Inhibits biotransformation of propafenone
	Local anesthetics	Increases risk of CNS adverse effects
	warfarin	Increases risk of bleeding
	cyclosporin	Increases serum levels and risk for nephrotoxicity
	rifampin	Decreases drug levels and effectiveness of propafenone

CLASS II ANTIARRHYTHMICS—BETA BLOCKERS		
acebutolol, esmolol	Antihypertensives, Diuretics, Phenothiazines	Increases risk for hypotension
	Sympathomimetics, Xanthines	Inhibits effects of acebutolol
	Insulin, Neuromuscular blockers, Oral hypoglycemics	Prolongs effects of interactive drug
	NSAIDs	Decreases antihypertensive effect of acebutolol
	cimetidine	Increases plasma levels of acebutolol
	MAO inhibitors	Significant hypertension
	digoxin	Increases serum digoxin levels
	morphine	Increases serum level of esmolol
propranolol	General anesthesia, IV phenytoin, verapamil	Causes additive myocardial depression
	Cardiac glycosides	Additive bradycardia
	Alcohol, Antihypertensives, Nitrates	Additive hypotension
	Amphetamines, cocaine, ephedrine, epinephrine, norepinephrine, phenylephrine, pseudoephedrine	Results in unopposed α stimulation leading to excessive hypertension and bradycardia
	Thyroid hormones	Decreases effectiveness of propranolol
	Beta agonists, Insulins, Oral hypoglycemics, theophylline	Alters effectiveness of interactive drug
	dopamine, dobutamine	Decreases beneficial β_1 cardiovascular effects of interactive drugs
	Anticholinergics, MAO inhibitors	May increase risk of hypertension
	Anticholinergics, cimetidine	Increases risk of toxicity to propranolol
	NSAIDs	Decreases antihypertensive action
CLASS III ANTIARRHYTHMICS—PROLONG ACTION POTENTIAL		
amiodarone	cyclosporine, digoxin, flecainide, lidocaine, mexiletine, phenytoin, procainamide, quinidine, warfarin	Increases serum levels of interactive drug and risk of toxicity
	cimetidine	Increases amiodarone levels
	cholestyramine, phenytoin	Decreases amiodarone blood levels
	Beta blockers, CCBs	Increases risk for bradyarrhythmias, sinus, arrest, or AV block
dofetilide	Amiloride, cimetidine, ketoconazole, metformin, megestrol, prochlorperazine, triamterene, trimethoprim, verapamil	Increases serum dofetilide levels
	bepridil, Phenothiazines, Tricyclic antidepressants	Prolongs QT interval
ibutilide	amiodarone, disopyramide, moricizine, procainamide, quinidine, sotalol	Additive antiarrhythmic action
	H_1 blockers, Phenothiazines, Tetracyclic antidepressants, Tricyclic antidepressants	Prolongs QT interval
sotalol	Antiarrhythmics, Phenothiazines, Tricyclic antidepressants	Increases prolonged QT interval
	digoxin	Increases proarrhythmic effects
	Calcium channel blockers	Increases effect on AV conduction and blood pressure
	Insulin, Oral hypoglycemics	Masks signs and symptoms of hypoglycemia; prolongs effect of interactive drugs
	Sympathomimetics	May inhibit effects of interactive drug
	clonidine	Potentiates rebound hypertension after stopping clonidine
CLASS IV ANTIARRHYTHMICS—Ca^{++} CHANNEL BLOCKERS		
diltiazem	Alcohol, Antihypertensives, fentanyl, Nitrates, quinidine	Additive hypotension when used concurrently
	NSAIDs	Decreases antihypertensive effects
	digoxin	Increases serum levels of interactive drug
	Beta blockers, digoxin, disopyramide, phenytoin	Results in bradycardia, conduction defects, or heart failure
	phenobarbital, phenytoin	Increases biotransformation and decreases effectiveness of diltiazem
	cimetidine, propranolol	Decreases biotransformation and increases risk of toxicity to diltiazem
	carbamazepine, cyclosporin, prazosin, quinidine	Decreases biotransformation of and increases the risk of toxicity to interactive drug
verapamil	rifampin	Decreases effectiveness of rifampin
	Nondepolarizing neuromuscular blockers	Increases muscle-paralyzing effects of interactive drug
	Calcium, vitamin D	Decreases effectiveness of verapamil with concurrent use
	lithium	Alters serum level of interactive drug
MISCELLANEOUS ANTIARRHYTHMICS		
adenosine	Xanthines	Decreases effect of adenosine
	dipyridamole	Increases effect of adenosine
	carbamazepine	Increases degree of heart block caused by adenosine
moricizine	theophylline	Decreases levels of interactive drug
	cimetidine, digoxin, propranolol	Decreases clearance and increases serum levels of moricizine

AV, Atrioventricular; *CCBs*, calcium channel blockers; *CNS*, central nervous system; *MAO*, monoamine oxidase; *NSAIDs*, nonsteroidal antiinflammatory drugs.

DOSAGE
TABLE 36-5 Antiarrhythmics

Drug	Use(s)	Dosage	Implications
CLASS I$_A$ ANTIARRHYTHMICS			
quinidine sulfate	Chronic supraventricular and ventricular arrhythmias	*Adult: PACs or PVCs:* 200–300 mg PO every 6–8 hr −or− 300–600 mg PO of ER formulation every 8–12 hr. Maintenance: <3–4 grams/day. *PSVT:* 400–600 mg PO every 2–3 hr until arrhythmia terminated. *Fibrillation:* 200 mg PO every 2–3 hr for 5–8 doses, then increase at daily intervals if necessary.	Sulfate formulation: 83% quinidine. Patient is usually digitalized before starting therapy. A test dose of a single 200-mg quinidine sulfate tablet may be administered before therapy to check for intolerance.
quinidine gluconate	Chronic supraventricular and ventricular arrhythmias	*Adult:* 324–660 mg PO every 6–12 hr as ER formulation −or− 325–650 mg PO every 6 hr if not ER. *Child:* 8.25 mg/kg 5 times daily.	Gluconate formulation: 62% quinidine. Patient is usually digitalized before starting therapy.
procainamide	Broad spectrum: suppression of chronic supraventricular and ventricular arrhythmias	*Adult: Supraventricular Arrhythmias:* 1.25 gram PO loading dose, then 750 mg 2 hr later, then 0.5–1 grams PO every 2–3 hr. Maintenance: 0.5–1 gram PO every 4–6 hr −or− 1 gram every 6 hr as ER. formulation. *Ventricular Arrhythmias:* 50 mg/kg/day PO in divided doses every 3 hr or every 6 hr for ER formulation. *Child:* 12.5 mg/kg PO 4 times daily.	**Not interchangeable with quinidine.** May cause lupuslike syndrome. Use lower doses or longer dosing intervals for older adults and patients with renal, hepatic, or cardiac insufficiency. ▲
disopyramide	Broad spectrum: used for ventricular arrhythmias	*Adult >50 kg:* 300 mg PO loading dose followed by 150 mg every 6 hr −or− 300 mg PO every 12 hr as ER formulation. Maintenance: 800 mg PO daily in divided doses. *Adult <50 kg:* 200 mg PO every 6 hr −or− 200 mg PO every 12 hr as ER formulation. *Child 12–18 yr:* 6–15 mg/kg/day in divided doses every 6 hr.	Loading dose should be eliminated in patients with cardiomyopathy or decompensated heart failure. Reduce dosage in renal insufficiency.
CLASS I$_B$ ANTIARRHYTHMICS			
lidocaine	Ventricular arrhythmias associated with acute MI, cardiac surgery, cardiac catheterization, cardioversion, digoxin toxicity	*Adult:* 1–2 mg/kg IV. Not to exceed 50–100 mg bolus. Continuous drip: 1–4 mg/min. Max: 300 mg/hr. *Child:* 1 mg/kg followed by IV drip of 20–50 mcg/kg/min.	**Preferred drug for digoxin-induced ventricular arrhythmias.** Lidocaine formulations containing catecholamines must never be given by IV route.
mexiletine	Ventricular arrhythmias including ventricular tachycardia and PVCs	*Adult:* Initial: 400 mg PO loading dose, then 200 mg 8 hr later, then 200–400 mg every 8 hr. If controlled on less than 300 mg every 8 hr, give same daily dose at 12-hr intervals. Not to exceed 1200 mg/day.	Continuous ECG monitoring required. Reduced dosage is necessary for patients with hepatic disease.
phenytoin	Narrow spectrum: digitalis-induced ventricular arrhythmias	*Adult:* 50–100 mg IV every 10–15 min until arrhythmia abolished or 15 mg/kg has been given. Rate not to exceed 50 mg over 1 min. Infusion rate may be as low as 5–10 mg/min in patients with hypotension or those on sympathomimetic drugs, who have cardiovascular disease, or are older adults.	**Not a first-line drug; lidocaine preferred.** Rapid administration may result in severe hypotension, cardiovascular collapse, or CNS depression. ▲
CLASS I$_C$ ANTIARRHYTHMICS—NA$^+$ CHANNEL BLOCKERS			
flecainide	Supraventricular and ventricular arrhythmias only	*Adult: Ventricular Tachycardia:* 100 mg PO every 12 hr initially. Increase by 50 mg twice daily until desired response or max total daily dose of 400 mg is reached. *PSVT–PAF:* 50 mg PO every 12 hr initially. Increase by 50 mg PO twice daily to desired response or until max total daily dose of 300 mg is reached.	Some patients may require every 8-hr dosing. Previous antiarrhythmic therapy (except lidocaine) should be withdrawn 2–4 half-lives before starting flecainide. Administer dopamine for circulatory depression if necessary, or diazepam or thiopental for seizures.
propafenone	Ventricular arrhythmias	*Adult:* 150 mg PO every 8 hr. Increase to 300 mg every 8–12 hr as needed. Allow 3–4 days before increasing interval.	Preexisting hypokalemia or hyperkalemia should be corrected before starting therapy.
CLASS II ANTIARRHYTHMICS—BETA BLOCKERS			
acebutolol	Premature ventricular contractions	*Adult:* 200 mg PO every 12 hr initially. Increase gradually to a max daily dose of 600–1200 mg twice daily.	Always check apical pulse before administering. If less than 60 bpm, hold drug.
esmolol	Atrial fibrillation, atrial flutter, sinus tachycardia	*Adult:* Loading dose of 500 mcg/kg over 1 min, followed by a 4-min maintenance infusion of 50 mcg/kg/min. May repeat loading dose if necessary. Maintenance: 100 mcg/kg/min over 4 min.	**Do not use longer than 48 hr.** Continuously monitor ECG. Titration of drug is complex. ▲
propranolol	PSVT, atrial fibrillation, atrial flutter, sinus tachycardia associated with excessive catecholamine release	*Adult:* 1–3 mg by slow IV push not to exceed 1 mg/min. Repeat after 2 min if needed and again in 4 hr if needed −or− 10–30 mg PO 3–4 times daily. Do not administer more often than every 4 hr. Maintenance: 10–80 mg PO 3–4 times daily. *Child:* 10–100 mcg/kg up to 1 mg/dose. May be repeated every 6–8 hr if needed.	IV doses are much smaller than PO doses. Continuous ECG monitoring required and patient may have PCWP or CVP monitoring during and for several hr after administration.

CLASS III ANTIARRHYTHMICS—PROLONG ACTION POTENTIAL

amiodarone	Life-threatening, recurrent ventricular arrhythmias, supraventricular tachycardia, ventricular fibrillation resistant to other drugs	*Adult:* Loading dose 800–1600 mg PO daily for 1–3 wk, then 600–800 mg/day in 1–2 doses for 1 mo, then 400 mg/day maintenance dose *–or–* 150 mg IV over 10 min followed by 360 mg over next 6 hr (1 mg/min), then 540 mg over the next 18 hr (0.5 mg/min). *Child:* 10 mg/kg/day for 10 days until desired response or adverse effects occur, then 5 mg/kg/day for several weeks, then decrease to 2.5 mg/kg/day or lowest effective dose.	Therapeutic effects delayed 5–30 days unless loading doses given. Effects persist several wk after drug is discontinued. Continue IV infusion at 0.5 mg/min until oral therapy is initiated. If duration of infusion was less than 1 wk, oral dose of amiodarone should be 800–1000 mg/day; if duration of infusion was 1–3 wk, oral dose should be 600–800 mg/day; if IV infusion extended past 3 wk, oral dose should be 400 mg/day.
dofetilide	Life-threatening, recurrent ventricular arrhythmias, supraventricular tachycardia, ventricular fibrillation resistant to other drugs	*Adult:* See manufacturer literature. Complex algorithm for dosing. In general, 500 mg PO twice daily based on creatinine clearance and QT interval.	Before administration of first dose, QT must be determined using an average of 5–10 beats. If QT >440 msec (500 msec in patients with ventricular conduction abnormalities), drug is contraindicated. If heart rate <60 bpm, QT interval should be used.
ibutilide	Rapid conversion atrial fibrillation, atrial flutter of recent onset	*Adult >60 kg:* 1 mg IV over 10 min. If arrhythmia still present 10 min after initial infusion, a second 1-mg infusion may be given 10 min after completion of first infusion. *Adult <60 kg:* 0.1 mg/kg given over 10 min. If arrhythmia still present 10 min after initial infusion, a second dose may be given 10 min after completion of first infusion.	Continuous ECG monitoring required for at least 4 hr following infusion or until QT interval has returned to baseline. Atrial fibrillation lasting longer than 2–3 days are treated with anticoagulants for at least 2 wk before ibutilide therapy.
sotalol	Life-threatening ventricular arrhythmias, sustained supraventricular tachycardia	*Adult:* 80 mg PO twice daily. Increase gradually at 2- to 3-day intervals to a range of 240–320 mg/day. Not to exceed 480–640 mg/day.	Increase dosage interval if CrCl <60 mL/min. Dosing more than twice daily usually not necessary because of long half-life. Patients who develop anaphylaxis may be more resistant to epinephrine.

CLASS IV ANTIARRHYTHMICS—CA⁺⁺ CHANNEL BLOCKERS

diltiazem	Paroxysmal supraventricular tachycardia, atrial flutter, atrial fibrillation	*Adult:* 30–120 mg PO 3–4 times daily *–or–* 60–120 mg PO twice daily if SR formulation *–or–* 0.25 mg/kg IV. May repeat in 15 min with a dose of 0.35 mg/kg. May follow with continuous infusion at 10 mg/hr (range 5–15 mg/hr) for up to 24 hr.	Most often used for prophylaxis. Empty tablets that appear in the stool are not significant.
verapamil	Paroxysmal supraventricular tachycardia, atrial flutter, atrial fibrillation	*Adult:* 80–120 mg PO every 6–8 hr. May increase as needed *–or–* 120–240 mg PO daily of ER formulation. Increase as needed to 480 mg/day *–or–* 75–150 mcg/kg/day. May repeat with 10 mg after 30 min. *Child >16 yr:* 4–8 mg/kg/day PO in divided doses. *Child 1–16 yr:* 100–300 mcg/kg. May repeat after 30 min. Initial dose not to exceed 5 mg. Repeat dose not to exceed 10 mg.	Contraindicated in digoxin toxicity because it worsens heart block. **Do not use IV form with IV propranolol because of potential for fatal bradycardia and hypotension.** Contact health care provider if pulse rate less than 50 bpm. ⚠

MISCELLANEOUS ANTIARRHYTHMICS

adenosine	Paroxysmal supraventricular tachycardia	*Adult:* 6 mg IV bolus. If first dose does not convert arrhythmia within 1–2 min, give 12 mg. May repeat 12-mg dose in 1–2 min if no response has occurred.	**Do not confuse adenosine with adenosine phosphate!** Continuous ECG monitoring required. ⚠
moricizine	Life-threatening ventricular arrhythmias refractory to other drugs	*Adult:* 600–900 mg/day every 8 hr. Within this range the dosage may be adjusted by 150 mg/day every 3 days as required and tolerated. Some patients may tolerate every-12-hr dosing, not to exceed 900 mg/day.	Necessitates continuous ECG monitoring. Previous antiarrhythmic therapy should be withdrawn 1–2 half-lives before starting moricizine. Dosage adjustments should be 3 days apart because of the long half-life of moricizine.

Bpm; Beats/min; *CNS,* central nervous system; *CrCl,* creatinine clearance; *CVP,* central venous pressure; *ECG,* electrocardiogram; *ER,* extended release formulation; *IV,* intravenous; *MI,* myocardial infarction; *PACs,* premature atrial contractions; *PCWP,* pulmonary capillary wedge pressure; *PO,* by mouth; *PVCs,* premature ventricular contractions; *PSVT–PAF,* paroxysmal supraventricular tachycardia–paroxysmal atrial fibrillation.

ventricular tachycardia. Phenytoin is used for arrhythmias associated with digoxin toxicity, although it has not been approved by the FDA for this use.

Pharmacodynamics

Lidocaine decreases depolarization, automaticity, and excitability of the ventricles during diastole. It has little effect on atrial tissues and therefore is of little use for atrial arrhythmias.

Mexiletine shortens the duration of action potential, thereby decreasing the effective refractory period (ERP) in the bundle of His and Purkinje fibers. These effects are mediated by blocking Na⁺ transport across myocardial cell membranes.

Phenytoin decreases abnormal ventricular automaticity to shorten the refractory period, the QT interval, and the duration of the action potential. Automaticity is decreased, and conduction through the AV node is improved. With the exception of phenytoin, class I$_B$ drugs produce no significant action on the autonomic nervous system. Most effects of phenytoin arise from actions within the central nervous system (CNS). Vagal nerve activity is tempered and outgoing traffic from the myocardium reduced.

Pharmacokinetics

Lidocaine is well absorbed from the GI tract; however, it is subject to extensive first-pass effect. Only about one third of the drug reaches the general circulation. Systemically, it is widely distributed throughout the body to concentrate in adipose tissue. It crosses the blood-brain barrier and placental membranes. Lidocaine is variably bound to plasma proteins depending on blood level of the drug. Lidocaine biotransformation takes place in the liver. Clearance of lidocaine approximates the rate of hepatic blood flow and is thus sensitive to changes in blood flow. It is important to note that lidocaine has a pronounced redistribution phase as well as a biotransformation phase. This is why the effects of a bolus dose of lidocaine are short-lived. Prolonged infusions of lidocaine reduce drug clearance (see Table 36-3).

Mexiletine is readily absorbed after oral administration, with a relatively low first-pass effect. Urinary acidification accelerates elimination, whereas alkalinization retards elimination of the drug.

Phenytoin is slowly absorbed from the GI tract and erratically and unreliably absorbed when given by intramuscular (IM) route. The bioavailability differs among the formulations. About 90% is bound to plasma proteins, with less binding found in patients with uremia. Distribution takes place quickly, with biotransformation occurring through hepatic hydroxylation. The CYP450 enzyme system responsible for phenytoin biotransformation becomes saturated at therapeutic concentrations of the drug; hence the half-life of phenytoin is dose dependent. Unexpected toxicity may occur in some patients.

Adverse Effects and Contraindications

Class I$_B$ antiarrhythmics have fewer adverse cardiac effects than do those in class I$_A$. The most common adverse effects of lidocaine include drowsiness, confusion, and stinging at the administration site. Although serious adverse effects of lidocaine are uncommon, high dosages cause cardiovascular depression (i.e., bradycardia, somnolence, hypotension, arrhythmias, heart block, cardiovascular collapse, and cardiac arrest).

Lidocaine is contraindicated for use in patients with hypersensitivity or advanced AV block. Use it cautiously in patients with liver disease or heart failure, in those weighing less than 110 pounds (50 kg), and in older adults. The presence of respiratory depression, shock, and heart block also necessitate cautious use. Safe use during pregnancy and lactation has not been established.

The most common adverse effects of mexiletine are predominantly neurologic and include tremor, blurry vision, nervousness, dizziness, and lethargy. Heartburn, nausea, and vomiting are also common effects. Arrhythmias, palpitations, chest pain, blood dyscrasias, headache, changes in sleep habits, confusion, and edema have been noted. The most serious adverse effect is hepatic necrosis.

Mexiletine is contraindicated for use in patients with hypersensitivity, cardiogenic shock, or second- or third-degree heart block (if a pacemaker has not been inserted). Exercise caution when using it in patients with sinus node or intraventricular conduction abnormalities, hypotension, heart failure, or severe hepatic involvement. Safe use during pregnancy and lactation and in children has not been established.

The most common adverse effects of phenytoin include nystagmus, ataxia, diplopia, gingival hyperplasia, nausea,

hypotension, hypertrichosis, and skin rashes. Life-threatening adverse effects include aplastic anemia, agranulocytosis, and Stevens-Johnson syndrome.

Phenytoin is contraindicated for use in patients with hypersensitivity to the drug or to propylene glycol (injection only), alcohol intolerance (injection and liquid only), sinus bradycardia, and heart block. There are a number of patients in whom phenytoin should be used with caution, including those with severe liver, severe cardiac, or respiratory disease, as well as older adults, obese patients, and pregnant patients. Fetal hydantoin syndrome may result if used chronically, and hemorrhage in the newborn may occur if the drug is used at term. Safe use during lactation has not been established.

Drug Interactions

Class I$_B$ drugs can exhibit additive or antagonistic effects when administered with other antiarrhythmic drugs. Few drug interactions have been reported with lidocaine. Basic drugs displace lidocaine from its binding sites. Plasma concentrations are higher in patients who are concurrently receiving cimetidine or propranolol (see Table 36-4).

Biotransformation of mexiletine can be increased with concurrent administration of phenytoin or rifampin. Drugs that drastically alter urinary pH may affect serum levels of mexiletine. Alkalinization increases the reabsorption and the serum levels of mexiletine. Acidification increases drug elimination and decreases effectiveness.

Concurrent use of beta blockers may precipitate heart failure in susceptible patients. Numerous drug interactions occur with phenytoin and are too numerous to discuss here.

Phenytoin decreases the absorption of folic acid. Foods that alter urinary pH may affect the serum levels of mexiletine. Concurrent administration of enteral tube feedings may decrease the absorption of phenytoin.

Dosage Regimen

Information on dosages of class I$_B$ antiarrhythmic drugs is found in Table 36-5.

Lab Considerations

In view of the potential for toxicity, closely monitor serum blood levels of antiarrhythmic drugs and evaluate for signs and symptoms of toxicity. Therapeutic serum lidocaine levels range from 2 to 5 mcg/mL. Monitor drug levels periodically throughout prolonged or high-dose therapy. Lidocaine has been shown to increase creatine phosphokinase values.

The incidence of adverse effects is greater with serum levels of mexiletine above 2 mcg/mL. Mexiletine occasionally causes positive ANA test results as well as a transient increase in AST concentrations. Thrombocytopenia may occur a few days after initiation of therapy but returns to normal about 1 month after discontinuation of therapy.

Phenytoin can cause increased serum alkaline phosphatase and glucose levels. Perform CBC and platelets, serum Ca^{++}, urinalysis, and hepatic and thyroid testing before therapy. Monitor serum folate levels. Glucose, alkaline phosphatase, and bromosulfophthalein laboratory values are elevated with phenytoin, with decreased values for the dexamethasone suppression test, metyrapone (cortisol), protein-bound iodine, and urinary steroids. Monitor serum phenytoin levels on a routine basis. Therapeutic blood levels are 10 to 20 mcg/mL.

Class I$_C$ Antiarrhythmics

◆ flecainide (Tambocor); ◆ Tambocor
◆ propafenone (Rhythmol); ◆ Rhythmol

Indications

Class I$_C$ drugs are used in managing severe refractory ventricular arrhythmias, including ventricular tachycardia, paroxysmal supraventricular tachycardia (PSVT), paroxysmal atrial flutter, and paroxysmal atrial fibrillation. Class I$_C$ drugs are reserved for hospitalized patients with malignant ventricular arrhythmias, symptomatic heart failure, sinus node dysfunction, or heart block.

Pharmacodynamics

Class I$_C$ drugs primarily block the inward movement of Na$^+$ through the fast Na$^+$ channel of the myocardial membrane. Spontaneous depolarization is thus decreased. Unlike class I$_A$ drugs, class I$_C$ drugs do not produce a significant change in the ERP or in the action potential duration.

Flecainide has little effect on normal SA or AV nodes or atrial cells; it depresses conduction and function of dysfunctional cells. Flecainide exerts negative inotropic effects. Flecainide is similar to procainamide except that it lacks the lupuslike syndrome seen frequently with procainamide.

Propafenone has weak beta-blocking actions and structurally resembles propranolol. Like flecainide, propafenone prolongs intracardiac conduction, produces minor effects on the capacity of the heart to be restimulated, and has little effect on normal SA node function. It also lengthens AV-nodal functioning and the effective refractory period. Propafenone modifies pacing and sensing thresholds of artificial pacemakers.

Pharmacokinetics

Flecainide is almost completely absorbed after oral administration. Absorption is prolonged in the presence of food but its bioavailability is not altered. Flecainide is moderately bound to plasma proteins. It is biotransformed in the liver, with the metabolites exerting little or no antiarrhythmic activity. Flecainide is eliminated unchanged by the kidneys; however, the drug can accumulate in patients with renal failure (see Table 36-3).

Although propafenone is almost completely absorbed from the GI tract, the bioavailability is reduced because of an extensive first-pass effect. Propafenone undergoes extensive oxidative biotransformation with 11 metabolites produced. Two of the 11 metabolites have known antiarrhythmic properties. Because of the variability between rapid acetylators (2 to 10 hours) and slow acetylators (10 to 32 hours), plasma concentration measurements have limited usefulness in adjusting dosage. Overall, the pharmacokinetic properties of propafenone are dose dependent. For example, an increase in dosage from 300 to 900 mg/day may result in as much as a tenfold increase in plasma concentrations.

Adverse Effects and Contraindications

Class I$_C$ drugs all have similar adverse cardiac effects. Proarrhythmic effects occur in 8% to 15% of patients with malignant ventricular arrhythmias. The most common adverse effects of flecainide include dizziness, nervousness, headache, fatigue, tremor, blurred vision, and nausea. Flecainide increases the pacing threshold, so pacemaker-dependent patients may need their pacemakers reprogrammed. New or worsening heart failure occurs in a small but significant percentage of patients receiving flecainide. The life-threatening adverse effects of flecainide include arrhythmias, heart failure, palpitations, chest pain, edema, and ECG changes. SA node dysfunction and second- and third-degree AV heart block can occur. Compared to class I$_A$ drugs, flecainide less commonly causes GI or urinary tract distress (see Evidence-Based Pharmacotherapeutics box).

Flecainide is contraindicated for use in patients with hypersensitivity or cardiogenic shock. Use it with caution in patients with heart failure, preexisting sinus node dysfunction, second- and third-degree heart block (without a pacemaker), and renal impairment. Flecainide has also been associated with bronchospasm. Safe use during pregnancy and lactation or in children has not been established.

The most common adverse effects of propafenone include a metallic taste in the mouth, GI distress (e.g., constipation, nausea, vomiting), dizziness, fatigue, and conduction abnormalities. Exacerbation of heart failure and proarrhythmic effects (e.g., supraventricular arrhythmias) is possible. Agranulocytosis is rare but has occurred.

Drug Interactions

Evidence suggests that cimetidine, digoxin, and propranolol all have the potential to cause clinically important drug interactions with flecainide and propafenone (see Table 36-4). Cimetidine increases blood levels owing to the decreased biotransformation of flecainide. Propafenone modestly increases serum digoxin levels. Use it cautiously with propranolol, metoprolol, and warfarin because the levels of these drugs may rise. Propafenone may have additive beta blocking effects, so it is contraindicated for use in individuals with bronchospastic disorders. Quinidine can inhibit the biotransformation of propafenone.

Patients on a strict vegetarian diet consume foods that increase the urinary pH to over 7. The rise in pH increases flecainide serum levels. Conversely, a diet of foods or beverages that decrease urinary pH to less than 5 increases the renal elimination of flecainide and decreases its effectiveness.

Dosage Regimen

The dosages of class I$_C$ drugs vary. To reduce the incidence of adverse effects, keep initial flecainide dosing low. The dosage may then be increased every 4 days and given in divided doses. Withdraw previous antiarrhythmic therapy (except lidocaine) 2 to 4 half-lives before starting flecainide.

Preexisting hypokalemia or hyperkalemia should be corrected before instituting propafenone therapy. Table 36-5 provides a summary of dosages for class I antiarrhythmic drugs.

Lab Considerations

The therapeutic serum level for flecainide is 0.2 to 1 mcg/mL. The probability of toxicity exists with serum levels exceeding 1 mcg/mL. Creatine phosphate levels are elevated in the presence of flecainide or propafenone. For patients on long-term therapy, periodically evaluate renal, pulmonary, and hepatic functions and CBC. Note also that flecainide may cause elevations in serum alkaline phosphatase

EVIDENCE-BASED PHARMACOTHERAPEUTICS

Cardiac Arrhythmia Suppression Trial

■ Background

A surrogate end point is a laboratory or physical sign used in therapeutic trials as a substitute for a clinically meaningful end point that is a direct measure of how a patient feels, functions, or survives and that is expected to predict the effect of the therapy. For a surrogate to be useful, one must identify the clinical end point, the class of intervention, and the population in which substitution of a biomarker for a clinical end point is considered reasonable.

The presence of asymptomatic ventricular ectopic beats is known to be a surrogate marker for an increased risk of sudden death due to ventricular fibrillation in patients who are convalescing from a myocardial infarction. And yet, there is disagreement about whether arrhythmias should be treated if they are found on ECG but are creating no symptoms in the patient.

■ Research Article

Echt, D., Liebson, E., Mitchell, L., et al. (1991). Mortality and morbidity in patients receiving encainide, flecainide, or placebo: The Cardiac Arrhythmia Suppression Trial. *New England Journal of Medicine, 324* (12), 781–788.

Purpose

The CAST study was designed to evaluate how encainide, flecainide, and moricizine affect the survival of patients who experienced a myocardial infarction and had over 10 premature ventricular beats per hour in relation to incidence of sudden death.

Design

This was a randomized, placebo-controlled study to examine mortality and morbidity after randomization to active drug or their respective placebos.

Methods

Of 1498 subjects with ectopic rhythms, 857 were assigned to receive encainide* (a potent Na^+ channel blocker) or its placebo (432 to active drug and 425 to placebo), and 641 were assigned to receive flecainide or its placebo (323 to active drug and 318 to placebo).

Findings

Early results were startling. There were 33 sudden deaths in patients taking either encainide or flecainide, compared to 9 in the placebo arm. A total of 56 patients died in the encainide and flecainide arms of the study, compared to 22 in the placebo arm. At final analysis, 63 patients died in the encainide or flecainide arms, compared to 26 in the placebo arm. Later results showed increased risk of death for the moricizine arm of the study, also.

At follow-up 10 months later, 89 subjects had died: 59 of arrhythmia (43 were receiving the drug vs.16 receiving placebo; p = 0.0004); 22 of nonarrhythmic cardiac causes (17 were receiving the drug vs. 5 receiving the placebo; p = 0.01); and 8 of noncardiac causes (3 were receiving the drug vs. 5 receiving the placebo). Virtually all deaths unrelated to an arrhythmia were caused by an acute myocardial infarction with cardiogenic shock (11 subjects were receiving the drug, and 3 the placebo), or to chronic heart failure (4 subjects were receiving the drug, and 2 the placebo).

There were no differences in subjects who received the active drug and those taking the placebo in the incidence of nonfatal, disqualifying, ventricular tachycardia, proarrhythmia, syncope, the need for a permanent pacemaker, heart failure, recurrent myocardial infarction, angina, or the need for coronary-artery bypass grafting or angioplasty.

Conclusions

The drugs encainide and flecainide were effective in suppressing ventricular arrhythmias (the surrogate marker) in patients following a myocardial infarction, but they nonetheless increased mortality. Nonlethal events, however, were equally distributed between the active-drug and placebo groups. The mechanisms underlying the high mortality rate during treatment with encainide or flecainide remains unknown.

■ Implications for Practice

A biologic marker is a candidate for surrogate end point if it is expected to predict clinical benefit (or harm, or lack of benefit or harm) based on epidemiologic, therapeutic, pathophysiologic, or other scientific evidence. Although collection of information on surrogate end points is encouraged, and provides additional insight into the reality of clinical research, it often provides evidence into the reliability of an observed association. When used as supplementary information, surrogate end points provide improvement in study design; however, investigators should be cautioned about drawing associations and inferences from this type of study.

*The manufacturer of encainide (Enkaid) capsules voluntarily withdrew the drug from market on December 16, 1991. Flecainide (Tambocor) remains on the market for the treatment of atrial and ventricular arrhythmias. It carries a black box warning of excessive mortality or nonfatal arrest rate of 5.1% vs. 2.3% for the matched placebo in asymptomatic non–life-threatening ventricular arrhythmias with MI 5 days to 2 years prior. There is no survival benefit for patients without life-threatening arrhythmias.

---

values during prolonged therapy. Propafenone may cause elevated ANA titers that are usually asymptomatic and reversible.

Class II Antiarrhythmics
◆ acebutolol (Sectral); ♣ Monitan, Sectral
◆ esmolol (Brevibloc)
◆ propranolol (Inderal, Inderal LA); ♣ Apo-Propranolol, Detensol, Novo-Pranol, PMS-Propranolol

▥ Indications

Beta-blocking drugs make up class II antiarrhythmics and include acebutolol, esmolol, and propranolol. Acebutolol is used primarily in the management of PVCs. Esmolol is an ultra–short-acting drug used for the rapid, short-term control of ventricular rate in patients with supraventricular arrhythmias and sinus tachycardia. Propranolol is used in the management of paroxysmal supraventricular tachycardia, atrial fibrillation, atrial flutter, and sinus tachycardia associated with excessive catecholamine release.

Class II antiarrhythmic drugs are not typically considered initial drugs of choice to treat arrhythmias except in intraoperative areas, where beta blockers are the mainstay with evidence to support reduced mortality with combined therapy. This is in part because of their multiple effects and because of possible breakthrough ectopy. The use of these drugs with other antiarrhythmics remains to be evaluated.

▥ Pharmacodynamics

Class II antiarrhythmic drugs exert antiarrhythmic effects by antagonizing SNS stimulation of β receptors in the heart. Blockade of β receptors at the SA node and ectopic pacemakers decreases automaticity. All beta blockers cause a substantial increase in the ERP of the AV node. This action is the basis for the use of these drugs as antiarrhythmics.

Class II antiarrhythmic drugs also exert significant negative inotropic effects. By decreasing myocardial oxygen demand, myocardial ischemia is decreased. As ischemia abates, myocardial cells lose their automaticity and suppress atrial and ventricular ectopy.

Acebutolol predominantly blocks β_1 receptors to slow sinus heart rate and decrease cardiac output and blood pressure. It slows AV conduction and reduces the rate of spontaneous firing of the SA node. In large doses it may block β_2 receptors, thus increasing airway resistance.

Esmolol also selectively blocks β_1 receptors to slow the heart rate, decrease cardiac output, and lower blood pressure. The exact mechanism for reducing blood pressure is unknown, but esmolol may block peripheral adrenergic receptors, thus decreasing sympathetic output from the CNS or may act by decreasing renin release from the kidney. Its antiarrhythmic effect is due to blocking stimulation of cardiac pacemaker potentials.

Propranolol is a nonselective beta blocker with effects on both β_1 and β_2 receptors. It also has substantial local anesthetic (membrane stabilizing) actions. It has no intrinsic sympathomimetic activity. Like acebutolol and esmolol, propranolol blocks β_1 receptors, thus slowing the heart rate, decreasing cardiac output, and reducing the blood pressure. However, by blocking β_2 receptors located in the respiratory tract, airway resistance is increased.

Pharmacokinetics

The pharmacokinetics of class II antiarrhythmics are identified in Table 36-3. Acebutolol is eliminated through the kidneys and the feces.

Esmolol is quickly and widely distributed, with peak concentrations reached quickly. Most of an esmolol dose is biotransformed to an inactive metabolite and eliminated in the urine.

Propranolol is almost completely absorbed from the GI tract after oral administration, but an extensive first-pass effect reduces bioavailability. As with lidocaine, the hepatic extraction of propranolol is high, and elimination is significantly reduced when hepatic blood flow decreases. Propranolol may decrease its own rate of elimination by decreasing cardiac output and hepatic blood flow, particularly in patients with left ventricular dysfunction. Liver disease decreases the plasma protein–bound fraction of propranolol and increases the amount of free drug in the circulation. Hyperthyroidism increases the clearance of propranolol by the liver. Propranolol is eliminated through the urine and the feces.

Adverse Effects and Contraindications

The most common adverse effects of class II antiarrhythmics usually occur with initial use of the drugs. **Because they inhibit SA node stimulation, class II drugs may produce bradycardia.**

The most common adverse effects include mild, transient hypotension, dizziness, nausea, diaphoresis, headache, cold extremities, fatigue, constipation, and diarrhea. Insomnia, flatulence, urinary frequency, and impotence or decreased libido occasionally occurs. A rash, arthralgia, myalgia, confusion (especially in the older adult), and a change in taste can occur but are rare. An overdose produces profound bradycardia and hypotension.

Acebutolol may precipitate heart failure or MI in patients with heart disease, thyroid storm in patients with thyrotoxicosis, and peripheral ischemia in patients with peripheral vascular disease. Hypoglycemia may occur in patients with previously controlled diabetes because the drugs mask its symptoms. Thrombocytopenia is possible but rare.

Esmolol is generally well tolerated. The most common adverse effects are transient and mild, including hypotension, dizziness, nausea, diaphoresis, headache, cold extremities, and fatigue. IV infusions of esmolol cause inflammation and induration at the injection site in about 80% of patients. Somnolence and confusion occasionally occur. Bronchospasm, bradycardia, and peripheral ischemia are rare.

The adverse effects of IV propranolol are more common and more severe than with oral dosage forms, especially in older adults and azotemic patients. Bradycardia is frequent. A Raynaud's type of peripheral vascular insufficiency, dizziness, and fatigue occur occasionally. Although rare, sedation, behavioral change, hypotension, GI upset, peripheral skin necrosis, rash, and rhythm and/or conduction disturbances have occurred.

Beta blockers are contraindicated for use in patients with hypersensitivity, sinus bradycardia, second- or third-degree heart block, cardiogenic shock, heart failure, asthma, and COPD, and during lactation. Use these drugs with caution in patients with thyrotoxicosis, and hepatic or renal impairment.

There is controversy regarding the safety of beta blockers in pregnancy. Reports of an increased incidence of growth retardation, delayed neonatal respirations, bradycardia, hypoglycemia, and blunting of accelerations of the intrapartum fetal heart rate have all been described. Whether this phenomenon is dose related or caused by the underlying disease for which the therapy is indicated is unclear. No evidence exists to suggest that beta blockers are teratogenic.

Drug Interactions

Class II antiarrhythmic drugs interact with a number of other drugs, sometimes increasing and at other times decreasing the drug effects (see Table 36-4).

Dosage Regimen

Check the apical pulse before administering class II antiarrhythmics and hold the drug if the pulse is less than 60 bpm (see Table 36-5). Once ventricular rate control is achieved, begin long-term oral therapy with an appropriate drug. As with other IV-administered antiarrhythmic drugs, the blood pressure and ECG should be continuously monitored.

Lab Considerations

Lab values that may be altered in the presence of acebutolol are numerous. Acebutolol may increase ANA titers and AST, ALT, bilirubin, alkaline phosphatase, lactate dehydrogenase, BUN, creatinine, K^+, uric acid, lipoproteins, and triglycerides values. There are no significant laboratory values altered with esmolol. Propranolol may cause increased ANA, glucose, BUN, K^+, serum lipoproteins, triglycerides, and uric acid levels. Beta adrenergic blockers may reduce symptoms associated with increased sympathetic output.

Class III Antiarrhythmics

◆ amiodarone (Cordarone); ✦ Cordarone
◆ dofetilide (Tikosyn)
◆ ibutilide (Corvert)
◆ sotalol (Betapace); ✦ Sotacor

Indications

Amiodarone is used to treat ventricular arrhythmias. Because of its long half-life and life-threatening adverse effects, amiodarone is indicated only for recurrent ventricular fibrillation and recurrent, hemodynamically unstable sustained ventricular tachycardia. Treatment should always be initiated in the hospital with efficacy and response assessed.

Dofetilide has restricted access in the United States but is approved for the conversion and maintenance of NSR in patients with atrial fibrillation or atrial flutter of longer than 1 week's duration. According to the Symptomatic Atrial Fibrillation Investigative Research on Dofetilide (SAFIRE-D) study (Singh et al., 2000), approximately 6%, 10%, and 30% of patients receiving 125 mg, 250 mg, and 500 mg of dofetilide, respectively, converted to sinus rhythm. Because dofetilide can cause life-threatening ventricular arrhythmias, reserve it for patients in whom atrial fibrillation or atrial flutter is highly symptomatic.

Ibutilide is approved for the acute termination of atrial fibrillation or atrial flutter, restoring sinus rhythm in approximately 50% of patients with these arrhythmias. It is, however, more effective in managing atrial flutter than atrial fibrillation. Arrhythmias of longer duration are less likely to respond to therapy. Ibutilide also appears to be effective in facilitating direct-current cardioversion of atrial fibrillation.

Sotalol is a first-line consideration in the treatment of malignant ventricular arrhythmias. Sotalol appears to be effective in the treatment of sustained supraventricular tachycardia and atrial fibrillation and in some patients with Wolff-Parkinson-White syndrome. Sotalol can reduce cardiac function in patients dependent on SNS activity to maintain a normal cardiac output.

Because of their adverse effects, class III drugs are typically considered second- or third-line drugs. These drugs can convert unidirectional block to bidirectional block, but they have little or no effect on depolarization.

Pharmacodynamics

Although the drugs in this class possess diverse pharmacologic properties, they all share the common property of prolonging the action potential duration and refractory period in Purkinje fibers and ventricular muscle, thus decreasing the automaticity rate of ventricular ectopic foci. The exact mechanism most responsible for the antiarrhythmic effects of class III drugs remains uncertain.

Amiodarone, a benzofuron derivative (much of the drug is iodine), exhibits electrophysiologic activity of each class within the Vaughan Williams classification system. Amiodarone demonstrates effectiveness for most tachycardias and has a relatively low proarrhythmic potential. Amiodarone causes potent blockade of Na^+ and Ca^{++} channels. It prolongs repolarization, reduces automaticity of the SA node, increases conduction time and refractory period of the AV node, and reduces conduction velocity in Purkinje fibers and the myocardium. Amiodarone may decrease intracardiac conduction, as shown by increased PR and QT intervals. The QRS complex may be unchanged or widened. Amiodarone also decreases myocardial oxygen demand and enhances cardiac performance, because it relaxes vascular smooth muscle and decreases systemic and coronary vascular resistance. It is also a weak, noncompetitive, alpha- and beta-blocking drug.

Dofetilide is a selective K^+ channel blocker that prolongs repolarization without affecting conduction velocity. It does so by blocking time-dependent K^+ currents. Dofetilide also increases the action potential duration in a concentration-dependent manner, primarily as the result of delayed repolarization. These actions and the associated increase in the ERP are noted in both atria and ventricles in both the resting and contraction modes. Increases in the QT interval are the result of prolongation of both effective and functional refractory periods at the bundle of His and Purkinje fibers and the ventricles. Dofetilide has no effect on Na^+ channels, α receptors, or β receptors.

Ibutilide prolongs both atrial and ventricular action potential durations and increases both atrial and ventricular refractory periods. Ibutilide activates the slow, inward movement of Na^+, producing mild slowing of sinus rate and AV conduction. There is a dose-related prolongation of the QT interval.

Sotalol prolongs the action potential, ERP, and QT interval. It decreases automaticity presumably by blocking β1- and β2-adrenergic receptors. It lengthens the action potential duration in myocardial fibers without producing significant effects on membrane responsiveness or conduction through Purkinje fibers. Conduction through the AV node is significantly reduced. Sotalol is also thought to terminate reentry arrhythmias by markedly prolonging refractoriness without affecting the propagation of the electrical impulse. At therapeutic drug levels, sotalol decreases heart rate.

Pharmacokinetics

Absorption of orally administered amiodarone is slow and variable, with 35% to 65% of the drug bioavailable. The time to peak plasma concentrations after an oral or IV dose is unknown. Amiodarone is distributed to and accumulates slowly in body tissues. High drug levels are reached in body fat, muscle, liver, lungs, and spleen. During long-term treatment with amiodarone, the active metabolite accumulates in the plasma, and its concentration may exceed that of the parent compound. Amiodarone is biotransformed in the liver. One metabolite, N-desethylamiodarone, has antiarrhythmic activity. Amiodarone is eliminated from the body via the bile. The half-life is biphasic, with a mean of 53 days. It can be detected in plasma for up to 9 months after administration.

Dofetilide is well absorbed following oral administration. Dofetilide is biotransformed in the liver by CYP 3A4, but it has a low affinity for this enzyme. There are no quantifiable metabolites circulating in plasma. Eighty percent of a single dose of dofetilide is eliminated unchanged in the urine; the remaining 20% is composed of inactive or minimally active metabolites.

Ibutilide is widely distributed following IV administration. Most of a dose is biotransformed, with the metabolites eliminated in the urine and the feces. The half-life is 2 to 12 hours, with a mean of 6 hours. Patients with atrial fibrillation of over 2 to 3 days' duration must be treated with anticoagulants for at least 2 weeks before ibutilide therapy. Observe the patient with continuous ECG monitoring for at least 4 hours following the infusion or until the QT interval has returned to baseline. If any arrhythmic activity is noted, continue ECG monitoring.

Sotalol is rapidly absorbed after oral administration, with a bioavailability of nearly 100%. Maximum plasma concentrations are reached 2 to 3 hours after administration, with approximately 50% of the drug bound to plasma proteins. The half-life is 12 hours. Sotalol is almost entirely eliminated in the urine as unchanged drug.

Adverse Effects and Contraindications

The adverse effects of class III antiarrhythmics vary widely and commonly lead to discontinuance of the drug. More than 75% of patients treated with amiodarone for 1 to 2 years experience adverse effects, and 25% to 33% of this number discontinue treatment. Hypotension, nausea, and anorexia are not uncommon. Twenty percent to 40% of patients develop CNS reactions, including malaise, fatigue, and tremor, involuntary movements, ataxia, abnormal gait, lack of coordination, dizziness, and paresthesias. Corneal microdeposits occur in almost all patients receiving the drug; however, only about 10% have vision disturbances. The deposits will disappear with reduction in dosage or when the drug is discontinued. Peripheral neuropathy and proximal myopathy may occur. Because amiodarone contains iodine, which is ultimately released into systemic circulation, it inhibits the conversion of thyroxine (T_4) to triiodothyronine (T_3). It can cause hypothyroidism or hyperthyroidism, with the latter a greater threat to cardiovascular status.

The adverse effects of amiodarone of greatest concern, however, are exacerbations of arrhythmias, worsening of heart failure, pulmonary fibrosis, and pneumonitis. Symptomatic pulmonary toxicity occurs in 10% to 15% of patients for treated 1 to 3 years with amiodarone. Death results in about 10% of patients with pulmonary involvement. Pulmonary toxicity is characterized by cough and progressive dyspnea. The disorder is thought to result from indirect toxicity (i.e., hypersensitivity pneumonitis) or direct toxicity (i.e., interstitial alveolar pneumonitis). Preexisting pulmonary disease does not seem to increase the risk of pulmonary toxicity. However, patients with pulmonary disease have a poor prognosis if pulmonary toxicity does develop. Substantial increases in low-density lipoprotein concentrations are frequently observed. Many patients on amiodarone develop photosensitivity.

Dofetilide can cause serious ventricular arrhythmias, including torsades de pointes. Prolongation of the QT interval is directly connected to the plasma concentrations of dofetilide. Reduced creatinine clearance or certain drug interactions are factors that can increase dofetilide plasma concentrations. Carefully monitoring the ECG for increased QT intervals and controlling drug dosages and plasma concentrations based on creatinine clearance values helps to reduce the risk of torsades de pointes.

Ibutilide is generally well tolerated. The most common adverse effect is an occasional episode of ventricular extrasystole, ventricular tachycardia, headache, and hypotension. Torsades de pointes has also been described. Overdosage results in CNS toxicity and may exaggerate expected prolongation of repolarization. It may worsen existing arrhythmias or produce new arrhythmias. Bundle branch block, AV block, bradycardia, and hypertension are rare. Ibutilide is contraindicated for use in patients with hypersensitivity to the drug or its ingredients. Cautious use is warranted in patients with abnormal liver function or heart block.

The most common adverse effects of sotalol include bradycardia and palpitations. Anxiety, nervousness, nausea, vomiting, diarrhea, constipation, nightmares, transient hypotension, heart failure, bronchospasm, peripheral ischemia (i.e., cold hands, feet), and unusual tiredness or weakness have also been noted. Although rare, skin rashes, chest pain, and depression may occur. The most severe adverse effects include prolonged QT interval, torsades de pointes, ventricular tachycardia, and premature ventricular complexes.

Drug Interactions

There are a number of drug interactions with class III drugs (Table 36-4). In general, because these drugs are slowly eliminated from the body, the potential for drug interactions and other adverse effects persists for many weeks after amiodarone is discontinued.

Dosage Regimen

Because it takes amiodarone several months to reach full effect, loading doses are used. Treatment effectiveness is evaluated after 2 to 8 weeks. Long-term effective treatment has been associated with plasma concentrations of 1 to 2.5 mcg/mL.

Before initiating dofetilide therapy, carefully withdraw previous antiarrhythmic therapy over a period of at least 3 half-lives. Do not start dofetilide immediately following amiodarone therapy because of the unpredictable pharmacokinetics of amiodarone. Dofetilide can be initiated after amiodarone plasma levels are below 0.3 mcg/mL, or after amiodarone has been withdrawn for at least 3 months.

The dosage of dofetilide must be individualized using a seven-step algorithm based upon the creatinine clearance and QT interval measurements. Use the QT interval if the heart rate is less than 60 bpm. There are no data on use of the drug when the heart rate is less than 50 bpm. Dofetilide treatment must be started in an environment that provides uninterrupted ECG monitoring and where personnel are educated in the management of ventricular arrhythmias. Continue patient monitoring for at least 3 days. Patients should not be discharged within 12 hours of an electrical or pharmacologic conversion to normal sinus rhythm.

Treat atrial fibrillation lasting longer than two to three days with anticoagulants for at least two weeks before ibutilide therapy is initiated. Maintain continuous ECG monitoring for at least 4 hours following infusion of ibutilide or until QT interval has returned to baseline.

Dosing more than twice daily with sotalol is usually not necessary because of its long half-life.

Lab Considerations

Amiodarone may cause elevated ALT, AST, and alkaline phosphatase concentrations. Monitor liver, lung, thyroid, and neurologic functions before and periodically throughout therapy. ANA titer concentrations may be elevated, but the patient is not usually symptomatic. The long elimination half-life of amiodarone causes persistent drug effects long after dosage adjustment or the drug is discontinued.

Perform regular creatinine clearance testing for the patient taking ibutilide and dofetilide. Routinely monitor hepatic and renal function and CBC in patients receiving prolonged sotalol therapy. Correct hypokalemia and hypomagnesemia before initiating therapy with sotalol.

CARDIOVASCULAR

Class IV Antiarrhythmics

- ◆ diltiazem (Cardizem, Cardizem SR, Cardizem CD, Dilacor XR); ♣ Novo-Diltiazem, Syn-Diltiazem
- ◆ verapamil (Calan, Calan SR, Isoptin, Isoptin SR, Verelan); ♣ Novo-Veramil, Nu-Verap

▥ Indications

Although there are other calcium channel blockers (CCBs), verapamil and diltiazem are the only drugs in this class approved by the FDA for treatment of arrhythmias. Diltiazem and verapamil are approved for the management of rapid ventricular rate in atrial fibrillation and atrial flutter and paroxysmal supraventricular tachycardia. Verapamil has been used successfully in the transplacental cardioversion of fetal paroxysmal atrial tachycardia.

▥ Pharmacodynamics

Class IV drugs are CCBs in that they inhibit Ca^{++} movement across cell membranes of cardiac and vascular smooth muscle. Inhibition of Ca^{++} movement slows the conduction rate between atria and ventricles and greatly increases the ERP of the AV node and slows the spontaneous firing of pacemaker cells in the SA node. However, heart rate slows minimally because this direct effect is balanced by increased reflex sympathetic activity resulting from arterial vasodilation. Depression of the AV node is responsible for slowing the ventricular response to atrial flutter or fibrillation and termination of paroxysmal supraventricular tachycardia. Neither verapamil nor diltiazem has cholinergic or beta blockade properties. Verapamil does, however, have appreciable alpha-blocking activity.

▥ Pharmacokinetics

The pharmacokinetics of class IV antiarrhythmics are identified in Table 36-3. The pharmacokinetics are also discussed in Chapter 37.

▥ Adverse Effects and Contraindications

The most common adverse effects of diltiazem therapy are peripheral edema, facial flushing, dizziness, headache, asthenia (i.e., weakness, loss of strength), and bradycardia. Diarrhea, constipation, and a rash are possible although rare. Occasionally, patients note hypotension, pruritus, burning at an IV injection site, vasodilation, atrial flutter, bradycardia, and diaphoresis. The most severe adverse effects include second- and third-degree heart block, increased frequency and duration of anginal pain, and heart failure.

Diltiazem is contraindicated for use in patients with sick sinus syndrome, second- and third-degree heart block (except in the presence of a pacemaker), severe hypotension (systolic blood pressure less than 90 mm Hg), acute MI, and pulmonary congestion. Cautious use is warranted in patients with renal or hepatic disorders.

The most common adverse effect of verapamil is constipation. Dizziness, hypotension, peripheral edema, bradycardia, headache, and fatigue are frequent occurrences. Hypotension, bradycardia, dizziness, and headache are occasionally noted when verapamil is given by IV route. Severe tachycardia is rare, although verapamil can increase ventricular rate because of reflex increases in SNS activity.

Like diltiazem, verapamil is contraindicated for use in patients with sick sinus syndrome, second- and third-degree heart block (except in the presence of a pacemaker), severe hypotension (systolic blood pressure less than 90 mm Hg), acute MI, and pulmonary congestion. In addition, use of verapamil is contraindicated in cardiogenic shock and severe heart failure (unless secondary to supraventricular tachycardia). Cautious use is warranted in patients with renal or hepatic disorders.

IV use of CCBs is contraindicated in patients who have hypotension, severe heart failure, sick sinus syndrome, AV block, atrial fibrillation, Wolff-Parkinson-White syndrome, or ventricular tachycardia.

▥ Drug Interactions

The major interaction of class IV antiarrhythmics is with digoxin, with the clearance of digoxin being reduced. Because of the additive effect of the CCBs on SA or AV node function, the negative inotropic effect of verapamil may negate the advantages of positive inotropic action of digoxin, thereby requiring a dosage adjustment. In addition, verapamil interacts with digoxin in a manner not unlike the quinidine-digoxin reaction, in which digoxin serum levels are increased. Concurrent use of verapamil or diltiazem with antihypertensive drugs that depress the SA node can intensify sinus bradycardia. Highly protein-bound drugs displace or could be displaced by CCBs.

▥ Dosage Regimen

The dosage of class IV antiarrhythmics are identified in Table 36-5. Chapter 37 also contains dosage information.

▥ Lab Considerations

Total serum Ca^{++} levels are not affected by class IV antiarrhythmics. Monitor serum K^+ levels periodically throughout therapy, because hypokalemia increases the risk of arrhythmias. Monitor renal and hepatic functions during long-term therapy. Liver function test values may increase after several days of therapy but return to normal on discontinuation of the drug.

Miscellaneous Antiarrhythmics

- ◆ adenosine (Adenocard, Adenoscan); ♣ Adenocard
- ◆ moricizine (Ethmozine)

Adenosine

Adenosine is an unclassified antiarrhythmic used for converting paroxysmal supraventricular tachycardia to sinus rhythm. It is ineffective for other arrhythmias.

Adenosine is a naturally occurring component of all body cells that is an important physiologic mediator in different organ systems. It is produced in myocardial cells by dephosphorylation of adenosine monophosphate (AMP) and by degradation of s-adenosylhomocysteine. Adenosine activates K^+ channels and, by increasing outflow of K^+ current, hyperpolarizes the membrane potential, decreasing spontaneous SA nodal depolarization. The nucleoside may also decrease inward Ca^{++} channel by blocking adenylate cyclase, which normally increases the inward Ca^{++} current. Automaticity and conduction are inhibited in the SA and AV nodes.

Absorption of adenosine is essentially complete after IV administration. It is taken up by erythrocytes and vascular endothelium and rapidly converted to inosine and adenosine monophosphate. Adenosine has a short duration of action. Its serum half-life is less than 10 seconds; thus it must be given as a rapid bolus injection, preferably through a central venous IV line. If given slowly, it is eliminated before it can reach cardiac tissues and exert cardiac action.

The frequent adverse effects of adenosine include facial flushing, headache, new arrhythmias (e.g., PVCs, sinus bradycardia), discomfort in the chest, arm, jaw, and throat, and shortness of breath. Cough, dizziness, nausea, and numbness and tingling in the arms are occasionally noted. Sinus arrest can also occur. However, because of adenosine's short half-life of 10 seconds, these adverse effects are short-lived. Adenosine is contraindicated for use in patients with second- and third-degree heart block, sick sinus syndrome (except with functioning pacemaker), atrial flutter or atrial fibrillation, and ventricular tachycardia. Use it with caution in patients with heart block, arrhythmias at the time of conversion, asthma, and hepatic or renal failure. Safe use during pregnancy and lactation and in children is unclear.

The dosing regimen of IV adenosine is identified in Table 36-5. Dosages over 12 mg decrease blood pressure by decreasing peripheral vascular resistance.

Moricizine

Moricizine (Ethmozine) shares many of the properties of class I drugs, but it does not cleanly fit into the existing subclasses. It is used in the management of life-threatening ventricular arrhythmias such as sustained ventricular tachycardia that have not responded to other drugs. Its antiarrhythmic effects are similar to those of class I_A drugs, but its uses and adverse effects are more similar to those of class I_C drugs.

Moricizine suppresses abnormal automaticity and prolongs the PR and QRS intervals and AV-nodal, bundle of His, and Purkinje fiber conduction times by blocking Na^+ channels in myocardial tissues. The drug has minimal effects on the amplitude of the action potential and on normal automaticity.

Moricizine is well absorbed but rapidly biotransformed following oral administration. Administration after a meal delays the rate of absorption but not the extent of absorption. Less than 1% of unchanged drug is eliminated in the urine. The metabolites may have antiarrhythmic action.

The most common adverse effects of moricizine include anxiety, dizziness, euphoria, headache, perianal numbness, fatigue, and nausea. Drug-induced arrhythmias are the most life-threatening adverse effects.

Moricizine is contraindicated for use in patients with hypersensitivity, cardiogenic shock, second- and third-degree heart block, or bundle branch block (unless a pacemaker is present). Exercise caution when using it in patients with electrolyte disturbances, heart failure, and severe renal or hepatic dysfunction. Use extreme caution in patients with sick sinus syndrome. Safe use during pregnancy or lactation and in children has not been established.

CLINICAL REASONING

Treatment Objectives

There are three general objectives for the management of arrhythmias. These include abolishing the abnormal rhythm,

restoring normal sinus rhythm, and preventing a recurrence of the arrhythmia. Overall desired outcomes of antiarrhythmic therapy include maintaining cardiac output, increasing activity tolerance, and reducing patients' fear and anxiety.

Determining the cause and type of the arrhythmia is essential to selecting the most appropriate drug. Identifying the circumstances in which the arrhythmia occurs helps determine if acute or chronic, long-term therapy is required. For example, the appearance of ventricular fibrillation in a patient with an acute MI may not necessitate long-term therapy to alleviate the arrhythmia, because the chance of recurrence is negligible. However, patients who have disabling symptoms such as dizziness, orthostatic hypotension, or palpitations may benefit from long-term therapy. Note that rhythm disturbances that are well tolerated in persons with structurally normal hearts may not be tolerated in those with heart disease.

There is a general consensus among health care providers that appropriate treatment for arrhythmias includes also treating the underlying disease processes contributing to the arrhythmia. However, there are some arrhythmias that should not be treated. The mere detection of an abnormality should not always be equated with the need for drug therapy (Box 36-2).

Establish the frequency and reproducibility of the arrhythmias before starting drug therapy, since inherent variability in the occurrence of arrhythmias can be confused with a beneficial or adverse drug effect. For example, a marked decrease in the duration of paroxysms of atrial fibrillation may be sufficient to render a patient asymptomatic, even if an occasional episode can still be detected.

Factors contributing to the choice of drug therapy include not only symptoms but also the type and extent of structural heart disease, the QT interval before drug therapy, the coexistence of conduction system disease, and the presence of noncardiac conditions and diseases such as diarrhea, lung disease, asthma, hypoglycemia, prostatism, glaucoma, arthritis, and tremors, among others.

Treatment Options

▥ Patient Variables

As with the patient who takes digoxin or antianginal drugs, the perceived susceptibility to disease and its seriousness influences the plan of care. Because many antiarrhythmic drugs have unpleasant or undesirable adverse effects, the likelihood of adherence is an important consideration. The health care provider must appreciate that many patients will not continue

---

BOX 36-2

Identifying an Arrhythmia*

- What is the site and the type (mechanism) for the arrhythmia?
- Is it supraventricular or ventricular?
- Is it passive (due to escape) or active (due to enhanced automaticity)?
- Is impaired conduction the problem?

*If unable to identify the baseline rhythm, begin treatment based on the width of the QRS complex. Rapid rates with narrow QRS complexes are treated as paroxysmal supraventricular tachycardias (PSVTs). Rapid rates with wide QRS complexes are treated as ventricular tachycardia (VT).

CARDIOVASCULAR

maintenance therapy with an antiarrhythmic because of unmanageable adverse effects. Once the importance is understood, the majority of patients usually understand the importance of medication adherence and of follow-up. The fact that the patient is often recovering from a life-threatening event, such as an MI, sometimes also motivates adherence to therapy.

Life-Span Considerations

Pregnant and Nursing Women. Pregnancy is accompanied by significant physiologic changes in the maternal cardiovascular system. Pregnancy-related changes in blood volume, cardiac output, pulse, blood pressure, and peripheral vascular resistance are discussed in Chapter 6. In the majority of individuals, these changes pose no significant threat to maternal or fetal well-being and are well tolerated. Even in women with preexisting rheumatic heart disease and with most forms of congenital heart disease, the physiologic changes of pregnancy do not result in a significant threat. However, sudden cardiac decompensation may occur in certain individuals during pregnancy. Included in this group are persons previously diagnosed with cardiac dysfunction as well as those who demonstrate decompensation for the first time during pregnancy. It is important to have a clear understanding of the normal changes of pregnancy so that normal complaints can be well managed. Symptoms suggesting significant underlying cardiac dysfunction can then be recognized as early as possible.

In general, do not use antiarrhythmic drugs during pregnancy unless the anticipated benefits outweigh the risks arising from failure to treat the arrhythmia or the possible risks to the fetus. Arrhythmias otherwise treated with quinidine or procainamide should also be treated during pregnancy without fear of adverse reaction to the fetus or newborn. Fetal hydantoin syndrome occurs in approximately 10% of fetuses chronically exposed to phenytoin. Lidocaine may increase uterine tone and decrease uterine blood flow when used as an anesthetic drug in a paracervical block. Fetal bradycardia has also been reported, secondary to either direct myocardial suppression or to changes in uterine perfusion and tone. There is no evidence of a teratogenic potential with lidocaine, and it may be safely administered in pregnancy as the drug of choice for certain acute ventricular tachyarrhythmias.

Children and Adolescents. Antiarrhythmic drugs are needed less often in children than in adults. Supraventricular tachycardias (often occurring with anxiety, fever, or hypovolemia) are the most common arrhythmias in children. The onset of supraventricular tachycardia is often sudden, and the duration is variable. Infants and young children with this arrhythmia may be unable to communicate the rapid heart rate, and the clinical course may progress to heart failure. Important signs of arrhythmia in the infant and young child include poor feeding, extreme irritability, and pallor.

As with adults, use antiarrhythmic drugs only when clearly indicated. Propranolol, quinidine, or verapamil may be used as prophylaxis or treatment. Lidocaine may be used to treat ventricular arrhythmias precipitated by cardiac surgery or digoxin toxicity. Monitor the child closely, because all antiarrhythmic drugs can cause adverse effects including hypotension and the development of new arrhythmias.

Older Adults. During the third and fourth decades of life, pacemaker cells decrease in number as myocardial fat, collagen, and elastin fibers increase. This change affects the SA node, which shows evidence of acceleration through the sixth decade. The number of SA cells at age 75 years is 10% of those that existed at age 20 years. Similarly, the AV node and the bundle of His lose a number of conductive cells into the fourth decade, and the left bundle between the fifth and seventh decades. Alteration in the excitation and contraction mechanisms is an adaptive rather than a degenerative change, because they maintain contractile function of the aged heart. The majority of rate irregularities in the older adult are attributed to myocardial damage (see Case Study).

CASE STUDY | Atrial Fibrillation

ASSESSMENT

History of Present Illness	BG is a 62-year-old white female in mild distress with vague complaints of intermittent but increasing episodes of dyspnea and fatigue. The dyspnea has progressively worsened over the past month, and she is now afraid to go out for her usual 1-mile walk each day. She finds herself sleeping with two pillows but occasionally awakens at night to sit by the open window "to catch my breath." She follows a 1500-calorie low-fat diet.
Past Health History	BG denies allergies to drugs or food. Her last ECG was 4 years ago during a routine physical exam. She denies history of other hospitalizations, illness, alcohol use or smoking, heart disease, thyroid disorders. Positive family history of CAD. Current drugs: Premarin 0.3 mg PO daily for menopausal symptoms.
Life-Span Considerations	BG retired this year to spend time with her husband, who retired 7 years ago. She believes in natural foods and tries to eat nutritious meals. She expressed on several occasions the concern that she will become a burden to this 72-year-old husband, who is physically unable to assume responsibility for her care. They have an adult son and daughter who live six blocks away. BG lives on Social Security and retirement benefits. She has Medicare parts A, B, and D; uses AARP pharmacy mail services for routine drugs. Will need to obtain new drug from local pharmacy until response to therapy is determined; therefore cost is greater than what she pays through AARP.
Physical Exam Findings	*Ht:* 5'4". *Wt:* 175 lbs (3 lbs above usual). *BP:* 160/70, respirations 26, increasing to 32 with minimal exertion; apical pulse 120 bpm resting and 130 to 140 bpm with exertion; radial pulse

	104 bpm. No carotid bruits noted. Bibasilar fine crackles on auscultation. Diaphragmatic excursion 4 cm. Irregularly irregular rhythm on auscultation of heart with variation in intensity of S_1. No S_3 or S_4. Abdomen soft, NT. Skin pale without cyanosis. Appears anxious.
Diagnostic Testing	Chest x-ray: Left ventricular enlargement with congestion of pulmonary vasculature. ECG: No previous tracing: Normal axis. Tachycardic at 164 bpm. Rhythm: irregularly irregular. P wave: present. QRS 0.8 s. PR interval: 0.16 s. QT interval: 0.38 s. Lytes: Na^+ 134 mEq/L; K^+ 3.6 mEq/L; Cl^- 92 mEq/L; BUN 34 mg/100 mL; creatinine 1.3 mg/100 mL.

DIAGNOSIS: Arrhythmia

MANAGEMENT

Treatment Objectives	1. Restore normal sinus rhythm. 2. Prevent development of other arrhythmias. 3. Prevent or reduce frequency of recurrent episodes of atrial fibrillation. 4. Maintain adequate tissue perfusion and cardiac output.
Treatment Plan	**Pharmacotherapy** • diltiazem SR 240 mg PO daily. • warfarin 10 mg PO today, 5 mg tomorrow; then recheck PT and INR • digoxin 0.125 mg PO daily **Patient Education** 1. Meaning of diagnosis of atrial fibrillation, treatment modalities 2. Name of the drug, the dose, and the reason it is needed; adverse effects to watch for 3. Importance of adherence to drug therapy 4. Avoidance of concurrent drugs without first checking with health care provider, to minimize potential drug interactions 5. Importance of follow-up appointments with health care provider and of wearing a form of medical alert identification. **Evaluation** 1. Normal sinus rhythm is restored. 2. Other arrhythmias were prevented from developing. 3. Recurrent episodes of atrial fibrillation have been prevented. 4. Adequate tissue perfusion and cardiac output have been maintained.

CLINICAL REASONING ANALYSIS

Q1. Why is it that she has to take three drugs for atrial fibrillation? Isn't one drug enough given her age?

A. She needs the diltiazem to create AV-nodal blockade, which in turn slows her heart rate. The warfarin is to reduce the risk of clots that arises because of the atrial fibrillation and the turbulent blood flow, and the digoxin is to help slow and strengthen myocardial contractions.

Q2. How do we know if the diltiazem is working?

A. A couple of ways: by monitoring her heart rate and rhythm on the ECG, looking for normal sinus rhythm, and checking to see if she has symptoms. The reason we treated her in the first place was because she was symptomatic from the atrial fibrillation.

Q3. What about drug interactions with diltiazem?

A. And there are many. We will give her the list of drugs that interact with all of her drugs.

Q4. While I was in talking with BG, she told me she can't afford the Cardizem SR. Is that another drug she is also taking?

A. No, Cardizem SR is the brand name for diltiazem. It appears after looking at her coverage that Medicare Part D prescription plan does not cover the brand name. We will change her prescription upon discharge to the generic formulation of diltiazem SR. It should be just fine and will be about one third the price of the brand name drug.

Q5. In talking with BG, she sounds like she understands the importance of taking her drugs as prescribed, but what will happen if she forgets to take the diltiazem for a day or two?

A. We can facilitate her taking her drugs regularly by giving her our little drug box. She will be able to fill it for each day of the week, and hopefully she won't forget. We need to emphasize the importance of taking her drugs regularly since an abrupt withdrawal of diltiazem may increase the risk for a return of her arrhythmia or precipitate others.

Arrhythmias are not uncommon in older adults, but in general, only arrhythmias causing symptoms of circulatory impairment should be treated. Hypotension and heart failure may occur from the myocardial depressant effects of antiarrhythmic drugs. Cautious use is required, and dosage generally has to be reduced to compensate for heart disease or impaired drug elimination processes. Several expert panels, such as Beers and colleagues (Fick et al., 2003), have developed criteria for helping health care providers evaluate the risk and benefit of these drugs in older adults, as well as providing safer alternatives to specific high-risk drugs.

▥ Drug Variables

Use of antiarrhythmics is appropriate when the patient has an acute life-threatening rhythm disturbance. After the acute phase has resolved, the need for antiarrhythmic therapy may end. In spite of this, there is some disagreement about the appropriateness of long-term antiarrhythmic therapy for patients with recurrent symptomatic episodes (see Controversy box). Rational antiarrhythmic therapy requires the health care provider to possess the knowledge, skill, and ability to do the following:

- Identify if the fast (or slow) rate is making the patient symptomatic.
- Accurately identify the arrhythmia (see Box 36-2).
- Interpret the mechanisms causing the arrhythmia.
- Interpret the ECG and the hemodynamic effects of the arrhythmia.
- Understand antiarrhythmic drug actions, including the desired onset of drug action, the suitability of the various routes of administration, adverse effects, the need for a stable serum concentration, and the likelihood of tolerance, proarrhythmic effects, and toxicity.

- Expect that the drug's therapeutic effects outweigh the potential adverse effects.

The therapeutic/toxic ratio of most antiarrhythmics is relatively narrow; therefore knowledge of pharmacokinetics is important to avoid toxic peak and subtherapeutic trough concentrations. Remember, however, that therapeutic response to one drug in a particular class does not guarantee a therapeutic response to another drug of the same class. Also note that many antiarrhythmics produce toxicity at therapeutic doses. Pay close attention to symptom reports, and assess for signs of toxicity even if plasma levels of a specific drug are within a generally accepted normal range.

The general trends and recommendations for the management of arrhythmias are identified in Table 36-6. Note that the premature atrial contractions are usually not treated with antiarrhythmic drugs.

Knowledge as to when peak plasma levels are reached for the various antiarrhythmic drugs may be helpful in determining when therapeutic effects are most likely to appear. However, there are many other factors that influence therapeutic effects, including the dose, frequency of administration, presence of conditions that alter drug biotransformation, arterial blood gases, serum electrolyte levels, and myocardial status. Antiarrhythmic drugs can accumulate in patients with renal or hepatic dysfunction, so carefully monitor patients for signs and symptoms of increasing impairment. Drug dosages may have to be adjusted based on these data.

Because some antiarrhythmics have proarrhythmic effects, remain alert to the development of new arrhythmias. The proarrhythmic effects of some antiarrhythmic drugs are of special concern in patients with compromised left ventricular function or who have sustained ventricular arrhythmias. Although they

---

Controversy

Antiarrhythmics: Good versus Harm

Jonathan J. Wolfe

On the surface, the concept of adding an antiarrhythmic drug to therapy in the patient with a history of MI appears reasonable and natural. This is so because we recognize that the post-MI patient is most vulnerable to development of arrhythmias. These irregularities of heart function constitute a leading cause of mortality in the recovery phase after surviving an MI.

Reality has proven that antiarrhythmics are problematic in actual practice. Part of the difficulty arises from their nature. Local anesthetic agents (class I) represent the most potent antiarrhythmics, but they are best administered parenterally. This is not practical for long-term treatment, and indeed, use of lidocaine infusions is best ended as soon as possible. None of these drugs is free of hazard.

The search for an ideal, orally administered antiarrhythmic has produced several classes of such drugs. The best-studied and still first-line drug is quinidine. The advent of sustained-release dosage forms has simplified the issue of adherence to treatment, once an effective dose is established. The patient who cannot tolerate quinidine may be tried on procainamide and other drugs. Metaanalysis does not yet permit certainty about the relative value of drugs in classes I, I_A, and III. In each case the health care provider must also consider the interactions of these drugs with other drugs the patient likely will use.

The antiarrhythmics remind us powerfully that there are no pure drugs. In every case, significant adverse effects accompany even the most

valuable product. The patient with preexisting heart disease and the patient who has survived an MI must be monitored closely in assessing the risk and benefit of add-on drug therapy.

CLINICAL REASONING ANALYSIS

- Your patient has survived an MI, lengthy cardiopulmonary resuscitation, and a stay in the intensive care unit. In addition to being depressed, this 64-year-old-man is extremely apprehensive and fearful of dying. He has searched the Internet for information about cardiac arrhythmias. Now he returns to the clinic demanding a prescription for flecainide. What is your first response? Do you feel it is proper for patients to request particular treatments?

- An 80-year-old woman in your cardiac care unit has just been cardioverted for the fourth time in 2 days. She has significant comorbid conditions (i.e., diabetes mellitus, chronic renal failure, and hypertension). Her orders include prophylactic IV boluses of lidocaine 50 mg for treatment of PVCs or other arrhythmias. Is she at significant risk for complications? Is a continuous infusion of lidocaine appropriate for her?

- A 72-old-man cared for in your clinic has been taking amiodarone for 2 weeks. His history includes two previous MIs. His wife calls, reporting that she found him dead in the back yard. She had not seen him for an hour. The EMS team was unable to resuscitate him from the unwitnessed arrest. His wife asks if the new drug caused him to die. What is your response?

TABLE 36-6 Overview of Arrhythmia Management

Arrhythmia	Acute Therapy*	Chronic Therapy*
SUPRAVENTRICULAR ARRHYTHMIAS		
Premature atrial, nodal, or ventricular depolarizations	Usually not treated	None indicated
Atrial tachycardia	1. Create AV-nodal blockade with adenosine, CCB, BB, or digoxin.	1. Control ventricular response with adenosine, CCB, BB, or digoxin. 2. Maintain NSR by K+ and Na+ channel blockade. 3. Extinguish focus with ablation.†
Atrial flutter	1. Create AV-nodal blockade with adenosine, CCB, BB, or digoxin. 2. Restore NSR with cardioversion.‡	1. Maintain NSR by K+ and Na+ channel blockade. 2. Create AV-nodal blockade with adenosine, CCB, BB, or digoxin. 3. Extinguish focus with ablation (in selected cases).
Atrial fibrillation	1. Create AV-nodal blockade with adenosine, CCB, BB, or digoxin. 2. Restore NSR.	1. Control ventricular response. 2. Maintain NSR by K+ and Na+ channel blockade.
PSVT	1. adenosine DOC 2. AV-nodal blockade with adenosine, CCB, or BB 3. Increase vagal tone with digoxin or phenylephrine.	1. Extinguish focus with ablation. 2. Create AV-nodal blockade with flecainide or propafenone.
AV reentry (PSVT)	1. adenosine DOC 2. Create AV-nodal blockade with adenosine, CCB, or BB. 3. Increase vagal tone with digoxin or phenylephrine.	1. Maintain NSR by K+ and Na+ channel blockade. 2. Extinguish focus with ablation.
Atrial fibrillation with AV conduction via accessory pathway	1. procainamide DOC 2. Synchronized cardioversion DOC	1. Extinguish focus with ablation. 2. Maintain NSR by K+ and Na+ channel blockade.
VENTRICULAR ARRHYTHMIAS		
Ventricular tachycardia after MI (unstable)	1. lidocaine 2. amiodarone 3. procainamide 4. Synchronized cardioversion§	1. ICD 2. amiodarone 3. Maintain NSR by K+ and Na+ channel blockade.
Ventricular tachycardia without structural heart disease (stable)	1. Beta blocker 2. lidocaine 3. amiodarone 4. procainamide 5. sotalol 6. Synchronized cardioversion§	1. verapamil 2. Beta blocker
Ventricular tachycardia or ventricular fibrillation without a pulse	1. Defibrillation × 3 at increasing voltage 2. epinephrine every 3–5 min or vasopressin once followed by defibrillation 3. amiodarone 4. magnesium sulfate 5. procainamide	
Prolonged QT (torsades de pointes)	1. magnesium 2. isoproterenol 3. phenytoin 4. lidocaine 5. Overdrive pacing	

*Acute therapy administered intravenously; chronic therapy implies long term use.
†Ablation is the use of high-frequency radio-wave destruction of tissue responsible for maintenance of the tachycardia.
‡When cardioversion is indicated, consider using sedative (e.g., diazepam, midazolam, barbiturates, etomidate, ketamine, methohexital) with or without an analgesic (e.g., fentanyl, morphine, meperidine). Anesthesia recommended if readily available.
§May go directly to cardioversion if ventricular rate >150 bpm. May give brief trial of drugs based on specific arrhythmia. Immediate cardioversion is not needed if heart rate >150 bpm.
Adapted from American Heart Association. (2003). *ACLS Provider Manual.* Dallas, TX: Author; and Hardman, J., Limbird, L., and Gilman, A. (Eds.). (2001). *Goodman and Gilman's the pharmacologic basis of therapeutics* (10th ed.). New York: McGraw-Hill.
AV, Atrioventricular; *BB,* beta blocker; *CCB,* calcium channel blocker; *DOC,* drug of choice; *ICD,* implanted cardioverter-defibrillator; *NSR,* normal sinus rhythm; *PSVT,* paroxysmal supraventricular tachycardia.

are effective drugs and are usually well tolerated, in some cases the arrhythmia is worsened. For example, a torsades de pointes arrhythmia may develop in patients receiving quinidine, procainamide, disopyramide, amiodarone, or sotalol. Women are more at risk for torsades de pointes than men, especially during administration of cardiovascular drugs that prolong depolarization. Liquid protein diets and electrolyte disturbances (e.g., hypokalemia, hypomagnesemia) may also precipitate development of this arrhythmia. By prolonging the QT interval, certain noncardiac drugs such as some antihypertensives, antibiotics, diuretics, antihistamines, tricyclic antidepressants, and phenothiazines may also set the stage for torsades de pointes. This arrhythmia and other proarrhythmic events often occur within a few days of initiating antiarrhythmic therapy, but they may also develop unexpectedly later in the course of long-term treatment.

Patient Education

As with all drugs, antiarrhythmics should be taken as prescribed, with the dosage regimen individualized to maximize therapeutic effects and minimize adverse reactions. Teach the patient and/or the family the name of the drug, the dose, and the reason it is needed. For patients on several drugs, explain the risks associated with multidrug therapy, such as the potential for drug interactions, altered drug responses, and increased risk of adverse effects.

Abrupt discontinuance of an antiarrhythmic drug has been associated with reappearance of arrhythmia. Encourage the patient not to miss a dose and to carry information regarding the prescribed drugs in written form. Teach the patient and family members to recognize and report signs and symptoms of bradycardia, hypotension, arrhythmia, heart failure, pulmonary and peripheral embolism, and cardiac arrest. Teach the patient to avoid sudden changes in position to reduce the severity of postural hypotension. Monitor blood pressure frequently, particularly in patients with known ventricular dysfunction or hypertrophy. The antiarrhythmic drug may have to be discontinued if severe hypotension occurs.

Advise patients to notify their health care provider or dentist of their drug regimen before dental treatment or surgery. Advise patients to avoid concurrent use of other drugs without first checking with their health care provider to minimize potential drug interactions. In addition, advise patients to avoid alcohol, smoking, excess Na^+ intake, caffeine, and sunlight (for those on amiodarone). Caution them to avoid hazardous activities until the effects of the antiarrhythmic drug are known. Encourage patients to keep follow-up appointments and to wear a form of medical alert identification.

Evaluation

Criteria that can be used to evaluate the therapeutic outcome of antiarrhythmic therapy include the following: (1) the impulse is generated at the SA node; (2) conduction occurs within a uniform, normal time period; (3) contraction takes place at regular, equally spaced intervals at a rate of 60 to 100 bpm in an adult and 130 to 160 bpm in a newborn; and (4) AV and intraventricular conduction take place via the appropriate conduction tissues. The data required for evaluating the therapeutic effectiveness relate to cardiac output, activity tolerance, fear and anxiety, tissue perfusion status, adherence or lack of adherence to the treatment regimen, and incidence of absence of complications resulting from antiarrhythmic therapy.

KEY POINTS

- Cardiac arrhythmias, the most common complication of MI, arise from disruptions in the spontaneous initiation of an impulse (automaticity), the conduction of the impulse (conductivity), or both.
- Arrhythmias may originate in any part of the conduction system: SA node, atria, AV node, bundle of His, Purkinje fibers, bundle branches, or ventricular tissues.
- Supraventricular arrhythmias are viewed along a continuum of rate acceleration and a progressive reduction in atrial function: premature atrial contractions, atrial tachycardia, atrial flutter, and atrial fibrillation.
- Nodal arrhythmias involve tachycardia, with increased workload for the heart or bradycardia from heart block. Heart block results from impaired conduction of the electrical impulse through the AV node.
- Ventricular arrhythmias may progress to ventricular tachycardia, ventricular flutter, ventricular fibrillation, or asystole.
- Management of the patient with an arrhythmia is focused on relieving the acute episode of cardiac irregularity, establishing normal sinus rhythm, and prevention of further attacks.
- Any arrhythmia that causes symptomatic hypotension or sudden death should be treated.

- Certain antiarrhythmic drugs are known to be more effective for one type of arrhythmia than another. Much of antiarrhythmic drug therapy remains a trial-and-error proposition.
- It is important to remember that the potential adverse effect of any antiarrhythmic drug is an exacerbation of the arrhythmia or the development of new rhythm disturbances.
- Class I antiarrhythmic drugs (quinidine, procainamide, disopyramide) depress cardiac action by blocking the Na^+ channel in the myocardial membranes. They exert negative inotropic, chronotropic, and dromotropic effects.
- Class II antiarrhythmic drugs (propranolol, esmolol, acebutolol) are beta blockers.
- Class III antiarrhythmic drugs (amiodarone, dofetilide, ibutinide, sotalol) alter the cardiac arrhythmia by slowing heart action, prolonging the duration of the action potential, or prolonging myocardial repolarization.
- Class IV antiarrhythmic drugs (verapamil, diltiazem) are calcium channel blockers.

Bibliography

Aerssens, J., and Paulussen, A. (2005). Pharmacogenomics and acquired long QT syndrome. *Pharmacogenomics, 6*(3), 259–270.

Dubin, D. (2000). *Rapid interpretation of EKG's: A programmed course* (6th ed.). Tampa: Cover.

Echt, D., Liebson, E., and Mitchell, L. et al. (1991). Mortality and morbidity in patients receiving encainide, flecainide, or placebo: The Cardiac Arrhythmia Suppression Trial. *New England Journal of Medicine, 324*(12), 781–788.

Fick, D., Cooper, J., and Wade, W., et al. (2003). Updating the Beers criteria for potentially inappropriate medication use in older adults: Results of a US consensus panel of experts. *Archives of Internal Medicine, 163*(22), 2716–2724.

Hilleman, D., and Bauman, J. (2001). Role of antiarrhythmic therapy in patients at risk for sudden cardiac death: An evidence based review. *Pharmacotherapy, 21*(5), 556–575.

Kowey, P. (1998). Pharmacological effects of antiarrhythmic drugs: Review and update. *Archives of Internal Medicine, 158*(4), 325–332.

Lip, G., and Tello-Montoliu, A. (2006). Management of atrial fibrillation. *Heart, 92*(8), 1177–1182.

Ross, D., Cooper, M., and Koo, C., et al. (1990). Proarrhythmic effects and antiarrhythmic drugs. *Medical Journal of Australia, 153* (1), 37–47.

Sanguinetti, M., and Bennett, P. (2003). Antiarrhythmic drug target choices and screening. *Circulation Research, 93*(6), 491–499.

Singh, B. (1999). Current antiarrhythmic drugs: An overview of mechanisms of action and potential clinical utility. *Journal of Cardiovascular Electrophysiology, 10*(2), 283–301.

Singh, S., Zoble, R., and Yellen, L., et al. (2000). Efficacy and safety of oral dofetilide in converting to and maintaining sinus rhythm in patients with chronic atrial fibrillation or atrial flutter: The Symptomatic Atrial Fibrillation Investigative Research on Dofetilide (SAFIRE-D) study. Available on line athttp://circ.ahajournals.org/cgi/content/full/102/19/2385. Accessed May 7, 2007.

Siddoway, L. (1995). Pharmacologic principles of antiarrhythmic drugs. In Podrid, P., Kowey, P. (Eds.). *Cardiac arrhythmias: Mechanisms, diagnosis, and management.* Baltimore: Williams & Wilkins.

Vaughan Williams, E. (1984). A classification of antiarrhythmic actions reassessed after a decade of new drugs. *Journal of Clinical Pharmacology, 24*(4), 129–147.

Working Group on Arrhythmias of the European Society of Cardiology. (1991). A new approach to the classification of antiarrhythmic drugs based upon their actions on arrhythmogenic mechanisms. *Circulation, 84*(1), 1831–1851.

Zipes, D. (1999). An overview of arrhythmias and antiarrhythmic approaches. *Journal of Cardiovascular Electrophysiology, 10*(2), 267–271.

CARDIOVASCULAR

37

Antihypertensive Drugs

Despite progress in prevention, detection, treatment, and control of high blood pressure (BP), hypertension (HTN) remains a significant public health problem. Approximately 30% of adults aged 20 years and over and living in the United States meet the current criteria for a diagnosis of HTN.

HYPERTENSION

EPIDEMIOLOGY AND ETIOLOGY

Hypertension is defined as a systolic blood pressure (BP) over 140 mm Hg or a diastolic BP over 90 mm Hg, or the requirement of taking antihypertensive drugs. Approximately 20 million of the estimated 43 million persons with HTN are not being treated, and almost 12 million of the nearly 23 million for whom drug therapy is prescribed have inadequately controlled BP. Suboptimal treatment by the health care provider is the most common cause of the lack of effect. In addition, 11 months after antihypertensive therapy is started, half of the patients stop taking their drugs. HTN is responsible for over 30,000 deaths annually. However, there is evidence that the morbidity and mortality associated with HTN decreases with effective management.

A classification for BP has been developed by the Seventh Report of the Joint National Committee on Prevention, Detection, Evaluation, and Treatment of High Blood Pressure (JNC VII), restaging the disorder for persons older than 18 years of age. The classification changes are based on the understanding that as both systolic and diastolic BP increases, so does the risk of cardiovascular complications. Optimal BP readings with respect to cardiovascular risk are less than 120 mm Hg systolic and less than 80 mm Hg diastolic (Table 37-1). A diagnosis of

HTN is assigned when the patient's BP exceeds 140/90 mm Hg on two or more visits following an initial screening.

Essential HTN (i.e., primary or idiopathic HTN) is polygenic in inheritance. Over 90% of HTN falls into this category. Several factors may contribute to essential HTN: environmental factors (e.g., obesity, dietary sodium, and stress), hyperinsulinemia, defective natriuresis, abnormal neural and peripheral autoregulation, and defects in the renin-angiotensin-aldosterone system (RAAS).

Secondary forms of HTN almost always involve the RAAS, although a specific cause for secondary HTN can be identified in only 10% to 15% of patients. There are several other terms used in relationship to HTN; these terms are identified in Box 37-1.

Nonmodifiable Risk Factors
Nonmodifiable factors contributing to the risk for HTN include age, sex, family history, and ethnicity. First-degree relatives (i.e., parents, sibling) of patients with HTN have 3

TABLE 37-1 JNC VII Classifications of Blood Pressure*

Stage	Systolic (mm Hg)		Diastolic (mm Hg)
Optimal†	<120	**AND**	<80
Prehypertension	120–139	**OR**	80–89
Stage 1	140–159	**OR**	90–99
Stage 2	≥160	**OR**	≥100

*Based on average of two or more readings taken at each of two or more visits following an initial screening in adults over age 18. The patient is not taking antihypertensive drugs and is not acutely ill.

†Optimal blood pressure with respect to cardiovascular risk is less than 120/80 mm Hg. However, unusually low values should be evaluated for clinical significance. When systolic and diastolic pressures fall into different categories, the higher category should be used to classify the patient's blood pressure status.

From Chobanian, A., Bakris, G., Black, H., et al. and the Joint National Committee on Detection, Evaluation, and Treatment of High Blood Pressure. (2003). The Seventh Report of the Joint National Committee on the Prevention, Detection, Evaluation, and Treatment of High Blood Pressure (JNC VII). *Hypertension, 42*(6), 1206–1252.

BOX 37-1

Terms Associated with Hypertension

Primary hypertension	Hypertension characterized by a slow, progressive elevation in blood pressure over several years; etiology uncertain
Secondary hypertension	Hypertension related to underlying renal or endocrine cause; etiology known
Resistant hypertension	Diastolic blood pressure readings consistently above 90 mm Hg while under treatment with antihypertensive drugs
Malignant hypertension	Severely elevated diastolic blood pressure over 140 mm Hg associated with papilledema; a medical emergency
Isolated systolic hypertension	Systolic blood above 160 mm Hg in patients over the age of 60
Complicated hypertension	Arterial hypertension of any cause in which there is evidence of cardiovascular damage related to BP elevation
White-coat hypertension	Blood pressure that is elevated when taken by health care provider but normal when measured outside of the health care environment
Refractory hypertension	Hypertension that fails to respond to therapy
Preeclampsia	Blood pressure elevation 15 mm Hg above normal pressure during pregnancy and characterized by increased blood pressure, albuminuria, and edema
End-organ damage	Damage occurring in major organs fed by the circulatory system (i.e., heart, kidneys, brain, eyes), due to uncontrolled hypertension

times the risk of developing the disorder. The onset of HTN ordinarily occurs between the ages of 25 and 55 years. A diagnosis of HTN is uncommon before the age of 20. However, compared with normotensive children, children younger than 16 years of age with BP readings in the 90th percentile have 3 times the relative risk of developing HTN as an adult. Further, the younger the patient is when HTN is detected, the greater the reduction in life expectancy.

Systolic BP is a more significant risk factor for cardiovascular disease (CVD) in persons over 50 years of age. Men are affected more often by HTN than women until women reach menopause. After menopause, women are affected more often than men. Hypertension is 2 to 3 times more common in women taking oral contraceptives, particularly in women who are also smokers. An increase in BP with increased age is primarily attributable to arteriosclerosis. The rise in systolic BP accounts for the isolated systolic HTN often seen in the older adult.

The incidence of HTN in Native Americans is the same or higher than in the general population. Among Hispanics, BP is generally the same as or lower than that of whites, despite a high incidence of obesity and type 2 diabetes. The prevalence of HTN among blacks is among the highest in the world. Compared with whites, HTN develops earlier in life, and BP elevation is much higher in blacks, causing a greater burden of complications in this population. The earlier onset, higher prevalence, and increased rate of HTN is accompanied by an 80% higher mortality rate from stroke, a 50% higher rate of heart disease, and a 320% incidence of HTN-related end-stage renal disease than in the general population.

Modifiable Risk Factors

Modifiable factors associated with the development of HTN include stress, socioeconomic and nutritional status, obesity, smoking, alcohol use, physical inactivity, high salt intake, and decreased calcium intake.

PATHOPHYSIOLOGY

Essential Hypertension

Essential hypertension is the most common form, affecting 90% to 95% of patients with HTN, although most persons are asymptomatic. The cause is unknown, although a variety of physiologic mechanisms are under investigation for their role in high BP. Patients with essential HTN appear to have abnormalities in Na^+ reabsorption in the kidneys; the RAAS and the mechanisms controlling Na^+ elimination are of particular interest. This system is usually activated in response to low renal perfusion. There is renal retention of Na^+ and water, which increases vascular volume, renal perfusion, and BP. Approximately 15% of patients with HTN have high levels of renin activity. With situations of hypovolemia and Na^+ deficiency, renin activity is stimulated, thus causing Na^+ and water retention and vasoconstriction.

In contrast, 30% of patients with HTN, including blacks, have low renin levels. The low renin level is linked to Na^+ excess, which reduces renin activity. However, the effect is the same as in patients with high renin activity: there is increased vascular volume and elevated BP.

Aldosterone is released when the RAAS is stimulated. In response to aldosterone, the kidneys retain Na^+ ions and

excrete K^+ ions. The possibility of reducing BP by increasing potassium intake rather than restricting Na^+ is being evaluated.

The role of vasopressin in the development of primary HTN has also been explored. A heightened sensitivity in blacks to vasopressin has been identified. This knowledge may help, in part, to explain some of the ethnic variability in BP.

Type 2 diabetes mellitus has been recognized as a risk factor for primary HTN. The prevalence of HTN in these patients is as high as 50%. Obesity in patients with type 2 diabetes explains part of the increased risk of HTN. Type 2 diabetes, obesity, and HTN may be accompanied by insulin resistance and hyperinsulinemia. Hypotheses being explored for the hypertensive mechanisms of insulin resistance include increased release of norepinephrine, Na^+ retention, and increased vascular tone. The increased vascular tone may be related to Na^+ transport mechanisms in the blood vessels. In black persons who have diabetes, BP declines as the blood sugar levels are reduced (independent of a change in antihypertensive drugs).

Secondary Hypertension

Secondary hypertension affects less than 5% to 10% of persons with the disease and is related to an identifiable cause (Box 37-2). When present, it usually develops before age 35 or after 55. Renal, adrenal, vascular, and neurologic disorders, pheochromocytoma, and exogenous compounds (e.g., certain drugs) are primarily responsible for secondary HTN.

Isolated Systolic Hypertension

Isolated systolic hypertension is defined as systolic BP greater than or equal to 140 mm Hg, with diastolic BP less than 90 mm Hg. It occurs in approximately 10% of persons aged 65 to 74 years and in 24% of patients older than 80 years of age. Decreased elasticity of the aorta and large arteries occurs as arteriosclerosis progresses with age. The reduced distensibility of arteries causes an elevated systolic BP without an increase in diastolic BP.

BOX 37-2

Common Causes of Secondary Hypertension

Systolic and Diastolic Hypertension
- Coarctation of the aorta
- Cushing's syndrome
- Diabetes mellitus
- Pheochromocytoma
- Drugs—Antidepressants, Apppetite suppressants, cyclosporin, erythropoietin, Glucocorticoids, Monoamine oxidase inhibitors, Mineralocorticoids, Nasal decongestants, Nonsteroidal antiinflammatory drugs, Oral contraceptives, Phenothiazines, Sympathomimetics, tyramine

Isolated Systolic Hypertension
- Aging, with associated aortic rigidity
- Decreased peripheral vascular resistance
- Anemia
- Aortic valvular insufficiency
- Thyrotoxicosis

CARDIOVASCULAR

Preeclampsia

Preeclampsia is characterized by elevated BP, proteinuria, and edema. Several theories have been proposed for its cause. An increased sensitivity to angiotensin II, hormonal changes that increase vasoconstriction, and a tendency toward reduced Ca^{++} intake during pregnancy may combine to cause a hypertensive state. Generalized vasospasm, due to an imbalance in the production of thromboxane A_2 (a vasoconstrictor) and prostacyclin (a vasodilator), may contribute to high BP.

Preeclampsia most often develops after the twentieth week of gestation in susceptible women, although it can occur earlier in the pregnancy. Onset of preeclampsia during the second trimester is associated with increased risk of maternal and fetal harm. The disorder occurs during first and subsequent pregnancies, with BP returning to normal between pregnancies.

Malignant Hypertension

Malignant hypertension is a rapidly progressing, potentially fatal form of HTN. In this form of HTN, the diastolic pressure exceeds 120 mm Hg. Approximately 1% of all patients with HTN develop malignant HTN. Left untreated, the 1-year mortality rate for malignant HTN is almost 90%. Males, middle-aged adults, and blacks are most likely to develop this form of HTN. The most common mechanism of the disorder is bilateral renal artery stenosis (RAS). Severe emotional stress, excessive salt intake, and abruptly stopping antihypertensive drug therapy are other causes of malignant HTN. Further, secondary causes of HTN may result in this accelerated form of high BP.

End-Organ Damage

End-organ damage (EOD) is associated with all forms of HTN. EOD or target-organ damage (TOD) usually refers to damage resulting from uncontrolled HTN that occurs in major organs fed by the circulatory system (i.e., heart, kidneys, brain, eyes); it is the major cause of morbidity and mortality associated with HTN. Any organ can be damaged, but the kidneys are most often affected. Damage to afferent arterioles produces thick, stiffened arterioles that are less responsive to changes in perfusion and may result in renal failure. BP variability is a more critical determinant than BP level for cardiac damage, renal lesions, and aortic hypertrophy.

The incidence of HTN as a cause of end-stage renal disease (ESRD) has doubled in the past 2 decades. There are geographic differences in the incidence of HTN as a cause of ESRD, from 6% in Japan to 28% in the United States and 13% in Europe. HTN was found to be an underlying cause in 29% of patients with ESRD, second only to diabetes mellitus (36%). In both the United States and South Africa, HTN is the most common cause of ESRD, but it is not clear whether this is related to a higher incidence and severity of HTN in blacks. Moreover, BP control in black patients does not necessarily lead to improved renal function. Other TOD that results from arterial destruction includes severe retinopathy, encephalopathy, heart failure, and dissecting aortic aneurysm (Box 37-3).

PHARMACOTHERAPEUTIC OPTIONS

Drugs from a number of different classifications are used in the management of chronic HTN (Fig. 37-1). The drug groups include diuretics, beta blockers, angiotensin-converting

---

BOX 37-3

End-Organ Damage of Hypertension

Kidneys
- Accelerated atherosclerosis, decreased renal perfusion
- Increased renin aldosterone, increased blood pressure
- Edema
- Decreased cellular oxygenation with resultant damage to renal parenchyma and renal filtration
- Renal insufficiency, prerenal azotemia
- Nephrosclerosis, renal failure

Eyes
- Retinal vascular sclerosis
- Exudates
- Blurring of vision, spots before eyes
- Blindness
- Hemorrhage

Brain
- Accelerated atherosclerosis, decreased cerebral perfusion
- Cerebral ischemia, transient ischemic attacks, stroke
- Weakened blood vessels, aneurysms
- Hemorrhage

Cardiovascular
- Coronary artery disease
- Increased myocardial workload
- Left ventricular hypertrophy, heart failure
- Decreased myocardial perfusion and ischemia, angina, myocardial infarction
- Sudden death

Peripheral
- Increased atherosclerosis

Vessel
- Weakened arterial walls, aneurysms
- Intermittent claudication, peripheral vascular disease
- Gangrene

---

enzyme inhibitors (ACEIs), angiotensin II receptor blockers (ARBs), alpha blockers, combined alpha and beta blockers, calcium channel blockers (CCBs), and direct-acting peripheral vasodilators.

Diuretics

Diuretics have had a large amount of data to show that they prevent cardiovascular complications in patients with HTN. The best evidence available justifying this recommendation comes from the ALLHAT (2002) study. Moreover, when combination therapy is needed in HTN, a diuretic is recommended. Four subclasses of diuretics are used in the treatment of HTN: thiazides and thiazide-like diuretics, potassium-sparing drugs, aldosterone antagonists, and loop diuretics.

Thiazides (e.g., hydrochlorothiazide and chlorothiazide) are the most commonly used in the diuretic class of drugs. They are most effective against HTN in patients with normal renal function (estimated glomerular filtration rate [GFR] >30 mL/min). In patients with reduced renal function, consider using a loop diuretic. Thiazides decrease BP by reducing blood volume and arterial resistance. The initial antihypertensive effects are the result of reduced blood volume. The long-term effects

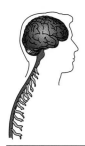

- Central alpha₂ receptors
- Alpha₁ blockers

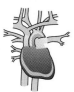

- Beta blockers
- Calcium channel blockers
- Combined alpha and beta blockers

- Angiotensin II receptor blockers
- Alpha₁ blockers

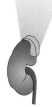

- ACE inhibitors
- Beta blockers
- Loop diuretics
- Potassium sparing diuretics
- Combined alpha and beta blockers

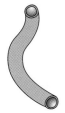

- Alpha blockers
- Angiotensin II receptor blockers
- Calcium channel blockers
- Direct acting peripheral vasodilators
- Thiazide diuretics

FIGURE 37-1 Sites of Action of Antihypertensive Drugs. Note that some antihypertensive drugs act at more than one site.

of these drugs are the result of changes in sodium balance and decreased sensitivity of the vessels to norepinephrine secondary to the sodium changes. As kidney function declines, a more potent diuretic is needed to counteract the associated increase in sodium and water retention.

Loop diuretics (e.g., furosemide and bumetanide) are approximately 10 times as potent as the thiazides, producing much greater diuresis. Similar to thiazides, loop diuretics reduce BP by reducing blood volume. Loop diuretics have no effect on vasculature. However, the loop diuretics are not routinely used in the management of HTN because the amount of fluid lost may be greater than desired. However, loop diuretics are used for patients who need greater diuresis than thiazides can provide (e.g., patients with heart failure, or who do not respond to thiazide diuretics).

Potassium-sparing diuretics are weak antihypertensives when used alone, but provide an additive effect when used in combination with a thiazide or loop diuretic (e.g., amiloride plus

hydrochlorothiazide). In combination therapy, these drugs may play an important role in balancing K^+ loss caused by thiazides or loop diuretics. Moreover, K^+-sparing diuretics can cause hyperkalemia, particularly in patients with chronic kidney disease or diabetes, and in patients receiving concurrent therapy with an ACEIs, ARBs, nonsteroidal antiinflammatory drugs (NSAIDs), or K^+ supplements. Because of a significant risk of hyperkalemia, avoid concurrent use of K^+-sparing diuretics with these drugs.

Aldosterone antagonists may be considered K^+-sparing drugs but are more potent antihypertensives with a slow onset of activity. However, they are viewed by the JNC VII, in its "compelling indications table," (see Fig. 37-2) as an independent class because of evidence supporting their express use in particular circumstances.

Beta-Adrenergic Blockers

SELECTIVE BETA BLOCKERS
- ◆ acebutolol (Sectral); ◆ Monitan, Sectral
- ◆ atenolol (Tenormin); ◆ Tenolin, Tenormin
- ◆ betaxolol (Kerlone)
- ◆ bisoprolol (Zebeta); ◆ Monocor
- ◆ metoprolol (Lopressor, Toprol-XL); ◆ Betaloc, Lopressor, Novo-Metoprol

NONSELECTIVE BETA BLOCKERS
- ◆ carteolol (Cartrol)
- ◆ nadolol (Corgard); ◆ Corgard
- ◆ penbutolol (Levatol)
- ◆ pindolol (Visken); ◆ Novo-Pindol, Syn-Pindolol
- ◆ propranolol (Inderal); ◆ Apo-Propranolol
- ◆ timolol (Blocadren); ◆ Apo-Timol, Gen-Timolol, Novo-Timol

COMBINED ALPHA₁ AND BETA BLOCKERS
- ◆ carvedilol (Coreg)
- ◆ labetolol (Normodyne, Trandate); ◆ Trandate

▓ *Indications*

Selective, nonselective, and combined alpha and beta blockers are among the most widely used antihypertensive drugs, second only to diuretics. They are also used in the management of angina pectoris, tachyarrhythmias, myocardial infarction, and glaucoma. These uses for beta blockers are discussed in Chapter 14 but are discussed here in relation to HTN therapy only. Chapter 61 discusses the use of beta blockers for the treatment of glaucoma.

Propranolol, a nonselective drug, is the oldest beta blocker and is considered the prototype of this class. With the advent of selective beta blockers, however, it is rarely used today because of its adverse effects and the consequently poor patient adherence to the treatment regimen. In addition to using beta blockers for HTN, beta blockers are also often used for angina pectoris, tachyarrhythmias, myocardial infarction, hypertrophic obstructive cardiomyopathies, pheochromocytoma, and hyperthyroidism and in the prevention of migraine headaches.

▓ *Pharmacodynamics*

The exact mechanism by which beta blockers reduce BP is not clear. Nonselective beta blockers (e.g., propranolol) block both β_1 (cardiac) and β_2 (smooth muscle of the bronchi and

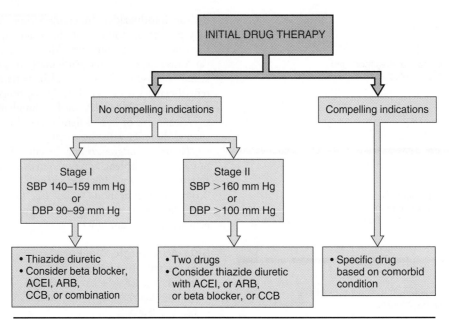

FIGURE 37-2 Compelling Indications for Individual Drug Classes. (ACEI, Angiotensin-converting enzyme inhibitor; ARB, angiotensin II–receptor blocker; CCB, calcium channel blocker.) (Adapted from Chobanian, A., Bakris, G., Black, H., et al. and the Joint National Committee on Detection, Evaluation, and Treatment of High Blood Pressure. [2003]. The Seventh Report of the Joint National Committee on the Prevention, Detection, Evaluation, and Treatment of High Blood pressure [JNC VII]. *Hypertension, 42*[6], 1206–1252.)

the blood vessels). Beta-selective drugs (e.g., atenolol, metoprolol) have more effect on β_1 receptors than on β_2 receptors.

Beta blockers in general impede the action of catecholamines at adrenergic receptors. β_1 Blockade reduces the heart rate (negative chronotropic effect), the force of myocardial contraction (negative inotropic effect), and the velocity of impulse conduction through the AV node (negative dromotropic effect). The automaticity of ectopic pacemakers is also decreased, as well as the BP in supine and standing positions. They also provide blockade of β_1 receptors on the juxtaglomerular apparatus of the kidneys to reduce the release of renin. Thus, angiotensin II–mediated vasoconstriction and aldosterone-mediated volume expansion are reduced and BP is reduced.

Carvedilol competitively blocks α_1, β_1, and β_2 receptors. Both the alpha and beta blocking actions contribute to the BP lowering effects of the drug. Beta blockade prevents the reflex tachycardia seen with most alpha-blocking drugs and significantly decreases plasma renin activity.

Labetolol is a combination alpha$_1$ and beta blocker. It promotes arteriolar and venous dilation through α_1 blockade. Heart rate and myocardial contractility are reduced by blocking β_1 receptors in the heart. Labetolol also suppresses the release of renin by blocking β_1 receptors in the juxtaglomerular apparatus of the kidneys.

Pharmacokinetics

The pharmacokinetics of beta blockers is identified in Table 37-2. Most of the drugs taken by mouth have varying bioavailabilities ranging from 25% to as much as 100% for metoprolol and labetolol given by intravenous (IV) route. The high protein binding of some drugs and a long duration of action increases the likelihood of once-daily dosing for

some patients. Most beta blockers are biotransformed by the liver. The remainder is eliminated via the kidneys.

Adverse Effects and Contraindications

Blockade of β_1 receptors is associated with adverse effects such as bronchoconstriction, peripheral vasoconstriction, and interference with glycogenolysis. Compared with the nonselective beta blockers, selective beta blockers cause less bronchospasm, less peripheral vascular insufficiency, and less impairment of glucose metabolism.

Despite beta blockers overall usefulness, they should not be used in patients with a history of sick sinus syndrome, heart failure, or second- or third-degree heart block. This is because blockade of β_1 receptors in the heart reduces myocardial contractility and atrioventricular (AV) conduction, and produces bradycardia. Blockade of α_1 receptors produces postural hypotension.

Avoid using beta blockers in patients with asthma or chronic obstructive pulmonary disease. They are potentially hazardous to the patient because they block β_2 receptors in the lungs, which cause constriction of the bronchioles. Beta blockers must be used with caution in patients with diabetes receiving hypoglycemic treatment, because they inhibit the usual sympathetic responses to hypoglycemia. Further, do not use beta blockers in patients with a history of depression because their drug actions can have an adverse effect on the CNS (see Evidenced-Based Pharmacotherapeutics). They also can cause vivid dreams, insomnia, depression, and sexual dysfunction.

Drug Interactions

The drug interactions of beta blockers are identified in Table 37-3. All beta blockers, both selective and nonselective drugs, interact with a wide variety of drugs. The unopposed α-

PHARMACOKINETICS
TABLE 37-2 Beta Blockers

Drug	Route	Onset	Peak	Duration	PB (%)	t½	BioA (%)
SELECTIVE BETA BLOCKERS							
acebutolol	PO	60 min	4–6 hr	10 hr	26	3–4 hr; 8–13 hr*	<50
atenolol	PO	60 min	2–4 hr	24 hr	6–16	6–9 hr	50–60
betaxolol	PO	3–4 hr	7–14 days†	24 hr	50–55	15–20 hr	UA
bisoprolol	PO	UA	1–4 hr	24 hr	24 hr	26–33	80
metoprolol	PO	15 min	UA	UA	12	3–7 hr	UA
	ER	UA	6–12‡	6–12 hr			
	IV	Immed	20 min	5–8 hr	12	3–7 hr	100
NONSELECTIVE BETA BLOCKERS							
carteolol	PO	UA	1–3 hr	>24 hr	23–30	6–8 hr; 8–12 hr§	85
nadolol	PO	5 days	6–9 days	24 hr	4–30	10–24 hr	30
penbutolol	PO	60 min	1.5–3 hr‖	24 hr	80–98	5 hr	UA
pindolol	PO	7 days	2 wk	8–24 hr	40	3–4 hr	UA
propranolol	PO	30 min	60–90 min	6–12 hr	93	3–5 hr	25
timolol	PO	UA	1–2 hr‖	12–24 hr	<10	3–4 hr	UA
COMBINED ALPHA AND BETA BLOCKERS							
carvedilol	PO	60 min	3–4 hr	8–10 hr	98	5–9 hr	UA
labetolol	PO	20–120 min	1–4 hr	8–12 hr	50	3–8 hr	25
	IV	2–5 min	5–15 min	2–24 hr	50	3–8 hr	100

*Acebutolol's half-life is biphasic.
†Betaxolol's peak cardiovascular effects with multiple dosing.
‡Metoprolol's maximal cardiovascular effects on blood pressure with chronic therapy may not occur for 1 wk. Hypotensive effects may persist for up to 4 wk after the drug is discontinued.
§Carteolol's half-life of parent drug and metabolite respectively.
‖Penbutolol and timolol's peak cardiovascular effects following a single dose. Full effects not seen until after several wk of therapy.
BioA, Bioavailability; *ER*, extended release; *Immed*, immediate; *IV*, intravenous; *PB*, protein binding; *PO*, by mouth; *t½*, half-life; *UA*, unavailable.

DRUG INTERACTIONS
TABLE 37-3 Beta Blockers

Drug	Interactive Drugs	Interaction
BETA BLOCKERS		
Beta blockers, in general	General anesthesia, phenytoin (IV), verapamil	Additive myocardial depression
	digoxin	Additive bradycardia
	Alcohol, antihypertensives, nitrates	Additive hypotension
	Amphetamines, cocaine, ephedrine, epinephrine, norepinephrine, phenylephrine, pseudoephedrine	Unopposed alpha-adrenergic stimulation, leading to excessive HTN, bradycardia
	Thyroid preparations	Decreases effectiveness of beta blocker
	NSAIDs	Decreases antihypertensive action of beta blockers
	Insulin, oral hypoglycemics	May alter effectiveness of interactive drug; may mask symptoms of hypoglycemia
	dopamine, dobutamine, theophylline	Decreases effectiveness of interactive drug
	MAO inhibitors	May result in HTN
labetolol, propranolol, timolol	cimetidine	May increase toxicity from beta blocker

HTN, Hypertension; *IV*, intravenous; *MAO*, monoamine oxidase; *NSAIDs*, nonsteroidal antiinflammatory drugs.

adrenergic stimulation caused by concurrent use of amphetamines, cocaine, ephedrine, epinephrine, norepinephrine, phenylephrine, and pseudoephedrine can lead to excessive HTN and bradycardia. Most NSAIDs reduce the antihypertensive action of beta blockers.

▥ Dosage Regimen

Once daily dosing with beta blockers is common. There are selected drugs that must be given on a twice-daily basis (Table 37-4). Increase dosages slowly at no less than weekly intervals. Some drugs (e.g., pindolol) may be titrated upward every 2 to 3 weeks as needed. Also, abrupt discontinuation may cause rebound HTN.

▥ Lab Considerations

Nonselective beta blockers may elevate the blood-urea-nitrogen (BUN), serum lipoproteins, potassium, triglyceride, uric acid, ANA, and blood glucose levels. Acebutolol, metoprolol, and labetolol, specifically, may cause increased serum alkaline phosphatase, lactate dehydrogenase (LDH), aspartate transaminase (AST), and alanine transaminase (ALT) levels.

Angiotensin-Converting Enzyme Inhibitors

- ◆ benazepril (Lotensin); ✦ Lotensin
- ◆ captopril (Capoten)
- ◆ enalapril (Vasotec); ✦ Vasotec
- ◆ fosinopril (Monopril); ✦ Monopril

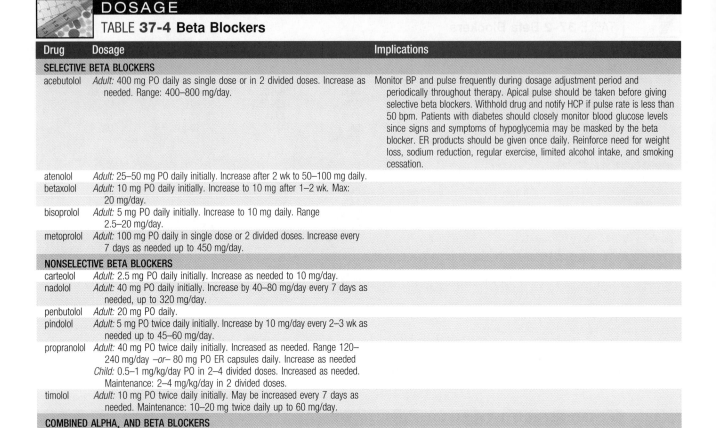

DOSAGE
TABLE **37-4** Beta Blockers

Drug	Dosage	Implications
SELECTIVE BETA BLOCKERS		
acebutolol	*Adult:* 400 mg PO daily as single dose or in 2 divided doses. Increase as needed. Range: 400–800 mg/day.	Monitor BP and pulse frequently during dosage adjustment period and periodically throughout therapy. Apical pulse should be taken before giving selective beta blockers. Withhold drug and notify HCP if pulse rate is less than 50 bpm. Patients with diabetes should closely monitor blood glucose levels since signs and symptoms of hypoglycemia may be masked by the beta blocker. ER products should be given once daily. Reinforce need for weight loss, sodium reduction, regular exercise, limited alcohol intake, and smoking cessation.
atenolol	*Adult:* 25–50 mg PO daily initially. Increase after 2 wk to 50–100 mg daily.	
betaxolol	*Adult:* 10 mg PO daily initially. Increase to 10 mg after 1–2 wk. Max: 20 mg/day.	
bisoprolol	*Adult:* 5 mg PO daily initially. Increase to 10 mg daily. Range 2.5–20 mg/day.	
metoprolol	*Adult:* 100 mg PO daily in single dose or 2 divided doses. Increase every 7 days as needed up to 450 mg/day.	
NONSELECTIVE BETA BLOCKERS		
carteolol	*Adult:* 2.5 mg PO daily initially. Increase as needed to 10 mg/day.	
nadolol	*Adult:* 40 mg PO daily initially. Increase by 40–80 mg/day every 7 days as needed, up to 320 mg/day.	
penbutolol	*Adult:* 20 mg PO daily.	
pindolol	*Adult:* 5 mg PO twice daily initially. Increase by 10 mg/day every 2–3 wk as needed up to 45–60 mg/day.	
propranolol	*Adult:* 40 mg PO twice daily initially. Increased as needed. Range 120–240 mg/day –*or*– 80 mg PO ER capsules daily. Increase as needed *Child:* 0.5–1 mg/kg/day PO in 2–4 divided doses. Increased as needed. Maintenance: 2–4 mg/kg/day in 2 divided doses.	
timolol	*Adult:* 10 mg PO twice daily initially. May be increased every 7 days as needed. Maintenance: 10–20 mg twice daily up to 60 mg/day.	
COMBINED ALPHA, AND BETA BLOCKERS		
carvedilol	*Adult:* 6.25 mg PO twice daily initially. May be increased every 7–14 days up to 25 mg twice daily.	
labetolol	*Adult:* 100 mg PO twice daily initially. May be increased by 100 mg twice daily every 2–3 days as needed. Range: 400–800 mg/day in 2–3 divided doses.	

bpm, Beats/min; *ER,* extended release; *HCP,* health care provider; *PO,* by mouth.

- lisinopril (Prinivil, Zestril)
- moexipril (Univasc)
- quinapril (Accupril)
- ramipril (Altace)
- trandolapril (Mavik)

Indications

ACEIs are among the first-line drugs in the treatment of HTN because of their efficacy and tolerability. They are effective for all types and degrees of HTN. ACEIs are recommended when use of diuretics and beta blockers is contraindicated. There is compelling evidence to indicate that ACEIs reduce proteinuria associated with diabetic nephropathy and help slow the progression of neuropathy. Early administration of ACEIs may decrease the incidence, the duration, and the inducibility of ventricular arrhythmias during the course of ischemic myocardial injury. ACEIs salvage ischemic myocardium, improve left ventricular function, reduce neurohumoral activity, and lessen the likelihood of electrolyte abnormalities.

Pharmacodynamics

Angiotensin (AT) II is formed from angiotensin I by the angiotensin-converting enzyme (ACE). AT-II is the principal pressor agent of the RAAS, whose actions include vasoconstriction, synthesis and release of aldosterone, cardiac stimulation, and renal reabsorption of sodium. ACE dilates arteries and veins by blocking the vasoconstrictor and aldosterone-secreting effects of AT-II. The vasodilation decreases arterial pressure and preload and afterload on the heart.

ACEIs also down-regulate sympathetic nervous system activity by blocking the facilitating effects of AT-II on sympathetic nerve release and reuptake of norepinephrine.

ACEIs enhance natriuretic and diuretic processes (renal excretion of sodium and water) by blocking the effects of AT-II in the kidney and by blocking AT-II stimulation of aldosterone secretion. This reduces blood volume, venous pressure, and arterial pressure, and inhibits cardiac and vascular remodeling associated with chronic HTN, heart failure, and myocardial infarction. The entire RAAS exists in vascular walls and in cardiac myocytes. This fact may explain the effectiveness of ACEIs in patients with normal and low plasma renin activity and in patients who have had a kidney removed.

Heart rate and cardiac output do not increase in response to ACE inhibition, but renal blood flow improves, and GFRs remain stable, suggesting that reduced glomerular hydrostatic pressure results from efferent glomerular arteriolar dilation.

However, ACEIs have a paradoxical effect on renal function. On one hand, they cause renal vasodilation, preventing the slow deterioration of glomerular filtration; reduce proteinuria; and improve morbidity and mortality in diabetic nephropathy. On the other hand, in states of low renal artery stenosis, severe heart failure, and severe sodium and volume depletion, they can worsen renal function and even precipitate acute renal failure. The usual interpretation is that in severe heart failure, renal artery stenosis, and sodium and volume depletion, renal function is angiotensin dependent.

ACEIs also increase the synthesis of vasodilating prostaglandins and inhibit the degradation of bradykinin. The resulting increase in levels of bradykinin contributes to the vasodilator action of ACEIs. The elevation in bradykinin levels is also thought to cause the adverse effect of a dry cough.

Beneficial effects of ACEIs include improved responsiveness to insulin and no elevation in lipid levels. They significantly reduce left ventricular hypertrophy in patients with HTN. The renal protection offered by ACEIs has been demonstrated in patients with scleroderma crisis and diabetic nephropathy.

Pharmacokinetics

The majority of ACEIs are well absorbed, with the bioavailability of the various drugs ranging from 13% for moexipril to 100% for IV enalapril (Table 37-5). ACEIs and their metabolites are well distributed, entering breast milk in small amounts.

The majority of ACEIs are biotransformed in the liver to active metabolites. A large amount of the drug is eliminated through the urine, with the remainder eliminated in the stool. The half-life of all ACEIs is increased in the presence of renal impairment.

Adverse Effects and Contraindications

ACEIs are usually well tolerated with a low incidence of adverse effects. A nonproductive cough occurs in 10% of patients, but it usually subsides several days after the drug is discontinued. The cough is caused by the breakdown of bradykinin, which causes an inflammatory response in respiratory tissues and the subsequent cough. The incidence of coughing is higher in women than in men. Angioedema of the face, the extremities, the lips, the tongue, the glottis, and the larynx has been reported in patients taking ACEIs.

ACEIs can cause hypotension in patients who are volume- or salt-depleted as a result of prolonged diuretic therapy, dietary salt restrictions, dialysis, diarrhea, or vomiting. Although rare, ACEI have caused cholestatic jaundice, a syndrome that progresses to fulminant hepatic necrosis and death. The mechanism of this syndrome is not understood.

In patients with severe heart failure whose renal function depends on activity of the RAAS, treatment with an ACEI has been associated with oliguria and progressive azotemia. On rare occasions, renal failure and death have occurred.

ACEIs are associated with fetal and neonatal injury, including hypotension, neonatal skull hypoplasia, anuria, reversible or irreversible renal failure, and death. Oligohydramnios may develop, presumably from decreased fetal renal function, and in this setting is associated with contractures of fetal limbs, craniofacial deformities, and hypoplastic lung development. Intrauterine growth retardation, prematurity, and patent ductus arteriosus have also been reported, although it is not clear whether these occurrences were due to exposure to the drug. Therefore, ACEIs should be discontinued as soon as pregnancy is detected.

Sudden and potentially life-threatening anaphylactoid reactions have been reported in some patients on ACEIs who are receiving hemodialysis with high-flux membranes.

PHARMACOKINETICS
TABLE 37-5 ACEIs and ARBs

Drug	Route	Onset	Peak	Duration	PB (%)	t½	BioA (%)
ACEIs							
benazepril	PO	30 min	2–4 hr	24 hr	97; 95†	10–11 hr*	37
captopril	PO	15–60 min	60–90 min	6–12 hr	25–30	<3 hr	75
enalapril	PO	60 min	4–6 hr	24 hr	50–60†	11 hr*	60
	IV	15 min	1–4 hr	6 hr	50–60†	11 hr*	100
fosinopril	PO	<60 min	2–6 hr	24 hr	95†	11.5 hr*	36
lisinopril	PO	60 min	6 hr	24 hr	0	12 hr	25
moexipril	PO	<60 min	3–6 hr	To 24 hr	50†	12 hr*	13+
quinapril	PO	<60 min	2–4 hr	To 24 hr	97†	1–2 hr	60
ramipril	PO	1–2 hr	4–6.5 hr	24 hr	73; 56†	13–17 hr*	50–60
trandolapril	PO	UA	60 min	UA	UA	16–24 hr	UA
ANGIOTENSIN II–RECEPTOR INHIBITORS							
candesartan	PO	2–3 hr	3–4 hr	>24 hr	>99	9 hr	15
eprosartan	PO	Rapid	1–2	>24 hr	98	5–9 hr	13
irbesartan	PO	Rapid	UA	>24 hr	90	11–15 hr	UA
losartan	PO	Varies	6 hr	>24 hr	98	2 hr; 6–9‡	UA
olmesartan	PO	Rapid	1–2 hr	>24 hr	99	13 hr*	26
telmisartan	PO	Rapid	30–60 min	>24 hr	99.5	24 hr	42; 58§
valsartan	PO	Slow	2–4 hr	>24 hr	95	6 hr	25

*The half-life of metabolites.
†Protein binding of ACE inhibitor's active metabolite.
‡Half life of losartan, olmesartan, and valsartan is biphasic.
§Bioavailability of telmisartan at 40 mg and 160 mg, respectively.
ACEIs, Angiotensin-converting enzyme inhibitors; *ARBs,* angiotensin II–receptor blockers; *BioA,* bioavailability; *IV,* intravenous; *PB,* protein binding; *PO,* by mouth; *t½,* half-life; *UA,* unavailable.

Do not use ACEIs in conjunction with supplemental K$^+$ therapy or with K$^+$-retaining drugs, because severe hyperkalemia may result as a consequence of reduced aldosterone levels.

Drug Interactions

The drug interactions of ACEIs are many (Table 37-6). The antihypertensive effects of ACEIs are decreased if they are taken with NSAIDs. Antacids decrease absorption of captopril and most other ACEIs. Other antihypertensives and diuretics increase the risk of hypotension. Concurrent use of K$^+$ supplements, K$^+$-sparing diuretics, and cyclosporine increases the risk of hyperkalemia. Increased serum lithium levels and symptoms of lithium toxicity have been reported in patients receiving concomitant ACEIs. Simultaneous administration of tetracycline with quinapril reduces the absorption of tetracycline by approximately 37% because of the high magnesium content of quinapril.

Dosage Regimen

As with all other drugs, the dosage regimen for ACEIs is drug- and patient-specific (Table 37-7). The dosage for an individual drug may be reduced for the patient who is also taking a diuretic. A precipitous drop in BP during the first 1 to 3 hours following the first dose of an ACEI may require volume expansion with normal saline but is seldom an indication for stopping therapy.

Lab Considerations

ACEIs may increase K$^+$ levels and transiently elevate BUN and creatinine levels, whereas Na$^+$ levels may be decreased. They can cause elevated AST, ALT, alkaline phosphatase, serum bilirubin, uric acid, and glucose levels. Antinuclear antibody testing may be positive. Captopril may cause false-positive test results for urine acetone.

Perform renal function tests before treatment with captopril. Check urine for protein in patients with prior renal disease and those who are receiving high dosages of an ACEI. Obtain a complete blood count (CBC) and differential before starting therapy, then every 2 weeks for 3 months, and periodically thereafter. Stop therapy if the neutrophil count falls to below 1000/mm^3. Although such cases are rare, ACEIs can produce a slight decrease in hemoglobin and hematocrit values.

Fosinopril may cause a falsely low serum digoxin level when the Digi-lab RIA kit is used. Use other testing kits to monitor digoxin levels.

Angiotensin II–Receptor Blockers
- candesartan (Atacand); ♣ Atacand
- eprosartan (Tevetan); ♣ Tevetan
- irbesartan (Avapro); ♣ Avapro
- losartan (Cozaar); ♣ Cozaar
- olmesartan (Benicar)
- telmisartan (Micardis); ♣ Micardis
- trandolapril (Mavik)
- valsartan (Diovan)

Indications

Angiotensin II–receptor blockers (ARBs), also known as AT-II inhibitors, are very similar to ACEI and are used for the same indications (i.e., HTN and heart failure). ARBs have not yet been approved for post–myocardial infarction therapy, although research is underway.

Pharmacodynamics

ARBs block type 1 AT-II receptors on blood vessels and other tissues such as the heart to stimulate vascular smooth muscle contraction. Since ARBs do not inhibit ACE, they do not elevate levels of bradykinin, which promotes the vasodilation produced by ACE and causes several of the adverse effects (i.e., dry cough) associated with ACEI use. Like the ACEIs, ARBs improve insulin sensitivity and reduce plasma levels of catecholamines.

DRUG INTERACTIONS
TABLE 37-6 ACEIs and ARBs

Drug	Interactive Drugs	Interaction
ACEIs		
ACEIs	alcohol, Antihypertensives, Diuretics, Nitrates, Phenothiazines	Excessive or additive hypotension
	cyclosporin, K+-sparing diuretics, Potassium supplements	Hyperkalemia possible with concurrent use
	indomethacin, NSAIDs	Response to ACEI may be blunted
	Antacids	Decreases absorption of ACEI
	digoxin, lithium	Increases risk of toxicity of interactive drug
	allopurinol	Increases risk of hypersensitivity reactions
	capsaicin	Increases incidence of cough
captopril	probenecid	Increases level of captopril
enalapril	rifampin	Decreases effectiveness of enalapril
quinapril	tetracycline	Decreases absorption of interactive drug
ANGIOTENSIN II–RECEPTOR BLOCKERS		
irbesartan, losartan, valsartan	phenobarbital	Decreases phenobarbital levels and effectiveness
	cimetidine	Increases losartan levels and effectiveness
	K+ supplements, K+-sparing diuretics	Increases the risk of hyperkalemia
	lithium	Increases risk of lithium toxicity
	rifampin	Decreases serum levels of ARB
losartan	fluconazole	Reduces conversion of losartan to its active form

ACEIs, Angiotensin-converting enzyme inhibitors; *ARBs,* angiotensin II–receptor blockers; *NSAIDs,* nonsteroidal antiinflammatory drugs.

DOSAGE
TABLE 37-7 ACEIs and ARBs

Drug	Dosage	Implications*
ACEIs		
benazepril	*Adult:* Initial: 5–10 mg PO daily. Increase gradually to maintenance dose of 20–40 mg/day as single dose or 2 divided doses.	Initiate therapy at 5 mg/day for patients taking diuretics.
captopril	*Adult:* Initial: 12.5–25 mg PO 2–3 times daily. Increase at 1- to 2-wk intervals up to 150 mg 3 times daily. Usual dose: 50 mg PO 3 times daily. Max: 450 mg/day. *Child:* Initial: 0.3 mg/kg 3 times daily. May be increased by 0.3 mg/kg every 8–24 hr.	Administer on empty stomach. Tablets may have sulfurous odor. Initiate therapy at 6.25–12.5 mg 2–3 times daily for patients taking diuretics. Start at 0.15 mg/kg in children receiving diuretics or who have renal impairment.
enalapril	*Adult:* Initial: 5 mg PO daily –or– 0.625–1.25 mg IV every 6 hr. Usual oral dosage range 10–40 mg/day in 1–2 divided doses.	Initiate therapy at 2.5 mg PO/day –or– 0.625 mg IV for patients on diuretics.
fosinopril	*Adult:* Initial: 10 mg PO daily. Dosage range: 20–40 mg daily. Maximum: 80 mg/day.	Monitor for neutropenia and agranulocytosis.
lisinopril	*Adult:* 10 mg PO daily. Increase to 20–40 mg/day.	Initiate therapy at 5 mg/day in patients taking diuretics.
moexipril	*Adult:* Initial: 7.5 mg PO daily. Usual dose: 7.5–30 mg/day in 1–2 divided doses.	Take on empty stomach. Initiate therapy at 3.75 mg in patients taking diuretics.
quinapril	*Adult:* Initial: 5–10 mg PO daily. Increase at 2-wk intervals. Dosage range: 20–80 mg/day in 1–2 divided doses.	Initiate therapy at 5 mg/day in patients taking diuretics.
ramipril	*Adult:* Initial: 2.5 mg PO daily. Increase slowly to 20 mg/day in 1–2 divided doses.	Initiate therapy at 1.25 mg/day for patients taking diuretics.
trandolapril	*Adult:* Initial: 1–2 mg PO daily. Usual dosage: 2–4 mg/day.	Initiate therapy at 0.5 mg/day for patients taking diuretics.
ANGIOTENSIN II-RECEPTOR BLOCKERS		
candesartan	*Adult:* 16 mg PO daily. May give in divided doses 8–32 mg daily.	Volume-depleted patients should be stabilized before receiving. Give lower dosages in patients taking diuretics or who have severe renal impairment.
eprosartan	*Adult:* 600 mg PO daily. Range: 400–800 mg/day.	Also available with hydrochlorothiazide 400 mg/12.5 mg.
irbesartan	*Adult:* Initial: 150 mg PO daily. Range: 150–300 mg PO daily.	Volume-depleted patients should be stabilized before receiving.
losartan	*Adult:* 50 mg PO daily alone –or– 25 mg daily in combination with other antihypertensives. Range: 25–100 mg PO once-twice daily.	Volume-depleted patients should be stabilized before receiving. May take without regard to meals.
olmesartan	*Adult:* 20 mg PO daily. Increase after 2 wk if needed to 40 mg/day.	Volume-depleted patients should be stabilized before receiving.
telmisartan	*Adult:* 40 mg PO daily. Range: 20–80 mg daily.	May be given concurrently with other antihypertensives.
valsartan	*Adult:* 80 mg PO daily. Gradually increase to 320 mg daily.	No dosage adjustment needed for concurrent use of a diuretic, in older adults, or mild-to-moderate liver disease or renal insufficiency.

*A precipitous drop in BP 1–3 hr following the first dose of ACE inhibitor may require volume expansion with normal saline but is not normally an indication for stopping therapy. Discontinuing diuretic therapy or increasing salt intake 1 wk before initiation of therapy decreases the risk of hypotension. Monitor patient closely for at least 1 hour after BP has stabilized. Resume diuretics if BP is not controlled.
ACEIs, Angiotensin-converting enzyme inhibitors; *ARBs,* angiotensin II–receptor blockers; *IV,* intravenous; *PO,* by mouth.

▥ Pharmacokinetics

Some ARBs need to be converted to an active form in the body before they can act. ARBs are generally well absorbed and distributed from the gastrointestinal (GI) tract, independent of food intake, reaching peak plasma concentrations in hours (see Table 37-5). ARBs differ in how they are eliminated from the body and the extent to which they are distributed throughout the body, but overall, elimination of the drugs and their metabolites is through the urine and feces.

▥ Adverse Effects and Contraindications

The frequency of cough with losartan is significantly lower than that seen with ACEIs. Losartan also appears to produce less angioedema than is associated with the ACEIs. Valsartan rarely, if ever, causes a cough.

The most frequently reported adverse effects with ARBs use are fatigue, headache, dizziness, insomnia, nasal congestion, and sinus disorders. Diarrhea, dyspepsia, and elevated liver enzymes and renal function tests, muscle cramps, myalgia, and back and leg pain have also been documented.

ARBs are contraindicated for use in patients with bilateral renal artery stenosis; renal failure may result. ARBs are also contraindicated for use during pregnancy.

Clinical experience thus far indicates no clinically significant age-, sex-, or ethnicity-related differences in the overall safety profile of ARBs. There is no evidence of rebound HTN if the drug is withdrawn suddenly.

▥ Drug Interactions

ARBs interact with few other drugs (see Table 37-6). Because ARBs can elevate serum K^+ levels, the use of K^+ supplements, salt substitutes (which often contain K^+), or other K^+-containing drugs (e.g., potassium penicillin) may result in hyperkalemia. ARBs also raise serum concentrations of lithium, possibly leading to adverse effects of the lithium. Rifampin decreases serum levels of losartan, and fluconazole reduces the conversion of losartan to its active metabolite. Whether NSAIDs interact with ARBs as they do with ACEIs is not yet known.

▥ Dosage Regimen

As with most other antihypertensive drugs, ARBs are given on a once-daily schedule (see Table 37-7). Correct volume depletion before patients receive an ARB. Use a lower dose of losartan when giving it concurrently with another antihypertensive. Slowly adjust the dosage according to patient response.

▥ *Lab Considerations*

Lab considerations for ARBs are similar to those of ACEIs. Although such cases are rare, ARBs can cause elevations in BUN and creatinine levels. Minimal decreases in hemoglobin and hematocrit values are usually insignificant. ARBs occasionally elevate liver enzymes and serum bilirubin levels.

Calcium Channel Blockers

DIHYDROPYRIDINES

- amlodipine (Norvasc); ◆ Norvasc
- felodipine (Plendil); ◆ Renedil
- isradipine (DynaCirc, DynaCirc CR)
- nicardipine (Cardene, Cardene SR)
- nifedipine (Adalat CC, Procardia XL); ◆ Adalat FT, Adalat PA, Apo-Nifed, Novo-Nifedin
- nisoldipine (Sular)

NONDIHYDROPYRIDINES

- diltiazem (Cardizem, Cardizem SR, Cardizem CD, Dilacor, Tiazac); ◆ Cardizem CD
- verapamil (Calan, Calan, SR, Covera HS, Isoptin SR, Verelan); ◆ Apo-Verap, Novo-Veramil)

As a class of drugs, the calcium channel blockers (CCBs) have many beneficial effects and relatively few adverse effects. Although other CCBs are used for other indications (e.g., antianginals, antiarrhythmics), those listed above are used predominantly in the management of HTN. Because of their effectiveness and safety, CCBs have been added as first-line drugs in the treatment of HTN. CCBs are effective as monotherapy and are particularly effective in treating black patients with HTN, and for treating HTN-associated with ischemic heart disease. The long-acting dihydropyridines are second-line therapy for older adults with isolated systolic HTN. Short-acting CCBs are not approved for the management of HTN owing to the increased risk of MI.

CCBs' effectiveness in treating HTN is related to their ability to cause smooth muscle relaxation by blocking the binding of calcium to its receptors. The effects on the cardiovascular system include depression of mechanical contraction of myocardial and smooth muscle and depression of both impulse formation and conduction velocity. The result is vascular smooth muscle relaxation and vasodilation. The dihydropyridine CCBs are potent vasodilators. The vasodilation is most profound with nifedipine. **Do not use short-acting nifedipine for treating essential HTN or hypertensive emergencies because of its association with erratic fluctuations in blood pressure and reflex tachycardia.**

The most common adverse effects of CCBs are headache, peripheral edema, and bradycardia. The dihydropyridine drugs produce symptoms of vasodilation, such as headache, flushing, palpitations, and peripheral edema. Other adverse effects of nifedipine include dizziness, gingival hyperplasia, mood changes, and various GI complaints. Diltiazem and verapamil can also cause GI upset, peripheral edema, and hypotension. Rare adverse effects include bradycardia, AV block, and heart failure. Verapamil can cause constipation in older adults. Because of their ability to compromise cardiac performance, diltiazem and verapamil must be used with caution in hypertensive patients who have a history of bradycardia, heart failure, or AV block.

Alpha₁ Receptor Blockers

- doxazosin (Cardura)
- phenoxybenzamine (Dibenzyline)
- phentolamine (Regitine); ◆ Rogitine
- prazosin (Minipress); ◆ Minipress
- terazosin (Hytrin)

Alpha blockers were discussed in Chapter 14. The primary use for this group of drugs is mild to moderate HTN. **This class of drugs should not be used as initial monotherapy for HTN.** The first-generation, nonselective drugs (i.e., phenoxybenzamine and phentolamine) are also useful in the diagnosis and treatment of pheochromocytoma and in other clinical situations associated with exaggerated release of catecholamines (e.g., phentolamine may be combined with propranolol, a beta blocker, to treat clonidine withdrawal syndrome).

Alpha₁ blockers reduce arterial pressure by dilating both resistance and capacitance vessels. As expected, BP is reduced more in the upright than in the supine position. Retention of salt and water occurs when these drugs are administered without a diuretic. Selectivity for α_1 receptors may explain why these drugs produce less reflex tachycardia than the nonselective alpha blockers. The receptor selectivity allows norepinephrine to exert unopposed negative feedback (mediated by presynaptic α_2 receptors) on its own release. In contrast, phentolamine blocks both synaptic and postsynaptic α receptors, resulting in reflex stimulation of sympathetic neurons and greater release of neurotransmitters onto β receptors, and correspondingly greater cardioacceleration.

The most significant adverse effect of alpha₁ blockers is orthostatic hypotension. It can be particularly severe with the initial dose of the drug. Significant hypotension continues with subsequent dosing, although it is less profound. Alpha₁ blockers are contraindicated for use in patients with a known hypersensitivity. They are classified as pregnancy category C drugs.

Central Alpha₂-Receptor Agonists

- clonidine (Catapres); ◆ Dixarit
- guanabenz (Wytensin)
- guanfacine (Tenex)
- methyldopa (Aldomet); ◆ Apo-methyldopa, Novomedopa

Central alpha₂–receptor agonists are discussed in Chapter 14. Do not use these drugs as initial monotherapy for HTN. Although less commonly used today, guanabenz and guanfacine are useful in the treatment of mild to moderate HTN. Methyldopa is not generally considered a first-line drug for the management of HTN, although it is widely used for HTN that develops during pregnancy (Table 37-8).

Central alpha₂ agonists work by stimulating α_2 receptors in the brainstem, thus subduing sympathetic outflow to the heart, kidneys, and peripheral vasculature. The resulting lack of norepinephrine production reduces systolic and diastolic BP, and slows the pulse rate slightly. The stimulation of α_2 receptors also affects the kidneys by reducing the activity of renin.

The adverse effects of centrally acting alpha₂ agonists include drowsiness, sedation, dizziness, weakness, sluggishness, dyspnea, restlessness, nervousness, hallucinations, and depression. Adverse effects on the GI tract include dry mouth, constipation, abdominal pain, and pseudoobstruction

PHARMACOKINETICS
TABLE 37-8 Vasodilators

Drug	Route	Onset	Peak	Duration	PB (%)	t½	BioA (%)
CENTRAL ALPHA₂-RECEPTOR AGONISTS							
clonidine	PO	30–60 min	2–4 hr	8 hr	20–40	12–16 hr	UA
	IV	Immed	2–20 min	24 hr	20–40	12–16 hr	100
ADRENERGIC ANTAGONISTS							
reserpine	PO	Slow	2–3 wk	14 days	0	5 days; 200 hr*	50
DIRECT-ACTING PERIPHERAL VASODILATORS							
diazoxide	IV	Immed	5 min	3–12 hr	>90	21–45 hr	100
hydralazine	PO	45 min	2 hr	3–8 hr	87	2–8 hr	UA
	IM	10–30 min	1 hr				UA
	IV	10–20 min	15–30 min				100
minoxidil	PO	30 min	2–3 hr	2–5 days	0	4.2 hr	UA
nitroprusside	IV	Immed	Rapid	1–10 min	UA	2 min†	100

*An initial half-life of reserpine is approximately 5 hr followed by a terminal half-life of the order of 200 hr. The clinical significance of the long terminal half-life is unknown.
†The half-life of metabolites of nitroprusside.
BioA, Bioavailability; *IM*, intramuscular; *Immed*, immediate; *IV*, intravenous; *PB*, protein binding; *PO*, by mouth; *t½*, half-life; *UA*, unavailable.

of the large bowel. Hepatitis, hyperbilirubinemia, and sodium retention with weight gain has been noted. Impotence and reduced libido are not uncommon. Also, first-dose hypotension and syncope are possible.

Adrenergic Antagonists

The only currently available adrenergic antagonist is reserpine (Serpasil), an alternative drug for HTN emergencies. Although unlabeled, reserpine has also been used to treat agitated psychotic patients, to reduce vasospastic attacks in patients with Raynaud's phenomenon, and for the short-term symptomatic treatment of thyrotoxicosis.

Reserpine acts to inhibit the sympathetic nervous system by depleting norepinephrine stores in the vesicles of adrenergic nerve endings. The inhibition results in a decrease in peripheral vascular resistance and a reduction in BP. Reserpine is plant-derived; its active ingredient is an alkaloid from the rauwolfia plant. Because this alkaloid promotes Na⁺ and water resorption, its antihypertensive effect diminishes with continued use. Reserpine is often combined with diuretics in an attempt to offset this effect.

Reserpine also interferes with the binding of serotonin at receptor sites. Reserpine decreases the synthesis of norepinephrine by depleting dopamine, its precursor, and competitively inhibiting reuptake in storage granules.

Forty percent to 50% of reserpine is absorbed following oral administration. It is widely distributed in tissues, especially adipose tissue. Reserpine crosses the blood-brain barrier and the placenta, and it is widely distributed in breast milk. There is no protein binding, and reserpine is biotransformed in the liver, with at least 50% eliminated in feces as unabsorbed drug. Small amounts are eliminated unchanged by the kidneys. The half-life of reserpine is 11 days.

It is used less often today because of its potentially severe adverse effects. Reserpine can produce severe depression that persists months after the drug is withdrawn and can increase the risk of suicide. Reserpine can also cause a parkinson-like syndrome with tremors and muscle rigidity. Respiratory depression, seizures, and hypothermia may also occur. The adverse effects of reserpine on the cardiovascular system include orthostatic hypotension, increased AV conduction

time, angina, and arrhythmias. Impotence, impaired sexual function, breast engorgement, and menstrual irregularities may also occur with reserpine.

Use of reserpine is contraindicated for patients with a history of depressive disorders, active peptic ulcer, ulcerative colitis, and gallstones, as well as for patients receiving electroconvulsive therapy. Use it with caution in patients with cardiac, cerebrovascular, or renal insufficiency. Safe use during pregnancy and lactation or in children has not been established.

Reserpine produces additive hypotension when used with other antihypertensive drugs. Nitrates and alcohol ingestion potentiate hypotension. An increased risk of arrhythmias may occur with cardiac glycosides, quinidine, procainamide, and other antiarrhythmic drugs. Concurrent use of monoamine oxidase (MAO) inhibitors may cause excitement and HTN. Reserpine may decrease the therapeutic response to ephedrine or levodopa. Patients receiving direct-acting sympathomimetic amines such as dopamine, dobutamine, metaraminol, and phenylephrine may demonstrate increased responses to those drugs.

Direct-Acting Peripheral Vasodilators

- ◆ diazoxide (Hyperstat, Proglycem); ◆ Hyperstat
- ◆ hydralazine (Apresoline); ◆ Apresoline, Novo-Hylazin
- ◆ minoxidil (Loniten, Rogaine); ◆ Apo-Gain, Loniten
- ◆ nitroprusside; ◆ (Nitropress)

▌ Indications

All peripheral vasodilators can be used to treat HTN, either alone or in combination with other antihypertensives, but reserve them for patients with essential or severe HTN. Use nitroprusside and diazoxide for rapid reduction of BP in hospitalized patients with hypertensive crisis. Nitroprusside is consistently effective even in refractory HTN and can be used to produce a controlled hypotension during surgery to reduce blood loss.

Diazoxide is commonly used along with a diuretic such as furosemide to counteract diazoxide-induced sodium and water retention, and to elevate blood glucose levels in hypoglycemic patients with hyperinsulinism caused by pancreatic islet cell adenoma or carcinoma, extra pancreatic malignancy, and other conditions.

Hydralazine is indicated for use in essential HTN. Hydralazine can be used in early malignant HTN that persists after sympathectomy.

Minoxidil is used in the management of severe symptomatic HTN associated with end-organ damage refractory to other drug therapy. Use of minoxidil in mild cases of HTN is not recommended.

Pharmacodynamics

Direct-acting peripheral vasodilators promptly reduce BP by eliciting peripheral vasodilation of arterioles. In general, the most noticeable effect is their hypotensive effect, which promptly reduces BP by relaxing smooth muscle of the arterioles. Cardiac output increases as BP is reduced. Coronary blood flow and cerebral blood flow are maintained, and renal blood flow is increased. Postural hypotension is minimized through preferential dilation of arterioles over other vasculature.

Nitroprusside is potent and rapid-acting, with effects similar to those of nitrates. The mechanism of action involves interference with the influx and intracellular activation of calcium. It relaxes vascular smooth muscle, promoting vasodilation. Thus, both arterial and venous BP is lowered, reducing preload and afterload.

Hydralazine increases renin activity in plasma. Increased renin activity leads to the production of angiotensin II. The result is stimulation of aldosterone and consequent sodium reabsorption. Hydralazine maintains or increases renal and cerebral blood flow. Hydralazine affects diastolic pressure more than systolic pressure.

Pharmacokinetics

Oral formulations of direct-acting peripheral vasodilators are well absorbed from the GI tract (see Table 37-8). Diazoxide and hydralazine are highly bound to plasma proteins. Minoxidil does not bind to plasma proteins. The known metabolites of minoxidil exert much less pharmacologic effect than minoxidil itself. Fifty percent of diazoxide is biotransformed in the liver, with 50% eliminated unchanged in the urine. Hydralazine is mostly biotransformed by the GI mucosa and the liver. Biotransformation of nitroprusside occurs rapidly in the liver and tissues to cyanide and subsequently by the liver to thiocyanate. Thiocyanate has a half-life of 2 minutes.

Adverse Effects and Contraindications

Adverse effects of direct-acting peripheral vasodilators vary with the specific drug. The adverse effects of nitroprusside include profound hypotension, nausea, retching, abdominal pain, nasal stuffiness, and diaphoresis. Restlessness, headache, dizziness, and muscle twitching occur. Retrosternal discomfort, palpitations, an increase or transient lowering of pulse rate, electrocardiogram (ECG) changes, decreased platelet aggregation, and methemoglobinemia have been noted. Further, nitroprusside use has occasionally resulted in accumulation of lethal amounts of cyanide. Cyanide toxicity is most likely to occur in patients with liver disease who have low levels of thiosulfate, a cofactor needed for cyanide detoxification. The risk of cyanide poisoning can be minimized by avoiding prolonged use.

Nitroprusside is contraindicated for use in persons with known hypersensitivity or compensatory HTN related to an arteriovenous shunt or coarctation of the aorta. Avoid using this drug in patients with increased intracranial pressure. Cautious use is warranted in patients with hepatic insufficiency, hypothyroidism, severe renal impairment, and hyponatremia, and in older adults with low vitamin B_{12} plasma levels or Leber's optic atrophy. (See Box 37-4.)

BOX 37-4

Nitroprusside Toxicity

Nitroprusside is widely considered the drug of choice for most cases of refractory HTN, but it can be problematic. Nitroprusside is biotransformed to cyanide; cyanide is an intracellular toxin—thus plasma or whole blood levels do not correlate with total body burden. Photodegradation releases cyanide from nitroprusside (hence the importance of protecting the solution from light), which then combines with endogenous thiosulfate to form thiocyanate, which is eliminated in the urine.

Endogenous thiosulfate is normally present in small concentrations, enough to metabolize the cyanide from about 50 mg of nitroprusside. However, thiocyanate is itself toxic and has half-life of 2.7 days, and longer in patients with renal failure. Cyanide toxicity occurs when body stores of thiosulfate are depleted. The overall incidence of toxicity appears to be infrequent; however, certain patients may be at high risk.

Risk factors for cyanide toxicity include hypoalbuminemia, hepatic or renal impairment, cardiopulmonary bypass procedures, or with nitroprusside infusion rates over 2 mcg/kg/min, or any nitroprusside infusion whose duration is greater than 72 hours. Dosages of nitroprusside are safe and unlimited when concurrent administration of sodium thiosulfate is added to the treatment regimen (1 gram for each 100 mg of nitroprusside). Without sodium thiosulfate, the recommended dosage of nitroprusside can cause toxicity in as little as 35 minutes after the infusion is started. A prophylactic infusion of hydrocobalamin, a form of vitamin B_{12}, at 25 mg/hr, decreases thiocyanate concentration.

Making a diagnosis of cyanide toxicity according to liver function testing takes too long, therefore diagnosis must be made by assessing the patient's clinical state and thiocyanate levels. **Normal thiocyanate levels are less than 4 mg/L, or less than 8 mg/L if the patient is a smoker. Toxicity exists at levels over 100 mg/L. Thiocyanate toxicity is life threatening at levels of 200 mg/L.**

Symptoms of cyanide toxicity are easily missed or are manifested late in the clinical course and include decreased mental status, agitation, lethargy, disorientation, seizures, tachycardia, HTN (which can lead health care personnel to administer increased doses of nitroprusside), shock, arrhythmias, coma, and death. Cardiovascular signs include early tachycardia and increased BP with hypotension, bradycardia, and arrhythmias later. Tachypnea progresses to apnea. Treatment for thiocyanate toxicity includes the following:

- Stop the drug and give 100% oxygen.
- Provide a buffer for cyanide by using sodium nitrite (contained in a commercial antidote kit) to convert as much hemoglobin as possible into methemoglobin, but only as the patient can tolerate.
- Infuse sodium thiosulfate to convert cyanide to thiocyanate. The necessary drugs are found in commercially available cyanide antidote kits.
- Perform hemodialysis, if needed. Hemodialysis is ineffective in removing cyanide, but it will eliminate most thiocyanate from the body.

Adverse effects of diazoxide include sodium and water retention, which can lead to heart failure. Shock levels of hypotension, angina, myocardial ischemia, and infarction can occur. Atrial and ventricular arrhythmias, transient cerebral ischemia, cerebral infarction, and ECG changes have been noted. Neurologic findings include throbbing headaches, dizziness, lightheadedness, lethargy, euphoria, momentary hearing loss, and weakness. Hyperglycemia can occur in diabetic patients and transient hyperglycemia in nondiabetic patients. Renal adverse effects include decreased urinary output, nephrotic syndrome, hematuria, increased nocturia, proteinuria, and azotemia.

Intravenous diazoxide is contraindicated for use in patients with coarctation of the aorta and arteriovenous shunt, and in patients known to be hypersensitive to diazoxide, thiazide diuretics, or sulfonamide-derived drugs. Use diazoxide cautiously in patients with diabetes mellitus, impaired cerebral or cardiac circulation, impaired renal function, and uremia, and in those taking corticosteroids or estrogen-progestin combinations. Safe use of diazoxide during pregnancy has not been established. Intravenous use during labor can cause cessation of uterine contractions.

Adverse effects of hydralazine include headache, tremors, dizziness, anxiety, palpitations, reflex tachycardia, angina, shock, and rebound HTN. Adverse GI effects include anorexia, nausea, vomiting, and diarrhea. Sodium and water retention, urinary retention, blood dyscrasias, reduction in hemoglobin and red blood cell counts, leucopenia, agranulocytosis, and impotence have been noted. Discontinue therapy if blood dyscrasias develop.

Common adverse effects of minoxidil include drowsiness, dizziness, and sedation. Potentially life-threatening effects include severe rebound HTN, heart failure, pulmonary edema, pericardial effusion, pericarditis, thrombocytopenia, and leukopenia. The possibility of minoxidil-associated cardiac damage cannot be excluded, with changes in the direction and magnitude of T waves noted on the ECG. An initial decrease in hematocrit, hemoglobin, and red blood cell count values can occur. Respiratory adverse effects include bronchitis and upper respiratory infection.

Dermatologic adverse effects of minoxidil include temporary edema and hypertrichosis. Elongation, thickening, and enhanced pigmentation of body hair are seen 3 to 6 weeks after initiation of therapy. The changes are first noticed on the temples and between the eyebrows, extending to other parts of the face, the scalp, the back, the arms, and the legs. Other adverse effects include Stevens-Johnson syndrome, rash, and bullous skin eruptions.

Avoid using hydralazine and minoxidil in hypertensive patients with a history of MI, angina pectoris, cardiac failure, dissecting aortic aneurysm, or renal disease. Hydralazine is also contraindicated for use in patients with coronary artery disease, rheumatic heart disease, and tachycardia. The myocardial stimulation produced by hydralazine can cause myocardial ischemia and anginal attacks. In doses greater than 300 mg/day, hydralazine produces a clinical picture resembling systemic lupus erythematosus.

Drug Interactions
There are several drug interactions with direct-acting peripheral vasodilators (Table 37-9). Because diazoxide is

highly bound to serum proteins, it can be expected to displace other substances that are also protein bound.

Dosage Regimen
The dosage regimen for direct-acting vasodilators is individualized based on patient response. Table 37-10 provides an overview of the dosage regimens.

Lab Considerations
Nitroprusside causes a decrease in bicarbonate concentrations, $PaCO_2$, and pH and an increase in lactate concentrations. Monitoring blood thiocyanate levels is recommended in patients receiving nitroprusside therapy or in patients with severe renal dysfunction; levels should not exceed 1 mmol/L. Obtain plasma cyanogen levels after 1 to 2 days of therapy, particularly in patients with impaired hepatic function. Monitor serum methemoglobin concentrations in patients receiving over 10 mg/kg of nitroprusside or patients who exhibit signs of impaired oxygen delivery despite adequate cardiac output and arterial $PaCO_2$.

Diazoxide may cause increased serum glucose, BUN, alkaline phosphatase, AST, sodium, and uric acid levels. It may cause decreased creatinine clearance, hematocrit, and hemoglobin values.

Hydralazine may cause a positive direct Coombs' test. CBC, electrolytes, and antinuclear antibodies titer determinations are needed before and periodically throughout prolonged therapy.

Minoxidil elevates BUN, serum creatinine, alkaline phosphatase, plasma renin activity, and sodium levels. Decreased red blood cell (RBC), hemoglobin, and hematocrit counts may also occur. Hematologic and renal values usually return to pretreatment levels with continued therapy. Monitor renal and hepatic function, CBC, and electrolytes before and periodically throughout therapy.

Newer Antihypertensives
Three new antihypertensives have reached the U.S. marketplace: eplerenone, bosentan, and treprostinil. All three drugs are currently approved for adult use only.

Aldosterone Inhibitor
Eplerenone (Inspra) is an aldosterone inhibitor. It binds to the mineralocorticoid receptor in both epithelial (e.g., kidney) and nonepithelial (e.g., heart blood vessels, brain) tissues and blocks the binding of aldosterone at its corresponding receptors. Eplerenone improves survival of stable patients with left ventricular systolic dysfunction (ejection fraction <40%) and clinical evidence of heart failure after an acute MI. It may be used as monotherapy or with other antihypertensive drugs.

Mean peak plasma concentrations of eplerenone are reached in 1.5 hours following oral administration; the absolute bioavailability of eplerenone is unknown. Plasma protein binding is primarily to alpha$_1$-acid glycoproteins at about 50%. Eplerenone's biotransformation is mediated by CYP 3A4 enzymes. No active metabolites of eplerenone have been identified in plasma. Less than 5% of the drug is recovered as unchanged drug in the urine and the feces. The elimination half-life of eplerenone is 4 to 6 hours.

DRUG INTERACTIONS

TABLE 37-9 Vasodilators

Drug	Interactive Drugs	Interaction
CENTRAL ALPHA₂-RECEPTOR AGONISTS		
clonidine	MAO inhibitors, TCAs	Decreases antihypertensive response or results in HTN crisis
	azelastine, tizanidine, cetirizine, Cold remedies	May increase risk of CNS depression, psychomotor impairment
	Beta blocker–thiazide combinations; Ophthalmic beta blockers; Systemic beta blockers; sotolol	Decreases antihypertensive response to interactive drugs; risk of severe rebound HTN of clonidine with withdrawal
	mirtazapine	Decreases antihypertensive effects of clonidine; increases risk for CNS depression
	digoxin, diltiazem, verapamil	Increases risk for bradycardia
	methylphenidate	Decreases antihypertensive effect; rare reports of sudden death
	Many others	Check drug reference
ADRENERGIC ANTAGONISTS		
reserpine	Other antihypertensives	Additive effects
	digoxin, quinidine, procainamide, Other antiarrhythmic drugs	Increases risk for arrhythmias
	MAO inhibitors	May cause excitement and HTN
	ephedrine, levodopa	Decreases response to ephedrine or levodopa
	dopamine, dobutamine, metaraminol, phenylephrine	Increases response to interactive drug
	Alcohol, Nitrates	Potentiates hypotension
DIRECT ACTING PERIPHERAL VASODILATORS		
diazoxide	Diuretics	Potentiates hyperglycemia, hyperuricemia, and hypotensive effects
	phenytoin	Increases biotransformation of interactive drug
	Corticosteroids, phenytoin, Estrogens, Progesterones	May increase hyperglycemia
	warfarin	Increases effects of interactive drug
	Insulins, Oral hypoglycemics	May alter effects of interactive drug
hydralazine	Alcohol, Antihypertensives, MAO inhibitors, Nitrates	Produces additive or exaggerated hypotension
	epinephrine	Reduces pressor response of interactive drug
	NSAIDs	Decreases antihypertensive response
	Beta blockers	Decreases tachycardia caused by hydralazine
	metoprolol, propranolol	Increases blood levels of hydralazine; hydralazine increases blood levels of interactive drugs
minoxidil	guanethidine	Severe hypotension
	NSAIDs	Decreases antihypertensive effects of minoxidil
	Alcohol, Antihypertensives, Nitrates	Additive hypotension
nitroprusside	Antihypertensives, Ganglionic blockers, General anesthetics	Increases hypotensive effects

CNS, Central nervous system; *HTN,* hypertension; *MAO,* monoamine oxidase; *NSAIDs,* nonsteroidal antiinflammatory drugs; *TCA,* tricyclic antidepressants.

Many commonly used drugs inhibit CYP 3A4 enzymes, including several antibiotics (e.g., erythromycin) and antifungal (e.g., ketoconazole, fluconazole) and antiviral drugs (e.g., saquinavir). Drinking grapefruit juice causes a small increase (about 25%) in eplerenone drug levels.

Treatment with eplerenone is initiated at 25 mg once daily and titrated as tolerated to the target dose of 50 mg, preferably within 4 weeks.

Endothelin Inhibitor

Bosentan (Tracleer) belongs to a class of pyrimidine derivatives known as endothelin₁ (ET-1) inhibitors. The actions of bosentan are mediated by binding to ET$_A$ and ET$_B$ receptors in the endothelium and vascular smooth muscle. Plasma concentrations of ET-1 are elevated and present in the lungs of patients with pulmonary arterial hypertension (PAH). Its presence suggests that this neurohormone may play a role in the pathogenesis of the PAH. Bosentan is a competitive antagonist at ET-1 receptor types ET$_A$ and ET$_B$.

The absolute bioavailability of bosentan after oral administration is about 50%, with peak plasma concentrations reached in 3 to 5 hours. Bosentan is an inducer of CYP 2C9 and CYP 3A4 enzymes, and possibly CYP 2C19 also. One of the three metabolites of bosentan is active, contributing 10% to 20% of drug action. Bosentan is eliminated through

the bile, with less than 3% of an administered oral dose recovered in urine.

Patients have also been hospitalized during the first 4 to 8 weeks of treatment with bosentan because of the weight gain, peripheral edema, and worsening heart failure. There have been several reports of hepatotoxicity with bosentan. Bosentan also causes a dose-related decrease in hemoglobin and hematocrit values after 1 to 3 months of use and therefore requires close monitoring of these parameters.

Begin treatment at 62.5 mg twice daily for 4 weeks and then increase to the maintenance dose of 125 mg twice daily. Dosages over 250 mg/day increase the risk for liver injury. Massive overdosage results in pronounced hypotension requiring active cardiovascular support.

Slowly rising, dose-dependent elevations of AST and ALT levels from bosentan use occur both early and later in treatment, and are typically asymptomatic. They ordinarily return to normal with discontinuance of the drug, or they may spontaneously reverse while treatment continues.

Direct Vasodilator

Like bosentan, treprostinil (Remodulin) is approved specifically for patients with PAH who have moderate to severe heart failure. Direct vasodilation of both pulmonary and systemic arterial vascular beds lowers blood pressure and inhibits

DOSAGE
TABLE 37-10 Vasodilators

Drug	Use(s)	Dosage	Implications
CENTRAL ALPHA₂-RECEPTOR AGONIST			
clonidine	Hypertension	*Adult:* 0.1–0.3 mg PO twice daily. *Child:* 5–25 mg/kg/day in 4 divided doses. Max: 0.9 mg/day. Increase gradually every 5–7 days.	**Watch for rebound HTN.** Decrease dose in patients with renal impairment.
ADRENERGIC ANTAGONIST			
reserpine	Hypertensive crisis	*Adult:* 0.1–0.25 mg PO daily orally if adjunct therapy or older adults. Maximum. 0.5 mg/day. *Child:* 5–20 mcg/kg/day.	Many contraindications and drug interactions. Check carefully before giving.
DIRECT-ACTING PERIPHERAL VASODILATORS			
diazoxide	Hypertensive crisis	*Adults and Child:* 1–3 mg/kg (not to exceed 150 mg/dose) IV every 5–15 min until BP lowered to desired level. May be repeated every 4–24 hr.	Administer undiluted over 30 sec or less only into a peripheral vein to prevent arrhythmias.
hydralazine	Moderate to severe hypertension	*Adult:* Initial: 10 mg PO 4 times daily –or– 20–40 mg IM or IV repeated as needed. May increase after 2–4 days to 25 mg PO 4 times daily for remainder of first wk. May increase to 50 mg PO 4 times daily up to 300 mg/day. *Child:* 0.75 mg/kg/day PO in 4 divided doses –or– 0.1–0.2 mg/kg/day IM or IV every 4–6 hr, as needed. May gradually increase to 7.5 mg/kg/day 4 times daily.	Twice-daily dosing may be used once maintenance dose is established. Administer with meals to enhance absorption. Give IV formulation through Y-tubing or 3-way stopcock.
minoxidil	Severe symptomatic hypertension or refractory hypertension	*Adult:* Initial: 5 mg PO daily. Increase at 3-day intervals to 10 mg/day, then 20 mg/day, then 40 mg/day in 2 divided doses. Usual dose: 10–40 mg/day. *Child <12 yr:* Initial: 0.2 mg/kg/day. Increase gradually at 3-day intervals until desired response reached. Usual dose: 0.25–1 mg/kg/day in 1–2 divided doses.	Dosages of 100 mg/day have been used in adults. For rapid BP control in children doses may be adjusted every 6 hr. Daily dose not to exceed 50 mg. Discontinue drug gradually to prevent rebound HTN. May be administered without regard to meals or food.
nitroprusside	Hypertensive crisis	*Adults and Child:* Initial dose 0.25–0.3 mcg/kg/min. Increase to 10 mcg/kg/min as needed. Usual dose 3 mcg/kg/min. Not to exceed 10 min of therapy at 10 mcg/kg/min.	Drug effects quickly reversed in 1–10 min by decreasing infusion rate or temporarily stopping the infusion. Monitor plasma thiocyanate levels and ECG in patients on prolonged infusions.

BP, Blood pressure; *ECG*, electrocardiogram; *HTN*, hypertension; *IM*, intramuscular; *IV*, intravenous; *PO*, by mouth.

platelet aggregation. Vasodilation also reduces ventricular afterload and increases cardiac output and stroke volume. Treprostinil produces dose-related negative inotropic actions.

Treprostinil is rapidly absorbed after subcutaneous infusion. Steady-state levels are reached in approximately 10 hours. Substantial biotransformation takes place in the liver, but the precise CYP enzymes responsible for the changes are unknown. The biologic activity and fat of the five metabolites are also unknown. Treprostinil has a biphasic elimination pattern, with a half-life of about 4 hours. Seventy-nine percent of an administered drug is eliminated unchanged and as metabolites in the urine, with the remainder eliminated in the stool. Treprostinil's only contraindication for use is a known drug allergy.

Treprostinil is infused subcutaneously, but the drug can be given via a central IV line if the subcutaneous route is not tolerated. If the initial dose is not tolerated, the infusion rate may be reduced. Sudden large reductions in dosage of treprostinil or an abrupt withdrawal of the drug result in worsening PAH symptoms.

CLINICAL REASONING

Treatment Objectives
The immediate goal of antihypertensive therapy is to reduce arterial pressure, minimize TOD, and prolong life. Ultimately, the goal of HTN prevention and management is to decrease cardiovascular and renal morbidity and mortality. By reaching and maintaining a target systolic blood pressure below 140 mm Hg and a diastolic blood pressure below 90 mm Hg, the goal may be realized. Treatment interventions to lower BP levels below 140/90 mm Hg prevent stroke, preserve renal function, and prevent or slow progression of heart failure. Drug therapy used appropriately can enhance the patient's quality of life.

Treatment Options
HTN is a multifactorial disease. As yet, no absolute clinical indicators (e.g., age, race, renin status) are available to guide the decision as to which drug to use for which patient. Individualizing treatment is essential in order to achieve a successful outcome, although there is a 60% to 80% chance the patient will respond to a particular drug group. Include lifestyle changes as early as possible in the treatment plan.

It is important to understand that the rate of BP increase may be more important than the absolute BP reading. **Patients with longstanding HTN may tolerate systolic BPs of 200 mm Hg or diastolic BPs of up to 150 mm Hg without developing hypertensive encephalopathy, whereas children or pregnant women may develop encephalopathy with diastolic BPs of 100 mm Hg.** The characteristic symptoms of hypertensive encephalopathy are headache and altered level of consciousness.

Lifestyle Changes
Although therapeutic lifestyle changes (TLC) are only discussed in this section on treatment options, such changes

are extremely important aspects of the management plan, particularly for patients with concurrent hypertension, hyperlipidemia, or diabetes. Lifestyle changes have been shown to prevent HTN, are effective in lowering BP, and reduce cardiovascular risk factors at little cost and with minimal risk. Even when changes in lifestyle are not sufficient to reduce BP, the changes may reduce the need for multidrug therapy.

Weight loss of even 10 pounds reduces BP in a large proportion of overweight patients. Furthermore, weight loss augments the BP-lowering effects of antihypertensive drugs and significantly reduces cardiovascular risk factors.

Na^+ intake is linked to BP elevation in some patients. Patients with HTN or diabetes, older adults, and blacks are more responsive to changes in Na^+ intake than other persons in the general population. Diets containing less than 2.4 grams of Na^+ daily are associated with reduced need for antihypertensive drugs, reduced diuretic-associated K^+ loss, and possible regression of left ventricular hypertrophy.

Regular aerobic activity enhances weight loss and functional health status and reduces cardiovascular risk factors and other causes of morbidity and mortality. BP can be reduced with 30 to 45 minutes of moderately intense exercise carried out daily.

Excessive alcohol intake causes resistance to antihypertensive drugs and is a risk factor for stroke. Advise patients to limit their daily intake of alcohol to no more than 24 ounces of beer, 10 ounces of wine, or 2 ounces of 100-proof whiskey. Significant elevations in BP can develop in patients with heavy alcohol intake who abruptly stop consumption.

Altering the dietary levels of Ca^{++}, K^+, magnesium, or Na^+ may improve BP in some patients. However, there is not strong evidence to suggest that supplements of any combination of potassium, magnesium, or calcium reduce mortality, morbidity, or BP in adults. Additional clinical studies are needed to determine whether use of potassium and magnesium is effective in lowering BP.

Hyperlipidemia is a significant independent risk factor for CAD. In spite of this factor, low-fat diets and those with a low proportion of saturated to unsaturated fats have had little, if any, direct effect on BP reduction. In some patients, the intake of omega-3 fatty acids lowers BP. However, some patients experience belching and abdominal discomfort with a large intake of these fatty acids.

Tobacco use in any form should be avoided by patients with HTN. Patients who continue to smoke while on antihypertensive therapy do not receive the full benefit of therapy. Further, the benefits to the cardiovascular system can be seen in all age groups within 1 year of discontinuing tobacco use. Advise smokers clearly and repeatedly to stop tobacco use of any kind. Interventions directed at minimizing weight gain after smoking cessation are often required.

Although caffeine raises BP acutely, tolerance to the pressor effects of caffeine develops quickly. No direct relationship has been found between caffeine intake and HTN.

▥ Patient Variables

Drug treatment of primary HTN is usually lifelong. Thus it is important to use a flexible approach to drug therapy. Patients respond differently to individual drugs or combinations of drugs. Further, simplified drug regimens make life easier for patients and increase adherence to treatment plans.

Monotherapy with once-daily or twice-daily dosing is likely to achieve adequate BP control in the patient adhering to prescribed treatment. However, effective dosages of antihypertensive drugs are often lower than those recommended in most texts. For example, drug therapy in the older adult should begin at one half the average starting dosage. Titration dosages should be small and spaced at longer intervals than those used for a younger patient.

JNC VII guidelines stress that drug choice should be based on what is most likely to benefit the individual patient. Factors to consider include the following:

- Age and ethnicity
- Severity of disease and extent of end-organ damage
- Concurrent risk factors and comorbid disease
- General lifestyle, including diet and exercise patterns
- Impact of HTN and drug therapy on quality of life (e.g., physical state, emotional well-being, sexual and social functioning, cognitive acuity)
- Previous response to drug therapy, if any

Nonetheless, patients may not adhere to their treatment regimen for a variety of reasons. The idea of lifelong treatment is a difficult adaptation for some people. For some patients, it is difficult to realize that treatment now, when they feel well, will prevent future complications. For others, drugs interfere with their quality of life. The cost of drugs may also be an issue for patients who have to pay for their drugs out of their pocket (see Case Study).

The JNC VII continues to recommend that all patients with stages 1 and 2 HTN attempt to make alterations in their lifestyle while drug therapy is started. JNC VII also recommends that patients with systolic BPs exceeding 160 mm Hg (after complying with vigorous TLC) receive drug therapy, even if the diastolic BP is normal (Fig. 37-2). Patients with systolic pressures ranging from 140 to 159 mm Hg are candidates for drug therapy, particularly when there is evidence of TOD. However, rigidly controlled HTN (i.e., diastolic pressure less than 85 mm Hg) can result in a fatal MI. BP readings within these ranges realize the greatest reduction in mortality and morbidity and are consistent with patient safety and tolerance.

Life-Span Considerations

Pregnant and Nursing Women. During normal pregnancy, systolic pressure changes very little. Diastolic pressure decreases by 10 mm Hg in early pregnancy and rises to prepregnancy levels in the third trimester. The initial fall is due to the general vasodilation that occurs with pregnancy. An increase in renin and aldosterone levels occurs in normal pregnancy.

HTN may be an indication of underlying maternal disease aggravated by pregnancy. HTN may also be the first sign of preeclampsia. Diagnostic criteria for HTN in pregnancy include a rise in BP of 20 to 30 mm Hg from preconception values or first trimester values, and an absolute level of BP greater than 140/90 mm Hg at any stage of pregnancy. Severe HTN is present when BP readings are greater than 170/110 mm Hg.

Preeclampsia occurs in 7% of all pregnancies and varies based on patient characteristics. Of these women, 70% have first-time pregnancies, while 30% have had multiple pregnancies. Preeclampsia is also exhibited in 70% of molar pregnancies. Severe preeclampsia is characterized by visual defects, severe headaches, seizures, altered consciousness, cerebrovascular accidents, severe right upper quadrant abdominal pain, heart

CASE STUDY Antihypertensive Drugs

ASSESSMENT

History of Present Illness	MD is a 57-year-old white asymptomatic female who presents for a routine employment physical because of an upcoming midlife career change. MD's preferred health care provider is a naturopath; however, she comes today to the internal medicine clinic because the future employer does not believe in naturopathy. She would prefer to receive all health care from this individual, particularly because he will be able to meet all of her health care needs with naturopathy.
Past Health History	No known allergies. Nonsmoker, nondrinker. Quit smoking 7 years ago but gained 50 lb. Stopped smoking because of an exacerbation of her asthma. Diagnosed with type 2 diabetes 10 years ago. Blood sugars poorly controlled by diet. Denies previous personal or family history of cardiovascular disease and renal or hepatic disorders, although patient is a poor historian. Medical records indicate patient not always adherent with recommended treatment plans regardless of state of health. Her last physical and eye exams were 2 years ago. Has no regular exercise program.
Life-Span Considerations	MD lives with her husband, who is a traveling architect. Their three adult children have recently moved into an apartment of their own. Husband and wife feel "like our nest is empty." MD is covered for prescriptions under her current health plan. Copayments range from $5–10 per drug. MD is an accountant and does not rely on her husband for income.
Physical Exam Findings	*Height:* 5'5". *Weight:* 182 lbs. *BP:* 210/118 right arm sitting and 206/114 left arm sitting. Apical pulse 100 and regular. Previous three readings ranged from 152/88 to 194/96 per patient BP log. PMI not discernable. No lifts, heaves, thrills, murmurs, rubs, or gallops noted. Negative for extra heart sounds. No carotid bruits noted. Breath sounds clear to auscultation bilaterally. Abdomen negative for HSM, bruits, or palpable masses. Pulses +2 all four extremities, 1+ peripheral edema. Neurologic exam negative. Fundoscopic exam unremarkable.
Diagnostic Testing	Chest x-ray unremarkable. Urinalysis: glycosuria, no protein. CBC: unremarkable. Hgb: 12.9, Hct: 42.0. Serum Ca^{++}: 9.0 mg/dL. Cl^-: 102 mmol/L. Random blood sugar: 180 mg/dL. BUN: 14 mg/dL. Creatinine: 1.2 mg/dL. Uric acid: 4.8 mg/dL. ALT: 28 U/L, AST: 34 U/L. Total cholesterol: 228 mg/dL. HDL: 36 mg/dL. Triglycerides: 186 mg/dL. LDL: 147 mg/dL. ECG: normal sinus rhythm, normal axis.

DIAGNOSIS: Hypertension

MANAGEMENT

Treatment Objectives	1. Reduce arterial pressure safely and effectively. 2. Prevent adverse effects and maintain quality of life. 3. Control type 2 diabetes mellitus. 4. Minimize end-organ complications such as stroke, cardiovascular disease, and renal failure.
Treatment Plan	**Pharmacotherapy** • lisinopril 20 mg PO once daily at bedtime • aspirin 81 mg daily • lovastatin 20 mg PO at dinner • metformin 500 mg PO twice daily **Patient Education** 1. Lifestyle modifications related to diet, sodium intake, regular aerobic exercise, stress management strategies, hyperlipidemia, and diabetes mellitus 2. Home monitoring of BP and blood sugar levels, and the importance of regular follow-up with health care provider 3. Ability to identify prescribed drugs by generic and trade names, the mechanism(s) of action, and adverse effects. Patients should know the dosing frequency and what to do if a dose is forgotten. 4. Importance of not abruptly stopping antihypertensive or antilipid drugs 5. Encourage contact with health care provider before using over-the-counter cold remedies, because many of these products contain sympathomimetic ingredients 6. Medical alert identification for hypertension and diabetes

Continued

CARDIOVASCULAR

CASE STUDY   Antihypertensive Drugs—Cont'd

Evaluation

Evaluation of the patient with HTN and diabetes mellitus is based on whether BP and blood sugars have been reduced and/or controlled and end-organ damage from either disease prevented or minimized.

CLINICAL REASONING ANALYSIS

Q1. So why did you not use a thiazide diuretic for MD? Aren't they first-line drugs for hypertension?

A. The thiazides are usually first-line drugs for hypertension, however, MD has a compelling indication for the ACEI or ARB, given her diabetes. Further, use of beta blockers is contraindicated for her, given her asthma and elevated triglyceride levels.

Q2. What is the difference between an ARB like losartan and an ACEI such as lisinopril?

A. ARBs generally have less risk for angioedema and respiratory adverse effects than ACEI. Their mechanisms of action are similar.

Q3. Isn't MD's hyperlipidemia a separate concern? I feel sorry for MD. Does she really need to start cholesterol therapy now? Can't she wait until her blood pressure is controlled?

A. Of course she can wait until her blood pressure is controlled to start the lovastatin. However, the sooner she gets her cholesterol levels down through drugs, diet, and exercise, the better controlled her diabetes and hypertension will be, and the lower her risk for stroke or heart attack.

Q4. My grandpa takes a multiple vitamin, an aspirin each day, and calcium, magnesium, and potassium to help reduce his blood pressure. He is also taking a blood pressure medicine. Is he wrong to be taking all of these supplements?

A. Epidemiologic studies suggest that altering the dietary levels of calcium, potassium, magnesium, or sodium can affect BP in some patients. However, there are no robust research studies suggesting that supplements of any combination of potassium, magnesium, or calcium reduce BP, mortality, or morbidity in adults.

---

failure, and oliguria. The condition's progression can only be stopped by delivery of the fetus.

Hydralazine is typically used to control HTN in the treatment of patients with eclampsia. Labetalol or nicardipine are preferred to hydralazine once the patient has been admitted to the intensive care unit. Labetalol and nicardipine, in both oral and IV formulations, appear to be safe and effective drugs for pregnant patients with HTN.

If taken before pregnancy occurs, diuretics and most other antihypertensive drugs (except ACEIs and ARBs, which are pregnancy category D drugs) may be continued. Methyldopa has been most extensively evaluated and is recommended for women whose HTN is first diagnosed during pregnancy. The use of beta blockers in early pregnancy is associated with intrauterine growth retardation. However, beta blockers (e.g., atenolol and metoprolol) can be effective alternatives and are considered safe for use during the latter half of pregnancy.

Diuretics are recommended for chronic HTN if they are prescribed before pregnancy, or if the patient appears to be salt-sensitive. They are not recommended for patients with preeclampsia. Hydralazine, a direct-acting vasodilator, is the parenteral drug of choice based on its long history of safety and effectiveness. The aim of antihypertensive therapy in the pregnant woman is to keep mean arterial pressure below 120 mm Hg but not less than 105 mm Hg. Hypotension may result in acute placental insufficiency.

Chronic HTN during pregnancy may be mild or severe. Pregnant women with chronic HTN are at risk for superimposed preeclampsia and abruptio placenta. Accelerated HTN may result in disseminated intravascular coagulation and resultant TOD to the mother. Fetal death or intrauterine growth restriction may occur as a result of uteroplacental insufficiency from HTN and can cause both maternal and fetal problems. Control of moderate and severe HTN results in a lower rate of perinatal morbidity and mortality.

Children and Adolescents. Criteria used for categorizing HTN in adults are not applicable to children. BP normally increases in children at a rate of 1.5 mm Hg systolic and 1 mm Hg diastolic values per year. BP readings level off at 18 to 20 years of age (Table 37-11).

The prevalence of HTN in children is 13%. Frequent causes of persistent HTN in children are renal HTN and coarctation of the aorta. Children have a higher risk of HTN if both parents are hypertensive. There is a striking increase in sustained new HTN between the ages of 15 and 25 years.

It is not clear if hypertensive adolescents continue to be hypertensive as adults. However, children whose BP is consistently above the 95th percentile for height, weight, and age should be closely evaluated and treated. Adherence to treatment regimens can be a major problem with adolescents who are asymptomatic. Children and adolescents do not want to be different from peers in regard to diet and lifestyle. Premature labeling of adolescents as hypertensive may later interfere with some career choices and the ability to obtain life insurance. Although the recommendations for choice of drugs are similar in children and adults, dosages of antihypertensives are smaller and adjusted very carefully for children.

TABLE 37-11 Average BP in Girls and Boys by Age

Age (Years)	BP in mm Hg			
	50th Percentile	90th Percentile	50th Percentile	90th Percentile
1	91/54	105/67	90/56	105/69
3	91/56	106/69	92/55	107/68
6	96/57	111/70	96/57	111/70
9	100/61	115/74	101/61	115/74
12	107/66	122/78	107/64	121/77
15	111/67	126/82	114/65	129/79
18	112/66	127/80	121/70	136/84

BP, Blood pressure. Data from the National High Blood Pressure Education Program Working Group on Hypertension Control in Children and Adolescents, 1996. Update on the 1987 Task Force Report on High Blood Pressure in Children and Adolescents. A working group report from the National High Blood Pressure Education Program. *Pediatrics, 98*(4 Pt 1), 649–658.

Older Adults. The prevalence of HTN among older adults is extremely common. Among Americans aged 60 years and older, elevated BP occurs in about 60% of whites, 71% of blacks, and 61% of Hispanics. Especially among older adults, systolic BP is a more accurate predictor of adverse events (i.e., coronary artery disease, heart failure, stroke, and end-stage renal disease) than is diastolic BP. Isolated systolic HTN is the most common form of HTN in older adults.

Blood pressure must be measured with special care in older adults because some persons have *pseudohypertension,* a falsely high BP reading, due to excessive vascular stiffness. In addition, older persons with HTN and excessive variability in systolic BP values may have white-coat HTN. Further, older adults are more likely to experience orthostatic changes in BP than younger patients. Thus, always measure BP readings with the patient standing as well as in the seated and supine positions.

The older adult is at increased risk for adverse drug effects because of the physiologic changes associated with aging. These changes can affect the concentration and distribution of drugs. The effects of drugs at their sites of action may also be affected. Renal blood flow decreases with age, which affects the dosing of antihypertensive drugs that are eliminated by the kidneys. Lean muscle mass decreases, whereas the proportion of fat in the body increases. This factor may extend the effects of fat-soluble drugs.

Further, older adults often take multiple drugs obtained from several different physicians. Eye drops might not be mentioned when patients are asked to list drugs taken. Nonetheless, certain drugs (e.g., ocular beta blockers) may cause systemic effects.

In older adults, begin antihypertensive therapy with lifestyle modifications. Older adults may respond to weight loss and a modest reduction in salt intake. If BP values do not respond, drug therapy is warranted. The starting dose of antihypertensive drugs is about half of that used in young patients. When compared with each other, diuretics (e.g., hydrochlorothiazide with amiloride) are superior to the beta blocker atenolol. Thiazide diuretics or beta blockers in combination are recommended because they reduce morbidity and mortality.

In older adults with isolated systolic HTN, the drugs of choice are diuretics, because they significantly reduce multiple end-organ complications. The goal of treatment is the same as in young patients: a systolic value less than 140 mm Hg and a diastolic value under 90 mm Hg. That being said, an interim goal of systolic values less than 160 mm Hg may be acceptable in patients who have marked systolic HTN. However, any reduction in BP confers benefit, and the closer the BP is to normal, the greater the benefit. Exercise caution when using antihypertensive drugs that may cause orthostatic BP changes (i.e., high-dose diuretics, alpha₁ blockers, and peripheral vasodilators), or drugs thatcause cognitive dysfunction (i.e., central sympathomimetics).

Consider using drugs that have been proven to reduce mortality and morbidity (i.e., beta blockers, diuretics). Remember, however, that reducing BP with multidrug therapy does not necessarily equate with an equal reduction in end-organ damage.

Drug Variables

The decision to start antihypertensive drug therapy requires careful consideration of several factors including the following:

- Stage and degree of BP elevation
- Presence of clinical cardiovascular or other risk factors
- Presence of EOD
- Safety profile of the specific drug or drugs
- Efficacy and convenience of specific drug or drugs
- Potential for drug interactions
- Treatment costs, including laboratory testing, and follow-up visits to health care provider

The following describes what would be the ideal antihypertensive drug: is effective in lowering BP to recommended goals; is efficacious as monotherapy; has a rapid onset of effect; has convenient once-daily dosing regimen to maximize adherence; provides 24-hour BP control with once-daily dosing, and with 50% of peak effects remaining at the end of the 24 hours; elicits an increase in response at higher doses (i.e., a clear dose-response effect); and has an optimum tolerability profile.

In contrast to this idealized picture, in actuality even the best drug is less than 70% effective on a long-term basis. Still, 80% of patients adhering to therapy eventually achieve adequate control with the use of one or two drugs. Only a small number of patients will require multidrug therapy.

The choice for initial therapy depends on the degree of BP elevation and the presence of compelling indications (discussed in next section). Current management approaches to HTN, as reported by JNC VII, continue to call for diuretics and beta blockers as initial therapy for uncomplicated HTN. (see Controversy box). As shown in Table 37-12, there are also unequivocal reasons for using specific drugs in certain clinical

CARDIOVASCULAR

Controversy

Initial Use of Diuretics and Beta Blockers

Jonathan J. Wolfe

The Seventh Report of the Joint National Committee on Prevention, Detection, Evaluation, and Treatment of High Blood Pressure (JNC VII) advocates choosing diuretics and beta blockers for initial treatment in patients when lifestyle changes are inadequate for blood pressure control. However, not all authorities agree with these recommendations. At present, diuretics and beta blockers are the only agents for which long-term data are available. The advantages over the long term cannot be compared with those of the newer drugs because of the limitations of previous studies.

Critics have questioned the scientific basis on which JNC VII selected diuretics and beta blockers as preferred agents. Studies used as a basis for these recommendations do not include high-risk populations, women, or blacks. Critics of JNC VII go on to argue that the guidelines underplay the importance of flexibility for patients with other diseases or risk factors. Flexibility in treatment regimens becomes an important issue when increasingly aggressive strategies are used by managed care programs and insurers to control what health care providers prescribe.

Direct costs are among the easiest medical costs to calculate. As insurers take steps that range from offering financial incentives to requiring prior authorization for the prescription of certain drugs, they encourage health care providers to use lower-cost drugs, especially low-dose diuretics and beta blockers. JNC VII guidelines are cited as the rationale.

The second controversy that occurs is the practice of giving sublingual nifedipine for hypertensive emergencies and urgencies. The practice of puncturing a nifedipine capsule and expressing the contents under the tongue is common. However, this practice is neither safe nor effective. Nifedipine is not absorbed sublingually. Most absorption takes place in the intestinal mucosa. Serious, even fatal adverse effects have been reported when nifedipine was administered for acute treatment of severe hypertension. Uncontrolled reduction in blood pressure with sublingual nifedipine can result in coma, stroke, myocardial infarction, acute renal failure, and death. Given the serious nature of its adverse effects and the lack of documentation as to its benefit, the use of nifedipine capsules for hypertensive emergencies should be abandoned.

CLINICAL REASONING ANALYSIS

- Critique the Seventh Report of the Joint National Committee on Prevention, Detection, Evaluation, and Treatment of High Blood Pressure (JNC VII, 2003). How will you interpret and use the results of this report?
- Is there reasonable evidence in this report to warrant discontinuing the practice of using sublingual nifedipine? Why or why not? What additional information, if any, do you need to make an informed decision about using nifedipine by the sublingual route?
- Does the report provide sufficient support for the unequivocal use of beta blockers, diuretics, and angiotensin-converting enzyme inhibitors (ACEIs) for selected groups of patients? How does the health care provider individualize therapy in light of the compelling indications for drugs in these categories?

TABLE 37-12 Perceived Advantages and Disadvantages of Antihypertensives

Perceived Advantages	Perceived Disadvantages
ACEIs	
• Effective in older adults with low cardiac output, reduce total blood volume*, high peripheral vascular resistance, low plasma renin activity, and high catecholamine activity (unequivocal indication)	• Concurrent NSAID use blunts action of ACEIs and may accelerate renal failure
• Slow development of nephropathy in type 1 and type 2 diabetes (unequivocal indication)	• Less effective in blacks (although not necessarily ineffective) and in patients with low renin states
• Increase survival after MI in patients who have HF or left ventricular dysfunction (unequivocal indication)	• May increase sodium and potassium levels, produce dry cough (bradykinin-induced), angioedema, and tracheobronchial irritation
• Reduce proteinuria in combination with nondihydropyridine CCBs more than either drug alone	• Cough contributes to likelihood of nonadherence
• Improve responsiveness to insulin	• Patients with renovascular HTN with renal perfusion maintained by high levels of angiotensin II and who have serum creatinine levels exceeding 3 mg/dL may develop ARF
• Do not elevate lipid levels	• Patients with high renin levels (i.e., volume-depleted, using diuretics, renovascular disease) may experience excessive hypotension
• Well tolerated and highly effective alone or with diuretics	• Although rare, associated with cholestatic jaundice that can progress to fulminant hepatic necrosis and death
• Less pedal edema in combination with dihydropyridine CCBs than CCBs used alone	
• Acceptable for patients with bronchospastic disease	
• Use of generic formulations acceptable	
ANGIOTENSIN II–RECEPTOR BLOCKERS	
• Produce effects similar to ACEIs while avoiding adverse effect of dry cough	• May increase sodium, potassium levels, angioedema, tracheobronchial irritation
• Useful in patients unable to tolerate ACEIs	• Decrease blood pressure if patient has low preexisting volume, is on diuretics, has HF, or has renal failure
• Useful in treating and preventing nephropathy from type 1 and type 2 diabetes	• Concurrent NSAID use may accelerate renal failure
• Improve insulin sensitivity and reduces plasma levels of catecholamines	• Usually more expensive as newest drugs on the market
• Losartan does not alter lipids, glucose, or other metabolic parameters	• May be less effective (but not ineffective) for blacks.
• Generic formulations acceptable	
DIURETICS (THIAZIDES, THIAZIDE, LOOP, POTASSIUM-SPARING)	
• Effective in blacks with HTN characterized by low renin state, low cardiac output, expanded total blood volume*, and high peripheral vascular resistance	• Cannot use in patients with symptomatic gout, poorly controlled diabetes, or severe hyperlipidemia

- Reduce M&M associated with HTN, MI, HF, renal failure (unequivocal indication)
- Relative reduction in frequency of fatal and nonfatal strokes (unequivocal indication)
- Have long, proven track record of effectiveness

- Enhances effects of other antihypertensive drugs without producing adverse effects
- Thiazides produce beneficial effects in patients with osteoporosis
- Loop diuretics produce greater diuresis than thiazides and do not promote vasodilation compared to thiazides
- Bumetanide less likely to cause hypercalcemia than other loop diuretics
- Indapamide produces little or no hypercholesterolemia
- Metolazone and indapamide may be effective in patients with impaired renal function when thiazides are not
- Considerably less expensive than other drugs; generic formulations acceptable

- May potentiate digoxin toxicity
- Increases risk of death if baseline ECG abnormalities

- Cannot use K+-sparing diuretics concurrently with ACEIs or K+ supplements owing to risk of hyperkalemia
- Amount of fluid lost with loop diuretics is greater than needed or desirable in most cases
- NSAIDs blunt the action of diuretics, reducing effectiveness

CENTRAL-ACTING ALPHA$_1$ BLOCKERS

- Decrease SNS outflow to reduce heart rate and peripheral vascular resistance
- Guanfacine produces fewer withdrawal symptoms than clonidine
- Methyldopa preferred for HTN during pregnancy
- Generic formulations acceptable

- Abruptly stopping drug causes rebound HTN
- Significant sedation, dry mouth, depression
- Impotence possible
- Concurrent NSAID use may accelerate renal failure

BETA BLOCKERS (SELECTIVE, NONSELECTIVE)

- Effective in young patients with HTN who have high cardiac output; normal total blood volume; normal peripheral vascular resistance; and high plasma renin activity (unequivocal indication)
- Decrease incidence of sudden death, stroke, MI, renal failure, and LVH associated with HTN (unequivocal indication)
- Appropriate for patients with migraine headaches
- May have favorable effects for patients with angina, atrial tachycardia, atrial fibrillation, essential tremor, hyperthyroidism
- Less likely to delay recovery from hypoglycemia or cause severe HTN when hypoglycemia leads to an increase in circulating catecholamines
- Labetolol decreases blood pressure more promptly than other drugs because of nonselective beta and alpha blockade
- Labetolol equally effective in blacks and whites, and does not elevate serum lipid levels
- Generic formulations acceptable

- Cannot use for patients with diabetes, asthma, HF (except for carvedilol), peripheral vascular disease, second- or third-degree heart block
- Drugs with nonintrinsic sympathomimetic action worsen GI upset and triglyceride levels
- May mask signs of hypoglycemia
- Can cause insomnia, depression, bizarre dreams, sexual dysfunction (impotence)
- Concurrent NSAID use blunts effects of beta blockers
- Becomes less effective as dosage is increased

CALCIUM CHANNEL BLOCKERS (DIHYDROPYRIDINES, NONDIHYDROPYRIDINES)

- Effective in older adult patients who have low cardiac output, reduced total blood volume, high peripheral vascular resistance, low plasma renin activity, and high catecholamine activity
- Decrease left ventricular hypertrophy
- Limited to no effect on insulin sensitivity, glycemic control, lipids, K+, and C++ levels
- May use in blacks, and those with chronic airflow limitation, variant angina, arrhythmias
- Decreased incidence of drug-induced orthostatic hypotension
- Effective for isolated systolic HTN in older adults
- Diltiazem and verapamil modestly reduce blood pressure following non–Q wave MI and after MI with preserved left ventricular dysfunction
- Verapamil, diltiazem, and amlodipine cause little or no change in heart rate
- Generic formulations acceptable

- Cautious use with concurrent beta blockers needed because they alter AV conduction
- Cannot use short-acting CCBs in patients with heart failure, sick sinus syndrome, second- or third-degree heart block
- Can cause reflex tachycardia and ischemic events, especially with immediate-release nifedipine, diltiazem, and verapamil
- May be associated with stroke, angina, vascular problems (specifically isradipine)
- Dihydropyridine formulations cause initial reflex tachycardia

ALPHA BLOCKERS (ALPHA-SELECTIVE, ALPHA- AND BETA-SELECTIVE)

- Cause vascular dilation and reduces peripheral vascular resistance
- Increase peak urine flow in men with benign prostatic hypertrophy
- Have no effects on lipid levels
- Less tachycardia than direct-acting peripheral vasodilators
- May increase HDL/total cholesterol ratio
- Improve responsiveness to insulin
- Provide symptomatic relief from prostatism
- Generic formulations acceptable

- Produce significant orthostatic hypotension, especially in older adults with first dose (first-dose phenomenon)
- Can cause stress incontinence in women
- Concurrent NSAID use may accelerate renal failure

ADRENERGIC NEURONAL BLOCKERS

- Reduces catecholamine release to decrease peripheral vascular resistance, cardiac output, and systolic blood pressure (more than diastolic)

- Exacerbate or causes depression
- Increased vasodilation and orthostatic hypotension with exercise, alcohol use, hot environment
- Decrease libido, may cause diarrhea

Continued

CARDIOVASCULAR

TABLE 37-12 Perceived Advantages and Disadvantages of Antihypertensives—Cont'd

Perceived Advantages	Perceived Disadvantages
DIRECT-ACTING VASODILATORS	
• No significant venous dilation so little orthostatic hypotension	• Need concurrent use of beta blocker and diuretic, or centrally acting drugs to help offset adverse effects
• Diazoxide and hydralazine acceptable for use during pregnancy	• Stimulate reflex sympathetic action of cardiovascular system and fluid retention
• Generic formulations acceptable	• Lupuslike syndrome with hydralazine, hirsutism with minoxidil

*Most prominent diagnostic finding of this age group.
ACEIs, Angiotensin-converting enzyme inhibitors; *ARF,* acute renal failure; *AV,* atrioventricular; *CCBs,* calcium channel blockers; *Cr,* creatinine; *ECG,* electrocardiogram; *GI,* gastrointestinal; *HF,* heart failure; *HTN,* hypertension; *LVH,* left ventricular hypertrophy; *MI,* myocardial infarction; *M&M,* morbidity and mortality; *NSAID,* nonsteroidal antiinflammatory drug; *SNS,* sympathetic nervous system.

situations. In most other situations, the choice of drug is individualized and the drug used that is most suitable to the patient's needs. Diuretics and beta blockers cause a 40% relative reduction in the frequency of fatal and nonfatal strokes over 5 years of treatment. Evidence also suggests that diuretics and beta blockers reduce the incidence of cardiovascular complications of HTN (i.e., sudden death, stroke, myocardial infarction, left ventricular hypertrophy, and renal failure).

If the initial drug of choice does not adequately control BP after reaching the full dosage, consider these two options for subsequent therapy: If the patient is tolerating the drug of first choice, a second drug from a different class may be added. If the patient is having significant adverse effects or there is no response to the first drug, a drug from a different class can be substituted. Using two drugs from the same classification is not advised. If a diuretic was not used first-line, use it as the second step, because it enhances the effects of the first drug. Keep the dosages of both drugs low to minimize adverse effects. If addition of the second drug controls BP, consider withdrawing the first drug.

There are increasing numbers of fixed-dose, combination antihypertensive drugs on the market (Box 37-5). Although combination antihypertensive drugs are convenient, many health care providers prefer to adjust the dosage of each drug individually. When optimum maintenance doses coincide to the ratio of drugs in a fixed-combination formulation, taking fewer tablets may help improve adherence to antihypertensive therapy and reduce cost.

Compelling Indications. The JNC VII report identifies six compelling indications (Fig. 37-2). Compelling indications represent specific comorbid conditions where evidence from clinical trials supports using specific antihypertensive classes to treat both the compelling indication and HTN. Drug for compelling indications are recommended for use either in combination with or in place of a thiazide diuretic. For example, patients with diabetes (especially those with nephropathy) or heart failure may benefit most from an ACEI. For patients with elevated lipid levels, an ACEI, alpha₁ blocker, or CCB may be a good choice.

In both whites and blacks, diuretics are proven to reduce the mortality and morbidity associated with HTN. Thus, diuretics are the drug of first choice in whites and blacks unless there are conditions prohibiting their use. CCBs and alpha₁ and beta blockers are also effective in lowering BP in this population. Monotherapy with beta blockers or an ACEI is less effective, but not necessarily ineffective. Black patients

BOX 37-5

Fixed-Dose Combination Antihypertensives

Thiazide Diuretic + Beta Blocker
- bendroflumethiazide + nadolol (Corzide)
- chlorthalidone + atenolol (Tenoretic)
- hydrochlorothiazide + bisoprolol (Ziac)
- hydrochlorothiazide + metoprolol (Lopressor HCT)
- hydrochlorothiazide + propranolol (Inderide)
- hydrochlorothiazide + timolol (Timolide)

Thiazide diuretic + ACEI
- hydrochlorothiazide + benazepril (Lotensin HCT)
- hydrochlorothiazide + captopril (Capozide)
- hydrochlorothiazide + enalapril (Vaseretic)
- hydrochlorothiazide + lisinopril (Prinzide, Zestoretic)
- hydrochlorothiazide + moexipril (Uniretic)
- hydrochlorothiazide + quinapril (Accuretic)

Thiazide Diuretic + ARB
- hydrochlorothiazide + candesartan (Atacand HCT)
- hydrochlorothiazide + eprosartan (Teveten HCT)
- hydrochlorothiazide + irbesartan (Avalide)
- hydrochlorothiazide + losartan (Hyzaar)
- hydrochlorothiazide + olmesartan (Benicar HCT)
- hydrochlorothiazide + telmisartan (Micardis HCT)
- hydrochlorothiazide + valsartan (Diovan HCT)

Thiazide Diuretic + Alpha Blocker
- polythiazide + prazosin (Minizide)

Thiazide Diuretic + Alpha₂ Receptor Agonist
- hydrochlorothiazide + methyldopa (Apresazide)

Thiazide Diuretic + Potassium-Sparing Diuretic
- hydrochlorothiazide + spironolactone (Aldactazide)
- hydrochlorothiazide + amiloride (Moduretic)
- hydrochlorothiazide + triamterene (Maxzide)

ACE inhibitor + CCBs
- benazepril + amlodipine (Lotrel)
- enalapril + felodipine (Lexxel)
- trandolapril + verapamil (Tarka)

ACEI, Angiotensin-converting enzyme inhibitor; *ARBs,* angiotensin II–receptor blockers; *CCBs,* calcium channel blockers.

often require multidrug therapy because of the higher incidence of complicated HTN in this population. A diuretic markedly improves the response of black patients to antihypertensive therapy.

A beta blocker without intrinsic sympathomimetic activity may be indicated for hypertensive patients with a history of angina or migraine headaches. Beta blockers are also effective in reducing mortality and morbidity in patients who have had an MI. ACEIs are used for patients with diabetic nephropathy or left ventricular systolic dysfunction.

Patient Education

It is important to develop and implement an individualized teaching plan for each patient. Teaching patients how to monitor BP at home enables them to become more active participants in care, treatment goals are reinforced, and adherence with therapy is enhanced. Advise patients to check the BP weekly and report significant changes to the health care provider. Reinforce the notion that HTN may not produce symptoms but is a chronic disease that requires lifelong interventions. Discuss patient beliefs about personal susceptibility to complications of HTN, treatment effectiveness, and consequences of nontreatment. Help patients understand that drug therapy controls, but does not cure, HTN.

Stress the importance of TLC at all visits. This includes discussion regarding the importance of a low sodium–low fat diet, weight reduction, limited alcohol consumption, smoking cessation, and increased physical activity. Not all patients are motivated to make the required changes for the management of HTN. However, patients who believe they play an active part in controlling their disease are more likely to adhere to the treatment regimen. Adherence is more likely when patients understand the plan, it makes sense to them, and it is consistent with their own cultural beliefs. Adequate information enables the patient to make informed choices about lifestyle changes.

HTN and obesity frequently coexist, so give dietary recommendations to all hypertensive patients. Weight control permits reduced dosages of antihypertensive drugs in patients receiving drug therapy. Dietary restriction of cholesterol and saturated fats is advised and helps reduce the incidence of arteriosclerotic complications. Excessive alcohol intake is related to nonadherence to the antihypertensive treatment program and should be avoided.

Na^+ restriction continues to be controversial. Na^+ intake of 2.4 grams/day elevates BP in some patients with essential HTN. In other patients, Na^+ restriction may limit drug effectiveness. Thus, a trial of mild Na^+ restriction is the most practical approach. Teaching the patient to eliminate, or at least restrict, the use of certain frozen, canned, or processed foods can reduce sodium intake considerably. Advise patients to avoid caffeine and tobacco intake as well.

A long-term regular exercise program helps control abnormally elevated BP. BP will increase if the patient returns to a sedentary lifestyle after as little as 3 months of exercise; however, subsequent BP readings will still be lower than preexercise levels. Isotonic exercises (e.g., jogging or walking) may reduce BP by 30% to 50%. Isometric exercises (e.g., weight lifting) may raise arterial pressure. Exercise lowers BP in blacks more dramatically than in whites. In older adults, low-intensity training results in a 20-mm Hg decrease in systolic pressure and a 12-mm Hg fall in diastolic pressure. Review the patient's individualized exercise plan and provide continuing encouragement.

Teach patients stress management techniques. These methods have been shown to decrease catecholamine release, oxygen consumption, respiratory rate, heart rate, and acute BP elevation. Use of a combination of biofeedback and stress management techniques has been shown to be better than either strategy alone.

Provide the patient written instructions about the treatment regimen, including identification of prescribed drugs by generic and trade names, the mechanism(s) of action, and adverse effects. Patients should know the dosing frequency and what to do if a dose is forgotten. Encourage the patient to contact the health care provider before using over-the-counter cold remedies, or any dietary supplement or herbal product, because many of these products contain sympathomimetic ingredients. Also, advise the patient to inform other health care providers and dentists of the diagnosis and treatment regimen of HTN before procedures or surgery.

Advise patients that abruptly stopping antihypertensive drugs may result in withdrawal syndrome characterized by sweating, palpitations, headache, tremulousness, and rebound HTN. Withdrawal syndrome can precipitate heart failure and MI in patients with cardiac disease; a thyroid storm in patients with thyrotoxicosis; peripheral ischemia in patients with peripheral vascular disease; and hypoglycemia in patients with previously controlled diabetes.

Although education has a substantial effect on the patient's knowledge and a positive effect on adherence with therapy, the effect of knowledge tends to diminish over time. It is beneficial to reinforce education periodically. Dialogue between the health care provider and the patient tends to reinforce treatment goals and positive behaviors.

Evaluation

Evaluation of the patient with HTN is based on whether BP has been reduced and TOD prevented or minimized. Reassess the patient if BP has not decreased after 4 to 8 weeks of therapy (Fig. 37-3). Discontinue the present drug, and restart treatment with a different drug at low dosage. If the BP has decreased but not to the level desired, and if the patient has no adverse drug effects, the initial drug can be continued but a second drug added at low dosage. Titrate the dosage of the second drug based on patient response. If, however, the patient's pressure has been reduced but not to the desired level, *and* the patient is experiencing adverse effects, *or* if the patient cannot tolerate the treatment regimen, discontinue the drug and start another. Another option for the patient who is responding to drug therapy is to decrease the dosage to a tolerable level of adverse effects. If the patient is still unable to tolerate the adverse effects, stop the drug and change to another.

If a patient's diastolic BP exceeds 115 mm Hg, reevaluate after 48 hours of therapy to ensure that at least a 5- to 10-mm Hg drop in pressure has occurred. Patients whose pressures fall below this number should be followed up on in 1 to 2 weeks. Recheck BP every 4 weeks, after each dosage change, or until controlled. Once BP is controlled, monitor the patient 2 to 4 times yearly. If BP remains controlled and there are no comorbid conditions, the serum creatinine, blood sugar, cholesterol values, and urinalysis should be checked a minimum of every 5 years; however, annual visits are preferred to monitor for TOD (Table 37-13).

CARDIOVASCULAR

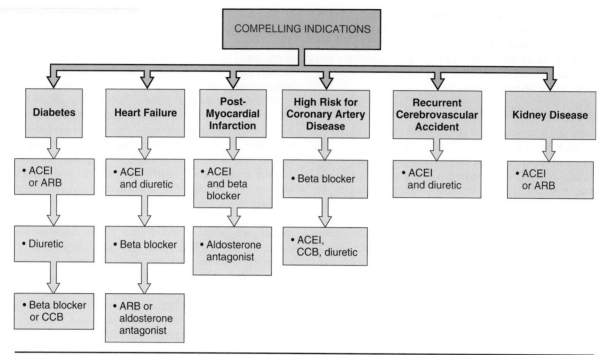

FIGURE 37-3 Algorithm for Patients Not at BP Goal. (*ACEI*, Angiotensin-converting enzyme inhibitor; *ARB*, angiotensin II–receptor blocker; *CCB*, calcium channel blocker. (Adapted from Chobanian, A., Bakris, G., Black, H., et al. and the Joint National Committee on Detection, Evaluation, and Treatment of High Blood Pressure. [2003]. The Seventh Report of the Joint National Committee on the Prevention, Detection, Evaluation, and Treatment of High Blood pressure [JNC VII]. *Hypertension, 42*[6], 1206–1252.)

TABLE 37-13 Recommendations for Blood Pressure Follow-Up

Initial Blood Pressure Reading*	Recommended Follow-up
Normal	Recheck in 2 years
Prehypertension	Recheck in 1 year†
Stage I hypertension	Confirm within 2 months
	Provide information about therapeutic lifestyle changes
Stage II hypertension	Evaluate or refer to health care provider within 1 month
	For those with higher pressures, evaluate and treat immediately or within 1 wk based on clinical situation

*If systolic and diastolic values are different, follow recommendations for shorter follow-up period. For example, a measurement of 160/86 should be evaluated within 1 month or referred to specialist
†Modify the follow-up schedule according to reliable information about past blood pressure measurements, other cardiovascular risk factors, or end-organ disease.
From Chobanian, A., Bakris, G., Black, H., et al. and the Joint National Committee on Detection, Evaluation, and Treatment of High Blood Pressure. (2003). The Seventh Report of the Joint National Committee on the Prevention, Detection, Evaluation, and Treatment of High Blood Pressure (JNC VII). *Hypertension, 42*(6), 1206–1252.

Step-down therapy may be considered for patients whose BP has been well controlled during the previous few visits. The drug dosage for these patients can be reduced by 50% and the patient reevaluated in 2 weeks. If the patient's condition is stable, the dosage may be decreased another 50% and the patient again evaluated in 2 weeks. If the patient is stable at this point, the drug may be discontinued and the patient again evaluated in 2 weeks. The following describes patients who may successfully withdraw from antihypertensive therapy, among others:

- The BP has been well controlled over the last few visits with the health care provider
- Pretreatment diastolic BP was less than 100 mm Hg
- No evidence of end-organ disease present
- BP has been controlled on monotherapy
- Those who have lost weight, are following a Na⁺ restricted diet, have decreased their alcohol intake, and have increased their exercise regimen

EVIDENCE-BASED PHARAMACOTHERAPEUTICS

Depression and Hypertension

■ Background
It is known that there are psychologic factors related to hypertension (HTN) and coronary artery disease. There is growing evidence that suggests a significant association, mediated through obesity, between symptoms of depression and HTN.

■ Research Article
Kabir, A., Whelton, P., Khan, M., et al. (2006). Association of symptoms of depression and obesity with hypertension: The Bogalusa Heart Study. *American Journal of Hypertension, 19*(6), 639–645.

Purpose
The purpose of this study was to evaluate the direct and indirect relationships between symptoms of depression, body mass index (BMI), and HTN in a biracial (blacks and whites) rural population.

Design
This was a cross-sectional study with 1017 study participants from 561 families of the Bogalusa Heart Study. Subjects were aged 12 to 62 years. Sixty percent of subjects were white and 52% were women. Mean BMI of the study population was 28. Roughly one third had presumptive depression, and 13.4% had hypertension.

Methods
A two-stage modeling approach was used to evaluate the relationship between symptoms of depression, BMI, and HTN. Generalized estimating equation methods (GEE) were used to account for within-family correlations. Adjusted coefficients (95% confidence interval [CI]) and odds ratios (OR) were used to explore relationships.

Findings
Mean (± standard error [SE]) BMI of the subjects was 28 (±7). Thirty-two percent of subjects had presumptive depression, and 13.4% had HTN. The indirect effect of a 5-unit-higher symptoms-of-depression score was associated with a 14% (OR: 1.14; 95% CI: 1.01–1.28; $p < 0.02$) higher likelihood of being hypertensive due to presence of a higher level of BMI in both whites and blacks. The direct effect of a 5-unit-higher symptoms-of-depression score was found to be nonsignificant (OR: 1.05; 95% CI: 0.92–1.20; $p < 0.22$) in whites and significant (OR: 0.81; 95% CI: 0.68–0.95; $p < 0.004$) in blacks.

Conclusions
This study shows a probable pathway between depression and development of HTN. If we know the causal pathways, effective prevention strategies can be developed. The presence of a significant indirect effect of symptoms of depression (mediated through higher level of BMI) in both whites and blacks suggests that BMI can be an intermediate variable linking symptoms of depression and HTN.

■ Implications for Practice
Because depressed individuals are more likely to be overweight, special care should be taken to address the symptoms of depression in the general population. Intervention strategies for depression may be helpful in developing an effective weight-reduction program and subsequently HTN-prevention programs. Further studies of HTN and depression in other cultural groups are warranted, using any of the antihypertensive drug classes. A confirmed diagnosis of depression should be used.

KEY POINTS

- Twenty-five percent of the adult population has HTN, and a significant number of people remain undiagnosed.
- The morbidity and mortality associated with HTN decreases when HTN is managed effectively.
- The exact etiology of essential HTN is unknown; several theories suggest complex hormonal and neural mechanisms.
- Modifiable risk factors for HTN include socioeconomic factors, nutrition, obesity, smoking, alcohol, physical activity, and stress levels. Nonmodifiable risk factors include age, sex, family history, and ethnicity.
- The initial evaluation of the patient is directed at detection of correctable forms of secondary HTN and determining baseline patient status.

- The majority of patients with essential HTN have no specific symptoms. The symptoms leading the patient to consult a health care provider are often related to TOD.
- The goal of treatment is to reduce arterial BP, minimize organ damage, and prolong life.
- Drug groups used to treat HTN include diuretics, beta blockers, ACEIs, ARBs, CCBs, central-acting alpha$_1$ blockers, alpha$_2$ agonists, and direct-acting vasodilators.
- It is important to incorporate lifestyle changes, individualized drug therapy, patient education, and follow-up into the treatment plan.
- Evaluation of the patient with HTN is based on whether BP has been reduced and TOD prevented or minimized.

Bibliography

ALLHAT Officers and Coordinators for the ALLHAT Collaborative Research Group. (2002). Major outcomes in high-risk hypertensive patients randomized to angiotensin-converting enzyme inhibitor or calcium channel blocker vs. diuretic: The Antihypertensive and Lipid-Lowering Treatment to Prevent Heart Attack Trial (ALLHAT). *Journal of the American Medical Association, 288*(23), 2981–2997.

Berenson, G., Srinivasan, S., Bao, W., et al. (1998). Association between multiple cardiovascular risk factors and atherosclerosis in children and young adults: The Bogalusa Heart Study. *New England Journal of Medicine, 338*(23), 1650–1656.

Beyer, F., Dickinson, H., Nicolson, D., et al. (2006). Combined calcium, magnesium, and potassium supplementation for the management of primary HTN in adults. *Cochran Database of Systematic Reviews.* 2006, Issue 3. Art. No. CD004805. DOI: 10.1002/14651858.CD004805.pub2.

Centers for Disease Control and Prevention. National Center for Health Statistics. Third National Health and Nutrition Examination Survey. Available online: www.cdc.gov/nhanes.htm. Accessed May 7, 2007.

Chobanian, A. (2006). Prehypertension revisited. *Hypertension, 48*(5), 812–814.

CARDIOVASCULAR

Chobanian, A., Bakris, G., Black, H., et al. and the Joint National Committee on Detection, Evaluation, and Treatment of High Blood Pressure. (2003). The Seventh Report of the Joint National Committee on the Prevention, Detection, Evaluation, and Treatment of High Blood pressure (JNC VII). *Hypertension, 42*(6), 1206–1252.

Dickinson, H., Nicolson, D., Campbell, F., et al. (2006). Potassium supplementation for the management of primary hypertension in adults. *Cochrane Database of Systematic Reviews.* 2006, Issue 3. Art. No. CD004641. DOI: 10.1002/14651858.CD004641.pub2.

Dickinson, H., Nicolson, D., Campbell, F., et al. (2006). Magnesium supplementation for the management of essential hypertension in adults. *Cochrane Database of Systematic Reviews.* 2006, Issue 3. Art. No. CD004640. DOI: 10.1002/14651858.CD004640.pub2.

Freedman, D., Dietzm, W., Srinivasan, S., et al. (1999). The relation of overweight to cardiovascular risk factors among children and adolescents: The Bogalusa Heart Study. *Pediatrics, 6*(Pt 1), 1175–1182.

Kim, M. (2005). Pediatric hypertension. *Circulation, 111*(5), e97–e98.

Luma, G., and Spiotta, R. (2006). Hypertension in children and adolescents. *American Family Physician, 73*(9), 1158–1168.

National Cholesterol Education Program. (2002). Third report of the Expert Panel on Detection, Evaluation, and Treatment of High Blood Cholesterol in Adults (Adult Treatment Panel III) final report. NIH Publication 02–5215. Bethesda, MD: National Heart, Lung, and Blood Institute, National Cholesterol Education Program.

National High Blood Pressure Education Program Working Group on High Blood Pressure in Children and Adolescents. (2004). The Fourth Report on the Diagnosis, Evaluation, and Treatment of High Blood Pressure in Children and Adolescents. *Pediatrics, 114*(Suppl 2), 555–576.

Nelson, L. (2000). Nitroprusside toxicity. *Emergency Medicine, 32*(10), 71–75.

Richard, V., Galie, N., Sitbon, O., et al. (2003). From endothelin to endothelin receptor antagonism: An innovative approach to pulmonary artery hypertension. Scientific Update. *Cardiology.* Presented at the Satellite Symposium at the European Society of Cardiology Congress 2003. Vienna, Austria.

Suresh, S., Mahajan, P., and Kamat, D. (2005). Emergency management of pediatric hypertension. *Clinical Pediatrics, 44*(9), 739–745.

Varon, J., and Marik, P. (2000). The diagnosis and management of hypertensive crises. *Chest, 118*(1), 214–227.

Zannad, F. (2003). EPHESUS: Eplerenone post-acute myocardial infarction heart failure efficacy and survival study. Presented at the European Society of Cardiology Congress 2003. Vienna, Austria.

Antilipidemic Drugs

38

Diseases of the heart and the blood vessels are the principal cause of death in the industrialized countries of the world. The main diseases to which these deaths are attributed are coronary artery disease (CAD), cerebrovascular disease, and peripheral arterial disease.

In the United States, as well, more people die from heart and blood vessel disease than any other illness, including cancer. More than three fourths of the deaths resulting from cardiovascular disease can be attributed to hyperlipoproteinemia and the resultant atherosclerosis. There are several risk factors that contribute to CAD, including hyperlipidemia. Hyperlipidemia is a modifiable risk factor, and intervening to do so can reduce CAD.

Effective treatment for hyperlipoproteinemia must be directed at causative factors and prevention rather than reversal, because it is a slowly developing disorder. Clinical investigation has shown that vigorous drug therapy slows progression, and in some cases produces regression, of atherosclerotic lesions that lead to CAD. In addition, a recent meta-analysis of "statin" trials has shown that for every 10% reduction in total cholesterol, CAD mortality risk is reduced by 15% and total mortality risk, in general, by 11%.

HYPERLIPOPROTEINEMIA

EPIDEMIOLOGY AND ETIOLOGY

Hyperlipidemia is a general term for elevated concentrations of any or all of the lipids contained in plasma. *Hyperlipoproteinemia* is a more specific term referring to an excess of lipoproteins in the blood, a disorder of lipoprotein metabolism that may be acquired or hereditary. The acquired form occurs secondary to another disorder or as a result of environmental factors (e.g., diet, smoking). The hereditary form has been classified into five phenotypes on the basis of clinical features (the Frederickson-Levy classification system) (Table 38-1). They are essentially organized according to underlying cause and characteristic lipid and lipoprotein values. There is no known increase in the incidence of CAD with type I hyperlipoproteinemia. Types IIA, IIB, and III hyperlipoproteinemia are positively correlated with CAD. The risk of CAD from Types IV and V hyperlipoproteinemia is unclear at this time.

Hyperlipoproteinemia has reached epidemic proportions in the United States. Twenty percent of adults over age 20 have total serum cholesterol levels over 240 mg/dL, a level associated with greater risk for CAD. Recommended lipid levels are identified in Box 38-1. Risk factors associated with hyperlipoproteinemia are variables of age, sex, genetic factors, diet, exercise, weight, smoking, comorbid diseases, and specific drugs. Table 38-2 provides an overview of CAD risk factors.

PATHOPHYSIOLOGY

Cholesterol is a waxy, fatlike substance found in all animal fats and oils. Cholesterol enters the body in the form of dietary fat but is also manufactured by the liver from saturated fats. Cholesterol is an essential element contained in all human cell membranes; it is a structural component of steroid hormones and bile acids, myelin sheath, and vitamin D. Triglycerides (TGs) are important in helping to transfer energy from food into body cells. The liver produces about 1000 mg of cholesterol per day, enough for the body to maintain its required functions. The highest rate of cholesterol synthesis occurs between midnight and 5 AM.

The production of atherogenic lipoproteins and atheromatous plaque involves both an exogenous and an endogenous pathway (Fig. 38-1). The exogenous pathway involves absorption of dietary fat from the intestine to the tissue and back to the liver. Essentially no feedback mechanism exists within the exogenous pathway. The endogenous pathway, however, exerts feedback inhibition through receptors on cell surfaces. The endogenous pathway involves the formation of lipoproteins within the liver, their metabolism in other parts of the body, and the return of lipoproteins to the liver. In order to facilitate transportation of lipids from the liver through the blood stream to other tissues, cholesterol and TGs are bound to specialized proteins called *apoproteins*. The apoproteins move through the plasma, distributing and picking up lipid components.

The four major classes of apoproteins are A (apos A-I, A-II, A-III, A-IV), B (apos B-48, B-100), C (apos C-I, C-II, C-III), and E (Table 38-3). Apoproteins are responsible for metabolic interactions and sometimes act as catalysts for enzyme reactions (e.g., lipoprotein lipase) that allow the transfer of lipid components to and from cells. Other apoproteins serve as cellular receptors for the metabolism of lipoproteins.

Lipoproteins are classified according to density, a reflection of relative protein and lipid content: chylomicrons, very-low-density lipoprotein (VLDL), intermediate-density lipoprotein, low-density lipoprotein (LDL), and high-density lipoprotein (HDL) (Fig. 38-2).

Chylomicrons

Chylomicrons, the largest lipoproteins, are composed primarily of TGs. TGs are synthesized primarily from carbohydrates in the liver and cholesterol that has been solubilized by bile acids (exogenous pathway) and make up 85% to 95% of each chylomicron. Triglycerides are removed from the chylomicrons by the action of the enzyme lipoprotein lipase. Patients deficient in this enzyme or its cofactors (insulin and apo C-II) have very high TG levels and a greater risk of pancreatitis. Normally, chylomicrons are not present in the blood after a 12- to14-hour fast. Chylomicrons

TABLE 38-1 Classification of Hyperlipoproteinemias

Type	Common Name	Abnormality						CAD Risk	Etiology
		Chyl*	Chol†	VLDL‡	LDL§	HDL‖	TG		
I	Exogenous hypertriglyceridemia	↑	N	NC	↓	↓	↑↑	Not known	Dietary fat not cleared from plasma
IIA	Familial hypercholesterolemia	—	↑	NC	↑	↓	N	Yes	Autosomal dominant
IIB	Combined hyperlipidemia	—	↑	↑	↑	NC	↑	Yes	Autosomal dominant
III	Familial dysbeta-hyperlipoproteinemia	↑	↑	↑	↑¶	NC	↑	Yes	Autosomal recessive
IV	Endogenous hypertriglyceridemia	—	N or ↑	↑	NC	NC or ↓	↑	Unclear	Excessive carbohydrate intake
V	Mixed hypertriglyceridemia	↑	↑	↑	NC	NC or ↓	↑↑	Unclear	Possible metabolic defect

*Chylomicrons: 85%-95% triglycerides, 3%-5% cholesterol esters, 1% free cholesterol, 8% phospholipids, 1% protein.
†Cholesterol. Most cases of elevated cholesterol values are multifactorial: genetics, nutrition, and metabolic disease.
‡Very-low-density lipoproteins: 64%-80% triglycerides, 7%-14% cholesterol esters, 6% free cholesterol, 18% phospholipids, 7% protein.
§Low-density lipoproteins: 7%-10% triglycerides, 40%-50% cholesterol esters, 7% free cholesterol, 23% phospholipids, 21% protein.
‖High-density lipoproteins: 1%-7% triglycerides, 17%-20% cholesterol esters, 2% free cholesterol, 26% phospholipids, 46% protein.
¶Beta VLDL particles.
CAD, Coronary artery disease; Chol, cholesterol; Chyl, chylomicrons; HDL, high-density lipoprotein; LDL, low-density lipoprotein; N, normal; NC, no change; TG, triglycerides; VLDL, very-low-density lipoprotein.

BOX 38-1

ATP III Classification of Total Cholesterol, LDL, and HDL (mg/dL)

Total Cholesterol

<200	Desirable
200–239	Borderline high
>240	High

LDL Cholesterol

<100	Optimal
100–129	Near optimal or above optimal
130–159	Borderline high
160–189	High
>190	Very high

HDL Cholesterol

<40	Low
>60	High

Adapted from Grundy, S., Cleeman, J., Bairey, C., et al. (2004). Implications of recent clinical trials for the National Cholesterol Education Program Adult Treatment Panel III Guidelines. Journal of the American College of Cardiology, 44(3), 720–732.

have the lowest density of all lipoproteins; they can be found floating on a plasma specimen left in the refrigerator overnight.

Very-Low-Density Lipoproteins

VLDLs contain about 75% TGs and 25% cholesterol. VLDLs are the major carrier of endogenous TGs from the liver and intestines to capillary beds that service adipose and muscle cells. VLDLs also serve as acceptors of cholesterol transferred from HDL, possibly accounting for the inverse relationship between HDL cholesterol and VLDLs. As the TGs are removed from VLDLs, the remnants become progressively smaller, with a higher percentage of cholesterol (45%), and are now referred to as an intermediate density lipoprotein (IDL).

IDLs are short-lived lipoproteins that are converted to LDLs or are taken up by the LDL receptors on the liver. IDLs are now made up of about 70% cholesterol. In normally healthy individuals, IDLs are not found in significant amounts.

TABLE 38-2 Risk Factors for CAD Other Than High LDL Levels

Variables	Comments
POSITIVE RISK FACTORS*	
Males over age 45 years	Men have higher total cholesterol levels than women until age 50 years
Females over age 55 without estrogen replacement	Women have a higher proportion of cholesterol as HDL than men. There is an increase in LDL levels with the onset of menopause.
Definitive MI or sudden death in first-degree male relative before age 55 or in female first-degree relative before age 65	Monogenic (a characteristic controlled by one gene or a pair of genes) mechanisms account for a small fraction of patients with hyperlipidemia. Familial hypercholesterolemia affects 5% of general population.
Current cigarette smoking (particularly if more than 10 cigarettes a day)	Reduces HDL cholesterol levels
An HDL less than 40 mg/dL	Proven to contribute to CAD
Treated or untreated systolic blood pressure over 140 mm Hg or diastolic pressure over 90 mm Hg	Other components also contribute to development of HTN and thus increase the risk for CAD related to hyperlipidemia.
Diet high in saturated fats	Raises total and LDL cholesterol levels
Treated or untreated diabetes mellitus	Elevates total cholesterol, TGs, and LDL levels
NEGATIVE RISK FACTOR†	
An HDL level over 60 mg/dL	Proven to be protective against CAD

*Obesity is not listed as a separate risk factor, because it operates through a variety of other risk factors that are included (e.g., HTN, hyperlipidemia, low HDL levels, and diabetes). Being overweight or obese elevates triglyceride levels more than cholesterol levels and decreases HDL levels. Both obesity and inactivity are targets for intervention.
†Net risk status is determined by adding the number of positive risk factors and then subtracting one risk factor if HDL level exceeds 60 mg/dL. High HDL levels protect against CAD.
CAD, Coronary heart disease; HDL, high-density lipoprotein; HTN, hypertension; LDL, low-density lipoprotein; MI, myocardial infarction; TGs, triglycerides.
Adapted from the Summary of the Third Report of the National Cholesterol Education Program Adult Treatment Panel. (2001). National Heart, Lung, and Blood Institute, National Institutes of Health. NIH Pub. No. 01–3670 and the ATP III update from Grundy, S., Cleeman, J., Bairey, C. et al. (2004). Implications of recent clinical trials for the National Cholesterol Education Program Adult Treatment Panel III Guidelines. Journal of the American College of Cardiology, 44(3), 720–732.

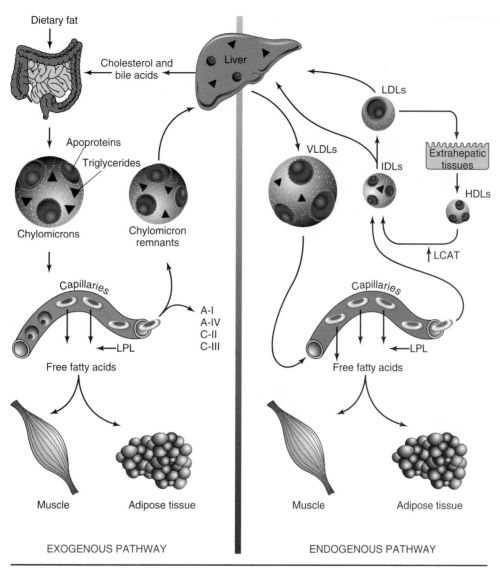

FIGURE 38-1 Metabolic Pathways for Lipoproteins. The exogenous and endogenous pathways that allow transportation of lipids, in the form of plasma-soluble lipoproteins, from the intestine and liver to body tissues and back to the liver. Apoproteins, which bind with cholesterol and triglycerides to form lipoproteins, sometimes act as catalysts for enzymatic reactions. Apoproteins A-1, A-IV, C-II, and C-III activate lipolytic enzymes to remove lipids from lipoproteins. Lecithin-cholesterol acyltransferase (LCAT) converts high-density lipoprotein (HDL) to intermediate-density lipoprotein (IDL) and low-density lipoprotein (LDL) for return to the liver. LPL, Lipoprotein lipase; VLDL, very-low-density lipoprotein.

Low-Density Lipoproteins

LDLs are responsible for supplying cholesterol to the tissues and therefore carry proportionally more cholesterol than other lipoproteins. High levels of LDLs, "the bad cholesterol," have been clearly implicated in atherogenesis. The core of LDLs is composed almost entirely of cholesterol and a relatively small amount of TGs (7% to 10%). Although most LDL receptors are found in the liver, extrahepatic tissues (e.g., endothelial cells, lymphoid cells, smooth muscle cells, and adrenal glands) use the receptor-dependent pathways to obtain the cholesterol needed for the synthesis of cell membranes and hormones. The extrahepatic tissues regulate cholesterol uptake by adding or deleting LDL receptors.

LDL levels are increased in persons who consume large amounts of saturated fats or cholesterol, have defects in either their LDL receptors or in the structure of the LDL apoprotein apo B, or have a familial form of increased LDLs. LDL can become trapped in the arterial vasculature at extremely high

TABLE 38-3 Major Classes of Lipoproteins

Lipoprotein Class	Major Lipid	Major Apoproteins
Chylomicrons and chylomicron remnants	Dietary TGs	A-I, A-II, B-48, C-I, C-II, C-III, E
Very-low-density lipoproteins	Endogenous TGs	B-48, C-I, C-II, C-III, E
Intermediate-density lipoproteins	Cholesterol esters, TGs	B-100, C-III, E
Low-density lipoproteins	Cholesterol esters	B-100
High-density lipoproteins	Cholesterol esters	A-1, A-II

TGs, Triglycerides.

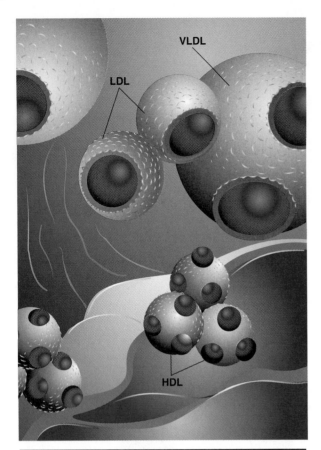

FIGURE 38-2 Density and Function of Lipoproteins. Lipoproteins are classified according to density, which reflects protein and lipid content. Lipids are transported in plasma as components of these particles. The larger VLDL particles contain a higher percentage of lipids and are less dense, whereas the smaller HDL particles have fewer lipids and a higher percentage of protein, and are denser. VLDLs and LDLs transport cholesterol and TGs away from the liver to organs and tissues. HDL particles move cholesterol toward the liver and away from tissues.

levels. The association of serum cholesterol with CAD is predominantly a reflection of LDL levels. Reducing LDL cholesterol remains the cornerstone of hyperlipidemia therapy.

Many of the mechanisms by which LDL increases the risk for atherosclerosis occur beneath the arterial wall. After traversing the tunica intima, LDL is oxidized by endothelial and smooth muscle cells. Oxidation of LDLs results in an accumulation of circulating monocytes, which take up the modified LDLs via alternative scavenger receptors. The monocytes become lipid-filled macrophages that further oxidize LDLs. Continued oxidation of LDLs appears to inhibit macrophage motility, and the first visible lesion of atherosclerosis, the "fatty streak," appears. The return of LDLs from peripheral tissues to the liver involves HDLs.

High-Density Lipoproteins

HDLs are synthesized in the liver and the intestine. HDLs contain relatively little lipid and much protein, and thus are the smallest and most dense of the lipoproteins. The primary function of HDL is to remove LDL from peripheral cells and to remove TGs that result from the degradation of

chylomicrons and VLDL particles. The HDL then transports these particles to the liver for metabolism. For this reason, HDLs are often referred to as "good cholesterol." The "reverse transport" system from the periphery to the liver may explain why patients with very high HDL levels have a lower risk for CAD, even if LDL levels are elevated. There are two subfractions of HDL: HDL_2 and HDL_3. HDL_2 levels are the single most powerful indicators of CAD risk. In addition to the protective effect of reverse transport, HDLs may be beneficial because they inhibit binding of LDL to matrix proteins, oxidation of LDL, and receptor uptake of oxidized LDL. Women have higher levels of HDL than men, in part because of higher estrogen levels. Exercise increases HDLs, whereas obesity, hypertriglyceridemia, and smoking are associated with lower HDL levels. Low HDL cholesterol is a strong independent predictor of CAD.

Triglycerides

Hypertriglyceridemia is associated with increased risk of CAD events; however, the association is not as strong as that of LDL cholesterol. Because elevated TGs may be considered an independent CAD risk factor, some suggest that some TG-rich lipoproteins are atherogenic.

Lipoprotein (a)

"Lipoprotein little a" (Lp[a]) is an LDL-like lipoprotein that contains additional apolipoprotein, apo A. Lp(a)'s unique structural features suggest that this lipoprotein has both thrombogenic and atherogenic potentials. Lp(a) associates with the vessel wall and inhibits binding of plasminogen to the cell surface. This association reduces the extent of plasmin generation, thereby interfering with clot lysis. Although the physiologic role of Lp(a) is not known, it has been speculated to deliver cholesterol to cells at wound sites, a function that may become pathologic when plasma levels of Lp(a) are high. Efficient delivery of cholesterol to cells requires the presence of receptors to mediate lipoprotein endocytosis; the identity of endocytic receptors responsible for the uptake of Lp(a) is a topic of current debate. Lp(a) has been noted to bind to the LDL receptor, and like LDL, it is removed more rapidly from plasma. Experiments indicate that the LDL receptor can mediate cellular catabolism of Lp(a). Drugs that increase LDL receptor activity do not appear to lower Lp(a) plasma levels.

Consider screening for Lp(a) when any of the following circumstances exist: (1) a patient or family history of premature atherosclerotic heart disease, (2) familial history of hyperlipidemia, (3) established atherosclerotic heart disease with a normal routine lipid profile, (4) hyperlipidemia refractory to therapy, and (5) history of recurrent arterial stenosis.

Atherogenesis

Atherogenesis and subsequent atherosclerosis is characterized by development of cholesterol-based lesions in the blood vessel wall. Atherosclerosis primarily affects larger arteries, including coronary arteries.

Atherogenesis begins with oxidation of LDLs in the arterial intimal space, by an as yet undefined process. As LDLs accumulate, circulating monocytes attach to the endothelial lining and penetrate between the endothelial cells into the subendothelial spaces. Upon entry into the subendothelial space, the monocytes form macrophages, which then ingest LDLs.

Macrophages, in particular, have a high affinity for oxidized LDL. Thus, by preventing the oxidation of LDL, antioxidants such as vitamin E (see Chapter 10) may be beneficial in preventing CAD. However, the efficacy of antioxidants remains unproven.

As macrophages ingest oxidized LDLs, they are converted to foam cells and form the fatty streak, the initial lesion of atherogenesis. Fatty-streak formation begins in the midteens, with the lesions growing as the person ages.

Oxidized LDLs and macrophages also act in other ways to promote the progression of atherogenic lesions once the fatty streak has been formed. Oxidized LDL acts as a chemotactic agent, recruiting other circulating monocytes and preventing macrophages from leaving subendothelial spaces. Macrophages produce chemotactic factors as well as growth factors (e.g., tumor growth factor beta [TGF-β]). The growth factors cause proliferation of smooth muscle cells from the intima media into the fatty streak, leading to the formation of fibrous plaque. Fibrous plaques protrude into the arterial lumen, compromising blood flow.

As foam cells grow, the endothelium stretches and becomes damaged. The damaged areas attract platelets, and clots are formed. In some cases, the fissures incorporate the thrombi inside the plaque and heal. Complicated lesions result over time from multiple episodes of damage and healing. The formation of complicated lesions is the primary cause of acute cardiovascular events. In some instances, however, rupture of a small, unstable plaque may cause the formation of a single large clot that entirely obstructs the vessel. The complicated, fibrous plaques of most concern for rupture are those that have a large lipid core and a thin fibrous cap (the larger of smooth muscle cells directly over the lipid core). Large plaques that have a strong fibrous cap are less likely to rupture because they are more stable.

PHARMACOTHERAPEUTIC OPTIONS

Several drug therapies are currently available in the United States for the treatment of hyperlipoproteinemia. First-line therapy uses hydroxymethylglutaryl coenzyme A (HMG-CoA) reductase inhibitors. Second-line therapy may use a cholesterol absorption inhibitor, bile acid resins; or as a third line, fibric acid derivatives and niacin may be used. All of these drugs reduce LDL levels. In some patients, a combination of drugs may be required.

HMG-CoA Reductase Inhibitors

◆ atorvastatin (Lipitor); ◆ Lipitor
◆ fluvastatin (Lescol); ◆ Lescol
◆ lovastatin (lovastatin, Mevacor); ◆ lovastatin, Mevacor, Altoprev
◆ pravastatin (Pravachol); ◆ pravastatin, Pravachol
◆ rosuvastatin (Crestor); ◆ Crestor
◆ simvastatin (simvastatin); ◆ simvastatin, Zocor

▓ Indications

The HMG-CoA reductase inhibitors (otherwise known as "statins") are the most heavily prescribed lipid-lowering drugs in the United States because of their ability to lower cholesterol and LDL by 30% to 55%, and more importantly, the associated morbidity and mortality rates. There is emerging evidence of their ability to affect plaque progression, even

when used alone. HDL levels increase 8% to 23% in response to these drugs.

▓ Pharmacodynamics

These drugs are selective inhibitors of the enzyme HMG-CoA reductase. HMG-CoA reductase is an enzyme required in the initial and rate-limiting step in cholesterol synthesis. They lower total cholesterol, LDL, and apo B lipoprotein levels by inhibiting HMG-CoA reductase and thus cholesterol synthesis in the liver.

The action of statins goes beyond inhibiting endogenous cholesterol synthesis. The reduction in cholesterol levels causes upregulation of the LDL receptor, which leads to increased clearance of LDLs from the blood stream. As greater catabolism of LDL occurs, plasma concentrations of LDL fall, and less LDL is available.

Aside from lipid-lowering action, statins demonstrate additional activity in the prevention of atherosclerosis. According to research, it is believed that statins may reduce cardiovascular events via four proposed mechanisms: improving endothelial function; modulating inflammatory responses; maintaining plaque stability; and preventing thrombus formation (Rosenson and Tangey, 1998).

▓ Pharmacokinetics

Statins differ in their bioavailability and in the effect of food on their absorption. Food reduces the bioavailability of these drugs (except lovastatin and simvastatin) but not their efficacy. All of these drugs are subject to significant first-pass effects (60%) by the liver.

Maximum plasma levels for most statins are seen in approximately 1 to two 2 hours, although their cholesterol-lowering effects may not be noted for several weeks (Table 38-4). Plasma concentrations are lower with evening than with morning dosing of the drug; however, LDL reduction is the same regardless of the time of day the drug is taken.

Metabolites of these drugs are also active reductase inhibitors. The drugs and their metabolites are primarily eliminated in the bile following hepatic and extrahepatic biotransformation. Small amounts (less than 20%) of the unchanged drugs are eliminated in the urine.

▓ Adverse Effects and Contraindications

The statins are well tolerated by most patients, and long-term therapy does not appear to have any serious risks. Headache and gastrointestinal (GI) complaints are the most common adverse effects (noted by <10% of patients) of the statins, although they are usually transient and mild. In addition, asymptomatic elevations in liver function tests (LFTs) may occur. Hepatotoxicity has been reported in a small percentage of patients taking statins, although jaundice and other clinical signs were absent. Cautious use of these drugs is warranted in patients with liver disease and in those who consume alcohol to excess. Possible adverse consequences of long-term suppression of cholesterol synthesis are not known.

Other adverse effects of statins include muscle weakness and pain, which may be a sign of myopathy; much of this is dosage related. If myopathy is suspected, check the patient's creatinine phosphokinase (CK) level, and stop the drug if levels exceed 10 times the upper limits. **If the statin drug is not withdrawn in the presence of myopathy, the myopathy**

CARDIOVASCULAR

PHARMACOKINETICS
TABLE 38-4 Antilipidemic Drugs

Drug	Route	Onset	Peak	Duration	PB (%)	t½	BioA (%)
HMG-CoA REDUCTASE INHIBITORS							
atorvastatin	PO	1 hr	1–2 hr	UA	>98	20 hr	12–14
fluvastatin	PO	Slow	UA	4–6 wk	>98	UA	29
lovastatin (prodrug)	PO	3 days	2–4 hr; 4–6 wk†	UA	>95	1–2 hr	<5
pravastatin	PO	1 hr	1–1.5 hr; wk†	48 hr	40–55	77 hr	10–26
rosuvastatin	PO	UA	3–5 hr	UA	88	19 hr	20
simvastatin (prodrug)	PO	1 hr	1.3–2.4 hr	UA	>95	UA	<5
CHOLESTEROL ABSORPTION INHIBITOR							
ezetimibe	PO	1–2 hr	4–12 hr	UA	>90	22 hr	UA
BILE ACID RESINS							
cholestyramine	PO	24–48 hr	1–3 wk	2–4 wk	NA	UA	NA
colesevelam	PO	Immed	2 wk	UA	NA	UA	NA
colestipol	PO	24–48 hr	4 wk	4 wk	NA	UA	NA
FIBRIC ACID DERIVATIVES							
gemfibrozil	PO	1–2 hr; 2–5 days*	4 wk*	Months	95	1.3–1.5 hr	UA
fenofibrate	PO	Varies	3–6 hr	Weeks	99	10–35 hr	42
OTHER ANTILIPEMIC DRUGS							
nicotinic acid	PO	Hr–days	1 hr; UA‡	UA	UA	1 hr	UA

*Time for gemfibrozil's onset and reduction of triglyceride–VLDL levels, respectively.
†The biphasic peaks of lovastatin and pravastatin, respectively.
‡Peak drug levels of niacin are reached in 1 hour, however, its peak effects on lipids is unknown.
BioA, Bioavailability; *HMG-CoA*, hydroxymethylglutaryl coenzyme A; *NA*, not applicable; *PB*, protein binding; *PO*, by mouth; *UA*, unavailable

progresses to *rhabdomyolysis.* **The principal result of this process is acute renal failure due to accumulation of muscle breakdown products in the blood stream.** Treatment is with intravenous (IV) fluids and dialysis, if necessary.

Cross-sensitivity has been reported with statins. They are also contraindicated for use in patients with active liver disease. Cautious use is warranted in patients with a history of liver disease, alcoholism, severe acute infection, hypotension, major surgery, trauma, uncontrolled seizure activity, visual disturbances, myopathy, or severe metabolic, endocrine, or electrolyte disorders. There is no compelling reason to use these drugs during pregnancy. Advise women of child-bearing age about the potential for fetal harm and warn them against becoming pregnant while taking these drugs. Statins are also contraindicated for use during lactation.

▥ Drug Interactions

Niacin, erythromycin, gemfibrozil, fenofibrate, cyclosporin, and azole antifungal drugs interact with statins to raise the risk of myopathy and rhabdomyolysis (Table 38-5). Since pravastatin biotransformation is not dependent on CYP 3A4 or CYP 2C9 isoenzymes, there is much lower risk for drug interactions; this is actually the drug of choice for patients taking cyclosporin. Warfarin and digoxin doses may have to be adjusted owing to their increased serum drug levels. When a statin is coadministered with an antacid, the plasma concentration of the inhibitor is reduced but not its ability to reduce LDL levels.

▥ Dosage Regimen

The dosage for statins varies with the specific drug (Table 38-6). Fluvastatin, pravastatin, and simvastatin are taken once daily at bedtime. These three drugs may be administered without regard to food. Lovastatin, on the other hand, should be administered with food, because an empty stomach decreases absorption by

as much as 30%. If needed, the dosages of these drugs can be increased at 4-week intervals.

▥ Lab Considerations

Check LFT values before starting therapy, at 6 and 12 weeks after starting or titrating therapy, and periodically thereafter. Discontinue treatment if two consecutive LFTs show values 3 times the upper limits of normal. Statins may also raise alkaline phosphatase and bilirubin levels.

Cholesterol Absorption Inhibitor
◆ ezetimibe (Zetia); ✦ Zetia

▥ Indications

Ezetimibe is used as an adjunct to diet and a statin in reducing elevated total cholesterol, LDL, and TG levels, and to increase HDL levels. Research has shown it reduces these parameters more than diet or each drug alone. Risk of cardiovascular morbidity and mortality has not been established for ezetimibe use, whether administered alone or concurrently with a statin. Ezetimibe is available in combination with simvastatin as Vytorin.

▥ Pharmacodynamics

The mechanism of action of ezetimibe differs from those of other classes of cholesterol-reducing compounds. Ezetimibe is concentrated at the brush border of the small intestine where it inhibits the absorption of cholesterol, thereby leading to a reduction in the delivery of intestinal cholesterol to the liver. Hepatic cholesterol stores are thus decreased, and cholesterol clearance from the blood stream is increased; this mechanism is distinct from and complementary to that of the statins.

In a study of hypercholesterolemic patients, ezetimibe inhibited intestinal cholesterol absorption by 54%, compared

DRUG INTERACTIONS
TABLE 38-5 Antilipidemic Drugs

Drug	Interactive Drugs	Interaction
HMG-COA REDUCTASE INHIBITORS		
All statins	Azole antifungals, cyclosporin, erythromycin, niacin, Fibrates	Increases risk for myopathy, rhabdomyolysis
atorvastatin, fluvastatin	cholestyramine, colestipol	Additive cholesterol-lowering effects
atorvastatin, simvastatin	digoxin, warfarin	Increases levels of interactive drug
fluvastatin	cimetidine, omeprazole, ranitidine	Increases fluvastatin levels
CHOLESTEROL ABSORPTION INHIBITOR		
ezetimibe	cholestyramine	Decreases AUC of ezetimibe
	gemfibrozil	Increases ezetimibe concentration
	Antacids	Decreases C_{max} by 30%
	cholestyramine	Decreases AUC by up to 80%
	cyclosporin	Increases AUC
BILE ACID RESINS		
cholestyramine, colesevelam, colestipol	acetaminophen, amiodarone, Antibiotics, Cardiac glycosides, Corticosteroids, Fat-soluble vitamins, folic acid, Iron preparations, methotrexate, naproxen, Oral anticoagulants, phenobarbital, piroxicam, propranolol, Thiazide diuretics, thyroxine, ursodiol	Decreases absorption of interactive drug
FIBRIC ACID DERIVATIVES		
gemfibrozil	warfarin	Increases effects of interactive drug
	lovastatin	Increases risk of myositis, myalgia
fenofibrate	Insulins, Sulfonylureas, warfarin	Increases effects of interactive drug
	probenecid	Increases risk for toxicity to fenofibrate
	rifampin	Decreases effects of fenofibrate
OTHER ANTILIPEMIC DRUGS		
nicotinic acid	All statins	Increases risk of myopathy, rhabdomyolysis
	guanethidine, guanadrel	Additive hypotension
	probenecid, sulfinpyrazone	Large doses may decrease uricosuric effects of interactive drugs

AUC, Area under the curve; *C_max,* maximum concentration; *HMG-CoA,* hydroxymethylglutaryl coenzyme A.

with placebo. There are no clinically important effects on plasma concentrations of the fat-soluble vitamins A, D, and E resulting from ezetimibe use. Ezetimibe also does not impair adrenocorticosteroid hormone production.

Pharmacokinetics
Ezetimibe is absorbed and extensively conjugated to a pharmacologically active metabolite following oral administration. Biotransformation of ezetimibe occurs primarily in the small intestine and the liver via glucuronide conjugation (a phase II reaction), with ensuing biliary and renal excretion.

Adverse Effects and Contraindications
The more common adverse effects of ezetimibe used as monotherapy include fatigue, back and joint pain, abdominal pain and diarrhea, sinusitis, viral infections, and cough. Myopathy and rhabdomyolysis are rare with monotherapy. When ezetimibe is combined with a statin drug (as in Vytorin), the adverse effects include fatigue, upper respiratory infections and headache, back pain and myalgias, abdominal pain and diarrhea. Ezetimibe is a pregnancy category C drug.

Drug Interactions
Ezetimibe is neither an inhibitor nor an inducer of the CYP450 enzymes, and it is improbable that ezetimibe will affect the biotransformation of drugs influenced by these enzymes. Ezetimibe should be given either 2 hours before or 4 hours after administration of a bile acid resin.

Dosage Regimen
Place the patient on a standard cholesterol-lowering meal plan before starting ezetimibe, and continue this diet during treatment with ezetimibe. Concomitant food administration, whether high-fat or nonfat meals, does not have an effect on the extent of ezetimibe absorption.

Bile Acid Resins
- cholestyramine (Questran, Questran Light, Cholybar); ◆ cholestyramine, Questran
- colestipol (Colestid); ◆ Colestid
- colesevelam (WelChol); ◆ WelChol

Indications
Bile acid resins are approved for the treatment of type II hypercholesterolemia. When used in conjunction with a low-cholesterol diet, they reduce LDL levels by 15% to 30%. They are useful for patients who have some risk for CAD but in whom diet therapy alone has failed to reduce LDL levels. By lowering plasma LDL levels, the bile acid resins significantly decrease morbidity and mortality from CAD. The resins tend to cause a transient rise in TG levels already over 250 mg/dL and are therefore not particularly useful in the treatment of mixed lipid disorders.

DOSAGE

TABLE 38-6 Antilipidemic Drugs

Drug/Type	Dosage	Implications
HMG-COA REDUCTASE INHIBITORS		
atorvastatin	*Adult:* 10 mg PO daily. Range: 10–80 mg/day. Max: 80 mg/day	Once-daily dose is taken at HS.
fluvastatin	*Adult:* Initial, 20 mg PO daily. Maintenance: 20–40 mg/day PO. Max: 40 mg PO twice daily	Once-daily dose is taken at HS.
lovastatin	*Adult:* 20 mg PO daily. Increase at 4-wk intervals to max of 80 mg/day in single or divided doses.	Once-daily dose is taken with the evening meal.
pravastatin	*Adult:* 10–20 mg PO daily. Increase at weekly intervals to a max of 80 mg/day.	Older adults start at 10 mg PO daily.
rosuvastatin	*Adult:* 10 mg PO daily. Increase every 2–4 wk to max of 40 mg/day.	10 mg/day if also on gemfibrozil, 5 mg to start if close to LDL goal, hypothyroid, or >65 yrs or Asian descent.
simvastatin	*Adult:* 5–10 mg PO daily. Increase at 4-wk intervals to a max of 80 mg/day.	Start with 20 mg/day for patients with LDL values >190 mg/dL; 5 mg/day if also on cyclosporin.
BILE ACID RESINS		
cholestyramine	*Adult:* 4 grams PO twice daily. Max: 24 grams/day. May dose 1–6 times daily *Child >6 yr and Adolescent:* 80 mg/kg PO 3 times daily. Increase to 8 grams/day in 2 or more divided doses.	Take before meals. Pediatric dosage typically based on cholesterol level rather than body weight. Increase dosage as needed and tolerated.
colesevelam	*Adult:* 6–7 tablets PO daily –or– 4–6 tablets if combined with statin.	1 tablet = 625 mg. Take in divided doses with meals, follow dose with liquid.
colestipol	*Adult:* 2–16 grams PO in divided doses once-twice daily. Increase 2–4 grams every 1–2 mo.	Take at separate times from other drugs. Mix granular formulation in over 4 oz liquid.
FIBRIC ACID DERIVATIVES		
gemfibrozil	*Adult:* 600 mg PO twice daily. Max: 1200 mg daily	Do not confuse with Levbid or Lorabid.
fenofibrate	*Adult:* 100 mg PO in divided doses.	Dose may vary depending on formulation used.
OTHER ANTILIPEMIC DRUGS		
niacin	*Adult:* IR formulation: 50–100 mg PO twice daily for 7 days. Increase gradually by doubling dose every wk up to 1–1.5 grams/day in 2–3 divided doses. Max: 3 grams/day *Adult:* ER formulation: 500 mg PO daily in divided doses twice daily for 1 wk. Increase to 500 mg PO twice daily. Maintenance: 2 grams/day	Once-daily dose is taken after the evening meal. **Take one adult aspirin 30 min before dose of niacin, eat the evening meal, and then take niacin dose to minimize hot flush.**
omega-3-acid ethyl esters (Lovaza)	*Adult:* *Reduce TG:* 2–4 grams/day PO *Cardiovascular health:* 1 gram/day PO *Rheumatoid arthritis:* >3 grams/day PO	Each 1-gram capsule contains 465 mg of EPA and 375 mg of DHA. Take with meals; withdraw therapy if no response in 2 mo.
red yeast rice	*Adults:* 600–1200 mg standardized extract PO 2–4 times daily	Not recommended for persons under 20 years of age.

DHA, Docosahexaenoic acid; *EPA,* eicosapentaenoic acid; *ER,* extended-release; *HMG-CoA,* hydroxymethylglutaryl coenzyme A; *HS,* bedtime; *IR,* immediate-release; *LDL,* low-density lipoprotein; *TG,* triglycerides.

▥ *Pharmacodynamics*

Bile acid resins are anion-exchange resins that reduce LDL levels by binding bile salts in exchange for chloride ions. These drugs form an insoluble complex with bile acids in the intestine. The bile acid–drug complex prevents the reabsorption of the bile acids, thus increasing their elimination. In an attempt to compensate for the loss of bile salts, the liver raises the rate of bile acid synthesis.

The ability of liver cells to increase their numbers of LDL receptors is vital for the therapeutic effects of bile acid resins to be realized. To benefit from the presence of LDL, liver cells increase the number of LDL receptors, thereby enlarging their capacity for LDL uptake. The resultant increase in LDL uptake is the mechanism responsible for lowering serum LDL levels. Unfortunately, this process also leads to increased production of VLDL particles. As a result, TG levels rise, particularly in patients whose baseline TG levels are already elevated. Patients genetically incapable of increasing the number of LDL receptors on their liver cells are unable to benefit from bile resins.

▥ *Pharmacokinetics*

The onset of hypocholesterolemic effects occurs in 24 to 48 hours, with peak action in 1 to 3 weeks (see Table 38-4). Once bound to the bile acids, the drugs are eliminated in the feces. The duration of action for the bile acid resins is 2 to 4 weeks. The dose-response curves for bile acid resins are not linear, and when given in doses above the maximum recommended doses, these drugs have demonstrated little additional cholesterol-lowering effect.

▥ *Adverse Effects and Contraindications*

Because bile acid resins are not absorbed, there are no systemic adverse effects. However, bile acid resin therapy is not without problems. Resins are insoluble powders with the consistency of fine sand. They must be mixed with fluids to be ingested. They tend to cause bloating, nausea, indigestion, flatulence, and constipation. Because of the exchange of chloride ions for bile acids, greater chloride absorption may result in hyperchloremic metabolic acidosis. Further, excess fat may appear in the stool because of the binding of bile acids by the resins and the resultant loss of their emulsifying action. Although it is possible that bile acid resin therapy may interfere with the absorption of fat-soluble vitamins (i.e., A, D, E, K), there is some disagreement as to whether vitamin supplementation is warranted.

Bile acid resins are contraindicated for use in patients with complete or partial biliary obstruction. Exercise caution when using them in patients with steatorrhea or preexisting constipation. Although these drugs can be used in the treatment of hypercholesterolemia in children and pregnant women, clear-cut data as to the safety of their long-term use in children or their use during pregnancy and lactation are not available.

Drug Interactions

Bile acid resins diminish the absorption of many orally administered drugs (see Table 38-5). The resulting decrease in absorption of antibiotics, cardiac glycosides, folic acid, and warfarin reduces their effects. The effect of bile acid resins on many other drugs has not been well studied.

Dosage Regimen

For maximal efficacy, bile acid resins should be taken with the largest meal of the day if once-daily dosing is used (see Table 38-6). Cholestyramine comes as a powder and colestipol as granules. These formulations should be mixed with water, noncarbonated beverages, soups, or applesauce. The resins are not to be taken dry because of the risk of esophageal irritation. Tablets are swallowed whole. Drugs such as thyroid hormones, antibiotics, and fat-soluble vitamins should be taken at least 1 hour before or 4 hours after the bile acid resin because of the resins ability to bind with the drugs and decrease their bioavailability.

Lab Considerations

Evaluate serum cholesterol and TG levels at the start of therapy and periodically thereafter. Transient elevations of alkaline phosphatase, aspartate transaminase (AST), and chloride levels have been reported. Decreases in serum calcium, sodium, and potassium levels may occur, but they are not severe enough for the drug to be discontinued. Bile acid resins can also cause prolonged prothrombin and international normalized ratio (INR) times.

Fibric Acid Derivatives

◆ fenofibrate (Antara, Lipofen, Lofibra, Tricor, Triglide); ◆ fenofibrate, Antara, Tricor, Triglide, Lofriba, Lipofen
◆ gemfibrozil (Lopid); ◆ gemfibrozil, Lopid

Indications

Fibric acid derivatives are not considered first-line cholesterol-lowering drugs because they have minimal effects on LDL levels. However, gemfibrozil is used for treatment of patients with TG concentrations exceeding 750 mg/dL who have not responded to dietary therapies. Gemfibrozil decreases serum TG levels by up to 60%, with variable reductions in total cholesterol. Gemfibrozil does not reduce LDL levels. Although gemfibrozil has minimal effects on LDL, fenofibrate decreases LDL levels by up to 20%. High TG levels pose a risk not only for atherogenesis but also more often for the development of pancreatitis.

Pharmacodynamics

The exact mechanism of action of fibric acid derivatives is unclear, but the principal action appears to result from the stimulation of extrahepatic lipoprotein lipase, which enhances the breakdown of VLDL to LDL. There is no explanation for how gemfibrozil raises HDL levels.

Pharmacokinetics

The onset of VLDL-TG reduction from gemfibrozil takes 2 to 5 days, although the drug reaches peak blood levels in 1 to 2 hours (see Table 38-4). Biotransformation takes place in the liver, with elimination in the urine. Fenofibrate absorption is increased when taken with food.

Adverse Effects and Contraindications

Fibric acid derivatives are generally well tolerated. The most common adverse effects are GI related and include epigastric distress, nausea and vomiting, dyspepsia, flatulence, and constipation. Flulike symptoms, including myopathy and arthralgias, are also common. The incidence of myopathy increases with concurrent use of statins or niacin. Contraindications to the use of fibric acid derivatives are hepatic or renal disease and primary biliary cirrhosis. Use these drugs cautiously in patients with a history of peptic ulcer disease.

Drug Interactions

As with other antilipemic drugs, there are interactions with fibric acid derivatives (see Table 38-5). The action of warfarin is enhanced in the presence of gemfibrozil and fenofibrate; thus it is wise to monitor liver function and prothrombin times periodically when the two drugs are used concurrently. Increased bleeding tendencies have been noted if oral anticoagulants are given with fenofibrate. A dosage reduction of as much as 50% is often required.

Dosage Regimen

Gemfibrozil is taken twice daily, 30 minutes before meals (see Table 38-6). Fenofibrate now has many formulations, so dosing is dependent on which formulation is used (e.g., Tricor dose is 145 mg/day).

Lab Considerations

As with other cholesterol-lowering drugs, hepatotoxicity can occur, thus monitor LFTs at 6 and 12 weeks after starting therapy and then periodically thereafter. And as with other cholesterol-lowering drugs, stop the drug if LFT values increase to more than 2 to 3 times the upper limit of normal.

Fibric acid derivatives increase the results of liver function, creatine phosphokinase, bromosulfophthalein (BSP), and thymol turbidity tests. In addition, gemfibrozil raises glucose levels and may cause a mild reduction in hemoglobin, hematocrit, and white blood cell measurements. Gemfibrozil may also decrease serum potassium concentration.

Niacin

◆ niacin (nicotinic acid, Vitamin B$_3$; Niaspan, Nia-bid, Niacor, Nicobid, Nicolar, Nicotinex, Slo-Niacin); ◆ Vitamin B$_3$ Flush Free, Niaspan

Indications

The lipid-lowering effects of nicotinic acid (niacin) were shown more than 30 years ago. Because it lowers both LDL

CARDIOVASCULAR

and VLDL, niacin has been used successfully in a variety of hyperlipidemic conditions. It is the drug of choice for patients at risk for pancreatitis and for those with concurrent elevations of LDL and VLDL. Niacin reduces plasma TG levels by 30% to 40% and total cholesterol levels by 15% to 20%, respectively. LDL levels may be reduced 15% to 20% or more, whereas HDL levels may be increased by up to 35%.

Pharmacodynamics

The mechanism of action of niacin is unclear; however, this water-soluble vitamin (B_3) is incorporated into nicotinamide coenzymes, which are required for many oxidative-reduction reactions to reduce VLDL synthesis in the liver, inhibit lipolysis in adipose tissues, and increase lipoprotein lipase activity. Both coenzymes act as hydrogen carriers for glycogenolysis, tissue respiration, and lipid metabolism.

The action of niacin in lowering lipid levels is independent of its vitamin activity. It also acts as a vasodilator in pharmacotherapeutic doses (more than 250 mg/day). The mechanism by which it lowers cholesterol levels and affects vasodilation is unclear at this time. However, the greater clearance of chylomicrons and VLDL from the plasma decreases LDL and an increases HDL. Central to the action of niacin is its ability to inhibit the release of free fatty acids from fatty tissue stores.

Pharmacokinetics

Niacin is well absorbed in the intestine following oral administration. It is widely distributed following rapid conversion to niacinamide. (Niacinamide has no effect on lipid levels.) When it is taken by mouth, peak drug concentrations are reached within 1 hour, but the time to peak effects on lipid levels is unknown (see Table 38-4). The half-life of niacin in plasma is approximately 1 hour. Large doses of niacin are eliminated unchanged in the urine.

Adverse Effects and Contraindications

Many patients are unable to tolerate the drug-induced intense flushing and pruritus of the trunk, the face, and the arms. The flushing is mediated by the release of prostaglandin E_1 and histamine and can be partially inhibited by the ingestion of 325 mg of aspirin 30 to 60 minutes before taking niacin, and taking the drug with the evening meal. The flushing usually decreases with prolonged administration, but this tolerance may not occur in warm climates. There is evidence that sustained-release formulations of niacin help minimize the flushing. There are also data that short-acting niacin has a higher incidence of hepatotoxicity.

The GI adverse effects of niacin include dyspepsia, vomiting, and diarrhea with activation of peptic ulcer disease in some patients. The GI problems are due, at least in part, to the increases in GI motility and gastric acid secretion stimulated by the released histamine. Less common adverse effects are a hyperpigmentation of the skin, usually in the axillae, the neck, or the groin (acanthosis nigricans), headaches of the vascular type, orthostatic hypotension (especially in older adults), and reversible blurred vision resulting from macular edema. Niacin also inhibits the tubular elimination of uric acid, thus predisposing the patient to hyperuricemia and gout. There is also a higher incidence of arrhythmias, including but not limited to atrial fibrillation. Anaphylaxis is more likely with IV use.

Elevations in plasma glucose levels, attributed to the rebound in fatty acid concentrations, may occur after each dose of niacin in susceptible individuals. The larger amounts of free fatty acids may compete with the use of glucose by peripheral tissues.

Hepatotoxicity may manifest as cholestatic jaundice, with marked elevations of LFTs. Fulminant hepatic failure has been reported in patients who were changed from immediate-release formulations to sustained-release formulations of niacin.

Niacin is contraindicated for use in patients with known hypersensitivity, hepatic dysfunction, or active peptic ulcer disease. Some formulations may contain tartrazine (FD&C Yellow No. 5 dye) and should be avoided in patients with aspirin allergy. Exercise caution using niacin in patients with arterial bleeding, gout, glaucoma, and diabetes mellitus.

Drug Interactions

Large doses of niacin may decrease the uricosuric effects of probenecid or sulfinpyrazone and cause a rise in uric acid levels (see Table 38-5). There is a higher risk of myopathy with concurrent use of any statin drug. Additive hypotension is associated with the concurrent use of adrenergic neuronal blocking drugs (i.e., guanethidine, guanadrel).

Dosage Regimen

The patient's ability to tolerate niacin may be increased by starting therapy at low doses. The short-acting dose of niacin is 1.5 to 3 grams per day in three divided doses; titrated upward every 1 to 2 weeks as needed. The extended-release formulation of niacin is dosed as 1 to 2 grams/day and titrated monthly to allow the patient to develop tolerance to flushing. The total dosage should not exceed 6 grams per day (see Table 38-6). Although the higher dosages increase the lipid-altering effects, they also increase the incidence of adverse effects. Administer the drug immediately after the evening meal for best results.

Lab Considerations

Monitor serum cholesterol, triglycerides, serum glucose, uric acid, and LFT values before and periodically throughout therapy, especially with prolonged high-dose therapy. Niacin may increase the prothrombin (PT) and INR levels and decrease serum albumin levels. High-dose therapy may cause falsely elevated values for catecholamine and urine glucose if they are measured using the copper sulfate method (Clinitest).

Omega-3 and Omega-6 Fatty Acids
◆ omega-3 acid ethyl esters (Lovaza); ✦ Lovaza

Indications

Over the last 2 decades, there has been a significant increase in the use of omega-3 and omega-6 fatty acids by patients attempting to reduce their risk of cholesterol-related heart problems. Omega-3 fatty acids significantly reduce the risk of sudden death caused by known CAD and arrhythmias. They are also used in the treatment of hyperlipidemia (specifically, elevated TGs), and appear to have a dose-related hypotensive response in patients with hypertension. They have little to no effect in patients with normal blood pressure.

Fish oil, in dosages of at least 3 grams/day, has also been used to reduce the morning stiffness and the number of tender, swollen joints in patients with rheumatoid arthritis.

By decreasing the dietary intake of omega-6 fatty acids and increasing the intake of omega-3 fatty acids, the proinflammatory mediators of rheumatoid arthritis are reduced. By altering the ratio of omega-3 fatty acids to omega-6 fatty acids, some patients have been able to reduce or discontinue their use of nonsteroidal antiinflammatory drugs (NSAIDs).

Pharmacodynamics

Omega-3 and omega-6 fatty acids are not synthesized by the body, and therefore must be acquired through diet or the use of supplements. Alpha-linoleic acid (ALA), an omega-3 fatty acid present in seeds and vegetable oils, produces eicosapentaenoic acid (EPA), a precursor to eicosanoids (e.g., prostaglandins, thromboxanes, and leukotrienes). ALA is antiinflammatory, antithrombotic, antiarrhythmic, and vasodilatory in action. Arachidonic acid, another precursor to eiconsanoids, is a longer-chain fatty acid derivative of linoleic acid. Since ALA and linoleic acid use the same enzymes to produce EPA, arachidonic acid, and other longer-chain fatty acids, competition for the enzymes results. The competition can be lessened by ingestion of fish and fish oil, which provide EPA and the polyunsaturated fatty acid docosahexaenoic acid (DHA) directly. Both fish and fish oil are rich sources of EPA and DHA. DHA is present in fatty fish (salmon, tuna, mackerel) and mother's milk. Box 38-2 identifies the common oils that contain omega-3 and omega-6 oils.

The benefit of omega-3 fatty acids is greater in patients with elevated TG levels. Omega-3 fatty acids produce a sustained reduction in plasma TG levels by inhibiting VLDL and apo B-100 synthesis and decreasing postprandial lipemia. The effects on LDL, apo B, and HDL levels are not as clear, but the effect on LDL appears to be dose dependent. Higher doses produce greater effects on lipid levels. Studies conclude that approximately 4 grams/day of omega-3 fatty acids reduces triglyceride concentrations by 25% to 30%, increases

LDL levels by 5% to 10%, and increases HDL levels by 1% to 3% (Volker, 2000).

Adverse Effects and Contraindications

Omega-3 fatty acids alter the process of atherogenesis, most particularly as precursors to the prostaglandins that interfere with coagulation. If taken in excess, omega-3 fatty acids inhibit platelet activity, thereby producing prolonged blood clotting and increasing the risk for bleeding. A prolonged bleeding time is common to Eskimo populations, who ordinarily have high dietary intake of omega-3 fatty acids and a low incidence of CAD.

Other risks associated with the intake of omega-3 fatty acids are vitamin A and vitamin D toxicity (from fish oil contained in cod liver oil), and increased weight gain from the 9 calories per gram in fish oil. Fishy aftertaste and GI upset (nausea, bloating, belching), all of which appear to be dose dependent, can also result.

Drug Interactions

There are no known drug interactions with omega-3 fatty acids.

Dosage Regimen

The recommended dosage of omega-3 fatty acids for the treatment of elevated TG levels is 2 to 4 grams/day, significantly higher than the dosage recommended for cardiovascular protection. Most over-the-counter (OTC) 1-gram fish oil capsules contain 180 mg of EPA and 120 mg of DHA. Therefore, 3 grams of fish oil daily, in divided doses, provides the recommended daily intake of omega-3 fatty acids. A dietary intake of up to 3 grams/day of omega-3 fatty acids from marine sources is "generally recognized as safe." Each 1-gram prescription capsule of Lovaza contains 465 mg of EPA and 375 mg of DHA.

There are reports of mix-ups between Omacor (omega-3- ⚠ **acid ethyl esters), and Amicar (aminocaproic acid), which inhibits plasminogen activators and is used in the treatment of bleeding from various causes. The risk of thrombosis is increased if patients inadvertently receive Amicar instead of Omacor. In turn, substitution of Omacor for Amicar may lead to serious bleeding. To reduce the likelihood of error, include the reason for use on all prescriptions or drug orders and set an alert in the computer order-entry system.**

Lab Considerations

There is conflicting evidence as to the effect of omega-3 fatty acids on glucose control; available evidence suggests that fish oil does not significantly elevate glucose or A1$_c$ levels.

Miscellaneous Antilipidemic Drugs
Red Yeast Rice
Indications

Belonging to the statin class of antilipidemic drugs, red yeast rice (sometimes known as Mevastatin) is a drug, not a food, as the name would imply. It was the first compound isolated in the 1970s during research into HMG-CoA reductase inhibitors produced by the mold *Penicillium citrinum*. Because of multiple adverse effects, it has only been in the last few years

---

BOX 38-2

Essential Fatty Acids in Common Oils

Omega-3 Oils
- Canola oil
- Fish oil
- Flaxseed oil
- Soybean oil*
- Walnut oil

Omega-6 Oils
- Borage oil
- Corn oil
- Cottonseed oil
- Grapeseed oil
- Peanut oil
- Primrose oil
- Safflower oil
- Sesame oil
- Soybean oil*
- Sunflower oil

*Soybean oil is included in both categories because it is higher in omega-6 fatty acids than most omega-3 oils.

that red yeast rice has been used; it is the only source for production of another statin—pravastatin.

Pharmacodynamics

Red yeast rice is made by fermenting *Monascus purpureus*, a type of yeast, over red rice. In so doing, the yeast acquires the ability to inhibit the action of the enzyme HMG-CoA reductase, an enzyme known to raise cholesterol levels, and which, in turn, increases the risk for CAD.

Adverse Effects and Contraindications

The adverse effects of red yeast rice include headache, abdominal distress, flatulence, dizziness, and heartburn, although these are rare. Do not use red yeast rice in patients who have or are at risk for having liver disease because, like prescription cholesterol-lowering drugs, red yeast rice can affect liver function. Persons who consume more than two alcoholic beverages per day, those with a serious infection or physical disorder, and those who have had an organ transplant are also advised to avoid red yeast rice. Further, because there is limited evidence about the safety of red yeast rice, particularly during pregnancy and lactation, it is best to limit its use to the short term.

Drug Interactions

Do not use red yeast rice concurrently with statins because it may enhance the effect of these drugs, thereby increasing the risk of liver damage. Grapefruit, or grapefruit juice, or marmalade taken concurrently with red yeast rice causes a significant increase in serum levels of the statin, leading to a greater risk for adverse effects and liver damage.

Dosage Regimen

The appropriate adult dosage may vary, given the formulation of the supplement, but is usually 600 mg of the standardized extract 2 to 4 times daily. Red yeast rice is available OTC as a single ingredient formulation and in combination supplements marketed to promote heart health. Lovaza is available by prescription.

Lab Considerations

Check LFT values before starting treatment, at 6 weeks, and again at 12 weeks after starting or titrating therapy, and twice annually thereafter.

Psyllium

Psyllium (found in Metamucil and other products) has also been shown to be effective in some patients with hyperlipidemia at a dose of 10 grams per day. Psyllium lowers LDL and total cholesterol levels by 5% to 10%. It is a logical drug of choice to treat moderately elevated LDL levels (130 to 159 mg/dL) when HDL levels are above 45 mg/dL, especially in older adults. Additionally, psyllium promotes bowel regularity, and sometimes causes flatulence, but has no serious adverse effects. Psyllium is discussed in more depth in Chapter 46.

CLINICAL REASONING

Treatment Objectives

The ultimate goal for treatment of hyperlipoproteinemia is to prevent the progression of coronary atherosclerosis and reduce the risk of CAD and other vascular disorders. The immediate goal is to reduce LDL levels while keeping the management regimen affordable.

Treatment Options

Effective reduction of CAD risk requires identifying and aggressively treating all risk factors responsive to intervention, including smoking, hypertension, diabetes, and obesity (Table 38-7). The approach to treatment is guided by an assessment of total CAD risk, not just the lipid abnormality. For a given LDL elevation, the threshold for initiation of therapy decreases and the intensity of therapy increases. Test lipid levels every 5 years beginning at age 20 as long as they remain in the normal range.

Risk Assessment

Most patients with lipid disorders display no overt signs and symptoms for decades. A myocardial infarction (MI) or stroke is often the first sign of a lipid problem. Therefore, screen patients for CAD risk factors at an early age, before these problems arise. Include a complete history and physical exam and perform a lipid profile for any symptomatic or asymptomatic patient with risk factors or risk equivalents for CAD. Further, determinations of total cholesterol, triglycerides, HDL, and LDL levels allow for a reasonable estimate of CAD risk. Although not routinely measured, apo B is a major component of LDL and is a more sensitive indicator of CAD in men than standard cholesterol measures. Apo A, a major component of HDL, is a much more sensitive predictor of CAD in women. As a rule of thumb, for every 10 mg/dL rise in total cholesterol levels, there is a 10% increase in risk for CAD.

Decisions about which tests to order requires consideration of test accuracy, cost, and availability as well as the significance and presence of other CAD risk factors. Results obtained with desktop analyzers using finger-stick blood samples are often erroneous. If the patient is hypothyroid with a normal cholesterol level, consider the possibility of a lab error, since patients with hypothyroidism generally have elevated total cholesterol levels.

Advise the patient to abstain from alcohol for 48 hours before testing. An 8- to 12-hour fast before testing is required. Water intake is acceptable. Without fasting, TG levels will be falsely elevated because of the circulating chylomicrons.

Each risk factor identified is thought by some health care providers to double the risk of CAD. For example, a 49-year-old male (first risk factor) who smokes (second risk factor) and has diabetes (third risk factor), hypertension (fourth risk factor), and a low HDL level (fifth risk factor) will have more than a thirtyfold increase (five risk factors: $2 \times 2 \times 2 \times 2 \times 2 = 32$) in risk for CAD compared with a female with no risk factors. Some health care providers "subtract" one risk factor in persons with an HDL level exceeding 60 mg/dL, and two risk factors for patients with an HDL level exceeding 70 mg/dL.

Patient Variables

THERAPEUTIC LIFESTYLE CHANGES. Therapeutic lifestyle changes (TLCs) are required of all patients with hyperlipidemia. Dietary modification, weight reduction, and exercise, is the core of lipid management, with drug therapy reserved for patients at highest risk (Box 38-3). Diet remains the

TABLE 38-7 Guidelines for Management of Hyperlipoproteinemia

Risk Category*	LDL Goal	Recommended Interventions†
LOW RISK FOR CAD		
0–1 risk factors	<160 mg/dL *Aim:* Slow risk for coronary atherosclerosis‡	1. TLC is first-line therapy. 2. After 3 mo, if LDL <160 mg/dL, continue TLC. 3. If after 3 mo, LDL 160–189 mg/dL, drug therapy is optional. 4. If after 3 mo, LDL is 190 mg/dL; consider drug therapy.
MODERATE RISK FOR CAD		
2+ risk factors (10-yr risk <10%)	<130 mg/dL *Aim:* Reduce short-term and long-term risk for CAD	1. TLC for 3 mo 2. After 3 mo, if LDL <130 mg/dL on TLC alone, continue TLC. 3. After 3 mo, if LDL >130 mg/dL, consider drug therapy.§ 4. After 3 mo of drug therapy, if LDL <130 mg/dL, TLC alone may be continued. 5. After 3 mo of TLC, if LDL >160 mg/dL, consider drug therapy.
MODERATELY HIGH RISK FOR CAD		
2+ risk factors (10-yr risk 10%–20%)	<130 mg/dL *Optimal goal:* <70 mg/dL *Aim:* Reduce long-term risk for CAD	1. TLC for 3 mo 2. After 3 mo, if LDL <130 mg/dL on TLC alone, continue TLC. 3. After 3 mo, if LDL ≥130 mg/dL, consider drug therapy. 4. After 3 mo of drug therapy, if LDL 130 mg/dL, TLC alone may be continued.
HIGH RISK FOR CAD		
CAD or CAD risk equivalents‖ (10-yr risk >20%)	<100 mg/dL *Optimal goal:* <70 mg/dL (particularly for patients at very high risk) *Aim:* Reduce risk for major coronary events and stroke	1. If baseline LDL <100 mg/dL, further lipid-lowering therapies are not required, but patients should follow TLC. 2. If LDL 100–129 mg/dL, initiate or intensify TLC and emphasize weight reduction and increased activity in persons with metabolic syndrome; delay use or intensification of LDL-lowering therapies and institute treatment of other lipid or nonlipid risk factors; consider use of other lipid-modifying drugs (e.g., fibrates, niacin) if patient has low HDL or elevated TG. 3. If LDL >130 mg/dL, intensify TLC, control risk equivalents, and start drug therapy.

*Factors favoring use of lipid-lowering drugs include men over 45 years and women over 55 years of age; heavy cigarette smoking; poorly controlled hypertension (BP >140/90 or on antihypertensive drugs); low HDL; strong family history of premature CAD (CAD in first-degree male relative over 55 yr and CAD in first-degree female relative over 65 yr); 10-yr risk approaching 10%.

†When starting drug therapy to lower LDL, it is advised that intensity of therapy be sufficient to achieve at least a 30%–40% reduction in LDL levels.

‡May conflict with cost-effectiveness considerations, thus clinical judgment is required.

§Lipid-lowering drug generally not recommended because the patient is not at high, short-term risk. Cost effectiveness is marginal.

‖CAD and CAD risk equivalents include diabetes; obesity; metabolic syndrome (abdominal obesity, elevated TG, small LDL particles, low HDL; elevated BP, insulin resistance with or without glucose intolerance; prothrombotic or proinflammatory states); abdominal aortic aneurysm; peripheral arterial disease; symptomatic carotid artery disease.

Note: Some authorities recommend use of LDL-lowering drugs in this category if an LDL cholesterol <100 mg/dL cannot be achieved by TLC. Others prefer use of drugs that primarily modify TGs and HDL (e.g., niacin or fibrate). Clinical judgment also may call for deferring drug therapy in this subcategory. Almost all persons with 0–1 risk factors have a 10-yr risk <10%, thus 10-yr risk assessment in persons with 0–1 risk factors is not necessary.

BP, Blood pressure; *CAD,* coronary artery disease; *HDL,* high-density lipoprotein; *LDL,* low-density lipoprotein; *TLC,* therapeutic lifestyle changes; *TG,* triglycerides.

BOX 38-3

AHA 2006 Diet and Lifestyle Recommendations for Cardiovascular Disease Risk Reduction

- Balance calorie intake and physical activity to achieve or maintain desirable body weight and to prevent weight gain.
- Limit intake of saturated fat to <7% of total calories; polyunsaturated fat up to 10% of total calories; monounsaturated fat up to 20% of total calories (for a total of 25% to 35% of total calories), *trans* fat to <1% of total calories, and cholesterol to <200 mg per day by the following means:
  - Choosing lean meats and vegetable alternatives
  - Selecting fat-free (skim), 1%-fat, and low-fat dairy products
  - Minimizing intake of partially hydrogenated fats
- Limit carbohydrates to 50% to 60% of total calories using the following, predominantly:
- Vegetables and fruits
- Whole-grain, high-fiber foods
- Twenty percent to 30% of total calories/day should consist of fiber.
- Protein intake should be approximately 15% of total calories.
- Consume fish, especially oily fish, at least twice a week.
- Minimize intake of beverages and foods with added sugars.
- Choose and prepare foods with little or no salt.
- If consuming alcohol, do so in moderation.
- When eating food prepared outside of the home, follow the AHA Diet and Lifestyle Recommendations.

American Heart Association. (2006). Diet and lifestyle recommendations revisions: A scientific statement from the American Heart Association Nutrition Committee. *Circulation,* *114*(1), 82–96.

cornerstone of treatment, effective for both prevention and treatment lipid disorders. Hospitalized patients who reduce their intake of cholesterol and saturated fat see a reduction in total cholesterol and LDL levels by as much as 30%. In contrast, however, the same drug therapy, used in outpatients, reduces cholesterol and LDL levels only about 10%, perhaps because outpatients are not as rigorous in adopting TLCs as those supported to do so during a hospital stay. The argument for dietary therapy as the initial step in treatment is based on the following considerations: (1) diet is the most physiologic approach, (2) TLCs should be lifelong, (3) no drugs are without known or potential adverse effects, and (4) in most cases, and drug therapy is expensive (see Controversy box).

LIFE-SPAN CONSIDERATIONS

Pregnant and Nursing Women. Avoid lipid-lowering therapy in women who are pregnant unless the benefits outweigh the risks. Metabolic changes during pregnancy elevate cholesterol, lipoproteins, and TGs. Cholesterol levels can increase by as much as 40% to 60% during pregnancy. The higher lipid levels needed for cellular metabolism, carbohydrates, lipids, proteins, vitamins, and inorganic substances are derived from ingested foods. These substrates are used to form new cells and synthesize new substances, and are also burned as fuel for energy.

During pregnancy, the use of glucose accelerates because of rapid fetal cell and organ growth. In addition, maternal sensitivity to insulin is diminished. As a result, pregnancy is said to produce a diabetes-like state. This diabetes-like state may contribute to the upset in lipid values, at least during the pregnancy. Although pregnancy occurs most often in young, healthy individuals, the risk of lipid disorders, especially those that are genetically determined, remains. Statins are classified as category X drugs and should not be used during pregnancy, given the risk for fetal abnormalities.

Children and Adolescents. Childhood cholesterol levels appear to be a major predictor of elevated cholesterol levels as an adult. Children with cholesterol levels in the upper percentiles of normal have a higher risk of retaining cholesterol levels in the upper percentiles of normal into adulthood. The more seriously affected children are customarily those for whom dietary and possibly drug management is warranted (i.e., children over 10 years of age in whom TLCs have not lowered lipid levels). On the other hand, children whose cholesterol levels are in the lower percentiles of normal are unlikely to have elevated cholesterol values as adults.

Older Adults. The age limit at which lipid-lowering therapy should or should not be initiated is highly debated. Cholesterol levels have been reported to gradually increase with age in both men and women. Women have high levels of HDL in all age groups. The postmenopausal drop in estrogen triggers a rise in cholesterol levels. With changes in lipid metabolism, cholesterol levels rise to a maximum at 65 years and then decrease, but never fall to levels as low as those in young adults. LDL and HDL levels in combination with elevated systolic blood pressures are significant in predicting coronary risk in the older adult. TG values also rise with age. The increase is greater in females than males at age 50; the TG level then decreases in men and rises significantly higher with aging in women. There is no strong evidence to support initiating lipid-lowering therapy in patients over 75 years of age.

Patients who have hypothyroidism, nephrotic syndrome, or liver disease have increased total cholesterol and LDL levels. Similarly, patients taking thiazide diuretics may have increased LDL levels. The concurrent use of antilipemic drugs with beta blockers generally reduces HDL levels, and in combination with estrogen increases HDL levels. Estrogen replacement therapy also increases TG levels.

Drug Variables

The range of available drugs is extensive, and they vary greatly in cost, effect on cholesterol fractions, efficacy, and adverse effects. No drugs currently available are effective in lowering all types of hyperlipoproteinemia, and all have adverse effects. Drug therapy is started when diet therapy

---

Controversy

Diet Versus Drugs in Treating Hyperlipidemia

Jonathan J. Wolfe

Health care providers universally recognize the central role of hyperlipidemia in cardiovascular disease. This set of diseases poses difficulties in treatment. On the one hand, a minority of patients have an inherited metabolic predisposition to high levels of cholesterol or triglycerides. Dietary and lifestyle interventions may not suffice for these persons with familial hyperlipidemia. They may meet tragically early cardiac deaths if their disorder is not diagnosed and aggressively treated.

In the United States, many people expose themselves to predictable disorders simply by rejecting a healthful diet and reasonable levels of exercise. This second group of patients would not seem to need lipid-lowering drugs. Indeed, their unhealthy lifestyle choices may also expose them to hepatic dysfunction related to therapy with lipid-lowering drugs. The issue becomes one of the cost and risk of using lipid-lowering drugs versus the cost and risk of cardiovascular disease. Are we, as a society, more apt to choose a drug than to alter our comfort index by adopting a low-fat diet and regular exercise plan?

In addition, nontraditional approaches to hyperlipidemia are available from a thriving dietary supplement industry. These dietary supplements exist outside U.S. Food and Drug Administration regulation; a product may be legally marketed so long as no therapeutic claims are made about it. Advice touting such dietary supplements for health promotion has proliferated in print and broadcast media, advertising, and busy retail outlets.

CLINICAL REASONING ANALYSIS

- Why do you think patients are quick to seek alternatives to traditional medicine in preventing cardiovascular disease related to elevated serum lipids?
- Why do you think patients so commonly prefer to take drugs rather than to alter their lifestyle choices regarding diet and exercise?
- What counseling would you provide to a patient who comes to the health care provider for a routine check-up and volunteers that she has stopped taking prescription drugs for hypercholesterolemia, but now takes an herbal tea that has the same effects and for lower cost?
- Why do patients consider herbal and other natural products to be safer than mainstream pharmaceuticals?
- What issues of social justice are involved when a patient on a fixed income says he no longer adheres to drug treatment regimens because it means a choice between buying groceries for the last 10 days of the month or buying his medication?

CASE STUDY — Antilipemic Drugs

ASSESSMENT

History of Present Illness	MM, a 56-year-old black male, is here for follow-up of hyperlipoproteinemia, type 2 diabetes mellitus, and hypertension. His last visit was 6 months ago, at which time he reports using dietary interventions and an exercise regimen to control his cholesterol and diabetes. He reports feeling "a little sluggish" recently but attributes it to stress in the workplace, the need for a part-time second job, and perhaps an elevation in his blood pressure. His work requires him to travel 3 to 4 times a month, and he admits to nonadherence with the diet and exercise regimen during his travels. He reports smoking one to two packs of cigarettes per day for last 30 years, and consuming 3 to 4 ounces of alcohol daily for the past 5 to 6 months. His current drugs include hydrochlorothiazide, 50 mg PO daily, and potassium chloride, 20 mEq PO daily, which he has used since diagnosed with hypertension 3 years ago.
Past Health History	Except for hypertension and diabetes, MM has an otherwise negative past health history. MM has a positive family history for heart disease and hypertension. His father died at 53 of an MI. Mother is alive and well at 71. Brother has diabetes mellitus and a history of alcoholism.
Life-Span Considerations	MM is attempting to support his family with two sons in their late teens and to care for MM's aging mother, who is trying to remain independent at home. MM admits he has a type A personality with a strong need to be the breadwinner in the family. His wife died 10 years ago in a motor vehicle accident.
Psychosocial Considerations	MM has health insurance and pharmacy coverage for his sons but does not carry his own insurance because of the expense. He is concerned about the cost of his own health care needs but feels unable to obtain personal health insurance at this time. He pays cash for visits to health care provider and hopes hospitalization will not be necessary.
Physical Exam Findings	*Height:* 5"9". *Weight:* 208 lb (up 25 lb from previous visit). *BP:* 168/90, 98.6° F-80–24. ENT negative. No carotid bruits, thyromegaly, lymphadenopathy, or JVD. HRRR without LTH$_M$. Abdomen soft, round, NT, no HSM, masses, or bruits. Pedal pulses 2+.
Diagnostic Testing	Total cholesterol: 290 mg/dL; LDL: 179 mg/dL; HDL: 34 mg/dL; TGs: 559 mg/dL; FBS: 180 mg/dL; A$_{1c}$: 11%. Serum potassium: 5.5 mg/dL. Proteinuria on urinalysis. CBC, other electrolytes, BUN and creatinine, and thyroid function tests are within normal limits.

DIAGNOSIS Hyperlipidemia

MANAGEMENT

Treatment Objectives	1. Improve adherence to concurrent drug, dietary, and exercise regimen. 2. Reduce lipid levels while keeping the treatment regimen affordable. 3. Regain control of type 2 diabetes. 4. Reduce the risk for progression of coronary atherosclerosis, myocardial infarction, and end-organ damage from CAD and diabetes.
Treatment Plan	**Pharmacotherapy** • Stop hydrochlorothiazide and potassium supplement. • lisinopril 20 mg PO once daily • ezetimbe 10 mg with 20 mg simvastatin (Vytorin 10/20 mg) PO once daily after evening meal • omega-3 fatty acids 2000 mg PO twice daily with meals (standardized extract) • rosiglitazone 4 mg PO daily • Enteric-coated aspirin 81 mg PO daily **Patient Teaching** 1. Significance of therapeutic lifestyle changes including weight loss, exercise, dietary modifications, and monitoring glucose levels at least once daily 2. The purpose and proper administration of prescribed drugs; do not stop drugs without first consulting health care provider 3. Adverse effects of drugs taken and when to contact health care provider if adverse effects develop 4. Importance of keeping regular appointments for follow-up visits and of having cholesterol, liver function tests, and A$_{1c}$ values done every 3 months

Continued

CARDIOVASCULAR

CASE STUDY   Antilipemic Drugs—Cont'd

5. Check BP and glucose levels are directed and bring log with him to each appointment.
6. Importance of and how to perform daily foot care
7. Importance of annual dilated eye exams and regular dental care
8. May place fish oil capsules in freezer to reduce fish oil taste and frequency of belching, if any

Evaluation

1. BP is controlled at less than 120/85 mm Hg.
2. A_{1c} is kept at 6.5% to 7% (135 to 170 mg/dL).
3. Lipid levels are returned to desirable limits: TC <200 mg/dL; TGs to <150 mg/dL, HDL to a minimum of 50 mg/dL, and LDL to <100 mg/dL (preferably 70 mg/dL).
4. Dietary goals and exercise regimens are reached and maintained.
5. Patient tolerates and adheres to drug therapy as prescribed.
6. Patient keeps follow-up appointments with health care provider and for lab work as directed.
7. Patient is able to verbalize understanding and importance treatment regimen as well as adverse effects of drugs taken.

CLINICAL REASONING ANALYSIS

Q1. I know MM has a type A personality and is way too stressed, but how do you decide what drug to use for him?
A. Choosing the best regimen for MM will take some time because of his many health problems, but will be individualized and based on his clinical status, the type of hyperlipoproteinemia he has, the amount of lipid-lowering that is required, and an assessment of his potential adherence to therapy. We also need to consider the drugs' adverse effects, costs, MM's health beliefs that support the need to lower his lipid levels, and his understanding that whatever we do for treatment will likely be lifelong.

Q2. I heard you say you want MM to stop taking his hydrochlorothiazide diuretic. Why is that? Isn't it cheap enough?
A. Thiazide diuretics tend to increase LDL levels. MM does not need any other cause for his elevated lipids. His lifestyle and family history are bad enough.

Q3. Can't MM just take the fish oil capsules or niacin to lower his cholesterol?
A. Some patients may be able to do that but not MM. Indeed, research has shown that at high enough dosages of niacin, his triglyceride levels could be reduced by 30% to 40% but the adverse effects at the high dosages can be miserable and there is a risk for elevated liver enzyme values. The fish oil capsules will also help somewhat but by themselves will not lower his lipid levels enough to be meaningful. However, in combination with a statin such as lovastatin and ezetimbe, his lipid values should come down nicely. Here, let me give you this table of the lipid-lowering effects of the various drug classes. It will help you to better understand why we do what we do.

Q4. What about the fish oil capsules? Besides reducing triglyceride levels, why should MM take them?
A. Omega-3 fatty acids have been shown to significantly reduce the risk of sudden death caused by arrhythmias and all-cause mortality in patients with known CAD. Studies also show that taking about 4 grams/day of omega-3 fatty acids reduces triglyceride levels by 25% to 30%. We have to watch his LDL closely, though, since the fatty acids can increase those levels.

Q5. If changes in lipid levels are not immediately apparent, why do we have to check him in 6 weeks as well as check his liver function and lipid levels?
A. Well, first of all, statin use carries with it a risk for rhabdomyolysis. Rhabdomyolysis is the breakdown of skeletal muscle due to injury, either mechanical, physical, or chemical. The principal result of this process is acute renal failure due to accumulation of muscle breakdown products in the blood stream, several of which are injurious to the kidneys. Should he develop myalgias, we will check a CK level as well as his LFTs to evaluate for rhabdomyolysis and elevated liver enzymes. Although we could check his LFTs and lipid levels in 3 months, I prefer to be a bit more cautious because of his other health issues. I want to watch him more closely than a patient with no risk factors for CAD and to support him in his attempts to adhere to therapy.

and exercise for 3 to 6 months have been ineffective. Conditions known to increase serum lipid levels (i.e., diabetes, hypothyroidism, liver disease, long-term corticosteroid use) may impose the need for drug therapy. Thus, clinical decisions regarding drug therapy are based on a number of factors.

Choosing the best management regimen to use and in which order is individualized and based on the patient's clinical status, the type of hyperlipoproteinemia the patient has, the amount of lipid-lowering that is required, and an assessment of potential patient adherence to therapy (Table 38-8 and 38-9). Factors affecting adherence include the drug's adverse effects, cost of

TABLE 38-8 Lipid-Lowering Effects of Antilipemic Drug Classes*

Drug	TC (%)	LDL (%)	HDL (%)	TG (%)
Bile acid resins	↓ 15–30	↓ 15–35	↑ 10–38	↑ 5–40
Fibric acid derivatives	↓ 2–10	↓ 5–18	↑ 17–25	↓ 40–50
HMG-CoA reductase inhibitors	↓ 20–45	↓ 20–45	↑ 8–23	↓ 8–25
niacin	↓ 15–30	↓ 15–30	↑ 10–30	↓ 30–40
probucol	↓ 10–20	↓ 10–15	↓ 10–15	NE

*Dose dependent reductions
HDL, High-density lipoprotein; *HMG-CoA*, hydroxymethylglutaryl coenzyme A; *LDL*, low-density lipoprotein; *NE*, no significant effect; *TC*, total cholesterol; *TG*, triglycerides.

TABLE 38-9 Additive Effect of Optimal Monotherapy vs. Combination Therapy*

	Change from Baseline			
	TC	TG	LDL	HDL
All atorvastatin doses	−32	−24	−44	+4
All atorvastatin doses + ezetimibe	−41	−33	−56	+7
All simvastatin doses	−26	−20	−36	+7
All simvastatin doses + ezetimibe	−37	−29	−51	+9
All pravastatin doses	−17	−14	−25	+7
All pravastatin doses + ezetimibe	−27	−21	−39	+8
All lovastatin doses	−18	−12	−25	+4
All lovastatin doses + ezetimibe	−29	−25	−40	+9
fenofibrate 160 mg + ezetimibe 10 mg	−22	−44	−20	+19
simvastatin 20 mg + fenofibrate 20 mg	—	−43	−31	+19
lovastatin 40 mg† + niacin ER 2 grams	—	−43	−42	+30
simvastatin 10 mg + colesevelam 3.8 grams	—	−12	−42	+10
atorvastatin 10 mg + colesevelam 3.8 grams	−31	−1	−48	+11
lovastatin 10 mg + colesevelam 2.3 grams	−21	−1	−34	+4
omega-3 ethyl esters	−9.7	−44.9	+ 44.5	+9.1

*Source of data is product information unless otherwise stated.
†−25 and −19; effect of niacin and lovastatin + niacin ER in Lp(a) reduction, respectively.
HDL, High-density lipoproteins; *LDL*, low-density lipoproteins; *TC*, total cholesterol; *TG*, triglycerides.

therapy, the patient and health care provider's health beliefs supporting the need to lower lipid levels, and the understanding that lipid therapy is lifelong. Studies have shown that 15% to 46% of patients who start a lipid-lowering drug discontinue treatment within 1 year. Always involve the patient in treatment decisions and advise of the absolute benefits and risks of the various management options.

STATINS. Statins have moved quickly to first-line status by virtue of their effectiveness, patient acceptability, and increasingly favorable safety records (Table 38-9). Most experts agree that the benefits of treatment with statins are a class-wide effect. They are more effective than all other drugs in lowering total cholesterol, LDL, and triglyceride levels. They also have proven efficacy in reducing cardiovascular mortality and morbidity. Further, they are better tolerated than bile acid resins or nicotinic acid. The choice of drug depends on the amount of LDL-lowering required to reach goal. The least expensive of these drugs can be chosen, because they are equal in effectiveness and patient tolerance.

In some cases, although these drugs are expensive, the selection of a specific drug may also be based on price. However, when cost is considered as a function of LDL-lowering capacity, only niacin is more cost-effective.

CHOLESTEROL ABSORPTION INHIBITOR. Ezetimibe, the only cholesterol absorption–inhibiting drug on the market at this time, can be used alone or in combination with statins. When used in combination, LDL-lowering of approximately 60% has been noted.

BILE ACID RESINS. Bile acid resins have been used for hyperlipoproteinemias for many years and have an established safety record. Bile acid resins are not systemically absorbed and can be used in patients who cannot tolerate the effects of statins, or used in combination with statins for patients unable to reach their LDL goal when receiving statin monotherapy. Though not as effective as statins or nicotinic acid, they are effective for patients with a low CAD risk but in whom diet alone failed to lower LDL to desired levels. There is some evidence that combination therapy reduces LDL levels to such an extent that there may be actual regression of atherosclerotic plaque.

Cholesterol levels start to decline 48 hours after the start of therapy but may take 1 year to stabilize. Bile resin therapy is usually discontinued if the patient's clinical response remains poor after 3 months of treatment. The resins may be used, however, in combination with gemfibrozil or nicotinic acid for patients who develop myopathy with a combination of gemfibrozil and a statin. Further, the resins modestly increase HDL levels.

NIACIN. Niacin has beneficial effects on each of the lipoproteins, but most patients are unable to tolerate the adverse effects of the drug. Niacin may be considered a first-line drug for patients with hypercholesterolemia in whom cost is a limiting factor; it is less expensive than statins and bile acid resins. Niacin may also be chosen when drugs from other drug groups are ineffective or not well tolerated. However, the effect of niacin on lipid-lowering can be enhanced by coadministration of bile acid resins. A full dose of niacin reduces LDL concentrations by 15% to 30%. When niacin is taken in combination with one of the bile acid resins, however, a 60% to 70% reduction is often reported.

Niacin is not as effective in reducing TGs as fibric acid derivatives. However, it is much less expensive, and should be considered if fibric acid derivatives are not effective or not tolerated.

FIBRIC ACID DERIVATIVES. Fibric acid derivatives are recommended in the treatment of elevated TGs because of their proven efficacy in reducing the incidence of cardiovascular disease and their TG-lowering effect. Unless there is a significant cost advantage, use gemfibrozil rather than fenofibrate, because there is no long-term study evaluating fenofibrate's effect on cardiovascular morbidity and mortality.

Fibric acid derivatives generally reduce LDL levels less than statins, bile acid resins, or niacin, and in some cases may even raise the levels. Therefore, consider them only if all other drugs have failed. Gemfibrozil can actually raise LDL levels in patients with very elevated TG levels, but decreases LDL levels in patients with normal or moderately elevated TG levels.

If after 3 months of treatment with any of the antilipemic drugs, the drug is tolerated and there has been at least a

CARDIOVASCULAR

15%, decrease in lipids but not to the desired level, the first drug can be continued or the dosage increased. If, on the other hand, the patient is not tolerating the drug, or there is less than a 15% decrease in total cholesterol levels, stop the first drug and start a second-line drug. In either case, monitor the patient as if it is the first use of the drug.

Treatment options for patients with elevated Lp(a) and risk factors for CAD include (1) lowering the LDL with statins (which are generally effective in CAD but have no effect on Lp[a] levels); (2) taking 1 to 2 grams of an extended-release form of niacin daily (although most effective in lowering Lp [a]); (3) folic acid (reduces homocysteine levels); and (4) a daily aspirin. There is no evidence to suggest that reducing homocysteine levels reduces cardiovascular events, however. Some health care providers feel antibiotics may be effective when C-reactive protein levels are high.

Patient Education

Patient education and discussion with family members are vital to foster an understanding of the importance of long-term commitment to therapy. Explanations of the lipid disorder, its consequences, treatment regimens, and required lifestyle modifications are important. Equally important is thorough teaching about the need for regular lab testing to evaluate drug effectiveness on body systems and organs, such as the liver.

Advise patients that antilipemic drugs are used together with dietary modifications of fat, cholesterol, calories, and alcohol. Include the importance of exercise, smoking cessation, weight reduction, and control of comorbid diseases in the teaching.

Constipation is possible with bile resins and other antilipemic drugs. Thus explaining the importance of fluids and fiber in the diet as well as exercise and the use of stool softeners and laxatives (if necessary) is vital. Tell the patient to report persistent constipation, nausea, flatulence, and heartburn, or frothy and foul-smelling stools. The patient should also report unusual bleeding or bruising, petechiae, or black, tarry stools. Treatment with vitamin K may be necessary.

It is important to work with the members of the patient's household who cook and shop for groceries, so they understand how to select and prepare "heart-healthy" meals. Eating less saturated fat and cholesterol can usually lower total cholesterol levels by 10% to 20%. Less pork and beef should be eaten, and more fish, chicken, turkey, and nonfat or low-fat milk. Minimal amounts of other whole-milk dairy products, such as cheese, butter, ice cream, and sour cream, are acceptable. Margarines and cooking oils containing polyunsaturated fats (e.g., safflower, corn, and soybean) or monounsaturated oil products (e.g., olive oil) should be used. Oat bran, consumed as cereal or muffins, helps reduce total cholesterol and LDL levels an average of 5% to 10%. Remind the patient to avoid regular intake of grapefruit and grapefruit juice if they are taking statin drugs (except for pravastatin).

Useful information for patients is available through the American Heart Association website (www.americanheart. org) and the Department of Health and Human Services National Heart, Lung, and Blood Institute website (www. nhlbi.nih.gov). The patient can calculate his or her 10-year risk of having a heart-related event at the latter web site.

Evaluation

The prognosis for patients with lipid disorders can be greatly improved through lasting lifestyle changes and, in many cases, long-term drug therapy. Drug therapy usually continues for many years and possibly a lifetime. However, the health care provider may consider reducing the dosage or even stopping drug therapy if the desired LDL level is maintained for a period of 2 years, to reestablish the diagnosis, and to check the efficacy of non–drug measures. Continue dietary therapy regardless. Measure lipid levels 4 to 6 weeks after drugs are stopped and again at 3 months. If the levels are again elevated, restart therapy.

KEY POINTS

- Hyperlipoproteinemia is an increase in the concentration of protein-lipid cholesterol, triglycerides, and phospholipids.
- Elevations of cholesterol and LDL and a reduction in HDL are strongly positive independent risk factors for the development of CAD in persons younger than 65 years of age.
- Most patients with lipid disorders display no overt signs and symptoms for decades. An MI or stroke often is the first sign of a lipid problem. Patients should be screened for CAD risk factors before cardiovascular problems arise.
- The ultimate goal for treatment of elevated lipids is a reduction in cardiovascular risk.
- The immediate treatment goal is a reduction in LDL cholesterol levels.
- Therapeutic lifestyle changes, including diet, exercise, smoking cessation, and drug therapy, if needed, effectively reduce total and LDL cholesterol levels and raise HDL levels.

- Treatment options include HMG-CoA reductase inhibitors, a cholesterol absorption inhibitor, bile acid resins, fibric acid derivatives, and a small number of miscellaneous drugs. Each group carries its own advantages and disadvantages for the individual patient.
- Patient education and discussion with family members are vital to foster an understanding of the importance of a long-term commitment to therapy.
- Explanations of the disorder, its consequences, treatment regimens, and the importance of lifestyle modifications are vital to successful management.
- The health care provider may consider reducing the dosage or even stopping drug therapy if the desired lipid levels are maintained for a period of 2 years to reestablish the diagnosis, and to check the efficacy of non–drug measures.

Bibliography

American Heart Association. (2006). Diet and lifestyle recommendations revisions: A scientific statement from the American Heart Association Nutrition Committee. *Circulation*, *114*(1), 82–96.

ALLHAT Collaborative Research Group. (2002). The antihypertensive and lipid-lowering treatment to prevent heart attack trial (ALLHAT-LLT): Major outcomes in moderately hypercholesterolemic, hypertensive patients randomized to pravastatin vs. usual care. *Journal of the American Medical Association*, *288*(23), 2998–3007.

Ballantyne, C., Abate, N., and Yuan, Z. (2005). Dose-comparison study of the combination of ezetimbe and simvastatin (Vytorin) versus atorvastatin in patients with hypercholesterolemia: The Vytorin versus atorvastatin (VYVA) study. *American Heart Journal*, *149*(3), 464–473.

Brown, B., Zhao, X., Chait, A., et al. (2001). Simvastatin and niacin, antioxidant vitamins, or the combination for the prevention of coronary disease. *New England Journal of Medicine*, *345*(22), 1583–1592.

Burr, M., Fehily, A., Gilbert, J., et al. (1989). Effects of changes in fat, fish, and fibre intakes on death and myocardial reinfarction: Diet and reinfarction trial (DART). *Lancet*, *2*(8666), 757–761.

Cheng, A., and Leiter, L. (2006). Implications of recent clinical trials for the National Cholesterol Education Program Adult Treatment Panel III guidelines. *Current Opinion in Cardiology*, *21*(4), 400–404.

Colhoun, H., Betteridge, D., Durrington, P. (2004). Primary prevention of cardiovascular disease with atorvastatin in type 2 diabetes in the Collaborative Atorvastatin Diabetes Study (CARDS): Multicenter randomized placebo-controlled trial. *Lancet*, *364*(9435), 685–696.

Covington, M. (2004). Omega-3 fatty acids. *American Family Physician*, *70*(1), 133–140.

Davidson, M., Ballantyne, C., Kerzner, B., et al. (2004). Efficacy and safety of ezetimbe coadministered with statins: Randomized, placebo-controlled, blinded experience in 2382 patients with primary hypercholesterolemia. *International Journal of Clinical Practice*, *58*(8), 746–755.

Dunbar, R., and Rader, D. (2005). Demystifying triglycerides: A practical approach for the clinician. *Cleveland Clinic Journal of Medicine*, *72*(8), 661–680.

Durrington, P., Bhatnager, D., Mackness, M., et al. (2001). An omega-3 polyunsaturated fatty acid concentrate administered for one year decreased triglycerides in simvastatin treated patients with coronary heart disease and persisting hypertriglyceridemia. *Heart*, *85*(5), 544–548.

Expert Panel on Detection, Evaluation, and Treatment of High Blood Cholesterol in Adults. (2001). Summary of the Third Report of the National Cholesterol Education Program Adult Treatment Panel. *Journal of the American Medical Association*, *285*(19), 2486–2497.

FIELD Study Investigators. (2005). Effects of long-term fenofibrate therapy on cardiovascular events in 9795 people with type 2 diabetes mellitus (the FIELD study): Randomized controlled trial. Available online: www.thelancet.com. Accessed May 7, 2007.

Frick, H., Elo, O., Kaapa, K., et al. (1987). Helsinki Heart Study: Primary prevention trial with gemfibrozil in middle-aged men with dyslipidemia: Safety of treatment, changes in risk factors, and incidence of coronary heart disease. *New England Journal of Medicine*, *317*(20), 1237–1245.

Frick, M., Heinonen, O., Huttunen, J., et al. (1993). Efficacy of gemfibrozil in dyslipidaemic subjects with suspected heart disease. An ancillary study in the Helsinki Heart Study frame population. *Annals of Medicine*, *25*(1), 41–45.

Gau, G., and Wright, S. (2006). Pathophysiology, diagnosis, and management of dyslipidemia. *Current Problems in Cardiology*, *31*(7), 445–486.

Grundy, S., Cleeman, J., Bairey, C., et al. (2004). Implications of recent clinical trials for the National Cholesterol Education Program Adult Treatment Panel III Guidelines. *Journal of the American College of Cardiology*, *44*(3), 720–732.

Heart Protection Study Collaborative Group. MRC/BHF heart protection study of cholesterol lowering with simvastatin in 20,536 high-risk individuals: A randomized placebo-controlled trial. *Lancet*, *360*(9326), 7–22.

Howe, P. (1997). Dietary fats and hypertension: Focus on fish oil. *Annals of the New York Academy of Science*, *827*, 339–352.

Joint National Committee on Detection, Evaluation, and Treatment of High Blood Pressure. (1997). The Sixth Report of the Joint National Committee on Detection, Evaluation, and Treatment of High Blood Pressure. *Archives of Internal Medicine*, *157*(21), 2413–2446.

Jones, P., Davidson, M., Stein, E., et al. (2003). Comparison of the efficacy and safety of rosuvastatin versus atorvastatin, simvastatin, and pravastatin across doses (STELLAR Trial). *American Journal of Cardiology*, *92*(2), 152–160.

Law, C., Morley, K., and Belch, J. (1993). Effects of fish oil supplementation on non-steroidal antiinflammatory drug requirement in patients with milk rheumatoid arthritis: A double-blind placebo controlled study. *British Journal of Rheumatology*, *32*, 982–989.

Law, M., Wald, N., and Rudnicka, A. (2003). Quantifying effect of statins on low density lipoprotein cholesterol, ischemic heart disease, and stroke: Systemic review and meta-analysis. *British Medical Journal*, *326*(7404), 1423.

McKenney, J., Jones, P., Adamczyk, M., et al. (2003). Comparison of the efficacy of rosuvastatin versus atorvastatin, simvastatin, and pravastatin in achieving lipid goals: results from the STELLAR trial. *Current Medical Research and Opinion*, *19*(8), 689–698.

Morris, M., Sacks, F., and Rosner, B. (1993). Does fish oil lower blood pressure? A meta-analysis of controlled trials. *Circulation*, *88*(2), 523–533.

O'Keefe, J., Cordain, L., Harris, W., et al. (2004). Optimal low-density lipoprotein is 50 to 70 mg/dL: Lower is better and physiologically normal. *Journal of the American College of Cardiology*, *43*(11), 2142–2146.

Pederson, T., Faergeman, O., Kastelein, J., et al. (2005). High-dose atorvastatin vs. usual-dose simvastatin for secondary prevention after myocardial infarction. The IDEAL study: A randomized controlled trial. *Journal of the American Medical Association*, *294*(19), 2437–2445.

Rhoads, G., Dahlen, K., Berg, N., et al. (1996). Lp(a) lipoprotein as a risk factor for myocardial infarction. *Journal of the American Medical Association*, *256*(18), 2540–2544.

Rosenson, R., and Tangey, C. (1998). Antiatherothrombotic properties of statins: Implications for cardiovascular event reduction. *Journal of the American Medical Association*, *279*(20), 1643–1650.

Sever, P., Dahlof, B., Poulter, N., et al. (2004). Prevention of coronary and stroke events with atorvastatin in hypertensive patients who have average or lower-than-average cholesterol concentrations, in the Anglo-Scandinavian Cardiac Outcomes Trial–Lipid Lowering Arm (ASCOT-LLA): A multicentre randomised controlled trial. *Drugs*, *64*(Suppl 2), 43–60.

Shepherd, J., Blauw, G., Murphy, B., et al. (2002). Pravastatin in elderly individuals at risk for vascular disease (PROSPER): A randomized controlled trial. *Lancet*, *360*(9346), 1623–1630.

Sheridan, S., Pignone, M., and Mulrow, C. (2003). Framingham-based tools to calculate the global risk of coronary heart disease: A systematic review of tools for clinicians. *Journal of General Internal Medicine*, *18*(12), 1039–1052.

Vasudevan, A., Hamirai, Y., and Jones, P. (2005). Safety of statins: Effects on muscle and the liver. *Cleveland Clinic Journal of Medicine*, *72*(11), 990–993, 996–1001.

Volker, D., Fitzgerald, P., Major, G., et al. (2000). Efficacy of fish oil concentrate in the treatment of rheumatoid arthritis. *Journal of Rheumatology*, *27*(110), 2343–2346.

CARDIOVASCULAR

Anticoagulant and Antiplatelet Drugs

Thromboembolic disease and risk factors for thromboemboli are seen frequently in ambulatory patients with deep vein thrombosis (DVT) of the lower extremities and occur in a significant number of hospitalized patients. Atrial fibrillation, ischemic stroke, valvular heart disease, prosthetic cardiac valves, coronary and peripheral vascular disease, and hypercoagulable states all contribute to the risk for thromboembolic events and the need for anticoagulant and/or antiplatelet therapy.

Drugs discussed in this chapter disrupt normal hemostasis, thereby reducing the risk of clotting but also increasing the risk of bleeding. These drugs include anticoagulants and antiplatelet drugs. Unlike thrombolytic drugs (see Chapter 40), which are used to dissolve blood clots, anticoagulant and antiplatelet drugs prevent the development or extension of clots. An understanding of the pathogenesis of thromboembolic disorders is essential for determining appropriate treatment.

THROMBOEMBOLIC DISEASE

EPIDEMIOLOGY AND ETIOLOGY

DVT affects one in 1000 persons and is more common in women (especially during pregnancy), although men have a 50% higher risk for DVT than women following anticoagulant therapy. Further, there is a 50% risk of a silent pulmonary embolism (PE) in patients with a proximal DVT; PE contributes to more than 200,000 deaths/year. The mortality rate associated with untreated PE ranges from 25% to 42%. However, survival rates are as high as 92% when the patient is adequately treated.

Thrombus formation that obstructs blood flow through both superficial and deep veins is usually attributed to *Virchow's triad:* venous stasis, damage to venous epithelium, and a hypercoagulable state. Two of the three factors must be present for thrombi to form. However, a patient may develop a clot from just one risk factor, such as the presence of an inherited hypercoagulable condition or cancer.

Venous stasis is usually associated with restricted mobility or a lack of the use of calf muscles. Other conditions contributing to venous stasis include prolonged bed rest, surgery with general, spinal, or epidural anesthesia that lasts longer than 30 minutes, pregnancy, obesity, paralysis, and heart failure. Researchers who compared markers of anticoagulation and fibrinolysis in people who spent 8 hours on an aircraft with those of people who spent 8 sedentary hours watching movies at sea level, or just going about their daily lives note that factors like low oxygen levels and reduced atmospheric pressure may help explain the increased thrombin generation on aircraft.

Damage to venous epithelium can be caused by intravenous (IV) injections, lack of attentive care of indwelling IV insertion sites, chemical injury from sclerosing drugs (see Chapter 40), imaging studies requiring IV contrast media, thromboangiitis obliterans (Buerger's disease), fractures, and dislocations. Hypercoagulable states (e.g., protein C or S deficiency, factor V Leiden mutation) often accompany thromboembolic events. All types of cancers increase clot risk, particularly those associated with visceral and ovarian tumors. Estrogen therapy and use of oral contraceptives increase the risk of a hypercoagulable state. Dehydration and blood dyscrasias raise platelet counts, reduce fibrinolysis, increase clotting factors or blood viscosity, and contribute to the risk of thrombus formation (see Box 39-1).

PHYSIOLOGY AND PATHOPHYSIOLOGY

Hemostasis, the ability of the body to manage blood flow following injury, has four mechanisms. Although initiated by distinctly different mechanisms, the intrinsic and extrinsic coagulation pathways come together in the following clot formation process: (1) vasoconstriction limits blood flow to the injured area; (2) platelets migrate to the injury site to form a temporary platelet plug; (3) fibrin meshwork is formed, which entraps the platelet plug; and finally (4) the clot is broken down through the action of plasmin, and normal blood flow resumes in the injured area (see Fig. 39-1). The coagulation factors for both the intrinsic and extrinsic pathways are identified in Table 39-1.

Intrinsic Pathway

In the absence of injury, the intrinsic coagulation pathway triggers clot formation whereby factor XII comes into contact with the foreign surface of an abnormal or injured vessel wall (e.g., the presence of atherosclerotic plaques). The contact begins a cascade of reactions that lead to conversion of inactive factor X to factor Xa ("a" means active) at the common pathway, and then to the conversion of prothrombin to thrombin and, finally, of fibrinogen to fibrin.

Extrinsic Pathway

The extrinsic coagulation pathway is triggered by tissue injury. The extrinsic pathway produces fibrin in seconds, much more quickly than the intrinsic pathway, by skirting the beginning stages of the cascade. The extrinsic pathway begins with tissue damage outside the vessel. Damaged tissues circulate factor III, or thromboplastin, which launches the clotting cascade to form factor Xa and the concluding pathway of clot development. In addition, a platelet plug forms when a vessel wall is injured as a result of collagen stimulation. When platelet adhesion occurs, adenosine diphosphate (ADP), thrombin, thromboxane A_2 (TXA_2), and prostaglandin H_2 are released into circulation. Platelets collect at the site of injury, forming a weak clot in an attempt to repair the injured site. The

Risk Factors for Thromboembolic Disease

- Abdominal and pelvic surgery, surgery on long bones
- Advanced age (particularly patients over 40 years of age)
- Bed rest, prolonged immobility, travel with limited ability to move about
- Cardiovascular disease (atrial fibrillation, heart failure, AMI, hypertension, stroke)
- Cigarette, cigar, or pipe smoking
- Dehydration or malnutrition
- Diabetes mellitus
- Estrogen therapy, use of oral contraceptives
- Fractured hip, joint replacement
- Intravenous therapy, venous catheterization
- Neoplasms, especially hepatic and pancreatic
- Obesity
- Pregnancy, particularly the postpartum period
- Previous history of thrombophlebitis, varicosities
- Blood dyscrasias (e.g., polycythemia vera and other acquired and inherited thrombophilias)
- Sepsis
- Surgery lasting more than 30 minutes with general, spinal, or epidural anesthesia
- Trauma, spinal cord injury

AMI, Acute myocardial infarction.

addition of fibrin results in the stable fibrin-platelet plug (see Fig. 39-2).

Drugs that prevent the formation of the clot (i.e., stable fibrin-platelet plug) by inhibiting certain clotting factors are known as *anticoagulants*. These drugs are given prophylactically; they have no direct effect on a clot already formed, or on tissues that become ischemic as a result of inadequate blood supply distal to the clot.

PHARMACOTHERAPEUTIC OPTIONS

Anticoagulants
Oral Anticoagulant
◆ warfarin (Coumadin, Jantoven); ✦ Warnerin, Warfilone

Parenteral Anticoagulants
◆ dalteparin (Fragmin); ✦ Fragmin
◆ enoxaparin (Lovenox); ✦ Klexane
◆ fondaparinux (Arixtra)
◆ tinzaparin (Innohep); ✦ Innohep
◆ unfractionated heparin calcium and heparin sodium (Calciparine, Liquaemin Sodium); ✦ Hepalean Leo, Heparin Leo

▦ *Indications*
Warfarin, a coumarin derivative, is the prototype and the oldest oral anticoagulant. It is the most frequently used oral anticoagulant for the long-term prevention and prophylaxis of DVT and PE. It is also used in the prophylaxis and treatment of thromboembolic complications associated with atrial fibrillation, and/or cardiac valve replacement. It reduces the risk of death, recurrent MI, and thromboembolic events such as stroke or systemic embolization after MI.

Unfractionated heparin (UFH), a parenteral anticoagulant, is used for the prevention and treatment of DVT and PE, in the treatment of atrial fibrillation with embolization, and with percutaneous coronary interventions (PCI), as adjunct treatment with thrombolytics in patients without and with ST-segment elevation myocardial infarction (MI; STEMI), as well as in the prevention of cerebral thrombosis in patients with an evolving stroke. Heparin is also used in the diagnosis and treatment of disseminated intravascular coagulation (DIC) and for prevention of clotting in blood samples and heparin locks, and during dialysis procedures.

The low–molecular weight heparin (LMWH) dalteparin is used in the treatment of unstable angina and non–Q-wave MI to prevent ischemic events. It is also used for prophylaxis of DVT in patients undergoing hip replacement or abdominal surgery who are at risk for thromboembolic complications (Box 39-1). Dalteparin is also used to prevent DVT or PE in acutely ill patients with severely restricted mobility.

Enoxaparin, a LMWH, is commonly used for the prevention of postoperative DVT following hip and knee replacement surgery and abdominal surgery; for long-term prevention follow hip replacement surgery; as DVT prophylaxis in patients with severely restricted mobility or acute illness; and in the treatment of unstable angina, non–Q-wave MI, and acute DVT (with warfarin).

Tinzaparin, a newer LMWH, is used in the treatment of acute symptomatic DVT with or without PE (concurrently with warfarin). Although still relatively new, fondaparinux has the potential to be used in the prevention and treatment of DVT after orthopedic surgery, and for the treatment of acute coronary syndromes.

Current guidelines support the use of warfarin, LMWH, or fondaparinux for thromboembolic prophylaxis following lower limb major orthopedic surgery. For prophylaxis in hospitalized medical patients or patients undergoing general surgery, use of UFH and LMWH is supported; however, recent data on fondaparinux suggest that it is also effective in these patient populations. The use of UFH or LMWH (both in conjunction with warfarin) for treatment of acute DVT or nonmassive PE is recommended. Recent data suggest that fondaparinux (in conjunction with warfarin) is also effective for the treatment of venous thromboembolic events.

▦ *Pharmacodynamics*
All anticoagulants work within the clotting cascade but do so at different points (see Fig. 39-1). Warfarin, a racemic mixture of two active isomers (the R and S forms), suppresses coagulation by inhibiting the production of vitamin K–dependent clotting factors in the liver. By reducing the amount of available vitamin K, clotting factors II, VII, IX, and X are reduced. The result is that these vitamin K–related clotting factors are also dysfunctional, and therefore the risk for clot formation is decreased.

Factors XI and XII are also inactivated, but these factors do not have as significant a role as the others. Of these, thrombin is the most sensitive to the action of UFH. In low dosages, UFH prevents the conversion of prothrombin to thrombin by its effects on factor Xa. In higher doses, UFH neutralizes thrombin, thus preventing the conversion of fibrinogen to fibrin. UFH is a large molecule, and because of its structure, only a small portion of the entire structure is necessary for binding with antithrombin III (AT-III). Platelet function that is dependent on the von Willebrand factor is also inhibited.

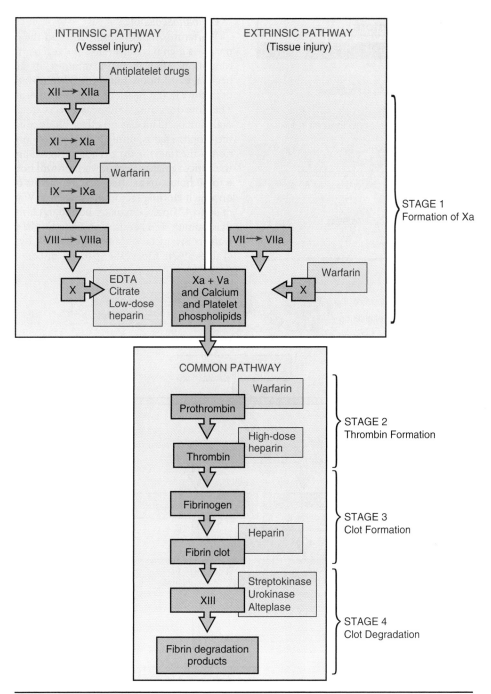

FIGURE 39-1 Clotting Cascade. The clotting cascade is a series of enzymatic reactions that produces a fibrin blood clot. Damage to blood vessels or, in some cases, hypercoagulability of the blood initiates the intrinsic pathway. The extrinsic pathway is activated by tissue injury. Anticoagulant and antiplatelet drugs can act at various locations throughout the cascade.

LMWHs such as dalteparin, enoxaparin, and tinzaparin are partial depolymerizations of UFH resulting in fragments approximately 33% the size of the parent compound. They are much more selective and work mostly on Xa and AT-III, without much effect on thrombin. Thus they don't affect the activated partial thromboplastin time (aPTT).

Fondaparinux is a pure AT-III-dependent factor Xa inhibitor. The binding of factor Xa to factor Va on platelets is responsible for the conversion of prothrombin to thrombin.

Fondaparinux has no actions on platelet functioning. Recombinant factor VIIa reverses the effects of anticoagulation from fondaparinux administration.

HEPARIN RESISTANCE. Heparin resistance is seen in patients receiving high dosages of heparin. Variables contributing to heparin resistance include the factor VIII levels, AT deficiency, increased clearance of heparin, and increases in fibrinogen and heparin-binding proteins. However, heparin dosage can be adjusted to achieve the desired anti–factor Xa concentrations.

TABLE 39-1 Coagulation Factors

Factor	Pathway	Common Names
I	Common	Fibrinogen
II	Common	Prothrombin
III	Extrinsic	Tissue thromboplastin, tissue factor
IV	Common	Calcium
V	Common	AC-Globulin, proaccelerin
VI	—	Accelerin (NOTE: This is really Factor Va, redundant to Factor V)
VII	Extrinsic	Prothrombin conversion accelerator, stable factor, cothromboplastin
VIII	Intrinsic	Antihemophilic factor A, antihemophilic globulin
IX	Intrinsic	Christmas factor, antihemophilic factor B, plasma thromboplastin
X	Common	Stuart-Prower factor
XI	Intrinsic	Plasma thromboplastin antecedent
XII	Intrinsic	Hageman factor
XIII	Common	Fibrin-stabilizing factor

▮▮ *Pharmacokinetics*

Warfarin is rapidly absorbed from the gastrointestinal (GI) tract, has high bioavailability, and reaches maximal serum concentrations after about 90 minutes. Its anticoagulant effects begin 8 to 12 hours following administration with inhibition of factor VII, but peak effects do not appear for 48 to 72 hours. The slow drug onset and peak effects are delayed because this oral anticoagulant has no effect on existing clotting factors in the blood. That is, until clotting factors present in the circulation at the time the drug is administered break down naturally, the anticoagulant effect of warfarin will not be evident. It takes 6 to 60 hours for existing clotting factors to decay, depending on which clotting factors are involved. Warfarin has a half-life of 36 to 42 hours, circulates bound to plasma proteins (primarily albumin; 97%) and accumulates in the liver, where the two isomers are metabolically transformed by different pathways (Table 39-2). Once the patient discontinues warfarin, the

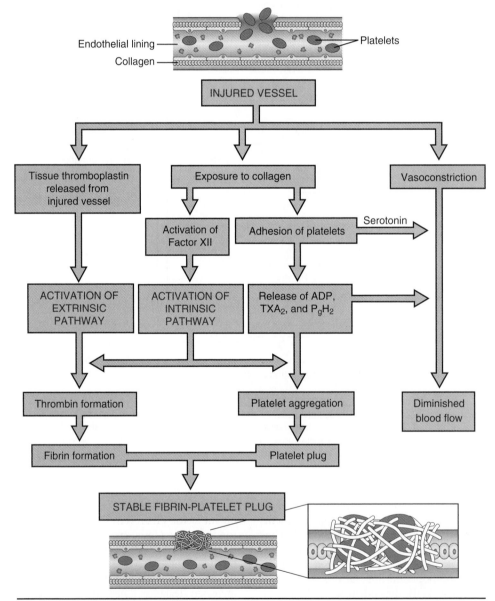

FIGURE 39-2 Events Leading to Formation of Stable Fibrin-Platelet Plug. When the endothelial lining of a blood vessel is damaged, physical and biochemical mechanisms work together to produce a stable fibrin-platelet plug, and prevent blood loss.

PHARMACOKINETICS
TABLE 39-2 Anticoagulant and Antiplatelet Drugs

Drugs	Route	Onset	Peak	Duration	PB (%)	t½	BioA (%)
ANTICOAGULANTS							
dalteparin	SubQ	20–60 min	3–5 hr	12 hr	High	2–5 hr	87
enoxaparin	SubQ	20–60 min	3–5 hr	12 hr	High	4.5 hr	91
fondaparinux	SubQ	Rapid	2 hr	UA	UA	17 hr	100
heparin	SubQ	20–60 min	2–4 hr	8–12 hr	High	1–2 hr*	100
	IV	Immed	5–10 min	2–6 hr	High	1–2 hr*	100
tinzaparin	SubQ	Rapid	4–5 hr	UA	UA	3–4 hr	86.7
warfarin	PO	Slow	0.5–3 days	2–5 days	95–97	0.5–3 days	85–99
NEWER ANTICOAGULANTS							
argatroban	IV	Immed	1–3 hr	6 days	54	39-51 min	100
bivalirudin	IV	Immed	10 min	60 min	0	25 min	100
desirudin	SubQ, IV	Immed	1–3 hr	UA	UA	2–3 hr	100
lepirudin	IV	Immed	10 min	1 hr	UA	60 min	100
ANTIPLATELET DRUGS							
abciximab	IV	Rapid	2 hr	14 days	UA	10 min; 30 min†	100
aspirin	PO	5–30 min	30–40 min; 3–4 hr‡	3–6 hr	Varies	15–20 min; 15–30 hr‡	Varies
clopidogrel	PO	Rapid	2 hr	7 days	UA	8 hr§	Varies
dipyridamole	PO	Varies	75 min	3–4 hr	91–99	10–15 hr	30–60
	IV	Immed	6.5 min	30 min	91–99	10 hr	100
pentoxifylline	PO	2–4 wk	8 wk	UA	UA	24–48 min	UA
eptifibatide	IV	Immed	UA	UA	UA	3.5–7.5 min	100
ticlodipine	PO	48 hr	7 days	14 days	High	24–36 hr; 4–5 days‖	90
tirofiban	IV	Immed	UA	4 hr	UA	1.6 hr	100
ANTICOAGULANT ANTAGONISTS							
protamine sulfate	IV	30–60 sec	UA	2 hr¶	UA	UA	100
phytonadione	PO	1–2 hr	1–2 hr**	12–24 hr	UA	UA	UA

*Half life of heparin increases with increasing dosage.
†Biphasic half-life of abciximab. Platelet function generally returns within 48 hr.
‡Peak serum levels of enteric coated aspirin; half-life of aspirin with low doses and large doses respectively.
§Half-life of clopidogrel active metabolite is 8 hr.
‖Half life of ticlopidine with single dose is 24–36 hr, with multiple dosing over 4–5 days.
¶Duration of action of protamine sulfate depends on body temperature.
**Peak action of phytonadione for control of bleeding when given PO. Duration of drug action of phytonadione to achieve normal INR value. Bleeding is usually controlled within 3–6 hr, and a normal INR may often be obtained 12–24 hr after administration.
BioA, Bioavailability; *Immed*, immediate; *INR*, international normalized ratio; *IV*, intravenous; *PB*, protein binding; *PO*, by mouth; *subQ*; subcutaneous; *t½*, half-life; *UA*, unavailable.

anticoagulant effects remain for up to 120 hours, not because of warfarin's half-life, but because of the time it takes to manufacture new vitamin K-dependent clotting factors, some of which have long half-lives.

UFH, on the other hand, is a protein destroyed by enzymes in the GI tract; therefore parenteral administration is necessary. UFH is well absorbed following subcutaneous (subQ) administration, with an immediate onset of action and peak levels occurring 2 to 4 hours after administration, depending on the dose. It is administered by intravenous (IV) route when rapid anticoagulation is needed, as in acute DVT, PE, or unstable angina. UFH is biotransformed by liver heparinase and removed by the reticuloendothelial system (i.e., lymph nodes and spleen) and secondarily by the kidneys. It is then excreted in the urine as unchanged drug. The half-life lengthens with increasing dosage. UFH does not cross the placenta or enter breast milk.

UFH is highly bound to plasma proteins and cellular components, including endothelial cells and macrophages, which reduces its therapeutic effect and increases the risk of immunologic reactions. Some patients develop heparin resistance characterized by no measureable changes in anticoagulant response despite receiving large doses (e.g., 35,000 units) daily.

UFH also has a nonlinear dose response, meaning that small changes in dosage can result in large changes in anticoagulant effects. For this reason, the use of UFH is usually restricted to inpatient settings where frequent laboratory monitoring can be done.

After subQ administration, the absolute bioavailability of tinzaparin is 86.7% on the basis of anti–factor Xa activity. The half-life of tinzaparin is longer than that of UFH. This longer half-life, together with higher bioavailability and less binding to plasma proteins, allows for once-daily administration. Unlike UFH, tinzaparin is primarily eliminated through an unsaturable renal mechanism, and its rate of clearance is dose-independent.

Glycosaminoglycans, the main components of LMWHs, cannot be used to directly measure LMWH pharmacokinetics, since glycosaminoglycans are normally present in tissues and biologic fluids. As a result, the pharmacokinetics of tinzaparin and all LMWHs are determined by using indirect measures, specifically anti–factor Xa and anti–factor IIa activity. The pharmacokinetics of LMWHs are identified in Table 39-2. LMWH does not cross placental membranes or enter breast milk; they are considered safe for use in pregnancy.

▥ *Adverse Effects and Contraindications*

Bleeding is the principal concern with anticoagulants, occurring in approximately 10% of patients. **The danger of bleeding increases as the dosage of the anticoagulant increases and with the addition of other platelet-altering drugs** (e.g., aspirin).

Potentially unfavorable reactions to warfarin include GI disturbances, skin necrosis, dermatitis, hair loss, urticaria, fever, and orange-red urine discoloration. Warfarin is contraindicated for use in patients with vitamin K deficiency, hemorrhagic disorders, subacute bacterial endocarditis, uncontrolled hypertension, and severe thrombocytopenia. Warfarin may be used in patients with hepatic disease provided they are closely monitored. Patients requiring indwelling catheter placement and those undergoing lumbar puncture, regional anesthesia, and surgery of the eye, brain, or spinal cord should avoid warfarin and may require temporary warfarin discontinuation. If they have a high thromboembolic risk during this time, they may also require bridging with heparin or LMWH during the period when the effects of warfarin are wearing off. When warfarin is reinitiated after the procedure, it may be initiated with heparin or LMWH until the international normalized ratio (INR) is therapeutic again.

Exercise caution when using warfarin in patients with bleeding tendencies such as hemophilia; increased capillary permeability, dissecting aneurysm, duodenal, gastric, or esophageal ulcers; active tuberculosis; diabetes; or heparin-induced thrombocytopenia, as well as patients at risk for hemorrhage, necrosis, and gangrene, and in women contemplating abortion. Also use caution with warfarin in patients with heart failure, diarrhea, fever, and thyrotoxicosis, since these situations all alter INR response. Warfarin administration during pregnancy and lactation is contraindicated. Warfarin crosses the placental membranes and can result in fetal injury, such as malformation, central nervous system (CNS) defects, optic atrophy, hemorrhage, and death. Warfarin also enters breast milk; do not use it during lactation. Contraindications to the use of warfarin include severe hepatic or renal damage, uncontrolled bleeding, open wounds or ulcers, severe hypertension, and neurosurgical procedures.

The adverse effects of UFH are similar but less extensive than those of warfarin. Bleeding tendencies, hyperkalemia, osteoporosis, and hair loss are possible. In addition, suppression of renal function occurs with high-dose, long-term therapy.

Heparin-induced thrombocytopenia (HIT_1 and HIT_2) is predominantly a clinical adverse effect characterized not only by thrombocytopenia (defined as a 50% fall in platelets or less than 150,000/mL, or acute systemic reactions occur within 5 to 30 minutes of IV administration of heparin), but also by thromboses, and thromboembolic complications. The immune-mediated form of HIT, HIT_2, occurs in 30% of patients treated with heparin. HIT can be thought of as an allergy-like reaction and is most common in patients receiving IV UFH, but also occurs in patients receiving LMWH, heparin flushes, and hemodialysis, and in patients with heparin-coated catheters. Of patients receiving UFH, up to 10% will develop detectable levels of HIT antibody. **Of the approximately 30% to 50% of patients who form HIT antibodies and develop thrombocytopenia, 30% to 80% go on to develop a thrombosis.**

HIT places patients at risk for life- and limb-threatening consequences, including peripheral arterial occlusion, ischemic stroke, limb gangrene, acute myocardial infarction, and pulmonary embolism. Although the anticoagulant effects of heparin may be reversed with the use of the antagonist, protamine sulfate, reversal of these effects is not an effective treatment for HIT.

Although it typically appears 4 to 14 days after the start of heparin therapy, HIT can also occur as early as 10 hours after administration if the patient has been exposed to heparin within the previous 100 days (reexposure), or can occur several days after withdrawal of all forms of heparin.

Because there is no way to identify patients at high risk for HIT before administration of heparin, maintaining a high index of suspicion is critical; immediate cessation of heparin upon strong clinical suspicion of HIT is mandatory.

Contraindications to use of UFH are similar to those of warfarin. Avoid use of UFH in patients with severe thrombocytopenia or uncontrolled bleeding. Avoid IV administration of UFH in any patient who cannot be regularly monitored or who is in labor or in the immediate postpartum period. It may, however, be used as prophylaxis in low doses. If an anticoagulant is needed during pregnancy for prophylaxis or treatment, UFH and LMWH may be used since they do not cross placental membranes.

The adverse effects, contraindications, and precautions of enoxaparin, dalteparin, and tinzaparin are also similar to those of UFH; however, there is a lower incidence of HIT with LMWH, as well as a lower incidence of osteoporosis. They are contraindicated for use in the presence of hypersensitivity, heparin-induced thrombocytopenia, and uncontrolled bleeding. In addition, these drugs are contraindicated for use in patients with an allergy to pork.

While the most commonly reported adverse effect of tinzaparin is bleeding, the frequency of major bleeding (1%) is low compared with that with UFH. Other bleeding events associated with tinzaparin and occurring less than 2% of the time include epistaxis, hemorrhage, and hematuria. Thrombocytopenia has been reported in approximately 1% of patients; the rate of severe thrombocytopenia (platelet count less than 50,000 cells/mcL) is less than 1%. Other commonly reported adverse events in controlled clinical trials were injection-site hematomas, abnormal elevations of aspartate transaminase (AST) and alanine transaminase (ALT), urinary tract infection, PE, and chest pain. Less common adverse events include headache, nausea, fever, back pain, and constipation (occurring in <2% of patients). Priapism has been reported as a rare occurrence during postmarketing surveillance.

Tinzaparin is contraindicated for use in patients with active major bleeding, patients with (or with a history of) HIT. There is a black box warning, shared by all LMWHs and heparins, regarding concomitant use with spinal or epidural anesthesia or spinal puncture and the increased risk of a spinal or epidural hematoma. As with other anticoagulants, tinzaparin should be used with extreme caution in patients predisposed to hemorrhage. Patients with known hypersensitivity to heparin, sulfites, benzyl alcohol, or pork products should not be treated with tinzaparin. Tinzaparin is in pregnancy category B. It is not known if tinzaparin is excreted in human milk.

▌ Drug Interactions

Numerous drug interactions can occur with anticoagulants, particularly warfarin. Avoiding drugs that interfere with INR controls is recommended. If this is not possible, close monitoring of the INR is required. Table 39-3 summarizes just a few of the extensive drug interactions for anticoagulants.

Alterations in vitamin K levels alter the effects of warfarin. A diet high in green leafy vegetables reduces the effectiveness of warfarin. Consistency in patient intake of high vitamin K foods is recommended. There are no major drug-food interactions with parenteral anticoagulants.

▌ Dosage Regimens

Patient response to warfarin is unpredictable. The average daily dosage ranges from less than 1 mg/day to over 20 mg/day. To avoid complications, dosages are adjusted based on the INR value every few days and then weekly for the first month, and then monthly if they are stable. Checking the

DRUG INTERACTIONS
TABLE 39-3 Selected Anticoagulant and Antiplatelet Drugs

Drug	Interactive Drugs	Interaction
ANTICOAGULANTS		
warfarin	allopurinol, amiodarone, Anabolic steroids, Androgens, aspirin, bumetanide, Cephalosporins, chloral hydrate, clofibrate, chloramphenicol, cimetidine, clofibrate, cotrimoxazole, danazol, disulfiram, erythromycin, ethacrynic acid, famotidine, fenoprofen, furosemide, garlic, gemfibrozil, gingko biloba, ginseng, glucagon, glucosamine-chondroitin, indomethacin, methimazole, meclofenamate, mefenamic acid, metronidazole, moxalactam, nalidixic acid, nizatidine, oxyphenbutazone, Oral hypoglycemics, phenytoin, phenylbutazone, plicamycin, propylthiouracil, quinidine, quinine, ranitidine, Salicylates, sulfinpyrazone, Sulfonamides, sulindac	Increased effects of anticoagulant and risk for bleeding
	American ginseng, aminoglutethimide, Barbiturates, carbamazepine, cholestyramine, colistopol, estramustine, Estrogens, griseofulvin, Oral contraceptives, primidone, rifampin, St. John's wort, vitamin E, vitamin K	Decreased effects of anticoagulants
	phenytoin	Increases effects of interactive drug
	methimazole, propylthiouracil	Alters effects of warfarin
heparin	Antiplatelet drugs, Cephalosporins, NSAIDs, Penicillins, probenecid, Oral anticoagulants	Increases effects of heparin
	nitroglycerin	Decreases effects of heparin
enoxaparin, dalteparin	Oral anticoagulants, Platelet-inhibiting drugs, Salicylates	Increases effects of anticoagulant and risk for bleeding
tinzaparin	Anticoagulants, Platelet inhibitors, gingko biloba	Increases risk for bleeding
argatroban	Antiplatelet drugs, Thrombolytics, Other anticoagulants	Increases risk for bleeding
bivalirudin	Antiplatelet drugs (other than aspirin), gingko biloba, Thrombolytics, warfarin	Increases risk for bleeding
desirudin	abciximab, Antiplatelet drugs, clopidogrel, dextran, dipyridamole, GPIIb-III drugs, Glucocorticoids, NSAIDs, Other anticoagulants, ticlopidine, Thrombolytics	Increases risk for bleeding
ANTIPLATELET DRUGS		
abciximab	Anticoagulants, Platelet aggregation inhibitors (e.g., aspirin, dextran, thrombolytic drugs)	Increases risk of bleeding and hemorrhage
aspirin	Antiplatelet drugs, heparin, Insulins, Oral anticoagulants, methotrexate, NSAIDs, GPIIb-IIIa antagonists, Sulfonylureas, Valproates	Increases effect of interactive drugs
	Beta blockers, ACE inhibitors, furosemide, probenecid, spironolactone, sulfinpyrazone	Decreases effect of interactive drugs
	Alcohol, Corticosteroids, NSAIDs, phenylbutazone	Increases risk of GI ulceration
	ammonium chloride, ascorbic acid, furosemide, Carbonic anhydrase inhibitors	Increases serum salicylate levels
	acetazolamide, Antacids, Alkalinizers, Corticosteroids, methazolamide	Decreases serum salicylate levels
clopidogrel	atorvastatin, fluvastatin, simvastatin	Inhibits clopidogrel biotransformation
	fluvastatin, NSAIDs, phenytoin, tamoxifen, tolbutamide, torsemide, warfarin	Interferes with biotransformation of interactive drug
eptifibatide	Anticoagulants, Platelet aggregation inhibitors (e.g., aspirin, dextran, thrombolytic drugs)	Increases risk of bleeding and hemorrhage
dipyridamole	theophylline	Decreases coronary vasodilation effects
pentoxifylline	Anticoagulants, Salicylates, Thrombolytics	Increases risk for bleeding
	cimetidine	Increases effects of pentoxifylline
ticlopidine	digoxin	Decreases effects of interacting drug
	Anticoagulants, aspirin, NSAIDs, theophylline	Increases effects of interacting drug
	cimetidine	Increases effects of ticlopidine
	Antacids	Decreases effects of ticlopidine
tirofiban	Anticoagulants, NSAIDs, Thrombolytics	Affects hemostasis

ACE, Angiotensin-converting enzyme; GI, gastrointestinal; NSAIDs, nonsteroidal antiinflammatory drugs.

INR within 2 weeks of a dosage change in an otherwise stable patient is also recommended (Table 39-4). The risk of bleeding is not usually increased if the INR is in the target range of 2 to 3; higher INRs are associated with a greater risk of bleeding.

In contrast to warfarin, UFH is dosed based on weight and then on the aPTT. Dosages are adjusted based on aPTT levels.

The therapeutic dosage range is usually a aPTT value 1.5 to 2 times the control value or to a target PTT based on the institution's thromboplastin (see Table 39-4). If the aPTT is too high, decrease the dosage; if the aPTT is too low, increase the dosage. Unlike UFH, the dosages of LMWH are not routinely monitored, but consider dosage adjustments for renal

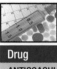

DOSAGE
TABLE 39-4 Selected Anticoagulant and Antiplatelet Drugs

Drug	Use(s)	Dosage	Implications
ANTICOAGULANTS			
dalteparin	DVT prophylaxis after general or orthopedic surgery, venous thromboembolism	*Adult:* 2500 units subQ each day starting 1–2 hr before surgery and repeating once daily for 5–10 days postop	Dosage for general surgery patients based on potential for thrombus formation. Approximate cost: $72/day
enoxaparin	DVT prophylaxis after hip replacement, general or orthopedic surgery	*Adult:* 30 mg subQ twice daily as initial dose as soon as possible after surgery, not more than 24 hr later. Up to 14 days may be needed.	Treatment continued throughout postop period. Approximate cost: $98/day
fondaparinux	Prophylaxis DVT in joint replacement or hip fracture; acute PE	*Adult:* 2.5 mg subQ daily for 5–9 days postop. Initial dose given 6–8 hr after surgery	Renal dosing considerations required.
heparin	Treatment of thromboembolism DVT, PE	*Adult Treatment:* 80 units/kg IV bolus then 18 units/kg/hr IV infusion –or– 15,000–20,000 units subQ every 12 hr *Postoperative Prophylaxis:* 5000 units subQ 2 hr before surgery and every 8–12 hr thereafter for 7 days or until patient ambulatory *Child >12 mo:* 50 units/kg IV bolus then 50–100 units/kg IV every 4 hr, or 75 units/kg bolus then 20 units/kg/hr continuous IV infusion	Dosage determined by patient weight initially and then changes made based on aPTT values. Adjust dosage of heparin by the measuring of aPTT, or, when very high doses are given, by ACT. These tests are sensitive mainly to the AT effects of heparin.
	Unstable angina; non-STEMI	*Adult:* 70 units/kg IV bolus. Max: 5,000 units. Follow by 12–15 unit/kg/hr IV infusion. Max: 1,000 units/hr	
	Patients receiving t-Pa for acute STEMI	*Adult:* 60 unit/kg IV bolus. Max: 4000 units. Follow by 12 units/kg/hr IV infusion.	
	PCI	*Adult:* 70 units/kg IV bolus. Additional doses to keep ACT in 200s.	Given together with GPIIb-IIIa therapy
tinzaparin	Acute symptomatic DVT with or without PE	*Adult:* 175 anti-Xa international units deep subQ once daily for at least 6 days and until patient sufficiently anticoagulated with warfarin	Injection site reactions common. Available as a 2-mL multiple-dose vial containing 20,000 anti–factor Xa units of tinzaparin sodium/mL. Approximate cost: $59/day
warfarin sodium	Prophylaxis against thrombus formation	*Adult:* 5–10 mg PO daily initially. Maintenance: 2–10 mg PO daily	Dosage determined by PT and INR values. Lower dosages needed for older adults
NEWER ANTICOAGULANTS			
argatroban	HIT prophylaxis and treatment	*Adult:* 2 mcg/kg/min IV as continuous infusion. Max: 10 mcg/kg/min. Adjust dosage based on aPTT.	Stop heparin and obtain aPTT before starting argatroban. Renal dosing considerations required. Approximate cost: $6275 for 7 days of therapy
	PCI	*Adult:* 25 mcg/kg/min initially plus bolus of 350 mg/kg over 3–5 min. Give additional bolus of 150 mg/kg if ACT <300 sec; if longer than 300 sec, decrease infusion to 15 mg/kg/min.	Check ACT at 5–10 min following bolus. Infusion rate based on body weight at 2 mcg/kg/min.
bivalirudin	Adjunct for patient with unstable angina undergoing PTCA; patients with HIT undergoing PCI	*Adult:* 1 mg/kg IV bolus followed by 4-hr infusion at 2.5 mg/kg/hr. May give additional IV infusion at rate of 0.2 mg/kg/hr for 20 hr or less if needed.	Renal dosing considerations required. ACT checked 5 min after bolus dose. Continue up to 4 hr. Use with 300–325 mg aspirin daily.
desirudin	Prophylaxis DVT for patients undergoing hip or knee surgery	*Adult:* 15 mg subQ twice daily for 9–12 days	Does not require routine lab monitoring unless high dosages are used.
lepirudin rDNA	HIT	*Adult:* 0.4 mg/kg IV bolus followed by 0.15 mg/kg/hour infusion as long as needed	Duration of therapy usually 2–10 days.
ANTIPLATELET DRUGS			
abciximab	Percutaneous coronary intervention	*Adult:* 0.25 mg/kg IV 10–60 min before angioplasty or atherectomy, then 12-hr IV infusion of 0.125 mcg/kg/min. Max: 10 mcg/min	Contraindicated for use in patients with active internal bleeding, GI, GU bleeding in last 6 wk, history of CVA within 2 yr of CVA with residual neurologic defect, PO anticoagulants within 7 days unless PT <1.2 × control; thrombocytopenia, recent surgery, or trauma in last 6 wk, intracranial neoplasm, severe uncontrolled HTN, AV malformation or aneurysm, history of vasculitis, prior IV dextran use before or during PTCA
	Percutaneous coronary intervention; unstable angina	*Adult:* 0.25 mg/kg IV followed by 18- to 24-hr infusion of 10 mcg/min; end 1 hr after procedure	

aspirin	TIA prophylaxis, thromboembolic event prophylaxis, unstable angina	*Adult:* 81 mg PO daily	**Low doses do not change lab values; high dosages do not confer added risk reduction.**
	Acute ischemic stroke; myocardial infarction	*Adult:* 160 mg PO daily	
clopidogrel	Risk reduction of MI, stroke, vascular death in patients with documented atherosclerosis; treatment of ACS.	*Adult:* 75 mg PO once daily in combination with aspirin *Adult ACS:* 300 mg loading dose once, then 75 mg PO daily in combination with aspirin	**Check platelet counts before drug therapy, every 2 days during the first week of treatment,** and weekly thereafter until therapeutic maintenance dose is reached.
dipyridamole	After valvular surgery	*Adult:* 75–100 mg PO 4 times daily	Used as an adjunct to warfarin therapy
eptifibatide	Acute coronary syndrome; PCI	*Adult as adjunct to PCI:* 180 mcg/kg IV bolus or infusion before PCI initiation, then continuous drip of 2 mcg/kg and a second 180 mcg/kg bolus 10 minutes after the first. Max: 15 mg/hr *Adult ACS:* 180 mcg/kg IV bolus or infusion, then 2 mg/kg/min until discharge or CABG, up to 72 hr. Max: 15 mg/hr.	Renal dosing considerations required. Continue until hospital discharge or for up to 18–24 hr. Minimum of 12 hr recommended. Concurrent aspirin and heparin therapy recommended.
pentoxifylline	Intermittent claudication associated with occlusive PVD	*Adult:* 400 mg PO 3 times daily	Tablets should not be crushed, broken, or chewed.
ticlopidine	CVA prophylaxis	*Adult:* 250 mg PO twice daily	Safety and efficacy in children under age 18 yr not established.
tirofiban	ACS, patients undergoing PCTA or atherectomy	*Adults:* 0.4 mcg/kg/min for 30 min, then 0.1 mcg/kg/min throughout procedure and for 12–24 hours following procedure	Renal dosing considerations required.
ANTICOAGULANT ANTAGONISTS			
protamine sulfate	Acute management heparin overdose, neutralize heparin after dialysis and other procedures, bleeding and hemorrhage	*Adult:* 1 mg/1000 units of heparin IV if given within 30 min of heparin dose. If after 30 min, give 0.5 mg/100 units of heparin	1 mg protamine sulfate neutralizes 90–115 units of heparin. Heparin disappears rapidly from circulation, reducing the dosage demand for protamine as time elapses. Further doses determined by aPTT values
phytonadione	Oral anticoagulant OD; hypoprothrombinemia	*Adult:* 2.5–10 mg PO or IM. May repeat in 6–8 hr if given IV or subQ –or– 12–48 hr if given PO. Max: 25–50 mg *Child:* 5–10 mg PO, subQ, or IM *Infant:* 1–2 mg PO, subQ, or IM	Monitor INR before and throughout therapy.

ACS, Acute coronary syndrome; *ACT,* activated clotting time; *AT,* antithrombin; *AV,* atrioventricular; *CABG,* coronary artery bypass graft; *CVA,* cerebrovascular accident; *DVT,* deep venous thrombosis; *GI, GU,* gastrointestinal, genitourinary; *HIT,* heparin-induced thrombocytopenia; *IM,* intramuscular (route); *INR,* international normalized ratio; *IV,* intravenous (route); *STEMI,* ST-segment elevation myocardial infarction; *OD,* overdose; *PCI,* percutaneous coronary intervention; *PTCA,* percutaneous transluminal coronary angiography; *PVD,* peripheral vascular disease; *t-PA,* recombinant tissue plasminogen activator; *subQ,* subcutaneous (route); *TIA,* transient ischemic attack.

dysfunction, and consider anti–factor Xa level monitoring in those with renal dysfunction or obesity, and during pregnancy.

The recommended initial dosage of enoxaparin is indication-specific. Treatment is usually continued throughout the postoperative period. Up to 14 to 35 days of therapy may be needed depending on the patient's situation.

Because of differences in manufacturing processes, anti–factor Xa and anti–factor IIa properties, and molecular weight distributions, tinzaparin cannot be used interchangeably with other LMWHs or UFH.

▌▍ *Lab Considerations*

The aPTT is the most common test for monitoring anticoagulant response to UFH. Blood is drawn 6 hours after an IV bolus dose of UFH, and the dosage is adjusted accordingly. Anti–factor Xa levels are available for LMWH monitoring in special populations, such as the obese, those with renal dysfunction, and the pregnant. Because tinzaparin theoretically may affect the PT and the INR, patients receiving both tinzaparin and warfarin should have their PT and INR measured before the next scheduled dose of tinzaparin.

The warfarin-caused red-orange discoloration of urine may interfere with the results of some lab tests. UFH, enoxaparin, and dalteparin can increase ALT and AST levels and thyroid function test results. UFH also causes prolonged bromosulfophthalein (BSP) levels and a false-negative ^{125}I fibrinogen uptake. Further, UFH decreases serum triglyceride and cholesterol levels and increases plasma free fatty acid concentrations.

Newer Anticoagulants

UFH and warfarin have been used for more than 50 years. LMWHs were developed 25 years ago and have been used clinically for more than a decade. Since the early 1990s, several new anticoagulants targeting almost every step in the coagulation pathways have been developed. Four parenteral direct thrombin inhibitors (DTIs) have been approved by the FDA: argatroban and lepirudin for the treatment of HIT, bivalirudin as an alternative to heparin in PCI, and desirudin as prophylaxis against DVT in hip replacement. Four other anticoagulants (i.e., activated protein C, a tissue factor pathway inhibitor, a synthetic pentasaccharide, and idraparinux) are in phase 2 or 3 clinical trials.

DTIs inhibit thrombin bound to fibrin or products of fibrin degradation. Argatroban and dabigatran are univalent DTIs that inactivate fibrin-bound thrombin and thrombin-mediated platelet activity. The bivalent DTIs include hirudin and bivalirudin. Because DTIs do not bind to plasma proteins, they elicit a more predictable response than UFH and should be more effective than LMWH.

⚠ There is no antagonist for anticoagulant drugs that rapidly reverse the action of DTIs; therefore monitoring of the aPTT is important for patients who have a high risk of bleeding. The anticoagulant effects of DTIs disappear 12 to 24 hours after the last dose.

Argatroban

Argatroban (Novastan) is used for prophylaxis and treatment of thrombosis in patients with heparin resistance and for patients at risk for HIT who will be having a percutaneous coronary intervention.

Argatroban does not require AT-III for antithrombotic activity; rather it exerts anticoagulant effects by inhibiting thrombin-catalyzed or thrombin-induced reactions, including fibrin formation; activation of factors V, VIII, and XIII; activation of protein C; and platelet aggregation. It inhibits the action of free and clot-associated thrombin. Argatroban does not interact with heparin-induced antibodies and has little or no effect on related proteases (i.e., trypsin, factor Xa, plasmin, and kallikrein).

Following IV administration, argatroban is distributed primarily to extracellular fluids. It is biotransformed in the liver and excreted primarily in the feces, presumably through biliary secretion. Argatroban requires dosage adjustments for patients with hepatic dysfunction. The primary metabolite is 3 to 5 times weaker than the parent drug. Unchanged argatroban is the major component in plasma.

Because argatroban is a DTI, coadministration of argatroban and warfarin produces a combined effect on the INR. There is no additional activity on vitamin K-dependent factor Xa activity. An aPTT is used to monitor treatment with argatroban. The dosage can be adjusted as needed (not to exceed 10 mcg/kg/min), until the steady-state aPTT is 1.5 to 3 times the initial baseline value (not to exceed 100 sec). Check the aPTT 2 hours after starting therapy to confirm that the desired range has been reached.

When starting warfarin therapy, the parental and oral anticoagulant dosing should overlap. Begin the oral anticoagulant (i.e., warfarin) with the anticipated daily dosage and recheck the INR in 4 to 6 hours. The duration of overlap of the two drugs has not been described. Combined oral and anticoagulant therapy using argatroban can be discontinued once the INR is over 4.

Bivalirudin

Bivalirudin (Angiomax) has been approved as a PCI adjunct for patients undergoing coronary angioplasty who are at high risk for a thromboembolic event. It is intended for use with aspirin and has been studied only in patients receiving concomitant aspirin.

Bivalirudin directly inhibits thrombin by binding specifically to both the catalytic site and to the anion-binding substrate of circulating and clot-bound thrombin. The binding of bivalirudin to thrombin is reversible since thrombin slowly cleaves the bivalirudin amino acid (Arg$_3$-Pro$_4$) bond, resulting in recovery of thrombin active site functions. Bivalirudin was no more effective than UFH for patients undergoing percutaneous coronary angioplasty.

Bivalirudin is partially eliminated by the kidneys and liver. Proteolysis at other sites of action contributes to its biotransformation. Dosages may need to be adjusted in patients with severe renal impairment. Monitoring of bivalirudin is done with the ACT.

Although bivalirudin causes less bleeding than high-dose UFH, it is better than UFH in patients at high risk with post-MI angina. The 90-minute patency of an infarct-related artery was higher when bivalirudin was used as an adjunct to streptokinase than when UFH was given (see thrombolytics discussion in Chapter 40). Bivalirudin continues in phase 3 studies for acute coronary syndromes.

Most bleeding associated with the use of bivalirudin in PCI occurs at the arterial puncture site, although hemorrhage can occur at any site. An unexplained fall in blood pressure or hematocrit, or any unexplained symptom, may signal a hemorrhagic event requiring cessation of drug administration. There is no known antagonist to bivalirudin, and the drug is only 25% cleared through hemodialysis. Exercise caution when using bivalirudin as the antithrombin during brachytherapy procedures such as that used for prostate or uterine cancers, where radioactive sources are positioned inside the target tissues and left permanently in the tissue. An increased risk of thrombus formation has also been associated with the use of bivalirudin in gamma brachytherapy, including fatal outcomes.

Lepirudin rDNA

Lepirudin rDNA (Refludan) has approval for use in patients with HIT. Lepirudin rDNA was developed from hirudin, a polypeptide originally found in the saliva of the medicinal leech *(Hirudo medicinalis)*. As the leech fastens onto the patient's skin, its salivary glands secrete a powerful anticoagulant, thus preventing blood clotting that would deprive the leech of its meal. To date, nearly 60,000 patients worldwide have been treated with lepirudin rDNA for HIT and associated thromboembolic disease so as to prevent further thromboembolic complications.

Lepirudin rDNA is a bivalent, highly potent, and specific DTI of both circulating and clot-bound thrombin, and has been proven as effective and safe anticoagulant therapy for patients with HIT. It promotes rapid recovery of platelet counts, provides effective anticoagulation, and prevents further thromboembolic events. Lepirudin rDNA was evaluated in phase 3 studies for DVT prophylaxis in postoperative patients, and for the treatment of acute coronary ischemic indications such as percutaneous coronary angioplasty, coronary thrombolysis, and unstable angina or non–Q-wave infarction. In separate studies, hirudin was found to be more effective than low-dose UFH and LMWH for the prevention of DVT in high-risk orthopedic patients. Lepirudin rDNA was more effective than UFH after coronary angioplasty, but the benefit was not sustained.

The most frequently occurring adverse effect of lepirudin rDNA is bleeding from puncture sites and wounds, anemia, and hematoma. As with other anticoagulants, hemorrhage can occur at any site in patients receiving the drug. There have been reports of intracranial bleeding in the absence of concomitant thrombolytic therapy. An unexplained fall in blood pressure or hematocrit, or any unexplained symptom, may signal a hemorrhagic event requiring cessation of drug administration.

Lepirudin rDNA is eliminated unchanged through the kidneys, thus caution is warranted in patients with renal impairment. Serious liver disease may contribute to the risk of bleeding. Forty percent to 74% of patients taking lepirudin rDNA develop antibodies after 4 or more days of use. Fatal anaphylaxis has occurred in patients who again receive lepirudin rDNA within 3 months of a previous exposure to the drug. Lepirudin rDNA is contraindicated for use in patients with hypersensitivity to the drug.

In general, lepirudin rDNA therapy is monitored using the aPTT. Dosage can be adjusted as needed until the steady-state aPTT is at the desired level above baseline. Check the aPTT shortly after starting therapy to confirm that the patient has attained the desired therapeutic range.

Desirudin

Desirudin (Iprivask), a recombinant hirudin used in the prevention and management of thromboembolic disease, is a DTI that binds directly and with high affinity to clot-bound and fluid phase thrombin. As a prophylaxis in patients undergoing hip replacement surgery, desirudin is significantly more effective in reducing the incidence of DVT than either UFH or LMWH. However, results in patients with acute coronary syndromes are less conclusive; furthermore, desirudin has not been shown to improve the long-term clinical benefit compared with heparin. However, it is as well tolerated as heparin, with a similar incidence of moderate and severe bleeding, intracranial hemorrhage, or stroke when used in the prevention of DVT associated with hip replacement surgery or the in treatment of acute coronary syndrome (ACS).

Desirudin is a selective inhibitor of free and clot-bound thrombin. The anticoagulant properties of desirudin are demonstrated by its ability to prolong the clotting time of plasma. One molecule of desirudin binds covalently and tightly to one molecule of thrombin and thereby blocks the thrombogenic activity of thrombin. As a result, all thrombin-dependent coagulation assays are affected. aPTT is used to measure the anticoagulant activity of desirudin. At therapeutic concentrations, desirudin has no effect on other enzymes of the hemostatic system such as factors IXa, Xa, kallikrein, plasmin, tissue plasminogen activator (t-PA), or activated protein C. In addition, it does not display any effect on other proteases, such as the digestive enzymes trypsin and chymotrypsin, or in complement activation by the classic or alternative pathways.

Desirudin is completely absorbed following subQ and IV administration and distributed to extracellular fluids. Free or protein-bound drug binds immediately to circulating thrombin. The elimination of desirudin is rapid, with 90% of the dose disappearing from the plasma 2 hours after administration. The half-life of desirudin is 2 to 3 hours.

Although desirudin is not significantly biotransformed by the liver, hepatic impairment or liver disease may alter the anticoagulant effect of the drug as a result of coagulation defects secondary to reduced generation of vitamin K–dependent coagulation factors. Desirudin should be used with caution in patients with these conditions.

Desirudin is contraindicated for use in patients with known hypersensitivity to natural or recombinant hirudins, and in patients with active bleeding and/or irreversible coagulation disorders. An aPTT should be monitored daily in patients at increased risk for bleeding and those with renal impairment.

Peak aPTT values should not exceed 2 times the control. Dosage reduction may be required until the aPTT falls to an acceptable level. Serum creatinine should also be monitored. If a patient is switched from oral anticoagulants to desirudin, or from desirudin to oral anticoagulants, the anticoagulant activity should be closely monitored.

Antiplatelet Drugs

- abciximab (ReoPro); ◆ ReoPro
- aspirin (ASA, Ecotrin, Empirin, others); ◆ Apo-ASA, Entrophen, Asaphen-EC
- clopidogrel (Plavix)
- dipyridamole (Persantine); ◆ Apo-Dipyridamole
- dipyridamole + aspirin (Aggrenox); ◆ Aggrenox
- eptifibatide (Integrilin); ◆ Integrilin
- pentoxifylline (Trental)
- ticlopidine (Ticlid)
- tirofiban (Aggrastat); ◆ Aggrastat

Indications

Antiplatelet drugs are used primarily for the prevention of arterial thrombus. Aspirin is the most commonly used antiplatelet drug and is used to reduce the risk of recurrent transient ischemic attacks (TIAs) or stroke in men and women with a history of TIA due to fibrin platelet emboli. It is also used for stroke prevention in patients with atrial fibrillation. Aspirin also reduces the risk of death or nonfatal MI in patients with a history of infarction or unstable angina pectoris.

Clopidogrel is used to reduce the risk of a thrombotic even in patients with a recent MI, stroke, or peripheral arterial disease. The drug is also indicated for patients with ACS managed medically or through PCI.

Dipyridamole is used to reduce the risk for a thromboembolic event and as an adjunct in the treatment of patients with artificial heart valves, exercise testing, and angina prophylaxis. Although unlabeled, dipyridamole has also been used in the prevention of myocardial reinfarction and the reduction of post-MI mortality; also, when the combination agent dipyridamole and aspirin (Aggrenox) is chosen, it helps to prevent the occlusion of coronary artery bypass grafts.

Eptifibatide is used to treat patients with ACS, including those managed medically and those undergoing PCI.

Pentoxifylline is used in the management of intermittent claudication and diabetic angiopathies.

Ticlopidine is used to reduce the risk of thrombotic stroke in patients who have experienced strokelike symptoms (i.e., TIAs) or those with a history of thrombotic stroke, and to reduce the risk of stent thrombosis in the patient whose condition is subacute. Its use has been reserved for patients who are intolerant to aspirin because of the risk for neutropenia. Its unlabeled uses include treatment of intermittent claudication, chronic arterial occlusion, and subarachnoid hemorrhage, as well as management of arteriovenous shunts or fistulas in patients with uremia, open heart surgery, coronary artery bypass grafts, primary glomerulonephritis, and sickle cell disease.

The newest of the antiplatelet drugs are the glycoprotein (GP) IIb and IIIa inhibitors, which include tirofiban, eptifibatide, and abciximab. They are used for thrombus prophylaxis during acute cardiovascular events such as MI. Abciximab is also used as an adjunct to PCI and as an adjunct treatment for refractory, unstable angina. Eptifibatide and tirofiban are used for acute coronary syndromes and PCI.

▥ Pharmacodynamics

The mechanisms of action of antiplatelet drugs vary depending on the drug, but in general they either block platelet activation or prevent their aggregation.

Aspirin acetylates and irreversibly inhibits cyclooxygenase (COX) in the platelet; the effects of aspirin then last the life of a platelet, or about 7 days. Aspirin is 50 to 100 times more potent in inhibiting platelet COX-1. The irreversible nature of aspirin's action prevents dilation of blood vessels and platelet aggregation. However, in high dosages, not only is COX inhibited, but also the formation of prostacyclin, a beneficial substance that causes blood vessel dilation and inhibits platelet aggregation. If prostacyclin formation is inhibited, vessels constrict and platelet aggregation takes place.

Aspirin's anti–vitamin K_1 actions inhibit thrombin production for the entire circulatory system. Aspirin dosages over 1500 mg/day contribute to its antithrombotic actions. A single 500-mg dose of aspirin reduces the total amount of thrombin formed. In contrast, thrombin generation is suppressed with repeated 300-mg doses of aspirin. The interaction of aspirin with platelet phospholipids, which is blunted in patients with elevated cholesterol levels, may explain the action of aspirin on thrombin production.

The mechanism of action for ticlopidine and clopidogrel is different from that of aspirin in that they inhibit platelet aggregation by altering platelet membranes, and as a result, the platelet does not receive the signal to aggregate and form a clot. The signal is sent by fibrinogen, which attaches to the GPIIb-IIIa receptor on the surface of the platelet. It takes 24 to 48 hours for this action to take effect, which suggests that the therapeutic effects may be produced by metabolites rather than the parent drug itself. The addition of aspirin (which blocks TXA_2 synthesis) to either ticlopidine or clopidogrel therapy produces additive or synergistic effects because these drugs block complementary pathways of platelet aggregation. However, this combination does not inhibit aggregation in response to thrombin.

Dipyridamole inhibits platelet aggregation by preventing the release of ADP, platelet factor 4 (Pf_4), and TXA_2. It is also thought that the compounds directly stimulate the release of prostacyclin and inhibit the formation of TXA_2. The drug is known to decrease coronary vascular resistance and increase coronary blood flow without increasing myocardial oxygen consumption.

Pentoxifylline is a methylxanthine derivative with characteristics similar to that of caffeine, theophylline, and other methylxanthines, but it has few cardiac effects. It does, however, produce many other effects such as increasing the flexibility of red blood cells (RBCs) and reducing the aggregation of platelets. The antiplatelet actions are from the inhibition of ADP, serotonin, and Pf_4. The antiplatelet effect of pentoxifylline also stimulates the synthesis and release of prostacyclin from vessels. It decreases fibrinogen concentration in the blood, although the precise mechanism is unknown. However, this may result from raising plasma concentrations of t-PA.

Despite the initiating factor for clotting, GPIIb-IIIa on the surface of platelets has become the target of newer antiplatelet drugs. The thrombin activity of the older antiplatelet drugs (e.g., aspirin, ticlopidine, and clopidogrel) is unaffected. The GPIIb-IIIa antagonists such as abciximab inhibit platelet aggregation by preventing fibrinogen-mediated platelet aggregation at receptors of the same name. This protein is important in promoting the aggregation of platelets in preparation for fibrin clot formation. The aggregation of platelets is significantly inhibited at dosages that reduce the number of receptors to 50% or less. When 80% of receptors are blocked, platelet aggregation is almost entirely halted; however, bleeding times are only mildly affected. Receptor blockade over 90% causes the bleeding time to be prolonged.

Eptifibatide is a synthetic disulfide-linked cyclic heptapeptide. It is patterned after an amino acid sequence found in the snake venom disintegrin. It has a high specificity, but not absolute specificity, for inhibition of GPIIb-IIIa and produces rapid inhibition of platelet aggregation by preventing binding of fibrinogen to receptor sites on platelets.

Tirofiban is a nonpeptide derivative of tyrosine that selectively inhibits the GPIIb-IIIa receptor to inhibit platelet aggregation and fibrinogen binding.

▥ Pharmacokinetics

The pharmacokinetics of antiplatelet drugs is identified in Table 39-2. Most are moderately well absorbed and widely distributed, although distribution sites are not always known. The majority are biotransformed in the liver, or in the RBCs, in the case of dipyridamole. Elimination of antiplatelet drugs is primarily through the urine.

Clopidogrel is biotransformed by the CYP 3A4 and 3A5 enzymes. Patients with end-stage renal function experience prolonged inhibition of platelet function that increases the risk for bleeding.

The mean plasma half-life of tirofiban is 1.6 hours. Bleeding times return to normal approximately 4 hours after discontinuing tirofiban therapy, with platelet aggregation declining to approximately 20% of normal. When administered with aspirin, the mean bleeding time increases fourfold to sixfold, even though tirofiban plasma levels are unaffected. Serum levels of tirofiban needed to inhibit platelet aggregation decrease 50% if the drug is used concurrently with aspirin.

▥ Adverse Effects and Contraindications

The potential adverse effects of the antiplatelet drugs can be serious. Like UFH and LMWH, they all pose a risk for serious bleeding. Contraindications to the use of antiplatelet drugs include known allergy to a specific antiplatelet drug, thrombocytopenia, active bleeding, leukemia, traumatic injuries, and a recent hemorrhagic stroke.

Most of the common adverse effects of antiplatelet drugs subside when the drug is discontinued; however, renal and liver damage caused by these drugs may be permanent. Acute salicylate overdose from aspirin is possible and manifests as respiratory alkalosis, hyperpnea, tachypnea, confusion, asterixis, seizures, tetany, and metabolic acidosis. Fever, coma, cardiovascular collapse, and dose-related renal and respiratory failure are possible.

Few adverse effects are associated with dipyridamole; however, fatal and nonfatal MIs, ventricular fibrillation, and bronchospasm have been noted. Thrombocytopenia, pancytopenia, and other blood dyscrasias have been documented with pentoxifylline.

The adverse effects of ticlopidine include diarrhea, nausea, and dyspepsia in less than 13% of patients. Vomiting, flatulence, pruritus, and dizziness are rare. Neutropenia occurs in approximately 2% of patients. Thrombotic thrombocytopenia purpura (TTP), agranulocytosis, hepatitis, cholestatic jaundice, and tinnitus occur rarely.

Drug Interactions

Several serious drug interactions are possible with antiplatelet drugs (see Table 39-3). When antiplatelet drugs are administered concurrently with anticoagulants, there is an increased risk for hemorrhage. Alcohol intake in conjunction with dipyridamole may potentiate hypotension. In addition, serum salicylate levels may be enhanced when dipyridamole is taken with foods such as cheese, cranberries, and fish, which acidify the urine. Furthermore, absorption of ticlopidine is enhanced when it is administered with food.

Dosage Regimens

Typical dosage regimens of the antiplatelet drugs are identified in Table 39-4.

Lab Considerations

Aspirin prolongs bleeding time for 4 to 7 days, and in large doses may cause prolonged bleeding times, false-negative urine glucose test results using Clinistix or Tes-Tape, or a false-positive urine glucose test result with the copper sulfate method (Clinitest). As with aspirin, no test of platelet function is currently recommended to assess the effects of clopidogrel in the individual patients.

CLINICAL REASONING

Treatment Objectives

Treatment objectives for the patient at risk for a thromboembolic event are directed toward prevention or progression of the disorder, regardless of the site or sequelae. In addition, treatment is directed at speedy resolution of pain, inflammation, patient discomfort, and reduction in morbidity and mortality.

Treatment Options

Patient Variables

The ability of the patient to adhere to the prescribed treatment regimen must be taken into account. The patient must be able to safely administer long-term anticoagulant or antiplatelet therapy at home. It is important that the patient and the caregivers understand and be able to adhere to the lab testing required for adequate monitoring of therapeutic as well as adverse effects.

LIFE-SPAN CONSIDERATIONS

Pregnant and Nursing Women. The risk of thromboembolic disease in pregnancy is about 6 times greater than in the nonpregnant state, with 3 to 12 occurrences per 1000 pregnancies. The true incidence may be significantly higher during the postpartum period. Risk factors for thromboembolic disease during pregnancy, in addition to those previously identified, include advanced maternal age (older than 40 years); collagen-vascular disease; grand multiparity (more than four previous term pregnancies); homocystinuria (predisposes to arterial and venous thrombosis); nephrotic syndrome; and a Cesarean section or instrumented delivery.

Pregnancy-related alterations in the coagulation system also predispose the woman to thrombus and related complications. Treatment for DVT and PE in pregnancy centers on anticoagulation. The incidence of TIA and stroke are relatively rare in pregnancy.

Older Adults. The use of anticoagulant and antiplatelet drugs in older adults has its own risks. Normal changes of aging affect use, required monitoring, and therapeutic effectiveness of the drugs.

CASE STUDY — Anticoagulant and Antiplatelet Drugs

ASSESSMENT

History of Present Illness	GR is a 75-year-old white male who is having a left total hip replacement tomorrow.
Past Health History	GR has no known allergies. He has been treated for atherosclerosis and mild hypertension for the past 2 years. He states that he has had pain in his left hip for several years that has limited his mobility. Current meds: furosemide 20 mg PO daily; Klor-Con 20 mEq PO daily.
Life-Span Considerations	GR lives alone and relies on Social Security income. He is unable to drive owing to his hip pain; therefore he relies on friends and neighbors for transportation to the grocery store and medical appointments. The rest of the time he is a "loner." Each of his four children calls him once weekly to see how he is but they all live in another state. He also smokes one pack of cigarettes per day. GR has a small retirement pension in addition to Social Security benefits.
Physical Exam Findings	VSS. GR is unable to read small print. ENT unremarkable except for a full set of dentures. No carotid bruits or lymphadenopathy. HRRR, no S_3 or S_4 heart sound. Breath sounds diminished bilateral lower lobes but no crackles, rhonchi, wheezes or E >A changes. No fremitus. Abdomen round, soft, NT. No HSM, masses, or bruits. Pain with abduction left hip. DP and PT pulses 1+. Trace pedal edema. Gait steady.

Continued

CASE STUDY — Anticoagulant and Antiplatelet Drugs—Cont'd

Diagnostic Testing	CBC, comprehensive metabolic profile, thyroid, lipids, PT and INR, and PTT within normal limits. Glucose, BUN, and creatinine within normal limits.

DIAGNOSIS: Deep DVT Prophylaxis

MANAGEMENT

Treatment Objectives	The risk for thromboembolic events will be reduced before and during recovery from hip replacement surgery.
Treatment Plan	**Pharmacotherapy** • Enoxaparin 30 mg subQ twice daily for 14 days • Start warfarin 5 mg PO, during last 3–4 days of enoxaparin therapy. **Patient Education** 1. Importance of adhering to anticoagulant therapy during recovery period 2. Purpose of anticoagulation therapy 3. Proper administration technique for enoxaparin 4. Importance of monitoring INR on regular basis once taking warfarin **Evaluation** Thromboembolic events were avoided during recovering from hip replacement surgery.

CLINICAL REASONING

Q1. I'm used to working with continuous IV heparin drips. When will he start the subcutaneous enoxaparin after surgery?

A. Enoxaparin is started as soon as possible after surgery. The first dose is often administered as soon as he leaves the PACU as part of the standard of care. However, GR also has large number of risk factors for development of DVT postoperatively, so we want to get him started as quickly as possible once he returns.

Q2. We learned in class that anticoagulation therapy should be avoided in older adults. GR is 75 years old, isn't he? Isn't that a concern?

A. Well, yes…but, enoxaparin is the drug of choice for postoperative hip replacement patients like GR. Secondly, no dosage adjustment is needed for patients with mild to moderate renal impairment, that is, a creatinine clearance of ranging from 30 mL/min to 80 mL/min. GR's creatinine clearance immediately postop was 55 mL/min. We will still watch his kidney function, however.

Q3. (Nurse to student): So now that we have started GR on enoxaparin, are there any lab tests needed to monitor his dosage?

A. (Student to nurse): No. Enoxaparin does not require laboratory monitoring, which will be good for GR since he is unable to drive and won't be able to get to a draw site to have an INR done. When given at the recommended dosages, routine coagulation tests such as a PTT or aPTT are relatively insensitive measures of enoxaparin activity, and therefore they are unsuitable for monitoring. If, during treatment, bleeding should occur or abnormal coagulation parameters develop, anti–factor Xa levels can be used to monitor the anticoagulant effects of the enoxaparin.

▥ Drug Variables

ANTICOAGULANTS. Before starting anticoagulant therapy, obtain a baseline complete blood count (CBC), renal function tests, baseline INR, and aPTT values as appropriate. Because many of the anticoagulant and antiplatelet drugs cause an elevation in liver function tests, it is important to establish a baseline for those values also.

The intervention of choice for prophylaxis of thromboembolic events is primarily drug therapy. The specific drug used depends on the possible location of the thrombus and the administration route most likely to be tolerated by the patient. The occurrence and recurrence of thromboembolic events can be decreased to less than 5% if adequate anticoagulation or antiplatelet regimen is maintained. Twenty-nine percent to

47% of patients have a recurrence of a thromboembolic event unless adequate anticoagulation is maintained after the initial treatment regimen has been completed.

LMWH differs from UFH in a number of ways. Compared with standard UFH, LMWH has more predictable anticoagulant activity; has better bioavailability; binds less to plasma proteins, platelets, and endothelial cells; and thus has better bioavailability and a longer half-life. LMWHs differ in the inhibition of specific factors in the coagulation cascade. Their dosages also differ, although they are generally administered in fixed doses adjusted for body weight. IV access is not needed, and no monitoring is required because the drug dosages are weight-based. They may be given once or twice a day with the same efficacy, and there is less incidence of

HIT, and faster regression of the thrombus. Other advantages they offer over UFH include the following: warfarin resistance (i.e., development of recurrent DVT while on warfarin) is avoided; LMWHs are not influenced by dietary habits; LMWHs don't have the many drug interactions (e.g., increased or inhibited liver biotransformation, antibiotics that decrease gut flora and thus vitamin K); there is no lag time between administration and effective levels; and there is no increase in vascular calcification. A major advantage of LMWHs over continuous IV infusions of UFH is that their simplified dosage regimen allows for the possibility of outpatient treatment and reduces costs.

Dosage Monitoring. As discussed preciously, because PT test results vary greatly from lab to lab, an INR is used to monitor warfarin therapy. Table 39-5 provides a brief overview of recommended ranges in INR values for monitoring oral anticoagulant therapy. An INR of 2 to 3 is sufficient for the majority of patients.

Therapeutic values for UFH therapy are similar to those of warfarin (Table 39-6). The aPTT therapeutic range is usually 1.5 to 2.5 times the normal value. Blood is drawn to establish

TABLE 39-6 Heparin Monitoring

Drug	Test*	Normal Values	Therapeutic Value
heparin	aPTT	16–25 sec	24–50 sec†

*The activated partial thromboplastin time, or aPTT, is a more sensitive test than PTT and has replaced the PTT in most laboratories. Normal ranges for aPTT vary with the phospholipid used. aPTT values >100 sec signify spontaneous bleeding.
†Therapeutic value usually calculated as 1.5–2.5 times the normal value.

baseline levels and then 6 hours after the start of the UFH infusion or dosage change. If the patient's baseline value is already elevated, hold the UFH until values normalize. Patients on low-dose UFH therapy may not require routine lab monitoring. The exceptions to this are in the cases of patients who are malnourished, those who have had prior coagulation difficulties, and those who are receiving broad-spectrum antibiotics (e.g., cephalosporins).

Management of Overdose. Withholding one or more doses of warfarin is usually sufficient if the patient's INR is excessively prolonged or if minor bleeding occurs. If overdose occurs and anticoagulation must be reversed, the administration of phytonadione (vitamin K_1) can be used. Phytonadione is an antagonist to warfarin. The dosage and route of phytonadione is dependent on the patient's situation and the severity of bleeding. The anticoagulation actions of warfarin should normalize within 24 hours following phytonadione administration (Table 39-7).

In the past phytonadione was administered parenterally to reverse the effects of warfarin. However, new information suggested that oral vitamin K_1 has advantages over the parenteral formulation. IV administration is not practical in the ambulatory setting because of the risk of anaphylaxis and hypersensitivity reactions. In addition, there are concerns about the erratic absorption of subcutaneously administered vitamin K_1. The advantages of oral vitamin K_1 include a decreased risk of allergic reactions, convenience, and low cost.

TABLE 39-5 Therapeutic INR Values for Prophylaxis and Treatment

Condition or Procedure	Desirable Range
Atrial fibrillation	2.0–3.0
Acute myocardial infarction	
Most cases of antiphospholipid antibody syndrome	
Prevention and treatment of systemic embolism	
Prevention and treatment of pulmonary embolism	
Prevention and treatment of venous thrombosis	
Tissue heart valves	
Valvular heart disease	
Recurrent systemic embolism	
Mechanical prosthetic heart valves	2.5–3.5

Controversy

How Safe Is Anticoagulation Therapy?

Jonathan J. Wolfe

Ambulatory anticoagulant therapy using warfarin has demonstrated its worth in prophylaxis against cardiac disease and stroke. When properly monitored, this anticoagulant therapy is safe, effective, and certainly less risky than embolization of the heart, the lungs, or the brain.

Monitoring anticoagulant therapy, however, presents special challenges. On one hand, it involves proper acquisition of clinical specimens and correct handling in both the clinic, office, or hospital, and the laboratory. Once results are known, they are correlated with the patient's clinical status and the desired therapeutic outcomes. For this reason, reliance on prothrombin time (PT) has been replaced by use of the international normalized ratio (INR). This test uses the international sensitivity index (ISI) as an exponent to relate a particular patient's PT (versus the mean normal PT) to the sensitivity of the reagent used. It is a robust and readily applied system that minimizes differences among laboratories and operators.

The other special challenge derives from the effect of both drugs and diet on warfarin pharmacokinetics. Drug interactions may bring the patient to disastrously low or high levels of anticoagulation, depending on the drugs

involved. Seasonal variations in dietary intake of vegetables rich in vitamin K, or taking an over-the-counter drug such as cimetidine may similarly send INR values sharply out of control. Therefore, patients must be educated about the seriousness of possible drug and diet interactions when taking warfarin.

CLINICAL REASONING ANALYSIS

- What problems had to be overcome in order to secure acceptance of INR as the successor to decades of reliance on PT?
- What information about dietary habits should you elicit from a patient who is to be placed on anticoagulant therapy?
- What cautions should you give patients who will be taking anticoagulants about consulting other physicians or having prescriptions filled in multiple pharmacies?
- What cautions are appropriate in choosing how to respond to a reported INR that is far out of line with a patient's past history?
- What assurance would you offer a reluctant patient who has been told that warfarin is really rat poison?

The effects of phytonadione can last up to 168 hours. Therefore, if warfarin must be restarted, resistance to its anticoagulant effects will continue until the effects of the phytonadione have subsided. If phytonadione does not control bleeding, or if quicker results are needed, clotting factor levels may be increased by giving plasma or clotting factor concentrates (see Chapter 38).

The antagonist to UFH and LMWH is protamine sulfate (see Table 39-4). The dosage of protamine sulfate is calculated based on the amount of heparin given and the time interval since administration, but in general, 1 mg of protamine sulfate is given for every 100 units of heparin to be neutralized. The antagonistic effects begin with the administration of the drug and last for up to 2 hours. However, because of the short half-life of heparin, overdose can often be treated by withholding the drug. Protamine only partially reverses the effects of LMWH; further, the newer injectable anticoagulants do not have antagonists to reverse their effects.

Antiplatelet Drugs. Before starting drug therapy, stabilize the condition of patients with diabetes mellitus, angina, heart failure, and hyperlipidemia. In selected cases, patients with signs and symptoms extending over 12 months may have a better response to antiplatelet therapy than those with symptoms of shorter duration. Improvement should be noted in 2 to 4 weeks after treatment is started. If improvement is apparent at 8 weeks, it is usually continued for approximately 6 months, followed by a 2-month drug-free period. If an improvement of at least 25% to 50% is not evident after 8 weeks, discontinue drug therapy and reassess the patient's condition.

Long-term use of clopidogrel significantly reduces the risk for major cardiovascular events following PCI. The combination of aspirin and clopidogrel is the recommended treatment after coronary stent implantation. Ticlopidine is not likely to be used for these purposes because of safety concerns regarding adequate loading dosage of the drug. In addition, ticlopidine also is associated with a higher risk for bone marrow toxicities compared with clopidogrel, and has no current indication for the long-term management of patients after MI.

Patient Education

Provide the patient and family with written instructions about all drugs they are receiving, including the name, prescribed dose, reasons for receiving the drug, and adverse effects. Advise them to use the drug exactly as prescribed and at the same time(s) each day. The health care provider should be told of any missed doses at the time of check-up or lab testing.

Instruct the patient to notify the health care provider if signs of bleeding or bruising occur. Early signs of bleeding include bleeding gums, black, tarry-looking stools, nosebleeds, excessively heavy menstrual flow, and hematuria. Teach patients to avoid alcohol and over-the-counter (OTC) drugs, especially those containing aspirin, ibuprofen, or other nonsteroidal antiinflammatory drugs (NSAIDs) without first consulting with the health care provider or pharmacist.

Caution patients to avoid intramuscular (IM) injections, contact sports, and other activities that may lead to injury. Instruct them to use a soft toothbrush, and to shave with an electric razor during anticoagulant therapy. Also, advise the patient to notify dentists or other health care providers of the anticoagulation therapy. Emphasize the importance of frequent follow-up lab tests, when appropriate, to monitor therapy.

Advise patients taking aspirin for antiplatelet therapy that one OTC aspirin formulation is generally as good as another. They need not pay a high price to get the desired effects. Most oral antiplatelet drugs should be taken with food or after meals to avoid GI upset. Further, if postural hypotension occurs, as is sometimes the case with dipyridamole use, instruct the patient to change positions slowly, or to lie down for a short time after taking the drug to reduce the risk of falling.

Evaluation

Clinical response to UFH anticoagulant therapy is indicated by an aPTT that is 1.5 to 2.5 times the normal, without signs

TABLE 39-7 Guidelines for Reversing Anticoagulant Effects of Warfarin

INR Value	Recommended Action*
INR value above desired range but <5.0; no significant bleeding	Reduce the dosage or hold the dose as appropriate; monitor INR more frequently; and resume treatment at lower dosage when the INR returns to the desired level. If the INR is marginally over the desired level, no dosage reduction may be required.
INR >5.0 but <9.0 with no significant bleeding	Hold the next 1–2 doses; monitor the INR more frequently. When the INR returns to the desired level, resume treatment at a lower dosage. Alternatively, omit the dose and give vitamin K_1 (≤5 mg orally), particularly if patient is at increased risk for bleeding. If more rapid reversal is required, administer 2–4 mg of vitamin K_1 orally, with the expectation that the INR will be lowered in 24 hr. If the INR remains high, administer an additional 1 to 2 mg of vitamin K orally.
INR >9.0 but no significant bleeding	Hold warfarin and give 5–10 mg of vitamin K orally with the expectation that the INR will be substantially lower in 24–48 hr. Monitor INR more frequently, and give additional vitamin K_1 if necessary. Resume treatment at a lower dose when the INR reaches desired level.
Significant bleeding at any INR level	Hold warfarin and give 10 mg of vitamin K_1 by slow IV infusion, supplement with fresh frozen plasma or prothrombin complex concentrate, depending on the urgency of the situation. Recombinant factor VIIa may be used as an alternative to prothrombin complex concentrate. Dose of vitamin K can be repeated every 12 hr if needed.
Life-threatening bleeding	Hold warfarin and give prothrombin complex concentrate supplemented with vitamin K_1 (10 mg by slow IV infusion). Recombinant factor VIIa may be used as an alternative to prothrombin complex concentrate. Repeat as necessary depending on INR value.

*If warfarin must be continued after high dosages of vitamin K_1 have been administered, use heparin or LMWH until the effects of vitamin K_1 have been reversed and the patient is once again responsive to warfarin therapy. Note that INR values over 4.5 are less reliable than values in or near the desired range.
INR, International normalized ratio; *IV*, intravenous; *LMWH*, low–molecular weight heparin.
From Ansell, J., Hirsh, J., Poller, L., et al. (2004). The pharmacology and management of the vitamin K antagonists: The seventh ACCP conference on antithrombotic and thrombotic therapy. *Chest, 126*(3), 204–233.

of bleeding. Clinical response to oral anticoagulants is evaluated using the INR range.

Antiplatelet therapy is considered successful if the patient experiences no further signs and symptoms of the disorder and negative sequelae have been avoided. The prevention and control of thromboembolic disease and its associated complications is evidence of overall treatment success.

KEY POINTS

- Thrombus development begins when red blood cells, white blood cells, platelets, and fibrin adhere to exposed collagen fibers in the affected vessel. The intrinsic pathway and the extrinsic pathway require certain clotting factors to produce a fibrin clot.
- The goal of anticoagulant and antiplatelet therapy is to prevent the formation and progression of intravascular blood clots and their sequelae.
- Treatment options for thromboembolic disease include oral anticoagulants, such as warfarin, and parenteral anticoagulants, UFH, or the LMWHs such as tinzaparin, dalteparin, and enoxaparin.
- Antiplatelet drugs are used primarily for prevention of arterial thrombus.
- Antiplatelet drugs include aspirin, dipyridamole, combination of aspirin and dipyridamole, pentoxifylline, ticlopidine, and tinzaparin.
- INR values are used to monitor therapeutic and potential adverse effects of oral anticoagulants. aPTT values are used to monitor UFH therapy. There is no routine laboratory monitoring for LMWH, although anti–

factor Xa levels may be performed in high-risk patients and those requiring high dosages.
- Protamine sulfate and phytonadione are the antagonists to heparin and warfarin, respectively. They are used in the event of dosage excess or if there is a need to quickly reverse the effects of the anticoagulant.
- Signs and symptoms of bleeding are monitored during administration of anticoagulants and antiplatelet drugs.
- Care of the patient receiving anticoagulant and antiplatelet drugs includes education about the drug's purpose and possible adverse effects, with the potential for bleeding noted primarily.
- Successful prophylaxis against thrombus formation is noted by its absence. Successful therapeutic UFH therapy is noted by an aPTT value 1.5 to 2.5 times the normal value. INR values for warfarin therapy ordinarily range from 2 to 3.

Bibliography

Ansell, J., Hirsh, J., Poller, L., et al. (2004). The pharmacology and management of the vitamin K antagonists: The seventh ACCP conference on antithrombotic and thrombotic therapy. *Chest, 126*(3), 204–233.

Daugherty, N., and Smith, K. (2006). Dietary supplement and selected food interactions with warfarin. *Orthopaedics, 29*(4), 309–314.

DiNisio, M., Middeldorp, S., and Buller, H. (2005). Direct thrombin inhibitors. *New England Journal of Medicine, 353*(10), 1028–1040.

Eichler, P., Friesen, H., Lubenow, H., et al. (2000). Antihirudin antibodies in patients with heparin-induced thrombocytopenia treated with lepirudin: Incidence, effects on aPTT, and clinical relevance. *Blood, 96*(7), 2373–2378.

Gage, B., and Milligan, P. (2005). Pharmacology and pharmacogenetics of warfarin and other coumarins when used with supplements. *Thrombosis Research, 117*(1–2), 55–59.

Goodin, S. (2005). Selecting an anticoagulant for recurrent venous thromboembolism in cancer. *American Journal of Health System Pharmacists, 62*(22 Suppl 5), S10–S13.

Greinacher, A., Eichler, P., Lubenow, N., et al. (2000). Heparin-induced thrombocytopenia with thromboembolic complications: Meta-analysis of 2 prospective trials to assess the value of parenteral treatment with lepirudin and its therapeutic aPTT range. *Blood, 96*(3), 846–851.

Greinacher, A., Janssens, U., Berg, G., et al. for the Heparin-Associated Thrombocytopenia Study (HAT) investigators. (1999). Lepirudin (recombinant hirudin) for parenteral anticoagulation in patients with heparin-induced thrombocytopenia. *Circulation, 100*(6), 587–593.

Hirsh, J., Dalen, J., Anderson, D., et al. (2001). Oral anticoagulants: Mechanism of action, clinical effectiveness, and optimal therapeutic range. *Chest, 119*(Suppl 1), 8S–21S.

Ho, W., Hankey, G., Quinlan, D., et al. (2006). Risk of recurrent venous thromboembolism in patients with common thrombophilia: A systematic review. *Archives of Internal Medicine, 166*(7), 729–736.

Holbrook, A., Pereira, J., Labiris, R., et al. (2005). Systematic review of warfarin and its drug and food interactions. *Archives of Internal Medicine, 165*(10), 1095–1106.

Levi, M. (2006). Male sex, first idiopathic deep vein thrombosis, and oral contraception were risk factors for recurrent venous thrombotic events. *Evidence Based Medicine, 11*(2), 59–69.

McRae, S., Tran, H., Schulman, S., et al. (2006). Effect of patient's sex on risk of recurrent venous thromboembolism: A meta-analysis. *Lancet, 368*(9533), 371–378.

McRae, S., and Ginsberg, J. (2005). New anticoagulants for the prevention and treatment of venous thromboembolism. *Vascular Health and Risk Management, 1*(1), 41–53.

Neeley, J., Carlson, S., and Lenhart, S. (2002). Tinzaparin sodium: A low-molecular-weight heparin. *American Journal of Health-System Pharmacies, 59*(15), 1426–1436.

Nutescu, E., Shapiro, N., Ibrahim, S., et al. (2006). Warfarin and its interactions with foods, herbs and other dietary supplements. *Expert Opinion on Drug Safety, 5*(3), 433–451.

Nutescu, E., Whittkowski, A., Dobesh, P., et al. (2006). Choosing the appropriate antithrombotic agent for the prevention and treatment of VTE: A case-based approach. *Annals of Pharmacotherapy, 40*(9), 1558–1570.

Nutescu, E., Shapiro, N., Chevalier, A. (2005). A pharmacologic overview of current and emerging anticoagulants. *Cleveland Clinic Journal of Medicine, 72*(Suppl 1), S2–S26.

Nutescu, E., Helgason, C., Briller, J., et al. (2004). New blood thinner offers first potential alternative in 50 years: Ximelagatran. *Journal of Cardiovascular Nursing, 19*(6), 374–383.

O'Conner, E., and Fraser, J. (2006). Heparin-induced thrombocytopenia without thrombosis: An evidence-based review of current literature. *Critical Care Resuscitation*, 8(4), 345–352.

Pengo, V., and Prandoni, P. (2006). Sex and anticoagulation in patients with idiopathic venous thromboembolism. *Lancet, 368* (9533), 342–343.

Patrono, C., Collier, B., Garret, A., et al. (2004). Platelet-active drugs: The relationships among dose, effectiveness, and side effects: The Seventh ACCP Conference on Antithrombotic and Thrombolytic Therapy. *Chest, 126*(3), 234–264.

Weitz, J. (2006). Emerging anticoagulants for the treatment of venous thromboembolism. *Thrombosis and Haemostasis, 96*(3), 274–284.

40

Thrombolytic and Sclerosing Drugs

Thrombolytic therapy was first introduced in 1958 for the treatment of acute myocardial infarction (AMI). It attracted little support, however, because it was believed that thrombosis was not the primary problem of AMI. In the last 2 decades, there has been a resurgence of interest in thrombolytic therapy for use during coronary angiography. The realization that, in many cases, thrombosis is in fact a primary cause of infarction has also added to the interest. Thrombolytic therapy is now the standard of care for patients with acute ST-elevation MI (STEMI), and it is emerging as a treatment modality for other disease processes related to thrombosis (e.g., pulmonary embolus [PE], deep vein thrombosis [DVT], peripheral arterial occlusive disease, and ischemic cerebrovascular accident).

Sclerosing drugs are used primarily for the treatment of bleeding esophageal varices and uncomplicated superficial varicose veins of the lower extremities.

CARDIOVASCULAR DISORDERS

CEREBROVASCULAR ACCIDENT

EPIDEMIOLOGY AND ETIOLOGY

A cerebrovascular accident (stroke, CVA, cerebrovascular occlusion) is the clinical term for acute loss of circulation to an area of the brain, resulting in ischemia and a corresponding loss of neurologic function. Stroke is one of the primary neurologic problems associated with high rates of morbidity, mortality, and disability in the world. Stroke, which leads to permanent neurologic damage, should be distinguished from a transient ischemic attack. A *transient ischemic attack* (TIA, often colloquially referred to as "ministroke") is caused by the temporary disturbance of blood supply to a restricted area of the brain, resulting in brief neurologic dysfunction that persists for less than 24 hours (Box 40-1).

Although the number of stroke-related deaths has declined in the past several years, stroke remains the third leading cause of death in the United States and the number one cause of death in the world. It also leaves a large number of people disabled each year. Treatment costs of stroke in the United States exceed $15 billion per year.

PATHOPHYSIOLOGY

In an *ischemic stroke*, circulation to the affected part of the brain is partially or totally blocked. These strokes are more common in patients with a history of valvular disease, prosthetic valve replacement, atrial fibrillation, ischemic heart disease, or rheumatic heart disease.

A *hemorrhagic stroke* generally evolves from the rupture of a saccular aneurysm, rupture of an arteriovenous malformation, or more commonly, uncontrolled hypertension.

Thrombotic strokes cause ischemia as a result of a clot forming around atherosclerotic plaques. The growing clot eventually obstructs the lumen. Because occlusion of the circulation is usually slow, the onset of symptoms is also slow.

Thrombotic strokes may involve small or large vessels. Large vessel thrombotic strokes involve the common and internal carotid arteries, vertebral vessels, and the circle of Willis. Small-vessel thrombotic strokes involve branches of the middle cerebral artery, the lenticulostriate arteries, or branches of the circle of Willis or vertebral or basilar arteries.

*Embolic stroke*s refer to the mechanism of the stroke, a blockage of arterial access to a part of the brain by an embolus. An embolus is most frequently the result of a thrombus, but it may be plaque dislodged from an atherosclerotic lesion. An embolus may also be made up of fat, air, or even cancer cells. Because an embolus arises from elsewhere in the body, the source of the embolus must be identified. Embolic strokes may result from a known cardiac disorder (e.g., atrial fibrillation). Symptoms may be transient as the embolus travels to another site or is lysed.

Regardless of the cause or location, as blood flow decreases, neurons stop functioning, and irreversible neuronal ischemia and injury begins. Further, brain metabolism is disrupted both in the involved area and in the opposite hemisphere.

MYOCARDIAL INFARCTION

EPIDEMIOLOGY AND ETIOLOGY

AMI has been the leading cause of death in the United States since the 1940s. Approximately 1.5 million AMIs occur annually in the United States, with a mortality rate exceeding 30%. AMI affects arteries that provide blood, oxygen, and nutrients to the myocardium. Death of myocardial tissue is permanent, resulting from sudden cessation of oxygen supply to the muscle, which contributes to heart failure and complicates the patient's care.

The underlying cause of AMI is usually atherosclerosis, or a narrowing of coronary vessels because of a build-up of plaque. Plaque develops, in part, as a result of chronic endothelial inflammation. Approximately 80% of AMIs, however, are the direct result of an embolus. Since the 1980s, there has been a major shift in the understanding of the causes of AMI and therefore the use of thrombolytics, which in turn has been shown in clinical studies to significantly reduce mortality.

BOX 40-1

Signs and Symptoms of Stroke by Area Affected

Spinothalamic Tract, Corticospinal Tract, and Dorsal Column of CNS
Muscle weakness or numbness (hemiplegia)
Reduction of pain or temperature sensation
Reduction in sensory or vibratory sensation

Brainstem and Cranial Nerves
Altered smell, taste, hearing, or vision (total or partial)
Drooping of eyelid (ptosis) and weakness of ocular muscles
Decreased reflexes: gag, swallow, pupil reactivity to light
Decreased sensation and muscle weakness of the face
Balance problems and nystagmus
Altered breathing and heart rate
Weakness in sternocleidomastoid muscle (SCM) with inability to turn head to one side
Weakness in tongue (inability to protrude and/or move from side to side)

Cerebral Cortex
Aphasia (Broca's or Wernicke's area)
Apraxia (altered voluntary movements)
Disorganized thinking, confusion, hypersexual gestures (frontal lobe)
Altered vision (occipital lobe)
Memory deficits (temporal lobe)
Hemineglect (parietal lobe)

Cerebellum
Trouble walking
Altered movement coordination
Dizziness

PATHOPHYSIOLOGY

The heart muscle receives its nutritive and oxygen-carrying blood supply through two major vessels located on the surface of the heart, the right and the left coronary arteries (Fig. 40-1). These arteries originate from the aorta, dividing into smaller arterioles that penetrate the heart muscle. The left coronary artery is further divided into two parts. Although there are certainly physiologic variants, in general, the left anterior descending artery supplies blood to the anterior surface of the left ventricle, and the left circumflex artery supplies blood to the lateral wall of the left ventricle. In about 20% of the population, however, the left circumflex artery supplies blood to the posterior portion of the heart. The right coronary artery supplies the inferior aspect of the left ventricle and the right ventricle. The right coronary artery also supplies the posterior aspect of the right and left ventricles. An obstruction in any one of the vessels impedes the flow of blood carrying oxygen and nutrients to that area of the myocardium.

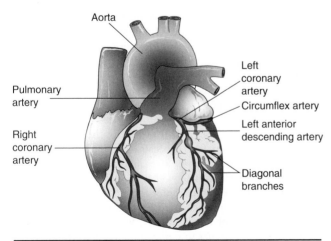

FIGURE 40-1 Obstructed Coronary Circulation. Right and left coronary arteries, through which the heart muscle receives its major blood supply.

In patients with coronary artery disease (CAD), atherosclerotic plaque builds up slowly over time. Because plaque has a rough surface, platelets begin to adhere, fibrin is deposited, and blood cells become trapped. A clot eventually forms that occludes the vessel. In some cases, the clot breaks away, traveling to smaller vessels, where it causes an occlusion. The degree of occlusion in the coronary arteries, turbulence of circulatory blood flow, and the fragility of plaque formation all influence the likelihood of emboli.

Immediately after an acute coronary event, blood flow ceases to the area beyond the occlusion. There may be small amounts of collateral blood flow available from surrounding vessels; however, in areas with no oxygen available to the affected tissues, myocardial cells die.

Infarction is a dynamic process that occurs over several hours. Obvious physical changes do not begin in the heart muscle until approximately 6 hours after the infarct. The infarcted area appears blue and swollen. Approximately 48 hours later, neutrophils invade to remove necrotic cells, and the area turns gray with yellow streaks. Granulation tissue forms at the edges by the eighth to tenth day after the infarct. Over the next 2 to 3 months, the necrotic area is reduced to a shrunken, thin, firm scar. The presence of scar tissue permanently changes the structure and the function of the affected muscle, which, in turn, increases morbidity and mortality.

PULMONARY EMBOLISM

EPIDEMIOLOGY AND ETIOLOGY

PE is the obstruction of the pulmonary artery by a thrombus originating in the venous system or in the right side of the heart. Ordinarily, a PE is caused by a blood clot that has broken loose from a peripheral clot. Populations at risk for thromboembolic disease were discussed in Chapter 39. DVT and PE are responsible for more than 250,000 hospitalizations and approximately 50,000 deaths each year in the United States. The immediate cause of death in the patient who develops PE is right-sided heart failure.

PATHOPHYSIOLOGY

Stasis of blood flow, damage to the endothelial lining of the vessel, and changes in the mechanics of coagulation are the three primary causes of DVT (Virchow's triad). Once a clot is formed, blood flowing past the clot may cause it to break loose from the artery lumen to become one or more emboli. When the embolus is dislodged, it is transported to the right ventricle and then to the pulmonary arterial system, where it becomes lodged and obstructs circulation.

Platelets accumulate behind the embolus, triggering release of serotonin and thromboxane A_2, which in turn causes vasoconstriction, and circulation decreases further. An imbalance results, with areas where the lung is ventilated but not perfused and resulting in hypoxia. The larger the affected vessel, the more serious the consequences. By definition, a massive PE obstructs more than 50% of blood flow to the lungs.

The hemodynamic consequence of this process is an increase in pulmonary vascular resistance. The increased peripheral vascular resistance is related to a decrease in the size of the pulmonary vascular bed, resulting in greater pulmonary arterial pressures. In turn, an increase in right ventricular workload is needed to maintain pulmonary blood flow. When myocardial work load requirements exceed capacity, right ventricular failure occurs. There is a subsequent decrease in cardiac output, and shock may occur.

PERIPHERAL VASCULAR OCCLUSION

EPIDEMIOLOGY AND ETIOLOGY

Peripheral vascular occlusions result in an acute loss of perfusion to tissues distal to blockage of a major artery or vein. Arterial emboli most often develop in the chambers of the heart as a result of atrial fibrillation or flutter. They also occur more commonly in the lower extremity than in the upper extremity; however, cerebral, mesenteric, and renal arteries can be affected. Emboli originating in the arterial system or that come from the left side of the heart are most common. Whereas chronic peripheral venous disease is a slow process, the onset of arterial occlusion is more sudden.

PATHOPHYSIOLOGY

Following obstruction of an artery, a soft coagulum forms proximal and distal to the area of stagnant flow. As the clot extends, collateral pathways are involved and the process becomes self-propagating. Ultimately, venous circulation can be involved. **The extent of vascular compromise is critical and determines the "golden" period of 4 to 6 hours. After this time, the profound ischemia leads to cellular death and is irreversible.**

Inadequate emptying of the atria allows blood flow to stagnate and predisposes to clotting. When clots detach, they are propelled into the arterial system and become lodged when they reach an area smaller in size than the embolus. The result is the immediate cessation of blood flow below the area of occlusion. Clots typically lodge at arterial bifurcations and in narrowed vessels. Secondary vasospasm contributes to ischemia.

An arterial aneurysm, a weakness in the intimal layer of an artery, permits stasis of blood with eventual clotting. The force of the arterial pressure can propel the clot from the aneurysm into arterial circulation.

CENTRAL VENOUS ACCESS OCCLUSION

Central venous access devices may, on occasion, become occluded by fibrin clots and other plasma proteins. Occlusions are a serious potential complication of central venous access device catheters.

Clots normally form when thrombin, an enzyme made from prothrombin, converts fibrinogen to fibrin. The conversion typically occurs in response to trauma to the vascular wall. Insertion of a large catheter would cause such trauma. The body's natural response is for activated plasminogen to form plasmin, a proteolytic enzyme that dissolves the clot and keeps fibrinogen from making new fibrin. This process cannot occur within the lumen of a central venous catheter. Therefore, blood adhering to the catheter wall has a tendency to form fibrin clots.

PHARMACOTHERAPEUTIC OPTIONS

Thrombolytics

FIRST-GENERATION THROMBOLYTICS
◆ streptokinase (Streptase, Kabikinase)
◆ urokinase (Abbokinase)

SECOND-GENERATION THROMBOLYTICS
◆ alteplase (recombinant tissue plasminogen activator [t-PA], Activase)
◆ anistreplase (anisoylated plasminogen streptokinase activator complex [APSAC], Eminase)

THIRD-GENERATION THROMBOLYTICS
◆ reteplase recombinant (Retavase)
◆ tenecteplase (TNKase)

▥ Indications

Thrombolytic therapy is indicated in the treatment of AMI, PE, DVT, ischemic CVA, and arterial occlusions. Thrombolytics are also used to restore patency to occluded central venous catheters. Some thrombolytic drugs have been found more effective in specific clinical syndromes or patient populations. Streptokinase, the prototype thrombolytic, was the first drug available for clinical use. Thrombolytics differ in their mechanisms of action, ease of preparation and administration, and cost.

With prompt use of thrombolytic drugs and reperfusion following an AMI, reduction in the size of the infarct, improvement in left ventricular function, and reduction in mortality rate have been seen. A thrombolytic drug is indicated for the patient who has chest pain consistent with an AMI for at least 30 minutes but not longer than 6 hours and who has at least 0.1 mV of ST-segment elevation in at least two contiguous electrocardiographic leads. Figure 40-2 shows the changes in electrocardiographic patterns associated with ischemia, injury, and infarction.

Alteplase (t-PA), streptokinase, and urokinase may be used in the treatment of acute massive PE. Rapid dissolution of the clot helps to normalize the patient's hemodynamic status.

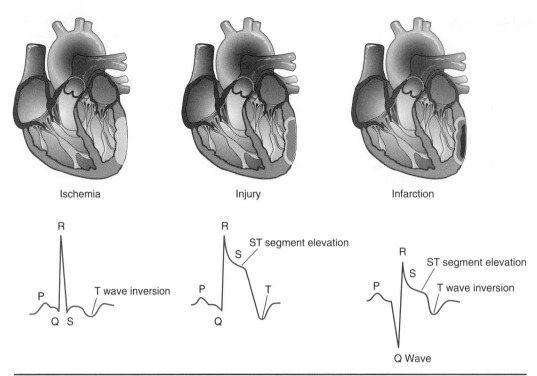

FIGURE 40-2 ECG Patterns. ECG patterns illustrate how ST-segment elevation progresses through each stage of ischemia, injury, and infarction.

Thrombolysis has been life-saving in patients with cardiogenic shock due to massive PE. In acute PE, these drugs restore patency of the pulmonary artery but do not improve long-term outcomes.

Streptokinase and urokinase have also been used in the treatment of DVT. Thrombolysis is indicated for patients with DVT who present with limb gangrene unresponsive to anticoagulation therapy. The role of locally delivered thrombolytic therapy for DVT is still unclear; however, potential benefits associated with thrombolysis include (1) preventing the downhill spiral of right-sided heart failure by physical dissolution of anatomically obstructing pulmonary arterial thrombus; (2) preventing the continued release of serotonin and other neurohumoral factors that might otherwise lead to worsening pulmonary hypertension; and (3) dissolving much of the source of the thrombus in the pelvis or deep leg veins, thereby decreasing the likelihood of recurrent large PEs.

Restoring patency of occluded arteriovenous (AV) shunts is another possible use for urokinase. Urokinase has been used in a pulse spray method via a multi–holed catheter placed in a crisscross pattern in the graft. Other suggested uses of thrombolytics include the prevention of fibrin build-up in peritoneal dialysis catheters. The treatment of thrombosis of prosthetic valves in the left side of the heart is also being explored.

▌▌ Pharmacodynamics

Unlike anticoagulants, which prevent the formation or extension of blood clots, thrombolytic drugs dissolve thrombi after formation. These drugs catalyze the formation of the serine protease plasmin from its precursor, plasminogen. Plasmin, in turn, degrades fibrin present in the clots. When thrombolytics are given intravenously, they produce a generalized lytic state which breaks down both protective hemostatic thrombi as well as pathologic thromboemboli.

Streptokinase comes from group C beta hemolytic streptococcus. This enzyme acts indirectly to break down clots by joining with plasminogen. The joining leads to the formation of activator complexes that convert inactive plasminogen into active plasmin. When streptokinase is acetylated and then combined with purified human plasminogen, the complex is known as APSAC.

Recombinant DNA technology is used to produce t-PA, which is fibrin-specific. When administered at appropriate dosages, t-PA binds to fibrin in the thrombus, converting plasminogen to plasmin. This binding starts a local fibrinolysis with limited systemic proteolysis. There are few effects on circulating plasminogen.

Like t-PA, APSAC is an active complex of streptokinase and plasminogen that was developed initially as a clot-specific drug; however, it seems to work equally well on systemic plasminogen conversion. APSAC is an inactive derivative of a fibrinolytic enzyme, with the center of the activator complex temporarily blocked by an anisoyl group. In solution, the anisoyl group is removed and the enzymatically active plasminogen streptokinase complex is activated.

Tenecteplase is pharmacologically related to t-PA but has a longer half-life than t-PA, is more selective of fibrin, and displays greater resistance to plasminogen activator inhibitors. Because it can be administered as a single, weight-adjusted bolus, care of acutely ill patients is greatly simplified.

Escherichia coli cells are used to produce the newest thrombolytic drug, reteplase. Reteplase also catalyzes the conversion of plasminogen to plasmin, with the activation stimulated by the presence of fibrin. Plasmin then degrades the fibrin matrix of the thrombus. Reteplase has a lower affinity for fibrin, which may result in better clot penetration. Reteplase has a longer half-life, less of an affinity for fibrin, and greater thrombolytic activity when compared to t-PA.

Urokinase is a protein initially isolated from human urine. It activates plasminogen directly. Because it is not a derivative of streptococci, as is streptokinase, there is less incidence of allergic reaction with urokinase than with streptokinase.

Thrombolytics activate plasminogen directly. Fibrinogen levels are decreased for 24 to 36 hours after therapy. Direct and indirect effects of thrombolysis are prolonged because of the drug's extended presence in the circulation and because of the elevated concentrations of fibrinogen degradation products in the plasma.

Pharmacokinetics

Information about all aspects of the pharmacokinetics of thrombolytic drugs is incomplete; however, Table 40-1 provides a summary of what is known. Streptokinase is cleared from the circulation by antibodies. It does not cross placental membranes, but the antibodies produced in response to the streptokinase do cross over to the fetus.

Urokinase is biotransformed and eliminated primarily by the liver; however, small amounts are eliminated in the urine. The half-life of the drug is 20 minutes or less but is prolonged if there is liver impairment.

t-PA is rapidly absorbed, with an immediate onset of action. t-PA crosses the placental barrier and may pass into breast milk. Biotransformation takes place in the liver, with small amounts eliminated in the urine.

APSAC crosses the placenta and may pass into breast milk. Biotransformation occurs in the plasma, with inactivation caused by binding to plasmin inactivators.

Reteplase is biotransformed in the liver and eliminated in the urine. It is not known whether it is excreted in human milk.

Adverse Effects and Contraindications

Overall, bleeding represents the most common complication of thrombolytic therapy; it is more common in women than men and occurs in 8% to 16% of patients. Major bleeding requiring treatment with blood transfusion occurs in 12% to 15% of patients. Bleeding may occur in the gastrointestinal (GI) tract, the genitourinary tract, and retroperitoneal, ocular, or intracranial spaces. Bleeding from puncture sites may also occur.

Hemorrhagic strokes, which occur in 0.5% to 1% of patients, present a serious risk associated with thrombolytic therapy and are associated with high mortality rates. The risk of intracranial hemorrhage is higher in patients receiving thrombolytics for the treatment of strokes than those receiving the drugs for treatment of MI. Hemorrhagic bleeding occurs most often with the an accelerated t-PA protocol. Drug-induced hypotension occurs infrequently but is reported more often with streptokinase and APSAC.

Other adverse effects of thrombolytic drugs include reperfusion arrhythmias, nausea and vomiting, and hypersensitivity reactions; hypotension and shivering have been noted with streptokinase. Streptokinase is also the thrombolytic most associated with hypersensitivity reactions, with symptoms ranging in severity from minor breathing difficulty to bronchospasm, periorbital swelling, or angioedema. Other, milder allergic effects such as urticaria, itching, flushing, nausea, headache, and musculoskeletal pain have been observed. Anaphylaxis is rare. Approximately 33% of patients experience an increase in temperature.

Cross-sensitivity of APSAC with streptokinase may occur. Streptokinase is an antigenic bacterial protein. It can cause a hypersensitivity response in any patient who has had a streptococcal infection in the previous year. These patients develop streptococcal antibodies that neutralize the streptokinase, causing severe allergic reactions.

Because thrombolytic therapy carries serious risks, care must be taken to exclude patients who are at high risk for complications and those in whom the risks outweigh the benefits that they would receive (Box 40-2). Thrombolytic therapy is generally contraindicated during pregnancy. Urokinase has been classified as pregnancy category B; the remaining thrombolytics are category C drugs.

Drug Interactions

The concurrent administration of antiplatelet drugs, anticoagulants, dipyridamole, indomethacin, and phenylbutazone increases the risk of bleeding. Further, there are many drug interactions with thrombolytics (Box 40-3). The use of low-dose aspirin with thrombolytics has been shown to reduce the incidence of reinfarction and CVA. Aspirin use produces a slight increase in the incidence of minor bleeding but not in major bleeding.

Dosage Regimen

Dosage regimens of thrombolytic drugs are different for each drug, depending on the patient's diagnosis (Table 40-2). Use caution when checking references, because some list dosages based on body weight in pounds while others do so in kilograms.

PHARMACOKINETICS
TABLE 40-1 Thrombolytics

Drug	Peak	Duration	t½	Patency at 90 min	Fibrinogen Depletion
alteplase	5–10 min	2.5–3 hr	5 min	75%	Mild
anistreplase	45 min	4–6 hr*	1–2 hr	UA	Mild
reteplase	5–10 min	UA	13–16 min	75%	Moderate
streptokinase	30–60 min†	4–12 hr	16 min	50%	Marked
tenecteplase	End of inf	UA	20–24 min	75%	Minimal
urokinase	End of inf	Up to 12 hr	20 min	UA	Mild

*Systemic hyperfibrinolytic state may persist for 48 hr after administration of anistreplase.
†Clearance and thrombolytic activity of streptokinase appear to decline with continuous infusion.
BioA, Bioavailability; *inf,* infection; *PB,* protein binding; $t_{1/2}$, half-life; *UA,* unavailable.

BOX 40-2

Contraindications to Use of Thrombolytics for Acute Ischemic Stroke

Absolute Contraindications

- Evidence of intracranial hemorrhage on pretreatment evaluation
- Suspicion of subarachnoid hemorrhage
- Intracranial surgery within the previous 14 days
- Serious head trauma within previous 3 months
- CVA within previous 3 months
- History of intracranial hemorrhage
- Uncontrolled hypertension (e.g., systolic BP >185 mm Hg or diastolic >110 mm Hg)
- Blood glucose value <50 or >400 mg/dL
- Seizure at onset of CVA
- Active internal bleeding
- Gastrointestinal or urinary bleeding within the past 21 days
- Intracranial neoplasm, AV malformation, or aneurysm

- Known bleeding diathesis including but not limited to current use of anticoagulant with a prothrombin time exceeding 15 seconds; administration of heparin within 48 hours preceding onset of CVA; an elevated aPTT upon arrival at health care facility
- Platelet count under 100,000 mm^3
- Recent MI

Ablative Contraindications

Patients with severe neurologic deficit over 22 on National Institute of Health Scale

Patients with early infarct signs on CT scan (e.g., substantial edema, mass effect, or midline shift)

---

aPTT; Activated partial thromboplastin time; *AV,* arteriovenous; *CT,* computed tomography; *CVA;* cardiovascular accident; *MI,* myocardial infarction.

BOX 40-3

Drug Interactions With Thrombolytics

- abciximab
- acenocoumarol
- alteplase (t-PA)
- ancrod
- anisindione
- anistreplase (anisoylated plasminogen streptokinase activator complex [APSAC])
- antithrombin III (human)
- ardeparin
- argatroban
- aspirin (moderate, established)
- bivalirudin
- certoparin
- cilostazol
- clopidogrel
- dalteparin
- danaparoid
- defibrotide
- dermatan sulfate
- desirudin

- dipyridamole
- enoxaparin
- eptifibatide
- fondaparinux
- heparin
- lamifiban
- lepirudin
- nadroparin
- parnaparin
- pentosan polysulfate sodium
- phenindione
- phenprocoumon
- reteplase
- reviparin
- sibrafiban
- tenecteplase
- tinzaparin
- tirofiban
- urokinase
- warfarin
- xemilofiban

▥ Lab Considerations

Before beginning thrombolytic therapy, obtain a baseline complete blood count (CBC), fibrinogen level, thrombin time, partial thromboplastin time (PTT) (or activated partial thromboplastin time, aPTT), prothrombin (PT) time, and blood type. Abnormalities in these laboratory values may prevent the patient from being considered as a candidate for thrombolytic therapy. During therapy, there will be an increase in the thrombin time, the PTT, and the PT values, which should normalize within 12 to 24 hours. There will be a decrease in the fibrinogen and plasminogen levels (Table 40-3).

CLINICAL REASONING

Treatment Objectives

Overall treatment objectives for the patient receiving a thrombolytic include minimizing loss of tissue and minimizing drug-induced morbidity and mortality. In addition, treatment objectives include prevention of ischemia-related arrhythmias; opening the occluded artery as soon as possible; and maintaining patency after blood flow is reestablished.

Treatment Options

▥ Patient Variables

AMI, PE, and ischemic strokes are generally considered urgent or emergent conditions that warrant treatment with thrombolytics. Because health care team members are often focused on the urgency of the situation, psychosocial aspects of care are often overlooked. Take extra care to address these needs, and ensure that informed consent is obtained and adequate education provided.

The patient must be screened carefully for contraindications to thrombolytic therapy. When a patient falls into the category of having relative contraindications, the risks must be weighed carefully against the benefits before a treatment decision is made. Although there is no age limit in the contraindications, the age of the patient must be considered when deciding whether the benefits of thrombolytic therapy outweigh the risks.

LIFE-SPAN CONSIDERATIONS. Safety and efficacy of thrombolytic drugs have not been established for pregnant and nursing women, or children or adolescents. Further, patients 75 years of age or older are at higher risk for bleeding from stroke and the comorbid disease processes that accompany thrombolytic therapy.

▥ Drug Variables

There are advantages and disadvantages to each of the thrombolytic drugs. At times, the differences in pharmacodynamic or pharmacokinetic profiles influence drug selection.

DOSAGE

TABLE 40-2 Thrombolytics

Drug	Use(s)	Dosage*	Implications
alteplase (t-PA)	Ischemic CVA	*Adult:* 0.9 mg/kg IV over 60 min. Give 10% of dose bolus over 1 min. Max: 90 mg IV.	Initiate heparin at end of infusion. Estimated cost per 100-mg vial: $3212
	AMI	*Adult >65 kg:* *Standard dosage regimen:* 15 mg IV bolus then step-down infusion *Accelerated protocol >65 kg:* 100 mg IV bolus then step-down infusion *Accelerated protocol <65 kg:* 15 mg IV bolus then step-down infusion	**Doses over 150 mg have higher risk of intracranial bleeding.** Initiate heparin at end of infusion. Check agency policy regarding step-down infusion therapy.
	CT-confirmed PE	*Adult:* 100 mg IV over 2 hr	Initiate heparin at end of infusion.
	AV cannula occlusion	*Adult:* 2 mg IV. May repeat every 2 hr or more	Superficial bleeding at puncture site. Estimated cost per 2-mg vial: $77
anistreplase (APSAC)	AMI	*Adult:* 30 units IV bolus over 2–5 min	**Antigenic. Avoid if history of strep infection in last year.**
reteplase	AMI	*Adult:* 10 units IV bolus over 2 min, then second bolus 30 min later	Estimated cost per dose: $2196
streptokinase	AMI	*Adult:* 1.5 million units IV over 30–60 min followed by 100,000 units/hr for 24–72 hr	**Antigenic. Avoid if strep infection within previous year.** Estimated cost per single dose using 100,000-unit vial: $568
	DVT, PE, embolism, or thrombosis	*Adult:* 250,000 units IV loading dose over 60 min followed by 100,000 units/hr for 24 hr	
	AV cannula occlusion	*Adult:* 100,000–250,000 units to each occluded limb of cannula, clamp for 2 hr, then aspirate	Flush line with normal saline after aspiration.
tenecteplase	AMI	*Adult <60 kg:* 30 mg or 6 mL IV bolus over 5 sec based on patient weight and symptoms ≥60 to <70 kg: 35 mg or 7 mL; ≥70 to <80 kg: 40 mg or 8 mL	Concentrate: 200 units/mg. Max dosage: 50 mg. Estimated cost per dose using 50-mg vial: $2750
urokinase	PE, DVT	*Adult:* 4400 units/kg loading dose over 10 min followed by 4400 units/kg/hr for 12 to 24 hr	Estimated cost per dose using 5-mL vial: $431.82
	AV cannula occlusion	*Adult:* 5000 units/mL to occluded catheter, then aspirate. Repeat every 5 min for 30 min. Volume instilled is equal to or slightly less than volume of catheter.	If no result, cap and leave in catheter for 30–60 min; then aspirate.

⚠ *Some references list dosage based on body weight in pounds rather than kilograms. Check dosage carefully.*
AMI, Acute myocardial infarction; *AV,* arteriovenous; *CT,* computed tomography; *DVT,* deep vein thrombosis; *IV,* intravenous (route); *PE,* pulmonary embolism.

Other times, formulary status or the availability of the drug in a given institution may limit the thrombolytic alternatives. Patients who meet the selection criteria for the administration of thrombolytics must also be carefully screened for contraindications before a final decision is made to treat the patient with a thrombolytic (Table 40-4). Compared with streptokinase, the thrombolytic drugs are more costly and carry a slightly greater risk of cerebral hemorrhage (about 0.2% absolute excess), especially among older adult hypertensive women with a low body weight. Heparin must be used along with fibrin-specific drugs to maintain antithrombotic effects.

There is little risk of antigen-antibody response with t-PA; however, there is an increased risk for cerebral bleeding.

TABLE 40-3 Test Results After Thrombolytic Therapy

Lab Test	Results
Protime (PT)	Increased
Activated partial thromboplastin time (aPTT)	Increased
Thrombin time	Increased
Fibrinogen level	Decreased
Plasminogen level	Decreased

Reteplase is also indicated for the treatment of the patient with an acute MI. The primary advantage of reteplase is the simple method of administration, which allows for quicker initiation of therapy and decreases opportunity for dosage errors.

Health care facilities that administer thrombolytics must have qualified health care providers who are experienced in the use of thrombolytics as well as access to cardiac catheterization labs. Institutions that do not have catheterization labs begin treatment for patients who fit the established protocol and then transfer the patient to a facility that can provide coronary angiography and angioplasty.

The possibility of bleeding exists up to 24 hours after thrombolytic therapy has been discontinued. Avoid unnecessary venipunctures or injections during that time. ⚠ When they are necessary, pressure should be applied manually for 10 minutes at venous sites and 30 minutes at arterial sites. Pressure dressings are then applied. Avoid venipunctures in noncompressible sites such as subclavian or internal jugular sites. Type and cross-match the patient in advance for possible blood replacement.

CEREBROVASCULAR ACCIDENT. Initiation of thrombolytic therapy for the treatment of acute ischemic stroke cannot begin until the possibility of a hemorrhagic stroke has been ruled out. Facilities that do not have the ability to perform

---

TABLE 40-4 Indications for Effective Thrombolytic Therapy*

CLASS I: EVIDENCE OR OPINION FAVORS SAFETY, EFFICACY, AND BENEFIT OF THROMBOLYTIC THERAPY

- Administer a thrombolytic within 12 hr of STEMI-symptom onset in patients who have an ST elevation over 0.1 mV in at least two contiguous precordial leads, or at least two adjacent limb leads, and in the presence of a new, or presumably new, LBBB.

CLASS IIA: EVIDENCE OR OPINION FAVORS EFFICACY OF THROMBOLYTIC THERAPY

- Administer a thrombolytic within 12 hr of STEMI-symptom onset and 12-lead ECG findings consistent with a true posterior MI.
- Administer a thrombolytic to patients with symptoms of STEMI beginning within the prior 12–24 hours who have continuing ischemic symptoms and ST elevation over 0.1 mV in at least two contiguous precordial leads, or at least two adjacent limb leads.

---

*Recommendation made in the absence of contraindications to thrombolytic therapy.
ECG, Electrocardiogram; *LBBB,* left bundle branch block; *MI,* myocardial infarction; *STEMI,* ST-elevated myocardial infarction.
From Antman, E., Anbe, D., Armstrong, P., et al. (2004). ACC/AHA Guidelines for the management of patients with ST-elevation myocardial infarction: A report of the American College of Cardiology/American Heart Association Task Force on Practice Guidelines (Committee to Revise the 1999 Guidelines for the Management of Patients with Acute Myocardial Infarction). Available online: www.acc.org/clinical/guidelines/stemi/index.pdf. Accessed May 16, 2007.

---

head computed tomography (CT) scans must transfer the patient to a facility that does before treatment can be begun. ▲ **The only thrombolytic presently approved the treatment of ischemic stroke is t-PA, which must be administered within 3 hours of onset of symptoms.**

MYOCARDIAL INFARCTION. The purpose for treating an acute myocardial infarction in a timely fashion is to reduce myocardial muscle damage and restore the contractile function of the atria and ventricles. The critical time for effective treatment of an AMI is 6 hours from onset of chest pain. The American College of Cardiology–American Heart Association (ACC-AHA) guidelines for treatment of STEMI note that prehospital thrombolytic therapy is reasonable if a physician is present in the ambulance of a well-organized emergency medical service (EMS) (e.g., 12-lead electrocardiogram [ECGs] in the field with transmission capability) and when transport times exceed 60 minutes.

Patients are referred for angioplasty if at least half of ST-segment elevations do not resolve and pain relief is not seen in 60 to 90 minutes after the thrombolytic drug is administered. Aspirin is a standard adjunct to all reperfusion drug regimens.

The low cost makes streptokinase the most widely prescribed thrombolytic drug. Third-generation thrombolytics are more easily administered compared with streptokinase and carry an average mortality rate of 1% but they are much costlier (see Table 40-2).

PULMONARY EMBOLISM. Thrombolytics have been shown to decrease the mortality rate associated with PE. Begin the administration of thrombolytics in the treatment of PE as soon as possible after the onset of symptoms. Thrombolysis can be given for severe PEs when surgery is not immediately available or possible. However, the use of thrombolytics in moderate PEs is still debatable. The aim of the therapy is to dissolve the clot, but there is an attendant risk of bleeding or stroke. Some benefit may be derived if administered up to 2 weeks after symptom onset. Therefore, rapid recognition of the patient who has experienced a PE is key to maximizing drug benefit. Any of the thrombolytics, except APSAC, can be used. APSAC is FDA-approved only for the treatment of acute MI. Therapy may be started up to 7 days after the thrombotic event.

PERIPHERAL ARTERIAL OCCLUSION. The systemic use of thrombolytics in peripheral arterial occlusion has been disappointing because bleeding complications outweigh the benefits. However, local intraarterial thrombolytic therapy with urokinase has emerged as an alternative to surgery in the treatment of selected patients. It is important to remember that thrombolytics may break up the clot and cause emboli to be released into the circulation. To be most effective, therapy must begin within 5 days of the onset of the symptoms.

Streptokinase is commonly used and is recommended for thrombolytic treatment of DVT. However, urokinase has been most extensively studied, and although it is used almost exclusively for restoring patency to occluded central venous lines, there are dosage recommendations for AMI, DVT, and PE.

COMORBID STATES. There are several variables to consider when deciding which thrombolytic to use. The risks of allergic reactions, increased risk of intracerebral bleeding, and the efficacy of each drug must be considered. In studies performed to determine the "best" thrombolytic, several concurrent therapies have been recommended. The use of low-dose aspirin with concurrent use of thrombolytics has been shown to increase the efficacy of the drug in treating MI. The accelerated t-PA protocol provides for a better patency rate when intravenous (IV) heparin is used in conjunction with the t-PA. The greatest advantage of t-PA seems to be prevention of valvular damage and consequent venous insufficiency, as well as postphlebotic syndrome.

The drug of choice for patients who have previously received streptokinase, who have been given APSAC, or who have been treated for a streptococcal infection within the previous year is t-PA. These patients develop streptococcal antibodies that neutralize the streptokinase, causing severe allergic reactions. Careful consideration must also be given to the time that has elapsed from the onset of symptoms to the beginning of treatment, especially in the patient with an acute MI or acute ischemic stroke. Once tissue death has occurred, even though patency of the vessel is restored, there is little that can be done to improve function of the affected tissues. **The risks associated with late use of thrombolytic** ▲ **therapy heavily outweigh possible benefits.**

Patient Education

Research has demonstrated that patients and family members wait as much as 90 minutes before seeking medical attention for their symptoms. Further, the time-sensitive issues involved in using thrombolytics place additional pressure on patients, family, and the health care providers. Education and emotional support is essential and patients and family usually benefit from a clear, easy-to-understand explanation of the benefits and risk of thrombolytics.

Explain thrombolytic therapy and possible complications to the patient and family before starting treatment. Instruct the patient to report any adverse effects, such as lightheadedness, dizziness, palpitations, or nausea. Explain the probability that bruising will occur as a result of the therapy, and that bed rest and minimal handling of the patient are therefore required. Instruct the patient to report developing or intensifying pain.

Community education regarding the signs and symptoms of a heart attack and stroke and the importance of the need to seek help immediately should be a high priority for health care providers. It is common for patients having an AMI to put off getting help as they work through their denial of what is happening. However, the sooner they seek help, the greater benefit thrombolytic therapy will be. Community initiatives to ensure first responders are trained to transport patients to an appropriate center, in the event thrombolytic or invasive procedures are probable, is key. Delays in treatment often lead to worsening outcomes for patients.

Risk factors and preventive measures for AMI, PE, and DVT should also be taught to the community because most of these disease processes can be prevented or their incidence decreased. Certain risk factors have been linked to the occurrence of CAD. Major risk factors include advancing age, male sex, family history of heart disease, diabetes mellitus, smoking, elevated blood pressure, elevated serum cholesterol, excess weight, excess alcohol intake, sedentary lifestyle, and left ventricular hypertrophy. All risk factors, with the exception of age, sex, and family history of heart disease, can be modified somewhat to reduce the risk of cardiovascular disease and decrease the associated mortality. The risk factors of CAD are the same factors that are linked to peripheral artery occlusive disease. Essentially, it is the same disease process, only in different vessels.

Evaluation

Evaluate the patient receiving thrombolytic therapy for the effectiveness of treatment. In general, therapy is deemed effective if the patency of the vessel is restored, circulation to the area beyond the occlusion is restored, and the viability of tissues maintained.

The desired outcome for the patient with a stroke is that there is minimal or no disability in the short term and for at least 3 months after the event. Careful monitoring and management of blood pressure is necessary, especially for the patient with an acute stroke. An elevated blood pressure is likely to contribute to the development of intracranial bleeding and can worsen ischemia. Frequent monitoring of the patient's neurologic status is imperative. If there is a sudden decrease in level of consciousness, cerebral hemorrhage should be suspected.

Indications that treatment reperfusion therapy for the patient with STEMI has been successful include cessation of chest pain, the onset of reperfusion arrhythmias, resolution of ST-segment elevation, and a peak in the creatine kinase value at 12 hours.

The patient treated for a PE should experience resolution of the chest pain and a return of pulmonary hemodynamics to a normal range. Patients with occluded arteries or veins should note a cessation of the accompanying symptoms. If thrombolytics are used for the treatment of DVT, monitor closely for symptoms of PE.

LOWER EXTREMITY AND ESOPHAGEAL VARICES

EPIDEMIOLOGY AND ETIOLOGY

Varicosities are most frequently found in the saphenous veins in the lower extremities. It is estimated that varicose veins affect 1 in 5 persons worldwide. They are most prevalent in women and in persons whose occupations require prolonged standing or sitting. Primary varicosities are those in which the superficial veins are dilated. The valves may or may not be incompetent. The primary form tends to be familial and is probably caused by a congenital weakness of the veins. Secondary varicosities are usually the result of a previous injury such as thrombophlebitis of a deep femoral vein with subsequent valvular incompetence. Secondary varicosities may also occur in the esophagus (esophageal varices), in the anorectal area (hemorrhoids), and as abnormal arteriovenous connections.

Esophageal varices are dilated, tortuous veins that are usually found in the submucosa of the lower esophagus; however, they may develop more proximally or extend into the stomach. The development of esophageal varices or alternate circulation routes from the portal to the systemic circulation is the major complication of portal hypertension. Although varices can be present at any level of the GI tract, those connecting the left gastric vein with esophageal circulation are the most clinically significant. The mortality rate resulting from initial variceal bleeding is 45% to 50%. They are one of the major causes of death in patients with cirrhosis.

PATHOPHYSIOLOGY

Varicosities develop most often as a result of increased hydrostatic pressure or obstruction of venous blood flow. Continually elevated venous pressure weakens venous walls. The constant pressure also prevents the valves from closing completely. As pressure elevation continues, valves are damaged and the veins become tortuous and enlarged. There is an accompanying increase in the capillary pressure, and perfusion is decreased. Painful weak muscles and edema ensue. Stasis ulcers and gangrene can develop.

Esophageal varices are almost always related to portal hypertension. There is a backflow of blood into esophageal vessels and an increased amount of pressure within the vessels. The vessels become tortuous, brittle, and bleed easily. Varices usually produce no symptoms until the pressure suddenly increases, and then massive hemorrhage can occur.

Factors contributing to hemorrhage from esophageal varices include straining, coughing, sneezing, heavy lifting, vomiting, poorly chewed foods, or irritating foods or fluids. Nonsteroidal antiinflammatory drugs (NSAIDs), bisphosphonates, and any drugs that erode esophageal mucosa may increase the risk of bleeding.

PHARMACOTHERAPEUTIC OPTIONS

Sclerosing Drugs
◆ ethanolamine oleate (Ethamolin)
◆ morrhuate sodium (Scleromate)
◆ sodium tetradecyl sulfate (Sotradecol)
◆ Hypertonic saline (20%)

Indications

Sclerosing drugs are used in the treatment of superficial varicose veins of the lower extremities. Other possible uses for sclerosing drugs include treatment of internal hemorrhoids, closure of hernial rings, and the removal of condylomata acuminata. Sclerosing of varicose veins is an adjunct to, rather than a primary treatment for, varicosities. There have been some cases in which sclerosing drugs were used in place of surgery for varicose veins; however, the risk-to-benefit ratio must be heavily weighed.

Endoscopic sclerotherapy is indicated in both acute and chronic cases of esophageal varices. Prophylactic sclerotherapy may be performed on distended but nonbleeding veins.

Morrhuate sodium and sodium tetradecyl sulfate are used in both the treatment of varicose veins and esophageal varices. Ethanolamine oleate is not recommended for the treatment of varicose veins.

Pharmacodynamics

Sclerosing drugs thrombose and obliterate distended veins. They traumatize the endothelial lining, causing inflammation of the intima of the vessel with subsequent formation of a thrombus. The thrombus occludes the vein, and fibrous tissue develops, obliterating the vein.

Pharmacokinetics

Sclerosing drugs are usually cleared from the circulation within minutes via the portal vein. There seems to be a delayed response, especially with ethanolamine oleate, and complete sclerosing and obliteration of the vein may take up to 3 months.

Adverse Effects and Contraindications

A common adverse effect of sclerosing drugs is burning or cramping at the varicosity injection site. Sloughing of tissue occurs if the drug is allowed to extravasate. Mild systemic responses include headache, dizziness, nausea, and vomiting. Significant adverse effects include cellulitis, phlebitis, thrombophlebitis, urticaria, tissue sloughing and necrosis, and anaphylaxis. Allergic reactions may occur within a few minutes of the injection. Allergic reactions are more common when therapy is reinstituted after an interval of several weeks.

With endoscopic sclerotherapy the patient may experience chest pain for up to 72 hours. The pain is not cardiac in nature but related to the procedure. Local reactions, which include esophagitis, tearing of the esophagus, and sloughing of the mucosa, contraindicate further treatment with sclerosing drugs. Pleural effusion or infiltrate, esophageal perforation, ulceration, and strictures have been noted. **Overdosage or overtreatment of esophageal varices results in severe necrosis of the esophagus.**

Sclerosing drugs are contraindicated for use in patients with a known hypersensitivity to the drug, acute superficial thrombophlebitis, valvular or deep vein incompetency, and large superficial veins that communicate freely with deep veins. Embolism can occur as late as 4 weeks after an injection. Sclerosing drugs are also contraindicated for use in patients with underlying arterial disease, varicosities caused by abdominal and pelvic tumors, uncontrolled diabetes mellitus, thyrotoxicosis, tuberculosis, a neoplasm, asthma, sepsis, blood dyscrasias, or acute respiratory or skin disease, as well as in bedridden patients. The sclerosing drugs are classified as pregnancy category C. It is not known whether they are excreted in human breast milk.

Drug Interactions

There are few documented drug interactions with sclerosing drugs. Heparin is incompatible with sclerosing drugs; do not admix in the syringe with a sclerosing drug.

Dosage Regimen

The usual dosage of sclerosing drugs depends on the reason for their use. Dosages are usually decreased in patients with a history of liver or heart disease. Ethanolamine oleate is administered at the time of the bleed, and then repeated at 1 week, 6 weeks, 3 months, and 6 months after the initial dose. It is indicated for the prevention of recurrent bleeding of esophageal varices. Do not use it as a prophylactic therapy.

The dosage of morrhuate sodium depends on the size of the varicosity. The usual dose for obliteration of small to medium-sized veins is 50 to 100 mg (1 to 2 mL) of a 5% solution. The dosage for larger vessels is 150 to 250 mg (3 to 5 mL). The injection may be repeated at 5- to 7-day intervals as needed.

The dosage for sodium tetradecyl sulfate also depends on the size of the varicose vein, although the strength of the solution also varies with the size of the varicosity being treated. A 1% solution is used for small to medium varicosities, and a 3% solution is used for larger veins. The dosage is kept small, with 0.5 to 2 mL used for each injection. The quantity of a single dose should not exceed 1 mL. Do not exceed the maximum dosage of 10 mL.

Lab Considerations

Because there is a significant risk for DVT and PE with the administration of sclerosing drugs, use angiography or Doppler venous examination to evaluate the degree of valvular incompetence before injection.

CLINICAL REASONING

Treatment Objectives

Treatment of varicose veins is directed toward improving circulation, relieving discomfort and swelling, and avoiding complications. The objective of sclerotherapy for esophageal varices is to control the bleeding and avoid hemorrhage. It does not eliminate the possibility that the varicosities will recur.

Treatment Options

Patient Variables

The psychosocial considerations related to peripheral varicosities may be significant. The disease can be exacerbated in patients whose employment requires excessive periods of standing or sitting. If the patient is unable to work because of the discomfort or because the varicosities are unsightly, feelings of powerlessness and changes in self-image have an impact on the patient's state of wellness.

Typically, sclerotherapy is used as an adjunct to surgery. However, patients who are at very high risk for surgery may be possible candidates for treatment solely with sclerosing drugs. Because the use of sclerosing drugs has not been studied during pregnancy, use sclerotherapy only when it is absolutely necessary and the benefits greatly outweigh risks.

Esophageal varices are often a complication of cirrhosis of the liver, which in turn may be the result of chronic alcohol use. Often, these patients have not admitted to themselves or others just how extensive their drinking problem is until they are diagnosed with cirrhosis. The efficacy of sclerotherapy for patients with habitual alcohol use is less than would otherwise be desired.

LIFE-SPAN CONSIDERATIONS. The normal changes associated with pregnancy may predispose the woman to varicosities in the lower extremities. These varicosities usually do not require sclerotherapy. Both esophageal varices and peripheral varicosities are typically progressive states that occur when the primary problem has been present over a prolonged period. Hence the older population may be at increased risk given the associated risk factors for the disorders (see Case Study).

▥ Drug Variables

There seems to be less incidence of anaphylaxis with ethanolamine oleate than with the other drugs, even though it is still a possible adverse effect. Ethanolamine oleate requires a much longer course of therapy than the other drugs, putting the patient at risk for complications for an extended period of time. It also is rapidly diffused through the vein to produce an extravascular inflammatory response that is not present with the other drugs. Sclerosing drugs control active esophageal bleeding in 70% to 80% of patients having one treatment and in 90% to 95% with an additional injection.

These patients require close physiologic monitoring before, during, and after treatment because bleeding can occur for up to 24 hours after the treatment is completed.

Patient Education

Prevention is a key factor related to varicose veins. Tell the patient predisposed to varicose veins to avoid occupations that require prolong periods of standing or sitting. They should also avoid wearing tight girdles or garters and not cross the legs at the knee. Any activity that increases venous stasis or increases pressure in the venous system in the lower extremities can lead to the formation of varicose veins. Patients who are obese have a higher incidence of varicose veins; dietary teaching about weight loss may be warranted.

As with all interventions, patient education is vital to the success of the treatment. Tell patients what to expect during the procedure and what unusual sensations or adverse effects may occur. Also, advise them of the behaviors and or activities that should be avoided after therapy and when to return for follow-up care. For example, most patients having treatment for varicosities will be required to wear compression stockings after therapy. The amount of compression therapy necessary following sclerotherapy for telangiectasias and reticular veins, however, is a controversial issue. Use of at least a minimally graduated compression stocking is recommended for the first few days and possibly for 7 to 10 days. The compression theoretically helps improve results and minimizes adverse effects such as edema and postinflammatory hyperpigmentation. Using class I (20–30 mm Hg) or class II (30–40 mm Hg) compression is best. For patients who cannot tolerate the compression, a class I fashion support hose can be prescribed. After treatment, the patient can continue low-impact exercises such as walking or riding bicycles, but withhold direct isometric exercise to the lower legs for at least 1 week.

Instruct patients with esophageal varices to avoid alcohol, NSAIDs, and irritating foods. These substances irritate varices and cause bleeding. After sclerotherapy for esophageal varices, achiness and a feeling of stiffness develop that may persist for 48 hours. Varices have a tendency to recur, so the need for follow-up endoscopy must be stressed. Offer assistance finding support groups for patients who use alcohol.

Evaluation

After treatment for varicose veins, the vein will be hard, edematous, and tender for the first 24 hours. The surrounding skin will be a light bronze color, which is temporary. However, there may be a permanent but barely discernible discoloration that remains along the path of the sclerosed vein.

When sclerosing drugs are administered for esophageal varices, bleeding should stop 2 minutes after the introduction of the drug. If bleeding continues, a second injection attempt is made below the bleeding site. Conduct a follow-up examination to determine whether or not assistance with alcohol abuse has been obtained.

CASE STUDY   Thrombolytics

ASSESSMENT

History of Present Illness	(Paramedic report) JH is a 66-year-old anxious-appearing obese white male arriving by ambulance with complaints of substernal chest pain radiating to the left arm, shortness of breath, and nausea. ST-segment elevation of 2–4 mm V_1-V_5. Midsternal pain started 1 hr ago while in a meeting at work. Pain increasing from 4/10 to 8/10. A&O × 3. Diaphoretic. BP 94/70, pulse weak, thready. O_2 started 8 L/min/NC; IV lactated Ringer's right antecubital; sublingual nitroglycerin spray × 1 without relief. MI-protocol labs drawn.
Relevant Past Health History	No known allergies. Hypertension taking lisinopril. Type 2 diabetic taking pioglitazone. High lipids. Strep throat several times in past year, treated 1 time with antibiotics. No regular exercise; 43 pack/year smoking history. Strong family history of CAD before age 50 and other risk factors, including smoking, hypertension, and elevated lipids.

Continued

CASE STUDY Thrombolytics—Cont'd

DIAGNOSIS: Acute myocardial infarction in patient with type 2 diabetes

MANAGEMENT

Treatment Objectives	1. Maintain airway. 2. Prevent myocardial damage. 3. Restore patency of occluded vessel. 4. Preserve myocardial function.
Treatment Plan	**Pharmacotherapy** • Continue O₂/NC • Continue lactated Ringer's • Continuous 12-lead monitoring • Accelerated protocol alteplase (t-PA): 100 mg IV bolus, followed by 50 mg over next 30 min, then 35 mg over the next hr **Patient Education** 1. Teach patient about timely use of thrombolytic: benefits and risks. 2. Advise of possibility of bruising and of seepage from IV sites. 3. Treatment with ASA (81–160 mg/day), a beta blocker, ACE inhibitor, and a statin will be needed upon discharge. **Evaluation** 1. Vital signs have returned to normal limits. 2. Patency of occluded vessel has been restored, and ST-segment elevation in V₁-V₅ have returned to normal. 3. Myocardial function has been preserved in the short term.

CLINICAL REASONING ANALYSIS

Q1. Our community hospital is 90 minutes away from St. James. Is it a good idea to treat JH in our community hospital rather than sending him to St. James (Regional Medical Center)?

A. Yes. The decision had to be made within the first hour after symptoms developed for the best outcomes. Because transfer for PCI (percutaneous coronary interventions) would impose a further treatment delay, considerably exceeding 60 minutes, thrombolysis was the best option. Reperfusion in STEMI limits myocardial damage and reduces mortality by about 30%, or maybe more in his case since the ischemic time has been relatively short. St. James was too far away.

Q2. Before you administered the t-PA you said JH had no contraindications to receiving the drug. What are those contraindications? Things around here were moving too fast before for me to ask.

A. Here is a pocket card with the contraindications to thrombolytic therapy listed (see Box 40-2). Note that there are absolute and relative contraindications. You can also check your textbook.

Q3. How long will JH be monitored for bleeding from the thrombolytic?

A. Typically they will watch him closely for the next 24 to 36 hours. However, t-PA is fibrin-specific; therefore once it is injected, bound to fibrin, and converted to plasmin, there is less effect on the circulating plasminogen and less risk of bleeding.

Q4. You said he would also be on a heparin drip? Why is that?

A. Heparin is given along with the t-PA in order to sustain the fibrinolytic effects.

Q5. Will he be taking any other drugs?

A. Yes. Aspirin alone reduces mortality by 20% to 25%, and chewing the tablets ensures a rapid effect. Adequate pain management with morphine relieves discomfort and its deleterious effect on myocardial demand. Finally, an IV beta blocker will be given—in the absence of contraindications, of course—with an aim for an optimal heart rate of 50 to 60 beats/min and a systolic blood pressure of not less than 90–100 mm Hg. Our standard protocol is three 5-mg boluses of IV metoprolol every 5–10 minutes.

Q6. What if the patient's symptoms or ST-segment elevation do not resolve?

A. Had reperfusion not been successful and there was continuing evidence of myocardial ischemia, prompt transfer to St. James for consideration of rescue PCI would have been a reasonable option. Angioplasty would be considered if the ST-segment elevation did not decrease by at least 50%, or if there was no resolution of the pain.

KEY POINTS

- Thrombolytic drugs are used in the treatment of AMI, DVT, PE, peripheral arterial occlusion, ischemic CVAs, and occluded central venous catheters.
- Thrombolytic drugs have subtle differences in their mechanism of action for dissolving thrombi after formation.
- Assessment of the patient should include special attention to a history of streptococcal infection within the previous year.
- Treatment objectives include opening the occluded artery as soon as possible, maintaining patency after flow is reestablished, and preventing complications related to bleeding.
- First-generation thrombolytic drugs include streptokinase and urokinase. Second-generation drugs include t-PA and APSAC. Reteplase and tenecteplase are the newest thrombolytic drugs.
- Close attention should be paid to relative and absolute contraindications of thrombolytic drugs, as well as to how much time has passed since symptom onset.
- Patient monitoring during thrombolytic therapy should include CBC, thrombin time, partial thromboplastin time, and prothrombin time values, and other laboratory testing specifically required for the disorder being treated.
- In general, thrombolytic therapy is deemed successful if the patency of the vessel is restored, circulation to the area beyond the occlusion is restored, the viability of tissues is maintained, and morbidity and mortality has been decreased.
- Sclerosing drugs are used in the management of varicose veins or esophageal varices to occlude tortuous, weakened veins.
- Sclerosing drugs act to thrombose and obliterate distended veins by traumatizing the endothelial lining of the vessels.
- Treatment objectives for varicose veins are directed toward improvement of circulation, relief of discomfort and swelling, and avoidance of complications of sclerotherapy.
- Treatment objectives for esophageal varices are to control bleeding and prevent hemorrhage.
- Sclerosing drugs for varicose veins are administered directly into the affected vein.

Bibliography

Antman, E., Anbe, D., Armstrong, P., et al. (2004). ACC/AHA Guidelines for the management of patients with ST-elevation myocardial infarction: A report of the American College of Cardiology/American Heart Association Task Force on Practice Guidelines (Committee to revise the 1999 Guidelines for the Management of Patients With Acute Myocardial Infarction). Available online:www.acc.org/clinical/guidelines/stemi/index.pdf. Accessed May 16, 2007.

Arcasoy, S., and Kreit, J. (1999). Thrombolytic therapy of pulmonary embolism: A comprehensive review of current evidence. *Chest, 115* (6), 1695–1707.

ASSENT-2 Investigators. (1999). Single-bolus tenecteplase compared with front-loaded alteplase in acute myocardial infarction: The ASSENT-2 double-blind randomized trial. *Lancet, 354*(9180), 716–722.

Boersma, E., Maas, A., Deckers, J., et al. (1996). Early thrombolytic treatment in acute myocardial infarction: Reappraisal of the golden hour. *Lancet, 348*(9030), 771–775.

Bogaty, P., Buller, C., Dorian, P, et al. (2004). Applying the new STEMI guidelines: 1. Reperfusion in acute ST-segment elevation myocardial infarction. *Canadian Medical Association Journal, 171*(9), 1039–1041.

Braunwald, E., Zipes, D., Libby, P., et al. (2005). *Heart disease: A textbook of cardiovascular medicine* (7th ed.). Philadelphia: WB Saunders.

Dalen, J. (2002). Pulmonary embolism: What we have learned since Virchow? Treatment and prevention. *Chest, 122*(5), 1801–1817.

Dorian, P., Bogaty, P., Buller, C., et al. (2004). Applying the new STEMI guidelines: 2. Disturbances of cardiac rhythm after ST-segment elevation myocardial infarction. *Canadian Medical Association Journal, 171*(9), 1042–1044.

du Breuil, A., and Umland, E. (2007). Outpatient management of anticoagulation therapy. *American Family Physician, 75*(7), 1031–1042.

Dundar, Y., Hill, R., Dickson, R., et al. (2003). Comparative efficacy of thrombolytics in acute myocardial infarction: A systematic review. *QJM, 96*(2), 103–113.

Hambleton, J. (2004). Drugs used in disorders of coagulation. In Katzung, B. *Basic and clinical pharmacology.* (9th ed.). New York: McGraw-Hill.

McSweeney, J., Cody, M., O'Sullivan, P., et al. (2003). Women's early warning symptoms of acute myocardial infarction. *Circulation, 108*(21), 2619–2623.

Menen, V., Harrington, R., Hockman, J., et al. (2004). Thrombolysis and adjunctive therapy in acute myocardial infarction: The Seventh ACCP Conference on Antithrombotic and Thrombolytic Therapy. *Chest, 126*(Suppl 3), 549S–575S.

Monagle, P., Chan, A., Massicotte, P., et al. (2004). Antithrombotic therapy in children: The Seventh ACCP Conference on Antithrombotic and Thrombolytic Therapy. *Chest, 126*(Suppl 3), 645S–687S.

Rich, M. (2003). Thrombolytic therapy is indicated for patients over 75 years of age with ST-elevation acute myocardial infarction: Protagonist viewpoint. *American Journal of Geriatric Cardiology, 12*(6), 344–347.

Roy, P., Meyer, B., Vielle, C., et al. (2006). Appropriateness of diagnostic management and outcomes of suspected pulmonary embolism. *Annals of Internal Medicine, 144*(3), 157–164.

Suzuki, Y., Kano, T., Katayama, Y., et al. (2003). Reduction of infarction volume by bolus injection of pamiteplase, a modified tissue plasminogen activator with a longer half-life. *Neurological Research, 25*(5), 477–480.

Vale, L., Steffens, H., and Donaldson, C. (2004). The costs and benefits of community thrombolysis for acute myocardial infarction: A decision-analytic model. *Pharmacoeconomics, 22*(14), 943–954.

Wood, K. (2002). Major pulmonary embolism: Review of a pathophysiologic approach to the golden hour of hemodynamically significant pulmonary embolism. *Chest, 121*(3), 877–905.

41

Urinary Antimicrobials and Related Drugs

Urinary tract infection (UTI, cystitis) is a common health problem among all age groups. UTIs account for over 9.1 million annual visits to health care providers. It is a common malady in women of child-bearing age. In the past, terms such as acute, chronic, and recurrent have been commonly used to describe the spectrum of UTIs. These words have been replaced by terminology considered more descriptive of the clinical presentation of a UTI (Box 41–1).

A variety of antimicrobial drugs are available for the treatment of UTI. The focus of this chapter is the treatment of UTI with quinolones, sulfonamides, or urinary-tract antiseptic drugs. Drugs in these groups target the urinary system and have proven to be efficacious against bacteria that typically cause UTIs. They are also among the most widely prescribed drugs for UTIs. Beta-lactam antibiotics, including penicillin and cephalosporin drugs, and tetracyclines are also used for treatment of UTI although less often. Information about the beta-lactams is found in Chapter 27.

URINARY TRACT INFECTIONS

EPIDEMIOLOGY AND ETIOLOGY

UTIs encompass a variety of conditions including cystitis, pyelonephritis, urethritis, and catheter-related bacteriuria. The incidence of UTIs depends on the patient's age and sex. UTIs are 30 times more common in women up to the age of 50 because of the relative shortness of the female urethra. By the age of 24, one third of all women will have had at least one UTI. Approximately 10% to 20% of women experience a symptomatic UTI during their lifetime. The highest prevalence of UTIs is among women of lower socioeconomic groups who have a high parity, a history of UTI, and sickle cell disease or sickle cell trait.

The occurrence of UTI in nonpregnant women correlates with the commencement of sexual activity. The use of a diaphragm or spermicidal gel for birth control tends to increase susceptibility to bacteriuria. Many women with a symptomatic UTI report having had intercourse 24 to 48 hours before the onset of symptoms. In fact, the relative odds of acute UTI occurring during the 48 hours after sexual intercourse increase by a factor of 60. UTIs become a problem in men after the age of 50 because of prostate enlargement and urinary stasis. Although UTI is far less prevalent in men, it is almost always a more serious condition than in women.

There are drugs associated with varying degrees of urinary retention and observation (Fig. 41-1). Other factors commonly linked to the development of UTIs, but not scientifically substantiated, include inadequate fluid intake, the use of occlusive undergarments or tight-fitting pants, frequent tub baths, the use of bubble bath or tampons, and wiping from the back to front after urination or defecation. Because users of oral contraceptives also have an increased risk of UTI, the higher prevalence rates may reflect estrogen-mediated dilation of the urethra. Another risk factor for the development of UTI is the voluntary retention of urine for an hour or longer beyond one's usual strong urge to urinate. This practice contributes to a pattern of infrequent bladder emptying, repeated bladder overdistention, and urinary stasis.

The significance of bacteriuria in older adults is in question. The prevalence of UTI increases with age, with bacteriuria present in approximately 6% to 8% of women over the age of 60 and 20% of women over 80 years. There is also an increased prevalence of bacteriuria in 1% to 3% of men between 60 and 65 years of age. The rate of infection increases to over 10% for men over 80 years of age. Institutionalization dramatically increases the prevalence of bacteriuria among both sexes because of functional deficits and coexisting illnesses such as cerebrovascular accidents, Alzheimer's disease, and Parkinson's disease.

Fifty percent of the severely impaired institutionalized elderly have bacteriuria. The rate rises to nearly 100% with long-term indwelling catheterization. The presence of pyuria has been used traditionally to differentiate infection from colonization in the older adult, but this is not helpful since virtually all patients who have bacteriuria also have pyuria.

Factors contributing to bacteriuria in noninstitutionalized older women include the decreased influence of estrogen on the urinary tract mucosa, ineffective bladder emptying with increased residual urine, and the presence of cystocele, rectocele, and bladder diverticula. The primary factors contributing to bacteriuria in noninstitutionalized older men include lower urinary tract obstructions such as urethral strictures and benign prostatic hyperplasia. These disorders result in increased residual urine and persistent bacterial prostatitis. Risk factors common to older adults of both sexes include prior bladder catheterization, previous antibiotic use, alterations in cognition, and diseases that compromise the immune system such as cancer or diabetes. In fact, diabetes itself appears to predispose patients to UTI. Women with type 2 diabetes are not at any higher a risk of developing asymptomatic bacteruria than nondiabetic women. Independent and significant risk factors for infection are macroalbuminuria and elevated serum creatinine levels. Finally, there are conditions that predispose persons of all ages to UTIs. Included in this category are urinary tract instrumentation or surgery, the presence of urinary calculi, neurogenic voiding dysfunction, preexisting chronic renal disease, immunosuppression, and malnutrition. Because risk factors are shared by many and bacteriuria frequently resolves spontaneously as well as with therapy, the cumulative prevalence of bacteriuria is actually higher.

BOX **41-1**

Commonly Confused Terms

- **Acute urinary tract infection:** Symptomatic infection caused by a single pathogen. For most persons the occurrence will be their first documented urinary tract infection.
- **Unresolved bacteriuria:** The presence of bacteria in the urine after initial treatment for urinary tract infection is completed
- **Bacterial persistence:** Recurrence of infection by the same organism several days after antimicrobial therapy has been discontinued and urine culture shows sterile urine
- **Reinfection:** Recurrence of infection by a different pathogen after a previous infection has been eradicated. It is estimated that 80% to 95% of all recurrent infections are reinfections.
- **Uncomplicated urinary tract infection:** An afebrile infection, usually of the lower urinary tract, in a young, sexually active, nonpregnant, immunocompetent woman with no known structural abnormalities or urinary dysfunction
- **Complicated urinary tract infection:** Infection occurring in patients who have structural or functional abnormalities of the urinary tract, or who have coexisting illness.

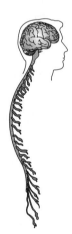

- baclofen
- carbamazepine
- clonazepam
- Opioids and opioid-like drugs
- phenytoin

- Anticholinergics
- Antihistamines
- Antiparkinson drugs
- Beta adrenergic drugs
- Calcium channel blocking drugs
- Diuretics
- Ganglionic blocking drugs
- Muscle relaxants
- Prostaglandin inhibitors
- Phenothiazines
- Tricyclic antidepressants

- Alpha adrenergic agonists
- Amphetamines
- Beta adrenergic blocking drugs
- Estrogen combinations
- levodopa
- Tricyclic antidepressants

FIGURE 41-1 Drugs Associated with Varying Degrees of Urinary Retention and Obstruction.

PATHOPHYSIOLOGY

Cystitis

UTIs are classified as lower urinary tract infections (i.e., cystitis) and upper urinary tract infection (i.e., pyelonephritis). UTI is predominantly a localized infection, whereas pyelonephritis produces systemic symptoms as well as the dysuria, frequency, and urgency commonly associated with lower UTI.

Although the lower urinary tract is constantly exposed to pathogenic bacteria, a symptomatic infection necessitating treatment may not always result. Several host defense mechanisms work to protect the bladder from bacterial invasion. Regular, spontaneous voiding with complete bladder emptying promptly clears invading bacteria and is the urinary tract's principal line of defense against infection. Another important defense are the natural antibacterial properties of urine. Extremes in urinary pH, high urine osmolality, and high concentrations of urea nitrogen and ammonium inhibit bacterial growth. The presence of specific antibodies (immunoglobulins A and G [IgA, IgG]) and antibacterial enzymes (lysozyme and lactoferrin) in the urine are also thought to deter bacterial growth.

An intact bladder wall readily resists bacterial invasion. However, when the mucosa is altered from its normal state by infrequent voiding, repeated overdistention, obstruction, pregnancy, or ischemia, it is more susceptible to bacterial adherence and infection.

Current evidence suggests that most episodes of UTI in adult women are secondary to ascending infection (Fig. 41-2). Bacteria reach the bladder primarily by traveling upward from the urethra. Infection of the lower urinary tract in females is typically caused by bacteria that first colonize the vagina. With sexual activity, bacteria are forced through the characteristically short female urethra to reach the bladder. In males, bacteria colonize the urethra and can infect not only the bladder but also the epididymis and the prostate.

Under normal circumstances, organisms do not navigate the length of the male urethra, and the organisms that do settle in the male urinary tract tend to be different from those that plague women. In men, an antibacterial substance produced by the prostate acts as a natural defense, thus prohibiting the further migration of pathogenic organisms into the bladder. Men with a history of bacterial prostatitis appear to be more susceptible to UTI because zinc, a key component of prostatic secretions, is either present in significantly reduced amounts or absent. Men who have a UTI are always assumed to have a complicated infection.

Bacteria must adhere to mucosal cells to colonize and infect the lower urinary tract. Bacterial cells typically possess long, filament-like appendages called pili or fimbriae that bind the bacteria to the mucosal cell. Bacterial adherence also requires the availability of receptors in host cells. Adherence further depends on host susceptibility, as well as the strains, the numbers, and the virulence of the organism. On occasion, the number of organisms alone sometimes overwhelms intrinsic defense mechanisms of the urinary tract and produce infection. Microorganisms that commonly cause lower urinary tract infection are frequently normal inhabitants of the intestinal tract. *Escherichia coli* cause 80% to 90% of uncomplicated UTIs. Other urinary tract pathogens are listed in Table 41-1.

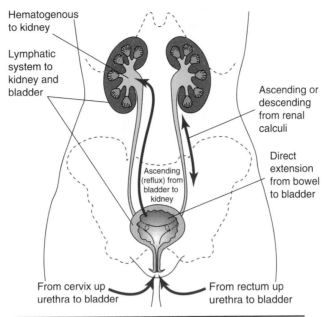

FIGURE 41-2 Route for Bacteria Entering the Female Urinary Tract.

Pathologic changes in the bladder in the early stages of an acute infection include edema, hyperemia, and neutrophil infiltrates. Eventually the surface of the bladder takes on a granular texture, and the tissue becomes friable. Hemorrhagic and visible ulcerations containing exudate appear. With bacterial persistence, the submucosal layer of the bladder becomes involved, causing the bladder wall to become thick, fibrotic, and inelastic.

A urine culture is considered diagnostic when there are greater than 100,000 (10^5) colony-forming units (CFU) of a single pathogen per milliliter of urine. Contaminated urine cultures usually contain fewer than 10,000 (10^4) CFU/mL. However, a count of 100 to 10,000 CFU/mL may be clinically significant, especially if a single known organism has been isolated and the patient is symptomatic, because frequent voiding slows the doubling or incubation time for bacteria in the urine.

Pyelonephritis

It is estimated that pyelonephritis accounts for more than 250,000 office visits to health care providers and nearly 200,000 hospital admissions annually in the United States. Pyelonephritis typically results from bacteria ascending up the ureters to the kidneys. On rare occasions, bacteria spread to the kidney through the blood stream from a distant focus of infection such as infections of the teeth, gums, ears, or throat. More unusual, although possible, is the lymphatic spread of bacteria from the large intestines to the kidney.

TABLE 41-1 UTI Antimicrobials and Susceptible Organisms

Drug Class	Susceptible Organisms
FLUOROQUINOLONES	
ciprofloxacin	Most strains of gram-positive and gram-negative micro-organisms including *E. coli,* as well as most anaerobic bacteria.
gatifloxacin levofloxacin	Most strains of gram-positive and gram-negative microorganisms including *E. coli*
lomefloxacin	*S. saprophyticus* (gram-positive) and several gram-negative including *E. coli*
norfloxacin ofloxacin	Most strains of gram-positive and gram-negative microorganisms including *E. coli.* Inactive against *T. palladium* and obligate anaerobes.
SULFONAMIDES	
sulfamethoxazole-trimethoprim	Most strains of gram-positive and gram-negative microorganisms including *E. coli.*
sulfisoxazole	*E. coli, Klebsiella, Enterobacter, Staphylococcus aureus, Proteus mirabilis, Proteus vulgaris, Staphylococcus saprophyticus*
URINARY TRACT ANTISEPTICS	
methenamine	*E. coli, Klebsiella, Serratia, Citrobacter*
nalidixic acid	*E. coli, Proteus, Enterobacter* *Pseudomonas* species are generally resistant
nitrofurantoin	*E. coli, S. aureus,* Enterococci Some strains of *Enterobacter* and *Klebsiella* are resistant; most strains of *Proteus* species are resistant. Not effective against *Pseudomonas.*
sulfamethoxazole/trimethoprim	Most strains of aerobic gram-positive and gram-negative organisms but not against anaerobic bacteria or *Pseudomonas aeruginosa*

Pyelonephritis is often secondary to an established infection in the bladder. The migration of bacteria to the kidney is facilitated by vesicoureteral reflux, ineffective ureteral peristalsis, susceptibility of the renal medulla to infection, and bacterial virulence. *E. coli, Klebsiella, Proteus, Enterobacter, Pseudomonas, Serratia,* and *Citrobacter* are pathogens commonly cultured from the urine in patients with pyelonephritis. On occasion, *Enterococcus faecalis* and *Staphylococcus aureus* are the infection-causing organisms.

Pathologic changes with acute pyelonephritis include a grossly enlarged kidney with yellow-colored abscesses throughout the renal parenchyma. Mucosal surfaces of the renal pelvis and calices are congested, thickened, and covered by exudate. With bacterial persistence, the kidney becomes scarred and pitted. Fibrosis and thinning are evident in portions of the parenchyma. In some instances, glomeruli become fibrotic and the tubules atrophied.

PHARMACOTHERAPEUTIC OPTIONS

Sulfonamides

◆ sulfamethoxazole-trimethoprim (Bactrim, Cotrim, Septra, Sulfatrim);
  ✦ Apo-Sulfatrim, Novotrimel
◆ sulfisoxazole (Gantrisin); ✦ Sterine, Pediazole, Renazoner

⁞⁞⁞ Indications

The combination of sulfamethoxazole and trimethoprim is recommended for the initial treatment of uncomplicated, acute UTIs caused by *E. coli, Morganella morganii, Proteus mirabilis, Proteus vulgaris, Klebsiella,* and *Enterobacter.* The combination drug is also used for extended periods in the treatment of persistent bacteriuria and recurrent infections. Sulfonamides used for other purposes are discussed in Chapter 27.

⁞⁞⁞ Pharmacodynamics

Sulfonamides are broad-spectrum and bacteriostatic; that is, they restrict reproduction of the pathogens without killing them. They act by competitively inhibiting para-aminobenzoic acid (PABA), a necessary element in bacterial folate synthesis. By blocking the synthesis of dihydrofolic acid, there is a decrease in tetrahydrofolic acid, which interferes with the

synthesis of purines, thymidine, and DNA in the bacteria. Therefore, the bacteria most sensitive to sulfonamides are those that synthesize their own folic acid (i.e., *E. coli, Rickettsia rickettsii*). *Pseudomonas aeruginosa* is not sensitive to sulfonamides.

The combination of sulfamethoxazole-trimethoprim acts synergistically to reduce the emergence of bacterial resistance more than when either drug is used separately, which is why it is more commonly prescribed. Trimethoprim's mechanism of action is similar to that of the sulfonamides.

The solubility and efficacy of sulfamethoxazole and sulfisoxazole is enhanced in alkaline urine. The presence of serum, purulent exudate, and necrotic tissue interferes with the activities of sulfonamides because PABA is present in such materials.

⁞⁞⁞ Pharmacokinetics

Most orally administered sulfonamides are rapidly absorbed from the GI tract and are distributed throughout all body tissues. Bioavailability ranges from 82% to 100% (Table 41-2). Biotransformation occurs in the liver primarily through acetylation, with elimination through the kidneys.

Most sulfonamides are reabsorbed to some extent by the kidney. Small quantities of sulfonamides are also eliminated in other bodily secretions such as stool, bile, and breast milk. Some of the sulfonamides and especially their acetyl derivatives are relatively insoluble in neutral or acid media. Thus, as the kidney concentrates urine (which becomes more acidic), there is a danger that the sulfonamide will precipitate, causing crystalluria, hematuria, renal stones, and even renal failure.

Trimethoprim is rapidly absorbed when taken orally, reaching peak urine concentrations within the first 4 hours after a single dose. Less than 20% of the drug is biotransformed; 80% is eliminated unchanged in the urine; and 4% is eliminated in the stool. When trimethoprim is combined with sulfamethoxazole, there is a synergistic effect; yet combining these two drugs does not affect the biotransformation or excretion patterns of either.

⁞⁞⁞ Adverse Effects and Contraindications

Adverse effects occur infrequently with sulfonamides but include headaches, nausea, vomiting, abdominal pain, crystalluria, hematuria, drug fever, and chills. One of the most serious

PHARMACOKINETICS

TABLE 41-2 Selected Urinary Antimicrobials

Drug	Route	Onset	Peak	Duration	PB (%)	t½	BioA (%)
SULFONAMIDES							
sulfamethoxazole-trimethoprim	PO	Rapid	1–4 hr	To 24 hr	44–70	8–10 hr	100
sulfisoxazole	PO	Rapid	1–4 hr	To 48 hr	85	4.6–7.8 hr	82–100
QUINOLONES							
ciprofloxacin	PO	Rapid	1–2 hr	To 24 hr	20–40	3–4 hr	70
gatifloxacin	PO	Rapid	1–2 hr	To 24 hr	20	7–14 hr	96
levofloxacin	PO	Rapid	1–2 hr	To 48 hr	24–38	6–8 hr	99
lomefloxacin	PO	Rapid	1–1.5 hr	To 48 hr	10	8 hr	95–98
norfloxacin	PO	Rapid	1 hr	To 48 hr	10–15	3–4 hr	30–40
ofloxacin	PO	Rapid	1–2 hr	To 36 hr	32	4–5 hr	98
URINARY ANTISEPTICS							
methenamine	PO	<30 min	2 hr	To 8 hr	NA	3–6 hr	UA
nitrofurantoin	PO	Rapid	30 min	6–12 hr	60	20–60 min	<40

BioA, Bioavailability; *NA,* not applicable; *PB,* protein binding; *PO,* by mouth; *t½,* half-life; *UA,* unavailable.

adverse effects of sulfonamides is hypersensitivity, including generalized skin eruptions, urticaria, pruritus, photosensitivity, periorbital edema, and erythema multiforme.

Stevens-Johnson syndrome is a severe and sometimes fatal form of erythema multiforme. The syndrome is a skin- and mucous-membrane reaction in which macular, bullous, papular, or vesicular lesions develop in the oral and anogenital mucosa, the eyes, and the viscera. The characteristic lesion is the iris, or bull's eye, or target lesion. It consists of a central papule with two or more concentric rings.

Constitutional symptoms such as malaise, headache, fever, arthralgia, and conjunctivitis are also seen with this syndrome. Blood dyscrasias and hematologic effects are other serious adverse reactions and include leukopenia, neutropenia, and thrombocytopenia. However, these adverse effects are reversible upon discontinuation of the drug. Additionally, patients should avoid dehydration while taking sulfonamide antibiotics to avoid crystalluria. Determine if the patient has a history of blood dyscrasias, glucose-6-phosphate dehydrogenase (G6PD) deficiency, or porphyria, since these disorders contraindicate the use of sulfonamides.

Do not use sulfonamides in infants under 2 months old or in pregnant or lactating women (category C). They are also contraindicated for use in patients with a hypersensitivity to sulfa or other chemically related drugs.

The most frequent adverse effects of trimethoprim include rashes, pruritus, and exfoliative dermatitis. Other potential adverse effects include epigastric distress, nausea, vomiting, and thrombocytopenia. Trimethoprim is contraindicated for use in patients with hypersensitivity to the drug and in patients with folate deficiency–induced megaloblastic anemia. It is not recommended for use during pregnancy (category C) and should be used with caution in lactating mothers, since trimethoprim interferes with folic acid biotransformation.

Drug Interactions

Table 41-3 lists drug interactions for the sulfonamides commonly used for UTIs. Sulfonamides increase the risk of toxicity from oral anticoagulants, oral hypoglycemic drugs, phenytoin, methotrexate, and leucovorin. When sulfonamides are used concurrently with methenamine, there is an increased risk of crystalluria. Concurrent use of sulfonamides with methotrexate contributes to increased bone marrow depression. **Because sulfonamides enhance the action of warfarin, close monitoring of prothrombin time (PT) and international normalized ratio (INR) values is warranted.**

Dosage Regimen

A 3-day regimen is recommended for the treatment of uncomplicated UTIs. Treatment may be extended from 3 to 7 or 10 days in patients with bacterial persistence or reinfection. A loading dose is needed to establish therapeutic levels of sulfamethoxazole in the urine (Table 41-4). There are dosing considerations for patients with renal or hepatic insufficiency or failure.

DRUG INTERACTIONS
TABLE 41-3 Selected Urinary Antimicrobials

Drugs	Interactive Drugs	Interaction
SULFONAMIDES		
sulfamethoxazole-trimethoprim	leucovorin	Increases rate of treatment failure and morbidity in patients with HIV who have *Pneumocystis jirovecii* pneumonia (previously *Pneumocystis carinii* pneumonia [PCP])
	warfarin	May prolong prothrombin time
	phenytoin	Inhibits biotransformation of phenytoin
sulfisoxazole	methotrexate	Increases risk of hematologic toxicity
	warfarin	May prolong prothrombin time
QUINOLONES		
ciprofloxacin	Aluminum antacids	Reduces bioA of ciprofloxacin by 90%
	theophylline	Elevates serum theophylline levels, increasing risk of adverse reactions such as seizures.
	Caffeine	Decreases clearance of caffeine
gatifloxacin	Aluminum antacids	Reduces bioA of gatifloxacin by 69%. Separate by at least 2 hr for minimal interaction.
	Iron supplements	Reduces bioA of gatifloxacin by 35%–54%
	probenecid	Increases AUC of gatifloxacin by 42%, extends $t_{1/2}$ by 44%
levofloxacin	Aluminum antacids	Reduces bioA of levofloxacin
lomefloxacin	Aluminum antacids	Reduces bioA of lomefloxacin by 48%. Separate the 2 by at least 2 hr for minimal interaction.
	probenecid	Increases AUC of lomefloxacin by 50%–63%
norfloxacin	theophylline	Elevates serum theophylline levels, increasing risk of seizures
	probenecid	Increases AUC of norfloxacin
	Caffeine	Decreases clearance of caffeine
	Aluminum antacids	Reduces bioA of norfloxacin
ofloxacin	Aluminum antacids	Reduces bioA of ofloxacin. Separate by at least 2 hr for minimal interaction.
	theophylline	Elevates serum theophylline levels, increasing risk of adverse reactions such as seizures
URINARY TRACT ANTISEPTICS		
methenamine hippurate	Sodium bicarbonate, Diuretics	Reduces efficacy of methenamine
methenamine mandelate	Sodium bicarbonate	Reduces efficacy of methenamine
nitrofurantoin	Hemolytics	Increases potential for toxic adverse effects
	probenecid	Increases serum levels of nitrofurantoin in presence of high doses of interactive drug
	Neurotoxic drugs	Increases potential for neurotoxicity

AUC, Area under the curve; *BioA,* bioavailability; *HIV,* human immunodeficiency virus; $t_{1/2}$, half-life.

DOSAGE
TABLE **41-4 Selected Urinary Antimicrobials**

Drug	Use(s)	Dosage*	Implications
SULFONAMIDES			
sulfamethoxazole-trimethoprim	Acute, persistent, or reinfection UTI, UTI prophylaxis	*Adult:* *Acute:* 1 DS tablet PO every 12 hr for 3 days *Persistent or Reinfection:* 1 DS tablet PO every 12 hours for 7–10 days *Prophylaxis:* 1 DS tablet PO per day *Child;* *Acute:* trimethoprim 6–12 mg/kg and 30–60 mg/kg sulfamethoxazole PO in divided doses every 12 hr up to 10 days *Prophylaxis:* trimethoprim 1–2 mg/kg/day and 5–10 mg/kg/day sulfamethoxazole PO every evening	SS tablets: 80 mg trimethoprim and 400 mg sulfamethoxazole. DS tablets: 800 mg sulfamethoxazole and 160 mg trimethoprim. IV formulations are available.
sulfisoxazole		*Adult:* 2–4 grams PO initially then 4–8 grams/day PO in 4–6 divided doses for 3–7 days *Child >2 mo:* 75 mg/kg PO, then 25 mg PO every 4 hr *–or–* 37.5 mg/kg or 120–150 mg/kg/day in divided doses every 4–6 hr every 6 hr	Child maintenance dose should not exceed 6 grams/day.
QUINOLONES			
ciprofloxacin	Uncomplicated and complicated UTI in adults	*Uncomplicated:* 250 mg PO every 12 hr for 3 days *Complicated:* 400–500 PO or IV every 12 hr for 7–10 days	Most effective when caused by gram-negative bacilli resistant to other drugs. Continue at least 2 days after signs and symptoms of infection have disappeared.
gatifloxacin		*Uncomplicated:* 200 mg PO or IV daily for 3 days *Complicated:* 400 mg PO or IV daily for 7–10 days	Gatifloxacin may disturb blood glucose. Monitor patients with diabetes for elevated glucose levels. Continue antibiotic for 2 days after signs and symptoms have disappeared.
levofloxacin		*Uncomplicated:* 250 mg PO or IV daily for 3 days *Complicated:* 250 mg PO or IV daily for 10 days	
lomefloxacin		*Uncomplicated* Escherichia coli *in females:* 400 mg PO daily for 3 days *Uncomplicated (Klebsiella pneumoniae, Proteus mirabilis, or Staphylococcus saprophyticus):* 400 mg PO daily for 10 days *Complicated:* 400 mg PO daily for 14 days	Doses should be taken at least 1 hr before or 2 hr after a meal or ingestion of milk.
norfloxacin		*Uncomplicated (E. coli, K. pneumoniae, P. mirabilis):* 400 mg PO every 12 hr for 3 days *Uncomplicated (for other organisms):* 400 mg PO every 12 hr for 7–10 days *Complicated:* 400 mg PO every 12 hr for 10–21 days	
ofloxacin		*Uncomplicated (E. coli or K. pneumoniae):* 200 mg PO every 12 hr for 3 days *Uncomplicated (other organisms):* 200 mg PO every 12 hr for 7 days *Complicated:* 200 mg PO every 12 hr for 10 days	
URINARY ANTISEPTICS			
methenamine	Long-term suppression or elimination of bacteriuria	*Adult and Child >12 yr:* 1 gram PO twice daily for hippurate form; 1 gram 4 times daily for mandelate formulation *Child 6–12 yr:* 0.5–1 gram PO twice daily for hippurate form; 0.5 grams 4 times daily for mandelate formulation	**Effective only in acid urine with pH range of 5–5.5.** Patient adherence needed to maintain acid urine.
nitrofurantoin	Uncomplicated acute UTI, persistent bacteriuria, reinfection, and bacteriuria in pregnancy	*Adult and Child >12 years:* 50–100 mg PO 4 times daily for 7 days of Macrodantin formulation	Not suitable for children <12. Not available in extended-release

*Be sure to specifically check dosage adjustments for patients with renal insufficiency or failure.
DS, Double-strength; *IV,* intravenous (route); *PO,* by mouth; *SS,* single-strength; *UTI,* urinary tract infection.

▮▮▮ *Lab Considerations*

Sulfonamides can cause false-positive urine glucose results when Benedict's solution is used. Sulfisoxazole, in particular, may interfere with urine dipstick test results and produce false-positive results using sulfosalicylic acid tests for proteinuria. Trimethoprim interferes with serum methotrexate assays if procedures other than radioimmunoassay are used.

Quinolones

- ciprofloxacin (Cipro); ✦ Cipro
- gatifloxacin (Tequin, Zymar); ✦ Tequin
- gemifloxacin (Factive)
- levofloxacin (Levaquin, Quixin); ✦ Levaquin
- lomefloxacin (Maxaquin)
- moxifloxacin (Avelox); ✦ Avelox

◆ norfloxacin (Noroxin, Chibroxin); ◆ Noroxin
◆ ofloxacin (Floxin) ◆ ofloxacin

Indications

Quinolones are used for adults who have complicated UTIs. Bacteria sensitive to quinolones include most Enterobacteriaceae, gram-positive organisms (e.g., staphylococci), some enterococci, and most strains of *P. aeruginosa*. Quinolone antibiotics are also discussed in Chapter 27.

There are fears about inappropriate use of quinolones and the development of resistant bacterial pathogens (e.g., *S. aureus*, *P. aeruginosa*, and *Serratia marcescens*). Therefore, restrict the use of oral quinolones to patients with complicated UTIs that are bacterial-resistant, patients who are unable to take or tolerate other oral agents, those with a UTI that was not previously cleared using other antibiotics, and for patients in whom use of intravenous (IV) antibiotics may be the only alternative.

Pharmacodynamics

Quinolones are broad-spectrum, bacteriocidal drugs that kill bacteria. Quinolones inhibit DNA gyrase, which in turn interferes with DNA replication, repair, and transcription. In high concentrations, they produce a dose-dependent inhibition of RNA synthesis. In addition, quinolones have postadministration activity against gram-positive and gram-negative bacteria; as a result, bacterial growth does not resume for several hours. This postadministration inhibition of bacterial growth means that orally administered quinolones can be given in shorter dosage regimens.

Pharmacokinetics

Quinolones differ in their absorption (e.g., ofloxacin is highly absorbed; norfloxacin is the least absorbed) from the GI tract (see Table 41-2). High concentrations of ciprofloxacin and ofloxacin are found in urine and most tissues (i.e., kidneys, prostate).

Norfloxacin concentrates well in urine and the GI tract even though it does not achieve high serum concentrations. Protein binding does not significantly vary and ranges from 10% to 15% for norfloxacin to 40% for ciprofloxacin.

Ofloxacin is eliminated primarily by renal excretion. Ciprofloxacin is removed from the body via renal, biliary, and transintestinal routes; whereas norfloxacin undergoes biotransformation in the liver, with subsequent biliary and renal elimination.

Adverse Reactions and Contraindications

Overall, quinolones are fairly well tolerated; gastrointestinal (GI) adverse effects are most common. The typical complaints include dry mouth, nausea, vomiting, dyspepsia, diarrhea, abdominal pain, and flatulence. Central nervous system (CNS) adverse reactions occur in fewer than 7% of patients but include headache, dizziness, fatigue, insomnia, agitation, restlessness, and hallucinations, and seizures (with ciprofloxacin). Gatifloxacin may cause hyperglycemia or hypoglycemia. Skin disorders, occurring in fewer than 2% of patients, usually manifest as either a rash or pruritus.

Long-term use of quinolones is associated with cartilage erosion and joint disease in juveniles. Although quinolones are highly effective, data on the safety of quinolone use in children and adolescents with complex comorbid conditions or multidrug

resistance are limited. These drugs are not recommended for children or women who are pregnant (category C) or lactating.

Drug Interactions

Quinolones interact with a number of other drugs including theophylline, aluminum antacids, calcium, iron, anticoagulants, and caffeine. Toxicity to these drugs is possible because of increased serum concentrations. **Because quinolones enhance the action of warfarin, close monitoring of PT and INR values is warranted. Levofloxacin used concomitantly with warfarin may cause QT prolongation.** Table 41-3 lists drug interactions for the quinolones.

Dosage Regimen

Once-daily dosing is possible because of the long duration of action of most quinolones. The dosage varies with the specific quinolone and whether or not the UTI is complicated or uncomplicated, and acute or persistent (see Table 41-4). A 14-day treatment regimen is recommended for complicated UTIs.

Lab Considerations

Because quinolones increase the effect of anticoagulants, regular monitoring of PT and INR values is recommended. Taking quinolones concurrently with theophylline places patients at risk for theophylline toxicity; therefore check serum theophylline levels frequently. Gatifloxacin disturbs blood glucose levels in patients with diabetes.

Urinary Tract Antiseptics

◆ methenamine (Hiprex, Mandelamine, Mandameth, Urised, Urex); ◆ Hip-Rex
◆ nitrofurantoin (Furadantin, Macrobid, Macrodantin); ◆ Novo-Furan

Indications

Urinary tract antiseptics exert antibacterial action in the urine but have little or no systemic antibacterial action (see Table 41-1). Rather than for acute, symptomatic infections, methenamine is used for long-term prophylaxis and as suppressive therapy for patients at risk for reinfection. It is effective against *E. coli*, *Klebsiella*, *Enterobacter*, *P. mirabilis*, *M. morganii*, *Serratia* species, and *Citrobacter* species. Use methenamine once the original UTI has resolved, and prophylaxis or suppressive therapy is needed.

Uncomplicated, acute UTIs and symptomatic bacteriuria during pregnancy are safely treated with nitrofurantoin. It is effective also for the long-term treatment of persistent bacteriuria, or reinfection caused by *E. coli*, enterococci, some strains of *Klebsiella* and *Enterobacter*, and *S. aureus*. It is not effective against *Proteus, Pseudomonas, and Serratia*.

Pharmacodynamics

The pharmacodynamics of urinary tract antiseptics vary with the individual drug. The effectiveness of methenamine depends on the concentration of formaldehyde in the urine. Formaldehyde and ammonia are formed when methenamine decomposes in the urine. For methenamine to be effective, the urinary pH must be less than 5.5. To reach this level, methenamine is combined with acid salts (i.e., methenamine hippurate, methenamine mandelate). In contrast, nitrofurantoin is bacteriostatic and acts by inhibiting bacterial enzymes, and then interferes with the formation of a bacterial cell wall.

Pharmacokinetics

Methenamine is well absorbed following oral administration (see Table 41-2). It is biotransformed in the liver to ammonia and formaldehyde, with the formaldehyde appearing in the urine. Formaldehyde levels stabilize within 2 to 3 days after treatment is started.

Orally administered nitrofurantoin is absorbed in its entirety from the GI tract. The microcrystalline formulation of nitrofurantoin (i.e., Macrodantin) disintegrates more slowly, causing the absorption rate to also be slower. When taken with food, there is less GI upset and the bioavailability of nitrofurantoin is improved. Twenty percent to 25% of the drug is excreted unchanged in the urine (Table 41-5). The efficacy of nitrofurantoin is reduced in alkaline urine.

Adverse Reactions and Contraindications

Adverse effects reported with methenamine include nausea, vomiting, cramps, and anorexia. Genitourinary symptoms such as dysuria, frequency and/or urgency, hematuria, and proteinuria also may be noted. When taken in large doses, urinary flow rates are reduced, and crystalluria is possible. Methenamine is contraindicated for use in patients with renal insufficiency, severe dehydration, or severe hepatic insufficiency. Although empiric evidence suggests that methenamine may be safely administered to women during the last trimester of pregnancy (category C), use caution when giving the drug to pregnant women.

Anorexia, nausea, and vomiting are the predominant adverse reactions associated with nitrofurantoin. Toxicity is associated with prolonged use of the drug. Although rare, the adverse effects of nitrofurantoin include pulmonary fibrosis, acute and chronic hepatotoxicity, and peripheral neuropathy. Because of the severity and irreversible nature of these conditions, continuously and carefully monitor patients taking nitrofurantoin.

Use caution when prescribing nitrofurantoin for patients with peripheral neuropathy because it may worsen the condition. In patients with pulmonary disease, the drug may cause pulmonary reactions, including pneumonitis. Nitrofurantoin is contraindicated for use in patients with anemia, vitamin B

deficiency, diabetes, kidney disease, electrolyte imbalance, or debilitating disease.

Although nitrofurantoin is generally regarded as safe for use during pregnancy (category B), it is contraindicated for use in pregnant women at term and during labor and delivery when there is a risk of hemolytic anemia due to immature erythrocyte enzyme systems.

Drug Interactions

Table 41-3 lists drug interactions for commonly used urinary tract antiseptics. Many of the urinary tract antiseptics interact with probenecid to decrease the elimination of the urinary tract antiseptics.

Dosage Regimen

For suppressive or preventive therapy for UTIs, administer a total daily adult dose of 1 gram of methenamine in two divided doses for the hippurate salt, and 1 gram 4 times daily after meals, and at bedtime for the mandelate salt formulation (see Table 41-4). Methenamine may be administered safely to children 6 to 12 years of age, but in reduced dosages.

The usual dose of nitrofurantoin (Macrobid) is 100 mg every 12 hours; dosage for Macrodantin is 50 to 100 mg 4 times daily. Continue treatment for 7 days. Lower doses of nitrofurantoin may be taken nightly for many months in patients requiring long-term prophylaxis. The drug can actually be used for the length of the pregnancy, if needed, but the drug must be stopped before delivery.

Lab Considerations

Nitrofurantoin causes false-positive reactions for urine glucose when the test is performed using Benedict's or Fehling's solution.

CLINICAL REASONING

Treatment Objectives

Treatment objectives for patients with a UTI are to (1) eradicate symptomatic infection, (2) identify and correct predisposing factors, (3) prevent reinfection, and (4) stop the infection's upward movement toward the kidneys.

TABLE 41-5 Urinary Concentrations of Antimicrobials

Drug	Single Dose	Urinary Antimicrobial Concentration (mcg/mL)	Eliminated in Urine (%)
ciprofloxacin	250 mg	Over 200 during first 2 hr, 30 in 8–12 hr	40–50
gatifloxacin	400 mg	UA	>70
levofloxacin	250 mg	166 in first 2 hr	87
lomefloxacin	400 mg	>300 first 4 hr; thereafter 35 for 24 hr	65
methenamine	1 gram	25%–85%*	90
nitrofurantoin	100 mg	50–150	20–25
norfloxacin	400 mg	>200	26–32
ofloxacin	200 mg	220	65–80
sulfisoxazole	200 mg	UA	52
sulfamethoxazole (SMZ)–trimethoprim (TMP)	800 mg SMZ and 160 mg TMP (1 DS tablet)	400/150	50 (0%–37% active)

*Formaldehyde concentration in urine.
DS, Double-strength; UA, unavailable.

CASE STUDY Urinary Antimicrobial and Related Drugs

ASSESSMENT

History of Present Illness	MR is a 23-year-old Caucasian woman who is concerned that her urine contains blood. She complains of burning on urination, suprapubic discomfort, and the need to urinate every 30 to 60 minutes. Symptoms have intensified over the last 24 hours. Feels her symptoms may be related to recent sexual activity and is extremely embarrassed about needing to contact her health care provider. She admits to intercourse with a new partner 2 days ago.
Past Health History	MR usually voids every 4 to 8 hours during the day, and rarely at night. Denies previous history of genitourinary or gynecologic problems, and practices good hygiene habits. Diaphragm and spermicidal gel are used for contraception. Takes vitamin C daily, otherwise uses no prescription or other OTC drugs. No known allergies.
Life-Span Considerations	Sexually active about 4 years.
Psychosocial Considerations	Full-time college student. Single. Lives with a roommate in an apartment. Admits to being relatively noncompliant with taking medicine: "I never have time to remember." Enrolled in a health care plan through her employer; all drug prescriptions require a copayment of $20.
Physical Exam Findings	Temp 98.6° F. Exam unremarkable, except for slight discomfort on deep palpation of suprapubic region. No CVA tenderness. Pelvic exam is unremarkable.
Lab Testing	Urine dipstick positive for nitrites and leukocytes. Microscopic examination of urinary sediment shows numerous white and red blood cells. Gram stain reveals *E. coli*. Culture pending.

DIAGNOSIS: Acute uncomplicated urinary tract infection

MANAGEMENT

Treatment Objectives	1. Alleviate symptoms. 2. Identify and correct predisposing factors. 3. Eliminate bacteriuria. 4. Prevent reinfection. 5. Prevent complications.
Treatment Plan	**Pharmacotherapy** • Sulfamethoxazole-trimethoprim DS by mouth twice daily for 3 days **Patient Education** 1. Increase fluid intake to 2 L/day. 2. 480 mL cranberry juice daily 3. Regular, complete bladder emptying; void after intercourse **Evaluation** Evaluate for relief of irritative symptoms, absence of urine odor, return of urine to its characteristic clear, light yellow color and decrease in urgency, frequency, and dysuria.

CLINICAL REASONING ANALYSIS

Q1. **My health care provider always gives me levaquin for UTIs. Why did you choose the combination of sulfamethoxazole-trimethoprim instead?**

A. Both drugs cover most strains of gram-positive and gram-negative organisms including *E. coli*, a common organism of UTIs, as well as a number of other organisms. Sulfamethoxazole-trimethoprim is rapidly absorbed following oral administration. Both drugs exist in the blood as unbound, bound, and biotransformed compounds. The free forms of sulfamethoxazole-trimethoprim are therapeutically active forms.

Q2. **Don't we have to worry about her compliance? She admits she is not good at taking medications.**

A. Uncomplicated, acute UTIs can be effectively treated with this drug. We want to avoid using a drug that she will need to take for an extended period.

Q3. **Don't we need to worry about bacterial resistance?**

A. By using both drugs, we block two consecutive steps in the biosynthesis of nucleic acids and proteins necessary to many bacteria. Sulfamethoxazole inhibits bacterial synthesis of dihydrofolic acid by competing with PABA. Trimethoprim blocks the production of tetrahydrofolic acid from dihydrofolic acid by binding to and reversibly inhibiting the

Continued

required enzyme, dihydrofolic reductase. In vitro studies have also shown that the combination reduces the risk of bacteria resistance compared with either drug alone.

Q4. MR is already taking vitamin C daily. Does she need to also consume cranberry juice or pills?

A. Cranberry juice inhibits the adherence of *E. coli* cells to cells lining the bladder. The vitamin C she takes will help to keep the urine pH in an acidic range of 5–6, thus also reducing the likelihood that bacteria will take up residence in the bladder mucosa.

Treatment Options

▓ *Patient Variables*

LIFE-SPAN CONSIDERATIONS

Pregnant and Nursing Women. Asymptomatic bacteriuria, defined as repeated recovery of greater than 10^5 CFU/mL in voided urine, occurs in approximately 5% of pregnancies. The risk of bacteriuria is greatest between the ninth and seventeenth weeks of gestation. Increasing levels of progesterone and an enlarging uterus produce physiologic changes in both the upper and lower portions of the urinary tract, creating an environment that favors bacteriuria. Without prophylaxis, 25% to 40% of pregnant women with untreated asymptomatic bacteriuria will develop pyelonephritis. Untreated asymptomatic bacteriuria can result in preterm labor. Women with bacteriuria are also twice as likely to deliver a low–birth weight infant. If a pregnant woman develops an acute UTI, especially with high fever, amniotic fluid infection may develop and retard the growth of the placenta. The relative risk of perinatal infant mortality is estimated to be 1:6.

Complicated UTIs are found during pregnancy and in women who are immunosuppressed, have diabetes, chronic kidney disease, and urinary tract abnormalities, as well as those who undergo urinary tract instrumentation. For these women, empiric therapy is recommended. A longer course of treatment with a broad-spectrum antibiotic is used until the diagnosis of UTI is confirmed and antibiotic sensitivities identified.

Uncomplicated UTIs are ordinarily treated with a 3-day course of sulfamethoxazole-trimethoprim, or with a 3-day course of a quinolone if resistance to *E. coli* is suspected. Although they are quite effective, do not use quinolones during pregnancy because of the risk for cartilage abnormalities in the fetus.

Sulfamethoxazole-trimethoprim use in pregnancy is debatable since it interferes with the biotransformation of folic acid. These drugs tend to raise the level of free bilirubin in the serum, thus increasing the risk of kernicterus in the neonate. Avoid sulfonamides, particularly late in the third trimester.

Treat catheter-related infections for 5 days. Prophylaxis for recurrent lower UTIs extends for 6 months. Treatment is then discontinued and the patient reassessed.

Children and Adolescents. During the first 6 months of life, all healthy girls and boys are susceptible to UTIs. This is due in part to immature immune systems and intense bacterial colonization of the periurethral area in females and the foreskin in males. Uncircumcised infants seem to have significantly more UTIs than circumcised infants. By 4 months of age, UTIs are 10 times more common in girls than in boys. Pyelonephritis is usually preceded by a UTI. The risk of developing an acute pyelonephritis before puberty is approximately 3% for girls and 1% to 2% for boys. Beyond the newborn and infant periods, the prevalence of UTIs in childhood and adolescence is less than 1%. However, the increased incidence of UTIs in girls continues throughout childhood and extends into adulthood.

Children troubled by bacterial persistence or repeated reinfection are thought to have some pathophysiologic predisposition to UTIs. Additionally, congenital conditions such as vesicoureteral reflux, ureteropelvic junction obstruction, megaureter, and spina bifida contribute to the incidence of urinary infection in children. Other factors such as the use of bubble bath and constipation also have been suggested as contributing factors in the development of UTIs.

Children with an uncomplicated UTI respond as well as adults to 3-day treatment with oral culture-sensitive antibiotics. However, if they are seriously ill, with a high fever, are unable to tolerate oral fluids, or are infected with a highly resistant pathogen, start treatment with the parenteral form of a broad-spectrum antimicrobial drug. Continue treatment for approximately 10 days once the child is able to take adequate fluids and an oral antibiotic formulation. Because children are sometimes less tolerant of acute symptoms, systemic analgesia with acetaminophen, warm sitz baths, or warm abdominal compresses may be used for pain relief.

Because the onset of UTI symptoms closely coincides with sexual intercourse, young women with acute postcoital UTIs are often embarrassed and may be reluctant to seek help. It is important that these patients understand that UTIs are commonly associated with normal sexual activity and does not imply that the patient engaged in unusual or abnormal sexual acts.

Older Adults. There is a high incidence of asymptomatic bacteriuria, bacteremia, and mortality in older adults. Long-term use of an indwelling urinary catheter almost guarantees a UTI. Atypical presentations of UTI in the older adult are common. The older adult may have a blunted fever response, anorexia, nausea, and vomiting, and abdominal pain may be present. Confusion and changes in behavior also are very common in older adults and can be seen in early infection. Fever, chills, and flank pain in the older adult are considered medical emergencies because septicemia may develop.

There is no demonstrable benefit in treating asymptomatic UTIs in older adults, except when there is a history of renal disease or urinary tract abnormalities; when the patient is to undergo an invasive genitourinary procedure; or if there is evidence of sepsis. UTI symptoms, a change in mental status, loss of appetite, increased white blood cell (WBC) count, or fever indicates the need for a urine culture.

Indiscriminate use of broad-spectrum antibiotics to treat asymptomatic bacteriuria invites the emergence of resistant organisms, especially among institutionalized older adults. On occasion, suppressive drugs such as methenamine or acidifying drugs such as vitamin C are used. Fewer than 1% of nursing home deaths are attributed to UTIs. Adjuvant drugs such as urinary antiseptics and antispasmodic drugs can be used to treat symptoms associated with UTI (see Chapter 43).

Older adults with symptomatic UTIs usually do not respond to short-course therapy and should be treated for 7 to 14 days. Institutionalized older adults are exposed to a wide range of organisms; therefore a broad-spectrum antibiotic is recommended. Sulfamethoxazole-trimethoprim is an effective broad-spectrum antibiotic that can be used for initial treatment and long-term prophylaxis in older adults. In some cases, a quinolone is the drug of choice. However, there are no studies demonstrating their superiority over other oral drugs for this population. Restrict the use of quinolones in the older adult to when infection is caused by an organism resistant to other oral agents. Lower dosages may be needed since the older adult is more likely to have impaired renal and hepatic function and is more susceptible to adverse effects. Regardless of the drug and dosage prescribed, renal function must be monitored.

Drug Variables

A 1- to 2-week course of an antibiotic for acute UTIs was once considered the standard treatment. In recent years, however, considerable effort has been devoted toward decreasing the emergence of resistant pathogens. Now, UTI treatment with an appropriate antimicrobial for 3 days has dramatically reduced the cost of treatment and reduced the incidence of antibiotic resistance. Some antibiotics cost considerably more than others but have an efficacy equal to that of less costly drugs, even when treatment is limited to 3 days. In all cases, selection of an appropriate antibiotic should be guided initially by (1) culture and sensitivity reports; (2) by the overall efficacy and risk for adverse reactions; and (3) by cost-effectiveness of the treatment (see Evidence-based Pharmacotherapeutics box).

Sulfonamide-trimethoprim is often the best drug for patients who have a first-time UTI because of its safety profile, efficacy, ease of administration, and low cost. A quinolone can be used if the patient is allergic to sulfamethoxazole-trimethoprim. Also, consider a quinolone for patients with upper urinary tract infections (i.e., pyelonephritis) that have systemic manifestations.

 ## EVIDENCE-BASED PHARMACOTHERAPEUTICS

Antibiotic Therapies for Urinary Tract Infections

■ Background

Uncomplicated urinary tract infection (UTI) is a frequent malady in sexually active young women. UTIs can be treated with a variety of antibiotics, each with a different cure rate and adverse effects. In years past, antibiotic treatment regimens lasting 7 to 10 days were used. Today's practice is to treat an uncomplicated UTI using a 3-day antibiotic treatment regimen.

■ Research Article

Milo, G., Katchman, E., Paul, M., et al. (2005). Duration of antibacterial treatment for uncomplicated urinary tract infection in women. *The Cochrane Database of Systematic Reviews.* 2005, Issue 2. Art. No. CD004682.pub2. DOI: 10.1002/14651858.CD004682.pub2.

Purpose

The purpose of this study was to compare 3-day antibiotic therapy with a 5-day or longer antibiotic treatment regimen for bacteriologic and symptomatic treatment failure rates, the development of pyelonephritis, and adverse effects of antibiotic treatment. These parameters were examined in light of the short- versus the long-term effects.

Design

A meta-analysis of studies that examined uncomplicated UTIs in otherwise healthy 18- to 65-year-old sexually active female subjects treated with 3- and 10-day antibacterial therapies was done.

Methods

A meta-analysis was undertaken by two independent reviewers who extracted data from 32 randomized, controlled studies ($N = 9605$) found in the Cochrane Library (2004), EMBASE (1980–2003) and MEDLINE (1966–2003). Information about symptomatic treatment failure rates, bacteriologic failure rates, and adverse effects were analyzed. Heterogeneity was first evaluated by examining graphic presentations, and then by using Chi^2 and I^2 measurements. Subgroup analyses looked at any impact that heterogeneity had within the main results.

Findings

Symptomatic failure rate: Short-term vs. long-term follow-up: There were no significant differences between 3-day and 5- to 10-day treatment regimens (short-term values: relative risk [RR] 1.06, 95% confidence interval [CI] 0.88–1.28, p= 0.52). There was no significant heterogeneity observed for this comparison ($Chi^2 = 27.14$, degrees of freedom [df] = 23, p = 0.25, $I^2 = 15.3\%$).

Bacteriologic failure: Short-term vs. long-term follow-up: The 5- to 10-day antibiotic regimens appeared to be superior to the 3-day regimens, although the results were not significant using the random effects model (RR 1.19, 95% CI 0.98–1.44, p = 0.08). No significant heterogeneity was observed for this comparison.

Adverse Effects: Short-term vs. long-term treatment regimen: Subjects treated with 5- to 10-day regimens had significantly more adverse drug reactions (ADRs) than those treated with 3-day regimens (RR 0.83, 95% CI 0.74–0.93, p = 0.001).

Conclusions

The 5- to 10-day treatment regimens were more effective than 3-day therapies, keeping the patients' urine sterile 2–15 days after the end of treatment. Another advantage of 5- to 10-day over 3-day treatment regimens in preventing bacteriologic failure was observed after 4–10 weeks (RR 1.43, 95% CI 1.19–1.73, P = 0.0002). The advantage of the longer therapy in terms of bacteriologic success appeared to be independent of the antibiotic class chosen for UTI treatment including quinolones. The 3-day regimens were similar to the 5- to 10-day regimens in achieving symptomatic cure.

■ Implications for Practice

The present practice of treating uncomplicated UTIs in young women for only 3 days to achieve symptomatic relieve is probably sufficient for the majority of patients. However, it leaves a significant risk of recurrent or persistent bacteriuria independent of the class of the drug. Future research in this area should address the question of the link between bacteriuria and symptomatic UTIs.

Controversy

Cranberry Juice: Effective or Ineffective?

An older adult gentleman with atrial fibrillation, hypertension, and recurrent cystitis is taking warfarin. He is well, but his international normalized ratio (INR) level is fluctuating between 1 and 10. An assessment is conducted asking the patient various questions centers on habits, prescription drugs taken, and the use of over-the-counter drugs and vitamins or herbs. The patient responds, "No," to each question. When asked if he drinks cranberry juice, the gentleman responds, "Yes."

Patients often drink cranberry juice to help prevent or fight urinary tract infections (UTIs). It contains various antioxidants and in fact, many people do not think of it as a drug. Cranberries contain a nondialyzable polymeric substance that prevents bacteria from adhering to the mucosa of the bladder walls, thus allowing the flow of urine to wash away the bacteria.

However, cranberry juice can cause fluctuations in the INR of patients taking warfarin. Cranberry juice contains flavonoids that inhibit CYP450 activity. Warfarin is predominantly biotransformed by CYP450, so the interaction is biologically plausible.

CLINICAL REASONING ANALYSIS
- What evidence supports the use of cranberry juice in preventing or treating UTIs?
- Are there antimicrobial drugs used to treat UTIs that have interactions with warfarin?
- What actions should be taken by the health care provider to ensure a patient's INR stays within a therapeutic range?

Health care providers and experts concerned about the development of resistance recommend that quinolones not be used to treat uncomplicated UTIs, if other viable alternatives exist. However, 15% to 20% of all pathogens causing uncomplicated, acute UTIs show resistance to nitrofurantoin, 33% are resistant to sulfonamides, and 5% to 15% are resistance to trimethoprim, and sulfamethoxazole-trimethoprim.

Numerous studies have evaluated the overall effectiveness and safety of various quinolone dosing regimens compared with other urinary antimicrobial drugs. Ciprofloxacin is as effective as sulfamethoxazole-trimethoprim and superior to trimethoprim alone, and is better than sulfamethoxazole-trimethoprim for the treatment of complicated UTIs.

Methenamine use may be prolonged for 6 months or more, because the risk of toxicity is small.

Patient Education

First and foremost, teach patients about nonpharmacologic approaches that help keep the bladder healthy (Box 41-2). Dark, concentrated urine suggests a need for more adequate hydration. Fluid intake of 6 to 8 or more 8-oz glasses per day should be maintained even after antibiotic treatment is complete. Cranberry juice has been used for years to keep bacteria from imbedding in the mucosa of the bladder wall and causing recurrent infections. Cranberry juice (or cranberry pills) is more effective for prophylaxis than for treatment of UTIs.

Teach the patient to finish the entire course of antibiotics. Although shorter treatment regimens considerably enhance patient adherence with treatment, the inclination to stop the drug once UTI symptoms have resolved remains. Emphasize that infections will persist and reoccur without adherence with the treatment regimen. Explaining the basic principles of antibiotic drug action (i.e., the ability of the drug to reach peak concentrations in the urine) helps increase adherence to treatment. Teach patients taking methenamine to monitor the pH of their urine to ensure drug efficacy.

Also teach patients about the potential benefits and adverse effects of the prescribed drugs. Explain the reasons

---

BOX 41-2

Patient Teaching for Preventing UTIs

- Make regular urination a habit (i.e., at 3- to 4-hour intervals); avoid long waits.
- Increase fluid intake, especially water, to a minimum of 6 to 8 8-oz glasses daily.
- Avoid bladder irritants such as caffeine, alcohol, and carbonated beverages.
- Avoid prolonged bicycling, motorcycling, horseback riding, and traveling involving long periods of sitting, which can contribute to irritation of the urethral meatus.
- Practice good hygiene, including wiping from front to back after urination and bowel movements.
- Avoid bubble bath, perfumed soap, and feminine hygiene spray.
- Urinate before and after intercourse to empty the bladder and cleanse the urethra. Be aware that vigorous or frequent sexual activity may contribute to urinary tract infection.
- Do not ignore vaginal discharge or other signs of vaginal infection.
- Wear cotton underwear. Avoid wearing nylon pantyhose, tight slacks, or any clothing that traps perineal moisture and prevents evaporation.
- Complete prescribed drug treatment regimens even though symptoms are diminished.
- Do not use drugs left over from previous infections.
- Drink 480 mL of cranberry or blueberry juice daily to acidify the urine and relieve symptoms.
- Use Credé's maneuver (pressing on the bladder suprapubically) to facilitate bladder emptying when appropriate.
- Prevent constipation through the use of adequate dietary fiber and fluids, activity, and timely toileting.
- When an indwelling catheter is required, use the smallest size possible; maintain a closed sterile drainage system and unobstructed urine flow.
- Reevaluate frequently the need for indwelling catheters and remove as soon as possible.

UTIs, Urinary tract infections.

for prophylaxis or long-term suppressive therapy and the importance of taking their drug immediately before retiring for the night. Urinary antibiotics are efficacious only if peak urine concentrations are reached during the longest natural period of urinary retention, that is, while the patient sleeps.

Teach patients about the signs and symptoms of a hypersensitivity reaction, along with information about treatment. Ordinarily, treatment of a hypersensitivity reaction includes having the patient stop the drug, taking diphenhydramine (Benadryl), and contacting the health care provider.

Evaluation

Expect the patient with an uncomplicated UTI to respond quickly to treatment. Urgency, frequency, and dysuria disappear within 24 to 48 hours when the appropriate antibiotic is used. Although not routinely recommended, the ideal time to perform the "test of cure" urine culture is 4 to 7 days after the completion of drug therapy. The patient undergoing treatment for a complicated UTI requires closer monitoring and prolonged treatment to ensure that bacteria are completely eradicated.

Should a reinfection occur after a 3- or 7- to 10-day course of an antibiotic, restart treatment, perhaps with a different antibiotic, while having the patient take the antibiotic for an additional 2 weeks. Be sure to check the culture and sensitivities to confirm the appropriate drug is used. If another relapse occurs after 2 weeks, continue treatment for 6 weeks. If the patient has another relapse after 6 weeks of antibiotic therapy, the appropriate antibiotic regimen should be used for 6 months. Use low-dose, long-term prophylaxis for women who have more than three symptomatic, recurrent infections in a year. In these cases, reinfection with the same or a different organism should be suspected.

Follow-up cultures should be done 1 to 2 weeks after the antibiotic regimen is completed. The follow-up cultures are mandatory, within 1 to 2 weeks of completion of treatment, in children, pregnant women with recurrent symptoms of upper UTIs, and patients who are at high risk for renal damage (even if they are asymptomatic). A child who requires long-term UTI prophylaxis should receive a different antibiotic from that used to treat the acute infection.

GENITOURINARY

KEY POINTS

- The prevalence of UTIs is greater in females than in males and tends to increase with age.
- Bacteria enter the urinary system primarily by ascending from the urethra. In rare instances, the mode of entry may be by hematogenous or lymphatic spread.
- Children older than 6 months of age who are troubled by persistent bacteriuria in the absence of any congenital condition may have a pathophysiologic predisposition to UTI.
- The prevalence of UTIs in women of child-bearing age is primarily related to sexual activity, use of the diaphragm or spermicidal gel, inadequate hygiene, and poor voiding habits.
- Institutionalized older adults have a higher prevalence of UTIs than noninstitutionalized older adults because of functional deficits, coexisting illnesses, and greater exposure to microorganisms.
- The primary factor contributing to bacteriuria in older females is the decreased influence of estrogen on the urinary tract mucosa. The primary factor contributing to bacteriuria in older men is benign prostatic hyperplasia.
- Pathogens infecting the urinary tract are frequently normal inhabitants of the intestinal tract. *E. coli* causes about 80% to 90% of acute UTIs.
- Urinary frequency, urgency, dysuria, and sometimes hematuria are classic signs of acute UTI. Voiding may be as frequent as every 15 to 30 minutes and associated with suprapubic discomfort or urethral burning. Flank pain also may be reported. The presence of pyuria, with or without hematuria, is indicative of UTI.

- A urine culture is diagnostic of UTI when there are greater than 100,000 CFU/mL of a single pathogen. A culture reporting 100 to 10,000 CFU/mL may be clinically significant if a single pathogen is isolated and the patient is symptomatic.
- Treatment objectives include the prompt eradication of symptoms of the UTI and the prevention of disease progression to the kidneys.
- The selection of an antibiotic for the treatment of a UTI is based on culture and sensitivity reports, overall drug efficacy, the risk for adverse reactions, and the cost-effectiveness of treatment. Empiric choice of antimicrobial is based on common pathogens, age group, and patient risk factors.
- Sulfamethoxazole-trimethoprim and nitrofurantoin are equally efficacious and less costly alternatives to quinolones for the treatment of acute UTIs.
- The use of oral quinolones is reserved for the treatment of complicated UTIs caused by bacteria resistant to other antibiotics, or for instances when a parenteral drug is needed, or when other drug therapies have failed.
- Teach patients to complete the entire course of treatment, of the need for regular bladder emptying and adequate hygiene, and of the importance of recognizing signs and symptoms of UTIs.
- Evidence that the UTI has been treated effectively include the patient's verbalization of the relief of frequency, urgency, and dysuria; the absence of urine odor; return of urine to its clear, light-yellow color, and absence of pyuria.

Bibliography

Colgan, R., and Powers, J. (2001). Appropriate antimicrobial prescribing. *American Family Physician*, 64(6), 999–1004.

Drug Watch: Cranberry juice reduces bacteruria and pyuria. (1994). *Bandolier Journal*, July, 6–3, Available online: www.jr2.ox.ac.uk/bandolier/band6/b6-3.html. Accessed May 16, 2007.

Dulczak, S., and Kirk, J. (2005). Overview of the evaluation of diagnosis, and management of urinary tract infections in infants and children. *Urologic Nursing*, 25(3), 185–191.

Ebel, M. (2006). Point of care guides: Treating adult women with suspected urinary tract infection. *American Family Physician*, 73(2), 293–296.

Fihn, S. (2003). Acute uncomplicated urinary tract infection in women. *New England Journal of Medicine*, 349(3), 259–266.

Griebling, T. (2004). In Litwin, M., and Saigal, C. (Eds.). *CDC: Urologic disease of America: Interim compendium*. US Government Publishing office.

Griebling, T. (2005). Urologic disease in America project: Trends in resource use for urinary tract infection in women. *The Journal of Urology, 173*(4), 1281–1287.

Ishay, A., Lavi, I., Luboshitzky, R. (2006). Prevalence and risk factors for asymptomatic bacteriuria in women with type 2 diabetes mellitus. *Diabetic Medicine, 23*(2), 185.

Karlowicz, K. (1999). Pharmacologic therapy for acute cystitis in adults: A review of treatment options. *Urologic Nursing, 17*(3), 106–116.

Kahan, N., Chinitz, D., Waitman, D., et al. (2004). Empiric treatment of uncomplicated UTI in women: Wasting money when more is not better. *Journal of Clinical Pharmacy and Therapeutics, 29*(5), 437–441.

Kahan, N., Friedman, N., Lomnisky, Y., et al. (2005). Physician specialty and adherence to guidelines for the treatment of unsubstantiated uncomplicated urinary tract infection among women. *Pharmacoepidemiology and Drug Safety, 14*(5), 357–361.

Midthun, S., Paur, R., Bruce, A., et al. (2005). Urinary tract infections in the elderly: A survey of physicians and nurses. *Geriatric Nursing, 26*(4), 245–251.

Milo, G., Katchman, E., and Paul, M., et al. (2005). Duration of antibacterial treatment for uncomplicated urinary tract infection in women. *The Cochrane Database of Systematic Reviews.* Issue 2. Art. No. CD004682.pub2. DOI: 10.1002/14651858.CD004682.pub2.

Nickel, J. (2005). Management of urinary tract infections: Historical perspective and current strategies: Part 2–Modern management. *The Journal of Urology, 173*(1), 27–32.

NKUDIC. (2004). National Kidney and Urologic Disease Information Clearinghouse. *Kidney and urologic disease statistics for the United States.* Available online: www.kidney.niddk.nih.gov/kudiseases/pubs/kustats/index.htm#up. Accessed May 17, 2007.

Scholes, D., Hooton, T., Roberts, P., et al. (2005). Risk factors associated with acute pyelonephritis in healthy women. *American College of Physicians, 142*(1), 20–27.

Walsh, K. (2005). Getting to yes. *The American Geriatrics Society, 53*(6), 1072.

Zore, J., Kiddoo, A., and Shaw, K. (2005). Diagnosis and management of pediatric urinary tract infections. *Clinical Microbiology Reviews, 18*(2), 417–422.

Diuretics

42

There are five classes of diuretics: thiazides, thiazide-like diuretics, loop diuretics, potassium-sparing agents, carbonic anhydrase inhibitors, and osmotics. Before discussing the drug classes and the drugs themselves it is important to review how fluids function within the body and, in particular, the roles of filtration and elimination in the kidneys.

Body fluids promote health and wellness. They serve as media for the transport of substances to, from, and across cell membranes. They are the media in which most metabolic reactions take place. Body fluid also provides lubrication for body parts and assists in heat regulation. A chemical equilibrium must be maintained if these functions are to occur. The equilibrium is reflected in normal urine volume, and composition, distribution, and pH of body fluids. Equilibrium is achieved through fluid, electrolyte, and acid-base balances, with the volume and composition of fluid controlled by three processes: glomerular filtration, tubular reabsorption, and tubular secretion.

RENAL FUNCTION

Urine formation begins with filtration of the plasma by the glomeruli. Renal blood flow is about 25% of cardiac output, or about 1200 mL/min. Water and crystalloids are readily filtered, whereas blood cells and large molecules such as proteins are restrained by the filtration membrane. As fluid is forced through glomeruli, plasma proteins (primarily albumin) remain in the circulation, maintaining *oncotic pressure* (the sum of protein osmotic pressure and osmotic pressure of obligate cations). Albumin tends to pull water into the blood vessels.

Hydrostatic pressure, the pressure a solution exerts against the wall of its container, is maintained by contractions of the heart. Blood vessels have greater hydrostatic pressure than interstitial spaces, and therefore there is a tendency for water to be forced out. At the arterial end, nutrients diffuse out of blood vessels. At the venous end, owing to oncotic pressure, water and waste products diffuse into blood vessels.

Three classes of substances are filtered at the glomerulus: electrolytes, nonelectrolytes, and water. The electrolytes filtered include sodium, potassium, calcium, magnesium, bicarbonate, chloride, and phosphate. The ultrafiltrate also contains other small–molecular weight solutes. Nonelectrolytes filtered include glucose, amino acids, and the metabolic end products of protein metabolism: urea, uric acid, and creatinine.

After passing through the glomerulus, the filtrate travels through renal tubules, where 99% is reabsorbed. The composition of the reabsorbed filtrate approximates that of extracellular fluid. Through reabsorption, sodium passively enters tubule cells down an electrochemical gradient. Sodium also moves against a concentration gradient into the blood by active transport using adenosine triphosphate (ATP). ATP moves sodium out of the cell and potassium into the cell across the basilar membranes. In addition, sodium diffuses back into peritubular capillaries through pericellular pathways, where it recaptures the filtrate.

Tubular secretion refers to the active and passive processes that move substances from peritubular capillaries into the interstitial fluid and then into tubular lumens. Thus, substances that are secreted are eliminated from the body.

In a healthy individual, these processes work well, and equilibrium is maintained. However, alterations in the volume, the composition, the distribution, or the pH of body fluids cause disequilibrium and, in some cases, illness. The disequilibrium may occur as a result of disorders of intake, elimination, or regulation of body fluid components, or as a part of a pathophysiologic response to other illnesses. A fluid shift from the extracellular compartment to the interstitial compartment results in edema.

Fluid volume excess, also referred to as *edema,* results from a number of disease states and is organized according to the mechanisms involved (Box 42-1). Alterations in cardiac, renal, hepatic, or endocrine function are primary etiologies, although edema may be seen with other states such as the edema associated with pregnancy and premenstrual tension. Edema may also be drug-induced.

FLUID VOLUME EXCESS

EPIDEMIOLOGY AND ETIOLOGY

A number of disorders can lead to increased fluid retention in the intravascular and interstitial spaces, resulting in fluid volume excess (edema). The organs most often involved with disorders producing fluid volume excess are the heart, the liver, and the kidneys.

The causes of heart failure can be divided into three groups. The first group includes conditions that result in direct damage to the heart (e.g., myocardial infarction, myocarditis, myocardial fibrosis, ventricular aneurysms). The second group includes problems that result in ventricular overload (e.g., left ventricular hypertrophy), and in the third group are conditions leading to ventricular constriction (e.g., cardiac tamponade, constrictive cardiomyopathies, and pericarditis).

Severe liver problems can result from a variety of causes such as infective organisms, neoplastic growths, toxic agents, and trauma. The pathologic states that result can be categorized as focal or diffuse.

Nephrotic syndrome (nephrosis) is associated with allergic reactions, systemic disease, circulatory problems, and

Common Causes of Peripheral Edema

MECHANISM	DISORDERS AND STATES
Direct damage to the heart	• Myocardial infarction • Myocarditis • Myocardial fibrosis • Ventricular aneurysms
Ventricular overload	• Left ventricular hypertrophy
Ventricular constriction	• Cardiac tamponade • Constrictive cardiomyopathies • Pericarditis
Increased capillary pressure	• Allergic responses • Cardiogenic pulmonary edema • Environmental heat stress • Heart failure • Hepatic obstruction • Increased levels of ACTH • Idiopathic edema in women • Inflammation • Pregnancy • Premenstrual sodium retention • Prolonged standing • Thrombophlebitis
Increased capillary permeability	• Immune responses • Neoplastic diseases • Noncardiogenic pulmonary edema • Tissue injury and burns
Decreased colloidal osmotic pressure	• Liver disease • Protein-losing enteropathy • Starvation
Obstruction of lymphatic flow	• Infection or disease of lymph nodes • Surgical removal of lymph nodes
Drug-induced	• *NSAIDs*: ketoprofen, flurbiprofen, naproxen, phenylbutazone, tolmetin • *Antihypertensives*: diltiazem, labetolol, nifedipine, pindolol • *Hormones*: Androgenic steroids, Corticosteroids, Estrogens • *Others*: estramustine, etretinate, interferon alfa-2a, Phenothiazines, tamoxifen

ACTH, Adrenocorticotropic hormone; *NSAIDs*, nonsteroidal antiinflammatory drugs.

pregnancy. Glomerular disease is the most common precipitating event in adults. Fifty percent to 75% of adults who develop nephrosis progress to renal failure within 5 years. No specific treatment exists for nephrotic syndrome. Diuretics may be prescribed but are often ineffective.

PATHOPHYSIOLOGY

Edema is caused by a disruption in Starling forces. This very basic principle of cardiac function states that the force of the contraction is proportional to the length of the contracting fibers, somewhat like the stretch of a rubber band. When ventricular filling is increased or decreased by a given volume of blood, the displacement of the heart increases or decreases with this volume. Effectively, this means that the force of contraction will increase as the heart is filled with more blood and is a direct consequence of the effect of an increasing load on a single muscle fiber. The force that any single muscle fiber generates is proportional to the initial sarcomere length (known as preload), and the stretch on individual fibers is related to the end-diastolic volume (EDV) of the ventricle.

Edema results from increases in capillary hydrostatic pressure, capillary permeability, or interstitial oncotic pressure, or it may be due to a decrease in plasma oncotic pressure. The presence of edema indicates an excess amount of sodium, which is accompanied by an obligatory water load. Sodium excess may serve as either an initiating event or as a secondary factor in the development of edema. Excess sodium levels are most often caused by increased retention or a decreased ability to eliminate the ion. The sodium and water retention is often a compensatory mechanism serving to restore and maintain circulatory volume while fluid accumulates in interstitial spaces. Retention of sodium and water is illustrated in conditions such as cardiac failure, liver disease, and chronic kidney disease (Fig. 42-1).

Heart Failure

Heart failure begins when the heart is unable to maintain effective pumping action. Compensation for ineffective pumping occurs via the sympathetic nervous system (SNS). Stimulation of the SNS leads to an increased heart rate acutely, and decreased cardiac contractility and constriction of peripheral arteries over time. Vasopressin, which is released through sympathetic stimulation, leads to a constriction of the arteries. A decrease in peripheral arterial blood flow and renal blood flow results.

Decreased perfusion of the kidneys leads to the release of renin and the conversion of circulating angiotensin I to angiotensin II. Angiotensin II is a powerful vasoconstrictor that stimulates the adrenal glands to release aldosterone. Aldosterone, in turn, stimulates the kidney to reabsorb sodium and water. Thus blood pressure is maintained by constricting the blood vessels and increasing intravascular volume. In the process, glomerular filtration rate (GFR) also decreases, resulting in the retention of sodium and water.

As the process continues, a point is reached at which the compensatory mechanisms no longer work. The circulatory and respiratory systems become overloaded with increasing hydrostatic pressure, causing edema, either in the pulmonary tissues or in peripheral tissues.

As pulmonary edema develops, it inhibits oxygen and carbon dioxide exchange at the alveolar capillary membranes. There is a mild increase in respiratory rate and a decrease in both PaO_2 and $PaCO_2$. If pulmonary venous pressure continues to increase, more fluid moves into the interstitial lung spaces than the lymphatic drainage system can handle. The patient develops severe tachypnea and worsening blood gas status. Alveolar edema worsens even more as pulmonary venous pressure increases. As the disruption at the alveolar-capillary membranes worsens, the alveoli and airways become flooded with fluid.

Clinical signs and symptoms of pulmonary edema are unmistakable. The patient is agitated and cold and clammy, and has severe dyspnea. There is orthopnea, the use of accessory muscles, and a respiratory rate greater than 30 breaths/min. There may be wheezing and coughing with the production of frothy, blood-tinged sputum. The heart rate and

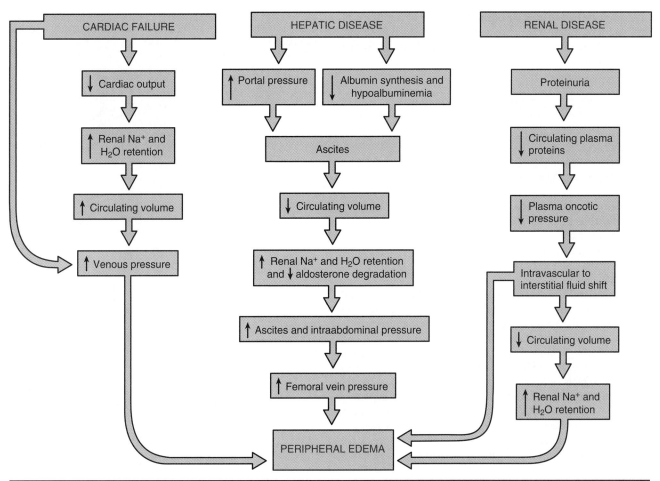

FIGURE 42-1 Mechanisms leading to peripheral edema, a primary manifestation of alteration in capillary hemodynamics and sodium and water balance caused by cardiac failure, hepatic disease, and renal disease.

blood pressure are elevated or at shock level depending on the severity of the condition.

The process may progress to affect the right ventricle also. The hydrostatic pressure of the venous system increases, leading to peripheral edema. The edema of right-sided heart failure is seen in the lower extremities as pitting edema. Right-sided heart failure can progress to hepatomegaly. Liver lobules become congested, with venous blood causing impaired liver function. Eventually, liver cells die, fibrosis occurs, and cirrhosis can develop.

Hepatic Disease

Much like heart failure, liver disease is characterized, in part, by a disruption in capillary hemodynamics. There is increased pressure within the portal vein, which in turn causes increased hydrostatic pressure. In addition, albumin synthesis is decreased and hypoalbuminemia develops. As albumin is lost, oncotic pressure decreases, and fluid leaks out of the vasculature into interstitial spaces. The result of these changes is *ascites,* an accumulation of fluid within the peritoneal cavity. As the accumulation of fluid progresses, the patient develops hypovolemia and the kidneys are underperfused. When kidney perfusion decreases, renin and angiotensin activities are initiated and the degradation of aldosterone is decreased. The response is to retain sodium and water, further

contributing to the accumulation of fluid in the abdomen and to increases in intraabdominal pressure. The ascites and the abdominal pressure increase because of increased femoral vein pressure, leading to peripheral edema.

Peripheral edema and ascites are but two of the complications of liver disease. In time, jaundice, gastrointestinal (GI) distress, skin lesions, hematologic disorders, endocrine disturbances, and peripheral neuropathies also appear.

Renal Disease

Nephrotic syndrome, also known as renal edema, is not a single disease entity but a constellation of symptoms that involve the loss of protein in the urine. Damaged glomeruli permit sodium and plasma proteins to leak into the tubules to be lost in the urine. In some cases, protein loss may exceed 3 grams/day. Increased permeability of glomerular membranes is responsible for the massive loss of protein in the urine.

The loss of circulating plasma proteins reduces plasma oncotic pressure. There is a fluid shift from the extracellular compartment to interstitial spaces, thereby reducing circulating volume. The kidneys respond by increasing the retention of sodium and water; peripheral edema results.

Hypoalbuminemia, hyperlipidemia, and hyperlipiduria are seen in patients with nephrotic syndrome. Generalized edema results from the hypoalbuminemia, and this condition, in turn, leads to hypoperfusion of the kidney. Poor perfusion of the kidney stimulates the renin-angiotensin-aldosterone response. Water and sodium are retained, and edema formation continues.

PHARMACOTHERAPEUTIC OPTIONS

Thiazides
- chlorothiazide (Diuril)
- hydrochlorothiazide (Esidrix, Hydrodiuril); ♣ Apo-Hydro
- methyclothiazide (Aquatensen, Enduron)

Thiazide-Like Diuretics
- chlorthalidone (Hygroton, Thalitone); ♣ Apo-Chlorthalidone
- indapamide (Lozol); ♣ Lozide
- metolazone (Zaroxolyn, Mykrox)

▐▐ Indications
Thiazide and thiazide-like diuretics are mild diuretics and the first choice in treating most patients with hypertension (HTN), particularly salt-sensitive patients. They are frequently used to control the edema associated with mild fluid overload secondary to right-sided heart failure and to chronic hepatic or renal disease. Removing the excess fluid volume produces beneficial effects. Along with sodium restriction, thiazides are usually sufficient to control mild to moderate hypertension (see Chapter 37). In addition, thiazides are the only drugs available to decrease urine volume in patients with nephrogenic diabetes insipidus, in whom the drugs produce a fall in urine volume and a rise in urine osmolarity.

▐▐ Pharmacodynamics
Because inhibiting sodium reabsorption in a given portion of the nephron affects electrolyte elimination, the site of action provides information as to the relative potency of the drug (Fig. 42-2). Thiazide and thiazide-like diuretics act by inhibiting the reabsorption of sodium and chloride in the early distal tubule and the thick ascending limb (the diluting segment) of the ascending Loop of Henle, increasing the elimination of sodium and water. They increase potassium and chloride excretion and decrease excretion of calcium, bicarbonate, and uric acid. They have a relatively moderate potency and lead to elimination of 5% to 8% of the filtered load. Sodium and chloride ions pass into the collecting ducts, taking water with them.

▐▐ Pharmacokinetics
Thiazides are readily, but incompletely, absorbed by the GI tract. The drugs are variably plasma protein bound. The onset of drug action, peak effects, and the duration of action vary with the various drugs (Table 42-1). They all differ in half-life. The differences in thiazides appear to be proportional to plasma protein binding and the degree of reabsorption in the renal tubule. They differ also in their degree of biotransformation and elimination.

▐▐ Adverse Effects and Contraindications
The most common adverse effects of thiazide and thiazide-like diuretics are electrolyte imbalances, including hypokalemia, hypomagnesemia, hypercalcemia, and hyperuricemia

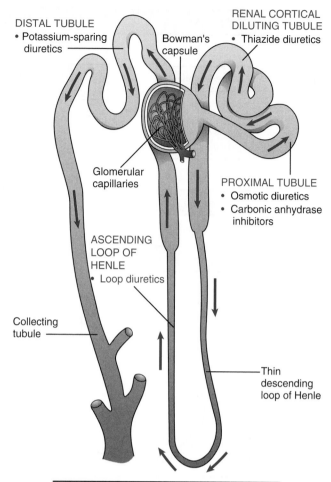

FIGURE 42-2 Sites of Diuretic Actions in the Nephron.

(see Evidence-Based Pharmacotherapeutics box). The increased quantity of sodium reaching the distal tubule site is the primary reason for the potassium loss in the urine. **Fifteen percent to** ▲ **20% of patients taking low-dose thiazide diuretics develop hypokalemia; therefore potassium supplements may be needed by some patients.** Serum potassium levels can fall below 3 mEq/L to 3.5 mEq/L with long-term therapy. Serum calcium levels may be elevated in the presence of thiazides because of the increased protein-bound fraction of calcium.

Like uric acid, thiazides occupy an organic acid transport system, and competition may result in hyperuricemia and gout in susceptible individuals. In addition, contraction of plasma volume also serves to increase uric acid reabsorption in the proximal tubule.

Although hyperlipidemia and hyperglycemia have been reported with thiazides, such increases are relatively small, and their clinical significance is controversial. There may be interference with the conversion of proinsulin to insulin. Thiazides have also been reported to reduce libido and cause impotence.

Some patients experience tinnitus, paresthesias, abdominal cramping, nausea, vomiting, diarrhea, muscle cramps, weakness, and sexual dysfunction. Blood dyscrasias have also been reported that include leukopenia, thrombocytopenia, agranulocytosis, and aplastic anemia. Mild dizziness, headache, and paresthesias have been seen. In the case of overdose, lethargy

PHARMACOKINETICS

TABLE 42-1 Diuretics

Drug	Route	Onset	Peak	Duration	PB (%)	$t_{1/2}$	BioA (%)
THIAZIDES							
chlorothiazide	PO	2 hr	4 hr	6–12 hr	95	1–2 hr	10
hydrochlorothiazide	PO	2 hr	4 hr	6–12 hr	65	1–2 hr	UA
methyclothiazide	PO	2 hr	1–2 hr	24 hr	55	14	UA
THIAZIDE-LIKE DIURETICS							
chlorthalidone	PO	2 hr	4–6 hr	24–72 hr	UA	40 hr*	UA
indapamide	PO	Minutes	2 hr	56 hr	71–79	14 hr	UA
metolazone	PO	1 hr	2 hr	12–24 hr	33	14 hr	UA
POTASSIUM-SPARING DRUGS							
amiloride	PO	2 hr	6 hr	24 hr	40	6–9 hr	20
spironolactone	PO	8 hr	2–4 hr	48 hr	90	17–22 hr	UA
eplerenone	PO	Minutes	1.5 hr	16 hr	50	4–6 hr	UA
triamterene	PO	2–4 hr	2–4 hr	72 hr	60	2–4 hr	UA
LOOP DIURETICS							
bumetanide	PO	<1 hr	1–2 hr	4–6 hr	95	1–1.5 hr	100
	IV	Minutes	15–30 min	0.5–1 hr	95	UA	100
ethacrynic acid	PO	30 min	2 hr	6–8 hr	95	<1 hr	UA
	IV	5 min	15–20 min	2 hr	95	UA	100
furosemide	PO	60 min	1–2 hr	6–9 hr	95	2 hr	60
	IV	5 min	30 min	2 hr	95	UA	100
torsemide	PO	1 hr	1–2 hr	6–8 hr	>99	3.5 hr	80
	IV	10 min	1 hr	6–8 hr	>99	2–4 hr	100
OSMOTIC DRUGS							
mannitol	IV	30–60 min	*IOP:* 30–60 min *Diuresis:* 6–12 hr	4–8 hr	UA	15 min–1.5 hr	UA

*Chlorthalidone is sequestered in red blood cells; the $t_{1/2}$ is longer if blood rather than plasma is analyzed.

BioA, Bioavailability; *IOP,* intraocular pressure; *IV,* intravenous; *PB,* protein binding; *PO,* by mouth; *SR,* sustained-release; $t_{1/2}$, half-life; *UA,* unavailable.

EVIDENCE-BASED PHARMACOTHERAPEUTICS

Thiazides and the Risk for Hip Fracture

■ Background

Thiazide diuretics decrease the urinary elimination of calcium and increase the density of bone mass. Given this statement, it would appear logical that their use may prevent fractures. Because most fractures of the hip are secondary to osteoporosis, treating the osteoporosis is an important component of patient care.

■ Research Article

Schoofs, M., van der Klift, M., Ron, A., et al. (2003). Thiazide diuretics and the risk for hip fracture. *Annals of Internal Medicine, 139*(6), 476–482.

Purpose

The purpose of this study was to (1) explore the relationship between duration of thiazide and thiazide-like diuretic use and the risk for hip fracture, and (2) to explore the risk for hip fracture once the drug is discontinued.

Design

This study was undertaken as part of the prospective, population-based Rotterdam (Netherland) study, a cohort study on the incidence and determinants of disease and disability in older adults. Subjects were followed from mid-1991 until they had an incident hip fracture, died, or reached the end of the study in late 1999, whichever came first. All residents living in a suburb of Rotterdam who were 55 years of age or older were asked to participate; 78% of the eligible subjects (10, 275) did so.

Methods

Thiazides, thiazide-like diuretics, and combination thiazide–potassium-sparing diuretics, and potassium were drugs of interest. Chlothalidone, a thiazide-like diuretic, was also included because of its affect on calcium elimination. Detailed reports regarding all dispensed drugs were made available to the investigators on a daily basis through a network of pharmacies.

Subjects were organized into seven groups based on their thiazide or thiazide-like drug use. The categories were as follows: (1) subjects who never used a thiazide or thiazide-like diuretic; (2) those who took the drug for at least 6 weeks; (3) those who took the drug for at least 6 weeks up to 1 year; (4) those taking the drug over 1 year; (5) those who stopped the drug in the last 2 months; (6) those who stopped the drug after 2 or more months of use; (6) those who stopped the drug after 2 months but less than 4 months after use; and (7) subjects who stopped the drug after 4 months of use.

Subject risks for hip fracture related to thiazides and thiazide-like diuretics were computed using the Cox proportional hazards model, which compared drug exposure on the index date with the incidence of hip fracture with the risk for hip fracture in subjects in a cohort group. Categorical variables were used to compute the length of time the drug was used with the time since last documented use of the thiazide or thiazide-like drug.

Findings

The relationship between hip fracture and thiazide or thiazide-like diuretic use was found to be statistically significant in the reduction of hip fractures, relative to subjects who never used the drug (relative risk for hip fracture, 0.46; 95% confidence interval, 0.21 to 0.96). For subjects who took the thiazide or thiazide-like diuretic for 1 year or longer, the better the adjusted relative risk for hip fracture.

Conclusions

The protective effect of thiazide and thiazide-like diuretics in reducing the risk for hip fracture fades within 4 months after the drug is discontinued. Even though the risk for hip fracture was increased with short-term use of the diuretic, risk reduction reached statistical significance after 1 year of continuous use.

■ Implications for Practice

Study investigators were attentive to extraneous and confounding variables when designing and carrying out the study, including numerous examples of variables to be considered in future studies.

Whether or not similar additive benefits exist with other bone protective drugs requires additional review.

GENITOURINARY

and even coma may occur. Cardiac function and respiratory rate are not significantly depressed, although orthostatic hypotension unrelated to volume changes may be experienced.

▲ **Thiazide diuretics exhibit cross-allergenicity with sulfonamide drugs and therefore are contraindicated for use in patients with a sulfa allergy.** Allergic reactions are usually mild, although anaphylaxis has occurred. Use of thiazide diuretics during pregnancy is not recommended because they cross the placental membranes (category B drugs). Newborns may develop thrombocytopenia and bone marrow depression. The drugs also appear in breast milk.

Thiazides are relatively contraindicated for use in patients with a creatinine clearance less than 30 mL/min because the efficacy is diminished.

Drug Interactions

Thiazide and thiazide-like diuretics potentiate the actions of antihypertensive drugs; especially those with actions at ganglionic or peripheral adrenergic sites (Table 42-2). **Patients on digoxin are more susceptible to digoxin toxicity because of the potassium loss. The situation is worsened when thiazides are used concurrently with corticosteroids or adrenocorticotropic hormone.** Thiazide diuretics enhance the effects of depolarizing skeletal muscle relaxants such as tubocurarine, a drug frequently used in surgery. Lithium elimination is decreased by thiazides, predisposing the patient to lithium toxicity. Because thiazide diuretics produce alkaline urine, the effectiveness of

methenamine is decreased. Anion exchange resins delay the absorption of thiazides if they are taken concurrently.

Dosage Regimens

The dosage of thiazide and thiazide-like diuretics should be individually adjusted (Table 42-3). The drug may be administered daily as a single dose or in divided doses when treating edema, or in divided doses when treating hypertension. Most antihypertensive dosing is once daily. **Use of any thiazide warrants caution in patients who have renal or hepatic disease.** ▲

Lab Considerations

Lab considerations include monitoring serum electrolytes (especially potassium), blood glucose, blood urea nitrogen (BUN), and serum uric acid levels before and periodically throughout therapy. Some thiazide diuretics are not as effective in patients with a creatinine clearance less than 30 mL/min. Elevation in serum cholesterol, low-density lipoprotein, and triglyceride concentrations may be noted on lipid panels.

For more information, see the Evolve Resources Bonus Content "Influence of Selected Drugs on Laboratory Values," found at http://evolve.elsevier.com/Gutierrez/pharmacotherapeutics.

Calcium levels may rise as a result of the decrease in calcium elimination. In a few patients who have been on long-term therapy, both hypercalcemia and hypophosphatemia have occurred. The imbalance may lead to suppression of parathyroid gland activity. In these patients, calcium, phosphate, and

DRUG INTERACTIONS
TABLE 42-2 Selected Diuretics

Drugs	Interactive Drugs	Interaction
THIAZIDE AND THIAZIDE-LIKE DIURETICS		
Thiazide and thiazide-like diuretics	Antihypertensives	Increases action of the antihypertensive drug
	digoxin	Increases potential for digoxin toxicity due to potassium loss
	Oral hypoglycemic drugs, Insulins	May cause hyperglycemia and hyponatremia, resulting in thiazide resistance
	Corticosteroids, ACTH	Increases loss of potassium
	probenecid	Decreases uric acid elimination; may precipitate gout
	Lithium, Salicylates	Decreases elimination of lithium, salicylates; lithium toxicity, salicylate toxicity
	NSAIDs	Decreases antihypertensive effect of thiazide
	Depolarizing skeletal muscle relaxants	Increases responsiveness to skeletal muscle relaxants
	methenamine	Methenamine requires acid urine to be effective; thiazides cause alkaline urine
	kayexalate	Decreases absorption of thiazides
POTASSIUM-SPARING DIURETICS		
Potassium-sparing diuretics	Other potassium-sparing diuretics and potassium supplements, ACEIs, lithium	Increases risk of hyperkalemia
	Salicylates, NSAIDs	Decreases effectiveness of spironolactone
	Antihypertensives	Increases effectiveness of antihypertensive
eplerenone	conivaptan, itraconazole, ketoconazole, telithromycin	Increases eplerenone levels and risk of hyperkalemia and serious arrhythmias
LOOP DIURETICS		
Loop diuretics	Oral hypoglycemic drugs	Increases potential for hyperglycemia
	Aminoglycosides, cisplatin	Increases potential for ototoxicity
	lithium	Decreases elimination of lithium, increasing risk of lithium toxicity
	digoxin	Increases potential for digoxin toxicity related to potassium loss
	NSAIDs	Decreases antihypertensive and diuretic effect of diuretic
	Neuromuscular blockers	Increases effects of neuromuscular blockade
	Theophyllines	Increases diuresis from furosemide
OSMOTIC DIURETICS		
mannitol	lithium	Decreases effectiveness of lithium in presence of mannitol

ACEI, Angiotensin-converting enzyme inhibitor; *ACTH*, adrenocorticotropic hormone; *NSAIDs*, nonsteroidal antiinflammatory drugs.

DOSAGE
TABLE **42-3 Diuretics**

Drug	Use	Dosage	Implications
THIAZIDE DIURETICS			
chlorothiazide	Edema of cardiac, renal or hepatic failure; hypertension	*Adult: Edema:* 500–1000 mg PO or IV daily once-twice daily *Hypertension:* 250–500 mg PO once-twice daily *Child <6 mo:* 20–40 mg/kg/day PO in 2 divided doses *Child >6 mo:* 10–20 mg/kg/day in 2 divided doses	May not be administered IM or subQ. Use cautiously in patients with severe renal disease.
hydrochlorothiazide	Edema of cardiac, renal or hepatic failure; hypertension	*Adult: Edema:* 25–100 mg PO daily or intermittently. Max: 200 mg/day *HTN:* 12.5–50 mg PO daily *Child <6 mo:* 2–3 mg/kg/day PO in 2 divided doses *Child >6 mo:* 2 mg/kg/day PO in 2 divided doses	Adjust dose based on patient response. **Use cautiously in patients with severe renal disease, impaired hepatic function, or progressive hepatic disease.**
methyclothiazide	Edema of cardiac, renal or hepatic failure; hypertension	*Adult:* 2.5–5 mg PO daily	Long-acting drug
THIAZIDE-LIKE DIURETICS			
chlorthalidone	Edema, hypertension	*Adult: Edema:* 50–100 mg PO daily –or– 100 mg on alternate days *HTN:* 25–100 mg PO daily –or– 100 mg 3 times/wk or on alternate days. May require up to 200 mg/day for therapeutic effect	Long-acting drug. Use cautiously in patients with severe renal disease, impaired hepatic function, or progressive hepatic disease
metolazone	Hypertension and edema secondary to heart failure, hepatic disease, renal disease	*Adult:* 5–20 mg PO daily *HTN:* 2.5–5 mg PO daily	Effective if GFR < 20 mL/ min. Use cautiously in patients with hyperuricemia or impaired renal or hepatic function.
POTASSIUM-SPARING DRUGS			
amiloride	Adjunct to thiazide or loop diuretics in HTN or edema associated with HF. Maintenance of serum potassium levels in patients with hypokalemia	*Adult:* 5–10 mg PO daily. May increase up to 20 mg/day	**Contraindicated for use in patients with elevated serum potassium levels**
eplerenone	Post-MI heart failure, HTN	*Adult:* 25 mg PO daily. Increase to 50 mg in 4 wk. *HTN:* 50 mg PO once-twice daily	Monitor K+ at baseline, 1 wk, 1 mo, and then periodically. Full therapeutic effect apparent within 4 wk
spironolactone	Refractory edema, hypertension, idiopathic edema, cirrhosis, nephrotic syndrome, hirsutism, primary aldosteronism	*Adult: Edema:* 25–200 mg PO daily *HTN:* 25–50 mg PO daily as a single dose or 2 divided doses *Primary aldosteronism:* 100–400 mg/day PO in 1–2 divided doses *CHF severe:* 12.5–25 mg daily. Max: 50 mg daily	**Use cautiously in fluid and electrolyte disturbances, renal insufficiency, and hepatic disease.**
triamterene	Adjunct to other diuretics for HTN, edema associated with HF, cirrhosis, nephrotic syndrome, idiopathic edema, steroid-induced edema, and edema of hyperaldosteronism	*Adult:* 100–300 mg/day PO in 1–2 divided doses	**Use cautiously in patients with hepatic disease or diabetes mellitus, and during pregnancy and lactation.**
LOOP DIURETICS			
bumetanide	Edema, hypertension	*Adult:* 0.5–2 mg PO or IV daily. May repeat every 4–5 hr up to 10 mg/day	Use supplemental potassium or potassium-sparing diuretics to prevent hypokalemia.
ethacrynic acid	Acute pulmonary edema, other forms of edema	*Adult:* 50–100 mg/day PO in 1–2 divided doses. Max: 400 mg/day –or– 0.5–1 mg/kg/dose IV. May repeat doses every 8–12 hr only if indicated. Max: 100 mg/dose *Child: Edema:* 1 mg/kg/dose PO once daily; increase every 2–3 days as needed. Max: 3 mg/kg/day	Use cautiously in patients with electrolyte imbalance, azotemia, or oliguria. May be substituted for other diuretics in patients with sulfa allergy.
furosemide	Acute pulmonary edema, other forms of edema, HTN crisis, ARF, CRF, HTN, hypercalcemia	*Adult: HTN:* 20–80 mg PO once-twice daily –or– 20–40 mg IV. Max single dose: 160–200 mg *Child:* 1–2 mg/kg PO every 6–8 hr. Max: 6 mg/kg/dose IM or IV no more often than every 6 hr. Increase by 1 mg/kg after 2 hr.	May cause profound water and electrolyte depletion.

GENITOURINARY

Continued

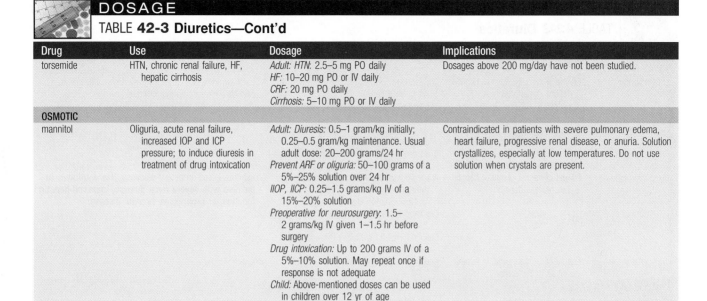

DOSAGE
TABLE 42-3 Diuretics—Cont'd

Drug	Use	Dosage	Implications
torsemide	HTN, chronic renal failure, HF, hepatic cirrhosis	*Adult: HTN*: 2.5–5 mg PO daily *HF*: 10–20 mg PO or IV daily *CRF*: 20 mg PO daily *Cirrhosis*: 5–10 mg PO or IV daily	Dosages above 200 mg/day have not been studied.
OSMOTIC			
mannitol	Oliguria, acute renal failure, increased IOP and ICP pressure; to induce diuresis in treatment of drug intoxication	*Adult: Diuresis*: 0.5–1 gram/kg initially; 0.25–0.5 gram/kg maintenance. Usual adult dose: 20–200 grams/24 hr *Prevent ARF or oliguria*: 50–100 grams of a 5%–25% solution over 24 hr *IIOP, IICP*: 0.25–1.5 grams/kg IV of a 15%–20% solution *Preoperative for neurosurgery*: 1.5–2 grams/kg IV given 1–1.5 hr before surgery *Drug intoxication*: Up to 200 grams IV of a 5%–10% solution. May repeat once if response is not adequate *Child*: Above-mentioned doses can be used in children over 12 yr of age	Contraindicated in patients with severe pulmonary edema, heart failure, progressive renal disease, or anuria. Solution crystallizes, especially at low temperatures. Do not use solution when crystals are present.

ARF, Acute renal failure; *CRF*, chronic renal failure, *CNS*, central nervous system; *FDA*, Food and Drug Administration; *GFR*, glomerular filtration rate; *HF*, heart failure; *HTN*, hypertension; *ICP*, intracranial pressure; *IICP*, increased intracranial pressure; *IIOP*, increased intraocular pressure; *IM*, intramuscular (route); *IOP*, intraocular pressure; *IV*, intravenous; K^+, potassium; *MI*, myocardial infarction; *PE*, pulmonary edema; *PO*, by mouth; *subQ*, subcutaneously.

parathyroid hormone levels may have to be monitored. For accurate results, stop the thiazide drug before obtaining samples for parathyroid function tests.

Thiazide diuretics interact with digoxin and lithium. Therefore monitor serum levels of digoxin and lithium on a regular basis to reduce the risk of toxicity.

Potassium-Sparing Diuretics
- amiloride (Midamor); ♣ Midamor
- eplerenone (Inspra)
- spironolactone (Aldactone); ♣ Novospiroton
- triamterene (Dyrenium)

▥ Indications
Potassium-sparing drugs (i.e., aldosterone antagonists) are weak diuretics when used alone. However, their ability to protect against potassium loss makes them beneficial as adjunct therapy with other, more effective diuretics. They are generally used in combination with a thiazide diuretic or an antihypertensive drug. These drugs preserve both hydrogen and potassium, counteracting the metabolic alkalosis produced when sodium and potassium are eliminated with chloride.

Spironolactone and triamterene are used to treat primary aldosteronism and edema secondary to cirrhosis, nephrotic syndrome, idiopathic edema, and hirsutism. Although once widely used in the treatment of hypertension, spironolactone has lost its popularity because of its adverse effects (i.e., hyperkalemia, gynecomastia). Breast cancer and fibroadenomas have been reported in a few male patients during and after spironolactone therapy. No cause-and-effect relationship has been established, however.

▥ Pharmacodynamics
This class of diuretics is divided into two categories based on their effectiveness in the presence of aldosterone: a portion of the sodium-potassium exchange in the distal tubule is aldosterone dependent and a portion is aldosterone independent. Spironolactone is the major aldosterone antagonist. Competitive antagonism of aldosterone results in inhibition of the sodium-potassium exchange. Spironolactone is effective when mineralocorticoid activity is high, but it has little activity in the absence of aldosterone. The result is an increase in the elimination of 2% to 3% of filtered sodium and chloride. Because spironolactone is a competitive inhibitor, its action is overcome by higher concentrations of aldosterone. Calcium elimination is increased through the direct effect of aldosterone on tubular transport mechanisms.

The aldosterone-independent sodium-potassium exchange is inhibited by triamterene and amiloride, drugs that directly block the uptake of sodium into the distal tubule cell.

Triamterene is effective from the peritubular side. Amiloride acts at the luminal surface of the tubule cell. The voltage-dependent process results in a decrease in sodium permeability and sodium loss without potassium loss.

Eplerenone brings about sustained increases in plasma renin and serum aldosterone, consistent with inhibition of the negative feedback mechanism of aldosterone on renin secretion. The result is an increase in renin activity, with the aldosterone levels not overcoming the effects of the drug on blood pressure. Eplerenone is relatively selective, binding more to mineralocorticoid receptors than to receptors for corticosteroid, progesterone, or androgens, and therefore fewer adverse effects are noted.

▥ Pharmacokinetics
All potassium-sparing diuretics are given by mouth and are absorbed by the GI tract (see Table 42-1). Their onset of action is relatively rapid, and the duration of action increases with multiple doses. Maximum benefits may not be seen for several days after the start of therapy.

The absorption of potassium-sparing diuretics is variable in the GI tract. Spironolactone, as a steroid derivative, is extensively biotransformed by the liver, where it is converted to the metabolite canrenone. Both the spironolactone and its metabolite are 90% protein bound in the plasma. The metabolites of spironolactone appear in both the urine and bile.

Adverse Effects and Contraindications

Because of the potassium-sparing characteristics of these drugs, there is an increased potential for hyperkalemia with chronic use. Other general adverse effects include headache, dizziness, orthostatic hypotension (related to volume depletion), dry mouth, and sore throat. Megaloblastic anemia and folic acid deficiency are sometimes seen with triamterene use. In rare instances, agranulocytosis has occurred with spironolactone. Both spironolactone and amiloride may cause GI distress. A dose-related increase in triglyceride levels is noted with eplerenone.

Spironolactone may also contribute to breast tenderness, menstrual abnormalities, and gynecomastia. Some men who take spironolactone have reported impotence.

Hypersensitivity reactions may occur in some patients and include urticaria, pruritus, rash, erythematous eruptions, and photosensitivity. Anaphylaxis has been reported.

⚠ **Potassium-sparing diuretics are contraindicated for patients with anuria, renal impairment, and severe hepatic dysfunction**. Exercise caution when using in patients with diabetes mellitus and in patients who are either pregnant or lactating.

Drug Interactions

The potassium-sparing diuretics have few drug interactions (see Table 42-2). Those that do occur are related to the use of potassium supplements. ⚠ **Patients receiving a second potassium-sparing diuretic, an angiotensin-converting enzyme inhibitor (ACEI), or an angiotensin II–receptor blocker (ARB) are at higher risk for hyperkalemia and should be monitored closely.**

Dosage Regimens

Dosing with potassium-sparing diuretics is once daily (see Table 42-3). Dosages may be titrated upward as needed.

Lab Considerations

Monitor electrolytes routinely. For patients taking digoxin, have digoxin levels drawn before and periodically throughout therapy to monitor for toxicity.

Loop Diuretics

◆ bumetanide (Bumex); ♣ Burinex
◆ ethacrynic acid (Edecrin); ♣ Edecrin
◆ furosemide (Lasix); ♣ Apo-furosemide, Lasix
◆ torsemide (Demedex)

Indications

Furosemide, the prototype loop diuretic, is the one most commonly used. Loop diuretics are used in the management of edema related to heart failure, renal disease, and hepatic cirrhosis. This class of drugs is useful when greater diuretic potential is desired. Reserve loop diuretics for hypertensive patients who are unresponsive to thiazides or who have chronic renal insufficiency. The ability of loop diuretics to inhibit calcium reabsorption makes them useful in hypercalcemic crises. Loop diuretics may be used in combination with potassium-sparing diuretics to prevent hypokalemia. Furosemide is used in conjunction with mannitol to treat severe cerebral edema.

Torsemide is approved for use in patients with hypertension, chronic renal failure, heart failure, and hepatic cirrhosis.

Pharmacodynamics

Loop diuretics are a group of chemically dissimilar compounds that have similar mechanisms and sites of action. In order for a loop diuretic to be effective, some degree of renal function must exist. Loop diuretics act in the ascending limb of the Loop of Henle to inhibit sodium and chloride reabsorption. The dose-dependent diuresis produced is characterized by increased water, sodium, potassium, chloride, calcium, and magnesium elimination. Twenty percent to 25% of the sodium filtered is eliminated. The increased potassium loss is primarily due to the increase in volume flow rate through distal tubules and increased delivery of sodium to the sodium-potassium exchange pumps.

Loop diuretics decrease left ventricular filling pressure and increase venous capacitance. Increased renal vasodilation permits an increase in the inner cortical and medullary blood flow. Increased medullary flow leads to a decrease in medullary hypertonicity and decreased water reabsorption in the collecting ducts. Evidence suggests this is a prostaglandin-induced process. The use of loop diuretics leads to increased amounts of the vasodilator prostaglandin E_2 by inhibiting the enzyme prostaglandin dehydrogenase. Prostaglandin E_2 also acts directly on the ascending limb to inhibit chloride transport. Hence hemodynamics seem to improve even before significant diuresis has occurred.

Pharmacokinetics

In general, loop diuretics maintain their efficacy in patients with impaired renal function. They are well absorbed with a steep dose-response curve, have a rapid onset of action, and are widely distributed. Although loop diuretics are extensively bound to plasma proteins, they have a strong affinity for an excretory transporter of organic acids, accounting for their relatively short half-lives (see Table 42-1). Furosemide is eliminated essentially unchanged through the kidneys. Loop diuretics cross the placental membranes and also appear in breast milk.

Bumetanide is structurally related to furosemide and is comparable in activity and maximal effects, but it is considerably more potent (40 times) on a weight basis. Bumetanide is biotransformed by the liver. One third of ethacrynic acid is eliminated in the bile and the remainder in the urine.

Torsemide is well absorbed with oral administration, with minor first-pass effect. Serum concentrations reach a peak within 1 hour of administration. Eighty percent of torsemide is removed from the circulation by biotransformation in the liver and clearance of the remainder (about 20% in healthy adults) in the urine. The major metabolite is inactive.

Adverse Effects and Contraindications

Most adverse effects and contraindications to the use of loop diuretics are related to fluid and electrolyte imbalances as a result of diuresis. Volume contraction and loss of electrolytes leads to hypovolemia, hyponatremia, hypokalemia, hyperuricemia, and hyperglycemia. Because potassium is lost along with the water, hypokalemia is a frequent problem. If a patient is also taking digoxin, there is an additional risk for digoxin toxicity (see Chapter 34) and development of arrhythmias (see Chapter 36).

Ototoxicity is most often related to rapid intravenous (IV) administration of loop diuretics. The mechanism involved in the ototoxicity is unclear, but it is thought to result from alterations in electrolytes in the inner ear. Ototoxicity usually manifests as tinnitus, vertigo, hearing impairment, and (rarely) deafness. The potential for ototoxicity is greater with ethacrynic acid and lower with furosemide. Bumetanide is the least ototoxic of the three drugs. The potential for toxicity is of particular concern in patients who are concurrently receiving other ototoxic drugs (e.g., aminoglycoside antibiotics). In general, ototoxicity is a reversible event, disappearing upon withdrawal of the drug. Permanent hearing loss has been reported with ethacrynic acid.

Hyperuricemia is related, in part, to the contraction of fluid volume. However, it is also due to interference with the elimination of uric acid by the excretory transport system of organic acids.

A decrease in glucose tolerance has been reported occasionally. The rationale for its development is unclear; however, it may be associated with diuretic-induced hypokalemia or with insulin activity.

Occasionally, allergic reactions, photosensitivity, leukopenia, anemia, granulocytopenia, and thrombocytopenia occur. All loop diuretics, except ethacrynic acid, have a sulfa component, so patients with sulfa allergy may also have some component of an allergic reaction. Allergic reactions manifest as skin eruptions, exfoliative dermatitis, and jaundice.

Use torsemide with caution in patients who have liver disease, since unanticipated alterations in fluid and electrolyte balance may precipitate mental status changes and hepatic coma. Diuretic use is safer for these patients when carried out in an acute care environment. To reduce the risk for hypokalemia and metabolic alkalosis, an aldosterone antagonist such as spironolactone should be used concurrently.

Loop diuretics must be used cautiously in pregnant women (category B). Only when the potential benefits significantly outweigh the risks would the drug be indicated. The safe use of bumetanide in children younger than 18 years of age has not been established.

Drug Interactions

There are a number of drugs that interact with loop diuretics, resulting in fluid and electrolyte imbalance, altered renal function, and enhancement of the other drugs' effects (see Table 42-2). Although rarely, loop diuretics interact with oral hypoglycemic drugs, increasing the risk for hyperglycemia. When used with aminoglycosides, cisplatin, or other drugs with ototoxicity potential, they may cause additive ototoxicity. Patients taking lithium carbonate or salicylates may experience a decrease in drug elimination, resulting in lithium or salicylate toxicity.

Hypokalemia-induced arrhythmias may develop when digoxin is used concurrently with loop diuretics. When they are used with nonsteroidal antiinflammatory drugs (NSAIDs), the antihypertensive and diuretic characteristics of loop diuretics are reduced. Furosemide interacts with neuromuscular blocking drugs to enhance neuromuscular blockade and with phenytoin to decrease the absorption and effectiveness of furosemide.

Dosage Regimens

Because of their efficacy and potency, keep initial doses of loop diuretics relatively low (see Table 42-3). Although loop diuretics are effective in treating renal impairment, higher than normal doses may be needed as creatinine clearance declines.

For most conditions, the dosage of loop diuretic is reduced as blood pressure falls. Continue therapy until the lowest possible dose of furosemide is reached that is compatible with maximum symptom relief.

Lab Considerations

Loop diuretics can lead to toxicity if taken concurrently with digoxin or lithium. Periodically monitor patients taking these drugs for serum digoxin and lithium levels. Check theophylline levels if the patient is taking both theophylline and furosemide.

Monitor electrolytes, renal and hepatic functioning, and glucose and uric acid levels before and periodically throughout the course of therapy. Patients may develop metabolic alkalosis, hypokalemia, hyponatremia, and hypochloremia because potassium, sodium, and chloride are lost. Calcium and magnesium levels may reflect hypocalcemia and hypomagnesemia. Glucose and uric acid levels may also be elevated.

Osmotic Diuretics

◆ mannitol (Osmitrol)

Indications

The primary use of osmotic diuretics is in preventing acute renal failure. When the GFR falls, as when surgical procedures result in a large blood loss, there is more complete reabsorption of tubular fluid, which can lead to anuria. Maintenance of tubular flow also prevents the precipitation of toxins in the kidneys, as in drug overdose. Decreased tubular flow also favors precipitation of compounds having low solubility and may cause physical damage to the nephrons. In drug overdose, increasing the urine flow rate increases drug elimination. Mannitol is the most commonly used osmotic diuretic.

Osmotic diuretics are also useful in conditions requiring dehydration of cells. For example, intraocular and intracranial pressure elevations can be alleviated with mannitol. Water is drawn toward the osmotically active drug in the plasma.

Avoid osmotic diuretics in the management of heart failure because the addition of osmolar substances to the plasma contributes to edema. Expansion of the extracellular fluid is undesirable as well as risky.

Pharmacodynamics

Osmotics have no specific cellular receptors. Osmotic diuretics are low–molecular weight inert substances that remain in renal tubules to increase plasma osmolality, glomerular filtrate, and tubular fluid (i.e., they increase the osmolality of plasma). The presence of the additional solute and the resulting increase in tubular flow rate interferes with the reabsorption of filtrate and normal urinary concentration. The result is elimination of large amounts of solute and water. Although sodium and water reabsorption is inhibited in the proximal tubule, there are also major effects noted in the thick ascending limb of the loop of Henle.

Pharmacokinetics

Mannitol is rapidly distributed when given intravenously (see Table 42-1), filtered by glomeruli and eliminated unchanged in the urine. The elimination rate is reduced in patients with renal insufficiency.

⫶ Adverse Effects and Contraindications

The common adverse effects of the osmotic diuretic are a transient expansion of plasma volume and an increase in extracellular osmolality. These increases can result in circulatory overload. Patient responses include tachycardia, electrolyte imbalance, volume depletion, and cellular dehydration. The degree of volume expansion is dose dependent.

Other adverse effects of mannitol include headache, nausea, and vomiting. Mannitol can produce rebound elevations of intracranial pressure 8 to 12 hours after diuresis. Chest pain, blurred vision, rhinitis, thirst, and urine retention have been reported. The osmotics cause local irritation at the IV site. If extravasation occurs, thrombophlebitis may result.

In patients with renal impairment, mannitol may accumulate in the blood, causing dangerous shifts in salt and water balance. Mannitol is contraindicated in severely renal impaired patients. Other contraindications to the use of mannitol include active intracranial bleeding and marked dehydration. Safe use of the drugs during pregnancy, lactation, or in children has not been established.

⫶ Drug Interactions

There are no significant drug interactions with mannitol except for its interaction with lithium. Mannitol enhances the elimination of lithium, decreasing its effectiveness (see Table 42-2).

⫶ Dosage Regimens

The toxicity of mannitol depends on how much drug is administered and how much the drug affects fluid balance.

⫶ Lab Considerations

Mannitol increases the elimination of lithium; thus patients should have lithium levels monitored. Monitor serum electrolyte levels before and periodically throughout therapy because mannitol creates the potential for fluid and electrolyte disturbances.

For more information, see the Evolve Resources Bonus Content "Influence of Selected Drugs on Laboratory Values," found at http://evolve.elsevier.com/Gutierrez/pharmacotherapeutics.

CLINICAL REASONING

Treatment Objectives

Treatment objectives for the patient with fluid volume excess are to bring about a negative fluid balance, mobilize excessive extracellular fluid, reduce fluid volume excess, and improve hemodynamics, exercise tolerance, and the quality of care, as well as to prolong survival.

Treatment Options

Nowhere in health care is the axiom "treat the underlying cause" more important than in the treatment of edematous

CASE STUDY	Diuretics

ASSESSMENT	
History of Present Illness	JR is a 65-year-old white male in moderate distress who reports recurring dyspnea and increased edema in his lower extremities. He notes dyspnea on exertion (after ambulating 3 or 4 feet on level surface), orthopnea, and peripheral edema. Harder to breathe when lying down and is up all night urinating. Reports he is adherent with his drug regimen but has problems staying on his sodium-restricted diet; loves his Mexican food and a beer a couple of times a week. No complaints of chest pain (except that caused by dyspnea), diaphoresis, lightheadedness.
Past Health History	JR denies food or drug allergies. He has a previous history of hospitalizations for cardiomyopathy and heart failure, the last one 4 weeks ago. No known history of hypertension. Current drugs: enalapril, 5 mg PO daily; digoxin, 0.25 mg PO daily; furosemide, 80 mg PO twice daily. JR has a past history of smoking but stopped 2 years ago. Denies alcohol use.
Life-Span Considerations	Illnesses that appear relatively minor in older adults may precipitate decompensation that can rapidly progress to a severe state. Patients with history of heart failure and weight gain of as little as 1 pound per week require attention. JR retired at age 58 from a private postal service secondary to health problems. Receives retirement benefits from the postal service and from retired military service. Visits his health care provider on a regular basis. First began having health problems at age 52. Before this, he rarely sought medical care. JR is married and has two children and six grandchildren. Patient receives much emotional support from his family. JR gets his drugs through the Veterans Administration pharmacy.
Physical Exam Findings	*Height:* 5′11″. *Admission weight:* 189 pounds (up 20 pounds up in last 4 weeks). *VS:* BP 118/82, respirations 28/min and shallow, apical heart rate regular but weak. SpO_2 89%, P-96. Wet crackles at the bases of the lungs, jugular vein distention, and 4+ peripheral edema extending to the mid-thigh. S_3 heart sound present.
Diagnostic Testing	Serum Na^+: 142 mg/dL; serum K^+: 2.9 mg/dL; Cl: 95 mg/dL; BUN: 52 mg/dL; creatinine 2.2 mg/dL. Digoxin level 1.2 mg/dL. CXR unchanged from previous hospitalization; left ventricular hypertrophy with curly-B lines noted.

Continued

CASE STUDY Diuretics—Cont'd

DIAGNOSIS: Heart Failure with Peripheral Edema

MANAGEMENT

Treatment Objectives	1. Relieve symptoms of fluid volume excess. 2. Improve exercise tolerance and the quality of life. 3. Improve hemodynamics and prolong survival.
Treatment Options	**Pharmacotherapy** • Furosemide 80 mg IV bolus now • Increase furosemide to 120 mg PO twice daily, assess urine output after each dose, and increase dosage at direction of health care provider if no response. • Continue enalapril at 10 mg PO twice daily. • Metoprolol 50 mg PO twice daily • Potassium chloride 30 mEq PO twice daily **Patient Education** 1. Teach JR about the effects of his cardiomyopathy and heart failure on fluid and electrolyte balance in layman's terms, and the role of sodium and potassium. 2. Advise patient his urine will be draining through the catheter into the bag at the side of the bed. He is to ask for help when getting out of bed so as not to pull on the catheter. 3. Teach JR to take the furosemide as ordered first thing in the morning and again before 6 PM to avoid interrupting sleep to urinate (upon discharge). 4. At times, peak drug action will interfere with work or leisure plans. Help JR to adjust his schedule accordingly. 5. Advise him to take the potassium supplement by mouth each time he takes the furosemide. 6. If he has difficulty taking the drug, work with JR to find a potassium formulation he is willing to take. 7. Provide JR a list of potassium-rich foods and foods with large amounts of sodium that should be avoided. Involve nutritional services if necessary. Caution him to avoid salt substitutes without first contacting the health care provider. 8. Teach JR to keep a daily record of his weight. Report weight gain greater than 2 pounds per day or 5 pounds per week unless otherwise instructed. **Evaluation** After 3 days of IV furosemide, JR's respiratory rate and depth has improved, the 4+ peripheral edema is now 1+, and he has lost 14.6 pounds. Fluid volume excess has improved. He can ambulate with assistance around the hall with minimal dyspnea and without the need to sit down after 10 feet. He no longer needs the bedside table with which to prop his arms when sitting.

CLINICAL REASONING ANALYSIS

Q1. Why did you choose furosemide for JR rather than a thiazide? Doesn't the JNC VII recommend thiazides first-line?

A. Yes. However, furosemide causes fewer metabolic changes than thiazides, and we need to get some fluid off in a short period. Thiazides are mild diuretics and have a longer onset of action; in contrast, a loop diuretic like furosemide has a steep dose-response curve, a rapid onset of action (within 5 minutes when we give it IV), and is widely distributed. It will reach peak efficacy in about 30 minutes. Watch JR's urinary catheter bag after we give him the drug. It will start to fill in within about 30 minutes.

Q2. Couldn't he simply take the furosemide by mouth?

A. JR had a 20-pound weight gain and was having worsening signs and symptoms of heart failure. A fast-acting IV drug was needed.

Q3. But what about his potassium level? Don't we need to worry about that with furosemide?

A. We do. You see his liter of IV fluids? It contains 30 mEq of KCl to help offset the potassium loss from the furosemide. And besides, his potassium level is a bit low. He will also go home on a potassium supplement.

Q4. What do we do about his Mexican food and beer? He is not going to stop them.

A. JR does have problems staying on a sodium-restricted diet. Loop diuretics remain effective in circumstances in which salt intake is high. Let's have nutrition services meet with him before discharge. Perhaps they can help him find a way to reduce the salt intake in his meal while still enjoying his intake.

Q5. His digoxin level was normal. What is the significance of his electrolyte levels?
A. Initial findings of increased BUN and creatinine were indicative of decreased renal blood flow related to his cardiomyopathy and heart failure. The major consideration during diuresis is the loss of potassium. That's why we have KCl in his IV. JR is also on digoxin and would be at risk for digoxin toxicity if he becomes hypokalemic; then we have an entirely different problem on our hands.

Controversy

Diuretics: Drugs of Abuse?

Patients obsessed with weight loss may abuse diuretics. The acute weight loss produced by these drugs has been exploited by some diet clinics that may initiate a program with a diuretic so that dramatic weight loss will occur early. However, this weight loss is short-lived since it is related only to water loss, and returns as soon as the person rehydrates. Such acute weight loss is also occasionally exploited in high school and college wrestling programs. Diuretic use before a match enables a wrestler to meet a weight limit at weigh-in with the athlete rehydrating before wrestling. Such patients may also abuse laxatives.

CLINICAL REASONING ANALYSIS

- A 17-year-old high school student comes to you as a new patient with a request for diuretics. You learn that the patient has been receiving diuretics and other drugs from more than one health care provider. You advise him that use of these drugs for weight control is unjustified, particularly in healthy young athletes with no preexisting conditions. He storms out of your office. What do you do now?

- You are working as a provider in a local urgent care clinic when an obviously very pregnant 19-year-old wobbles in with complaints of ankle and leg edema. During the exam she asks for a diuretic so that her legs and hands don't look like sausages. You note that her BP is 150/90. She has no obstetrician. Is there a best way to address this person's request?

- You are attending your son's college football game. It is hot, with no shade for a reprieve. The mother next to you confides that her athlete son has been abusing drugs but she isn't sure which ones. She says he seems to be always in the bathroom urinating and is complaining of muscle weakness and cramps, constipation, nighttime voiding (the toilet is always flushing), impaired ability to concentrate. He hasn't told his coach because he doesn't want to be benched. What do you do?

states. Diuretics are used as adjuncts to specific other therapies. General measures used to promote mobilization of edematous fluid include bed rest and moderate sodium restriction (i.e., 1 to 2 grams of sodium chloride per day).

▮ Patient Variables

The use of diuretics for quick weight control is not justified in the absence of edematous conditions. This abuse has been observed in some obese individuals and in athletes who must meet a weight limit.

Some patients are at risk for hypokalemia, an inevitable consequence of the effective action of thiazide and loop diuretics. Patients with high circulating aldosterone levels, such as those seen in primary hyperaldosteronism, are already eliminating too much potassium. Patients with heart disease who are taking digoxin may have arrhythmias related to hypokalemia. High doses of long-acting diuretics may be a problem because the patient is already potassium-depleted. Concurrent therapy with corticosteroids or potent laxatives further contributes to potassium loss. To make matters worse, hypokalemia impairs glucose tolerance in patients with diabetes mellitus.

Consider drug therapy for patients with mild to moderate heart failure, after the disorder is diagnosed and acute reversible precipitating factors are ruled out. Symptoms warranting therapy include shortness of breath, decreased exercise tolerance, orthopnea, and nocturnal polyuria.

Preexisting conditions that necessitate caution in the use of diuretics include a history of gout, renal calculi, and seizure disorders. Furthermore, because most patients receive diuretics for a chronic condition, their exposure to the drugs is extended, increasing the potential for fluid and electrolyte imbalances and toxicity.

LIFE-SPAN CONSIDERATIONS

Children and Adolescents. In infants and children, the most common causes of heart failure are congenital heart disorders and rheumatic fever. These conditions result in decreased renal blood flow and urinary insufficiency. Dosage considerations include the age and size of the child with attention directed toward treating the underlying cause of the edema.

Older Adults. Owing to altered physiology and underlying comorbid diseases, older adults are more sensitive to diuretics and tend to experience more adverse effects than younger people. The renal function of the older adult is diminished because of the normal changes of aging, and thus he or she may be unable to handle shifts in fluid and electrolyte balance. Check serum electrolyte levels (especially potassium) at least every 3 to 4 months.

▮ Drug Variables

Thiazides are the preferred drug to reduce blood pressure unless there are compelling or specific indications for using another drug. The antihypertensive action requires several days to produce effects. The duration of action of thiazides requires a single daily dose to control blood pressure. Combination therapy with thiazide and a potassium-sparing diuretic may be prudent when potassium levels are less than 4 mEq/L, or when a low potassium level may potentiate toxicity, as in patients concurrently taking the cardiac glycoside digoxin (Box 42-2).

Hydrochlorothiazide is useful only when heart failure exists concomitantly with hypertension. The diuretic effect of hydrochlorothiazide is not always maintained for an extended period. Metolazone, on the other hand, is useful in diuretic-resistant states. Even in low doses, when metolazone is combined with furosemide, a dramatic diuresis may occur.

BOX 42-2

Combination Diuretics

Thiazide and Thiazide-Like Diuretic Combinations
ACEIs
- captopril + hydrochlorothiazide (Capozide)
- benazepril + hydrochlorothiazide (Lotensin HCT)
- enalapril + hydrochlorothiazide (Vaseretic)
- fosinopril + hydrochlorothiazide (Monopril HCT)
- lisinopril + hydrochlorothiazide (Prinzide, Zestoretic)
- moexipril + hydrochlorothiazide (Uniretic)
- quinapril + hydrochlorothiazide (Accuretic)

Angiotensin II–Receptor Blockers
- candesartan + hydrochlorothiazide (Atacand HCT)
- eprosartan + hydrochlorothiazide (Teveten HCT)
- irbesartan + hydrochlorothiazide (Avalide)
- losartan + hydrochlorothiazide (Hyzaar)
- olmesartan + hydrochlorothiazide (Benicar HCT)
- telmisartan + hydrochlorothiazide (Micardis HCT)
- valsartan + hydrochlorothiazide (Diovan HCT)

Beta Blockers
- atenolol + chlorthalidone (Tenoretic)
- labetalol + hydrochlorothiazide (Normozide)
- metoprolol + hydrochlorothiazide (Lopressor HCT)
- pindolol + hydrochlorothiazide
- propranolol + hydrochlorothiazide (Inderide)
- timolol + hydrochlorothiazide (Timolide)

Centrally Acting Antihypertensives
- clonidine + chlorthalidone (Combipress)
- guanethidine + hydrochlorothiazide (Esimil)
- methyldopa + chlorothiazide (Aldoclor)
- methyldopa + hydrochlorothiazide (Aldoril)

Potassium-Sparing Diuretics
- amiloride + hydrochlorothiazide (Moduretic)
- spironolactone + hydrochlorothiazide (Aldactazide, Spiractazide)
- triamterene + hydrochlorothiazide (Dyazide, Maxzide)

Vasodilator
- hydralazine + hydrochlorothiazide (Apresazide, Apresoline-Esidrix)

Much depends on the lipid-solubility of thiazides and their volume of distribution. There is a flat dose-response curve with thiazides, which means that the toxic and therapeutic levels never meet. As a result, these drugs have a wide margin of safety. The greater volume of distribution leads to lowered renal clearance and longer duration of action. Although chlorthalidone has a slightly longer duration of action than others, no real benefit is achieved because thiazide diuretics are all dosed once daily and are well tolerated.

The disadvantages of thiazides include a relatively low potency and resistance to its effects in the presence of renal impairment. Furthermore, they have no therapeutic value in patients with a GFR of less than 25 to 30 mL/min. Drug-induced hyperuricemia may produce gouty arthritis or uric acid stones.

Combination diuretic therapy is based on the principle of sequential blockade of nephron sites. For example, a diuretic that works at the loop of Henle or in the early distal tubules combined with one that works at the late distal tubules reduces the loss of potassium caused by loop and thiazide diuretics. The combination diuretics are most often used for patients who develop resistance to one diuretic, or when it

is desirable to nullify potassium loss by adding a drug that acts at another site.

Potassium-sparing diuretics, such as spironolactone, may be used as monotherapy or in addition to other diuretics in the treatment of heart failure or cirrhosis. They are particularly useful when hypokalemia persists despite the use of ACEI. In treatment of hypertension, combination therapy with thiazide and triamterene or amiloride is most common. In addition, these drugs have fewer adverse effects and are less likely to cause hyperkalemia.

Furosemide, a loop diuretic, is usually preferred over thiazide diuretics for fluid volume excess because it is more effective, has a broader dose-response curve, faster onset, and greater diuresis, and causes fewer metabolic changes than thiazides when given in equivalent natriuretic dosages. These variables allow for greater accuracy in titrating a dose to a particular patient, and there are fewer GI adverse effects. Administer IV loop diuretics slowly, following the manufacturer's recommendations for administration time. Slow administration rates decrease the risk of ototoxicity.

There are several other drug groups, in addition to diuretics, that should not be used alone to treat heart failure but in combination with other life-saving therapies. Diuretics relieve symptoms and prolong life, much as ACEIs (see Chapter 37) and beta blockers do. ACEIs taken with digoxin improve cardiac output; however, the use of ACEIs in the absence of furosemide may be ineffective. ACEIs, in combination with hydralazine and isosorbide prolong survival, although ACEIs have been found to be superior to either hydralazine or isosorbide alone. Diuretics, ACEIs, digoxin, and nitrates all reduce preload.

Patient Education

Adherence is best encouraged by teaching the patient about the disease process and the drug used to treat the problem. Include family members or significant others in the teaching. Information to be included is the name of the drug, the dose, why the drug is being given, and what can be expected to occur as a result of taking the drug. Instruct the patient on any special precautions and adverse effects. Lastly, advise the patient to expect an increase in urinary frequency, and in the amount of urine produced.

All diuretics are best taken in the morning or early after- ▲ **noon so the effects are complete before the patient's normal sleep time.** By taking it early in the day, the drug has generally dissipated before bedtime, thus avoiding interruption of sleep patterns. If the dosage regimen seems to interfere with sleep patterns or if there appears to be no improvement in the patient's condition, a review of the drug regimen may be needed.

Advise the patient to remain close to bathroom facilities the first few hours after taking the drug. At times, the peak period of drug activity interferes with work or leisure plans. Help patients adjust their schedules so as not to be caught in embarrassing situations. A patient caught in an embarrassing situation is not likely to adhere with therapy for long. Statistically, diuretics are associated with urinary incontinence, particularly in older adult women.

Patients on diuretics are at risk for electrolyte imbalance; therefore, it is important that they recognize the signs and symptoms that may occur with these disturbances. Rapid heart rate, rapid respirations, dizziness, muscle weakness, abdominal cramps, nausea, and vomiting are all symptoms that should be reported.

Postural hypotension can occur in patients taking diuretics. This problem may be related to the drug itself or to hypovolemia. It is important that the patient sit up a few minutes before standing to minimize these effects. Advise patients to protect themselves from the sun and to report any episodes of delayed sunburn or the development of a rash.

With the exception of the potassium-sparing diuretics, potassium is depleted with diuretic therapy. Therefore, dietary teaching is an important part of the patient teaching plan. A dietitian may assist with the teaching in some cases. Hypokalemia can be avoided by consuming foods high in potassium and by using potassium supplements. In patients receiving potassium-sparing diuretics or ACEIs, these same foods need to be avoided or eaten only in moderation. Salt substitutes are high in potassium and should be avoided also. Teach the patient to identify and avoid foods high in sodium content. Fast foods, canned foods, and prepackaged foods are often high in sodium and sugar. Many of the beneficial foods require more time and effort for preparation and are more costly.

Give the patient guidelines to help identify his or her response to therapy. Daily weights can be used to monitor diuretic response. Instruct patients to weigh themselves on the same scale first thing in the morning, after voiding but before eating, and while wearing similar clothing each day. The patient should have an idea of the target weight and when to notify the health care provider. A weight gain of more than 2 pounds daily should be reported; in older adults, 1 pound/week may be significant. Always evaluate for continuous weight gain.

Evaluation

Evaluation of the effectiveness of diuretic therapy is based on the original treatment objectives. In most cases, the criteria include an informed patient and family who understand the disease processes and the treatment regimen; a reduction in symptoms as a result of compliance with the plan of care; dietary controls; and minimum adverse effects related to therapy. The decrease in uncomfortable symptoms such as swollen feet and legs, puffy hands, or dyspnea on exertion may be sufficient incentive to comply with the regimen.

Evaluate the patient for fluid volume deficit as well as for drug resistance. In the face of a shrunken intravascular volume, the part of the tubular system not affected by the diuretic reacts by reabsorbing more sodium. For this reason, it is important to obtain answers to the following questions:

- Is the patient adherent with sodium restriction guidelines?
- Are the optimal drug and dosage being used?
- Is complete bed rest required?
- Are there any electrolyte imbalances that should be corrected?
- Is the patient's general cardiovascular status optimal?

Also check for signs of fluid deficit, particularly if the patient has overresponded to the diuretic therapy. Changes in blood pressure or vital signs may be the first indication that the patient is having excessive diuresis. Orthostatic hypotension may be a problem, putting the patient at a greater risk of falling. Other signs and symptoms of fluid volume deficit include poor skin turgor, dry skin and mucous membranes, weight loss, tachycardia, reduced urine output, and rapid respirations.

KEY POINTS

- The volume and composition of body fluid is controlled by three processes: glomerular filtration, tubular reabsorption, and tubular secretion.
- Electrolytes filtered through the glomeruli include sodium, potassium, calcium, magnesium, bicarbonate, chloride, and phosphate.
- Alterations in cardiac, renal, hepatic, or endocrine function are primary etiologies of edema. Other causes include pregnancy, premenstrual tension, and drug-induced causes.
- Fluid volume excess causes an abnormal accumulation of fluid in tissues or cavities of the body, resulting in peripheral and periorbital edema, a bounding pulse, pulmonary crackles, and dyspnea without exertion.
- Heart failure decreases renal blood flow, which, in turn, decreases the GFR, resulting in the retention of sodium and water.
- Liver disease increases the pressure within the portal vein. Along with decreased albumin synthesis, the result is decreased oncotic pressure, which leads to underperfused kidneys, which in turn respond by retaining sodium and water.
- The damaged glomeruli of nephrotic syndrome hold back sodium and permit plasma proteins to leak into the tubules. Generalized edema results from hypoalbuminemia, and this problem, in turn, leads to hypoperfusion of the kidney.
- Before and throughout diuretic therapy, hemoglobin and hematocrit, electrolytes, glucose, blood urea nitrogen, creatinine, serum protein levels, uric acid, cholesterol, and triglyceride levels should be measured.
- Combination diuretic therapy is based on the principle of sequential blockade of nephron sites.

- Combination therapy is most often used for patients who develop resistance to one diuretic or when it is desirable to nullify potassium loss by adding a drug that acts at a different site.
- Dietary restrictions of salt and adequate intake of potassium are essential.
- Hydrochlorothiazide is used as first line drug for hypertension. The drug may be useful in patients with heart failure and only mild edema.
- Loop diuretics are usually preferred over thiazides because they are more effective, have a broader dose-response curve and faster onset, provide greater diuresis, and cause less metabolic changes when given in equivalent doses for patients with heart or renal failure.
- Potassium-sparing diuretics such as spironolactone may be used in addition to other diuretics. Spironolactone is used at low dosages in treatment of heart failure and often at low or high dosages to manage ascites associated with liver failure.
- Patients at risk for hypokalemia include those with high circulating aldosterone levels; those with hypokalemia who are taking digoxin, or who have diabetes; and those on long-acting diuretics or who are receiving concurrent corticosteroids or potent laxatives.
- All diuretics are best if taken in the morning or early afternoon so the effects are complete before the patient's normal sleep time.
- Information to be included in the teaching plan are the name of the drug, the dose, why the drug is being given, and what can be expected to occur as a result of taking the drug.
- Hypokalemia can be avoided by consuming foods high in potassium and the possible use of potassium supplements. In patients on potassium-sparing diuretics or ACEI these same foods need to be avoided or eaten only in moderation. Teach the patient to identify and avoid foods high in potassium.

■ Patients receiving diuretics are at risk for fluid and electrolyte imbalance; therefore, it is important that they recognize the signs and symptoms of disturbances and be aware of appropriate interventions.

■ Effectiveness of diuretic therapy is evaluated by accurately monitoring physical exam parameters, blood pressure, weight, fluid and electrolyte balance, and laboratory values.

Bibliography

Burger, H., de Laet, C., and van Daele, P., et al. (1998). Risk factors for increased bone loss in an elderly population: the Rotterdam study. *American Journal of Epidemiology, 147*(9), 871–879.

Hardman, J, Limbird, L., and Gilman, A. (Eds.). (2001). *Goodman and Gilman's the pharmacologic basis of therapeutics* (10th ed.). New York: McGraw-Hill.

LaCroix, A., Ott, S., and Ichikawa, L. (2000). Low-dose hydrochlorothiazide and preservation of bone mineral density in older adults: A randomized, double-blind, placebo-controlled trial. *Annals of Internal Medicine, 133*(7), 516–526.

Lindon, M., Wing, M., and Christopher, M., et al. (2003). A comparison of outcomes with angiotensin-converting–enzyme inhibitors and diuretics for hypertension in the elderly. *New England Journal of Medicine, 348*(7), 583–592.

Logan, A. (2006). Dietary sodium intake and its relation to human health: A summary of the evidence. *Journal of the American College of Nutrition, 25*(3), 165–169.

Katzung, B. (2005). *Basic and clinical pharmacology* (9th ed.). New York: Lange Medical Books.

McCance, K., and Huether, S. (2002). *Pathophysiology: The biologic basis for disease in adults and children* (4th ed.). St. Louis: Mosby.

NHLBI's National High Blood Pressure Education Program. (2003). The Seventh Report of the Joint National Committee on Prevention, Detection, Evaluation, and Treatment of High Blood Pressure. Available online: www.nhlbi.nih.gov/guidelines/hypertension/index.htm. Accessed May 8, 2007.

Reid, I., Ames, R., and Orr-Walker, B., et al. (2000). Hydrochlorothiazide reduces loss of cortical bone in normal postmenopausal women: A randomized controlled trial. *American Journal of Medicine, 109*(5), 362–370.

Sawicki, P., and McGauran, N. (2006). Have ALLHAT, ANBP2, ASCOT-BPLA, and so forth improved our knowledge about better hypertension care? *Hypertension, 48*(1), 1–7.

Shah, S., Anjum, S., and Littler, W. (2004). Use of diuretics of cardiovascular diseases: (1) Heart failure. *Postgraduate Medical Journal, 80*(942), 201–205.

Starling, H., and Vischer, M. (1927). The regulation of the output of the heart. *Journal of Physiology, 62*, 243–261.

43

Drugs Used for Bladder, Prostate, and Erectile Dysfunction

Urinary incontinence can be arranged into two categories to better define its cause. Distinguishing between the failure to store urine and the failure to empty it is a simple method by which to classify bladder dysfunction. This system conceptualizes lower urinary tract function as depending on the interaction of the bladder and bladder outlet (sphincter) for normal urine storage and elimination. A defect in either bladder or sphincter function results in either failure to store or failure to empty. Mixed bladder and sphincter dysfunction may also be responsible for patient symptoms.

Incontinence can also be fixed or transient. Transient incontinence ordinarily has a defined, sudden onset and often has a discrete cause. Fixed or established causes of incontinence can be subdivided into several broad headings with differential diagnoses based on patient sex. These etiologies can affect urine storage, bladder emptying, or both (Table 43-1).

OVERACTIVE BLADDER

EPIDEMIOLOGY AND ETIOLOGY

Overactive bladder (OAB) is also known as detrusor instability, detrusor hyperreflexia, spasmodic bladder, unstable bladder, and urge incontinence. OAB is a syndrome of increased urinary urgency, daytime frequency, and nocturia, with or without urge incontinence. The key symptom is urgency, a sudden urge to urinate that interrupts all other activities until the bladder is emptied or incontinence occurs. Daytime frequency (i.e., more than eight episodes daily, or urinating every 2 hours or less while awake) and nocturia (i.e., three or more episodes nightly) are also seen in the majority of patients.

According to the National Overactive Bladder Evaluation Program, OAB affects almost 17% of the U.S. adult population, or an estimated 33 million people. Of these individuals, approximately 37% meet the criteria for OAB with urge incontinence. Although OAB can develop in anyone at any age, it is more common in women and older adults. Despite the high prevalence of urinary incontinence, fewer than one half of community-dwelling persons with OAB consult a health care provider about the problem.

When patients do seek help, the majority of cases are classified as idiopathic, although identifiable underlying causes of OAB include nerve damage caused by abdominal or pelvic trauma or surgery; bladder calculi; adverse effects of drugs (Box 43-1); and neurologic diseases such as multiple sclerosis, Parkinson's disease, stroke, and spinal cord lesions. Other conditions can produce symptoms similar to overactive bladder, including urinary tract infection (UTI) and normal pressure hydrocephalus.

PATHOPHYSIOLOGY

The ability to retain urine relies on normal function of the nervous system, the kidneys, the bladder, the bladder sphincters, and the physical and psychologic ability to recognize and appropriately respond to the urge to urinate. The bladder's ability to fill and store urine requires a functional sphincter and a stable bladder wall muscle (i.e., detrusor muscle).

Unlike the smooth muscle of the gastrointestinal (GI) tract or ureters, the detrusor muscle has a nearly 1:1 ratio of nerve receptors to smooth muscle cells. Normally, the detrusor muscle remains in a relaxed state during bladder filling and storage, with contraction during voluntary micturition. On average, the bladder holds 350 mL to 550 mL of urine. When approximately 200 mL of urine fills the bladder, the first stimulus to void occurs. While the bladder continues to fill, the nervous system alerts the patient of the need to urinate. Contraction of the detrusor muscle forces urine out of the bladder. Simultaneously, the urinary sphincter must be able to relax to allow the urine to exit. In patients with OAB, however, the layered, smooth detrusor muscle contracts spastically before the bladder has reached the filling capacity necessary to stimulate micturition, increasing the risk of urge incontinence.

There are several interventions that can be used to manage OAB with urge incontinence. The treatment option chosen varies depending on symptom severity and the extent to which symptoms interfere with the activities of daily living. There are three primary treatment modalities for OAB: antimuscarinic therapy, bladder retraining, and surgery.

PHARMACOTHERAPEUTIC OPTIONS

Antimuscarinic Drugs

FIRST-GENERATION ANTIMUSCARINIC DRUGS
- oxybutynin (Ditropan, Ditropan XL, Oxytrol); ◆ Ditropan, Ditropan XL
- tolterodine (Detrol, Detrol LA); ◆ Detrol, Detrol LA

SECOND-GENERATION ANTIMUSCARINIC DRUGS
- darifenacin (Enablex); ◆ Enablex
- solifenacin (Vesicare); ◆ Vesicare
- trospium (Sanctura); ◆ Sanctura

Indications

Antimuscarinics have been the drugs of choice for management of OAB over the last 30 years. Generic oxybutynin was the most commonly prescribed drug through the late 1990s. Immediate-release tolterodine appeared soon thereafter followed by an extended-release and a transdermal formulation of oxybutynin. Unlike first-generation drugs, second-generation antimuscarinic drugs specifically target the bladder and produce potentially fewer adverse effects and safety concerns.

TABLE 43-1 Types of Incontinence

	Failure to Store	Failure to Empty
Females	Bladder dysfunction • Detrusor instability or hyperreflexia • Decreased bladder compliance • Fistula • Urgency-related bladder decompensation Outlet dysfunction • Stress incontinence • Intrinsic sphincter deficiency	Bladder dysfunction • Detrusor decompensation • Bladder denervation; absent or poorly sustained contraction Outlet dysfunction • Neurogenic sphincter dysfunction • Iatrogenic urethral obstruction

Males	Bladder dysfunction
	• Detrusor instability or hyperreflexia
	• Detrusor instability secondary to outlet obstruction
	• Decreased bladder compliance
	• Bladder decompensation with overflow incontinence
	Outlet dysfunction
	• Stress incontinence
	    • Iatrogenic (after prostatectomy)
	    • Neurogenic denervation
		Bladder dysfunction
		• Bladder decompensation
		• Bladder denervation
		Outlet dysfunction
		• Benign prostatic hyperplasia with obstruction
		• Neurogenic sphincter dysfunction

BOX 43-1

Drugs Affecting Bladder Function

Irritant Adverse Effects

ACEIs	Cough (stress incontinence)
Antidepressants, Antipsychotics, Sedative-hypnotics	Sedation, retention, overflow incontinence
Alcohol	Sedation, frequency, OAB
Alpha blockers	Decreased urethral tone (stress incontinence)
Alpha agonists	Increased urethral tone, retention (overflow incontinence)
Anticholinergics	Retention (overflow incontinence)
Beta agonists	Inhibited detrusor function, retention (overflow incontinence)
Caffeine	Frequency, OAB with urge incontinence
Calcium channel blockers	Retention (overflow incontinence)
Diuretics	Frequency, OAB with urge incontinence
Opioid analgesics	Retention, constipation, sedation, OAB with overflow incontinence

ACEI, Angiotensin-converting enzyme inhibitor; OAB, overactive bladder.

Pharmacodynamics

Although the majority of cholinergic receptors found in the detrusor muscle are of the M_2 subtype, normal micturition and urinary bladder contraction is primarily the responsibility of the M_3 receptors. Most of the approved drugs for OAB target these M_3 receptors. Antimuscarinics exert an antispasmodic effect on the detrusor muscle, inhibiting the muscarinic action of acetylcholine and thereby preventing unwanted contractions and urine leakage. In patients with involuntary contractions, antimuscarinic drugs increase the volume allowed to accumulate before the first contraction occurs, decrease the amplitude of this abnormal contraction, and increase total bladder capacity.

The role of M_2 receptors has not been completely established, but they are thought to functionally oppose sympathetic-mediated detrusor relaxation. All current anticholinergic drugs lack true specificity for only the muscarinic receptors in the bladder, although some manufacturers claim the drugs have functional selectivity and specificity to target the bladder over other end-organs, such as the salivary glands. Blocking effects do not occur at skeletal neuromuscular junctions or autonomic ganglia (antinicotinic effects).

Pharmacokinetics

Food has no effect on the multidose pharmacokinetics on darifenacin. It is 98% bound to plasma proteins and extensively biotransformed by the liver with oral dosing. Darifenacin is biotransformed primarily by the CYP450 enzyme systems, particularly CYP 3A4 and 2D6. Sixty percent of the metabolites are eliminated in the urine and 40% in the feces (Table 43-2).

Transdermal oxybutynin is a racemate of (+) and (−) isomers. It is transported across intact skin and into the systemic circulation by passive diffusion. Absorption of oxybutynin is bioequivalent when the patch is applied to the abdomen, the buttocks, or the hip. Steady-state conditions are reached during the second application. The transdermal formulation bypasses the first-pass GI and hepatic biotransformation, thereby reducing the formation of the metabolite.

After oral administration of oxybutynin, presystemic first-pass effects result in a bioavailability of approximately 6% with higher plasma concentrations of the metabolite compared to the parent drug. The CYP450 enzyme systems, especially CYP 3A4, are responsible for the biotransformation of oxybutynin, which occurs primarily in the liver and the intestinal wall. Less than 0.1% of the administered dose is eliminated unchanged in the urine.

Tolterodine is highly bound to α1-acid glycoproteins. It is gradually, but more extensively biotransformed in slow metabolizers than in rapid metabolizers, resulting in significantly higher serum levels of the parent drug compared with metabolites. Tolterodine is eliminated primarily through the urine, with a small amount in the feces.

Like tolterodine, solifenacin is primarily bound to α1-acid glycoproteins. It is highly distributed to non–central nervous system (CNS) tissues. The drug is extensively biotransformed in the liver by way of CYP 3A4 system; however, alternate

PHARMACOKINETICS
TABLE 43-2 Drugs for Bladder, Prostate, and Erectile Dysfunction

Drug	Route	Onset	Peak	Duration	PB%	t ½	BioA %
ANTIMUSCARINICS							
darifenacin	PO	2–4 hr	7 hr	UA	98	13–19 hr	15–19
oxybutynin ER	Patch	48 hr	72 hr	96 hr	UA	12.4–13.2 hr	156; 187*
oxybutynin XL	PO	30–60 min	4–6 hr	6–10 hr	UA	2–5 hr	156; 187*
solifenasin	PO	Slow	3–8 hr	UA	UA	45–68 hr	90
tolterodine	PO	Slow	2–6 hr	UA	96	8.8–9.9 hr; 5.9 and 4.0 hr†	77
trospium	PO	Slow	5–6 hr	UA	50–85	15–21 hr	5–10
ALPHA BLOCKERS							
alfuzosin	PO	Rapid	8 hr	UA	82–90	10 hr	49
doxazosin	PO	1–2 hr	2–6 hr	24 hr	98	22 hr	UA
prazosin	PO	Rapid	3 hr	UA	>90	2–3 hr	90
tamsulosin	PO	UA	5 days	UA	94–99	9–15 hr	>90
terazosin	PO	2–6 wk	UA	24 hr	94	12 hr	UA
5α-REDUCTASE INHIBITORS							
dutasteride‡	PO	24 hr	—	3–8 wk	99	5 wk	UA
finasteride	PO	24 hr	1–2 days	5–7 days	90	6–8 hr	UA
DIRECT-ACTING CHOLINERGIC							
bethanecol	PO	30–90 min	1 hr	6 hr	UA	3.5 hr	Low
PHOSPHODIASTERASE INHIBITORS							
sildenafil	PO	Rapid	30–120 min	<4 hr	96	4 hr	40
tadalafil	PO	30 min	30 min–6 hr	36 hr	94	17.5 hr	UA
vardenafil	PO	Rapid	30–120 min	<4 hr	95	4–5 hr	15

*The relative bioavailabilities of R- and S-oxybutynin are 156% and 187%, respectively. Antimuscarinic effects of oxybutynin resides primarily with the R-isomer. Efficacy begins to decline 1–2 hr after removal of patch.
†Mean half-life of tolterodine with half-life of metabolites.
‡Outcomes of effective dutasteride therapy may not be known for up to 6 months.
BioA, Bioavailability; *PB,* protein binding; *PO,* by mouth; *t½,* half-life; *UA,* unavailable.

pathways exist. Less than 15% is eliminated in the urine as unchanged drug. It is not known whether tolterodine is eliminated in breast milk.

Administration of trospium with a high-fat meal results in reduced absorption, with the area under the curve (AUC) and maximum concentration (C_{max}) values 70% to 80% lower than those seen when trospium is administered on an empty stomach. Of the dose absorbed, metabolites account for approximately 40% of the eliminated dose. The mean renal clearance for trospium is 4 times higher than the average glomerular filtration rate (GFR), indicating that active tubular secretion is a major route of elimination for trospium.

⦀ Adverse Effects and Contraindications

Most treatment-related adverse events of antimuscarinics are described as mild or moderate in intensity but include the typical anticholinergic adverse effects of blurry vision, cognition impairment, dry mouth, dizziness, fatigue, constipation, dyspepsia, and possible urinary retention. **High environmental temperatures may cause heat intolerance, fever, and diaphoresis. Antimuscarinics must be used with great caution in patients with QT prolongation, although the occurrence of QT abnormalities is primarily related to plasma concentration of the drug.** Antimuscarinics are contraindicated for use in patients who have urinary or gastric retention, gastroparesis or other GI mobility problems, or uncontrolled narrow-angle glaucoma, and in patients at risk for these conditions. Antimuscarinics are also contraindicated for use in patients with known hypersensitivity to these compounds and should be used with caution in patients with

dementia and Alzheimer's disease. Antimuscarinics are pregnancy category B and C drugs.

⦀ Drug Interactions

Antimuscarinics, when used concomitantly with other anticholinergic drugs or with drugs that cause dry mouth, constipation, somnolence, and other anticholinergic-like effects, can cause increased frequency and/or severity of the effects (Table 43-3). Anticholinergic drugs may also affect the absorption of drugs administered concurrently, owing to the anticholinergic effects on GI motility.

⦀ Dosage Regimen

Dosages of the antimuscarinics used for OAB are identified in Table 43-4. Most of the drugs are dosed once to twice daily. Overall, patients tend to tolerate extended-release better than immediate-release formulations. Regardless of the drug and formulation chosen, adjust the dosage to achieve a balance between efficacy and tolerability.

⦀ Lab Considerations

No lab monitoring is necessary with oxybutynin formulations.

CLINICAL REASONING

Treatment Objectives

The goal in the treatment of OAB with urge incontinence is aimed at increasing the storage ability of the bladder, relaxing involuntary contractions, and improving bladder function. An overview of OAB management is summarized in Box 43-2.

GENITOURINARY

DRUG INTERACTIONS

TABLE **43-3** Drugs for Bladder and Erectile Dysfunction

Drug	Interacting Drugs	Interaction
ANTIMUSCARINICS		
darifenacin	Azole antifungals, clarithromycin, flecainide, midazolam, nelfinavir, nefazodone, ritonavir, TCAs, thioridazine, Other anticholinergic drugs	Increases AUC for darifenacin
	digoxin	Increases digoxin levels
oxybutynin chloride	amitriptyline, Anticholinergics, Azole antifungals, Antiparkinsonian drugs, chlorpromazine, digoxin, diphenhydramine, Macrolides, Muscle relaxants, Sedative-hypnotics	Increases anticholinergic adverse effects of both drugs
solifenasin	Azole antifungals	Increases mean AUC of solifenasin
tolterodine	fluoxetine	Inhibits biotransformation of tolterodine
	Azole antifungals, cyclosporine, Macrolide antibiotics, vinblastine	Increases C_{max} and AUC of tolterodine
ALPHA BLOCKERS		
alfuzosin	Alpha blocking drugs (prazosin, terazosin, doxazosin, tamsulosin)	Additive effects
	cimetidine	Increases concentration alfuzosin
doxazosin	Alcohol, Antihypertensive drugs, Nitrates	Additive hypotension
	NSAIDs, Estrogens	Decreases antihypertensive effects
	clonidine	Decreases antihypertensive effects of clonidine
prazosin	NSAIDs, Estrogens, Sympathomimetics	Decreases effect of prazosin
	Alcohol, Antihypertensive drugs, Nitrates	Additive hypotension
	Licorice	Sodium and water retention and potassium loss
tamsulosin	Alpha blocking drugs (prazosin, terazosin, doxazosin, alfuzosin)	Additive effects
	cimetidine	Increases effects of tamulosin
	warfarin	Alters effects of warfarin
terazosin	Alcohol, Antihypertensive drugs, Nitrates	Additive hypotension
	NSAIDs, Estrogens, Sympathomimetics	Decreases effects of terazosin
MUSCARINIC AGONIST		
bethanechol	Cholinesterase inhibitors	Synergistic effects with risk of toxicity
	atropine, procainamide, quinidine	Decreases effect of bethanechol
	Ganglionic blockers	Severe hypotension
PHOSPHODIASTERASE INHIBITORS		
sildenafil, tadalafil, vardenafil	Nitrates	Potentiates effects of nitrates
	cimetidine, erythromycin, itraconazole, ketoconazole, Protease inhibitors	Significant increase in sildenafil levels
	Alpha blockers	Increases risk for symptomatic hypotension
	rifampin	Reduces sildenafil levels

AUC, Area under the curve; C_{max}, maximum concentration; NSAIDs, nonsteroidal antiinflammatory drugs; TCA, tricyclic antidepressant.

DOSAGE

TABLE **43-4** Drugs for Bladder, Prostate, and Erectile Dysfunction

Drug	Dosage	Implications
ANTIMUSCARINICS		
darifenacin	*Adult:* 7.5 mg ER formulation PO daily. May titrate in 2 wk to 15 mg daily based on patient response	No dosage adjustment needed for older adults or those with renal disorders.
oxybutynin	*Adult:* 5 mg IR formulation PO 2–4 times daily. Max: 20 mg/day –or– ER formulation: 5 mg PO daily. Maximum: 30 mg/day –or– 39 cm³ patch formulation applied every 3–4 days	Adjust dosage to achieve balance between efficacy and tolerability. Biologically inert portion of XL formulation remains intact during intestinal transit and is visible in stool.
solifenasin	*Adult:* 5–10 mg ER formulation PO once daily	Do not exceed 5-mg daily dosage in patients with renal disease.
tolterodine	*Adult:* 1–2 mg IR formulation PO once-twice daily based on patient response –or– 2–4 mg ER formulation PO daily	May take without regard to food.
trospium	*Adult:* 20 mg IR formulation PO twice daily	Take at least 1 hr before meals or on an empty stomach.
ALPHA BLOCKERS		
alfuzosin	*Adult:* 10 mg PO once daily	Give 30 min after same meal each day.
doxazosin	*Adult:* 1 mg PO initially.	May increase to 16 mg daily (especially in hypertensive patients).
prazosin	*Adult:* 1 mg PO 2–3 times daily initially	Dosage adjusted based on patient response.
tamsulosin	*Adult:* 0.4 mg PO once daily. May increase to 0.8 mg if inadequate response in 2–4 wk	Take 30 min after same meal each day.
terazosin	*Adult:* 1–5 mg PO daily. Max: 20 mg/day. May give in divided doses	Take at HS. If therapy is interrupted, retitrate using 1 mg dose at HS.
yohimbine	*Adult:* 5.4 mg PO 3 times daily	Yohimbine is indicated as a sympatholytic and mydriatic. It may have activity as an aphrodisiac.

5α-REDUCTASE INHIBITORS		
dutasteride	*Adult:* 0.5 mg PO daily	**Because of risk to male fetus, women who are or may become pregnant should not handle tablets or capsules or be exposed to patient's semen.**
finasteride	*Adult:* 5 mg PO daily	
MUSCARINIC AGONIST		
bethanechol	*Adult:* 10–50 mg PO 3–4 times a day *Child:* 0.6 mg/kg/day in 3–4 divided doses	Minimum effective dose determined by starting with 5–10 mg and repeating the same amount at 1- to 2-hr intervals until desired response is achieved.
PHOSPHODIASTERASE INHIBITORS		
sildenafil	*Adult:* 50–100 mg PO based on patient response. Max: 100 mg/day. 25-mg dose may be used for patients receiving an alpha blocker or ritonavir.	**Should not be taken with nitrates.** Take 30 min–4 hr before sexual activity. Patients taking alpha blockers should take no more than 25 mg, and the two should be taken at least 4 hr apart. High-fat meal delays absorption.
tadalafil	*Adult:* 5–20 mg PO based on patient response. Max: 20 mg/72 hr	**Should not be taken with nitrates or alpha blockers** (except tamsulosin, 0.4 mg daily). Dosage should not exceed 10 mg, and drug should not be taken more frequently than once every 72 hr. Food has no effect on absorption.
vardenafil	*Adult:* 5–20 mg PO based on patient response. Max: 20 mg/day	**Should not be taken with nitrates or alpha blockers.** Take 25–60 min before sexual activity. High-fat meal delays absorption.

ER, Extended-release formulation; *HS,* bedtime; *IR,* immediate-release formulation; *PO,* by mouth; *XL,* extended-release formulation.

BOX 43-2

Management of OAB With Incontinence

Patient History
- Urinary, with bladder diary
- Medical-surgical
- Obstetric and gynecologic; pelvic
- Drug history
- Quality of life

Physical Exam
- Abdominal
- Pelvic exam including pelvic musculature, and vaginal pH
- Rectal
- Neurologic

Diagnostic Testing
- Urinalysis and urine culture
- Serum creatinine; PSA
- PVR
- Urodynamic studies
- Cystoscopy

Pharmacotherapeutic Options
- First- or second-generation antimuscarinics
- Antidepressants (TCAs)
- Estrogen

Non–Drug Treatment Modalities
- Lifestyle interventions
- Fluid and dietary modifications
- Constipation prevention
- Weight reduction
- Scheduled voiding
- Urge-control techniques
- Pelvic floor muscle training (Kegel exercises)
- Surgery

PSA, Prostate-specific antigen; *PRV,* postvoid residual volume; *TCAs,* tricyclic antidepressants.

Treatment Options

Patient Variables

For some patients, discussing OAB symptoms is simply too embarrassing to bring up in conversation with anyone, even a health care provider. Those who do seek help wait an average of 3 years to do so. Half of the patients who do not seek treatment consider incontinence a normal part of aging.

It is important to determine if the patient has incontinence, frequency, or urgency, and associated lower urinary tract symptoms such as hesitancy, pain or dysuria, a feeling of incomplete bladder emptying, and urine leakage following urgency, a cough, sneeze, or exercise. Ask about the use of absorbent pads, duration of symptoms, and when incontinence started.

LIFE-SPAN CONSIDERATIONS

Pregnant and Nursing Women. In women it is important to consider the number of pregnancies, mode of delivery, use of instrumentation and/or episiotomy, and the presence of fibroid tumors. Find out if there is a history of breast cancer or use of hormone replacement therapy, and whether estrogen therapy might be used in the future. Consider hematuria, pelvic organ prolapse, and pain and itching in the vaginal area before selecting estrogen as a treatment (see Drug Variables).

Children and Adolescents. Childhood bedwetting (enuresis) is linked to incontinence in adulthood. Among women with a childhood history of enuresis, the risk of developing daytime incontinence or nocturnal enuresis is increased more than tenfold. Enuresis is possibly a heritable predisposition that spans generations.

Older Adults. Studies of urinary incontinence and depressive symptoms in women and older adults suggest that OAB can result in depression. Other studies suggest there is an association between the two and that reduced production of serotonin observed in depression may cause detrusor overactivity and bladder dysfunction. Still other research suggests that increased production of corticotropin-releasing factor, implicated in panic and anxiety disorders, is associated with increased voiding frequency.

▥ Drug Variables

The once-popular generic oxybutynin is considered to have good efficacy but poor tolerability for many patients. The newer patch formulation of oxybutynin seems to be more tolerable.

Solifenacin is a long-acting antimuscarinic with a selective affinity for M_3 receptors. As such, there are no significant CNS or cardiac events identified. Because of its low lipophilic affinity, tolterodine is less likely to penetrate a normal blood-brain barrier, which may explain the low incidence of cognitive adverse effects associated with its use.

The extended-release formulation of tolterodine allows for once-daily dosing and offers improvement over the immediate-release form in efficacy and tolerability. Trospium is also less likely to cross a normal blood-brain barrier. The drug is not highly biotransformed and for the most part is eliminated unchanged through the kidneys.

In addition to the drugs previously mentioned, transvaginal estrogen administered with or without progesterone is sometimes prescribed for incontinence, but there are conflicting data regarding its efficacy. Transvaginal hormone replacement therapy restores the integrity of the urethral mucosa and increases resistance to outflow (see Chapter 58). Antidepressants such as imipramine and duloxetine have been used off-label to treat stress incontinence and nocturia with some success. Surgery is reserved for patients who are severely debilitated by their incontinence, who have an unstable bladder (severe inappropriate contraction), and poor ability to store urine. Further, many patients who are incontinent have dementia and therefore may not put nonpharmacologic approaches into practice.

Patient Education

It is important for patients to understand that there may be a "trial-and-error" process involved in finding an effective drug and dosage. Teach patients the adverse effects of antimuscarinic use and the drug interactions.

Establishing a routine schedule for voiding is a major factor in the patient's ability to be independent and to function in the community. Distribute fluid intake throughout the course of the day so that the bladder does not receive a large volume of urine all at once. Avoid drinking large quantities of fluids with meals; limit intake to less than 8 oz at any 1 time, and take small sips of fluids between meals. Stop fluid intake 2 to 3 hours before bedtime. In addition, eliminate foods and fluids that are bladder irritants (i.e., artificial sweeteners, caffeine, spicy foods, carbonated drinks, and highly acidic foods such as citrus fruits and juices).

Pelvic muscle training, also known as Kegel exercises, is used to treat stress incontinence. However, these exercises may also be beneficial in relieving the symptoms of urge incontinence. The principle behind Kegel exercises is to strengthen the muscles of the pelvic floor, thereby improving the urethral sphincter function. The success of Kegel exercises depends on proper technique and adherence to a regular exercise program. Seventy-five percent of patients who use biofeedback to enhance performance of Kegel exercises report symptom improvement, with 15% considered cured.

Evaluation

Successful treatment of OAB with urge incontinence is evidenced by a reduction in daytime frequency, that is, less than eight episodes a day or voiding less frequently than every 2 hours while awake. There is also a reduction in nocturia.

BENIGN PROSTATIC HYPERPLASIA

The cause of benign prostatic hyperplasia (BPH) is not well understood, and no definitive information exists on risk factors. BPH occurs primarily in older men and not in men whose testes were removed for another reason prior to puberty. This information has led some health care providers to think that BPH development may be stimulated by factors tied to both aging and functioning testes.

EPIDEMIOLOGY AND ETIOLOGY

BPH is an enlargement of the prostate. Because hyperplasia, and not hypertrophy, causes the major prostatic changes, the term *benign prostatic hyperplasia* is preferred over benign prostatic hypertrophy. Although the exact cause of BPH is unknown, urination becomes increasingly more difficult, and the bladder never feels completely empty. Prostatic enlargement may eventually obstruct urinary outflow completely.

Many patients are uncomfortable discussing problems with urination and the prostate's role in it, since the prostate plays a role in both intercourse and urination. Nevertheless, prostate enlargement is a very normal part of male aging. More than half the men over age 55 years and as many as 90% of men in their 70s and 80s exhibit symptoms of BPH; symptoms rarely develop before age 40. Increases in life expectancy cause simultaneous increases in the occurrence of BPH. Worldwide, BPH is more common in black men.

PATHOPHYSIOLOGY

With maturation, the prostate experiences two primary growth periods. During the first growth period, which occurs in puberty, the prostate doubles its size. Growth starts again at approximately age 25, and this second growth phase often produces symptoms of BPH years later.

Throughout the life span, men produce testosterone and estrogen, but quantities of active testosterone decrease with age. This results in a higher proportion of estrogen than was previously available in younger years. Some health care providers feel BPH develops because the higher amount of estrogen within the gland increases the activity of substances that promote cell growth.

Dihydrotestosterone (DHT), a substance derived from testosterone in the prostate, is the subject of a different theory on BPH development. Although testosterone production decreases with age, older men continue to produce and accumulate high levels of DHT in the prostate. This accumulation of DHT may encourage hyperplasia. Researchers have also found that men who do not produce DHT do not develop BPH.

With aging, the periurethral glands undergo hyperplasia (abnormal increase in the number of normal cells). Because of its position around the urethra, enlargement of the prostate gland

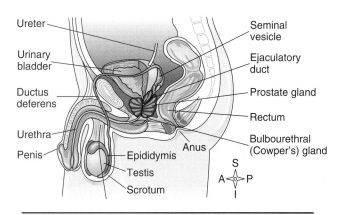

FIGURE 43-1 Anatomical Illustration Showing Enlarged Prostate of BPH.

quickly causes it to compress the urethra and interfere with the normal outflow of urine from the bladder (Fig. 43-1). The bladder wall becomes thicker and irritable, and begins to contract even when it contains only small amounts of urine, resulting in frequency. Over time, the detrusor muscle weakens with the bladder loosing the ability to contract to empty urine. Urinary retention results. A narrowed urethra and incomplete emptying of the bladder contributes to many of the symptoms of BPH.

The usual remedy for BPH is prostatectomy. However, in many cases, peripheral alpha blocking drugs and 5α-reductase inhibitors are used to relieve symptoms and improve urination.

PHARMACOTHERAPEUTIC OPTIONS

Alpha Blockers

NONSELECTIVE ALPHA BLOCKERS
◆ tamsulosin (Flomax); ◆ Flomax

SELECTIVE ALPHA BLOCKERS
◆ alfuzosin (Uroxatrol); ◆ Uroxatrol
◆ doxazosin (Cardura, Cardura XL); ◆ Cardura, Cardura XL
◆ prazosin (Minipress); ◆ prazosin
◆ terazosin (Hytrin); ◆ Hytrin

▦ Indications
Alpha blockers are used for the treatment of obstructive uropathy resulting from BPH.

▦ Pharmacodynamics
Alpha blockers selectively block receptors to relax the smooth muscle of the prostate and bladder neck without interfering with bladder contractility, thereby decreasing bladder resistance to urinary outflow. Tamsulosin is a nonselective alpha-1_A blocker developed to avoid the adverse effects of the selective alpha blockers.

▦ Pharmacokinetics
The majority of alpha blockers have a short onset of action, with peak effects reached anywhere from 2 hours to 6 or 8 weeks. Prazosin and tamulosin are over 90% bioavailable after oral administration. The alpha blockers are widely distributed, with biotransformation taking place in the liver with elimination through the kidneys (see Table 43-2).

▦ Adverse Effects and Contraindications
Adverse effects of alpha blockers are of concern, especially in light of the potential for hypotension. **Of the drugs used for BPH, prazosin has the greatest potential for causing orthostatic hypotension.** On the other hand, cardiac output may actually improve, thus preventing heart failure.

Adverse effects such as postural hypotension, fatigue, dizziness, and asthenia affect fewer than 10% of patients treated with nonselective alpha blockers (e.g., doxazosin, prazosin). The adverse effects can be minimized by slowing titration of the drug and taking it at bedtime.

▦ Drug Interactions
Drug interactions with alpha blockers are identified in Table 43-3. Alcohol, antihypertensive drugs, nitrates and other drugs that cause vasodilation increases the risk of orthostatic hypotension. Alpha blockers used for BPH taken along with other alpha blockers for hypertension, for example, may result in additive effects.

▦ Dosage Regimen
Alpha blockers used in the management of prostatic hyperplasia are usually taken on a daily basis, with the dosage adjusted based on patient response (see Table 43-4). Alfuzosin and tamsulosin should be taken daily about 30 minutes before the same meal of the day. In most cases, if an alpha blocker is stopped, retitration will be necessary.

▦ Lab Considerations
Terazosin may decrease serum albumin, total protein, hemoglobin, and hematocrit values and white blood cell count. The other alpha blockers have no effects on lab values.

5α-Reductase Inhibitors
◆ dutasteride (Avodart); ◆ Avodart
◆ finasteride (Proscar); ◆ Propecia, Proscar

▦ Indications
5α-Reductase inhibitors (androgen hormone inhibitors) are used in the symptomatic management of BPH. 5α-reductase inhibitors prevent the progression of BPH and reduce the likelihood that surgery will be needed, particularly in men with large-volume prostates.

▦ Pharmacodynamics
Anabolic hormone inhibitors competitively inhibit the steroid 5α-reductase, the intracellular enzyme that normally converts testosterone to the potent androgen 5α-dihydrotestosterone. These drugs block the production of DHT, thus reducing prostatic tissue growth and diminishing symptoms of BPH. **It can take 3 to 6 months of therapy with a 5α-reductase inhibitor before a satisfactory patient response is achieved.**

▦ Pharmacokinetics
Finasteride and dutasteride are well absorbed by mouth and are biotransformed in the liver. Finasteride is biotransformed into active metabolites with a half-life of 6 hours (see Table 43-2). The plasma half-life of dutasteride is highly variable and dose dependent. These drugs are eliminated in the feces and the urine.

GENITOURINARY

⫶ *Adverse Effects and Contraindications*

The adverse effects associated with finasteride include impotence, decreased libido, and smaller volume of ejaculate. Exercise caution when using the drug in patients with liver

⚠ disease. **Advise the male patient not to expose a female sex partner to a crushed tablet of finasteride, because of the potential for teratogenic effects in a male fetus.** Dutasteride remains in the blood stream for an extended period, and consequently blood donations should be avoided until 5 months after the last dose to avoid passing the drug to pregnant women through transfusion.

Finasteride and dutasteride are contraindicated for use in women and children. Advise pregnant women or women who may become pregnant not to handle or touch the tablets or capsules.

⫶ *Drug Interactions*

Finasteride decreases the clearance of theophylline (see Table 43-3). In addition, serum concentrations of prostate-specific antigen (PSA) are decreased in a patient taking finasteride, even in the presence of prostate cancer. There have been no significant metabolic studies conducted for drug interactions with dutasteride. However, caution is always advised when managing multiple drugs and unknown interactions.

⫶ *Dosage Regimen*

Dutasteride and finasteride are taken by mouth once daily without regard to meals. Inform patients that effective therapy may take up to 6 months (see Table 43-4).

⫶ *Lab Considerations*

Finasteride and dutasteride decrease PSA levels, even in the presence of prostate cancer. Finasteride reduces PSA levels by 40% to 50%.

For more information, see the Evolve Resources Bonus Content "Influence of Selected Drugs on Laboratory Values," found at http://evolve.elsevier.com/Gutierrez/pharmacotherapeutics.

CLINICAL REASONING

Treatment Objectives

The objective in drug therapy for BPH is to relieve symptoms of obstructive uropathy, improve urination, prevent the progression of BPH, and reduce the risks of BPH-related surgery, especially in men with large-volume prostates (see Evidence-Based Pharmacotherapeutics box, The MTOPS Trial).

Treatment Options

⫶ *Patient Variables*

The American Urologic Association (AUA) created a Symptom Index (SI) Scale (Table 43-5) to correlate symptom severity with prostate size. The AUA recommends that the scale be used at initial patient assessment and then when the patient returns for periodic follow-up. Follow-up enables the health care provider to initiate acute or intensive therapy when the score increases. Do not use this scale for patients with severe symptoms.

TABLE **43-5 AUA Symptom Index***

	AUA Symptom Score (Circle one number on each line)					
Over the Past Month:	Not at All	Less than 1 in 5 Times	Less than Half the Time	About Half the Time	Over Half the Time	Almost Always
1. How often have you had a sensation of not emptying your bladder completely after urinating? *(Incomplete emptying)*	0	1	2	3	4	5
2. How often have you had to urinate again less than 2 hours after you finished urinating? *(Frequency)*	0	1	2	3	4	5
3. How often have you found you stopped and started again several times when you urinated? *(Intermittency)*	0	1	2	3	4	5
4. How often have you found it difficult to postpone urination? *(Urgency)*	0	1	2	3	4	5
5. How often have you had a weak urinary stream? *(Weak stream)*	0	1	2	3	4	5
6. How often have you had to push or strain to begin urination? *(Straining)*	0	1	2	3	4	5
7. How many times did you most typically get up to urinate from the time you went to bed at night until the time you got up in the morning? *(Nocturia)*	0	1	2	3	4	5
	(None)	(1 time)	(2 times)	(3 times)	(4 times)	(5 times)
QUALITY OF LIFE DUE TO URINARY SYMPTOMS						
If you were to spend the rest of your life with your urinary condition, just the way it is now, how would you feel about that?						
0	1	2	3	4	5	6
Delighted	Pleased	Mostly satisfied	Neither satisfied nor dissatisfied	Mostly dissatisfied	Unhappy	Terrible

*The American Urology Association Symptom Score (AUA) is based on responses to 7 questions concerning urinary symptoms. Each question allows patients to choose one of several responses that indicate symptom severity. The total score can therefore range from 0 to 35 (asymptomatic to very symptomatic). 0–7 points = mild symptoms; 8–19 points = moderate symptoms; 20–35 points = severe symptoms.
From Barry, M., Williford, W., Chang, Y., et al. (1995). Benign prostatic hyperplasia specific health status measures in clinical research: How much change in the American Urological Association Symptom Index and the Benign Prostatic Hyperplasia Impact Index is perceptible to patients? *The Journal of Urology, 154*(5), 1770–1774.

EVIDENCE-BASED PHARMACOTHERAPEUTICS

The MTOPS Trial

■ Background

As noted in the 1994 AHCPR treatment guidelines, prostate surgery offers the best chance for symptom improvement in patients with BPH, but surgery also has the highest rate of significant complications. Alpha blockers generally cause a small increase in urinary flow rates, and a small but perceptible reduction in BPH symptoms but with unknown long-term efficacy. Finasteride, on the other hand, results in a small increase in urinary flow rates and a small but perceptible reduction in symptoms. However, finasteride must be taken long-term, and, as with alpha blockers, there is no evidence of long-term efficacy in reduction of BPH, complication rates, or the need for surgery.

■ Research Article

Bautista, O., Kusek, J., Nyberg, L., et al. (2006). Study design of the Medical Therapy of Prostatic Symptoms (MTOPS) trial. *Controlled Clinical Trials, 24*(2), 224–243.

Purpose

The primary purpose of the study was to determine if the long-term drug therapy of BPH using finasteride, doxazosin, or the combination of both drugs could prevent or postpone clinical progression of BPH and the need for surgery or other invasive therapies. The secondary purpose was to gain insight into the molecular-level prostate pathophysiology of men with moderate to severe BPH symptoms who are either on watchful waiting status or on drug therapy.

Design

The MTOPS trial was a 4-year multicenter, randomized, placebo-controlled, double-masked clinical trial. Subjects were randomized and double-masked to one of the following treatment groups ($N = 688$ per treatment group): (1) placebo; (2) 5-α reductase inhibitor finasteride (5 mg daily); (3) alpha-adrenergic blocker doxazosin (in a titration to response to either 4 or 8 mg); or (4) a combination of finasteride (5 mg) and doxazosin (4 or 8 mg daily).

After stratification by clinical site, the urn randomization method was used to allocate subjects to one of the four treatment groups. Men at least 50 years old with moderate to severe symptoms based on the AUA-SI who had not had medical, surgical, or experimental interventions for BPH were eligible to participate in the trial. Inclusion criteria included providing a signed informed consent before initiation of any study procedure; male subject over age 50 years of age who had four peak urinary flow rate measurements of less than 15 mL and a voided volume over 125 mL; and an AUA-SI symptom score less than 30.

Methods

Health care providers at 17 MTOPS medical centers across the country treated 3047 men with BPH for an average of 4.5 years. Subjects had vital signs, urinary symptoms, urinary flow, adverse effects, and drug use assessed every 3 months. A DRE, serum PSA level, and urinalysis were performed yearly. Prostate size was determined via ultrasound at the start and at the end of the study. To assess the natural history of BPH, subjects were followed prospectively with respect to BPH symptoms, peak urinary flow rate, prostate volume, sexual function, and quality of life. BPH symptoms were quantified using the AUA-SI and BPH impact index questionnaires. Subjects were defined as having reached BPH progression if any of the following events occurred:

- Four-point rise from baseline in the AUA-SI score
- A rise in serum creatinine attributable to BPH
- An acute urinary retention event
- Recurrent UTI or urosepsis event
- Incontinence event

Each of the three active treatment groups was compared to the placebo group allowing for a 0.05 type I error rate for the three pairwise comparisons. Two-sided tests were used at all times. Using a standard Bonferroni adjustment to maintain a studywise error rate of 0.05, each pairwise comparison was tested using a 0.0167 level of significance.

Findings

When used together, finasteride and doxazosin reduced the overall risk for progression of BPH by 66% compared with placebo. The combination provided the greatest symptom relief and improvement in urinary flow rates. Monotherapy with doxazosin reduced the overall risk of disease progression by 39% and finasteride alone by 34% relative to placebo. Combination therapy and finasteride alone significantly reduced the risk of invasive therapy by 67% and 64% respectively. Doxazosin did not reduce the long-term risk of invasive therapy.

BPH progression occurred in 5% of men receiving combination therapy, in 10% of men taking doxazosin, in 10% of men taking finasteride, and in 17% of men taking placebo. The events signaling disease progression included worsening symptoms (78%), but also included acute urinary retention (12%), and incontinence (9%).

The risk of urinary retention was reduced 81% with combination therapy and by 68% with finasteride monotherapy. Doxazosin alone did not reduce the risk of urinary retention. The risk of incontinence was reduced 65% with combination finasteride-doxazosin therapy.

Twenty-seven percent of men taking doxazosin, 25% of men taking finasteride, and 18% of men taking combination therapy stopped treatment early because of adverse effects. The most common complaint of men treated with finasteride was sexual dysfunction; the most common complaints of men treated with doxazosin were dizziness and fatigue.

Conclusions

There is evidence supporting the premise that the combination of doxazosin and finasteride is more efficacious in relieving and preventing progression of symptoms than either of the two drugs alone. Patients most likely to benefit from combination therapy are those in whom baseline risk of progression is significantly higher, generally patients with larger glands and higher PSA values.

MTOPS is the largest randomized, controlled clinical trial to simultaneously compare the long-term BPH progression of men treated with an alpha blocker, a 5α-reductase inhibitor, or a combination of both, against men treated with placebo. During the trial, the finasteride study group found that men with BPH treated with 5 mg per day had a significant decrease in total urinary symptoms scores, increased peak urinary flow rates, and decreased prostatic volume compared to men treated with placebo.

■ Implications for Practice

The implications of this study are simple: finasteride therapy alone is effective in the treatment of BPH symptoms in men over 50 years of age, although combination therapy may be more efficacious than monotherapy. A head-to-head study using finasteride with dutasteride may provide similar outcomes but would be worth exploring. Studies comparing the other alpha blockers should also be considered.

AHCPR, Agency for Health Care Policy and Research (now the Agency for Healthcare Research and Quality [AHRQ]); *AUA-SI,* American Urologic Association Symptom Index; *BPH,* benign prostatic hyperplasia; *DRE,* digital rectal exam; *MTOPS,* Medical Therapy of Prostatic Symptoms (trial); *PSA,* prostate-specific antigen; *UTI,* urinary tract infection.

GENITOURINARY

LIFE-SPAN CONSIDERATIONS

Older Adults. BPH is the most common benign tumor in men, and its incidence is age-related. The main risk factors are increasing age and the presence of androgens, family history of BPH, environment, and diet. Men who consume a diet high in animal fats are more likely to develop this problem.

▍ *Drug Variables*

If symptoms are mild (AUA-SI score less than 7), no drug therapy is recommended. Recommend that the patient limit fluid intake after dinner, avoid decongestants such as pseudoephedrine, massage the prostate after intercourse, and void frequently. Drug therapy is started when the AUA-SI score is over 7.

Medical treatment for BPH consists of alpha blockers and 5α-reductase inhibitors. Long-term 5α-reductase inhibitor monotherapy, although slow to onset, is a viable therapy for symptom relief in men with mild to moderate symptoms. Patients who do not respond to a nonselective alpha blocker may respond to tamsulosin, a highly selective alpha-1_A blocker, and because of the selectivity, may experience fewer adverse effects. With alpha blockers, results are often apparent in 3 to 7 days.

The results of multiple studies of BPH indicate that 5α-reductase inhibitors may be more efficacious in men with a prostate size over 40 grams, whereas alpha blockers are effective across the range of prostate sizes. To reduce the risk of polypharmacy, it may be prudent to use an alpha blocker in the patient who also has hypertension. When required, combination therapy may show greater improvement.

Patient Education

Advise patients that improvement in urine does not occur overnight, but will begin within 1 to 2 weeks with noticeable improvement in 3 to 4 weeks. Teach the importance of getting up slowly from lying or sitting positions and to quickly sit down or recline if abrupt dizziness occurs. Avoid tasks that require alertness or motor skills until response to the drug is completely established.

Teach patients with BPH to decrease fluid intake several hours before bedtime, and to avoid alcohol and diuretics.

Other drugs to avoid include anticholinergics, antihistamines, and some antidepressants (e.g., tricyclic antidepressants such as doxepin and amitriptyline; selective serotonin reuptake inhibitors, such as fluoxetine, are acceptable).

Many men use herbal or nutritional supplements to support prostate health. Supplements often used include saw palmetto, pygeum, and zinc (Table 43-6). Other protective factors include diets rich in isoflavonoids, especially genistein; cruciferous vegetables (containing isothiocyanate sulforaphane); retinoids, especially lycopene; vitamin E; and selenium. Caution patients to follow the manufacturer's recommendations.

Evaluation

The efficacy of drug therapy for BPH is demonstrated through the relief of obstructive uropathy symptoms, improved urination, a reduction in the risks of BPH-related surgery, and the reduced progression of BPH. Because BPH develops over a prolonged period, the changes within the urinary tract are slow. Reversing progressive BPH is not possible.

URINARY RETENTION

EPIDEMIOLOGY AND ETIOLOGY

Urinary retention is a condition in which urine is retained in the bladder. Urine production continues, but the accumulated urine is not released. The incidence of urinary retention varies with the etiology. It occurs in 10% to 15% of patients who receive general anesthesia and 20% to 25% of patients following spinal anesthesia. More than half the men over the age of 50 have BPH, which contributes to urinary retention. Urinary retention can be serious because of the risk of urinary tract infection and stone formation. There is also a risk of direct damage to the bladder, the ureters, or the kidneys. Further, continued bladder distention leads to loss of bladder tone.

Patients who have received epidural anesthesia may develop urinary retention. Furthermore, opioid analgesics are

---

TABLE 43-6 Complementary and Alternative Therapies for BPH

Saw palmetto	• From dark berries of palm tree native to Florida and North Carolina • Inhibits testosterone conversion to DHT, resulting in prevention of prostate enlargement. Stops DHT binding to receptor sites; general inhibitor effects on both estrogen and androgen receptors • Inhibits 5α-reductase more effectively than finasteride • Effective in reducing symptoms of BPH. Efficacy in treating chronic prostatitis not established. • Adverse effects: gastrointestinal upset, constipation, diarrhea, dizziness, nausea, vomiting (infrequent) • No known drug interactions • Does not affect PSA levels or interfere with diagnosis of prostate cancer • Dosages vary—most studies used 160 mg twice daily or 320 mg once daily
Pygeum	• Ground, powdered bark of pygeum tree, a type of evergreen from Africa • Compounds in pygeum bark exert antiinflammatory effects, and others are thought to influence testosterone metabolism. • Significantly more effective than placebo with respect to urinary frequency, urgency, dysuria, and urinary flow rate • Widely used in Europe for symptom relief of BPH and to postpone use of stronger drugs or surgery. Also used for impotence and male infertility • Adverse effects: gastrointestinal upset (infrequent) • Dosage: 50–100 mg of extract standardized to contain 14% triterpenes and 0.5% n-docosanol twice daily • Combine pygeum with nettle root for increased effectiveness.
Zinc sulfate	• Stimulates activity of approximately 100 enzymes to promote biochemical reactions in body • Inhibits 5α-reductase to prevent conversion of testosterone to DHT • Improves urinary symptoms and reduces the size of the prostate • Dosage: 150 mg daily for 2 mo followed by maintenance dose of 50–100 mg/day

BPH, Benign prostatic hyperplasia; *DHT,* dihydrotestosterone; *PSA,* prostate-specific antigen.

commonly used for pain management, and the level of voiding reflex inhibition is directly related to the level of analgesia. In other words, the more effective the pain control, the greater the risk of urinary retention. These effects are observed with both epidural and parenteral routes of administration. Depending on the dosage, opioid analgesics may impair bladder function for as long as 14 to 16 hours.

Preoperative drugs, anesthetics, and surgical manipulation, either alone or in combination, can also cause urinary retention. Because general anesthetics have an inhibitory effect on bladder function, the longer the patient is under general anesthesia, the greater the risk of urinary retention. Circumstances associated with surgery that affect the patient's ability to void include the length of the procedure and the amount of intravenous fluid administered. The patient may have an overfull bladder on completion of the procedure or may not be alert enough to recognize the need to void. Thus the bladder becomes distended, increasing the likelihood of retention.

Anorectal disorders such as hemorrhoids, abscess, or fecal impaction also contribute to urinary retention. The retention is caused by obstruction or spasms of perineal muscles, hampering the ability to relax. Anorectal surgery is associated with a particularly high incidence of postoperative urinary retention. Stimulation of the vesicoanal reflex inhibits contraction of the detrusor muscle, resulting in urinary retention. The reflex may be activated by physically stimulating the anus or rectum by the presence of packing materials in the anus or the rectal vault, or by pain associated with examination or procedures.

Autonomic dysfunction secondary to spinal cord injury initially results in an areflexive bladder that later leads to urinary retention and a neurogenic bladder. Immobility also contributes to urinary retention. Patients confined to bed, particularly those unable to sit upright, may find it difficult if not impossible to void using a bedpan. In an effort to avoid movement and the possibility of increased pain, patients may ignore the sensation of a full bladder. Anxiety that someone will see or hear them using a bedpan or bedside commode may inhibit their ability to relax enough to void. Because privacy is an uncommon commodity in institutional settings, urinary retention may escalate.

PATHOPHYSIOLOGY

Urinary retention produces a series of adverse consequences. As urine accumulates, hydrostatic pressure against the bladder wall increases. Hyperplasia of the detrusor muscle, development of connective tissue in the bladder wall, or development of diverticula may result. Ureteral peristalsis also increases as pressure against the accumulating urine rises. The ureters gradually distend and elongate, becoming fibrotic and tortuous. The pressure is transmitted through the renal pelvis and calices to the parenchyma. In turn, the resulting hydronephrosis exerts pressure on renal vasculature, causing ischemia and parenchymal damage. Without interruption, the process can progress to renal failure and death.

In addition, as pressure within the bladder continues to rise, the pressure overcomes the restraint of the sphincter and incontinence results. Urine is released until the intravesicular pressure is reduced, but only to the extent that the external sphincter can regain control. The cycle is repeated as the bladder continues to overfill. Prolonged high intravesicular pressures predispose the patient to diverticula. A diverticulum is an outpocketing of the mucous membrane lining due to weakness in the bladder wall. Bladder diverticula contribute to the risk of urinary tract infections and malignancy. Infections are related to urinary stasis; malignancy is thought to be related to chronic irritation.

Drug therapy can be used to treat urinary retention and thus reduce the likelihood of complications. Muscarinic agonist drugs may be used to facilitate voiding in select patients.

PHARMACOTHERAPEUTIC OPTIONS

Muscarinic Agonist
◆ bethanechol chloride (Urecholine); ◆ Duvoid, Myotonachol

▌▌▌ Indications
Bethanechol chloride is used for the short-term treatment of postoperative or postpartum urinary retention. The drug is also used on a long-term basis to treat patients who have urinary retention as a result of neurogenic bladder. Because bethanechol chloride also acts on the GI tract, it may be used to treat gastroesophageal reflux disease and megacolon (i.e., dilation and hypertrophy of the colon). The drug is also used as an adjunct in the treatment of tricyclic antidepressant–related bladder dysfunction.

▌▌▌ Pharmacodynamics
Muscarinic agonists (i.e., direct-acting cholinergics) are structurally and pharmacologically similar to acetylcholine (ACh). Drug effects are the result of direct stimulation of cholinergic receptors in postsynaptic membranes. Bethanechol is a synthetic choline ester; however, unlike naturally occurring ACh, bethanechol is not destroyed in the synapse by acetylcholinesterase. Thus the drug enhances the activity of naturally occurring ACh. Muscarinic receptors are strongly stereoselective, that is, the (−) isomer is almost 1000 times more potent than the (+) isomer. The enhancement results in contraction of the detrusor muscle and emptying of the bladder. There is also stimulation of intestinal peristalsis, resulting in bowel elimination.

▌▌▌ Pharmacokinetics
Bethanechol chloride is poorly absorbed when taken by mouth, and thus larger doses are needed. The peak response by the detrusor muscle occurs in 1 hour, with drug effects lasting up to 6 hours. The onset of drug effects occurs 5 to 15 minutes after subcutaneous (subQ) administration. Peak drug effects are reached in 15 to 30 minutes and last up to 2 hours (see Table 43-2).

▌▌▌ Adverse Effects and Contraindications
The most common adverse effects of bethanechol chloride are associated with the GI and urinary systems. Urinary urgency, nausea, vomiting, salivation, abdominal cramps, and diarrhea are frequent. Headache, malaise, increased lacrimation, increased bronchial secretions, miosis, flushing of the skin, and diaphoresis has also been reported. **The most life-threatening adverse effects of bethanecol chloride include syncope, heart block, and cardiac arrest. Do not use**

bethanechol chloride in patients with urethral obstruction, or if the urethral sphincter is unable to dilate. In these instances, intravesical pressure increases against an obstructed outlet, which in turn causes ureterovesical reflux and the risk of a ruptured bladder.

Bethanechol chloride is also contraindicated for use in patients in whom the strength or the integrity of the bladder wall or GI tract is compromised. Because of the risk of damage to the GI tract, do not use bethanechol chloride in patients with a mechanical obstruction or acute inflammatory lesions of the GI tract, a history of peptic ulcers, spastic disturbances, or peritonitis.

Patients with latent or active asthma may have life-threatening bronchial constriction in the presence of bethanechol chloride. The drug is also contraindicated for use in patients with pronounced bradycardia, hypotension, cardiac disease, vasomotor instability, hypertension, or marked vagotonia (irritability of the vagus nerve). The drug causes significant changes in blood vessel diameter and resulting changes in cardiac function and blood pressure. Patients with hyperthyroidism or seizure disorders may have an exacerbation of their disease and are at increased risk for cardiac complications. Patients suffering from Parkinson's disease may notice an increase in tremors because of the cholinergic effect of bethanechol chloride. Bethanechol chloride is a pregnancy class C drug. It is not known if the drug passes into breast milk.

▥ Drug Interactions

Atropine, an anticholinergic drug, reverses the muscarinic effects of bethanechol chloride (see Table 43-3). Although this phenomenon is useful in cases of toxicity, it can interfere with treatment if atropine or other anticholinergic drugs are used concurrently with bethanechol chloride. Procainamide and quinidine have similar effects. Cholinergic drugs and cholinesterase inhibitors produce synergistic effects that can result in toxicity if they are given concurrently. Concurrent use of ganglionic blocking drugs (e.g., mecamylamine) may result in severe hypotension. Patients typically complain of severe abdominal cramping and diarrhea before the hypotension becomes profound.

▥ Dosage Regimen

The initial adult dose of bethanechol chloride is determined by orally administering 5 to 10 mg of the drug every 1 to 2 hours until the desired response is obtained or a total of 50 mg has been given (see Table 43-4).

▥ Lab Considerations

Monitoring serum levels of bethanechol chloride is not ordinarily required. However, bethanechol chloride may increase aspartate transaminase (AST), serum amylase, and serum lipase concentrations.

CLINICAL REASONING

Treatment Objectives

The treatment objective for the patient with urinary retention is to stimulate complete bladder emptying. Muscarinic agonists are used on a short-term basis until the effects of surgery, childbirth, or other drugs have diminished.

Treatment Options

▥ Patient Variables

Urinary retention typically develops while a patient is hospitalized rather than being an illness that brings the patient to the health care system. The patient may complain of bladder fullness or generalized pelvic discomfort. The patient reports a need to void but is unable to do so. The patient may also complain of overflow incontinence, or a feeling that the bladder is not emptying with each voiding. Pay particular attention to patients who lack normal sensory function of the bladder and those who have received local, epidural, or spinal anesthetics. Patients with neurogenic atony may not complain of urinary symptoms.

Be sure to elicit information regarding a past history of peptic ulcer disease, asthma, cardiovascular disease, or hyperthyroidism. A previous history of mechanical obstruction of the GI or the urinary tract may contraindicate use of these drugs. Also note patient allergies.

Patients voiding more than once per hour or in amounts smaller than 50 mL are probably experiencing urinary retention with overflow. Patients may become diaphoretic or restless owing to discomfort from the distended bladder. Always consider urinary retention when fluid intake is considerably greater than urinary output.

If urinary retention is suspected despite the patient's having voided, postvoiding catheterization is performed. Measuring the amounts of urine voided allows comparison of the amount of urine voided spontaneously and the amount of urine obtained through catheterization. Patients may think they are voiding adequately, when in reality only a small amount of urine is voided and the majority remains in the bladder.

Life-Span Considerations

Pregnant and Nursing Women. The normal physiologic changes accompanying pregnancy predispose women to postpartum urinary retention. During pregnancy and the weeks immediately following the delivery, smooth muscle tone is reduced owing to increased levels of progesterone. A dilated bladder with poor muscle tone is less likely to empty itself effectively. The pressure within the bladder nearly doubles during pregnancy and then rapidly returns to prepregnancy levels during the first postpartum week. This rapid change in pressure results in hypotonia of bladder muscles.

Bladder tone and sensation may be reduced as the result of operative vaginal procedures and the effects of analgesia and anesthesia. Epidural analgesia is frequently used for vaginal deliveries and cesarean sections. The duration of the voiding difficulty is also influenced by analgesic drugs. For example, use of long-acting bupivacaine can result in decreased detrusor strength for up to 8 hours after administration. Further, pain or fear of pain interferes with the ability to relax. These factors in combination with postpartum diuresis frequently lead to bladder distention or to incomplete emptying of the bladder. Edema and increased blood flow to the bladder mucosa and the urethra can interfere with free passage of urine.

Postpartum urinary retention is usually a short-lived complication. However, with recent decreases in the length of hospital stay following childbirth, patients not only need to be assessed for the problem but also need to be taught about the possibility of urinary retention once they return home.

Children and Adolescents. The psychosocial impact of neurogenic atony once the patient has successfully attained bladder control can be significant. Children may feel ashamed if they can no longer control bladder function. This problem is compounded if the child's peers learn about the use of absorbent undergarments or episodes of incontinence.

Older Adults. Urinary retention in the older adult is not uncommon. Causes include phimosis, meatal stenosis, urethral trauma or stricture, BPH, prostate cancer, and bladder tumors. Bleeding with clot formation, uterine prolapse, fecal impaction, spinal cord injuries, and neurologic impairment (e.g., diabetes mellitus, nerve damage from neoplasms) may also contribute to urinary retention.

▮ Drug Variables

Not all cases of urinary retention require intervention. Using a drug to stimulate bladder contraction is generally not advised if swelling of perineal tissues is obstructing urine flow. If the patient is unable to void because of positioning or privacy concerns, stimulating bladder contractions probably will not help. However, for patients whose bladders are not contracting adequately, use of a muscarinic agonist may be appropriate.

Bethanechol is the only drug in this class prescribed for urinary retention. Oral administration results in a longer duration of action. Bethanechol is not suitable for patients who have questionable structural integrity of the urinary or the GI tract. Use it very cautiously in patients with a previous history of bronchial asthma or cardiac disease.

Patient Teaching

Teach the patient methods to stimulate voiding. If the patient has a neurogenic bladder, he or she can be taught to exert pressure on the abdomen by learning forward or pressing on the abdomen. A Valsalva maneuver increases intraabdominal pressure on the bladder, which may assist with voiding. Some patients will learn Credé's maneuver. The patient places the fingers over the bladder and presses downward slowly toward the symphysis pubis, as though "milking" urine out of the bladder. Credé's maneuver is often combined with intermittent self-catheterization. A straight urethral catheter is inserted into the bladder at specified intervals, the urine is drained, and the catheter is removed.

Encourage patients with bladder atony to learn self-catheterization, because it increases independence and mobility. The patient or another person who has been properly educated about the technique may insert the catheter. Intermittent catheterization is not a panacea, however. This intervention requires the patient to assume a great deal of personal responsibility; some patients are not sufficiently motivated to fulfill the responsibility.

Evaluation

The expected outcome for patients using bethanechol chloride is regular, complete emptying of the bladder. For hospitalized patients, this would be observed as relative balance between fluid intake and urine output, no distention of the bladder, and no complaints of pelvic discomfort. Expect urinary output to exceed 50 mL per void. For patients using bethanechol chloride on a regular basis, the expectation is regular emptying of the bladder without incontinence.

MISCELLANEOUS URINARY DRUGS

Urinary Tract Antispasmodics

- ◆ flavoxate (Urispas); ✦ Urispas
- ◆ hyoscyamine (Anaspaz, Cystospaz, Levbid, Levsin, others);
  - ✦ hyoscyamine

Flavoxate

Flavoxate is a urinary tract antispasmodic. It is used for the symptomatic relief of the dysuria, urgency, nocturia, frequency, and incontinence associated with cystitis. It also has been used in the management of prostatitis, urethritis, and urethrocystitis. It acts by relaxing the detrusor muscle and other smooth muscle through cholinergic blockade. It produces anticholinergic, local anesthetic, and analgesic effects.

Flavoxate is well absorbed when taken by mouth; however, the onset of drug action is relatively slow. Duration of drug action is approximately 6 hours, with a half-life of 2 to 3 hours. Drug excretion is through the urine.

Flavoxate is generally well tolerated. Common adverse effects are usually mild and transient. Drowsiness and dry mouth and throat are common. Occasionally constipation, difficult urination, blurred vision, dizziness, headache, photophobia, nausea, vomiting, and abdominal pain have occurred. Confusion, hypersensitivity, increased intraocular pressure, and leukopenia are rare occurrences. Use caution when prescribing flavoxate in patients with glaucoma. Flavoxate is contraindicated for use in the presence of hypersensitivity, pyloric or duodenal obstruction, obstructive intestinal lesions or ileus, achalasia, GI bleeding, or obstructive uropathies of the lower urinary tract. The usual dose of flavoxate is identified in Table 43-4.

Hyoscyamine

Hyoscyamine is an anticholinergic used as an aid in controlling spastic bladder. It also is used as an adjunct in the treatment of GI hypermotility, neurogenic bowel syndrome, and visceral spasm. Hyoscyamine inhibits the action of acetylcholine at muscarinic receptor sites, thus reducing the motility of the urinary and GI tracts.

As discussed in Chapter 15, there are numerous contraindications to and warnings regarding the use of anticholinergics. The most frequent adverse effects include dry mouth (sometimes severe), decreased sweating, and diaphoresis. Occasionally there may be blurred vision, bloating, urinary hesitancy, and drowsiness (with high dosage), headache, intolerance to light, loss of taste, nervousness, flushing, insomnia, impotence, and mental confusion. **Toxic dosages of hyoscyamine ▲ causes adverse effects in the cardiac, respiratory, and CNS systems.**

Hyoscyamine is well absorbed from the GI tract to be widely distributed. It is 50% protein bound. Biotransformation is primarily through the liver, with a half-life of 3 to 4 hours. Excretion is primarily in the urine.

Hyoscyamine interacts with antacids, and antidiarrheal drugs may decrease drug absorption. When anticholinergic drugs are taken concurrently with hyoscyamine, anticholinergic drug effects will be enhanced. Hyoscyamine may decrease the absorption of ketoconazole. There are no significant laboratory considerations. The dosage of hyoscyamine is identified in Table 43-4.

Urinary Tract Analgesic

◆ phenazopyridine (Pyridium, Azo-Standard, Urogesic, Urodine);
◆ Pyridium

Phenazopyridine is a nonopioid urinary tract analgesic that provides relief of UTI symptoms such as pain, itching, burning, urgency, and frequency. It is intended for short-term use only because the underlying reason for the irritation should be determined and appropriately treated. Phenazopyridine's exact mechanism of action is unknown, but it appears to produce topical analgesic and local anesthetic effects on the urinary tract mucosa. It has no antimicrobial activity.

Phenazopyridine is well absorbed after oral administration; onset time to urinary analgesia is unknown. Peak effects are reached in 5 to 6 hours, with a duration of action of 6 to 8 hours. It is biotransformed in the liver and other body tissues. Almost 90% is excreted by the kidneys within 24 hours. No significant drug interactions are noted with phenazopyridine. The dosage of phenazopyridine is noted in Table 43-4.

The adverse effects of phenazopyridine are few but include headache, vertigo, nausea, abdominal pain, cramps or gas, and a rash. Its most common adverse effect is the bright reddish-orange color it produces in the urine and other body fluids (discolored tears can stain soft contact lenses). **Phenazopyridine also causes a blue to purple skin discoloration, due to methemoglobinemia, and may cause hemolytic jaundice, although both are rare.** It is contraindicated for use in patients with glomerulonephritis, severe hepatitis, renal insufficiency, renal failure, uremia, and a glucose-6-phosphate dehydrogenase (G6PD) deficiency. Safe use during pregnancy and lactation has not been established.

Phenazopyridine interferes with urine tests based on color reactions (glucose, ketones, bilirubin, nitrites, leukocytes, steroids, and protein). Use glucose enzymatic testing methods (Clinistix, Tes-Tape) to test urine glucose concentrations in patients taking this drug.

ERECTILE DYSFUNCTION

EPIDEMIOLOGY AND ETIOLOGY

Erectile dysfunction (ED) is the total inability to achieve and sustain a penile erection firm enough for intercourse, an inconsistent ability to do so, or a tendency to sustain only brief erections. The term "impotence" may also refer to other issues that interfere with intercourse and reproduction (e.g., decreased libido, ejaculation, or orgasm problems). For this reason, the preferred term is ED.

It is estimated that at least 10 to 30 million men in the United States suffer from ED. In one population survey ($N = 1400$ men ages 18 to 59), researchers found the prevalence of ED to approach 31%. The National Ambulatory Medical Care Survey (NAMCS) data on new drugs show an estimated 2.6 million mentions of sildenafil (Viagra) during health care provider visits in 1999, and one third of those occurred during visits for a purpose other than ED (Hing, et al., 2006). The survey was conducted annually from 1973

to 1981, in 1985, and annually since 1989. Seven of every 1000 male visits to a health care provider in 1985 were made for ED. By 1999, the rate almost tripled to 22.3. The prevalence rates continue to increase as men age. One third to one half of men with diabetes have ED. And, although ED is common, it is still underreported, primarily owing to patient embarrassment. However, discussing ED with health care providers has gradually become more acceptable, presumably because vacuum devices and injectable drugs to assist with erectile difficulties have become widely available.

Approximately 70% of cases of ED result from damage to nerves, arteries, smooth muscles, and fibrous tissues, often as the consequence of diabetes, kidney disease, neurologic disorders (e.g., multiple sclerosis), atherosclerosis, and peripheral vascular disease. Lifestyle choices (i.e., smoking, alcoholism) that contribute to heart disease and vascular problems also raise the risk for ED. Other possible causes include hormonal abnormalities, such as low levels of testosterone. Being overweight or obese and a lack of exercise are also contributing causes of ED.

Radical prostatectomy and bladder surgery injures nerves and arteries near the penis, causing ED. Injury to the penis, the spinal cord, the prostate, the bladder, and the pelvis lead to ED by damaging nerves, smooth muscles, arteries, and fibrous tissues of the corpora cavernosa of the penis.

Approximately 25% of common drugs such as antidepressants, antianxiety drugs, antihypertensives, histamine₂ antagonists, antihistamines, and appetite suppressants may produce ED as an adverse effect.

Many psychologic factors (e.g., stress, anxiety, guilt, low self-esteem, fear of sexual failure) are contributing factors in 10% to 20% of ED cases. Men with an organic cause for ED may experience similar psychologic distress.

The most popular intervention for ED came about with the launching of sildenafil citrate in 1998. Sildenafil is now prescribed by more primary care providers for ED than by urologists. Since 1998, vardenafil and tadalafil have also reached the marketplace.

PATHOPHYSIOLOGY

Anatomically, the penis contains three chambers. The two dorsal chambers each contain one of a pair of erectile bodies (i.e., corpora cavernosa) and the ventral chamber a spongy tissue cylinder (i.e., corpus spongiosum). Each chamber has an arterial blood supply, a venous drainage system, and neural innervation that contribute to normal physiologic function (Fig. 43-2).

Each corpus cavernosa contains venous sinusoids that trap blood when filled. Each sinusoid increases in volume as blood enters the penis. When the cylinders reach maximum volume, the pressure rises, and the penis becomes rigid. Penile rigidity facilitates vaginal penetration.

The corpus spongiosum, located ventrally within the penis, contains the urethra. This chamber mushrooms out on the distal end of the penis to form the glans. The spongiosum becomes engorged with blood during sexual arousal. Venous communication often exists between the corpus spongiosum and the corpora cavernosa.

The penis is innervated by both the autonomic and the somatic nervous systems. An erection begins with sensory or

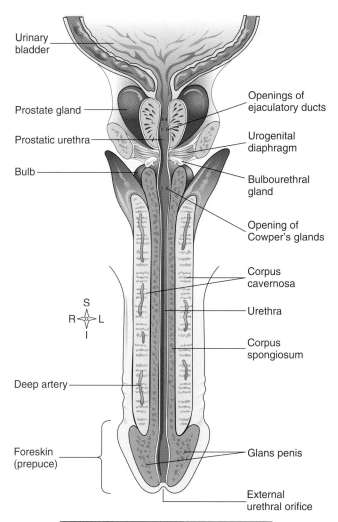

Urinary bladder

Prostate gland

Prostatic urethra

Bulb

Openings of ejaculatory ducts

Urogenital diaphragm

Bulbourethral gland

Opening of Cowper's glands

Corpus cavernosa

Urethra

Corpus spongiosum

Deep artery

Foreskin (prepuce)

Glans penis

External urethral orifice

FIGURE 43-2 Illustration Showing Penile Anatomy.

mental stimulation, at the level of the penis itself, or both. Transmission of impulses from parasympathetic nerves and nonadrenergic-noncholinergic nerves is facilitated by nitric acid, the most potent neurotransmitter for the erectile process. Nitric acid increases intracellular levels of type 5-cyclic guanosine monophosphate (cGMP) in the cavernosal smooth muscle, which acts to relax cavernosal tissue, and stimulates phosphorylation of the proteins (e.g., protein kinase G) that regulate smooth muscle tone. These actions bring about relaxation of the corpora cavernosa, thus permitting blood to fill the spaces. The inward flow of blood creates pressure in the corpora cavernosa, causing the penis to enlarge. Thick fascial tissue, the tunica albuginea, traps blood in the corpora cavernosa to sustain the erection, which is maintained until ejaculation. After ejaculation the penis contracts to stop the inflow of blood and open drainage channels.

Smooth muscle cells line both the cavernosal sinuses and the afferent arterioles. When the smooth muscle relaxes, the lumina increase in size and blood flow increases. When the smooth muscle lining the cavernosal sinuses relaxes, the sinuses accommodate more blood. Thus they increase in size, with subsequent compression of venules causing venous trapping. However, if inadequate venous trapping occurs, even with good inflow the penis does not become rigid.

PHARMACOTHERAPEUTIC OPTIONS

Phosphodiasterase Inhibitors
◆ sildenafil (Viagra, Revatio);   ◆ Revatio, Viagra
◆ tadalafil (Cialis);   ◆ Cialis
◆ vardenafil (Levitra);   ◆ Levitra

▥ Indications
Phosphodiasterase (PDE) inhibitors are used in the treatment of ED. It helps many men with ED associated with diabetes mellitus (57%), spinal cord injuries (83%), and radical prostatectomy (43%) to effect an erection. Sildenafil has also been used in the treatment of pulmonary hypertension (see Evidence-Based Pharmacotherapeutics box, Sildenafil for Pulmonary Hypertension).

▥ Pharmacodynamics
Taken before sexual activity, PDE inhibitors block the degradative action of type 5-cGMP, the predominant PDE enzyme in the corpus cavernosa. PDE inhibitors enhance the effects of nitric oxide that relax smooth muscles in the penis during sexual stimulation. The relaxation permits increased blood flow into the penis. PDE inhibitors are ineffective without sexual stimulation.

▥ Pharmacokinetics
PDE inhibitors are rapidly absorbed following oral administration. The absorption rate is reduced if the drugs are taken with a fatty meal. The pharmacokinetics of PDE inhibitors are dose dependent over the recommended dosage range. Plasma concentrations are approximately 40% of the parent drug. Protein binding is independent of total dose concentrations. PDE inhibitors are primarily eliminated by hepatic biotransformation, particularly by CYP 3A4, and are converted to active metabolite with properties similar to the parent drug. Elimination is through the feces and to a lesser extent in the urine.

Tadalafil remains in the body longer than the other two PDE inhibitors. Because of its 36-hour duration of action, tadalafil is also known as the "weekend pill." Vardenafil has a relative short duration of action compared with tadalafil (see Table 43-2).

▥ Adverse Effects and Contraindications
The common adverse effects of PDE inhibitors include headache, flushing, indigestion, nasal congestion, back pain, and muscle aches. Patients who have back pain and muscle aches usually note the symptoms 12 to 24 hours after taking the drug; the symptoms usually resolve in 48 hours. Dyspepsia and abnormal vision are noted at high dosages.

The vision changes are ordinarily mild and transient and primarily include changes in color vision (a blue tinge to objects viewed), but also light sensitivity and blurry vision. **A loss of vision in one or both eyes may be a sign of nonarteritic, anterior ischemic optic neuropathy (NAION). NAION may cause permanent loss of vision.** Men at higher risk for NAION include those with heart disease and those who are over 50 years of age, who have diabetes, hypertension, hyperlipidemia, or certain eye problems (retinitis pigmentosa), or who smoke.

Because these drugs have systemic vasodilator properties, transient decreases in supine blood pressure may occur. This

GENITOURINARY

EVIDENCE-BASED PHARMACOTHERAPEUTICS

Sildenafil for Pulmonary Hypertension

■ Background

Pulmonary hypertension (PH) is high blood pressure within the pulmonary circulation. Pulmonary hypertension can be of unknown cause (i.e., primary pulmonary hypertension [PPH]) or due to a known underlying cause (secondary pulmonary hypertension [SPH]). Pulmonary arteriolar vasoconstriction is an important finding of PH. Drug therapy is aimed at vasodilation of pulmonary vasculature.

Sildenafil (Viagra, Revatio) works on the pulmonary blood vessels the same way it works in the penile vessels. The increase in 5-cyclic guanosine monophosphate (5-cGMP) within the pulmonary vasculature smooth muscle cells results in relaxation. In patients with pulmonary hypertension, this can lead to vasodilation of the pulmonary vascular bed and, to a lesser extent, vasodilation in systemic circulation. Revatio is indicated for WHO group 1 patients (i.e., mean pulmonary artery pressure [PAP] over 25 mm Hg at rest and pulmonary capillary wedge pressure [PCWP] less than 15 mm Hg during right heart catheterization), and all New York Heart Association (NYHA) functional classes, to improve exercise ability. It is the first oral drug to be approved for an early stage of the disease.

■ Research Article

Kanthapillai, P., Lasserson T., and Walters, E. (2004). Sildenafil for pulmonary hypertension. *The Cochrane Database of Systematic Reviews.* 2004, Issue 4. Art. No. CD003562. DOI: 10.1002/14651858.CD003562.pub2.

Purpose

The purpose of the study was to determine the clinical efficacy of sildenafil, a vasodilator that works by inhibiting the enzyme type V phosphodiesterase, administered by any route to subjects with primary or secondary forms of PH.

Design

Randomized, controlled trials were considered for inclusion in the review. Trials included in the study assessed the effects of sildenafil in subjects diagnosed with PPH and SPH.

Methods

Two investigators independently assessed, reviewed, and extracted data from 4 clinical trials ($N = 77$). Data were entered in the computer program RevMan Analyses 1.0.2. Continuous data were pooled with an estimate on either weighted mean difference (WMD) or standardized mean difference (SMD) scales. Dichotomous data were pooled and relative risks (RR) were calculated.

Findings

Two studies looked at the "acute effects" of sildenafil. Two small crossover studies assessed the effects of long-term administration of sildenafil. The "acute effect" studies indicated that sildenafil has a pulmonary vasodilatory effect. The two crossover studies showed improvement in symptoms. One study showed improvement in fatigue domains from a validated health status questionnaire. Both crossover studies reported that the drug was well tolerated. One small longer-term study found some favorable effects in terms of symptoms of PH, but in the absence of longer-term outcomes, it could not be established whether this meant that the people given the drug felt that their levels of daily activity were better.

Conclusions

The validity of the observed effects is questionable because of the small participant numbers and inadequate exploration of the different disease etiologies.

■ Implications for Practice

The effects on long-term outcome such as NYHA functional class, symptoms, mortality, and exercise capacity require further validation. More studies of sufficient size are necessary before the long-term effects of sildenafil on clinically important outcomes can be established.

---

effect would be of minor significance in most patients, but consider carefully whether patients with underlying cardiovascular disease could be adversely affected. Prolonged erections and priapism (painful erections lasting longer than 4 hours) are infrequent.

Cardiovascular adverse effects such as angina, atrioventricular (AV) block, migraine, syncope, tachycardia, palpitations, abnormalities on electrocardiogram (ECG), hypotension, postural hypotension, prolonged QT interval, heart failure, cardiomyopathy, myocardial ischemia, and cerebral thrombosis are reported in fewer than 2% of patient taking PDE inhibitors. Most, but not all, of these patients had underlying cardiovascular disease before using a PDE inhibitor. Sensitivity to the effects of PDE inhibitors is increased in patients with an underlying condition such as left ventricular outflow obstruction (e.g., aortic stenosis, idiopathic hypertrophic stenosis) and those with severely impaired autonomic control of blood pressure. Vardenafil was not linked with clinically relevant prolongations of the QT interval, the time it takes the heart to electrically recharge itself. Prolonged QT intervals sometimes lead to dangerously irregular heart beats and death. **Do not prescribe a PDE inhibitor to men with a history of myocardial infarction or stroke within the past 6 months,** **those with uncontrolled high blood pressure, severe low blood pressure, or liver disease, or those with unstable angina.** Administration of a PDE inhibitor to patients using any form of organic nitrate, either regularly or intermittently, is contraindicated because the combination can cause a precipitous drop in blood pressure.

▓ Drug Interactions

Taking a PDE inhibitor and an alpha blocker (e.g., doxazosin) within 4 hours of each other can cause a sudden drop in blood pressure (see Table 43-3). It is recommended that at least 24 hours be allowed to elapse between doses of a PDE inhibitor and a nitrate drug. When used concurrently with CYP 3A4 inhibitors such as erythromycin, ketoconazole, and itraconazole, as well as the nonspecific inhibitor cimetidine, increased plasma levels of sildenafil can result.

▓ Dosage Regimen

None of the PDE inhibitors are to be used more than once a day (see Table 43-4). Reduce drug dosages in patients with kidney or liver disorders. No dosage adjustment is needed for patients with diabetes mellitus.

▥ Lab Considerations

There are no known lab considerations with PDE inhibitors.

Miscellaneous Drugs for Erectile Dysfunction

Yohimbine

Yohimbine blocks presynaptic α_2 receptors. It is to be noted that in male sexual performance, erection is linked to cholinergic activity and to $alpha_2$ blockade, which theoretically results in increased penile inflow, decreased penile blood outflow, or both. Yohimbine's action on peripheral blood vessels resembles that of reserpine, though it is weaker and of short duration. Yohimbine's peripheral autonomic nervous system effect is to increase cholinergic and decrease adrenergic activity. Yohimbine also exerts a stimulating action on the mood and may increase anxiety. Such actions have not been adequately studied or related to dosage, although they appear to require high dosages of the drug. Yohimbine has a mild anti-diuretic action, which it probably achieves by stimulation of hypothalamic centers and release of posterior pituitary hormone.

Reportedly, yohimbine exerts no significant influence on cardiac stimulation or other effects mediated by beta-adrenergic receptors. Its effect on blood pressure, if any, would be to lower it; however, no adequate studies are at hand to quantify this effect in terms of yohimbine dosage. Occasional adverse effects require the dosage to be reduced to one half a tablet 3 times a day, followed by gradual increases to one tablet 3 times a day. Therapy should not extend more than 10 weeks.

Alprostadil

Alprostadil (Muse), prostaglandin E_1 pellet, is used in the treatment of ED due to neurogenic, vasculogenic, or psychogenic causes. Alprostadil acts on vascular smooth muscle of the penis to dilate cavernosal arteries, allowing blood flow to and entrapment in the lacunar spaces of the penis.

Using a prefilled applicator, the man is able to place a pellet in the urethra. Within 8 to 10 minutes, the drug causes an erection, which can last between 30 and 60 minutes. A few adverse effects have been noted with the use of alprostadil, such as aching in the penis, the testicles, and the area between the penis and the rectum; warmth or a burning sensation in the urethra; redness from increased blood flow to the penis; and minor urethral bleeding or spotting.

Alprostadil is also available as Caverject (✦ Caverject), an injectable method. The drug is injected into the corpus cavernosa of the penis using a fine needle. Erection occurs within 2 to 5 minutes. Penile pain, prolonged erection, localized pain, penile fibrosis, and injection site hematoma and ecchymosis may be noted, along with a headache, respiratory infection, and flulike symptoms. **This method is not used if the female partner is pregnant (unless a condom barrier is also used).**

Alprostadil interacts with vasodilator drugs and can increase the risk for hypotension. In patients taking anticoagulants or thrombolytics, the risk for bleeding is increased.

CLINICAL REASONING

Treatment Objectives

The objective in using a PDE inhibitor for a patient with ED is to assist him in establishing an erection sufficient for vaginal penetration and lasting long enough for satisfactory intercourse.

Treatment Options

▥ Patient Variables

Most health care providers begin treatment of ED using the least invasive strategy and then move on to more invasive strategies. For some men, making a few healthy lifestyle changes may solve the problem. Quitting smoking, losing excess weight, and increasing physical activity helps some men regain sexual function. The next consideration is reducing the use of drugs with potential adverse effects. For example, antihypertensive drugs act in different ways (see Chapter 37). If a particular drug is causing erectile problems, perhaps a different drug can be prescribed. Psychotherapy and behavior modification may also be considered for some patients.

▥ Drug Variables

Although orally administered PDE inhibitors improve response to sexual stimulation, they do not trigger the automatic erection as injections do. Orally administered testosterone may help men who have low levels of natural testosterone; however it is often ineffective and can cause liver damage. There are also claims that drugs such as yohimbine, dopamine and serotonin agonists, and trazodone are effective, but the effects are inconsistent and the claims, to date, have not been substantiated.

Patient Education

Teach patients the physiology of an erection and what happens with ED. However, explaining the concept can be difficult. A simple analogy of attempting to fill a tire connected to an air hose helps describe the process more easily. If the tire does not fill when air is being pumped, there can either be a kink in the air hose (i.e., an arterial problem), or a leak in the tire (i.e., a venous trapping problem).

Tell patients who are adversely affected by use of a PDE inhibitor to discuss the situation with their health care provider before taking another dose of the drug. A patient experiencing an erection lasting longer than 4 hours is advised to see medical assistance. Priapism can result in penile tissue damage and permanent loss of potency if not immediately treated.

Advise the patient that use of a PDE inhibitor offers no protection from sexually transmitted diseases. These drugs have no effect on sperm motility or morphology.

Evaluation

Successful treatment of ED is manifest by the patient's self-report of the ability to establish an erection sufficient for vaginal penetration. Using a global improvement question, 83%

of patients reported improved erections on sildenafil versus placebo. Data from erection diaries indicated that 59% of patients using sildenafil who attempted sexual intercourse were successful compared to 13% on placebo (Tarig, et al., 2003). Sildenafil improves erection in 43% of patients who had radical prostatectomies compared with 14% for placebo.

KEY POINTS

OVERACTIVE BLADDER

■ In patients with OAB, the layered, smooth detrusor muscle contracts spastically before the bladder has reached the filling capacity necessary to stimulate micturition, increasing the risk of urge incontinence.

■ There are three primary treatment modalities for OAB: antimuscarinic therapy, bladder retraining, and surgery.

■ Antimuscarinics exert an antispasmodic effect on the detrusor muscle, inhibiting the muscarinic action of acetylcholine and thereby preventing unwanted contractions and urine leakage.

BENIGN PROSTATIC HYPERPLASIA

■ Although the exact cause of BPH is unknown, urination becomes increasingly more difficult and the bladder never feels completely empty. Prostatic enlargement eventually obstructs urinary outflow completely.

■ The usual remedy for BPH is prostatectomy. However, in many cases, alpha blocking drugs and 5α-reductase inhibitors are used to relieve symptoms and improve urination.

■ Alpha blockers relax the smooth muscle of the prostate and the bladder neck without interfering with bladder contractility, thereby decreasing bladder resistance to urinary outflow.

■ 5α-reductase inhibitors (also known as androgenic hormone inhibitors) block the production of DHT, thus reducing prostatic tissue growth and diminishing symptoms of BPH.

URINARY RETENTION

■ Urinary retention is a common occurrence following surgery or childbirth and in patients with neurogenic atony of the bladder.

■ The objective of treatment for urinary retention is regular and complete emptying of the bladder.

■ Direct-acting cholinergics such as bethanecol enhance the activity of naturally occurring ACh to cause bladder contraction.

ERECTILE DYSFUNCTION

■ Erectile dysfunction is the repeated inability to get or maintain an erection firm enough for sexual intercourse. If there is inadequate venous trapping of blood, even with good inflow, the penis does not become rigid.

■ PDE inhibitors block the degradative action of type 5-cGMP, the predominant enzyme in the corpus cavernosa. They enhance the effects of nitric oxide, a chemical that relaxes smooth muscles in the penis during sexual stimulation and allows increased blood flow.

■ A loss of vision in one or both eyes may be a sign of nonarteritic, anterior ischemic optic neuropathy (NAION). NAION may cause permanent loss of vision.

■ Patients with an underlying condition such as left ventricular outflow obstruction (e.g., aortic stenosis, idiopathic hypertrophic stenosis) and those with severely impaired autonomic control of blood pressure are more sensitive to the effects of the PDE inhibitors.

■ Men who have had a myocardial infarction or stroke within the past 6 months and those with uncontrolled high blood pressure, severe low blood pressure, liver disease, or unstable angina should not take a PDE inhibitor.

Bibliography

American Urological Association. (2003). Guideline on the management of benign prostatic hyperplasia: Chapter 1: Diagnosis and treatment recommendations. *The Journal of Urology, 170*(2 pt 1), 530–537.

Anderson, B., and Khadra, A. (2006). Acute urinary retention: Developing an A&E management pathway. *British Medical Journal, 15*(8), 434–438.

Appell, R. (2006). Pharmacotherapy for overactive bladder: An evidence-based approach to selecting an antimuscarinic agent. *Drugs, 66*(10), 1361–1370.

Barnett, C., and Machado, R. (2006). Sildenafil in the treatment of pulmonary hypertension. *Vascular Health and Risk Management, 2*(4), 411–422.

Barry, M., Williford, W., Chang, Y., et al. (1995). Benign prostatic hyperplasia specific health status measures in clinical research: How much change in the American Urological Association Symptom Index and the Benign Prostatic Hyperplasia Impact Index is perceptible to patients? *The Journal of Urology, 154*(5), 1770–1774.

Bautista, O., Kusek, J., Nyberg, L., et al. (2006). Study design of the Medical Therapy of Prostatic Symptoms (MTOPS) trial. *Controlled Clinical Trials, 24*(2), 224–243.

Cardozo, L., Lisec, M., Millard, R., et al. (2004). Randomized, double-blind placebo controlled trial of the once daily antimuscarinic agent solifenacin succinate in patients with overactive bladder. *Journal of Urology, 172*(5 pt 1), 1919–1924.

Chapple, C., Martinez-Garcia, R., Selvaggi, L., et al. for the STAR Study Group. (2005). A comparison of the efficacy and tolerability of solifenacin succinate and extended-release tolterodine at treating overactive bladder syndrome: Results of the STAR trial. *European Urology, 48*(3), 464–470.

Desgrandchamps, F. (2004). Who will benefit from combination therapy? The role of 5 alpha reductase inhibitors and alpha blockade: A reflection from MTOPS. *Current Opinion in Urology, 14*(1), 17–20.

Diokno, A., Appell, R., Sand, P., et al. (2003). Prospective, randomized, double-blind study of the efficacy and tolerability of the extended-release formulations of oxybutynin and tolterodine for overactive bladder: Results of the OPERA trial. *Mayo Clinic Proceedings, 78*(6), 687–695.

Fagelman, E. (2002). Herbal medicines to treat benign prostatic hyperplasia. *Urology Clinics of North America, 29*(1), 23–29.

Herbison, P., Hay-Smith, J., Ellis, G., et al. (2003). Effectiveness of anticholinergic drugs compared with placebo in the treatment of overactive bladder: Systemic review. *BMJ*, *326*(7394), 841–844.

Hing, E., Cherry, D., and Woodwell, D. (2006). National Ambulatory Medical Care Survey: 2004 Summary. *Advance Data*, *23* (374), 1–33.

Kreder, K. (2006). Solifenacin. *Urology Clinics of North America*, *33*(4), 483–490.

Ishani, A., MacDonald, R., Nelson, D., et al. (2000). *Pygeum africanum* for the treatment of patients with benign prostatic hyperplasia: A systematic review and quantitative meta-analysis. *American Journal of Medicine*, *109*(8), 654–664.

Lam, J., Cooper, K., and Kaplan, S. (2004). Changing aspects in evaluation and treatment of the patient with benign prostatic hyperplasia. *Medical Clinics of North America*, *88*(2), 281–308.

Middleton, K., and Hing, E. (2006). National Hospital Ambulatory Medical Care Survey: 2004 Outpatient department summary. *Advance Data*, *23*(373), 1–27.

Mikhail, N. (2005). Management of erectile dysfunction by the primary care physician. *Cleveland Clinic Journal of Medicine*, *72*(4), 293–311.

National Kidney and Urologic Diseases Information Clearinghouse. (2006). Prostatic enlargement: Benign prostatic hyperplasia. NIH Publication No. 06–3012. Available online: http://kidney.niddk.nih.gov/kudiseases/pubs/prostateenlargement/index.htm. Accessed May 12, 2007.

Nickle, J., Fradet, Y., Boake, R., et al. (1996). Efficacy and safety of finasteride therapy for benign prostatic hyperplasia: Results of a 2-year randomized controlled trial (the PROSPECT study). *Canadian Medical Journal*, *155*(9), 1251–1259.

Noe, L., Becker, R., Williamson, T., et al. (2002). A pharmacoeconomic model comparing two long-acting treatments for overactive bladder. *Journal of Managed Care Pharmacy*, *8*(5), 343–352.

Rossi, R., Nuzzo, A., and Lattanzi, A., (2007). Sildenafil improves endothelial function in patients with pulmonary hypertension. *Pulmonary Pharmacology and Therapeutics*, *20*(4). Available online: www.ncbi.nlm.nih.gov/sites/entrez?db=PubMed&term=%22Pulm%20Pharmacol%20Ther%22%5BJournal%5D. Accessed June 24, 2007.

Sandu, J., and Te, A. (2004). The role of 5-alpha-reductase inhibition as monotherapy in view of the MTOPS data. *Current Urologic Reports*, *5*(4), 274–279.

Simon, H. (2006). On call: I know that Viagra is safe for men with high blood pressure, but is it also safe for men with high eye pressures? *Harvard Men's Health Watch*, *11*(3), 8.

Stefel, A. (2004). Erectile dysfunction: Etiology, evaluation, and treatment options. *Medical Clinics of North America*, *889*(2), 387–416.

Steers, W. (2006). Darifenacin: Pharmacology and clinical usage. *Urology Clinics of North America*, *33*(4), 475–482.

Tarig, S., Omran, M., Kaiser, F., et al. (2003). Erectile dysfunction: Etiology and treatment in young and old patients. *Clinical Geriatric Medicine*, *19*(3), 539–551.

Vasavada, S., and Rackley, R. (2006). How effective is pharmacotherapy for overactive bladder? *Patient Care*, *2006*, 40–43.

Zinner, N., Gittelman, M., Harris, R., et al. (2004). Trospium chloride improves overactive bladder symptoms: A multicenter phase III trial. *Journal of Urology*, *171*(6 pt 1), 2311–2315.

Zinner, N. (2006). Darifenacin: A muscarinic M_3-selective receptor antagonist for the treatment of overactive bladder. *Expert Opinion in Pharmacotherapy*, *8*(4), 511–523.

GENITOURINARY

Drugs Used for Renal Dysfunction

The kidneys receive 20% to 25% of the cardiac output every minute and are very sensitive to changes in blood supply. A number of prerenal and intrarenal events can cause a critical fall in renal perfusion pressure (supplied by the arterial pressure of the blood), which may reduce renal blood flow (RBF). When RBF is diminished, the nutrients and oxygen for basic renal cellular metabolism and tubular transport systems are also diminished. Further, when RBF decreases, the fundamental driving force for glomerular filtration, the arterial blood pressure, is reduced. A reduction in renal perfusion pressure may result in a further decline in RBF because vasoconstrictive hormones, including angiotensin, vasopressin, and catecholamines, will have been released in response to the fall in perfusion pressure. As a result, glomerular filtration may no longer be maintained. A failure of glomerular filtration reduces urine flow and causes blood urea nitrogen (BUN) and creatinine (Cr) levels in the blood to rise. Correcting the factors that contribute to reduced RBF helps reestablish adequate circulation, thereby preventing ischemic injury.

ACUTE RENAL FAILURE

EPIDEMIOLOGY AND ETIOLOGY

Acute renal failure (ARF) is a sudden, rapid, partial or complete loss of renal function occurring over a matter of hours or, at most, a few days. The failure may be *oliguric* (less than 500 mL of urine excreted per day) or *nonoliguric* (more than 800 mL of urine per day) and usually, but not always, is accompanied by azotemia. *Azotemia* is a build-up of nitrogenous waste in the blood.

ARF can occur in seriously ill people of any age, sex, or community, and in any hospital unit or extended-care facility. Numerous renal insults can cause ARF, but the acute syndrome, unlike chronic renal failure, is usually reversible.

The etiologies of ARF are divided into three groups based on anatomic location: prerenal, intrarenal, and postrenal (Fig. 44-1 and Table 44-1). *Prerenal failure* occurs when there are losses or shifts of circulating blood volume, decreased cardiac output, decreased peripheral vascular resistance, and/or renal vascular obstruction.

Acute tubular necrosis (ATN) is the most common cause of *intrarenal azotemia* and of ARF in general. ATN is basically ARF caused by ischemia or toxins, or both. Urinary output in ATN is related to the number of injured nephrons and the location of the injury (i.e., cortex versus medulla). Approximately 50% of patients with ATN have oliguric renal failure.

A **Intrarenal causes of ARF are the most serious, and carry the greatest morbidity and mortality**. Other intrarenal causes of ARF include trauma, infection, glomerulonephritis, and vascular lesions.

Postrenal obstruction is the major cause of postrenal azotemia; it accounts for 2% to 15% of all cases of ARF, and is the second most common cause of ARF in infants.

PATHOPHYSIOLOGY

ARF is characterized by an initial oliguric phase (less than 500 mL of urine/day), followed in 10 or 14 days to a few weeks by a diuretic phase. Problems seen during the oliguric phase include an inability to eliminate solute loads, regulate electrolytes, and eliminate metabolic waste products. During the diuretic phase, large amounts of fluids (4 to 5 L/day) and electrolytes are lost. The recovery phase, before renal function returns to a normal range, may take as long as 6 months to a year. The prognosis is better for patients who have nonoliguric ARF than those with the oliguric form.

CHRONIC RENAL FAILURE

EPIDEMIOLOGY AND ETIOLOGY

In patients with chronic renal failure (CRF), the kidney is unable to remove metabolic wastes and excess water from the circulation. CRF develops insidiously over many years, or as a result of ARF from which the patient fails to recover. More than 100 different disease processes contribute to progressive loss of renal function, but diabetes mellitus and hypertension account for over 60% of the cases of end-stage renal disease (ESRD) in the United States. The third most common cause of CRF is glomerulonephritis, an inflammation of the glomeruli that frequently follows streptococcal infections of the upper respiratory tract. Acute glomerulonephritis may resolve completely or progress to chronic glomerulonephritis and eventual renal failure.

Genetics play a major role in the development of CRF and ESRD. The incidence of renal failure in the black population is 4 times as great as in the white population. In addition, blacks have a 6.2 times greater chance of developing ESRD secondary to hypertension. Focal and segmental glomerulosclerosis that occurs in association with intravenous (IV) drug use and acquired immunodeficiency syndrome (AIDS) is the most common cause of renal failure in young black adult males. These figures represent a 10 times greater risk for developing CRF than whites. Hispanics and Native Americans are at increased risk for renal failure secondary to type 2 diabetes mellitus (T2DM).

When renal failure progresses to ESRD, kidney impairment is permanent. The incidence of CRF is continually growing in the United States as a result of our increasing ability to prolong life using technical replacements for renal function (e.g., dialysis). It is estimated that more than one third of people on

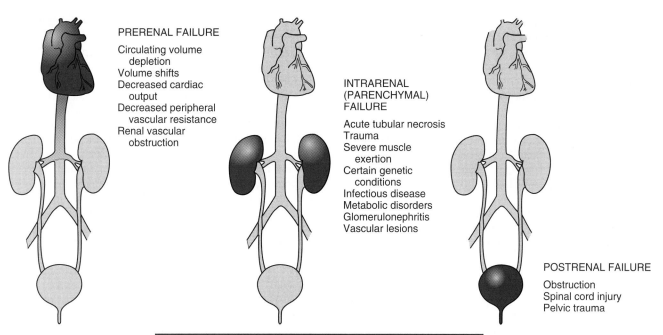

FIGURE 44-1 Anatomic Location of Prerenal, Intrarenal, and Postrenal Failure.

TABLE 44-1 Causes of Renal Failure

PRERENAL CONDITIONS	
Hypovolemia	Hemorrhage, burns, shock, excessive sweating, GI losses, peritonitis, nephrotic syndrome, Diuretics, diabetes insipidus
Altered peripheral vascular resistance	Antihypertensive drugs, sepsis, drug overdose, anaphylaxis, neurogenic shock
Cardiac disorders	Heart failure, myocardial infarction, cardiac tamponade, arrhythmias
Renal artery disorders	Emboli, thrombi, stenosis, aneurysm, occlusion, trauma
Drug-induced; hepatorenal syndrome	ACEIs, NSAIDs
INTRARENAL CONDITIONS	
Inflammatory processes	Bacterial, viral, preeclampsia
Immune processes	Autoimmunity, hypersensitivity, rejection
Trauma	Penetrating (e.g., knife, bullet), nonpenetrating (e.g., fall, crushing injury, motor vehicle accident, sports injury)
Obstruction	Neoplasm, stones, scar tissue
Systemic and vascular disorders	Diabetes mellitus, systemic lupus erythematosus, sickle cell disease, multiple myeloma, renal vein thrombosis
Drug-induced	Anesthetics, Antimicrobials, NSAIDs, Antineoplastics, contrast media
Nephrotoxins	Tumor toxins, heme pigments (e.g., hemoglobin, myoglobin), pesticides, fungicides, organic solvents, heavy metals, mushrooms, snake venom
POSTRENAL CONDITIONS	
Obstruction	Congenital anomalies (e.g., ureteropelvic stricture), benign prostatic hyperplasia, pelvic cancer, trauma, surgical injury

ACEIs, Angiotensin-converting enzyme inhibitors; *GI,* gastrointestinal; *NSAIDs,* nonsteroidal antiinflammatory drugs.

hemodialysis have diabetes, and that 25% to 50% of patients with insulin-dependent diabetes will develop ESRD within 10 to 20 years of starting insulin therapy.

PATHOPHYSIOLOGY

CRF is characterized by histologic evidence of irreversible renal damage, which progresses in three stages. Initially, there is diminished renal reserve without accumulation of metabolic wastes. The unaffected kidney compensates for the decreased function of the diseased kidney. The failure progresses from mild to severe renal insufficiency, involving the steady accumulation of metabolic waste products in the

blood. Severe fluid and electrolyte imbalances develop. The four stages of CRF include (1) diminished renal reserve without accumulation of metabolic wastes; (2) mild loss of renal function (GFR 40% to 80% of normal); (3) moderate loss of renal function (GFR 15% to 40% of normal); and (4) severe loss of renal function (GFR 2% to 20% of normal).

As renal failure goes forward, the progressive failure of multiple systems leads to anemia, uremia, disorders of calcium and phosphorus biotransformation, and acidosis. Anemia, an expected complication of advanced renal failure, primarily results from the inability of diseased kidneys to manufacture erythropoietin (EPO). However, it can be further aggravated by deficiencies of iron and certain vitamins. Although iron deficiency is uncommon in renal failure alone, it is common in patients who are maintained on hemodialysis for long periods. The anemia is a consequence of continued blood sampling for diagnostic studies and losses associated with the dialysis.

The uremic state is associated with abnormal platelet function that manifests as prolonged bleeding times and a predisposition to bleeding. A number of abnormal mechanisms contribute to the potential for bleeding. Platelet factor III activity is decreased; there are decreased levels of thromboxane A_2, increased levels of the platelet inhibitor prostacyclin, and suboptimal activity of factor VIII (von Willebrand's factor). The defects in platelet function can be partially corrected by repeated dialysis. Desmopressin (trade name DDAVP), a synthetic analogue of antidiuretic hormone (ADH), increases von Willebrand's factor concentrations and shortens bleeding times.

Disorders of calcium and phosphorus metabolism, including hypocalcemia, hyperphosphatemia, secondary hyperparathyroidism, bone disease, and metastatic calcification, are common findings in patients with advanced renal failure. These disturbances are largely a consequence of the kidneys' inability to eliminate phosphate, synthesize the active metabolite of vitamin D (1,25[OH]2D3), and eliminate hydrogen ions. Retention of phosphorus results in hyperphosphatemia, promoting soft tissue calcification and suppressing serum calcium levels. The hypocalcemia, in turn, causes secondary hyperparathyroidism and promotes bone disease. The hyperparathyroid state is further intensified by an inability of the diseased kidney to synthesize 1,25(OH)2D3, which normally exerts a suppressive effect on parathyroid hormone synthesis. Therapy is directed at normalizing serum phosphorus levels and suppressing the hyperparathyroid state. This goal can be accomplished by the administration of phosphate-binding drugs and calcitriol, a vitamin D supplement.

Acidosis compounds the genesis of bone disease. The patient with CRF has a positive hydrogen ion balance as a result of the inability to eliminate diet-derived acids. The retained hydrogen ions are thought to be buffered by bone salts, resulting in the dissolution of bone. Orally administered sodium bicarbonate effectively corrects the acidosis and prevents the dissolution of bone.

PHARMACOTHERAPEUTIC OPTIONS

The management of a patient with renal failure ordinarily includes multidrug therapy, diet therapy, and dialysis in some form. Drug classes used in the management of renal failure include angiotensin-converting enzyme inhibitors (ACEIs), angiotensin II–receptor blockers (ARBs), antianemic drugs (e.g., EPO, B_{12}, folate), iron supplements, antihemorrhagic drugs, phosphate binders, vitamin D supplements, heavy metal antagonists (chelating drugs), systemic antacids, loop diuretics, renal vasodilators, and cation-exchange resins.

Angiotensin-Converting Enzyme Inhibitors

The major objectives in the management of patients with CRF are to slow or prevent the progression of renal failure to ESRD, and to alleviate the complications and consequences of advanced renal failure. ACEIs (see Chapter 37) are most useful in patients with type 1 diabetic nephropathy who have decreasing renal function; however, the ACEIs are thought to exert similar effects in all types of proteinuric renal diseases. The most commonly used ACEI approved by the FDA for these purposes is captopril.

ACEIs block the conversion of angiotensin I to angiotensin II. By blocking the formation of angiotensin II, efferent arteriolar vasoconstriction is reduced and the stimulus for secretion of the mineralocorticoid hormone, aldosterone, is diminished. Withdrawal of angiotensin-II–induced constriction of efferent arterioles reduces filtration pressure, which, when high, damages the glomerular basement membrane and increases the permeability of the membrane to proteins, resulting in proteinuria. Consequently, ACEIs reduce proteinuria and help restore normal glomerular filtration. Decreased aldosterone secretion reduces sodium retention caused by the hormone, promotes the excretion of excess salt and water, and normalizes arterial blood pressure. Overall, the ACEIs slow the rate of renal deterioration in CRF. The pharmacokinetic characteristics of ACEIs are identified in Chapter 37.

Adverse reactions of ACEIs include skin rash, hypotension, angioedema, and cough. Black women are at the highest risk for angioedema. **A major adverse effect noted in patients** ▲ **who have renal failure who are taking ACEIs is hyperkalemia.** Hyperkalemia results from reduced circulating aldosterone concentrations. Hyperkalemia secondary to captopril administration results from reduced circulating aldosterone concentrations and a reduced GFR. A loss of taste perception (i.e., dysgeusia) may also occur and is usually reversible in 2 to 3 months.

ACEIs are contraindicated for use in patients with hypersensitivity to the drugs. Cross-hypersensitivity among ACEIs may occur. Use caution when giving ACEIs to patients with renal impairment, hepatic impairment, hypovolemia, hyponatremia, hyperkalemia, renal artery stenosis, or cerebrovascular or cardiac insufficiency; older adults; and patients receiving concurrent diuretic therapy. ACEIs are also contraindicated for use in patients with hypersensitivity to the drugs, in patients with bilateral renal artery stenosis, and in pregnant women. Use during pregnancy may cause fetal malformation or death, and hypotension, oliguria, or hyperkalemia may occur in the newborn. Safety during lactation and in children has not been established.

There is a higher incidence of life-threatening neutrope- ▲ **nia and agranulocytosis in patients with impaired renal function. Therefore, it is recommended that white blood cell counts (WBC) with differential be obtained before starting therapy and monitored periodically thereafter. Discontinue ACEI therapy if the neutrophil count falls below 1000/mm³.**

BUN and creatinine levels are measured because ACEIs, as a consequence of reducing glomerular filtration pressure, can cause the BUN and creatinine to be transiently increased. Patients who may have elevated levels are those who are volume- or sodium-depleted, who have bilateral renal artery stenosis, or who had a rapid reduction in chronic or severe hypertension. Monitor WBCs before initiation of therapy and periodically throughout treatment.

Angiotensin II–Receptor Blockers

Angiotensin II–receptor blockers (ARBs) are advocated by the American Diabetes Association as first-line treatment for patients with diabetic nephropathy. Although there are no adequate head-to-head studies comparing ARBs and ACE inhibitors in patients with diabetic nephropathy, there is support for recommendations based on each of the following three observations: (1) ARBs delay the progression of nephropathy in patients with type 2 diabetes, hypertension, microalbuminuria, and renal insufficiency (i.e., serum creatinine >1.5 mg/dL); (2) ARBs and ACEIs delay the progression of microalbuminemia in patients with type 2 diabetes, hypertension, and microalbuminuria; and (3) ACE inhibitors delay the progression of nephropathy in patients with type 1 diabetes, hypertension, and any degree of albuminuria.

As discussed in Chapter 37, ARBs block type 1 angiotensin II–receptors on blood vessels and other tissues such as the heart that stimulate vascular smooth muscle contraction. They are generally well tolerated and have a relatively low incidence of adverse effects. When adverse effects are present, they most often involve fatigue, headache, dizziness, insomnia, nasal congestion, and sinus congestion. Diarrhea, dyspepsia, elevated liver enzymes and renal function test results, muscle cramps, myalgia, and back and leg pain have also been documented. Because ARBs do not increase bradykinin levels like ACEIs, the dry cough associated with ACEIs is less of a problem. The frequency of cough with losartan is significantly lower than that seen with ACEIs. Losartan also appears to produce less angioedema than ACEIs. Valsartan rarely, if ever, causes a cough.

⚠ **ARBs contribute to renal failure in patients with bilateral renal artery stenosis and therefore are to be avoided.** The reason for avoiding ARBs in these patients is that the elevated circulating and intrarenal angiotensin II constricts efferent arterioles more than afferent arterioles within the kidney, which helps to maintain glomerular capillary pressure and filtration. Removing this constriction by blocking angiotensin II–receptors on the efferent arterioles can cause an abrupt fall in GFR. This is not usually an issue in patients who have unilateral renal artery stenosis, because the unaffected kidney usually maintains sufficient filtration after AT_1 receptors are blocked; however, with bilateral renal artery stenosis, it is especially important to ensure that renal function is not compromised. ARBs are contraindicated for use in pregnancy.

ARBS have few drug interactions with other drugs (see **⚠** Table 37–6). **Because ARBs may increase blood levels of potassium, the use of potassium supplements, salt substitutes (which often contain potassium), or other drugs that increase potassium may result in excessive blood potassium levels.** Slowly adjust the dosage of ARBs based to patient response.

Antianemics
◆ darbepoetin alfa (Aranesp)
◆ epoetin alfa (erythropoietin, EPO, Epogen, Procrit)

▥ Indications
Anemia universally accompanies CRF. In fact, hematocrit values of 16% to 22% (normal hematocrit range: males, 41% to 50%; females, 36% to 44%) were common in the days before epoetin alfa was available. Epoetin alfa is a well-accepted drug for the treatment of the anemia associated with CRF. It is used for patients who are not on dialysis, as well as for those undergoing the various dialytic therapies. Epoetin alfa is not a substitute for blood transfusions and is not intended as an emergency treatment for severe anemia or blood loss. However, it has decreased the transfusion dependency of many patients with CRF. Patients treated with this drug have an increase in hematocrit, improved energy, and less fatigue. Other favorable outcomes include improvements in cardiovascular status and cognitive function, exercise tolerance, and quality of life.

Epoetin alfa is also used for the management of anemia secondary to zidovudine therapy in human immunodeficiency virus (HIV)–positive patients. Patients with nonmyeloid malignancies who have anemia secondary to antineoplastic drug therapy may also be candidates for epoetin alfa.

Recombinant darbepoetin alpha is a second-generation recombinant EPO-stimulating protein used for treating the anemia associated with CRF and that found in patients with cancer. It is sometimes known as NESP (novel erythropoiesis–stimulating protein).

▥ Pharmacodynamics
Darbepoetin alfa and epoetin alfa induce erythropoiesis by stimulating the division and differentiation of erythroid progenitor cells. Newly formed reticulocytes are released from the bone marrow and mature to erythrocytes. Erythropoietin production in the kidney occurs in interstitial cells in the inner cortex that are in immediate proximity to the proximal tubules. Cells are activated to produce EPO as the hematocrit drops. Clinically significant increases in the reticulocyte count occur within 7 to 10 days of starting treatment with epoetin alfa, with a rise in hemoglobin and hematocrit occurring in 2 to 6 weeks. Darbepoetin alfa produces a dose-dependent increase in hemoglobin.

However, the increased hemoglobin and hematocrit levels increase blood viscosity and peripheral vascular resistance. Blood pressure increases in 25% to 30% of patients, and thus changes in antihypertensive therapy may be required. Furthermore, increased red blood cell (RBC) volume shortens bleeding time. Patients on hemodialysis often require increased anticoagulation to prevent blood clotting in the dialyzer or vascular access device. The stimulation of erythropoiesis also increases the demand for iron, making iron supplementation necessary for many patients.

▥ Pharmacokinetics
Epoetin alfa and darbepoetin alfa are well absorbed following subcutaneous (subQ) or IV administration, although their distribution, biotransformation, and elimination are unknown (Table 44-2). An increase in reticulocyte count is observed in 7 to 14 days, with peak activity noted in 2 to 6 weeks. The increase in RBC counts lasts approximately 2 weeks once the drug has been discontinued.

▥ Adverse Effects and Contraindications
Hypertension is the most common adverse effect of darbepoetin alfa (occurring in 23% of patients) and epoetin alfa, but these drugs are also associated with hypotension, arrhythmias and cardiac arrest, angina and chest pain, heart failure, acute myocardial infarction, and stroke and transient ischemic attacks. Headache, transient rashes, arthralgias, and thrombotic events (in patients on dialysis) are also possible. Female patients may resume menses and fertility may be restored; therefore, evaluate the risk of pregnancy.

PHARMACOKINETICS

TABLE 44-2 Drugs Used to Treat Renal Dysfunction*

Drug	Route	Onset	Peak	Duration	PB (%)	t½	BioA (%)
ANTIANEMICS							
darbepoetin alfa	IV, subQ	Immed	24–72 hr; 71–123	Weeks	UA	27–89 hr	100
epoetin alfa	IV, subQ	7–14 days	2–6 wk†	2 wk	UA	4–13 hr	UA
IRON SUPPLEMENTS							
Iron formulations	PO	4 days	7–10 days‡	2–3 mo	UA	UA	UA
iron dextran	IM	Slow	1–2 wk	Months	UA	6 hr	UA
ANTIHEMORRHAGIC DRUG							
desmopressin	IV, subQ	Minutes	15–30 min	1.5–2 hr	UA	75 min	100
	IN	1 hr	1–5 hr	8–20 hr	UA	75 min	10–20
PHOSPHATE-BINDING DRUGS							
aluminum hydroxide§	PO	Hours–days	Days–weeks	Days	UA	UA	UA
Calcium salts	PO	UA	UA	UA	45	UA	UA
	IV	Immed	Immed	0.5–2 hr	45	UA	100
VITAMIN SUPPLEMENTS							
calcitriol	PO	2–6 hr	2–6 hr	1–5 days	Variable	3–8 hr	UA
paricalcitol	IV	Immed	UA	2 hr	>99	15 hr	100%
HEAVY METAL ANTAGONIST							
deferoxamine	IM, IV, subQ	Immed	UA	UA	UA	1 hr	UA
CATION-EXCHANGE RESIN							
sodium polystyrene sulfonate	PO	2–12 hr	UA	6–24 hr	UA	UA	0
	PR	2–12 hr	UA	4–6 hr	UA	UA	0
SYSTEMIC ANTACID							
sodium bicarbonate	PO	Immed	30 min	1–3 hr	UA	UA	UA
	IV	Immed	Rapid	UA	UA	UA	100
LOOP DIURETIC							
furosemide	PO	30–60 min	1–2 hr	6–8 hr	95	30–60 min	60
	IV	5 min	30 min	2 hr	95	UA	100
RENAL VASODILATOR							
dopamine	IV	1–2 min	10 min	Duration of inf	UA	2 min	100

*ARBs and ACEIs are used in the treatment of renal failure. They are discussed in Chapter 37 and thus pharmacokinetic data is not repeated here.
†The subQ route for epoetin alfa produces peak plasma concentrations in patients with CRF in 24–72 hours, whereas in cancer patients, peak plasma concentrations are seen in 71–123 hours. Although the IV route provides a more rapid peak, the delayed systemic absorption from the subQ route provides for a more sustained response. Peak effect, which is the targeted hematocrit level, may be achieved in 8 wk with adequate dosing. Elevation in RBC count lasts approximately 2 wk following discontinuation of the drug.
‡Peak levels and the amount of iron absorbed are approximately in linear relationship to dose ingested.
§Hypophosphatemic effects of aluminum hydroxide given orally.

BioA, Bioavailability; *CRF*, chronic renal failure; *Immed*, immediate; *IM*, intramuscular; *IN*, intranasal; *inf*, infection; *IV*, intravenous; *PB*, protein binding; *t½*, half-life; *subQ*, subcutaneous; *UA*, unavailable.

▲   **Although rare, seizures are the most serious adverse effect of darbepoetin alfa and epoetin alfa,** occurring in about 1% of the patients receiving epoetin alfa. If the hematocrit increases more than 4 points in a 2-week period, the likelihood of a hypertensive reaction and seizures increases.

Epoetin alfa is contraindicated for use in patients with hypersensitivity to albumin or mammalian cell–derived products or in those with uncontrolled hypertension. It is also contraindicated for use in patients with erythropoietin levels exceeding 200 milliunits/mL. Use the drug cautiously in patients with a history of seizures. Safe use during pregnancy and lactation and in children has not been established.

▥ Drug Interactions

There are few drug interactions with epoetin alfa. The drug may increase the requirement for heparin anticoagulation in patients on hemodialysis (Table 44-3).

▥ Dosage Regimen

Before starting therapy, evaluate the patient's iron and ferritin levels, because the efficacy of epoetin alfa is decreased if iron stores are insufficient to promote erythropoiesis. Iron deficiency may occur with the use of epoetin alfa owing to an internal shift of iron stores to RBCs during the correction of acute anemia, or the external loss of RBC iron during both the acute and maintenance phases of therapy. Because iron is necessary for continued RBC production, virtually all patients receiving epoetin alfa eventually require supplemental iron.

A poor initial response or a loss of response may be due to other factors such as infection, iron deficiency, or occult bleeding. Serum ferritin levels should be greater than 100 mcg/mL and transferrin saturation greater than 20%. If iron stores fall below these levels, administer supplemental iron before starting epoetin alfa. Oral iron preparations may be adequate for peritoneal dialysis patients; however, hemodialysis patients may require parenteral iron because there is a continuous loss of blood with the hemodialysis procedure (1 mL of blood loss is equal to 1 mg of iron loss).

▥ Lab Considerations

Epoetin alfa has been reported to cause an increase in WBC and platelet counts, and may decrease bleeding times. It can cause elevations in BUN, creatinine, phosphorus, potassium, sodium, and uric acid levels. It is unclear if the

DRUG INTERACTIONS
TABLE 44-3 Drugs Used to Treat Renal Dysfunction*

Drug	Interactive Drug	Interaction
ANTIANEMIC		
epoetin alfa, darbepoetin alfa	heparin	Increases heparin requirement for anticoagulation during dialysis
IRON SUPPLEMENTS		
ferrous fumarate, gluconate, sulfate, iron dextran	ciprofloxacin, enoxacin, norfloxacin, ofloxacin, penicillamine	Decreases effects of interactive drug
	levodopa	Decreases effects of iron supplement
	chloramphenicol, vitamin E	Impairs hematologic response to iron therapy
	tetracycline	Decreases absorption of interactive drug
	Antacids	Inhibits absorption of iron by forming insoluble compounds
	Vitamin C	Increases absorption of oral iron reparations
ANTIHEMORRHAGIC DRUGS		
desmopressin	chlorpropamide, clofibrate, carbamazepine	Enhances antidiuretic response to desmopressin
	demeclocycline, lithium, norepinephrine	Diminishes antidiuretic response to desmopressin
PHOSPHATE-BINDING DRUGS		
Calcium formulations	ciprofloxacin, digoxin, Quinolones, Iron salts, phenytoin, tetracyclines	Decreases absorption of interactive drugs
	digoxin	Hypercalcemia increases the risk of digoxin toxicity
	Antacids	Chronic use may lead to milk-alkali syndrome
	atenolol, CCB drugs	Excessive amounts of calcium may decrease the effects of interactive drugs
	Thiazide diuretics	Concurrent use may result in hypercalcemia
	sodium polystyrene sulfonate	Decreases ability of interactive drugs to decrease serum potassium levels
aluminum hydroxide	chlorpromazine, digoxin, Quinolones, Iron salts	Decreases absorption of interactive drug
	calcium citrate, sodium citrate	Markedly enhances absorption of aluminum leading to toxicity
	amphetamine, mexilitine, quinidine	Interactive drug levels may be increased if enough AlOH is ingested such that urinary pH is increased
	Salicylates	Decreases interactive drug blood levels
VITAMIN SUPPLEMENTS		
calcitriol	Magnesium containing antacids	Increases risk of hypermagnesemia
	cholestyramine, mineral oil	Decreases absorption of fat-soluble vitamins
	Thiazide diuretics	Increases risk of hypercalcemia
	Barbiturates, Hydantoins, primidone	Increases biotransformation of calcitriol and decreases effects
paricalcitol	digoxin	Increases risk of digoxin toxicity
HEAVY METAL ANTAGONIST		
deferoxamine	ascorbic acid	Increases effectiveness of deferoxamine but also may increase cardiac iron toxicity
CATION-EXCHANGE RESIN		
sodium polystyrene sulfonate	Magnesium and calcium-containing antacids and laxatives	Increases risk of metabolic alkalosis
	digoxin	Increases risk of digoxin toxicity
SYSTEMIC ANTACID		
sodium bicarbonate	ketoconazole	Decreases absorption of ketoconazole
	demeclocycline, doxycycline, lithium, Salicylates, Sulfonylureas, Tetracyclines	Increases excretion of interacting drug
	flecainide, mexilitine, quinidine	Decreases excretion of interacting drug
	Anorexiants, Sympathomimetics	Increases effects of interacting drug
	amphetamine, ephedrine, pseudoephedrine	Increases half-lives and duration of action of interacting drugs
LOOP DIURETIC		
furosemide	Oral hypoglycemic drugs	Increases potential for hyperglycemia
	Aminoglycosides, cisplatin	Increases potential for toxicity
	lithium, Salicylates	Decreases secretion of lithium, salicylate; increases risk of toxicity
	digoxin	Increases potential for digoxin toxicity related to potassium loss
	NSAIDs	Decreases antihypertensive effect of furosemide
	Neuromuscular blocking drugs	Increases effects of neuromuscular blockade
	phenytoin	Decreases absorption and effectiveness of furosemide
	theophylline	Increases diuresis from furosemide
RENAL VASODILATOR		
dopamine	Beta blockers	Decreases therapeutic effects of dopamine
	General anesthetics	Increases risk of arrhythmias
	Monoamine oxidase inhibitors	Increases intensity and prolongs cardiac stimulant and vasopressor effects of dopamine
	phenytoin	May cause sudden hypotension and bradycardia

*Angiotensin II–receptor blockers (ARBs) and angiotensin-converting enzyme inhibitors (ACEIs) are discussed in Chapter 37 and thus drug interactions are not repeated here.
AlOH, Aluminum hydroxide; CCB, calcium channel blockers; NSAIDs, nonsteroidal antiinflammatory drugs.

GENITOURINARY

elevations are the result of drug action or the efficacy of dialysis, or if they are caused by lack of adherence with dietary restrictions. Monitor the patient for an additional 2 to 6 weeks following a change in dosage or until the hematocrit has stabilized. Once stable, monitor the hematocrit at monthly intervals throughout the course of therapy.

Iron Supplements

- ferrous fumarate (Femiron, Feostat, Fumasorb, Fumerin, Hemocyte, Ircon); ◆ Palafer
- ferrous gluconate (Fergon, Ferralet, Simron); ◆ Apo-Ferrous Gluconate
- ferrous sulfate (Feosol, Fer-In-Sol, Slow Fe); ◆ Apo-Ferrous Sulfate, Fer-in-Sol, Slow-Fe
- iron dextran (Imferon, InFeD); ◆ Dexiron
- iron polysaccharide (Niferex, Niferex-PN, Fe-Tinic Hytinic, Nu-Iron 150)

Indications

Patients on dialysis are prone to iron deficiency because of repeated blood testing, surgical interventions, and blood loss during hemodialysis. A minority of dialysis patients will have an increase in hematocrit and symptomatic improvement with correction of iron deficiency alone. However, because iron is a necessary component of erythropoiesis, therapy with epoetin alfa will be hindered if patients do not have adequate iron stores.

Niferex is an oral iron preparation used in the treatment and prevention of iron-deficiency anemia, and for nutritional supplementation when iron intake in the diet is inadequate to meet body needs.

Pharmacodynamics

Iron is an essential mineral found in hemoglobin, myoglobin, and a number of enzymes and is necessary for effective erythropoiesis and for transport and utilization of oxygen. It elevates serum iron concentration and is then converted to hemoglobin or trapped in the reticuloendothelial cells for storage and eventual conversion to a usable form of iron. Parenteral iron enters the blood stream and organs of the reticuloendothelial system (i.e., liver, spleen, bone marrow), where it is separated from the dextran complex and becomes part of the body's iron stores.

Niferex is formulated with two types of iron: ferrous bisglycinate chelate (Ferrochel) and polysaccharide iron complex. Neither formulation is an iron salt. One mg of polysaccharide-iron complex is equivalent to one mg of elemental iron. Ferrochel provides 0.75 mg of elemental iron/mg and is more easily absorbed than other iron salts.

Pharmacokinetics

In general, 5% to 10% of dietary iron is absorbed. In deficiency states, this may increase to 30%. Iron supplements are well absorbed following intramuscular (IM) administration. Because iron is over 90% protein bound, it remains in the body for many months (see Table 44-2), crosses placental membranes, and enters breast milk. Iron supplements undergo hepatic biotransformation, with small daily losses occurring through desquamation and the production of sweat, urine, and bile.

Adverse Effects and Contraindications

Oral iron formulations are usually well tolerated, although nausea, epigastric pain, constipation, diarrhea, abdominal cramping, gastrointestinal (GI) bleeding, and black stools

may result. Contact irritation of the throat may occur with oral formulations, particularly liquids. Hypotension is the most common adverse effect of parenterally administered iron supplements. Headache, dizziness, syncope, tachycardia, urticaria, flushing, arthralgias, and phlebitis have also been reported. Impotence has been reported in young men, and amenorrhea in young women. The impotence and amenorrhea result from iron-loading in the anterior pituitary gland. Seizures and anaphylaxis are the most serious adverse effects. It has been suggested that the repletion of iron stores may serve as a growth medium for certain microorganisms.

Iron supplements are contraindicated for use in patients ▲ **with primary hemochromatosis, hemolytic anemias, and other anemias not associated with iron deficiency. Use extreme caution when administering iron supplements to patients with severe liver impairment.** Caution should also be used when iron supplementation is used for patients with peptic ulcers, ulcerative colitis, or regional enteritis; these conditions may be aggravated. Some products contain alcohol or tartrazine and should be avoided in patients with known intolerance or hypersensitivity. Patients with autoimmune disorders and arthritis are more susceptible to allergic reactions.

Arbitrary use of iron supplements can lead to iron overload and toxicity, which is characterized by anorexia, oliguria, diarrhea, hypothermia, shock, metabolic acidosis, and death. In addition, the patient may experience vascular congestion of the GI tract, the liver, the kidneys, the heart, the brain, the spleen, the adrenals, and the thymus. Cirrhosis develops as a result of excess iron storage in the liver. **Hepatoma, the primary** ▲ **cancer of the liver, has become the most common cause of death among patients with hemochromatosis. Accidental overdose of iron-containing products is a leading cause of fatal poisoning in children less than 6 years of age.**

Drug Interactions

Iron decreases the actions of quinolone antibiotics when taken concurrently (see Table 44-3). Iron absorption is decreased when it is taken with antacids, and the effectiveness of levodopa is decreased. Ascorbic acid taken concurrently enhances absorption of iron in a ratio of 200 mg ascorbic acid per 30 mg iron. Serum iron levels may increase when iron preparations are taken with chloramphenicol. Because there are no physiologic means of removing toxic amounts of iron from the body, a heavy metal antagonist (e.g., deferoxamine) may be needed to chelate the iron.

Dosage Regimen

Dosage regimens of iron formulations are identified in Table 44-4.

Lab Considerations

Iron levels of patients on dialysis (especially those receiving epoetin alfa) should be evaluated monthly. Monitor total serum iron, total iron-binding capacity (TIBC), folate, and ferritin levels until the target hematocrit value is reached. Thereafter, perform iron studies every 2 to 3 months. An iron saturation of less than 20% and serum ferritin levels less than 60 mcg/mL are consistent with iron deficiency. Similarly, lack of hemoglobin and hematocrit response to epoetin alfa, and microcytic RBCs, are also strongly suggestive of iron deficiency. Occult blood in stools may be obscured by the black coloration of iron in stool. Guaiac test results may occasionally be false-positive.

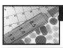

DOSAGE

TABLE **44-4 Drugs Used in Renal Dysfunction***

Drug	Use(s)	Dosage	Implications
ANTIANEMIC DRUGS			
darbepoetin alfa	Anemia of CRF	*Adult:* Initially, 0.45 mcg/kg subQ or IV once weekly. Adjust dosage to achieve and maintain target Hgb; not to exceed 12 grams/dL. Do not increase dosage more often than once monthly.	**Not interchangeable with epoetin alfa.** Dosages based on H&H. Check Hgb at least weekly during first 4 wk of therapy. ▲
	Anemia of cancer	*Adult:* 2.25 mcg/kg/dose once weekly	
epoetin alfa	Anemia related to CRF	*Adult:* 50–100 units/kg IV or subQ 3 times weekly. Increase by 25 units/kg if Hct does not rise 5–6 points, or has not reached target range after 8 wk of therapy. Maintenance: Decrease dosage by 25 units/ month until desired levels are achieved.	Determine endogenous serum erythropoietin level before using. Target hematocrit range for patients on dialysis: 30%–35%. If patient not on dialysis, should be given when Hct <30%.
	Anemia secondary to zidovudine therapy	*Adult:* 100 units/kg IV or subQ 3 times weekly for 8 wk. If inadequate response, may increase by 50–100 units/kg every 4–8 wk, up to 300 units/kg 3 times weekly	Determine serum EPO level before using; levels over 500 milliunits/mL may not respond to therapy. Monitor Hct weekly during dosage adjustment.
	Anemia secondary to antineoplastic therapy	*Adult:* 150 units/kg subQ 3 times weekly. May increase after 8 wk up to 300 units/kg 3 times weekly	Patients with lower baseline EPO levels may respond more rapidly. Not recommended if EPO levels exceed 200 milliunits/mL.
IRON SUPPLEMENTS			
ferrous fumarate	Iron supplementation: prevention and treatment of iron deficiency anemia, iron replacement for blood loss	*Adult: Prophylaxis:* 200 mg PO daily. *Therapeutic:* 200 mg PO 3–4 times daily. CR capsules twice daily *Child: Prophylaxis:* 3 mg/kg/day PO. *Therapeutic:* 3–6 mg/kg PO 3 times daily	6–10 mo required to raise iron stores before desired response achieved. Ferrous fumarate = 33% elemental iron.
ferrous gluconate		*Adult: Prophylaxis:* 325 mg PO daily. *Therapeutic:* 325–650 mg PO 4 times daily SR capsules may be given twice daily. *Child: Prophylaxis:* 8 mg/kg/day PO. *Therapeutic:* 16 mg/kg PO 3 times daily	Ascorbic acid enhances absorption of iron in ratio of 200 mg ascorbic acid/30 mg iron. Ferrous gluconate = 12% elemental iron.
ferrous sulfate		*Adult: Prophylaxis:* 300–325 mg PO daily. *Therapeutic:* 300 mg PO 2–4 times daily. TR tablets given twice daily. *Child: Prophylaxis:* 5 mg/kg/day PO. *Therapeutic:* 10 mg/kg PO 3 times daily	Ferrous sulfate = 20% elemental iron.
iron dextran		*Adult and Child >15 kg:* Total dose (mL) = 0.0476 × weight (kg) × (14.8 − Hgb) + 1 mL/5 kg up to 14 mL for iron stores. Divide and give in small daily doses IM or IV until total is reached. Not to exceed 100 mg/ day *Child:* Total dose (mL) = 0.0476 × (kg) × (12 − Hgb) + iron stores (not to exceed 25 mg/ day in children under 5 kg; 50 mg/day in children under 10 kg; or 100 mg/day in others)	Test doses of 0.5 mL (25 mg) should be given before therapy. Give only Z-track into upper, outer quadrant of buttocks. Total daily dose should not exceed 1.4 grams in adults.
polysaccharide iron complex	Anemia, iron-deficiency anemia, nutritional supplementation	*Adult:* One tablet or capsule PO daily	**Keep this product out of reach of children. Accidental overdose of iron-containing products is a leading cause of fatal poisoning in children <6 yr of age.** ▲
ANTIHEMORRHAGIC DRUG			
desmopressin	Bleeding associated with uremia; prevention of post–renal biopsy bleeding	*Adult and Child >3 mo:* 0.3 mcg/kg IV. May repeat as needed *Adult and Child:* 1 spray (150 mcg) in each nostril *Adult and Child <50 kg:* 1 spray (150 mcg) in one nostril *Child <10 kg:* 0.3 mcg/kg IV. May repeat as needed.	Reduction in bleeding usually occurs within 1 hr and lasts about 4 hr. Tachyphylaxis may occur if used more frequently than every 24–48 hr.
PHOSPHATE-BINDING DRUGS			
calcium acetate, calcium carbonate	Reduce serum phosphorus levels in uremia, secondary hyperparathyroidism; reduce severity of bone disease in uremic patients;	*Adult:* Dosage necessary to control calcium levels between 8 and 11 mg/dL and serum phosphate levels at 3.5–6 mg/dL	Separate administration of aluminum hydroxide and other oral drugs by at least 1–2 hr.

Continued

GENITOURINARY

DOSAGE

TABLE 44-4 Drugs Used in Renal Dysfunction*—Cont'd

Drug	Use(s)	Dosage	Implications
aluminum hydroxide	prevent development of metastatic calcification	*Adult:* 1.9–4.8 grams (30–40 mL) of regular suspension –or– 15–20 mL of concentrated suspension PO 3–4 times daily *Child:* 50–150 mg/kg/day PO in 4–6 divided doses	
VITAMIN D SUPPLEMENT			
calcitriol	Correction of hypocalcemia or uremia	*Adult: Prophylaxis:* 0.5–3 mcg PO daily. *Hyperparathyroidism of dialysis:* 2–3 mcg IV 3 times/wk at end of dialysis treatment. *Chronic peritoneal dialysis:* 1–3 mcg three times weekly *Child 1–5 yr:* 0.25–0.75 mcg PO daily *Child >6 yr:* 0.5–2 mcg PO daily	Dosage is limited by the development of hypercalcemia. Observe patient closely for evidence of hypocalcemia.
paricalcitol		*Adult:* 0.04–0.1 mcg/kg IV bolus every other day during dialysis. Dosage may be increased by 2–4 mcg at 2- to 4-wk intervals.	A Ca × P level over 75 indicates drug dosage should be reduced or the drug stopped until values normalize
HEAVY METAL ANTAGONIST			
deferoxamine	Acute iron toxicity; treatment of chronic iron overload. Unlabeled use: management of aluminum accumulation in bone in renal failure and aluminum-induced dialysis encephalopathy	*Adult: Acute toxicity:* 15 mg/kg/hr IV up to 90 mg/kg/8 hr (not to exceed 6 grams/day) –or– 90 mg/kg IM initially, then 45 mg/kg (up to 1 gram/dose) every 4–12 hr (not to exceed 6 grams/day). *Chronic overload:* 0.5–1 gram IM, IV, or intraperitoneal routes 4 times daily –or– 1–2 grams/day subQ. Not to exceed 15 mg/kg/day. *Adult and Child >3 yr:* 20–40 mg/kg/day by continuous subQ infusion given over 8–24 hr *Child <3 yr: Acute or chronic overload:* 10 mg/kg/hr IV. Not to exceed 6 grams/24 hr or 2 grams/dose	Increase in plasma aluminum or iron levels 12–24 hr after administration reflects binding to the drug. Spacing of dose determined by severity of signs and symptoms. Signs and symptoms take 2–3 mo to correct.
CATION-EXCHANGE RESIN			
sodium polystyrene sulfonate	Treatment of hyperkalemia secondary to ARF and CRF	*Adult:* 15 grams PO once to 4 times daily –or– 30–50 grams as enema every 6 hr *Child:* Calculate dosage based on exchange ratio of 1 mEq potassium per gram of resin	Exchange ratio: 15 mEq potassium/15 mEq sodium. Patient should have 1–2 watery stools each day during the course of therapy.
SYSTEMIC ANTACIDS			
sodium bicarbonate	Treatment of metabolic acidosis associated with renal failure	*Adult:* 2–5 mEq/kg over 4–8 hr IV. *Acidosis of CRF:* 1 gram 3 times daily. Maintenance: 1 gram 3 times daily *Child:* 0.5–1 mEq/kg	Rate and dosage determined by ABGs and estimate of base deficit.
LOOP DIURETIC			
furosemide	ARF; CRF; HTN crisis related to ARF	*Adult: CRF:* 80–120 mg PO daily –or– 240–500 mg IV every 4–6 hr PRN until desired response is achieved. *HTN crisis:* 100–200 mg IVP over 1–2 min. *Child:* 2 mg/kg PO as a single dose. Increase by 1–2 mg/kg every 6–8 hr, then 1–2 mg/kg/day up to 5–6 mg/kg/day –or– 1 mg/kg IV. May increase by 1 mg/kg every 2 hr. Not to exceed 6 mg/kg/day	May cause profound water and electrolyte depletion. Use cautiously in patients with anuria and hepatic coma. Doses up to 6 grams/day have been used.
RENAL VASODILATOR			
dopamine	Hemodynamic imbalances associated with renal failure	*Adult:* 0.3–5 mcg/kg/min IV. Increase by 5–10 mcg/kg/min IV to a rate of 20–50 mcg/kg/min.	Check urine output frequently when dosages over 16 mcg/kg/min. Safety and efficacy in children has not been established.

*ARBs and ACE inhibitors are used in the treatment of renal failure. They are discussed in Chapter 37 and thus dosing information is not repeated here.
ABGs, Arterial blood gases; *ARF*, acute renal failure; *CR*, controlled-release; *CRF*, chronic renal failure; *EPO*, erythropoietin; *Hct*, hematocrit; *Hgb*, hemoglobin; *H&H*, hemoglobin and hematocrit; *HTN*, hypertension; *IVP*, intravenous push; *PR*, per rectum; *PRN*, as needed; *SR*, sustained-release; *TR*, time-release.

Antihemorrhagic Drugs

◆ desmopressin (DDAVP, Stimate); ◆ DDAVP

▌ *Indications*

Desmopressin is effective in reversing the bleeding disorder present in uremia and is useful for the prevention of post–renal biopsy bleeding. It is also used in the management of diabetes insipidus caused by a deficiency of vasopressin and to control bleeding in certain types of hemophilia and von Willebrand's disease (Factor VIII deficiency).

▌ *Pharmacodynamics*

Desmopressin is a synthetic polypeptide that is structurally related to the posterior pituitary hormone ADH (see Chapter 55). The mechanism for antihemorrhagic action is unclear, but desmopressin is thought to increase factor VIII activity. Desmopressin-induced vasoconstriction may also aid in reducing the tendency to bleed. The antidiuretic effect increases the permeability of the collecting duct, thereby enhancing water reabsorption by the nephrons.

▌ *Pharmacokinetics*

Ten percent to 20% of desmopressin is absorbed from the nasal mucosa when the drug is administered intranasally, and it is 100% bioavailable when given IV (see Table 44-2). Distribution sites are unknown. Desmopressin is biotransformed by the kidneys and has a half-life of 75 minutes.

▌ *Adverse Effects and Contraindications*

▲ **The major adverse effects of desmopressin is mild hypertension** (caused by constriction of vascular smooth muscle) and water retention (caused by increased permeability of the renal collecting ducts to water). Milder adverse effects include rhinitis, headache, nausea, and abdominal or stomach cramps. Large IV doses can cause tachycardia. Phlebitis at the IV injection site is possible. Water intoxication and hyponatremia are possible after long-term use.

Desmopressin is contraindicated for use in patients with hypersensitivity to the drug or hypersensitivity to chlorobutanol, and in patients with type IIB or platelet-type (pseudo)
▲ von Willebrand's disease. **Use desmopressin with caution in patients with angina pectoris or hypertension.** Safe use during pregnancy and lactation has not been established.

▌ *Drug Interactions*

Desmopressin enhances diuresis when used in the presence of chlorpropamide, clofibrate, or carbamazepine (see Table 44-3). Demeclocycline, lithium, or norepinephrine may diminish the antidiuretic response to desmopressin.

▌ *Dosage Regimen*

The dosage and route of administration for desmopressin varies with the reason for use (see Table 44-4). It can be given either by intranasal or parenteral routes (IV or subQ). The parenteral route is usually recommended, although intranasal administration has also been used for antihemorrhagic action.

▌ *Lab Considerations*

Desmopressin may cause concentrated urine with increases in specific gravity and osmolality. As a result of water retention, hyponatremia and a decrease in serum osmolality may occur in patients with normal renal function. These effects are minimal in patients with chronic renal disease.

Phosphate-Binding Drugs

◆ aluminum hydroxide (AlternaGEL, Alu-Cap, Alu-Tab, Amphojel, Basaljel, Dialume, Nephrox); ◆ AmphoGel
◆ calcium acetate (Phos-Ex, PhosLo)
◆ calcium carbonate (Caltrate, Maalox Antacid Caplets, Nephro-Calci, Os-Cal, Rolaids, Tums, Titralac, others); ◆ Apo-Cal, Caltrate 600, Maalox Quick-Dissolve, Os-Cal

▌ *Indications*

Phosphate-binding drugs are used in renal failure to normalize serum phosphorus levels, decrease the severity of secondary hyperparathyroidism, and decrease the incidence and severity of bone disease. The major calcium compounds include calcium carbonate and calcium acetate. Aluminum hydroxide may be used as a phosphate binder in adults when calcium compounds prove ineffective. Overall, the use of aluminum hydroxide as a phosphate binder is largely discouraged.

▌ *Pharmacodynamics*

Patients with renal failure often have a buildup of phosphate. Calcium salts prevent absorption of dietary phosphorus from the GI tract by combining with phosphorus to form the insoluble compound calcium phosphate. Aluminum hydroxide binds phosphate in the GI tract to lower serum phosphate levels.

▌ *Pharmacokinetics*

Absorption of calcium salts from the GI tract requires the presence of vitamin D. Elimination is mostly through the feces, with only 20% eliminated by the kidneys. The half-life of calcium salts has not been determined (see Table 44-2).

Aluminum salts are poorly absorbed when taken orally, ▲ **but over time substantial amounts of aluminum may accumulate. Absorbed aluminum distributes widely into the body, concentrating in the central nervous system (CNS).** Aluminum is mostly eliminated in the feces.

▌ *Adverse Effects and Contraindications*

The major adverse effects of calcium salts are mild GI complaints such as diarrhea, gas, and constipation. Hypercalcemia may also occur but is unusual if the patient takes the calcium compounds with meals and is not receiving vitamin D supplements. **Arrhythmias have been noted with excess calcium** ▲ **intake.** Phosphate depletion resulting in osteopenia or osteoporosis can be induced with excessive use of phosphate binders.

Calcium salts are contraindicated for use in patients with hypercalcemia, renal calculi, or ventricular fibrillation. Use them cautiously in patients receiving digoxin, and in patients who have severe respiratory insufficiency or renal or cardiac disease.

Aluminum is retained in patients who have uremia causing severe skeletal, hematopoietic, and neurologic toxicity. **Because of the risk of aluminum toxicity, do not administer** ▲ **aluminum-containing phosphate-binding compounds to children with renal failure.**

Aluminum hydroxide is contraindicated for use in patients with severe abdominal pain of unknown cause. Exercise caution when using it in patients with hypercalcemia or hypophosphatemia. Use during pregnancy is generally considered safe, but chronic use of high dosages should be avoided.

Drug Interactions

Calcium compounds prevent the absorption of other elements (e.g., iron), antibiotics (i.e., tetracyclines, fluoroquinolone antibiotics), and digoxin. Do not give calcium acetate concurrently with other calcium supplements (see Table 44-3).

⚠ **Do not prescribe concurrent use of aluminum hydroxide with compounds containing citrate (i.e., sodium citrate, calcium citrate) because they markedly enhance the absorption of aluminum.**

Dosage Regimen

Dosages of calcium salts are expressed in milligrams, grams, or milliequivalents (mEq) of calcium. The dosage of calcium salts is adjusted to maintain serum phosphorus levels between 3.5 to 6 mg/dL (see Table 44-4).

Lab Considerations

The efficacy and safety of the phosphate binders are determined by monitoring serum phosphorus and calcium levels. Maintain serum phosphorus levels between 3.5 and 6 mg/dL and serum calcium levels between 8 and 11 mg/dL. Monitor plasma aluminum levels in patients receiving aluminum-containing binders. If aluminum levels exceed 25 mcg/L, reduce the dose or discontinue the drug.

Vitamin D Supplements
- calcitriol (Rocaltrol); ◆ Rocaltrol
- paricalcitol (Zemplar)

Indications

Calcitriol, a fat-soluble vitamin and a synthetic form of vitamin D_3, is well accepted in the treatment of CRF. It replaces a hormone that can no longer be synthesized by the diseased kidney. Calcitriol is also effective, especially when given by IV route, in suppressing parathyroid hormone (PTH) production and improving bone disease that results from secondary hyperparathyroidism.

Paricalcitol is indicated for the prevention and treatment of secondary hyperthyroidism associated with CRF. It is a synthetic vitamin D analogue. To achieve maximum suppression of PTH levels and improve bone disease, a treatment regimen of a year or more may be needed. The desired outcome is reduced bone pain, elimination of fractures, and improvement of muscle strength.

Pharmacodynamics

Calcitriol is a synthetic steroid hormone identical to that synthesized by the renal proximal tubule cells. Calcitriol is the active form of vitamin D and binds to receptors in the small intestine to promote the production of calcium-binding protein. The calcium-binding protein is essential for the absorption of dietary calcium and phosphorus. Paricalcitol suppresses PTH levels and has no significant effect on the incidence of hypercalcemia or hyperphosphatemia.

Pharmacokinetics

Calcitriol is readily absorbed from the small intestine following oral administration. It is bound in the serum to α-globulins (see Table 44-2). Biotransformation and elimination of the drug is primarily through biliary mechanisms.

Adverse Effects and Contraindications

Hypercalcemia is the primary adverse effect associated with calcitriol. However, because of the relatively short duration of action of calcitriol, any hypercalcemia associated with its administration is also of brief duration and is usually associated with minimal symptoms. Manifestations of hypercalcemia include weakness, nausea, vomiting, and muscle and bone pain.

Calcitriol is contraindicated for use in patients with hypersensitivity, hypercalcemia, and vitamin D toxicity, and during lactation (in large doses). Use it with caution in patients with sarcoidosis and hyperparathyroidism, and in those receiving cardiac glycosides. Safe use of large doses during pregnancy has not been established.

Do not use paricalcitol in patients who have vitamin D toxicity, hypercalcemia, or hypersensitivity to its ingredients. Signs of vitamin D toxicity associated with hypercalcemia include weakness, headache, somnolence, nausea, vomiting, dry mouth, constipation, muscle pain, bone pain, and a metallic taste. Later signs are anorexia, weight loss, calcific conjunctivitis and photophobia, rhinorrhea, pruritus, hyperthermia, decreased libido, overt psychoses, and alterations in BUN, cholesterol, and liver function test values.

Drug Interactions

Barbiturates, primidone, and hydantoin are CYP450 inducers and thus reduce the effect of calcitriol by accelerating its biotransformation (see Table 44-3). Calcitriol-induced hypercalcemia potentiates the effect of digoxin, causing arrhythmias. Aluminum hydroxide precipitates bile acids in the small intestine, decreasing absorption of calcitriol and other fat-soluble vitamins. In addition, calcitriol promotes the absorption of phosphorus from dietary sources, resulting in hyperphosphatemia.

Digoxin toxicity is potentiated by hypercalcemia of any cause; therefore exercise caution when digoxin is prescribed concurrently with calcitriol and paricalcitol.

Dosage Regimen

The usual oral dose of calcitriol for patients who are hypocalcemic during chronic dialysis is 2.5 to 3 mcg/day (see Table 44-4), although larger dosages have been used. Dialyzed patients with secondary hyperparathyroidism respond to 2 to 3 mcg/day by IV route 3 times a week, given at the end of dialysis. For treatment of secondary hyperparathyroidism in patients receiving chronic peritoneal dialysis, it can be administered in an oral dose of 1 to 3 mcg 3 times weekly. The dosage of calcitriol, however, is limited by the development of hypercalcemia.

Hypercalcemia related to acute overdose of paricalcitol ⚠ necessitates emergency action. During dosage adjustment, closely monitor serum calcium and phosphorus levels (e.g., evaluate twice weekly). If clinically significant hypercalcemia develops, reduce or interrupt the dosage. Chronic administration of paricalcitol increases patient risk for hypercalcemia and metastatic calcification. Bone lesions arise from suppressed PTH levels.

Lab Considerations

The efficacy of calcitriol therapy is documented by suppression of PTH levels, normalization of serum calcium, and reduction of alkaline phosphatase levels. Histologic and radiologic evidence of improved hyperparathyroid bone disease can also be documented. Monitor serum calcium levels monthly because of the possibility of hypercalcemia. Overdosage is associated with a serum (Ca × P) level over 75 and elevated BUN, alanine aminotransferase (ALT) and aspartate aminotransferase (AST) values. Falling alkaline phosphatase levels may also signal the onset of hypercalcemia. Closely monitor serum phosphorus levels to prevent hyperphosphatemia and production of soft tissue calcification. Calcitriol may also cause elevated serum cholesterol levels.

Heavy Metal Antagonist
◆ deferoxamine (Desferal); ✦ Desferal

▥ Indications
Deferoxamine alleviates bone pain, muscle weakness, and the anemia that result from iron and aluminum toxicities. It is also used in the management of secondary iron overload syndrome associated with multiple transfusion therapy. Musculoskeletal symptoms and anemia are ordinarily corrected in 2 or 3 months. Deferoxamine is also used as an adjunct with gastric aspiration and lavage with sodium bicarbonate for acute iron ingestion. Aluminum neurotoxicity is more resistant to treatment, with months to 1 year of continuous therapy required before improvement is noted.

▥ Pharmacodynamics
The key characteristic shared by all chelators is that the metal ion bound to the chelator is chemically inert. Because chelators are diffusely dispersed throughout the body, they bind the target metal ion preferentially over other metals. Deferoxamine has a particularly strong affinity for trivalent iron and aluminum, forming soluble inert complexes that are readily eliminated by the kidney or removed with dialysis. Deferoxamine removes between 30 and 70 mg of iron per day.

▥ Pharmacokinetics
Deferoxamine is poorly absorbed by the GI system following oral administration; therefore, it must be given by IM or subQ route. It is rapidly biotransformed by tissue and plasma enzymes, with a serum half-life of approximately 1 hour (see Table 44-2). The chelated complexes have an extended plasma half-life. Elimination of iron is dependent on either renal function or removal by dialysis, with an additional 33% removed through biliary elimination.

▥ Adverse Effects and Contraindications
The most common adverse effects of deferoxamine are fever, tachycardia, diarrhea, and abdominal discomfort. A red coloration to the urine, anaphylactic reactions, auditory neurotoxicity, and ocular toxicity have also been reported with deferoxamine. Hypotension, shock, skin rash, hives, itching, and wheezing can result and are often due to a too-rapid infusion of deferoxamine. **In susceptible individuals, deferoxamine increases the proliferation and virulence of fungal organisms, resulting in severe, often fatal, infection.** Because deferoxamine is a naturally occurring iron siderophore (a molecule facilitating iron uptake), it acts as a growth factor for *Yersinia* and *Rhizopus* (mucormycosis).

▥ Drug Interactions
Ascorbic acid improves the chelation action for iron and increases the amount of iron eliminated (see Table 44-3). However, use deferoxamine judiciously because concurrent use enhances tissue iron toxicity, especially in the heart, causing cardiac decompensation.

▥ Dosage Regimen
The dosing of deferoxamine is determined by the severity of symptoms associated with the iron toxicity (see Table 44-4). Rapid infusion may cause hypotension, erythema, urticaria, wheezing, convulsions, tachycardia, and/or shock.

For acute iron ingestion, gastric aspiration and lavage with sodium bicarbonate is used. A trial dose of deferoxamine is administered 2 to 4 hours after the acute ingestion but after the GI tract has been cleansed. The urine is monitored for color change. Orange-rose-colored urine indicates significant iron ingestion.

▥ Lab Considerations
Serum deferoxamine levels are not directly monitored. However, an increase in plasma aluminum or iron levels 12 to 24 hours following deferoxamine administration reflects binding to the drug. Monitor liver function studies to assess damage from iron poisoning.

Cation-Exchange Resins
◆ sodium polystyrene sulfonate (Kayexalate, SPS)

▥ Indications
Sodium polystyrene sulfonate is used for the treatment of hyperkalemic states in both ARF and CRF (see also Chapter 48) when renal mechanisms for eliminating these ions fail.

▥ Pharmacodynamics
Sodium polystyrene sulfonate is a cation-exchange resin. When used as an enema, the resin exchanges sodium ions in the large intestine for potassium and, to a lesser extent, other cations (e.g., calcium and magnesium), which are then eliminated in the feces. After oral administration of the resin, sodium ions are exchanged for hydrogen ions in the stomach. The hydrogen ions are subsequently exchanged for potassium cations in the large intestine.

▥ Pharmacokinetics
Sodium polystyrene sulfonate is nonabsorbable and not biotransformed. The exchange efficiency is approximately 33%. One gram of resin has the capacity to exchange 1 mEq of potassium for 1 mEq of sodium. Virtually 100% of administered doses, oral or rectal, are eliminated in the feces.

▥ Adverse Effects and Contraindications
Because sodium polystyrene sulfonate exchanges sodium for potassium, fluid retention caused by the added sodium and hypokalemia may occur. This risk is decreased with rectal administration of the resin.

▥ Drug Interactions
Avoid concurrent use of antacids and laxatives containing magnesium because of the risk of metabolic alkalosis. Hypokalemia enhances cardiac glycoside toxicity.

Dosage Regimen

Sodium polystyrene sulfonate may be administered either orally or rectally (see Table 44-4). Rectal administration is recommended when the patient is receiving nothing by mouth or is vomiting, or if there is an upper GI tract disorder. However, the rectal route is less effective in reducing potassium levels than the oral method of administration. Further, constipation, fecal impaction, and colonic necrosis have been reported either as the result of the omission of cleansing enemas before or after the resin enema, or because of failure to give sorbitol with the oral formulation.

Lab Considerations

Monitor serum electrolytes, including calcium and magnesium levels, when therapy continues for more than 1 day. Serum potassium levels should be monitored at least daily to determine the effectiveness of therapy. Monitor bicarbonate levels at least weekly with chronic therapy, especially if the resin is prescribed concurrently with laxatives and antacids.

Systemic Antacids

◆ sodium bicarbonate (Citrocarbonate, Neut, Soda Mint); ✦ Neut
◆ sodium citrate (Bicitra, Oracit, Shohl Modified Solution); ✦ Oracit, PMS-Dicitra

Indications

Correction of acidosis results in improvement of the GI symptoms associated with uremia. In addition, by buffering the retained dietary acids, sodium bicarbonate saves bone buffers and retards the development of renal osteodystrophy. Chronic correction of acidosis in uremia is accomplished by the oral administration of either sodium bicarbonate or sodium citrate. Both are equally effective in correcting the acidotic state. However, because of citrate's ability to enhance the absorption of toxic elements, namely aluminum, bicarbonate is the preferred drug.

Pharmacodynamics

Sodium bicarbonate is a systemic alkalinizing drug. The logic for its use in the treatment of ARF also applies to the treatment of CRF. By increasing plasma bicarbonate levels, excess hydrogen ions are buffered and blood pH is raised, thus reversing the clinical manifestations of acidosis.

Pharmacokinetics

Given intravenously, sodium bicarbonate has a rapid onset of onset with wide distribution in the body (see Table 44-3). The increase in serum pH results in translocation of intracellular potassium with a corresponding acute fall of serum potassium levels. It is eliminated through the kidneys.

Adverse Effects and Contraindications

Administration of sodium bicarbonate can result in modest sodium and fluid retention. The retention of sodium and fluids has the potential for aggravating heart failure, hypertensive states, and edema formation.

Dosage Regimen

Rate and dosage of bicarbonate is determined by arterial blood bases (ABGs) and estimates of base deficit (see Table 44-4). Bicarbonate replacement is calculated based on the difference between the actual serum bicarbonate level and the desired bicarbonate level. With acute acidosis, the volume of distribution of bicarbonate is assumed to be 50% of body weight. In most cases, half of the calculated bicarbonate deficit is initially replaced. Replacement therapy is monitored by serial determinations of serum CO_2 content and arterial pH. Sodium citrate dosage is calculated based on urinary pH.

Diuretics

◆ furosemide (Lasix); ✦ Lasix
◆ mannitol (Osmitrol)

In patients with renal failure, diuretics are mostly used for the conversion of oliguric ATN to nonoliguric ATN. Loop diuretics (e.g., furosemide) and osmotics (e.g., mannitol) are most often used, although the efficacy of diuretics in renal failure varies. Owing to reduction in renal function, large doses of the diuretic are usually required. Administer diuretics only after vital signs are stabilized and extracellular fluid volume is optimized. Diuretics are discussed in greater detail in Chapter 42.

Loop diuretics are used in the early stages of renal insufficiency and in the ATN type of ARF. The nonoliguric form of ATN rarely requires dialysis and has a better prognosis than oliguric ATN. Osmotic diuretics are used for the prevention of radiocontrast media–induced ATN.

Although diuretics have some effect on RBF, possibly by increasing prostaglandin synthesis, their major therapeutic efficacy is in improving tubule flow rate. A loop diuretic may not improve renal function, but it can increase diuresis and facilitate patient management. As kidney function deteriorates, diuretics become increasingly nephrotoxic, and they are seldom used in patients with ESRD after dialysis has been initiated.

Renal Vasodilator

◆ dopamine (Intropin)

Low-dose dopamine has been used to improve RBF, GFR, and renal salt and water elimination. In hypotensive states associated with increased renal vasoconstriction, dopamine improves RBF, thereby reducing oliguria and preventing the development of ARF. Additional uses of dopamine are discussed in Chapter 14.

Dopamine has two distinct actions. It stimulates adrenergic receptors to cause vasoconstriction and acts on dopaminergic receptors to cause vasodilation. In addition, dopamine causes a decrease in sodium reabsorption and increases the rate of sodium elimination in the urine (a natriuretic effect). Low-dose dopamine (0.5 to 2 mcg/kg/minute by IV route) causes renal vasodilation. In so doing, it increases RBF, GFR, and sodium elimination, with minimal effect on the vasoconstrictive adrenergic receptors.

There are few adverse effects with low-dose dopamine. However, at doses of 2 to 10 mcg/kg/min, dopaminergic and β receptors are stimulated, producing cardiac stimulation and greater renal vasodilation. Hypotension and arrhythmias are potentially problematic at higher doses.

CLINICAL REASONING

Drug therapy in patients with impaired renal function is complex. Health care providers must consider four major factors when using multidrug therapy. First, the deterioration of renal function results in major changes in the bioavailability, the distribution, the biotransformation, and the activity of drugs. Most drugs or their metabolites are at least partially removed by the kidneys; therefore, reduced renal function influences both therapeutic and toxic responses. Secondly, drugs may adversely affect renal function by causing a physiologic alteration in RBF and GFR, or by causing parenchymal injury. Third, there are increasing numbers of drugs being used to prevent or retard the progression or development of ARF. Drug therapy has been used in an attempt to retard the progression of CRF, specifically in the treatment of diabetic nephropathy. Finally, several drugs can be used to manage the complications related to loss of renal function.

Treatment Objectives

▲ **The primary objective in the management of renal failure is prevention. The avoidance or removal of nephrotoxic drugs, along with rapid correction of cardiovascular alterations that lead to renal ischemia, will prevent or minimize the progression of renal failure.** Once renal failure has developed, however, treatment objectives are directed at supporting the patient and maintaining existing system functioning. Achieving and maintaining acceptable fluid and electrolyte balance, and minimizing the risk of complications from fluid and electrolyte imbalances are also relevant objectives. Maintenance of adequate nutritional status and compliance with the plan of care are also desirable outcomes.

One of the risk-reduction objectives listed in the *Healthy People 2000* and *Healthy People 2010* documents of the United States Public Health Service and the Department of Health and Human Services relates to ESRD. The objective is to reverse the increase in incidence of ESRD (requiring maintenance dialysis or transplantation) to attain an incidence of no more than 13 per 100,000 cases.

Treatment Options

▥ *Patient Variables*

The patient with renal failure responds to many drugs differently from the patient with healthy kidneys. Because of variations in response, an assortment of regimens provides the best results. The major patient variable encountered is the degree of renal impairment. Because many drugs are eliminated through the kidneys, the potential for toxicity is increased as renal function decreases. If patients with slower than normal elimination rates (e.g., those with renal disease and older adults) are given normal doses of drugs, accumulation and toxicity can occur. Toxicity is potentially preventable with proper modification of dose.

LIFE-SPAN CONSIDERATIONS

Pregnant and Nursing Women. In general, renal disease is not affected by pregnancy if it is mild and the patient is not hypertensive at time of conception. However, in the presence of renal disease and hypertension, pregnancy is often complicated with worsening hypertension or a decline in renal function, or both.

Renal disease can be caused by a urinary tract infection before or during pregnancy, can be the result of other diseases such as diabetes, or can occur during pregnancy from complications ranging from preeclampsia and HELLP (i.e., *h*emolysis,

*e*levated *l*iver enzymes, and *l*ow *p*latelets) syndrome, to abruptio placenta or sepsis. Treatment of sudden ARF during pregnancy resembles that of the nonpregnant population. The aim is to retard the development of uremic symptoms and restore acid-base and electrolyte balance and volume homeostasis.

Children and Adolescents. Renal disease affects children in many of the same ways it affects adults. However, because the child's body, character, and personality are still forming, the effects on maturation are even more pronounced. Further, because childhood illness often results in stunted physical, psychologic, and educational development, it is generally true that the older the child is when he or she becomes ill, the better the chances are of having established a secure sense of self.

Growth failure is an important consequence of childhood renal disease. The growth rate may be somewhat improved with control of acidosis and calcitriol supplementation. Recombinant human growth hormone has been used in children with uremia and in those with transplants who experienced substantially decreased growth rates. In addition, adequate peritoneal dialysis, especially continuous cycle–assisted peritoneal dialysis, is the therapy of choice for improved growth rate. However, none of the above-mentioned therapies produce catch-up growth.

The recurrent hospitalizations and lengthy treatment regimens often make the child's reintegration to school and social activities a challenge. However, the return to school and activities helps minimize the depression, isolation, and low self-esteem associated with chronic illness. The child needs encouragement to assume as much responsibility for self-care as possible. The child's ability to cope with what may be a complex drug regimen can foster self-esteem and improve the outcomes of the treatment regimen. However, the age and maturity of the child will determine the degree to which he or she participates in the drug therapies used.

Older Adults. Owing to the normal physiologic changes of aging, older adults are more susceptible to dehydration, hypotension, fever, and acute renal insufficiency. Advanced age also represents an additional risk factor for the development of ARF secondary to antimicrobial use (e.g., aminoglycosides) as well as contrast media.

The incidence of ESRD increases dramatically with advanced age. Between the ages of 20 and 44 years, the incidence of ESRD is 91 per million people compared with 680 per million people between the ages of 65 and 75 years. The etiology of renal failure also changes with aging.

As a consequence of social, financial, psychologic, and comorbidity factors, older patients frequently do not cope well with chronic dialysis and the drug therapies that are associated with renal failure. These factors result in chronic fatigue, depression, concerns regarding quality of life, and suicidal ideations. Over 40% of patients 65 years and older discontinue dialysis for the above-mentioned reasons.

▥ *Drug Variables*

Estimate the degree of renal function and the effects of renal impairment on drug elimination and half-life. The effects of dialysis on drug removal and the appropriate method for altering drug doses or dosage intervals to achieve desired blood levels are also important factors to be considered.

▲   **ARBs and ACEIs are highly effective in slowing the progression of diabetic nephropathy. Because over 30% of patients with ESRD have diabetes, there is a major impact on ESRD treatment programs.** In addition, there is reasonable evidence that other types of proteinuric renal disease may also benefit from the use of ACE inhibitors. The average cost of treating a patient with ESRD is over $70,000 annually, but preventive therapy with ACE inhibitors at the recommended dose would be less than $2000 annually. Further, the use of an ACE inhibitor in patients with type 1 diabetic nephropathy could reduce national health care costs by $3 billion over the next 10 years.

In contrast, recent advances in therapies directed at improving the quality of life of patients with ESRD have done little to improve rehabilitation but have markedly increased costs. For example, epoetin alfa, the antianemic drug, has increased the cost of treating a patient with ESRD by $5000 to $7000/year. It is also estimated that the cost of recombinant human growth hormone for treatment of growth failure in children with renal disease will be even more expensive than epoetin alfa.

Drug administration regimens are adjusted based on the degree of functional impairment imposed by using interval-extension and dose-reduction strategies (Table 44-5). Using the *interval-extension* method, the time between each dose is lengthened while the dose remains the same. Interval extension is useful for drugs that have wide therapeutic ranges and long plasma half-lives. With the *dose-reduction* method, the size of the individual dose is reduced, but the interval between each dose remains unchanged. Dose reduction is preferred when constant blood levels of a drug are required, and for drugs with narrow therapeutic ranges and rather short half-lives. At times, both methods are employed to achieve maximum therapeutic benefits. Guidance regarding dosage reduction and interval modification for most drugs can be found in a number of references.

Measuring peak and trough serum drug levels is useful in documenting the effectiveness of the dosing schedule. The levels are indicators of drug elimination and reflect potential drug accumulation. Peak levels are most useful when they are obtained 30 minutes to 1 hour after the third dose of the drug. Trough levels are obtained immediately before the next dose. Reliable clinical assessment of changes in the patient's condition and knowledge of drug interactions must be used to aid

▲   in the interpretation of test results. **Consider these principles when adjusting dosages for patients with renal failure:**

- Loading doses given to a patient with renal insufficiency are usually the same as the initial dose of a drug given to a patient with normal renal function.
- The maintenance dosage of a drug for patients with renal insufficiency can be adjusted using the interval-extension or the dose-reduction method.
- The initial dose may be somewhat higher in patients with substantial edema or ascites than that usually given to achieve desired blood levels.

The importance of consistency in obtaining peak and trough values cannot be overstated. Regardless of the sampling procedure used, it is important that the same time interval between sampling and dose administration be used consistently when comparing results from serial samples on the same patient.

Patient Education

The majority of patients with renal failure receive care as outpatients; therefore, the most important role of the health care provider is patient teaching. Whenever possible, encourage the patient to take the major responsibility for adherence with the treatment plan. However, owing to the changes in the cognitive functioning of the patient or the level of understanding due to age limitations, it is important to involve friends and family members in the teaching process.

Include friends and family in the plan of care from the beginning, and consider their goals and objectives for treatment. Not only should they be educated about the medical regimen but also the consequences if they choose not to adhere to the prescribed treatment plan. Ongoing support by friends and family with management by the health care provider is of primary importance in assisting the patient to achieve personal goals.

Ensure that all involved have a thorough understanding of the consequences of renal disease so as to adjust to the numerous limitations of renal failure. An understanding of the reasons for dietary restrictions, drug regimens, and adherence to the dialysis schedule, when applicable, is necessary for acceptance and compliance with the medical regimen.

All patients with decreased renal function must limit their protein consumption to some degree because the accumulation of nitrogenous waste products from protein metabolism is the primary cause of uremia. Protein is restricted based on the degree of renal insufficiency and the severity of the symptoms. The GFR, albumin, creatinine, and BUN levels are often used as a guide to safe levels of protein consumption.

Low-protein diets are usually deficient in vitamins, and water-soluble vitamins are removed from the blood during dialysis. In addition, anemia is a chronic problem owing to the limited iron content of low-protein diets and decreased erythropoietin production by the kidneys. For these reasons, all patients with renal failure are given vitamin and mineral supplements. Teach patients to take the vitamin and mineral supplements after dialysis rather than before because they will be dialyzed out of the body.

Phosphate-binding drugs, often referred to by the patient as antacids, are necessary because the metabolism of calcium and phosphorus is altered in renal failure. Teach the patient the reason for use of these drugs and to avoid preparations containing magnesium. Patients' inability to metabolize magnesium predisposes them to dangerous levels of magnesium toxicity. Further, instruct the patient how to monitor for signs and symptoms of hypophosphatemia, including muscle weakness, anorexia, malaise, tremors, and bone pain.

Emphasize the importance of taking antihypertensive drugs (see Chapter 37) on a regularly scheduled basis. Uncontrolled elevations in blood pressure further compromise renal perfusion and worsen renal failure.

Diuretics are often used in the early stages of renal failure and should be taken early in the day to avoid disturbing sleep. The diuresis produced is useful in treating fluid overload in patients who still have some urinary function. Careful intake and output records should be kept because as kidney function deteriorates, these drugs become increasingly nephrotoxic. Diuretics are seldom used in patients with ESRD once dialysis has been initiated.

TABLE 44-5 Antibiotic Dosing in Renal Dysfunction*

Drug	Method of Dose Adjustment	CrCl >50 mL/min	CrCl 10–50 mL/min	CrCl <10 mL/min	Dialysis H or P
AMINOGLYCOSIDES					
amikacin	Dose	60%–90%	30%–70%	20%–30%	H and P
	Interval†	12 hr	12–18 hr	24 hr	
gentamicin	Dose	60%–90%	30%–70%	20%–30%	H and P
	Interval	8–12 hr	12 hr	24 hr	
netilmicin	Dose	60%–90%	30%–70%	20%–30%	H and P
	Interval	8–12 hr	12 hr	24 hr	
tobramycin	Dose	60%–90%	30%–70%	20%–30%	H and P
	Interval	8–12 hr	12 hr	24 hr	
CEPHALOSPORINS					
cephalexin	Interval	6 hr	6–8 hr	6–12 hr	H
cefadroxil	Interval	8 hr	12–24 hr	24–48 hr	H
cephradine	Dose	—	50%	25%	H and P
cephapirin	Interval	6 hr	6–8 hr	12 hr	H and P
cefazolin	Interval	8 hr	12 hr	18–48 hr	H
cefaclor	Dose	—	50%	33%	H
cefmetazole	Interval	12 hr	24 hr	48 hr	H
cefotetan	Interval	12 hr	24 hr	48 hr	H
cefoperazone	Interval	—	—	—	H
ceftriaxone	Dose	—	—	—	No
ceftazidime	Interval	8–12 hr	8–12 hr	18–24 hr	H
TETRACYCLINES					
doxycycline	Interval	12 hr	12–18 hr	18–24 hr	No
minocycline	Dose	—	—	—	No
FLUOROQUINOLONES					
norfloxacin	Interval	—	24 hr	24 hr	H and P
ciprofloxacin	Interval	—	12 hr	24 hr	H and P
ofloxacin	Dose	—	50%	25%–50%	H and P
PENICILLINS					
amoxicillin	Interval	6 hr	6–12 hr	12–16 hr	H
ampicillin	Interval	6 hr	6–12 hr	12–16 hr	H
carbenicillin	Interval	8–12 hr	12–24 hr	24–48 hr	H and P
cloxacillin	Dose	—	—	—	No
dicloxacillin	Interval	—	—	—	No
methicillin	Interval	4–6 hr	6–8 hr	8–12 hr	No
oxacillin	Dose	—	—	—	No
penicillin G	Dose	—	75%	20%–50%	H
	Interval	6–8 hr	8–12 hr	12–16 hr	—
piperacillin	Interval	4–6 hr	6–8 hr	8 hr	H
ticarcillin	Interval	6–8 hr	12–24 hr	12–24 hr	H and P
MISCELLANEOUS					
aztreonam	Dose	—	50%–75%	25%	—
chloramphenicol	Dose	—	—	—	H
clindamycin	Dose	—	—	—	No
erythromycin	Dose	—	—	—	No
metronidazole	Dose	—	—	50%	H
	Interval	8 hr	—	—	—
trimethoprim-sulfamethoxazole	Interval	12 hr	12 hr	24 hr	H
vancomycin	Interval	24–72 hr	72–240 hr	240 hr	No
ANTIFUNGALS					
amphotericin B	Interval	24 hr	24 hr	24–36 hr	No
flucytosine	Dose	50%	30%–50%	20%–30%	H and P
fluconazole	Dose	—	50%	25%	H
ketoconazole	Dose	—	—	—	No
itraconazole	Dose	—	—	—	UA
miconazole	Dose	—	—	—	No
	Interval	6 hr	12–24 hr	24–48 hr	H and P
ANTITUBERCULOSIS					
ethambutol	Dose	—	50%	30%–50%	H and P
	Interval	24 hr	24–36 hr	48 hr	—
isoniazid	Dose	—	—	65%–75%	H and P
rifampin	Interval	—	—	—	No
ANTIVIRALS					
acyclovir	Interval	8 hr	24 hr	48 hr	H
amantadine	Interval	12–24 hr	48–72 hr	168 hr	No
ganciclovir	Dose	50%	25%	25%	H
	Interval	24 hr	24 hr	24 hr	—

*See also Chapters 27–30. Dosage is given as percentage administered to an adult with normal renal function.
†The interval refers to the hours between dosing.
CrCl, Creatinine clearance; H, removed by hemodialysis; P, removed by peritoneal dialysis; UA, unavailable.

EVIDENCE-BASED PHARMACOTHERAPEUTICS

BMI and Risk for ESRD

■ Background

The risk factors for chronic renal failure (CRF) and end-stage renal disease (ESRD) include hypertension, diabetes mellitus, smoking, and obesity. It is unclear if being overweight or obese itself contributes to the risk for ESRD, or if other independent risk factors play a role. The risk for death from the earlier stages of CRF is greater than the risk for progression toward ESRD, but the reasons for this remain unclear. Because obesity may contribute to risk in patients with CRF, it is important to evaluate these variables

■ Research Article

Hsu, C., McCulloch, C., Iribarren, C. (2006). Body mass index and risk for end-stage renal disease. *Annals of Internal Medicine, 144*(1), 21–28.

Purpose

The purpose of this study was to determine if overweight or obesity in subjects with renal disease contributes to their risk for ESRD.

Design

This was a 21-year longitudinal study. The adult, volunteer subjects ($N = 350,252$) were recruited from a large northern California health maintenance organization. The subjects all received annual health examinations between 1964 and 1985.

Methods

The investigators considered subjects with body mass indices of 25 kg/m^2 to be overweight and subjects with BMIs of 30 kg/m^2 or higher to be obese. Serial measurements of other variables such as kidney function, blood sugar levels, blood pressure, and whether or not the subjects smoked were analyzed, taking into account the time it took for ESRD to develop in normal, overweight, and obese subjects.

Findings

ESRD developed in 1471 of the subjects. Thirty percent of the subjects were overweight; 10% were obese. Subjects who were overweight and obese subjects developed ESRD 2 to 5 times faster than subjects whose BMI was in a normal range. The risk increased even though diabetes, hypertension, and smoking variables were accounted for in the analyses.

Conclusions

Independent of the common risk factors of diabetes, hypertension, and smoking, being overweight or obese may be a risk factor for ESRD.

■ Implications for Practice

In this study the BMI, the blood pressure, the blood sugar levels, and the smoking history were measured only once for many of the subjects. The severity of the variables of diabetes, hypertension, and smoking could easily have changed over this longitudinal study. Further, many of the overweight and obese subjects took antihypertensive and antidiabetic drugs to treat their disorders. If these subjects' blood pressure and blood sugar readings were normal because of drug therapy, obesity may appear to be a more important risk factor for ESRD than it truly is. Further, these findings may not be generalizable to persons who do not have regular health examinations.

BMI, Body mass index.

Because a large percentage of patients with renal failure also have diabetes, include the need for close monitoring of blood glucose levels in the patient education. As renal disease progresses, the patient with diabetes requires a decrease in insulin dosage because insulin is partially biotransformed by the kidneys. Urinary glucose measurements may be inaccurate owing to the renal disease and, if possible, should not be used.

Inform patients and their families of the resources that are available. Home care nurses are often required to monitor the patient's status and evaluate maintenance of the prescribed treatment regimen. Social services personnel are usually involved because of the complex process of paying for the required care and in applying for financial aid. Physical and occupational therapists often work with patients who have renal failure, depending on their needs. The patient and family may benefit from joining support groups or obtaining other services locally. Resources such as The National Kidney Foundation and the American Kidney Fund are good initial contacts.

Evaluation

Successful achievement of treatment objectives is indicated by a number of factors. The patient is free from peripheral edema, hypertension, respiratory distress, and other signs of fluid and electrolyte imbalance. There are no signs of infection, and the patient is feeling more rested and less fatigued. Blood pressure is maintained within an acceptable range. There are no signs of bleeding; anorexia, nausea, and pruritus are controlled; and there is no muscle cramping. The patient demonstrates mental clarity and an ability to perform activities of daily living independently and safely. Any comorbid illness, including heart failure, anemia, and dehydration, is controlled or resolved. Furthermore, the patient should be able to correctly describe the nature of his or her illness, treatment and drug regimens, and plans for follow-up care. In evaluating patient outcomes it is important to inquire about understanding of the diagnosis, its implications, and treatment regimens (e.g., diet, drugs, and dialysis).

KEY POINTS

- Prerenal factors associated with ARF cause hypoperfusion, intrarenal factors cause injury to renal parenchyma, and postrenal factors obstruct urine flow.
- The most common cause of ARF is renal hypoperfusion; the second most common cause is nephrotoxins.
- With ARF, there is usually a recent history of infection, severe trauma, a complicated surgical procedure, an episode of sepsis, or the administration of nephrotoxic drugs, such as contrast media, antimicrobials, or antineoplastic drugs.

- Four stages characterize CRF: (1) diminished renal reserve without accumulation of metabolic wastes; and (2) mild (40% to 80% of normal function), (3) moderate (15% to 40%), or (4) severe (2% to 20%) renal insufficiency.
- Multiple system dysfunction occurs as renal failure progresses, leading to anemia, uremia, disorders of calcium and phosphorus biotransformation, and acidosis, and finally, ESRD.
- The objectives in the management of renal failure are prevention, removal of nephrotoxic drugs, rapid correction of cardiovascular

alterations leading to renal ischemia, and reduction of the severity and duration of established ARF.

■ The management of a patient with renal failure includes drug therapy, diet therapy, and dialysis in some form.

■ Adjust the drug dosage to correlate with the severity of the patient's renal failure by using the interval-extension and dose-reduction methods.

■ ARBs and ACEIs are most useful in decreasing functional deterioration in diabetic renal disease, but they are also thought to exert similar beneficial effects in all types of proteinuric renal diseases.

■ Epoetin alfa is a well-accepted drug for the treatment of the anemia associated with CRF.

■ Because iron is necessary for continued RBC production, virtually all patients receiving epoetin alfa eventually require supplemental iron.

■ Desmopressin, an antihemorrhagic drug, is effective in reversing the bleeding associated with uremia and is useful for the prevention of post–renal biopsy bleeding.

■ Phosphate-binding drugs (e.g., calcium carbonate) normalize serum phosphorus levels and decrease the severity of secondary hyperparathyroidism and the incidence and the severity of bone disease.

■ Calcitriol, a vitamin D supplement, is effective in suppressing parathyroid hormone production and improving bone disease resulting from the secondary hyperparathyroidism.

■ Deferoxamine, a heavy metal antagonist, is effective in alleviating bone pain, muscle weakness, and the anemia that results from iron and aluminum toxicities.

■ Furosemide, a loop diuretic, is used primarily in the ATN type of ARF to convert oliguric ATN to nonoliguric ATN, as well as in the early stages of renal insufficiency.

■ In hypotensive states associated with increased renal vasoconstriction, dopamine, a renal vasodilator drug, may improve RBF, preventing the development of ARF and reducing oliguria.

■ Sodium polystyrene sulfonate, a cation-exchange resin, is used in the treatment of hyperkalemic states in both ARF and CRF.

■ Sodium bicarbonate is a systemic alkalizing drug used for the treatment of metabolic acidosis caused by the impaired acid elimination in renal failure.

■ Evaluation of patient outcomes includes a patient who is free of peripheral edema, hypertension, respiratory distress, or other signs of fluid and electrolyte imbalance. Also, the patient should demonstrate mental clarity and an ability to perform his or her activities independently and safely.

GENITOURINARY

Bibliography

Agraharkar, M., and Safirstein, R. (2001). Pathophysiology of acute renal failure. In Greenberg, A., and Coffman, T. (Eds.). *Primer on kidney diseases* (3rd ed.). San Diego: Academic Press.

Corsonello, A., Pedone, C., and Corica, F. (2005). Concealed renal insufficiency and adverse drug reactions in elderly hospitalized patients. *Archives of Internal Medicine, 165*(7), 790–795.

Djamali, A., Samaniego, B., Muth, R., et al. (2006). Medical care of kidney transplant recipients after the first post-transplant year. *Clinical Journal of the American Society of Nephrology, 1*(4), 623–640.

Hsu, C., McCulloch, C., and Iribarren, C. (2006). Body mass index and risk for end-stage renal disease. *Annals of Internal Medicine, 144*(9), 701–702.

Johansen, K., Kutner, N., Young, B., et al. (2006). Association of body size with health status in patients beginning dialysis. *American Journal of Clinical Nutrition, 83*(3), 543–549.

Johnson, D., and Usherwood, T. (2005). Chronic kidney disease: Management update. *Australian Family Physician, 34*(11), 915–923.

Keith, S., Nichols, G., Gullion, C., et al. (2004). Longitudinal follow-up and outcomes among a population with chronic kidney disease in a large managed care organization. *Archives of Internal Medicine, 164*(6), 659–663.

Kent, P. (2005). Integrating clinical nutrition practice guidelines in chronic kidney disease. *Nutrition in Clinical Practice, 20*(2), 213–217.

Porter, J., Rafique, R., Srichairatanakool, S., et al. (2005). Recent insights into interactions of deferoxamine with cellular and plasma iron pools: Implications for clinical use. *Annals of the New York Academy of Sciences, 1054*, 155–168.

Ruilope, L. (2003). Proven benefits of angiotensin receptor blockers in the progression of renal disease. *European Heart Journal Supplements, 5*(Suppl C), C9–C12.

Schrier, R., Wang, W., Poole, B., et al. (2004). Acute renal failure: Definitions, diagnosis, pathogenesis, and therapy. *Journal of Clinical Investigation, 114*(1), 5–14.

Summary of notifiable diseases, United States. (2005). Morbidity and Mortality Weekly Report (MMWR), *52*(54), 7.

United States Renal Data System. *USRDS 2005 Annual Data Report.* Bethesda, MD: National Institute of Diabetes and Digestive and Kidney Diseases (NIDDK), National Institutes of Health (NIH), U.S. Department of Health and Human Services (DHHS); 2005. Available online: www.usrds.org Accessed May 10, 2007.

45

Drugs for Hyperacidity, Gastroesophageal Reflux Disease, and Peptic Ulcer Disease

Management of hyperacidity, gastroesophageal reflux disease (GERD), and peptic ulcer disease (PUD) relies on four classes of drugs: (1) drugs that inhibit gastric acid production, including proton pump inhibitors (PPIs), histamine₂-receptor antagonists (H₂RAs), and prostaglandins; (2) antacids that neutralize gastric acids; (3) prokinetic drugs that stimulate gastric motility; and (4) cytoprotective drugs. Optimal management of hyperacidity, GERD, and PUD requires knowledge of these drug classes, normal gastrointestinal (GI) physiology, and the pathophysiology of hyperacidity states. To understand how the drugs work, it is important to understand the normal physiology of gastric acid secretion.

Secretion of gastric acid by parietal cells is regulated by three substances: histamine, acetylcholine (ACh), and gastrin. The sight and smell of food and the presence of food in the mouth and the stomach stimulate acid secretion. The secretion is mediated by the vagus nerve. ACh stimulates muscarinic receptors (M_3) on parietal cells to increase calcium concentrations in the cell. When food is present in the stomach, the pH is raised, causing gastrin to be released from the mucosa. Gastrin then circulates through the blood stream to parietal and paracrine cell receptors.

Paracrine cells release histamine, which acts on parietal cell H_2 receptors to increase amounts of intracellular adenosine monophosphate (cAMP). This action in turn increases the activity of a protein kinase that activates the hydrogen–potassium–adenosine triphosphatase enzyme (H^+-K^+-ATPase) at the luminal border of the parietal cell. The H^+-K^+-ATPase enzyme serves as the so-called proton pump that secretes H^+ into the gastric lumen. Although the H_2, M_3, and gastrin receptors interact to augment acid secretion, histamine is considered the most important of the three and may serve as the final common pathway in the regulation of gastric acid secretion.

Excessive gastric secretions or gastric secretions with a pH less than 2 is known as *hyperacidity*. Hyperacidity may be an acute, chronic, episodic, or a relatively continuous problem. The problem has clinical significance because it predisposes the patient to gastric and intestinal irritation, ulcerations, and the risk for perforation.

GASTROESOPHAGEAL REFLUX DISEASE

EPIDEMIOLOGY AND ETIOLOGY

GERD (also known as reflux) symptoms have a great impact on the patient's quality of life, greater than that of PUD, untreated hypertension, mild heart failure, angina, or menopause. Epidemiology studies suggest that 65% of adults suffer from heartburn at least once a month; 24% have had symptoms for over 10 years; 17% of adults use indigestion aids at least once weekly; and as many as 10% have symptoms on a daily basis. Even so, only 24% of patients have previously consulted a health care provider about the problem. Of those who experience heartburn, 30% to 79% will have esophagitis. On the other hand, many patients with esophagitis do not have symptoms, or they may present with atypical symptoms. GERD is particularly common during pregnancy, with an increased incidence in patients over age 40. Mortality associated with GERD is rare (1 death per 100,000 patients).

The prevalence of GERD varies with geography, but is highest in Western countries. Apart from pregnancy-induced GERD and, possibly, nonerosive reflux disease, there does not seem to be a major difference in incidence between sexes. And, although sex does not play a key role in the development of GERD, it is a crucial factor in the development of Barrett's esophagus, a complication of GERD in which the normal squamous epithelium is replaced with specialized columnar epithelium.

Many patients self-treat with over-the-counter (OTC) drugs, with as many as 46% of patients with mild disease healing spontaneously; another 31% will show significant improvement. The true incidence and prevalence of GERD is difficult to know because patient symptoms do not correlate perfectly with disease severity, and there is no uniform definition or universal gold standard for diagnosing the disorder.

Risk Factors

There are numerous factors that place patients at risk for GERD and esophagitis; they are listed in Box 45-1.

PATHOPHYSIOLOGY

The term GERD refers to any symptomatic clinical condition or histologic alteration resulting from gastroesophageal reflux, the upward movement of gastric contents from the stomach into the esophagus. Under normal circumstances, the lower esophageal sphincter (LES) provides an antireflux barrier. Reflux develops when there is transient LES relaxation. Abdominal strain from increased gastric volume (secondary to delayed gastric emptying) along with impaired esophageal epithelial defense mechanisms contributes to mucosal damage.

Chronic reflux can progress to erosive esophagitis and transformation of esophageal mucosa from epithelial cells into the columnar gastric type of mucosal cells (Barrett's esophagus). Barrett's esophagus is a premalignant condition associated with gastric distention, transiently reduced LES pressure, and diminished esophageal peristalsis. This upward movement is in contrast to what happens in persons without GERD, where reflux results in increased esophageal peristalsis and rapid emptying of the esophagus. Severe erosive

BOX 45-1

Risk Factors for GERD, Esophagitis, and PUD

Risk Factors for GERD
- Foods that lower LES pressure: high-fat foods, yellow onions, chocolate, and mint
- Foods that irritate esophageal mucosa: citrus fruits such as orange juice and grapefruit juice and tomatoes
- Hiatal hernia: contributes to acid trapping
- Chronic belching, aerophagia
- Drugs that lower LES pressure: theophylline, Anticholinergics, progesterone, Calcium channel blockers (nifedipine, verapamil), Alpha adrenergic drugs, diazepam, meperidine
- Indwelling nasogastric tube
- Chest trauma
- Down syndrome, mental retardation, cerebral palsy, repaired tracheoesophageal fistula
- Eradication of *Helicobacter pylori*: results in increased acid production, loss of acid buffering

Risk Factors for Esophagitis
- White male who has a hiatal hernia
- Body mass index >30 mm^2
- Chronic NSAID use

Risk Factors Strongly Associated with PUD
- Family history of ulcer
- Chronic lung disease, renal failure, Zollinger-Ellison syndrome, hyperparathyroidism
- Smoking more than half a pack per day

Risk Factors Possibly Associated with PUD
- High-dose and/or prolonged corticosteroid therapy
- Blood group type O (30% greater risk than other blood types)
- HLA-B12, B5, Bw35 phenotypes
- Lower socioeconomic status; manual labor

GERD, Gastroesophageal reflux disease; *LES*, lower esophageal sphincter; *NSAID*, nonsteroidal antiinflammatory drug; *PUD*, peptic ulcer disease.

esophagitis may occur in the absence of reduced LES pressure. Neutralization of esophageal contents by esophageal and salivary secretions is an important protective mechanism.

There is an uncertain and complex relationship between GERD and the *Helicobacter pylori* organism. Studies have shown that the symptoms of GERD may actually worsen in some patients when *H. pylori* are eliminated (see discussion that follows).

PEPTIC ULCER DISEASE

EPIDEMIOLOGY AND ETIOLOGY

Peptic ulcer disease (PUD) is defined as a break in the continuity of gastric or duodenal mucosa. It can develop in any part of the GI tract that comes in contact with hydrochloric (HCl) acid and pepsin. PUD is clinically significant because of the loss of integrity of the gastric or duodenal walls, the actual or the potential hemorrhage, and the impact on nutritional balance.

Duodenal ulcers are 4 times more common than gastric ulcers, with a life-time prevalence of about 10% in men and 5% in women, although the gender gap is slowly closing.

There are 200,000 to 400,000 new cases of duodenal ulcers annually. The dominant age range for duodenal ulcers is 25 to 75 years. Gastric ulcers account for 87,500 new cases annually, with 50 persons out of 100,000 afflicted. The peak incidence occurs between the ages of 55 to 65 years.

No firm prevalence figures exist about PUD in children. Duodenal ulcers are rare before age 15. Gastric ulcers are rare under age 40. One percent to 2% of hospitalized children have peptic ulcerations. Male children are affected more often than female children, and the disorder is more common in late school-age children and adolescents than in younger children.

PUD is chronic and reoccurring, affecting at least 10% of populations in developed countries. An even greater number of persons suffer from dyspeptic symptoms without ever having ulcers (nonulcer dyspepsia). Of the adult population worldwide, 50% to 80% is infected with *H. pylori*. If the infection is left untreated, it can persist for decades, although only 10% to 20% of patients go on to develop peptic ulcer disease or neoplasia; however, many more have low-grade gastritis.

Risk Factors

Use of nonsteroidal antiinflammatory drugs (NSAIDs) increases the risk of recurrence and of GI complications 2 to 6 times, depending on the dose, the half-life of the drug, the dosing frequency, and the duration of use. Twenty percent to 40% of patients with duodenal ulcers have a positive family history, with a 50% concordance in identical (monozygotic) twins, compared with a 14% concordance in fraternal (dizygotic) twins. The rate of ulcer recurrence and complications increase more than 3 times with continued cigarette smoking of more than half a pack per day. High-dose or prolonged corticosteroid therapy is a possible risk factor for PUD. Persons with type O blood group have a 30% greater risk for duodenal ulcers than persons with other blood types.

A number of diseases are associated with PUD, including chronic lung disease or renal failure, Zollinger-Ellison syndrome, and hyperparathyroidism. The connection of these diseases to PUD relates to the hypercalcemia that develops; hypercalcemia stimulates gastrin secretion and, therefore, acid secretion. Other contributing factors to PUD are the stresses associated with head injuries and burns (Cushing's and Curling's ulcers, respectively); in patients who have experienced respiratory failure, major surgical procedures, or shock; and in those who are septic.

PATHOPHYSIOLOGY

PUD results when the normal balance of those factors that damage and those that protect the GI mucosal barrier is disturbed. Acute ulcers are associated with minimal inflammation and superficial erosion. They are of short duration and quickly resolve once the cause is identified and removed. Chronic ulcers are at least 4 times as common as acute erosions. Although defined as peptic ulcers, gastric and duodenal ulcers are distinctly different in their etiology and incidence (Fig. 45-1).

Most peptic ulcers occur downstream from the source of acid secretion. Ninety-eight percent of duodenal ulcers are located in the first portion of the duodenum within 2 cm of the pyloric ring. Duodenal ulcers are associated with increased numbers of parietal cells in the stomach, elevated gastrin levels, and rapid gastric emptying. Hypersecretion of HCl acid

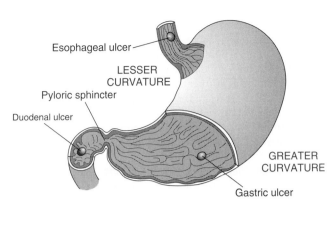

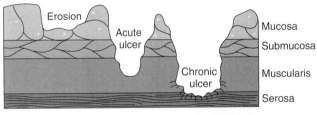

FIGURE 45-1 Location and Depth of Ulcers.

and pepsin appear to be the most important factors in their development, although an inadequate secretion of bicarbonate by the duodenal mucosa may also be related.

Other factors contributing to ulcer formation include failure of the feedback mechanism by which acid in the gastric antrum inhibits gastrin release. Thus, serum gastrin levels after eating remain high longer than normal, stimulating further acid secretion. It has been postulated that high serum gastrin levels are caused by the *H. pylori* organism. Rapid gastric emptying overcomes the buffering capacity of the bicarbonate-rich pancreatic secretions, which contribute to inflammation. The presence of multiple ulcers distal to the bulb raises the possibility of Zollinger-Ellison syndrome.

Gastric ulcers can appear in any portion of the stomach but are most often on the lesser curvature in close proximity to the antral junction (see Fig. 45-1). They arise as a result of backward diffusion of acid or pyloric sphincter dysfunction. Normally, the thick, tenacious barrier of gastric mucus acts as the first line of defense against autodigestion, protecting the stomach from mechanical trauma and chemical agents. Although the exact nature of the mucosal barrier is unclear, and even though a large concentration gradient exists (gastric acid has a pH of 1 to 2; the blood, 7.45), there is very little backward diffusion of hydrogen ions from the lumen to the blood.

In addition to mucosal and epithelial barriers, the resistance of tissues to ulceration depends on an abundant blood supply and continued, rapid regeneration of epithelial cells. Gastric ulcers are usually slow to heal, in part, because of poor circulation to the ulcerative site. Further, gastric epithelial cells are normally replaced every 3 days. Failure of the replacement mechanism may also play a part in the pathogenesis of PUD.

Complications

Simply stated, intractability means that conservative treatment of hyperacidity and PUD failed to adequately control the patient's symptoms. One third of all patients with ulcers

have a single episode of intractability with no recurrence. Sleep is interrupted by the pain, time is lost from work, hospitalization may be required, or patients are just unable to follow the treatment regimen. Intractability is the most common reason for recommending surgery.

Only approximately 5% of all ulcers perforate, but perforations account for 65% of deaths from PUD. Perforations are usually found on the anterior wall of the duodenum or the stomach because this area is covered only by peritoneum. Perforation occurs when an ulcer infiltrates serosal surfaces, spilling the gastric or duodenal contents into the peritoneum. A chemical peritonitis develops as a result of escaping gastric acid, pepsin, food, air, saliva, bile, pancreatic juices, and bacteria. A bacterial peritonitis develops 6 to 12 hours after the perforation, followed by a paralytic ileus. The intensity of the peritonitis is proportional to the amount and duration of the spillage through the perforation.

Bleeding is a common complication of PUD, occurring in more than 25% of patients at some time during the course of the disease. The most common site for hemorrhage is the posterior wall of the duodenal bulb. The left gastric artery may be penetrated by a gastric ulcer, and the superior pancreatic-duodenal artery by a duodenal ulcer.

Gastric outlet obstruction is the result of inflammation and edema, pylorospasm, or scarring in about 5% of patients. It is more common in patients who have duodenal ulcers but occasionally occurs if a gastric ulcer is located close to the pyloric sphincter.

PHARMACOTHERAPEUTIC OPTIONS

Proton Pump Inhibitors

◆ esomeprazole (Nexium); ◆ Nexium
◆ lansoprazole (Prevacid); ◆ Prevacid
◆ omeprazole (Prilosec, Prilosec OTC); ◆ Prilosec, Losec
◆ pantoprazole (Protonix); ◆ Pantoloc
◆ rabeprazole (Aciphex); ◆ Aciphex, Pariet

▌ Indications

PPIs are used to treat GERD, esophagitis, gastritis, active PUD, and Zollinger-Ellison syndrome. A large proportion of patients with severe esophagitis who do not respond to H2RAs (see discussion that follows) can be healed with PPIs. PPIs have been shown time and again to be better than H2RAs for symptom relief and mucosal healing. PPIs reduce dyspepsia and have been shown to prevent endoscopically-detected ulcers, but there is no compelling evidence to date that they prevent serious NSAID-related GI complications. Although PUD treated with PPIs heals rapidly, recurrence is frequent unless *H. pylori* are eliminated.

▌ Pharmacodynamics

PPIs produce a profound, long-lasting suppression of gastric acid secretion (in >90% of patients) and thus are able to maintain the gastric pH above 4, even during the acid surges that occur after eating. The parent drug is inactive, but under the highly acidic conditions inside the parietal cell, it is converted to sulfonamide. The sulfonamide combines irreversibly with the H^+-K^+-ATPase proton pump system that prevents hydrogen secretion into the gastric lumen. Thus the final step in basal, nocturnal, and stimulated acid production is blocked. Sulfonamide does not readily cross biologic membranes, and because of the unique nature of the proton pump, PPIs have little action on other ion pumps in the body.

Suppressing gastric acid secretion results in reduced blood flow to the antrum, the pylorus, and the duodenal bulb; pepsin activity decreases, and serum pepsinogen levels increase (Fig. 45-2). In patients with gastric ulcers there is an increase in nitrate-producing bacteria and an elevation of nitrate concentrations in gastric juices. There are initial compensatory increases in serum gastrin levels, but no additional increase occurs with continued treatment, and there do not appear to be ill effects from this increase. Tolerance to the antisecretory effect of a PPI has not been reported.

Pharmacokinetics

PPIs are well absorbed following oral administration, typically within 1 hour. Concurrent intake of a cola beverage may improve absorption. Although the half-lives for all PPIs range from 1 to 2 hours, the durations of action are longer

and more varied (Table 45-1). All PPIs are biotransformed by the liver to inactive metabolites that are eliminated primarily in the urine. The elimination of these drugs is slower in patients who have mild liver impairment or in older adults; however dosage adjustments are not needed.

Because PPIs are degraded in the acidic environment of the stomach, they are formulated in a delayed-release capsule or tablet formulation. Lansoprazole, esomeprazole, and omeprazole contain pH-sensitive granules in a capsule form.

Adverse Effects and Contraindications

PPIs are generally well tolerated, with few adverse effects. The most frequent adverse effects include headache and diarrhea. A rash, inflammation, urticaria, pruritus, alopecia, and dry skin have been seen. Also, although rarely, PPIs have been associated with blood dyscrasias, hepatic dysfunction, Stevens-Johnson syndrome, toxic epidermal necrolysis, erythema multiforme, and pancreatitis. Anaphylaxis is possible but also rare.

The danger of long-term acid suppression with a PPI has been debated. Atrophic changes have been reported in the

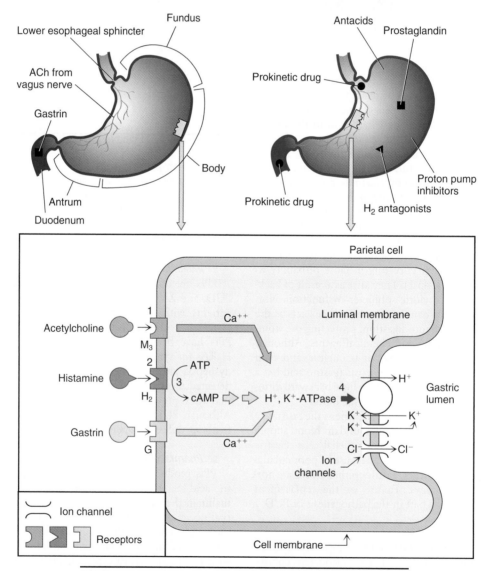

FIGURE 45-2 Mechanisms Regulating HCl Secretion by Gastric Parietal Cells.

PHARMACOKINETICS

TABLE **45-1** Drugs for Hyperacidity, GERD, and PUD

Drug	Route	Onset	Peak	Duration	PB%	$t_{1/2}$	BioA %
PROTON PUMP INHIBITORS							
esomeprazole	PO	<60 min	1.5 hr	24 hr	97	1–1.5 hr	64–69
lansoprazole	PO	2–3 hr for 15-mg dose; 1–2 hr for 30-mg dose*	1.7 hr	24 hr for 15-mg dose; >24 hr for 30-mg dose	97.5	1–1.5 hr; 3.2-7.2†	>80
omeprazole	PO	<60 min	0.5–3 hr	72 hr	95	0.5–1 hr; 3 hr‡	30–40
pantoprazole	PO	UA	2.5 hr	24 hr	>98	1–2 hr	77
	IV	Immed	2.5 hr	24 hr	>98	1–2 hr	100
rabeprazole	PO	60 min	2.5 hr	24 hr	96	1–2 hr	52
HISTAMINE₂-RECEPTOR ANTAGONISTS							
cimetidine	PO	40–90 min	4.5 hr; <1.5 hr§	UA	13–25	2 hr	60–70
	IV	Immed	UA	UA	13–25	2 hr	100
famotidine	PO	1–2 hr	1 hr	1–4 hr‖	15–20	2.5–3.5 hr	45–50
	IV	Immed	1 hr	8–15 hr‖	17	1.3–2.6 hr	100
nizatidine	PO	60 min	0.5–3 hr‖	UA	35	1–2 hr	>90
ranitidine	PO	60 min	1–3 hr	1–3 hr	15	2–3 hr	50–60
	IV	Immed	15 min	1–3 hr	15	2–3 hr	100
PROSTAGLANDIN							
misoprostol	PO	30 min	1–1.5 hr	3–6 hr	80–90	20–40 min	UA
PROKINETIC DRUG							
metoclopramide	PO	30–60 min	1–2 hr	20 hr	30	4–6 hr	65–95
	IM	10–15 min	2.2 hr	20 hr	30	4–6 hr	65–95
	IV	1–3 min	1–2 hr	20 hr	30	4–6 hr	65–95

*Antisecretory activity of lansoprazole.
†Elimination half–life of lansoprazole lengthened in patients with hepatic disorders.
‡Elimination half-life of omeprazole in patients with hepatic disorders.
§At concentrations of cimetidine that inhibit gastric acid secretion by 50% and 90% respectively.
‖Concentration of famotidine or nizatidine that inhibit gastric secretion by 50%.
BioA, Bioavailability; *IM*, intramuscular; *Immed*, immediate; *IV*, intravenous; *PB*, protein binding; *PO*, by mouth; $t_{1/2}$, half-life; *UA*, unavailable.

gastric corpus after 36 months of treatment, especially if gastritis or GERD was present before PPI administration. The major concern is the potential for overproduction of gastrin, which can cause gastric enterochromaffin-like (ECL) cell hyperplasia, neuroendocrine cell tumors, liver adenomas and carcinoma in animals. Even after 10 years of experience, this concern retains theoretical status in humans rather than that of an observed risk. More experience with these drugs is needed to assess long-term safety. PPIs have also been shown to cause achlorhydria in some patients because of the profound acid suppression. Safe use in children has not been established.

Drug Interactions

All PPIs are biotransformed by the CYP450 system to some extent; specifically the CYP 2C19 and CYP 3A4 enzymes. For this reason, careful monitoring is needed when using PPIs with other drugs also biotransformed in the liver (Table 45-2). Similarly, omeprazole and esomeprazole inhibit the biotransformation of diazepam and phenytoin leading to elevated serum levels of these drugs.

▲ **PPIs inhibit the biotransformation of oral anticoagulants, diazepam, theophylline, and phenytoin, leading to elevated serum levels of these drugs. Pantoprazole is less likely to have significant drug interactions compared with the other PPIs.**

PPIs also interfere with the absorption of other drugs requiring an acid gastric pH to be effective. Examples of such drugs include ketoconazole, ampicillin, digoxin, and iron salts. The absorption of B_{12} may be reduced.

Dosage Regimen

Treatment of hyperacidity and GERD lasts 4 to 8 weeks. Patients who do not respond to standard PPI dosages may require higher dosages (Table 45-3). The usual treatment period for erosive esophagitis is 8 weeks. For these patients and those who have erosive disease, higher dosages and/or dosing more often provides better acid control, particularly after meal-associated acid surges. Comparable doses of PPIs are omeprazole, 20 mg = esomeprazole, 20 mg = lansoprazole, 30 mg = rabeprazole, 20 mg = pantoprazole, 40 mg/day.

Lab Considerations

Serum levels of theophylline may be elevated in the presence of lansoprazole. Lansoprazole is known to cause increased liver function test (LFT) and gastrin levels, but can also cause abnormal albumin to globulin ratios, hyperlipidemia, and increased or decreased cholesterol levels.

Histamine₂-Receptor Antagonists

◆ cimetidine (Tagamet); ♣ Tagamet, Peptol
◆ famotidine (Pepcid); ♣ Pepcid
◆ nizatidine (Axid); ♣ Axid
◆ ranitidine (Zantac); ♣ Zantac

Indications

H₂RAs, also known as H₂-blocking drugs, are used for short-term management of active duodenal ulcers and benign gastric ulcers. In low doses, H₂RAs can be used for duodenal

DRUG INTERACTIONS

TABLE 45-2 Clinically Significant GI Drug Interactions

Drug	Interactive Drugs	Interaction
PROTON PUMP INHIBITORS		
lansoprazole	diazepam	Decreases biotransformation with increased serum levels of digoxin
	theophylline*	Increases clearance of theophylline and decreases serum concentrations
omeprazole	clarithromycin	Increases plasma levels of both drugs
	diazepam*	Effects 103% increase in half-life of diazepam
	phenytoin*	Effects 15% reduction in clearance
	warfarin*	Prolongs elimination
lansoprazole, omeprazole	sucralfate	Decreases absorption of PPI
	ketoconazole, itraconazole, ampicillin, digoxin, Iron salts	Decreases absorption of interactive drug
rabeprazole	digoxin*	Increases digoxin levels by ~20%
HISTAMINE₂-RECEPTOR ANTAGONISTS		
H₂RAs in general; cimetidine in particular	Benzodiazepines,* Tricyclic antidepressants; propranolol, metformin, mexilitine, nifedipine, phenobarbital, theophylline,* warfarin*	Prolongs half-life of interactive drug, thereby increasing its effects and risk of toxicity
NONSYSTEMIC ANTACIDS		
aluminum hydroxide, magnesium hydroxide	allopurinol, Corticosteroids, diflunisal, digoxin, iron, isoniazid, penicillamine, Phenothiazines, Quinolones, ranitidine, Tetracyclines	Decreases effects of interactive drug
	Amphetamines, Benzodiazepines, Salicylates	Increases effects of interactive drug
	Amphetamines, flecainide, quinidine	Reduces elimination
calcium compounds	digoxin	Increases risk for digoxin toxicity
PROSTAGLANDIN		
misoprostol	Magnesium containing antacids	Increases risk for diarrhea
CYTOPROTECTIVE DRUG		
sucralfate	Antacids	Decreases effectiveness of sucralfate
	phenytoin, tetracycline, Vitamins A, D, E, and K	Increases absorption of interactive drug
	Quinolones	Decreases bioavailability of interactive drugs

*Clinically significant interactions.
H₂RAs, Histamine₂-receptor antagonists; *PPI,* proton pump inhibitor.

DOSAGE

TABLE 45-3 Drugs for Hyperacidity, GERD, and PUD

Drug	Uses	Dosage	Comments *
PROTON PUMP INHIBITORS			
omeprazole	GERD, erosive esophagitis	*Adult:* 20–40 mg PO daily for 4–8 wk. Max: 80 mg/day *Child 2–16 yr:* 0.6-0.7 mg/kg PO once-twice daily for 3–6 mo; then taper. Max: 80 mg/day	30 generic 20-mg capsules = $94
	Gastric ulcer	*Adult:* 40 mg PO daily for 4–8 wk. Max: 80 mg/day	
	Hypersecretory conditions	*Adult:* 60 mg PO daily. Max:120 mg 3 times daily	
	Helicobacter pylori treatment	*Adult:* 20 mg PO twice for 10 days if triple therapy with clarithromycin and amoxicillin; 40 mg daily for 14 days if dual therapy with clarithromycin	
	Ulcer prophylaxis associated with NSAIDs	*Adult:* 20–40 mg PO once daily	
esomeprazole	GERD, erosive esophagitis	*Adult:* 20–40 mg PO once daily for 4–8 wk. Max: 80 mg/day	30 brand-name 40-mg capsules = $258
	H. pylori treatment	*Adult:* 40 mg PO once daily for 10 days	
lansoprazole	GERD	*Adult:* 15–30 mg PO once daily for 8 wk *Child 12–17 yr:* 15 mg PO once daily for 8 wk. Max: 30 mg twice daily	30 brand-name 30-mg capsules = $246
	Erosive esophagitis	*Adult:* 30 mg PO once-twice daily for 8 wk	
	Duodenal ulcer	*Adult:* 15 mg PO once-twice daily for 4–8 wk	
	Gastric ulcer	*Adult:* 30 mg PO once-twice daily for 8 wk	
	Ulcer prophylaxis with NSAID use	*Adult:* 15–30 mg PO once daily	
	H. pylori treatment	*Adult:* 30 mg PO twice daily for 10–14 days; 3 times daily for 14 days if dual therapy with amoxicillin; 3 times daily if triple therapy with clarithromycin and amoxicillin	
	Hypersecretory conditions	*Adult:* 60 mg PO once daily. Max: 90 mg twice daily. Divide doses if over 120 mg/day	
pantoprazole	Erosive esophagitis	*Adult:* 40 mg PO once-twice daily for 8 wk	30 brand-name 40-mg tablets = $107
	Hypersecretory conditions	*Adult:* 40 mg PO twice daily. Max: 240 mg/day	
	Acute PUD	*Adult:* 80 mg IV as 1-time dose.	

rabeprazole	GERD	*Adult:* 20 mg PO once-twice daily for 4–8 wk	30 brand-name 20-mg tablets = $122
	Duodenal ulcer	*Adult:* 20 mg PO once daily for 4 wk	
	Hypersecretory conditions	*Adult:* 60 mg PO once daily. Max: 120 mg daily	
	H. pylori treatment	*Adult:* 20 mg PO twice daily for 7 days if used with amoxicillin and clarithromycin	

HISTAMINE$_2$-RECEPTOR ANTAGONISTS

cimetidine	PUD	*Adult:* 300 mg PO 4 times daily. Max: 2400 mg/day. Alternate: 800 mg HS, or 400 mg twice daily	Many drug interactions. Check drug reference before prescribing. 120 generic 300-mg tablets = $33
		Neonate: 5–10 mg/kg daily in divided doses	
		Infant: 10–20 mg/kg daily in divided doses	
		Child: 20–40 mg/kg daily in divided doses	
	GERD	*Adult:* 400 mg PO before meals and HS	
		Neonate: 5–10 mg/kg daily in divided doses	
		Infants: 10–20 mg/kg daily in divided doses	
		Child: 20–40 mg/kg daily in divided doses	
	Zollinger-Ellison syndrome	*Adult:* 300–600 mg PO 4 times daily	
ranitidine	Duodenal ulcer, Gastric ulcer, GERD	*Adult:* 150 mg PO twice daily	60 generic 150-mg tablets = $20
		Child <1 mo: 2–4 mg/kg PO daily in divided doses	
		Child 1 mo–16 yr: 5–10 mg/kg PO daily in divided doses	
	Erosive esophagitis	*Adult:* 150 mg PO 4 times daily	
		Child <1 mo: 2–4 mg/kg PO daily in divided doses	
		Child 1 mo–16 yr: 5–10 mg/kg PO daily in divided doses	
	Dyspepsia	*Adult:* 75 mg PO twice daily	
famotidine	Active duodenal ulcer	*Adult:* 40 mg PO HS for 4–6 wk. Alternate: 20 mg twice daily	30 generic 40-mg tablets = $6
		Child 1–16 yr: 0.5–1 mg/kg PO daily in divided doses	
	Maintenance duodenal ulcer	*Adult:* 20 mg PO HS	
	Gastric ulcer	*Adult:* 40 mg PO HS	
	Zollinger-Ellison syndrome	*Adult:* 20–60 mg PO every 6 hr	
		Max: 160 mg every 6 hr	
	Intractable ulcers	*Adult:* 20 mg IV every 12 hr	
nizatidine	GERD	*Adult:* 150 mg PO twice daily	60 brand-name 150-mg tablets = $18
		Child 6 mo–11 yr: 6–10 mg/kg PO daily in divided doses	
		Child >11 yr: 150 mg PO twice daily	
	Maintenance duodenal ulcer	*Adult:* 150 mg PO HS	
	Active gastric ulcer	*Adult:* 300 mg PO HS	

NONSYSTEMIC ANTACIDS†

aluminum hydroxide (AlternaGEL, Amphojel, BasalGel)	Hyperacidity, GERD, PUD, gastritis, esophagitis, hiatal hernia, stress ulcerations	*Adult:* 5–30 mL *–or–* 2 tablets (500–1500 mg) PO 1 hr and 3 hr after meals and HS	12-oz suspension = $8
		Child: 5–15 mL PO every 1-2 hr	
magnesium + hydroxide	Hyperacidity, GERD, PUD, gastritis, esophagitis, hiatal hernia, stress ulcerations	*Adult:* 5–15 mL PO suspension every 1–2 hr *–or–* 650–1300 mg as tablets 4 times/day	120 generic 400-mg tablets = $12
calcium carbonate	Hyperacidity, GERD, PUD, gastritis, esophagitis, hiatal hernia, stress ulcerations	*Adult:* 1–2 tablets PO 4 times daily	96 generic 750-mg tablets = $5

PROSTAGLANDIN

| misoprostol‡ | NSAID ulcer prevention | *Adult:* 100–200 mcg PO 4 times daily | 120 generic 100-mg tablets = $65 |

PROKINETIC DRUG

metoclopramide	GERD	*Adult:* 5–15 mg PO before meals and HS	120 generic 10 mg-tablets = $21
		Child: 0.1–0.2 mg/kg PO 4 times daily. Max: 0.8 mg/kg in divided doses/24 hr	
	Diabetic gastroparesis	*Adult:* 10 mg PO or IV before meals and HS	

CYTOPROTECTIVE DRUG

sucralfate	Short-term treatment of duodenal ulcer; NSAID-related gastric erosion	*Adult:* 1 gram PO 4 times daily 1 hr before meals and HS	120 generic 1-gram tablets = $40
		Child: 10–20 mg/kg PO before meals and HS	
	Duodenal ulcer maintenance	*Adult:* 1 gram PO 4 times daily	
		Child 1–10 yr: 1 gram PO 1 hr before bedtime	
	Esophagitis	*Child >6 yr:* 1 gram PO 4 times/day	

*Approximate retail price for 30-day supply of drug in the United States. From www.drugstore.com
†Combinations of aluminum hydroxide and magnesium hydroxide are more commonly used for antacid effects than single formulations.
‡Pediatric dosing not applicable to this drug.
GERD, Gastroesophageal reflux disease; *HS, at* bedtime; *IV,* intravenous; *NSAID,* nonsteroidal antiinflammatory drug; *PO,* by mouth; *PUD,* peptic ulcer disease.

ulcer prophylaxis, and for the prevention and treatment of acute stress ulcerations, esophagitis resulting from GERD, and Zollinger-Ellison syndrome.

Pharmacodynamics

H_2RAs inhibit the action of histamine at H_2 receptors, thereby inhibiting gastric acid secretion and reducing total pepsin output. The resultant decrease in acid permits healing of ulcerated areas. The drugs are highly selective with little to no effect on H_1 or other receptors. (H_1 antagonists, the typical antihistamines, are discussed in Chapter 51.) H_1 antagonists prevent or reduce the effects of histamine but do nothing to block the production of gastric acid.

Pharmacokinetics

As a group, H_2RAs are rapidly and well absorbed following oral administration and have comparable volumes of distribution, serum half-lives, and clearance parameters (see Table 45-1). With the exception of nizatidine, the H_2RAs undergo extensive first-pass biotransformation, and therefore bioavailability is reduced to 30% to 80% of an orally administered dose. Active renal tubular secretion is the primary mechanism for elimination of these drugs, although elimination takes place through the liver. The half-life of H_2RAs is significantly prolonged in patients with liver disorders.

Adverse Effects and Contraindications

There are few adverse effects associated with H_2RAs, although dizziness, somnolence, headache, confusion, and hallucinations have been noted. Diarrhea is the most common GI adverse effect. Cimetidine, in particular, may act as an antiandrogen to cause reversible impotence and gynecomastia. The frequency of adverse effects is similar to that of PPIs.

There are no absolute contraindications to the use of H_2RAs except a history of allergy. However, the drugs should be used with caution in pregnant or lactating women,

children, and older adults, and in patients with impaired renal or hepatic function (see Controversy box).

Drug Interactions

All drugs that inhibit gastric acid secretion and thus change gastric pH alter the bioavailability and absorption rate of other drugs, although not all interactions are clinically significant (see Table 45-2). Cimetidine, but not the other H_2RA drugs, inhibits the activity of the CYP450 enzymes, thereby slowing the biotransformation and prolonging the half-life of the other drugs. For this reason, cimetidine is used less often. Cimetidine also inhibits the gastric biotransformation of alcohol. Such interactions require either dosage-reduction or interval-extension strategies and close patient monitoring. **H_2RAs prolong the half-life of benzodiazepines, phenytoin, and theophylline, thereby increasing the interactive drug effects and risk of toxicity.** ▲

The absorption of two cephalosporin antibiotics, cefpodoxime and cefuroxime, and ketoconazole and itraconazole in particular, are reduced unless they are taken at least 2 hours before the H_2RA drug. Vitamin B_{12} absorption also depends to some degree on a relatively acidic environment and may be compromised in the presence of an H_2RA drug.

Another potential site for drug interactions with H_2RA drugs is in the kidney. H_2RA drugs compete with other drugs for the renal tubular active transport system, decreasing the elimination of such drugs as metformin and leading to potential toxicity from that drug.

Dosage Considerations

H_2RAs heal more than 90% of duodenal ulcers and more than 70% of gastric ulcers in 4 to 6 weeks when dosing recommendations are followed; and despite short plasma half-lives, these drugs may often be taken only once or twice daily (see Table 45-3). H_2RAs are generally well tolerated and can be administered, if necessary, in doses well above those needed

---

Controversy

Self-Treating with OTC Antisecretory Drugs
Jonathan J. Wolfe

The advent of intravenous cimetidine in 1976 was universally acclaimed. Here was a drug that had no known adverse effects and could essentially rescue patients with gastric ulcerations from bleeding. Gone was the need for partial to total gastric resection, which too often led to dumping syndrome. Gone also were the desperate and often futile interventions (e.g., iced gavage with levarterenol) against uncontrollable hemorrhage. The commercial success of the drug has served as a benchmark for every product since that time.

The intervening years have brought change. The adverse effects of this original H_2-receptor antagonist (H_2RA) became clear. The effect of cimetidine on the CYP450 enzyme systems in the liver and its adverse effect profile limits its use in combination with many other drugs. Newer, more selective H_2RAs and proton pump inhibitors (PPIs) have come to market (e.g., ranitidine and omeprazole, respectively) that have a better adverse effects profile. And, as the patents for these drugs have expired, their costs have decreased compared with brand-name drugs requiring a prescription.

Perhaps the most stunning change has been the appearance of over-the-counter (OTC) forms of the H_2RAs and PPIs. What once was a miracle infusion in the intensive care unit is now hanging on racks in service stations next to breath mints, chewing gum, and condoms. Indeed, these wonder drugs are advertised directly-to-the-consumer on television and in print media as the answer to heartburn.

CRITICAL ANALYSIS DISCUSSION
- When prescription H_2RAs and PPIs were first introduced, patients were advised to take the drug regularly rather than in response to symptoms. Why do we now have OTC products for self-treatment?
- How do you respond to a patient who tells you that rather than pay for a new prescription for esomeprazole, he will simply "take 4 75-mg OTC tablets of ranitidine at bedtime "when the pain is bad.""
- What hazard is posed when the patient chooses to use an OTC H_2RA or PPI for several months before seeking the advice of a health care provider?
- What restrictions on the OTC sale of H_2RAs and PPIs would you consider reasonable?

to produce an effect (e.g., ranitidine, 150 mg 4 times daily; nizatidine, 150 mg 4 times daily; famotidine, 40 mg twice daily; cimetidine, 800 mg twice daily).

Lab Considerations

The complete blood count (CBC) and differential should be monitored periodically throughout therapy. White blood cell counts should be monitored while the patient is receiving cimetidine, especially if other drugs known to cause neutropenia are taken. H_2RA drugs may cause a transient increase in LFT results and in serum creatinine levels. Serum prolactin concentrations may be increased following an intravenous (IV) bolus of cimetidine. Cimetidine may also cause decreased parathyroid hormone (PTH) concentrations. False-negative results of allergy tests may be noted; therefore cimetidine should be discontinued 24 hours before testing. False-negative results for urine protein have been noted with ranitidine. Nizatidine has caused false-positive results on tests for urobilinogen.

Nonsystemic Antacids
* aluminum hydroxide
* calcium carbonate
* magnesium hydroxide

Indications

The most commonly used nonsystemic antacids are combinations of aluminum hydroxide and magnesium hydroxide (see Table 45-4 for the trade names). These days, antacids are typically used to treat symptoms of acid reflux or heartburn on an as-needed basis for symptom relief, but only if the patient describes symptomatic relief after use. Although antacids were once the only available treatments for PUD, the more efficacious and convenient PPIs and H_2RA drugs have become the primary choices for that condition.

Sodium bicarbonate, a systemically absorbed antacid, is discussed in more depth in Chapter 48. It is potent, but its effects are brief, and the potential for electrolyte imbalance is greater than with nonsystemic antacids. An ideal antacid is one that decreases acidity, is effective for prolonged periods, is pleasant to take by mouth, is not constipating or cathartic in effect, and does not cause systemic adverse effects.

Pharmacodynamics

Antacids are weak bases that neutralize hydrochloric acid secreted by parietal cells, increase gastric pH, and inhibit the conversion of pepsinogen to pepsin. Ninety-nine percent of gastric acid is neutralized when pH is increased from 1 or 2 to 3. Although their mechanism for increasing gastric pH differs and their effectiveness may be inferior to the PPIs and H_2RAs, the end result is similar.

A change in gastric pH also affects the activity of pepsin. Pepsin activity is greatest at a pH of 1.5 to 2.5. By increasing the pH, proteolytic activity is reduced, becoming minimal at a pH above 4. However, it is thought that by raising gastric pH, the potential for bacterial growth increases. Nevertheless, by increasing the pH and decreasing pepsin activity, symptomatic relief and healing is facilitated. Neither the amount nor the duration of neutralization required for optimal healing is known (Table 45-4). Most health care providers recommend that the gastric pH be maintained between 3.0 and 3.5 during the course of treatment.

Pharmacokinetics

Table 45-1 provides an overview of the pharmacokinetics of selected antacids. In general, antacids are nonabsorbable and therefore nonsystemic. Very small amounts of aluminum-based and up to 10% of magnesium-based antacids are absorbed from the GI tract. The remainder is excreted in the feces. However, with chronic use, 15% to 30% of magnesium and smaller quantities of the aluminum are absorbed. The absorbed magnesium and aluminum are widely distributed, crossing placental membranes. They are also found in breast milk.

When calcium carbonate reacts with hydrochloric acid in the stomach, it forms insoluble salts that are not well absorbed in the intestine. Small amounts of calcium are absorbed, however, which can cause hypercalcemia.

Adverse Effects and Contraindications

Antacids differ in the amount needed to raise gastric pH and in their adverse effects. Aluminum compounds generally have a slow onset of action and a low neutralizing capacity; therefore large doses are required. Ingestion of large amounts of aluminum-based antacids over a long period causes hypophosphatemia and osteomalacia. The aluminum combines

TABLE 45-4 Acid-Neutralizing Capacity of Selected Antacids

Brand Name*	Ingredient (mg/5 mL)				Na Content (mg)	ANC
	$Al(OH)_3$	$Mg(OH)_2$	$CaCO_3$	Simethicone		
Alternagel	600	0	0	—	<2.5	16
Amphogel	320	0	0	—	2.3	10
Basagel	400†	†	†	—	2.9	12
Gaviscon	31.7‡	‡	‡	—	4	13
Gelusil	200	200	0	25	0.7	12
Gelusil-M§	300	200	0	25	1.2	15
Maalox	225	200	0	0	1.4	13
Milk of Magnesia	0	390	0	0	0.12	14
Mylanta	200	200	0	20	0.7	13
Mylanta II	400	400	0	40	1.1	25

*These antacids are also available in solid dosage forms (i.e., tablets). Although the composition of these forms is similar to that of suspensions, there are variations.
†Basalgel: $Al(OH)CO_3$ is equivalent to 400 mg of AL $(OH)_3$.
‡Gaviscon: $Al(OH)_3$ plus 137 mg CO_3 plus sodium alginate.
§Therapeutic concentrate of Gelusil; *M*, medium strength.
ANC, Acid neutralizing capacity (5 mg/mL).

with phosphates in the GI tract, preventing phosphate absorption. Further, aluminum concentrates in the central nervous system (CNS) to contribute to encephalopathy, anemia, and anorexia. Because they have been known to cause constipation, aluminum compounds are often formulated in combination with magnesium.

Magnesium compounds have a rapid onset of action and a high neutralizing capacity but can cause diarrhea and hypermagnesemia. Because magnesium is excreted by the kidneys, it is contraindicated for use in patients with significant renal impairment or anuria. Magnesium compounds are contraindicated for use in patients with hypermagnesemia, hypocalcemia, and heart block, and in women in active labor. Magnesium hydroxide has the potential to cause drowsiness, hypothermia, decreased respiratory rates, bradycardia, arrhythmias, hypotension, flushing and sweating, decreased deeptendon reflexes, and paralysis.

Calcium carbonate has a greater potential for allowing acid rebound and leading to the formation of kidney stones. Furthermore, calcium compounds should not be used in patients with ventricular fibrillation, or hypercalcemia.

Drug Interactions

Most significant drug interactions alter the effects of other drugs rather than those of the antacids (see Table 45-2). **Antacids impede the absorption of certain drugs by binding to them (chelation) to form insoluble compounds. Drugs that have decreased absorption because of chelation include antibiotics such as tetracycline and the quinolones and oral thyroid replacement hormones. Antacids also cause decreased absorption of digoxin, captopril, and acetaminophen.** The absorption of drugs requiring a strong acid environment for absorption such as ketoconazole, itraconazole, and ampicillin may be reduced.

Calcium compounds alter urine pH (to make it more alkaline), which reduces the clearance of drugs such as quinidine and enhances the urinary elimination of salicylates. The elimination of amphetamines is markedly reduced, and toxicity is possible with large dosages of antacids and alkaline urine. Further, antacids remove the enteric coating on drugs, thereby causing the premature release of the drug into the stomach.

Dosage Regimen

Antacid dosages, including the frequency of administration, depend primarily on the purpose for the antacid's use, its buffering capacity, and the patient's response. Generally speaking, aluminum-containing antacids are the least potent and calcium carbonates the most potent. One gram of calcium carbonate equals 400 mg or 20 mEq of elemental calcium. Calcium-based antacids are safe only for intermittent use.

For a patient with a nasogastric tube in place, the antacid dosage may be titrated by aspirating stomach contents, determining the pH with phenaphthazine (Nitrazine) paper, and then basing the dose on the pH. Most gastric acid is neutralized at a pH above 3.5, with most pepsin activity eliminated at a pH above 5. If the pH is less than 5, the frequency or the dosage of the antacid may be increased.

Lab Considerations

Serum phosphate, calcium, and electrolyte levels should be monitored periodically in patients who use antacids chronically. Hypercalcemia increases the risk of cardiac glycoside toxicity, and hypocalcemia can create tetany, arrhythmias, and other adverse effects. Serum osmolarity, acid-base balance, and renal function testing may also be warranted, depending on the patient's response to therapy.

Prostaglandin

◆ misoprostol (Cytotec); ✦ Cytotec

Indications

Misoprostol is used to prevent gastric and duodenal ulcerations caused by NSAIDs. When they dissolve in the stomach, NSAIDs inhibit the synthesis of naturally occurring prostaglandins and therefore, with long-term use, gastric ulcers are a significant problem. Patients with arthritis who must take NSAIDs to relieve inflammation and pain are often prescribed misoprostol to replace the prostaglandins.

There is no evidence that misoprostol relieves the pain of ulcers or prevents ulcer complications or death; however, several placebo-controlled studies demonstrated that misoprostol significantly reduces duodenal ulcer development in patients taking NSAIDs. The MUCOSA Trial of 1994 demonstrated that misoprostol was markedly more effective than placebo, however, in preventing NSAID-induced ulcer complications in high-risk patients (Simon et al., 1996). When used to treat duodenal ulcers, misoprostol is no more effective than H_2RAs, and it has a worse adverse effects profile.

Pharmacodynamics

Misoprostol, an ester of prostaglandin E, inhibits the secretion of gastric acid, both basally and in response to food, histamine, pentagastrin, and coffee, by direct action on parietal cells. Prostaglandin E is a chemical relative of prostaglandins normally synthesized in the stomach, where they (i.e., the prostaglandins) block gastric acid secretion. Misoprostol also increases bicarbonate and mucus production (cytoprotective effects).

Pharmacokinetics

Misoprostol is well absorbed following oral administration and rapidly converted to an active form. Plasma steady state levels are achieved within 2 days. Misoprostol undergoes biotransformation in the liver and is eliminated by the kidneys (see Table 45-1).

Adverse Effects and Contraindications

Minor adverse effects such as mild nausea, abdominal discomfort, and dizziness are occasionally reported, but ordinarily misoprostol is well tolerated. Serious adverse effects include vaginal bleeding, spotting, cramping, hypermenorrhea, dysmenorrhea, and abortion in pregnant women, an action expected of a prostaglandin E analogue. Bleeding is reported in 50% of pregnant patients, with a 7% incidence of abortion. Therefore, it is important that misoprostol not be recommended for women of child-bearing age without the consistent use of effective birth control methods and a negative pregnancy test noted before beginning therapy.

Drug Interactions

No known drug interactions exist with natural or synthetic prostaglandin drugs. There is an increased risk of diarrhea when misoprostol is taken with a magnesium-containing antacid.

Dosage Regimen

The dose of misoprostol does not need adjustment in patients with renal impairment.

Prokinetic Drug

◆ metoclopramide (Reglan); ♣ metoclopramide, Reglan

Indications

Metoclopramide is used in conjunction with PPIs and H₂RAs for the management of GERD; however, data are lacking that it helps with endoscopic healing. Postsurgical and diabetic gastroparesis is also effectively treated with metoclopramide. Metoclopramide can also be useful in preventing antineoplastic drug-induced emesis. This drug facilitates small bowel intubation in radiographic procedures and is used in the prevention and treatment of postoperative nausea and vomiting when nasogastric suctioning is undesirable. Although not approved by the Food and Drug Administration (FDA) for such use, metoclopramide has also been used as treatment for hiccoughs.

Pharmacodynamics

Metoclopramide is a dopamine₂-receptor antagonist and a 5-HT₄–receptor stimulant that increases LES tone and the force of gastric contractions, improves the coordination of gastroduodenal contractions, and enhances gastric emptying. Metoclopramide acts by causing the release of ACh, thereby increasing gastric motility and gastric emptying. There is little evidence to date that metoclopramide heals esophageal erosions. It also has anticholinergic and CNS effects as a result of the dopamine blockade.

Pharmacokinetics

Metoclopramide acts relatively quickly to promote esophageal and gastric emptying (see Table 45-1). It is also well absorbed from the GI tract, from rectal mucosa, and from intramuscular (IM) administration sites. It is also widely distributed to body tissues and fluids, crossing the blood-brain barrier and placental membranes. Twenty-five percent of the original drug is eliminated unchanged in the urine. There is partial biotransformation in the liver.

Adverse Effects and Contraindications

Common adverse effects of metoclopramide include drowsiness, restlessness, fatigue, and anxiety. Insomnia, headache, dizziness, confusion, and depression have also been reported. The risk of adverse effects is much greater in patients with renal dysfunction, because the drug is primarily eliminated by the kidneys.

Contraindications to the use of metoclopramide include mechanical obstruction, GI bleeding, concomitant use of other dopamine antagonists, anticholinergic drugs, seizure disorder, and in patients who have pheochromocytoma. It should be used with caution in patients with depression, Parkinson's disease, hypertension, heart failure, cirrhosis, and nicotinamide adenine dinucleotide (NADH) methemoglobin reductase deficiency.

Drug Interactions

Metoclopramide interacts with a variety of other drugs (see Table 45-2).

Dosage Regimen

The dosage regimen for metoclopramide drug is identified in Table 45-3. Because this drug is used for a variety of purposes, dosages should be checked carefully before administration.

Lab Considerations

Metoclopramide may alter LFT results. It may also cause increased serum prolactin and aldosterone concentrations.

Cytoprotective Drug

◆ sucralfate (Carafate); ♣ Sulcrate

Indications

Sucralfate, as a locally acting drug, has been used in the management of PUD and hyperacidity when patients are unable to tolerate H₂RAs or a PPI, or when the H₂RA or PPI have been ineffective. Sucralfate is the only approved drug in this group. It has very limited value in the treatment of GERD and has no role in the eradication of *H. pylori*. It is the preferred drug for duodenal ulcers because it is less expensive than parenteral H₂RAs or PPIs, is not likely to increase the chance of nosocomial pneumonia, and does not require regular measurements of gastric pH.

Pharmacodynamics

Sucralfate is a complex of sulfated sucrose and aluminum hydroxide that binds electrostatically to positively charged tissue proteins and mucin within the ulcer crater. A viscous barrier is formed that protects the ulcer from the destructive action of the digestive enzyme pepsin. Sucralfate also inhibits pepsin, binds with bile salts, and stimulates mucosal prostaglandins. Unlike the H₂RAs and PPIs, sucralfate has no significant effect on gastric acid secretion.

Pharmacokinetics

Only 5% of sucralfate is absorbed systemically. It is well tolerated, producing few adverse effects (see Table 45-1). It is mostly eliminated in the feces.

Adverse Effects and Contraindications

Systemic effects to sucralfate are rarely observed because of the drug's minimal absorption. The adverse effects most often reported include dry mouth and constipation. Nausea, indigestion, and gastric discomfort have been noted in some patients. Concerns have been voiced about the retention of aluminum in patients with impaired renal function.

Drug Interactions

Because sucralfate binds digoxin, tetracycline, warfarin, phenytoin, quinidine, and theophylline, these drugs should be taken at different times. Antacids decrease the effectiveness of the sucralfate, whereas the absorption of phenytoin, fat-soluble vitamins, and tetracyclines is increased in the presence of sucralfate. Sucralfate also decreases the bioavailability of quinolones (see Table 45-2).

Dosage Regimen

A 4- to 8-week treatment regimen is recommended to ensure healing. By taking sucralfate before meals, it has time to form the protective coating over the ulcer before a high level of gastric acidity is reached (see Table 45-3). It requires an acidic

GASTROINTESTINAL

environment to be effective. If a nasogastric route is required, consultation with a pharmacist is needed. Information is necessary about the amount and type of diluent needed, because sucralfate is insoluble and a bezoar may form.

▥ Lab Considerations

There are no lab considerations associated with sucralfate. It is a locally acting drug and therefore has few systemic effects.

CLINICAL REASONING

Treatment Objectives

Until recently, control of acid secretion was the goal for treating GERD and PUD. Now control of acid secretion is simply part of the treatment regimen. Successful outcomes of treatment for hyperacidity, GERD, and PUD are measured in terms of three separate end points: (1) symptom relief, (2) healing injured mucosa, and (3) preventing complications. The short-term goal of therapy is to relieve symptoms to the point where they do not impair the patient's quality of life. As with all patient care, perceived susceptibility to disease and its seriousness influences treatment outcomes. The need for recurrent, long-term treatment regimens should raise questions regarding the patient's commitment to the plan of care. A plan that is relevant to the patient and the family, as appropriate, increases the level of adherence. The patient and family should be able to articulate an understanding of the treatment regimen and demonstrate an acceptable degree of compliance.

The second goal is to heal injured mucosa. Lifestyle modifications and the ability to follow through with the treatment regimen should be evaluated.

The long-term goal of therapy is to decrease the risk of complications such as esophagitis, strictures, and Barrett's esophagus. There are a small number of patients who may not respond to treatment despite high-dose PPI or H₂RA therapy. Inadequately treated severe esophagitis may lead to Barrett's esophagus and its related risk for adenocarcinoma.

Treatment Options

▥ Patient Variables

Prevention of GERD and PUD may be primary, secondary, or tertiary. For persons at high risk for PUD, identifying the contributing factors is paramount. Once those factors have been identified, the person can take primary preventative action. Smoking, although not a primary cause of GERD, PUD, or hyperacidity, has an irritating effect on the mucosa, increases gastric motility, and delays mucosal healing. The combination of inadequate rest and smoking accelerates ulcer development.

Secondary prevention involves the detection and treatment of the disease early in its course. For example, NSAID use should be stopped, when possible. Intervention is directed at detecting problems early in their course so that prompt treatment forestalls the serious consequences of advanced disease. When irritating drugs must be continued, enteric-coated or highly buffered preparations may be suitable.

Tertiary prevention of GERD and PUD is time-intensive. The management of GERD for the patient is lifelong. The

healing and subsequent cure of PUD requires many weeks of therapy. Although the pain of these two disorders may be alleviated in less than a week, healing is much slower. Complete healing may take 4 weeks to as many as 12 weeks, depending on treatment regimen and patient response.

Because recurrence of GERD and PUD is common, interruption or discontinuation of therapy can have detrimental results. Patients may stop the drug when they sense no further reflux or the ulcer has healed, or if therapy is continued, it is done so intermittently, based on reappearance of symptoms. Decisions regarding the most appropriate drug therapy should be made in light of the total patient; and in most cases, more than one approach is combined to provide the patient maximum healing capability in the shortest time.

Life-Span Considerations

Pregnant and Nursing Women. The pregnant patient has unique considerations. Nausea and vomiting during the first trimester is usually caused by the body's response to human chorionic gonadotropin secreted by the implanted fetus and reactions to changes in carbohydrate metabolism (see Chapter 6). However, gastric contents become more acidic during pregnancy as a result of elevated gastrin levels produced by the placenta. During the second and third trimesters, GI symptoms are attributable to the pressure from the growing uterus, as well as smooth muscle relaxation triggered by elevated progesterone levels. Relaxation of the cardiac sphincter frequently causes reflux. Gastric emptying time and intestinal motility are also delayed, which leads to frequent complaints of constipation and bloating.

Children and Adolescents. In newborns, reflux is normal because neuromuscular control of the LES is not fully developed. The frequency of reflux is highest in premature infants, decreasing during the first 6 to 12 months of life. Recurrent vomiting occurs in 50% of infants during the first 3 months of life. Physiologic reflux is distinguished from GERD by the presence of irritability, feeding problems, hematemesis, failure to thrive, and anemia. Fewer than 5% of infants with this disorder continue to have GERD into childhood.

Older children and adolescents have symptoms of GERD similar to those of adults (i.e., heartburn, epigastric pain, dysphagia, odynophagia). As in adults, erosive esophagitis can lead to hematemesis, melena, anemia, and hypoalbuminemia. Barrett's esophagus may develop in children and adolescents.

Ulcers occur mostly in children with genetic predisposition to PUD. They are most often solitary and deep in the gastric antrum or duodenum. Stress is a major factor in the development of ulcers in children. Chronic abdominal pain or weight loss may be the only signs of primary PUD. The abdominal pain may be nonspecific, but epigastric pain, especially if it penetrates to the back and is relieved temporarily by eating, points to the possibility of an ulcer. Anemia and the presence of blood in the stool are further indications of possible PUD.

Older Adults. Although PUD occurs most frequently at younger ages, the incidence is on the rise in older adults. An older adult experiencing a major body insult, whether medical or psychologic, is at risk for ulcer development, particularly if a preexisting gastritis is present. In addition to causes such as stress, diet, and genetic predisposition, other factors are believed to account for the increased incidence of ulcers in the aged. Longevity, more precise diagnostic evaluation, and the fact that ulcers can be a complication of chronic airway limitation disorders also increase the incidence.

Early symptoms commonly associated with PUD may not be as evident in the older patient. Epigastric pain is not a prominent feature. More frequently, the outstanding symptoms the older adult exhibits include poorly localized pain, decreased appetite, decreased general energy level, melena, weight loss, vomiting, and anemia. Even with a perforation, symptoms may be vague. Regardless of the etiology, the consequences of GI bleeding are much more severe in the elderly.

Drug Variables

The introduction of PPIs and H_2RAs in the past decade dramatically improved our ability to control acid secretion and promote healing. Antacids and anticholinergic drugs, once a mainstay of ulcer therapy, now play a less significant role. Mucosal protectant drugs also aid ulcer healing. The recognition that a bacterial cause underlies many ulcers led to therapies that include antibiotics for eradicating the *H. pylori* organism. Single antimicrobial therapy is not effective in eradicating *H. pylori*. A combination of antibiotics and an antisecretory drug must be used for effective eradication.

Initial treatment regimens for GERD are in part dependent on the patient's condition (frequency of symptoms, degree of esophagitis, and presence of complications). Otherwise healthy patients with a history of uncomplicated GERD can be treated empirically, using measures identified in steps 1 and 2 in Box 45-2. The steps are based on symptom relief and degree of esophageal damage. In many cases, these measures will suffice. If the patient fails to respond or if GERD is complicated by dysphagia, weight loss, and anemia, or if the stool tests positive for occult bleeding, a more comprehensive diagnostic evaluation by a gastroenterologist is warranted. In severe cases, surgery may be needed. Whatever method is used, every attempt should be made to aggressively control symptoms and prevent relapses early in the course of the patient's disease in order to prevent complications seen with long-standing, symptomatic GERD (Table 45-5).

The health care provider must weigh the risks and benefits of continuing any drugs known to worsen GERD and esophagitis. Smoking causes aerophagia, which leads to belching and regurgitation. However, data are lacking to show that symptoms improve in patients who quit smoking. Nevertheless, patients should be encouraged to quit smoking. Alcohol, although not thought to play a role in severe disease, decreases LES pressure and may exacerbate symptoms.

PROTON PUMP INHIBITORS. Proton pump inhibitors are the drugs of choice in moderate to severe GERD and esophagitis. Many independent clinical trials have shown the superiority of PPIs over H_2RAs or sucralfate both in their ability to control symptoms and to heal esophagitis in patients with GERD. They are more cost-effective in patients with severe disease.

As a rule, PPIs relieve symptoms in days and heal esophagitis in 4 to 8 weeks. In head-to-head PPI trials, healing rates among the PPIs were similar at 4 and 8 weeks; lansoprazole and rabeprazole, however, may relieve symptoms faster after the first dose when compared to omeprazole (van Pinxteren et al., 2004). This is particularly true when 30 mg of lansoprazole is compared to 20 mg of omeprazole. Both daytime and nighttime symptoms, as well as pain severity, were reported to be significantly better with lansoprazole, 30 mg, compared

---

BOX 45-2

Treatment for GERD

Step 1: Therapeutic Lifestyle Changes
- If obese, lose weight.
- Significantly reduce or eliminate all tobacco use (reduces LES pressure).
- Take advantage of gravity. Sleep with the head of the bed elevated on 4'' to 5'' blocks under the bedposts (pillows are not adequate for elevation).
- Avoid tight clothing around the waist.
- Reserve fluid intake for after or between meals.
- Avoid large meals within 2 to 3 hours of bedtime or before exercise.
- Avoid foods that irritate esophageal mucosa: alcohol, citrus fruits such as orange juice, grapefruit juice, and tomatoes.
- Avoid foods that lower LES pressure: yellow onions, peppermint, and high-fat foods and carbohydrates (chocolate is particularly problematic because it is high in both elements).
- Avoid, where possible, drugs that lower LES pressure: theophylline, anticholinergics, progesterone, calcium channel blockers (nifedipine, verapamil), alpha adrenergic drugs, diazepam, and meperidine.

- Avoid, where possible, drugs that may injure esophageal mucosa: tetracycline, wax-matrix potassium supplements, NSAIDs, and steroids.
- For infants, in addition to the above, maintain upright position during and for at least 20 minutes after feeding. Thicken feedings with 1 tablespoon of rice cereal per ounce of formula.

Step 2: Drug Therapy
- Continue step 1 therapy.
- Add an oral H_2RA. If not effective after 6 to 8 weeks, change to a PPI, but limit duration of therapy to no more than 3 to 6 months (drug of choice for erosive esophagitis).
- Add metoclopramide.

Step 3: Referral
- Continue steps 1 and 2 therapy, and confer with or refer to gastroenterologist.

Step 4: Surgical Intervention
- Consider antireflux surgeries (e.g., Roux-n-Y, Nissen fundoplication, crural tightening) for refractory disease.

H_2RA, Histamine$_2$-receptor antagonists; *LES,* lower esophageal sphincter; *PPI,* proton pump inhibitor.

TABLE 45-5 Treatment of GI Damage

Etiology of Damage	Treatment Modalities (In Addition to Therapeutic Lifestyle Changes)
Helicobacter pylori	Antibiotics + PPI or H₂RA
Increased acid secretion	PPI, H₂RA, or prostaglandin
Reduced viscosity of gastric mucus	Prostaglandins and sucralfate stimulate mucus secretion
Reduced bicarbonate levels	Prostaglandins and sucralfate stimulate production
Increase in pepsin	Antacids (particularly magnesium antacids) increase stomach pH and bind to aluminum salts, or sucralfate

H₂RA, Histamine₂-receptor antagonists; *PPI*, proton pump inhibitor.

with omeprazole, 20 mg or lansoprazole, 15 mg after the first dose. Symptom relief was similar with a 40 mg dose of omeprazole compared with 30 mg of lansoprazole.

Esomeprazole is the (−) isomer of omeprazole and may offer greater acid suppression and improved healing rates compared with the other PPIs. In one trial of 1,960 patients, more patients with erosive esophagitis were completely healed at 4 and 8 weeks with esomeprazole, 20 mg (70.5% and 89.9%) and 40 mg (75.9% and 94.1%) than with omeprazole, 20 mg (64.7% and 86.9%) (p < 0.05) (Hawkey, et al., 2005). Another study of 2425 patients found higher rates of healing. The median time to sustained resolution of symptoms was 5 days with esomeprazole, 40 mg; 8 days with esomeprazole 20 mg; and 9 days with omeprazole, 20 mg. Esomeprazole, 20 mg and 40 mg improve upper GI symptoms associated with continuous, daily NSAID therapy (DeVault and Castell, 2005).

Esomeprazole provided better control in intragastric pH than omeprazole, lansoprazole, and pantoprazole in studies of patients with GERD. Two large randomized, double-blind, multicenter trials showed that esomeprazole, 20 mg and/or 40 mg for 8 weeks produced higher healing rates for erosive esophagitis and better symptoms control than omeprazole, 20 mg. Esomeprazole also maintained healing compared with a placebo in patients with endoscopically confirmed healed erosive esophagitis. Similarly, symptom-driven, on-demand use of esomeprazole effectively controlled symptoms of GERD for 6 months (Gisbert, et al., 2004).

Rabeprazole, 20 mg was found to be equally as effective as omeprazole, 20 mg daily at 4 and 8 weeks in healing erosive esophagitis. Both the frequency and intensity of symptom relief was similar in both groups. However, rabeprazole offers no established advantage over omeprazole or lansoprazole for treatment of duodenal ulcers, GERD, or Zollinger-Ellison syndrome (Gisbert, et al., 2004).

To lessen the recurrence of PUD associated with *H. pylori* infection, treatment regimens must involve eradication of the organism (Box 45-3). Recurrence of duodenal ulceration after healing can be as high as 80% within 1 year if eradication of *H. pylori* is not part of treatment. The recurrence rate is less than 5% when *H. pylori* are eradicated. The effectiveness of the different drug combinations in eradicating the organism depends on the antibacterial activity of the drugs, the resistance patterns of the organism, the patient's history of antibiotic use, and the patient's ability to tolerate the drug's adverse effects and to take a large number of pills. For many patients, shorter treatment

regimens that require fewer pills per day are better tolerated and may prove to be more effective than more complicated regimens with higher eradication rates.

Esomeprazole-based 7-day triple therapy is as effective for eradication of *H. pylori* as a longer treatment period with omeprazole. Endoscopically confirmed ulcer healing 4 weeks after treatment initiated is found in 90% of patients with active duodenal ulcer. In general, duodenal ulcers are treated with night-time acid suppression, whereas gastric ulcers and GERD usually require 24-hour acid suppression.

The classic triple therapy includes 1 week of bismuth, metronidazole, and either tetracycline or amoxicillin. This regimen eliminates *H. pylori* in 90% of patients and heals ulcers in virtually all patients. However, this regimen tends not to be adhered to because of the adverse effects of the drugs. There is a chance for rapid development of resistance to clarithromycin and metronidazole, and there is the undesirable disulfiram-like reaction when alcohol is taken concurrently with metronidazole. These adjunct drugs are discussed in Chapters 26 and 27. Bismuth is discussed further in Chapter 46.

In contrast, dual therapy includes omeprazole given with a single antibiotic, usually either clarithromycin or amoxicillin. However, omeprazole has also been used with both antibiotics or as quadruple therapy with both antibiotics plus metronidazole.

Both metronidazole and tetracycline cause mild GI upset, and amoxicillin can cause diarrhea. Bismuth subsalicylate temporarily turns the tongue and stool black, and can cause tinnitus. Clarithromycin can also cause GI symptoms, although they are less frequent than those seen with metronidazole or tetracycline. Clarithromycin can cause taste disturbances that some patients find intolerable.

H₂RAs. All four H₂RAs suppress gastric acid and pepsin secretion, although the efficacy of these drugs is extremely variable and often less than desired. Response to an H₂RA depends on the severity of the disease, the dosage regimen used, and the duration of treatment. Although the relative secretory potencies differ, famotidine is the most potent and cimetidine the least potent of the four. H₂RAs suppress gastric acid equally when administered in equipotent dosages. These factors are important to remember when comparing the various clinical trials and/or assessing a patient's response to treatment.

The severity of esophagitis affects the patient's response to H₂RA treatment. For the patient with mild but symptomatic GERD, a low-dose, OTC formulation may be advantageous. For nonerosive disease, H₂RAs may be given at usual doses twice daily. Patients who do not respond to usual dosages may be secreting excessive amounts of gastric acid and therefore require higher dosages. Although higher dosages of an H₂RA may provide greater relief of symptoms and endoscopic healing rates, limited information is available about the safety of these drugs at high dosages, and they can be less effective and more costly than once daily PPIs. Because all H₂RAs have similar efficacy, selection of the drug to use in the management of GERD should be based on factors such as differences in pharmacokinetics, safety profile, and cost.

Ranitidine is the most widely studied H₂RA. Comparative, multicenter, randomized, double-blind studies of ranitidine with cimetidine, nizatidine, or famotidine have demonstrated equal efficacy and tolerability in treating and maintaining healed lesions of duodenal ulcers (Munoz, 2005).

BOX 45-3

Treatment Options for Peptic Ulcer Disease

Regimens	Duration of Therapy	Likelihood of Adherence
Active, _Helicobacter pylori_-associated PUD*†		
amoxicillin 1 gram PO twice daily **&** clarithromycin 500 mg PO twice daily **&** lansoprazole 30 mg PO twice daily (Prevpac therapy)	10–14 days	Likely
bismuth subsalicylate 525 mg PO 4 times daily **&** metronidazole 250 mg PO 4 times daily **&** tetracycline 500 mg PO 4 times daily (Helidac therapy)	14 days	Unlikely
omeprazole 20 mg PO twice daily **&** metronidazole 500 mg PO twice daily **&** clarithromycin 500 mg PO twice daily	10–14 days	Likely
clarithromycin 500 mg PO twice daily **&** metronidazole 500 mg PO twice daily **&** bismuth citrate 400 mg PO twice daily	14 days	Likely
tetracycline 500 mg PO 4 times daily **&** metronidazole 500 mg PO 4 times daily **&** bismuth subsalicylate 525 mg PO 4 times daily **&** omeprazole 20 mg PO twice daily	7–14 days	Unlikely
tetracycline 500 mg PO 4 times daily **&** clarithromycin 500 mg PO 3 times daily **&** bismuth subsalicylate 525 mg PO 4 times daily **&** omeprazole 20 mg PO twice daily	7–14 days	Unlikely
metronidazole 500 mg PO 4 times daily **&** clarithromycin 500 mg PO 3 times daily **&** bismuth subsalicylate 525 mg PO 4 times daily **&** omeprazole 20 mg PO twice daily	7–14 days	Unlikely
Uncomplicated, Active, Duodenal Ulcer not Attributed to _H. Pylori_ Infection†		
omeprazole 20 mg PO daily _–OR–_ lansoprazole 15 mg PO daily	4 wk	Likely
cimetidine 800 mg PO HS _–OR–_ ranitidine 300 mg PO HS or 150 mg twice daily _–OR–_ nizatidine 300 mg PO HS or 150 mg twice daily _–OR–_ famotidine 40 mg PO HS or 20 mg twice daily	4–6 wk	Likely to unlikely
sucralfate 1 gram PO 4 times daily	4–6 wk	UA
Uncomplicated, Active, Gastric Ulcer Not Attributed to _H. Pylori_†‡		
omeprazole 20 mg PO twice daily _–OR–_ lansoprazole 30 mg PO daily	6–8 wk	Likely
cimetidine 300 mg PO 4 times daily or 800 mg HS or 400 mg PO twice daily _–OR–_ ranitidine 150 mg PO twice daily or 300 mg HS _–OR–_ nizatidine 300 mg PO HS _–OR–_ famotidine 40 mg PO HS	8–12 wk	Likely to unlikely
Prevention of NSAID-Induced Ulcers§		
misoprostol 100 to 200 mcg PO 4 times daily	Indefinite	Likely
Proton pump inhibitor PO twice daily (for high-risk patients intolerant of misoprostol)	Indefinite	Likely
Chronic Maintenance Therapy‡‖		
cimetidine 400 to 800 mg PO HS _–OR–_ ranitidine 150 mg PO twice daily or 300 mg PO HS _–OR–_ nizatidine 150 to 300 mg PO HS _–OR–_ famotidine 20 mg PO HS	12 wk to indefinite	Likely to unlikely

NOTES: No single specific regimen for PUD is universally recognized. Eradication rates identified for regimens with good (80%–90%) to excellent rates (>90%).

*Any PPI may be used in its recommended dosage. In patients with an active ulcer, therapy with PPI should be extended to 28 days using conventional dosages.

†Give PPI before meals and the antibiotics and bismuth with meals. Do not use bismuth subsalicylate longer than 3 wk. Avoid metronidazole-based treatment regimens in areas of known metronidazole resistance or in patients who have failed a course of treatment that included metronidazole. The choice among the regimens should be based on convenience, potential for toxicity, and cost.

‡All H2 antagonists have equivalent efficacy and toxicity. If the patient is taking other drugs that interact with cimetidine, then ranitidine, famotidine, or nizatidine may be chosen, whichever is the least expensive.

§Prophylaxis for NSAID-induced ulcer is reserved for high-risk patients (i.e., prior ulcer disease or ulcer complications, use of corticosteroids or anticoagulants, patients older than age 70).

‖Chronic maintenance therapy is indicated for patients with recurrent ulcers who are _H. pylori_–negative or in whom attempts at elimination of the organism have failed, and in patients with a history of ulcer complications.

NSAID, Nonsteroidal antiinflammatory drug; _UA,_ unavailable.

Adapted from Carter, B. (Ed.). (2003). _Pharmacotherapy self-assessment program_ (3rd ed.). Kansas City, MO: American College of Pharmacology.

As a part of triple or quadruple _H. pylori_ therapy, the H₂RAs play in important role in treating PUD of an infectious origin. Symptom relief occurs more readily, and efficacy rates may be higher, when an H₂RA is added to the regimen. Further, like the PPIs, H₂RAs may also improve the activity of some antibiotics by increasing gastric pH.

ANTACIDS. Antacids are not used to heal PUD or relieve GERD, but they may be helpful used in combination with other antiulcer drugs for intermediate, rapid relief of pain or dyspepsia, even though documentation of their efficacy in placebo-controlled clinical trials is lacking. The choice of antacid for uncomplicated hyperacidity problems depends

EVIDENCE-BASED PHARMACOTHERAPEUTICS

Short Term Treatment of Gastroesophageal Reflux

■ Background

Epidemiology studies suggest that 65% of adults suffer from heartburn at least once a month; 24% have had symptoms for over 10 years; 17% of adults have used indigestion aids at least once weekly, and as many as 10% have symptoms on a daily basis. Even so, only 24% of patients have previously consulted a health care provider for the problem. Most heartburn is diagnosed as gastroesophageal reflux (GERD), a term referring to both symptoms and the resultant esophageal mucosal damage from reflux of gastric acid into the esophagus. The majority of people treat themselves with antacids, but other drugs are also available.

■ Research Article

Van Pinxteren, B., Numans, M., Bonis, P. et al. (2004). Short-term treatment with proton pump inhibitors, H₂-receptor antagonists and prokinetics for gastro-oesophageal reflux disease-like symptoms and endoscopy negative reflux disease. *The Cochrane Database of Systematic Reviews. 2004,* Issue 3. Art. No. CD002095. DOI: 10.1002/14651858.CD002095. pub2.

Purpose

The purpose of this study was to compare the effectiveness of proton pump inhibitors (PPIs), histamine₂-receptor antagonists (H₂RAs), and prokinetic drugs for the short-term treatment for adults with GERD and reflux disease with no endoscopic abnormalities. The primary outcome was heartburn remission (defined as no more than 1 day per week with mild heartburn). The secondary outcome was (partial) symptom relief, thus, quality of life.

Design

Meta-analysis was carried out of 27 randomized, controlled trials (*N* = 8402) conducted in North America, Europe, and Australia. Single- or double-blind and parallel group designs were analyzed where one of the intervention types was contrasted with placebo or another intervention. Thirteen of the studies were empiric, 10 studies were in the reflux disease group with no endoscopic abnormalities, and four studies included both. Studies were organized into an empiric treatment group (no endoscopy) and a reflux group with no endoscopic abnormalities.

Methods

The meta-analysis studied the following comparisons for both the empiric treatment group and the endoscopically normal reflux disease group: PPI versus placebo, H₂RA versus placebo, prokinetic versus placebo, PPI versus H₂RA, PPI versus prokinetic, and H₂RA versus prokinetic. The relative risks (RR) at a 95% confidence interval (CI) were used when examining the influences of the treatment interventions.

The empiric group included 8 trials using PPIs; 12 studies used an H₂RA; and 5 studies used prokinetic drugs. In the group without endoscopic abnormalities, PPIs were studied in 12 trials; H₂RAs in 6 trials; and a prokinetic drug in 1 trial.

Findings

Heartburn remission: Two of the empirical placebo-controlled PPI-trials favored a PPI for heartburn remission (RR 0.37, CI 0.32-0.44). The two trials comparing a H₂RA with a placebo (RR 0.77, CI 0.60-0.99), and the one study comparing prokinetic drug with a placebo (RR 0.86, CI 0.73-1.01) favored the H₂RA. In the six endoscopically normal reflux groups versus placebo-controlled PPI, the RR was 0.68 (CI 0.59-0.78). For the two trials of H₂RA versus placebo, the RR was 0.84 (CI 0.74-0.95). In the three trials that directly compared PPIs with H₂RAs, no significant difference in effectiveness was found (RR 0.74, CI 0.53-1.03). In the only trial comparing a PPI with a prokinetic, the RR favored the PPI (RR 0.72, CI 0.56-0.92).

Overall symptom improvement: In the four empiric placebo-controlled H₂RA and two prokinetic trials the RRs were 0.72 (CI 0.63-0.81) and 0.71 (CI 0.56-0.90), respectively. In the one trial directly comparing a PPI with an H₂RA, the RR was 0.29 (CI 0.17-0.51).

In the four endoscopically normal reflux groups comparing PPIs with placebo, the RR was 0.63 (CI 0.55-0.72). In the two trials comparing H₂RA with placebo the RR was 0.41 (CI 0.13-1.33). In the only trial directly comparing the two groups for overall symptom improvement, a PPI was superior to an H₂RA (RR 0.83, CI 0.76-0.91).

Daytime heartburn relief: In the four empirical trials comparing H₂RA versus placebo the RR was 0.80 (CI 0.71-0.89). The two studies that compared a prokinetic drug with a placebo, the RR was 0.63 (CI 0.51-0.77). In the only direct comparison trial there was no significant difference in efficacy between H₂RA and prokinetic drug. No PPI trials were included.

The only trial in the endoscopically normal reflux group included in the meta-analysis compared H₂RA with placebo (RR 0.75, CI 0.61-0.93).

Nighttime heartburn relief: In the three empiric trials comparing H₂RA with placebo, the RR was 0.77 (CI 0.63-0.94). In the one trial comparing a prokinetic drug with placebo, the RR was 0.51 (CI 0.41-0.64). No PPI trials were included.

The only trial in the endoscopically normal reflux group included in the meta-analysis comparing H₂RA versus placebo, the RR risk was 0.80 (CI 0.59-1.08).

Conclusions

Antisecretory drugs are effective in the empiric treatment of GERD and in treatment of endoscopically normal reflux disease for relieving heartburn. Furthermore, PPIs are superior to H₂RAs for the empiric treatment of typical GERD symptoms.

■ Implications for practice

More data are needed comparing PPIs with H₂RAs in patients with endoscopically normal reflux disease. The metaanalysis suggests PPIs are superior, but significance was not reached for the primary outcome measure of heartburn remission. Whether a PPI is worth the extra expense, in terms of heartburn remission and quality of life, should be explored in pharmacoeconomic studies.

---

on characteristics of both the patient and the drug. As a general rule, single-compound antacids are preferable to combinations; however, the most commonly used antacids are combinations of aluminum and magnesium. Although the basic anions in antacids include carbonate, bicarbonate, citrate, phosphate, or trisilicate, the hydroxide formulation is most commonly used. Combining an antacid with a laxative adverse effect (e.g., magnesium hydroxide) with one having a constipating adverse effect (e.g., aluminum hydroxide) tends to prevent or reduce the incidence of diarrhea or constipation. By combining rapid-acting and slow-acting formulations, antacids prolong the neutralization of gastric acid. Combinations usually also permit smaller dosages of individual ingredients, thereby preventing or reducing adverse effects.

Some antacids contain simethicone. Simethicone does not affect gastric acidity but instead is an antiflatulent. Simethicone is reported to decrease the surface tension of gas bubbles, thereby reducing GI distention and abdominal discomfort. However, simethicone does not prevent the formation of gas. Simethicone has an immediate onset, with antiflatulent effects lasting up to 3 hours. There is no systemic absorption, and the drug is eliminated unchanged in feces.

MISOPROSTOL. Misoprostol has been used in several placebo-controlled studies that demonstrated a reduction in the development of duodenal ulcers in patients taking NSAIDs. Convincing data that misoprostol is effective in patients taking NSAIDs is limited. In addition, misoprostol does not relieve ulcer pain. Misoprostol is not more effective than the H_2RAs and it has a worse adverse effects profile. However, the MUCOSA trial showed that misoprostol was significantly more effective than placebo in preventing NSAID-induced ulcer complications in high-risk patients (Simon et al., 1996). Duodenal ulcers heal faster when the NSAID is discontinued but can be managed with a H_2RA or with a PPI if NSAID therapy must continue.

SUCRALFATE. Sucralfate at 4 grams/day is as effective as cimetidine or ranitidine in promoting healing of duodenal and gastric ulcers and in rapidly relieving symptoms. Although sucralfate is FDA-approved for the treatment and maintenance of duodenal ulcers, there is no role for sucralfate in the eradication of *H. pylori*.

Patient Education

Provide patient education with regard to the disease state, lifestyle modifications, and drug therapy. Counsel the patient on what causes hyperacidity, GERD, or PUD. A thorough explanation of the mechanisms of hyperacidity, reflux, or ulcer disease and their aggravating factors helps provide a rational basis for patient action.

Counsel the patient on lifestyle modifications that improve symptoms. These include avoiding foods and drugs that worsen GERD, avoiding tight-fitting clothes, eating smaller meals, raising the frame of the bed, losing weight, and avoiding tobacco use (see Box 45-2).

Teach the patient and family members, as appropriate, the name of the drug, the dose, and the purpose for the drug, benefits anticipated from therapy, and the period over which therapy is anticipated to extend. Halting therapy when symptoms improve is a major cause for exacerbation of symptoms.

Take an active role in educating patients about potential adverse effects and drug interactions that may occur with therapy. Advise patients which drugs may interact with their therapy and what warning signs they should report to their health care provider. The use of other potentially ulcerogenic drugs should be avoided.

Instruct the patient and family that any change in symptoms or the appearance of blood, tarry stools, coffee-ground emesis, unexplained weight loss, dysphagia, or odynophagia signals the need to contact the health care provider. Patients must be encouraged to continue with follow-up care for at least 1 year.

Teach the patient that no single measure will alleviate the discomfort of hyperacidity, GERD, or PUD, but when all of the interventions are performed together, relief is extremely likely. Non–drug measures such as relaxation and stress management help prevent or minimize symptoms and often are as effective as drugs when they are used concurrently.

There is no practical way to avoid psychologic stress because it is a part of everyday life, but it is possible to reduce the stress.

Evaluation

Outcome evaluation targets relief of symptoms. Evaluation also includes the other goals of therapy including healing injured mucosa, and preventing complications. Relapse rates are high for patients with GERD, esophagitis, and PUD but can be significantly reduced with eradication of *H. pylori* and appropriate maintenance therapy. Recently, the practice of obtaining serial immunoglobulin A (IgA) titers has proven helpful. A drop in serum IgA titers from baseline at 3 months confirms eradication. Patients who do not respond to antimicrobial therapy for *H. pylori* eradication should be offered a second course of therapy with a different combination of drugs.

Patients with GERD, esophagitis, or PUD who remain symptom-free require no more frequent follow-up than their annual physical exam. Those who are not responsive to therapy or who develop complications of their disease require consultation with or referral to a gastroenterologist.

In addition to the traditional end points that show a certain therapy has been effective, we must also evaluate the cost-effectiveness of that therapy in relation to the planned outcomes and its effects on the patient's quality of life. The most expensive therapy is the one that is ineffective, meaning that if a drug does not accomplish treatment goals, it costs

CASE STUDY | Proton Pump Inhibitors

ASSESSMENT

History of Present Illness	GH, a 58-year-old female, comes to the office today with complaints of increasing gastric distress over the past 4 weeks. One week ago she had an abscessed tooth and has been taking 600 mg of ibuprofen 3 times daily for the discomfort. She self-treats with Maalox with short-term relief of her gastric distress. GH also notes that she has had a cough that is particularly bad at night and worsens if she eats before bedtime. Her current drugs include HRT and verapamil for hypertension.
Past Health History	GH denies a past history of PUD. She had a cholecystectomy 5 years ago and is pleased that she can now eat tomatoes and drink orange juice; she was unable to do so until she had her gallbladder removed. GH does not consume alcohol but she has a 15 pack/year smoking history. The remainder of her past health history is unremarkable. There is no family history of GI disorders.

Continued

CASE STUDY — Proton Pump Inhibitors—Cont'd

Life-Span Considerations	GH is a housewife who lives on a farm with her husband of 34 years. They raise tomatoes, turnips, broccoli, and spinach to sell at the local farmer markets. She sucks on cinnamon Altoid breath mints when out in the field because it helps with dry mouth. GH has two grown children who live in a distant city and are "too busy to help out with the farm." Her 57-year-old husband was hospitalized 3 months ago with an MI. Although his health has improved, GH still worries about him a great deal, particularly now that harvest season is in full swing.
Psychosocial Considerations	Because GH and her husband are self-employed, they carry only catastrophic health insurance and have no pharmacy coverage. GH is worried that with her GI distress she will be admitted to the hospital and not be available to help her husband on the family farm. When not in the fields, she is active in community and church affairs.
Physical Exam	VS stable. *Height:* 63". *Weight:* 184 pounds. *BMI:* 29.7. Bowel sounds present in all quadrants. There is palpable tenderness over the epigastrium. No palpable HSM, masses, or abdominal bruits. Her stool is negative for occult blood.
Lab Testing	CBC, electrolytes, BUN, creatinine, and ESR are within normal limits. *Helicobacter pylori* antibody negative. A colonoscopy 10 years ago was negative for polyps or diverticuli.

DIAGNOSIS: Gastroesophageal reflux disease

MANAGEMENT

Treatment Goals	1. Alleviate symptoms. 2. Promote healing. 3. Prevent complications. 4. Prevent recurrence of reflux.
Treatment Plans	**Pharmacotherapy** • Stop ibuprofen • esomeprazole 40 mg PO daily on empty stomach first thing in the morning **Patient Education** 1. Be sure to take esomeprazole on an empty stomach first thing in the morning so as to shut down the acid pumps in the stomach. 2. Avoid NSAIDs. 3. No tight clothing around the waist. 4. Remain upright for 2 to 3 hours after eating. 5. Avoid alcohol, caffeine, mint (including cinnamon Altoids, which contain peppermint), grapefruit and orange juice and fruit, yellow onions, tomatoes in any form (pizza, salsa, spaghetti, soup, etc.). 6. Six small meals a day rather than three larger meals. 7. Regularly participate in stress reduction activities such as yoga, patterned breathing, or meditation. 8. Follow up in office in 2 weeks. Arrange for EGD in next 1 to 2 months, once the current flare has resolved. **Evaluation** 1. GH's abdominal symptoms are relieved. 2. Healing has been promoted without complications of therapy. 3. Life style changes may have helped to reduce the risk of reoccurrence.

CLINICAL REASONING ANALYSIS

Q1. What risk factors does GH have for GERD?

A. Her intake of tomatoes and orange juice... the verapamil she takes for hypertension... She has a high-fat diet; as a farm wife she cooks and eats "meat and potatoes with gravy" on a regular basis for her family and the farm hands. The verapamil, as a calcium channel blocking drug, relaxes the esophageal sphincter as well as peripheral vessels. We may need to consider changing her blood pressure drug to another at the next visit.

Q2. **Earlier you mentioned something to GH about things in her life that could contribute to her symptoms? What were you referring to?**

A. Her weight... She smokes.... GH worries about her husband and his risk for another MI, and the cost of his health care. She uses cinnamon Altoids (which contain peppermint)... Her recent intake of ibuprofen...

Q3. **My clinical instructor wants me to teach GH about lifestyle changes that will help reduce her symptoms. I'm not sure what to teach. Would you review the things she should do to help?**

A. Stop or reduce her intake of orange juice and tomatoes. Discuss the possibility of changing her blood pressure medicine to another drug class. Avoid using straws. A low-fat diet and weight loss helps reduce reflux. Avoid tight clothing around her waist and reclining within 2 to 3 hours of eating. Consider raising the head of the bed 4 to 5 inches to facilitate gastric emptying.

Q4. **What do you tell GH that will help her to avoid the nighttime coughing episodes she is having?**

A. Avoid tight clothing around her waist and reclining within 2 to 3 hours of eating. Consider raising the frame of the bed 4 to 5 inches to facilitate gastric emptying.

Q5. **Why did you prescribe esomeprazole for GH rather than an H₂RA?**

A. The PPI esomeprazole. Despite the fact that only a small number of placebo-controlled empiric treatment trials were identified, research studies suggest that antisecretory drugs are effective in the empiric treatment of GERD and endoscopically normal reflux disease. Provided that the diagnostic probability of GERD is high, PPIs appear to be superior to H₂RAs for the empiric treatment of GERD, but not in the treatment of endoscopy normal reflux disease. Although prokinetic drugs are considered to be equally effective as H₂RAs, the evidence base for their use in treatment of GERD and endoscopically normal reflux disease is weak.

Q6. **What adverse effects of esomeprazole would cause you to change GH's treatment regimen?**

A. Although rare, if GH developed signs and symptoms associated with blood dyscrasias, hepatic dysfunction, Stevens-Johnson syndrome, toxic epidermal necrolysis, erythema multiforme, or pancreatitis, the drug should be stopped. A headache and diarrhea, unless severe, would not necessarily cause the drug to be stopped. And, although this is not an adverse effect, if the drug were cost-prohibitive it might need to be changed to one that is less expensive.

CASE STUDY *H. pylori* Drug Therapy

ASSESSMENT

History of Present Illness	NJ, a 27-year-old male, reports to the medical clinic today with increasing weakness, dark stools, and epigastric tenderness for past 48 hours. He has tried an occasional dose of Maalox with some relief. He had been taking two ibuprofen several times a day for the discomfort and for headaches. The pain sometimes wakes him at night and seems to get better after eating. He has a daily bowel movement without difficulty. He considers self otherwise healthy.
Past Health History	NJ had an appendectomy at age 16 without sequelae. A blood test drawn at the time of his appendectomy shows type O blood. The remainder of past medical history is unremarkable except for infrequent bouts of exercise-induced asthma for which he intermittently uses an albuterol inhaler. Once or twice yearly he needs a prednisone taper to treat a flare of his asthma.
Life-Span Considerations	Along with the daycare center, NJ is the sole caregiver for his 2-year-old daughter. NJ is a construction worker who lives on the outskirts of town with his wife of 5 years. His wife is a stay-at-home mom who was hospitalized recently after a serious motor vehicle accident. Although her condition has improved, NJ worries about how much longer she will be hospitalized. NJ is worried that he will be admitted to the hospital for the abdominal pain and not be able to care for his daughter. NJ is active in community and church affairs. He has been smoking now for the last 8 years and is up to one ppd. He reports that he does not drink alcohol and until recently hasn't taken OTC drugs. NJ and his wife have been financially strained since her motor vehicle accident. They carry only catastrophic health insurance and have no pharmacy coverage. NJ is worried about the cost of daycare, his wife's medical bills, and any long-term rehabilitation costs that will be needed once she is discharged.
Physical Exam	VSS. *Height:* 5'7". *Weight:* 135 lbs. Breath sounds clear to auscultation. Bowel sounds present all four quadrants. Epigastrium is tender to light and deep palpation. No hepatosplenomegaly, masses, or bruits noted.
Diagnostic Testing	CBC and electrolytes WNL. *Helicobacter pylori* antibodies are present on analysis. Stool positive for occult blood. UGI reflects small ulcer on posterior aspect of duodenal bulb.

Continued

CASE STUDY   *H. pylori* Drug Therapy—Cont'd

DIAGNOSIS: *H. pylori* peptic ulcer disease

MANAGEMENT

Treatment Goals	1. Alleviate symptoms. 2. Promote healing. 3. Prevent complications. 4. Prevent recurrence.
Treatment Plans	**Pharmacotherapy** • Stop OTC antacids and aspirin use. • Helidac therapy per package instructions for 14 days • Continue bismuth subsalicylate daily after Helidac therapy complete, and continue for 6 wk. **Patient Education** 1. Avoid alcohol, spicy foods, caffeine. 2. Elevate head of bed 30 degrees. 3. Learn stress-reduction strategies such as walking, yoga, and meditation. 4. Follow guidelines for self care identified in handout (see Box 45-3). **Evaluation** 1. NJ's abdominal symptoms are relieved. 2. Healing has been promoted without complications of therapy. 3. Lifestyle changes may have helped to reduce the risk of reoccurrence.

CRITICAL ANALYSIS QUESTIONS

Q1. What risk factors does NJ have for PUD?

A. Family history of ulcer, chronic lung disease, smoking more than half a ppd, high-dose and/or prolonged corticosteroid therapy, blood group type O, NSAID use.

Q2. What factors in NJ's life may be contributing to his symptoms?

A. Worry about his wife, child, and finances.

Q3. What information does NJ need regarding lifestyle changes that will help reduce his symptoms? How is this information similar or dissimilar to the patient with GERD?

A. Stop smoking. Explore stress-reduction strategies. Stop aspirin use. PUD is associated with the *H. pylori* organism. The symptoms of GERD and PUD are very similar and thus the measures that help reduce GERD symptoms also help to reduce PUD symptoms (in addition to drug therapy).

Q4. What is the cost of a Prevpac compared with Helidac therapy for the 14-day treatment period? Is the Prevpac the most cost-effective means for treating GH's *H. pylori* infection? What other options are there for treating NJ's PUD other than Prevpac or Helidac therapy?

A. Look here at this table I have. It gives the cost of the various therapies. As you can see, it is less expensive to write a prescription for the generic formulations of drugs in GH's regimen (Helidac) than to use the prepackaged therapy.

Q5. Yes, I see you ordered the generic drugs contained within Helidac therapy for NJ. What are the mechanisms of action of the drugs contained in this regimen?

A. Bismuth subsalicylate possesses topical mucosal and antimicrobial effects, reduces secretions, and binds bacterial toxins for elimination. Metronidazole is bacteriocidal and enters anaerobic cells, disrupts DNA, and inhibits nucleic acid synthesis in the organism. Tetracycline is bacteriostatic, inhibiting the organism's protein synthesis.

Treatment Regimen	14-Day Therapy	Total Drug Costs*
Prevpac (lansoprazole + amoxicillin + clarithromycin)	—	$267
lansoprazole 30 mg twice daily (Prevacid)	$120	$302
amoxicillin 500 mg twice daily	$32	
clarithromycin 500 mg twice daily (Biaxin)	$150	
Helidac (bismuth subsalicylate + metronidazole + tetracycline)	—	$200
bismuth subsalicylate 2 tabs 4 times daily	$20	$70
metronidazole 250 mg 4 times daily	$34	
tetracycline 500 mg 4 times daily	$16	

*Prices from www.drugstore.com. Does not include costs of laboratory testing.

Q6. What are the parameters for monitoring success of treatment?

A. Outcome evaluation targets symptom relief. Evaluation also includes the other goals of therapy including healing injured mucosa and preventing complications. Relapse rates are high for patients with GERD, esophagitis, and PUD, but can be significantly reduced with eradication of *H. pylori* and appropriate maintenance therapy. Recently, the practice of obtaining serial IgA titers has proven helpful. A drop in serum IgA titers from baseline at 3 months confirms eradication. Patients who do not respond to antimicrobial therapy for *H. pylori* eradication should be offered a second course of therapy with a different combination of drugs.

more because the patient must be retreated. For example, for the patient with GERD one must consider the primary goals of treatment: to relieve symptoms, heal injury, prevent recurrence, and prevent complications. These factors must be evaluated separately since different costs are associated with achieving each end point. The drug that is the least expensive and provides the greatest benefit relative to dosing interval and number of tablets taken is the optimal one.

KEY POINTS

- Hyperacidity is defined as an excess of gastric secretions or gastric secretions with a pH less than 2.
- GERD refers to any symptomatic clinical condition or histologic alteration resulting from gastroesophageal reflux, the upward movement of gastric contents from the stomach into the esophagus.
- Chronic GERD can progress to erosive esophagitis and transformation of esophageal mucosa from epithelial cells into the columnar gastric type of mucosal cells (Barrett's esophagus).
- PUD is characterized by circumscribed areas of mucosal inflammation and ulceration caused by excessive secretion of gastric acid, disruption of the protective mucosal barrier, or both. *H. pylori* are identified as an etiologic factor in PUD in both adults and children.
- The primary objectives in the treatment of hyperacidity, GERD, and PUD are to relieve symptoms, promote healing, and prevent complications.
- Duodenal ulcers are the most common and are associated with increased numbers of parietal cells (acid-secreting), the presence of *H. pylori* organisms, and elevated gastrin levels. Duodenal ulcers are treated with night-time acid suppression.
- Gastric ulcers develop in the antrum of the stomach and tend to become chronic. Gastric secretions may be increased or decreased, with pain occurring after eating. *H. pylori* are usually not present. Gastric ulcers and GERD usually require 24-hour acid suppression.

- Treatment of hyperacidity, GERD, and PUD includes therapeutic lifestyle modifications and administration of PPIs, H_2RAs, prostaglandin, misoprostol, and a cytoprotective drug.
- PPIs bind with the H^+-K^+-ATPase enzyme to prevent the release of gastric acid into the stomach lumen more than H_2RAs. Independent clinical trials have shown the superiority of PPIs over H_2RAs or sucralfate in their ability to control symptoms and to heal esophagitis in patients with GERD.
- H_2RAs inhibit the action of histamine at H_2 receptors, which in turn suppresses gastric acid and pepsin secretion. The efficacy of H_2RAs is extremely variable and often less than desired.
- Antacids raise the pH of gastric secretions to a level less acidic, or neutral. They do not coat the stomach lining and are not particularly effective.
- The prostaglandin misoprostol inhibits gastric acid secretion (antisecretory effect) and increases bicarbonate and mucus production (cytoprotective effect).
- The cytoprotective agent sucralfate and bismuth increase prostaglandin, mucus, and bicarbonate secretion and reduce the number of *H. pylori*.
- Successful outcomes of treatment for hyperacidity, GERD, and PUD are measured in terms of three separate end points: (1) symptom relief, (2) healing injured mucosa, and (3) preventing complications.

Bibliography

Abramowicz, M. (Ed.). (2003). Prilosec, Nexium, and stereoisomers. *The Medical Letter on Drugs and Therapeutics, 45*(1159), 51.

Aronson, B. (2000). Applying clinical practice guidelines to a patient with complicated gastroesophageal reflux disease. *Gastroenterology Nursing, 23*(4), 143–147.

Chey, W., Inadomi, J., Booher, A., et al. (2005). Primary care physicians' perceptions and practices on the management of GERD: Results of a national survey. *American Journal of Gastroenterology, 100*(6), 1237–1242.

Delaney, B., Moayyedi, P., Forman, D. (2003). Initial management strategies for dyspepsia. *The Cochrane Database of Systematic Reviews. 2003*, Issue 2. Art. No. CD001961. DOI: 10.1002/14651858. CD001961.

DeVault, K., Castell, D. (2005). Updated guidelines for the diagnosis and treatment of gastroesophageal reflux disease. *American Journal of Gastroenterology, 100*(1), 190–200.

DeVault, K. (2000). Guidelines for the diagnosis and treatment of gastroesophageal reflux disease. *American Journal of Managed Care, 6*(9 Suppl), S476–S479, S508–S511.

Duggan, A., Tolley, K., Hawkey, C., et al. (1998). Varying efficacy of *Helicobacter pylori* eradication regimens: Cost effectiveness study using a decision analysis model. *BMJ, 316*(7145), 1648–1654.

Ford, A., Delaney, B., Forman, D., et al. (2003). Eradication therapy for peptic ulcer disease in *Helicobacter pylori* positive patients. *The Cochrane Database of Systematic Reviews. 2003*, Issue 4. Art. No. CD003840.pub2. DOI: 10.1002/14651858.CD003840.pub2.

GASTROINTESTINAL

Gisbert, J., Khorrami, S., Carballo, F., et al. (2004). *H. pylori* eradication therapy vs. antisecretory non-eradication therapy (with or without long-term maintenance antisecretory therapy) for the prevention of recurrent bleeding from peptic ulcer. *The Cochrane Database of Systematic Reviews*. 2004, Issue2. Art No. CD004062. pub2. DOI: 10.1002/14651858.CD004062.pub2.

Hawkey, C., Talley, N., Yeomans, N. (2005). Improvements with esomeprazole in patients with upper gastrointestinal symptoms taking non-steroidal antiinflammatory drugs, including selective COX-2 inhibitors. *American Journal of Gastroenterology*, *100*(5), 1028–1036.

Kahrilas, P., Howden, C. (2002). *Contemporary diagnosis and management of dyspepsia and GERD*. Newtown, PA: Handbooks in Health Care.

Moayyedi, P., Soo, S., Deeks, J., et al. (2005). Eradication of *Helicobacter pylori* for non-ulcer dyspepsia. *The Cochrane Database of Systematic Reviews*. 2005, Issue 1. Art No. CD002096.pub2. DOI: 10.1002/14651858.CD002096.pub2.

Moayyedi, P., Soo, S., Deeks, J., et al. (2005). Pharmacological interventions for non-ulcer dyspepsia. *The Cochrane Database of Systematic Reviews*. 2005, Issue1. Art. No. CD001960.pub2. DOI: 10.1002/14651858.CD001960.pub2.

Munoz, J. (2005). *H. pylori* eradication therapy vs. antisecretory non-eradication therapy (with or without long-term maintenance antisecretory therapy) for the prevention of recurrent bleeding from peptic ulcer. (Cochrane Review). *The Cochrane Library*. Chichester, UK: John Wiley & Sons.

National Digestive Diseases Information Clearinghouse. (2003). *Gastroesophageal reflux in children and adolescents*. Available online: http://digestive.niddk.nih.gov/ddiseases/pubs/gerinchildren. Accessed May 17, 2007.

National Digestive Diseases Information Clearinghouse. (2003). *Heartburn, hiatal hernia, and gastroesophageal reflux disease (GERD)*. Available online:http://digestive.niddk.nih.gov/ddiseases/pubs/gerd. Accessed May 17, 2007.

Rostom, A., Dube, C., Wells, G., et al. (2005). Prevention of NSAID-induced gastroduodenal ulcers. *The Cochran Database of Systematic Reviews*. 2005, Issue 4. Art No. CD002296.DOI: 10.1002/14651858.CD 002296.

Simon, L., Hatoum, H., Bittman, R., et al. (1996). Risk factors for serious nonsteroidal-induced gastrointestinal complications: Regression analysis of the MUCOSA trial. *Family Medicine*, *28*(3), 204–210.

Soll, A. (1996). Consensus conference. Medical treatment of peptic ulcer disease. Practice guidelines. Practice Parameters Committee of the American College of Gastroenterology. Medical treatment of peptic ulcer disease: Practice guidelines. *Journal of the American Medical Association*, *275*(8), 622–629.

Spencer, C., Faulds, D. (2000). Esomeprazole. *Drugs*, *60*(2), 321–329.

Take, S., Mizuno, M., Ishiki, K. (2005). The effect of eradicating *Helicobacter pylori* on the development of gastric cancer in patients with peptic ulcer disease. *American Journal of Gastroenterology*, *100*(5), 1037–1042.

Van Pinxteren, B., Numans, M., Bonis, P., et al. (2004). Short-term treatment with proton pump inhibitors, H_2-receptor antagonists and prokinetics for gastro-oesophageal reflux disease-like symptoms and endoscopy negative reflux disease. *The Cochrane Database of Systematic Reviews*. 2004, Issue 3. Art. No. CD0020995.pub2. DOI: 10.1002/14651858.CD002095.pub2.

Webb, D. (2000). New therapeutic options in the treatment of GERD and other acid-peptic disorders. *American Journal of Managed Care*, *6*(9 Suppl), S467–S475, S508–S511.

46

Laxatives and Antidiarrheal Drugs

ormal physiologic functions of the lower gastrointestinal (GI) tract include motility, absorption, and secretion. Alterations in one or more of these functions result in constipation or diarrhea. Although various drugs are used for symptomatic relief, drug therapy does not correct the underlying cause and, in some cases, may contribute to the problem. This chapter focuses on drugs used to prevent or alleviate constipation and diarrhea.

CONSTIPATION

EPIDEMIOLOGY AND ETIOLOGY

Constipation is defined as infrequent defecation, a hardened or reduced caliber of stool, a sensation of incomplete evacuation, or the need to strain with bowel movements. Defecation less than 3 times a week is a commonly accepted criterion for the diagnosis of constipation. Approximately 4 million people in the United States have constipation on a frequent basis. This figure corresponds to a prevalence of 2%, making constipation the most frequent GI problem seen in ambulatory care settings. The prevalence is highest in the southern United States and is reported more often by patients over age 65. In this age group, the problem is more often a result of physical inactivity rather than of intrinsic bowel changes related to aging.

Constipation is 3 times more common in women than in men. Nonwhite patients report constipation 13 times more often than white patients. In some cultures, patients believe that autointoxication occurs if bowel movements do not occur on a regular basis. Patients from low-income families report constipation more often than patients with higher incomes. An estimated 900 people die each year in the United States from diseases associated with constipation.

Constipation of recent onset is usually related to changes in lifestyle or health status. Inadequate fluids or fiber in the diet is the most common cause of chronic constipation. Dietary changes such as restrictive weight loss diets, dietary changes related to aging, and poor dentition are other culprits. In contrast, constipation of long duration indicates a functional etiology (i.e., not responding to the urge to defecate) or chronic organic disease. Busy schedules with no established time for regular elimination contribute to constipation. Disorders that may originally present as constipation include hypothyroidism, diabetes mellitus, hypokalemia, hypercalcemia, and neurologic disorders. Drugs that commonly inhibit GI motility include antidepressants and anticholinergics, and excessive use of antacids or opiates can do the same (especially codeine) (Box 46-1).

Chronic laxative and enema use causes the mesenteric plexus to be less sensitive to stimulation. Chronic constipation can also result from degenerated or absent neural pathways to the large intestine from neurogenic disorders such as spinal cord trauma or cerebral vascular disease. Functional or mechanical conditions such as muscle weakness, pain, anal lesions, low-residue diet, sedentary lifestyle, lack of exercise, depression, or even lack of toilet facilities can lead to constipation problems.

PATHOPHYSIOLOGY

The primary function of the colon is to absorb water, sodium, and other minerals. By removing 90% of the fluid, the colon converts 1000 to 2000 mL of isotonic chyme from the ileum to about 150 grams of semisolid stool each day, which contain an additional 100 to 150 mL of water. In general, the first remnants of a meal reach the hepatic flexure in 6 hours, the splenic flexure in 9 hours, and the pelvic colon in 12 hours. Transport is much slower from the pelvic colon to the anus. As much as 25% of the meal's residue may still be in the rectum 72 hours later.

The fundamental mechanism of constipation involves decreased transit time of stool through the colon and increased reabsorption of fluid. Regardless of the cause, prolonged retention of stool in the rectum results in drying because of the reabsorption of water. The harder and drier the stool, the more difficult it is to expel.

PHARMACOTHERAPEUTIC OPTIONS

Symptomatic relief of constipation is often accomplished by drugs often classified as laxatives, cathartics, or purgatives. The same drug can produce any of the three effects depending on the dosage and the patient's sensitivity to the drug. *Laxatives* slightly increase water content in the stool and encourage evacuation of soft stool. *Cathartics* and *purgatives* promote intense elimination activity and loss of water. A diet rich in fiber such as bran is a nonpharmacologic and very effective method for alleviating sporadic constipation. However, chronic constipation might necessitate occasional use of a laxative. Laxatives are divided into five groups: bulk-forming laxatives; stool softeners; osmotic laxatives; stimulant laxatives; and miscellaneous laxatives.

Bulk-Forming Laxatives
- methylcellulose (Citrucel)
- polycarbophil (Fiberall, Fibercon, Fiber-Lax, Mitrolan)
- psyllium (Effer-Syllium, Metamucil, Perdiem, many others); ◆ Metamucil, others

▌ Indications
Bulk-forming laxatives such as psyllium and methylcellulose may be safely used for the long-term management of simple, chronic constipation, particularly when related to a low-fiber diet. They are useful in situations in which straining should be avoided (e.g., myocardial infarction, rectal surgery) and are

BOX 46-1

Drugs Likely to Cause Constipation

- Activated charcoal
- Analgesics (Opioids, NSAIDs)
- Aluminum-containing antacids, cimetidine, ranitidine, sucralfate
- Anticholinergic drugs, atropine
- Antidiarrheal drugs
- Antihistamines (first-generation agents)
- Antiparkinson drugs
- barium sulfate
- Beta blockers, Calcium-channel blockers, clonidine
- Bile-acid sequestrants, HMG-CoA reductase inhibitors ("statins")
- Calcium supplements
- Cation-exchange resins
- Diuretics
- Heavy metals (especially lead)
- Iron supplements
- MAO inhibitors
- Muscle relaxants
- Osmotic laxatives, Stimulant laxatives (habitual use), sodium polystyrene sulfonate
- Phenothiazines
- phenylephrine, pseudoephedrine
- trazodone
- terbutaline
- Tricyclic antidepressants

HMG-CoA, Hydroxymethylglutaryl–coenzyme A; MAO, monoamine oxidase; *NSAIDs,* nonsteroidal antiinflammatory drugs.

useful in the management of chronic watery diarrhea (see Evidence-Based Pharmacotherapeutics box). Polycarbophil is used in the management of constipation or diarrhea associated with diverticulosis or irritable bowel syndrome.

Pharmacodynamics

Bulk-forming laxatives are natural and semisynthetic polysaccharides and cellulose derivatives. They combine with water in the intestine to form an emollient gel or viscous solution. The result is an increase in peristalsis and a reduced transit time. Bulk-forming laxatives produce the same action as 6 to 10 grams/day of dietary fiber. Antidiarrheal activity occurs because the drug takes on water within the intestinal lumen.

Bulk-forming laxatives are the least harmful of the different kinds of laxatives. They do not hinder absorption of nutrients and are less likely to be habit-forming than other types. Compared with stimulant laxatives that empty the entire bowel, bulk-forming laxatives have a longer onset of drug action, and because they evacuate only the descending colon, the sigmoid colon, and the rectum, the potential for dependency is reduced.

Pharmacokinetics

Bulk-forming laxatives are indigestible and not absorbed from the GI tract. Onset of action occurs in about 12 hours. No distribution occurs, and elimination is through the stool (Table 46-1). Bulk-forming laxatives produce a soft, formed stool in 2 to 3 days.

Adverse Effects and Contraindications

Bloating and flatulence are common but undesirable adverse
A effects of bulk-forming laxatives. **Bowel obstruction may occur**

if fluid intake is inadequate. In addition, allergic reactions such as urticaria, dermatitis, rhinitis, and bronchospasm can result from inhaling the powder. Esophageal obstruction has occurred in patients who have dysphagia or esophageal strictures. These laxatives are not recommended for patients with conditions that cause the esophageal or intestinal lumen to be narrowed.

Drug Interactions

Bulk-forming laxatives decrease the absorption of warfarin, salicylates, and cardiac glycosides (Table 46-2). Polycarbophil may decrease the absorption of tetracycline when the two drugs are taken concurrently. There are no known direct drug interactions with methylcellulose.

Dosage Regimen

The usual dosages of bulk-forming laxatives in adults and children are identified in Table 46-3.

Lab Considerations

Bulk-forming laxatives may cause elevated blood glucose levels with prolonged use of formulations containing sugar. Sugar-free formulations are available.

Stool Softeners

- docusate calcium (Pro-Cal-Sof, Surfak); ✦ Selax
- docusate potassium (Diocto-K)
- docusate sodium (Colace, Correctol Extra Gentle, Dialose, Modane, many others)

Indications

Orally administered stool softeners prevent constipation in patients who should avoid straining such as those with a myocardial infarction or those who have had rectal surgery. When administered as an enema, they help soften fecal impactions.

Pharmacodynamics

Stool softeners incorporate water and lipids into the stool, producing an emollient action that reduces surface tension. The drugs act primarily in the jejunum and the colon. By incorporating water into the stool, a softer fecal mass results (Fig. 46-1).

Pharmacokinetics

Small amounts of docusate may be absorbed from the small bowel following oral administration. The extent of absorption from the rectum is unknown. The onset time of drug action varies from 2 to 15 minutes for the rectal formulation to 24 to 72 hours for the orally administered tablets or capsules (see Table 46-1). One to 2 days or more may be needed before a softened fecal bolus reaches the rectum and evacuation occurs.

Adverse Effects and Contraindications

The adverse effects of orally administered stool softeners include throat irritation, mild cramps, and rashes. Diarrhea is certainly a possibility with excessive use. Stool softeners are contraindicated for use in patients with hypersensitivity, abdominal pain, nausea, or vomiting, especially if the constipation is associated with fever or other signs of an acute abdomen. **Excessive or prolonged use of stool softeners can lead to** **A** **dependency.**

EVIDENCE-BASED PHARMACOTHERAPEUTICS

Therapy for Irritable Bowel Syndrome

■ Background

Irritable bowel syndrome (IBS) is a common health problem, particularly among young women. Treatment has typically included bulk-forming laxatives, antispasmodics, and antidepressants; however, uncertainly remains about the effectiveness of these drugs.

■ Research Article

Quartero, A., Meineche-Schmidt, V., Muris, J., et al. (2005). Bulking agents, antispasmodic and antidepressant medication for the treatment of irritable bowel syndrome. *The Cochrane Database Systematic Reviews.* 2005, Issue 2. Art. No. CD003460.pub2. DOI: 10.1002/14651858.CD003460.p2.

Purpose

The primary purpose of this study was to evaluate the efficacy of bulk-forming laxatives, antispasmodic drugs, and antidepressants in the treatment of IBS using the outcomes of (1) relief of abdominal pain (i.e., dichotomous and continuous), (2) global assessment of improvement (i.e., dichotomous), and (3) symptom improvement score. (i.e., dichotomous and continuous).

Design

A meta-analysis of 41 randomized trials (i.e., 11 studies on bulk-forming laxatives, 24 studies on antispasmodic drugs, and 6 studies on antidepressants) compared the efficacy of each class of drugs to a placebo in patients over 12 years of age with IBS.

Method

The investigators examined 687 studies; 66 met the criteria for inclusion in the meta-analysis. After eliminating studies that did not report separately, data from 40 studies remained for analysis. Pooled risk ratios (RR),* risk differences (RD), standardized mean differences (SMD), and 95% confidence intervals (CI) were calculated for all subgroups. When appropriate, the number needed to treat (NNT) was also calculated.

Findings

Bulk-producing laxatives:

$N = 59$ Dichotomous outcome for relief of abdominal pain (3 studies); (RR 1.22; 95% CI 0.86–1.73)

$N = 128$ Continuous outcome for relief of abdominal pain (3 studies); (SMD 0.68; 95% CI 0.86–2.33)

$N = 482$ Dichotomous outcome on global assessment of improvement (9 studies); (RR 1.09; 95% CI 0.78–1.50)

$N = 253$ Dichotomous outcome for symptom improvement score (5 studies); (RR 0.93; 95% CI 0.56–1.54)

$N = 70$ Continuous outcome for symptom improvement score (2 studies); (SMD 0.44; 95% CI 1.20–0.31)

Antispasmodic Drugs:

$N = 1260$ Dichotomous outcome for relief of abdominal pain (11 studies); (RR 1.34; 95% CI 1.13–1.59) (RD = 0.17; 95% CI 0.06–0.28); (NNT = 6; 95% CI 4–15)

$N = 467$ Continuous outcomes for relief of abdominal pain (7 studies); (SMD 0.65; 95% CI 0.94–0.35)

$N = 1236$ Dichotomous outcome on global assessment of improvement (16 studies); (RR 1.42; 95% CI 1.17–1.72); (RD = 0.2, 95% CI 0.09–0.30); (NNT = 5; 95% CI 3–11)

$N = 34$ Dichotomous variable for improvement of symptom score (1 study); (RR 1.33; 95% CI 0.96–1.85)

$N = 66$ Continuous outcome for improvement of symptom score (pooled data of 2 studies) (SMD 0.37; 95% CI -0.85–0.12)

Antidepressants Drugs:

$N = 81$ Dichotomous outcome relief of abdominal pain (2 studies); (RR 0.83; 95% CI 0.33–2.12)

$N = 101$ Continuous outcomes for relief of abdominal pain (2 studies); (SMD 0.53; 95% CI 2.29–1.23)

$N = 241$ Dichotomous variable for global assessment of improvement (4 studies); (RR 1.16; 95% CI 0.78–1.73)

■ Conclusions

As a whole, the findings as to the effectiveness of treatment of IBS with various gastrointestinal (GI) drugs are less than robust. Even though there are data to suggest that GI antispasmodics may be efficacious in relieving abdominal pain associated with IBS and improve symptoms, it remains uncertain whether GI antispasmodics are effective for IBS. No evidence has been found to suggest that antidepressants and bulk-producing laxatives are beneficial in the treatment of IBS.

■ Implications for Practice

Bulk-producing laxatives may help improve constipation and can be used empirically for the treatment of IBS, but their use should be evaluated early in treatment. Valid outcome measures should be used in future research of treatment for IBS. Using the SMD requires the assumption that the differences in the two groups are the same. Unintentional consequences of treatment may reduce the variability of the treatment group on the measured outcome. The SMD uses the standard deviation of the control group to provide a cautious estimate of effect size. In contrast, findings that resulted in substantial variation in the estimate of effect size warrant further investigation. Additional exploration of these differences is recommended.

*The pooled RR is the risk of an event (i.e., abdominal pain, global assessment of improvement, symptom improvement score) in treated subjects divided by the risk of the same event in untreated subjects. The more likely or the less likely an event is to happen in one group compared with another is the relative risk. If the treatment (i.e., drug therapy) has nothing to do with the outcomes, the two rates are the same and the relative risk is 1.0 (which is equal to a proportion of 1:1). If the treated subjects have a higher rate of outcomes, the relative risk is greater than 1, suggesting that treatment may have something to do with outcome.

Note that standardized means difference (SMD) is not the same as the standard error in the differences in means. The SMD value does not depend on the measurement scale. By and large, the SMD is ordinarily recommended for use in clinical trials to gauge effect size, as well as the outcomes of treatment on outcomes measured on a continuous scale. It is the difference between two normalized means—i.e., the mean values divided by an estimate of the within-group standard deviation. The SMD is used for comparing data obtained at different scales.The numbers of subjects that are needed to treat (NNT) to avoid a single additional adverse outcome is but one way of expressing the benefit of one treatment over another.

PHARMACOKINETICS
TABLE **46-1** Selected Laxatives

Drug	Route	Onset	Evacuation	Site	Stool Type
BULK-FORMING LAXATIVES					
psyllium	PO	12 hr	2–3 days	SB-C	SF
polycarbophil	PO	12 hr	2–3 days	SB-C	SF
methylcellulose	PO	12 hr	2–3 days	SB-C	SF
STOOL SOFTENERS					
docusate calcium	PO	24 hr–5 days	3–5 days	SB-C	SF
docusate potassium	PO	24–72 hr	3–5 days	SB-C	SF
docusate sodium	PO	24–72 hr	3–5 days	SB-C	SF
	PR	2–15 min	Hours	C	SF
OSMOTIC LAXATIVES					
magnesium sulfate	PO	3–6 hr	3–6 hr	SB-C	W
magnesium hydroxide and magnesium citrate	PO	0.5–3 hr	3–6 hr	SB-C	W
magnesium citrate	PO	0.5–3 hr	3–6 hr	SB-C	W
sodium phosphate, sodium biphosphate	PO	0.5–3 hr	3–6 hr	C	W
	PR	2–15 min	<60 min	C	W
polyethylene glycol electrolyte solution	PO	30–60 min	60 min	SB-C	W
STIMULANT LAXATIVES					
bisacodyl	PO	6–10 hr	6–12 hr	C	SS
	PR	15–60 min	15–60 min	C	SS
castor oil	PO	2–6 hr	2–3 hr	SB	W
cascara sagrada	PO	6–10 hr	6–10 hr	C	SS
senna	PO	6–24 hr	1–3 days	SB-C	SF
MISCELLANEOUS LAXATIVES					
glycerine	PR	0.25–5 hr	15–30 min	C	SF
lactulose	PO	24–48 hr	1–3 days	C	SF
lubiprostone	PO	1.4 hr	24 hr	UA	UA
mineral oil	PO, PR	6–8 hr	6–8 hr	C	SS

C, Colon; *PO,* by mouth; *PR,* per rectum (i.e., suppository); *SB,* small bowel; *SF,* soft, formed stool in 1–3 days; *SS,* semisoft stool in 6–12 hr; *UA,* unavailable; *W,* watery stool in 2–6 hr.

DRUG INTERACTIONS
TABLE **46-2** Selected Laxatives and Antidiarrheal Drugs

Drug	Interactive Drugs	Interaction
BULK-FORMING LAXATIVES		
psyllium, polycarbophil	digoxin, Salicylates, tetracycline, warfarin	Decreases absorption of interactive drug
OSMOTIC LAXATIVES		
magnesium salts	Neuromuscular blockers	Potentiates effects of interactive drug
	Quinolone antibiotics	Decreases absorption of interactive drug
STIMULANT LAXATIVES		
bisacodyl	Antacids	Removes enteric coating from bisacodyl
cascara	disulfiram	Disulfiram-like reaction
OPIOID ANTIDIARRHEALS		
diphenoxylate, loperamide	Alcohol, Antihistamines. Opioids, Sedative-hypnotics	Additive CNS depression
	Anticholinergics, disopyramide, Tricyclic antidepressants	Additive anticholinergic effects
	MAO inhibitors	Hypertensive crisis
ABSORBENT ANTIDIARRHEALS		
attapulgite, bismuth subsalicylate	aspirin	Potentiates salicylate toxicity
	tetracycline, enoxacin	Decreases absorption of interactive drug
	heparin, warfarin, Thrombolytics	Increases risk of bleeding

CNS, Central nervous system; *MAO,* monoamine oxidase.

▥ *Drug Interactions*

There are no significant drug interactions with docusate laxatives. Do not, however, administer docusate sodium concurrently with mineral oil.

▥ *Dosage Regimen*

The dosage regimen for stool softeners varies with the specific drug, although they are usually administered only once daily (see Table 46-3). Drug effectiveness is assessed after 3 days and the dosage increased as needed (maximum of 500 mg daily for docusate sodium; 300 mg daily for docusate potassium).

Osmotic Laxatives

◆ magnesium sulfate (Epsom Salts)
◆ magnesium hydroxide (Phillips' Milk of Magnesia [MOM])
◆ magnesium citrate (Citrate of Magnesia); ◆ Citro-Mag

DOSAGE

TABLE **46-3 Selected Laxatives and Antidiarrheal Drugs**

Drug	Use(s)	Dosage	Implications
BULK-FORMING			
psyllium	Simple, chronic, atonic, or spastic constipation, particularly related to low fiber diets. Chronic watery diarrhea.	*Adult:* 1–2 tsp, packets, or wafers (3–6 grams) PO in a full glass of liquid 2–3 times daily. Not to exceed 30 grams daily *Child >6 yr:* 1 tsp, packet, or water (1.5–3 grams) PO in 4–8 oz of liquid 2–3 times daily. Not to exceed 15 grams daily in divided doses	Must be followed by 8 oz liquid. **Not to be taken HS, to prevent obstruction**
polycarbophil	Diverticulosis, IBS	*Adult:* 1–4 grams PO daily PRN. Not to exceed 6 grams /24 hr *Child 2–6 yr:* 500 mg PO daily PRN. Not to exceed 1.5 grams/24 hr *Child 6–12 yr:* 500 mg PO one-3 times daily PRN; not to exceed 3 grams/24 hr	For severe diarrhea, may repeat every 30 min. Follow with 8 oz of liquid. Can be given throughout the day to minimize abdominal fullness
methylcellulose	Simple, chronic constipation	*Adult:* 4–6 grams PO daily *Child >6 yr:* 1–3 grams PO daily	Follow with 8 oz of liquid
STOOL SOFTENERS			
docusate calcium	Constipation in patients unable to strain	*Adult:* 240 mg PO once daily *Child >6 yr:* 50–150 mg PO once daily	Docusate calcium and potassium available as capsules; sodium formulation available as tablets, capsules, syrup, liquid, solutions, or enema
docusate potassium		*Adult:* 100–300 mg PO once daily. Max: 300 mg daily *Child >6 yr:* 100 mg PO once daily	
docusate sodium		*Adult:* 50–500 mg PO daily *–or–* 50–100 mg PR once daily. Max: 500 mg daily *Child <3 yr:* 10–40 mg PO daily *Child 3–6 yr:* 20–60 mg PO daily *Child 6–12 yr:* 40–120 mg PO daily	
STIMULANT LAXATIVES			
bisacodyl	Constipation related to immobility, drugs, slowed transit times, IBS, SCI, neurologic disorders	*Adult:* 5–15 mg PO *–or–* 10 mg PRN single dose. Max: 30 mg/day *Child <2 yr:* 5 mg PRN as single dose *Child >6 yr:* 5–10 mg PO or PRN as single dose	Retain enema or suppository 15–30 min before evacuating. Give oral formulations early in the day with a full glass of water
cascara sagrada		*Adult:* 0.5–1.5 mL of fluid extract (200–400 mg) PO as single dose	**Disulfiram reaction if taken concurrently**
senna		*Adult:* Dosage varies with formulation *Child >5 yr:* 50% of adult dose	Available as tablets, granules, liquid concentrate, and syrup
OSMOTIC LAXATIVES			
magnesium sulfate	Radiographic or surgical procedures. Intermittently chronic constipation	*Adult:* 10–15 grams PO as single dose *Child 6–11 yr:* 5–10 grams PO as single dose	Best if chilled, mixed with cold fruit juice, or ice. 8.1 mEq magnesium/gram
magnesium hydroxide		*Adult:* 30–60 mL PO as single dose or in divided doses *–or–* 10–20 mL of concentrate *Child 6–11 yr:* 15–30 mL PO as single dose or in divided doses	34.3 mEq magnesium/gram
magnesium citrate		*Adult:* 240 mL PO as single dose *Child 2–6 yr:* 4–12 mL PO as single dose *Child 6–12 yr:* 50–100 mL PO as single dose	Best if chilled, mixed with cold fruit juice or ice. 4.4 mEq magnesium/gram
sodium phosphate/ biphosphate		*Adult:* 20–30 mL PO as single dose *–or–* 120 mL enema *Child >2 yr:* 50% of adult dose PRN as single dose *Child 5–9 yr:* 2.5–10 mL PO as single dose *Child 10–11 yr:* 5–10 mL PO as single dose	Each 20 mL of oral solution contains 96.4 mEq of sodium. Enema contains 4.4 grams sodium/ 118 mL. Do not administer near bedtime.
polyethylene glycol electrolyte solution		*Adult:* 240 mL of solution PO every 10 min to 4 L until fecal discharge appears clear and has no solid material *Child:* 25–40 mL/kg/hr until fecal discharge is clear and has no solid material	Fast 3–4 hr before taking; avoid solid food within 2 hr of administration. May be given through NG tube
MISCELLANEOUS LAXATIVES			
glycerine	Constipation secondary to reduced gastrocolic reflex activity	*Adult:* 2–3 grams PRN as suppository *–or–* 5–15 mL as enema *Child <6 yr:* 1–1.7 grams as suppository *–or–* 2–5 mL as enema	Evacuation of colon usually in 15–30 min

GASTROINTESTINAL

Continued

DOSAGE
TABLE 46-3 Selected Laxatives and Antidiarrheal Drugs—Cont'd

Drug	Use(s)	Dosage	Implications
lactulose	Chronic constipation	*Adult:* 15–30 mL/day PO up to 60 mL/day	Mix with 240 mL of fruit juice, water, milk, or carbonated citrus beverage to improve flavor. May be given on empty stomach for rapid results.
lubiprostone	Chronic idiopathic constipation	*Adult:* 24 mcg PO with food twice daily	Periodically assess the need for continued therapy.
mineral oil	Constipation related to impaction, fissures, hemorrhoids	*Adult and Child >12 yr:* 5–45 mL PO as single dose or in divided doses –or– 60–150 mL PR as single dose *Child 2–11 yr:* 30–60 mL PRN as single dose *Child 6–12 yr:* 5–20 mL PO as single dose or in divided doses	Avoid giving within 2 hr of meals, or to patients in a reclining position. Moisten suppositories with water rather than lubricant to prevent interfering with action of the suppository.
OPIOID ANTIDIARRHEALS			
diphenoxylate with atropine	Adjunct treatment for diarrhea	*Adult:* 5–20 mg/day PO *Child 2–12 yr:* Initially 0.075–0.1 mg/kg PO 4 times daily in liquid dosage form; decrease dosage as condition permits	One tablet or 5 mL of liquid contains 2.5 mg diphenoxylate with 0.025 mg of atropine.
loperamide	Adjunct treatment of acute diarrhea. Chronic diarrhea associated with IBD. Decrease volume of ileostomy drainage	*Adult:* 4 mg initially PO, then 2 mg after each loose stool. Maintenance: 4–8 mg PO per day. Not to exceed 8 mg/day if OTC; 16 mg/day if prescription *Child 6–8 yr or 24–30 kg:* 1 mg initially, then 1 mg with each loose stool. Not to exceed 4 mg/24 hr *Child 9–11 yr or 30–47 kg:* 2 mg initially, then 1 mg with each loose stool. Not to exceed 6 mg/24 hr	OTC use in children not to exceed 2 days. Give with clear fluids to help prevent dehydration that accompanies diarrhea.
	Adjunct in symptomatic management of mild-to-moderate acute diarrhea	*Adult:* 1.2–1.5 grams PO after each loose stool. Not to exceed 9 grams/24 hr *Child 3–6 yr:* 300 mg PO after each loose stool. Not to exceed 2.1 grams/24 hr *Child 6–12 yr:* 600 mg PO after each loose stool. Not to exceed 4.2 grams/24 hr	Increases risk of dehydration if used in children younger than age 3 yr or in older adults
camphorated tincture of opium	Diarrhea	*Adult:* 5–10 mL (the equivalent of 2–4 mg of anhydrous morphine) 1–4 times a day until diarrhea is controlled *Child >2 years of age:* 0.25–0.5 mL PO (the equivalent of 100–200 mcg [0.1–0.2 mg] of anhydrous morphine) per kg of body weight 1–4 times a day	**Paregoric contains 45% alcohol, which is an undesirable ingredient in drugs used for children.** ⚠
ABSORBENT ANTIDIARRHEAL			
bismuth subsalicylate	Adjunct mild-to-moderate diarrhea. Traveler's diarrhea (not FDA approved for this use)	*Adult:* 2 tablets PO every 30 min –or– 30 mL every 30–60 min up to 8 doses/24 hr *Child 3–6 yr:* 5 mL every 30–60 min up to 8 doses/24 hr *Child 6–9 yr:* 10 mL every 30–60 min up to 8 doses/24 hr *Child 9–12 yr:* 1 tablet –or– 15 mL every 30–60 min up to 8 doses/24 hr	Contains aspirin. **CDC warns against giving drug to children or teenagers during or after recovery from chickenpox (varicella) or flulike illness because of possibility of Reye's syndrome.** ⚠

CDC, Centers for Disease Control and Prevention; *FDA,* Food and Drug Administration; *HS,* at bedtime; *IBS,* irritable bowel syndrome; *NG,* nasogastric; *OTC,* over the counter; *PO,* by mouth; *PRN,* as needed; *SCI,* spinal cord injuries

◆ polystyrene glycol electrolyte solution (Colovage, Colyte, Golytely, Halflytely, Miralax, Nulytely, OCL, Peglyte); ◆ Klean-Prep
◆ sodium phosphate or biphosphate (Phospho-Soda, Fleet Enema)

▥ Indications

Depending on the laxative in use, osmotic laxatives can produce an overnight laxative effect (such as with magnesium hydroxide) or produce a cathartic effect, which results in complete evacuation of the colon. The latter effect is useful in preparation for a bowel exam, to flush poisons from the system, or to remove parasites.

▥ *Pharmacodynamics*

Osmotic laxatives act by drawing water into the intestinal lumen and causing peristalsis; the greater the concentration of solutes, the greater the osmotic activity. Hypertonic solutions cause diffusion of fluid from the plasma into the intestine to dilute the solution to an isotonic state. Magnesium salts cause an increase in the secretion of cholecystokinin from the duodenum. This activity is thought to increase the secretion and motility of the small bowel and the colon, contributing to the cathartic effects.

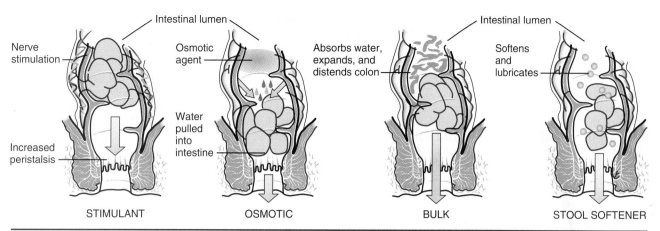

FIGURE 46-1 Mechanism of Action of Laxatives. Stimulant laxatives act on intestinal walls of the small bowel or the colon to increase the amount of fluid and electrolytes within the lumen. Osmotic laxatives draw water into the intestinal lumen to stimulate peristalsis. The greater the concentration of solutes, the greater the osmotic activity. Bulk-forming laxatives combine with water to form an emollient gel or viscous solution, resulting in an increase in peristalsis. Stool softeners produce an emollient action that reduces surface tension and thus facilitates penetration of water and lipids into the stool.

▥ *Pharmacokinetics*

The onset of osmotic laxatives when taken by mouth varies from 30 minutes to 6 hours depending on the preparation (see Table 46-1). Most osmotic laxatives produce a watery stool in 3 to 6 hours.

▥ *Adverse Effects and Contraindications*

The most common adverse effect of osmotic laxatives is diarrhea. However, the greater the concentration of solutes, the more likely it is that these laxatives may cause nausea. Drowsiness, bradycardia, arrhythmias, hypotension, flushing, sweating, and hypothermia are most likely to occur with parenteral administration of magnesium salts (i.e., treatment and prevention of hypomagnesemia, pregnancy-induced hypertension).

▲ **All osmotic laxatives are contraindicated for use in patients with nausea and vomiting of unknown origin, abdominal pain, impaction, and intestinal obstruction.** Magnesium salts are contraindicated for use in renal disease because magnesium ions may be retained. Use caution when giving them to patients with renal disease because of their sodium content. Patients who are receiving central nervous system (CNS) depressants for seizure activity may experience a significant drop in serum calcium levels that could precipitate additional seizure activity.

▥ *Drug Interactions*

Magnesium salts potentiate the action of neuromuscular blocking drugs (see Table 46-2). The absorption of quinolone antibiotics is reduced in the presence of magnesium salts. Polyethylene glycol electrolyte solutions interfere with the absorption of orally administered drugs by decreasing transit time through the bowel. Do not give oral drugs within 1 hour of starting laxative therapy.

▥ *Dosage Regimen*

The dosages of osmotic laxatives vary with the specific drug, but most are given as a single dose (see Table 46-3). The greater the concentration of solutes, the more likely the patient is to become nauseated; therefore it is important that all preparations be accompanied by at least 8 oz of water. The water also assists the laxative to leave the stomach.

Stimulant Laxatives

- ◆ bisacodyl (Dulcolax, Fleet Laxative, Correctol, Feen-a-Mint); ♣ Dulcolax
- ◆ castor oil (Purge, Fleet Flavored Castor Oil)
- ◆ cascara sagrada
- ◆ senna (Black-Draught, Ex-Lax, Fletcher's Castoria, Senexon, Senokot, Senolax)

▥ *Indications*

Stimulant laxatives are used for constipation associated with prolonged bed rest, constipating drugs, slowed transit times, and irritable bowel syndrome. They are also used to evacuate the bowel before radiologic studies or surgery. Stimulants are included as part of a bowel regimen for patients with spinal cord injuries or neurologic disorders. Castor oil is used less often today than in the past owing to its many adverse effects and poor palatability.

▥ *Pharmacodynamics*

Stimulant laxatives are obtained from the roots, the bark, and the seed pods of a number of plants. They act on the intestinal wall of the small bowel and colon to increase fluids and electrolytes within the intestinal lumen. In addition, they cause the release of prostaglandins and produce an increase in cyclic adenosine monophosphate (cAMP) concentration. The increase in cAMP concentration, in turn, increases the secretion of electrolytes and contributes to cathartic effects.

Specifically, bisacodyl, cascara, and senna stimulate the submucosal and mesenteric plexus to produce semisoft or soft formed stool. Castor oil combines with lipase in the small bowel to produce ricinoleic acid (the active component of castor oil), which in turn stimulates the smooth muscle of the small bowel. Castor oil is classified as a cathartic because it draws more water into the bowel, producing a more watery stool. Cascara produces propulsive movements of the colon by direct chemical irritation. It is converted to an active metabolite in the colon. Similarly, docusate is a prodrug that is converted by intestinal bacteria into the desurcetyl metabolite, which is the active form. Consequently, bisacodyl is dispensed in enteric-coated tablets, which must never be crushed, so as to prevent early activation of bisacodyl.

Pharmacokinetics

The pharmacokinetics of stimulant laxatives is identified in Table 46-1. Their onset times vary from less than 15 minutes for bisacodyl suppositories to more than 24 hours for senna preparations. Less than 5% of bisacodyl is absorbed following oral administration.

Cascara is minimally absorbed when taken orally. Cascara circulates throughout the body to be eliminated in the bile, the urine, the saliva, the colonic mucosa, and breast milk. Evacuation of the bowel occurs in 6 to 10 hours.

Senna is also minimally absorbed following oral administration. Its distribution, biotransformation, elimination, and half-life are unknown. It produces soft, formed stools in 1 to 3 days.

Adverse Effects and Contraindications

The most common adverse effects of stimulant laxatives include mild cramping, nausea, vomiting, diarrhea, and even dehydration in susceptible individuals. **Continued use of these stimulant laxatives produces an irritable bowel syndrome–like diarrhea that can be severe enough to cause fluid and electrolyte imbalances. Stimulant laxatives can cause proctitis in males. Hypokalemia, tetany, and protein-losing enteropathy also occur with long-term use of stimulant laxatives.**

Stimulant laxatives are contraindicated for use in patients with hypersensitivity, abdominal pain of unknown cause (especially when associated with fever), rectal fissures, and ulcerated hemorrhoids. Castor oil is contraindicated for use in the presence of infestation with fat-soluble worms, during pregnancy, and in breastfeeding mothers. Cascara sagrada contains alcohol; avoid use in patients with known intolerance to alcohol. Excessive or prolonged use of stimulant laxatives may lead to dependence.

Drug Interactions

Stimulant laxatives decrease the absorption of other orally administered drugs because of increased motility and decreased transit times (see Table 46-2). The enteric coating of bisacodyl is prematurely removed if taken with antacids or within 1 hour of consuming dairy products. Cascara is compounded with magnesium oxide (to make it less bitter), flavoring agents, sweeteners, and alcohol (18%). **Do not use cascara in patients taking disulfiram for control of alcoholism because of the risk of a disulfiram-like reaction.**

Dosage Regimen

The dosage regimen for stimulant laxatives varies with the specific drug and formulation, but in general, they are administered at bedtime for evacuation 6 to 12 hours later (see Table 46-3). For more rapid results, oral formulations can be given on an empty stomach with a full glass of water. Suppository formulations can cause proctitis and rectal burning. If prescribing castor oil, advise patient to take it early in the day, mixed with a carbonated beverage or fruit juice to increase palatability.

Miscellaneous Laxatives

- glycerine (Fleet Babylax, Sani-Supp)
- lactulose (Cephulac, Cholac, Chronulac, others); ✦ Acilac, Laxilose
- lubiprostone (Amitza)
- mineral oil

Glycerine

Glycerine is used for conditions in which the rectum is filled with stool but the defecation reflex is not triggered or transit time is severely delayed. Glycerine acts by drawing water from the extravascular spaces into the lumen of the colon. Diarrhea is the most common adverse effect, although nausea, vomiting, and dehydration have also occurred. The usual dosage is 2 to 3 grams as a suppository or 5 to 15 mL as an enema, administered 30 minutes after a meal to take full advantage of the gastrocolic reflex. In children, 1 to 1.7 grams as a suppository or 2 to 5 mL as an enema is given after meals.

Lactulose

Lactulose is a semisynthetic, hyperosmotic disaccharide used in the treatment of chronic constipation in adults and older adults. Its superiority to conventional laxatives has not been established. It is also used to restore regular bowel movements in patients who have had a hemorrhoidectomy, but it is not approved for such use. Lactulose is also used in the management of hepatic encephalopathy (see Chapter 48) because it lowers the pH of the colon, which in turn inhibits diffusion of ammonia across colonic membranes.

Less than 3% of lactulose is absorbed from the small intestine following oral administration. Resident bacteria in the colon biotransform lactulose to lactic acid and small amounts of acetic and formic acids. The acids exert mild osmotic actions and produce soft-formed stools in 1 to 3 days. The effects of lactulose are decreased in the presence of antimicrobial drugs.

The most common adverse effects of lactulose include cramps, distention, flatulence, belching, and diarrhea. Lactulose is contraindicated for patients with hypersensitivity and in those who are on a low-galactose diet. Use with caution in patients with diabetes mellitus because of the risk of hyperglycemia. It is also used with caution in older adults or debilitated patients. Lactulose carries a pregnancy category C designation. It is not known if lactulose is distributed to breast milk.

Lubiprostone

Lubiprostone, the first drug of its chemical type, has received FDA approval to treat chronic constipation in adults. Lubiprostone, a chloride channel activator, increases intestinal motility by increasing fluid secretion and the passage of stool without altering sodium and potassium concentrations in the serum. The symptoms of chronic idiopathic constipation are thus alleviated. Lubiprostone is administered twice daily with food.

The most common adverse effects of lubiprostone include headache, fatigue, nausea, abdominal pain, diarrhea, and flatulence. Whether these events are directly related to the drug is not yet known. The drug is contraindicated for patients with a known sensitivity to the drug or its ingredients, and in patients with a history of mechanical obstruction of the GI tract.

There are few drug interactions with lubiprostone because the CYP 3A4, 2D6, 2A6, 2B6, and 2C19 enzymes are not involved in the biotransformation.

Mineral Oil

Mineral oil is the only lubricant laxative in use today. It is used to soften impacted stool during management of constipation. Mineral oil coats the surface of the stool and the intestine with a film and retards water reabsorption to allow passage of the stool through the intestine. It does not stimulate intestinal peristalsis. Distribution is to the liver, the spleen, mesenteric lymph nodes, and the intestinal mucosa. It produces a semisoft stool in 6 to 8 hours (see Table 46-1).

The adverse effects of mineral oil are few; however, anorexia, nausea, vomiting, and nutritional deficiencies can occur. Anal irritation can occur with rectal administration.

⚠ **Lipid pneumonia is possible in patients who aspirate mineral oil. Chronic use decreases the absorption of fat-soluble vitamins (A, D, E, and K), food, and bile salts.** However, there is some evidence to suggest that only the precursor of vitamin A (carotene) is affected, and that natural vitamin A is absorbed in the intestine in the presence of mineral oil.

Mineral oil is contraindicated in the presence of hypersensitivity. The rectal route is contraindicated for children younger than 2 years of age, and the oral route is contraindicated for children younger than 6 years of age. Use mineral oil cautiously in older adults or debilitated patients because of the

⚠ increased risk of lipid pneumonia. **Use mineral oil with caution in pregnancy because mineral oil decreases the absorption of fat-soluble vitamins and may cause hypoprothrombinemia in the newborn.**

The absorption of fat-soluble vitamins is decreased in the presence of mineral oil (see Table 46-2). Similarly, concurrent use of mineral oil with stool softeners may increase the absorption of mineral oil.

As with most other laxatives, a single dose is administered, usually at bedtime (see Table 46-3). Routine use is discouraged. Children's doses vary with the age of the child and the route of administration.

CLINICAL REASONING

Treatment Objectives

The primary treatment objective for patients with constipation is to reestablish a normal bowel pattern and to effect comfortable stooling. Treatment modalities address three main areas: (1) correction of the underlying condition causing the constipation; (2) patient education, (3) and non–drug therapies. Prevention is the best overall approach.

Treatment Options

Although there are valid uses for laxatives, constipation is generally resolved with attention to lifestyle changes, including increasing exercise, fluids, and fiber in the diet, and appropriate bowel training. According to the National Center for Health Statistics, Americans eat 5 to 14 grams of fiber daily, far short of the recommended 20 to 35 grams recommended by the American Dietetic Association. Both soluble and insoluble fiber in the form of fruits, vegetables, and whole grains are recommended for most persons without fear of colon obstruction. Another lifestyle consideration includes establishing a regular pattern for bathroom visits while heeding the urge to defecate. Ignoring the urge to defecate increases the time available for absorption of fluid from the stool, contributing to constipation. Drug therapy is used in cases resistant to simple treatment measures; optimally, this means using

the least number of drugs in the lowest dosages for the shortest duration of time.

▮▮ Patient Variables

Elicit a careful description of usual and current elimination patterns, including information about the onset, the frequency, the duration, precipitating or aggravating factors, and stool consistency, size, and color. Ask about related symptoms such as abdominal pain, fever, flatulence, or a sensation of incomplete evacuation. It is also helpful to inquire about the patient's perception of normal bowel patterns, because many patients describe themselves as constipated if they do not have a daily bowel movement. When questioning the patient about drug use, it is important to include over-the-counter (OTC) drugs, especially laxatives and enemas. Chronic use of laxatives or enemas causes dilation and hypertrophy of the colon (megacolon).

Ask if there is a history of colorectal disease, hemorrhoids, or rectal fissures. Neurologic diseases and spinal cord lesions that disrupt colon and abdominal motor nerves may provide insight into the cause. An abrupt onset of constipation or onset in patients 45 to 50 years old suggests an organic cause and requires immediate attention. If abdominal cramping is relieved by defecation, irritable bowel syndrome may be the cause of the constipation.

A history of intermittent or partially obstructing bowel lesions or metabolic disorders such as diabetes mellitus, hypothyroidism, hypokalemia, hypercalcemia, and uremia contribute to constipation. Straining to have a stool (i.e., a *Valsalva maneuver*) produces changes in intrathoracic pressure, leading to reduced coronary, cerebral, and peripheral circulation. Other potential outcomes of straining include the development of hernias and worsening symptoms of gastroesophageal reflux.

Signs of constipation include abdominal masses with palpable tenderness, silent or abnormal bowel sounds, external hemorrhoids, strictures, anal tears or abrasions, and impaction. Anal sphincter tone is increased in patients with functional problems and strictures but decreased with constipation of neurologic etiology.

Constipation resistant to ordinary interventions may require testing to establish the cause of the problem. Abdominal radiographs may demonstrate stool in the colon. Although fecal occult blood testing (FOBT) carries a 50% to 90% sensitivity rate, this procedure is an inexpensive way to screen for bleeding lesions that contribute to constipation. Occult testing is not indicated if the patient has hemorrhoids or fissures because the lesions may cause misleadingly positive results.

LIFE-SPAN CONSIDERATIONS

Pregnant and Nursing Women. Constipation during pregnancy is common. The effects of progesterone on smooth muscle relaxation reduce gastric emptying time and intestinal motility, which contributes to constipation. Constipation is also caused by mechanical compression of the bowel by the enlarging uterus and the effects of iron supplements. The increase in electrolyte and water absorption during pregnancy adds to the problem.

For pregnant women, the drugs of choice are usually ⚠ **bulk-forming laxatives or stool softeners, those without systemic absorption.** Ducosate sodium is not associated with fetal malformations and may be safely used during pregnancy, as well as lactulose and sorbitol. Castor oil is not recommended during pregnancy because it may cause uterine contractions. Mineral oil is also not recommended because it interferes with the absorption of fat-soluble vitamins in the mother and results in deficiencies in the neonate.

Children and Adolescents. Stool patterns of children vary widely; parents usually pay little attention to a child's frequency of bowel movements unless there is incontinence. Normally, neonates pass more than four stools daily during the first week of life. The frequency declines to one to two stools daily by the age of 4 years. Factors such as emotional distress, family conflict, dietary changes, febrile illness, or recent travel can alter the child's bowel habits.

Constipation and incontinence in children is disturbing, both to the child and the parents. Toilet training or painful stools secondary to constipation can result in avoidance behaviors to toileting. In turn, the avoidance results in larger, harder, and more painful stools. Eventually, soiling results, there is even greater stress, parental anger, and worsening constipation and soiling.

A significant number of children have chronic functional constipation that often begins in infancy and tends to be self-perpetuating. Large, hard stools are retained because elimination is difficult. Chronic distention of the rectum and colon gradually decrease a child's awareness of the need to defecate. This problem results in more retention, more water reabsorption, and hardening of the stool. As the rectum becomes dilated, liquid stool oozes around the hard mass as involuntary soiling.

Girls and women with anorexia nervosa or bulimia may abuse laxatives as a means for reducing nutrient absorption to effect weight loss. Bulimia is 10 times more common in women than men; affecting up to 3% of young women. The health care provider should consider whether the patient could be depressed or socially isolated and thus less active.

Few, well-designed placebo-controlled studies have been conducted in children looking at the use of osmotic laxatives, fiber, switching formulas, juices containing sorbitol, rectal stimulation, or the use of glycerine suppositories. Electrolyte disturbances, dehydration, and cardiac arrest have been reported when sodium phosphate enemas were used in children under the age of 2 years.

Older Adults. The concern about regular bowel movements is particularly common in older adults. Although intestinal motility decreases with age, constipation is not necessarily a problem of older adults. Inactivity, poor appetite, tooth loss, and poor-fitting dentures contribute to the risk of constipation. Further, many older adults habitually use laxatives or enemas to effect bowel movements.

Overuse of laxatives is of special concern because this age group is likely to be more intolerant of the fluid and electrolyte imbalances that accompany laxative abuse. Bulk-forming laxatives are recommended for older adults as supplements to dietary fiber and fluids. Stool softeners can be used on a short-term basis. **Use osmotic and stimulant laxatives sparingly because of the significant fluid and electrolyte loss produced. Lubricants are discouraged because of the potential danger of aspiration and lipid pneumonia, especially with immobile patients**. Further, some laxatives may exacerbate existing disease states (e.g., heart failure, hypertension).

▌ Drug Variables

The initial drug of choice for constipation depends on the type and severity of constipation, the effect desired, and the underlying cause of the condition. In cases of drug-induced constipation, correction is accomplished by adjusting the drug dosage or by using alternative drugs before resorting to concurrent laxative use.

Bulk-forming Laxatives. As long as no contraindications exist to their use, bulk-forming laxatives are chosen as first-line therapy for constipation. These drugs are not absorbed systemically and may be an appropriate choice for patients in whom a rapid response is not necessary. Further, their pharmacologic effect is that of the natural effect of fiber from food on the GI tract. Their adverse effects are usually mild, and if necessary they can be taken safely for long durations compared to other classes of laxatives such as the stimulants.

Bulk-forming laxatives are usually effective in 2 to 3 days, are safe for long-term use, and are least likely to cause laxative dependency. The choice of the product depends on the patient's acceptance of texture and taste (e.g., orange flavored, minty, tasteless), its other ingredients (e.g., low sodium, sugar-free), and cost.

Lactulose may be considered if bulk-forming laxatives are contraindicated, ineffective, or not tolerated. It can also be used for long-term management of chronic constipation, whereas osmotic and stimulant laxatives, and stool softeners are for short-term use.

Stool Softeners. There is little therapeutic difference in docusate stool softeners. If hard dry stools are the problem, or in situations where straining should be avoided, consider a stool softener such as ducosate sodium for first-line therapy. Like bulk-forming laxatives, stool softeners are not absorbed systemically, and they have minimal adverse effects. They are primarily suitable for short-term use. Evidence suggests that docusate can be hepatotoxic and may increase the absorption of hepatobiliary toxins, because it injures and increases the permeability of intestinal mucosa. Stool softeners can be used if lactulose is ineffective or not tolerated.

Glycerine suppositories are probably the safest of all laxative formulations. They cause an irritation of rectal mucosa and are preferred as first-line agents in infants.

Osmotic Laxatives. When more rapid action is needed, magnesium hydroxide may be chosen. Osmotic laxatives are equally effective and have adverse effects similar to those of stimulant laxatives. Magnesium hydroxide is usually preferred over magnesium citrate or magnesium sulfate because of its milder action. Even though the onset of action of osmotic laxatives is faster than that of bulk-producing laxatives or stool softeners, dehydration is a concern if there is excessive use. This is especially true of patients unable to tolerate excessive fluid loss. Patients with renal insufficiency and older adults should avoid magnesium-containing formulations. Base the choice between drugs in this group and stimulant laxatives on patient preference, availability, and cost.

The drug of choice for radiologic bowel preps is most often polyethylene glycol electrolyte solution. It produces the most complete evacuation of the GI tract of all the available laxatives. Ordinarily, patients prefer this osmotic laxative over enemas or cathartic drugs because it is more convenient, acts quickly, and causes less discomfort. Sodium phosphate and sodium biphosphate enemas, in combination with bisacodyl, can be used if polyethylene glycol electrolyte solution cannot be tolerated.

Stimulant Laxatives. When bulk-forming or osmotic laxatives fail to produce stool, a stimulant laxative may be chosen. All stimulant laxatives are equally effective and less expensive than lactulose when a rapid response is desired. Some health care providers advocate the use of senna instead of the other stimulants, claiming it to be the mildest and most physiologic of all the non–fiber laxatives. However, there are no good studies to confirm or deny this claim. Stimulant laxatives have the highest potential for abuse compared to the other laxative classes. Therefore, use them only for short-term treatment. The decision about which stimulant laxative to use can thus be based in part on availability and cost. **Castor oil is a potent cathartic; do not use it routinely for managing constipation.**

Patient Education

Correct misconceptions about bowel function. Advise patients that laxatives are temporary measures and are not intended for long-term treatment of constipation. Inform the patient that autointoxication does not occur if bowel movements are less frequent. Teach the patient to use non–drug therapies such as increasing bulk in the diet, increasing fluid intake, and increasing physical activity before resorting to a laxative. Patients with abdominal pain, nausea, vomiting, or fever should be advised not to use laxatives without first consulting their health care provider.

Drug therapy may be warranted if constipation has not been relieved after 2 to 4 weeks of non–drug management. Bulk-forming laxatives should be taken early in the day to minimize the possibility of intestinal obstruction that may occur with nighttime administration. Additionally, teach patient to take these laxatives 1 hour before or 2 hours after other drugs to promote absorption. All laxatives are taken with a full glass of water. Psyllium formulations should be diluted at the bedside with 8 oz of water, milk, or juice. The mixture is taken immediately after mixing because it will congeal in a few minutes.

Advise patients not to chew psyllium granules or take them at bedtime. **Do not give psyllium granules to patients who are unable to sit upright, because they may cause esophageal or intestinal obstruction.** Some dosage forms of psyllium contain sugar, aspartame, or excessive sodium. Avoid these in patients on restricted diets.

Enteric-coated laxatives (e.g., bisacodyl) should not be taken within 1 hour of drinking milk or taking an antacid. Do not give cascara sagrada and docusate potassium to patients who abuse alcohol.

Do not give mineral oil to bedridden patients or children, because it can cause lipid pneumonia should the patient aspirate. It should be administered to patients in an upright position. Avoid giving mineral oil within 2 hours of stool softeners. Do not lubricate suppositories containing mineral oil before administration because the lubricant interferes with the action of the suppository. Moisten the suppository with water or a water-soluble lubricant.

Evaluation

Normal bowel patterns are individually determined, and the frequency of evacuation may vary from 3 times a day to 3 times a week. Clinical response to treatment is demonstrated by the passage of a soft, formed bowel movement, usually within 12 to 24 hours. In some cases, 3 days of therapy may be required to produce results. Fifty percent of patients who regularly use laxatives reestablish normal bowel habits once the laxative administration is discontinued.

DIARRHEA

EPIDEMIOLOGY AND ETIOLOGY

Diarrhea is not a disease but a symptom experienced by most people at some point in their lifetime. Diarrhea is the leading cause of death in developing countries, where over 10,000 children under the age of 6 years are affected daily. In the United States, diarrhea accounts for over 250,000 hospitalizations per year and 7.9 million office visits. Forty-eight million diarrheal episodes lasting over 48 hours occur annually.

True *diarrhea* is defined as an increase in the frequency of loose, watery stools (three or more daily), usually over a period of 24 to 48 hours. Box 46-2 identifies microorganisms, drugs, and diseases that are likely to cause diarrhea.

Acute diarrhea is self-limiting, lasting 1 to 14 days, and characterized by watery, loose stools of less than 2 weeks' duration; it is usually of viral or bacterial origin. Viral gastroenteritis is the most common cause of diarrhea in the United States, with

---

BOX 46-2

Drugs, Bugs, and Diseases Likely to Cause Diarrhea

DRUGS	BUGS	DISEASES
Antimicrobials	*Aeronomas* species	AIDS
Antineoplastics	*Bacillus cereus*	Bowel resection
Bile acids	*Campylobacter*	Colon cancer
Cardiac glycosides	*Chlamydia trachomatis*	Diverticulitis
Cholinergic drugs	*Clostridium difficile*	Enteral feedings
Cholinesterase inhibitors	*Cryptosporidium*	Gastroenteritis
guanethidine	*Escherichia coli*	Hyperthyroidism
Magnesium-based antacids	*Entamoeba histolytica*	Inflammatory bowel disease
methyldopa	*Giardia*	Irritable bowel syndrome
Osmotic laxatives	*Mycobacterium avium-intracellulare*	Lactose intolerance
quinidine	*Salmonella*	Malabsorption
reserpine	*Shigella*	Pheochromocytoma
Stimulant laxatives	*Staphylococcus aureus*, viruses, *Yersinia*	

AIDS, Acquired immunodeficiency syndrome.

outbreaks linked to the Norwalk virus in adults and the roto-virus in children. Common food contaminants are produced by bacteria and bacterial toxins, such as *Staphylococcus aureus, Clostridium perfringens, Escherichia coli,* and *Salmonella.* Drugs can also cause diarrhea (see Box 46-2).

Traveler's diarrhea is primarily caused by *E. coli* and trans-mitted by poor food-handling practices and contaminated water. The enterotoxin promotes diarrhea by increasing fluid secretion in the small bowel. Some parasites, such as *Giardia lamblia,* are responsible for inducing diarrhea after a person drinks from a contaminated water source.

Persistent diarrhea lasts longer than 14 days but less than 30 days. *Chronic diarrhea* lasts more than 30 days. Diarrhea can also be categorized as osmotic, secretory, or exudative (inflam-matory), or it may be related to the transit of stool through the colon (intestinal motility).

PATHOPHYSIOLOGY

Osmotic diarrhea (retention of water in the stool) develops when nonabsorbable solutes are retained in the intestinal lumen. The result is a hyperosmolar state that pulls water and ions into the intestines. Poorly absorbed salts such as magnesium sulfate, lac-tose, and large amounts of sorbitol (a sugar substitute found in gum, diet foods, and soft drinks) draw fluids into the lumen, resulting in an overload of fluid in the colon.

Secretory diarrhea (secretion of water into the stool) develops secondary to the active transport of sodium through the sodium-potassim–adenosine triphosphatase (Na^+-K^+-ATPase) pump in the epithelium of the colon. Chloride ions are exchanged for HCO_3 ions, and there is an uptake of sodium chloride. Any drug that increases the concentration of cAMP in colonic cells inhibits sodium chloride uptake and causes secretion of chloride. The result is secretion of fluid into the colonic lumen. Cholinergics and cholinesterase-inhibiting drugs (see Chapter 15) cause secretion of sodium chloride and water, resulting in loose stools.

Exudative diarrhea can be caused by ulcerative colitis, Crohn's disease (regional enteritis), tuberculosis, and cancers such as lymphoma and adenocarcinoma. This type of diarrhea develops when the mucosa of the large intestine becomes inflamed or ulcerated. The mucosal surfaces release proteins, blood, mucus, and other fluids into the lumen of the intes-tine. The patient may have a pressing need to have a bowel movement; the frequency of the bowel movements is related to the sensitivity of the colon to distention by the stool.

Normal intestinal motility allows fluids, electrolytes, and nutrients to pass through the colon with sufficient contact time for absorption to take place. However, *altered intestinal motility,* that is, any factor increasing or decreasing the movement of contents through the intestines, may result in decreased absorption of fluids and electrolytes. Although avoiding laxatives in the presence of diarrhea seems all too obvious, concealed abuse of stimulant laxatives is a surpris-ingly frequent cause of chronic diarrhea. Other common causes of chronic diarrhea include bacterial overgrowth; malabsorption, such as with celiac sprue and Whipple's dis-ease; inflammatory bowel disease, such as ulcerative colitis and Crohn's disease; tumors; postsurgical diarrhea as in postgastrectomy dumping syndrome; functional issues such as irritable bowel syndrome and diverticulitis; and

drug-induced causes (e.g., prokinetic drugs, serotonin, prostaglandins).

Diarrhea stool mixed with mucus and red blood cells is associated with typhus, typhoid, cholera, amebiasis (e.g., *Entamoeba histolytica*), or large bowel cancers. Diarrhea mixed with mucus and white blood cells may be indicative of ulcer-ative colitis, regional enteritis, shigellosis, salmonellosis, or intestinal tuberculosis. A pasty stool with high-fat content is indicative of a malabsorption disorder. Any changes in stool are of concern and warrant further investigation.

PHARMACOTHERAPEUTIC OPTIONS

Opioid Antidiarrheals
◆ diphenoxylate with atropine sulfate (Lomotil, Lofene, Logen, Lonox); ♣ Lomotil
◆ loperamide (Imodium, Imodium A-D, Kaopectate II Caplets, Maalox Anti-Diarrheal Caplets, Pepto Diarrhea Control); ♣ Diarr-Eze, Loperacap
◆ camphorated tincture of opium (Paregoric)

▦ Indications
Opioids, as systemic antidiarrheal drugs, are the most effective antidiarrheal drugs. Although hydroalcoholic solutions of opium powder have long been used to treat diarrhea, synthetic opioids are now preferred. The systemic antidiarrheals are much more effective than local preparations (e.g., absorbents, intestinal flora modifiers) in treating and controlling diarrhea. Atropine, an anticholinergic drug, is combined with diphenoxylate in subther-apeutic doses to discourage abuse of the preparation.

Camphorated tincture of opium is a systemic opioid drug with antispasmodic and antiperistaltic actions. Although both drugs are used less often today, camphorated tincture of opium has been particularly useful in the management of diarrhea associated with human immunodeficiency virus (HIV) infection. Opium tincture has been added to enteral feedings to help reduce the diarrhea typically caused by such feedings. In addition, the preparation (in dilute form) may be given to suppress symptoms of withdrawal in opioid-dependent neonates.

▦ Pharmacodynamics
Opioids such as diphenoxylate act at the mu (μ) and, pos-sibly, the delta (Δ) receptors to decrease intestinal motility and slow transit time. This prolonged transit time facilitates absorption of fluid, electrolytes, and solutes throughout the intestinal tract. Stimulation of the opioid receptors decreases the secretion of fluid into the small intestine, reducing the frequency, the volume, and the liquid nature of the stools.

Loperamide inhibits peristalsis, prolonging transit time through direct effects on nerves in the intestinal muscle wall. Thus fecal volume is reduced, viscosity and bulk are increased, and the loss of fluid and electrolytes is lessened. Loperamide reduces the volume of discharge from an ileostomy and can be used in the treatment of traveler's diarrhea and the chronic diarrhea associated with inflammatory bowel disease, and pro-vides symptomatic relief of acute nonspecific diarrhea.

The antidiarrheal activity of camphorated tincture of opium is related to the opioid content and thus is available only by pre-scription. **Camphorated tincture of opium is a Schedule III** ⬩

drug containing 0.04% morphine (0.4 mg/mL) and 45% alcohol. Opium tincture is an alcohol-based, Schedule II solution that contains 10% opium by weight. Opium tincture is 25 times more concentrated than camphorated tincture of opium and carries a high potential for abuse.

Camphorated tincture of opium is quickly absorbed from the GI tract, with distribution to parenchymal tissues including the kidneys, the lungs, the liver, and the spleen. Biotransformation occurs in the liver, with approximately 90% of the metabolites eliminated through the kidneys. The remainder is eliminated in the stool.

▒ Pharmacokinetics

Diphenoxylate is well absorbed from the GI tract. Its distribution is unknown. Most of the drug is biotransformed in the liver, with some conversion to an active antidiarrheal metabolite, difenoxin (see Table 46-1).

Loperamide is slowly and incompletely absorbed following oral administration. It crosses the blood-brain barrier relatively slowly. Loperamide is 97% protein bound, undergoing enterohepatic recirculation. It is biotransformed in the liver, with 30% of the drug eliminated in the stool and only minimal elimination in the urine.

Camphorated tincture of opium is well absorbed from the GI tract but undergoes rapid biotransformation, so the effect of oral formulations is less than after parenteral administration.

▒ Adverse Effects and Contraindications

Diphenoxylate's adverse effects are caused by both μ-agonist activity and nonselective muscarinic antagonism. The most common adverse effects of opioid antidiarrheal drugs include constipation and dizziness. Blurred vision, dry mouth and dry eyes, tachycardia, epigastric distress, nausea and vomiting, ileus, drowsiness, headache, insomnia, nervousness, and confusion are also possible. Urinary retention and flushing may also occur.

Although diphenoxylate is effective in the treatment of mild to moderate diarrhea, do not use it in patients with chronic ulcerative colitis, acute bacillary or amebic dysentery, dehydration, narrow-angle glaucoma, or alcohol intolerance, or in children under 2 years of age. Diphenoxylate may potentiate an ulcerating process in the colon and provoke the development of a toxic megacolon. Opioids are contraindicated for patients with drug hypersensitivity, severe liver disease, infectious diarrhea (due to *E. coli, Salmonella,* or *Shigella*), and in diarrhea associated with pseudomembranous colitis *(Clostridium difficile).* **Avoid using diphenoxylate in patients who are dehydrated or who have narrow-angle glaucoma, children younger than 2 years of age, and those with alcohol intolerance.**

The adverse effects of loperamide are fewer than those of diphenoxylate with atropine; drowsiness and constipation are the most common, but dizziness, nausea, and dry mouth also may occur. Loperamide is contraindicated for patients with drug hypersensitivity, abdominal pain of unknown cause (especially if associated with fever), or alcohol intolerance. Use loperamide cautiously in patients with liver disease, during pregnancy and lactation, and in older adults. Opioids should also be used cautiously in patients with inflammatory bowel disease or prostatic hypertrophy, during pregnancy, and in children.

Euphoria, analgesia, or dependence are unlikely to occur with camphorated tincture of opium as long as recommended doses are used for short periods of time. Adverse effects are typically dose-related and include nausea, vomiting, dysphoria, constipation, and increased biliary tract pressure. Large doses can cause dizziness, drowsiness, fainting, flushing, and CNS depression. Anaphylaxis is rare. Patients older than 60 years of age tend to be more sensitive to these drugs than younger patients.

Opium tincture and camphorated tincture of opium are contraindicated for patients with hypersensitivity and in those who have pseudomembranous colitis or severe ulcerative colitis (toxic megacolon may develop). Use the drugs with caution in patients with liver disease or severe prostatic hypertrophy and during pregnancy (Category B), as well as in patients who are prone to opioid dependency.

▒ Drug Interactions

Table 46-2 lists the drug interactions with opioid antidiarrheal drugs. The interactions are similar to those found when the opioid is used for analgesia (see Chapter 16).

▒ Dosage Regimen

Doses of diphenoxylate with atropine are stated in terms of the diphenoxylate content. Each tablet of diphenoxylate with atropine contains 2.5 mg diphenoxylate and 0.025 mg of atropine. The dosage may be decreased as symptoms improve. Use a calibrated measuring device for liquid preparations. Diphenoxylate is a Schedule V controlled drug.

The oral adult dose of loperamide for the treatment of diarrhea is 4 mg initially, then 2 mg after each loose stool up to 16 mg/day. Children's dosages initially range from 1 to 2 mg orally, followed by 1-mg tablets with each loose stool. Depending on the child's weight, the dosage should not exceed 4 to 6 mg/day.

▒ Lab Considerations

Evaluate liver function tests periodically during prolonged therapy with antidiarrheal drugs. Diphenoxylate with atropine may cause increased serum amylase concentrations.

Absorbents

- ◆ activated attapulgite (Kaopectate, Parepectolin, Diar-Aid)
- ◆ bismuth subsalicylate (Pepto-Bismol, Bismatrol, Pink Bismuth)

▒ Indications

Attapulgite is a nonspecific antidiarrheal drug. Although this absorbent clay produces stools with a more normal appearance, fluid loss may remain unchanged, and electrolyte losses may actually increase. The claim that attapulgite facilitates removal of bacterial toxins has not been supported.

Bismuth subsalicylate (BSS) has multiple uses. It is used in the adjunctive treatment of traveler's diarrhea and in treatment of gastritis and peptic ulcer disease associated with *Helicobacter pylori,* and it is sometimes used as a local protectant for the skin. The availability of this relatively inexpensive OTC drug fosters its overuse and increases the potential for toxicity to both the salicylate and bismuth components. Caution patients that the drug may cause tongue and/or stool darkening.

GASTROINTESTINAL

Pharmacodynamics

Attapulgite is thought to act by absorbing bacteria and toxins, thus decreasing water loss by decreasing the number and water content of the stools.

BSS is a relatively insoluble compound and has absorbent, demulcent, astringent, and weak antacid characteristics. Although this mechanism is poorly understood, BSS is broken down in the GI tract to salicylate, which is thought to produce local antiinflammatory actions and thus decrease the synthesis of intestinal prostaglandins. The antibacterial actions of bismuth may contribute to the prevention of traveler's diarrhea.

Pharmacokinetics

Attapulgite acts locally. The pharmacokinetics of distribution, biotransformation, and elimination routes are unknown.

Bismuth is not absorbed; however, the salicylate is hydrolyzed from the parent compound, and 90% is absorbed from the small intestine (Table 46-4). Salicylates are highly bound to plasma proteins, with distribution to the placenta. They also enter breast milk. The salicylate component undergoes significant hepatic biotransformation. The half-life of the salicylate component is 2 to 3 hours at low doses, and 15 to 30 hours for larger doses.

Adverse Effects and Contraindications

The adverse effects of attapulgite are few. It may increase the fecal elimination of sodium and potassium, but the most common adverse effect is constipation.

The adverse effects of BSS include constipation, a gray-black tongue and stools, and tinnitus. It is contraindicated for older adults and debilitated patients who may suffer from bowel impactions, and in patients who are hypersensitive to aspirin. Use cautiously in patients who have diabetes mellitus or gout.

⚠ **The Centers for Disease Control and Prevention (CDC) recommends that BSS not be used in children or teenagers during or after recovery from chickenpox (varicella) or flu-like illnesses because of the association of salicylates with Reye's syndrome.** Because bismuth is radiopaque, it is generally not used in patients who will be undergoing radiologic examination of the GI tract. Safe use for infants or during pregnancy and lactation has not been established.

Drug Interactions

Much like BSS, attapulgite decreases the GI absorption of concurrently administered drugs. Administer other drugs 2 to 3 hours before or 2 to 4 hours after taking attapulgite.

BSS taken concurrently with aspirin may potentiate salicylate toxicity (see Chapter 17). It decreases the absorption of tetracycline antibiotics or enoxacin (chewable tablets only).

⚠ **Large dosages of BSS may increase the risk of bleeding in the presence of thrombolytics, warfarin, or heparin.** For example, a 2-oz dose of bismuth salts produces the same salicylate blood level as one 5-grain aspirin tablet. Large doses also increase the risk of hypoglycemia from insulin or oral hypoglycemics, and may decrease the effectiveness of probenecid.

Dosage Regimen

Table 46-3 identifies the usual dosing regimens for absorbent laxatives.

Lab Considerations

Chronic high doses of BSS may cause false-positive urine glucose tests (using copper sulfate methods), false-negative test results with enzymatic glucose tests, and falsely increased uric acid levels. It can also cause alterations in vanillylmandelic acid concentrations and liver function tests. It decreases serum potassium and triiodothyronine (T_3 and T_4) concentrations, and elevates the international normalized ratio (INR) times.

Miscellaneous Antidiarrheal Drugs

◆ belladonna alkaloids (Donnagel)
◆ lactobacillus acidophilus (Lactinex, Bacid)
◆ octreotide (Sandostatin); ✦ Sandostatin, Sandostatin LAR

Belladonna Alkaloids

Belladonna alkaloids are classified as anticholinergic drugs and include atropine and hyoscyamine. However, there is no conclusive evidence that drugs in this class are effective in the treatment of diarrhea. They do, however, prevent the spasms and cramping frequently associated with acute or chronic diarrhea when given in a sufficient dose.

A single 30-mL dose of a belladonna alkaloid formulation contains a combination of kaolin and pectin, atropine, hyoscyamine, scopolamine hydrobromide, and alcohol. Because of the multiple ingredients in these products, the patient is at risk for combined adverse effects and added expense. Single-ingredient drugs are recommended to control specific symptoms. Belladonna is contraindicated for patients with narrow-angle glaucoma and intestinal obstruction because of the addition of atropine and hyoscyamine. It is given cautiously in patients with urinary tract obstruction because of its ability to cause obstruction uropathy. Patients with respiratory or cardiac disease may experience tachycardia.

Lactobacillus Acidophilus and Lactobacillus Bulgaricus

Lactobacillus acidophilus and *Lactobacillus bulgaricus* are OTC products thought to promote the growth of normal intestinal flora, particularly *E. coli*. There is also the notion that increased dietary intake of products containing lactobacillus as well as lactose and dextrose (e.g., milk, buttermilk, yogurt) are all equally effective in recolonizing the intestine. However, recent research has suggested that adjustments in dietary intake may be more effective than ingestion of the actual lactobacillus organism.

Octreotide

Octreotide is identical to the natural hormone somatostatin and is used most often in the treatment of acromegaly (see Chapter 55). It also is used in the treatment of vasoactive intestinal peptide (VIP)–oma-associated diarrhea, for symptoms of carcinoid tumors, in the acute treatment of carcinoid crisis, and for secretory diarrhea. It is described as a universal inhibitor of secretory cells, acting to increase absorption of fluid and electrolytes from the GI tract and decrease transit time. It has been used as an investigational drug to control severe, refractory diarrhea. Refractory diarrhea may occur with dumping syndrome, severe enterotoxic infections, short-gut syndrome, graft-versus-host disease, and acquired immunodeficiency syndrome (AIDS).

Octreotide acetate is a cyclic octapeptide drug that inhibits growth hormone, glucagon, and insulin more effectively than the natural hormone, somatostatin. Its suppression of luteinizing hormone's (LH's) response to gonadotropin-releasing hormone (GnRH) and inhibition of the release of serotonin, gastrin, vasoactive intestinal peptide (VIP), secretin, motilin, and pancreatic polypeptide are similar to somatostatin's actions. The drug also reduces growth hormone and/or insulin-like growth factor I (IGF-I; somatomedin C) in acromegaly, inhibits gallbladder contractions, reduces bile secretion, and suppresses the secretion of thyroid-stimulating hormone (TSH).

Octreotide is administered subcutaneously, with a time to peak concentration of minutes. It is about 65% protein bound, with an elimination half-life of 1.7 hours, although the half-life may be increased by 46% in older adults.

Common adverse effects of octreotide include transient nausea, diarrhea, abdominal cramping, and fat malabsorption. Headache, drowsiness, dizziness, fatigue, and weakness have been reported. Palpitations and orthostatic hypotension are possible. Gallstones may develop because octreotide decreases the emptying of the gallbladder. It also alters the secretion of insulin and glucagon, leading to hyperglycemia or hypoglycemia.

CLINICAL REASONING

Treatment Objectives

The loss of fluid and electrolytes as well as stool that characterizes diarrhea is an important aspect of many infectious and noninfectious GI disorders. Although acute-onset diarrhea is most often of infectious origin, it is usually self-limiting, and specific drug therapy is seldom warranted. Thus treatment objectives for the patient with acute diarrhea include the maintenance of adequate hydration and skin integrity, with the limited use of select antidiarrheal drugs. Treatment objectives for the patient with chronic diarrhea include treating the underlying cause of the diarrhea, then reestablishing bowel patterns.

Treatment Options

▦ *Patient Variables*

The American culture is very bathroom-oriented. Status, and even assessed valuation of a house for tax purposes, is determined by the number of bathrooms per household. Indeed, persons from foreign countries have totally different experiences with toilet facilities. Nevertheless, toileting is a private activity for most people, taking place behind closed doors. During illness or hospitalization, this formerly private activity suddenly may be exposed for all to view and discuss, and perhaps even worse, for others to smell.

As with the patient with constipation, ask the patient complaining of diarrhea about usual and current elimination patterns including information about the frequency, consistency, size, and color of the stools. Explore related symptoms such as abdominal pain and flatulence, onset and duration of the problem, and any precipitating, aggravating, or mitigating factors. Some patients describe themselves as having diarrhea if they have more than one stool per day regardless of the consistency. Alternating periods of constipation and diarrhea

are not unusual with irritable bowel syndrome. Systemic manifestations of acute diarrhea include fever, nausea, vomiting, and malaise.

Pertinent lifestyle factors to assess for the patient with diarrhea include usual activities, the usual elimination patterns, occupation, type and frequency of exercise, stress level, and dietary habits. A sexual history is important when the patient complains of diarrhea because in males it may be a manifestation of gay bowel syndrome. Determine if there has been an increase in the consumption of laxative-like foods such as bran, lactose, sorbitol, fructose, brassica vegetables (e.g., broccoli, cabbage), coffee, or tea. Has the patient had unexplained weight loss or been exposed to carriers of enteric infection? Has the patient consumed potentially contaminated food or water or traveled recently? Often there is a history of eating raw seafood or shellfish. Patients may report eating in restaurants or fast-food restaurants, attending a picnic or banquet, or having been in close contact with ill children or family members.

It is important to ask about use of laxatives, magnesium-containing antacids, excess alcohol, caffeine-containing beverages, and herbal teas. Note also if the patient has recently taken antibiotics, digitalis, quinidine, loop diuretics, or antihypertensive drugs.

Perform a urinalysis for all patients with diarrhea; it may reveal early dehydration. Stool examination includes the size, shape, consistency, color, and odor, as well as the presence or absence of blood, mucus, pus, tissue fragments, food residues, bacteria, or parasites. Alterations in the size or shape of the stool indicate altered motility or abnormalities in the colonic wall. Assess the gross appearance of the stool before administration of barium or antidiarrheal drugs.

LIFE-SPAN CONSIDERATIONS

Pregnant and Nursing Women. Diarrhea during pregnancy mirrors the range of GI disease in the population. Ordinarily, gastroenteritis in pregnancy does not pose significant risk to the fetus if maternal hydration is maintained. Most infections (viral, bacterial, or parasitic) tend to be localized to the bowel mucosa and do not present a risk for infection of the fetus. Diarrhea during pregnancy usually resolves in several days without antibiotic therapy; consider antibiotics for severe infections. Use of opioids, which cause CNS depression, is particularly undesirable. Avoid BSS because of the salicylate component and the potential for bleeding (see Case Study).

Children and Adolescents. Over 500 million children worldwide suffer from diarrhea each year. Acute diarrhea is the leading cause of illness in children under 5 years of age. Dehydration, electrolyte disturbances, and the malnutrition that diarrhea causes are fatal in approximately 400 children each year in the United States. Diarrhea occurs more often when there is overcrowding, substandard sanitation, inadequate facilities for preparation and refrigeration of food, and generally inadequate health care education.

As a general rule, the younger the child, the greater the susceptibility, and the more severe the diarrhea. The frequency of diarrhea in infancy is closely related to the ingestion of contaminated milk. There is a lower incidence of diarrhea in breastfed infants. Most cases of diarrhea in children are caused by bacterial, viral, or parasitic pathogens. Rotovirus is very common in day care situations. Simple teething can be a source of limited acute diarrhea. Malnutrition contributes

CASE STUDY Laxatives

ASSESSMENT

History of Present Illness	SB is a 26-year-old G_1 P_0 at 28 weeks' gestation who comes to the OB clinic today with complaints of constipation. Her last BM was 3 days ago, and it was hard and dry. She ordinarily has one soft, formed bowel movement a day. She acknowledges not drinking enough fluids and eating primarily carbohydrates, "fast-food stuff. It's quick and easy." Her activity level has declined since it started snowing. She is afraid of falling and so has given up her daily walk. She takes a daily prenatal vitamin with iron, but she thinks the iron in her vitamins is contributing to her constipation and adding to her hemorrhoidal discomfort.
Past Health History	SB's past health history is unremarkable. She had an appendectomy at age 13 and an episode of mononucleosis at age 18.
Life-Span Considerations	Constipation for SB is related to a combination of issues: intestinal smooth muscle relaxation associated with progesterone secretion, mechanical compression of the bowel by an enlarging uterus, and the effects of iron supplements and inactivity.
Psychosocial Considerations	SB has become less active with the approach of winter and advancing gestation. SB reports that her husband is excited about the pregnancy but is worried about SB's increasing constipation. SB and her husband carry health insurance that covers perinatal care and pharmacy needs.
Physical Exam Findings	VS WNL. Skin pink and warm. Mucous membranes moist. Abdominal exam reveals 28-week pregnancy. Rectal exam reveals several small, external hemorrhoids, other wise unremarkable. Stool heme negative.
Diagnostic Testing	Serum electrolytes, hemoglobin, hematocrit, and thyroid functions WNL.

DIAGNOSIS: Constipation in Pregnancy

MANAGEMENT

Treatment Objectives	Reestablish regular, comfortable stooling that empties rectum, using the least number of drugs in the lowest dosage possible for the shortest duration of time.
Treatment Plan	**Pharmacotherapy** • psyllium 2 to 3 tsp in a full glass of water twice daily; follow with another full glass of water • docusate calcium 240 mg PO once daily **Patient Education** 1. Increase fluid intake to 64 oz or more daily. 2. Increase fiber in diet to at least 20 grams daily in the form of whole grains, fruits, and vegetables. 3. Increase activity within the home; consider going to a shopping mall to walk. 4. Continue prenatal vitamin despite constipation. **Evaluation** Regular, comfortable stooling that empties rectum has been reestablished using non–drug therapies and least number of drugs in the lowest dosage possible for the shortest duration of time.

CLINICAL REASONING ANALYSIS

Q1. Why did you choose ducosate calcium and psyllium rather than castor oil or mineral oil?

A. Bulk-forming laxatives and stool softeners are acceptable in the treatment of constipation during pregnancy because they are not absorbed systemically. Castor oil is an FDA category X drug, and it can cause uterine contractions. Mineral oil, a category C drug, interferes with absorption of nutrients needed for fetal growth.

Q2. But isn't diarrhea an adverse effect of stool softeners?

A. The most common adverse effect of stool softeners is indeed diarrhea. Bulk-forming laxatives may offset that, and they do not hinder absorption of nutrients. There are no absolute contraindications to the use of stool softeners or bulk-forming laxatives during pregnancy.

Q3. Stimulant laxatives are used for constipation associated with prolonged inactivity, constipating drugs such as her prenatal vitamins, and slowed transit times. SB has all of these. Wouldn't a stimulant laxative be even better? How about senna–I heard it's a natural laxative?

A. Stimulant laxatives act on the intestinal wall of the small bowel and the colon to increase fluids and electrolytes within the intestinal lumen. Continued use of these laxatives produces an irritable bowel syndrome–like diarrhea that can be severe enough to cause significant fluid and electrolyte imbalances. The imbalances place both mother and fetus at risk for complications. Senna is a category C drug.

to the severity and may be a consequence of diarrheal disease due to reduced dietary intake, malabsorption, or the catabolic response to infection. Because a child's metabolic rate is higher than an adult's, the child is predisposed to a more rapid depletion of nutritional reserves. Metabolic acidosis can result from severe diarrhea and dehydration.

Older Adults. The causes of diarrhea in older adults are not unlike those of diarrhea in other age groups. Fifteen percent of diarrhea in older adults is related to infection, with 19% of the cases caused by bacterial infection, 68% by viral infections, and 3% by parasitic infections. Fecal impaction accounts for 16% of cases of diarrhea, antibiotic use for 11%, laxative abuse for 6%, and inflammatory bowel disease for 4%. Impaction may be mistaken for diarrhea because liquid stool comes around the impaction and is eliminated frequently. Dietary indiscretions (e.g., too much fruit, especially bananas) and hyperosmolar tube feedings, protein-calorie malnutrition and anxiety are also culprits in older ▲ adults. **Mortality increases dramatically in patients with severe diarrhea who are over age 74 years**. Dehydration is less likely to occur in a middle-aged group than in young children and older adults.

▦ Drug Variables

▲   **The therapeutic effects of antidiarrheal drugs do not alleviate the underlying cause of the diarrhea**. These drugs only reduce the interference with daily activities that the diarrhea causes. The mainstay of nonspecific prescription drug therapy for diarrhea continues to be the opioids such as loperamide. This drug reduces the amount of fluid present in the colon, primarily by slowing transit time and thus promoting reabsorption of water and electrolytes. Loperamide is ordinarily well tolerated and has few drug interactions. Do warn patients, however, about the potential for drowsiness. Further, loperamide does not eliminate the need for fluids and electrolytes, and should be avoided in patients with high fever, bloody stools, liver failure, and antibiotic-associated pseudomembranous colitis.

For patients unable to tolerate loperamide, an absorbent such as BSS, or an antisecretory drug, may be used. BSS provides substantial relief in mild to moderate diarrhea and is useful in the prophylaxis of traveler's diarrhea caused by ▲ a variety of infectious organisms. **However, use BSS with caution in patients taking warfarin, and do not use the drug in children or adolescents who have a viral illness or in patients with a documented hypersensitivity to salicylates.**

Diphenoxylate and camphorated tincture of opium are Schedule V drugs with a potential for abuse and as such ▲ are restricted to third-line therapy for diarrhea. Further, **the atropine component of diphenoxylate-atropine combination can cause significant anticholinergic adverse effects in some patients and exacerbate certain comorbid conditions.** Exercise caution when using combination drugs such as diphenoxylate with atropine in older adults who have glaucoma or prostatic hypertrophy.

Antidiarrheal drugs have limited value in children, primarily because of concerns about possible toxicity. And although pediatric dosages are identified for diphenoxylate with atropine and loperamide, the World Health Organization does not recommend giving either of these drugs to

children. **The CDC and the American Academy of Pediat-** ▲ **rics (AAP) recommends that oral fluid and electrolyte replacement therapy be used as the treatment of choice for most cases of diarrhea-caused dehydration** (CDC, 2006; AAP, 2007).

Patient Education

Most acute diarrhea is self-limiting, and although an otherwise healthy adult may not be harmed by dietary abstinence during an episode of mild to moderate diarrhea, the ingestion of soft, easily digested foods and the oral administration of solutions containing electrolytes, glucose, and amino acids usually suffices. In some cases, parenteral fluids may be needed to achieve adequate hydration.

After diarrhea is relieved, it is usually best to have the patient avoid milk and dairy products for another 7 to 10 days because mild lactose intolerance commonly accompanies many cases of diarrhea. Begin with bananas, rice, applesauce, tea, and toast (BRATT) and an electrolyte-rich drink diet, and slowly progress to a normal diet. Continued replacement of fluids is important.

Many people think that taking fluids will worsen their diarrhea; therefore they request opiates. Discuss the proper role of these drugs. Educate the patient as to the role of antibiotics and the emergence of resistant bacterial strains, the potential complications of antibiotic use, and the efficacy of antidiarrheal preparations.

When prescribing opioid antidiarrheal drugs, caution patients to take the drug exactly as directed and to avoid using alcohol or taking other CNS depressants concurrently. Avoid taking more than the prescribed amount because of the habit-forming potential and, in children, the risk of overdose. If the patient is on a scheduled dosing regimen, missed doses should be taken as soon as possible. Double doses should be avoided. Advise patients to avoid driving or other activities that require alertness until response to the drug is known. Instruct the patient to notify the health care provider if diarrhea persists or if fever, abdominal pain, or abdominal distention occurs.

Perianal discomfort associated with diarrhea can be relieved by washing with warm water or absorbent cotton after each stool in lieu of using irritating toilet paper. Avoiding soap decreases perianal irritation. A short course of hydrocortisone cream may be useful when there is considerable perianal irritation. Some patients report that cleansing gently with cotton pads soaked in witch hazel (Tucks) provides considerable relief.

Evaluation

The therapeutic outcome of antidiarrheal treatment is relief of diarrhea. Treatment effectiveness is noted by the return to normal bowel function and absence of abdominal cramping, flatulence, and other discomforts associated with diarrhea. However, if symptoms of acute diarrhea continue, fever persists, or blood or mucus appears in the stool, discontinue antidiarrheals and reevaluate the patient. Patients unable to maintain oral hydration or who have become significantly volume-depleted (as evidenced by postural hypotension) require serious consideration for parenteral fluid replacement or possible hospital admission.

GASTROINTESTINAL

Controversy

Pepto-Bismol, Loperamide, and Diarrhea

Jonathan J. Wolfe

Diarrhea has compelling characteristics that no patient can ignore. The definition may vary among patients. In some, it is represented by a greater than normal number of bowel movements, and in others, it may be the passage of ill-formed or liquid stools. Close definition may not matter much because diarrhea is usually self-limiting. Because the problem is acute and understandable, the patient is likely to manage it without medical consultation.

Not all diarrhea, however, is benign. In some cases, diarrhea is caused by overuse of laxatives. Many patients express concern if a daily evacuation does not occur. However, reliance on stimulant laxatives to promote daily regularity may prove harmful, particularly in an older, inactive patient with small dietary intake. Diarrhea also may be a symptom of disease. If it does not subside shortly but persists, use of antidiarrheals is inappropriate. Over-the-counter (OTC) products are intended to treat only uncomplicated minor disorders. Finally, diarrhea in both the very young and the very old can have severe consequences. Dehydration and loss of electrolytes may quickly progress to life-threatening levels.

Many OTC antidiarrheals are available. The simplest are absorbent products like pectin. These drugs take up excess water in the lumen of the large intestine, minimizing watery stools. Bismuth salts are very popular for both indigestion and diarrhea are but not for prolonged use. Finally, opioid derivatives such as loperamide may be used. Their temporary effect on opioid receptors in the bowel wall is effective, but again these drugs are only appropriate for short-term use.

The choice of an antidiarrheal is too often made on the basis of trade name or price. Even trade names are not foolproof. For instance, loperamide is present in Imodium A-D Caplets, Kaopectate II Caplets, and Maalox Antidiarrheal Caplets, as well as in the liquid Pepto Diarrhea Control. The customer accustomed to these trade names may well think that he or she is purchasing a known and relatively innocuous product, when in fact loperamide is the active ingredient.

CRITICAL REASONING ANALYSIS

- What groups of patients are at risk and need to be evaluated promptly when diarrhea occurs?
- Do you experience personal difficulties when discussing diarrhea with a patient? Does this problem vary when the patient is younger than you, or older, or of a different cultural background?
- How may a patient characterize a present episode of diarrhea? What important factors may she not tell you at first?
- Why is persistent diarrhea in an older adult who is taking digoxin or warfarin a critical matter?
- What concerns would you have if a patient on intravenous total parenteral nutrition (TPN) reports a sudden occurrence of diarrhea? What if the flow is from an ileostomy rather than from the rectum?
- What concerns would you have if a patient being treated with gentamicin experienced a sudden onset of profuse watery diarrhea flecked with matter that looks like mucosa?

KEY POINTS

- Constipation is the most frequent GI problem encountered in ambulatory care settings and is most often caused by inadequate fluid and fiber intake, lack of exercise, busy schedules with no established elimination patterns, excessive use of laxatives, and the use of certain other drugs.
- The fundamental mechanism of constipation involves the decreased transit time of stool through the colon, along with increased reabsorption of fluid.
- Patient assessment should include information about the patient's usual elimination patterns, activity levels, concomitant disease, and drug use.
- The primary treatment goal for constipation is to reestablish a normal pattern of bowel functioning and to effect comfortable elimination of the stool, using the least number of drugs in the lowest dosages for the shortest duration of time.
- Drugs used to treat or manage constipation include one or more of the following: stimulants, stool softeners, bulk-forming laxatives, osmotics, and a few miscellaneous drugs.
- Oil-based laxatives should not be given to bedridden patients or children because of the possibility of lipid pneumonia should the patient aspirate.
- Clinical response to treatment for constipation is demonstrated by the passage of a soft, formed bowel movement, usually within 12 to 24 hours. However, normal bowel patterns are individually determined, and the frequency of evacuation may vary from 3 times a day to 3 times weekly.

- Diarrhea is a symptom of an underlying disorder and affects most people at some point during their lifetime. It can be caused by bacterial, viral, or parasitic infestation. An important cause of diarrhea is the concealed use of stimulant laxatives.
- Diarrhea results from any factor that decreases fluid absorption in the bowel, increases fluid secretion, or alters bowel motility.
- The primary treatment goal for diarrhea is to reestablish a normal pattern of bowel functioning using the least number of drugs in the owest dosages for the shortest duration of time.
- The mainstay of nonspecific drug therapy for diarrhea continues to be opioids. Bismuth subsalicylate has been used to prevent traveler's diarrhea with some success.
- Miscellaneous remedies for diarrhea include the belladonna alkaloids, *L. acidophilus,* and octreotide, although these drugs are not considered first-line agents.
- Care of the patient with diarrhea is also directed toward relieving fluid and electrolyte imbalances, perianal irritation, and reoccurrence of the diarrhea.
- Treatment effectiveness of antidiarrheal drugs is noted by a return to normal bowel patterns, and the absence of abdominal cramping, flatulence, and other discomforts associated with diarrhea.

Bibliography

American Academy of Pediatrics (AAP). (2007). *Treating diarrhea and dehydration*. Available online:www.aap.org/pubed/ZZZA-HYUYQ7C.htm?&sub_cat=107. Accessed May 20, 2007.

Brandt, L., Schoenfeld, P., Prather, C., et al. (2005). An evidence-based approach to the management of chronic constipation in North America. *American Journal of Gastroenterology, 100*(Suppl 1), S1S4.

Camilleri, M. (2003). Chronic constipation. *The New England Journal of Medicine, 349*(14), 1360–1368.

Centers for Disease Control (CDC) and Prevention. Division of Parasitic Diseases. (2006). *Fact Sheet: Diarrhea*. Atlanta: Author.

Gilbert, D., Moellering, R., Jr. Eliopoulos, G., et al. (2007). *The Sanford guide to antimicrobial therapy*. (37th ed.). Hyde Park, VT: Antimicrobial Therapy, Inc.

Gutierrez, K., and Queener, S. (2004). *Pharmacology for nursing practice*. Philadelphia: Mosby.

Hardman, J., Limbird, L., and Gilman, A. (Eds.). (2001). *Goodman and Gilman's the pharmacologic basis of therapeutics*. (10th ed.). New York: McGraw-Hill.

Hsieh, C. (2005). Treatment of constipation in older adults. *American Family Physician, 72*(11), 2277–2285.

Katzung, B. (2005). *Basic and clinical pharmacology*. (9th ed.). New York: Lange Medical Books.

McCance, K., and Huether, S. (2002). *Pathophysiology: The biologic basis for disease in adults and children*. (4th ed). St. Louis: Mosby.

National Digestive Diseases Information Clearinghouse (NDDIC). (2003). *Diarrhea*. Bethesda, MD: Author.

GASTROINTESTINAL

47

Antiemetics and Related Drugs

Nausea and vomiting is a commonly experienced phenomenon. *Nausea* is defined as an unpleasant sensation of impending vomiting. *Vomiting* is the forceful expulsion of stomach contents through the mouth. The severity can range from a slight queasiness to uncontrollable vomiting. The causes of nausea and vomiting include a great many stimuli that range from overindulgence in rich and abundant food and drink to drugs, toxins, inflammation or infection, vestibular disorders, pregnancy, psychogenic issues, and metabolic derangements. Treatment goals for the patient with nausea and vomiting include preventing or relieving symptoms associated with the emetogenic event. Treating the nausea and vomiting helps avoid potentially life-threatening complications such as dehydration, electrolyte imbalances, and malnutrition.

NAUSEA AND VOMITING

EPIDEMIOLOGY AND ETIOLOGY

There are many causes of nausea and vomiting, but the most common stem from ingestion of drugs, alcohol intake, GI upset, neurologic processes, and metabolic disorders. Although nausea and vomiting may occur with any drug, it is commonly associated with alcohol, aspirin, opioids, some antibiotics, cardiac glycosides, antineoplastic therapy, and theophylline drugs. Table 47-1 provides an overview of the most common causes of nausea and vomiting.

Sporadic cases of nausea and vomiting are fairly common, but epidemic occurrences suggest environmental exposure to viral or bacterial infections or food poisoning (e.g., staphylococcal enterotoxin). Sensory experiences that may induce nausea and vomiting include pungent odors or gruesome events.

PATHOPHYSIOLOGY

Vomiting is a complex, reflexive pathologic process under central nervous system (CNS) control and involves modulation of medullary sites and neurotransmitters. The vomiting center in the lateral reticular formation of the medulla receives stimulation from the sympathetic nervous system, the cerebral cortex, the limbic system, the vestibular system or the chemoreceptor trigger zone (CTZ). Distention of the stretch receptors from motility disorders or obstruction in the stomach, the duodenum, the colon, or the biliary tract sends impulses to the vomiting center via the peripheral afferent neurons of the vagus nerve (Fig. 47-1). Irritation, inflammation, or cardiac or gastrointestinal (GI) tract ischemia can stimulate the vomiting center. Vestibular dysfunction sends impulses to the vomiting center by way of vestibular nerve connections.

The CTZ is rich in dopamine, opiate, and serotonin receptors. It is stimulated by metabolic derangements (e.g., electrolyte disorders, diabetic ketoacidosis, uremia), drugs (e.g., glycosides, antineoplastics, opiates), and toxins circulating in the blood and cerebral spinal fluid. When stimulated, the vomiting center sends an efferent impulse that initiates a cascade of events. The glottis closes, the diaphragm and abdominal muscles contract, the gastroesophageal sphincter relaxes, and reverse peristalsis moves stomach contents upward toward the mouth for expulsion.

PHARMACOTHERAPEUTIC OPTIONS

Drugs used in the management of nausea and vomiting are in several different classifications, including antihistamines, phenothiazines, prokinetic drugs, cannabinoids, serotonin antagonists, and a variety of miscellaneous agents. Benzodiazepines and corticosteroids are also used in the management of nausea and vomiting. Most of the antiemetic drugs produce anticholinergic and antidopaminergic effects.

Antihistamines
- cyclizine (Marezine)
- dimenhydrinate (Dramamine); ♣ Gravol
- diphenhydramine (Benadryl); ♣ Apo-Dimenhydrate, Benadryl, Buckley's Jack and Jill's Bedtime, Gravel, Nytol, Sleep-Ez D
- hydroxyzine (Vistaril, Atarax); ♣ Apo-Hydroxyzine, Atarax
- meclizine (Antivert, Bonine); ♣ Bonamine, Antivert

▥ Indications
Antihistamines are used most often in the management of the nausea and vomiting associated with vestibular disturbances such as motion sickness. In addition, antihistamines such as diphenhydramine are used in the management of allergic reactions, insomnia, parkinson-like reactions, and some nonallergic conditions. Antihistamine use for patients with allergies, including rhinitis, urticaria, and angioedema, is discussed in Chapter 51.

▥ Pharmacodynamics
Antihistamines suppress nausea and vomiting through their ability to interrupt visceral afferent pathways responsible for stimulating nausea and vomiting. Not all antihistamines are effective as antiemetics, however. There is no correlation between their ability to prevent motion sickness and their potency as antihistamines or anticholinergics. Nevertheless, the mechanism by which they suppress motion sickness is unclear.

▥ Pharmacokinetics
Table 47-2 illustrates the pharmacokinetics of the various antihistamines. The antihistamines are well absorbed orally, with onset times of 15 to 60 minutes. Peak activity occurs in

TABLE **47-1 Causes of Nausea and Vomiting**

Category	Drugs and Disorders
Drugs	aspirin, Nonsteroidal antiinflammatory drugs (NSAIDs), Opioids
	Antineoplastic drugs (e.g., cisplatin, carboplatin, cyclophosphamide)
	digoxin, quinidine
	erythromycin, tetracycline, nitrofurantoin
	levodopa, lithium, phenytoin
	theophylline, bromocriptine
	Hormonal therapies
Gastrointestinal	Achalasia, cholecystitis, gastric outlet obstruction, gastroparesis, gastric stasis, irritable bowel syndrome, hepatitis, after gastric surgery, incarcerated hernia, small bowel obstruction, pancreatic disease, pyelonephritis, volvulus
Metabolic	Adrenal insufficiency, diabetic ketoacidosis, electrolyte imbalances
	hypercalcemia, pregnancy, thyrotoxicosis, uremia, water intoxication
Neurologic	Cerebellar hemorrhage, drug withdrawal, increased intracranial pressure, migraine, head trauma, severe hypertension
Psychogenic	Anorexia nervosa, physical or sexual abuse, posttraumatic stress disorder, unpleasant sights or sounds, pain; anticipatory nausea and vomiting
Toxins	Staphylococcal enterotoxin
Vestibular disorders	Labyrinthitis, Meniere's disease, motion sickness, benign positional vertigo

1 to 4 hours with a 3- to 8-hour duration. The protein binding capacity of the majority of the drugs is unknown. Half-lives vary from 2 to 7 hours. Biotransformation occurs in the liver, with elimination via the urine.

▌ *Adverse Effects and Contraindications*

The most significant adverse effect of antihistamines is sedation. Anticholinergic adverse effects include dry mouth, blurred vision, and urinary retention. Antihistamines are contraindicated for use in patients with known hypersensitivity or narrow-angle glaucoma, and in premature or newborn infants. Older adults are more susceptible to the drug's anticholinergic effects. Use these drugs cautiously in patients with cardiovascular disease, thyroid and liver disease, pyloric obstruction, and benign prostatic hyperplasia.

▌ *Drug Interactions*

There are several drug interactions with antihistamines (Table 47-3). Additive sedation can occur with the concurrent use of alcohol, antidepressants, opioids, and sedative-hypnotics; monoamine oxidase (MAO) inhibitors intensify and extend the anticholinergic effects of antihistamines. Erythromycin, clarithromycin, ketoconazole, and itraconazole can increase the risk of serious arrhythmias with prolonged QT intervals.

GASTROINTESTINAL

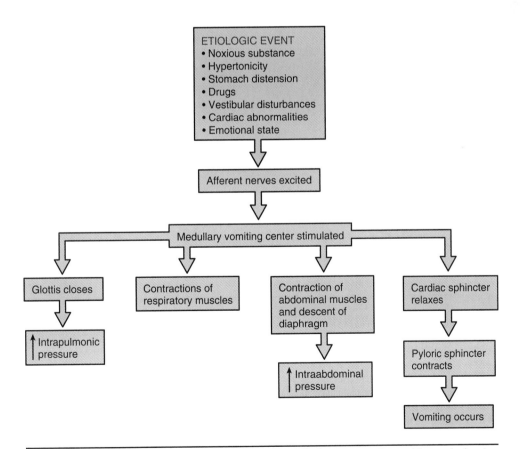

FIGURE 47-1 The vomiting center receives input from the sympathetic nervous system and the cerebral cortex, the limbic and vestibular systems, and the chemoreceptor trigger zone (CTZ). Distention of the stomach, the duodenum, the colon, or the biliary ducts sends impulses to the vomiting center via the peripheral afferent of the vagus nerve.

PHARMACOKINETICS

TABLE **47-2** Selected Antiemetic Drugs

Drug	Route	Onset	Peak	Duration	PB (%)	$t_{1/2}$
ANTIHISTAMINES						
cyclizine	PO	UA	UA	4–6 hr	UA	UA
dimenhydrinate	PO	15–60 min	1–2 hr	3–6 hr	UA	UA
	PO, ER	UA	UA	To 12 hr		
	IM	20–30 min	1–2 hr	3–6 hr		
	IV	Rapid	UA	3–6 hr		
diphenhydramine	PO	15–60 min	1–4 hr	4–8 hr	98–99	2.4–7 hr
	IM	20–30 min	1–4 hr	4–8 hr		
	IV	Rapid	UA	4–8 hr		
hydroxyzine	PO, IM	15–30 min	2–4 hr	4–6 hr	UA	3 hr
meclizine	PO	60 min	UA	8–24 hr	UA	6 hr
SEROTONIN ANTAGONISTS						
dolasetron	IV	Rapid	10 min	UA	69–77	7.3 hr
granisetron	PO	Rapid	60 min	To 12 hr	UA	0.9–31 hr*
	IV	Rapid	30 min	To 24 hr	UA	0.9–31 hr*
ondansetron	PO, IV	Rapid	15–30 min	4 hr	70–76	3.5–5.5 hr
palonosetron	IV	Rapid	Dose-related	UA	62	40 hr
PHENOTHIAZINES						
chlorpromazine	PO, ER	30–60 min	UA	4–6 hr; 10–12 hr†	>90	30 hr
	PR	1–2 hr	UA	3–4 hr		
	IM	UA	UA	4–8 hr		
	IV	Rapid	UA	UA		
prochlorperazine	PO, ER	30–40 min	UA	10–12 hr	>90	UA
	PR	60 min	UA	3–4 hr		
	IM	10–20 min	10–30 min	3–4 hr		
	IV	Rapid	10–30 min	3–4 hr		
promethazine	PO, PR, IM	10 min	UA	12 hr	65–90	UA
	IV	3–5 min	UA	12 hr		
thiethylperazine	PO	30 min	UA	UA	UA	UA
	IM, PR	UA	UA	UA	UA	UA
PROKINETIC DRUGS						
metoclopramide	PO	30–60 min	UA	1–2 hr	30	2.5–5 hr
	IM	10–15 min	UA	1–2 hr		
	IV	1–3 min	Immed	1–2 hr		
CANNABINOIDS						
dronabinol	PO	UA	2 hr	4–6 hr	97–99	25–36 hr
MISCELLANEOUS						
aprepitant	PO	Slow	4 hr	UA	95	9–13 hr
benzquinamide	IM	15 min	30 min	3–4 min	58	30–40 min
droperidol	IM, IV	3–10 min	30 min	2–4 hr‡	UA	2.2 hr
trimethobenzamide	PO	30–50 min	UA	3–4 hr	UA	UA
	PR	10–40 min	UA	3–4 hr		
	IM	15–35 min	UA	2–3 hr		
scopolamine	PO, IM, subQ	30 min	60 min	4–6 hr	Low	8 hr
	Patch	4 hr	UA	72 hr		

*The half–life of granisetron in patients with cancer is 8–9 hr, with a range of 0.9–31.1 hr; in healthy individuals, the half-life is 4.9 hr, with a range of 0.9 hr.
†Duration of the extended-release formulation of chlorpromazine.
‡Droperidol listed duration of tranquilization effects; alterations in consciousness may last up to 12 hr.
ER, Extended-release formulation; *IM*, intramuscular (route); *Immed*, immediate; *IV*, intravenous (route); *PB*, protein binding; *PO*, by mouth; *PR*, per rectum; subQ, subcutaneous (route); $t_{1/2}$, half-life; *UA*, unavailable.

▥ *Dosage Regimen*

The dosage regimens for antihistamines used to treat nausea and vomiting are identified in Table 47-4. A single dose is often all that is required when used in the management of motion sickness, although dosing 3 to 4 times a day may be necessary. For motion sickness, the antihistamine should be taken 1 to 2 hours in advance of the activity.

▥ *Lab Considerations*

Skin testing results for allergies may be falsely negative in patients taking dimenhydrate, diphenhydramine, and meclizine at the time of testing. Discontinue dimenhydrinate 72 hours before any skin testing; discontinue diphenhydramine 4 days before testing.

Serotonin Antagonists

- ◆ dolasetron (Anzemet); ♣ Anzemet
- ◆ granisetron (Kytril); ♣ Kytril
- ◆ ondansetron (Zofran); ♣ ondansetron, Zofran
- ◆ palonosetron (Aloxi)

▥ *Indications*

Serotonin antagonists are the most potent agents for the management of nausea and vomiting. The four drugs in this

DRUG INTERACTIONS
TABLE **47-3** Selected Antiemetics

Drug	Interactive Drugs	Interaction
ANTIHISTAMINES		
cyclizine, dimenhydrinate, diphenhydramine, hydroxyzine	Alcohol, Antihistamines, Opioids, Sedative-hypnotics	Additive CNS depression
Antihistamines in general	MAO inhibitors	Prolongs action and anticholinergic effects of antihistamine
Antihistamines in general	erythromycin, clarithromycin, ketoconazole, itraconazole	Increases risk for QT prolongation
PHENOTHIAZINES		
chlorpromazine, prochlorperazine	Alcohol, Nitrates	Additive hypotension
promethazine	acetaminophen-propoxyphene, amiodarone, apomorphine, class 1A antiarrhythmics, dofetilide, dolasetron, duloxetine, ephedra, fluoxetine, olanzapine, ibutilide, imatinib, lopinavir-rotinavir, Macrolides, palonsetron, pimozide, pindolol, propafenone, propranolol, Quinolones, solifenacin, sotalol, SSRIs, terbinafine, tipranavir, yohimbe, ziprasidone	Increases risk of QT prolongation, arrhythmias, CNS depression, psychomotor impairment
thiethylperazine	CNS depressants	Additive CNS depression
Phenothiazines in general	Oral anticoagulants	Antagonizes effects of interacting drug
PROKINETIC DRUGS		
metoclopramide	Alcohol, antidepressants, Antihistamines, General anesthetics, Opioids, Sedative-hypnotics	Additive CNS depression
	Insulins	Requires insulin adjustment
	haloperidol, Phenothiazines	Increases risk of EPS
	Anticholinergics, Opioids	Antagonizes GI effects of metoclopramide
	cyclosporine	Increases risk of cyclosporine toxicity
	MAO inhibitors	Increases risk of hypertensive crisis
	succinylcholine	Increases risk of NMB
SEROTONIN ANTAGONISTS		
dolasetron	atenolol, cimetidine	Increases serum levels of dolasetron
	rifampin	Decreases serum levels of dolasetron
granisetron, ondansetron	Phenothiazines and other drugs causing EPS	Increases risk for EPS
CANNABINOIDS		
dronabinol	Alcohol, Amphetamines, Antihistamines, cocaine, Opioids, Sedative-hypnotics, Sympathomimetics, Tricyclic antidepressants	Additive CNS depression
	Anticholinergics	Increases risk for tachycardia
MISCELLANEOUS		
aprepitant	Drugs biotransformed by CYP 3A4 system; e.g., antineoplastic drugs	Increases serum levels of interacting drug
benzquinamide	Alcohol	Additive CNS depression
droperidol	Antihypertensives, Nitrates	Additive hypotension
	Alcohol, Antihistamines, Antidepressants, Opioids, Sedative-hypnotics	Additive CNS depression
trimethobenzamide	Alcohol	Additive CNS depression
scopolamine	Antihistamines, Antidepressants, Opioids, Sedative-hypnotics	Additive CNS depression
	disopyramide, quinine	Additive anticholinergic effects

CNS, Central nervous system; *EPS*, extrapyramidal symptoms; *GI*, gastrointestinal; *MAO*, monoamine oxidase; *NMB*, neuromuscular blockade; *SSRIs*, selective serotonin-reuptake inhibitors.

GASTROINTESTINAL

class are available in the United States and have been approved to prevent the nausea and vomiting associated with emetogenic antineoplastic therapies, including high-dose cisplatin. They are also approved for the prevention and treatment of postoperative nausea and vomiting.

Research suggests that serotonin antagonists are more effective than prokinetic drugs (see following discussion) in relieving the nausea and vomiting associated with antineoplastic drug treatment. These drugs are well tolerated by most patients and are even more effective when combined with dexamethasone.

▌ Pharmacodynamics

Serotonin receptors (5-HT$_3$) are located in the endings of the vagus nerve in the GI tract. It is through these that antineoplastics cause the release of serotonin from the enterochromaffin cells of the GI tract, where it is stored, signaling serotonin receptors in the CTZ to cause nausea and vomiting.

Serotonin antagonists block 5-HT$_3$ receptors in the CTZ and peripherally in the vagal and splanchnic afferent fibers from the enterochromaffin cells in the upper GI tract.

▌ Pharmacokinetics

The pharmacokinetics of serotonin antagonists are shown in Table 47-2. The onset of drug action of these drugs is rapid when taken orally or given intravenously, with a duration of action of 4 to 24 hours. Serotonin antagonists are biotransformed by the CYP450 enzyme system; therefore inhibitors or inducers of this enzyme system may affect drug clearance. The half-lives of these drugs vary depending with the specific patient.

▌ Adverse Effects and Contraindications

There are many adverse effects to dolasetron, although overall the adverse effects are much like those of granisetron and ondansetron. The most common adverse effects are

DOSAGE
TABLE **47-4 Selected Antiemetics**

Drug	Use(s)	Dosage	Implications
ANTIHISTAMINES			
cyclizine	Motion sickness, prophylaxis for postoperative N/V	*Adult:* Motion sickness: 50 mg PO every 4–6 hr; not to exceed 200 mg/day. Postop vomiting: 50 mg IM 30 min before termination of surgery, then every 4–6 hr PRN	Give deep IM in well-developed muscle. Avoid inadvertent IV administration.
dimenhydrinate	Motion sickness	*Adult:* 50 mg PO, IM, or IV every 4 hr starting *–or–* 25 mg ER capsules PO every 12 hr *–or–* 50 to 100 mg PR every 6–8 hr PRN. Max: 400 mg/day *Child >12 yr:* 50 mg PR every 8–12 hr PRN *Child 6–12 yr:* 25–50 mg PO every 6–8 hr. Not to exceed 150 mg/day *Child 8–12 yr:* 25–50 mg PR every 8–12 hr PRN *Child: 6–8 yr:* 12.5–25 mg PR every 8–12 hr PRN	**Do not confuse with diphenhydramine.** Give at least 30 min before and preferably 1–2 hr before exposure to precipitating factors.
diphenhydramine	Motion sickness	*Adult:* 25–50 mg PO every 3–4 hr *–or–* 10–50 mg IM or IV every 2–3 hr PRN. Maximum: 400 mg/day. *Child:* 1–1.5 mg/kg PO every 4–6 hr PRN. Not to exceed 300 mg/day *–or–* 1.25 mg/kg IM or IV 4 times daily. Maximum: 300 mg/day	**Do not confuse with dimenhydrinate.** Give at least 30 min before and preferably 1–2 hr before precipitating factors. Give IM into well-developed muscle. Avoid subQ injections.
hydroxyzine	Antiemetic	*Adult:* 25–100 mg PO or IM 3–4 times daily *Child:* 0.5 mg/kg PO every 6 hr PRN *–or–* 1 mg/kg IM *Child <6 yr:* 12.5 mg PO every 6 hr PRN *Child 6–12 yr:* 12.5–25 mg every 6 hr PRN	Give deep IM into well-developed muscle using Z-track technique. Do not use deltoid site. **Tissue damage may occur from subQ or intraarterial injections.**
meclizine	Motion sickness	*Adult:* 25–50 mg PO 60 min before activity. May repeat in 24 hr	Avoid concurrent use of alcohol or other CNS depressants.
PHENOTHIAZINES			
chlorpromazine	Antiemetic	*Adult:* 10–25 mg PO every 4 hr PRN *–or–* 50–100 mg PR every 6–8 hr PRN *–or–* 25 mg IM initially, then 25–50 mg IM every 3–4 hr PRN *–or–* up to 25 mg IV *Child >6 mo:* 0.55 mg/kg PO every 4–6 hr PRN *–or–* 1 mg/kg PR every 6–8 hr PRN	Remain recumbent at least 30 min following IM or IV administration to minimize hypotensive effects.
prochlorperazine	Antiemetic	*Adult and Child >12 yr:* 5–10 mg PO 3–4 times daily. May be increased every 2–3 days up to 40 mg/day *–or–* 5–10 mg IM every 3–4 hr PRN *–or–* 25 mg PR twice daily *Child 18–39 kg:* 2.5 mg PO or PR 3 times daily *–or–* 5 mg twice daily not to exceed 15 mg/day *Child 14–17 kg:* 2.5 mg PO 2–3 times daily; Not to exceed 10 mg/day *–or–* 2.5 mg PR 2–3 times daily. Not to exceed 10 mg/day *Child 9–13 kg:* 2.5 mg PO or PR once-twice daily. Not to exceed 7.5 mg/day	Give with full glass of water to minimize GI upset. Inject deep IM into well-developed muscle. Dilute syrup in citrus- or chocolate-flavored drinks.
promethazine	Motion sickness; treatment and prevention of N/V	*Adult:* Motion sickness: 25 mg PO 30–60 min before departure; May repeat in 8–12 hours. Antiemetic: 10–25 mg PO, PR, IM, or IV every 4 hr PRN. Initial PO dose should be 25 mg. *Child >2 yr: Motion sickness:* 0.5 mg/kg 30–60 min before departure. May be given twice daily PO. *Antiemetic:* 0.25–0.5 mg/kg every 4–6 hr *–or–* 12.5–25 mg PO, PR, or IM every 4–6 hr	Give with food or milk to minimize GI upset. Tablets may be crushed and mixed with food or fluids. Give deep IM into well-developed muscles. SubQ route can cause tissue necrosis. Rapid IV administration can cause transient hypotension.
thiethylperazine	Antiemetic	*Adult:* 10 mg PO, PR, or IM 1–3 times daily PRN	Remain recumbent at least 60 min to minimize hypotensive effects. May cause severe hypotension if inadvertently given by IV.
PROKINETIC DRUG			
metoclopramide	Antineoplastic-induced N/V	*Adult:* 1–2 mg/kg IV 30 min before treatment. May repeat 1–2 mg/kg every 2 hr for 2 doses, then every 3 hr for 3 additional doses *Child:* 0.1–0.2 mg/kg/dose 30 min before meals and HS	Give IV doses slowly over 1–2 min. Rapid infusion causes transient but intense anxiety and restlessness followed by drowsiness.
	Postoperative N/V	*Adult:* 10–20 mg IM	Give near the end of surgery.
SEROTONIN ANTAGONISTS			
dolasetron	Antineoplastic-induced N/V	*Adult and Child 2–16 yr:* 1.8 mg/kg IV as single dose 30 min before emetogenic event *Child <2 yr:* Not determined	No dosage adjustment needed for older adults or patients with renal or hepatic dysfunction.

	Prevention and treatment of postoperative N/V	*Adult:* 12.5 mg IV 15 min before cessation of surgery *Child 2–16 yr:* 0.35 mg/kg with max of 12.5 mg as a single dose 15 min before cessation of surgery –or– 1.2 mg/kg to a max of 100 mg 2 hr before surgery	Injectable formulation may be mixed with apple or apple-grape juice for oral dosing.
granisetron	Antineoplastic induced N/V	*Adult:* 1 mg PO twice daily. First dose at least 30 min before treatment; second dose 12 hr after the first	Give only on days of antineoplastic therapy. Single dose provides 24–hr antiemetic effects in most cases.
ondansetron	Prophylaxis for postoperative N/V	*Adult:* 4 mg IV before induction of anesthesia or postoperatively	Single dose usually provides 24–hr effects.
	Prevention of acute and delayed N/V with initial and repeated courses of moderate to highly emetogenic antineoplastics	*Adult and Child >12 yr:* 8 mg PO 30 min before treatment and repeated 8 hr later; then 8 mg every 12 hr for 1–2 days PRN –or– 0.15 mg/kg IV 15–30 min before treatment, and every 4 hr for 2 doses –or– until N/V subside –or– 32-mg single dose 30 min before treatment *Child 4-11 yr:* 4 mg PO 30 min before treatment, and repeated 4 and 8 hr later; 4 mg PO every 8 hr may be given for 1–2 days following treatment *Child >3 yr:* 0.15 mg/kg IV 15–30 min before treatment, repeated 4 and 8 hr later	Give only on days antineoplastic treatment is given. Give each dose as IV infusion over 15 min. Given direct IV over 2–5 min.
palonosetron	Prevention of acute and delayed N/V with initial and repeated courses of moderate to highly emetogenic antineoplastics	*Adult:* 0.25 mg IV as a single dose 30 min before start of antineoplastic therapy *Child:* Not established	Repeated dosing within 7 days not suggested because safety and efficacy have not been established.
CANNABINOIDS			
dronabinol	Antineoplastic-induced N/V. Appetite stimulant in HIV/AIDS	*Adult and Child:* 5–7.5 mg/m^2 PO 1–3 hr before antineoplastic drug then every 2-4 hr after treatment with total of 4–6 daily doses. Not to exceed 15 mg/m^2 *Adult: Appetite stimulant:* 2.5 mg PO twice daily before lunch and dinner to max of 20 mg in divided doses	Keep capsules refrigerated but not frozen. Do not double doses. Use once-daily dosing if patient intolerant to twice daily regimen.
MISCELLANEOUS			
aprepitant	Antineoplastic-induced N/V	*Adult:* Day 1: 125 mg PO 60 min before antineoplastic; days 2 and 3: 80 mg before therapy; day 4: none	Given along with a corticosteroid and 5-HT$_3$ antagonist
droperidol	Postoperative and postprocedural N/V	*Adult:* 0.625–1.25 mg IM or IV every 3–4 hr PRN. Max 2.5 mg/dose. Give by slow IV over 2–5 min.	Monitor BP and P throughout. **Observe for EPS. R/O prolonged QT before use.**
trimethobenzamide	Mild to moderate nausea and vomiting	*Adult:* 250 mg PO 3–4 times daily –or– 200 mg PR or IM 3–4 times daily *Child 15-45 kg:* 100-200 mg PO or PR 3-4 times daily *Child <15 kg:* 100 mg PR 3-4 times daily	IM painful. Give deep IM using Z-track technique. **Avoid use in children who may have a viral illness (Reye's syndrome)**
scopolamine	Prophylaxis and treatment motion sickness	*Adult:* 0.5 mg Transderm-Scop patch 4 hr before effect desired. Transderm-V 1.5 mg patch started 12 hours before travel. *Antiemetic/anticholinergic effects:* 0.3-0.65 mg IM, IV, or subQ 3-4 times daily	Transderm-Scop delivers 0.5 mg over 72 hr. Transderm-V delivers 1.5 mg over 72 hr.

BP, Blood pressure; *EPS*, extrapyramidal symptoms; *ER*, extended-release; *HS*, at bedtime; *IM*, intramuscular (route); *IV*, intravenous (route); *N/V*, nausea and vomiting; *P*, pulse; *PO*, by mouth; *PR*, per rectum; *PRN*, as needed; *subQ*, subcutaneous (route); *R/O*, rule out.

headache and diarrhea. Weakness, somnolence, agitation, anxiety, and CNS stimulation have also occurred. Fever, fatigue, abnormal liver function, abdominal pain, hypertension, pain, dizziness, and chills and shivering occur in fewer than 4% of patients. Although rare, dolasetron has been associated with atrioventricular (AV) block, chest pain, orthostatic hypotension, myocardial ischemia, syncope, severe bradycardia, and palpitations. Fever and anaphylactoid reactions have been documented. Because serotonin antagonists do not block dopamine receptors, they do not produce extrapyramidal effects characteristic of some antiemetics. Serotonin antagonists are contraindicated for use in patients with hypersensitivity to the drug. Use with caution during pregnancy (category B) and in children.

▓ Drug Interactions

Cimetidine increases serum levels of dolasetron, whereas rifampin decreases serum levels when used concurrently. Atenolol decreases the clearance of dolasetron by one fourth.

Concurrent use of granisetron with other drugs that cause extrapyramidal reactions may increase the risk of such reactions from granisetron (see Table 47-3). There are no significant drug interactions with ondansetron or palonosetron.

▓ Dosage Regimen

Table 47-4 provides the recommended dosages for serotonin antagonists. Dolasetron, granisetron, and palonosetron are administered only on days the patient receives antineoplastic therapy. Ondansetron, when used for prophylaxis and treatment of postoperative nausea and vomiting, is given 15 to 30 minutes before surgery.

Lab Considerations

Monitoring parameters for serotonin antagonists include baseline and follow-up liver function tests. Dosage reductions may be needed in patients with severe hepatic dysfunction. To reduce the risk of arrhythmia-related complications, monitor electrolytes for hypokalemia and hypomagnesemia.

Phenothiazines

◆ chlorpromazine (Thorazine); ◆ Chlorpromanyl, Largactil, Novo-Chlorpromazine
◆ prochlorperazine (Compazine); ◆ prochlorperazine
◆ promethazine (Anergan, Pentazine, Phencen-50, Phenergan, Prorex, Prothazine); ◆ Phenergan
◆ thiethylperazine (Torecan)

Indications

Phenothiazines are used most often to suppress nausea and vomiting associated with antineoplastic therapy, radiation therapy, and toxins. Chlorpromazine is particularly useful in the management of intractable hiccough; prochlorperazine is available in suppository form if the oral route is unavailable. The basic discussion of the phenothiazines is found in Chapter 21.

Pharmacodynamics

The phenothiazines suppress nausea and vomiting by blockade of dopamine receptors in the CTZ. To varying degrees, these drugs also produce blockade of muscarinic, histamine, and norepinephrine receptors. The blockade of these receptors is responsible for the action and major adverse effects of the phenothiazines.

Pharmacokinetics

The pharmacokinetics of phenothiazines is identified in Table 47-2. Onset of drug action occurs 30 minutes to 1 hour after the drugs are taken by mouth, with a more rapid onset from other routes. Most phenothiazines are over 90% protein bound. Peak action times are unknown.

Adverse Effects and Contraindications

The antiemetic actions of phenothiazines occur at dosages much lower than those used in the management of schizophrenia. Although unusual when used for nausea and vomiting, phenothiazines have a variety of serious adverse effects, including extrapyramidal reactions such as pseudoparkinsonism, dystonia, akathisia, and tardive dyskinesia. Anticholinergic actions include hypotension and sedation. Phenothiazines may mask diagnostic symptoms of acute surgical conditions or neurologic syndromes.

Because of the additional risk of additive CNS depression, use phenothiazines cautiously in patients taking other CNS depressants. Phenothiazines may exacerbate parkinsonian symptoms. The safety of phenothiazines during pregnancy is controversial; most are pregnancy category C drugs. The drugs can also reduce the seizure threshold in patients with seizure disorders.

Drug Interactions

Drug interactions of phenothiazines are numerous and are identified in Table 47-3. There are a wide variety of interactions, with each interacting drug producing distinct effects. In general though, phenothiazines potentiate CNS depression with alcohol and other CNS depressants. They also potentiate the action of alpha blockers, and levels of the drug can be increased with the beta blocker propranolol. The dosages of antiepileptic drugs may have to be adjusted. Phenothiazines antagonize oral anticoagulants.

Dosage Regimen

Dosage regimens of phenothiazines used as antiemetics are identified in Table 47-4. When comparing dosage requirements, potency is compared with that of 100 mg of chlorpromazine. Low-potency phenothiazines are more likely to produce sedative and orthostatic hypotensive effects. Medium-potency phenothiazines vary in their ability to produce sedation and extrapyramidal effects. High-potency phenothiazines are most likely to produce extrapyramidal effects and least likely to cause sedation and orthostatic hypotension.

Lab Considerations

Lab considerations with phenothiazines include periodic complete blood counts and liver function tests. Chlorpromazine causes decreased hematocrit, hemoglobin, leukocytes, granulocytes, and platelet values and may elevate bilirubin, alanine transaminase (ALT), aspartate transaminase (AST), and alkaline phosphatase values. False-positive or false-negative pregnancy tests and false-positive urine tests for bilirubin are noted during phenothiazine use.

Thiethylperazine may increase prolactin levels, may interfere with gonadorelin test results, and may also cause false-positive or false-negative pregnancy tests.

Prokinetic Drug

◆ metoclopramide (Reglan); ◆ Apo-Metoclop

Indications

Prokinetic drugs are helpful in treating motility disorders such as the gastroparesis associated with diabetic autonomic neuropathy and postvagotomy states, in the management of esophageal reflux, and in the treatment and prevention of postoperative nausea and vomiting when nasogastric suctioning is undesirable. Metoclopramide is the drug of choice for suppressing nausea and vomiting related to highly emetic antineoplastic drugs (e.g., cisplatin, dacarbazine). It has also been used in the treatment of hiccoughs with some success, although it has not been approved by the Food and Drug Administration (FDA) for such use. (See also Chapter 45.)

Pharmacodynamics

Metoclopramide blocks dopamine receptors in the CTZ, thereby suppressing nausea and vomiting. It increases upper GI motility, the resting tone of the esophageal sphincter, gastric contractions, and peristalsis of the duodenum and jejunum by enhancing the actions of acetylcholine. Although it is structurally related to procainamide (see Chapter 36), an antiarrhythmic drug, metoclopramide lacks significant local anesthetic or antiarrhythmic actions.

Pharmacokinetics

Metoclopramide is well absorbed from the GI tract and from rectal mucosa and intramuscular (IM) tissue sites. It is widely distributed to body tissues and fluids crossing the blood-brain barrier and placenta. It enters breast milk in concentrations greater than plasma. Metoclopramide is partially biotransformed in the liver, with 25% eliminated unchanged in the urine (see Table 47-2).

Adverse Effects and Contraindications
Sedation and diarrhea are common with high doses of metoclopramide. Metoclopramide does not have useful antipsychotic effects; however, it can cause significant extrapyramidal symptoms, especially at high doses and particularly in children. Twenty-five percent of adults ages 18 to 30 years develop dystonia after receiving high-dose metoclopramide (i.e., 2 mg/kg/dose) for antineoplastic-induced nausea and vomiting. The extrapyramidal symptoms can be prevented and controlled by giving diphenhydramine, a drug with prominent anticholinergic actions. Other reversal drugs include benztropine (an antiparkinson's drug) and diazepam. Because of its ability to increase GI motility, metoclopramide is contraindicated for use in the presence of obstruction, hemorrhage, and perforation of the GI tract. Metoclopramide is a pregnancy class B drug thought to be safe to breastfeeding infants if the mother is taking less than 45 mg/day.

Drug Interactions
Drug interactions with metoclopramide are rather extensive and vary with the specific drug (see Table 47-3). Metoclopramide accelerates intestinal transit, thus decreasing the absorption and bioavailability of other drugs. In addition, the absorption of food nutrients to the intestine may be decreased to such an extent that diabetic patients may need insulin dosage adjustments.

Dosage Regimen
The dosage regimen for metoclopramide varies with the use for the drug (see Table 47-4). When used for the prevention of antineoplastic-induced nausea and vomiting, the dose is 1 to 2 mg/kg intravenous (IV) 30 minutes before the treatment. Additional doses of 1 to 2 mg/kg may be given every 2 hours for two doses, then every 3 hours for three additional doses.

Lab Considerations
Metoclopramide may alter liver function test results and cause increased serum prolactin and aldosterone concentrations.

Cannabinoids
◆ dronabinol (Marinol)

Indications
Dronabinol is a cannabinoid antiemetic approved by the FDA for managing the nausea and vomiting associated with antineoplastic therapy. Dronabinol is also used as an appetite stimulant to prevent or reverse weight loss in patients with acquired immunodeficiency syndrome.

Dronabinol (Δ-9-tetrahydrocannabinol, THC) is the primary active ingredient in marijuana. In general, this drug is used only if other treatments for nausea, such as metoclopramide or a serotonin antagonist, have failed. To be effective, dronabinol should be used at least 6 to 12 hours before antineoplastic therapy. The use of this drug has declined

somewhat because of its incidence and severity of adverse effects and because serotonin antagonists are now available.

Pharmacodynamics
Dronabinol activates receptors in the vomiting center that are responsible for suppressing nausea and vomiting.

Pharmacokinetics
Dronabinol is extensively biotransformed following absorption, resulting in a bioavailability of 10% to 20%. The time to onset is unknown, but drug effects appear to peak in 2 hours, with a duration of action of 4 hours (see Table 47-2). Dronabinol is highly lipid-soluble, entering breast milk in high concentrations.

Adverse Effects and Contraindications
Dronabinol produces subjective effects similar to those evoked by marijuana: dysphoria, detachment, depersonalization, and temporal deterioration. Generally, younger patients tolerate and respond better to these drugs than older patients. **Dronabinol can cause tachycardia, hypotension, and CNS effects. Therefore use it cautiously in patients with cardiovascular disease.**

Dronabinol is contraindicated for use in patients with psychiatric disorders and also in patients with hypersensitivities to dronabinol, marijuana, or sesame oil; nausea and vomiting due to other causes; and during lactation. Dronabinol is a Schedule II drug. Chronic use may lead to abuse and withdrawal syndrome on discontinuation. Safety in children under the age of 18 has not been established.

Drug Interactions
Drug interactions are identified in Table 47-3. Dronabinol causes additive CNS depression when used concurrently with alcohol, antihistamines, opioids, tricyclic antidepressants, and sedative-hypnotics. It increases the risk for tachycardia when combined with amphetamines, cocaine, sympathomimetics, anticholinergics, antihistamines, and tricyclic antidepressants.

Dosage Regimen
Twice-daily dosing of dronabinol is recommended (see Table 47-4). The dosage can be reduced if the patient experiences CNS toxicity.

Miscellaneous Drugs
◆ aprepitant (Emend)
◆ droperidol (Inapsine)
◆ trimethobenzamide (Tigan)
◆ scopolamine (Transderm Scop, Transderm-V); ♣ Transderm-V

Aprepitant
Aprepitant is the first drug in a class known as neurokinen$_1$ (NK$_1$) antagonists. Aprepitant is an add-on drug used for prevention of the acute and delayed nausea and vomiting associated with moderate and highly emetogenic antineoplastic drugs. Its action is to selectively antagonize Substance P and NK$_1$ receptors, which in turn reduces nausea and vomiting. The pharmacokinetics of aprepitant as currently understood are identified in Table 47-2. Inhibiting the CYP 3A4 enzyme

system (e.g., with antineoplastic drugs) could result in elevated plasma concentration of the interacting drug.

The adverse effects of aprepitant are many, with a reported incidence over 0.5%. Isolated cases of serious adverse effects include dehydration, enterocolitis, febrile neutropenia, hypertension, hypoaesthesia, neutropenic sepsis, pneumonia, and sinus tachycardia. Aprepitant is contraindicated for use in patients who are hypersensitive to the drug, and chronic continuous use for prevention of nausea and vomiting is not recommended.

Droperidol

Droperidol is a butyrophenone antiemetic used postoperatively or after procedures, for nausea and vomiting. It is also useful for the nausea and vomiting associated with antineoplastic or radiation therapy and toxins. Like the phenothiazines, this butyrophenone suppresses emesis by blocking dopamine receptors in the CTZ.

The adverse effects of droperidol are similar to those with phenothiazines, including extrapyramidal reactions, sedation, and hypotension. **Droperidol is contraindicated for use in patients with hypersensitivity, narrow-angle glaucoma, bone marrow depression, CNS depression, severe liver or cardiac disease, and known intolerance**. Exercise caution when using droperidol in older adults and in debilitated or severely ill patients. Cautious use is also warranted in patients with diabetes, respiratory insufficiency, prostatic hyperplasia, CNS tumors, intestinal obstruction, or seizures (may lower seizure threshold), and during pregnancy or lactation. Safe use has not been established in children younger than 2 years of age, although droperidol has been used during cesarean section without respiratory depression in the newborn.

Trimethobenzamide

Trimethobenzamide, an unclassified antiemetic, is used in the management of mild to moderate nausea and vomiting. Although its mechanism of action is unknown, the relatively weak antiemetic effects appear to result from dopamine blockade. Trimethobenzamide is not as effective as serotonin antagonists, phenothiazines, or metoclopramide, but it can be given by IM route to treat nausea and vomiting associated with antineoplastic drugs that have mild to moderate emetogenic potential.

Adverse effects other than pain at the injection site are fairly uncommon and may include drowsiness, dizziness, allergy-type skin eruptions, extrapyramidal symptoms, and seizures. It is contraindicated for use in newborn or premature infants and patients with a hypersensitivity to benzocaine suppositories. **Cautious use of trimethobenzamide in children with viral illnesses is needed because of the increased risk of Reye's syndrome.** Safe use during pregnancy and lactation has not been established.

Additive CNS depression may occur with trimethobenzamide if the drugs are taken concurrently with other CNS depressants, such as alcohol, antidepressants, antihistamines, opioids, and sedative-hypnotics.

Scopolamine

Scopolamine is an anticholinergic (muscarinic antagonist) that is moderately effective for prophylaxis and treatment of motion sickness. Scopolamine acts by inhibiting the muscarinic activity of acetylcholine, thus reducing vestibular hyperstimulation (see also Chapter 15). Transdermal scopolamine should be applied 4 to 12 hours before travel. Its use is not recommended for use in children. Advise the patient that it may dilate the pupil on the same side where the patch is worn. Prolonged use of scopolamine contributes to tolerance.

Scopolamine is well absorbed following IM, subcutaneous, and transdermal administration. Protein binding is low, with a half-life of 8 hours. Scopolamine is primarily biotransformed and eliminated through the liver.

Dry mouth, blurry vision, drowsiness, and urinary retention are the most common adverse effects of scopolamine. Use scopolamine cautiously in patients with suspected intestinal obstruction, prostatic hyperplasia, and chronic renal, hepatic, pulmonary, or cardiac disease. It is contraindicated for use in patients hypersensitive to bromides (injection formulation only) and those with narrow-angle glaucoma, acute hemorrhage, or tachycardia secondary to cardiac insufficiency or thyrotoxicosis. Safe use during pregnancy and lactation has not been established.

Benzodiazepines

Benzodiazepines such as diazepam and lorazepam are also used to alleviate anticipatory nausea and vomiting associated with antineoplastic therapy. The beneficial effect of diazepam is primarily related to its reduction of anxiety and therefore is given 12 hours before antineoplastic therapy. Lorazepam is often combined with metoclopramide and dexamethasone. The benzodiazepines are discussed in Chapter 19.

Corticosteroids

Corticosteroids confer a positive benefit when added to antiemetic therapy for the patient receiving antineoplastic therapy. Although many health care providers use dexamethasone, other corticosteroids such as methylprednisolone are also likely to be useful. Dexamethasone is an add-on drug to serotonin antagonists for the prevention of cisplatin-induced nausea and vomiting. Corticosteroids generally help patients feel better overall.

The mechanism by which corticosteroids suppress vomiting is unknown, but one theory suggests perhaps there is an inhibition of the prostaglandins involved in cerebral edema. In situations of nausea and vomiting secondary to increased intracranial pressure, corticosteroids provide relief by reducing inflammation. Of the corticosteroids studies, dexamethasone was superior to prochlorperazine and comparable to high-dose metoclopramide when used in conjunction with mild to moderately emetogenic antineoplastic regimens.

Modern antiemetic therapy for the prevention of antineoplastic-induced nausea and vomiting uses a combination of drugs. The foundations are the 5-HT$_3$ receptor antagonists, to which corticosteroids, benzodiazepines, or NK$_1$–receptor antagonists are added to achieve high levels of protection from nausea and vomiting.

CLINICAL REASONING

Treatment Objectives

Potentially life-threatening complications can result from nausea and vomiting, including dehydration, electrolyte imbalances, and malnutrition. Therefore treatment goals include preventing or relieving it and its distressing symptoms, and maintaining hydration. The aim is to determine whether empiric therapy with an antiemetic drug, a gastric-acid suppressing drug, or a prokinetic drug would be beneficial or whether the patient should be admitted to an acute care setting for correction of fluid and electrolyte imbalances.

Treatment Options

The treatment objective is directed at finding and correcting the underlying cause of the nausea and vomiting. Most cases are self-limiting and require no special treatment. Patients are encouraged to take clear liquids in small, frequent amounts. In some cases, however, IV rehydration and administration of an antiemetic drug is needed. Hospitalization is required for patients with recalcitrant vomiting, hypokalemia, or metabolic concerns, especially those who are very young or very old.

▥ *Patient Variables*

For ambulatory patients, drugs causing minimal sedation are generally preferred. Some sedation, however, does occur even with therapeutic doses. For prophylaxis, plan administration so that peak drug effects correspond to the time of anticipated nausea. For example, antiemetics used in the prevention of motion sickness are usually taken at least 30 minutes to an hour before travel, and then as needed. Pretravel administration allows time for drug dissolution and absorption to take place.

Excessive sedation may occur even with therapeutic doses of antiemetics but is more likely to occur with high doses. The risk of sedation can be reduced by avoiding high doses when possible and assessing the patient for responsiveness before each dose to adjust dosage or frequency of administration. Small doses of phenothiazines produce antiemetic effects; large doses produce antipsychotic effects.

Nausea and vomiting prophylaxis for patients receiving antineoplastic drugs is imperative, because nausea and vomiting may curtail effective, ongoing treatment. Because the risk of nausea and vomiting usually worsens with each treatment cycle, up to 30% of patients refuse further treatment. Adequate prophylaxis and treatment eliminate symptoms in up to 82% of patients (Table 47-5). Patients receiving antineoplastics that have a low emetogenic potential (Table 47-6) but who have had nausea or vomiting during a previous course of therapy should receive prophylaxis.

Anticipatory nausea and vomiting can occur any time. It is seen more commonly in patients who previously received antineoplastic drugs with high emetogenic potential. Patients younger than 50 years who report any of the following experiences may be at risk for anticipatory nausea and vomiting: susceptibility to motion sickness; prior nausea or vomiting; and feelings of flushing or diaphoresis after previous treatment sessions. Anticipatory nausea and vomiting can develop rapidly, often appearing after only one infusion and escalating in

TABLE 47-5 Combination Antiemetic Regimens According to Emetogenic Potential

COMBINATION ANTIEMETIC REGIMENS FOR DRUGS WITH LOW TO MODERATE EMETOGENIC POTENTIAL	
A	• Oral dronabinol every 6 hr starting 24 hr before treatment • Oral prochlorperazine every 6 hr starting 24 hr before treatment until 24 hr after last treatment
B	• Oral prochlorperazine "spansules" twice daily PO on day 1 and days 3–6 • IV dexamethasone daily for 5 days –or– PO twice daily on days 1–5 (tapered dose) • Oral diphenhydramine 1 hr before treatment • Oral lorazepam 1 hr before treatment • IV metoclopramide 1 hr before treatment
C	• IV lorazepam or IV diphenhydramine 45 min before treatment • IV metoclopramide 30 min before and 90 min after treatment • IV dexamethasone 30 min before and 90 min after treatment

COMBINATION ANTIEMETIC REGIMENS FOR DRUGS WITH MODERATE EMETOGENIC POTENTIAL	
A	• IV metoclopramide 20 min before and 90 min after treatment • IV dexamethasone 20 min before treatment • IV diphenhydramine 30 min before treatment
B	• IV metoclopramide 20 min before and 90 min after treatment • IV dexamethasone 40 min before treatment • IV lorazepam 35 min before treatment

COMBINATION ANTIEMETIC REGIMENS FOR DRUGS WITH HIGH EMETOGENIC POTENTIAL	
A	• IV granisetron immediately before treatment • IV dexamethasone 5 min before treatment • IV ondansetron 30 min before treatment and every 4 hr, with 3 doses after treatment • IV dexamethasone 5 min before treatment
B	• IV metoclopramide 20 min before and 90 min after treatment • IV dexamethasone 20 min before treatment • IV lorazepam 30 min before treatment
C	• IV metoclopramide 30 min before and 90 min after treatment • IV diphenhydramine 45 min before treatment • IV dexamethasone 45 min before treatment
D	• IV ondansetron 30 min before treatment • IV dexamethasone 30 min before treatment • Oral prochlorperazine SR at bedtime • Oral lorazepam at bedtime • Oral diphenhydramine at bedtime

IV, Intravenous; *PO,* by mouth; *SR,* slow-release.

GASTROINTESTINAL

TABLE 47-6 Emetogenic Potential

Drugs with Low Emetogenic Potential	Drugs with Moderate Emetogenic Potential*	Drugs with High Emetogenic Potential*
bleomycin	carboplatin	cisplatin
chlorambucil	carmustine	cyclophosphamide
etoposide	cytarabine	dacarbazine
fluorouracil	daunorubicin	dactinomycin
hydroxyurea	doxorubicin	mechlorethamine
methotrexate	ifosfamide	streptozocin
mitomycin C	lomustine	
vinblastine	procarbazine	
vincristine		
vindesine		

*Emetogenic potential of some drugs is dose-dependent.

severity during subsequent treatments. Many patients find their first treatment to be much easier than they expected. However, as treatment continues, patients begin to notice the anticipatory adverse effects. With repeated treatments, the problem becomes worse.

Psychogenic vomiting is associated with a physical syndrome, sexual abuse, posttraumatic stress, and eating disorders. Formal psychiatric assessment and psychologic testing (e.g., Minnesota Multiphasic Personality Inventory) may be helpful.

The expense associated with antiemetic therapy is closely related to the cause of the nausea. When the nausea and vomiting is self-limited, the expense is relatively small. However, for patients receiving antineoplastic therapies, the cost of antiemetic regimens can be high (see Case Study).

LIFE-SPAN CONSIDERATIONS

Pregnant and Nursing Women. Morning or daily nausea or vomiting is a typical complaint during the first 12 to 14 weeks of a normal pregnancy. It is usually self-limited and intermittent, beginning at about 6 weeks' and disappearing at about 12 weeks' gestation. It is commonly worse in the morning. If severe (hyperemesis gravidarum), electrolyte imbalances, dehydration, or starvation may occur.

▲ **Routine prophylaxis or treatment of nausea and vomiting is not recommended because of the potential for teratogenic effects. Treatment is warranted if hyperemesis gravidarum or protracted vomiting occurs, or if non–drug measures have failed, such as ingesting crackers and tea before morning rising, taking small, light, appetizing meals, and keeping head movement to a minimum.** The usefulness of pyridoxine (vitamin B$_6$) as an antiemetic has not been confirmed, but it is the least likely drug to be toxic. Meclizine (pregnancy category B) may be considered if pyridoxine is ineffective.

Children and Adolescents. Children in general have nausea and vomiting more often than adults. Repetitive vomiting during or soon after a meal suggests different causes in children than adults. If there is no fever, no weight loss, and no abdominal distention and the child does not appear sick, the cause may be a feeding disorder (i.e., overfeeding or too-rapid feeding). Vomiting in infants and children may be associated with acute gastroenteritis or an acute illness (e.g., urinary tract infection, otitis media, and asthma), feeding disorders, hypertrophic pyloric stenosis, or intussusception.

Older Adults. Older adults are at risk for fluid volume depletion and electrolyte disturbances, with the changes of aging

sometimes contributing to the potential for nausea and vomiting. Esophageal motility is decreased and the distal esophagus becomes slightly dilated. Esophageal emptying is slower, and there is reduced gastric motility and emptying. Nausea and vomiting may be the only symptom of an underlying urinary tract infection.

▮ *Drug Variables*

Antiemetics are more effective for prophylaxis of symptoms than treatment. However, given the complexity of the various pathways that control and stimulate vomiting, no single drug is effective in all patients. Most antiemetic drugs are available in oral, parenteral, and rectal dosage forms. As a general rule, oral dosage forms are preferred for prophylaxis, and rectal or parenteral forms preferred for treatment. Further, the antiemetic drug of choice depends on the primary cause of the nausea and vomiting. For example, if nausea and vomiting is related to a specific drug, discontinue that drug, if possible. With motion sickness, counsel the patient to avoid the initiating event when able, thereby avoiding the trigger for the nausea and vomiting.

The costs of serotonin antagonists notwithstanding, these drugs are often chosen for concurrent use with antineoplastic drugs that have a high emetogenic potential. Compare the expense of a serotonin antagonist to the cost of preparing the three or four parenteral drug regimens and the cost of related antiemetic rescue drugs. Serotonin antagonists are usually well tolerated and, in combination with dexamethasone, may be more effective than any other drug alone.

Drugs with anticholinergic and antihistaminic properties are preferred for motion sickness caused by travel by land, sea, or air, especially if sedation is desired. For rough seas and extended journeys, transdermal scopolamine is more convenient than oral dimenhydrinate or promethazine. Treatment is also warranted for patients with prolonged nausea (longer than 30 minutes) or repeated episodes of vomiting unrelieved by decreased vestibular stimulation (head movement). Meclizine is inexpensive and can be taken once a day. Prophylaxis with scopolamine or promethazine is effective in 90% of patients.

Unless sedation is desired, choose dimenhydrinate instead of diphenhydramine, because it is more effective for motion sickness and produces less sedation. Dimenhydrinate causes less sedation than diphenhydramine but has a higher incidence of anticholinergic effects.

In certain patients, combinations of drugs from different classes may provide better symptom control with less toxicity. For example, treatment of a patient with anticipatory, acute, or delayed forms of vomiting may receive a benzodiazepine (e.g., lorazepam), a serotonin antagonist (e.g., ondansetron), and a corticosteroid (e.g., dexamethasone). Combination strategies take advantage of the synergistic mechanisms afforded by each drug. This is advantageous because lower doses of individual drugs generally produce fewer adverse effects. The decision as to the specific drug to use is thus based, in part, on potential adverse effects, because no one drug has proven to be more effective than any other drug.

Provide prophylaxis for patients at high risk for aspiration (e.g., patients with wired jaws, patients with a history of moderate to severe postoperative vomiting). The incidence of nausea and vomiting associated with anesthesia is about 30%; therefore prophylaxis is useful and more comforting for the

CASE STUDY   Antiemetics

ASSESSMENT

History of Present Illness	CM is a 52-year-old male who reports to the office today for a required annual employment physical. He is also requesting a prescription for motion sickness. He reports he will be crossing "the treacherous Drake Passage by ship" on his way to Antarctica and is worried he will not be able to perform his job as engineer should he experience motion sickness. The Drake Passage takes 3 days to cross. Although he has not previously crossed the passage, he reports having motion sickness anytime a body of water is rocky. He has tried OTC Benadryl and other "motion sickness pills" but has found them to be less than effective.
Past Health History	CM's medical history is unremarkable except for "hay fever" and early benign prostatic hypertrophy that causes occasional urinary hesitancy. He had an intramedullary rod inserted in his right femur without sequelae after an MVA at age 25. He takes no OTC or prescription drugs.
Life-Span Considerations	CM is single and feels he must remain so because of the extended periods of time he is away from home.
Psychosocial Considerations	No history of psychiatric disorders. Denies smoking and use of tobacco, or alcohol since the MVA at age 25. The cost of CM's annual physical exam is covered by his employer. Prescription costs are covered by employer using an in-house formulary if drugs are required. Special permission is required if a non–formulary drug is required.
Physical Exam Findings	CM's physical exam is unremarkable. *Cardiac:* RRR. Breath sounds clear bilaterally. CN II-XII intact. Strength bilateral upper and lower extremities equal. Bowel sounds present all four quadrants. Prostate approximately 35 grams. Negative hernia exam. Healed incision right buttock from intramedullary rod insertion.
Diagnostic Testing	CM agreed to participate in a research study about allergic responses to chemicals contained within the living quarters in Antarctica. He will be having allergy testing upon arrival and again in 3 months. Routine laboratory testing reveals CBC, electrolytes, UA, and EKG are within normal limits. Drug screen negative. PSA within normal limits.

DIAGNOSIS: Nausea and Vomiting Prophylaxis

Management	**Treatment Objectives** 1. Prevent or relieve distressing symptoms associated with nausea and vomiting. 2. Prevent complications such as electrolyte imbalances, dehydration, and malnutrition.
Treatment Plan	**Pharmacotherapy** • 0.5 mg Transderm-Scop patch placed behind ear 4 hr before boarding ship. Change to other ear on day 3 if patch still needed. **Patient Teaching** 1. Teach proper application of patch. Use only one patch at a time. Do not cut patch. 2. Wash hands after applying patch. 3. Slowly sip clear liquids and to consume foods served cool or at room temperature. 4. Minimize visual, auditory, and olfactory stimulation as much as possible. 5. Decrease physical activity during episodes of nausea. **Evaluation** 1. Nausea and vomiting were prevented while crossing Drake Passage. 2. Fluid and electrolyte balance were maintained.

CLINICAL REASONING ANALYSIS

Q1. Why did you choose scopolamine patch rather than oral meclizine as prophylaxis?

A. Scopolamine is the most effective drug against motion sickness. However, toxicity following oral administration has limited its use. Even if the antiemetic effects were maintained and the adverse effects reduced with smaller dosages, the duration of action at lower dosages is relatively short. The patch, however, alleviates these problems by allowing a constant delivery of drug to maintain a safe and effective blood level over a prolonged period of time.

Continued

GASTROINTESTINAL

CASE STUDY   Antiemetics—Cont'd

Q2. Can he wear the patch anywhere on the body?
A. We will instruct CM to wear the patch behind his ear for the first 3 days and then remove it. He will use a new patch behind his other ear for the next 3 days if it is still needed. We will also tell him that it may dilate the pupil on the same side where the patch is worn.

Q3. Wouldn't it be easier to take a pill such as meclizine once a day rather than wearing a patch for 3 days?
A. Not necessarily. Besides, CM is to have allergy testing performed upon arrival in Antarctica. Meclizine can cause false-negative skin test results.

Q4. If the scopolamine does not keep him from being nauseated and vomiting, what alternatives are there?
A. If he is actively nauseated and vomiting sometimes, the ship's health care provider will order metoclopramide to facilitate gastric emptying. The alternatives include antihistamines such as dimenhydrate and cyclizine, which exert central anticholinergic activity, but we have to be careful because of the allergy testing he will be having upon arrival. If we do have to use an antihistamine, it will delay the allergy testing for at least 3 days.

patient. Postoperative nausea requires treatment in only about 5% of patients. Routine prophylaxis after surgery is discouraged because of hypotension and sedative effects.

As a general rule, use of antiemetics is contraindicated when it prevents or delays diagnosis or when signs and symptoms of drug toxicity may be masked (e.g., during digoxin therapy); routine use to prevent postoperative vomiting is also discouraged. If appropriate diagnostic tests have been obtained and no specific diagnosis has been made, a therapeutic trial of a prokinetic drug may be justified.

Patient Education

To help minimize nausea and vomiting, patients are advised to slowly sip clear liquids and to consume foods served cool or at room temperature. Milk and milk products, as well as very sweet, fatty, salty, or spicy foods are generally avoided. Some patients receiving antineoplastic therapy may be unable to tolerate plain water or red meat. Advise the patient to minimize visual, auditory, and olfactory stimulation, and remove noxious stimuli from the environment. Physical activity should be decreased during episodes of nausea. A cool wet washcloth to the face and neck may help the patient feel more comfortable. Because pain can cause nausea and vomiting in some patients, administration of analgesics is appropriate.

Good oral hygiene with frequent rinsing after an emesis helps relieve bad taste and reduces corrosion of tooth enamel by gastric acid. Dry mouth can be relieved with frequent rinsing, sugarless gum or candy, and adequate fluid intake.

Inform patients that drowsiness is a common occurrence with antiemetics and that driving and other activities requiring alertness should be avoided until response to the drug is known. Advise patients that tolerance to drowsiness develops but tolerance to response time does not.

Caution patients against sudden position changes, which may cause a drop in blood pressure. Advise the patient to avoid concurrent use of alcohol or other CNS depressants. Advise the patient taking a cannabinoid to do so only when supervised because of its tendency to cause mood changes. Other drugs should not be taken without the knowledge or consent of the health care provider.

Evaluation

Antiemetic efficacy is noted by verbal reports of decreased nausea and an absence of vomiting, adequate intake and retention of fluids, a decrease in specific gravity, return of normal electrolytes, and an increase in patient well-being. Determine if the dosage and frequency of administration is the most effective for an individual patient.

KEY POINTS

- Nausea and vomiting are common symptoms and may accompany almost any illness, drug therapy, or stressful situation; they are the most common adverse effect of antineoplastic drugs.
- Common states associated with nausea and vomiting include GI inflammation, infection, obstruction, motility disorders, vestibular or intracranial disorders, metabolic derangements, toxins, and psychogenically caused conditions.
- Treatment goals include preventing or relieving the distressing symptoms associated with nausea and vomiting. Potentially life-threatening complications such as electrolyte imbalances, dehydration, and malnutrition necessitate immediate intervention.
- The treatment of vomiting is first directed at finding and correcting the underlying cause. Most causes of acute vomiting are self-limited and necessitate no special treatment.

- Choice of an antiemetic depends primarily on the cause of the nausea and vomiting and the patient's condition. Antiemetics are generally more effective for prophylaxis than for treatment.
- Treatment options include antihistamines, phenothiazines, prokinetics, serotonin antagonists, cannabinoids, and a number of miscellaneous drugs. Benzodiazepines and corticosteroids have also been used as adjuncts in the treatment of nausea and vomiting.
- Combinations of drugs from different drug classes often provide better symptom control with less toxicity for the patient receiving antineoplastic drugs and take advantage of the synergistic mechanisms afforded by each drug.
- Plan administration times so that peak effects correspond to the time of anticipated nausea.
- Therapeutic effects are assessed by verbal reports of decreased nausea, observed absence of vomiting, and a general sense of improved well-being.

Bibliography

de Wit, R., Herrstedt, J., Rapoport, B., et al. (2003). Addition of the oral NK1 antagonist aprepitant to standard antiemetics provides protection against nausea and vomiting during multiple cycles of cisplatin-based chemotherapy. *Journal of Clinical Oncology, 21*(22), 4105–4111.

Ernest, A., Weiss, S., Park, S., et al. (2000). Prochlorperazine versus promethazine for uncomplicated nauseas and vomiting in the emergency department: A randomized, double-blind clinical trial. *Annuals of Emergency Medicine, 36*(2), 89–94.

García-Miguel, F., Montaño, E., Martín-Vicente, V., et al. (2000). Prophylaxis against intraoperative nausea and vomiting during spinal anesthesia for cesarean section: A comparative study of ondansetron versus metoclopramide. *The Internet Journal of Anesthesiology, I4N2*, Available online: www.ispub.com/journals/IJA/Vol4N2/nvpo.htm. Accessed May 21, 2007.

Golding, J., Gresty, M. (2005). Motion sickness. *Current Opinions in Neurology, 18*(1), 29–34.

Gutierrez, K., Queener, S. (2003). *Pharmacology in nursing practice.* Philadelphia: Mosby.

Haughney, A. (2004). Nausea and vomiting in end-stage cancer: These symptoms can be treated most effectively if the underlying cause is known. *American Journal of Nursing, 104*(11), 40–48.

Hesketh, P., Grunberg, S., Gralla, R., et al. (2003). The oral neurokinin-1 antagonist aprepitant for the prevention of chemotherapy-induced nausea and vomiting: A multinational, randomized, double-blind, placebo-controlled trial in patients receiving high-dose cisplatin: The aprepitant-protocol 052 study group. *The Journal of Clinical Oncology, 21*(22), 4112–4119.

National Comprehensive Cancer Network. (2006). Antiemesis: Clinical practice guidelines in oncology. Vol. 1. Available online: www.nccn.org/professionals/physician_gls/PDF/antiemesis.pdf. Accessed May 21, 2007.

Parkman, H., Hasler, W., Fisher, R. (2004). American Gastroenterological Association technical review of the diagnosis and treatment of gastroparesis. *Gastroenterology, 127*(5), 1592–1622.

Colorado State University. (1998). Physiology of vomiting. Available online: http://arbl.cvmbs.colostate.edu/hbooks/pathphys/digestion/stomach/vomiting.html. Accessed May 20, 2007.

GASTROINTESTINAL

48

Cation-Exchange Resins and Ammonia-Detoxifying Drugs

This chapter considers the drugs used to counteract two dangerous imbalances: increased levels of potassium (K^+) and excess ammonia (NH_3^+). K^+, the major intracellular ion, and other electrolytes such as sodium (Na^+), chlorine (Cl^-), calcium (Ca^{++}), and magnesium (Mg^-) are closely involved in the regulation of body fluids. Elevation of serum K^+, also known as hyperkalemia, is rare in people with normal kidney function but often occurs with renal impairment. Hyperkalemia must be corrected because dangerously high serum K^+ levels lead to cardiac, gastrointestinal (GI), renal, and neurologic dysfunction.

NH_3^+ is formed in the body as part of several cellular processes and from enteric bacteria in the GI tract. Under normal conditions, it is quickly removed from the blood, converted into urea, and eliminated in the urine. However, if the liver is damaged or seriously diseased, NH_3^+ accumulates in the blood, with severe toxic consequences.

HYPERKALEMIA

EPIDEMIOLOGY AND ETIOLOGY

A normal serum K^+ level ranges between 3.5 to 5.5 mEq/L. Serum K^+ levels that exceed 5.5 mEq/L are considered *hyperkalemia*. There are three primary causes for hyperkalemia: first, when there is movement of K^+ out of cells, which occurs whenever severe tissue damage is present, as in crushing injuries, sepsis, fever, or surgery. K^+ movement out of cells also occurs in metabolic acidosis, hyperglycemia, insulin deficiency, and adrenal insufficiency. Secondly, hyperkalemia can be caused by increased dietary intake of K^+ that exceeds the ability of the kidneys to eliminate it, the concurrent use of K^+-sparing diuretics and K^+ supplements, or adrenal insufficiency. Patients with untreated adrenal insufficiency have increased K^+ levels because of a related aldosterone deficiency. Administration of stored blood further contributes to elevated K^+ levels. A third cause of hyperkalemia is decreased elimination of K^+, which occurs with renal failure (Box 48-1). Patients who slowly develop severe hyperkalemia seem to adjust to the excess K^+ with few symptoms. Shock and the reduced renal function it entails also promote hyperkalemia. Even the common practice of repeatedly clenching and unclenching the fist during venipuncture can raise serum potassium levels by 1 or 2 mEq/L. The elevation is due to the local release of K^+ from forearm muscles.

PATHOPHYSIOLOGY

K^+ is the major intracellular *cation;* a positively charged ion important in maintaining the balance between intracellular and extracellular fluid compartments. During *anabolism* (tissue build-up) or when glucose is converted to glycogen, K^+ enters the cell. With *catabolism* (tissue breakdown or injury) K^+ leaves the cell. The body conserves K^+ less effectively than it conserves Na^+, and the kidneys excrete K^+ even when the body needs it. Normally, about 5% of total body K^+ is eliminated each day. Serum K^+ levels do not necessarily reflect total body K^+ levels because most of the K^+ is intracellular.

An active transport system for Na^+ and K^+ is found in all cells; the Na^+-K^+–adenosine triphosphatase (ATPase) pump. The pump system moves Na^+ out of the cell and K^+ into the cell. Approximately 60% to 70% of the adenosine triphosphate (ATP) synthesized by cells, particularly muscle and nerve cells, is used to maintain this transport system. Excitable tissues (e.g., muscle, nerves, kidneys, and salivary glands) have a high concentration of $Na+$, K^+, and ATPase. For every ATP molecule, there are three molecules of Na^+ transported out of the cell, whereas only two molecules of K^+ move into the cell. This leads to creation of a membrane potential, with the inside of the cell more negative than the outside (Fig. 48-1).

In the presence of hyperkalemia, membrane potentials are decreased and the cells become more excitable. Patients develop muscle irritability, numbness, and tingling because

---

BOX 48-1

Causes Of Hyperkalemia

Diminished Renal Elimination
- Reduced glomerular filtration
- Acute oliguric renal failure
- Chronic renal failure

Reduced Tubular Secretion
- Addison's disease
- Hyporeninemia
- Use of angiotensin-converting enzyme inhibitors
- Hypoaldosteronism
- Use of potassium-sparing diuretics
- Voltage-dependent renal tubular acidosis
- Use of trimethoprim-sulfamethoxazole

Transcellular Shifts
- Acidosis
- β-adrenergic blockade
- Trauma, burns
- Rhabdomyolysis
- Hemolysis
- Tumor lysis

Diabetic Hyperglycemia
Depolarizing Muscle Paralysis (succinylcholine)
Hyperkalemic Periodic Paralysis

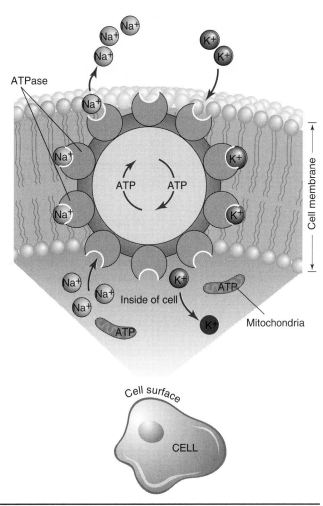

FIGURE 48-1 Sodium-potassium exchange system. Three Na$^+$ ions are exchanged for two K$^+$ ions using adenosine triphosphate (ATP) to pump Na$^+$ out of the cell and K$^+$ into the cell against a steep electrochemical gradient. An energy-containing ATP molecule, produced by the mitochondria, binds to the transporter protein, ATPase (adenosine triphosphatase).

of overstimulation by nerve impulses. Skeletal muscle spasms, nausea, colic, and diarrhea are common. Muscles become weak as K$^+$ is lost to the cells and because the overstimulation causes lactic acid to accumulate.

Overstimulation of the myocardium occurs if hyperkalemia is not controlled. Electrocardiogram (ECG) tracings reflect high-peaked T waves. Hyperkalemia does not prolong the QT interval. The QRS complex continues to widen; atrial arrest occurs as K$^+$ levels continue to increase. A sudden rise of only 1 to 3 mEq/L of K$^+$ can be fatal.

Another cause of hyperkalemia is the chronic acidosis that is a consequence of uncontrolled diabetes. Insulin insufficiency leads to hyperkalemia, because the action of insulin to promote K$^+$ movement into cells is diminished. Metabolic acidosis, which is a consequence of uncontrolled diabetes, causes hyperkalemia by shifting K$^+$ out of cells. For each 0.1 unit fall in pH, serum K$^+$ rises by approximately 0.6 mEq/L.

Physical exam findings of the patient with hyperkalemia include a slow, weak pulse rate; a low blood pressure; and

evidence of weakness and flaccid paralysis; in addition, bowel sounds are hyperactive, with frequent audible rushes and gurgles. Abdominal distention and frequent, explosive, watery diarrhea may be noted. Behavioral changes are not usually seen with hyperkalemia because cardiac abnormalities cause the patient to seek help before serum K$^+$ levels become high enough to produce neurologic manifestations.

PHARMACOTHERAPEUTIC OPTIONS

Cation-Exchange Resins

◆ sodium polystyrene sulfonate resin (Kayexalate, SPS); ♣ Kayexalate

▌ Indications

Sodium polystyrene sulfonate resin is used for the treatment of mild to moderate hyperkalemia (K$^+$ level over 6 to 8 mEq/L). It aids in the removal of excess K$^+$ from the body but is considered an adjunct to other measures such as restriction of K$^+$ intake, control of acidosis, and a high-calorie diet.

PHARMACOKINETICS
TABLE 48-1 Cation-Exchange Resins and Ammonia-Detoxifying Drugs

Drug	Route	Onset	Peak	Duration	PB (%)	$t_{1/2}$
CATION-EXCHANGE RESIN						
sodium polystyrene sulfonate resin	PO	2–12 hr	UA	6–24 hr	NA	UA
	PR	2–12 hr	UA	4–6 hr	NA	UA
AMMONIA-DETOXIFYING DRUGS						
lactulose	PO	24–48 hr	UA	UA	UA	UA
neomycin	PO	Rapid	1–4 hr	4–6 hr	UA	2–3 hr

NA, Not applicable; *PB*, protein binding; *PO*, by mouth; *PR*, per rectum; $t_{1/2}$, half-life; *UA*, unavailable.

▥ Pharmacodynamics

Following rectal administration of sodium polystyrene sulfonate resin, Na^+ ions are partially released from the resin in exchange for other ions. Clinically, much of the exchange capacity is used for ions other than K^+ such as Ca^{++}, Mg^-, Fe, organic cations, lipids, steroids, and proteins. These resins can be repeatedly given by mouth to maintain low plasma potassium concentration.

▥ Pharmacokinetics

The onset of rectally administered sodium polystyrene sulfonate resin is approximately 30 minutes, whereas that of orally administered drug is 2 to 12 hours, with peak drug action unknown (Table 48-1). The resin is not absorbed but rather distributed throughout the intestines to be eliminated in 6 to 24 hours. A single enema removes enough K^+ to reduce potassium by 0.5 to 2 mmol/L within 1 hour. The duration of action of the drug when administered rectally is 4 to 6 hours.

▥ Adverse Effects and Contraindications

The adverse effects of orally administered sodium polystyrene sulfonate resin include gastric irritation; anorexia, nausea, vomiting, and constipation may occur, especially with large doses. Large oral doses can cause fecal impaction, especially in older adults. Occasionally, the resin causes diarrhea. Extensive intestinal necrosis is a rare occurrence but has been noted in patients with chronic renal failure or those who have had a kidney transplant. In all cases, the patients were azotemic, with the necrosis usually developing about 36 hours after

therapy was started. Thus the use of sodium polystyrene sulfonate resin is contraindicated in patients with azotemia or those who have had a kidney transplant.

Hypokalemia and clinically significant Na^+ retention are possible. Because the cation-exchange action of the resin is not selective for K^+, increased elimination of other cations also occurs, resulting in other electrolyte disturbances such as hypocalcemia and hypernatremia. **Because sodium polystyrene sulfonate resin provides a clinically significant Na^+ load, use caution with patients whose Na^+ intake must be restricted** (e.g., patients with heart failure, severe hypertension, or marked edema). In these patients, compensatory restriction of Na^+ intake from other sources may be indicated.

▥ Drug Interactions

Concurrent use of antacids containing Mg^- or Ca^{++} decreases the resin-exchanging ability of sodium polystyrene sulfonate resin. Concurrent use also increases the risk of metabolic alkalosis (Table 48-2). Hypokalemia also increases the risk of toxicity to digoxin.

▥ Dosage Regimen

Sodium polystyrene sulfonate resin may be taken by mouth or given as a retention enema (Tables 48-3 and 48-4). Resin cookie or candy recipes are available from a pharmacist or dietician for use in children.

▥ Lab Considerations

Monitor serum K^+ levels daily during therapy. The duration of treatment is individually determined based on patient

DRUG INTERACTIONS
TABLE 48-2 Cation-Exchange Resins and Ammonia-Detoxifying Drugs

Drug	Interactive Drugs	Interaction
CATION-EXCHANGE RESIN		
sodium polystyrene sulfonate	Calcium- or magnesium-containing antacids	Decreases resin-exchanging ability; increases risk of systemic alkalosis
	digoxin	Hypokalemia enhances risk of toxicity with interactive drug.
AMMONIA-DETOXIFYING DRUGS		
lactulose	Antimicrobial drugs	Prevents acidification of colon contents
	Antacids	Inhibits decrease in fecal pH in colon
neomycin	cyclopropane, halothane, nitrous oxide, tubocurarine, succinylcholine, decamethonium	Increases risk of respiratory paralysis
	ethacrynic acid, furosemide	Increases risk of ototoxicity
	azlocillin, cisplatin, carbenicillin, methoxyflurane, mezlocillin, piperacillin, ticarcillin	Increases risk of nephrotoxicity

TABLE 48-3 Adjunct Treatments for Hyperkalemia*

Drug or Procedure	Mechanism
sodium bicarbonate	Increases serum pH
dextrose 50%	Increases insulin release
regular insulin	Intracellular uptake of potassium
albuterol	β_2 adrenergic stimulation
calcium gluconate	Raises threshold potential; reestablishes cardiac excitability
furosemide	Removes potassium from the plasma
Hemodialysis	Extracorporeal potassium removal
Peritoneal dialysis	Removes potassium from peritoneal cavity

*Adjunctive treatments for hyperkalemia other than sodium polystyrene sulfonate.

response. Closely monitor the patient's clinical condition since intracellular K^+ deficiency is not always reflected in serum K^+ levels or ECG tracings.

CLINICAL REASONING

Treatment Objectives
The treatment objectives for hyperkalemia are to normalize serum K^+ levels and prevent complications. In addition, the patient with chronic hyperkalemia will be able to prepare and administer the resin and maintain normal bowel function with neither diarrhea nor constipation.

Treatment Options

▥ Patient Variables
Ask patients with hyperkalemia if they have palpitations, skipped heartbeats, or other cardiac irregularities, muscle twitching, or numbness and tingling in the hands, feet, or around the mouth. Muscle weakness ascends from the distal to proximal areas affecting the muscles of the arms and the legs. Trunk, head, and respiratory muscles are unaffected until serum K^+ levels reach fatal levels.

Note recent changes in bowel habits, especially diarrhea, colic, and explosive bowel movements. Ask about recent medical or surgical interventions and about urinary output, including frequency and amount of voiding. Elicit specific information about the intake of foods laden with K^+ (especially those eaten raw) and salt substitutes (because many of the substitutes contain K^+ salts).

Note any past history of diabetes mellitus and renal or adrenal insufficiency. A drug history remains vital, with attention to drugs that contribute, from whatever means, to K^+ retention. For example, patients taking trimethoprim, a K^+-sparing diuretic (combined with sulfamethoxazole or dapsone), have K^+ levels that progressively rise. Over 25% of these patients have K^+ levels over 5 mEq/L, and 10% have life-threatening hyperkalemia. K^+ levels return to normal after the drug has been discontinued. Hyperkalemia in the older adult may manifest as depression, confusion, lethargy, impaired mental functioning, anorexia, and weakness.

Hyperkalemia associated with renal failure is usually accompanied by elevations of serum creatinine and blood urea nitrogen (BUN) levels, a decreased blood pH, and normal or low hematocrit and hemoglobin levels.

▥ Drug Variables
Cation-exchange therapy is most beneficial when hyperkalemia is not life-threatening and when other interventions have reduced the dangers of hyperkalemia. Patients whose Na^+ intake must be restricted (e.g., those with heart failure, severe hypertension, or marked edema) may not be candidates for cation-exchange therapy. In these patients, compensatory restriction of Na^+ intake from other sources may be indicated.

Before treatment of hyperkalemia is started, determine the cause of the hyperkalemia and eliminate it, if possible. Hyperkalemia should be anticipated and prevented in persons who have a significant decrease in urinary output for any reason, especially if they are receiving oral or intravenous K^+. Because the action of the resin is slow, treatments that shift K^+ into the cells (e.g., sodium bicarbonate or dextrose, with or without insulin) or other treatments (e.g., calcium salts) are

DOSAGE
TABLE 48-4 Cation-Exchange Resins and Ammonia-Detoxifying Drugs

Drug	Use(s)	Dosage	Implications
CATION-EXCHANGE RESIN			
sodium polystyrene sulfonate resin	Mild to moderate hyperkalemia	*Adult:* 15 grams PO 1–4 times daily in water or sorbitol *–or–* 25–100 grams/100 mL sorbitol every 6 hr as retention enema. Increase to 40 grams PO 4 times daily. *Child:* 1 gram/kg/dose PO or PR	Each gram contains 4.1 mEq Na^+. Exchanges 1 gram of Na^+ ions for 0.5 to 1 mEq K^+ ions
AMMONIA-DETOXIFYING DRUGS			
lactulose	Portal-systemic encephalopathy, chronic constipation	*Adult:* 20–30 grams (30–45 mL) PO 3–4 times daily until stools are soft *–or–* 30–45 mL/100 mL of 0.9% NaCl or water PR every 4–6 hr	Titrate to 2–3 stools/day. *Syrup:* 10 grams lactulose = 15 mL. Decreases NH_3^+ concentrations by 25% to 50% *Enema:* Retain 30–60 min.
neomycin	Portal-systemic encephalopathy	*Adult:* 500 mg PO 4 times daily. Increase to 4–12 grams PO in divided doses daily. *Child:* 40–100 mg/kg/day in divided doses every 4–6 hr	Contraindicated for use in patients with renal dysfunction

PO, By mouth; *PR,* per rectum.

warranted (see Table 48-3). These other treatments are specifically indicated if the hyperkalemia is manifest by conduction defects (widening of the QRS complex) or arrhythmias. However, an ECG is an insensitive method for detecting hyperkalemia because 60% of patients with a serum K^+ level greater than 6.5 mEq/L will not manifest ECG changes.

Sodium bicarbonate promotes the movement of K^+ into the cells by increasing extracellular pH and also through direct action of the HCO_3 ion itself. Dextrose increases the release of endogenous insulin, promoting intracellular uptake of K^+. Insulin is often administered with dextrose to promote the effect of endogenous insulin. Insulin alone may be given to the patient with hyperglycemia. Calcium chloride changes the relationship between membrane and threshold potentials, restoring normal myocardial conduction. Calcium chloride does not lower serum K^+ levels in any way, and, because it is short acting, it must be repeated if symptoms recur until serum K^+ levels are lowered.

An osmotic laxative (i.e., sorbitol) is usually mixed with oral sodium polystyrene sulfonate resin to prevent constipation. It can be added to the resin powder, or a commercially prepared product may be used. Do not use magnesium-containing laxatives, however. The powdered resin should not be mixed with foods or liquids that contain large amounts of K^+ (e.g., bananas, orange juice, prune juice, apricot nectar, or milk).

When sodium polystyrene sulfonate resin is administered as a retention enema, the resin is retained in the colon for at least 30 to 60 minutes. To remove the resin, the colon is then irrigated with a solution that does not contain Na^+. Approximately 2 liters of solution may be needed to sufficiently flush out the resin. Monitor serum K^+ and Na^+ levels at least once daily for signs and symptoms of hypokalemia, including irritability, confusion, muscle weakness, and arrhythmias. Watch the patient with hypertension, heart failure, or edema for evidence of Na^+ and fluid overload.

Patient Education

Education is a key factor in the prevention of hyperkalemia. Diet education includes avoidance of foods laden with K^+ and instruction about which foods are permissible. Teach the patient to read food labels with attention to potassium content. It is also important to teach the person who does the shopping or who prepares the meals, as well as the patient. Further, **advise the patient taking sodium polystyrene sulfonate resin to avoid foods high in Na^+ such as processed foods and lunch meats, snack foods that are high in Na^+, and salt substitutes.**

Inform the patient of the signs and symptoms of hyperkalemia and which findings to report. When drug therapy is necessary, instruct the patient on the purpose and method of drug administration and that frequent laboratory tests will be needed to monitor the effectiveness of the drug. Demonstrate how to prepare and use the resin correctly if patient or family member will be administering the drug.

Because hypokalemia enhances the risk of toxicity to digoxin and diuretics, reeducate patients about the signs and symptoms of digoxin toxicity. Teach the patient how to accurately take the pulse and to determine its regularity and quality. Also advise the patient to avoid calcium or magnesium antacids because they reduce the effectiveness of the resin.

Inform the patient about the constipating effects of the resin and strategies to help prevent or reduce constipation. A high-fiber diet and 8 to 12 glasses of fluids per day will help. Contact the health care provider should constipation occur. Taking the drug early in the day helps prevent problems with diarrhea at night.

Evaluation

Evaluation of drug effectiveness is demonstrated by normalization of serum K^+ levels without adverse effects. The patient with chronic hyperkalemia is able to demonstrate how to prepare and administer the resin. Normal bowel function is established during therapy, with neither constipation nor diarrhea.

HEPATIC ENCEPHALOPATHY

EPIDEMIOLOGY AND ETIOLOGY

Hepatic encephalopathy is a state of disordered central nervous system (CNS) function. Also called portal-systemic encephalopathy, it is one of the major complications of cirrhosis. It results from failure of the liver to detoxify noxious substances of GI origin because of hepatocellular dysfunction or portal-systemic shunting. NH_3^+ is the most readily identified toxin but is not solely responsible for the patient's disturbed mental status.

PATHOPHYSIOLOGY

NH_3^+ is normally formed in the body in several ways: (1) by the liver during deamination of amino acids; (2) by epithelial cells of the proximal and distal tubules and collecting duct of the nephron, as part of the regulation of hydrogen ions; and (3) by bacteria of the GI tract acting on urea and dietary proteins. A normally functioning liver converts absorbed NH_3^+ to urea, a less toxic substance. Urea is then eliminated in the urine. However, damage to the liver or shunting of blood flow around the liver inhibits the conversion of NH_3^+ to urea. The elevated serum NH_3^+ level that results leads to hepatic encephalopathy with decreasing levels of consciousness, impaired neuromuscular functioning and, in some cases, death.

Several conditions result in or contribute to hepatic encephalopathy, including cirrhosis, high protein intake, old blood in the bowel from GI bleeding, alkalosis secondary to hyperventilation or hypokalemia, constipation, or infection. Patients with cirrhosis have a higher rate of urea breakdown in the GI tract than healthy persons. Dietary protein acts as a substrate for bacterial production of NH_3^+ or other nitrogenous toxins. Serious GI bleeding decreases perfusion to the liver, the brain, and the kidneys and also contributes 15 to 20 grams of protein/100 mL as NH_3^+ substrate.

Alkalosis leads to diffusion of NH_3^+ across the blood-brain barrier to cause lethargy, confusion, and irritability. Hypokalemia is a major precipitating metabolic factor. As serum levels decrease, K^+ shifts from the intracellular compartment to exchange for Na^+ and H^-. The shift of H^- ions into the intracellular compartment increases the acid level in that compartment, decreasing the pH and increasing the base in the extracellular compartment. The extracellular alkalosis liberates H^- from ammonium (NH_4^+) and NH_3^+. NH_3^+ is gaseous and readily crosses into cells, where it accumulates and exerts toxic effects. Increased accumulation of base in the extracellular compartment from other causes precipitates the same response.

Constipation allows for increased production and absorption of NH_3^+ resulting from the longer contact time for bacteria and substrates. Constipation may also provoke use of a Valsalva maneuver while stooling and thus precipitate bleeding from esophageal varices or hemorrhoids. Infection leads to increased tissue catabolism, which in turn contributes to a higher nitrogen load.

The patient with hepatic encephalopathy usually demonstrates a history of failing health including reports of anorexia, nausea, vomiting, indigestion, flatulence, and constipation. Reports of vague, dull, mild or steady, wavelike abdominal pain may be noted. The pain is usually in the right upper quadrant. The patient is often fatigued and does not tolerate activity.

The manifestations of hepatic encephalopathy vary and may occur rapidly or gradually over the course of a few days. Assessment findings reflect alterations in the level of consciousness, in intellectual function, behavior, and personality,

and in neuromuscular function (Box 48-2). Weight loss masked by water retention can also be seen.

Patients with hepatic encephalopathy have a number of abnormal lab test results including increased levels of total, unconjugated, and conjugated bilirubin; increased urine bilirubin and urobilinogen; and elevated liver enzymes (alanine transaminase [ALT], aspartate transaminase [AST], lactate dehydrogenase [LDH], and alkaline phosphatase). Increased international normalized ratio (INR) values, decreased platelets, decreased leukocyte count, decreased red blood cell count, decreased serum albumin and serum glucose levels, hypokalemia, and hyponatremia may also be noted. The first line of therapy is to limit protein intake; the second line of therapy is administration of nonsystemic antibiotics and lactulose.

PHARMACOTHERAPEUTIC OPTIONS

Ammonia-Detoxifying Drugs

◆ lactulose (Cephulac, Cholac, Chronulac, Constilac, Constulose, Duphalac, Enulose); ◆ Luculax
◆ neomycin (Mycifradin Sulfate)

▦ Indications

Lactulose is used as an adjunct to protein restriction and as supportive therapy for the prevention and treatment of hepatic encephalopathy. It is useful in the management of hepatic encephalopathy resulting from surgical placement of portacaval shunts or from chronic diseases such as cirrhosis. Lactulose reduces blood NH_3^+ concentrations and produces a corresponding improvement in the mental state of the patient.

Lactulose is also useful for the treatment of chronic constipation in adults and older adults, although its superiority to conventional laxatives has not been established (see Chapter 46). Lactulose has also been used to restore regular bowel movements in patients who have had a hemorrhoidectomy, but at present it is not approved by the FDA for such use.

In contrast, lactulose is not helpful when the encephalopathy is drug-induced or when it is caused by inborn errors of metabolism or electrolyte disturbances. It is not effective in the treatment of coma associated with hepatitis or other acute liver disorders.

Neomycin, an aminoglycoside antibiotic (see Chapter 27), is also used in the management of hepatic encephalopathy to decrease the population of enteric bacteria that generate NH_3^+ from the breakdown of protein and urea. It is also used to decrease the GI tract's bacterial count in preparation for surgery.

▦ Pharmacodynamics

Lactulose, as a semisynthetic disaccharide, is not absorbed by the GI tract but rather is broken down by enteric bacteria. It decreases NH_3^+ levels associated with the biotransformation of the sugar in the lower GI tract. The breakdown of lactulose to organic acids (i.e., lactic, formic, and acetic acids) causes a drop in colon pH from 7 to 5. This acidification of the colon inhibits the diffusion of NH_3^+ from the colon into the blood, because NH_3^+ is converted from a lipid-soluble gas into nondiffusible ammonium ions. In addition, lactulose causes fecal acidification, which reduces the production of ammonia by fecal bacteria.

BOX 48-2

Symptoms of Hepatic Encephalopathy

Stage 1—Prodromal Period
- Changes in sleep patterns
- Slowed responses
- Shortened attention span
- Depressed or euphoric mood
- Irritability
- Tremors
- Incoordination
- Impaired ability to write

Stage 2—Impending
- Disorientation to time
- Lethargy
- Impaired calculation ability
- Decreased inhibition
- Anxiety or apathy
- Inappropriate behaviors
- Slurred speech
- Decreased reflexes
- Ataxia and asterixis

Stage 3—Stuporous
- Disorientation to place
- Confused, somnolent
- Stuporous but capable of being aroused
- Anger, rage, paranoia
- Hyperreflexia
- Clonus
- Presence of Babinski's sign
- Asterixis

Stage 4—Coma
- No intellectual functioning
- Unconscious
- Loss of deep tendon reflexes
- Responsive only to deep pain
- Hyperventilation
- Fetor hepaticus
- Increased body temperature
- Increased pulse rate

CASE STUDY Ammonia-Detoxifying Drugs

ASSESSMENT

History of Present Illness	MM's wife accompanies her 59-year-old husband to this appointment. He has had 3 days of increasing confusion, lethargy, restlessness, and irritability. She notes his writing has been impaired; he has involuntary muscle tremors, especially in the hands; his speech is slurred; and he has "bad breath–like a diaper pail." She reports that he consumed 1 pint of whiskey per day for the last 15 years. He has not eaten much for the last 3 days, but ordinarily she sees that he follows a high-calorie, low-protein diet. His last drink was 3 days ago.
Past Health History	MM has a history of Laennec's cirrhosis with three previous hospitalizations for GI bleeding. His last bleed was 1 year ago. He is taking no other drugs at this time but has a history of not adhering to treatment regimens.
Life-Span Considerations	No specific age-related changes of aging; however, because of his history of cirrhosis has loss of liver function. MM's ability to progress through ages and stages of growth and development impaired as result of alcohol intake.
Psychosocial Considerations	MM has been a confectionery worker for 24 years. He was recently relieved of his duties because of his alcohol intake. MM's wife reports he has consistently lost time from work owing to his alcohol intake and hospitalizations. He has attempted several times to participate in a corporate-sponsored rehabilitation program but with little success. He acknowledges that the alcohol abuse started when he started going with fellow employees to the local saloon after work. He has been married 37 years to the same woman, who oversees his health care needs and drug regimens. MM receives financial assistance from the confectionery industry and union. Health care insurance is available through the union, but he has no supplementary insurance coverage or pharmacy program eligibility.
Physical Exam Findings	*Height:* 5'9". *Weight:* 167 lb (up 9 lb from previous visit). *BP:* 139/88. VSS. Spider angiomas over nose and cheeks; dilated vessels over upper body and lower extremities. Multiple ecchymotic areas on extremities with 1+ edema of lower extremities. Bowel sounds diminished all four quadrants; liver is not palpable. General body odor of urine. Irritable. CN II-XII intact. DTRs 1+ upper and lower extremities. Hands tremulous.
Diagnostic Testing	Electrolytes low-normal. Urine bilirubin and urobilinogen, total and conjugated bilirubin, ALT, AST, LDH, and alkaline phosphatase levels are elevated. Serum ammonia level elevated.

DIAGNOSIS: Hepatic Encephalopathy

MANAGEMENT

Treatment Objectives	1. Decrease blood ammonia levels by 25% to 50%. 2. Facilitate overall increase in cognition from baseline status.
Treatment Options	**Pharmacotherapy** • neomycin 500 mg PO 4 times daily until mental status improves, then discontinue and start lactulose • lactulose (started after finishing neomycin) 30–45 mL PO 3 to 4 times daily; titrate to two to three stools daily **Patient Education** 1. Strongly encourage MM to stop alcohol intake and provide support for his efforts. Encourage participation in an alcohol support group such as Alcoholics Anonymous. 2. Encourage a low-protein diet in consultation with dietitian. 3. Instruct wife about the use of neomycin and lactulose. Emphasize the importance of consistent use of lactulose, with titration to the number of stools. 4. Encourage MM and his wife to report changes in bowel habits, particularly diarrhea. 5. Increase fluid intake (not alcohol) to 1500 to 2000 mL/day. **Evaluation** 1. Ammonia levels decreased by 25% to 50%. 2. Overall improvement in cognition is seen from baseline status.

CLINICAL REASONING ANALYSIS

Q1. Given his nonadherence to treatment, wouldn't it be better for him to take one drug rather than two?
A. Adherence is a consideration, but given his declining mental status at this time, it is best for him to start with the neomycin under his wife's supervision, rid himself of some of the ammonia, and then start the second drug as maintenance.

Q2. But don't these drugs act the same way—to rid the body of ammonia?
A. No, lactulose and neomycin are differently. Ammonia is normally produced in the intestines by bacterial action on dietary proteins. Neomycin inhibits bacterial protein synthesis, thereby producing bactericidal effects and subsequent stooling. The lactulose inhibits diffusion of ammonia from the colon into the blood stream. Neomycin has a rapid onset but a relatively short duration of action

Q3. Shouldn't we do lab tests before we start the drugs?
A. Yes. No specific tests are required to use the lactulose, but we do have several tests to do before we start neomycin therapy. We have his current ammonia level, but we will repeat it along with obtaining BUN, creatinine, and creatinine clearance results. We will also monitor these parameters throughout his prolonged therapy. Keep in mind though that MM's signs and symptoms are more reliable to use in evaluating treatment success than ammonia levels.

Q4. Why can't he simply use neomycin for treatment rather than stopping it and starting lactulose?
A. Neomycin is an aminoglycoside antibiotic with the potential for ototoxicity and nephrotoxicity. It has a relatively narrow therapeutic index, hence the importance of BUN, creatinine, and creatinine clearance testing. We will also need to arrange for audiometry testing to establish his baseline hearing, as a precaution in light of the possibility of ototoxicity developing.

GASTROINTESTINAL

The laxative action of lactulose is probably caused by the osmotic effect of the drug's organic acid metabolites. The osmotic effect of lactulose and its metabolites causes an increase in the water content of stool and subsequent softening. The increased osmolarity of the bowel results in a laxative effect, manifested as diarrhea, which discharges the ammonium ions. The laxative effect takes 24 to 48 hours after administration to be seen.

Neomycin produces bactericidal effects by inhibiting protein synthesis by enteral bacteria at the level of the 30S ribosome, thus interfering with maintenance of the structure and the metabolic activity of the bacterial cell.

▥ Pharmacokinetics
Less than 3% of a dose of lactulose is absorbed from the small intestine following oral administration. Unabsorbed lactulose reaches the colon unchanged, where it is transformed by bacteria to lactic acid and small amounts of acetic and formic acids. The bacteria normally present in the colon that act on lactulose include *Lactobacilli, Bacteroides, Escherichia coli,* and *Clostridia.*

Neomycin is also minimally absorbed (less than 3%) following oral administration. Its distribution is unknown. The amounts that are systemically absorbed are eliminated unchanged through the kidneys (see Table 48-1).

▥ Adverse Effects and Contraindications
The adverse effects of lactulose primarily affect the GI tract. During the first few days of therapy, anorexia, nausea, vomiting, and abdominal cramping are common. These effects usually subside with continued therapy, although dosage reduction may be required in some cases. Diarrhea, flatulence, distention, and belching have been noted.

Lactulose is contraindicated for use in patients with hypersensitivity and in those on a low-galactose diet. Exercise caution when using the drug in patients with diabetes mellitus, older adults, and in debilitated patients. Lactulose carries a category C rating and thus is generally avoided during pregnancy. It is not known whether lactulose is distributed to breast milk.

The primary adverse effects of neomycin are ototoxicity and nephrotoxicity. Hypersensitivity reactions are always possible. Neomycin is contraindicated for use in patients with preexisting ototoxicity or nephrotoxicity, in patients with cross-allergenicity to aminoglycosides, and in patients with renal impairment.

▥ Drug Interactions
The effects of lactulose are decreased in the presence of neomycin and other oral antimicrobial drugs (see Table 48-2). Neomycin interacts with a number of drugs. There is an increased risk of ototoxicity with loop diuretics and of nephrotoxicity with nephrotoxic drugs.

▥ Dosage Regimen
The dosage of lactulose is titrated to maintain two to three stools a day (see Table 48-4). When lactulose is administered as a retention enema, 30 to 45 mL in 100 mL of fluid is used. The optimal dosing of neomycin is unknown.

▥ Lab Considerations
Lactulose reduces NH_3^+ levels by 25% to 50%. Closely monitor blood and urine electrolytes when lactulose is used for prolonged periods.

When neomycin is used in the treatment of encephalopathy, lab monitoring includes urinalysis with specific gravity, BUN and creatinine levels, and creatinine clearance, before and throughout therapy. There are no known lab test interferences with either lactulose or neomycin.

CLINICAL REASONING

Treatment Objectives

The treatment goal for hepatic encephalopathy is an overall increase in the patient's cognitive ability from baseline status. If the patient was comatose, a return to consciousness is the goal.

Treatment Options

Many patients tolerate increased dietary protein during lactulose therapy. However, the drug does not alter the course of the underlying liver disease. Therefore lactulose used in the treatment of hepatic encephalopathy does not obviate treatment of the underlying disease, nor does it preclude the use of other treatment measures.

An effective clinical response occurs in 75% to 85% of patients. Because lactulose is relatively nontoxic, it is a valuable alternative to neomycin, especially when prolonged therapy is required, or when use of neomycin is contraindicated. Patients who previously failed to respond to neomycin and dietary protein restriction may respond to lactulose, and vice versa.

Because neomycin destroys bacteria and lactulose requires bacterial degradation to be effective, concomitant therapy with these drugs is theoretically counterproductive. However, it appears that lactulose remains active when it is administered with neomycin, and there is some evidence that concomitant therapy may be more effective than the use of either drug alone. Some health care providers recommend neomycin for acute episodes of hepatic encephalopathy and lactulose for long-term management of chronic disease.

Patient Education

Teach the patient taking lactulose to dilute it to counteract the sweet taste and to take it on an empty stomach, thereby promoting drug action. It should be stored in a cool environment but not where the drug may freeze. The patient should report any change in bowel habits, particularly diarrhea, because diarrhea may indicate an overdose. Emphasize the importance of consistent use and titration to the number of stools.

Neomycin is ordinarily used in conjunction with a low-residue diet, and with a laxative or enema for preoperative bowel prep. Instruct the patient to take the neomycin as directed for the full course of therapy. Neomycin can be taken without regard to meals, but caution the patient that neomycin can cause nausea, vomiting, or diarrhea. The patient should be well hydrated (1500 to 2000 mL/24 hr) during therapy. Instruct the patient taking neomycin to report any signs of hypersensitivity, tinnitus, vertigo, rash, dizziness, or difficulty urinating.

Evaluation

A clearing of confusion, lethargy, restlessness, and irritability signals effective treatment of hepatic encephalopathy with lactulose. Passage of soft, formed stool usually occurs within 24 to 48 hours. Improvement may be seen within 2 hours following rectal administration and 24 to 48 hours following oral administration of lactulose. Improved neurologic status should be noted with effective neomycin therapy.

KEY POINTS

- Hyperkalemia may be caused by excessive K^+ intake, muscle injuries, sepsis, fever, surgery, metabolic acidosis, hyperglycemia, insulin deficiency, or shock.
- Hyperkalemia increases membrane potentials, and cells become more excitable. The cardiovascular system, the CNS, and the GI tract are most often affected.
- The treatment objectives for the patient with hyperkalemia are to normalize serum $K+$ levels and to prevent complications.
- Serum K^+ levels can be reduced by administering sodium polystyrene sulfonate, a cation-exchange resin. If K^+ levels must be dropped quickly because of conduction defects or arrhythmias, treatment options include sodium bicarbonate (to lower pH), dextrose (to provide insulin release), insulin, and calcium gluconate (for cardiac toxicity).
- Patient teaching includes the purpose for and the method of drug administration, the potential for constipation, and the importance of adequate fluid intake.
- Evaluation of drug effectiveness includes normalization of serum K^+ levels without adverse effects.

- Hepatic encephalopathy can be precipitated by increased NH_3^+ from GI bleeding (often secondary to alcohol abuse), increased protein in the diet, hypokalemia and alkalosis, and depressed CNS states such as hypoxia and sedation.
- Damage to the liver or shunting of blood around the liver inhibits the conversion of NH_3^+ to urea, leading to hepatic encephalopathy with decreased level of consciousness, impaired neuromuscular functioning, and in some cases, death.
- The treatment objective for hepatic encephalopathy is to produce an overall increase in the cognitive ability of the patient from baseline status. If the patient is comatose, a return to consciousness is the goal.
- Hepatic encephalopathy is treated with a low-protein diet, lactulose, and neomycin.
- Effective treatment with lactulose will manifest as a clearing of confusion, lethargy, restlessness, and irritability. Improvement usually occurs within 2 hours following rectal administration and 24 to 48 hours following oral administration.

Bibliography

Choate, K., Kahle, K., Wilson, F., et al. (2003). WNK1, a kinase mutated in inherited hypertension with hyperkalemia, localizes to diverse Cl^--transporting epithelia. *Proceedings of the National Academy of Science USA, 100*(2), 663–668.

Hollander-Rodriguez, J., and Calvert, J. (2006). Hyperkalemia. *American Family Physician, 73*(2). Available onlinehttp://www.aafp.org/afp/20060115/283.html. Accessed May 21, 2007.

Jolobe, O. (2006). Extreme hyperkalemia. *Southern Medical Journal, 99*(1), 96.

Juurlink, D., Mamdani, M., Lee, D., et al. (2004). Rates of hyperkalemia after publication of the randomized aldactone evaluation (RALES) study. *New England Journal of Medicine*, *351*(6), 543–551.

Kim, H., and Han, S. (2002). Therapeutic approach to hyperkalemia. *Nephron*, *92*(Suppl 1), 33–40.

Maddrey, W. (2005). Role of antibiotics in hepatic encephalopathy: Current status and future directions. *Review of Gastroenterological Disorders*, *5*(1), 1–9.

McVeigh, G. (2005). Management of hyperkalemia in adults. *Ulster Medical Journal*, *74*(2), 75–77.

Pallone, T., Zhang, Z., and Rhinehart, K. (2003). Physiology of the renal medullary microcirculation. *American Journal of Physiology and Renal Physiology*, *284*(2), 253–266.

Perazella, M. (2000). Drug-induced hyperkalemia: Old culprits and new offenders. *American Journal of Medicine*, *109*(4), 307–314.

Shawcross, D., and Jalan, R. (2005). Dispelling the myths in the treatment of hepatic encephalopathy. *Lancet*, *365*(9457), 431–433.

Stewart, C., and Cerhan, J. (2005). Hepatic encephalopathy: A dynamic or static condition. *Metabolic Brain Disease*, *20*(3), 193–204.

GASTROINTESTINAL

49

Alkalinizing and Acidifying Drugs

The basis for all acid-base relationships is *pH*, the hydrogen (H^+) ion concentration of body fluids. The normal pH range of blood is 7.35 to 7.45. Even a slight deviation in the H^+ ion concentration causes profound changes in the rate of chemical reactions. An increase in H^+ ions makes body fluids more acidic, and a decrease makes them more alkaline. Despite the day-to-day reliability of the body's pH-regulating processes, alkalinizing or acidifying drugs are sometimes needed to correct imbalances. To understand the use of alkalinizing and acidifying drugs in treating acid-base imbalances, an overview of normal regulatory mechanisms is needed.

ACID-BASE BALANCE AND IMBALANCE

To maintain acid-base balance, the body has four major lines of defense: (1) the bicarbonate-carbonic acid buffer system; (2) the respiratory system; (3) the renal system; and (4) the hemoglobin-phosphate system.

BICARBONATE-CARBONIC ACID BUFFER SYSTEM

The bicarbonate-carbonic acid buffer system can be thought of as a sponge. Depending on the specific situation, the sponge either soaks up surplus H^+ ions or releases them. It acts within seconds to prevent excessive changes in H^+ concentrations.

As the primary buffer system of the body, the bicarbonate-carbonic acid buffer system is composed of carbonic acid (H_2CO_3) and sodium bicarbonate ($NaHCO_3^-$) in the same solution. Carbonic acid is a very weak acid; thus its ability to dissociate into H^+ ions and bicarbonate (HCO_3^-) ions is less powerful than that of other acids. Most carbonic acid in solution dissociates to CO_2 and H_2O, with a net result of high concentrations of dissolved CO_2 but only a weak concentration of acid. Hydrolysis of HCO_3^- in solution yields the hydroxyl ion (OH^-) and thus increases the alkalinity of the solution. Normally, to maintain acid-base balance (pH of 7.35 to 7.45), the ratio of carbonic acid to base HCO_3^- must be 1:20. There are also small amounts of other buffers such as K^+, calcium bicarbonate ($CaHCO_3^-$), and magnesium bicarbonate ($MgHCO_3^-$) in the body.

HEMOGLOBIN

The hemoglobin-phosphate system also helps maintain the body's acid-base balance. Hemoglobin in red blood cells uses a process called the *chloride shift* to help maintain acid-base balance. The shift is regulated by the level of oxygen (O_2) in the plasma. There is a reciprocal exchange of chloride (Cl^-) for HCO_3^- ions.

PHOSPHATE BUFFER SYSTEM

The phosphate system acts in the same manner as the bicarbonate-carbonic acid system to regulate acid-base balance. Strong acids are neutralized to form a weak acid of sodium diphosphate and NaCl, resulting in a slight change in pH. When a strong base is added to the system, it is neutralized to a weak base and H_2O. This changes the pH slightly toward alkaline. The total buffering power of this system is less than that of the bicarbonate-carbonic acid system. However, the role of the bicarbonate-carbonic acid system in the kidney tubules (see later discussion) does increase the buffering power of the phosphate system.

RESPIRATORY SYSTEM

The respiratory system influences pH by controlling exhalation of CO_2. If a sudden change in pH occurs, the respiratory system, working alone, readjusts the concentration of H^+ within 1 to 3 minutes.

CO_2 is continuously formed by different metabolic processes. For example, the carbon in foods is oxidized to CO_2. CO_2 diffuses out of cells into interstitial fluids and then into intravascular fluids. It is transported to the lungs, where it diffuses into alveoli to be exhaled. An increase in the metabolic rate increases the concentration of CO_2 in extracellular fluids. If the respiratory rate increases, the expiration of CO_2 increases, lowering the amount of CO_2 in extracellular fluids.

Using a feedback mechanism, the respiratory system acts to control H^+ concentration through direct action on the medullary respiratory center. In addition, changes in ventilation rate and depth alter H^+ concentration of body fluids. When the H^+ ion concentration of the extracellular fluid increases, the rate and depth of respirations increase and more CO_2 is exhaled. CO_2 concentration in extracellular fluid thus decreases, leading to a drop in H^+ concentration and an increase in pH.

RENAL SYSTEM

Because the kidneys eliminate varying amounts of acid or base, they play a vital role in controlling pH. The kidneys can either generate H^+ ions or eliminate them by a variety of mechanisms; they adjust pH by regulating the elimination of bicarbonate (HCO_3^-). The amount of HCO_3^- entering the renal tubules changes in proportion to the extracellular HCO_3^- concentration. When HCO_3^- concentrations in extracellular fluid are normal, H^+ secretion and filtration of HCO_3^- normally balance and neutralize each other. Although the kidneys are the most powerful of the control mechanisms, when they work alone, several hours to a day or more is needed to restore balance.

In acidosis the kidneys eliminate H^+ by two major mechanisms. The first is by generating HCO_3^-, and the other is by increasing the secretion of ammonia. In the proximal tubule, the enzyme carbonic anhydrase catalyzes the conversion of $CO_2 + H_2O$ into H_2CO_3, which spontaneously breaks down into HCO_3^- and H^+. H^+ ions are secreted into the lumen of the proximal tubule, where they react with HCO_3^- to form H_2CO_3; continuing the cycle, H_2CO_3 is again broken down by carbonic anhydrase into CO_2 and H_2O. CO_2 diffuses into proximal cells to generate HCO_3^-. The secretion of ammonia (NH_3) neutralizes H^+ ions by incorporating them into ammonium (NH_4^+). This mechanism is vital to increase the urinary excretion of ketoacids in patients with diabetic ketoacidosis. Although the renal mechanism is slow to act, it differs from the respiratory mechanism in that it continues to respond until the extracellular pH reaches normal.

An inability of the body to maintain acid-base balance results in respiratory or metabolic alkalosis, respiratory or metabolic acidosis, or a combination of imbalances (Table 49-1). Furthermore, these imbalances can occur in three forms: primary, mixed, and compensated.

Primary imbalances originate from an acute condition such as respiratory alkalosis resulting from hyperventilation. *Mixed imbalances* occurs when one disorder results in acidosis and another disorder results in alkalosis, or when two

---

TABLE 49-1 Overview of Acid-Base Balance

Condition	Possible Etiology	Imbalance Mechanism
RESPIRATORY ACIDOSIS		
Reduced elimination of hydrogen ions	Airway obstruction Respiratory depression related to the following: • Anesthetics, drugs (especially opioids) • Poisons • Electrolyte imbalances • Trauma and spinal cord injury • Cerebral edema • Guillain-Barré syndrome • Poliomyelitis • Myasthenia gravis Alveolar-capillary obstruction related to the following: • Vascular occlusive disease • Pneumonia • Pulmonary edema • Tuberculosis • Cystic fibrosis • Atelectasis • Adult respiratory distress syndrome • Emphysema • Lung cancer • Inadequate chest expansion • Muscle weakness • Skeletal deformities	Acute acidosis: • Increases in carbon dioxide cause carbonic acid and hydrogen content to increase and the pH to decrease. Chronic acidosis: • Renal response to increase in carbon dioxide. Hydrogen ions eliminated. Reabsorption of sodium bicarbonate helps restore pH.
RESPIRATORY ALKALOSIS		
Excessive loss of carbon dioxide	Shock Hyperventilation related to the following: • Fear • Anxiety • Mechanical ventilation CNS stimulation related to the following: • Catecholamine • progesterone • Salicylates Hypoxemia related to the following: • Asphyxiation • Asthma • High altitudes • Pneumonia • Pulmonary emboli	Acute alkalosis: • Carbon dioxide blown off, causing a base excess and pH increases. Chronic alkalosis: • Renal response to decreased carbon dioxide. More bicarbonate excreted. Chloride retained to restore pH.
METABOLIC ACIDOSIS		
Overproduction of hydrogen ions	Excessive oxidation fatty acids related to the following: • Diabetic ketoacidosis • Starvation Hypermetabolism related to the following: • Heavy exercise • Seizure activity • Fever • Hypoxia, ischemia	Large amounts of fixed acids in blood results in loss of bicarbonate and decreased pH. Immediate respiratory response results in decreased carbon dioxide levels but not sufficiently to correct imbalance.

Continued

GASTROINTESTINAL

TABLE 49-1 Overview of Acid-Base Balance—Cont'd

Condition	Possible Etiology	Imbalance Mechanism
	Excessive ingestion acids related to the following: • Salicylate intoxication • Methanol ingestion • Ethanol intoxication	
Reduced elimination of hydrogen ions	Renal failure	
Reduced production of bicarbonate	Renal or liver failure Pancreatitis	
Increased elimination of bicarbonate	Dehydration Diarrhea Buffering of organic acids	
METABOLIC ALKALOSIS		
Increased base components	Administration parenteral base related to the following: • Blood transfusion • Parenteral nutrition • Sodium bicarbonate	Loss of acid or retention of base results in elevated pH and bicarbonate. Minimal respiratory response results in normal or elevated carbon dioxide levels. Bicarbonate-carbonic acid buffer system activated and respirations become slow and shallow. Kidneys retain more hydrogen and excrete more bicarbonate.
Increased base components	Excessive ingestion of base related to the following: • Antacids • Milk-alkali syndrome • Cushing's syndrome	
Decreased acid components	Gastric suctioning Hyperaldosteronism Prolonged vomiting Thiazide diuretics	

disturbances are both acidotic or both alkalotic. *Compensated imbalances* are the body's attempt to bring the pH back to normal after a primary imbalance has occurred. Compensated imbalances are usually found with chronic disorders (e.g., chronic obstructive pulmonary disease [COPD]). In essence, respiratory imbalances are compensated for by the renal system; metabolic imbalances are compensated for by the respiratory system.

PATHOPHYSIOLOGY OF ALKALOSIS AND ACIDOSIS

Because alkalosis and acidosis are manifestations of many conditions, rather than separate disease states, their actual incidence is unknown. Each acid-base imbalance is classified as respiratory or metabolic, then further broken down into the common disorders respiratory alkalosis, respiratory acidosis, metabolic alkalosis, or metabolic acidosis.

Alkalosis

Alkalosis is a decrease in H^+ concentration of the blood and is reflected by an arterial pH above 7.45. It is not a disease as such but a consequence of a pathogenic process. Alkalosis results from an actual or relative increase in the concentration or strength of base in the blood.

In an actual base excess, the concentration of the base components are proportionately higher than normal compared with the concentration of acid components. There is either an overproduction of base or reduced elimination of bases, usually HCO_3^-.

In a relative base excess, the concentration of acid components is decreased. The base excess (BE) results from either increased elimination of acids (as H^+) or reduced production of acids.

Alkalosis causes disturbances in metabolism and pulmonary respiration, with serious and potentially life-threatening results. The most common manifestations of alkalosis include stimulation of the central nervous system (CNS) and the neuromuscular and cardiovascular systems.

Respiratory Alkalosis
Respiratory alkalosis, occurring as a result of alveolar hyperventilation, results in decreased serum CO_2 levels *(hypocapnia).* The most common causes of respiratory alkalosis include fear caused by traumatic scenes and drugs (particularly aspirin and other salicylates). Excessive exhalation of CO_2 causes a reduction in serum CO_2 levels and decreased carbonic acid production. The body attempts to compensate by reducing the rate and depth of respirations to conserve CO_2 and by increasing renal elimination of HCO_3^-.

Metabolic Alkalosis
Metabolic alkalosis results from excessive accumulation of fixed bases or excessive loss of fixed acids in body fluids. The most common causes of metabolic alkalosis include vomiting or suctioning and the administration of alkalinizing salts (e.g., sodium bicarbonate [$NaHCO_3^-$]). A major cause of metabolic alkalosis is loss of fixed acids, such as hydrochloric acid (HCl), from the stomach, either through gastric suctioning or excessive vomiting. The loss of acid increases pH. Carbonic acid dissociates, and HCO_3^- concentration increases through renal absorption. This results in increased renal elimination of H^+, K^+, and Cl^-. Cl^- competes with HCO_3^- in combining with Na^+. Thus, when Cl^- levels fall, HCO_3^- levels rise. As pH increases, Ca^{++} binding increases and serum Ca^{++} levels decrease, creating hypocalcemia. Serum K^+ levels also decrease as a result of the body's attempt to maintain electrical neutrality. Most of the serious manifestations of alkalosis are attributed to the

accompanying hypocalcemia. The body attempts to compensate for metabolic alkalosis by hypoventilation and by increasing the urinary loss of HCO_3^- through decreased H^+ secretion.

Acidosis

Acidosis is an arterial blood pH below 7.35. Like alkalosis, acidosis is not a specific disease, but rather a symptom of a disease or pathologic process. Acidosis results from an actual or relative increase in the concentration of acids. In actual acidosis, the concentration of acid components does not increase. Instead, the concentration of base components is decreased (base deficit), which makes the fluid more acid than alkaline. An actual base deficit results from processes that cause increased elimination of base (usually HCO_3^-), reduced production, or overproduction of ketoacids (in the patient with diabetes).

Acidosis causes significant changes in physiologic functions. Many of the early signs and symptoms of acidosis manifest as depression of the CNS or the neuromuscular, cardiovascular, and respiratory systems.

Respiratory Acidosis

Low arterial pH and elevated serum CO_2 levels *(hypercapnia)*, usually from hypoventilation, constitute respiratory acidosis. Abnormally slow or shallow respirations, or poor alveolar ventilation resulting in inadequate gas exchange, causes CO_2 to accumulate in the lungs and serum, increasing carbonic acid levels in the circulating blood and lowering pH. It can be acute, as in sudden ventilatory failure in asthma, or chronic, as in emphysema. The body attempts to compensate by increasing the renal reabsorption of HCO_3^- by increasing the secretion of H^+ ions.

Metabolic Acidosis

Metabolic acidosis results from excessive production of acids (as in uncontrolled diabetes), or loss of base in body fluids. Fixed acids, such as HCl, are produced by metabolism or ingested foods. Organic acids (related to ketoacids) are produced when the muscles oxidize fatty acids instead of glucose to form adenosine triphosphate (ATP). The generation of organic ketoacids neutralizes HCO_3^-, thereby reducing pH. Metabolic acidosis never results from a respiratory problem, with the exception of lactic acidosis from anaerobic metabolism.

Increased levels of circulating H^+ result in stimulation of peripheral chemoreceptors and, within minutes, increases

the respiratory rate and brings about the onset of acidosis. The body attempts to compensate for metabolic acidosis by hyperventilating, which results in reduced CO_2 levels.

PHARMACOTHERAPEUTIC OPTIONS

Alkalinizing Drugs

- acetazolamide (Diamox); ◆ Diamox
- sodium acetate
- sodium bicarbonate (Neut)
- sodium citrate (Shohl's modified solution, Bicitra, Oracit); ◆ Oracit
- sodium lactate

▦ Indications

Alkalinizing drugs such as $NaHCO_3^-$, sodium acetate, sodium citrate or citric acid, and sodium lactate are used to increase blood pH and thus correct metabolic acidosis.

Acetazolamide is used to facilitate removal of phenobarbital or lithium after overdose. It is not recommended for use with salicylate overdose because both drugs can cause metabolic acidosis. It has also been used to offset the cerebral edema encountered with exposure to high altitudes.

$NaHCO_3^-$ is also used to increase urinary pH in patients with barbiturate, lithium, or salicylate toxicities so as to enhance elimination of these drugs. $NaHCO_3^-$ may be used as an adjunct to other therapies for treatment of hyperkalemia (to promote the reuptake of K^+ into the cells).

▦ Pharmacodynamics

Acetazolamide, a carbonic anhydrase inhibitor (see Chapter 42), raises urinary pH by increasing the urinary loss of HCO_3^- but paradoxically lowers blood pH by promoting the elimination of Na^+, K^+, bicarbonate, and H_2O. When HCO_3^- is lost, the reabsorption of Cl^- with Na^+ increases and causes hyperchloremic metabolic acidosis that self-limits the action of acetazolamide.

$NaHCO_3^-$ dissociates in the blood to increase HCO_3^- and decrease H^+ concentration. As the H^+ ions are eliminated in the urine, urinary pH rises. Sodium acetate, citrate, and lactate must first be converted to HCO_3^-, and then they act in the same fashion as $NaHCO_3^-$.

▦ Pharmacokinetics

$NaHCO_3^-$ is 100% bioavailable when administered intravenously. It is widely distributed to extracellular fluid, with an immediate onset of action and peak drug levels reached

PHARMACOKINETICS
TABLE 49-2 Selected Alkalinizing and Acidifying Drugs*

	Route	Onset	Peak	Duration	PB (%)	$t_{1/2}$	BioA (%)
ALKALINIZING DRUGS							
sodium bicarbonate	IV	Immed	15 min	1–2 hr	UA	UA	100
ACIDIFYING DRUGS							
ascorbic acid	PO, subQ	2 days–3 wks	UA	UA	UA	UA	UA
	IV	Immed					100
ammonium chloride	PO	UA	1–3 hr	UA	UA	UA	UA
HCl	IV	Immed	15 min	1 hour	—	—	100

*As noted in intracellular fluids.
BioA, Bioavailability; *IV*, intravenous; *PB*, protein binding; *PO*, by mouth; *subQ*, subcutaneous; t₁/₂, half-life; *UA*, unavailable.

GASTROINTESTINAL

in 15 minutes (Table 49-2). $NaHCO_3^-$ is eliminated in the urine and has an unknown half-life.

Adverse Effects and Contraindications

The adverse effects of alkalinizing drugs are usually related to large dosages. Excessive $NaHCO_3^-$ causes metabolic alkalosis that manifests as hyperirritability, tetany, or both. When administered too rapidly to correct diabetic ketoacidosis, the result can be tissue hypoxia, cerebral dysfunction, and lactic acidosis. **In general, sodium bicarbonate should not be used for the treatment of diabetic ketoacidosis (DKA). The underlying condition should be corrected, that is to say dehydration first, and then high glucose.**

Acetazolamide produces a wide range of adverse effects. CNS reactions include headache, sedation, confusion, and paresthesias. In a patient with severe liver disease, acetazolamide can raise the blood sugar, decrease uric acid elimination, produce metabolic acidosis, and precipitate hepatic coma. Hypersensitivity reactions and bone marrow depression can lead to aplastic anemia.

The high Na^+ content of $NaHCO_3^-$ (276 mg/gram) causes water retention and edema in some patients. Therefore use $NaHCO_3^-$ cautiously in patients with heart failure, renal failure, or other fluid balance disorders. Injection of $NaHCO_3^-$ is contraindicated in patients with Cl depletion from vomiting or from continuous gastrointestinal (GI) suction, as well as in patients taking diuretics that have been identified to produce hypochloremic alkalosis. Oral administration of $NaHCO_3^-$ produces gastric distention and flatus when it combines with HCl in the stomach and releases CO_2.

Sodium citrate produces fewer adverse effects than $NaHCO_3^-$, but in excess can also cause metabolic alkalosis or tetany, and may aggravate existing cardiovascular disease by increasing Ca^{++} levels. Orally administered sodium citrate has a laxative-like effect and can frequently cause hypocalcemia that manifests as perioral hypoesthesia. It should not be used in patients who are allergic to citrus products.

Sodium lactate also produces fewer adverse effects than $NaHCO_3^-$ but in excess can cause metabolic acidosis (rather than alkalosis). Because the Na^+ content is high (204 mg/gram), water retention and edema may develop. Do not use sodium lactate in patients with an acute disorder or in patients who have liver impairment, because the conversion of lactate to bicarbonate occurs in the liver.

Drug Interactions

Drugs interacting with alkalinizing drugs are identified in Table 49-3. The most common interactions are related to their ability to increase the reabsorption, or to facilitate elimination, of interacting drugs.

Dosage Regimen

The dose of a specific alkalinizing drug is individualized based on lab calculations of the HCO_3^- levels needed. $NaHCO_3^-$ is initially administered as 1 mEq/kg of body weight, to be followed by 0.5 mEq/kg every 10 minutes. The dosage is then based on the formula identified in Table 49-4. The dosages for sodium citrate and lactate are also individualized.

Lab Considerations

Check serum Na^+, K^+, Cl^-, HCO_3^-, and anion gap levels and kidney function before and throughout therapy. In emergent situations, obtain and monitor arterial blood gases (ABGs) frequently. When using these drugs for urinary alkalinization in drug overdose, monitor urinary pH every 4 hours.

$NaHCO_3^-$ antagonizes the effects of pentagastrin and histamine during testing of gastric acid secretion. Avoid using the drug in the 24 hours preceding the test.

Acidifying Drugs
◆ ammonium chloride
◆ ascorbic acid
◆ hydrochloric acid

Indications

Two acidifying drugs are used to correct metabolic alkalosis: ammonium chloride and hydrochloric acid (HCl). Ammonium chloride is specifically useful in correcting acidosis when use of NaCl is contraindicated (e.g., in a patient with a fluid overload). Ammonium chloride and ascorbic acid serve as urine-acidifying drugs. These two drugs can be used to increase the effectiveness of certain urinary antibacterial drugs (see Chapter 41) and to enhance drug elimination in drug overdose.

Pharmacodynamics

As an acidifying salt that has a fixed anion, ammonium chloride is converted to urea in the liver. H^+ and Cl^- ions are liberated, thus lowering blood pH. It lowers urinary pH by producing acid urine and changing the elimination rate of many drugs and drug metabolites.

Ascorbic acid directly acidifies the urine by producing H^+ ions and lowering urinary pH. Hydrochloric acid infusions are used to correct acute metabolic alkalosis refractory to other treatment. Hydrochloric acid for injection is prepared

DRUG INTERACTIONS
TABLE 49-3 Selected Alkalinizing and Acidifying Drugs

Drug	Interactive Drugs	Interaction
ALKALINIZING DRUGS		
sodium bicarbonate	Amphetamines, ephedrine, flecainide, mecamylamine, methadone, pseudoephedrine, quinidine, quinine	Increases reabsorption of interactive drugs
	aspirin, chlorpropamide, Salicylates, lithium, phenobarbital, Tetracyclines	Increases elimination of interactive drug
	Glucocorticoids	Excessive sodium retention

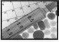

DOSAGE

TABLE 49-4 Selected Alkalinizing and Acidifying Drugs

Drug	Uses	Dosage	Implications
ALKALINIZING DRUGS			
acetazolamide	Alkalinize urine in phenobarbital or lithium overdose	Individualized dosage based on the overdosed drug	Check urinary pH frequently
sodium bicarbonate	Metabolic acidosis in cardiac arrest	1 mEq/kg IV to be followed by 0.5 mEq/kg every 10 min as needed	*Step 1:* Base deficit = desired HCO_3 level − patient's HCO_3 level.
	Less severe metabolic acidosis	2–5 mEq/kg IV over 4–8 hr	*Step 2:* Bicarbonate dosage (mEq) = 0.4 × kg × base deficit
	Chronic renal failure	20–36 mEq/kg PO daily in divided doses	Dosage necessary to achieve serum bicarbonate level of 18–20 mEq/L
	Alkalinize urine	48 mEq PO followed by 12–24 mEq PO every 4 hr	Check urinary pH frequently.
sodium citrate	Metabolic acidosis	*Adult:* Up to 5 mL/min IV of dilute solution. 10–30 mL PO 4 times daily and at bedtime. *Child:* 5–15 mL PO 4 times daily and at bedtime	Dosage based on patient's chloride deficit. 1 mL of solution = 1 mmol of sodium bicarbonate
	Alkalinize urine in drug overdose	4–12 grams PO daily in divided doses every 4–6 hr	Check urinary pH frequently.
sodium lactate	Metabolic acidosis in patients who cannot tolerate oral product	Dosage (mL of 1/6 molar solution) = 0.8 × body weight (lb) × (60 − plasma CO_2 value)	Converts to sodium bicarbonate in the liver
	Alkalinize urine in drug overdose	30 mL/kg IV of a 1/6 molar solution –*or*– PO in divided doses over 24 hr	
ACIDIFYING DRUGS			
ammonium chloride	Metabolic alkalosis	*Adult:* 100–200 mEq in 500–1000 mL IV solution. Dosage (mEq) = chloride deficit in mEq/L × 0.2 × kg body weight	Dosage based on chloride deficit. Each gram of ammonium chloride reduces CO_2–combining power of a 70-kg adult by about 16 mg/kg will lower the CO_2–combining power by 1%. Dilute solution not to exceed 5 mL/minute
	Acidify urine	*Adult:* 4–12 grams PO in divided doses every 4–6 hr *Child:* 75 mg/kg/day in four divided doses	
ascorbic acid	Acidify urine in drug overdose	4–12 grams PO daily in divided doses	
hydrochloric acid	Metabolic alkalosis unresponsive to fluid and electrolytes; decompensated CHF or renal failure with oliguria	Dose HCl (mEq) = (0.2 L/kg × kg body weight) × (103 − observed serum chloride) 0.1–0.2 molar solution IV at 0.2 mEq/kg/hr or less. Additional doses based on every-4-hr ABGs	Give through central venous IV line
sodium chloride	Metabolic alkalosis	250, 500, 1000 mL IV infused over 8–24 hr	Monitor serum sodium levels

ABG, Arterial blood gases; *CHF;* congestive heart failure; *IV,* intravenous (route).

GASTROINTESTINAL

as needed by the hospital pharmacist. It is administered at a rate of 100 mL/hr with pH monitoring done hourly.

Pharmacokinetics

Ammonium chloride taken orally is completely absorbed in 3 to 6 hours. Drug action peaks 1 to 3 hours after intravenous (IV) administration (see Table 49-2). Ammonium chloride is biotransformed to HCl and urea, which is then eliminated via the kidneys.

Adverse Effects and Contraindications

The adverse effects of acidifying drugs are usually mild. Ammonium chloride can cause anorexia, nausea, vomiting, and thirst when taken orally. Using enteric-coated tablets may reduce adverse GI effects; however, absorption of this dosage form is unpredictable.

▲ **Large doses of ammonium chloride can cause metabolic acidosis secondary to hyperchloremia, especially in patients**

with impaired renal function. Other adverse effects of large doses of ammonium chloride include rash, headache, hyperventilation, bradycardia, progressive drowsiness, confusion, and excitement alternating with coma. Tetany, hyperglycemia, glucosuria, twitching, hyperreflexia, and electroencephalogram changes have also been reported. Most of these adverse effects are related to NH_3 toxicity resulting from inability of the liver to convert NH_4 ions to urea. Because the acidifying action of ammonium chloride depends on its hepatic conversion to urea, the drug is contraindicated for use in patients with liver disease. Safe use in perinatal and pediatric populations has not been established.

High doses of ascorbic acid cause nausea, vomiting, diarrhea, abdominal cramps, flushing, headache, and insomnia. Hemolytic anemia can develop in patients with glucose-6-phosphate dehydrogenase (G6PD) deficiency after high doses of ascorbic acid.

▥ Drug Interactions

There are no known drug interactions with ammonium chloride or ascorbic acid.

▥ Dosage Regimen

As with the alkalinizing drugs, the dosage regimen of acidifying drugs is individualized. The dosage of ammonium chloride is calculated based on the patient's Cl^- deficit (see Table 49-4). To acidify urine in the treatment of drug overdose, ascorbic acid is dosed at 4 to 12 grams daily, given orally in divided doses.

▥ Lab Considerations

Monitor the patient's acid-base and electrolyte balance before and throughout treatment with acidifying drugs. Take blood urea nitrogen (BUN) and creatinine measurements before using arginine, because the drug contains large amounts of metabolizable nitrogen, which causes a temporary elevation in nitrogen levels. Also monitor liver function.

CLINICAL REASONING

Treatment Objectives

The treatment goals for alkalosis are directed at (1) increasing the level of H^+ ions; (2) preventing further H^+, K^+, Ca^{++}, and Cl^- losses; and (3) restoring fluid balance. Treatment goals for acidosis are directed at correcting the underlying cause of the acidosis and normalizing the acid-base balance. It should be evident that overtreating one type of imbalance may upset the balance in the opposite direction. Thus, use caution when determining specific treatment modalities.

Treatment Options

Interventions for the patient with alkalosis or acidosis are directed at maintaining and monitoring existing system functioning as well as correcting the acid-base imbalance. Review the patient's history of any preexisting condition that may contraindicate the use of alkalinizing or acidifying drugs, or warrant their cautious use.

Laboratory monitoring is required for initial dosage calculations and future adjustments. Thus, draw samples for ABGs using the correct technique, and immediately deliver them to the laboratory for analysis. Minimize errors in ABG analysis due to faulty specimen collection. Potential sampling errors and their implications are identified in Table 49-5.

▥ Patient Variables

Determine whether the patient has a recent history of vomiting or diarrhea; a history of heart or renal failure, cirrhosis, diabetes mellitus, or chronic airway limitation; or recent surgery. A drug history is important to elicit because drugs cause or contribute to acid-base imbalance. Request information from family members because some alterations in acid-base balance cause changes in the patient's cognitive function or emotional status.

ALKALOSIS. Whether the origin of alkalosis is respiratory or metabolic, the patient's symptoms are the result of the body's attempt to compensate for the imbalance. Many of the symptoms are also related to the hypocalcemia and hypokalemia that usually accompany alkalosis. Stimulation of the CNS appears in the patient's reports of lightheadedness, vertigo, agitation, and confusion. One of the earliest symptoms of

TABLE **49-5 Potential ABG Sampling Errors**

Sampling Error	Effects			Implications
	pH	PaCO$_2$	PaO$_2$	
Air bubbles in syringe	↑	↓	↑	Immediately expel all air bubbles. Do not agitate or use sample that appears frothy.
Inadvertent venous sample or venous contamination of arterial sample	↓	↑	↓	Avoid femoral artery. Use needle with short bevel. Do not overshoot artery and then withdraw to catch it. Watch for autofilling of syringe with arterial puncture. Verify questionable results with new sample.
Alteration of pH due to presence of anticoagulant	↓	–	–	Use lithium heparin, if possible. Use 1:1000 units/mL concentration. Use minimum 2-mL discard sample with arterial line aspiration.
Dilution of sample due to presence of anticoagulant	↑	↓	↓	Use syringe with minimum dead space. Use dried heparin if available.
Effects of metabolism on white blood cells in sample	↓	↑	↓	Place sample on ice immediately after drawing, with analysis occurring within 20 minutes. Have sample analyzed immediately if patient has leukocytosis.

ABG, Arterial blood gas.

alkalosis is a tingling sensation in the fingers and toes or around the mouth. The presence of Trousseau's and Chvostek's signs may be noted with hypocalcemia. Palpitations and dry mouth may also be noted.

In addition, carpopedal spasms, tetany, hyperactive deep tendon reflexes, skeletal muscle weakness, and muscle cramping and twitching are evident. Syncopal episodes, seizures, and coma are possible. Although skeletal muscles contract as a result of overstimulation, the muscles themselves become weaker because of the alkalosis and hypokalemia.

Hand-grasp strength is reduced, and the patient may be unable to support body weight or walk. Respiratory efforts become less effective as the skeletal muscles of respiration become weaker. Because alkalosis produces increased myocardial irritability, especially in the presence of an accompanying hypokalemia, the heart rate increases and the pulse becomes thready. The blood pressure may be normal or low.

ACIDOSIS. Clinical manifestations of acidosis are similar, whether the cause is respiratory or metabolic. Early complaints include general malaise and headache. The patient may also report nausea, vomiting, and abdominal pain. Depressed CNS function is common in patients with acidosis and may be manifested as lethargy progressing to confusion, especially in the older adult. The patient becomes stuporous as acidosis worsens or if it is accompanied by hyperkalemia. The acidotic state and accompanying hyperkalemia cause a decrease in muscle tone and deep tendon reflexes. The muscle weakness is bilateral and can progress to flaccid paralysis.

If the acidosis is of respiratory origin, breathing effectiveness is greatly diminished, with respirations rapid but shallow. If the acidosis has a metabolic origin, the rate and depth of respirations increase in proportion to the increase in H^+ concentration. Respirations are rapid, deep, and regular but not under voluntary control *(Kussmaul's respirations)*. Skin and mucous membranes are pale to cyanotic because respirations are ineffective.

However, in metabolic acidosis, in which respirations are essentially unaffected and the rate increased, the patient's skin is pink, warm, and dry. Cardiovascular manifestations of acidosis include tachycardia. As acidosis worsens or is accompanied by hyperkalemia, electrical activity through the heart is reduced and bradycardia results. As a result of changes in heart activity, peripheral pulses are difficult to locate and are easily obliterated with light pressure. Hypotension is the result of vasodilation.

The most common laboratory tests for the diagnosis and monitoring of acid-base balance are the pH, CO_2, HCO_3^-, and electrolyte levels. Knowledge of electrolyte concentrations is useful in determining pH imbalances because of the following rule: $Na^+ - ([Cl^-] + [HCO_3^-]) =$ anion gap. Normal values for anion gap are 8 to 16 mEq/L in plasma. In acidosis, the anion gap is over 16; in alkalosis the anion gap is less than 8.

A pH over 7.45 indicates alkalosis. Because the clinical manifestations of metabolic alkalosis are similar to those of respiratory alkalosis, it is important to monitor ABG values and serum electrolytes as well as patient signs and symptoms to determine the cause (Table 49-6).

The presence of acidosis is also detected by checking ABGs, as well as evaluating K^+ and Cl^- levels. Acidosis is present when arterial pH falls below 7.35. The patient with acidosis should have one or more electrocardiographic evaluations, primarily to detect changes associated with hyperkalemia such as peaked T waves, a wide QRS complex, and prolonged PR intervals. Ventricular arrhythmias are common.

LIFE-SPAN CONSIDERATIONS

Pregnant and Nursing Women. There is a slight degree of respiratory alkalosis throughout pregnancy. Because cell numbers increase, additional O_2 is required during pregnancy. Progesterone stimulates the respiratory rate. In addition, pregnancy causes a small degree of hyperventilation since tidal volume (amount of air breathed with ordinary respiration) decreases steadily throughout pregnancy. In the process, excess CO_2 is blown off, resulting in a decrease in carbonic acid and pH changes. Although the normal pH range remains between 7.35 and 7.45, the pH tends toward the upper range.

Children and Adolescents. Infants and children have acid-base buffering systems that are less well developed than those in adults, and they tend to develop acid-base imbalances more easily. Common conditions predisposing an infant to acid-base imbalances include fevers, upper respiratory infections, vomiting, and diarrhea. Further, infants and small children are less able to describe symptoms such as thirst or changes in sensation (e.g., paresthesias); therefore perform a careful evaluation of early changes in acid-base balance.

Older Adults. Age is an important variable in assessing the patient with an acid-base imbalance because the older adult is more vulnerable to conditions that cause imbalances. Conditions that contribute to acidosis or alkalosis include cardiac, renal, and pulmonary impairments, diabetes mellitus, persistent diarrhea, pancreatitis, and fever.

Alkalosis causes the myocardium to be more sensitive to digoxin, resulting in increased risk for digoxin toxicity. Many older adults take one or more cardiac drugs or diuretics; thus information about prescribed or over-the-counter drugs should be noted, since many of these alter acid-base, fluid, or electrolyte balance.

Because of decreased chest wall compliance, elasticity of lung tissues, number of alveoli, and respiratory muscle strength, the older adult cannot eliminate CO_2 as readily. This limits the patient's ability to compensate for metabolic alterations and predisposes the patient to respiratory acidosis.

The physical changes of aging also result in a decrease in nephrons. The older adult may take 18 to 48 hours to achieve acid-base balance after an upset, whereas a younger adult may

TABLE 49-6 Lab Findings in Acid-Base Imbalances

Imbalance	Compensation	Gas Parameters*			Electrolytes†		
		pH	PaCO₂	HCO₃	K⁺	Ca⁺⁺	Cl⁻
Respiratory alkalosis	Uncompensated	↑ 7.45	↓ 35	N			
	Partially compensated	↑ 7.45	↓ 35	↓ 22			
	Compensated	N	↓ 35	↓ 22	↓	↓	↑
Respiratory acidosis	Uncompensated	↓ 7.35	↑ 46	N			
	Partially compensated	↓ 7.35	↑ 46	↑ 26			
	Compensated	N	↑ 46	↑ 26	↑	N	↑↓
Metabolic alkalosis	Uncompensated	↑ 7.45	N	↑ 26			
	Partially compensated	↑ 7.45	↑ 26	↑ 26			
	Compensated	N	↑ 46	↑ 26	↓	↓	↓
Metabolic acidosis	Uncompensated	↓ 7.35	N	↓ 22			
	Partially compensated	N or ↓ 7.35	↓ 35	↓ 22			
	Compensated	N	↓ 35	↓ 22	↑	N	↑

*Arterial blood gas values at sea level:
pH   7.35–7.45
PaCO₂   35–46 mm Hg
HCO₃   22–26 mEq/L
†Electrolyte levels relative to sodium values. Normal electrolyte values:
Potassium   3.5–5.0 mEq/L
Chloride   98–106 mmol/L
Calcium   8.8–10.0 mg/dL
↑Lab values above normal range; ↓ lab values below normal range; *N*, normal.

need only 6 to 10 hours. By returning some substances to body fluids and eliminating others, the kidneys compensate (in several hours) for even large deviations from normal. However, as aging continues, compensatory abilities decline.

▥ Drug Variables

RESPIRATORY ALKALOSIS. Because alkalosis is a manifestation of other abnormal processes, treatment is most effective when first directed at the underlying abnormality. Mild asymptomatic alkalosis requires no specific treatment. With hysterical hyperventilation, symptoms are alleviated by having the patient rebreathe a mixture of CO_2 and O_2 from a large paper bag, or by giving inhalations of 5% CO_2 at intervals.

For patients ascending to high altitudes, 2 days of pretreatment with acetazolamide produces a mild metabolic acidosis. The mild acidosis offsets the initial respiratory alkalosis and thus minimizes symptoms related to hyperventilation.

RESPIRATORY ACIDOSIS. The only practical treatment for respiratory acidosis involves improvement of the basic underlying cause of the hypoventilation. Consider the possibility of drug abuse in otherwise healthy individuals who suddenly develop acute respiratory depression. Consider using naloxone, an opioid antagonist (see Chapter 16), in all comatose patients in whom no apparent cause of respiratory depression can be identified.

⚠ **Alkalinizing drugs have no place in the management of chronic respiratory acidosis**. If the underlying cause of respiratory acidosis is pneumonia, begin appropriate antimicrobial therapy. Patients with severe respiratory acidosis should be immediately ventilated. There is no role for sodium bicarbonate here—it won't help. **In patients with chronic hypercapnia**

⚠ **(e.g., related to COPD), O_2 should be used with extreme caution and in the lowest possible concentration to avoid serious tissue hypoxia. Hypoxemia may be the primary stimulus to respiration in this situation. Sudden increases in arterial CO_2 values from O_2 administration may result in cessation of respirations.**

METABOLIC ALKALOSIS. Treatment that is effective for metabolic alkalosis is different from that which is effective for respiratory alkalosis. Therefore, the health care provider must be able to distinguish between metabolic and respiratory alkalosis in order to prevent and manage the condition.

In most cases, acute metabolic alkalosis can be corrected by the IV administration of adequate amounts of NaCl solution. The ability of a neutral salt to correct an acid-base imbalance is based on physiologic rather than chemical mechanisms. For example, in alkalosis due to vomiting, the body is depleted of H_2O, H^+, Cl^-, and to a lesser degree, Na^+. Once an adequate extracellular volume is reestablished, normal renal mechanisms take over and Na^+, along with HCO_3^-, is eliminated in the urine.

In severe cases of metabolic alkalosis, ammonium chloride can be used when it is desirable to lower the systemic pH promptly and directly without reliance on either renal or hepatic mechanisms. The infused acid is immediately buffered by circulating blood, although mild hemolysis may occur. Think of this procedure as a heroic measure used only when more conventional therapy has failed.

In some patients, the primary purpose for therapy in metabolic alkalosis is to change the pH of the urine. When renal function is normal, this is readily accomplished by using either alkalinizing or acidifying salts. Their use produces a

modest distortion in systemic acid-base balance. However, in edema-forming states, when the renal reabsorption of Na^+ is inappropriately high, alkalinizing salts are poorly eliminated. Also, in the presence of renal insufficiency, the capacity of the kidney to compensate for acidosis is diminished, and acidifying salts may have harmful systemic effects.

METABOLIC ACIDOSIS. In most cases, the treatment for metabolic acidosis is aimed at the underlying cause. Disorders characterized by failure of bicarbonate regeneration or reduced elimination of inorganic acids represent acidosis. Thus, the treatment of these disorders requires administering relatively modest amounts of bicarbonate. For example, in chronic renal failure, alkali therapy is generally not required unless plasma HCO_3^- levels fall below 16 to 18 mEq/L. If the acidosis is more severe, HCO_3^- supplementation in the form of modified Shohl's solution can be used.

Treatment of patients with metabolic acidosis due to external bicarbonate loss varies with the nature of the disorder. For example, in acute acidosis due to GI losses, $NaHCO_3^-$ can be given cautiously to raise the plasma bicarbonate concentration to16 mEq/L over a 12 to 24 hour period rather than to repair the entire bicarbonate deficit. The use of bicarbonate in this manner is valid only if there are no further GI losses.

If the underlying cause is diabetic ketoacidosis, the usual treatment regimen includes fluids and insulin. Insulin promotes glucose utilization by the cells and thus completes oxidation of ketoacids, and ketogenesis is reduced. Therefore alkali therapy is ordinarily not necessary. In addition, because the hyperventilatory response to acidosis in some patients with diabetes is governed by arterial, rather than central medullary chemoreceptors, $NaHCO_3^-$ given intravenously may result in arterial alkalinization and a fall in the ventilation rate. In severe ketoacidosis, administration of $NaHCO_3^-$ may be necessary to increase $NaHCO_3^-$ levels and neutralize nonvolatile acid accumulation.

However, $NaHCO_3^-$ is seldom used alone in the treatment of metabolic acidosis. If hypokalemia is present, correct it with K^+ replacement before administering $NaHCO_3^-$. If $NaHCO_3^-$ is given in the presence of hypokalemia without taking this measure, the acidosis may be corrected using K^+ to shift back into the cells, but the resulting severe hypokalemia may culminate in cardiac arrest.

$NaHCO_3^-$ must be used with caution in patients with heart failure or other edematous or Na^+-retaining states, and in patients with oliguria or anuria, because of the potentially large amounts of Na^+ administered in each dose.

Patients with low levels of K^+ may be predisposed to metabolic alkalosis, and patients with coexistent hypocalcemia may exhibit carpopedal spasm as plasma pH rises. Appropriate treatment of electrolyte balances before or concomitantly with HCO_3^- infusion can diminish the risk of these situations.

In the case of alcoholic ketoacidosis, IV NaCl, K^+, thiamine, and glucose are usually ordered. Do not use alkali therapy unless the metabolic acidosis is in the lethal range (<7.1). The same considerations apply to starvation ketosis.

Patient Education

Advise patients of the importance of regular follow-up examinations to monitor serum electrolyte levels and acid-base balance. As with any other drug, teach the patient and family the name of the drug, its purpose, dosage, and frequency, and possible adverse effects. The patient taking $NaHCO_3^-$ on a prolonged basis may develop GI distress and flatulence. Because GI distress contributes to nonadherence to therapy and subsequent acute acidosis, a different alkalinizing drug may be required. Instruct patients and families how to prepare and administer the drug and to avoid certain activities if the alkalinizing drug is one that may cause drowsiness (e.g., acetazolamide).

Teach the patient on long-term therapy that $NaHCO_3^-$ should not be taken concurrently with milk products; the formation of renal calculi or hypercalcemia may result. Sodium citrate is more palatable when diluted with 60 to 90 mL of water and refrigerated before use. It should be taken 30 minutes after meals or as a bedtime snack to minimize its laxative effects.

Teach the patient to recognize signs of fluid retention such as rings that have gotten tighter, ankles that are swelling, or a weight gain of 2 to 3 pounds in a few days. Advise the patient to report these signs promptly.

Evaluation

The signs and symptoms of the acid-base imbalance should resolve without the appearance of the opposite disorder. Monitor the patient closely for signs and symptoms of overdosage of the alkalinizing or acidifying drug. In addition, monitor the respiratory rate, volume, and patterns, breath sounds, lab values, and ABGs. Observe the patient closely and provide care needed to ensure patient safety; restraints may be needed in some cases. Assess skin color, temperature, peripheral pulses, and capillary refill, and look for signs of CNS irritability or depression. The patient may need to be switched to a different drug or the drug may have to be discontinued.

Serum electrolyte values are monitored at least daily or every other day until a return to normal occurs, and then less frequently. Observe the patient carefully to make sure the original acid-base imbalance isn't overcorrected.

KEY POINTS

- The body uses three primary defense mechanisms to maintain acid-base balance: the bicarbonate-carbonic acid buffer system, the respiratory system, and the renal system.
- Respiratory alkalosis occurs when alveolar hyperventilation results in excessive loss of CO_2. Respiratory acidosis results primarily from decreased alveolar ventilation, leading to retention of CO_2.
- Metabolic alkalosis results from the loss of H^+ ions or the accumulation of base components such as HCO_3^-. Metabolic acidosis results from a decrease in base components, or through increased H^+ ion levels.
- Monitor patients for evidence of CNS stimulation or depression representative of alkalosis or acidosis, respectively.

- Always treat the underlying cause of acidosis. When appropriate, acidosis is corrected with $NaHCO_3^-$. Alkalosis may be corrected with ammonium chloride.
- Care must be taken when correcting acid-base imbalances not to overtreat and produce the opposite imbalance.
- Advise patients of the importance of regular follow-up examinations to monitor serum electrolyte levels and acid-base balance and to monitor progress.
- Resolution of the signs and symptoms of the acid-base imbalances should occur without the appearance of the opposite disorder.

Bibliography

American Gastroenterological Association Clinical Practice and Practice Economics Committee. (2001). AGA technical review on parenteral nutrition. *Gastroenterology, 121*(4), 970–1001.

Dominguez-Roldan, J., Jimenez-Gonzalez, P., Garcia-Alfaro, C., et al. (2005). Electrolytic disorders, hyperosmolar states, and lactic acidosis in brain-dead patients. *Transplantation Proceedings, 37*(5), 1987–1989.

Funk, G., Doberer, D., Osterreicher, C., et al. (2005). Equilibrium of acidifying and alkalinizing metabolic acid-base disorders in cirrhosis. *Liver International, 25*(3), 505–512.

Gennari, F. (2002). Disorders of potassium homeostasis: Hypokalemia and hyperkalemia. *Critical Care Clinics, 18*(2), 273–288.

Gutierrez, K., and Queener, S. (2003). *Pharmacology for nursing practice.* St. Louis: Mosby.

Hess, B. (2006). Acid-base metabolism: Implications for kidney stone formation. *Urology Research, 34*(2), 1–5.

Lin, S., Chiu, J., Hsu, C., et al. (2003). A simple and rapid approach to hypokalemic paralysis. *American Journal of Emergency Medicine, 21*(6), 487–491.

Martin, M., FitzSullivan, E., Salim, A., et al. (2006). Use of serum bicarbonate measurement in place of arterial base deficit in the surgical intensive care unit. *Archives of Surgery, 140*(8), 745–751.

McCance, K., and Heuther, S. (2002). *Pathophysiology: The biologic basis for disease in adults and children* (4th ed.). St Louis: Mosby.

Rosival, V. (2005). Diagnosis of acid-base derangements and mortality prediction in the trauma intensive care unit: The physiochemical approach. *Journal of Trauma-Injury Infection & Critical Care, 59*(2), 509.

Simons, P., Nadra, I., and McNally, P. (2003). Metabolic alkalosis and myoclonus. *Postgraduate Medical Journal, 79*(933), 414–415.

GASTROINTESTINAL

Antiasthmatic and Bronchodilator Drugs

Bronchodilator and antiasthmatic drugs are used in the treatment of respiratory disorders characterized by inflammation, bronchospasm or bronchoconstriction, mucosal edema, and excessive mucus production. The hallmark of asthma is hyperactivity of the airways caused by inflammation in response to various physical, chemical, environmental, or pharmacologic stimuli. Treatment is directed at preventing attacks when possible and normalizing the patient's lifestyle. Treatment involves both non–drug and drug measures. As a general rule, drug therapy for hypersensitive airway disorders is more effective in relieving symptoms than in curing the underlying disorder.

Primary health care providers can generally manage the spectrum of symptoms, but when conservative methods fall short, referral to an allergist or respiratory specialist is appropriate. Because inflammation plays a central role in the airway dysfunction of asthma, it is not surprising that national and international guidelines for asthma management have targeted inflammation as the specific therapeutic target. Antiinflammatory drugs treat asthma, whereas bronchodilators treat the symptoms of asthma.

ASTHMA

EPIDEMIOLOGY AND ETIOLOGY

Asthma falls within the top 10 conditions causing limitation of activity and increased health care costs. In the United States, the cost of asthma-related health care exceeds $16 billion annually. In 2004 alone, there were 13.6 million outpatient office visits, 1 million urgent care visits, and 1.8 million emergency room (ER) visits as a result of asthma. Further, 30% of patients who made visits to the ER for complaints of asthma did not have health insurance (compared with the mere 6% of patients who had private health insurance). Overall, the number of patients diagnosed with asthma tends to be highest in the South, in non-Hispanic Caucasians, in 18- to 44-year-olds, and in females.

There are two basic types of asthma—extrinsic and intrinsic. The majority of patients with *extrinsic asthma* are *atopic*; that is, they have a hereditary predisposition to produce immunoglobulin E (IgE) antibodies directed toward common allergens (e.g., molds, fungi, animal proteins). Extrinsic asthma is more common in childhood and accounts for nearly 15 million lost school days.

Intrinsic asthma, most often seen in adults, is caused by exposure to airway irritants such as perfumes, household cleaning products, insecticides, and cold air. Tobacco smoke is a major cause of asthma symptoms in children as well as adults. In addition to the inflammatory response that develops in the airways, asthma reduces lung function and increases the need for drug

therapy. Inhaled particulates from air pollution are another major trigger of asthma symptoms and have led to increased numbers of visits to ERs and hospitalizations. Other contributing factors to asthma are upper respiratory tract infections, purulent rhinitis, acute sinusitis, and gastroesophageal reflux disease (GERD). In addition, approximately 5% of patients in the United States who have asthma are sensitive to sulfite-containing foods (e.g., shrimp, processed foods, avocados, acidic juices, wine, and beer). Intrinsic asthma is not related to allergen exposure (Box 50-1).

Regardless of whether the asthma is extrinsic or intrinsic, in susceptible individuals, processes within the airways cause recurrent episodes of wheezing, breathlessness, chest tightness, and cough, particularly at night and in the early morning. Extensive airflow obstruction often characterizes these asthmatic episodes, but the effects often resolve, either spontaneously or with treatment.

PATHOPHYSIOLOGY

Although asthma was once regarded largely as a disease of airway smooth muscle, it is now known to be a chronic inflammatory disease of the airways, complicated by periodic exacerbations. In recent years, an increased understanding of the pathophysiology of asthma has exposed a complex network of interactions among a variety of inflammatory cells and the mediators they secrete.

Even patients with mild, asymptomatic asthma have obvious, although microscopic, inflammatory changes in their airways. The changes are distinguished by infiltration of the mucosa and epithelium by activated T cells, mast cells, and eosinophils. T cells and mast cells secrete an array of chemicals in asthma, the functions of which are to direct eosinophil growth and maturation and to prevent B cells from switching to IgE from IgM, which helps to explain the inflammatory responses of asthma. The aftereffects are increased capillary permeability, stimulation of local and central neural reflexes, epithelial disruption and stimulation of mucus-secreting glands, smooth muscle hypertrophy, and airway wall remodeling (Fig. 50-1).

The inflammation seen in patients with asthma is multifactorial; however, leukotrienes (LTs) play a major role in this process. The LT family includes metabolites of arachidonic acid, an essential fatty acid that must be obtained in the diet. Arachidonic acid is presented to the 5-lipoxygenase enzyme by 5-lipoxygenase–activating protein, a cofactor present in the nuclear membrane. The interaction leads to formation of LTA_4, an unstable intermediate LT (Fig. 50-2).

Depending on the cell type, further conversion of LTA_4 occurs by widespread enzyme actions in tissues and circulation. LTs induce numerous biologic effects including augmentation of neutrophil and eosinophil migration, monocyte

---

BOX 50-1

Asthma Triggers

Environmental Factors
- Air pollutants (e.g., aerosol sprays, smoke, exhaust fumes, oxidants, perfumes, sulfur dioxides)
- Animal dander (e.g., dogs, cats, rodents, horses), house-dust mite
- Environmental changes (e.g., moving to new house, starting a new school)
- Pollens, spores, and mold (e.g., trees, grasses, shrubs, weeds)

Occupational Exposures
- Industrial chemicals and plastics, metal salts, pharmaceuticals
- Wood and vegetable dusts

Foods and Food Additives
- Sulfites, bisulfites, and metasulfites
- Nuts, milk and dairy products

Drugs
- Antibiotics
- Beta blockers (e.g., propranolol)
- Nonsteroidal antiinflammatory drugs (e.g., indomethacin)

Diseases and Conditions
- Menses, pregnancy
- Paranasal sinusitis, history of nasal polyps, viral upper respiratory infections
- Thyroid disease, tracheoesophageal fistula

Other Triggers
- Exercise and cold, dry air
- Gastroesophageal reflux
- Strong emotions (e.g., fear, anger, laughing, crying)

---

aggregation, leukocyte adhesion, increased capillary permeability, and smooth muscle contraction. These effects contribute to inflammation, edema, mucus secretion, and bronchoconstriction of the airways.

Bronchial constriction induced by allergens or anti-IgE antibodies is primarily mediated by a specific group of LTs (i.e., LTC_4, LTD_4, and LTE_4). These three LTs are potent mediators that cause long-term contraction of bronchial smooth muscle. An antigen-IgE antibody complex is formed, causing the release of chemical mediators in the lower respiratory tract. Histamine plays a minor role in this response.

In 5% to 10% of patients with asthma, a cyclooxygenase inhibitor (e.g., aspirin) produces profound bronchoconstriction. This is particularly true in patients with late-onset intrinsic asthma. Patients with aspirin-sensitive asthma produce greater amounts of LTs and have increased airway sensitivity when challenged by these drugs.

Timing of symptoms varies greatly among patients. Bronchoconstriction can have an immediate, histamine type of pattern or may form a late response, with airway hypersensitivity lasting for days, weeks, or months. A second wave of symptoms sometimes appears 6 to 8 hours after initial antigen exposure. The classic manifestations of asthma are dyspnea, wheezing, and coughing in the absence of respiratory infection, especially at night.

Drug therapy for asthma centers on decreasing airway inflammation; relaxing smooth muscles to improve airflow into the lungs; and counteracting the allergy component, where possible. These drugs include inhaled corticosteroids, antiallergy drugs, beta agonists, LT antagonists, antimuscarinic drugs, and occasionally, xanthines. Current recommendations support the use of inhaled corticosteroids as primary drug therapy.

PHARMACOTHERAPEUTIC OPTIONS

Inhaled Corticosteroids
- beclomethasone (Beclovent, Beconase, Vanceril, Vancenase); ✦ Beclodisk, Becloforte
- budesonide (Rhinocort, Pulmicort); ✦ Rhinocort, Pulmicort

- flunisolide (Aerobid, Nasalide); ✦ Bronalide, Rhinalar
- fluticasone (Flovent, Flovent Diskus, Flovent HFA); ✦ Flovent Diskus, Flovent HFA
- mometasone (Asmanex); ✦ Asmanex
- triamcinolone (Azmacort); ✦ Azmacort

Indications
Inhaled corticosteroids were developed in an attempt to obtain the advantages of chronic corticosteroid therapy without the systemic adverse effects. Inhaled formulations are used in the long-term management of asthma. Long-term asthma control is necessary to prevent exacerbations and chronic symptoms for patients with persistent asthma at any level.

Systemic corticosteroids are used to gain prompt control of the disease and also to manage moderate to severe persistent asthma. Hydrocortisone, prednisone, and methylprednisolone are systemic drugs (see Chapter 56) given to patients with acute exacerbations of asthma who do not respond adequately to bronchodilators, and in those with severe persistent asthma who fail to respond adequately to nonsystemic (inhaled) corticosteroids.

Pharmacodynamics
The precise mechanism of drug action in the lungs is unknown. It is thought that inhaled corticosteroids act topically on the epithelial lining of the airways to decrease inflammation and reduce mucus secretion. Corticosteroids are also thought to increase the number and sensitivity of adrenergic receptors, which restores or increases the effectiveness of beta agonists.

Pharmacokinetics
Absorption of corticosteroids occurs rapidly from all respiratory tissues. Beclomethasone and flunisolide are rapidly absorbed from the lungs, whereas triamcinolone is absorbed more slowly.

The potential for systemic activity is established by the bioavailability and the potency of the inhaled corticosteroids (Table 50-1). Almost all of an inhaled corticosteroid dose is bioavailable. Approximately 80% of the dose from a metered-dose inhaler (MDI; without a spacer or holding chamber) is

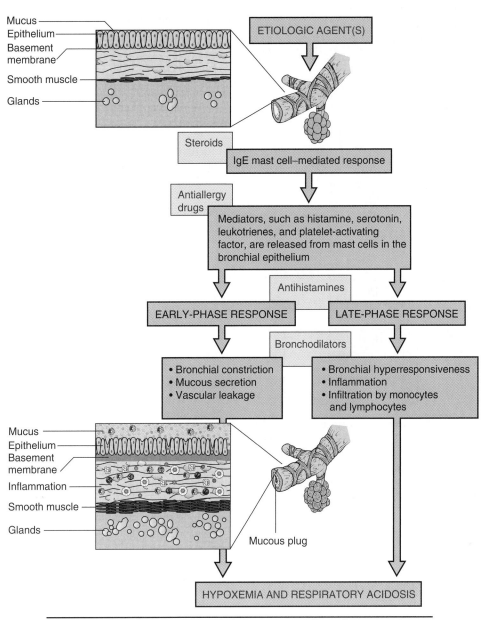

FIGURE 50-1 Pathophysiology of Bronchial Inflammation and Airway Hyperresponsiveness.

swallowed; more drug is delivered to the lungs (instead of the stomach) with the use of spacers. Those drugs with a high first-pass effect will cause fewer systemic effects because of their inactivation by the liver. Biotransformation in this case "neutralizes" the drug and thus has a protective effect from the systemic toxicities of corticosteroids. The onset time of most inhaled corticosteroids is a few days, although peak action may not occur for up to 4 weeks in some cases.

Adverse Effects and Contraindications

The most frequent adverse effects of inhaled corticosteroids includes headache (worse with triamcinolone more than others), throat itching (with budesonide), and wheezing, bronchospasm, and cough. Localized infections with *Candida albicans* or *Aspergillus niger* may be present in the mouth and pharynx. Oral candidiasis occurs in 75% of patients using inhaled corticosteroids, although the incidence of clinically

apparent infection is considerably lower. These infections may necessitate treatment with appropriate antifungal drugs, or use of the corticosteroid inhaler may have to be stopped.

A few patients complain of hoarseness and dry mouth after using an inhaled corticosteroid. Rare cases of immediate and delayed hypersensitivity reactions, including urticaria, angioedema, rash, and bronchospasm, have been reported following oral inhalation of corticosteroids.

Hypothalamic-pituitary-adrenal (HPA) axis suppression ▲ is noted in adults receiving 32 puffs/day (approximately 1600 mcg) of an inhaled steroid over a period of 1 month. Patients also exhibit signs of adrenal insufficiency when they are exposed to trauma, surgery, or infections (particularly gastroenteritis) while using inhaled corticosteroids. Although inhaled steroids provide control of asthmatic symptoms, they do not provide the quantity of systemic steroid necessary to cope with these stressors. **Deaths have occurred due to ▲**

RESPIRATORY

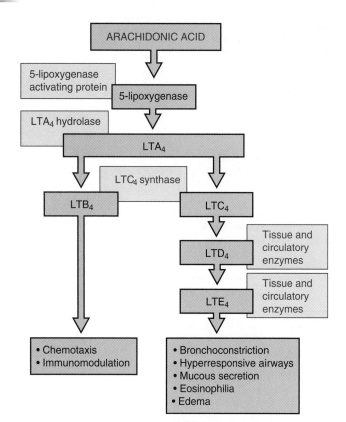

FIGURE 50-2 Leukotriene Synthesis and Activity. Leukotrienes are acidic, sulfur-containing lipids that produce effects similar to those of histamine. Five types of leukotrienes are generated from the arachidonic acid released from mast cell membranes by an intracellular phospholipase that acts on membrane phospholipids (LTA_4, LTB_4, LTC_4, LTD_4, and LTE_4). LTB_4 is a chemotactic agent that causes aggregation of leukocytes. LTC_4, LTD_4, and LTE_4 all cause contraction of smooth muscle, bronchospasm, and increased vascular permeability.

adrenal insufficiency during and after transfer from systemic corticosteroids to topical drugs. Several months are required for recovery of HPA axis function.

Corticosteroids are contraindicated for use as the primary treatment of status asthmaticus or other acute episodes of asthma in which intensive measures are required. Some inhaled corticosteroids contain alcohol, propylene, or polyethylene glycol; avoid these in patients with known hypersensitivity or intolerance.

Drug Interactions

There are no clinically significant drug interactions with recommended dosages of inhaled corticosteroids. However, for patients who must take oral corticosteroids, be alert to possible interactions.

Dosage Regimen

Inhaled corticosteroids are administered via oral inhalation using MDIs, breath-actuated MDIs, or dry-powder inhalers, or by using a nebulizer (Table 50-2). Once maximum response is achieved in 1 to 2 weeks, reduce the dosage to the lowest level that maintains control. Furthermore, there is no evidence that asthma control can be more effectively achieved by administration of inhaled corticosteroids in amounts exceeding the recommended dosages. Systemic dosing of corticosteroids is discussed in Chapter 52.

Lab Considerations

Inhaled corticosteroids can cause elevated serum and urine glucose levels if significant absorption occurs. In addition, periodic adrenal function tests for patients on chronic therapy may be necessary to assess for HPA suppression.

Beta Agonists

SHORT-ACTING BETA AGONISTS
* albuterol (ProAir, Proventil, Ventolin, others); ✦ Gen-Salbutamol, ProAir, Ventolin, others
* fenoterol; ✦ Berotec
* levalbuterol (Xopenex); ✦ Xopenex
* metaproterenol (Alupent)
* pirbuterol (Maxair)
* terbutaline (Bricanyl); ✦ Bricanyl Turbuhaler

LONG-ACTING BETA AGONISTS
* formoterol (Foradil); ✦ Foradil, Oxeze
* salbuterol (Salbuvent)
* salmeterol (Serevent)
* salmeterol and fluticasone (Advair Diskus); ✦ Advair Diskus

Indications

Short-acting beta agonists (e.g., albuterol, metaproterenol, and pirbuterol) are used to relieve bronchoconstriction and are the treatment of choice for acute exacerbations of asthma. They are effective prophylaxis for exercise-induced bronchospasm.

Long-acting beta agonists (e.g., salbuterol, salmeterol) are found most often in combination with an inhaled corticosteroid (e.g., Advair) and are used for long-term symptom control. The combination is particularly helpful for patients whose asthma symptoms occur during the night.

Pharmacodynamics

Beta agonists cause airway smooth muscle relaxation by activating adenylate cyclase and increasing cyclic adenosine monophosphate (cAMP). The action produces a functional antagonism of bronchoconstriction. The release of mast cell mediators is hindered by beta agonists; vascular permeability is reduced; and mucociliary clearance improves with the use of beta agonists. They do not inhibit the inflammatory response characteristic of the late phase or the ensuing hyperresponsiveness of the bronchial tree. All short-acting beta agonists (except for metaproterenol) are β_2-selective, although with sufficient dosage, beta agonists also exert effects on β_1 receptors, resulting in some of the adverse effects commonly seen in clinical practice.

Pharmacokinetics

The onset of drug action for short-acting beta agonists occurs in minutes, depending on the specific drug (see Table 50-1). Salmeterol has a slower onset of action than the short-acting beta agonists, but a longer duration of action. **Deaths have been reported in patients who used salmeterol ▲ as a rescue drug, not understanding that it takes a minimum of 20 minutes for the drug to become effective.**

PHARMACOKINETICS

TABLE 50-1 Selected Antiasthmatic and Bronchodilator Drugs

Drugs	Route	Onset	Peak	Duration	PB (%)	t½	BioA (%)
INHALED CORTICOSTEROIDS							
beclomethasone	INH, PO	Rapid	Up to 4 wk	3.25 days	91	3–15 hr	20
budesonide	INH	24 hr	3–7 days	UA	91	2 hr	11
flunisolide	INH	Rapid	UA	UA	91	1–2 hr	20
fluticasone	INH	Few days	1–2 wk	UA	91	UA	1
triamcinolone	INH	Few days	3–4 days	UA	91	4 hr	10.6
BETA AGONISTS							
albuterol	PO	30 min	2–2.5 hr	4–8 hr	UA	2–4 hr	UA
	INH	5 min	1.5–2 hr	3–8 hr			
metaproterenol	PO	15–30 min	60 min	4 hr	UA	UA	UA
	INH	1–4 min	60 min	3–4 hr			
pirbuterol	INH	5 min	1–5 hr	6–8 hr	UA	2 hr	UA
salmeterol	INH	10–25 min	3–4 hr	8–12 hr	UA	UA	UA
LEUKOTRIENE ANTAGONISTS							
montelukast	PO	UA	3–4 hr	UA	99	2.7–5.5 hr	63–73
zafirlukast	PO	UA	3 hr	UA	UA	10 hr	40
ANTIALLERGY DRUGS (MAST CELL STABILIZERS)							
cromolyn	INH	15 min	2–4 wk	4–6 hr	UA	80 min	2.5–3
nedocromil	INH	2 weeks	20–40 min	4–6 hr	89	1.5–2.3 hr	2.5–3
ANTIMUSCARINIC DRUGS							
ipratropium	INH, solu	5–15 min	1–2 hr	3–6 hr	UA	2 hr	UA
tiotropium	INH, solu	5–15 min	1–2 hr	3–6 hr	72	5–6 days	19.5; 2–3*
XANTHINE DERIVATIVES							
aminophylline	PO	1–6 hr	4–6 hr	6–8 hr	UA	3–15 hr	UA
	IV	Immed	30 min	4–8 hr	UA		100
theophylline	PO	Varies	1–2 hr	6 hr	60; 36; 35†	4–5 hr; 3–15 hr‡	UA
	PO, ER	Delayed	4–8 hr	8–24 hr	35†	3–13 hr	UA
	IV	Rapid	End of inf	6–8 hr	35†	3–13 hr	100
MONOCLONAL ANTIBODY							
omalizumab	SubQ	Slow	7–8 days	UA	UA	26 days	62

*Bioavailability of inhaled and solution formulations of tiotropium, respectively.
*Provided a loading dose of methylxanthine drug has been given and steady state serum levels exist.
†Protein binding of theophylline in healthy adults, neonates, and patients with cirrhosis, respectively.
‡Half-life of theophylline in patients who smoke and nonsmokers, respectively.
BioA, Bioavailability; *ER*, extended-release formulation; *inf*, infusion; *INH*, inhalation; *IV*, intravenous; PB, protein binding; *PO*, by mouth; *solu*, solution; *SubQ*, subcutaneous; *t½*, half-life; *UA*, unavailable.

DOSAGE

TABLE 50-2 Selected Bronchodilator and Antiasthmatic Drugs

Drug	Uses	Dosage	Implications*
INHALED CORTICOSTEROIDS			
beclomethasone	Chronic steroid dependent asthma; reduces need for oral corticosteroid	*Adult and Child >12 yr:* *Low dose:* 168–504 mcg daily = 4–12 puffs of 42-mcg/puff MDI – or– 2–6 puffs of 84-mcg/puff MDI *Med. dose:* 504–840 mcg daily = 12–20 puffs of 42-mcg/puff MDI – or– 6–10 puffs of 84-mcg/puff MDI *High dose:* Over 840 mcg daily > 20 puffs of 42 mcg/puff MDI –or– >10 puffs of 84-mcg/puff MDI *Child age 6–12 yr:* *Low dose:* 84–336 mcg daily = 2–8 puffs of 42 mcg/puff MDI –or– 1–4 puffs of 84-mcg/puff MDI *Med. dose:* 336–672 mcg daily = 8–16 puffs of 42-mcg/puff MDI – or– 4–8 puffs of 84-mcg/puff MDI *High dose:* >672 mcg daily = >16 puffs of 42-mcg/puff MDI –or– >8 puffs of 84-mcg/puff MDI	**Corticosteroid inhalers should not be used to treat an acute asthma attack but should be continued even if other inhalation drugs are used.** 16.8-gram canister contains 200 puffs. Instruct the patient in the correct use of the MDI. Advise patient to use peak flow monitoring to determine respiratory status. Rinse mouth with water after puff to prevent mouth and throat dryness and fungal infections of mouth.

Continued

DOSAGE
TABLE **50-2 Selected Bronchodilator and Antiasthmatic Drugs—Cont'd**

Drug	Uses	Dosage	Implications*
budesonide	Chronic steroid-dependent asthma; reduces need for oral corticosteroid	*Adults:* *Low dose:* 200–400 mcg daily = 1–2 puffs *Med. dose:* 400–600 mcg daily = 2–3 puffs *High dose:* >600 mcg daily > 3 puffs *Child: Low dose:* 100–200 mcg daily = 1 puff *Med. dose:* 200–400 mcg daily = 1–2 puffs *High dose:* >400 mcg daily > 2 puffs	Each Turbuhaler delivers 200 mcg/dose. Rinse mouth with water after puffs to prevent mouth and throat dryness and fungal infections of mouth. See above.
dexamethasone	Chronic steroid-dependent asthma; reduces need for oral corticosteroid	*Adult:* 3 metered sprays via inhalation aerosol 3–4 times daily. Not to exceed 12 metered sprays/day *Child:* 2 metered sprays via inhalation aerosol 3–4 times daily. Max: 8 sprays/day	12.6-gram canister contains 170 84-mcg puffs. Rinse mouth with water after puffs to prevent mouth and throat dryness and fungal infections of mouth. See implications under beclomethasone.
flunisolide	Chronic steroid-dependent asthma; reduces need for oral corticosteroid	*Adult and Child >6 yr:* *Low dose:* 500–1000 mcg daily = 2–4 puffs of a 250-mcg/puff MDI *Med. dose:* 1000–2000 mcg daily = to 4–8 puffs of a 250-mcg/puff MDI *High dose:* 2000 mcg daily > 8 puffs of a 250-mcg/puff MDI *Child:* *Low dose:* 500–750 mcg daily = 2–3 puffs of a 250-mcg/puff MDI *Med. dose:* 1000–1250 mcg daily = 4–5 puffs of a 250-mcg/puff MDI *High dose:* 1250 mcg daily > 5 puffs of a 250-mcg/puff MDI	7-gram canister delivers 100 250-mcg puffs. Rinse mouth with water immediately after puffs to prevent mouth and throat dryness and fungal infections of mouth. See implications under beclomethasone.
fluticasone	Chronic steroid-dependent asthma; reduces need for oral corticosteroid	*Adult:* *Low dose:* 88–264 mcg daily = 2–6 puffs of a 44-mcg/puff MDI –or– 2 puffs of a 110-mcg/puff MDI, –or– 2–6 puffs of 50-mcg/puff DPI *Med. dose:* 264–660 mcg daily = 2–6 puffs of a 110-mcg/puff MDI –or– 3–6 puffs of a 100-mcg/puff DPI *High dose:* >660 mcg daily = >6 puffs of a 110-mcg/puff MDI –or– >3 puffs of a 220-mcg/puff MDI –or– >6 puffs of a 100-mcg/puff DPI –or– >2 puffs of a 250-mcg/puff DPI *Child:* *Low dose:* 88–176 mcg daily = 2–4 puffs of a 44-mcg/puff MDI *Med. dose:* 176–440 mcg daily = 4–10 puffs of a 44-mcg/puff MDI –or– 2–4 puffs of a 110-mcg/puff MDI –or– 2–4 puffs of a 100-mcg/puff DPI *High dose:* >440 mcg daily = 4 puffs of a 110-mcg/puff MDI –or– >2 puffs of a 220-mcg/puff MDI –or– >4 puffs of a 100-mcg/puff DPI –or– >2 puffs of a 250-mcg/puff DPI	Initial dosage based on prior asthma drugs. Do not change dose schedule or stop taking the drug. Teach proper use of inhaler. Rinse mouth with water immediately after puffs to prevent mouth and throat dryness and fungal infections of mouth. See also implications under beclomethasone.
triamcinolone	Chronic steroid-dependent asthma; reduces need for oral corticosteroid	*Adult and Child >12 yr:* *Low dose:* 400–1000 mcg daily = 4–10 puffs of a 100-mcg/puff MDI *Med. dose:* 1000–2000 mcg daily = 10–20 puffs of a 100-mcg/puff MDI *High dose:* >2000 mcg daily > 20 puffs of a 100-mcg/puff MDI *Child:* *Low dose:* 400–800 mcg daily = 4–8 puffs of a 100-mcg/puff MDI *Med. dose:* 800–1200 mcg daily = 8–12 puffs of a 100-mcg/puff MDI *High dose:* >1200 mcg daily > 12 puffs of a 100-mcg/puff MDI	20-gram canister contains 240 puffs. Rinse mouth with water immediately after puffs to prevent mouth and throat dryness and fungal infections of mouth. See also implications under beclomethasone.

BETA AGONISTS[†]

albuterol	Reversible airway disease due to asthma or COPD	*Adult and Child >14 yr:* 2–6 mg PO 3–4 times daily; not to exceed 32 mg/day *–or–* 4–8 mg of ER formulation twice daily *–or–* 2 puffs every 4–6 hr *–or–* 2 puffs 15–20 min before exercise *–or–* 1.25–5 mg 3 times daily via nebulizer *–or–* 1–2 capsules (200–400 mcg) every 4–6 hr via Rotahaler *Child 6–14 yr:* 2 mg PO 3–4 times daily; not to exceed 24 mg/day *–or–* 1 capsule every 4–6 hr PRN via Rotahaler *Child 2–6 yr:* 0.1 mg/kg PO 3 times daily; not to exceed 2 mg 3 times daily, initially. May increase to 0.2 mg/kg 3 times daily; not to exceed 4 mg 3 times daily	17-gram MDI canister contains 200 90- to 100-mcg puffs. Albuterol is compatible with cromolyn and ipratropium in nebulizer. Take 15 min before exercise for exercise-induced asthma (EIA).
metaproterenol	Reversible airway disease due to asthma or COPD	*Adult and Child >9 yr and 27 kg:* 20 mg PO 3–4 times daily *–or–* 2–3 puffs every 3–4 hr; not to exceed 12 puffs/day *–or–* 5–15 inh of undiluted 5% solution 3–4 times daily via nebulizer. Not to exceed every-4-hr use *–or–* 0.2–0.3 mL of 5% solution *–or–* 2.5 mL of 0.4%-0.6% solution 3–4 times daily via IPPB. Not to exceed every 4 hr	Affects both β$_1$ and β$_2$ receptors. 14-gram MDI canister contains 200 650-mcg puffs. Aerosol solution container holds 5 mL or 100 650- to 750-mcg inhalations.
pirbuterol	Reversible airway disease due to asthma or COPD	*Adult:* 1–2 puffs every 4–6 hr; not to exceed 12 puffs/day	14-gram autoinhaler canister contains 300 200-mcg puffs; 25.6 gram autoinhaler canister contains 400 200-mcg puffs.
salmeterol	Long-term prevention of symptoms (not for acute attacks or exercise-induced bronchospasm)	*Adult:* 2 puffs by MDI *–or–* one blister twice daily, 12 hr apart	**If symptoms occur before next dose is due, use a rapid-acting inhaled bronchodilator to treat symptoms. Not for acute treatment or first-line for maintenance therapy.** 13-gram MDI canister contains 120 21-mcg puffs. MDI canister should be primed or tested before first use. Long-acting agent. ⚠

LEUKOTRIENE ANTAGONISTS

montelukast	Prophylaxis and chronic long-term treatment of asthma	*Adult and Child >15 yr:* 10 mg PO daily HS. *Child 6–14 yr:* 5 mg chewable tablet daily HS	Take on empty stomach. There is no evidence of improved efficacy with morning versus evening dosing.
zafirlukast	Prophylaxis and chronic long-term treatment of asthma	*Adult:* 40 mg PO twice daily	Take on an empty stomach. Bioavailability is decreased when taken with food.

ANTIALLERGY DRUGS (MAST CELL STABILIZERS)

cromolyn	Asthma prophylaxis	*Adult:* 2–4 puffs 3–4 times daily via MDI *–or–* 1 ampule 3–4 times daily via nebulizer *Child:* 1–2 puffs 3–4 times daily via MDI *–or–* 1 ampule 3–4 times daily	*MDI:* 1 mg/puff. *Nebulizer:* 20 mg/ampule. One dose before exercise or allergen exposure provides effective prophylaxis for 1–2 wk.
nedocromil		*Adult:* 2–4 puffs 2–4 times daily *Child:* 1–2 puffs 2–4 times daily	

XANTHINE DERIVATIVES[‡]

aminophylline	Management of reversible airway disease due to asthma or COPD, especially nocturnal symptoms	*Adult:* Loading dose: 5 mg/kg PO. Maintenance: 300 mg/day in divided doses every 6–8 hr. May increase after 3 days to 400 mg/day, and again after 3 more days to 600 mg in divided doses *Child <16 yr:* Loading dose: 5 mg/kg. Maintenance dose varies based on lean body weight.	**Narrow therapeutic index. Therapeutic range: 10–20 mcg/mL. Serum levels over 20 mcg/mL are associated with toxicity.** Anhydrous aminophylline is 86% theophylline by weight. Dihydrate aminophylline is 79% theophylline. Dosage is determined by serum drug levels. Healthy adults or young smokers may require every-6-hr dosing. Give ER formulation every 12–24 hr. ⚠

ANTIMUSCARINIC DRUGS

ipratropium	Asthma maintenance therapy	*Adult:* 1–2 puffs 3–4 times daily; not to exceed 12 puffs/24 hr or more often than every 4 hr *–or–* 250–500 mcg 3–4 times daily via nebulizer	**Not for acute bronchospasm or in persons with peanut allergy.** Use hard candy, frequent drinks, or sugarless gum to relieve dry mouth. ⚠
tiotropium		*Adult:* 1 capsule (18 mcg) daily via HandiHaler device	

MONOCLONAL ANTIBODY

omalizumab	Moderate to severe persistent asthma with perennial allergies that is poorly controlled with inhaled corticosteroid	*Adult and Child >12 yr:* 150–375 mg subQ every 2–4 wk	**Retesting of IgE levels during treatment cannot be used as guide for dosage determination.** SubQ dosage and frequency based on IgE levels and body weight (kg). ⚠

*The dosage of a metered-dose inhaler (MDI) is referred to as the *actuator dose,* the amount of drug leaving the device and delivered to the patient. Identifying actuator dose is a labeling requirement in the United States. An actuator dose is different from the *valve dose,* which is the amount of drug leaving the valve, part of which the patient does not receive. Reference to the valve dose is seen in many European countries and certain scientific literature. Dry-powder inhaler (DPI) dosages are expressed as the amount of drug remaining in the inhaler following activation.

[†]The potencies among and between beta agonists are different in short-acting inhaled beta$_2$ agonists, but they are essentially equipotent on a per-puff basis.

[‡]Doses of xanthines are expressed in theophylline equivalents. Because of differing theophylline content, the various salts and derivatives of theophylline are equivalent on a weight basis.

COPD, Chronic obstructive pulmonary disease; *DPI,* dry-powder inhaler; *ER,* extended release; *HS,* at bedtime; *inh,* inhalation; *IPPB,* intermittent positive pressure breathing (apparatus); *MDI,* metered-dose inhaler; *PRN,* as needed; *subQ,* subcutaneous (route).

RESPIRATORY

The systemic absorption of beta agonists is minimal since distribution of inhaled drugs is essentially limited to the respiratory tract. Biotransformation takes place in the liver, with elimination of beta agonists through the kidneys.

Adverse Effects and Contraindications

The adverse effects of short-acting beta agonists include headache, tachycardia, hypokalemia, hyperglycemia, and skeletal muscle tremors. Although rare, there is an increased risk for lactic acidosis. The adverse effects of long-acting beta agonists include tachycardia and hypokalemia and, with overdose, prolongation of the QT interval. Weakened bronchoprotection may occur within 1 week of chronic therapy. However, the clinical significance of this effect has not been established since symptom control and bronchodilation are retained despite the diminished bronchoprotective effect. The contraindications to usage of beta agonists include a history of hypersensitivity to adrenergic agonists.

Drug Interactions

Drug interactions of beta agonists are relatively few, but significant (Table 50-3). The additive effects of beta agonists when used concurrently with other adrenergic drugs or monoamine oxidase inhibitors can lead to hypertensive crisis. When used with beta blockers, the therapeutic effects of the beta agonist may be negated.

Dosage Regimen

The dosage of beta agonists is individualized based on patient response. In many cases, two puffs of the short-acting drugs 2 to 4 times daily are required. For exercise-induced asthma, two puffs are used 15 to 20 minutes before exercising. The longer-acting drugs such as salmeterol are administered twice daily, 12 hours apart (see Table 50-2).

Lab Considerations

Beta agonists can cause a transient decrease in serum potassium concentrations when administered via nebulizer or in higher than recommended doses. Increased serum glucose levels are rare but are more pronounced with frequent, high-dose use of salmeterol.

Leukotriene Antagonists

◆ montelukast (Singulair); ◆ Singulair
◆ zafirlukast (Accolate); ◆ Accolate

Indications

Zafirlukast is indicated for the prevention and treatment of mild persistent asthma in adults and children 5 years of age or older. It is an alternative to low-dose inhaled corticosteroids or antiallergy drugs. Montelukast is the only LT approved for prevention and treatment of asthma in adults and children 2 years of age and older.

Zafirlukast and montelukast therapy can be continued ⚠ **during acute exacerbations of asthma but are not appropriate for acute asthma attacks, including status asthmaticus. They are not bronchodilators.**

Pharmacodynamics

LTB_4 (a neutrophil chemo-attractant), LTC_4, and LTD_4 provoke symptoms consistent with those seen in asthma: bronchoconstriction, mucosal edema, mucus hypersecretion, and increased bronchial reactivity. Zafirlukast is a potent competitive cysteinyl LT antagonist. By inhibiting the action of LTC_4, further conversion to other LTs is prevented and the characteristic symptoms of asthma are reduced. It is more effective in the early phase of allergen-induced airway response, with lesser effects on the late response. It is less effective than inhaled beclomethasone.

Montelukast is an orally active compound that binds with high affinity and selectivity to the cysteinyl LT_1 receptor (in preference to other pharmacologically important airway receptors such as the prostanoid, cholinergic, or β receptors). It acts to inhibit physiologic actions of LTD_4 at the cysteinyl LT_1 receptor without causing agonist activity.

Pharmacokinetics

Zafirlukast is rapidly absorbed from the gastrointestinal (GI) tract, reaching peak serum concentrations in approximately 3

DRUG INTERACTIONS
TABLE **50-3 Selected Bronchodilator and Antiasthmatic Drugs**

Drug	Interactive Drugs	Interaction
BETA AGONISTS		
albuterol, metaproterenol, pirbuterol, salmeterol	Other adrenergic agonists, MAO inhibitors	Additive effects may lead to hypertensive crisis.
	Beta blockers	May negate therapeutic effect of adrenergic agonist
LEUKOTRIENE ANTAGONISTS		
montelukast, zafirlukast	aspirin, warfarin	Increases serum concentration of interactive drug, thereby increasing the risk of bleeding
	phenobarbital, rifampin	Induces biotransformation of montelukast and zafirlukast
	theophylline	Decreases effect of zafirlukast
XANTHINE DERIVATIVES		
aminophylline, oxytriphylline, theophylline	Adrenergic agonists	Additive CV and CNS effects
	allopurinol, Beta blockers, cimetidine, disulfiram, interferon, influenza vaccine, Macrolides, Quinolones, mexiletine, thiabendazole, ticlopidine	May decrease biotransformation and lead to toxicity
	halothane	Increased risk of arrhythmias
	carbamazepine, isoniazid, Loop diuretics	Increased or decreased theophylline levels

CV, Cardiovascular; *CNS*, central nervous system; *MAO*, monoamine oxidase.

hours (see Table 50-1). Taking the drug with food reduces bioavailability by 40%. Zafirlukast is biotransformed in the liver and eliminated primarily in the feces. The half-life may be twice as long in older adults.

Montelukast is rapidly absorbed following oral administration, with 99% protein binding. It is extensively biotransformed in the liver and eliminated almost exclusively in the feces.

Adverse Effects and Contraindications

The primary adverse effects of LT antagonists include headache, dry mouth, and somnolence. Unspecified pain, abdominal pain, dyspepsia, nausea, asthenia, and myalgias have been reported. Less common adverse effects include arthralgia, chest pain, conjunctivitis, constipation, dizziness, fever, flatulence, hypertonia, insomnia, lymphadenopathy, malaise, neck pain and rigidity, nervousness, pruritus, urinary tract infection, vaginitis, and vomiting. LT antagonists are contraindicated for use in patients with hypersensitivity to the drug or to any of its inactive ingredients. Safety and efficacy in children under 2 years of age have not been established.

Drug Interactions

Concurrent use of zafirlukast with warfarin increases the serum concentrations of warfarin, presumably because zafirlukast inhibits specific enzymes in the CYP450 system. Zafirlukast also inhibits an enzyme that catalyzes the biotransformation of corticosteroids. Table 50-3 lists other drugs that interact with zafirlukast. Phenobarbital and rifampin, which induces hepatic biotransformation, decrease the effectiveness of montelukast.

Dosage Regimen

The recommended dosages of LTs are identified in Table 50-2. Zafirlukast is taken 1 hour before or 2 hours after meals, whereas montelukast is given each day in the evening.

Lab Considerations

Alanine transaminase (ALT) and aspartate transaminase (AST) elevations have been noted in patients taking LT antagonists. Transaminase elevations greater than or equal to 3 times the upper limit of normal have been noted, although the elevations return to normal on discontinuation of therapy.

Antiallergy Drugs

◆ cromolyn (Nalcrom, Rynacrom, Vistacrom)
◆ nedocromil (Tilade); ◆ Tilade CFC-Free Inhaler

Indications

Antiallergy drugs (previously known as mast cell stabilizers) are approved only for asthma prophylaxis, allowing for reduced dosages of corticosteroids and bronchodilators. These drugs are effective for patients with mild persistent asthma, including allergic asthma and asthma induced by exercise, cold air, and sulfur dioxide. Cromolyn is more effective in reducing seasonal increases in bronchial reactivity (allergic asthma) but is less effective when compared with inhaled corticosteroids. They are mild to moderate antiinflammatory drugs used initially for long-term therapy in children. **Antiallergy drugs are not effective for treating acute bronchospasm or status asthmaticus.**

Pharmacodynamics

The antiallergy drugs cromolyn and nedocromil stabilize mast cells, whereby the activation and release of chemical mediators from eosinophils and epithelial cells are blocked. They block early and late reactions to allergens and alter the function of chloride channels. The alterations in chloride channels result in inhibition of cough as well as inhibition of the early (mast cells) and late (eosinophils) response to antigens. Cromolyn and nedocromil have no direct effect on airway smooth muscle tone and will not reverse asthmatic bronchospasm.

Pharmacokinetics

Antiallergy drugs do not cross biologic membranes; hence drug action is primarily local. The onset time of antiallergy drugs varies from 1 to 2 weeks, with peak activity ordinarily noted at 2 to 3 weeks (see Table 50-1). The duration of action of antiallergy drugs is generally 4 to 6 hours.

Small amounts of cromolyn reach systemic circulation after inhalation (10%). The small amounts that are absorbed are eliminated unchanged in the bile and urine. Two and one half percent to 3% of nedocromil is absorbed.

Adverse Effects and Contraindications

Headache is common with cromolyn or nedocromil use. Irritation of the trachea, bronchospasm, and cough have occurred. Although the incidence of adverse effects is relatively low, hypotension, chest pain, restlessness, dizziness, central nervous system (CNS) depression, seizures, anorexia, nausea, and vomiting have been reported. Arrhythmias are thought to be caused by the propellants (chlorohydrocarbons) used in aerosol formulations, and it has been suggested that the propellants in aerosols may aggravate coronary artery disease. Approximately 15% to 20% of patients note an unpleasant taste from inhaled nedocromil. Sedation and coma may occur with overdose.

Antiallergy drugs are contraindicated for use in patients with hypersensitivity to the drug. Use them with caution in patients who have impaired liver or kidney function. Safe use during pregnancy and lactation has not been established.

Drug Interactions

There are no known drug interactions with cromolyn or nedocromil.

Dosage Regimen

Cromolyn is available as a capsule for use in a Spinhaler and as a solution for inhalation (see Table 50-2). Some patients may select delivery via nebulizer (20 mg/ampule). Discontinue antiallergy drugs if a therapeutic response is not obtained with 4 weeks of therapy. Pretreatment with a bronchodilating drug may be required before using an antiallergy drug.

Xanthine Derivatives

◆ aminophylline (Phyllocontin); ◆ Phyllocontin
◆ oxtriphylline; ◆ Choledyl
◆ theophylline (Elixophyllin, Slo-Phylline, Theo-Dur, Theolair, Theospan, many others)

Indications

Xanthine derivatives such as theophylline are the most effective bronchodilator drugs. Although they are less effective as bronchodilators than beta agonists, they are principally

RESPIRATORY

used as adjuncts to inhaled corticosteroids for the prevention of nocturnal symptoms. Oxtriphylline is available in Canada but is no longer available in the United States.

Pharmacodynamics

Xanthines alleviate the early phase of asthma attacks and the bronchoconstrictive portion of the late-phase response. Through phosphodiesterase inhibition and adenosine antagonism, xanthines produce bronchial smooth muscle relaxation, but there is minimal bronchodilation at therapeutic concentrations. Diaphragmatic contractility and mucociliary clearance are increased and thus are responsible for reversing diaphragmatic fatigue in patients with chronic obstructive pulmonary disease (COPD). They also may have mild antiinflammatory effects but cause no reduction in bronchial hyperresponsiveness. Xanthines may affect the infiltration or eosinophils into bronchial mucosa, while also decreasing the numbers of epithelial T cells.

Pharmacokinetics

Aminophylline is well absorbed from oral dosage formulations, with slow but complete absorption from extended-release formulations (see Table 50-1). Aminophylline and oxtriphylline are widely distributed to body tissues, crossing the placental membranes. Breast milk concentrations are 70% those of plasma levels. The drugs are not distributed to adipose tissue.

Aminophylline and oxtriphylline are converted to theophylline in the liver; in turn, 90% of the theophylline is biotransformed to caffeine. Theophylline metabolites are eliminated through the kidneys. A febrile illness such as influenza, hypoxia, cor pulmonale, decompensated heart failure, cirrhosis, and renal disease decreases biotransformation of the xanthines. **⚠ Smoking increases the biotransformation of theophylline, thus decreasing its serum concentration.**

Adverse Effects and Contraindications

Therapeutic as well as toxic effects of theophylline are related to plasma concentration. Pulmonary function improvement is generally seen when effective plasma concentration range from 5 to 20 mg/L. At concentrations above 20 mg/L the patient may complain of headache, insomnia, nervousness, and nausea. At concentrations over 40 mg/L, seizures, neuromuscular irritability, tremors, arrhythmias (i.e., supraventricular tachycardia), hypokalemia, hyperglycemia, and vomiting have been ⚠ reported. **The risk for intentional or accidental overdose is ever present with theophylline bronchodilators.**

Other adverse effects include aggravation of ulcers or gastroesophageal reflux, difficulty urinating and proctitis (in older males with prostatism), and hyperactivity in some children.

Drug Interactions

Drug interactions with xanthines are many (see Table 50-3). Furthermore, regular but excessive intake of charcoal-broiled foods may decrease the effectiveness of xanthines. Excessive intake of xanthine-containing foods or beverages (e.g., colas, coffee, chocolate) increases the risk of cardiovascular and CNS effects. The absorption of xanthines is increased when the drugs are taken with food. A high-protein diet increases biotransformation, leading to decreased theophylline concentrations. Conversely, a diet high in carbohydrates decreases biotransformation and increases theophylline concentrations.

Dosage Regimen

The dosage regimen for xanthine derivatives is expressed in theophylline equivalents and varies with the specific drug, patient body weight (mg/kg), route of administration, and serum drug levels (see Table 50-2). Dosages are based on lean body weight since theophylline does not distribute to body fat. Regardless of the theophylline salt used, dosages should be calculated for equivalence based on anhydrous theophylline content.

Use dosage intervals to produce minimal fluctuations between peak and trough serum levels. When converting from an intermediate-release to a sustained-release formulation, keep the total daily dose the same, adjusting only the dosing interval. To achieve rapid effects, an initial loading dose is required

Lab Considerations

Monitor arterial blood gases and fluid and electrolyte balance in patients receiving parenteral xanthine therapy. Monitor serum drug levels for evidence of toxicity after initiating therapy, with dosage increase, and if the patient displays signs or symptoms of theophylline toxicity.

Antimuscarinic Drugs

- ◆ ipratropium (Atrovent); ✦ Atrovent
- ◆ tiotropium (Spiriva HandiHaler); ✦ Spiriva inhaler

Indications

The antimuscarinic drugs ipratropium and tiotropium are used as bronchodilators in maintenance therapy of bronchospasm associated with chronic obstructive pulmonary disease (COPD), including chronic bronchitis and emphysema. **Ipratropium is the drug of choice for beta blocker–induced bronchospasm. Antimuscarinic drugs are not designed for use in acute bronchospasm.** ⚠

Pharmacodynamics

Antimuscarinic drugs inhibit only that component of bronchoconstriction that is mediated by muscarinic$_3$ (M$_3$) receptors in the parasympathetic nervous system. The bronchodilation that follows tiotropium inhalation is predominantly a site-specific, rather than a systemic, effect. Muscarinic receptor activity in bronchial smooth muscle is inhibited, resulting in decreased concentrations of cyclic guanosine monophosphate (cGMP). Decreased levels of cGMP produce local bronchodilation. The end result is bronchodilation without systemic antimuscarinic adverse effects. Ipratropium produces most bronchodilation in larger airways, in contrast to beta agonists, which act primarily in smaller airways. Antimuscarinic drugs were discussed in Chapter 15.

Pharmacokinetics

There is minimal systemic absorption with ipratropium, whose action begins 5 to 15 minutes after inhalation, reaching a peak in 1 to 2 hours and with effects lasting up to 6 hours (see Table 50-1). Small amounts of the drug are biotransformed in the liver.

In common with other inhaled drugs, the majority of tiotropium is deposited in the GI tract and, to a lesser extent, the lung, the target organ. Food does not influence absorption. The absolute bioavailability of oral solutions is 2% to 3%. In light of this, the absolute bioavailability of 19.5% of inhaled tiotropium suggests that the fraction reaching the lungs is highly bioavailable but the portion reaching the GI tract is poorly absorbed. The extent of biotransformation appears to be small. Tiotropium is highly bound to tissues.

▥ *Adverse Effects and Contraindications*

Systemic adverse effects of ipratropium and tiotropium are uncommon because of their poor absorption; when present, however, the adverse effects include nervousness, dizziness, and headache. The most common adverse effect of tiotropium is dry mouth at initial stages of therapy, which usually resolves during continued treatment.

A   **Ipratropium is contraindicated for use in hypersensitive patients, and in those with allergy to atropine, belladonna alkaloids, bromide, fluorocarbons, or peanuts. Avoid the use of these antimuscarinic drugs during acute bronchospasm.** Tiotropium is contraindicated for use in hypersensitive patients. Use ipratropium and tiotropium with caution in patients who have bladder neck obstruction, glaucoma, or urinary retention. Safe use during pregnancy or lactation or in children has not been established.

▥ *Dosage Regimen*

The usual adult dose of ipratropium is one to two puffs via MDI, 3 to 4 times daily (see Table 50-2). The dosage of ipratropium should not exceed 12 puffs in 24 hours, and the drug should not be used more often than once every 4 hours. When ipratropium solution is used in a nebulizer, 250 to 500 mcg is given 3 to 4 times daily. The nebulizer route is used for children, with drug doses of 125 to 250 mcg given 3 to 4 times daily.

The usual dose of tiotropium is one capsule (18 mcg) once daily using the HandiHaler inhalation device.

Monoclonal Antibody

◆ omalizumab (Xolair)

▥ *Indications*

Omalizumab is used to decrease the incidence of exacerbation in patients with moderate to severe persistent asthma that is inadequately controlled with inhaled corticosteroids. Safety and efficacy has not been established in other allergic conditions. See Chapter 32 for additional information on monoclonal antibodies.

▥ *Pharmacodynamics*

Omalizumab is a recombinant DNA–derived human IgG$_1$κ monoclonal antibody that inhibits the binding of IgE to high-affinity IgE receptors on the surface of mast cells and basophils. Reduction in surface-bound IgE limits the degree of release of mediators of the allergic response. The concurrent use of omalizumab and allergen immunotherapy has not been evaluated.

▥ *Pharmacokinetics*

Omalizumab is slowly absorbed after subcutaneous (subQ) administration, with peak concentrations reached in 7 to 8 days. Mean serum concentration of free IgE is over 96% using

recommended dosages. The drug is eliminated through the liver, the reticuloendothelial system, and endothelial cells. Clearance of omalizumab involves IgG clearance processes, as well as clearance via specific binding and complex formation with IgE.

▥ *Adverse Effects and Contraindications*

The adverse effects of omalizumab occur in 4% to 11% of patients. Injection-site reactions are most common (ecchymosis, redness, warmth, stinging, hive formation) followed by viral infections, sinusitis, headache, and pharyngitis. Occasionally arthralgias, leg pain, fatigue, and dizziness occur. Arm pain, earache, dermatitis, pruritus, and anaphylaxis are possible, but rare. Malignant neoplasms occur in 0.5% of patients. **The drug is not for use in reversing acute broncho-** **A** **spasm, for acute exacerbations of asthma, and in patients with status asthmaticus.**

▥ *Drug Interactions*

There are no known drug interactions with omalizumab.

▥ *Dosing Regimen*

Dosing of omalizumab is complex but overall is based on the body weight (kg) and IgE levels (see Table 50-2). Be sure to check the package insert for information on preparation and administration. The drug is viscous, and subQ administration may take 5 to 10 seconds to administer. **When using omalizu-** **A** **mab, do not stop or change other asthma treatment regimens.**

▥ *Lab Considerations*

A baseline serum total IgE level is obtained before initiation of treatment since dosages are based on pretreatment levels.

CLINICAL REASONING

Treatment Objectives

Drug regimens are organized so as to gain long-term control of persistent asthma, and to effectively manage symptoms and exacerbations with quick-relief drugs to preserve normal to near normal pulmonary functioning. In addition, prevention of recurrent exacerbations of asthma while minimizing acute care interventions is also an objective.

Treatment Options

Asthma is clearly not a one-drug disease. Thus, multi–drug therapy is generally the rule rather than the exception. The type and amount of drug prescribed is determined by the seriousness of the asthma (Table 50-4).

Two documents set the standards for the diagnosis and treatment of asthma: *Guidelines for the Diagnosis and Management of Asthma* (National Asthma Education and Prevention Program Expert Panel, 1997, 2002) and the *International Consensus Report on Diagnosis and Treatment of Asthma* (National Asthma Education and Prevention Program Expert Panel, 1992). According to these documents, begin chronic asthma therapy when (1) bronchospasm-triggering events set off symptoms, (2) when symptoms are not controlled, or (3) when beta agonists are used more than twice daily for 1 week. Introduce prophylaxis before exercise in all patients with exercise-induced asthma (EIA), and in all patients with seasonal asthma (ideally

TABLE 50-4 Stepwise Approach for Managing Asthma in Adults and Children Over 5 Years Old

Goals of Asthma Treatment

- Prevent chronic and troublesome symptoms (e.g., coughing or breathlessness in the night, in the early morning, or after exertion)
- Maintain (near) "normal" pulmonary function
- Maintain normal activity levels (including exercise and other physical activity)
- Prevent recurrent exacerbations of asthma and minimize the need for emergency department visits or hospitalizations
- Provide optimal pharmacotherapy with minimal or no adverse effects
- Meet patients' and families' expectation of and satisfaction with asthma care

	Classification of Severity: Clinical Features Before Treatment*		
	Symptoms†	Nighttime Symptoms	Lung Function
STEP 4 **Severe Persistent**	• Continual symptoms • Limited physical activity • Frequent exacerbations	Frequent	• FEV_1 or PEF ≤60% predicted • PEF variability >30%
STEP 3 **Moderate Persistent**	• Daily symptoms • Daily use of inhaled short-acting beta₂ agonist • Exacerbations affect activity • Exacerbations ≥2 times a week; may last days	>1 time a week	• FEV_1 or PEF >60% ≤80% predicted • PEF variability >30%
STEP 2 **Mild Persistent**	• Symptoms >2 times a week but <1 time a day • Exacerbations may affect activity	>2 times a month	• FEV_1 or PEF ≥80% predicted • PEF variability 20%–30%
STEP 1 **Mild Intermittent**	• Symptoms ≤2 times a week • Asymptomatic and normal PEF between exacerbations • Exacerbations brief (from a few hours to a few days); intensity may vary	≤2 times a month	• FEV_1 or PEF ≥80% predicted • PEF variability <20%

*The presence of one of the features of severity is sufficient to place a patient in that category. An individual should be assigned to the most severe grade in which any feature occurs. The characteristics noted in this table are general and may overlap because asthma is highly variable. Furthermore, an individual's classification may change over time.
†Patients at any level of severity can have mild, moderate, or severe exacerbations. Some patients with intermittent asthma experience severe and life-threatening exacerbations separated

	Long-Term Control	Quick Relief	Education
	PREFERRED TREATMENTS ARE IN BOLD PRINT.		
STEP 4 **Severe Persistent**	Daily medications: • **Antiinflammatory: inhaled corticosteroid (high dose) and** • Long-acting bronchodilator: either long-acting inhaled beta₂ agonist, sustained-release theophylline, or long-acting beta₂ agonist tablets AND • Corticosteroid tablets or syrup long term (2 mg/kg/day, generally do not exceed 60 mg/day)	• Short-acting bronchodilator: **inhaled beta₂ agonists** as needed for symptoms • Intensity of treatment will depend on severity of exacerbation • Use of short-acting inhaled beta₂ agonists on a daily basis, or increasing use, indicates the need for additional long-term-control therapy	Steps 2 and 3 actions plus • Refer to individual education/counseling

STEP 3
Moderate Persistent
	Daily medication:
	• Either
	   – **Antiinflammatory: inhaled corticosteroid** (medium dose) OR
	   – Inhaled corticosteroid (low-medium dose) and add a long-acting bronchodilator, especially for nighttime symptoms: either **long-acting inhaled beta₂ agonist**, sustained-release theophylline, or long-acting beta₂ agonist tablets
	• If needed
	   – Antiinflammatory: inhaled corticosteroids (medium-high dose) AND
	   – Long-acting bronchodilator, especially for nighttime symptoms; either **long-acting inhaled beta₂ agonist**, sustained-release theophylline, of long-acting beta₂ agonist tablets
		• Short-acting bronchodilator: **inhaled beta₂ agonists** as needed for symptoms
		• Intensity of treatment will depend on severity of exacerbation
		• Use of short-acting inhaled beta₂ agonists on a daily basis, or increasing use, indicates the need for additional long-term-control therapy
			Step 1 actions plus
			• Teach self-monitoring
			• Refer to group education if available
			• Review and update self-management plan

STEP 2 **Mild Persistent**	Daily medication: • **Antiinflammatory: either inhaled corticosteroid (low doses) or cromolyn or nedocromil** (children usually begin with a trial of cromolyn or nedocromil) • Sustained-release theophylline to serum concentration of 5–15 mcg/mL is an alternative. Zafirlukast or zileuton may also be considered for patients ≥12 years of age, although their position in therapy is not fully established	• Short-acting bronchodilator: **inhaled beta₂ agonists** as needed for symptoms • Intensity of treatment will depend on severity of exacerbation • Use of short-acting inhaled beta₂ agonists on a daily basis, or increasing use, indicates the need for additional long-term-control therapy	Step 1 actions plus • Teach self-monitoring • Refer to group education if available • Review and update self-management plan

| STEP 1
Mild Intermittent | • No daily medication needed | • Short-acting bronchodilator: **inhaled beta₂ agonists** as needed for symptoms
• Intensity of treatment will depend on severity of exacerbation
• Use of short-acting inhaled beta₂ agonists more than 2 times a week may indicate the need to initiate long-term-control therapy | • Teach basic facts about asthma
• Teach inhaler, spacer, holding chamber technique
• Discuss roles of medications
• Develop self-management plan
• Develop action plan for when and how to take rescue actions
• Discuss appropriate environmental control measures to avoid exposure to known allergens and irritants (See component 4.) |

↓ Step down
Review treatment every 1 to 6 months; a gradual stepwise reduction in treatment may be possible.

↑ Step up
If control is not maintained, consider step up. First, review patient medication technique, adherence, and environmental control (avoidance of allergens or other factors that contribute to asthma severity).

Notes: • The stepwise approach presents general guidelines to assist clinical decision making; it is not intended to be a specific prescription. Asthma is highly variable; clinicians should tailor specific medication plans to the needs and circumstances of individual patients.
   • Gain control as quickly as possible; then decrease treatment to the least medication necessary to maintain control. Gaining control may be accomplished either by starting treatment at the step most appropriate to the initial severity of the patient's condition or by starting at a higher level of therapy (e.g., a course of systemic corticosteroids or higher dose of inhaled corticosteroids).
   • A rescue course of systemic corticosteroid may be needed at any time and at any step.
   • Some patients with intermittent asthma experience severe and life-threatening exacerbations separated by long periods of normal lung function and no symptoms. This may be especially common with exacerbations provoked by respiratory infections. A short course of systemic corticosteroids is recommended.
   • At each step, patients should control their environment to avoid or control factors that make their asthma worse (e.g., allergens, irritants); this requires specific diagnosis and education.

before the season for the known allergen). Corticosteroids, anti-allergy drugs, LT antagonists, long-acting beta agonists, and xanthine derivatives are used for long-term control of asthma. Short-acting beta agonists and anticholinergics are used for acute asthma attacks.

▐ Patient Variables

Many of the drugs used in the treatment of allergies and asthma are purchased by consumers over the counter. They are easily accessible to almost all persons, are easy to use, and in many cases, are generally effective. For these reasons, many patients with asthma have not been diagnosed or adequately treated. Family and societal health care beliefs and norms may keep the patient from seeking help (see Case Study).

Pulmonary function tests provide an objective and reproducible means of evaluating the presence and the severity of lung disease, as well as the response to therapy. A key measurement is *peak expiratory flow rate* (PEFR), or the greatest flow velocity that can be obtained during a forced expiration. PEFRs place the disease into physiologic categories: red, yellow, and green zones (Fig. 50-3). In general, spirometry testing can be reliably performed by adults as well as children by the age of 5 or 6. Arrange for the patient with persistent asthma who is exposed to perennial indoor allergens to have skin testing.

PEFRs are usually measured upon awakening and before bedtime, and before and after administration of a beta agonist. Use the same peak flow meter each time a measurement is taken to reduce the risk of measurement error. **PEFRs should be performed when symptoms appear, when there has been a change in therapy, and every 1 to 2 years thereafter.**

Teach the patient how to establish a personal best PEFR, that is, a minimum of twice-daily measurements and the best of three measurements on each occasion. Based on their personal best, patients may be instructed (1) to double the dose of the inhaled corticosteroid if their PEFR is less than 75% of their personal best; (2) to double the dose of the inhaled corticosteroid when starting a short course of oral corticosteroids if the PEFR is less than 50% of their personal best; and (3) to seek medical attention right away if the PEFR is less than 25% of personal best. When properly used, peak flow meter readings allow for early recognition of symptoms and prompt initiation or modification of therapy.

Assess the FEV_1 (forced expiratory volume in 1 second) once during an acute exacerbation to determine the reversibility of bronchoconstriction. Improvement in bronchoconstriction is considered an increase of 15% to 20% in FEV_1 after receiving a short-acting beta agonist. Obtain arterial blood gases if the PEFR is less than 40% of predicted, the FEV_1 is less than 1.2 L, or the patient is not responding to treatment. Consider hospitalization for patients who manifest any one of the following:

• Subjective report of severe difficulty breathing
• Failure to respond fully and promptly to inhaled beta agonist therapy that was followed promptly by full oral doses of prednisone
• Use of the accessory muscles of respiration
• The presence of pulsus paradoxus in excess of 10 mm Hg
• An FEV_1 less than 1 L/sec
• A $PaCO_2$ inappropriately high for respiratory rate
• The presence of an underlying cardiac condition
• An inadequate home situation or a history of poor adherence to therapy

RESPIRATORY

CASE STUDY   Antiasthmatic and Bronchodilator Drugs

ASSESSMENT

History of Present Illness	RL is a 25-year-old Native American female who has had moderate persistent asthma since age 7, resulting in recurrent episodes of acute attacks. RL has been treated in the emergency room or hospitalized for asthma attacks once a month for the last 10 months. She comes to the emergency room today stating that today's began when she awoke this morning, although she reports wheezing during the night and having a headache. She admits to using her inhaler intermittently. Symptoms of a URI had been present for the past 48 hours. RL has a 10-pack year history of smoking. Current drugs include cromolyn sodium 4 times daily and metaproterenol MDI PRN. Her wheezing this morning was not relieved by her metaproterenol MDI. She reports using up to 14 MDI canisters this month alone in an attempt to control her asthma.
Past Health History	RL was hospitalized at age 17 for severe respiratory distress and has used intermittent steroid therapy to maintain control ever since. Her family history reveals that both parents are diabetics, as well as three of her five siblings. Her mother has a 40-year history of asthma and eczema.
Life-Span Considerations	RL is in Erikson's stage of intimacy versus isolation. She is attempting to establish intimate bonds of love and friendship, although her attempts have been hindered by her asthma.
Psychosocial Considerations	RL was married at age 20, was divorced a year later, and has one child, a daughter now age 4 years. She is at present in college full-time and living with her parents until she completes her education. RL has no income of her own. Her parents are supporting RL and their grandchild while RL is in school. Health care needs are covered through her parents' insurance coverage.
Physical Exam Findings	*Height:* 5'2". *Weight:* 190 lbs. VS: *BP:* 120/80. 97.2° F- 90 and regular- 28 and labored. Audible wheezes on inspiration and expiration over bilateral lung fields. Altered ratio of inspiration to expiration. Heart sounds not audible because of the wheezes. Skin pink and diaphoretic.
Diagnostic Testing	Spirometry reveals an FEV_1 of 68% of predicted with a variable PEFR exceeding 30%.

DIAGNOSIS: Exacerbation of moderate persistent asthma

MANAGEMENT

Treatment Objectives	1. Resolve current asthma exacerbation; achieve peak flow levels in the green range and an FEV_1 over 90% upon discharge 2. Prevent chronic, troublesome symptoms (e.g., coughing or shortness of breath nocturnally, in the early morning, or after exercise) 3. Maintain near-normal pulmonary function exercise and other physical activities (SpO_2 over 92%)
Treatment Options	**Pharmacotherapy** • Stop cromolyn sodium and metaproterenol inhaler today. • Start oral prednisone burst regimen per written instructions. • Self-administer albuterol and ipratropium nebulizer treatment every 4 hours while awake until next visit in 48 hours. **Patient Teaching** 1. Acute care instructions: Increase fluid intake to 2 to 3 liters/day; monitor PEFR. 2. Stop smoking. 3. Begin or continue educational efforts to teach the patient about the nature of asthma and how this information can assist her in her treatment; specifically, the central role that inflammation plays in its pathogenesis and prognosis. 4. Rationale for use of steroids to gain long-term control of asthma; how to safely use oral steroids 5. Rationale for switch to inhaled steroid when stable 6. Refer to support group if available. 7. Review and update self-management plan at each office visit.

Evaluation

1. Patient perception of improvement, quality of life, and the ability to engage in activities of daily living
2. Peak flow levels in the green range and an FEV_1 over 90%
3. SpO_2 over 92% with activity

CRITICAL REASONING ANALYSIS

Q1. Why are you having her stop the cromolyn sodium?

A. She is having trouble using the drug 4 times a day, and there is a possibility the cromolyn is causing tracheal irritation. It may also not be effective because of RL's intermittent use.

Q2. I know there are several prednisone taper regimens. What prednisone taper regimen will you use, and why?

A. Personal preference really—and the fact that patients do well if they take the prednisone at the same time each morning. Many experts recommend a dose of 1 to 2 mg/kg of prednisone per day. I start with 50 mg of prednisone on day 1; 40 mg on day 2; 30 mg daily for 3 days; 20 mg daily for 4 days; and then 10 mg daily for 4 days. I always give the patient a written set of these instructions along with the prescription.

Q3. How will you manage her asthma after she completes this acute drug regimen for her asthma exacerbation?

A. I will prescribe a fluticasone-salmeterol inhaler (Advair) after her prednisone taper is completed. Advair is simple to use and should therefore facilitate her adherence with twice-daily puffs, and it does not require her to coordinate puffs with activation of the inhaler. The salmeterol component is a long-acting beta agonist and the fluticasone a corticosteroid. Together, they should control her symptoms. She can use the albuterol inhaler on a PRN basis.

Q4. Why did you change her from metaproterenol to albuterol?

A. Metaproterenol acts on both β_1 and β_2 receptors, which increases the risk of adverse effects. Albuterol is β_2-specific and acts to relax bronchioles without producing cardiovascular adverse effects.

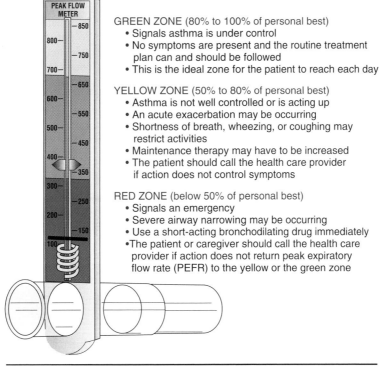

GREEN ZONE (80% to 100% of personal best)
- Signals asthma is under control
- No symptoms are present and the routine treatment plan can and should be followed
- This is the ideal zone for the patient to reach each day

YELLOW ZONE (50% to 80% of personal best)
- Asthma is not well controlled or is acting up
- An acute exacerbation may be occurring
- Shortness of breath, wheezing, or coughing may restrict activities
- Maintenance therapy may have to be increased
- The patient should call the health care provider if action does not control symptoms

RED ZONE (below 50% of personal best)
- Signals an emergency
- Severe airway narrowing may be occurring
- Use a short-acting bronchodilating drug immediately
- The patient or caregiver should call the health care provider if action does not return peak expiratory flow rate (PEFR) to the yellow or the green zone

FIGURE 50-3 Interpreting Peak Expiratory Flow Rates. Expiratory flow rate zones are based on the patient's personal best effort rather than on a set level of expiration. A baseline reading is required for accurate interpretation of peak expiratory flow rate (PEFR).

RESPIRATORY

BOX 50-2

Important History Questions for Patients with Asthma

- In the last 12 months, have you experienced sudden, severe, or recurrent episodes of coughing, wheezing, or shortness of breath?
- Have you had a cough or cold that settles in your chest or takes longer than 10 days to go away?
- Is coughing, wheezing, or shortness of breath more of a problem during specific seasons or time of year?
- Do your symptoms occur only when you are in certain places or when exposed to allergens such as animals, tobacco smoke, or perfumes?
- When do your symptoms occur? During the night? Early morning? After moderate exercise, running, or other physical activity?
- What drugs, if any, do you use that help you breathe better? If so, how often do you use the drugs?
- How many puffs of an inhaler do you use daily? How many inhalers have been used in the last month?
- Do you use inhaled cocaine, nasal or ocular decongestants, or antihistamines?
- What is your status between attacks (e.g., restrictions in activities of daily living)?
- Do you use a peak flow meter? If so, what are the highest and lowest readings since your last visit?
- What is the geographic location of your home? Is your home a frame, stucco, brick, or mobile home? What type of insulation do you have?
- What type of heating (e.g., wood-burning stove or fireplace) is used?
- What is the humidity level in your home?
- Do you have upholstered furnishings? What types of draperies and bedding do you have?
- Do you have any plants in your home? What kind of and how many pets do you have? What are their habits?
- What house-cleaning methods do you use?
- What chemical irritants or sensitizers, physical demands, and stressors do you encounter on the job?
- Do you cough or wheeze during the week but not on weekends when you are away from work?
- Do your eyes and nasal passages become irritated soon after arriving at work?

LIFE-SPAN CONSIDERATIONS. Box 50-2 provides additional information regarding the history-taking components to include for a patient with allergies and asthma.

Pregnant and Nursing Women. During pregnancy, a number of changes take place in the respiratory tract mediated by the mechanical effects of the enlarging uterus, increased oxygen demands, and the respiratory stimulant effect of progesterone. Estrogen causes hyperemia of nasopharyngeal mucosa, with edema and increased production of mucus. This leads to a feeling of stuffiness and an increased tendency for epistaxis. Warn pregnant women of this normal change and advise against using over-the-counter (OTC) drugs and nasal sprays to alleviate the symptoms. A normal saline spray may be helpful in reducing some of the discomfort and should be encouraged in women who find the stuffy feeling uncomfortable.

Although about 4% of pregnancies are complicated by asthma, the true prevalence may be much higher. Asthma may occur at any time during pregnancy. If it is diagnosed before pregnancy, it may be worsened by the pregnancy. One third of pregnant women with asthma are adversely affected, one third remain the same, and one third improve. Women with asthma usually return to their prepregnancy level of the disease by about 3 months postpartum.

Maternal and fetal morbidity and mortality are increased if asthma is uncontrolled during pregnancy. Maternal complications include preeclampsia, gestational hypertension, hyperemesis gravidarum, vaginal hemorrhage, and complications of labor. Fetal complications include increased risk of perinatal mortality, intrauterine growth retardation, preterm birth, low birth weight, and neonatal hypoxia. If asthma is controlled, the woman can maintain a normal pregnancy, with little or no increased risk to herself or the fetus.

Women with asthma who use inhaled bronchodilators or ▲ **corticosteroids have no greater risk of congenital anomalies in the fetus or adverse perinatal outcomes than the general population.**

As with any other patient, albuterol, a short-acting inhaled $beta_2$ agonist, is used as a rapid-relief drug to treat asthma symptoms. Patients with symptoms that occur at least 2 days a week or 2 nights a month need daily drug therapy to manage their symptoms and prevent a flare-up of their asthma. The preferred drug is a corticosteroid to control the underlying asthma-related inflammation. There is more safety data on budesonide use during pregnancy than on other inhaled corticosteroids. Alternatively, LT antagonists, cromolyn, or theophylline may be used.

Metaproterenol by inhalation and subQ terbutaline have been used extensively in pregnant women. If there is no satisfactory response from initial bronchodilators, give intravenous (IV) aminophylline for the patient with an acute asthma attack. Theophylline serum levels are closely followed. Use corticosteroids in patients with severe exacerbations and for patients who do not respond to beta agonists.

The asthma guidelines recommend either increasing the dose of inhaled corticosteroid or adding a long-acting beta agonist (e.g., salmeterol) to the regimen of patients whose persistent asthma is not well controlled on low doses of inhaled corticosteroids alone. Theophylline and cromolyn are also considered safe for use in pregnancy. The theophylline dosage may have to be reduced during the third trimester because of a decrease in drug clearance.

Children and Adolescents. A strong relationship exists between viral infections and the appearance of asthma in infants. Allergens play a less important role in this age group because it takes time for allergic sensitivity to develop. In children, however, allergy influences the persistence and severity of the disease (see Box 50-1).

Assessment of symptoms in the child is much like that of the adult but also includes a feeding history for a very young child, with attention to cow's milk, eggs, and wheat. Do not overlook the stability of family members' relationships and stress levels. Note information about the child's toys and bedroom and other rooms of the house where the child spends waking hours. Include the child's exposure level to babysitters, relatives, day care, and school environments, and the presence or absence of symptoms in all of these areas. The source of present and past health information (often the parents) is important because valid recall of times and events associated with symptoms is critical in providing clues to the causal antigen. As a rule, children who have asthma tend to have slow growth rates before reaching puberty, with males more affected than females. Treating children with high-dose inhaled corticosteroids for severe persistent asthma is less likely to affect linear growth than prolonged use of high-dose systemic corticosteroids. Short-term oral (i.e., 3 to 10 days) corticosteroid use is ordinarily effective in treating exacerbations of asthma.

The pulmonary function of adolescents is more comparable to the predicted norms in children than to those in adults. A trial with cromolyn is often used when initiating antiinflammatory therapy in an adolescent. Provide the child's school a written treatment plan, and ensure prompt access to the drugs.

Older Adults. Commonly, older adults who develop asthma late in life (1% to 2%) have intrinsic asthma, which does not have allergic or environmental triggers. Neither IgE nor skin testing is useful in the older adult, probably because of the decrease in allergic response associated with aging. Unfortunately, treatable airway disorders in older adults often go undiagnosed, perhaps because of the high prevalence of other forms of respiratory disease (e.g., emphysema, chronic bronchitis) and cardiac failure that have similar clinical presentations. Some older adults may not be able to perform spirometry testing reliably. Additional tests, such as symptom scores and distance walked without dyspnea and wheezing, can be used to evaluate the patient.

Because chronic bronchitis or emphysema may coexist with asthma, a trial of systemic corticosteroids can be used to establish the extent of reversibility and therapeutic benefit. Furthermore, many older adults have comorbid conditions (e.g., arthritis, heart disease, and hypertension) that are being treated with drug therapy (e.g., aspirin, beta blockers). Asthma drugs may aggravate comorbid conditions; therefore adjustments in the drug regimen may be needed. Be aware of the increased potential for drug interactions.

▊ Drug Variables

Owing to the life-threatening nature of severe exacerbations of asthma, treatment should be started immediately once an exacerbation is recognized. All patients with a severe exacerbation should immediately receive oxygen, systemic corticosteroids, and high doses of an inhaled short-acting beta$_2$ agonist.

SYSTEMIC CORTICOSTEROIDS. Oral corticosteroids are needed for urgent and emergent intervention. The oral dose is ordinarily 30 to 60 mg daily for 1 week, in addition to other drugs. Or, when a parenteral formulation is needed, 1 mg/kg of methylprednisolone (Solu-Medrol) may be given every 4 hours if needed. The antiinflammatory effect of corticosteroids is delayed at least 4 hours; therefore, IV administration provides little, if any, time advantage. Further, IV administration is significantly more expensive than using the oral route and appears to be no more effective. Parenteral hydrocortisone can be used in patients who are nauseated or have difficulty absorbing oral drugs. Discontinue systemic corticosteroid treatment in 7 to 10 days (some patients' asthma may worsen at this point).

Once the patient is past the acute bronchoconstriction, an MDI or nebulized formulation of albuterol may be used, along with the usual maintenance dosages of systemic corticosteroid. Based on patient response, the daily dosage of corticosteroid is gradually reduced. **As a general rule, dosage** ▲ **reductions do not exceed 2.5 mg of prednisone or its comparable equivalent. The importance of a slow withdrawal rate cannot be overemphasized.** A number of weeks to months are required for recovery of HPA axis function that was suppressed during original treatment regimens. Deaths have occurred as the result of adrenal insufficiency during and after transfer from systemic corticosteroids to inhaled corticosteroids.

Monitor the patient closely during the transition from systemic corticosteroid use to inhaled corticosteroids since the change may uncover allergies that until now were suppressed by the systemic steroids (e.g., conjunctivitis, rhinitis, eczema).

INHALED CORTICOSTEROIDS. During withdrawal from corticosteroids, some patients may note withdrawal symptoms (e.g., lassitude, joint or muscle pain, depression). The withdrawal symptoms may appear despite maintenance or even improvement in respiratory function during withdrawal. Encourage them to continue using the inhaler, but carefully monitor for signs of adrenal insufficiency (e.g., hypotension, weight loss). If evidence of adrenal insufficiency occurs, boost the systemic steroid dose temporarily and slow the continued withdrawal.

In line with national and international guidelines, earlier and more widespread use of inhaled corticosteroids is recommended. Regular use of inhaled corticosteroids (1) suppresses inflammation; (2) decreases bronchial hyperresponsiveness; (3) decreases asthma symptoms in patients with chronic disease; (4) improves pulmonary function in mild asthma; and (5) reduces or eliminates the need for oral corticosteroids. Bronchiolar reactivity is reduced, although maximal reduction may be delayed for 9 to 12 months after treatment begins.

Corticosteroids are the most effective antiinflammatory drugs available for the treatment of asthma. All of the inhaled corticosteroids are equally effective and have few systemic adverse effects at therapeutic dosages. In the United States and many other countries of the world, inhaled corticosteroids have become the first-line treatment, with inhaled beta$_2$ agonists used as needed. The small risk of adverse effects of corticosteroids is offset by their effectiveness in long-term suppression of inflammation.

Still, a number of concerns remain. There is a rising trend in prevalence, morbidity, severity, and mortality rates for asthma. Despite the well-recognized efficacy and safety of inhaled corticosteroids, many patients still have poorly controlled asthma and a poor quality of life. In addition, there are concerns about the long-term safety of inhaled corticosteroids (especially in high doses and at the extremes of age). Poor compliance with the treatment plan and poor administration technique (especially for inhaled formulations) contribute to the risk of exacerbations and adverse drug effects.

To reduce the adverse effects associated with long-term use of corticosteroids, a number of measures are recommended. Use the lowest possible dosage of inhaled corticosteroids and administer them through a spacer or holding chamber. Consider using a long-acting beta agonist with a low to medium dose of inhaled corticosteroid (e.g., salmeterol and fluticasone [Advair]) rather than using a higher dose of the inhaled corticosteroid. Evaluate whether adding calcium (1000 to 1500 mg/day) and vitamin D (400 units/day) supplements for postmenopausal women would be beneficial.

Estrogen replacement therapy (ERT) may be appropriate for some postmenopausal women who are taking more than 1000 mcg of inhaled corticosteroid per day to minimize the osteoporosis risk. Inhaled corticosteroids reduce the need for, and dosage of, systemic drugs; thus the likelihood of osteoporosis is reduced.

Beclomethasone and budesonide via MDI are comparable on a microgram-to-microgram basis. The effects produced by beclomethasone are comparable to twice the dose of triamcinolone on a microgram basis. Because the majority of patients with asthma require low corticosteroid dosages (300 to 400 mcg/day), beclomethasone is the most convenient and cost-effective preparation. Beclomethasone in high dosage (i.e., 2000 mcg/day) increases the output of urinary hydroxyproline. The increased output of this amino acid (produced in the digestion of hydrolytic decomposition of proteins, especially of collagens) reflects an increase in bone resorption, whereas budesonide does not cause this.

Budesonide has the highest inhaled-to-systemic ratio of the drugs available at present; however, it is less bioavailable than beclomethasone. In low dosages (i.e., less than 1000 mcg/day), the impact of differences in bioavailability between budesonide and beclomethasone is probably not significant. Budesonide administered via Turbuhaler achieved effects similar to twice the dose delivered by MDI. This suggests the efficacy of the drug is influenced by the delivery device. Thus, base the decision to use budesonide or beclomethasone on cost and the patient's preference.

Fluticasone achieves effects similar to 2 times the dosage of beclomethasone and budesonide via MDI on a microgram basis. Fluticasone has a significant first-pass effect and, therefore, a better efficacy-to-safety relationship; however, individual patients may respond differently to different drugs.

BETA AGONISTS. The morbidity and mortality associated with asthma have increased despite advances in drug therapy. The increased rates may be due to a false sense of security with beta agonists that cause the patient to delay seeking medical assistance. On the one hand, beta agonists are by far the most effective bronchodilators available. They relax airway smooth muscle from the trachea to the terminal bronchioles and play a role in increasing mucociliary clearance. However, they do not inhibit either the late-phase response or the subsequent bronchial hyperresponsiveness. Orally administered beta agonists are less useful because of the increased incidence of adverse effects. Excessive use of beta agonists may cause hypokalemia. These drugs may be useful for nocturnal asthma or severe asthma.

There have been a number of concerns about the long-term use of beta agonists. (1) The first concern is that beta agonists worsen asthma by inducing tachyphylaxis. This hypothesis has not been substantiated, although the regular use of beta agonists appears to lead to a greater decline in FEV_1 than does intermittent use. Therefore, regular use is not recommended. A beta agonist prescription that is refilled more often than every 30 days suggests a loss of control of symptoms. If the patient is not already using an inhaled corticosteroid, it is appropriate at this point to prescribe the drug. (2) The second concern is that there is an association between mortality risk from asthma and increased beta agonist use. At present, there is no apparent relationship between the risks of death from asthma with the use of beta agonist oral or metered-dose inhalers. The increased incidence of death probably reflects worsening of the disease. (3) Arterial oxygen tension decreases after beta agonist use. There is transient worsening of ventilation and perfusion mismatch, although the effect is usually small. Nonetheless, additional oxygen may be required. (4) Another concern was that beta agonist use enhances myocardial toxicity from the fluorocarbon propellants in the inhaler. There is sensitization of the myocardium at high fluorocarbon concentrations, above those obtained through normal inhaler use. For this reason and out of environmental concerns, inhalers today are now free of fluorocarbons. The newer inhalers have hydrofluoroalkane (HFA) as propellants, have a smaller particle size, and may deliver increased amounts of drug. In contrast, dry powder inhalers, those activated by inspiration, have no propellant.

Furthermore, subQ epinephrine (an adrenergic) for the initial treatment of acute asthma is no longer thought superior to inhaled $beta_2$ agonists. The inhaled form of epinephrine is not recommended for the initial treatment of acute asthma because it stimulates α and β receptors and because there are selective $beta_2$ agonists available that have fewer adverse effects. Although used less often, isoproterenol (a nonselective beta agonist) administered by oral inhalation may be used to treat bronchoconstriction, although a selective $beta_2$ drug is preferred because it causes less cardiac stimulation.

LEUKOTRIENE ANTAGONISTS. LT antagonists may be used as alternatives to low-dose inhaled corticosteroids or antiallergy drugs in patients over age 12 with mild, persistent asthma. Zafirlukast appears to be modestly effective for maintenance treatment of mild to moderate asthma, but taking the drug with food markedly decreases its bioavailability. Many other drugs may prove troublesome if taken concurrently with an LT antagonist.

Unlike theophylline, there is no need to monitor LT-antagonist drug concentrations. Asthma symptoms are reduced by one third, and use of inhaled corticosteroids and beta agonists fall one fourth to one third. However, the relative low potency and short half-lives of LT antagonists mean that dosing 4 times a day is required.

ANTIMUSCARINIC DRUGS. Antimuscarinic drugs are especially effective in the management of asthma in older adults. These drugs provide the additional benefit of bronchodilation, and they can be started along with the first dose of a beta agonist in patients with severe disease. Although they provide an additional small increase in PEFR when they are used with submaximum doses of beta agonists, antimuscarinics have not been shown to reduce other variables (e.g., the need for admission to a hospital, shorter length of stay).

On the other hand, antimuscarinic drugs are less effective than beta agonists and are ordinarily used in combination with other bronchodilators. They may be valuable alternatives even for patients who are partial responders and are valuable for patients who are intolerant of inhaled beta agonists. They may, however, be slightly less effective than beta agonists in reversing bronchospasm, but they are probably equally effective for patients with COPD (if it includes a partially reversible element). Add an antimuscarinic to the treatment regimen for chronic asthma only after the progression from high-dose corticosteroids and beta agonists fails to control symptoms. They should not be used before beta agonist therapy is tried because of concerns that they may cause bronchoconstriction.

ANTIALLERGY DRUGS. The chief advantage of antiallergy drugs lies in the low incidence of adverse effects, thus making them relatively safe drugs for use in children. When used on a daily basis, antiallergy drugs are effective in controlling persistent asthma symptoms. Nedocromil is as potent as standard doses of inhaled corticosteroids (in moderate asthmatics), and improved asthma control may be obtained by the addition of nedocromil to standard dosage of inhaled corticosteroids. Further, because viral infections are a common asthma trigger in children, antiallergy drugs may prevent the inflammation associated with these illnesses.

XANTHINES. Xanthines may be added as a third-line drug to the treatment regimen for patients with acute asthma, although they provide little additional benefit when used concurrently with optimal doses of inhaled beta agonists. Nevertheless, there is benefit to be gained when xanthines are used as adjuncts to inhaled corticosteroids for prevention of nocturnal asthma symptoms. Theophylline should be used only if the patient fails to improve after the first 12 hours of treatment with beta agonists, ipratropium, and prednisone. Theophylline may also be considered for patients who cannot tolerate beta agonist therapy and whose heart rate is less than 120 beats per minute.

Dosage adjustments of theophylline formulations are based on clinical response and improvement in pulmonary function with careful monitoring of serum concentrations. If the level is too low (i.e., 5 to 10 mcg/mL), increase the dosage by about 25% at 3-day intervals until either the desired clinical response or the desired serum concentration is achieved. The total daily dose may be given at more frequent intervals if asthma symptoms repeatedly occur at the end of a dosing interval. If the serum theophylline level is within the desired range (i.e., 10 to 20 mcg/mL), maintain the present dosage and check the serum levels at 6- to 12-month intervals. Finer dosage adjustments may be needed for some patients. Decrease theophylline dosage by 10% if serum levels are between 20 and 25 mcg/mL, and recheck levels in 3 days. If the level is between 25 and 30 mcg/mL, skip the next scheduled dose and reduce subsequent doses by about 25%. When serum levels exceed 30 mcg/mL, skip the next two doses and decrease subsequent doses by 50%. Again, the serum levels should be rechecked in 3 days. Once the patient is stabilized on a dosage, serum levels tend to remain constant. The risk for significant toxicity, the drug's narrow therapeutic range, and individual patient differences in biotransformation make routine monitoring of serum drug levels necessary.

Patient Education

Begin patient and family education at the time of asthma diagnosis, but tailor learning to the needs of the patient while maintaining sensitivity to cultural beliefs and practices. PEFRs guide therapeutic decisions; therefore, provide patients with a written care plan based on signs and symptoms and PEFRs.

Drug therapy should be increased when the PEFR is below 80% of the patient's personal best.

Because asthma is clearly not a one-drug disease, the patient must be familiar with a variety of treatment regimens. Combination therapy is generally the rule rather than the exception. Patients using inhaled corticosteroids are taught to observe for hoarseness, cough, throat irritation, and fungal infection of the mouth and throat. Patients receiving high-dosage corticosteroid therapy are advised to avoid exposure to chickenpox or measles. How the use of corticosteroids (i.e., the dose, the route, and the duration of use), the contribution of comorbid disease, and prior corticosteroid use affects the risk of disseminated infection is unknown. Advise patients to seek medical advice if they are exposed to infection.

Patients who experience a sudden change in stress levels or who have a severe asthma attack and patients who were withdrawn from oral corticosteroids should begin taking large dosages of the corticosteroid and contact their health care provider for further instructions. **Advise patients with asthma to carry medical alert identification that identifies their need for supplemental systemic corticosteroids during stressful periods or a severe attack.**

Administration Devices and Technique

There are several aerosol delivery devices: MDI, breath-actuated MDI, dry-powder inhalers, and nebulizers. Each has advantages and disadvantages. Match the decision for a particular delivery device with patient needs and the likelihood of adherence to the regimen. The technique, the advantages, and the disadvantages are outlined in Table 50-5.

The technique of drug administration varies with the specific aerosol delivery device and whether or not a spacer or holding chamber device is used. However, there are several problems encountered with the use of MDIs. Many patients are unable to coordinate activation with inhalation or activate the MDI in the mouth while breathing through their nose. Some patients do not have adequate strength to activate an MDI or are unable to hold their breath for the required length of time after use. Some patients inhale more than one puff with each inspiration or do not wait a sufficient amount of time between each puff (1 to 5 minutes is recommended). Not shaking the MDI before use, or holding the MDI upside down or sideways contributes to ineffective use. Not tilting the head back and opening the mouth causes the drug to bounce off the teeth, the tongue, or the palate, thus limiting the amount of drug reaching the patient's airways.

Some patients use both a bronchodilator inhaler and a corticosteroid inhaler. **Advise patients to use the bronchodilator drug before the corticosteroid to enhance penetration of the corticosteroid into the bronchial tree.** Further, several minutes should elapse after use of the bronchodilator before the corticosteroid inhaler is used.

Rinse the mouth with water or mouthwash after each use of an inhaled corticosteroid to minimize dry mouth and hoarseness. Rinsing the mouth and gargling after use is advised to reduce the frequent but mild candidiasis that may occur. When present, candidiasis responds well to antifungal drugs such as nystatin mouthwash or clotrimazole troches. The inhalation device (not the drug canister) should be washed at least daily in warm running water.

TABLE 50-5 Comparison of Delivery Devices

Advantage(s)	Disadvantage(s)
Metered-dose inhaler (MDI): Actuated during slow,* deep inhalation, followed by 10-second breath holding	
• Mouth rinsing may reduce systemic absorption	• Slow inhalation is difficult for some patients. • Some patients may have difficulty coordinating actuation with inhalation. • Patients may incorrectly stop inhalation at actuation; 80% of drug is deposited in oropharynx.
Breath-actuated MDI: Slow, deep inhalation, followed by 10-second breath holding	
• Helpful for patients who are unable to coordinate actuation with inhalation • Slow inhalation difficult for some patients. • Patients may incorrectly stop inhalation at actuation. • Device requires more rapid inspiration to activate than is optimal for deposition. • Shape of device restricts use with currently available spacer or holding devices.	
Dry-powder inhaler (DPI): Rapid, deep inhalation with mouth closed tightly around the mouthpiece	
• Can be used in children younger than 4 years • Most appear to have similar delivery efficacy as MDI with or without spacer or holding device • Mouth rinsing is effective in reducing systemic absorption • Dose is lost if patient exhales through device. • Some devices deliver greater quantity of drug than an MDI.	
Nebulizer: Slow tidal breathing with occasional deep breaths. Tightly fitting face mask is used if patient is unable to use mouthpiece.	
• Relies less on patient coordination or cooperation • Delivery method of choice for cromolyn in children • Delivery method of choice for high-dose beta$_2$ agonists and anticholinergics in all patients with moderate to severe exacerbations • Expensive, time-consuming, bulky • Significant variances in output between and among nebulizers	
Spacer or holding device: Slow inhalation or tidal breathing immediately after actuation. One actuation into device per inhalation. If face mask is used, 3 to 5 inhalations per actuation.	
• Easier to use than MDI alone • Using a face mask allows MDI to be used with small children • Large-volume devices (>600 mL) may deliver higher doses to the lungs compared with an MDI alone in patients with poor MDI technique • Reduces the deposit of drug in the oropharynx and the potential for systemic absorption of inhaled corticosteroids • Recommended for patients using medium to high doses of inhaled corticosteroids • As effective as a nebulizer in delivering high doses of a beta$_2$ agonist during exacerbations	• Does not eliminate the need to coordinate actuation with inhalation • Bulky; output from MDI may be reduced in some devices after cleaning • Output from MDI with spacer or holding device is dependent on both MDI and spacer type

*Slow inhalation means 30 L/min for a period of 3 to 5 sec. Rapid inhalation means 60 L/min for a period of 1 to 2 sec.
Adapted from the National Institutes of Health, National Heart, Lung and Blood Institute, National Asthma Education and Prevention Program. (2002). *Update on Selected Topics: Guidelines for the Diagnosis and Management of Asthma* (Pub. No. 02–5075). Bethesda, MD: U.S. Department of Health and Human Services.

Corticosteroid formulations are not the same on a microgram or per-puff basis. With newer delivery devices, and drug formulations that permit increased amounts of drug to reach the airways, dosages may be different than in the past. Instruct the patient as to the correct dosage and use of the delivery device.

Educate patients who have severe persistent asthma, nasal polyps, or documented sensitivity to aspirin or nonsteroidal antiinflammatory drugs (NSAIDs) about the risk for severe and potentially fatal exacerbations with corticosteroid use. Encourage patients with asthma to be treated for rhinitis, sinusitis, and gastroesophageal reflux, if present, in a timely manner to minimize the adverse effects of these disorders on their asthma. Advise patients with asthma to avoid aspirin use.

Patients with chronic lung disease (and other chronic conditions as well) are encouraged to receive the influenza vaccine annually and a single inoculation with pneumococcal vaccine. Advise patients to avoid sulfite-containing food and drinks (e.g., red wine, dried fruit, dried soup mixes) and other foods to which they are sensitive. The occurrence of sulfite reactions depends on the nature of the food, the level of residual sulfite, the sensitivity of the individual, and perhaps the form of residual sulfite and the mechanism of the reaction.

When bronchospasm is triggered by exercise, prophylaxis through prior inhalation of bronchodilating or antiallergy drugs is better than avoiding exercise altogether, especially in children. Further, teach the patient and family correct techniques for coughing, deep breathing, percussion, and postural drainage, when appropriate.

Evaluation

Evaluating treatment outcomes in terms of patient perception of improvement, quality of life, and the ability to engage in activities of daily living is of growing importance. Consider the role that pharmacogenomics, the study of patient response to drug therapy based on genetic make-up, may play when evaluating patient response to bronchodilators and antiasthmatic drugs.

Effectiveness of beta agonists is demonstrated by prevention or relief of bronchospasm and a reduction in the frequency of acute asthma attacks. Exercise-induced bronchospasm is prevented or reduced. Chronic asthma symptoms are relieved with corticosteroids or antiallergy drugs. Patients with asthma should strive for normal exercise tolerance, and sleep should not be interrupted by coughing or wheezing.

Monitoring of disease activity is done by measuring PEFRs and keeping symptom diaries. The peak-flow meter readings are used to identify the severity of an exacerbation and to help guide therapeutic decisions.

Pulmonary function tests can also be used to assess the effectiveness of long-term therapy. However, some patients given bronchodilators do not show a demonstrable effect on pulmonary function test results but improve clinically. Clinical improvement is demonstrated by an increase in the distance the patient can walk, decreases in the use of as-needed drugs, and fewer reports of shortness of breath, chest tightness, and wheezing. Continue either oral or inhaled corticosteroids only if a positive, measurable response is seen.

Patients with less frequent attacks and normal pulmonary function test results during the initial assessment also have increased rates of remission. However, remissions are less frequent in older patients. When a patient's asthma is controlled, discontinue oral corticosteroids first, then theophylline and ipratropium. Continue therapy for the duration of allergen exposure in patients with seasonal asthma. Thirty percent to 50% of children with chronic asthma markedly improve or become symptom-free by early adulthood. Although the health care provider manages a wide range of asthma-related problems, when conservative methods fail to control symptoms, one must consider referral to an appropriate allergist or respiratory specialist.

KEY POINTS

- Asthma is defined as a chronic, reversible, inflammatory disorder of the airways.
- Asthma is categorized by etiology: intrinsic asthma is provoked or worsened by infection, exertion, emotion, and nonspecific environmental factors; extrinsic asthma is related to a hereditary predisposition to allergy with symptoms caused by environmental allergens.
- Asthma severity is classified as mild intermittent, mild persistent, moderate persistent, and severe persistent.
- Because asthma is not a one-drug disease, combination therapy is generally the rule rather than the exception.
- Drug classifications used in the management of acute and chronic asthma include beta agonists, LT antagonists, xanthine derivatives, anticholinergics, inhaled (and systemic) corticosteroids, and antiallergy drugs.
- *Guidelines for the Diagnosis and Management of Asthma* and the *International Consensus Report on Diagnosis and Treatment of Asthma* set the standards for diagnosis and treatment of asthma.
- Inhaled corticosteroids are considered first-line drugs for patients with asthma and permit chronic steroid therapy with minimal systemic adverse effects.
- Short-acting beta agonists are used to relieve acute asthma symptoms. Long-acting beta agonists are used concurrently with corticosteroids in long-term symptom control, particularly nocturnal symptoms.

- LT antagonists are used for prophylaxis and chronic treatment of mild and moderate persistent asthma in adults and children.
- Although rarely used today, xanthines are mild to moderate bronchodilators used as adjunctive therapy to inhaled corticosteroids for the prevention of nocturnal asthma symptoms.
- Antimuscarinic drugs are used as bronchodilators during maintenance therapy of reversible airway obstruction due to asthma, but more commonly in chronic obstructive lung disease.
- Antiallergy drugs (previously known as mast cell stabilizers) are indicated only for prophylaxis of acute asthma attacks.
- Treatment objectives include the long-term control of persistent asthma, effective management of symptoms and exacerbations with quick-relief drugs so as to preserve normal to near-normal pulmonary functioning, and prevention of recurrent exacerbations of asthma while minimizing acute care interventions.
- Evaluate treatment outcomes in terms of patient perception of improvement, quality of life, and the ability to engage in activities of daily living.
- Consider hospitalization for patients with an acute attack of asthma refractory to initial treatment and in whom specific signs and symptoms exist.

Bibliography

American Lung Association. (2006). Trends in asthma morbidity and mortality. Available online: www.lungusa.org/site/pp.asp?c=dvLUK 9O0E&b=33347. Accessed May 21, 2007.

Bergner, A., and Bergner, R. (1994). The International Consensus Report on Diagnosis and Treatment of Asthma: A call to action for US practitioners. *Clinical Therapy, 16*(4), 694–706.

Centers for Disease Control and Prevention. (2004). *Pharmacogenomics of asthma.* Available online: www.cdc.gov/genomics/info. Accessed May 21, 2007.

Dombrowski, M. (2006). Asthma and pregnancy. *Obstetrics and Gynecology, 108*(3), 667–681.

Imbruce, R., and Selevan, J. (1997). Pharmacoeconomics and the quality of life in the diagnosis and management of asthma: What is your FEEVY? *Journal of Care Management, 3*(Suppl 3), 1–9.

International Consensus Report on Diagnosis and Management of Asthma. (1992). International Asthma Management Project. *Allergy, 47*(13 Suppl), 1–61.

Joint Task Force on Practice Parameters, American Academy of Allergy, Asthma and Immunology; American College of Allergy, Asthma and Immunology and Joint Council of Allergy, Asthma and Immunology. (2006). Attaining optimal asthma control: A practice parameter. *Journal of Allergy and Clinical Immunology, 116*(5), S3–S11. (Erratum in *Journal of Allergy and Clinical Immunology* [2006], *117*[2], 262).

National Asthma Education and Prevention Program Expert Panel. (1997). Report 2: Guidelines for the Diagnosis and Management of Asthma, National Institutes of Health. *International consensus report on the diagnosis and treatment of asthma.* (Pub. No. 92–3091). Bethesda, MD: U.S. Department of Health and Human Services.

National Asthma Education and Prevention Program Expert Panel. (2002). Report 2: Guidelines for the Diagnosis and Management of Asthma, National Institutes of Health. *Guidelines for the Diagnosis and Management of Asthma–Update on Selected Topics 2002.* Bethesda, MD: U.S. Department of Health and Human Services.

RESPIRATORY

National Asthma Education and Prevention Program Expert Panel. (2003). *Report 2: Stepwise Approach for Managing Asthma*. Bethesda, MD: U.S. Department of Health and Human Services.

National Institutes of Health, National Heart, Lung, and Blood Institute. (1997). *Highlights of the Expert Panel Report 2: Guidelines for the Diagnosis and Management of Asthma*. (Pub. No. 97–4051A.) Bethesda, MD: U.S. Department of Health and Human Services.

National Institutes of Health, National Heart, Lung and Blood Institute, National Asthma Education and Prevention Program. (2002). *Update on Selected Topics: Guidelines for the Diagnosis and Management of Asthma*. (Pub. No. 02–5075.) Bethesda, MD: U.S. Department of Health and Human Services.

National Institutes of Health, National Heart, Lung, and Blood Institute and World Health Organization. (2003). *Global Initiative for Asthma: Update 2003*. Bethesda, MD: U.S. Department of Health and Human Services. Available online: www.ginasthma.org. Accessed July 20, 2007.

National Institutes of Health, National Asthma Education Program Working Group Report: Considerations for diagnosing and managing asthma in the elderly. Available online: www.nhlbi.hib. gov/nhlib/lung/asthma/prof/as_elder.htm. Accessed May 21, 2007.

Omalizumab (Xolair). Package insert. San Francisco, CA: Genentech Pharmaceuticals.

Oppenheimer, J., and Li, J. (2006). Attaining asthma control. *Current Opinion in Allergy and Clinical Immunology*, 6(2), 119–123.

Taylor, D., Auble, T., Calhoun, W., et al. (1999). Current outpatient management of asthma shows poor compliance with International Consensus Guidelines. *Chest*, 116(6), 1638–1645.

51

Antihistamines and Related Drugs

The term *allergy* comes from the Greek *allos*, meaning "different from the normal," and *ergon*, referring "to work" or "energy." All persons come in contact with the same antigens, yet not all persons display allergic symptoms. The term *antigen* is often used interchangeably with the term *allergen*. Allergy symptoms appear when the immune response is exaggerated or inappropriate, causing inflammation and damage to affected tissues. In order to understand the antihistamines as used for allergic rhinitis, one must first understand histamine itself.

As discussed in previous chapters, histamine is a hydrophilic vasoactive amine produced by decarboxylation of the amino acid histidine. Histamine has involvement in local immune responses, regulates physiologic function in the gut, acts as a neurotransmitter, and plays a possible role in chemotaxis of white blood cells. Upon formation, histamine is either stored or undergoes rapid inactivation.

Histamine acts locally, with prominent and varied effect. In the vascular system, histamine dilates small blood vessels and increases capillary permeability. In the bronchi, histamine produces constriction. Histamine stimulates acid secretion in the stomach, and in the central nervous system (CNS), histamine acts as a neurotransmitter. Despite this array of actions, the clinical utility of antihistamines is limited. Yet histamine is still of great interest because of its involvement in two common pathologic states: allergies and peptic ulcer disease (see also Chapter 45).

RHINITIS

EPIDEMIOLOGY AND ETIOLOGY

Rhinitis is defined as inflammation of the lining of the nose; *rhinosinusitis*, as inflammation of the lining of the paranasal sinuses due to any etiology. Both conditions are extremely common and affect individuals during productive years of childhood and young adulthood. The symptoms of rhinitis include sneezing, itching, nasal congestion, and rhinorrhea. The patient may also complain of postnasal drip, cough, irritability, and fatigue. The distinguishing features of the five primary types of rhinitis are summarized in Table 51-1.

Rhinosinusitis

Rhinosinusitis has become the preferred term for rhinitis and sinusitis since inflammation of the sinuses is usually associated with concomitant disease of the nose and nasal mucosa. The most common types of rhinosinusitis are of allergic or viral etiology. Viral rhinitis due to pathogens such as rhinovirus and coronavirus usually precede the development of a secondary acute bacterial rhinosinusitis. Upper respiratory tract viruses lead to generalized mucosal edema,

up-regulation of proinflammatory mediators, and changes in binding sites whereby bacteria more readily attach to nasal and sinus mucosa. The nasal discharge may be clear or purulent, and yellow, and still be caused by a virus. Patients typically improve within 5 to 7 days, with resolution of symptoms in 10 to 14 days. Consider bacterial rhinosinusitis if symptoms persist beyond 10 days or worsen after 5 to 7 days.

Allergic Rhinitis

Allergic rhinitis (AR) is a heterogeneous disorder that despite its high prevalence often goes undiagnosed. AR appears in persons of all races, occurring most often in families with *atopy*, a hereditary predisposition for allergy. It is estimated to affect 40 million Americans, resulting in over 20 million visits to the health care provider each year. Boys are twice as likely to get AR as girls. Half of children develop the condition before age 10, and half after that time. With about 10 million prescriptions written for nasal corticosteroid ("steroids") sprays each year in the United States, and about 1 billion prescriptions for antihistamines worldwide, the direct treatment cost for rhinitis exceeds $5.3 billion. Further, there are significant indirect costs in terms of lost workdays (the average is 4 workdays/year) as well as restricted leisure activities.

AR can coincide with asthma and other atopic diseases, and is often associated with asthma exacerbations.

Seasonal Allergic Rhinitis

Seasonal allergic rhinitis (SAR) is fairly easy to identify because of the rapid and reproducible onset and offset of symptoms associated with pollen exposure. Symptoms of SAR are the worst after being outdoors. In the United States, SAR is triggered by tree pollens in the spring; grasses in midsummer; and weeds in the fall, a period that typically lasts from August until the first frost.

Perennial Allergic Rhinitis

Chronic or *perennial allergic rhinitis* (PAR) occurs during about 9 months of the year and is usually caused by airborne pollutants in the home (e.g., pet dander, dust mites, wool, and certain foods) and other places. Symptoms of PAR are the worst after spending time indoors. Exposure to dust mites and mold in upholstered furniture, mattresses, and pillows cause symptoms that are worse in the morning. PAR occurs about half as often as SAR.

Nonallergic Rhinitis with Eosinophilia Syndrome

Nonallergic rhinitis with eosinophilia syndrome (NARES) produces symptoms similar to those of PAR and does not respond to allergy skin testing. In this syndrome, as in AR, eosinophils are found in nasal secretions, but the patient does not have allergies. A similar observation is frequently made in patients with asthma: an abundance of eosinophils are found

TABLE 51-1 Rhinitis Syndromes

	Allergic Rhinitis	Rhinosinusitis	Vasomotor Instability	NARES	Rhinitis Medicamentosa
Age at onset	Childhood	All ages	Adults	All ages	Adults
Etiology	Allergens, hyperreactivity	Infection	Vascular	??	Overuse of intranasal decongestant sprays
Associated Factors	Family history; pale mucosa	URI	Pregnancy; thyroid disorders	Pale mucosa	Use topical decongestants; antihypertensives
Sneezing	Moderate	Absent	Absent	Marked	Absent
Pruritus	Moderate	Absent	Absent	Marked	Absent
Rhinorrhea	Moderate	Absent	??	Marked	Absent
Congestion	Mild	Mild	Marked	??	Moderate
PND	Slight	Moderate	Marked	??	Absent
Seasonal Variation	Seasonal or perennial	Perennial	Perennial	Perennial	Perennial
Eosinophilia Nasal Secretions	Slight	Absent	Absent	Slight	Absent
Skin Test Results	Positive	Negative	Negative	Negative	Negative
Total IgE	Increased	Normal	Normal	Normal	Normal
Treatment	Intranasal steroids; environmental control; immunotherapy	Antibiotics	Decongestant; nasal saline irrigations; exercise	Intranasal steroids	Stop decongestant

IgE, Immunoglobulin E; *NARES*, nonallergic rhinitis with eosinophilia syndrome; *PND*, postnasal drip; *URI*, upper respiratory infection.
Adapted from Slavin, R. (1982). Relationship of nasal disease and sinusitis to bronchial asthma. *Annals of Allergy, 49(2), 76–79*; and Hadley, J., Kavuru, M., Anon, J., et al. (2005). *Diagnosis and management of rhinitis and rhinosinusitis. West Islip*, NY: Professional Communications.

in bronchial secretions even though the patient does not have allergies (see Chapter 50).

NARES without evidence of atopy is a chronic entity. Seventeen percent of patients with asthma and/or AR have nasal polyps, whereas 70% of patients with nasal polyps had asthma. Nasal polyps associated with rhinitis and asthma is seen primarily in patients over the age of 40 years. Aspirin sensitivity is seen in over 30% of asthmatic patients who also have nasal polyps.

Vasomotor Rhinitis

Vasomotor rhinitis is a form of nonallergic rhinitis affecting a substantial number of patients with chronic rhinitis with rhinorrhea. Some patients have a hyperreactive nose that responds in an exaggerated way to nonspecific irritants without allergic sensitization. Exacerbation of symptoms results from changes in temperature and humidity, exposure to hot or cold foods, anxiety, exposure to smoke, air pollution, odors, occupational irritants and allergens, or the ingestion of vasoactive substances in food or drinks (Box 51-1). Many patients may simply be intolerant of the normal production of nasal mucus. In these patients, the usual itchy, watery eyes and nose are not found. The presence of conjunctivitis casts doubt on a diagnosis of AR.

Rhinitis Medicamentosa

Rhinitis medicamentosa is characterized by rebound nasal congestion brought about by extended use of intranasal decongestants. An otherwise intermittent rhinitis may become constant and unrelenting from rebound edema after a few days of use, resulting in a vicious cycle with more frequent use of the offending drug (e.g., oxymetazoline [Afrin]) and ongoing or worsening symptoms. Patients soon sense a dependence on the drug and characteristically have a great deal of difficulty abandoning its use.

PATHOPHYSIOLOGY

A triad of physical elements (i.e., mucus, cilia, and hairs that trap particles in the air) accomplishes the temperature regulation of air coming into the nose. Blood flow to nasal mucosa adjusts the size of turbinates, which in turn affect resistance to airflow. The characteristics of the filtered air particles affect the nasal mucosa. Mucosal irritants such as cigarette smoke or cold air can cause short-term rhinitis. However, allergens cause a cascade of events that can lead to more significant reactions.

Inflammation of the nasal mucosa is the result of intricate interactions among inflammatory mediators, primarily immunoglobulin E (IgE). There are approximately 500,000 IgE receptors on the surface of each mast cell (Fig. 51-1). Degranulation of mast cells releases histamine, tryptase, chymase,

---

BOX 51-1

Sources of Irritants and Allergens in Vasomotor Rhinitis

OCCUPATIONAL IRRITANTS	OCCUPATIONAL ALLERGENS
Acids	Acid anhydrides
Ammonia	Animals
Cleaning agents	Coffee beans
Chlorine	Colophony*
Cold air	Cotton fibers
Cooking odors	Enzymes
Cosmetic odors	Grains
Detergents	Green tea
Exhaust fumes	Latex
Formaldehyde	Papain
Hair spray	Platinum salts
Paint fumes	Toluene diisocyanate
Solvents	Wood dusts
Tobacco smoke	

*Colophony is a substance used in varnishes and inks and on the bows of stringed instruments.
Adapted from Hadley, J., Kavuru, M., Anon, J., et al. (2005). *Diagnosis and management of rhinitis and rhinosinusitis*. West Islip, NY: Professional Communications; and Slavin, R. (1982). Relationship of nasal disease and sinusitis to bronchial asthma. *Annals of Allergy, 49(2), 76–79*.

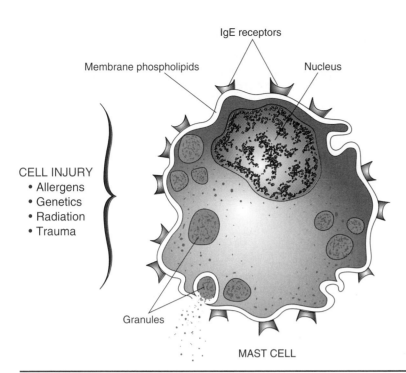

FIGURE 51-1 Mast Cell Degranulation. Mast cell degranulation releases histamines, prostaglandins, interleukins, and leukotrienes, causing local vasodilation and increased capillary permeability, hypotension, urticaria, and bronchoconstriction.

kinins, and heparin. Concurrently, the mast cells synthesize leukotrienes and prostaglandin D_2, which eventually prompt the symptoms of rhinorrhea (i.e., nasal congestion, sneezing, itching, redness, tearing, swelling, ear pressure, postnasal drip). Stimulated mucous glands produce increased secretions and nasal congestion. Vasodilation leads to congestion and pressure within the sinuses and nasal passages. The vascular permeability that is associated with inflammation is increased, which results in plasma exudation and edema. Tissue swellings are often referred to as hives or urticaria. When the swelling is enormous, it is referred to as *angioedema*. Sneezing and itching result from the stimulation of sensory nerves. The entire reaction process can occur very quickly, often in a matter of minutes, which is why the reaction has been named the *early-phase response*.

Over a period of 4 to 8 hours, the inflammatory mediators recruit other cells (i.e., neutrophils, eosinophils, lymphocytes, and macrophages) to the mucosal surface. The migration of these cells produces continued inflammation and is referred to as a *late-phase response*. There is reduced sneezing and itching, and increased mucous production and congestion in the late-phase response compared with that seen during an early-phase response. Late-phase responses can last for hours or days.

PHARMACOTHERAPEUTIC OPTIONS

Intranasal Corticosteroids

FIRST-GENERATION
◆ beclomethasone (Beconase AQ, Qvar); ♣ beclomethasone
◆ budesonide (Rhinocort Aqua); ♣ Entocort, Pulmicort

◆ flunisolide (Nasarel); ♣ Bronalide, Rhinalar
◆ triamcinolone (Nasacort AQ, Nasacort HFA); ♣ Azmacort, Nasacort AQ

SECOND-GENERATION
◆ fluticasone (Flonase); ♣ Flonase
◆ mometasone (Nasonex, Asmanex); ♣ Elocom

▥ Indications

The basic pharmacology of steroids is discussed in Chapter 56. Consideration here is limited to their use in AR. Intranasal steroids are the most effective drugs for the treatment of SAR and PAR. With proper use, over 90% of patients achieve symptom control; intranasal steroids do not cure the underlying disorder. In the past, intranasal steroids were reserved for patients whose symptoms were not controlled with more conventional drugs (e.g., adrenergics, antihistamines, intranasal cromolyn). However, because of their safety profile and superior efficacy, intranasal steroids have joined histamine₁ (H₁) antagonists as a first-line therapy. These drugs are of little value in acute therapy because drug action and patient response are not immediate.

▥ Pharmacodynamics

Intranasal steroids relieve congestion and rhinorrhea by limiting late-phase response and reducing inflammation. Steroids interrupt inflammation by inhibiting the synthesis of mediators (i.e., histamine, leukotrienes, and prostaglandins), which in turn reduces redness, warmth, edema, and discomfort. Phagocytic infiltration is suppressed, and damage from lysosomal enzyme release is averted. Further, steroids suppress lymphocyte proliferation to lessen the immune component of inflammation.

PHARMACOKINETICS
TABLE 51-2 Selected Antihistamines and Related Drugs

Drug	Route	Onset	Peak	Duration	Postnasal Dip (%)	$t_{1/2}$
INTRANASAL CORTICOSTEROIDS						
beclomethasone	NS	UA	Up to 4 wk	3.25 days	91	15 hr
budesonide	NS	24 hr	3–7 days	UA	91	2 hr
flunisolide	NS	Few days	Up to 3 wk	UA	91	1–2 hr
fluticasone	NS	Few days	1–2 days	UA	91	UA
triamcinolone	NS	UA	Up to 4 wk	UA	UA	4 hr
FIRST-GENERATION H_1 ANTAGONISTS						
brompheniramine	PO	15–30 min	1–2 hr	6–8 hr	UA	12–35 hr
chlorpheniramine	PO	15–30 min	6 hr	4–12 hr	72	14–25 hr
clemastine	PO	15–60 min	1–2 hr	12 hr	UA	UA
cyproheptadine	PO	15–60 min	1–2 hr	8 hr	UA	UA
dimenhydrinate	PO	15–60 min	1–2 hr	4–8 hr	UA	3.5 hr
diphenhydramine	PO	15–60 min	1–4 hr	4–8 hr	98–99	2.4–7 hr
hydroxyzine	PO	15–30 min	2–4 hr	4–6 hr	UA	3 hr
promethazine	PO	15–30 min	UA	4–25 hr	65–90	10–14 hr
SECOND-GENERATION H_1 ANTAGONISTS						
azelastine	NS	Rapid	2–3 hr	UA	88	22 hr; 54 hr*
cetirizine	PO	1–3 hr	1 hr	UA	UA	6.6–10.6 hr; 7 hr; 4.9 hr†
fexofenadine	PO	Rapid	2.6 hr	UA	60–70	14.4 hr
loratadine	PO	1–3 hr	8–12 hr	>24 hr	97; 73–77‡	8–11 hr; 20 hr‡
THIRD-GENERATION H_1 ANTAGONIST						
desloratidine	PO	Rapid	3 hr	UA	82–89	27 hr

NA, Not applicable; *NS*, intranasal spray; *PB*, protein binding; *PO*, by mouth; *$t_{1/2}$*, half-life; *UA*, unavailable.
*Azelastine's half-life is 22 hr; desmethylazelastine, the active metabolite, has a half-life of 54 hr.
†Cetirizine's half-life for adults, school-age children, and children younger than 4 years of age, respectively.
‡Loratadine's half-life is 7.8–11 hr, with 97% protein binding; descarboethoxyloratadine, the metabolite, has a half-life of 20 hr, with 73%–77% protein binding.

▥ Pharmacokinetics

The pharmacokinetics of intranasal steroids is identified in Table 51-2. Budesonide and fluticasone peak in a shorter time compared with other intranasal steroids, which can take 3 to 4 weeks to reach peak effectiveness.

▥ Adverse Effects and Contraindications

The adverse effects of intranasal steroids are mild. The most common are drying of the intranasal mucosa and a burning or itching sensation. These effects are caused by the vehicle used for administration and not by the drugs themselves. Formulations that use an aqueous vehicle are much less irritating than formulations using a nonaqueous vehicle (e.g., alcohol, poly-ethylene glycol, Freon). Although rare, systemic absorption of intranasal steroids can cause hypothalamic-pituitary-adrenal (HPA) axis suppression. There is ongoing research as to the sup-pressive effect of steroid intranasal sprays on bone growth in children (Juniper, et al., 2005). A small, but statistically signifi-cant effect on children's bone growth led the Food and Drug Administration (FDA) to require a warning notice on all intra-nasal steroid sprays in the United States.

▥ Drug Interactions

A   Budesonide and flunisolide interact with a number of different drugs to increase plasma concentrations of the intranasal steroid while decreasing serum cortisol levels; the result is HPA suppression and Cushing's syndrome (Table 51-3).

▥ Dosage Regimen

Intranasal steroids are administered using a metered-spray device. Full dosages are used initially (Table 51-4). Once symptoms have been controlled, the dosage can be reduced to the lowest effective amount. If intranasal passages are obstructed, clear them with nasal irrigations and/or an intrana-sal decongestant spray before intranasal steroid administration.

H_1 Antagonists
FIRST-GENERATION H_1 ANTAGONISTS
- azatadine (Optimine); ♣ Optimine
- brompheniramine (Bromfed, Dimetapp)
- chlorpheniramine (Chlor-Trimeton); ♣ Chlor-Tripolon
- clemastine (Tavist)
- cyproheptadine (Periactin); ♣ dexchlorpheniramine, Periactin
- diphenhydramine (Benadryl); ♣ Buckley's Jack and Jill Bedtime, Nytol, Sleep-Eze
- dimenhydrinate (Dramamine)
- hydroxyzine (Atarax, Vistaril); ♣ Apo-hydroxyzine, novohydroxyzin
- promethazine (Phenergan); ♣ Phenergan

SECOND-GENERATION H_1 ANTAGONISTS
- azelastine (Astelin)
- cetirizine (Zyrtec); ♣ Reactine
- fexofenadine (Allegra)
- loratidine (Claritin); ♣ Claritin

THIRD-GENERATION H_1 ANTAGONISTS
- desloratidine (Clarinex); ♣ Clarinex

Drugs used in the management of histamine-mediated disor-ders are referred to as antihistamines, but more specifically histamine₁ (H_1) antagonists or H_1 blockers. Antihistamines were the oldest drugs used for allergy. H_1 antagonists are avail-able as single-ingredient formulations (e.g., fexofenadine) or

DRUG INTERACTIONS

TABLE 51-3 Selected Antihistamines and Related Drugs

Drug	Interactive Drugs	Interaction
INTRANASAL CORTICOSTEROIDS		
budesonide, fluticasone	Azole antifungals, Protease inhibitors, clarithromycin, fluvoxamine, imatinib, nefazadone, quinupristin-dalfopristin, telithromycin	Increases plasma budesonide levels, decreasing serum cortisol levels and resulting in adrenal suppression and Cushing's syndrome
FIRST-GENERATION H₁ ANTAGONISTS		
brompheniramine, chlorpheniramine, cyproheptadine, dimenhydrinate, diphenhydramine, hydroxyzine	pramlintide	Combined with anticholinergics may further delay gastric emptying
	sodium oxybate, dexmedetomide	Combination increases risk of CNS depression and psychomotor impairment.
chlorpheniramine	MAO inhibitors, Other CNS depressants, Phenothiazines Tricyclic antidepressants	Combination increases risk of CNS depression and psychomotor impairment.
cyproheptadine	MAO inhibitors	Prolongs and intensifies anticholinergic effects of cyproheptadine
promethazine	Many interactions	Check reference
SECOND-GENERATION H₁ ANTAGONISTS		
azatadine	heparin, warfarin	Decreased effect of interacting agent
	MAO inhibitors	Increased effects of azatadine
	Alcohol, Barbiturates, Opioids, Sedative-hypnotics, Tricyclic antidepressants	Increased CNS depression with higher than recommended dosages
fexofenadine	Antacids	Reduces absorption of fexofenadine, reducing efficacy
	nevirapine	Induces biotransformation, and efficacy of fexofenadine is reduced
loratadine	Alcohol	Increases loratidine levels
THIRD-GENERATION H₁ ANTAGONISTS		
desloratidine	erythromycin, ketoconazole	Increases loratidine levels

CNS, Central nervous system; *MAO*, monoamine oxidase.

DOSAGE

TABLE 51-4 Selected Antihistamines and Related Drugs

Drug	Uses	Dosage	Implications
INTRANASAL STEROIDS			
beclomethasone	AR, chronic nasal inflammatory conditions	*Adult and Child >12 yr:* 1–2 sprays each nostril twice daily	42 mcg/spray; 200 metered sprays/16.8-gram canister
budesonide	AR, prophylaxis for nasal polyps	*Adult:* 1–4 sprays each nostril once daily. Max: 4 sprays/nostril/day	32 mcg/spray; 200 metered sprays/7-gram canister
flunisolide	AR, prophylaxis for nasal polyps	*Adult:* 2 sprays each nostril 2–3 times daily. Max: 8 sprays per nostril per day *Child 6–14 yr:* 2 sprays each nostril twice daily *–or–* Alternate: 1 spray/nostril twice daily. Maximum 4 sprays each nostril per day.	250 mcg/spray; 100 metered sprays/7-gram canister
fluticasone	AR, prophylaxis for nasal polyps	*Adult:* 2 sprays each nostril once daily *–or–* one spray each nostril twice daily. Max: 4 sprays/day *Child >4 yr:* 1–2 sprays each nostril daily. Max: 4 sprays/day	50 mcg/spray; 120 metered sprays/9-gram bottle. May decrease to 1 spray/nostril/day
triamcinolone	AR, prophylaxis for nasal polyps	*Adult and Child >12 yr:* 1–2 sprays each nostril once daily. Max: 2 sprays/nostril/day. *Child 6–12 yr:* 1–2 sprays each nostril daily. Max: 2 sprays/nostril/day	100 mcg/spray; 240 metered sprays/20-gram canister; *–or–* 55 mcg/spray; 100 metered sprays/15-gram canister
FIRST-GENERATION H₁ ANTAGONISTS			
brompheniramine	Nasal allergies	*Adult:* 4–8 mg PO 3–4 times daily *–or–* 8–12 mg twice daily of SR form. Max dose: 24 mg *Child 6–12 yr:* 0.5 mg/kg PO daily in divided doses *Child <6 yr:* 0.5 mg/kg/day PO in divided doses	Give oral doses with food or milk to decrease GI irritation. SR formulations should be swallowed whole; do not crush, break, or chew.
clemastine	SAR, PAR, urticaria	*Adult:* 1.34–2.68 mg PO 2–3 times daily. Max: 8 mg/day	Watch for hemolytic anemia, agranulocytosis, and thrombocytopenia.
chlorpheniramine	Nasal allergies	*Adult:* 2–4 mg PO 3–4 times daily *–or–* 8–12 mg PO 1–3 times daily of SR formulation *Child 6–12 yr:* 2 mg PO every 4–6 hr. Max: 12 mg/day *–or–* 8 mg PO every 24 hr of SR formulation *Child 2–6 yr:* 1 mg PO every 4–6 hr	Give oral doses with food or milk to decrease GI irritation. SR tablets should be swallowed whole; do not crush, break, or chew.

Continued

DOSAGE
TABLE 51-4 Selected Antihistamines and Related Drugs—Cont'd

Drug	Uses	Dosage	Implications	
cyproheptadine	Nasal allergies	*Adult:* 4 mg PO every 8 hr. Range: 4–20 mg/day in 3 divided doses. Max: 32 mg/day *Child 6–14 yr:* Initially 0.25 mg/kg PO every 8–12 hr daily in divided doses; then 4 mg PO every 8–12 hr. Max: 16 mg/day *Child 2–6 yr:* Initially 0.25 mg/kg PO every 8–12 hr daily in divided doses; then 2 mg PO every 8–12 hr. Max: 12 mg/day	Give with food or water to minimize GI irritation.	
dimenhydrinate	Motion sickness	*Adult:* 50–100 mg PO/IM/IV every 4 to 6 hours PRN	Take 0.5 to 1 hour before activity. **Do not confuse with diphenhydramine.**	▲
diphenhydramine	Nasal allergies	*Adult:* 25–50 mg PO every 4–6 hr *–or–* 10–50 mg IM or IV every 2–3 hr PRN. Max: 400 mg/day *Child >9.1 kg:* 12.5–25 mg PO every 4–6 hr PRN *Child <9.1 kg:* 6.25–12.5 mg PO every 4–6 hr PRN	**Risk of QT prolongation. Use with caution. Do not confuse with dimenhydrinate.**	▲
hydroxyzine	Pruritus	*Adult:* 25–100 mg PO 3–4 times daily *Child <12 yr:* 0.5 mg/kg PO every 6 hr PRN	Crush tablets or open capsules and mix with food for those with difficulty swallowing.	
promethazine	Allergic conditions	*Adult:* 25 mg PO HS *–or–* 10–12.5 mg 4 times daily. *Child >2 yr:* 0.5 mg/kg PO HS *–or–* 5–12.5 mg PO 3 times daily	Crush tablets and mix with food or fluids for those with difficulty swallowing.	
SECOND-GENERATION H₁ ANTAGONISTS				
azelastine	SAR, vasomotor rhinitis	*Adult and Child >11 yr:* 2 sprays in each nostril twice daily *Child 5–11 yr:* 1 spray in each nostril twice daily	One spray = 137 mcg. Over 10 mg/day may cause drowsiness.	
cetirizine	AR, chronic urticaria	*Adult and Child >5 yr:* 5–10 mg PO once daily or as 2 divided doses *Child 2–5 yr:* 2.5 mg PO daily. May increase to 5 mg as single dose or 2 divided doses. *Child: 12–23 mo:* 2.5 mg PO daily	Use humidifier if secretions thicken or nasal dryness becomes bothersome. Renal dosing consideration required.	
fexofenadine	SAR	*Adult and Child >12 yr:* 60 mg PO twice daily *–or–* 180 mg once daily.	Once-daily dosing for patients with impaired renal function	
loratadine	SAR	*Adult and Child >12 yr:* 10 mg PO once daily	**Do not confuse with desloratidine.** Use lower doses in presence of liver disease. Avoid alcohol; serious sedation can occur.	▲
THIRD-GENERATION H₁ ANTAGONIST				
desloratidine	AR	*Adult and Child >12 yr:* 5 mg PO daily *Child 6–11 yr:* 2.5 mg PO once daily *Child 1–5 yr:* 1.25 mg PO once daily	**Do not confuse with loratadine.** Desloratidine is an isomer of loratidine.	▲
MAST CELL STABILIZER				
cromolyn sodium	SAR, PAR	*Adult and Child >6 yr:* 1 spray each nostril 3–4 times daily. May increase to 6 times/day	Nasal passages should be clear. Patient may require nasal decongestant before use.	

AR, Allergic rhinitis; *GI,* gastrointestinal; *HS,* at bedtime; *IM,* intramuscular; *IV,* intravenous (route); *PAR,* perennial allergic rhinitis; *PO,* by mouth; *PRN,* as needed; *SAR,* seasonal allergic rhinitis; *SR,* sustained-release.

in combination with pseudoephedrine (fexofenadine with pseudoephedrine) or phenylephrine (brompheniramine with phenylephrine). H₁ antagonists fall into three major groups: first-generation H₁ antagonists, which are typically sedating, and second- and third-generation H₁ antagonists, which are usually not sedating. H₂ antagonists are used for peptic ulcer disease and are discussed in Chapter 45. H₃ receptors are responsible for regulation of the presynaptic activity of histamines and their synthesis and release into the synapse. Thus far, H₃ receptor drugs have only been used in experimental settings.

▌▌ Indications

All H₁ antagonists are used to treat allergic disorders, reducing symptoms in 75% to 95% of patients with AR. They relieve itchy eyes, nose, and throat, and reduce rhinorrhea and sneezing.

H₁ antagonists are also used to treat contact dermatitis, atopic dermatitis, drug-induced skin eruptions, pruritus ani, and pruritus vulvae. H₁ antagonists are used to reduce urticaria associated with mild transfusion reactions and contrast media. However, because mild allergic reactions are mediated by other substances as well as histamine, relief of symptoms may be incomplete (see Chapter 63).

Some H₁ antagonists are used for nonallergic disorders such as insomnia (e.g., diphenhydramine), motion sickness (e.g., dimenhydrinate), and nausea and vomiting (e.g., hydroxyzine, promethazine) (see Chapter 47). The CNS-depressant nature of first-generation H₁ antagonists makes these drugs useful for sedation and insomnia. Many of the over-the-counter (OTC) sleep aids contain diphenhydramine as an active ingredient.

The effectiveness of first- and second-generation H₁ antagonists in treating upper respiratory infections and otitis media remains controversial. **These drugs neither prevent** ▲ **upper respiratory infections and otitis media nor shorten the duration of symptoms. Moreover, because histamine does not mediate cold symptoms, H₁ blockade will not provide even symptomatic relief. The only benefit H₁ antagonists have in treating upper respiratory infections is to reduce rhinorrhea** (see Chapter 52).

Although H_1 antagonists are helpful in treating urticaria and pruritus associated with anaphylaxis, they are less effective in managing the major symptoms (hypotension, bronchospasm, laryngeal edema). Epinephrine, an adrenergic drug (see Chapter 14) used to open airways and reduce hypotension, is the drug of choice for anaphylaxis and other serious allergic reactions.

Pharmacodynamics

H_1 antagonists reversibly inhibit histamine receptors by binding selectively to H_1 receptors, thereby blocking the action of histamine. They do not prevent histamine release, nor do they reduce histamine release from basophils or mast cells. Blockade of nonhistamine, muscarinic receptors underlies the anticholinergic adverse effects of antihistamines.

The drugs fexofenadine, loratadine, and cetirizine are peripherally selective H_1 antagonists. As the name suggests, this group of drugs binds much more selectively to peripheral H_1 receptors. Moreover, they have a lower affinity for binding to the cholinergic and α receptor sites than do other antihistamines. Popularity for peripherally selective H_1 antagonists stems from the limited adverse effects associated with their use; in binding to the peripheral histamine receptor site, adverse effects such as CNS depression, dry mouth, blurred vision, and tachycardia are avoided.

Pharmacokinetics

H_1 antagonists are thoroughly absorbed after oral administration (see Table 51-2). Drug effects typically last 8 to 12 hours; however, the longer-acting drugs may be less effective owing to inadequate absorption and dissolution. All first-generation and most of the second-generation H_1 antagonists are biotransformed by the CYP450 enzyme system and eliminated through urine and stool. The half-lives and clearance rates of H_1 antagonists are extremely variable. H_1 antagonists used in children have shorter half-lives than those used in adults.

Adverse Effects and Contraindications

In many cases, the mild adverse effects of H_1 antagonists are often more of a nuisance than a source of serious discomfort or danger. Drowsiness is more common with first-generation H_1 antagonists than with second-generation drugs and is characterized by slowed reaction times, diminished alertness, and drowsiness in 20% of patients. Impaired performance occurs whether or not the patient feels drowsy. This is particularly of concern in older adults who are at high risk for falls. Fortunately, tolerance to the sedative effect of H_1 antagonists often develops within a few days or weeks.

H_1 antagonists can cause paradoxical excitement, headache, nervousness, tremors, and even seizures in some patients, particularly children, older adults, and patients with liver disease. Impaired cognition, confusion, dizziness, and tinnitus have occurred in older adults. Adverse effects of H_1 antagonists on the gastrointestinal (GI) tract are common and include anorexia, nausea, vomiting, diarrhea or constipation, and weight gain.

The cholinergic blockade produced by first-generation H_1 antagonists results in dry mouth, eyes, nasal passages, and throat. Vaginal dryness, urinary hesitancy, and palpitations have been reported. Second-generation H_1 antagonists are less likely to produce anticholinergic adverse effects.

First-generation H_1 antagonists also competitively and potently inhibit muscarinic receptors and may produce *anticholinergic syndrome*, which is marked by the appearance of symptoms such as sinus tachycardia, dry skin, dry mucous membranes, dilated pupils, ileus, urinary retention, and agitated delirium. "Dry as a bone, red as a beet, hot as a hare, mad as a hatter, and blind as a bat," has been used as a mnemonic device to describe the central and peripheral anticholinergic effects characteristic of antihistamine poisoning. Furthermore, H_1 antagonists obstruct fast sodium channels and disrupt cortical neurotransmission, worsening sedation and seizure activity.

Diphenhydramine may prolong the QT interval, presumably by inhibiting the delayed potassium rectifier channel. However, torsades de pointes has not been previously reported with use of diphenhydramine, probably because of the concurrent sinus tachycardia generated by the anticholinergic-induced tachycardia, which shortens repolarization. ◢

The arrhythmias usually appear with excessive antihistamine dosages but have been reported with concurrent use of macrolide antibiotics (i.e., erythromycin, clarithromycin), imidazole antifungals (i.e., itraconazole, ketoconazole), and other drugs that inhibit the cytochrome CYP450 system, as well as patients with severe hepatic disease. Accordingly, H_1 antagonists are relatively contraindicated for use in patients with liver disease or those who may be receiving macrolide antibiotics or imidazole antifungal drugs. In some cases, syncope preceded the development of arrhythmias.

H_1 antagonists are also contraindicated for use in patients with hypersensitivity, narrow-angle glaucoma, prostatic hypertrophy, stenosing peptic ulcers, or bladder neck obstruction, and in pregnant and nursing women (especially if the infant is premature). Safe use during pregnancy has not been established, although some formulations have been moved from pregnancy category C to category B in recent years. Piperidine H_1 antagonists such as azatadine and cyproheptadine are teratogenic; unlike the other H_1 antagonists, the piperidine group act on H_2 as well as H_1 receptors.

Second-generation H_1 antagonists do not cross the blood-brain barrier and therefore are unlikely to produce CNS depression. However, there are rare cases, and occasionally the health care provider encounters patients complaining of sedation. The likelihood of sedation increases when the manufacturer's recommended dosages of second-generation H_1 antagonists are exceeded. Adverse cardiovascular effects including tachycardia, arrhythmias, and occasionally myocardial depression refractory to vasopressor support have been reported with second-generation H_1 antagonists.

There are no major medicolegal implications linked to AR, but the health care provider should take note of some potentially serious issues. **Driving while under the influence of a ◢ first-generation H_1 antagonist is illegal in some states. Patients should be warned about the potentially sedating effects of H_1 antagonists and advised to use caution in driving and operating heavy machinery. Serious consequences can also result from failure to recognize and diagnose medical conditions that should be considered in the differential diagnosis of AR.** If it is not effectively treated, AR may also lead to chronic fatigue, impaired ability to perform usual activities of daily living, difficulty sleeping, sinus infections, postnasal drip, cough, and headache and should be evaluated. In addition, AR is a strong risk factor for asthma.

Drug Interactions

First-generation H_1 antagonists enhance the adverse effects of ethanol, diazepam, and other drugs with CNS activity (see Table 51-3). In recommended dosages, second-generation H_1 antagonists do not potentiate CNS effects. Taken concurrently with oral and parenteral anticoagulants, the second-generation H_1 antagonist azatadine may reduce the patient's response to these drugs. MAO inhibitors will increase the effects of azatadine. CNS depressants and tricyclic antidepressants used concurrently will cause increased CNS depression with higher than recommended dosages.

Dosage Regimen

Table 51-4 contains the selected dosage regimens for selected first- and second-generation H_1 antagonists. Follow the manufacturers' recommendations carefully to avoid misuse and overdose. Dosages for antihistamines used in motion sickness, nausea, and vomiting are identified in Chapter 47.

Lab Considerations

H_1 antagonists produce false-negative results in allergy skin testing; thus discontinue use 72 to 96 hours before testing. Serum amylase and prolactin concentrations increase with the concurrent use of cyproheptadine and thyrotropin-releasing hormone. Promethazine can cause false-positive or false-negative pregnancy tests.

Cromolyn Sodium

Cromolyn sodium (Nasalcrom) was originally discussed in Chapter 50 in the context of asthma management. Cromolyn sodium is generally the safest drug for treatment of allergies. The nasal spray formulation is effective in preventing seasonal and perennial AR. Cromolyn stabilizes mast cells to inhibit activation and release of chemical mediators from eosinophils and epithelial cells. It blocks the early and late reactions to allergens, and thus histamine and other chemicals are not released. It also alters the migration of eosinophils to the inflammatory site and decreases the number of end products of inflammation.

Small amounts of the intranasal formulation of cromolyn reach the circulation after inhalation, but less than from other routes. The small amounts of drug that are absorbed are eliminated unchanged in urine and feces.

The most commonly reported adverse effects of intranasal cromolyn are sneezing, nasal burning, epistaxis, throat irritation, hoarseness, and an unpleasant, bitter taste. The most serious adverse effect of cromolyn sodium is bronchospasm and coughing.

CLINICAL REASONING

Treatment Objectives

Treatment objectives for patients with allergies and nasal congestion primarily centers on relief of symptoms. Minimizing exposure to external allergens and ensuring adherence to treatment plans are also important.

Treatment Options

Patient Variables

A cost-contained approach to the treatment of allergic rhinitis consists of a first-generation H_1 antagonist and switching to a nonsedating formulation only if daytime sedation becomes a problem. Daytime sedation occurs in 10% to 25% of patients. Tolerance to the sedative effects of first-generation H_1 antagonists is common. Substituting an inexpensive, sedating drug for the nighttime dose of a twice-daily formulation may help. It is important to remember that some degree of psychomotor impairment occurs with use of a first-generation H_1 antagonist even without noticeable sedation. Second-generation H_1 antagonists (except for azatadine) are 15 to 30 times more expensive than many first-generation drugs.

Life-Span Considerations

Pregnant and Nursing Women. The changes of pregnancy are mediated by the enlarging uterus, increased oxygen demands, and the respiratory stimulant effect of progesterone. There is an estrogen-induced hyperemia of the nasopharynx mucosa with concurrent edema and increased mucus production. These changes lead to a sense of stuffiness and increased tendency for epistaxis. Warn women of this normal change and advise against using OTC decongestant intranasal sprays in hopes of alleviating symptoms. Normal saline nasal spray may be helpful in reducing some of the discomfort.

Limit antihistamine use in pregnancy, especially during the first trimester. However, H_1 antagonists (with the exception of brompheniramine) have not been shown to have deleterious effects in pregnancy or in the fetus.

Children and Adolescents. AR can manifest in people of all ages, but it primarily begins during childhood, adolescence, and the early adult years. The mean age of onset is reported to be between age 8 and 11 years, with as many as 80% of AR cases developing before age 20. In children, AR has a reported prevalence as high as 40%, with a subsequent decline with age. A child with atopy may have dark circles under the eyes ("allergic shiners") and have a transverse crease above the tip of the nose from frequent upward nose rubbing ("allergic salute"). Much of the time children can be effectively treated with saline nasal irrigations (see Evidenced-Based Pharmacotherapeutics box).

Older Adults. It is difficult to determine whether losses in somesthetic sensitivity is attributed to aging itself, to disease states that occur with greater frequency with aging, or as the results of other drugs taken. Local sinus and respiratory tract factors and comorbid diseases probably play a larger role in the allergic response than age-related changes in immunity. Clinically, older adults are more susceptible to respiratory tract and other infections, and are more likely to purchase OTC drugs for self-treatment. H_1 antagonists such as diphenhydramine cause dizziness, sedation, syncope, confusion, paradoxical CNS stimulation, and hypotension in older adults, putting them at greater risk for falls. Men with prostatic hypertrophy who are taking H_1 antagonists may have difficulty voiding because the drugs tend to cause spasm of the urethra (see Case Study).

Drug Variables

In general, drugs are more effective for allergic rather than nonallergic forms of rhinitis, and acute allergies usually respond more favorably than chronic allergies. Intranasal steroids are the most potent drugs available for the relief of most forms of rhinitis. Their efficacy is comparable to those of orally administered steroids, but they carry substantially reduced risk for adverse effects.

EVIDENCE-BASED PHARMACOTHERAPEUTICS

Pediatric Allergic Rhinitis and Nasal Irrigation

■ Background
Many health care providers recommend hypertonic nasal irrigations as an adjunct to drugs in the management of pediatric allergic rhinitis. However, there is limited evidence to suggest that the procedure is helpful in reducing symptoms.

■ Research Article
Garavello, W., di Berardino, F., Romagnoli, M., et al. (2005). Nasal rinsing with hypertonic solution: An adjunctive treatment for pediatric seasonal allergic rhinoconjunctivitis. *International Archives of Allergy and Immunology, 137*(4), 310–314.

Purpose
The purpose of this study was to determine if nasal irrigations using hypertonic saline solution are effective in children for relief of rhinoconjunctivitis caused by seasonal grass pollens.

Design
A randomized, controlled trial

Methods
Subjects ($N = 46$) with documented allergic rhinoconjunctivitis caused by seasonal grass pollens participated in the study, which was carried out over a 7-week period during allergy season. Half of the subjects ($N = 22$) were used as the control group and did not receive nasal irrigations, whereas subjects in the treatment group ($N = 22$) received nasal irrigations 3 times daily using hypertonic saline. Two subjects in each group were lost to follow-up. A mean symptom score for each subject was calculated weekly during pollen season. The symptoms of interest included the presence of nasal discharge and obstruction, reddening, and itching of the eyes. Subjects were permitted the use of orally administered antihistamines when needed. The average number of antihistamines taken per week was also tracked.

Findings
For the treatment group, the average weekly symptom score declined throughout the entire 7 weeks of pollen season. During weeks 6 and 7 of the study, the differences between the use of nasal irrigations and allergy symptoms became statistically significant. There was a markedly reduced intake of orally administered antihistamines in subjects in the group doing nasal irrigations. The finding was statistically significant in 5 of the 7 weeks of the study. No adverse effects were noted in the group doing nasal irrigations.

Conclusions
Subjects using nasal irrigations were less likely to use orally administered antihistamines compared with the control group, a finding that supports the use of nasal irrigations in children with seasonal allergic rhinoconjunctivitis. Hypertonic saline nasal irrigations were well tolerated, efficacious, and seen as a less costly alternative to orally administered antihistamines. If the findings are valid, nasal lavage would also be helpful in adults, reducing the use of antihistamines.

■ Implications for Practice
Because there is little evidence to date to support the use of saline nasal irrigations, additional studies should be conducted using a larger sample size and carried out over a longer time span and with consideration and control of extraneous variables.

CASE STUDY — Antihistamines

ASSESSMENT

History of Present Illness	JR, a 23-year-old female, comes to the outpatient clinic with complaints of recurrent headache, nasal congestion and sneezing, watery eyes, sore throat from postnasal drip, and intermittent dry cough. She is certain she has a sinus infection. She self-treated with saline nasal irrigations that "helped a little" and aspirin for headache, and used cold compresses to her forehead for the discomfort.
Past Health History	JR has two sisters and a brother who have hay fever and asthma of varying severity. JR denies a history of asthma or other respiratory disorders, hypertension, or heart disease. Except for fall hay fever, she is otherwise healthy. She denies food or drug allergies.
Life-Span Considerations	JR moved out of her parent's home after graduating from college. She rescued a puppy from the animal shelter as a "roommate." She finds it tough being on her own, and being a first-time third-grade elementary schoolteacher. Many children in her class have been ill.
Psychosocial Considerations	JR is on a tight budget; she is repaying several large student loans and has a high-rent apartment and a car payment.
Physical Exam Findings	*BP:* 124/72. 99.4° F-76-20. SpO$_2$: 94%. Skin warm and dry. TM landmarks identified; no redness, retraction or bulging. Nasal mucosa is pale, boggy, with clear discharge. No palpable sinus tenderness or lymphadenopathy. Oropharynx with clear mucoid drainage noted in posterior pharynx. Breath sounds clear to auscultation bilaterally.
Diagnostic Testing	No diagnostic testing indicated for JR at this time.

DIAGNOSIS: Seasonal Rhinitis

MANAGEMENT

Treatment Objectives	1. Relieve allergy symptoms. 2. Reduce exposure to allergens where possible. 3. Maintain control of seasonal allergic rhinitis.

Continued

RESPIRATORY

CASE STUDY   Antihistamines—Cont'd

Treatment Options

Pharmacotherapy
- OTC fexofenadine 180 mg PO daily until symptoms improve or fall allergy season has passed
- Saline nasal irrigations 3 times daily per written instructions; follow with once daily intranasal steroid
- budesonide two sprays in each nostril once daily (after saline nasal irrigations) until symptoms improve

Patient Teaching
1. Increase fluid intake.
2. Start fexofenadine and budesonide intranasal spray (if needed) at start of fall allergy season.
3. Brush hair and wash face to remove dust, pollens, allergens before bedtime.
4. Keep puppy off the furniture and out of the bedroom.

Evaluation
1. Headache, watery eyes, sore throat, nasal congestion, sneezing, and intermittent cough are relieved.
2. JR voices understanding of importance of using drugs prophylactically rather than after symptoms appear.
3. Puppy remains out of the bedroom.

CLINICAL REASONING ANALYSIS

Q1. How do you know she has allergic rhinitis as opposed to a sinus infection? Doesn't she have nasal congestion?

A. Yes, JR has nasal congestion, but it could be caused by a number of different agents including pollens, dust, weeds, and her puppy. Her nasal passages are pale and boggy, which suggests an allergic cause to her congestion rather than a bacterial cause, which usually causes edematous turbinates and a thick, mucopurulent discharge; and, there was no pain on palpation of the frontal and maxillary sinuses. Generally sinusitis causes frontal or maxillary tenderness. Allergies do not usually cause this discomfort.

Q2. What variables do you consider when deciding whether to use a first- or second-generation H$_1$ antagonist?

A. Second-generation H$_1$ antagonists are less likely to cross the blood-brain barrier, and their sedating and anticholinergic adverse effects are minimized. Also, second-generation drugs have dose-related bronchodilating effects and provide some protection against bronchospasm caused by histamine, allergens, exercise, hyperventilation, or cold, dry air.

Q3. I know JR won't be taking this, but what is the difference between Sudafed and Sudafed PE; and is one better than the other in treating head congestion?

A. Sudafed contains pseudoephedrine, whereas Sudafed PE contains phenylephrine. Both Sudafed and Sudafed PE are alpha-adrenergic agonists and as such they produce essentially the same actions and effects. Also, pseudoephedrine is now regulated and phenylephrine is not, so it makes Sudafed PE easier to obtain.

Q4. Why would you use budesonide intranasal spray rather than giving her oral steroids?

A. Intranasal steroids are now first-line therapy for allergic rhinitis. Steroid efficacy of budesonide nasal spray is comparable to that of orally administered formulations but carries substantially reduced risk for adverse effects. Also, it reaches peak effects in about 24 hours, whereas the other intranasal steroids take longer. Oral steroids carry with them potentially serious adverse effects.

Q5. What will you do if fexofenadine isn't effective in relieving her symptoms?

A. Not all patients respond to drugs in the same fashion. If one drug isn't effective in relieving her symptoms, or if excessive sedation or other adverse effects appear, another drug from the same or a different class may be tried.

For patients who do not adequately benefit from a full dosage of a second-generation H$_1$ antagonist and a maintenance dose of cromolyn sodium, an intranasal steroid may be used. If one drug is not effective in relieving symptoms, or if excessive sedation or GI distress results, another drug from a different class may be tried.

Second-generation H$_1$ antagonists are effective in controlling symptoms of AR but do not appreciably improve nasal congestion (Table 51-5). Consequently, second-generation H$_1$ antagonists are combined with a decongestant in several products. Because of their efficacy and safety profile, second-generation H$_1$ antagonists are often preferred for first-line treatment of AR, and SAR in particular. Because of the sedation and other adverse effects associated with the older, first-generation H$_1$ antagonists, second-generation H$_1$ antagonists are usually preferred. Second-generation H$_1$ antagonists are more highly protein

TABLE **51-5** Comparison of H₁ Antagonist Drug Effects

Drug Class (example)	H₁-Receptor Specificity	Anticholinergic Effects	Performance Impairment	Relieves Sneezing	Relieves Nasal Congestion	Relieves Rhinorrhea	Relieves Eye Symptoms	Rapid Allergy Relief
SINGLE-ENTITY FIRST-GENERATION H₁ ANTAGONISTS								
Alkylamines (e.g., chlorpheniramine	Effective	Moderate	Mild	Yes	No	Yes	Yes	Yes
Ethanolamines (e.g., dimenhydrinate)	Moderate	Significant	Marked					
Phenothiazines (e.g., promethazine)	Potent	Marked	Marked					
Piperidines (e.g., cyproheptadine)	Effective	Moderate	Slight					
SINGLE-ENTITY SECOND-GENERATION H₁ ANTAGONISTS								
azelastine	Moderate	Little or none	Mild	Yes	Yes	Yes	Yes	Yes
cetirizine	Moderate	Little or none	Mild					
fexofenadine	Moderate to high	Little or none	Little or none					
loratadine	Moderate to high	Little or none	Little or none					
SINGLE-ENTITY THIRD-GENERATION H₁ ANTAGONIST								
desloratidine	Moderate to high	Little or none	Little or none	Yes	Yes	Yes	Yes	Yes
COMBINATION H₁ ANTAGONIST AND DECONGESTANT								
First-generation	Moderate to potent	Mild to marked	Marked	Yes	Yes	Yes	Yes	Yes
Second-generation	Moderate to high	Mild to marked	Mild	Yes	Yes	Yes	Yes	Yes

bound and lipophobic than their predecessors. They are thus less likely to cross the blood-brain barrier, and thus their sedating and anticholinergic adverse effects are minimized.

In comparably low doses, the first-generation antihistamines brompheniramine and chlorpheniramine are useful and suitable for daytime use; however, individual responses vary, and drowsiness or stimulation can result. Clemastine, dimenhydrinate, and diphenhydramine are strong CNS depressants with a high incidence of drowsiness and are more appropriate for nighttime use. Azatadine and cyproheptadine provide prolonged antihistaminic activity with a relatively low incidence of drowsiness. Nevertheless, attentiveness is decreased, and the operation of machinery or driving may be unsafe.

Long-term use of first-generation H₁ antagonists is associated with a decrease in drug efficacy in some patients. This phenomenon is attributed to autoinduction of hepatic biotransformation and increases in drug clearance, with successively lower serum and, presumably, lower tissue concentrations.

Patient Education

The most important aspect of allergy care is patient education. Patients must understand the nature of their allergy and how to prevent and treat symptoms. Avoiding allergens has important clinical significance in limiting the severity of the disease. Advise patients to stop smoking and to avoid other irritants or precipitating factors. This aspect is often overlooked when teaching patients who have mild allergies.

Appropriate avoidance procedures are based on knowledge of the responsible allergens, which differ for SAR and PAR. Instruct patients with SAR not to take long walks in the woods during pollination periods. Remaining indoors with the windows closed when symptoms are severe and the pollen

count is high (e.g., hot, windy, sunny days) reduces allergen exposures. Some patients find air conditioners helpful, but the filter does little to remove pollen from the air. Air conditioning only makes staying indoors with the windows closed on a hot day more tolerable. The outside air intake on air conditioners should be closed to prevent bringing in pollinated air. Daisies, dahlias, and chrysanthemums should not be kept indoors because these flowers are cousins to ragweed. Advise patients with allergies to mold not to keep African violets or geraniums indoors. Minimizing dust accumulation in the bedroom and avoiding irritants such as tobacco smoke, chemical vapors, and strong perfumes lessens symptoms.

Housecleaning with a damp mop 2 to 3 times a week reduces dust. Dacron or polyester pillows should replace feather pillows. Advise that pillows and mattress covers be used to avoid contact with allergens though bed linens. Brushing hair before retiring reduces the risk of pollen and dust transfer to bed linens. Areas where mold can collect (e.g., damp basements and furniture) should be thoroughly cleaned. Furnishings made of synthetic fabrics are preferable to cotton and wool and minimize dust collection. Humidification reduces dust. Pets may have to be removed from the home if allergic symptoms become disabling; however, simply keeping the pet out of the home does not sufficiently reduce dander in the air. Carpets usually should be removed or at least cleaned often.

Teach patients that intranasal steroids are first-line drugs in the treatment of AR and sinus congestion but are more effective when used after saline nasal irrigations. Have patients blow their nose in advance of intranasal drug administration so as to not place the drug on the surface of secretions. When combination therapy is warranted, have the patient use an intranasal decongestant spray 5 to 15 minutes before the

RESPIRATORY

intranasal steroid spray. Using the decongestant first causes shrinkage of mucous membranes so the corticosteroid can better reach deeper intranasal passages. The patient should also be advised to contact the health care provider if allergic symptoms do not improve within 3 to 4 weeks or if nasal discharge becomes purulent.

Instruct patients to take H_1 antagonists only as prescribed or as instructed on the package. Alcohol and other drugs should not be consumed without first contacting the health care provider. CNS depressants can cause respiratory depression and even death in some patients when used along with H_1 antagonists. Advise patients to avoid driving or operating machinery until the sedative effects of the drugs are known or the period of drowsiness has worn off. As with all drugs, antihistamines should be stored out of the reach of small children to avoid accidental ingestion.

The anticholinergic properties of some H_1 antagonists limit their use in patients with prostatic hypertrophy, those with a predisposition to urinary retention, or those who have narrow-angle glaucoma. Instruct patients with these disorders to contact their health care provider before using an H_1 antagonist.

Instruct the patient as to the correct technique for using intranasal sprays and that some drugs may cause temporary stinging. Replace intranasal drug canisters or bottles every 3 months, even if not completely empty. The patient is thus assured that active drug will be available when it is needed. Proper cleaning of the canister or bottle done weekly helps to maintain patency of the device.

Advise patients to consume 2000 to 3000 mL of fluids daily to thin secretions and make them easier to remove. In addition, instruct them to maintain dental hygiene by brushing and flossing. The diminished salivary flow resulting from cholinergic blockade contributes to dental caries and gum disease. Appointments for regular dental check-ups should be made. Mouth dryness can be minimized by using ice, sugarless gum, or hard candy.

Patients may also consider immunotherapy, also called desensitization, for reduction of their symptoms and to decrease drug requirements. High-dose allergy shots have been effectively used in immunotherapy, with 80% to 90% success rates for some allergens. When considering this route, patients should be informed that immunotherapy does not show immediate results, and benefits may not be evident for 6 to 12 months after beginning therapy. Desensitization is a long-term process and can extend up to 5 years if the treatment has been beneficial. Be aware that immunotherapy may produce severe systemic allergic reactions, so therapy should be carefully evaluated in comparison with other treatment plans.

Evaluation

In patients using nasal corticosteroids, improvement in postnasal drip and congestion is usually apparent 1 to 4 weeks after the start of an intranasal corticosteroid. A referral to an allergist is appropriate when an allergic etiology cannot be distinguished from vasomotor rhinitis, after several interventions have been tried and symptoms are still not relieved, or when the antigen or antigens must be identified for management purposes. Patients using long-term nasal corticosteroids should have periodic otolaryngology exams to monitor nasal mucosa and passages for infection or ulceration. Referral to an otolaryngologist is also warranted for symptoms related to polyps or foreign bodies, tumors, a necrotizing inflammatory condition, or atrophic rhinitis.

Patients changing from systemic corticosteroids to nasal formulations should be monitored for signs of adrenal insufficiency (anorexia, nausea, weakness, fatigue, hypotension, and hypoglycemia) during initial therapy.

Effectiveness of treatment is demonstrated most often by patients' verbal statements of symptom improvement. If an H_1 antagonist was used for SAR or PAR, symptoms are relieved. If it was specifically used for its sedative characteristics, drowsiness or sleep resulted.

KEY POINTS

- An estimated 50% of the population suffers from chronic or recurrent allergies. Hyperactivity of the airways to various physical, chemical, environmental, or pharmacologic stimuli is the hallmark of allergy and asthma.
- Patient history is the most important component in the evaluation of a suspected or confirmed allergic disorder. A careful review of home, workplace, and environmental factors should be conducted. Allergy testing should be selective and based on clues provided by the patient's history whenever possible.
- The treatment objective for the use of intranasal steroids, H_1 antagonists, and cromolyn sodium is primarily symptom relief. No one drug completely abolishes symptoms.
- Corticosteroids are the drugs of choice for AR.
- H_1 antagonists are more effective for allergic rather than nonallergic forms of rhinitis. Acute forms respond more favorably to drug therapy than chronic rhinitis.
- First-generation H_1 antagonists are effective in relieving nasopharyngeal itching, sneezing, water rhinorrhea, and ocular manifestations of allergy such as itching, tearing, and erythema. However, they are less effective for nasal congestion.

- First-generation H_1 antagonists are sedating to various degrees, and their anticholinergic effects include visual disturbances, urinary retention, and even arrhythmias in some patients.
- Second-generation H_1 antagonists cause less sedation and anticholinergic adverse effects. These drugs have dose-related bronchodilating effects and provide some protection against bronchospasm caused by histamine, allergens, exercise, hyperventilation, and cold, dry air.
- Cromolyn sodium, a mast cell inhibitor, is essentially without adverse effects and is the only intervention of a prophylactic nature.
- H_1 antagonists can prevent nasal congestion but do not relieve existing congestion. Thus they are more effective taken before symptoms occur.
- Patient education should include the correct use of intranasal sprays, nebulizers, and drops.
- Efficacy of drug therapy is based on evidence of reduced inflammation, dilation of airways, and stabilization of mast cells, and patient verbal statements of symptom relief.
- Refer to an appropriate allergist when conservative methods fail to control symptoms.

Bibliography

Allergic Rhinitis and its Impact on Asthma Workshop Group–Independent Expert Panel. (2001). Allergic rhinitis and its impact on asthma. *Journal of Allergy and Clinical Immunology*, 108(5), S147–S334.

Alho, O., Karttunen, R., and Karttunen, T. (2004). Nasal mucosa in natural colds: Effects of allergic rhinitis and susceptibility to recurrent sinusitis. *Clinical Experiments in Immunology*, 137(2), 366–372.

Al Sayyad, J., Fedorowicz, Z., Alhashimi, D., et al. (2007). Topical nasal steroids for intermittent and persistent allergic rhinitis in children. *Cochrane Database of Systematic Reviews. 2007*, Issue 1. Art. No. CD003163. DOI: 10.1002/14651858.CD003163.pub4.

Becker, J. (2004). Allergic rhinitis. *eMedicine*. Available online: www.emedicine.com/ped/topic2560.htm. Accessed May 23, 2007.

CDC fast stats A-Z. (2004). *Advanced data from vital and health statistics, No. 346, Table 13*. August 26, 2004. Available online:www.cdc.gov/nchs/fastats/allergies.htm. Accessed May 23, 2007.

Corren, J., and Kachru, K. (2007). Relationship between nonallergic upper airway disease and asthma. *Clinical Allergy and Immunology*, 19, 101–114.

Dykewicz, M., Fineman, S., Skoner, D., et al. (1998). Diagnosis and management of rhinitis: Complete guidelines of the Joint Task Force on Practice Parameters in Allergy, Asthma and Immunology. American Academy of Allergy, Asthma, and Immunology. *Annals of Allergy Asthma Immunology*, 81(5 Pt 2), 478–518.

Juniper, E., Stahl, E., Doty, R., et al. (2005). Clinical outcomes and adverse effect monitoring in allergic rhinitis. *Journal of Allergy and Clinical Immunology*, 115(3 Suppl 1), S390–S413.

Garavello, W., Di Berardino, F., Romagnoli, M., et al. (2005). Nasal rinsing with hypertonic solution: An adjunctive treatment for pediatric seasonal allergic rhinoconjunctivitis. *International Archives of Allergy and Immunology*, 137(4), 310–314.

Garavello, W, Romagnoli, M., Sordo, L., et al. (2003). Hypersaline nasal irrigation in children with symptomatic seasonal allergic rhinitis: A randomized study. *Pediatric Allergy and Immunology*, 14(2), 140–143.

Hadley, J., Kavuru, M., Anon, J., et al. (2005). *Diagnosis and management of rhinitis and rhinosinusitis*. West Islip, NY: Professional Communications.

Hussain, I., and Kline, J. (2004). DNA, the immune system, and atopic disease. *Journal of Investigational Dermatology Symposium Proceedings*, 9(1), 23–28.

Liou, A., Grubb, J., and Schechtman, K. (2003). Causative and contributive factors to asthma severity and patterns of medication use in patients seeking specialized asthma care. *Chest*, 124(5), 1781–1788.

Long, A., McFadden, C., DeVine, D., et al. (2002). Management of allergic and non-allergic rhinitis (Evidence/Technology Assessment No. 54, Prepared by New England Medical Center Evidence-based Practice Center under Contract No. 290-97-0019). AHRQ Pub. No. 02-E024. Rockville, MD: Agency for Healthcare Research and Quality.

McCann, D., and Roth, B. (2006). Toxicity: Antihistamines. *eMedicine*. Available online: www.emedicine.com/emerg/topic38.htm. Accessed May 23, 2007.

Meltzer, E., Szwarcberg, J., and Pill, M. (2004). Allergic rhinitis, asthma, and rhinosinusitis: Diseases of the integrated airway. *Journal of Managed Care Pharmacy*, 10(4), 310–317.

National Jewish Hospital. (2006). Allergic and non-allergic rhinitis. Denver: Author. Available online. www.nationaljewish.org/disease-info/diseases. Accessed May 23, 2007.

Schwetz, S., Olze, H., Melchisedech, S., et al. (2004). Efficacy of pollen blocker cream in the treatment of allergic rhinitis. *Archives of Otolaryngology, Head, Neck Surgery*, 130(8), 979–984.

Sheikh, J. (2005). Allergic rhinitis. *eMedicine*. Available online: www.emedicine.com/med/topic104.htm#target1. Accessed May 23, 2007.

Slavin, R. (1982). Relationship of nasal disease and sinusitis to bronchial asthma. *Annals of Allergy*, 49(2), 76–79.

RESPIRATORY

52

Decongestants, Expectorants, Antitussives, and Mucolytics

Upper respiratory infections (URIs) are commonly seen in primary care. Whether the cause is viral, bacterial, or environmental in nature, URIs are usually self-limiting, and symptomatic relief is the goal of treatment. URI symptoms can be treated with expectorants, antitussives, decongestants, and mucolytic drugs. Most of these drugs are available over the counter (OTC) and are frequently self-initiated. Prescription strengths are also available for a variety of upper respiratory problems, including the common cold, cough, and rhinitis. Rhinosinusitis was discussed in Chapter 51.

COMMON COLD

EPIDEMIOLOGY AND ETIOLOGY

Acute infectious rhinitis (i.e., the common cold) is the most common acute infection, accounting for over 10% of primary care office visits each year in the United States. Patients visit their health care providers when symptoms become unresponsive to OTC drugs or the patient becomes frustrated with the illness. The cost of medical treatment of common colds is substantial, exceeding $10 billion per year, with over $500 million spent on OTC products. The result is approximately 26 million missed work and 22 million school days each year and 27 million visits to health care providers. In addition, there are 250 million days of restricted activities.

Most adults have an average of two to four common colds a year, with the incidence increasing in the fall, peaking in winter, and then slowly declining each spring. Peak incidence occurs around holidays because of the mobility of patient populations. Adult women are affected more often than men. Children experience an average of 6 to 10 episodes per year; colds occur more often in families with children ages 2 to 7 years who attend day care.

Most colds in the United States occur during the fall and winter months. The rate of incidence slowly increases beginning in late August or early September, and remains elevated through March or April of each year, when it declines. Ordinarily, there are more colds with the opening of schools in the fall and with the onset of cold weather. The change in temperature prompts people to stay indoors, which increases the risk that viruses will spread among household members, fellow employees, or students. The incidence and the severity of the common cold increase in relation to the stress levels of the patients, likely as the result of a weakened immune system.

The common cold can be caused by any of 200 different viruses. Rhinovirus is responsible for 30% to 40% of cases occurring predominantly in the fall and spring and is the most persistent cause of common colds. The rhinovirus actively replicates in temperatures below 95° F, but replicates poorly in temperatures above 99° F. This may explain why it causes the common cold and not pneumonia. Coronavirus is responsible for 10% to 15% of common colds and is more prevalent during the winter months. Other organisms causing upper respiratory symptoms include the parainfluenza virus, adenovirus, Coxsackie virus, and respiratory syncytial viruses (RSV).

Although almost all people experience an acute episode of coughing at some time in their lives, many studies report a prevalence of chronic cough in only 8% to 14% of the population. Viral infections producing a cough are particularly pronounced during the winter months, occurring more frequently in children than in adults. Common bacterial organisms associated with cough include *Streptococcus pneumoniae*, *Mycoplasma pneumoniae*, *Staphylococcus aureus*, *Haemophilus influenzae*, and mixed anaerobic bacteria.

PATHOPHYSIOLOGY

The common cold virus is transmitted by direct inoculation of the mucous membranes of the nose and eyes, usually from contaminated hands or by direct droplet exposure. If the body's upper respiratory tract defense mechanisms (i.e., cough, sneeze and gag reflexes, lymph nodes, immunoglobulin A [IgA] antibodies, and rich vasculature) fail, viral pathogens enter, causing nasopharynx complaints of "being all stuffed up and having a runny nose." Acute nasopharyngeal inflammatory reactions result in dilation of the blood vessels in the nasal mucosa. The dilation, in turn, causes engorgement of mucous membranes and an increase in mucus production. Characteristically, the copious nasal discharge progresses from being clear and watery to thickened within 24 hours. A scratchy throat, nonproductive cough, loss of taste and smell, and sneezing are common complaints. A key diagnostic finding of the common cold is the absence of systemic symptoms.

In general, the mechanisms associated with a cough are mechanical, inflammatory, or chemical in nature. Coughs can be stimulated from congestion or occur as the result of postnasal drip. The etiologic agent stimulates afferent fibers in the vagus, the trigeminal, the glossopharyngeal, or the phrenic nerve. These nerves convey information to the cough center in the medulla. Efferent fibers from the cough center, in turn, carry motor impulses to the larynx and the muscles of the diaphragm, the chest wall, and the abdomen, resulting in a cough. In patients with excessive sputum production, increased secretions stimulate coughing.

PHARMACOTHERAPEUTIC OPTIONS

Oral and Intranasal Decongestants

- desoxyephedrine (Vicks formulations)
- ephedrine (Pretz-D); ◆ Combination products
- pseudoephedrine (Sudafed, Novafed, Drixoral, many combination products); ◆ Sudafed, many combination products
- oxymetazoline (Afrin, Dristan Nasal Mist); ◆ Afrin Sinus, Dristan Nasal Mist, Claritin Nasal Spray
- xylometazoline (Otrivin, Natru-Vent); ◆ Otrivin Nasal Spray
- phenylephrine (Neo-Synephrine, Sudafed PE)

▥ Indications

Oral and intranasal decongestants are used to relieve symptoms associated with common colds, rhinitis, allergies, and sinusitis. Antihistamines and decongestants have been used widely to increase eustachian tube patency, particularly during air flights, though effectiveness is far from proven. Decongestants are also used by many to relieve nasal congestion resulting from scuba or deep sea diving, but are not indicated for such use.

▥ Pharmacodynamics

Oral and intranasal decongestants are adrenergic amines chemically related to norepinephrine, a major neurotransmitter of the sympathetic nervous system (see Chapter 14). They act as a decongestant by stimulating α receptors of vascular smooth muscle, thus constricting dilated arterioles within the nasal mucosa and reducing blood flow to the engorged area. Intranasal use produces a rapid and intense vasoconstriction. Vasoconstriction is delayed and less intense with oral formulations. Pseudoephedrine is the dextroisomer of ephedrine and is approximately one fourth as potent as a pressor drug.

▥ Pharmacokinetics

In general, the absorption of adrenergic nasal decongestants is minimal. The onset of drug action occurs in 1 to 2 minutes via the intranasal route, and 15 to 30 minutes if the drug is taken orally. Peak decongestant activity varies from 5 to 10 minutes to 1 to 2 hours, with duration of decongestant action ranging from 30 minutes for ephedrine, for example, to 12 hours for pseudoephedrine (Table 52-1).

Nasal decongestants may be systemically absorbed from both the nasal mucosa and the gastrointestinal (GI) tract after intranasal administration, resulting in systemic adverse effects, especially when excessive doses are used. Circulating drugs are biotransformed in the liver and intestines by the enzyme monoamine oxidase (MAO). The duration of decongestant effects following application to nasal mucosa is variable and may range from 30 minutes to 4 hours. The decongestants are generally eliminated through the urine and feces within 72 hours.

Although pseudoephedrine's half-life is dependent upon the pH of the urine, the half-life at a urine pH of 5.5 to 6 is 9 to 16 hours. In alkaline urine, the half-life may be prolonged to 50 hours, or it may be reduced to 1.5 hours with very acidic urine. In children, a half-life of 3.1 hours has been reported.

▥ Adverse Effects and Contraindications

Stinging, burning, and drying of nasal mucosa has occurred with intranasal decongestant drops or sprays. **Prolonged use ▲ of a topical nasal decongestant (for more than 3 days or 72 hours) produces a chronic congestion known as *rhinitis medicamentosa*. After 3 days of continuous use, response to these drugs becomes blunted *(tachyphylaxis)*, leading to increased use, often on an hourly basis.** Abrupt cessation results in marked rebound congestion, presumably due to marked reflex vasodilation and an erythematous mucosa. The congestion resolves in 2 to 3 weeks if intranasal decongestants are stopped, but can be extremely uncomfortable while

PHARMACOKINETICS

TABLE 52-1 Selected Decongestants, Expectorants, Antitussives, and Mucolytics

	Route	Onset	Peak	Duration	PB%	t½
DECONGESTANTS						
ephedrine	NS	1–2 min	5–10 min	30 min–4 hr	UA	UA
desoxyephedrine	NS	1–2 min	5–10 min	30 min–4 hr	UA	UA
oxymetazoline	NS	1–2 min	5–10 min	To 12 hr	UA	UA
phenylephrine	NS	1–2 min	5–10 min	30 min–4 hr	UA	UA
pseudoephedrine	PO	15–30 min	30–60 min	4–6 hr 8–12 hr*	UA	UA
xylometazoline	NS	1–2 min	5–10 min	30 min–4 hr	UA	UA
EXPECTORANTS						
guaifenesin	PO	30 min	UA	4–6 hr	UA	UA
dornase alpha	IV	15 min	3 days	UA	UA	UA
ANTITUSSIVES						
benzonatate	PO	15–20 min	UA	3–8 hr	UA	UA
codeine	PO	<30 min	60–90 min	4–6 hr	30–35	3 hr
dextromethorphan	PO	15–30 min	UA	3–6 hr	UA	UA
hydrocodone	PO	Rapid	30–90 min	4–8 hr	30–35	4 hr
MUCOLYTICS						
acetylcysteine	Inh	Rapid	UA	Brief	UA	UA
OTHER RESPIRATORY DRUGS						
alpha₁-proteinase inhibitor	IV	2–3 days	1–3 wk	1–2 wk	UA	4.5–5.2 days
beractant	INT	Immed	Hours	UA	UA	UA
colfosceril palmitate	INT	Immed	Hours	12 hr	UA	12 hr

*Pseudoephedrine's duration of action for sustained-action formulation is 8–12 hr.
Immed, Immediate; *Inh*, inhaled formulation; *INT*, intratracheal; *IV*, intravenous; *NS*, nasal spray; *PB*, protein binding; *PO*, by mouth; *t½*, half-life; *UA*, unavailable.

RESPIRATORY

DRUG INTERACTIONS

TABLE 52-2 Interactions: Decongestants, Antitussives, and Mucolytics

Drug	Interactive Drugs	Interaction
DECONGESTANTS		
Adrenergic decongestants	ergonovine, oxytocin, Tricyclic antidepressants	Increases cardiovascular effects of phenylephrine
	guanethidine, Phenothiazines	Decreases effect of interactive drug
	Beta blockers	Mutual inhibition
	digoxin, theophylline	Increases risk of arrhythmias
	MAO inhibitors, methyldopa	Increases vasopressor effects
ANTITUSSIVES		
codeine, hydrocodone, diphenhydramine	Alcohol, Antidepressants, Antihistamines, Opioids, Sedative-hypnotics	Additive CNS depression
diphenhydramine	disopyramide, quinidine, Tricyclic antidepressants	Additive anticholinergic properties
	MAO inhibitors	Intensifies and prolongs anticholinergic actions
dextromethorphan	MAO inhibitors, SSRIs	Serotonin syndrome, hypotension, hyperpyrexia
	quinidine	Increases blood levels and adverse effects of dextromethorphan
MUCOLYTICS		
acetylcysteine	Activated charcoal	Decreases effectiveness of acetylcysteine

CNS, Central nervous system; *MAO*, monoamine oxidase; *SSRIs*, selective serotonin reuptake inhibitors.

it lasts. However, a less drastic approach is to discontinue drug use in one nostril at a time. Rebound congestion and tachyphylaxis is not seen with pseudoephedrine.

Occasionally, mild central nervous system (CNS) stimulation (i.e., restlessness, nervousness, tremors, headache, and insomnia) occurs. Large dosages produce tachycardia and palpitations. Use them with caution in patients who have heart disease, marked hypertension, advanced arteriosclerotic disease, insulin-dependent diabetes mellitus, or hyperthyroidism. By stimulating α receptors on vasculature, adrenergic drugs cause widespread vasoconstriction. The generalized vasoconstriction is most likely to occur with oral decongestants; however, if taken in excess, even the nasal formulations can cause significant vasoconstriction.

Adrenergic decongestants can produce subjective effects similar to those of amphetamines. For this reason, these drugs **A** are subject to abuse. **Pseudoephedrine and ephedrine are the most commonly abused. Although these drugs are not regulated under the Controlled Substances Act, pharmacies have started keeping them behind the counter so as to impede inappropriate use. Cases of psychosis induced by pseudoephedrine have occurred in patients with an underlying psychiatric disorder and after deliberate overdose.**

Adrenergic decongestants are contraindicated for use in patients concurrently using MAO inhibitors and in those with known intolerance to active ingredients or its preservatives (bisulfites, thimerosal, aromatics, or chlorobutanol). Systemic reactions appear to be most prevalent in infants, young children, and older adults; some investigators do not recommend the use of intranasal decongestants in these age groups.

Pseudoephedrine causes minimal changes in pulse and blood pressure after single doses of 60 mg. Single doses of 180 mg cause minor elevations in systolic blood pressure (about 7 mm Hg), minor increases in heart rate (about 9 beats/min), and no changes in diastolic blood pressure in healthy individuals.

The American Academy of Pediatrics notes that pseudoephedrine is usually compatible with breastfeeding. However, symptoms of excessive stimulation in a breastfeeding infant have been observed; therefore nursing mothers should be advised to watch for these symptoms if they are taking pseudoephedrine.

▦ Drug Interactions

There are many drug interactions with decongestants. Table 52-2 provides an overview of specific interactions. Many of the interactions are related to drug effects on the cardiovascular or autonomic nervous systems. Concurrent uses of drugs that acidify urine decrease the therapeutic effects of decongestants, whereas concurrent uses of drugs that alkalinize the urine contribute to toxicity.

▦ Dosage Regimen

Dosages for intranasal decongestants typically are one to two drops/sprays from twice daily to a frequency of every 3 to 4 hours. Oral formulations are taken no more often than every 4 to 6 hours for immediate-release formulations. Extended-release formulations are ordinarily taken every 12 hours (Table 52-3).

Expectorants

- guaifenesin (Guiatuss, Halotussin, Humibid, Mucinex, Robitussin, others); ✦ Benylin-E Extra Strength, Mucinex, Vicks Chest Congestion Relief, others
- dornase alpha (recombinant human deoxyribonuclease or DNase; Pulmozyme)

▦ Indications

A variety of compounds are promoted for their expectorant actions (e.g., ammonium chlorides, terpin hydrate, and potassium guaiacolsulfonate), but in almost all cases, efficacy is doubtful. However, there are two exceptions, guaifenesin and dornase alpha. Guaifenesin is the only OTC expectorant recognized by the Food and Drug Administration (FDA) as safe and effective. It is also the only expectorant for which scientific evidence supports efficacy in decreasing the viscosity of sputum. Guaifenesin is used for the symptomatic management of cough associated with the common cold, laryngitis, bronchitis, pharyngitis, pertussis, or influenza, and for coughs provoked by chronic paranasal sinusitis. Guaifenesin is often found in combination with analgesics or antipyretics, antihistamines, and decongestants.

DOSAGE

TABLE 52-3 Selected Decongestants, Expectorants, Antitussives, and Mucolytics

Drug	Uses	Dosage	Implications	
DECONGESTANTS				
ephedrine	Relief of nasal congestion accompanying colds, allergies, or sinusitis	*Adult and Child >12 yr:* 2 or 3 NS (0.25% solution) every 4 or more hr PRN *Child 6–11 yr:* 1 or 2 NS (0.25% solution) every 4 or more hr PRN	**Potential for abuse. Rebound congestion if used too often or for longer than 72 hr.** Stress need to take as directed.	⚠
oxymetazoline	Relief of nasal congestion accompanying colds, allergies, or sinusitis	*Adult and Child >6 yr:* 2–3 NS or drops (0.05% solution) twice daily PRN *Child 2–5 yr:* 2–3 drops (0.025% solution) twice daily PRN	**Do not confuse with xylometazoline. Rebound congestion if used too often or for longer than 72 hr.** Stress need to take as directed.	⚠
phenylephrine	Nasal and/or sinus congestion of common cold, hay fever, allergies, or sinusitis	*Adult and Child >6 yr:* 2–3 drops (0.25%–1% solution) every 4 or more hr –or– 10 mg PO every 4 hr PRN *Child <6 yr:* 2–3 NS or drops (0.125% solution) every 4 or more hr –or– 1 mL (0.25% drops) every 4 hr PRN. *Adult and Child >12 yr:* 2–3 NS (0.25%-1% solution) every 4 or more hr PRN –or– 10–20 mg PO every 4 hr. *Child 6–12 yr:* 2–3 NS (0.25% solution) every 4 or more hr PRN.	**Potential for abuse. Rebound congestion if used too often or for longer than 72 hr.** Available as drops, sprays, and oral formulations. Stress need to take as directed.	⚠
pseudoephedrine	Relief of nasal congestion accompanying colds, allergies, or sinusitis	*Adult and Child >12 yr:* 60 mg PO every 4–6 hr PRN –or– 120 mg PO LA formulation every 12 hr PRN *Child 6–12 yr:* 30 mg PO of IA formulation every 4–6 hr PRN *Child 2–6 yr:* 15 mg every 4–6 hr PRN	**Potential for abuse.** Check package literature for dosing of combination products. Stress need to take as directed.	⚠
xylometazoline	Nasal congestion accompanying colds, allergies, or sinusitis	*Adult and Child >12 yr:* 1–3 drops or NS (0.1% solution) in each nostril every 8–10 hr PRN *Child 2–12 yr:* 2–3 drops or NS (0.05% solution) in each nostril every 8–10 hr PRN	**Do not confuse with oxymetazoline. Rebound congestion occurs if used too often or for longer than 72 hr.** Stress need to take as directed.	⚠
EXPECTORANTS				
guaifenesin	Symptomatic management of cough associated with URI	*Adult:* 200–400 mg PO every 4 hr –or– 600–1200 mg PO every 12 hr of SR formulation *Child 6–12 yr:* 100–200 mg PO every 4 hr –or– 600 mg PO every 12 hr of SR formulation. Max: 1.2 grams/day *Child 2–6 yr:* 50–100 mg PO every 4 hr. Max: 600 mg/day	Take each dose with full glass of water to decrease viscosity of secretions. SR formulations should be taken whole. Do not open, crush, break, or chew.	
dornase alpha	Cystic fibrosis	*Adult:* 2.5 mg (1 ampule) once daily via aerosol mist using a compressed-air nebulizer system	Twice-daily dosing may be beneficial for some patients.	
ANTITUSSIVES				
benzonatate	Nonproductive cough due to minor throat or bronchial irritation	*Adult:* 100–200 mg PO 3 times daily up to 600 mg daily	**Inadvertent release of drug from capsules causes local anesthetic effect and choking.**	⚠
codeine (with guaifenesin) (Robitussin AC)	Antitussive	*Adult:* 20 mL PO every 4 hr PRN; not to exceed 120 mg/day	**Potential for abuse.** Stress need to take as directed. Controlled substance.	⚠
dextromethorphan	Coughs associated with minor URI; chronic nonproductive cough	*Adult and Child >12 yr:* 10–20 mL PO every 12 hr PRN *Child 6–12 yr:* 5 mL PO every 12 hr PRN *Child 2–5 yr:* 2.5 mL PO every 12 hr PRN	15–30 mL is equivalent in cough suppression to 8–15 mg of codeine. **Potential for abuse.** Stress need to take as directed.	⚠
hydrocodone with homatropine (Hycodan)	Antitussive	*Adult:* 1–2 tabs PO every 4–6 hr PRN. Max: 6 tabs or 6 tsp/day	**Potential for abuse.** Controlled substance.	⚠
MUCOLYTICS				
acetylcysteine	Adjunctive therapy for abnormally viscous secretions in acute and chronic bronchopulmonary disease, cystic fibrosis	*Adult and Child:* 1–2 mL of 10%-20% solution –or– enough 10%–20% solution to produce heavy mist via nebulizer every 1–4 hr PRN	Instruct patient to clear airway completely before taking aerosol treatment. Encourage adequate fluid intake (2000–3000 mL) per day to decrease viscosity of secretions.	
	acetaminophen overdose	*Adult and Child:* 140 mg/kg initially followed by 70 mg/kg every 4 hr for 17 doses. Dilute with cola, juice, or water to a 5% concentration.	Drug reacts with rubber and metals (iron, nickel, and copper). Avoid contact with these substances.	
OTHER RESPIRATORY DRUGS				
alpha₁-proteinase inhibitor	Panacinar emphysema	*Adult:* 60 mg/kg IV once weekly. Infusion rate at least 0.08 mL/kg/min	Immunize for hepatitis B before beginning therapy.	
beractant	Prophylaxis and rescue of infants at high risk for IRDS or hyaline membrane disease	*Infants:* 4 mg/kg intratracheal; may repeat dose no sooner than 6 hr after preceding dose. Quarter doses are given with infant in various positions. Ventilate with positive pressure after each quarter dose.	Beractant is frozen; warm before giving. Do not instill drug into mainstream bronchus.	
colfosceril palmitate	Prophylaxis for infants at risk for IRDS	*Infants:* 2.5 mg/kg IT for 2 doses; may repeat in 12 hr in infants remaining on ventilator	Give through side port of IT tube. Check instructions for proper administration technique.	

ET, Endotracheal tube; *IA*, immediate-acting; *IRDS*, infant respiratory distress syndrome; *IT*, intratracheal tube; *IV*, intravenous (route); *LA*, long-acting; *NS*, nasal sprays; *PO*, by mouth; *PRN*, as needed; *SR*, sustained-release; *URI*, upper respiratory infection.

RESPIRATORY

Dornase alpha reduces the incidence of respiratory infections and improves pulmonary function in patients with cystic fibrosis. Dornase alpha is not a replacement for other components of therapy for cystic fibrosis (e.g., antibiotics, bronchodilators, daily physical exercise).

▌▌ Pharmacodynamics

Guaifenesin renders a cough more productive by stimulating the flow of respiratory tract secretions. The loosened secretions move upward toward the pharynx by ciliary movement and by coughing. A common misconception is that guaifenesin relieves irritated mucous membranes by preventing dryness. Evidence does not support this belief (Fig. 52-1). Dornase alpha is a genetically engineered enzyme (DNase) that hydrolyzes DNA in the sputum. It reduces the viscous elasticity of sputum.

▌▌ Pharmacokinetics

The pharmacokinetics of selected expectorants are listed in Table 52-1. Guaifenesin is well absorbed from the GI tract after oral administration. Distribution sites are unknown, but its metabolites are biotransformed and eliminated through the kidneys.

The onset of drug action for dornase alpha occurs within 15 minutes of nebulized administration. There is minimal systemic absorption after inhalation. Peak effects are not noted for 3 days, and the duration of drug action is unknown. It is unknown whether dornase alpha crosses the placenta or is distributed in breast milk.

▌▌ Adverse Effects and Contraindications

Adverse effects of guaifenesin include nausea, vomiting, diarrhea, and abdominal pain. Dizziness, headache, rashes, and urticaria have also been noted. Guaifenesin is contraindicated for use in patients with hypersensitivity to the drug. Some guaifenesin formulations contain alcohol; avoid these in patients with known intolerance to alcohol. Guaifenesin also inhibits platelet function, and its use should therefore be avoided in patients taking anticoagulants. Guaifenesin is a pregnancy category C drug. Safety of guaifenesin during lactation is unknown.

In general, expectorants should not be used for persistent coughs associated with smoking, asthma, or emphysema, or if the cough is accompanied by excessive secretions or fever. Safe use of expectorates during pregnancy has not been established, although guaifenesin has been used without adverse effects.

The adverse effects of dornase alpha are uncommon, but voice alteration, pharyngitis, rash, chest pain, and allergic reactions may occur. There are no contraindications to use of dornase alpha.

▌▌ Drug Interactions

There are no known drug interactions with guaifenesin or dornase alpha.

▌▌ Dosage Regimen

The dosage of guaifenesin depends on the specific formulation used (see Table 52-3). The dosage of extended-release formulations is higher than that for syrup, oral solutions, capsules, or tablet formulations. Sustained-release formulations should be taken whole.

Doses of dornase alpha are administered via aerosol mist using a compressed-air nebulizer system. Treatment should last 10 to 15 minutes. Twice-daily dosing may be beneficial for some patients.

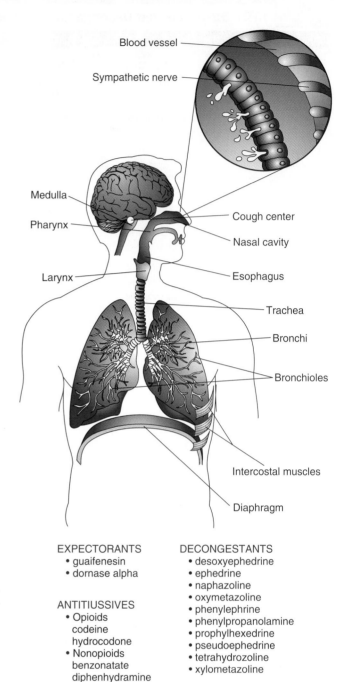

EXPECTORANTS
- guaifenesin
- dornase alpha

ANTITIUSSIVES
- Opioids
  codeine
  hydrocodone
- Nonopioids
  benzonatate
  diphenhydramine
  dextromethorphan

DECONGESTANTS
- desoxyephedrine
- ephedrine
- naphazoline
- oxymetazoline
- phenylephrine
- phenylpropanolamine
- prophylhexedrine
- pseudoephedrine
- tetrahydrozoline
- xylometazoline

FIGURE 52-1 Sites of Drug Action for Upper Respiratory Disorders. Decongestants stimulate α receptors, causing vasoconstriction, reduced blood flow, reduced fluid exudation, and shrinkage of edematous membranes. Expectorants and mucolytics stimulate the flow of respiratory tract secretions. Antitussives act centrally in the cough center or peripherally at the site of irritation to suppress coughing.

Antitussives

NONOPIOIDS

◆ benzonatate (Tessalon Pearls); ✦ Tessalon

◆ diphenhydramine (Benadryl, Compoz, Sominex, many others); ✦ Allerdryl, Benadryl

◆ dextromethorphan (Benylin DM, Robitussin Cough Calmers, Sucrets Cough Control, St. Joseph Cough Suppressant, Vicks Formula 44, many others); ✦ Balminil DM, Koffex, many others

Opioids
◆ codeine; ◆ Paveral
◆ hydrocodone-homatropine (Hycodan)

Indications

Antitussives are most appropriately used to suppress dry, hacking, nonproductive coughs that keep patients awake at night. Opioids and nonopioid drugs are used as antitussives. An opioid such as codeine is one of the more commonly used antitussives. Smaller doses are employed for coughs than doses used for pain relief. Hydrocodone is often formulated in combination with decongestants. In contrast, dextromethorphan is the most frequently used nonopioid antitussive. It is a chemical analogue of codeine without its analgesic or dependency features. Nonopioid antitussives are found in combination with antihistamines, decongestants, and expectorants in cough and cold remedies. Dextromethorphan is most effective for chronic nonproductive coughs. Diphenhydramine is the only antihistamine with proven efficacy as an antitussive in the treatment of coughs associated with the common cold or irritants (see Chapter 51). Overall, nonopioid antitussives are as effective as opioid antitussives in relieving cough.

Pharmacodynamics

In general, antitussive drugs act either centrally or peripherally. Centrally-acting drugs such as codeine, hydrocodone, and dextromethorphan act in the cough center in the medulla to suppress the cough. Dextromethorphan does not inhibit ciliary activity, whereas codeine does. Peripherally acting drugs such as benzonatate act at the site of the irritation that is producing the cough.

Pharmacokinetics

The pharmacokinetics of selected antitussives are similar overall (see Table 52-1). The onset of most drugs occurs in 15 to 30 minutes, reaching peak action in 30 to 90 minutes, with a duration of action of 3 to 8 hours.

Adverse Effects and Contraindications

Overall, opioids are limited in their usefulness because of adverse effects (see Chapter 16). **The major adverse effects of opioids are apparent in the CNS depression they cause.** At low dosages, the risk of dependency and undesired adverse responses is reduced but not eliminated. Sedation, confusion, and hypotension may occur, especially with high doses. The most serious adverse responses are respiratory depression, laryngeal edema, and anaphylaxis.

Opioids are contraindicated for use in patients with known hypersensitivity to the drug or to its other ingredients, and during pregnancy and lactation. Avoid products containing alcohol, aspartame, saccharine, sugar, or tartrazine dye (FD&C Yellow No. 5) in patients with hypersensitivity to these compounds. Cautious use is warranted in patients with head trauma, increased intracranial pressure, severe hepatic, renal, or pulmonary disease, hypothyroidism, adrenal insufficiency, or alcoholism. Older adults and debilitated patients are at greater risk for the CNS depression caused by opioids.

Nonopioid antitussives vary in their adverse effects. Benzonatate can produce sedation, headache, and mild dizziness. Nasal congestion, pruritus, and skin eruptions, as well as GI upset, have occurred. Benzonatate acts as a potent local anesthetic if the integrity of the capsule is compromised. This antitussive is contraindicated for use in patients with hypersensitivity to the drug. Cross-sensitivity with other local anesthetics of the ester type (tetracaine, procaine, and others) may occur.

The adverse effects of diphenhydramine are related to its antihistaminic characteristics. Drowsiness, dry mouth, and anorexia are most common, but the patient may also have blurry vision, photosensitivity, tinnitus, paradoxical excitement (greater in children), dizziness, and headache. It is generally contraindicated for use with acute attacks of asthma, in the presence of hypersensitivity and, because some of the liquid formulations contain alcohol, in patients with known alcohol intolerance.

The adverse effects of dextromethorphan are few. Nausea has been noted; with high doses, so have dizziness and sedation. It is contraindicated for use in the presence of hypersensitivity; in patients taking monoamine oxidase inhibitors or selective serotonin reuptake inhibitors (SSRIs); and, because of the high alcohol content, in patients with known alcohol intolerance. Use it cautiously in patients with a cough lasting more than 1 week or when the cough is accompanied by fever, rash, or headache. Safe use of dextromethorphan during pregnancy and lactation or in children under the age of 2 years has not been established.

Drug Interactions

CNS depressants, alcohol, sedative-hypnotics, and antidepressants provide additive CNS depression when they are used concurrently with opioid and nonopioid antitussives (see Table 52-2). There are many drug interactions with dextromethorphan. Concurrent use with MAO inhibitors or SSRIs results in serotonin syndrome (e.g., excitation, confusion, hypotension, and hyperpyrexia). Additive CNS depression is found with concurrent use of antihistamines, alcohol, sedative-hypnotics, other antidepressants, or opioids. Quinidine increases the blood levels and adverse effects of dextromethorphan.

Dosage Regimens

An antitussive dose, whether used for an adult or child, depends on the specific formulation (see Table 52-3). As with the antitussives, the dosage of extended-release formulations is higher than that of lozenges, syrups, oral solutions, capsules, or tablets. Older adults or debilitated patients may require a dosage reduction because they are more susceptible to CNS depression, anticholinergic effects, and constipation.

Mucolytics
◆ acetylcysteine (Mucomyst)
◆ sodium chloride nasal solution

Indications

Two compounds, sodium chloride nasal solution and acetylcysteine, are used as adjuncts for patients with abnormally thick mucous secretions. They are particularly helpful in patients with acute and chronic bronchopulmonary disease, atelectasis from mucous obstruction, or cystic fibrosis. Acetylcysteine is thought to protect the liver from damage caused by acetaminophen overdose (see Chapter 17).

RESPIRATORY

Pharmacodynamics

Acetylcysteine interrupts DNA and glycoprotein bonds at the molecular level through the process of mucolysis. It reacts directly with mucus by splitting the disulfide bonds of mucoproteins. Liquefaction occurs within minutes after administration. Thus sputum viscosity is reduced and pulmonary secretions are easier to cough up. Acetylcysteine is believed to protect the liver from damage caused by acetaminophen by maintaining or restoring the hepatic concentration of glutathione, a tripeptide that protects erythrocytes from oxidation and hemolysis. Glutathione is necessary for inactivation of acetaminophen metabolites.

Pharmacokinetics

Acetylcysteine is absorbed from the GI tract following oral administration. Action is local when the inhalation route is used. The remainder of the drug is absorbed from the pulmonary epithelium. The distribution, protein binding, and half-life are unknown, although acetylcysteine is biotransformed by the liver (see Table 52-1).

Adverse Effects and Contraindications

Acetylcysteine can trigger bronchospasm in susceptible patients, and therefore the drug is usually administered with or immediately after a bronchodilator. The most common adverse effects of acetylcysteine include burning in the back of the throat, stomatitis, nausea, rhinorrhea, and epistaxis. It can also cause drowsiness, increased respiratory secretions, urticaria, fever, and chills. Because of its sulfur content, acetylcysteine has the additional disadvantage of smelling like rotten eggs. The drug also corrodes iron, metal, copper, and rubber.

There are no known adverse effects to the intranasal use of sodium chloride. The adverse effects of sodium chloride are seen primarily with oral and intravenous (IV) use.

Drug Interactions

Drug interactions with acetylcysteine and sodium chloride are limited. Activated charcoal may absorb acetylcysteine, thus decreasing its effectiveness as an antidote. Do not mix it in solutions containing tetracycline, erythromycin, amphotericin B, or ampicillin (see Table 52-2).

Dosage Regimen

The method used for administration of acetylcysteine dictates the dosage used (see Table 52-3). Acetylcysteine, when used as an antagonist to acetaminophen overdose, is dosed based on body weight.

Miscellaneous Respiratory Drugs
Alpha₁-Proteinase Inhibitor

Alpha$_1$-proteinase inhibitor (Prolastin) is used for chronic replacement therapy for patients with clinically demonstrable panacinar emphysema. This chronic, hereditary, and usually fatal disorder manifests itself in the third or fourth decade of life. An imbalance between elastase and alpha$_1$-antitrypsin inhibitor is believed to be the basis for the disorder.

Absorption of the drug is essentially complete following IV administration. It achieves high concentrations in epithelial fluid of the lungs. The drug is broken down in the intravascular spaces, with a half-life of 4.5 to 5.2 days.

The adverse effects of alpha$_1$-proteinase inhibitor include a fever, occurring about 12 hours after drug administration. The fever resolves spontaneously. Lightheadedness, dizziness, and transient leukocytosis have also been reported.

There are no significant contraindications to the use of the drug, although caution is warranted when using it in patients at risk for circulatory overload. Although the drug is derived from pooled fresh human plasma and has been heat-treated to reduce the potential transmission of disease, safe use in children and during pregnancy has not been fully established. There are no known drug interactions.

Beractant and Colfosceril

Beractant (Survanta) and colfosceril palmitate (Exosurf) are surfactants. Surfactants are used to treat newborns at risk for infant respiratory distress syndrome (infants of gestational age under 32 weeks or birth weight under 1300 grams or both) and to treat hyaline membrane disease in premature infants. A deficiency of surfactant prevents reexpansion of small alveoli in the lungs. This problem causes the larger alveoli to enlarge. The result is a decrease in lung compliance and inadequate pulmonary perfusion.

These drugs replenish surfactant, restoring surface activity to the lungs. Surfactants lower the surface tension on alveolar surfaces during respiration and stabilize alveoli so they are less likely to collapse at resting transpulmonary pressures. Oxygenation improves within minutes of drug administration. Both beractant and colfosceril are distributed and biotransformed by lung tissues.

Surfactants can cause adverse effects such as pulmonary and intracranial hemorrhage, hypotension, apnea, and barotrauma. Infants receiving surfactants have a higher incidence of patent ductus arteriosus. Transient bradycardia, oxygen desaturation, and increased CO_2 tension has been reported with beractant. Beractant is contraindicated for use in infants who are at risk for circulatory overload. Nosocomial infections have occurred with beractant, with no increase in mortality.

Gagging is occasionally noted with colfosceril palmitate. Apnea, bradycardia, and tachycardia are rare. Failure to reduce peak ventilator inspiratory pressures after chest expansion and drug administration may result in overdistention of the lungs and a fatal pulmonary air leak. Hyperoxia can develop, with failure to reduce transcutaneous oxygen saturation to less than 95%. Hypocapnia and reduced blood flow to the brain may result if there is failure to reduce arterial or transcutaneous CO_2 levels to below 30 mm Hg.

CLINICAL REASONING

Treatment Objectives

Treatment objectives include strategies that prevent, minimize, or help improve symptoms. Societal expectations and pharmaceutical industries encourage about 90% of patients to treat the symptoms of a common cold at home.

Treatment Options

Despite patients insisting otherwise, the color, the consistency, and the purulence of nasal discharge are not diagnostic of bacterial or viral etiology. Only 1 of every 8 patients presenting with cold symptoms has a bacterial etiology to their complaint. **Treatment for a common cold is symptomatic; ▲ there is no justification for using antibiotics.**

If vital signs are normal, fever is under 102° F, and the patient can perform daily activities, prescription drugs are generally not required during the first 7 days of illness. Nonpharmacologic treatment includes eating a proper diet, getting adequate rest and sufficient fluid intake, humidifying room air (particularly during sleep), inhaling warm, moist heat (e.g., warm shower), and saline nasal irrigations. Preventive and self-care modalities include washing the hands often, especially when around people who have colds; keeping hands away from the mouth, nose, and eyes; reducing stress to a minimum as much as possible; and refraining from smoking. Cough suppression is generally not needed in patients with an uncomplicated common cold. Antihistamines are largely ineffective for treating cold symptoms. Use of antibiotics is appropriate if a cough has persisted for 3 weeks or longer, and a sputum culture and sensitivity demonstrates that a known bacterial infection is present.

▓ Patient Variables

There is a growing interest in treating common colds with alternative or complementary therapies. For example, echinacea's ability to inhibit microbial infections stems from its ability to stimulate the body's immune response. Zinc lozenges may be helpful in treating the common cold, although their mechanism of action is unknown. The more tradition alternatives of chicken soup and vitamin C may be helpful in improving cold symptoms and boosting the immune system. As grandma used to say: "They can't hurt . . ."

Choices between ethnomedical options and interventions of Western medicine vary among ethnic groups and vary from one patient experience to another. **At any given time, treatment of the common cold and other upper respiratory disorders reflects exclusive use of traditional herbal remedies or a combination of herbs and Western medicine.** In addition, it is often said that if families would familiarize themselves with herbs, their medicinal properties, and uses, many visits to the health care provider would be saved. Herbs, no matter what their modern name and no matter how unorthodox they are said to be, continue to be the treatment of choice by many who value their effects.

LIFE-SPAN CONSIDERATIONS

Pregnant and Nursing Women. Nasal stuffiness and epistaxis are common during pregnancy and result from estrogen-induced edema and vascular congestion of the nasal mucosa. Fetal respiratory depression is theoretically a possibility if a woman with severely impaired renal function chronically takes dextromethorphan during pregnancy and up to the time of delivery.

Children and Adolescents. Three annual waves of the common cold typically occur in children, with the greatest incidence occurring with the opening of school. The more severe cases, with a tendency toward complications, occur in midwinter. Another round of mild cases of the common cold occurs in the spring.

Cold symptoms in a young child pose additional problems. The obstruction of the upper airways causes difficulty in sucking, consumes energy, and increases oxygen needs. Restlessness, malaise, and anorexia result. Crankiness and an acetone breath odor appear as a result of secondary dehydration. In addition, a mild degree of ketoacidosis occurs when fever is present.

There is no good evidence that OTC drugs are effective for the common cold in preschool children. There is a risk of serious toxicities in this age group, especially when combination formulations are used. Caution is warranted when using combination cough and cold products, because many contain aspirin. Research demonstrated a relationship between influenza virus infection and Reye's syndrome. Use caution when giving antitussives to young children because of the risk for depression of the cough reflex and aspiration.

Orally administered decongestants can be used in older children to shrink engorged nasal mucosa. Decongestant sprays can be used by older children, but only with adult supervision. Use these vasoconstrictive drugs with caution in patients with heart disease, marked hypertension, advanced arteriosclerotic disease, insulin-dependent diabetes mellitus, or hyperthyroidism.

Half-strength decongestant nose drops such as pseudoephedrine or phenylephrine are available for children who are over 3 months of age. In younger infants, sterile saline nose drops are used because a sympathomimetic decongestant can cause irritability and tachycardia. The addition of corticosteroids and antibiotics has not been shown efficacious for the common cold.

Older Adults. Using the standard medical model of diagnosis, there is a 1:1 correspondence between clinical signs and symptoms and a pathologic process. However, the medical model does not accurately define the presentation of many illnesses in the older adult. Older adults and people with chronic debilitating diseases are especially vulnerable to complications associated with upper respiratory disorders.

▓ Drug Variables

Expectorants, antitussives, decongestants, and mucolytic drugs relieve symptoms, but no one drug relieves all cold symptoms. In general, treat a single symptom with a single-ingredient product; it permits flexibility for symptom treatment and offers the ability to individualize dosage. Combination formulations are generally discouraged, but it depends on the patient and symptoms. Many OTC formulations contain an antihistamine (e.g., chlorpheniramine), a nasal decongestant (e.g., pseudoephedrine), and an analgesic (e.g., acetaminophen). Table 52-4 provides a list of but a few combination products.

Histamine$_1$ (H_1) antagonists have been used as decongestants because they block the effects of histamine at various receptor sites in the body and thus helps reduce sneezing and rhinorrhea (see Chapter 51). Critics point out, however, that the use of antihistamines is irrational and has no place in the treatment of common colds. They base this statement on the premise that the drying effect of antihistamines may worsen symptoms by impairing mucus flow and causing upper airway obstruction. In rebuttal, on the other hand, antihistamines have been effective in controlling the symptoms of watery eyes, runny nose, and clogged ears.

Decongestants are more reliable than antihistamines in providing symptom relief; however, oral decongestants are generally less effective than topical formulations and can cause adverse systemic effects. Because decongestants cause systemic vasoconstriction, they may raise blood pressure if used in dosages sufficient to alleviate nasal congestion. Oral pseudoephedrine produces a dramatic reduction in nasal symptoms.

Few data are available to support efficacy of antitussives against the common cold. When cough significantly interferes with sleeping or eating, an opioid antitussive such as codeine could be used. In many cases, a single dose before bedtime

DOSAGE

TABLE 52-4 Comparative Examples of OTC Cough and Cold Remedies

Brand name	Antihistamine	Nasal Decongestant	Antitussive	Expectorant	Analgesic
Comtrex Maximum Strength Day and Night Cold and Cough		phenylephrine	dextromethorphan		APAP
Comtrex Maximum Strength Day and Night Severe Cold & Sinus	chlorpheniramine	phenylephrine			APAP
Contact Non-Drowsy		pseudoephedrine			
Contact Cold & Flu Maximum Strength	chlorpheniramine	phenylephrine			APAP
Contact Cold & Flu Non-Drowsy Maximum Strength	chlorpheniramine	phenylephrine			APAP
Coricidin HBP	chlorpheniramine				APAP
Coricidin D	chlorpheniramine				APAP
Dimetapp Elixir, Tablets, and Extentabs	brompheniramine				
Humibid ER				guaifenesin	
Multisymptom Tylenol Cold	chlorpheniramine	pseudoephedrine	dextromethorphan		APAP
Mucinex				guaifenesin	
Mucinex D		pseudoephedrine		guaifenesin	
Mucinex DM			dextromethorphan	guaifenesin	
Robitussin Cough Gels			dextromethorphan		
Robitussin Cough & Cold CF		phenylephrine	dextromethorphan	guaifenesin	
Robitussin Cough and Cold Long-Acting	chlorpheniramine		dextromethorphan		
Robitussin Cough and Cold Nighttime	chlorpheniramine	phenylephrine	dextromethorphan		
Robitussin Cough, Cold & Flu Nighttime	chlorpheniramine	phenylephrine	dextromethorphan		APAP
Robitussin Cough DM Syrup			dextromethorphan	guaifenesin	
Robitussin Cough Long-Acting			dextromethorphan		
Robitussin Head & Chest Congestion PE		phenylephrine		guaifenesin	
Theraflu Nighttime Severe Cold	pheniramine	phenylephrine			APAP
Theraflu Cold and Cough	pheniramine	phenylephrine	dextromethorphan		
Theraflu Cold & Sore Throat	pheniramine	phenylephrine			APAP
Theraflu Flu & Chest Congestion				guaifenesin	APAP

APAP, Acetaminophen; OTC, over-the-counter.

will suffice. Opioid liquid and tablet formulations are equally effective, but the potential for abuse and dependency of the opioid remain. The most popular and effective OTC antitussive is dextromethorphan.

Many patients expect to receive a syrup formulation for cough suppression, and it may provide some psychologic benefit. However, a cough lasting longer than 1 week or one that is accompanied by fever, rash, or headache necessitates further evaluation. Many cough formulations contain glucose or alcohol; exercise caution when using them in patients who have diabetes or alcoholism.

Patient Education

The best preventive measures to avoid catching a cold are simple: avoid exposure to others who are ill, engage in good handwashing, and keep the hands away from the face. A proactive approach to avoidance of coughs and colds is to send educational materials to patients at the beginning of the cold season. Pamphlets and other informational materials are usually appreciated by patients and can help cut down on unnecessary visits and telephone calls. The informational materials should include self-care hints and information about when to seek medical attention (e.g., high fever, marked pain or tenderness in an ear or sinus, increasingly purulent sputum, dyspnea, and pleuritic chest pain). Review the role of antibiotics in the treatment of a viral infection (i.e., only for complications such as otitis or sinusitis), as well as the risks of unnecessary antibiotic therapy (allergic reactions, alteration of bacterial flora, emergence of resistant strains). Unnecessary office visits and

telephone calls can be reduced by as much as 30% to 40% through well-designed educational efforts.

Because many patients self-treat coughs, colds, and rhinitis, it is important to discuss the dangers of indiscriminate use of OTC expectorants, antitussives, and decongestants. Help patients to understand which symptoms may be relieved with self-treatment and for which symptoms self-treatment is ill-advised (see Controversy and Evidence-based Pharmacotherapeutics boxes). Advise patients taking prescription drugs to contact their health care provider before taking OTC drugs.

Relief from cold symptoms and avoidance of complications are facilitated by rest, fluids, analgesia, and perhaps inhalation of steam. Vitamin C has no proven role in the prevention or alleviation of symptoms of the common cold. Recommend that at least 8 glasses or more (1500 to 2000 mL) of liquids be taken per day. Talk with patients about the benefits of a balanced diet. Instruct them about the need for additional rest and sleep during periods of illness. And, advise them to stop smoking. Limiting talking, maintaining adequate environmental humidity, and chewing sugarless gum or sucking on hard candy help alleviate the discomfort caused by a chronic nonproductive cough. Instruct the patient to contact the health care provider if a cough persists for more than 1 week or if it is accompanied by fever, rash, persistent headache, or sore throat.

Instruct the patient on the proper administration and use of nasal sprays or drops. **Do not use nasal decongestants (i.e., ⚠ oxymetazoline, phenylephrine, tetrahydrozoline, and xylometazoline) for longer than 72 hours or in excessive amounts to**

CASE STUDY — Common Cold

ASSESSMENT

History of Present Illness	JE, a 27-year-old female, comes to the urgent care clinic today with complaints of a "stuffy head" and a dry, hacking cough that is keeping her and her partner awake at night. She has had these symptoms for 3 days, and they are interfering with her work performance. She is requesting a diagnosis so that she can purchase the "right medicine at the drug store." She reports that fellow workers have also been sick with "head colds," and 12 children at the day care center where she works have been absent because of coughs and colds.
Past Health History	JE has a history of seasonal allergic rhinitis that she treats by avoiding suspected allergens as much as possible. She has an episode of sinusitis about twice yearly. She self-treats with OTC antihistamines only if sneezing becomes uncontrollable. She denies history of cardiovascular disease, hypertension, hyperthyroidism, asthma, or diabetes mellitus. JE denies drug or food allergies, or the use of home remedies.
Life-Span Considerations	JE believes she finally has a position in a stable company that maximizes her contributions and also provides her with long-lasting career opportunities. She expresses concern that the infection will progress to another bout of sinusitis and cost her time away from work.
Psychosocial Considerations	JE chooses to self-treat with OTC cough and cold remedies as much as possible to keep costs down. She does not have health insurance because of her recent job change. She will pay for the entire cost of treatment.
Physical Exam Findings	*BP:* 116/72 mm Hg. 99.2° F-88-24. SpO_2 96%. Skin warm and dry. Tympanic membranes without bulging or retraction or redness; landmarks visible. Nasal mucosa pink but edematous with clear discharge. Oropharynx slightly reddened with clear, mucoid postnasal drip. No palpable cervical adenopathy or sinus tenderness. Breath sounds clear bilaterally.
Diagnostic Testing	Diagnostic testing is not indicated for patients with common cold or rhinitis.

DIAGNOSIS: Common cold

MANAGEMENT

Treatment Objectives	Prevent, minimize, and relieve the uncomfortable symptoms of a common cold while allowing the illness to run its course naturally.
Treatment Options	**Pharmacotherapy** • Expectorant: guaifenesin 1200 mg PO twice daily followed by 8 oz water • Decongestant: oxymetazoline 0.05%, two sprays each nostril twice daily–not to exceed 3 days' use • Analgesic-antipyretic: acetaminophen 500 mg tabs 2 PO every 4 to 6 hours PRN aches and fever • Antitussive: promethazine with codeine 1 to 2 tsp PO HS (if OTC drug is ineffective) **Patient Education** 1. Increase fluid intake, humidity during sleep, rest. 2. Inhale warm, moist heat (e.g., warm shower, humidifier). 3. Saline nasal irrigations 2 to 3 times daily per written instructions. 4. Return to clinic if no improvement in 7 days or symptoms worsen. **Evaluation** 1. Patient remains afebrile and head stuffiness has lessened. 2. Cough frequency, severity, and productivity has lessened; sputum less viscous.

CLINICAL REASONING ANALYSIS

Q1. You didn't give her antibiotics–but isn't that why she came in today?

A. Yes, that is why she came to the office today. An important principle to remember is that just because a patient requests antibiotics, it doesn't mean that it is appropriate to prescribe them. And, given that she has a common viral infection, use of antibiotics would be inappropriate. They are not effective for viruses and inappropriate use contributes to resistance.

Continued

RESPIRATORY

CASE STUDY   Common Cold—Cont'd

Q2. So, if I understand you correctly, the appropriate treatment for the common cold is to treat its symptoms, right?

A. Absolutely. We recommend guaifenesin to help loosen mucus in her head and chest. She can take an OTC analgesic-antipyretic such as acetaminophen for muscle aches and fever; and we gave her promethazine with codeine to use for her cough. The nasal irrigations will help with sinus congestion.

Q3. Why did you tell her to use oxymetazoline nasal spray for only 3 days? Isn't it better to use it regularly while she is ill?

A. I suggested oxymetazoline nasal spray to help in the short term with her nasal congestion. It is important though that the drug not be used in excess or more than 3 days because of the risk for rhinitis medicamentosa.

Q4. I guess I don't understand what rhinitis medicamentosa is.

A. Rhinitis medicamentosa is defined as rebound nasal congestion caused by the extended use of topical decongestants such as oxymetazoline, phenylephrine, and xylometazoline nasal sprays. It typically develops after 3 days of use. Receptors in the blood vessels of the nose up-regulate after repeated use, consequently requiring increased frequency of use and higher doses to avoid the rebound congestion that results when the effects of the drug wear off. Nasal passage swelling associated with rebound congestion may in time cause polyps that block nasal airflow. Surgery is needed to remove the polyps for a return to nasal breathing.

avoid rebound congestion. Instruct the patient to blow the nose gently before instilling nasal solutions or sprays and to avoid contamination of nasal droppers or spray tips. Administration devices should be rinsed in hot water after use and allowed to dry.

Help patients learn proper cough techniques. Patients with a dry, hacking cough are encouraged to take fluids freely to promote thin, easily raised sputum. Although the risk is small, opioid antitussives can lead to habituation and dependency. Tell the patient not to exceed recommended dosages. Increasing the dose does not appreciably increase antitussive efficacy.

The potential for abuse, however, is increased with an increase in dosage. Further, opioid adverse effects (i.e., respiratory depression) are potentiated by concurrent use of barbiturates or alcohol. The alcohol content of some antitussives can be as high as 40%. Opioids also tend to cause constipation.

Advise patients to minimize caffeine intake, because it may cause increased nervousness, tremors, or insomnia in the presence of decongestants. Have the patient contact the health care provider if headache, nausea, vomiting, irregular pulse, extreme nervousness or restlessness, confusion, delirium, or

Controversy

Effectiveness of Over-the-Counter Drugs for Coughs and Congestion

Jonathan J. Wolfe

Coughs and congestion bring many patients to the clinic for diagnosis and treatment. The symptoms may have already led the patient to a display of over-the-counter (OTC) preparations for coughs and colds. Drugs may not be needed, because the best agent for reducing viscosity of mucus is water. Water is the chief constituent of healthy secretions. Secretions are thickened by dust and cellular debris, but the presence of microorganisms changes the picture. Thick, clinging mucus hinders breathing. People with asthma and other obstructive processes quickly become acutely ill in the presence of mucous plugs within their airways.

Patients often take cough products based on guaifenesin, which is widely available without prescription. They swallow a dose of 5 to 10 mL, but then do not drink any liquid for a time. This is thought to allow the medicine to coat the throat, but it is the wrong way to take cough syrup. The high concentration of sugar in the syrup draws water to itself and dilutes the dose rather than providing a protective coating. In fact, guaifenesin is effective in oral solid form, acting to moisten the mucosa systemically.

Other OTC formulations contain a variety of active ingredients. Some include antihistamines that dry the respiratory tree further. Other drugs contain codeine, an antitussive that suppresses the cough center. However, after 48 hours or so, the antitussive effect of codeine falls off drastically. Dextromethorphan, a nonopioid antitussive, is a preferable drug,

but continued use of either product is counterproductive. Patients also may overlook the sugar and alcohol content of cough remedies. Patients with diabetes are at particular risk here.

A vaporizer may be a better answer than many OTC preparations. Cool mist vaporizers are inexpensive and effective. Perhaps more effective and convenient is simply running hot water in a tub or shower with the bathroom door shut. Rapid humidification of air in a small space may bring faster relief and reduce anxiety.

CLINICAL REASONING ANALYSIS

- What caution would you offer a patient with thickened secretions who is constantly blowing her nose?
- What product or products would you recommend to the patient whose nostrils are reddened and cracked from discharge and blowing?
- What method of removing thickened secretions from the nares of an infant would you recommend to parents?
- What other benefits will a patient with congestion and a low-grade fever derive from increased hydration of the mucosa?
- What characteristics of sputum or sinus discharge indicate that the patient requires an evaluation by the health care provider and therapy with antibiotics?
- What inequities do you see if a low-income patient spends money for OTC remedies in an attempt to avoid the cost of medical care and prescription drugs?

EVIDENCE-BASED PHARMACOTHERAPEUTICS

Over-the-Counter Formulations for Acute Cough

■ Background

A cough is a common, yet taxing, malady associated with a common cold. Many health care providers recommend the use of over-the-counter (OTC) drugs and just as many people self-treat with OTC cough and cold remedies. Yet there is little evidence to suggest that these drugs are effective in relieving an acute cough.

■ Research Article

Schroeder, K., and Fahey, T. Over-the-counter medications for acute cough in children and adults in ambulatory settings. *The Cochrane Database of Systematic Reviews. 2004,* Issue 4. Art. No. CD001831. DOI: 10.1002/14651858CD001831.pub2.

Purpose

The purpose of this study was to evaluate the efficacy of OTC drugs for acute cough.

Design

This meta-analysis examined 24 randomized, controlled, comparative studies (17 in adults, 7 in children) carried out in ambulatory care settings. Each of the studies looked at the comparison between OTC cough formulations and placebo in adults ($N = 2876$) and children ($N = 516$) who had an acute cough. Data on cough relief and a variety of continuous and categorical data were gathered.

Methods

Two reviewers independently extracted study data from the Cochrane Central Register of Controlled Trials (CENTRAL) (*The Cochrane Library* Issue 2, 2004); MEDLINE (January 1966 to June Week 3, 2004); EMBASE (January 1990 to March 2004); and the UK Department of Health National Research Register (December 2003). Personal collections of references and reference lists of the reviewers were also searched. Inquiries to the authors of the studies and to pharmaceutical companies were made requesting information on additional published or unpublished studies.

Data from each of the 24 studies extracted were examined for pertinent references, and the quality of the studies was assessed. The authors of each of the studies analyzed were contacted for additional information. Quantitative analyses were performed when appropriate data were available.

Findings

Antitussives—6 of the 24 trials weighed antitussives against placebo. It was found that codeine showed no more efficacy than placebo in reducing cough. Two of the studies found dextromethorphan was more efficacious compared to placebo in relieving cough symptoms, whereas the third study showed no effectiveness. One of the studies suggested that antitussives were no more effective in children than a placebo.

Expectorants—There were no statistically significant differences between the treatment group and the control group in the use of guaifenesin to improve cough frequency and severity. In the larger of two studies, 75% of the subjects taking guaifenesin for a cough noted that the drug was helpful compared with 31% in the control group. In a second study, cough frequency and severity improved for both groups. Neither of the studies included children.

Mucolytics—In another trial, a mucolytic was compared with placebo. The treatment group noted reduced cough frequency and symptoms scores on days 4 and 8 of the study. Results of another study favored active use of a mucolytic over a placebo from days 4 through 10.

Antihistamine-decongestant combinations—In these two studies, antihistamine-decongestant combinations were compared with placebo. The group treated with a combination of antihistamine and decongestant showed significant symptom improvement when compared with placebo. In a second study, no differences were found between the treatment and the control groups. Two additional studies that included children also noted no differences between the treatment and the placebo groups.

Antihistamines—Three studies compared antihistamines with placebo for symptom reduction. Antihistamine use in children with colds showed that treatment with antihistamines was no more effective than placebo in relieving symptoms. The other two studies showed antihistamines were no more effective than placebo in relieving cough symptoms.

Conclusions

Results of this review suggest there is no good evidence for, or against, the efficacy of OTC drugs for acute cough. Review the results of this study with caution, considering the differences in the studies in terms of design, populations of interest, treatment, and outcomes. The studies were small in number, with results that were often contradictory. Also, the effect sizes of many of the studies were unclear, and the clinical relevancy of the positive results is questionable.

■ Implications for Research

Additional evidence about the effectiveness of OTC cough remedies would indeed be helpful. For the patient, the ability to judge the effectiveness of self-care modalities goes a long way not only in helping to manage symptoms, but also to reduce lost work days due to acute cough, and the time and cost of trips to the health care provider.

---

muscle tremors occur. Drowsiness is a common adverse effect of many cough and cold preparations. Also advise the patient to use caution when driving or operating machinery. Counsel patients on the management of opioid-induced constipation.

Evaluation

The effectiveness of topical nasal decongestants is dramatic, with efficacy noted within minutes. The patient often reports that breathing is easier, postnasal drip is relieved, and nasal discharge and sneezing are reduced. Oral decongestants are usually effective within 1 hour.

The effectiveness of expectorants is demonstrated by an ability of the patient to effect a productive cough with increased sputum clearance. The effectiveness of a mucolytic drug is demonstrated by decreased sputum viscosity and increased productivity.

The characteristics of the patient's cough (frequency, severity, productive, sputum volume, viscosity, and difficulty raising sputum) should improve with use of a mucolytic or antitussive. Monitor the patient for adverse reactions and hypersensitivity responses.

Antitussives produce cough suppression, a decrease in the frequency and duration of coughing spells, and improvement in the patient's ability to sleep. Check to be sure the secretions have not thickened. Although the dosage of an opioid antitussive is lower than that used for pain, the patient's level of consciousness and respiratory depth and rate should be noted before administration.

KEY POINTS

- Common colds are the most common acute infection in human beings, accounting for 10% of office visits to health care providers annually in the United States. It is estimated that 15% to 20% of the population suffer from chronic or recurrent nasal congestion.
- Etiologic agents associated with the common cold include rhinovirus, influenza virus, parainfluenza virus, respiratory syncytial virus, corona virus, adenovirus, echovirus, and Coxsackie virus.
- The virus of the common cold is transmitted by direct inoculation of the mucous membranes of the nose and eyes, usually from contaminated hands.
- Treatment objectives include strategies that prevent, minimize, or help correct symptoms associated with upper respiratory disorders.
- Adequate hydration should be maintained throughout therapy.

- Expectorants and mucolytics stimulate the flow and reduce the viscosity of respiratory tract secretions. The effectiveness of an expectorant is demonstrated by the patient's ability to effect a productive cough with increased sputum clearance.
- Nasal decongestants are adrenergic agents that shrink mucous membranes, thus reducing congestion and improving nasal drainage. The effectiveness of nasal decongestants is demonstrated by the patient's report that he or she can breathe easier, postnasal drip is relieved, and nasal discharge and sneezing are reduced.
- Opioid and nonopioid antitussives act centrally or peripherally to suppress cough, reducing the frequency and intensity of the cough. Antitussives should produce cough suppression, a decrease in the frequency and duration of coughing spells, and improvement in the patient's ability to sleep.

Bibliography

Agency for Health Care Policy and Research. (1999). *Diagnosis and treatment of acute bacterial rhinosinusitis.* Evidence report/technology assessment No. 9 (ACHPR Publication No. 9). Rockville, MD: Author.

Arroll, B. (2006). Common cold. *Clinical Evidence, 6*(13), 1853–1861.

Arroll, B. (2005). Common cold. *Clinical Evidence, 6*(15), 2006–2014.

Arroll, B. (2005). Antibiotics for upper respiratory tract infections: An overview of Cochrane reviews. *Respiratory Medicine, 99*(3), 255–261.

Arroll, B., and Kenealy, T. (2005). Antibiotics for the common cold and acute purulent rhinitis. *Cochrane Database of Systematic Reviews. 2005,* Issue 3. Art. No. CD000247. DOI: 10.1002/14651858. CD000247.pub2.

Charles, C., Yelmene, M., and Luo, G. (2004). Recent advances in rhinovirus therapeutics. *Current Drug Targets: Infectious Disorders, 4*(4), 331–337.

Eccles, R. (2006). Efficacy and safety of over-the-counter analgesics in the treatment of common cold and flu. *Journal of Clinical Pharmacy and Therapeutics, 31*(4), 309–319.

Eccles, R. (2006). Mechanisms of the placebo effect of sweet cough syrups. *Respiratory, Physiology, and Neurobiology, 152*(3), 340–348.

Gilbert, D., Moellering Jr., R, Sande, J., et al. (2007). *The Sanford guide to antimicrobial therapy* (37th ed.). Hyde Park, VT: Antimicrobial Therapy.

Goroll, A., and Mulley, A. (2005). *Primary care medicine: Office evaluation and management of the adult patient* (5th ed.). Philadelphia: Lippincott, Williams & Wilkins.

National Institute of Health. (2004). The common cold. Available online: www.niaid.nih.gov/factsheets/cold.htm. Accessed May 24, 2007.

Pratter, M. (2006). Cough and the common cold: ACCP evidence-based clinical practice guidelines. *Chest, 129*(1 Suppl), 72S–74S.

Turner, R. (2005). New considerations in the treatment and prevention of rhinovirus infections. *Pediatric Annals, 34*(1), 53–57.

Schroeder, K., and Fahey, T. Over-the-counter medications for acute cough in children and adults in ambulatory settings. *Cochrane Database of Systematic Reviews. 2004,* Issue 4. Art. No. CD001831. DOI: 10.1002/14651858.CD001831.pub2.

Sitzman, K. (2005). Managing the common cold. *AAOHN: The Official Journal of the American Association of Occupational Health Nurses, 53*(2), 96.

53

Drugs Used in the Treatment of Diabetes Mellitus

Diabetes mellitus is a metabolic disorder characterized by inappropriate hyperglycemia resulting from defects in insulin secretion, insulin action, or both. The incidence of diabetes mellitus is reaching epidemic proportions, affecting nearly 18.2 million people in the United States, with about 30% of these cases going undiagnosed. Approximately 20% of the population in the United States is at risk for the disease as a result of advancing age, obesity, and decreased physical activity.

Uncontrolled diabetes leads to long-term complications, including retinopathy, nephropathy, and neuropathy. The majority of patients who have type 2 diabetes mellitus (T2DM) also have hypertension and dyslipidemia, and also have 2 to 5 times the risk of cardiovascular disease. Seventy-five percent of patients with T2DM will die of diabetes-related cardiovascular disease (i.e., heart disease, stroke).

Pharmacologic therapies allow a patient with diabetes to achieve near-normal glycemic control when combined with appropriate lifestyle changes, specifically, diet and exercise. Landmark studies such as the Diabetes Control and Complications Trial (DCCT) (DCCT Research Group, 1990) for patients with T1DM and the United Kingdom Prospective Diabetes Study (UKPDS) (Clarke, 2004) for patients with T2DM, support that glycemic control postpones, prevents, or slows progression of retinal, renal, and neurologic complications.

DIABETES MELLITUS

EPIDEMIOLOGY AND ETIOLOGY

Type 1 Diabetes

Type 1 diabetes (T1DM) results from autoimmune destruction of pancreatic beta cells that leads to absolute insulin deficiency, and accounts for 5% to 10% of those diagnosed with diabetes. Markers of the immune destruction of beta cells are present in 85% to 90% of individuals when fasting hyperglycemia is first detected. The disease has strong human lymphocytic antigen (HLA) associations, with linkage to the *DQA* and *DQB* genes.

The rate of beta cell destruction is variable, rapid in some individuals (generally infants and children) and slower in adults. By and large, patients present to the health care provider with the classic complaints of diabetes (i.e., polyuria, polydipsia, polyphagia) and markedly elevated blood glucose levels. In some cases, ketoacidosis may be the first indication that diabetes is present. T1DM commonly occurs in childhood and adolescence, but can occur at any age.

Viral triggers such as congenital rubella and Coxsackie B_4 infection, as well as environmental toxins, or hormonal alterations during pregnancy and at puberty are thought to initiate the process of beta cell destruction.

Type 2 Diabetes

T2DM accounts for 90% to 95% of those diagnosed with diabetes. Previously known as non–insulin dependent diabetes or adult-onset diabetes, T2DM is characterized by insulin resistance and relative (rather than absolute) insulin deficiency; however, autoimmune destruction of beta cells does not occur. Insulin secretion is defective and insufficient to compensate for insulin resistance.

The onset of symptoms in T2DM is slower and generally not of an acute nature (Table 53-1). T2DM is frequently not diagnosed until complications appear. The risk of developing T2DM increases with age, obesity, and lack of physical activity. In the last 10 years, the incidence of T2DM in children and adolescents has risen sharply.

Gestational Diabetes

The carbohydrate intolerance that develops with the onset of pregnancy, or that is first recognized during pregnancy, is known as gestational diabetes (GDM). Approximately 7% of all pregnancies are complicated by GDM. Women with previously undiagnosed T2DM are included in this classification. Untreated or poorly treated GDM results in higher morbidity and mortality risks for mother and fetus. Congenital birth defects and macrosomia are more common in infants born to women with GDM. Both women with GDM and their offspring are at a higher risk for development of subsequent T2DM.

Prediabetes

The term prediabetes refers to elevated blood sugar levels that do not meet the diagnostic criteria for a diagnosis of diabetes but are elevated nonetheless. There are two forms of prediabetes: impaired fasting glucose (IFG) and impaired glucose tolerance (IGT). Patients with IGT have fasting glucose levels over 100 mg/dL but less than 125 mg/dL. Those with IGT have elevated 2-hour postprandial glucose levels ranging from 140 mg/dL up to 199 mg/dL. These prediabetic levels are potential risk factors not only for diabetes but also cardiovascular disease in the future.

Other Specific Types

Diabetes may also develop as the result of genetic defects in beta cell function; defects in the action of insulin; and diseases of the exocrine pancreas (such as cystic fibrosis). It can also be induced by drugs or chemicals. The second-generation antipsychotic drugs are associated with the development of T2DM.

PATHOPHYSIOLOGY

Insulin is a hormone produced in the beta cells of the islets of Langerhans: it is formed from a substance called *proinsulin*. When the pancreas is stimulated, proinsulin is broken apart;

TABLE 53-1 Comparisons of Type 1 and Type 2 Diabetes Mellitus

Features	T1DM	T2DM
Etiology	Viral infection	Unknown
Pathology	Autoimmune destruction of pancreatic beta cell	Insulin resistance Beta cell exhaustion
Symptoms	Abrupt onset: polyuria, polyphagia, polydipsia, fatigue	Frequently none: fatigue, blurred vision, presence of complications evident at time of diagnosis
Antigen patterns	HLA-DR4, HLA-DR3	None
Antibodies	Present at diagnosis	None
Endogenous insulin and C-peptide levels	None	Low, normal or high
Body weight at diagnosis	Nonobese	Obese in 85% of cases
Drug management	Insulin therapy	Oral therapy. Insulin required for 20% to 30% of patients
Medical nutrition therapy	Required	Required
Exercise program	Required	Required

HLA, Human lymphocytic antigen.

insulin and the connecting peptide (C-peptide) are both secreted and enter the blood stream. Insulin is released when blood glucose concentrations exceed 100 mg/dL.

Beta cell dysfunction leads to impaired insulin synthesis and/or release, and peripheral insulin resistance. *Insulin resistance* implies decreased sensitivity of target cells (i.e., muscle, adipose, and liver cells) to insulin and occurs with both the body's own insulin as well as to injected insulin. Insulin is necessary for the metabolism of carbohydrates, proteins, and fats. The actions of insulin include the following:

- Stimulating the entry of glucose into cells for use as an energy source
- Promoting storage of glucose as glycogen (glycogenesis) in muscle and liver cells
- Stimulating the entry of amino acid into cells, thereby enhancing protein synthesis
- Enhancing fat storage (lipogenesis) and preventing breakdown of fat for energy (lipolysis and ketogenesis)
- Inhibiting the production of glucose from liver or muscle glycogen (glycogenolysis)
- Inhibiting formation of glucose from noncarbohydrates, such as amino acids (gluconeogenesis)

Insulin deficiency impairs glucose uptake in peripheral tissues (primarily muscle) and liver, leading to hyperglycemia. Insulin deficiency also causes impaired protein synthesis and excessive protein breakdown. The resulting increase in amino acids leads to increased hepatic glucose production (by means of gluconeogenesis), and hyperglycemia. Severe insulin deficiency and increased counterregulatory hormones cause excessive hydrolysis of triglycerides, the stored form of fat, releasing greater amounts of free fatty acids and glycerol. In patients with T2DM, excessive amounts of ketone bodies can be formed in the liver from free fatty acids, resulting in ketonemia and metabolic acidosis. Hyperglycemia also leads to osmotic diuresis, causing hypotonic fluid losses, dehydration, and electrolyte depletion.

Diagnosis

There are three ways to diagnose diabetes. Each test result must be confirmed at a later date unless unmistakable symptoms of elevated blood sugar are present. The fasting blood sugar (FBS) is the preferred diagnostic test.

1. The presence of symptoms characteristic of diabetes (i.e., polyuria, polydipsia, polyphagia, blurry vision, and unexplained weight loss) and a random blood glucose level of 200 mg/dL or higher. A random blood glucose level is obtained any time of the day without regard to the time since the last meal.
2. An FBS over 126 mg/dL. Fasting is defined as no caloric intake for 8 hours.
3. Two-hour postprandial blood glucose levels are 200 mg/dL or higher during an oral glucose tolerance test using a 75-gram glucose load.

T1DM is diagnosed primarily by clinical signs and symptoms, but the diagnosis can also be supported by the absence of C-peptide and the presence of markers of beta cell destruction. These markers include islet cell autoantibodies, autoantibodies to insulin, autoantibodies to glutamic acid decarboxylase (GAD), and autoantibodies to tyrosine phosphatases.

Proinsulin is the precursor to insulin. It is composed of alpha and beta chains linked by a third polypeptide chain called the C-connecting peptide, or *C-peptide*. For every molecule of insulin in the blood, there is one C-peptide molecule. C-peptide levels can be measured and used as an indicator of insulin production. C-peptide test results can also be used to determine if hyperglycemia is the result of decreased insulin production or of a decline in the cellular uptake of glucose.

Patients with T1DM have little or no C-peptide in their plasma, whereas in patients with T2DM, C-peptide levels may be normal or decreased. Normal plasma C-peptide values in persons without diabetes range from 0.5 to 3 mcg/mL.

PHARMACOTHERAPEUTIC OPTIONS

Individuals with T1DM require insulin for *glycemic control.* Individuals with T2DM can be managed with a variety of approaches, including administration of insulin, stimulation of insulin release from beta cells, increasing peripheral tissue utilization of glucose, decreasing hepatic glucose production, and decreasing utilization of ingested carbohydrates. Drug treatment modalities for T1DM include rapid-, short-, intermediate-, and long-acting insulins. Several of these insulins are now available in combinations.

Insulins

▥ Indications

Insulin is required for all patients who have T1DM and for many with T2DM. For about 58% of persons with

T2DM, the gradual, progressive decline in beta cell function eventually leads to the need for supplemental insulin. Insulin is started when glucose and glycosylated hemoglobin A$_{1c}$ (now known simply as A$_{1c}$) goals are not met with other therapies.

Pharmacodynamics

Beta cells of the pancreatic islet cells monitor blood glucose levels constantly so that insulin secretion is closely linked to changes in glycemia (Fig. 53-1). Insulin is secreted in two major patterns: basal and postprandial. Basal secretion produces relatively constant, low levels of insulin that act to maintain normal blood glucose levels between meals. Insulin secretion at meals normally occurs in two phases: an early burst of "first-phase" insulin secretion, followed by a smaller but sustained peak of "second-phase" postprandial secretion. The first phase consists of a rapid secretion of insulin into portal circulation and serves to stop production of glucose in the liver; this first phase lasts only 20 to 30 minutes. The second phase of insulin secretion lasts 2 to 3 hours and serves to minimize postprandial glycemic elevations.

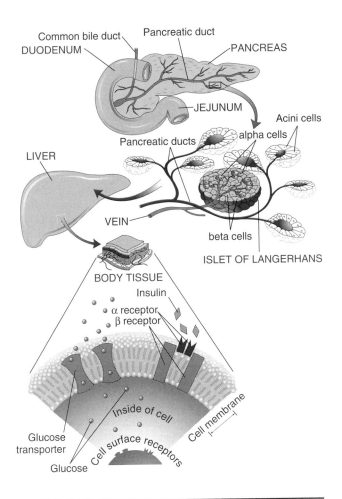

FIGURE 53-1 Insulin-Glucose Balance. Insulin is released in a pulsatile fashion by beta cells and enters portal circulation, where it travels directly to the liver. About 50% of the insulin is either used or degraded. Alpha cells in the islets of Langerhans secrete glucagon. Glucagon maintains blood glucose by increasing the release of glucose from the liver into the circulation.

Pharmacokinetics

The manufacturing of beef insulin for human use in the United States was discontinued in 1998. Beginning in January 2006, pork insulin for human use is no longer manufactured or marketed in the United States. Insulin is now produced through recombinant DNA (rDNA) technology using *Saccharomyces cerevisiae* (bakers' yeast), or a nonpathogenic laboratory strain of *Escherichia coli* as the production bacteria. Insulin analogues are genetically engineered human insulins in which the structure of the insulin molecule has been modified to alter the rate of absorption and the duration of action within the body. The pharmacokinetics of insulins are identified in Table 53-2.

INSULIN THERAPY. Insulin therapy can be divided into three types. *Bolus insulin* (or prandial insulin) doses using rapid- or fast-acting insulins are given before meals so as to prevent the rise in postprandial blood glucose levels that occur after eating. Corrections in blood glucose levels can only be made with rapid- or fast-acting insulins. *Basal insulin* dosages of longer-acting insulins suppress glucose production between meals and during the night. *Supplemental insulin* doses are added to a treatment regimen to make corrections for insufficient basal or bolus doses of insulin.

Rapid-Acting Insulin Analogues. There are three rapid-acting insulin analogues: insulin lispro (Humalog), insulin aspart (NovoLog), and insulin glulisine (Aprida). Rapid-acting insulins are absorbed faster and have a shorter duration of action compared to regular insulin. They are used for the bolus component of intensive insulin therapy. Rapid-acting insulin analogues should be injected 15 minutes before a meal or immediately after a meal. Rapid-acting insulins are used in insulin pump therapy. Inhaled insulin (Exubera) is a rapid-acting inhaled insulin new to the treatment armamentarium (see later discussion).

Fast-Acting Insulin. Regular insulin is produced by rDNA technology and is structurally identical to insulin produced by the human pancreas. Regular insulin has a short duration of action and is administered 30 minutes before eating a meal.

Intermediate-Acting Insulin. Humulin N is a crystalline suspension of human insulin with protamine and zinc and provides intermediate-acting insulin with a slower onset of action and longer duration of activity than that of regular insulin.

Fixed-ratio premixed insulins provide protamine for basal coverage in one injection and a rapid-acting insulin analogue for bolus coverage (see Table 53-2). These formulations include NovoLog mix 70/30 (70% insulin aspart–protamine suspension and 30% insulin aspart injection), Humalog Mix 75/25 (75% insulin lispro–protamine suspension and 25% insulin lispro injection), and Humalog Mix 50/50 (50% insulin lispro–protamine suspension and 50% insulin lispro injection). Premixed insulin helps with patients' adherence to therapy and reduces errors associated with mixing insulin.

Long-Acting Insulin. Insulin glargine is a human insulin analogue designed with a low aqueous solubility at a neutral pH. It is completely soluble at a pH of 4. After injection into subcutaneous (subQ) tissue, the acidic solution is neutralized, leading to formation of microprecipitates from which small amounts of insulin glargine are slowly released, which results in a relative concentration/time profile over 24 hours with no pronounced peak. This profile allows for once-daily dosing as the patient's basal insulin. The prolonged action of insulin detemir is mediated by slow systemic absorption of insulin detemir molecules from the injection (see Table 53-2).

PHARMACOKINETICS
TABLE 53-2 Insulins

Drug	Onset	Peak	Duration
RAPID-ACTING INSULINS			
lispro (Humalog)	15 min	30–90 min	3–5 hr
aspart (NovoLog)	15 min	40–50 min	3–5 hr
glulisine (Apidra)	20 min	55 min	3–5 hr
Inhaled insulin (Exubera)	15 min	1 hr	6 hr
SHORT-ACTING INSULIN			
Regular	30 min	2.5–5 hr	8 hr
INTERMEDIATE-ACTING INSULIN			
NPH	2–4 hr	4–10 hr	10–16 hr
LONG-ACTING INSULINS			
Insulin detemir (Levemir)	Slow	6–8 hr	12–24 hr†
Insulin glargine (Lantus)	1 hr	Peakless	>24 hr†
COMBINATION INSULINS*			
Humulin 70/30	15 min	Dual	10–16 hr
Humulin 50/50	15 min	Dual	10–16 hr
Novolin 70/30	15 min	Dual	10–16 hr
Humalog Mix 75/25	15 min	Dual	10–16 hr
Humalog Mix 50/50	15 min	Dual	10–16 hr
NovoLog Mix 75/25	15 min	Dual	10–16 hr

*Combination insulins have dual peaks, with the regular peaking in about 2.5 hr and the NPH peaking 4–10 hr later.
†Many patients will need to take insulin detemir or glargine twice daily.
NPH, Neutral protamine Hagedorn insulin.

Factors affecting the onset, the degree, and the duration of action of insulin activity include the type of insulin, dosage, the presence of insulin antibodies, injection technique, injection site, and individual patient response. The quickest absorption of the drug occurs through the abdomen, followed by absorption through the arms, the thighs, and the buttocks.

▥ Adverse Effects and Contraindications

The major adverse effect of insulin is hypoglycemia. Hypoglycemia occurs because of excess insulin as the result of insufficient or ill-timed food intake, increased physical activity, and increased insulin absorption rates.

Redness, swelling, or itching at the injection site may occur, but these symptoms typically diminish in a few days to a few weeks. Rare instances of insulin allergy have been reported. Symptoms of insulin allergy include generalized pruritus, shortness of breath, wheezing, hypotension, rapid pulse, and sweating. Patients having allergic symptoms should receive symptomatic treatment before switching to different insulin with the same duration of action (i.e., insulin lispro to insulin aspart). There are no contraindications to the administration of rDNA insulins.

Dawn phenomenon may occur in some patients taking insulin, with blood glucose levels remaining normal until approximately 3 AM, when nocturnal effects of growth hormone elevate blood glucose levels. In contrast, *Somogyi phenomenon* occurs during the night and consists of an insulin-induced hypoglycemic reaction with a rebound elevation in blood glucose levels. Compensatory mechanisms such as increased secretion of epinephrine, cortisol, and growth hormone are activated in the body's attempt to oppose the excessive insulin.

Lipodystrophies, lipohypertrophy (lumps) or lipoatrophy (depressions), occur as a result of insulin impurity and improper injection technique. *Lipoatrophy*, a pitting of fatty tissue, is an immune phenomenon that occurs in a small number of patients and is related to purity of insulin preparation. Using highly purified insulin preparations reduces the occurrence of atrophy. Lipoatrophy is treated by injecting rDNA insulin around the edge of the atrophied area. *Lipohypertrophy*, or fatty thickening of the lipid tissues, slows insulin absorption and is best prevented by rotation of injection sites.

▥ Drug Interactions

Glucose metabolism is affected by many substances, and therefore patients should be watched closely and may need insulin dosage to be adjusted. Many substances increase the blood glucose–lowering effects of insulin and increase the potential for hypoglycemia. The signs of hypoglycemia may be blunted or absent when sympatholytic drugs such as beta blockers, clonidine, guanethidine, and reserpine are used (Table 53-3).

▥ Dosage Regimen

Insulin is available in concentrations of 100 units/mL or 500 units/mL. Insulin dosage and the timing of the injection is based on the patient's glycemic response to food intake, exercise, and the type of insulin used (Table 53-4). U-500 insulin is used for patients with insulin resistance who require large doses. The time course of insulin action usually requires three or more doses per day to meet glycemic goals.

A single-injection regimen is commonly used for patients with T2DM who are also being treated with oral drug therapy. An intermediate- or long-acting insulin preparation is usually used. Bedtime administration improves FBS control by

DRUG INTERACTIONS
TABLE **53-3** Insulin

Interactive Drugs	Interaction
Corticosteroids, Estrogens, isoniazid, niacin, Oral contraceptives, Phenothiazines, Thyroid replacement hormones	Elevates blood glucose levels
ACEIs, Beta blockers, disopyramide, Fibrates, fluoxetine, MAOIs, Oral antidiabetic drugs, propoxyphene, Salicylates, somatostatin, Sulfonamide antibiotics	Increases potential for hypoglycemia
Beta blockers, clonidine, reserpine, guanethidine	Masks symptoms of hypoglycemia
Alcohol, Beta blockers, clonidine, lithium	Either increases or decreases blood glucose
pentamidine	Hypoglycemia followed by hyperglycemia

ACEIs, Angiotensin-converting enzyme inhibitors; *MAOIs,* monoamine oxidase inhibitors.

TABLE **53-4** Sample Plan for Preprandial Rapid-Acting Insulin*

Using an Insulin-to-Carbohydrate Ratio for Meal Insulin Dose	For a Constant-Carbohydrate Diet with a Fixed Insulin Dose for the Meal
If blood glucose is < 50 mg/dL • Delay injection until 10 to 15 min after starting to eat; –or– • Include at least 15 grams of rapidly available carbohydrate at the start of the meal.	• If the planned meal is larger than usual, increase insulin analogue by 1 to 2 units. • If the planned meal is smaller than usual, decrease the insulin analogue by 1–2 units.
If blood glucose is 70–130 mg/dL • Take prescribed pre-meal dose of insulin analogue.	*Adjustment for Exercise* • Do not exercise at the peak action time of insulin • Decrease insulin by 10%–20% for the meal before planned exercise; –or– • Eat additional carbohydrate at the meal preceding planned exercise; omit insulin for this additional food. • Eat additional carbohydrate if preexercise blood glucose level is less than 100 mg/dL. Eat 10–15 grams of carbohydrate for every hour of moderate physical activity. • Eat 15–30 grams of carbohydrate for every hour of intense physical activity.

*Target blood glucose level: 70–130 mg/dL or a mean target of 100 mg/dL; correction factor is 1 unit per 50 mg/dL.

suppressing nighttime hepatic glucose production. Once-daily injections of intermediate- or long-acting insulin may be used when dosages are less than 30 units per day. Twice-daily dosing of insulin may be required when larger doses are required owing to enhanced peak effect with larger doses.

In a two-injection regimen, insulin is administered in the morning, before breakfast, and before the evening meal. This may include only intermediate-acting insulin; rapid- or fast-acting insulin mixed with intermediate-acting insulin, or premixed formulations. Two-injection regimens using only intermediate-acting insulin are not appropriate for patients with T1DM. Two thirds of the daily dosage of insulin can be administered before breakfast and one third of the dose given before the evening meal for patients who eat three meals per day.

For patient using a three-injection regimen, rapid- or fast-acting insulin and intermediate-acting insulin is given before breakfast, rapid- or fast-acting insulin alone is given before the evening meal, and intermediate-acting insulin alone before bedtime. This regimen reduces the risk of nocturnal hypoglycemia (2 AM to 4 AM) and reduces early-morning (5 AM) hyperglycemia by providing insulin coverage for release of cortisol and growth hormone (dawn phenomenon).

In a four-injection regimen, rapid- or fast-acting insulin is administered before each meal, and long-acting insulin is administered once a day. The dosage of rapid- or fast-acting insulin is based on predetermined insulin/carbohydrate ratios.

Continuous subQ insulin administration is provided by an insulin pump. Pump therapy provides a continuous basal amount of insulin administered in addition to bolus doses given before meals. Bolus insulin formulas are based on insulin/carbohydrate ratios and adjusted based on evaluation of blood glucose monitoring results.

Correction-dose insulin may be added to any of these regimens to treat blood glucose elevation at the time of the meal. Blood glucose elevation is treated with rapid- or fast-acting insulin.

Lab Considerations

The effectiveness of insulin therapy is measured by FBS values, blood glucose values before meals, and blood glucose values measured 2 hours after eating. Blood glucose levels should return to preprandial levels 2 hours after eating. Quarterly measurement of the A_{1c} level is the standard of care for the monitoring of long-term glycemic control.

Recombinant Human Insulin Inhalation Powder

Indications

Human rDNA inhaled insulin (Exubera) was approved by the Food and Drug Administration (FDA) in January 2006 for the treatment of adult patients with diabetes mellitus for the control of hyperglycemia. For patients with T1DM, inhaled insulin is used in combination with basal insulin. In patients with T2DM, inhaled insulin can be used as monotherapy or in combination with oral diabetes drugs or longer-acting insulins.

Pharmacodynamics

Insulin delivered into pulmonary circulation by means of a nebulizer provides effective meal-related glycemic control.

ENDOCRINE

The pulmonary alveolar bed provides a large vascular bed for the absorption of the dry powdered insulin formulation.

Pharmacokinetics

Inhaled insulin has an onset of action similar to that of rapid-acting insulin analogues and is given just before a meal. Its peak effect and duration of action is similar to that of regular insulin. The prolonged duration of action of inhaled insulin relative to rapid-acting insulin is achieved by making use of the dependence of pulmonary absorption of insulin on the size and dissociation rate of insulin particles (see Table 53-2).

Adverse Effects and Contraindications

The most common adverse effect of inhaled insulin is hypoglycemia. Mild to moderate cough is seen in 2% to 30% of patients using inhaled insulin.

Inhaled insulin is contraindicated for use in patients hypersensitive to the insulin or any of its components. Do not prescribe it for patients who smoke or who have stopped smoking within the past 6 months. If a patient resumes smoking, inhaled insulin must be discontinued because of the increased risk of hypoglycemia. **Inhaled insulin is not recommended for use in patients with lung disease such as asthma or chronic obstructive pulmonary disease (COPD).**

Drug Interactions

Drug interactions for inhaled insulin are the same as for other insulin preparations (see Table 53-3). Bronchodilators and other inhaled drugs may alter absorption. Consistent timing of dosing of bronchodilators relative to the inhaled insulin administration, close monitoring of blood glucose concentrations, and dose titration, as appropriate, are recommended.

Dosage Regimen

Inhaled insulin is available in 1-mg or 3-mg unit dose blisters inserted into a handheld inhalation device about the size of an eyeglasses carrying case. Individual doses are released into the chamber for inhalation into the lungs by pumping the inhaler handle and pressing the button. Careful patient education is required to ensure that the patient is using the device correctly and is getting the correct dose (see Table 53-4). Inhaled insulin prescriptions are accompanied by a drug administration guide containing FDA-approved information written especially for patients.

Lab Considerations

Since inhaled insulin may affect lung function, perform spirometry (forced expiratory volume in 1 second [FEV_1]) testing before starting the drug, after the first 6 months of use, and annually thereafter. Repeat pulmonary function tests in patients who experience a decline of over 20% in FEV_1 from baseline. Discontinue the drug if there is a 20% decline from baseline FEV_1.

Biguanides

✦ metformin (Glucophage, Glucophage XR, Riomet); ✦ Fortamet, Glycon, Glucophage

Indications

Metformin is an insulin-sensitizing drug with potent antihyperglycemic properties. It is used in combination with diet and exercise therapy for lowering blood glucose levels in patients with T2DM. Metformin is effective as monotherapy or in combination with sulfonylureas, insulin, and thiazolidinediones. Clinically, metformin lowers fasting and postprandial hyperglycemia. Metformin also decreases plasma very low-density lipoprotein (VLDL) triglycerides, resulting in modest decreases in plasma triglycerides and total cholesterol. Metformin reduces FBS by 50 to 70 mg/dL and A_{1c} by 1.5% to 2%. Use of metformin is appropriate for patients who are overweight or obese and have insulin resistance.

Pharmacodynamics

Metformin acts primarily to reverse the defects of diabetes by reducing hepatic glucose production, but also by reducing intestinal glucose production and increasing insulin sensitivity (improved peripheral glucose uptake and utilization). Its major mode of action is to reduce hepatic glucose output, which is increased at least twofold in patients with T2DM. Metformin does not increase insulin secretion from the pancreas, and is not associated with hypoglycemia at therapeutic doses except in special situations. Metformin does not cause weight gain.

Pharmacokinetics

Metformin is not protein bound and is widely distributed through the body. Metformin does not undergo hepatic biotransformation or biliary excretion; rather it is excreted unchanged in the urine, with 90% of the drug eliminated within 24 hours. Peak serum levels are reached 1 to 3 hours after an oral dose. Bioavailability of metformin tablets is approximately 50% to 60%. Food decreases the extent and slightly delays the absorption of metformin; however, it is recommended that it be taken with food.

Adverse Effects and Contraindications

Diarrhea, nausea, vomiting, abdominal bloating, flatulence, anorexia may occur in about 30% of the patients during initiation of the drug. These effects are temporary and often diminish with continued treatment. To minimize effects, initiate therapy at low doses, and gradually increase at weekly or biweekly intervals. Hypoglycemia may occur if caloric intake is inadequate, with strenuous exercise, or in combination with other hypoglycemic drugs. Monitor patients for possible development of anemia since metformin can inhibit absorption of cyanocobalamin (vitamin B_{12}).

Metformin may increase blood lactate levels as a result of enhanced lactate production and carries an FDA-mandated black box warning regarding lactic acidosis. Metformin-associated lactic acidosis is common, but serious metabolic complications are more likely to occur in patients with renal insufficiency. Cardiovascular collapse from acute heart failure, myocardial infarction or other conditions characterized by hypoxia, or any other cause has been associated with lactic acidosis. Discontinue metformin if any of these events occur.

Radiologic studies (e.g., computed tomography [CT]) that use intravenous iodinated contrast material has been associated in metformin-treated patients with lactic acidosis and can lead to acute renal failure. Discontinue metformin temporarily before these procedures and withhold for 48 hours following the procedure. Restart metformin after kidney function has been revaluated and found to be normal.

▲ **Metformin is contraindicated for use in patients with renal disease, defined as serum creatinine levels greater than 1.5 mg/dL in men and greater than 1.4 mg/dL in women.** Impaired kidney function slows elimination and may cause metformin accumulation. Metformin use is also contraindicated for patients with heart failure that requires drug therapy, in patients with hypersensitivity to metformin, and in the presence of acute or chronic metabolic acidosis including ketoacidosis.

Drug Interactions

▲ **Alcohol is known to potentiate the effect of metformin on lactate metabolism. Caution patients against drinking excessive amounts of alcohol, whether acutely or on a chronic basis, while using metformin.** Cimetidine reduces the renal clearance of metformin. Other cationic drugs (amiloride, digoxin, morphine, procainamide, quinidine, quinine, ranitidine, triamterene, trimethoprim, and vancomycin) that compete for the common tubular transport system have the potential to increase plasma metformin levels and increase the risk for lactic acidosis. A number of other drugs may worsen hyperglycemia and lead to loss of glycemic control when taken with metformin (see Table 53-3). Close monitoring of blood glucose levels in patients who require these drugs will help to determine when dosage changes are needed for metformin.

Concurrent administration of furosemide, a loop diuretic, and metformin may increase serum concentrations of metformin and decrease concentrations of furosemide. Concurrent use of nifedipine may increase serum concentrations of metformin without an effect on the level of nifedipine. Use of either drug with metformin increases the risk of hypoglycemia.

Dosage Regimens

There is no fixed dosage regimen for management of patients with T2DM who take metformin or metformin extended-release tablets. Treatment must be individualized for each patient. Initiate metformin therapy with a single dose (usually 500 mg), taken with the patient's largest meal to prevent gastrointestinal (GI) symptoms. After initiation of therapy, metformin is taken in divided doses with meals. Dosages may be increased by 500 mg every 1 to 2 weeks until blood glucose goals are reached, or until the maximum dosage of 2000 to 2550 mg is reached (2000 mg daily for children 10 to 16 years of age). Significant responses are usually not seen at levels below 1500 mg per day.

The initial dose of extended-release metformin is 500 mg once daily with the evening meal. The dosage may be increased weekly in increments of 500 mg to a maximum dose of 2000 mg daily. In many cases the target dosage is 2000 mg daily.

Lab Considerations

The effectiveness of metformin therapy is determined through periodic measurements of blood glucose and A_{1c} levels. Measure serum creatinine levels before starting therapy and at least yearly thereafter to verify that they are normal. Discontinue metformin if serum creatinine level is greater than 1.5 mg/dL in men or greater than 1.4 mg/dL in women.

▲ Monitor liver functions periodically. **Avoid using metformin in patients with clinical or laboratory evidence of hepatic disease. Impaired hepatic function has been associated with some cases of lactic acidosis.**

Monitor serum vitamin B_{12} levels every 2 to 3 years in patients with inadequate vitamin B_{12} intake or absorption to assess for development of anemia.

Thiazolidinediones

◆ pioglitazone (Actos); ♣ Actos
◆ pioglitazone + metformin (Actoplus); ♣ Actoplus
◆ rosiglitazone (Avandia); ♣ Avandia
◆ rosiglitazone + metformin (Avandamet); ♣ Avandamet

Indications

Thiazolidinediones (TZDs; also known as "glitazones") are used in the treatment of T2DM alone or in combination with sulfonylureas, metformin or insulin. Both drugs are used as monotherapy, particularly in patients who are overweight, those who are obese with insulin resistance, or for whom use of metformin is contraindicated or it is not tolerated. TZDs decrease A_{1c} levels by 0.7% to 1% and FBS levels by 25 to 50 mg/dL.

Pharmacodynamics

TZDs are effective only in the presence of insulin. They decrease insulin resistance at peripheral sites and in the liver, resulting in increased insulin-dependent glucose disposal and decreased hepatic glucose output. They cause activation of insulin-responsive genes in the nucleus that regulate lipid and carbohydrate metabolism. Gene activation occurs through selective action of the drugs on the nuclear receptors called peroxisome proliferator–activated receptor-gamma (PPAR-gamma). PPAR receptors are found in tissues important for insulin action such as adipose tissue, skeletal muscle, and the liver.

Pharmacokinetics

Pioglitazone is rapidly absorbed after oral administration and is distributed bound, primarily to serum albumin. Pioglitazone is extensively biotransformed by CYP 3A4 to both active and inactive metabolites. It is eliminated in urine and feces. The active metabolites have a half-life of up to 24 hours (Table 53-5).

Rosiglitazone is well absorbed from the GI tract. Rosiglitazone is extensively biotransformed by the CYP 2C8. All circulating metabolites of rosiglitazone are considerably less potent than parent drug and therefore do not contribute to the insulin-sensitizing activity of rosiglitazone. Drug metabolites are eliminated in the urine and feces.

Adverse Effects and Contraindications

Rosiglitazone and pioglitazone may cause hypoglycemia, headache, weight gain, and anemia. They may also cause dizziness, GI disturbances, muscle cramps, dyspnea, paresthesias, and elevation of cholesterol levels.

Peripheral edema occurs within the first 6 months of therapy in some patients. The edema is unresponsive to diuretic therapy and frequently necessitates withdrawal of the TZD. TZDs are contraindicated for use in patients with New York Heart Association Class III and IV heart failure (see Chapter 34, Table 34-2).

Several cases of liver damage have been reported. Do not use TZDs in patients with clinical evidence of active liver

ENDOCRINE

PHARMACOKINETICS
TABLE 53-5 Selected Antidiabetic Drugs

Drug	Route	Onset	Peak	Duration	PB (%)	$t_{1/2}$
BIGUANIDE						
metformin	PO	UA	1–3 hr	8–12 hr	Negligible	1.5–6 hr
THIAZOLIDINEDIONES						
pioglitazone	PO	Weeks	2–4 hr	>24 hr	99	3–7 hr
rosiglitazone	PO	UA	1 hr	12–24 hr	99.8	3–4 hr
FIRST-GENERATION SULFONYLUREAS						
acetohexamide	PO	1 hr	2 hr	12–24 hr	90	1.3 hr
chlorpropamide	PO	1 hr	3–6 hr	24–72 hr	Highly	25–60 hr
tolazamide	PO	20 min	2–4 hr	10 hr	95	7 hr
tolbutamide	PO	1 hr	8 hr	6–12 hr	98	4.5–6.5 hr
SECOND-GENERATION SULFONYLUREAS						
glyburide	PO	2 hr	3–4 hr	24 hr	Highly	24 hr
glipizide	PO	90 min	2–3 hr	12–24 hr	99	2–4 hr
glimepiride	PO	1 hr	2–3 hr	24 hr	99.5	5 hr
MEGLITINIDE ANALOGUES						
repaglinide	PO	30 min	1 hr	4 hr	98	1 hr
nateglinide	PO	20 min	1 hr	4 hr	98	1.5 hr
ALPHA-GLUCOSIDASE INHIBITORS						
acarbose	PO	1 hr	2 hr	4–6 hr	Negligible	2 hr
miglitol	PO	5–15 min	2–3 hr	4–5 hr	<4	2 hr
AMYLIN AGONISTS						
pramlintide	subQ	Rapidly	20 min	UA	UA	30–50 min
INCRETIN MIMETICS						
exenatide	subQ	<60 min	3 hr	5 hr	UA	2.4 hr

PB, Protein binding; *PO,* by mouth; *subQ,* subcutaneous (route); $t_{1/2}$, half-life; *UA,* unavailable.

disease or alanine transaminase (ALT) concentrations greater than 2.5 times the upper limit of normal.

⚠ **According to a report in the British Medical Journal (Tanne, 2007), the US Food and Drug Administration has asked the manufacturers of rosiglitazone and pioglitazone to place "black box" warnings on their labels to warn of an increased risk of heart failure, as rosiglitazone and related drugs can cause fluid retention.** However, the new labels do not address whether these drugs pose an increased risk of heart attacks and strokes.

⚠ **In premenopausal, anovulatory women with insulin resistance, treatment with TZDs may result in resumption of ovulation. These patients may be at risk for pregnancy if adequate contraception is not used.**

Reduction in hematocrit and hemoglobin values has been noted in patients taking TZDs. These effects are attributed to dilutional effect from an increase in plasma volume.

TZDs exert their antihyperglycemic effects only in the presence of insulin; do not use them in the treatment of T1DM or diabetic ketoacidosis.

▧ Drug Interactions

⚠ **Contraceptives containing ethinyl estradiol or norethindrone may not be effective when used concurrently with TZDs. Alternative methods of contraception should be considered.** Pioglitazone has no clinical effect on prothrombin times (PT) and international normalized ratio (INR) when administered to patients receiving chronic warfarin therapy (Table 53-6).

Gemfibrozil, ketoconazole, and trimethoprim can increase plasma concentration of rosiglitazone. Rifampicin reduces

rosiglitazone concentrations. Use caution when giving these drugs to patients taking rosiglitazone, and monitor glycemic control.

▧ Dosage Regimen

Pioglitazone may be taken without regard to meals and the dosage increased if the patient does not respond by demonstrating the desired lowering of blood glucose levels (Table 53-7). Rosiglitazone may be taken with or without food. Consider combination therapy for patients not responding to the maximum dosage. Dosage adjustment is not necessary in patients with renal disease or in older adults.

▧ Lab Considerations

Response to TZD therapy is evaluated by measuring A_{1c} levels, which is a better measurement of long-term glycemic control than FBS measurements. Measure hemoglobin and hematocrit levels periodically during therapy to detect the development of anemia, should it occur.

Monitor serum transaminase levels before starting treatment, every 2 months for the first year, and periodically thereafter. Also obtain serum transaminase levels if symptoms of hepatic dysfunction develop (i.e., unexplained nausea, vomiting, abdominal pain, fatigue, anorexia, or dark urine). Discontinue pioglitazone if serum transaminase levels are greater than 3 times the upper limit of normal on repeat testing.

Sulfonylureas
FIRST-GENERATION DRUGS

◆ acetohexamide (Dymelor)
◆ chlorpropamide (Diabinese); ✦ Apo-chlorpropamide

DRUG INTERACTIONS
TABLE 53-6 Antidiabetic Drugs

Interaction	Interactive Drugs	Interaction
BIGUANIDE		
metformin	cimetidine	Reduces renal clearance of metformin
	alcohol, amiloride, digoxin, morphine, procainamide, quinidine, quinine, ranitidine, triamterene, trimethoprim, vancomycin	Increases plasma metformin levels and increases the risk for lactic acidosis.
	Calcium channel blockers, Corticosteroids, Diuretics, Estrogens, isoniazid, nicotinic acid, Oral contraceptives, phenytoin, Phenothiazines, Sympathomimetics, Thyroid hormones	Tends to elevate blood glucose levels
	furosemide	Increases serum level of metformin and decreases concentrations of furosemide
	nifedipine	Increases serum concentrations of metformin
THIAZOLIDINEDIONES		
pioglitazone, rosiglitazone	ethinyl estradiol, norethindrone	Interactive drug may be less effective
	gemfibrozil, ketoconazole, trimethoprim	Increases plasma concentration of rosiglitazone
	rifampicin	Reduces rosiglitazone concentration
SULFONYLUREAS		
All sulfonylureas	Beta blockers	Masks symptoms of hypoglycemia
	octreotide	Increases or decreases glucose level
	aminoglutethimide, chlorpromazine, Corticosteroids, diazoxide, epinephrine, Oral contraceptives, Rifamycins, Thiazide diuretics, Thyroid hormones	Elevates blood glucose levels
	ACEIs, alcohol, allopurinol, azapropazone, Beta blockers, chloramphenicol, cimetidine, clofibrate, fluconazole, Quinolones, heparin, ketoconazole, MAOIs, miconazole, phenylbutazone, ranitidine, Salicylates, Sulfonamides, sulfinpyrazone, Tetracyclines, Tricyclic antidepressants, warfarin	Increases potential for hypoglycemia
MEGLITINIDE ANALOGUES		
repaglinide, nateglinide	Drugs that induce or suppress the CYP450 system; highly-protein bound drugs	Alters expected effects of repaglinide
	ACTH, Amphetamines, Barbiturates, carbamazepine, Corticosteroids, corticotropin, Estrogens, glucagon, isoniazid, Oral contraceptives, Phenothiazines, phenytoin, rifampin, Salicylates, Sympathomimetics, Thiazide diuretics, Thyroid hormones	Increases risk of hyperglycemia
	Anabolic steroids, Androgens, Beta blockers, chloramphenicol, erythromycin, gemfibrozil, ketoconazole, MAOIs, miconazole, NSAIDs, probenecid, Sulfonamides, warfarin	Increases risk for hypoglycemia
ALPHA-GLUCOSIDASE INHIBITORS		
acarbose, miglitol	Intestinal absorbents, digestive enzymes	Reduces the effect of acarbose
	digoxin	Reduces bioavailability of digoxin
AMYLIN ANALOGUE		
pramlintide	Drugs effecting GI motility, alpha-glucosidase inhibitors	Delays absorption of interactive drugs
	Antidiabetic drugs	Increases risk for hypoglycemia
INCRETIN MIMETIC		
exenatide	Orally administered drugs	Reduces the extent and rate of absorption

ACEIs, Angiotensin converting enzyme inhibitors; *ACTH,* adrenocorticotropic hormone; *GI,* gastrointestinal; *NSAIDs,* nonsteroidal antiinflammatory drugs; *MAOIs,* monoamine oxidase inhibitors

- tolazamide (Tolinase)
- tolbutamide (Orinase)

SECOND-GENERATION DRUGS
- glyburide (Diabeta, Glynase Prestabs, Micronase); ♣ Diabeta, Daonil, Glynase, Micronase
- glyburide + metformin (Glucovance); ♣ Glucovance
- glipizide (Glucatrol, Glucatrol XL); ♣ Glucatrol, Glucatrol XL
- glipizide + metformin (Metaglip)
- glimepiride (Amaryl); ♣ Amaryl
- glimepiride + rosiglitazone (Avandaryl); ♣ Avandaryl

Indications
Sulfonylurea drugs are classified as insulin secretagogues and stimulate the pancreas to release insulin. Sulfonylurea drugs are effective as first-line drugs in the treatment of T2DM that does not respond to lifestyle changes. Their ability to lower blood glucose levels is dependent upon the presence of functioning pancreatic beta cells. Sulfonylureas are divided into two groups based on their potency and duration of action. Even though second-generation drugs have greater potency, there are no therapeutic differences between first- and second-generation sulfonylurea drugs. Second-generation drugs generally have fewer adverse effects, with the exception of hypoglycemia, and fewer drug interactions. First-generation drugs are still available for purchase in local pharmacies but are seldom used today. Sulfonylurea drugs are appropriate for average-weight adults without lipid abnormalities.

Approximately 60% to 70% of patients with T2DM initially respond to sulfonylurea therapy. On average, sulfonylurea drugs decrease FBS by 60 to 70 mg/dL and A_{1c} level by 0.8% to 2%.

Pharmacodynamics
Sulfonylureas reduce blood glucose levels by stimulating insulin release from functional pancreatic beta cells. The

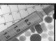

DOSAGE
TABLE 53-7 Oral Antidiabetic Drugs

Drug	Dosage	Implications	
BIGUANIDE			
metformin	*Adults:* Initial therapy: 500 mg PO once daily. Increase by 500 mg weekly until control achieved. Administer in divided doses. Max: 2550 mg daily.	**Monitor renal function before starting metformin therapy, and at least annually thereafter. Withhold drug if patient is scheduled for radiocontrast imaging studies.** Patients with serum creatinine levels above ULN for their age should not receive metformin. Temporarily stop drug if IV contrast studies are planned. Alcohol potentiates effect of metformin on lactate metabolism. Warn patients against excessive alcohol intake while taking metformin.	⚠
metformin XR	*Adult:* 500 mg PO twice daily or 850 mg once a day, given with meals. Increase by 500 mg weekly or 850 mg every 2 wk to total of 2000 mg per day in divided doses.		
THIAZOLIDINEDIONES			
pioglitazone	*Adult:* 15–30 mg PO once daily. May increase, if needed, to a max of 45 mg PO once daily after 8–12 wk.	**Black box warning of increased risk for heart failure. Check LFTs before start of therapy and periodically thereafter.** Do not start therapy if patient has active liver disease or ALT is 2.5 times the ULN. **Do not confuse pioglitazone with rosiglitazone.**	⚠ ⚠
rosiglitazone	*Adult:* 4 mg PO as single daily dose or divided doses. Max: 8 mg	**Black box warning of increased risk for heart failure.** LFT monitoring is recommended before start of therapy and periodically thereafter.	⚠ ⚠
FIRST-GENERATION SULFONYLUREAS			
acetohexamide	*Adult:* 250 mg PO daily. Usual dose: 250–1500 mg PO daily. Max: 1500 mg daily	Not recommended for patients with renal insufficiency because of potential for hypoglycemia. Use with caution in older adults, debilitated, or malnourished patients.	
chlorpropamide	*Adult:* 100–125 mg PO daily. Usual dose: 500 mg PO daily. Max: 750 mg PO daily	Hypoglycemia treatment may be necessary for several days because of the long-acting nature of the drug. Not recommended in older adults.	
tolbutamide	*Adult:* 1–2 grams daily with breakfast or in divided doses. Maintenance: 0.25–2 grams PO daily. Max: 1 gram daily	Do not use in patients with severe renal impairment.	
tolazamide	*Adult:* 100–250 mg PO daily. Maintenance: 100–1000 mg PO daily. Max: 1000 mg daily	Hypoglycemia is most common adverse effect. Hyponatremia and SIADH have been reported.	
SECOND-GENERATION SULFONYLUREAS			
glipizide	*Adult:* 5 mg PO daily. Usual dose: 10–15 mg PO once daily. Max: 40 mg PO IA formulation daily in divided doses. Max: 20 mg for XL formulation	Take on empty stomach. Give drug twice daily as dosage of increases. **Do not confuse glipizide with glyburide or glimeperide.**	⚠
glyburide	*Adult:* 2.5–5 mg PO daily. Usual dose: 1.25–20 mg PO daily. Max: 20 mg daily *Adult:* Micronized formulation: 1.5–3 mg PO daily; titrate to max of 12 mg/day	Proper patient selection required to prevent hypoglycemia. Give drug twice daily as dosage of micronized glyburide increases.	
glimepiride	*Adult:* 1–2 mg PO daily. Usual dose: 1–4 mg PO daily. Max: 8 mg daily	Take once daily with breakfast or the first main meal. Proper patient selection required to prevent hypoglycemia.	
MEGLITINIDE ANALOGUES			
repaglinide	*Adult:* 0.5–4 mg PO daily before each meal. Combination therapy: with metformin, pioglitazone, rosiglitazone, or insulin	Take no more than 30 min before eating a meal, but instruct patients to skip the dose if they skip the meal to reduce the risk for hypoglycemia. Renal and hepatic dosage considerations required. Combination therapy: with metformin or insulin. **Do not confuse repaglinide with nateglinide.**	⚠
nateglinide	*Adult:* Monotherapy: 60–120 mg PO before each meal. Usual daily dose: 120 mg PO 3 times daily		
ALPHA-GLUCOSIDASE INHIBITORS			
acarbose	*Adult:* 25 mg PO 3 times daily with first bite of food of each main meal. Titrate every 4–8 wk to max of 50–100 mg 3 times daily. *Maximum <60 kg* = 50 mg PO 3 times daily. *Maximum >60 kg* = 100 mg PO 3 times daily	Acarbose is administered with the first bite of each meal. Instruct patients to skip the dose if they skip the meal to reduce the risk for hypoglycemia.	
miglitol	*Adult:* 25 mg PO 3 times daily with first bite of food of each main meal. Titrate every 4–8 wk to max of 50–100 mg 3 times daily.	If not at A_{1c} goal in 3 months, titrate up to 100 mg 3 times daily. Maintain dosage once effective and tolerable dosage is established.	
AMYLIN ANALOGUE			
pramlintide	*Adults with T1DM:* 15 mcg subQ initially before meals. Target dose: 30–60 mcg before meals *Adults with T2DM:* 60 mcg subQ before meals. May increase after 3–7 days to 120 mcg subQ before meals. Max: 360 mcg subQ	**Black box warning for insulin-induced hypoglycemia. Reduce preprandial dose of rapid or fast-acting insulin by 50%.** Administer immediately before each major meal containing more than 250 kcal, or more than 30 grams of carbohydrate. Equivalence: 15 mcg = 2.5 units.	⚠
INCRETIN MIMETIC			
exenatide	*Adult:* 5 mcg subQ twice daily. May increase to 10 mg subQ twice daily after 1 mo	Give 60 min before morning and evening meals. **Not a substitute for insulin.** Not appropriate for patients with T1DM.	⚠

COMBINATION DRUGS		
glipizide + metformin (Metaglip)	*Naïve Adult:* 2.5/250 mg to 2.5/500 mg PO once-twice daily. Max: 10/1000 –or– 10/2000 mg PO twice daily. Max: 20/2000	Take with meals. Used when FBS > 280–320 mg/dL. See comments for glipizide and metformin, above.
glyburide + metformin (Glucovance)	*Naïve Adult:* 1.25/250 mg PO initially once-twice daily. May increase to 10/2000 mg daily in divided doses *Adult previously treated:* 2.5/500 or 5/500 mg PO twice daily with meals. May increase to 20/2000 mg daily in divided doses	Take with meals. See comments for glyburide and metformin, above.
rosiglitazone + metformin (Avandamet)	*Adult:* 1/500 mg –or– 2/500 mg –or– 4/500 mg PO twice daily. Max: 8/2000 mg daily	See comments for rosiglitazone and metformin, above.
rosiglitazone + glimepiride (Avandryl)	*Adult:* 4/1 mg –or– 4/2 mg –or– 4/4 mg PO daily. Max: 8/4 mg daily	See comments for rosiglitazone and glimepiride, above.
pioglitazone + metformin (Actoplus Met)	*Adult:* 15/500 mg to 15/850 mg PO once-twice daily. Max: 45/2550 mg daily	See comments for pioglitazone and metformin, above.
pioglitazone + glimepiride (Duetact)	*Adult:* 30/2 mg to 30/4 mg PO daily	See comments for pioglitazone and glimepiride, above

ALT, Alanine transaminase; *FBS,* fasting blood sugar; *IA,* intermediate-acting; *IV,* intravenous (route); *LFT,* liver function test; *PO,* by mouth; *SIADH,* syndrome of inappropriate antidiuretic hormone secretion; *subQ,* subcutaneous (route); *T1DM,* type 1 diabetes mellitus; *T2DM,* type 2 diabetes mellitus; *ULN,* upper limits of normal; *XL, XR,* extended-release.

drugs block adenosine triphosphate (ATP)–sensitive potassium channels that lead to membrane depolarization and to an increase in calcium influx, which in turn triggers the release of insulin from the beta cells. Sulfonylureas only stimulate phase I (initial rapid peak) release of insulin and have no effect on phase II (prolonged) insulin release.

Pharmacokinetics

Most sulfonylureas share similar kinetic properties for absorption, distribution, biotransformation, and elimination. Absorption is rapid and complete after oral administration, with distribution via plasma proteins to which the drugs are extensively bound. They are biotransformed in the liver and eliminated in the urine. Second-generation drugs, as well as the first-generation drug chlorpropamide, undergo enterohepatic circulation recycling, a process that contributes to the longer duration of action (see Table 53-5).

Adverse Effects and Contraindications

All sulfonylurea drugs can cause hypoglycemia. Risk factors for developing hypoglycemia include erratic eating habits, intense or prolonged exercise, alcohol ingestion, renal or hepatic disease, and advancing age. Renal or hepatic insufficiency may cause elevated blood levels of sulfonylurea drugs, thus increasing the risk for serious hypoglycemic reactions.

GI adverse effects tend to be dosage related but include nausea, epigastric fullness, heartburn, and weight gain, occurring in a small percentage of patients. These adverse effects usually decrease with a reduction in dosage. Liver function abnormalities, including isolated transaminase elevations, have been reported.

Allergic skin reactions (i.e., pruritus, erythema, urticaria, and maculopapular eruptions) occur in 1.5% of patients. These symptoms are transient and disappear with continued therapy.

Sulfonylurea drugs are contraindicated for use in patients with known hypersensitivity to the drug, and in the treatment of diabetic ketoacidosis. The use of drugs such as glyburide and chlorpropamide that are biotransformed to an active metabolite with significant renal excretion is contraindicated in patients with severe renal insufficiency because of risk of profound and prolonged hypoglycemia. Glyburide is not recommended for use in patients with creatinine clearance less than 50 mL/min because as much as 50% of the dose may be eliminated unchanged in the urine.

Chlorpropamide is associated with development of the syndrome of inappropriate antidiuretic hormone secretion (SIADH). It is also associated with a high incidence of hypoglycemia because of its prolonged duration of action, and is unsafe for use in older adults.

Drug Interactions

The hypoglycemic action of sulfonylureas may be potentiated by nonsteroidal antiinflammatory drugs (NSAIDs) and other highly protein-bound drugs (see Table 53-6). Observe patients for hypoglycemia when adding these drugs to a treatment regimen and for hyperglycemia when removing them. Oral contraceptives, corticosteroids, thiazide diuretics, and others can cause hyperglycemia when used with sulfonylureas, and lead to loss of glycemic control.

Dosage Regimen

Dosage recommendations for sulfonylurea drugs are listed in Table 53-7. Tolbutamide and tolazamide are fast-acting first-generation sulfonylureas. These drugs require multiple daily doses. Acetohexamide is generally administered twice a day. Chlorpropamide is the longest-acting first-generation sulfonylurea and is suitable for administration once a day. The second-generation drugs glyburide and glipizide are taken once or twice daily, and glimepiride once a day.

Initiate treatment with low dosages, and adjust every week as needed until desired glucose control is achieved or maximum dosage is reached. Dosage adjustments may be needed when sulfonylurea drugs are added to a treatment regimen containing other blood glucose–lowering drugs, when transferring from another oral drug, and for patients particularly susceptible to hypoglycemia.

ENDOCRINE

Lab Considerations

Oral hypoglycemic drugs may cause an increase in aspartate transaminase (AST), lactate dehydrogenase (LDH), and blood urea nitrogen (BUN) values. Monitor creatinine clearance in patients taking glyburide. Monitor serum sodium levels and plasma osmolality as well as serum potassium levels periodically throughout therapy in patients taking chlorpropamide.

Meglitinide Analogues

◆ nateglinide (Starlix)
◆ repaglinide (Prandin); ♣ Gluconorm

Indications

Meglitinide analogues are oral hypoglycemic drugs used as an adjunct to diet and exercise in the treatment of T2DM. Both repaglinide and nateglinide have a faster onset and shorter duration of action than sulfonylureas and both decrease fasting and postprandial blood glucose when given alone or in combination with metformin or a thiazolidinedione (see later discussion). Repaglinide has similar blood glucose–lowering effects as sulfonylurea drugs, with a 65- to 75-mg/dL reduction in FBS and 0.8% to 2% reduction in A_{1c}. Both drugs allow flexibility for patients who do not maintain regular meal schedules. Meglitinide analogues are appropriate for patients with T2DM who have postprandial hyperglycemia.

Pharmacodynamics

These rapid acting secretagogues lower blood glucose levels by stimulating the release of insulin from the pancreas. These drugs stimulate insulin secretion by interacting with the ATP-sensitive potassium channel on pancreatic beta cells. This action is dependent upon functioning beta cells in the pancreatic islets.

Pharmacokinetics

Repaglinide is rapidly absorbed after oral administration, with over 98% of the drug protein bound for distribution (see Table 53-5). Repaglinide is biotransformed to active metabolites in the liver by CYP 3A4 and excreted via feces.

Nateglinide has a more rapid onset and shorter duration of action than repaglinide. Nateglinide is biotransformed by CYP 2C9 and to a lesser extent by CYP 3A4 to both active and inactive metabolites. It is excreted in urine and feces.

Adverse Effects and Contraindications

Hypoglycemia is the major adverse effect of meglitinides. Risk factors for developing hypoglycemia include erratic eating habits, intense or prolonged exercise, alcohol ingestion, and use of one or more glucose-lowering drugs. Additional adverse effects include nausea, diarrhea, constipation, vomiting, and dyspepsia.

Both repaglinide and nateglinide are contraindicated for use in patients with hypersensitivity to each drug, insulin-dependent diabetes mellitus, and diabetic ketoacidosis, with or without coma.

Drug Interactions

Drugs that induce or suppress the CYP450 system may alter the expected hypoglycemic effects of repaglinide (see Table 53-6). There is an increased risk for hypoglycemia when repaglinide is administered with antifungal drugs such as ketoconazole or miconazole, and antibacterial drugs such as erythromycin.

Use of repaglinide with the CYP 2C8 inhibitor gemfibrozil (an antilipid drug) has resulted in marked repaglinide clearance and severe hypoglycemia. Use of this combination of drugs is contraindicated.

Highly bound-protein drugs potentiate the hypoglycemic effects of repaglinide. Beta blockers, chloramphenicol, monoamine oxidase (MAO) inhibitors, NSAIDs, probenecid, salicylates, sulfonamides, and warfarin may lower blood glucose levels when given with meglitinide analogues. Administration of anabolic steroids or androgens to a patient taking repaglinide increases the risk for hypoglycemia.

Monitor hyperglycemic symptoms in patients taking repaglinide, barbiturates, carbamazepine, and rifampin. Other interacting drugs are identified in Table 53-6. Closely monitor blood glucose levels when initiating therapy with one of these drugs.

Dosage Regimen

Meal patterns can be flexible with repaglinide, with the dose administered from 30 minutes before to immediately before meals (see Table 53-7). The dose is omitted if the meal is not eaten. An additional dose of repaglinide is given if an extra meal is eaten. The optimal time for administration of nateglinide appears to be 10 minutes before meals.

Allow at least 1 week between dosage adjustments to adequately assess blood glucose response. Take care when making dosage adjustments for patients with severe renal failure and for those with moderate to severe hepatic insufficiency.

Laboratory Considerations

Monitor therapeutic response to meglitinide analogues using periodic blood glucose testing. Evaluate renal and hepatic function at the start of therapy and periodically thereafter to identify patients for whom dosage adjustments have to be made.

Alpha-Glucosidase Inhibitors

◆ acarbose (Precose); ♣ Prandase
◆ miglitol (Glyset)

Indications

Acarbose and miglitol are antihyperglycemic drugs used as first-line or adjunctive drugs in the treatment of T2DM. Alpha-glucosidase inhibitors lower postprandial blood glucose when given alone or in combination with sulfonylureas, metformin, or insulin. Miglitol is an adjunct to diet in patients with T2DM who cannot be managed by diet alone. These drugs are appropriate for individuals with normal FBS levels but elevated postprandial readings.

Pharmacodynamics

Alpha-glucosidase inhibitors act to delay and decrease the absorption of complex carbohydrates from the GI tract. Normally, alpha-glucosidase enzymes, present in the brush border of the intestine, generate glucose in the GI tract by hydrolyzing the dietary oligosaccharides such as starch, dextrin, and maltose into simple sugars during the digestion process. Inhibition of the enzyme decreases the amount of glucose available for absorption from the GI tract and reduces postprandial blood glucose elevations. Alpha-glucosidase inhibitors reduce FBS levels by 35 to 40 mg/dL and A_{1c} levels by 0.7% to 1%.

Pharmacokinetics

The majority of acarbose remains in the lumen of the GI tract (see Table 53-5). It is degraded in the intestine by bacterial and digestive enzymes. About 35% of the dose is reabsorbed in the form of active metabolites. Acarbose is excreted in urine and feces.

Miglitol is completely absorbed at a dose of 25 mg, but only 50% to 70% absorbed at a dose of 100 mg. It is not biotransformed and is eliminated unchanged in the urine.

Adverse Effects and Contraindications

GI adverse effects are the most common reactions to acarbose and miglitol. Abdominal pain, diarrhea, and flatulence occur in a high percentage of patients taking acarbose. These symptoms occur because of the presence of undigested carbohydrate in the lower GI tract. The intensity of these symptoms tends to decrease with time.

⚠ Alpha-glucosidase inhibitors do not cause insulin secretion and do not cause hypoglycemia when administered as monotherapy. The potential for hypoglycemia increases when acarbose is given in combination with other blood glucose–lowering drugs. Because acarbose prevents the breakdown of table sugar, patients should have a ready source of glucose (glucose tablets or glucose gel) to treat symptoms of low blood sugar. High doses of acarbose cause transient increases in AST and/or ALT. Monitor patients with hepatic disease while they are receiving acarbose.

Alpha-glucosidase inhibitors are contraindicated for use in patients with known hypersensitivity to the drug and in patients with diabetic ketoacidosis. Both drugs are contraindicated for use in patients with inflammatory bowel disease, colonic ulceration, ileus, partial GI obstruction or predisposition to it, or GI disease involving disorders of absorption or digestion, as well as in patients who have conditions that may deteriorate as a result of increased gas formation in the intestine.

Acarbose and miglitol are excreted in breast milk and should not be administered to nursing mothers. Acarbose is contraindicated for use in pregnancy. Use miglitol during pregnancy only if clearly needed.

Drug Interactions

Intestinal absorbents (e.g., charcoal) and digestive enzyme formulations containing carbohydrate-splitting enzymes (amylase, pancreatin) may reduce the effect of acarbose and should not be taken concomitantly (see Table 53-6). Acarbose may affect digoxin bioavailability and necessitate a dosage adjustment.

Dosage Regimen

There is no fixed dosage for acarbose or miglitol (see Table 53-7). Daily dosage is individualized based both on effectiveness and tolerance of the drug without exceeding the maximum daily dose of 100 mg, 3 times a day. These drugs should be taken with the first bite of each main meal. Initiate therapy at the lowest level, with gradual increases in dosage until desired effect is achieved without disabling GI adverse effects. If a meal is skipped, the dose of acarbose or miglitol is skipped.

Lab Considerations

Check serum transaminases levels every 3 months during the first year of therapy, then periodically thereafter. Reduce the dosage or withdraw the drug if elevated transaminases levels are observed. Monitor therapeutic response to alpha-glucosidase inhibitors using periodic blood glucose testing.

Amylin Agonists
◆ pramlintide (Symlin)

Indications

Pramlintide is the first injectable antihyperglycemic drug for use in patients with diabetes treated with insulin. Pramlintide was approved for adults with T1DM and T2DM as an adjunct to mealtime insulin in patients who have been unable to achieve desired blood glucose control despite optimal therapy. On average, pramlintide decreases A_{1c} levels by 0.3% to 0.6%.

Pharmacodynamics

Pramlintide is a synthetic analogue of human amylin (a naturally occurring neuroendocrine hormone synthesized by pancreatic beta cells). It contributes to postprandial blood glucose control through several mechanisms: it slows gastric emptying (the rate at which food is released from the stomach to the small intestine), suppresses glucagon secretion after meals, thereby reducing endogenous glucose output from the liver, and regulates satiety so that less food is eaten.

Pharmacokinetics

Peak action of pramlintide is reached in about 20 minutes. Pramlintide has a half-life of 48 minutes. It is primarily biotransformed by the kidney. Pramlintide does not bind to blood cells or albumin. There is more variability after injection into the arm than after injection into the abdomen or thigh.

Adverse Effects and Contraindications

In general, pramlintide is well tolerated when started at very low dosages and titrated upward as needed. The most common adverse effect of pramlintide is mild to moderate GI upset including anorexia, nausea, vomiting, and abdominal pain, which is more likely to occur at the start of therapy and resolve over time. Symptoms can be alleviated by slow titration to therapeutic dosages. Nausea may also occur in patients who continue to eat beyond the point of fullness. Some weight loss may be noted. Other adverse effects include redness, swelling, or itching at the injection site, which typically resolves in a few days to a few weeks.

Pramlintide carries a black box warning for insulin-induced hypoglycemia. Hypoglycemia risk is higher in patients with T1DM, usually occurring within 3 hours of injection. **⚠ Do not use pramlintide if patients have gastroparesis or hypoglycemic unawareness and cannot identify when glucose levels fall.** The addition of any antihyperglycemic drug to a regimen containing pramlintide increases the risk of hypoglycemia and necessitates dosage adjustments and close monitoring of blood glucose.

Do not use pramlintide in patients who are allergic to the drug, metacresol, D-mannitol, acetic acid, or sodium acetate. The safety of pramlintide during pregnancy and lactation is unknown.

Drug Interactions

Because of the effects of pramlintide on gastric emptying, ⚠ do not use it in patients taking drugs that alter GI motility or who use alpha-glucosidase inhibitors (i.e., acarbose, miglitol). Pramlintide may cause delayed absorption of concomitantly administered oral drugs. When rapid action of an orally administered drug is needed (e.g., an analgesic; the drug should be ingested at least 1 to 2 hours before injection of pramlintide).

Concurrent use with other diabetic drugs increases the risk of hypoglycemia, owing to increased blood glucose–lowering effects. Drugs that increase the risk for hypoglycemia are listed in Box 53-1.

▓ Dosage Regimen

⚠ **The risk for drug errors involving pramlintide is great. The dosage of pramlintide is ordered in micrograms; however, it is drawn up in units using U-100 insulin syringes.** For example, 15 mcg of pramlintide equals 2.5 units. It is usually best to use a 3/10-mL (i.e., 30-unit syringe) U-100 syringe to get an accurate dose. Patients using pramlintide require extensive education in the administration and storage requirements of pramlintide.

Do not mix pramlintide with any type of insulin. Mixing pramlintide with insulin alters insulin activity. When administering pramlintide, always use a new syringe and needle, and give as a separate injection into a site distant from where insulin is injected. Administer each dose of pramlintide subcutaneously into the abdomen or thigh and rotate injection sites so that the same site is not used repeatedly. Administration of pramlintide in the arm is not recommended.

Pramlintide cannot be discontinued without accompanying dose adjustments of preprandial insulin. Instruct patients to seek guidance from their primary care provider for increasing preprandial insulin doses.

▓ Lab Considerations

Patients taking pramlintide should test blood glucose levels at least before and after each meal and at bedtime. Therapeutic response to pramlintide is determined be periodic blood glucose testing.

Incretin Mimetic

◆ exenatide (Byetta)

▓ Indications

Exenatide is indicated as adjunct therapy to enhance glycemic control in patients with T2DM who are using metformin, a sulfonylurea, or a combination of the two drugs, but who have not gained adequate glycemic control. Exenatide provides reductions in fasting and postprandial blood glucose concentrations, thereby increasing glycemic control; it is not a substitute for insulin and should not be used for the treatment of patients with T1DM (see Evidence-based Pharmacotherapeutics box).

▓ Pharmacodynamics

The incretin effect was discovered years ago when it was noticed that the pancreas releases more insulin when a person eats carbohydrate-containing foods than it does when a comparable amount of glucose is given intravenously. Based on this finding, it was hypothesized that factors in the GI tract play a role in blood glucose control. Researchers subsequently noted that a hormone found in the saliva from the Gila monster was similar to glucagon-like peptide 1 (GLP-1), an incretin hormone produced in the human digestive tract that is deficient in patients with diabetes mellitus.

Incretins act by improving the normal release of insulin from the pancreas by preserving beta cell function and increasing beta cell mass; suppressing the inappropriately elevated glucagon secretion; and delaying gastric emptying and reducing appetite. Exenatide increases both first-phase and second-phase insulin secretion in patients with T2DM.

▓ Pharmacokinetics

Exenatide reaches peak plasma concentration 2 hours after subQ injection. Exenatide is eliminated by glomerular filtration (see Table 53-2).

▓ Adverse Effects and Contraindications

Nausea is the most common adverse event. Because of the adverse effects of nausea, vomiting, and diarrhea, exenatide is not recommended in patients with severe GI disease.

Exenatide rarely causes hypoglycemia, and it tends to cause a gradual weight loss due to decreased calorie intake. However, **the incidence of hypoglycemia is higher in patients** ⚠ **concurrently receiving exenatide and a sulfonylurea.** It may be necessary to reduce the dosage of the sulfonylureas drug to reduce the risk of hypoglycemia when both drugs are given together.

Exenatide is not recommended for patients with end-stage renal disease or severe renal impairment (i.e., creatinine clearance less than 30 mL/min). Because of the adverse effects of

---

BOX 53-1

Drugs Influencing Plasma Glucose Levels

Drugs Increasing Plasma Glucose Levels
- allopurinol
- adrenocorticotropic hormone (ACTH)
- Amphetamines
- asparaginase
- Beta blockers
- Carbonic anhydrase inhibitors
- Caffeine (in large quantities)
- Calcium channel blockers
- cyclophosphamide
- Decongestants
- diazoxide
- epinephrine
- Estrogens
- furosemide
- glucagon
- Glucose gel and tablets
- Glucocorticosteroids
- Growth hormone
- lithium
- marijuana
- morphine
- nicotine (smoking)
- nicotinic acid

- Oral contraceptives
- phenytoin
- pentamidine
- Thiazide diuretics
- Thyroid hormones

Drugs Decreasing Plasma Glucose Levels
- Alcohol
- allopurinol*
- Anabolic steroids
- Beta blockers
- clofibrate*
- chloramphenicol*
- guanethidine
- Histamine₂ antagonists
- Insulin
- isoniazid
- Monoamine oxidase inhibitors
- Oral anticoagulants*
- oxytetracycline
- pentamidine
- phenylbutazone*
- probenecid
- Salicylates*
- Sulfonamides*

*Interact with sulfonylurea drugs only.

EVIDENCE-BASED PHARMACOTHERAPEUTICS

Interim Analysis of Effects of Exenatide

■ Background

Incretin mimetics, such as exenatide, represent a new class of drugs in the treatment of diabetes. Researchers noted that a hormone found in Gila monster saliva was similar to glucagon-like peptide 1 (GLP-1), an incretin hormone produced in the human digestive tract.

It is well known that obesity increases the risk for diabetes 10 to 90 times, with a 9% increase in risk for every kilogram of weight increase. Because the prevalence of obesity has doubled in the past 30 years, the prevalence of diabetes has also increased, with no reversal in sight. However, many current drug therapies for diabetes (i.e., sulfonylureas and thiazolidinediones, and insulins) result in weight gain; an estimated 2 kg for every 1% decrease in A_{1c}. In addition, many of the existing therapies are associated with hypoglycemia and edema and, despite treatment, the likelihood of eventual loss of glycemic control. These drawbacks led to the development of newer antidiabetic therapies.

■ Research Article

Blonde, L., Klein, E., Han, J., et al. (2006). Interim analysis of the effects of exenatide treatment on A_{1c}, weight, and cardiovascular risk factors over 82 weeks in 314 overweight patients with type 2 diabetes. *Diabetes, Obesity, and Metabolism, 8*(4), 436–447.

Purpose

The purpose of this two-phase study was to determine if exenatide, an incretin mimetic used as an adjunct in the treatment of T2DM, reduced A_{1c} levels and weight in subjects also treated with sulfonylurea and/or metformin.

Design

To enroll in the open-label, uncontrolled extension studies, subjects ($N = 1446$) had to complete an antecedent 30-week placebo-controlled study. These three, randomized, placebo-controlled, double-blind, stratified, balanced, parallel-group studies were designed to evaluate glycemic control, changes in A_{1c}, and safety in patients with T2DM. The first group of subjects was taking maximally effective doses of a sulfonylurea; the second group maximally effective dosages of metformin; and the third study group, maximally effective dosages of sulfonylureas *plus* metformin. Subject ages ranged from 16 to 77 years.

During this first phase, subjects were randomized to receive placebo or 5 or 10 mcg of exenatide subcutaneously twice daily. Subjects completing the 30-week study were asked to continue into the 52-week open-label extension study that followed. Subjects continued their previous antidiabetic regimen while receiving 5 mcg of exenatide subcutaneously twice daily for 4 weeks, followed by 10 mcg thereafter. Exenatide was self-administered into the abdomen 15 minutes before morning and evening meals. Study protocols for the open-label extension did not include guidelines regarding dosage adjustment of sulfonylureas; therefore any dosage adjustment was at the investigator's discretion. Subjects randomized to placebo groups in the first-phase studies were not included in this interim analysis.

Method

Plasma analyses of glucose levels and A_{1c} concentrations were measured. Changes in body weight were stratified by baseline body mass index (BMI) and characterized by weight-change quartile and concomitant antidiabetic drug. Changes in lipids were determined as a secondary endpoint. All safety analyses were performed using the 82-week intent-to-treat population (ITT; all subjects who received at least one injection of exenatide in time to complete the 82 weeks of exenatide therapy before the end of the study).

Findings

Of the subjects ($N = 1125$) who completed the first-phase studies, 87% chose to enter the open-label extension study. Three hundred fourteen subjects completed 82 weeks of exenatide treatment (63% males ages 46–56 years; weight 79–120 kg; BMI 28–40 kg/m², A_{1c} of 7.3%–9.3% with a mean +/− one standard deviation [SD]). The most common reasons for leaving the study were withdrawal of consent (11%); adverse effects (7%), and administrative reasons (10%). Of those who withdrew for an adverse event, 3.6% did so because of nausea, and 0.4% because of hypoglycemia.

Reduction in A_{1c} from baseline to week 30 (−0.9 +/− 0.1% [mean +/− standard error of the mean (SEM)]) was sustained to week 82 (−1.1 +/− 0.1%), with 48% of patients achieving A_{1c} levels less than or equal to 7%.

It was noted that subjects who used exenatide had lost weight (a secondary endpoint) from baseline (−2.1 +/− 0.2 kg) at week 30, in 81% of subjects with progressive reduction at week 82 (−4.4 +/− 0.3 kg). Reductions in A_{1c} and weight at week 82 (−0.8 +/− 0.1% and −3.5 +/− 0.2 kg, respectively) were found for the ITT group.

Significant improvements in some cardiovascular risk factors were noted in the 82-week cohort who completed the study. Statistically significant changes were noted for high-density lipoprotein (HDL) levels (0.12 mmol/L), triglyceride levels (−0.43 mmol/L), and sitting diastolic blood pressure (−2.7 mm Hg). Although they did not achieve statistical significance, total cholesterol, low-density lipoprotein (LDL), apolipoprotein B, and systolic blood pressure (−3.9 mm Hg) also demonstrated trends toward improvement.

Conclusions

Patients with T2DM who were already taking a sulfonylurea and/or metformin and adjunctive exenatide sustained a reduction in A_{1c} levels, progressive weight reduction, and improvement in some cardiovascular risk factors. The weight loss was notable, however, given that no specific diet or exercise counseling or calorie restriction was required by the study, and there was no apparent plateau in weight loss by week 82. As may be expected, the greatest reduction in cardiovascular risk factors was seen in subjects with the greatest weight loss. Whether the changes in cardiovascular risk factors seen with exenatide therapy will have a substantial impact on future cardiovascular outcomes is unknown.

■ Implications for Practice

This two-phase study adds to prior published data on exenatide by the addition of a much longer period of clinical follow-up for active drug therapy. However, there were several shortcomings in this study, including the absence of a comparator group, the changing nature of the study, and the selection of a small subset of subjects. After week 30, the study changed from double-blind, placebo-controlled to open-label, with approximately 50% of subjects receiving the higher dose of exenatide. These changes may account for the notable loss of weight and A_{1c} reductions observed with the transition. Ongoing studies of subjects who received exenatide for even longer periods may determine whether there will be further reductions in A_{1c} levels, weight reduction, and cardiovascular risk factors.

nausea, vomiting, and diarrhea, exenatide is not recommended in patients with severe GI disease. Exenatide is contraindicated for use in patients with hypersensitivity to the product or any of its components, during pregnancy or lactation, and in patients with severe kidney disease or gastroparesis.

Drug Interactions

Exenatide may limit the extent and rate at which orally administered drugs are absorbed because it slows gastric emptying time. Use exenatide with caution in patients receiving oral drugs that require rapid GI absorption.

⚠ **Drugs that depend on threshold concentrations for efficacy, such as contraceptives and antibiotics, should be administered at least 1 hour before injection of exenatide.** When such drugs must be administered with food, they should be taken without prior exenatide administration.

Dosage Regimen

Exenatide is available as a prefilled pen that delivers a fixed 5-mcg or 10-mcg dose which is administered subcutaneously in the thigh, the abdomen, or the upper arm. It is typically taken twice daily, one 60 minutes before breakfast and the other before the evening meal. If it is forgotten or missed before starting to eat, it should not be taken during or after the meal, but rather the missed dose should be skipped entirely and the next dose taken as scheduled.

For patients who do not eat a morning meal, exenatide may be administered before the two major meals of the day, provided the meals are separated by at least 6 hours. If the patient eats only one meal per day, exenatide can be given before that meal and before a snack as long as they are separated by at least 6 hours. Each pen provides 60 doses (30 days of twice-daily injections).

A separate prescription is needed for the needles used on exenatide insulin pens. Pen needle sizes vary between manufacturers but are compatible with the exenatide pen: 31-gauge, $^3/_{16}$-inch; 31-gauge, $^1/_4$-inch; 31-gauge, $^5/_{16}$-inch; and 29-gauge, $^1/_2$-inch. A new needle is needed for each injection.

Other incretin mimetics continue to be studied. Early clinical trial results suggest that a long-acting formulation of exenatide may be administered once weekly or once every other week.

Lab Considerations

Therapeutic response to exenatide is determined be periodic A_{1c} testing. A 5-mcg dose reduces A_{1c} levels by 0.4% to 0.6%. Patients using a 10-mcg dose see an average A_{1c} decrease of 0.8% to 0.9%. Each 1% drop in A_{1c} reduces the risk of microvascular complications by 20% to 30% and the risk of cardiovascular disease by 15% to 20%.

Evaluate renal function at the start of therapy and periodically thereafter to identify patients with severe renal impairment (i.e., creatinine clearance less than 30 mL/min).

Incretin Inhibitors

- sitagliptin (Januvia)
- vildagliptin (Galvus)

A number of newer approaches to diabetes therapy are currently undergoing clinical trials, including those involving stimulation of the pancreatic beta cell with the gut-derived insulinotropic hormones (incretins), gastric-inhibitory polypeptide (GIP) and glucagon-like polypeptides 1 and 2 (GLP-1, GLP-2). The current focus is on an approach based on the inhibition of dipeptidyl peptidase 4 (DPP-4), the major enzyme responsible for degrading the incretins in vivo (i.e., incretin inhibitors). The rationale for this approach is that blocking incretin degradation would increase their physiologic actions, including the stimulation of insulin secretion and the inhibition of gastric emptying. It is now clear that both GIP and GLP-1 also have powerful effects on beta cell differentiation, mitogenesis, and survival. By potentiating these pleiotropic actions (i.e., the phenomenon in which a single gene determines two or more apparently unrelated characteristics of the same organism) of the incretins, DPP-4 inhibition may preserve beta cell mass and improve insulin secretory function in diabetics.

GIP, also known as glucose-dependent insulinotropic polypeptide, is an amino acid hormone that stimulates insulin secretion in the presence of glucose. GIP is a member of a family of structurally related hormones that include secretin, glucagon, vasoactive intestinal peptide, and growth hormone–releasing factor. GLP-1, the so-called gluco-incretin, is a potent insulin secretagogue that plays a major role in the enteroinsular axis, which in turn accounts for the finding that plasma insulin levels following oral intake of glucose are greater than those seen when glucose is given intravenously.

It's not yet clear how widely used these newer drugs are, given the price tag of $3 to $6 a day when, by contrast, diabetes drugs cost 50 cents a day or less. Even using three to four drugs from different classes that are used today, the expected cost of these drugs will likely curtail their use.

Sitagliptin

Sitagliptin is taken once daily for the treatment of T2DM. Sitagliptin is well tolerated either as monotherapy or combination therapy (added to pioglitazone or metformin). If approved, sitagliptin would potentially be the first in a new class of oral drugs, DPP-4 inhibitors, used to enhance the body's own ability to lower blood glucose when it is elevated.

Multiple doses of sitagliptin are generally well tolerated. Sitagliptin is a weak inhibitor of CYP450 enzymes in vitro and is primarily eliminated through the kidneys, with a half-life of 8 to 12 hours. A single dose of 100 mg produces DPP-4 inhibition for 24 hours. Doses greater than 100 mg daily yield DPP-4 inhibition of 80% or higher 24 hours after the last dose.

Sitagliptin was not associated with a weight gain from baseline, and the incidence of hypoglycemia was similar to placebo. The most common adverse effects of sitagliptin were a stuffy or runny nose and sore throat, headache, diarrhea, and joint pain.

Vildagliptin

Vildagliptin appears to be a safe, very well tolerated, and efficacious DDP-4 inhibitor to be used in the treatment of T2DM as monotherapy or when added on to metformin. Throughout phase 3 studies, vildagliptin has shown clinically significant and consistent A_{1c} reductions both as monotherapy and in combination with other oral (i.e., pioglitazone) and injectable antidiabetic drugs. Some 67% of people on vildagliptin and pioglitazone achieved the American Diabetes Association (ADA)–defined A_{1c} goal of less than or equal to 7% versus 42% of those who achieved this goal on monotherapy (vildagliptin 42.5%; pioglitazone 42.9%). More importantly, a reduction of up to 2.8% in A_{1c} was seen among patients with poor glycemic control who had the highest mean baseline blood sugar levels (about 10%) as measured by A_{1c}.

Among the interesting findings was the fact that vildagliptin increased the levels of GLP-1 and GIP in patients with T1DM and T2DM. Vildagliptin therapy also has favorable effects on lipid profiles, including reductions in triglycerides. Vildagliptin stimulates insulin secretion after an oral glucose load, and also improves insulin sensitivity after 6 weeks of therapy in patients with T2DM. There was also evidence of improvement in the acute insulin secretory response to glucose and improved disposition of the patient's glucose.

The most common adverse effects of vildagliptin are cold-like symptoms, headache, and dizziness. The overall incidence of adverse effects including hypoglycemia and edema was similar to placebo.

Insulin Antagonist

◆ rDNA glucagon (Glucagon, rGlucaGen)

Indications

Glucagon is an insulin antagonist (i.e., an "antihypoglycemic" drug) produced through rDNA technology for the treatment of hypoglycemia. It is effective only if there are sufficient amounts of liver glycogen present. Parenteral administration of glucagon relaxes the smooth muscle of the stomach, duodenum, small bowel, and colon and is used in radiologic procedures requiring relaxation of these tissues. Patients with low blood sugar levels that are associated with starvation, adrenal insufficiency, or chronic hypoglycemia will not be effectively treated with glucagon; they are treated with glucose.

Pharmacodynamics

Glucagon is produced naturally by the alpha cells of the pancreas (see Fig. 53-1) but may also be synthesized by adding the gene for glucagon to genetically altered, nonpathogenic strains of *E. coli* or *S. cerevisiae* bacteria. This synthesized glucagon acts in the same fashion as naturally occurring glucagon. Administration of glucagon stimulates glycogenolysis, which results in an increase in blood glucose levels, relaxation of GI smooth muscle, and an increase in the rate and the strength of myocardial contraction. The mechanism by which glucagon exerts its effects on GI smooth muscle and cardiac muscle is unknown.

Glucagon increases the production of adenylate cyclase in liver and adipose tissue, which catalyzes the conversion of ATP to cyclic adenosine monophosphate (cAMP). cAMP catalyzes reactions that activate phosphorylase, an enzyme that promotes the breakdown of glycogen to glucose. The presence of phosphorylase and hepatic reserves of glucagon determine the extent to which glucose levels are raised. The increase in blood glucose levels is not as great in patients with T1DM as in those with T2DM.

Pharmacokinetics

The onset, the peak, and the duration of action of glucagon depend on the route of administration. Onset is within 1 minute following intravenous (IV) administration, and 4 to 7 minutes, or 8 to 10 minutes following 1-mg or 2-mg intramuscular (IM) doses, respectively. Blood glucose levels return to normal or hypoglycemic levels within 1 to 2 hours. Its duration of action varies between 9 and 25 minutes if given by IV route, and 12 to 32 minutes when given by IM route. Glucagon is extensively biotransformed by the liver and the kidneys and eliminated in the urine.

Adverse Effects and Contraindications

Adverse effects to glucagon are rare, with the exception of nausea and vomiting. Exercise caution when using glucagon in patients with insulinoma or pheochromocytoma. IV administration of glucagon produces an initial increase in blood glucose, resulting in an increase in insulin release from the insulinoma and hypoglycemia. Administration of glucagon can cause the pheochromocytoma to release catecholamines, resulting in marked increase in blood pressure. Hypersensitivity reactions are characterized by respiratory distress, urticaria, and hypotension.

Glucagon is contraindicated for use in patients with known hypersensitivity. Use is also contraindicated in patients with allergies to glycerin and phenol, ingredients found in the diluent for glucagon.

Drug Interactions

Large doses of glucagon increase the risk of bleeding when given with warfarin because of decreased production of clotting factors in the liver, or as a result of increased sensitivity of the anticoagulant for its receptor site. The dose of anticoagulant may have to be decreased for patients receiving glucagon in doses of 25 mg or more daily for 2 days.

Dosage Regimen

See Table 53-8 for dosing recommendations. Dosage adjustments for patients with hepatic or renal impairment is not available, although it appears that no dosage adjustments are needed. An unconscious patient should respond within 15 minutes, although a second dose may be given if the patient does not respond to the first. IV glucose must be given if there is no patient response to glucagon.

Lab Considerations

Conduct frequent blood glucose monitoring until the hypoglycemia has been treated and the patient is asymptomatic.

TABLE 53-8 Tips for Using Glucagon Emergency Kit

- Do not use glucagon after the expiration date stamped on the kit.
- Use the diluent provided in the kit to prepare glucagon for injection.
- Discard any unused solution after preparation.
- Do not use glucagon at concentrations over 1 unit/mL, or if the solution is cloudy.
- *Adults and children >55 lb:* 1 mg (1 international unit) subQ, IM, or IV.
- *Adults and children <55 lb or <6–8 yr:* 0.5 mg (0.5 international units) subQ, IM, or IV. Do not exceed 1 mg.
- *Dosage of rDNA glucagon for adults and children >44 lb:* 1 mg (1 international unit) subQ, IM, or IV.
- *Dosage of rDNA glucagon children <44 lb:* 0.5 mg (0.5 international units), or alternatively, 0.02–0.03 mg/kg (international units/kg) subQ, IM, or IV. Do not exceed 1 mg.
- Glucagon can be given in the abdomen, the buttocks, the upper thighs, the back, or the fatty part of the upper arm.
- Turn the patient on his or her side after administering glucagon. An adverse effect of glucagon is nausea with vomiting. This position will prevent the patient from choking and aspirating.
- Feed the patient as soon as he or she awakens and is able to swallow. Give the patient a fast-acting source of carbohydrate (such as regular soft drink or fruit juice) and a longer-acting source of sugar (such as crackers and cheese or meat sandwich) to avoid a second hypoglycemic episode.
- If the patient does not awaken within 15 minutes, give another dose of glucagon and *inform emergency services immediately.*
- Notify the patient's primary care provider after recovery from hypoglycemia.

IM, Intramuscular (route); *IV,* intravenous (route); *subQ,* subcutaneous (route).

ENDOCRINE

Monitor prothrombin times and INRs in patients taking warfarin who receive large doses of glucagon.

Nutritive Agents

◆ 50% dextrose (D$_{50}$)
◆ Oral glucose gel or tablets

▥ Indications

Dextrose, a monosaccharide, is given by mouth or IV infusion for the treatment of insulin-induced hypoglycemia. A 5% to 10% solution is used to prevent hypoglycemia associated with insulin infusion for the treatment of diabetic ketoacidosis once blood glucose concentrations have fallen below about 250 mg/L.

▥ Pharmacodynamics

Carbohydrate in the form of dextrose may minimize depletion of hepatic glycogen and may have a protein-sparing action. Direct absorption from the intestine results in rapid increase in blood glucose concentrations and is effective in small doses. Dextrose is not absorbed from the buccal cavity and must be swallowed to be effective.

▥ Pharmacokinetics

Peak plasma concentrations of D$_{50}$ occur about 40 minutes after oral administration. Dextrose is metabolized via pyruvic or lactic acid to carbon dioxide and water.

▥ Adverse Effects and Contraindications

Do not give oral glucose solutions or tablets to patients who are unconscious or unable to swallow. Significant hyperglycemia and possible hyperosmolar syndrome may result from too rapid administration of 50% dextrose (D$_{50}$). IV administration of D$_{50}$ can cause fluid and/or solute overloading and result in dilution of serum electrolyte concentrations, overhydration, congested states, or pulmonary edema. Avoid using concentrated dextrose solution when intracranial or intraspinal hemorrhage is present, or in a patient with delirium tremens if the patient is already dehydrated. D$_{50}$ is hypertonic and may cause phlebitis and thrombosis at the site of injection.

▥ Drug Interactions

Administer D$_{50}$ with caution to patients receiving corticosteroids or corticotropin, especially if the solution contains sodium ions.

▥ Dosage Regimen

The dose of dextrose is variable and dependent on individual patient requirements and response to treatment. Administer 10 to 20 grams of dextrose orally for treatment of insulin-induced hypoglycemia. Response should occur within 10 minutes. Additional doses of dextrose can be given to counter hypoglycemic effects caused by long-acting insulin preparations.

To minimize irritation, give D$_{50}$ slowly, preferably through a small-bore needle and into a large vein. Each mL of D$_{50}$ solution contains 0.5 grams of dextrose. IV injection of 10 to 25 grams of dextrose (20 to 50 mL of D$_{50}$) is usually adequate to treat insulin-induced hypoglycemia.

Caution patients to read the directions on their glucose tablet or gel product to determine the amount of carbohydrate provided. Patients need to clearly understand how much of the product is required to provide the 10- to 20-gram dosage needed to treat hypoglycemia.

▥ Lab Considerations

Conduct frequent blood glucose monitoring until the patient has been treated and is asymptomatic. Monitor INRs in patients taking warfarin who receive large doses of glucagon.

CLINICAL REASONING

Treatment Objectives

The primary goal of diabetes therapy is euglycemia: to reach and maintain blood glucose target goals in order to prevent long-term complications of diabetes and improve the quality of life. Both the American Diabetes Association (ADA) and the American Association of Clinical Endocrinologists (AACE) have similar primary goals. The most recent ADA target goals in general include the following:

* Preprandial blood glucose levels of 90 mg/dL to 130 mg/dL
* Two-hour postprandial blood glucose levels less than 180 mg/dL
* A$_{1c}$ levels lower than 7%

The AACE recommends the following general blood glucose testing goals for adults with T1DM and T2DM:

* Preprandial blood glucose levels less than 110 mg/dL
* Two-hour postprandial blood glucose levels less than 140 mg/dL
* A$_{1c}$ levels lower than 6.5%

In addition, other parameter goals include:

* Blood pressure readings consistently less than 130/80 mm Hg
* Low-density lipoprotein (LDL) cholesterol levels less than 100 mg/dL
* High-density lipoprotein (HDL) cholesterol levels over 40 mg/dL
* Triglyceride levels below 150 mg/dL

Treatment Options

Interventions that mimic normal physiology as closely as possible help to accomplish these goals. Treatment of diabetes is based on correcting underlying physiologic abnormalities of absolute or relative insulin deficiency and insulin resistance. Initial treatment starts with referring the patient for diabetic education, which includes information on dietary requirements, diabetes self-management, blood glucose monitoring, and recommendations for physical activity. Drug therapy is generally started when lifestyle modifications do not reduce blood glucose to target levels. However, drug regimens do not always address all metabolic derangements of diabetes (Fig. 53-2).

Insulin is required for patients with T1DM. The treatment choice for a patient with T2DM is based on patient history, present level of glucose control, presence of comorbid conditions, patient preference, and the mechanism of action and adverse effects profile of available drugs.

Secondary failure rates in patients with T2DM on monotherapy are high. A second blood glucose–lowering drug with a different mechanism of action may be needed to improve glucose control. Because of progressive beta cell failure, many patients with T2DM eventually require insulin therapy to achieve target blood glucose levels.

There is discussion regarding when insulin should be initiated in the treatment of T2DM. There are studies that suggest that combining insulin with oral drugs early in the disease may reduce insulin resistance, limit weight gain, and improve blood lipid profiles (Magee, et al., 2006). Insulin reverses glucose toxicity (a molecular mechanism of action for glucose toxicity has been identified in studies demonstrating decreased insulin gene expression), which in turn improves both insulin sensitivity and insulin secretion. However, two important issues have not been addressed. One is whether the adverse effects on insulin-secreting cells of chronic exposure to high glucose concentrations are related in a continuous manner to glucose concentration, or whether there is a threshold that must be reached before glucose toxicity is expressed. The other is whether successful reversal of glucose toxicity is related to the length of previous exposure to supraphysiologic glucose concentrations. **There is a general agreement that when insulin therapy is postponed until all oral drugs fail, the insulin program must be more aggressive; multiple daily injections may be required to reach target blood glucose levels.**

The clinical relevance of these two issues stems from the need to understand the intensity with which hyperglycemia should be treated in T2DM. It is often suggested that the more quickly and more completely glycemia is normalized through diet or drug treatment, the more likely that residual beta cell function will be sufficient to maintain euglycemia.

▮▮ *Patient Variables*

A history of dietary intake is equally important, for there is no therapy a patient can't outeat. Initial referral for medical nutrition therapy (MNT) is important for assessment of the patient's dietary intake as well as for instruction in his or her individualized diet plan. No drug that lowers blood glucose levels should be prescribed without first determining when the patient eats meals, and the composition of these meals.

Assessment of the ability of the patient to adhere to the treatment plan is essential. It is necessary that the patient and the health care provider set realistic goals that both of them understand and approve. The success of flexible insulin therapy depends on the ability of the patient to perform accurate carbohydrate counting.

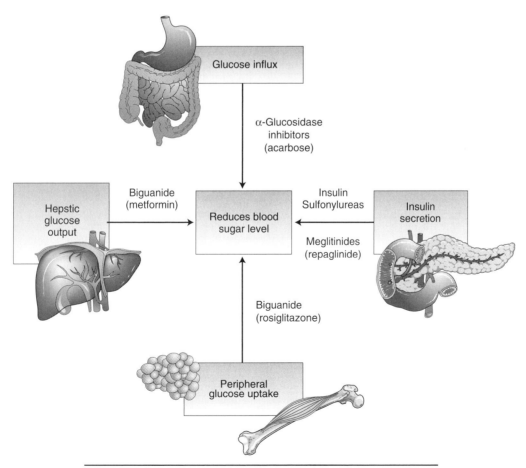

FIGURE 53-2 Current therapies for diabetes do not address all deranged pathways.

A treatment plan involving all aspects of diabetes therapy with individualized target blood glucose goals is developed for each patient with diabetes. Adjustments in drug dosages are based on trends and understanding of various factors that contribute to a specific blood glucose value. For example, hypoglycemia before the evening meal can occur because of excess intermediate-acting insulin at breakfast, excess rapid-acting insulin at lunch, insufficient carbohydrate intake at lunch, or an increase in exercise before the evening meal. Adjusting the dose of insulin without evaluating all other factors can result in hyperglycemia.

Blood glucose monitoring results are very important in pattern management. The effectiveness of a dose of intermediate-acting insulin given before breakfast is evaluated by the blood glucose value before the evening meal. The effectiveness of a dose of rapid-acting insulin given before breakfast is evaluated by the blood glucose value before lunch.

Life-Span Considerations

Pregnant and Nursing Women. The leading cause of mortality and morbidity in infants of mothers with T1DM and T2DM continues to be congenital malformations. The risk of malformation increases with increasing maternal hyperglycemia during the first 6 to 8 weeks of gestation. The standard of care for all women with diabetes with childbearing potential includes (1) education about the risks of malformations associated with unplanned pregnancy and poor metabolic control; and (2) use of effective contraception at all times unless the patient's diabetes is in good control and she is actively trying to conceive. A planned pregnancy with preconception care to achieve A_{1c} levels as near to normal as possible reduces the risk of congenital malformations.

Blood glucose testing done as early as possible in the pregnancy is necessary for women at high risk for GDM or those with marked obesity, a personal history of GDM, or a strong family history of diabetes. Screen women with GDM for diabetes 6 to 12 weeks after delivery and periodically thereafter for development of diabetes or prediabetes.

Metformin and acarbose are classified as category B drugs, with all other oral antidiabetic drugs classified as category C. Discontinue oral drug therapy during pregnancy since there are insufficient data to establish the safety of these products, and institute insulin therapy.

Children and Adolescents. Approximately 75% of all cases of T1DM are diagnosed in children and adolescents under 18 years of age. Further, the incidence of T2DM is increasing, especially in minority populations. It is important to accurately diagnose the type of diabetes, since the treatment of T1DM differs from that of T2DM.

Achievement of optimal blood glucose control is difficult in children because of changes in insulin sensitivity due to physical growth, limited ability to provide self-care, and susceptibility to hypoglycemia. Target blood glucose goals must be adjusted to prevent hypoglycemia. Most children under 7 years of age have hypoglycemic unawareness and lack the cognitive ability to recognize and treat hypoglycemia.

Family involvement is an important component of diabetes management in this age group. Adolescents present special challenges because of their search for autonomy. Evaluate behavioral, emotional, and psychosocial factors that may interfere with implementation of the treatment plan, and work with the individual and family members to resolve problems that occur. Modify goals as appropriate.

Older Adults. Diabetes is present in at least 20% of persons over the age of 65 years. There are higher rates of premature death, functional disability, and comorbid illness such as hypertension in older adults with diabetes than in older adults without diabetes. Many older adults with diabetes are frail and have underlying chronic disease states and substantial diabetes-related comorbidities.

Patient control of hyperglycemia is essential; however, older adults may experience a greater decline in morbidity and mortality by controlling cardiovascular risk factors. On the other hand, patients with complications from advanced diabetes are less likely to benefit from reducing the risk of macrovascular complications and are more likely to suffer from serious adverse effects of hypoglycemia. For the frail older adult with diabetes, it is important to set blood glucose targets at a level that will control symptoms of hyperglycemia but prevent acute complications of hyperglycemic hyperosmolar nonketotic syndrome (HHNS). Signs and symptoms of HHNS include a blood sugar level over 600 mg/dL; dry, parched mouth; extreme thirst (although this may gradually disappear); warm, dry skin that does not sweat; high fever; sleepiness or confusion; loss of vision; hallucinations; and weakness on one side of the body.

▮▮ *Drug Variables*

Oral Hypoglycemic Drugs. Oral drugs are used to treat relative insulin deficiency and insulin resistance characteristic of T2DM. Monotherapy is generally associated with A_{1c} reduction of 0.5% to 1.5%. Treatment for a patient with newly diagnosed T2DM can be initiated with either a sulfonylurea drug or metformin. Metformin is the preferred drug for overweight patients. When target blood glucose and A_{1c} levels are no longer achievable with a single drug, combination therapy is indicated; a sulfonylurea or TZD together with metformin is the most common regimen. Patients with blood glucose levels greater than 280 mg/dL will most likely not respond to sulfonylurea therapy and will require insulin for initial blood glucose control.

Treatment failure occurs when the patient is insensitive to the drugs' effects. Primary failure occurs in 20% of patients placed on sulfonylurea therapy. Secondary failure occurs in 5% to 10% of individuals whose blood glucose initially responded to a given drug.

Initiating Oral Therapy. Sulfonylurea drugs are appropriate for average-weight adults without lipid abnormalities. Initiate treatment using a low-dose sulfonylurea drug, given once daily, whose dosage is increased until the patient reaches the target blood glucose level. If target glucose levels are not reached with a maximum dosage of a sulfonylurea, a second oral drug with a different mechanism of action can be added. The choice of the second drug is based on individual patient characteristics and adverse effects profile of the drugs involved (see the Case Study).

Insulins. Insulin is required for treatment of T1DM, for treatment of gestational diabetes, and for diabetes associated with conditions such as pancreatic disease, chemical-induced diabetes, endocrinopathies, insulin-receptor disorders, and certain genetic disorders. The dose of insulin must be individualized and is balanced with MNT and exercise (see following discussion).

Initiating Insulin Therapy. Patients with T1DM who are within 20% of their ideal body weight and who are without infection

CASE STUDY | Drugs Used to Treat Diabetes

ASSESSMENT

History of Present Illness	You are seeing AB, a 78-year-old male with T2DM. He reports higher blood glucose levels since his metformin was discontinued 9 months ago because of severe diarrhea. He currently takes 12 units of NPH insulin twice daily and aspart insulin before each meal, 5 units before breakfast, 5 units at lunch, and 3 units at supper. AB has had diabetes for 12 years; it was initially treated with "pills" and then, for the past year, with insulin. AB's history includes coronary artery disease (metformin stopped in September 2005 because of a 49% ejection fraction). He reports no history of syncopal episodes. SMBG average according to glucometer is 164 mg/dL, with an A_{1c} of 8.5%. Of the readings less than 70 mg/dL, 10.2% were between 70 and 110 mg/dL, and 81.3% were over 110 mg/dL. Blood glucose values are highest in the evening and lowest at lunch. AB's weight is stable, and he has had no fever. Appetite is good, vision unchanged (last eye exam unknown), no chest pain, no dyspepsia, dysuria, and no paresthesias or numbness. Last dilated eye exam 3 months ago was normal. He has had occasional episodes of DOE. Other drugs taken include diltiazem SA 240 mg daily; metoprolol 50 mg daily; hydrochlorothiazide 12.5 mg daily before breakfast; lovastatin 80 mg every evening; and warfarin (generic formulation) 2.5 mg every Tuesday, Thursday, and Saturday, and 5 mg all other days.
Past Medical History	Atrial fibrillation for several years, treated with chronic anticoagulation, beta blockers, and calcium channel blockers. Myocardial infarction 13 years ago with a history of poorly controlled hypertension. Review of systems otherwise unremarkable.
Life-Span Considerations	AB lives with his wife in a neighboring city. He is a retired accountant who enjoys gardening and reading. His wife is supportive and is willing and able to prepare appropriate foods for Mr. B. He has frequent contact with his two children and seven grandchildren. Mr. B reports having sufficient funds to support his current lifestyle and medical needs.
Physical Exam Findings	*Ht:* 69 in. *Wt:* 75 kg. *BP:* 162/72. *VS:* 97.3° F-88-18. Snellen chart: 20/25 both eyes. ENT unremarkable, no fundus changes. No icterus, lymphadenopathy of neck or axillae, and no thyromegaly. HRRR without lifts, thrills, heaves, murmurs, or gallops; no S_3 or S_4. Abdomen soft, nontender, no HSM, masses, or bruits. No CVAT. No peripheral edema; DP and PT pulses 2+; 7-mm monofilament sensation intact; callus on right first toe, no other pressure areas or lesions noted.
Diagnostic Testing	Random finger stick blood sugar today: 144 mg/dL. UA: no protein, glucose, ketones. Serum creatinine: 1.0; A_{1c}: 8.6%. Total cholesterol: 96 mg/dL. Triglycerides, 148 mg/dL. HDL, 32 mg/dL. LDL, 153 mg/dL. Most recent INR 1 week ago: 2.4.

DIAGNOSIS: Insulin-Dependent T2DM

MANAGEMENT

Treatment Objectives	1. Set target blood glucose at level to avoid hypoglycemia in an active 78-year-old man. 2. Reduce percentage of blood glucose values that are over his target level. 3. Reduce the risk of the complications of diabetes.
Treatment Options	**Pharmacotherapy** • aspart insulin (Novolog) with each meal in a ratio of 1 unit per 10 grams of carbs • 37.5 units insulin glargine (Lantus) subcutaneously at bedtime • Start lisinopril, 20 mg PO twice daily for renoprotection. • Continue all other drugs as prescribed **Patient Education** 1. Drug formulation, administration, sites, and storage; disposal of syringes; travel advice 2. Glucose monitoring 3. Treatment of hypoglycemia 4. Meal planning 5. Exercise 6. Sick-day behaviors

Continued

ENDOCRINE

CASE STUDY   Drugs Used to Treat Diabetes—Cont'd

Evaluation

Blood glucose monitoring results determine if ratios of insulin to carbohydrate will have to be adjusted for each meal. Patient to follow-up in office next week for continued patient education and again in 3 months for routine diabetic check; sooner if SMBG rises above 160 mg/dL on regular basis.

CLINICAL REASONING ANALYSIS

Q1. How do you know what dosage of basal insulin to use for Mr. B?

A. The recommendation for basal insulin is based on 0.5 mg/kg of body weight. Therefore, his basal insulin requirement is 37 units.

Q2. And you are going to give him insulin before his meals, too? I don't understand. How do you know how much to give him?

A. He will use insulin aspart insulin (NovoLog) with each meal. It is dosed as 1 unit per 10 grams of carbohydrate for all meals and snacks. A 1:10 insulin to carbohydrate ratio is a reasonable starting point for Mr. B, although he will need lots of teaching about his regimen and the importance of SMBG in determining his dose at mealtimes.

Q3. What instructions would you provide for treatment of high blood glucose levels at mealtime?

A. Administer 1 additional unit of aspart insulin for every 50 points of blood glucose elevation over his target level of 130 mg/dL.

Q4. What education would you provide for Mr. and Mrs. B?

A. Instruction in carbohydrate counting provided by registered dietitian.

Q5. I just finished seeing Mr. B in the clinic for his 4-week check-up. His average SMBG increased to 180 mg/dL which continues to be highest in the evening and lowest at lunch. He is awaiting pacemaker placement and is less physically active than normal. I know we need to increase his glargine insulin dose, but how much? How do I figure this out?

A. Well, his daily blood glucose pattern has not changed overall; he seems to be accurate in carbohydrate counting according to his dietary log, and he is administering the premeal insulin bolus correctly. We will increase his basal rate of insulin glargine to 0.7 units/kg of insulin once daily. The rule of thumb for dosage increase is no more than 10% of previous dosage. His previous dosage was 0.5 units/kg, and at 75 kg, his revised dosage will be 40 units.

---

require 0.5 to 1.0 units/kg/day of insulin for glycemic control. The required dose during the "honeymoon period" (i.e., the period early in the disease when the pancreas is still producing insulin) is 0.2 to 0.6 units/kg/day. Dosage requirements increase markedly during illness, pregnancy, and the adolescent growth period (1.3–1.5 units/kg/day).

Approximately 40% to 50% of the total daily insulin (TDI) dose is used to provide basal insulin. The remainder is to provide meal-related coverage, and is administered according to the dietary practices of the individual. Meal-related insulin can be given as a fixed dose or as a ratio of insulin to carbohydrate intake. An initial dose of 0.8 to 1.2 units of insulin for every 10 grams of carbohydrate eaten is a reasonable starting place in adults. In children, the ratio of insulin to carbohydrate depends on age, body size, and activity, with a range of 0.3 to 1.0 units of insulin for every 10 grams of carbohydrate consumed.

Insulin is introduced into the treatment regimen of a patient with T2DM when blood glucose control can no longer be maintained with lifestyle changes and oral drug therapy, although some sources recommend adding insulin when the patient's A_{1c} level is over 7% with therapy. Insulin can be added gradually to the patient's current oral drug regimen. Possible choices include intermediate- or long-acting insulin at bedtime; human analogue insulin 70/30 or 75/25 mixtures before supper, before

breakfast, or both; and basal insulin glargine (Lantus) at bedtime, before supper, or in the morning.

Insulin requirements for individuals with T2DM may range from as little as 5 to 10 units per day to several hundred units per day, depending on the degree of insulin resistance. In patients with newly diagnosed T2DM who have significant hyperglycemia and glucose toxicity, insulin therapy can be started at a dose of 0.5 unit/kg/day. Premixed insulin can be given in two equally divided doses until specific glucose patterns are evident from self–blood glucose monitoring results. Patients with a more significant insulin deficiency may require a mixture of rapid- and intermediate-acting insulin at breakfast, rapid-acting insulin before supper, and intermediate-acting insulin at bedtime to control fasting hyperglycemia.

Patients with fasting hyperglycemia benefit from insulin administration at bedtime to suppress increased hepatic glucose production; this helps achieve lower blood glucose levels in the morning. Several insulin initiation formulas are available. The Treat-to-Target Trial recommends starting insulin therapy with one evening basal injection of 10 units of glargine or neutral protamine Hagedorn (NPH) insulin (Riddle, 2006). Weekly titration is accomplished by increasing the evening dose of basal insulin by two units for FBS levels between 100 mg/dL and 120 mg/dL, and the addition of one unit for each 20-mg/dL increment in blood glucose

▲ elevation over 120 mg/dL. **Insulin adjustments are made systematically, starting with the fasting, then the preprandial and, finally, the postprandial glucose levels. Avoid changing more than one insulin dose at a time, and do not change insulin doses more often than once a week to evaluate the results of insulin adjustments.**

If possible, the addition of insulin to a treatment regimen for patients with T2DM should be a planned event. The process of insulin initiation is smoother when the diabetic patient understands the progressive nature of T2DM and that he or she will more than likely require insulin for blood glucose control sometime in the future. Many patients are reluctant to start insulin therapy because of the fear that they have failed self-management or the perception that their disease is more severe. Involvement of a certified diabetes educator (CDE) will help the patient learn the skills needed to become more comfortable and proficient in insulin management.

Patient Education

▥ Glucose Monitoring

Blood glucose values provide important information about the adequacy of a treatment plan in achieving glycemic control. The frequency and timing of blood glucose testing is determined by the patient's needs and treatment goals. The recommendation for most patients with T1DM and pregnant women who have elevated blood glucose levels is to self-monitor blood glucose (SMBG) 3 or more times daily. SMBG should be carried out before each meal and at bedtime for patients taking multiple insulin injections. SMBG 2 hours after meals is often requested to evaluate postprandial blood glucose control.

The optimal frequency of SMBG for patients on oral drug therapy has not been determined; however, SMBG has to be performed with enough frequency to determine if treatment goals are being reached. The frequency of SMBG must be increased to evaluate any changes in therapy.

Many blood glucose meters are available for patient use. Because the accuracy of SMBG is instrument- and user-dependent, patients need careful instruction in procedures involved in blood glucose testing so as to obtain accurate results. All meters are accurate when used according to manufacturer's directions. It is helpful to review patients' technique from time to time to make certain that they are able to obtain accurate blood glucose monitoring results.

To achieve optimal glycemic control, teach patients how to use SMBG results to adjust dietary intake, how and when to exercise, and how to adjust pharmacologic therapy to achieve specific glycemic goals.

▥ Meal Planning

There is no standard "diabetic diet." Refer each person with diabetes to a registered dietitian for an assessment of his or her nutritional needs and the recommendation of a diet plan to meet them. Applicable to all persons with diabetes, the goals of MNT include the following:

- Attain and maintain blood glucose levels, lipid and lipoprotein profiles, and blood pressure readings in the normal range to help reduce the risk for macrovascular and cardiovascular disease.
- Prevent and treat chronic complications of diabetes. Modify intake as suitable for prevention and treatment

of obesity, dyslipidemia, cardiovascular disease, hypertension, and nephropathy.
- Improve overall health by learning to make healthy food choices and engaging in physical activity.
- Take into consideration the patient's nutritional, personal, and cultural preferences and lifestyle when addressing individual nutritional needs.

The preprandial insulin dose for persons receiving intensive insulin therapy is based on the total carbohydrate content of meals and snacks. Consistency in timing of meals and carbohydrate content is recommended for persons on fixed insulin regimens or receiving treatment with insulin secretagogues.

▥ Exercise

A daily minimum of 2 to 3 hours of moderate-intensity aerobic exercise improves glycemic control, reduces cardiovascular risk factors, contributes to weight loss, and improves well-being. Before increasing usual patterns of physical activity, patients with diabetes should undergo a detailed medical examination to screen for the presence of complications that may be worsened by exercise.

Drug dosage or carbohydrate intake may have to be altered in patients taking insulin and or secretagogues since physical activity may lead to hypoglycemia. Additional carbohydrates should be consumed if the preactivity blood glucose level is less than 100 mg/dL. Moderate-intensity exercise increases blood glucose uptake by 2 to 3 mg/kg/min above the usual requirements. A 70-kg person would need 8.4 to 12.6 grams (10 to 15) of carbohydrate per hour of moderate physical activity. Additional carbohydrate would be needed for intense activity.

▥ Annual Eye Exam and Regular Foot Checks

Patients with diabetes mellitus require annual eye exams by an ophthalmologist to monitor for retinal changes and other complications of diabetes. Teach patients to examine their feet daily for pressure areas, ingrown toenails, or lesions. Peripheral neuropathies associated with diabetes can lead to gangrene and amputation.

▥ Sick-Day Behaviors

Sudden loss of control in a previously stable patient leads one to suspect an underlying illness that may or may not present in a typical fashion. Glucose control usually worsens during illness because increased levels of counterregulatory hormones increase insulin requirements. It is important to teach patients that during illness they must increase glucose monitoring; drink adequate amounts of fluids, and ingest adequate amounts of carbohydrate, especially if blood glucose levels are less than 100 mg/dL. In adults, ingestion of 150 to 200 grams of carbohydrate daily (45 to 50 grams, or three to four carbohydrate choices every 3 to 4 hours) should be sufficient to maintain desired blood glucose levels and prevent starvation ketosis.

▥ Insulin Delivery Systems

There are a variety of insulin delivery systems on the market. Traditional insulin administration involves subQ injection using syringes calibrated in units. Disposable insulin syringes are manufactured with 0.3-, 0.5-, and 1-mL capacities and with different needle lengths.

Disposable syringes and needles are to be used only once. One potential issue is the inability to guarantee sterility of the insulin. A far more important reason to not reuse needles has arisen with the advent of new, smaller (30- and 31-gauge) needles: the needle tip may bend, forming a hook that can break off within the skin and lacerate tissues. Insulin delivery aids (e.g., nonvisual insulin measurement devices, syringe magnifiers, needle guides, and vial stabilizers) are available for people with visual impairment.

Several pen-like devices containing multidose insulin cartridges are also available. After attaching a disposable needle, the insulin dose is selected and a button depressed for each 1- to 2-unit increment desired, or once for the entire selected dosage. Although needles are used for the injection, there is no need for insulin to be drawn from multidose vials, adding to the convenience and accuracy of administration. The pen-like devices are helpful for patients who are visually or neurologically impaired, and who need multiple daily injections. In many patients, these devices have been shown to improve dosing accuracy and adherence to therapy.

Insulin can also be administered using a jet injector that delivers insulin as a fine stream into the skin. Jet injectors are available for those who are afraid of needles or for patients unable to use a syringe. The absorption and peak action of insulin delivered in this fashion may be altered, necessitating caution by the patient. The onset and peak action of the insulin occurs earlier when these devices are used. The injectors are expensive and may traumatize the skin if they are used incorrectly.

Insulin pumps are available as an alternative to conventional therapy and provide excellent glycemic control, but they require strong motivation on the part of the patient. The pumps deliver a constant basal rate of insulin throughout the day and night, with the capability of delivering a bolus dose of insulin at mealtimes. The needle, which is attached to a syringe via a length of plastic tubing, remains indwelling in the subQ tissue. The patient programs the pump unit to deliver the desired dose of insulin, based on SMBG levels. Patients must be alert to tenderness and erythema at the insertion site, which may indicate infection or abscess. The subQ insertion site, which is commonly on the abdomen, is ordinarily changed every 3 days.

Insulin may also be administered intravenously. This route is used for hospitalized patients in need of intense, around-the-clock monitoring of glucose levels.

Insulin Handling and Storage

Insulin deteriorates when exposed to excessive heat or cold (<36° F or >85° F; 2° to 8° C), light, or agitation. Constant refrigeration is not needed for the newer preparations, although patients should be instructed to refrigerate, not freeze, extra bottles until needed. Vials of insulin not in use should be refrigerated until the expiration date noted on the product label. Vials in current use should be kept at room temperature (59° to 86° F; 15° to 30° C) to minimize irritation at the injection site caused by cold insulin. Insulin may lose its potency after it has been in use for over 30 days. Any unused insulin should be discarded after that time. Because of variance of temperature, insulin should not be left in a car or checked through in airline luggage. Insulin vials should always be inspected for clumping before each use.

Some patients need to have their insulin syringes prefilled (e.g., the visually impaired, those dependent on others for drawing their insulin, those traveling or eating in restaurants).

A small number of syringes may be filled and stored in the refrigerator. Prefilled syringes may be stored for up to 30 days. Store the syringes with the needle pointing upward, to avoid clogging the needle with suspended insulin particles. Prefilled insulin syringes should be rolled between the hands to warm the insulin and to resuspend the insulin particles before administration.

Guidelines differ for the use and storage of prefilled insulin pens. Refer to manufacturer's guidelines for the specific product. Most cartridges or regular prefilled insulin pens may be kept unrefrigerated anywhere from 10 to 28 days.

Patients will ask if they can mix two insulins in one syringe to minimize the number of injections. This practice is acceptable under certain conditions, as long as the patient demonstrates accuracy in measurement techniques. Using insulins that have different durations of action elicits a more normal glycemic response than use of single insulin. The patient should prepare the insulin mixture in the same fashion for each injection. Commercially prepared insulin mixtures are available that help reduce the potential for the errors that occur when mixing insulin.

Consult the manufacturer's directions for each insulin formulation for mixing insulin. Once mixed, intermediate- and fast-acting insulin formulations can be used immediately or stored for future use. Rapid-acting insulin can be mixed with NPH insulin. This combination should be administered within 15 minutes of eating a meal. In contrast, insulin glargine should not be mixed with any other insulin because of the low pH of the diluent, and insulin detemir should not be diluted or mixed with any other insulin preparation.

Store inhaled insulin blister packs at room temperature (15° to 30° C, or 59° to 86° F). Do not refrigerate or freeze the blister packs; throw away the blister packs if they freeze. Use the blister packs within 3 months once the foil overwrap is opened. Keep unused blister packs in the foil overwrap. Store the inhaler and the release unit at room temperature.

Equipment Disposal

In December 2004 the Environmental Protection Agency (EPA) issued new recommendations for disposal of syringes used outside the hospital setting. The EPA no longer recommends use of sturdy household containers that are discarded into the trash when full. Current EPA guidelines recommend that needles and syringes be disposed of at a community drop-off center, at a household hazardous waste facility, by a residential "special waste" pick-up service, or at a syringe exchange program. A national disposal program such as a "sharps" mail-back program, or use of at-home-needle-destruction devices may be available in some communities. In many cases, used needles and syringes may be returned to the health care provider's office for disposal along with hazardous waste.

Treating Hypoglycemia

Hypoglycemia is the leading limiting factor in glycemic management. Whether the patient is using insulin or oral hypoglycemic drugs, treatment of hypoglycemia (blood glucose less than 70 mg/dL) requires ingestion of glucose or carbohydrate-containing foods. The acute glycemic response correlates more accurately with the glucose content of the food rather than with the carbohydrate content of the food. Any carbohydrate containing glucose raises blood glucose levels. Adding protein to carbohydrate does not affect the immediate glycemic response and will not prevent subsequent hypoglycemia in patients who are on insulin. Adding fat retards absorption of the carbohydrate and protein, thus prolonging the acute glycemic response, and is not recommended. However, for patients who notice the early symptoms of hypoglycemia, consuming a protein will be helpful.

For patients experiencing insulin-induced hypoglycemia, 10 grams of oral glucose raises blood glucose levels by about 40 mg/dL over 30 minutes, and 20 grams of oral glucose raises blood glucose levels by about 60 mg/dL over 45 minutes. In each case, glucose levels begin to fall within 60 minutes of the glucose ingestion. Carbohydrate portions containing 15 to 20 grams of glucose are used to treat hypoglycemia include the following:

- 3 to 4 glucose tablets
- 8 to 10 Lifesaver candies
- 2 tablespoons of raisins
- 4 to 6 ounces of non–diet soft drink
- 4 to 6 ounces of fruit juice
- 8 ounces of milk (no-fat or low-fat preferred)
- One dose tube of oral glucose gel

The increase in blood glucose levels may only be temporary; therefore a random glucose level should be drawn within 15 minutes of initial treatment and additional carbohydrate provided if necessary. Once the patient is stable, determine why the episode of hypoglycemia occurred to evaluate whether dosage adjustments of the patient's drugs are needed.

Patients with hypoglycemia who require the assistance of another person and who cannot be treated with an oral carbohydrate should be treated with emergency glucagon kits. Family members, roommates, and co-workers should be instructed in the use of glucagon for situations when the individual cannot be treated orally. Refer to Table 53-8 on how to use the glucagon emergency kit. Instruct all patients to carry medical identification to alert others of their diabetes in case of emergency.

Evaluation

Therapeutic response to pharmacologic treatment of diabetes is determined by periodic blood glucose and A_{1c} testing. Treatment success is determined by delay or prevention of diabetes complications and end-organ damage, and improvement in the quality of life.

KEY POINTS

■ Diabetes is a metabolic disorder characterized by inappropriate hyperglycemia from defects in insulin secretion, insulin action, or both.

■ Uncontrolled diabetes leads to long-term complications including retinopathy, nephropathy, and neuropathy. The landmark studies, DCCT and the UKPDS, concluded that glycemic control postpones, prevents, or slows progression of these complications.

■ T1DM results from autoimmune destruction of pancreatic beta cells that leads to absolute insulin deficiency. T1DM accounts for 5% to 10% of patients diagnosed with diabetes.

■ T2DM is characterized by insulin resistance and relative (rather than absolute) insulin deficiency. T2DM accounts for 90% to 95% of patients diagnosed with diabetes.

■ Diabetes can be caused by genetic defects in beta cell function, genetic defects in insulin action, or diseases of the exocrine pancreas, or can be drug- or chemical-induced.

■ Gestational diabetes (GDM) is defined as carbohydrate intolerance that occurs with the onset of pregnancy or that is first recognized during pregnancy. Approximately 7% of all pregnancies are complicated by GDM, placing the women at increased risk for future development of diabetes outside of pregnancy.

■ A treatment plan with individualized target blood glucose goals is developed for each patient with diabetes. Treatment of diabetes mellitus is based on correction of physiologic abnormalities of absolute or relative insulin deficiency created by diabetes.

■ Initial therapy for diabetes starts with referral for education in medical nutrition therapy, diabetes self-management, blood glucose monitoring, and recommendations for physical activity.

■ Insulin therapy is required for all patients with T1DM and for many patients with T2DM.

■ Treatment of T2DM focuses on therapeutic lifestyle changes (i.e., diet and exercise) combined with stimulation of insulin release from beta cells, increased peripheral tissue utilization of glucose, decreased hepatic glucose production, and decreased utilization of ingested carbohydrates, as well as replacement of insulin.

■ All patients taking blood glucose–lowering drugs should be instructed in the prevention and treatment of hypoglycemia.

■ All patients taking blood glucose–lowering drugs should be instructed in measures to prevent loss of blood glucose control during illness.

ENDOCRINE

Bibliography

American Diabetes Association. (2004). Insulin administration. *Diabetes Care, 27*(Suppl 1), S106–S109.

American Diabetes Association. (2004). Nutrition principles and recommendations in diabetes. *Diabetes Care, 27*(Suppl 1), S36–S46.

American Diabetes Association. (2004). Physical activity/exercise and diabetes. *Diabetes Care, 27*(Suppl 1), S58–S62.

American Diabetes Association. (2006). Diagnosis and classification of diabetes mellitus. *Diabetes Care, 29*(Suppl 1), S43–S48.

American Diabetes Association. (2006). Standards of medical care in diabetes–2006. *Diabetes Care, 29*(Suppl 1), S4–S42.

Byetta (exenatide) prescribing information. Amylin Pharmaceuticals. Available online:www.byetta.com. Accessed May 25, 2007.

Childs, B. (2006). Pramlintide use in type 1 diabetes resulting in less hypoglycemia. *Diabetes Spectrum, 19*(1), 50–51.

Clarke, P., Gray, A., Briggs, A., et al. (2004). A model to estimate lifetime health outcomes of patients with Type 2 diabetes: The United Kingdom Prospective Diabetes Study (UKPDS) Outcome Model (UKPDS, No. 68).

DCCT Research Group. (1990 Diabetes Control and Complications Trial [DCCT]). Update. *Diabetes Care, 13*(4), 427–433.

DeFronzo, R., Bergenstal, R., Cefalu, W., et al. (2005). Efficacy of inhaled insulin in patients with type 2 diabetes not controlled with diet and exercise. *Diabetes Care, 28*(8), 1922–1928.

Dungan, K., and Buse, J. (2005). Glucagon-like peptide-1 based therapies for type 2 diabetes: A focus on exenatide. *Clinical Diabetes, 23* (2), 56–62.

Engelgau, M. (2004). Diabetes diagnostic criteria and impaired glycemic states: Evolving evidence base. *Clinical Diabetes, 22*(2), 69–70.

Franz, M. (Ed.). (2003). *A core curriculum for diabetes education* (5th Ed). Chicago: American Association of Diabetes Educators.

Gleason, C., Gonzales, M., Harmon, J., et al. (2000). Determinants of glucose toxicity and its reversibility in the pancreatic islet β-cell line, HIT-T15. *American Journal of Physiology, Endocrinology, and Metabolism, 279*(5), E997–E1002.

Griffin, S., and Borders, J. (2006). Exenatide and pramlintide: New meds on the block. *Diabetes Self-Management, 23*(4), 74–76, 79.

Haas, L. (2005). An overview of insulin analogs and premixed insulin analogs in the management of diabetes. Available online: www. mededtoday.com. Accessed May 25, 2007.

Haas, L., Kulkarni, K., and Meece, J. (2005). An overview of insulin analogs and premixed insulin analogs in the management of diabetes. Available online: www.mededtoday.com. Accessed July 22, 2007.

Hirsh, I. (2005). Insulin analogs. *New England Journal of Medicine, 2* (352), 174–183.

Hirsh, I., Bergenstal, R., Parkin, C., et al. (2005). A real-world approach to insulin therapy in primary care practice. *Clinical Diabetes, 23*(2), 78–86.

Insulin for oral inhalation (Exubera). (2006). *Pharmacist's Letter/Prescriber's Letter, 22*(7), 37.

Kendall, D. (2006). Thiazolidinediones. *Diabetes Care, 29*(1), 154–157.

Kimmel, B., and Inzucchi, S. (2005). Oral agents for type 2 diabetes: An update. *Clinical Diabetes, 23*(2), 64–76.

Kulkarni, K. (2005). Carbohydrate counting: A practical meal-planning option for people with diabetes. *Clinical Diabetes, 23*(3), 120–122.

Magee, M., Shomali, M., Ahmann, A., et al. (2006). Initiating insulin therapy earlier: Rationale, strategies, and benefits. Available online: www.mededtoday.com. Accessed July 22, 2007.

Mehenna, A. (2005). Insulin and oral diabetic agents. *American Journal of Pharmacy Education, 69*(5), Article 89; 1–20. Available online: www.ajpe.org. Accessed May 25, 2007.

New drugs: Symlin and Byetta. (2005). *Pharmacist's Letter/Prescriber's Letter, 21*(6), 32.

Raskin, P., Brunton, S., and Magee, M. (2006). Insulin implementation strategies in action: Integrating evidence with practice. Available online: www.mededtoday.com. Accessed May 25, 2007.

Rave, K., Bott, S., Heinemann, L., et al. (2005). Time-action profile of inhaled insulin in comparison with subcutaneously injected insulin lispro and regular human insulin. *Diabetes Care, 28*(5), 1077–1082.

Riddle, M. (2006). The Treat-to-Target Trial and related studies. *Endocrine Practice, 12*(Suppl 1), 71–79.

Rolla, A., Cooppan, R., Tibaldi, J., et al. (2006). Insulin analogs: Implementation and strategies in type 2 diabetes. Available online: www. mededtoday.com. Accessed May 25, 2007.

Rolla, A., Steil, C., Hinnen, D., et al. (2005). Rationale for the development and clinical use of insulin analogs and premixed insulin analogs. Available online: www.mededtoday.com. Accessed May 25, 2007.

Skyler, J., Weinstock, R., Raskin, P., et al. (2005). Use of inhaled insulin in a basal/bolus insulin regimen in type 1 diabetic subjects. *Diabetes Care, 28*(7), 1630–1635.

Staels, B., and Fruchart, J. (2005). Therapeutic roles of peroxisome proliferator-activated receptor agonists. *Diabetes, 54*(8), 2460–2470.

Tanne, J. (2007). FDA places "black box" warning on antidiabetes drugs. *BMJ, 334*(7606), 1237.

Van de Laar, F., Lucassen, P., Akkermans, R., et al. (2005). Alpha-glucosidase inhibitors for patients with type 2 diabetes. *Diabetes Care, 28*(2), 154–163.

Zammitt, N., and Frier, B. (2005). Hypoglycemia in type 2 diabetes. *Diabetes Care, 28*(12), 2948–2961.

Thyroid and Parathyroid Drugs and Drugs for Calcium Disorders

54

The function of the thyroid gland is to take iodine from the circulation, combine it with the amino acid tyrosine, and convert it to the thyroid hormones triiodothyronine (T_3) and thyroxine (T_4) (Fig. 54-1). The thyroid gland stores T_3 and T_4 while they await release into the circulation under influence of thyroid-stimulating hormone (TSH). Thyroid hormones not bound to circulating plasma proteins provide the true determination of thyroid status for the patient. Alterations in thyroid and parathyroid gland function cause some of the most common endocrine disorders.

Hypothyroidism (myxedema) is caused by a deficiency of thyroid hormones, whereas *hyperthyroidism* (thyrotoxicosis) is the result of excessive production of thyroid hormones.

Hyperparathyroidism most often results from a parathyroid adenoma. The resulting increase in parathyroid hormone (PTH) secretion causes hypercalcemia and lowers serum phosphate. Loss of calcium from the bone occurs and may be sufficient to produce bone abnormalities. In contrast, reductions in PTH from *hypoparathyroidism* usually results from inadvertent removal during surgery on the thyroid gland. The subsequent lack of PTH results in hypocalcemia.

Osteoporosis, a loss of calcium from the bones, may be related to hyperparathyroidism as well as other causes, and is a major public health threat. Osteoporosis is responsible for more than 1.5 million fractures each year in the United States and an increased risk of death. Although it is widely recognized that 20% of patients die within the first year after a hip fracture, the mortality rate after vertebral fractures, even among healthy older women, is increased but underreported. Long-term studies of men and women with vertebral deformities confirm increased rates of mortality and hospitalization (especially for cardiovascular, pulmonary, and cancer-related deaths) in proportion to the number of vertebral deformities. Even clinically occult vertebral fractures increase the risk of mortality. Only three fourths of people who were ambulatory before a hip fracture are able to live independently afterward; the remainder require long-term care. Yet despite this evidence, osteoporosis continues to be underevaluated and undertreated.

HYPOTHYROIDISM

EPIDEMIOLOGY AND ETIOLOGY

More than 90% of patients with hypothyroidism have primary thyroid atrophy. In North America, Hashimoto's thyroiditis (i.e., chronic lymphocytic thyroiditis, autoimmune thyroiditis) is the most common cause. Prior treatments with radioiodine or thyroidectomy are the next most common causes of hypothyroidism. Hypothyroidism coexists with other autoimmune disorders such as rheumatoid arthritis, systemic lupus erythematosus, or pernicious anemia.

Fewer than 6% of patients with hypothyroidism have a secondary or central cause for their hypothyroidism. Secondary hypothyroidism is most often related to failure of the pituitary gland to synthesize sufficient quantities of TSH. Postpartum pituitary necrosis (Sheehan's syndrome) and a pituitary tumor are the most frequent causes of secondary hypothyroidism. A recently recognized cause of hypothyroidism is cancer therapy with interleukin-2 (IL-2), α-interferon, or granulocyte macrophage–colony stimulating factor (GM-CSF) (see Chapters 32 and 33).

Commonly used drugs such as lithium, iodine, amiodarone, and para-aminosalicylic acid also cause secondary hypothyroidism. Lithium interferes with the biosynthesis and release of thyroid hormone and may cause elevated serum TSH levels a few weeks after therapy is started (see Chapter 20). Iodine blocks the release of thyroid hormone. Amiodarone, a commonly used antiarrhythmic drug, is rich in iodine and is fat-soluble (see Chapter 36). It remains in the body for many weeks after therapy is stopped. Additionally, patients who use "health tonics" or eat kelp may be receiving too much iodine. Other goitrogenic (thyroid-stimulating) food substances include turnips, cabbage, spinach, soybeans, and seafood.

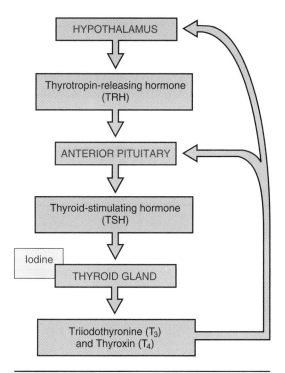

FIGURE 54-1 Thyroid hormone secretion is regulated through a negative feed back loop involving the hypothalamus, the anterior pituitary, and the thyroid gland.

Although the typical patient with hypothyroidism is a female over age 50 years, the disease can occur at any age and in either sex. Most cases occur between the ages of 30 and 60 years. Hypothyroidism is at least twice as prevalent as hyperthyroidism.

PATHOPHYSIOLOGY

In primary hypothyroidism, the production of the thyroid hormones T_4 and T_3 is inadequate. Insufficient quantities of thyroid hormones result in an overall decrease in the basal metabolic rate and a variety of signs and symptoms (Table 54-1). The thyroid gland enlarges in an attempt to compensate for the inadequacy, and a goiter is formed.

Reductions in stroke volume and heart rate lower cardiac output, with peripheral vascular resistance increasing to maintain systolic blood pressure. A variety of electrocardiographic (ECG) changes may be noted (e.g., bradycardia, prolonged PR interval, depressed P waves, and low amplitude). There is decreased cerebral blood flow, leading to hypoxia and mental status changes.

Total body water increases, and dilutional hyponatremia appears because of the reduced blood flow and the reduced renal elimination of water. There is a reduction in erythropoietin production and red cell mass, which leads to anemias and vitamin B_{12}, iron, and folate deficiencies.

There is a general slowing of gastrointestinal (GI) system functioning resulting in decreased appetite, constipation, weight gain, and fluid retention. Decreased protein metabolism leads to delayed skeletal and soft tissue growth and produces a slightly positive nitrogen balance. Abnormalities in lipid metabolism increase cholesterol and triglyceride levels. This increase is associated with the development of atherosclerosis and subsequent heart disease.

The metabolism of estrogen and androgens is altered. There is increased sensitivity to exogenous insulin but decreased absorption of glucose. Reduced secretions from sweat and sebaceous glands result in dry, flaky skin. Head and body hair become brittle. Nails are slow-growing, and there is delayed wound healing. An accumulation of hyaluronic acid in interstitial spaces causes the characteristic puffy appearance (*myxedema*) seen in hypothyroidism.

Myxedematous changes in respiratory muscles lead to hypoventilation and carbon dioxide retention. Dyspnea related to pleural effusions is possible, although the effusions may be asymptomatic. Muscle contraction and relaxation is slowed, and increased bone density contributes to muscle aching and joint stiffness. Deep tendon reflexes are decreased.

Many endocrinologists rely solely on high-sensitivity TSH measurements to monitor thyroid replacement therapy, and most suggest that a solid diagnosis of hypothyroidism can be made on the basis of free T_4 (fT_4) and ultrasensitive TSH values alone. However, total T_3 and T_4 levels may remain within a broad range of normal, even when the patient has true, but mild, hypothyroidism. Although the values may fall within the normal range, individually it is abnormal. Falsely low values may occur as the result of reduced serum thyroxine–binding globulins (e.g., nephrotic syndrome, protein loss by the gut, glucocorticoids), or drug-induced displacement of T_4 from binding proteins (e.g., high-dose salicylates, the use of furosemide in renal failure, phenytoin).

Total T_4 levels should not be relied upon to evaluate a patient's thyroid status. Total T_4 levels will fluctuate based upon the protein status of the patient and can easily be corrected for by measuring fT_4 instead of total T_4. Only fT_4 and free T_3 (fT_3) have metabolic activity. In mild hypothyroidism there is also a slight elevation in TSH values. The TSH level may be misleading in patients who have pituitary or hypothalamic hypothyroidism.

PHARMACOTHERAPEUTIC OPTIONS

Thyroid Replacement Hormones

- ◆ levothyroxine (Levothroid, Synthroid, Levoxyl, T_4); ✦ Eltroxin, Synthroid
- ◆ liothyronine (Cytomel, Triostat, T_3)
- ◆ liotrix (Thyrolar, $T_3 + T_4$)

▌▌▌ *Indications*

Inasmuch as hypothyroidism, myxedema, simple goiter, and cretinism result from hypofunction of the thyroid gland, the use of thyroid drugs represents true replacement therapy. Levothyroxine is the drug of choice for replacement

PHARMACOKINETICS

TABLE 54-1 Comparison of Hyperthyroidism and Hypothyroidism

Signs and Symptoms of Hyperthyroidism	Signs and Symptoms of Hypothyroidism
fT_4 levels elevated	fT_4 levels decreased
fT_3 levels elevated	fT_3 levels decreased
TSH levels decreased	TSH levels elevated
Goiter	Hoarseness, thick tongue
Nervousness, anxiety	Lethargy, slow speech, memory impairment
Dyspnea on exertion	Dyspnea
Tiredness	Weakness
Hot hands, sweaty palms, diaphoresis	Hair loss, coarseness of hair
Palpitations; rate over 90 bpm	Cardiac enlargement
Heat intolerance	Cold intolerance
Fine tremors of fingers	Dry, coarse, pale skin
Constipation, diarrhea	Constipation
Increased appetite but weight loss	Anorexia but weight gain
Exophthalmos, lid lag	Eyelid, facial, or peripheral edema
Scanty menses	Menorrhagia

bpm, Beats/min; *fT4,* free triiodothyronine; *fT3,* Free triiodothyronine; *TSH,* thyroid-stimulating hormone.

therapy in patients with diminished or absent thyroid functioning. **Since T_3 is produced as needed from T_4 at tissue sites, replacement of anything other than T_4 is usually not indicated.** T_3 is included in the therapeutic regimen only when there is a proven isolated T_3 deficiency. Thyroid hormones include both natural and synthetic derivatives. Natural products are derived from beef and pork and contain mixtures of both T_4 and T_3.

Pharmacodynamics

Thyroid hormones act to increase the metabolic rate of body tissues. They promote gluconeogenesis, thus increasing the utilization and mobilization of glycogen stores. The drugs also stimulate protein synthesis, cell growth and differentiation, and aid in the development of the central nervous system (CNS).

Pharmacokinetics

When given by mouth, levothyroxine is variably absorbed from the GI tract (Table 54-2). When taken on an empty stomach, preferably before breakfast, absorption is increased. It is well distributed to body tissues undergoing enterohepatic recirculation. Biotransformation of levothyroxine takes place in the liver, with metabolites eliminated in the feces. Levothyroxine is strongly bound to plasma proteins, making serum levels stable with once-daily dosing.

Adverse Effects and Contraindications

There are few adverse effects of levothyroxine other than those indicating overdosage. The most common adverse effects include irritability, insomnia, nervousness, headache, weight loss, and tachycardia. A few patients may be allergic to the tartrazine dye (FD&C Yellow No. 5) used in the yellow (100 mcg) or green (300 mcg) levothyroxine tablets. Although the incidence of tartrazine sensitivity in the general population is low, it is frequently found in patients who have aspirin hypersensitivity. Levothyroxine rarely results in clinical toxicity. **The most life-threatening adverse effect of levothyroxine is cardiovascular collapse; the risk is greater in older adults.**

PHARMACOKINETICS
TABLE 54-2 Thyroid and Parathyroid Drugs and Drugs for Calcium Disorders

Drugs	Route	Onset	Peak	Duration	PB (%)	$t_{1/2}$	BioA (%)
THYROID REPLACEMENT HORMONES							
levothyroxine (T_4)	PO	48 hr	3–4 wk	1–3 wk	99	6–71 days	93
liothyronine (T_3)	PO	48 hr	24–72 hr	72 hr	99.5	2 days	95
liotrix (T_3 and T_4)	PO	UA	T_3: 1–3 days; T_4: 1–3 wk	T_3: 72 hr; T_4: 1–3 wk	>99	T_3: 1–2 days; T_4: 7 days	41–79
SELECTED ANTITHYROID DRUGS							
propylthiouracil	PO	2–3 wk	6–10 wk	Weeks	75–80	1–2 hr	80–95
methimazole	PO	1 wk	4–10 wk	Weeks	0	4–6 hr	80–95
sodium iodide[131]	PO	3–6 days	UA	56 days	0	8 days	100
CALCIUM SALTS							
calcium carbonate	PO	UA	UA	UA	>90	UA	66
	IV	Immed	Immed	0.5–2 hr	45	UA	100
calcium gluconate	IV	Immed	Immed	UA	UA	UA	100
VITAMIN D ANALOGUES							
calcitriol	PO	2–6 hr	3–6 hr	3–5 days	99	5–8 hr	UA
dihydrotachysterol	PO	10–24 hr	2 wk	2 wk	UA	5–8 hr	UA
ergocalciferol	PO	12–24 hr	4 wk	2 mo	UA	5–8 hr	UA
BISPHOSPHONATES							
alendronate	PO	UA	1 hr	6 hr	78	10 yr	0.59–0.64
etidronate	IV	24 hr	3 days	11 days	UA	165 days	3
ibandronate	PO	UA	0.5–2 hr	UA	90–99	37–157 hr[†]	0.6
	IV	Immed	UA	UA	90–99	UA	100
pamidronate	IV	24 hr	5–7 days	120 hr	UA	2.5 hr; 27.2 hr[*]	100
risedronate	PO	UA	1 hr	UA	24	1.5; 480 hr[†]	0.63
zoledronic acid	IV	Slow	End of inf	UA	22	146	UA
SELECTIVE ESTROGEN-RECEPTOR MODULATORS							
raloxifene	PO	Slow	UA	UA	>95	27.7 hr	2
HORMONE MODIFIER							
teriparatide	SubQ	Rapid	30 min	3 hr	95	1 hr	95
MISCELLANEOUS HYPOCALCEMIC DRUGS							
calcitonin salmon	NS	Rapid	2–4 hr	6–8 hr	UA	43 min	3
	SubQ, IM	15 min	2–4 hr	6–8 hr	UA	70–90 min	100
gallium nitrate	IV	24 hr	5 days	7.5 days	UA	24–72 hr	100
plicamycin	IV	24–48 hr	72 hr	7–10 days	UA	UA	100

*Pamidronate's first- and second-phase half-life. Bone half-life is 300 days.
†The plasma elimination of ibandronate and risedronate is multiphasic.
BioA, Bioavailability; *Immed*, immediate; *inf*, infusion; *IV*, intravenous; *NA*, not applicable; *NS*, nasal spray; *PB*, protein binding; *PO*, by mouth; *subQ*, subcutaneous; $t_{1/2}$, half-life; *UA*, unavailable.

ENDOCRINE

DRUG INTERACTIONS

TABLE 54-3 Thyroid and Parathyroid Drugs and Drugs for Calcium Disorders

Drug	Interactive Drugs	Interaction
THYROID REPLACEMENT HORMONES		
levothyroxine, liothyronine, liotrix	Antacids, cholestyramine, colestipol	Impairs absorption of thyroid hormones
	epinephrine	Increases risk of coronary events
	warfarin	Increases INR and risk for bleeding
SELECTED ANTITHYROID DRUGS		
propylthiouracil	warfarin	Increases risk of bleeding
methimazole	theophylline, metoprolol, propranolol, digoxin	Increases risk of toxicity to interacting drug as patient moves from hyperthyroid to euthyroid state
CALCIUM SALTS		
Calcium salts	digoxin	Increases risk for digoxin toxicity
	Magnesium antacids	Competes with interacting drug for absorption
	atenolol, tetracycline, Iron salts, Quinolone antibiotics, phenytoin, Calcium channel blockers	Decreases effects of orally interacting drugs
	Thiazide diuretics	Concurrent use may result in hypercalcemia.
	sodium polystyrene sulfonate	Reduces ability of interacting drug to decrease serum potassium levels
VITAMIN D ANALOGUES		
Vitamin D analogues	cholestyramine, colestipol, mineral oil	Decreases absorption of analogue
	Thiazide diuretics	May result in hypercalcemia
	Glucocorticoids	Decreases effectiveness of vitamin D analogues
	digoxin	Increases risk of arrhythmias
	Barbiturates, Hydantoins, primidone, sucralfate	Increases vitamin D requirements
BISPHOSPHONATES		
alendronate	ranitidine	Doubles bioavailability of oral alendronate
	Calcium and multivalent ions	Interferes with absorption
ibandronate	Dietary supplements, Antacids with calcium, magnesium, aluminum, vitamin D	Interferes with absorption
etidronate, pamidronate	Calcium supplements, iron, Antacids, vitamin D	Antagonizes effects in treatment of hypercalcemia
	digoxin, neurotoxic drugs	Increases risk of glycoside toxicity
zoledronate	Calcium-containing drugs, vitamin D	Antagonizes effects of zoledronate
SELECTIVE ESTROGEN RECEPTOR MODULATORS (SERMS)		
raloxifene	cholestyramine	Reduces absorption of raloxifene and enterohepatic cycling of the drug
	warfarin	Decreases INR
HORMONE MODIFIER		
teriparatide	digoxin	Increases serum digoxin concentration
MISCELLANEOUS DRUG		
calcitonin	Calcium, Vitamin D analogues	Antagonizes calcitonin
gallium nitrate	Acetaminophen, Antibiotics, aspirin, cisplatin, cyclosporin, deferoxamine, Gold salts, lithium, methotrexate, penicillamine	May cause or worsen kidney problems
plicamycin	Live virus vaccines	Risk of virus transmission

INR, International normalized ratio.

▌▌ Drug Interactions

Drugs that lower cholesterol such as cholestyramine impair the absorption of thyroid hormones (Table 54-3). Several hours should separate administration of these drugs. Epinephrine used concurrently with levothyroxine increases the risk of coronary events in patients with coronary artery disease. Desiccated thyroid increases insulin or oral hypoglycemic requirements in patients with diabetes.

▌▌ Dosage Regimen

The dosages of thyroid hormones are individualized to approximate the patient's thyroid hormone deficit (Table 54-4). **⚠ Check serum TSH levels 4 to 6 weeks after starting therapy and adjust the dosage, if necessary.** Thereafter, obtain TSH and fT$_4$ levels once yearly.

▌▌ Lab Considerations

Periodic monitoring of TSH and fT$_4$ levels is warranted during thyroid hormone therapy. The concurrent use of thyroid hormones in patients with elevated biliary tract pressure may cause increases in plasma amylase and lipase. Further, the determination of these levels may be unreliable for 24 hours after administration of opioids.

CLINICAL REASONING

Treatment Objectives

The primary objective in the management of hypothyroidism is to restore the patient to a euthyroid state and to maintain plasma TSH levels in the low-normal range. Relief of the

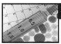

DOSAGE

TABLE 54-4 Thyroid and Parathyroid Drugs and Drugs for Calcium Disorders

Drug	Use(s)	Dosage	Implications
THYROID REPLACEMENT HORMONES			
levothyroxine (T₄)	Hypothyroidism	*Adult:* 50–75 mcg PO daily. Increase by 25–50 mcg PO every 2–3 wk. Maintenance: 0.075–0.125 mg PO daily	**Thyroid replacement hormone doses are ordered in micrograms (mcg) to avoid confusion with the decimals associated with milligrams (gm).** Slower onset but longer duration of action than T₃
	Myxedemic coma	*Adult:* 200–500 mcg IV. If no response in 24 hr, may give additional 100–300 mcg if needed	Continue at 75–100 mcg IV daily until switched to oral drug
	Congenital hypothyroidism	*Child 0–3 mo:* 10–15 mcg/kg PO daily *Child 3–6 mo:* 8–10 mcg/kg PO daily *Child 6–12 mo:* 6–8 mcg/kg PO daily *Child 1–5 yr:* 5–6 mcg/kg PO daily *Child 6–12 yr:* 4–5 mcg/kg PO daily *Child >12 yr:* 2–3 mcg/kg PO daily	Use lower dose and increase every 4–6 wk if at risk for heart failure. If given by IM or IV, use 50%–75% of oral dosage.
liothyronine (T₃)	Hypothyroidism	*Adult:* 25 mcg PO daily. Increase by 12.5–25 mcg every 1–2 wk to desired response. Maintenance: 25–75 mcg PO daily *Child, Older adult, Patient with CAD:* 5 mcg/day	Actions similar to T₄—onset more rapid, but shorter duration of action—allows for quicker dosage adjustment
	Simple goiter	*Adult:* 5 mcg PO daily. Increase by 5 to 10 mcg/day PO every 1–2 wk. Usual dose: 75 mcg/day	After 25–mcg dosage is reached, may increase by 12.5–25 mcg at weekly intervals to desired response.
	Myxedema	*Adult:* 5 mcg/day initially. Increase by 5–10 mcg/day every 1–2 wk. Maintenance: 50–100 mcg/day	After 25–mcg dosage is reached, may increase 12.5–25 mcg at weekly intervals to desired response.
	Congenital hypothyroidism	*Child <3 yr:* 5 mcg PO daily *Child >3 yr:* 5 mcg PO daily Increase by 5 mcg PO every 3–4 days to desired response.	20 mcg/day may be sufficient in infants.
liotrix (T₃ + T₄)	Hypothyroidism	*Adult:* 50 mcg T₃ + 12.5 mcg T₄ PO daily. Increase monthly to desired response. Maintenance: 50–100 mcg T₃ + 12.5–25 mcg T₄ daily *Older Adult:* 12.5–25 mcg T₃ + 3.1–6.2 mcg T₄ daily. Increase every 6–8 wk to desired response.	A constant fixed ratio of T₃:T₄ by weight. Represents thyroid hormone equivalents T₄ = 25 mcg T₃
SELECTED ANTITHYROID DRUGS			
propylthiouracil	Hyperthyroidism	*Adult:* 300–400 mg PO daily in 2–4 divided doses. Max: 900 mg/day *Neonate:* 10 mg/kg/day PO in divided doses *Child 6–10 yr:* 50–150 mg PO daily *Child >10 yr:* 150–300 mg PO daily	Can be compounded as enema or suppository if needed Maintenance dose is usually ½–⅔ of initial dose once patient is euthyroid.
methimazole	Hyperthyroidism	*Adult: Mild disease:* 15 mg PO daily. *Moderately severe disease:* 30–40 mg PO daily. *Severe disease:* 60 mg PO every 8 hr. Maintenance: 5–15 mg PO daily *Child:* 0.4 mg/kg every 8 hr in divided doses	Continue initial dosage until euthyroid state is achieved. May be given as single dose because of long half-life. Maintenance dose is ½ of initial dose.
sodium iodide¹³¹	Hyperthyroidism	*Adult:* 4–10 mCi PO as single dose based on TSH level and thyroid size	50%–60% of patients are cured by single dose. 20%–30% require a second dose.
	Thyroid cancer	*Adult:* 50–150 mCi PO	May repeat dosage in 6–12 mo based on patient response.
CALCIUM SALTS			
calcium acetate	Hyperphosphatemia of ESRD	*Adult:* 2 tablets 3 times daily with meals	25% elemental Ca⁺⁺
calcium carbonate	Osteoporosis Hypoparathyroidism, osteoporosis prevention	*Adult:* 1200 mg/day PO *Adult:* 1–2 grams/day PO in 3–4 divided doses, 1–2 hr after meals *Child:* 45–65 mg/kg/day PO in 3–4 divided doses	40% elemental Ca⁺⁺ (1 gram CaCo3 = 400 mg or 20 mEq Ca⁺⁺)
calcium chloride	Hypocalcemia	*Adult:* 0.5–1 gram repeated every 4–6 hr as needed *Child:* 2.5–5 mg/kg every 4–6 hr as needed	Give undiluted; or may dilute equal amounts of 0.9% saline or sterile water for injection.
calcium citrate	Treatment and prevention of calcium deficiency or hyperphosphatemia	*Adult:* Depends on specific brand	Cal-Citrate: 250 mg = 53 mg elemental Ca⁺⁺ Citracal: 950 mg = 200 mg elemental Ca⁺⁺
calcium gluconate	Hypocalcemic tetany	*Adult:* 100–1000 mg IV *Child:* 100–200 mg/kg IV over 5–10 min. May repeat in 6 hr; then begin maintenance	9% elemental Ca⁺⁺ Check IV site for patency. Extravasation causes cellulitis, necrosis, and sloughing of tissues.
VITAMIN D ANALOGUES			
calcitriol (D₃)	Hypoparathyroidism	*Adult:* 0.25–2.7 mcg PO daily Maintenance: 0.5–2.7 mcg/day PO *Child:* 0.04–0.08 mcg/kg/day PO	Dosages adjusted as needed to maintain serum Ca⁺⁺ levels at 8–10 mg/dL.
dihydrotachysterol	Hypocalcemia associated with hypoparathyroidism	*Adult:* 0.25–2.5 mg PO daily for 3 days. Maintenance: 0.25–1 mg/day PO	Give with Ca⁺⁺.
ergocalciferol (D₂)	Hypoparathyroidism	*Adult:* 50,000–200,000 units/day PO	Supplement with 500 mg elemental Ca⁺⁺ 6 times daily.

ENDOCRINE

Continued

DOSAGE

TABLE 54-4 Thyroid and Parathyroid Drugs and Drugs for Calcium Disorders—Cont'd

Drug	Use(s)	Dosage	Implications
BISPHOSPHONATES			
alendronate	Osteoporosis, Paget's disease	*Adult: Treatment:* 70 mg PO weekly *–or–* 10 mg PO daily; *Prevention:* 35 mg PO weekly or 5 mg PO daily; *Paget's Disease:* 40 mg/daily for 6 mo; *Steroid-induced:* 5 mg PO daily *–or–* 10 mg PO daily if postmenopausal and off estrogen	**Drugs *must* be taken *at least* half an hour before the first food, beverage, or drug of the day with 8 oz plain water only. Patients should remain upright for at least 30 minutes and until after their first food of the day.** Oral solutions should be followed by at least 2 oz water.
etindronate	Hyperthyroidism associated with malignancy	*Adult:* 7.5 mg/kg/day IV for 3 days; then switch to 20 mg/kg/day PO	
	Paget's disease	*Adult:* 5–10 mg/kg PO daily not to exceed 6 mo *–or–* 11–20 mg/kg/day; not to exceed 3 mo	
ibandronate	Osteoporosis	*Adult: Treatment and prevention:* 2.5 mg PO once daily *–or–* 150 mg once monthly	
pamidronate	Hyperparathyroidism, myeloma	*Adult:* 60–90 mg IV over 24 hr	
risedronate	Osteoporosis	*Adult:* 5 mg PO daily *–or–* 35 mg PO weekly	
	Paget's disease	*Adult:* 30 mg PO daily for 2 mo	
zoledronic acid	Osteoporosis	*Adult:* 4 mg IV once yearly	Zoledronic acid is 100 times more potent than pamidronate.
	Tumor-induced hypercalcemia melanoma, bony metastasis from solid tumors	*Adult:* 4 mg IV once monthly	
SELECTIVE ESTROGEN RECEPTOR MODULATORS (SERMS)			
raloxifene	Prevention and treatment of osteoporosis	*Adult:* 60 mg PO daily	High-fat meal increases the absorption.
HORMONE MODIFIER			
teriparatide	Postmenopausal osteoporosis with high risk for fracture; primary or male hypogonadal osteoporosis	*Adult:* 20 mcg subQ once daily into thigh or abdominal wall	Each injection pen can be used for up to 28 days including the first day of injection.
MISCELLANEOUS DRUGS			
calcitonin-salmon	Hypercalcemia	*Adult:* 4 international units/kg subQ or IM every 12 hr. Increase to 8 units/kg subQ or IM every 12 hr if no response in 2 days; may further increase to 8 international units/kg every 6 hr if no response in 2 days	Intradermal skin test should precede therapy. Watch for anaphylaxis. Do not confuse with calcitriol.
	Postmenopausal osteoporosis	*Adult:* 100 international units/day subQ or IM *–or–* 200 international units as once-daily nasal spray	Take with adequate Ca^{++} and vitamin D. Alternate nostrils daily.
	Paget's disease	*Adult:* 100 international units/kg subQ or IM daily initially. Maintenance: 50 units/day or 50–100 units every 1–3 days	Improvement in bone pain seen in first few months.
gallium nitrate	Hyperparathyroidism, hypercalcemia in malignancy	*Adult:* 100–200 mg/m^2 IV daily for 5 days	Allow 3- to 4-wk rest period between courses of therapy.
plicamycin	Hypercalcemia in malignancy	*Adult:* 15–25 mcg/kg IV once daily for 3–4 days. May be repeated after 7 days or 1–3 times weekly	Monitor closely for hypocalcemia. Use extreme caution if renal dysfunction is present.

CAD, Coronary artery disease; *ESRD,* end-stage renal disease; *HTN,* hypertension; *IM,* intramuscular (route); *IV,* intravenous (route); *PO,* by mouth; *subQ,* subcutaneous (route); T_3, triiodothyronine; T_4, thyroxine; *TSH,* thyroid-stimulating hormone.

symptoms of hypothyroidism is also a treatment objective. Management includes the gradual replacement of thyroid hormones and a low-calorie diet to promote weight loss. Lifelong therapy should be expected.

Treatment Options

▥ *Patient Variables*

In patients with signs and symptoms of hypothyroidism, TSH levels greater than 15 milliunits/L and fT$_4$ levels below normal can be effectively treated with either brand-name or generic thyroid hormone replacement (Box 54-1). Patients with mild or no symptoms of hypothyroidism, moderately elevated TSH levels (6 to 15 milliunits/L), and fT$_4$ levels within normal limits may be treated for subclinical hypothyroidism, although early treatment remains controversial.

Thyroid hormone replacement is not necessary for patients with normal TSH levels and fT$_4$ levels that are low or low-normal.

Health care providers frequently encounter patients who have been on thyroid hormone replacement for many years but for whom an initial diagnosis is not well documented. In such cases, determine whether replacement therapy is still warranted by decreasing the dose by 50% and check the TSH level in 6 to 8 weeks. If the TSH remains normal, the dose can be decreased by another 50% for 6 to 8 weeks and then, with normal TSH, discontinued entirely.

Life-Span Considerations

Pregnant and Nursing Women. Monitor pregnant women and newborns for potential thyroid abnormalities as a basic standard of care, although hypothyroidism is uncommon in pregnancy. However, if the condition is left untreated, it can

BOX 54-1

Levothyroxine vs. Brand-Name Products?

Until 2006, the bioavailability of levothyroxine was thought to differ between formulations, and patients were advised not to change levothyroxine brands with prescription refills. This warning is no longer valid.

According to the Food and Drug Administration, products evaluated as therapeutically equivalent can be expected to have equivalent clinical effects and the same potential for adverse effects when used as directed. However, differences in other characteristics such as shape, scoring configuration, release mechanisms, packaging, excipients (including colors, flavors, and preservatives), expiration date and time, and labeling may exist.

At times, such characteristic differences can result in patient confusion when replacing the originally used product. Patients may not readily accept a difference in tablet shape or a missing scoring configuration. One product may offer better stability under adverse storage conditions than the other. In rare cases, a patient may experience an allergic reaction caused by a coloring or preservative ingredient with use of one drug and not another. Be aware that therapeutically equivalent drugs may also have very different costs.

increase the rate of stillbirths, abortions, and congenital anomalies. Fetal thyroid hormone production starts at 12 weeks' gestation. Low T_4 levels in the mother during the first trimester may result in impaired fetal brain development.

Neonatal hypothyroidism occurs independently of maternal thyroid disease and is routinely screened via TSH testing 5 to 7 days after birth. **Left untreated, even for a relatively short time, neonatal hypothyroidism results in profound, lifelong mental retardation and cretinism.** In some cases, the fetal thyroid state may be monitored by measuring thyroid hormones in amniotic fluid. If breastfeeding is desired by mothers who are receiving thyroid hormones, monitor infant thyroid hormone levels.

Children and Adolescents. Thyroid disease may be congenital, with onset occurring from birth to 2 years. Left untreated, it affects growth and development and causes mental retardation. A delay of only 3 months in treatment of neonatal hypothyroidism causes irreversible mental retardation. Hypothyroidism occurring after 18 months of age is associated with reversible mental slowness. Ossification of the epiphyses and brain growth and development is particularly affected. It may be related to maternal iodine deprivation or congenital thyroid abnormalities.

The incidence of congenital hypothyroidism is approximately 1:4000, with a 1% to 3% prevalence reported in school children. Acquired hypothyroidism can be due to unknown causes, thyroiditis, or operative removal of the thyroid gland, or can be secondary to pituitary deficiency.

Thyroid disease is the most common endocrine disorder of adolescence. During adolescence, the prognosis of thyroid disease is usually good with appropriate therapy.

Older Adults. Clinical manifestations of hypothyroidism in the older adult are often subtle and can mistakenly be attributed to normal changes of aging. Hypothyroidism can present as carpal tunnel syndrome, dementia, pernicious anemia, or elevated cholesterol in addition to the common signs and symptoms previously discussed. Because clinical symptoms

of thyroid disease are unreliable in this age group, routine laboratory screening is recommended.

Drug Variables

Thyroid hormone replacement is the only treatment available for hypothyroidism. Levothyroxine provides standardized, predictable effects, thereby preventing the wide variety of symptomatic and metabolic disturbances (Box 54-2). However, the patient's response is greatly affected by age, the cause and duration of the goiter, and the degree of nodularity.

Although thyroid hormone formulations are economical, standardization of iodine content or bioassay is inexact. Synthetic derivatives are preferred over natural hormones because their composition is known and constant.

Levothyroxine has a number of advantages over other thyroid hormones including a uniform potency, relatively low cost, and lack of foreign protein antigenicity. It has been suggested that T_3 is safer than levothyroxine, but it is more potent and has a shorter half-life (2 to 3 days). Further, compared with levothyroxine alone, there are no beneficial changes in body weight, lipid levels, or hypothyroid symptoms with the use of a combination of T_4 and T_3. Serum drug levels fall more rapidly when T_3 is stopped, but its advantages are offset by difficulties in dosage regulation resulting in more frequent cardiovascular problems and symptoms of hyperthyroidism. In addition, more frequent dosing is required, making it less desirable for prolonged therapy than pure T_4 formulations. Other disadvantages include altered thyroid function tests and a higher cost.

A combination of T_3 and T_4 (liotrix) is available, but use of this product is controversial. There has been one randomized controlled trial involving a small number of patients ($N = 65$) that concluded that there was no difference in outcomes between the addition of T_3 in the treatment of hypothyroidism. There is also the potential for transient hyperthyroidism and the development of angina or arrhythmias.

Overdosage of any thyroid hormone is manifested as hyperthyroidism with similar signs and symptoms (i.e., tachycardia, chest pain, nervousness, insomnia, diaphoresis, tremors, and weight loss). If tachyarrhythmias or chest pain develop, the usual intervention is to withhold the thyroid hormone for 2 to 6 days. Acute overdose is treated by induction of emesis or gastric lavage.

Patient Education

Explain the disorder and the fact that treatment for hypothyroidism is lifelong. Tell the patient that response to treatment usually takes 4 to 6 weeks to manifest with maximal response not seen for several months.

Teach patients to take levothyroxine exactly as directed, on an empty stomach, and at the same time each day. Administration before breakfast is usually best. The drug should not be discontinued without first talking with the health care provider. The concurrent use of over-the-counter (OTC) drugs should be avoided unless otherwise instructed. Additive CNS and cardiac stimulation may occur with decongestants.

Teach the patient and family how to take a pulse and blood pressure. A resting pulse rate over 100 beats/min may indicate overdose. Thus, the drug should be withheld and the health care provider contacted. Blood pressure readings should remain in the normal range.

CASE STUDY   Thyroid and Parathyroid Drugs

ASSESSMENT

History of Present Illness	JC is a 35-year-old part-time secretary and mother who arrived at the clinic accompanied by her husband. She complains of fatigue, dry skin, hair loss, an inability to focus on her daily activities, and cold intolerance. JC also reports that she is gaining weight although she is eating little. She has had a noticeable change in the frequency and consistency of her bowel movements: "lots of constipation." Her menstrual flow and its frequency have increased over the last 3 months. In addition, JC states her neighbor thinks she is depressed because of the lack of interest in playing golf, a favorite activity. JC denies suicidal or homicidal ideations. JC's husband reports his wife is normally an out-going, well-organized individual, who finishes projects she starts, one who coordinates family activities very well. Over the last 3 months he reports she has become disorganized, and doesn't finish projects or activities she has started. He also reports that she does not like to take medicine of any kind. He has noticed her wearing heavy shirts and long pants even though the temperature has been in the 90s. They have been arguing recently because she wants the windows closed. He gets hot and wants them open.
Past Health History	JC denies a history of previous thyroid disorders but reports that her mother developed hypothyroidism at age 23. She denies a history of surgery or neurologic, musculoskeletal, or psychiatric illness, or other hormonal disorders.
Life-Span Considerations	JC is a part-time stay-at-home mom who cares for three children under the age of 10. Her husband is a well-paid bank executive. Until recently they both attended synagogue regularly, liked to play golf together, and spent time camping with the kids. Now, JC is "not interested in anything." He reports the family is enrolled in a health plan that covers clinic visits and hospitalizations. The prescription drug plan requires a copayment for prescription drugs.
Physical Exam Findings	*Height:* 5'7". *Present weight:* 188 lb (25 lb above her usual weight). *VS:* BP, 110/68 (BP 1 year ago 130/80); 98.2° F- apical pulse 70 -16. ENT negative except for palpable thyromegaly. No bruits noted over thyroid gland on auscultation. No exophthalmos but eyes puffy. EOMI, PERLA. No lymphadenopathy. Hair is coarse and thin; skin is dry. DTRs upper and lower extremities sluggish. 1+ pedal edema. No tremors. HRRR. BSCTA. Her decreased attention span is evident. Pelvic exam unremarkable.
Diagnostic Testing	TSH of 25.4 mg/dL, and decreased fT_3 and fT_4 levels. Total cholesterol, 225 mg/dL, up from 190 1 year ago; triglycerides, 170 mg/dL, up from 140 1 year ago, HDL and LDL normal range. Serum sodium, 130 mg/dL. Serum potassium, 4.2 mg/dL. ECG reflects low amplitude sinus bradycardia. Recent Pap smear negative.

DIAGNOSIS: Hypothyroidism

MANAGEMENT

Treatment Objectives	1. Provide symptom relief while waiting for therapeutic effectiveness of drug to be achieved. 2. Restore a euthyroid state by returning plasma TSH levels to a normal range.
Treatment Plan	**Pharmacotherapy** • levothyroxine 75 mcg daily first thing in the morning, on empty stomach. **Patient Education** 1. Recheck TSH in 6 weeks. Adjust levothyroxine dosage upward by 25 mcg if needed. 2. Schedule activities so as to allow for rest periods. 3. Eat balanced meals with increased high–biologic value protein. 4. Increase fluids. **Evaluation** Euthroid state is returning, with plasma TSH levels within the normal range. Symptoms have lessened or disappeared.

CLINICAL REASONING ANALYSIS

Q1. **We learned that patients with hypothyroidism can be treated with dessicated thyroid, levothyroxine, liothyronine, or liotrix. Why did you decide to use levothyroxine?**

A. First of all, levothyroxine is the drug of choice for replacement therapy in patients with diminished or absent thyroid functioning. It provides standardized, predictable effects compared with the other drugs and prevents the wide variety of symptomatic and metabolic disturbances seen with others. It is also less antigenic than natural products, which are derived from pork or beef. In addition, JC and her family uphold Jewish tradition, which includes dietary restrictions. Also levothyroxine is strongly bound to plasma proteins, making serum levels stable with once-daily dosing. T_3 replacement is unnecessary and inappropriate in the majority of patients because of the conversion of T_4 to T_3 in the circulation.

Q2. **I see. So, you started her on 75 mcg of levothyroxine daily, a synthetic drug. How did you know to start her on 75 mcg? Why not 100 mcg?**

A. Seventy-five mcg daily is an acceptable starting dose providing patients are healthy otherwise; that is, they have no risk factors for heart disease and don't have a long-standing history of thyroid disease. Dosage adjustments thereafter are usually made in 25 mcg or less. In older adults, we might start at 25 mcg/day initially and then adjust dosage as needed.

Q3. **What happens next, at the end of the 6 weeks? Will all of JC's symptoms be gone?**

A. We will recheck JC's TSH and fT_4 levels. Her TSH should be down toward normal, and she should have more energy, though she might not be herself yet. Her memory should have improved somewhat. Her other symptoms may still be present but to a lesser degree.

Q4. **If all that is true, will you increase her dose of levothyroxine to 100 mcg or leave it the way it is?**

A. It is likely that we will increase her dosage to 100 mcg/day and recheck the TSH again in 6 weeks. We will continue doing so until her symptoms have improved and her TSH is back into a normal range. After that we will check the TSH at least once a year or if she has any significant changes in her health.

BOX 54-2

Starting Levothyroxine Therapy in Adults*

Rapid: Full Estimated Replacement Dosage
- Healthy young patients with mild hypothyroidism; also most patients when hypothyroidism occurs shortly after surgery or RAI treatment for hyperthyroidism, unless known cardiac disease is present
- Begin at 100 mcg daily for 6-8 weeks; may be adjusted in 4-6 weeks based on TSH and fT_4 levels

Routine Replacement Dosage
- Most healthy patients younger than 45-50 years
- Begin at 75 mcg daily for first 4-6 weeks; may be increased in increments of 25-50 mcg every 4 to 6 weeks as tolerated

Cautious Use
- Patients over the age of 45-50 years
- Young patients with multiple risk factors for coronary artery disease
- Younger patients with severe or long-standing hypothyroidism
- Begin at 50 mcg daily for first 4 weeks; may be increased in increments 25-50 mcg every 4-6 weeks as tolerated

Extremely Cautious Use
- Patients with angina and arrhythmias, and elderly patients
- Patients over the age of 45 or 50 years with multiple risk factors for coronary artery disease
- Older patients with severe or long-standing hypothyroidism
- Begin at 25 mcg or less daily for first 4 weeks; may be increased in increments of 25-50 mcg or less every 4-6 weeks, if tolerated

*Clinical assessment of the patient takes precedence over arbitrary guidelines.
RAI, Radioactive iodine.

Stress the importance of follow-up. Explain that thyroid function tests will be performed regularly during the initial phase of treatment, with a change in overall health status, and at least yearly during therapy.

Evaluation

The patient's clinical response to levothyroxine can be evaluated by resolution of signs and symptoms of hypothyroidism. The expected response includes weight loss, an increased sense of well-being, and greater energy levels. The texture and characteristics of hair, skin, and nails should normalize, and constipation should be corrected.

TSH and, in some cases, T_4 levels can be used to monitor the effectiveness of therapy. If serum T_4 levels are low but the TSH is normal, measurement of fT_4 levels is warranted. The current standard of care is to achieve normal fT_4 and normal TSH levels in the patient regardless of clinical symptomatology. Even a mildly elevated fT4 with a below-normal TSH can result in significant toxicity to the patient. Persistent clinical and laboratory evidence of hypothyroidism in spite of adequate replacement indicates poor patient adherence with treatment, poor absorption, excessive fecal loss, or inactivity of the formulation. Intracellular resistance to thyroid hormones is rare.

HYPERTHYROIDISM

EPIDEMIOLOGY AND ETIOLOGY

Hyperthyroidism commonly affects women between the ages of 20 and 40. The incidence peaks between the ages of 50 and 60

ENDOCRINE

and is 7 times higher in persons over age 65. Hyperthyroidism is 4 times more prevalent in women than men, with approximately 1% of the women in the United States developing hyperthyroidism in their lifetime. Later in life, it affects men and women equally. Relapse after treatment and remission is most likely to occur during a postpartum period.

The most common cause of hyperthyroidism despite age or gender is Graves' disease (toxic diffuse goiter). Graves' disease accounts for about 8% of cases of hyperthyroidism. Further, about 15% of patients with this autoimmune disorder have a first-degree relative with the same disorder, and about half of the relatives have circulating thyroid autoantibodies. Another form of hyperthyroidism, toxic multinodular goiter (TMNG), is usually noted after the age of 50 and is more common in women than in men. Other causes include transient hyperthyroidism following any form of thyroiditis, thyroid adenoma, radiation-induced thyroiditis, thyroid carcinoma, trophoblastic tumors, and dermoid-secreting tumors of the ovary.

PATHOPHYSIOLOGY

Hyperthyroidism produces a hypermetabolic state with increased sympathetic nervous system activity. TMNG has one or more autonomous hyperfunctioning thyroid nodules. A toxic adenoma, the least common cause of hyperthyroidism, occurs when one or more of the adenomas function without TSH or other thyroid stimulation. Many of the signs and symptoms result from the action of certain IgG immunoglobulins (long-acting thyroid-stimulating hormones [LATS]) on the thyroid gland.

Excessive thyroid hormones affect carbohydrate, protein, and fat metabolism. There is increased absorption of glucose and diminished sensitivity to exogenous insulin. Protein breakdown exceeds protein synthesis, resulting in a negative nitrogen balance. Synthesis, mobilization, and breakdown of fats are increased. The net effect is lipid depletion and a chronic state of protein-energy malnutrition (PEM). Excess thyroid hormones increase the excretion of cholesterol in the feces, with an increase in transformation of cholesterol to bile salts. In addition, the conversion of B vitamins to their respective coenzymes is impaired.

Thyroid hormones increase the number of β receptor sites in the heart; not only are there more β receptors, but they are also more easily triggered as a result of the increase in thyroid hormones. Excess thyroid hormones increase heart rate and stroke volume, thus increasing cardiac output and peripheral blood flow. Systolic blood pressure is also elevated. This can explain both the signs and symptoms of the disorder as well as some of the complications. Hyperthyroidism also produces hypercalcemia and decreases the secretion of PTH hormones. This mechanism has implications for the development of osteoporosis.

The patient most often reports anxiety, diaphoresis, and fatigue, hypersensitivity to heat, nervousness, and palpitations, and may experience confusion about losing weight despite an increased appetite (see Table 54-1). Often there are reports of problems with the eyes such as difficulty focusing. The patient may also note peripheral edema, diarrhea, and oligomenorrhea or amenorrhea. The patient with hyperthyroidism may have a history of atrial fibrillation, angina, or heart failure.

Generally, the patient is nervous and thin. Muscle wasting may be evident. Vital signs reflect tachycardia, irregular pulse,

and a widened pulse pressure. The skin is moist and velvety and may show decreased pigmentation (*vitiligo*). Hair is often fine and thin. Spider angiomas and gynecomastia may be evident. Lid lag may be present, with a lack of accommodation; exophthalmos may be observed, and the patient may appear to stare. In severe cases, the patient may be unable to close the eyelids and must have the lids taped closed at night to protect the eyes. The ophthalmopathy of Grave's disease is a complex phenomenon. It occurs independently of the underlying thyroid disease. Resolution of the hyperthyroidism does not stop the progression of ophthalmopathy.

Drug-induced or spontaneous remissions may occur with hyperthyroidism. The rate of remission is greater for patients diagnosed early in their disease, and for those with mild hyperthyroidism or small goiters. The rate is also greater in those treated for extended periods with antithyroid drugs.

All forms of hyperthyroidism (except that caused by a rare pituitary TSH-secreting tumor) are associated with low or undetectable serum TSH concentrations. Most patients have elevated levels of T_3, T_4, and fT_4. A 24-hour radioiodine uptake test is neither sensitive nor specific for hyperthyroidism. It is, however, useful in distinguishing hyperthyroidism that may develop during the postpartum period from postpartum thyroiditis and in confirming the diagnosis of subacute thyroiditis.

If the patient has only one or two characteristic signs and symptoms of hyperthyroidism, the pretest probability of this condition is low, and no testing is required. The availability of ultrasensitive and reliable assays for serum TSH has made the laboratory diagnosis of hyperthyroidism rather straightforward. However, if the health care provider is compelled to test, the fT_4 level is a better reflection of the patient's true hormonal status. The serum TSH concentration alone cannot determine the degree of biochemical hyperthyroidism; fT_4 and fT_3 are required to provide this information. However, in laboratories using serum TSH assays with detection limits of 0.01 milliunits/mL (third generation), most patients with overt hyperthyroidism have values <0.05 milliunits/mL. Patients with subclinical hyperthyroidism can have undetectable or subnormal values, but values above 0.05 milliunits /mL, when associated with hyperthyroidism, are usually indicative of subclinical disease.

PHARMACOTHERAPEUTIC OPTIONS

Antithyroid Drugs
◆ propylthiouracil (PTU); ♣ Propyl-Thyracil
◆ methimazole (Tapazole); ♣ Tapazole

▥ Indications
The antithyroid drugs PTU and methimazole are first-line drugs for almost all patients with hyperthyroidism or thyrotoxicosis. They help the patient to regain a normal metabolic state until the natural course of the disease produces a spontaneous remission.

▥ Pharmacodynamics
By inhibiting the synthesis of thyroid hormones, PTU and methimazole reduce the signs and symptoms of hyperthyroidism. In addition to blocking the synthesis of thyroid hormones, PTU also reduces the peripheral conversion of T_4 to

the more potent T_3. In contrast, methimazole does not have this effect. In fact, methimazole antagonizes the inhibition produced by PTU if they are taken together. A *euthyroid* state is usually restored within 4 to 8 weeks. Remission usually occurs with 3 to 6 months of therapy.

PTU and methimazole also reduce serum concentrations of thyroid-stimulating immunoglobulins (TSIs) and increase suppressor T-cell activity. This finding suggests that the drugs have immunosuppressive activity.

Pharmacokinetics

Both PTU and methimazole are well absorbed from the GI tract, concentrating in the thyroid gland. Both drugs have similar onset times, peak, and duration of action (see Table 54-2). Note that previously synthesized body stores of thyroid hormones must be depleted before a clinical response is seen. Drugs and their metabolites are eliminated primarily through the kidneys.

PTU and methimazole are transported across placental membranes. Only about one fourth of the serum concentration of PTU crosses the placenta. PTU is present in breast milk in one tenth the concentration of methimazole.

Adverse Effects and Contraindications

The incidence of adverse effects is small, varying from 3% to 7%. A mild papular rash or urticaria, fever, arthralgias, and arthritis are all apparently dose related. Purpura and pruritus are occasionally seen. Skin reactions often subside spontaneously, whether or not the drug is withdrawn. Nausea and vomiting and nasal stuffiness are also common.

Benign transient leukopenia (i.e., white blood cells [WBCs] <4000/mm^3) develops in 12% of adult patients. However, leukopenia is not an antecedent to agranulocytosis, and its presence does not necessitate stopping the drug. The likelihood of cross-allergenicity between PTU and methimazole is approximately 50%. So, although the appearance of adverse effects to one drug may suggest that a substitution of the other is warranted, doing so might not prevent undesirable sequelae; if one drug causes them, the second is likely to do so as well.

Agranulocytosis is the most feared adverse reaction, although it occurs in only 0.2% of patients. It usually develops within 90 days of starting therapy and is characterized by high fever, bacterial pharyngitis, and an absolute granulocyte count below 250/mm^3. Fortunately, once the drug is stopped, the patient's WBC count normalizes in 7 to 10 days. Fatalities related to antithyroid drug use are rare.

Antithyroid drugs readily cross the placenta to inhibit fetal thyroid hormone secretion. Suppression of thyroid function in the fetus leads to fetal goiter and hypothyroidism. Administering thyroid hormones to the mother does not reverse the effects of the drugs on the fetus because T_3 and T_4 hormones do not cross the placenta. Furthermore, the long-term consequences of neonatal hypothyroidism are not clear. There is a 30% probability of mental retardation.

Drug Interactions

There is an increased risk of bleeding when antithyroid drugs are taken with oral anticoagulants (see Table 54-3). Increased therapeutic effects and toxicity of theophylline, metoprolol, propranolol, and cardiac glycosides may be noted as the patient moves from a hyperthyroid state to a euthyroid state.

Dosage Regimen

The dosage of antithyroid drugs is adjusted to achieve and maintain T_3, T_4, and TSH levels in the normal range (see Table 54-4). PTU generally cannot be given as a single daily dose owing to its short duration of action. Once a euthyroid state has been achieved, smaller dosages may be used. Once-a-day to twice-a-day dosing is also possible. In contrast, methimazole can be given as a single daily dose. Because it is 10 to 50 times as strong as PTU, initial doses of methimazole are 15 mg/day for mild disease, 30 to 40 mg/day for moderate disease, and 60 mg/day every 8 hours for severe disease.

Lab Considerations

Owing to the potential for blood dyscrasias, perform periodic monitoring of the complete blood count (CBC), liver function tests, protein, creatine kinase (CK), and TSH levels.

Radioactive Iodine
◆ sodium iodide^{131} (Iodotope Therapeutic)

Indications

Sodium iodide^{131} (^{131}I), a radioactive iodine (RAI), has its widest use in the treatment of hyperthyroidism in the older adult and in the diagnosis of certain thyroid disorders. It is clearly suggested for patients with a history of heart disease, although its use is contraindicated in patients with a recent myocardial infarction.

Pharmacodynamics

RAI is of use because the thyroid gland actively absorbs iodine, which is then used to produce thyroid hormones. The difference between RAI and the iodine present in foods, such as fish, seaweed, and iodized salt, is RAI's therapeutic action, which is created by its release of a beta particle. While in the thyroid gland, the RAI disrupts the function of some of the thyroid cells; the more RAI that is given, the more cells that cease to function. Thyroid hormones are no longer generated as a result of the disruption in cell function, and the signs and symptoms of thyroid overactivity start to resolve.

Pharmacokinetics

RAI is readily absorbed from the GI tract and taken up by the thyroid gland. Over 99% of its radiant energy is expended within 56 days (see Table 54-2).

Adverse Effects and Contraindications

There are few adverse effects with the use of RAI, and when present, they occur infrequently. Pharyngitis may develop a few days after beginning treatment, but is easily treated with a mild analgesic (e.g., acetaminophen). Parotiditis, which is rare, is caused by the iodine and not the radioactivity. Sucking hard candies for a few days may help to prevent this. RAI is best administered on an empty stomach (i.e., 2 hours before, or 2 hours after eating) because of the mild nausea that may develop.

The major adverse effect of RAI is iatrogenic hypothyroidism; it is so characteristic, in fact, that it is considered a consequence of therapy rather than a true adverse effect. Hypothyroidism develops in about 50% of patients within the first year of RAI therapy, with an annual increase of 2% to 3% each year. Within 10 to 20 years, nearly all patients

ENDOCRINE

treated with RAI will become hypothyroid. For this reason, it is mandatory that the patient receive close, lifelong follow-up care.

⠿ Drug Interactions

Antidiarrheal drugs containing kaolin will absorb the antithyroid drug, thereby reducing its absorption. Propranolol and antithyroid drugs help to control hyperthyroidism signs and symptoms in the period before the onset of RAI's therapeutic effects (see Table 54-3).

⠿ Dosage Regimen

RAI can be administered in capsule form or dissolved in water. The effective dosage of RAI is different for each patient depending on gland size, the uptake of iodine by the gland, and the rate of elimination of the RAI from the gland (see Table 54-4). Administering a higher dose of RAI ensures complete suppression of the gland. The trade-off is that permanent hypothyroidism is induced in nearly all patients within a short period. Some health care providers attempt to adjust the dosage to produce a euthyroid state while avoiding hypothyroidism. Depending to some extent on the dosage chosen, 50% to 60% of patients are cured of their hyperthyroidism with a single dose; 20% to 30% require two doses; and the remainder of patients require three or more doses before the disorder is controlled.

CLINICAL REASONING

Treatment Objectives

The treatment objective for hyperthyroidism is to reduce the levels of circulating thyroid hormones in anticipation of a spontaneous remission. Reducing the uncomfortable signs and symptoms is important.

Treatment Options

Historically, surgery was the first-line treatment for hyperthyroidism. Antithyroid drugs and RAI have replaced surgery as the treatments of choice. Surgery is not used as frequently today but may be appropriate for children, adolescents, pregnant women unable to tolerate PTU, and adults unresponsive to antithyroid drugs and who refuse RAI. Although these drugs are generally safe and effective, none of them are perfect. They do, however, provide satisfactory outcomes for most patients.

⠿ Patient Variables

The choice between the drugs available in the United States, methimazole and PTU, has traditionally been a matter of provider preference. Nevertheless, **methimazole, with its once-daily dosing schedule, has decided advantages over PTU, including better patient adherence and a more rapid improvement in serum concentrations of T_3 and T_4.**

Life-Span Considerations

Pregnant and Nursing Women. Minor changes in thyroid function occur during pregnancy. High estrogen levels during pregnancy stimulate the liver to increase production of thyroxine-binding globulins. Increased globulin levels result in elevated T_3 and T_4 levels, with elevated T_4 levels lasting 6 to 12 weeks postpartum. Serum concentrations of fT_3 and fT_4 are essentially unchanged. Serum TSH levels are normal to

slightly low during pregnancy. Human chorionic gonadotropin (hCG) produced by the placenta has weak thyroid-stimulating activity.

The incidence of hyperthyroidism in pregnancy is extremely low, affecting approximately 1 in every 500 to 2000 pregnancies; however, it is associated with a significant increase in neonatal mortality. Untreated hyperthyroidism results in premature labor, congenital anomalies, and low birth weight.

PTU is the drug of choice for pregnant hyperthyroid women because of its limited placental transfer and low potency. Another reason PTU is the drug of choice during pregnancy is the reported development of scalp defects in fetuses exposed to methimazole in utero. Both PTU and methimazole are pregnancy category D drugs. Antithyroid drugs are not teratogenic; however, neonatal thyroid function can be affected.

Children and Adolescents. Neonatal hyperthyroidism results from the transfer of maternal TSIs to the fetus. It is usually transient, lasting only 1 to 3 months. This is because the half-life of neonatal TSIs is approximately 2 weeks. TSIs stimulate the fetal thyroid to produce thyroid hormones, causing fetal or neonatal hyperthyroidism. Neonatal hyperthyroidism depends on maternal TSIs and not on the mother's thyroid status. Therefore, infants of euthyroid women with a previous history of hyperthyroidism are also at risk. Measurement of maternal TSI levels is useful to predict the likelihood of neonatal hyperthyroidism.

Older Adults. Hyperthyroidism frequently goes undetected in older persons for several reasons. The patient has fewer diagnostic signs and symptoms of hyperthyroidism, comorbid diseases may mask symptoms, and the symptoms that are commonly present in the younger population may be absent in older adults. Confirmation of hyperthyroidism, therefore, relies heavily on laboratory test results.

Older adults with hyperthyroidism may be apathetic, rather than having hyperactivity, tremor, and other symptoms of sympathetic overactivity. However, two thirds of such patients have symptoms similar to those in younger patients. An enlarged thyroid is present in 80% of those affected. More than 40% of older adults have cardiovascular symptoms such as palpitations, heart failure, atrial fibrillation, and angina pectoris. The most frequent patient reports relate to anorexia and a loss of ambition; weight loss is the most frequent objective finding. In addition, older adults often have persistent constipation. Classic eye manifestations are rare. Toxic multinodular goiter is more common in older adults, although the majority of hyperthyroid patients at any age have Graves' hyperthyroidism.

Laboratory reports indicate there is an age-related decrease in T_3 levels in healthy older adults. Male T_3 levels decrease by age 60. Female levels do not show a consistent decrease until age 70 or 80 years. These normal decreases in T_3 levels make the diagnosis of mild hyperthyroidism difficult. Circulating T_4 levels also decrease modestly with age. The reduction may be due to reduced metabolism of the aging thyroid gland, where most of T_4 is produced. There is also an age-related increase in TSH levels.

⠿ Drug Variables

Antithyroid drugs are deceptively easy to use, but because of the variability in the response of patients and the potentially serious adverse effects, all prescribing health care providers must have a working knowledge of the drugs' complex pharmacology. In the treatment of hyperthyroidism and other disorders, there is "a choice of treatments, not a treatment of choice." Antithyroid drugs such as PTU and methimazole continue to be important in the management of hyperthyroidism, some 60 years after they were introduced.

The advantage of using antithyroid drugs is that they provide an opportunity for spontaneous remission, and thus lifelong drug treatment is avoided. The disadvantage, on the other hand, is that permanent remissions occur in only about 30% of patients. Continuous and repeated therapy is usually required. Should a remission occur, lifelong follow-up is indicated. If a remission is not achieved, the patient may require additional treatment with antithyroid therapy or RAI.

⚠ **Methimazole, with its once daily dosing schedule, has decided advantages over PTU, including better patient adherence and a more rapid improvement in serum concentrations of T_3 and T_4.** The cost of low-dose generic methimazole is similar to that of PTU. In a recent search of Internet pharmacies, a 1-year supply of PTU (300 mg daily) was approximately $408 compared with a 1-year supply of methimazole (15 mg daily, $360; or 30 mg daily, $720). $720 is over 175% more expensive than $408. $312 is not a huge figure in an annual budget, but the proportion of the difference is significant.

Finally, differences in the adverse effect profiles of the two drugs favor methimazole. As discussed, PTU is preferred during pregnancy.

For bothersome symptoms of hyperthyroidism before treatment, long-acting beta-blocking drugs (e.g., propranolol, metoprolol, atenolol, nadolol) (see Chapter 35) are usually given as adjunctive therapy until the antithyroid drug restores the patient to a euthyroid state. The long-acting form of propranolol is preferred over the short-acting formulation of propranolol.

Serum T_3 and T_4 levels decrease more rapidly in patients treated with methimazole. Although the differences in PTU and methimazole serum levels are insignificant, moderate doses of methimazole pose a lower risk of agranulocytosis.

There are several advantages to using RAI. First, RAI is concentrated only in functional areas of the thyroid gland. Suppressed perinodular areas are spared radiation exposure. Therefore the risk of hypothyroidism, although it can occur, is less of a problem. However, eventual (decades later) hypothyroidism may be part of the natural history of the disease.

Secondly, no other body tissues are exposed to detectable amounts of ionizing radiation. Because RAI is taken by mouth, it is easy to administer; this is not done, though, until all other antithyroid drugs have been stopped.

Using PTU before RAI therapy decreases the efficacy of the iodine. It is important that the possibility of relapse be discussed with the patient so that a treatment strategy will be in place in the event of recurrence. If RAI is selected after a relapse, the outcome may be influenced by the prior use of ⚠ antithyroid drugs. **When used to normalize thyroid function before RAI therapy, PTU, but not methimazole, increases the failure rate of the RAI.** This "radioprotective" effect of PTU may be related to its ability to neutralize iodinated free radicals produced by radiation exposure, a property not shared by methimazole. The radioprotective effect can be overcome by increasing the RAI dosage.

Patient Education

Teach the patient and the family about the therapeutic and adverse effects of thyroid hormones and antithyroid drugs on the body and the signs and symptoms of imbalance. Inform the patient that he or she will begin to feel better after the initial few weeks of treatment. Because antithyroid drug therapy is lengthy, the patient needs encouragement to maintain adherence. Insufficient drug prolongs the period of thyrotoxicity, whereas too much drug may cause hypothyroidism. An interruption in therapy may result in symptoms reappearing. Lack of adherence also reduces the likelihood of a permanent remission. After the initial treatment period, manifestations of imbalance should be reported so that dosages can be changed.

Teach the patient to stop the antithyroid drug and notify the health care provider if symptoms of infection occur. Sore throat, enlarged lymph nodes, GI upsets, fever, rash, and jaundice are particularly important. Stress the importance of periodic blood tests and medical follow-up.

Further, caution the patient against taking OTC drugs such as decongestants that contain vasopressor compounds; these drugs are poorly tolerated by patients with hyperthyroidism. Antidiarrheal drugs containing kaolin will absorb the antithyroid drug, thereby reducing its absorption. Contact the health care provider before taking any drugs containing iodine.

Because a therapeutic response to antithyroid drugs cannot be expected for days to weeks, immediate interventions are sometimes required to help reduce or relieve symptoms of hyperthyroidism. Encourage the patient to continue wearing lightweight clothing and to use lightweight bed linens. The environment should be kept cool with high humidity.

Rest is important to conserve energy and reduce fatigue. However, because of the patient's high metabolic rate, it is often difficult to achieve. Teach the patient that control of environmental temperature, lighting, and noise levels minimizes unnecessary stimuli. Advise the use of all possible strategies to help induce sleep. In addition, persons working with, or around a patient with hyperthyroidism should maintain a calm but efficient manner because patients are unnecessarily stimulated by hustle and bustle. On the other hand, the patient may become impatient with slow responses.

Teach patients with a hyperthyroid state to consume a diet high in vitamins, minerals, and protein, and to include sufficient calories to prevent weight loss until their hypermetabolic rate decreases. More frequent meals or snacks are usually needed. Foods to avoid include those high in residue or those with laxative effects. Stimulants such as coffee, tea, cola drinks, chocolate, and foods containing caffeine should also be avoided. Recommend that patients monitor body weight 2 to 3 times weekly and gradually reduce calorie intake as symptoms of hyperthyroidism subside. A reduction in calories should not be difficult because the patient's appetite decreases with treatment. However, the intake of vitamins, minerals, and dietary nutrients should be maintained.

When RAI therapy is used, teach the patient to increase fluid intake to 3 to 4 L/day for 48 hours. Sufficient fluid intake helps remove RAI from the body. Instruct the patient to void frequently so as to not expose the gonads to radiation.

ENDOCRINE

The patient should report redness, swelling, sore throat, or the development of mouth lesions.

Since a small amount of radiation is emitted from the thyroid gland, where RAI is deposited after therapy, precautions are warranted with RAI treatment. Radiation benefits the patient, but preventive measures should be introduced to limit the amount of radiation exposure to family and friends. Advise the patient to remain at least one arm's length away from others, particularly pregnant women and children. Although brief interactions with the patient who has received RAI is permissible, extended periods of contact are ill-advised. Contact in excess of 2 hours in any 24-hour period should be avoided (e.g., sleeping side-by-side, traveling together, or watching a movie) for approximately 10 days. Contraception is advised during the 6-month period following treatment. Women must stop breastfeeding before starting RAI therapy since iodine will be concentrated and excreted during lactation.

The patient undergoing RAI treatment must refrain from sharing food and utensils including bottles, cans, and glasses. Tableware and eating utensils should be rinsed thoroughly before being put away with others. Immediately discard any used paper plates and plastic utensils outside of the home. Utensils handled during cooking, if used to taste the food, must be rinsed before next use.

Have the patient to drink lots of liquids to help remove the RAI from the system; void often, and flush twice after using the toilet; and be sure to thoroughly clean up any spilled urine. Personal clothing need not be laundered separately unless the patient has been diaphoretic, as occurs during exercise.

Advise patients to carry medical alert identification describing the treatment regimen. Further, dentists should be informed of the treatment regimen so as to minimize potentially adverse effects of any anesthetics used.

Evaluation

Treatment effectiveness for hyperthyroidism is demonstrated by a decrease in the severity of signs and symptoms, although these are slow to improve. It takes approximately 2 weeks before symptom improvement is noted. Tremors and irritability are lessened, muscle strength and heat intolerance improves, and sleep becomes more restful.

Thyroid function test results return to normal levels, and the patient ideally reflects a euthyroid state, rather than a hypothyroid state secondary to drug therapy. Reduced TSI levels generally suggest that a remission has taken place and that therapy can be modified or withdrawn.

If remission is not achieved, the patient may require an additional course of antithyroid therapy, or RAI. Approximately 20% of patients with a remission develop spontaneous hypothyroidism with antithyroid drug therapy alone; however, the need for lifelong follow-up remains.

HYPOPARATHYROIDISM

The function of the parathyroid gland is to secrete parathyroid hormone (PTH), whose main function is to control the level of ionized calcium in extracellular fluid and to defend the body against hypocalcemia. PTH stimulates osteolysis by osteoclasts that release calcium and phosphate into extracellular fluid. It increases the renal tubular reabsorption of calcium and magnesium and decreases the tubular reabsorption of phosphate and of bicarbonate, thereby enhancing urinary loss. It also increases the synthesis of the active form of vitamin D (i.e., calcitriol) from its precursor by activating a specific enzyme in the kidney. It directly enhances absorption of calcium in the intestines.

Alteration of parathyroid gland functioning produces hyperparathyroidism or hypoparathyroidism. Although not as common as thyroid disorders, parathyroid disorders can be life-threatening depending on their severity.

EPIDEMIOLOGY AND ETIOLOGY

Hypoparathyroidism has two primary causes. The most common, insufficient amounts of PTH (true hypoparathyroidism), is caused by inadvertent surgical removal of the gland. It is uncommon following a simple thyroid lobectomy, but the incidence of hypoparathyroidism following total thyroidectomy is 3% to 5%.

The idiopathic form of hypoparathyroidism is associated with absent or decreased PTH secretion from hypoplastic or damaged parathyroid glands. The average age of onset for the idiopathic form of the disorder is 16 years. Familial occurrences of idiopathic hypoparathyroidism are rare.

Pseudohypoparathyroidism is inherited, affecting females twice as often as males. The average age of onset for pseudohypoparathyroidism is 8.5 years. It is a rare familial disorder characterized by target-tissue resistance to PTH.

A functional hypoparathyroidism may occur as the result of magnesium deficiency. Magnesium deficiency, most often caused by malabsorption or alcoholism, prevents the secretion of PTH.

Prolonged administration of antiepileptic drugs such as phenytoin and phenobarbital, the antibiotic drug rifampin, glutethimide, and other enzyme-inducing drugs may also induce hypoparathyroidism (Box 54-3).

PATHOPHYSIOLOGY

PTH release normally occurs in response to low serum Ca^{++} levels, and secretion is suppressed by elevated levels. True hypoparathyroidism is associated with low levels of intact PTH in light of low total and ionized Ca^{++} concentrations and hyperphosphatemia. When there is insufficient Ca^{++} to meet metabolic needs, Ca^{++} stores in the bones are reduced. Chronic Ca^{++} insufficiency results in bone demineralization. Low levels of PTH also cause decreased renal clearance of phosphorus, thereby enhancing its tubular reabsorption and raising serum levels. Ca^{++} reabsorption in the intestines is decreased. There are several factors that depress Ca^{++} transport across the small intestine. For example, phytate, oxalate, and probably phosphate in the bowel promote the formation of a complex that is not absorbed from the wall of the gut.

Because Ca^{++} is responsible for neuromuscular integrity, the clinical manifestations of hypocalcemia become evident. In most cases, the neuromuscular irritability may be demonstrated by tapping over the facial nerve just in front of the ear. A unilateral contraction of facial muscles occurs (*Chvostek's*

BOX 54-3

Comparison of Hyperparathyroidism and Hypoparathyroidism

Signs and Symptoms of Hyperparathyroidism

- Serum calcium >10.5 mg/dL on three successive measurements
- Elevated PTH levels
- Low serum phosphorus (<2.5 mg/dL)
- Fatigue, apathy, anxiety, depression
- Syncope, arrhythmias, hypertension
- Decreased muscle tone, hypotonia, joint pain
- Dysphagia, polyphagia, anorexia, vomiting
- General abdominal distress, constipation
- Polyuria, nephrolithiasis, nephrocalcinosis
- Weight loss
- Osteopenia and osteoporosis

Signs and Symptoms of Hypoparathyroidism

- Total and ionized serum calcium <8.5 mg/dL
- Decreased PTH levels
- Elevated serum phosphorus (>5.4 mg/dL)
- Numbness and/or tingling of lips or fingers
- Dry hair and skin, brittle nails
- Twitching
- Laryngospasm, carpopedal spasms
- Seizures
- Muscle spasms

sign). Carpopedal spasms may be induced by placing a blood pressure cuff on the arm and inflating it above systolic pressure *(Trousseau's test)* for a period of 3 minutes. *Tetany* refers to the involuntary muscle spasms that affect muscles of the upper and lower extremities. When respiratory muscles are involved, respiratory distress may result. Deep tendon reflexes may be hyperactive. Serum and urinary Ca^{++} levels are low, with high serum and urinary phosphate levels. Alkaline phosphatase levels are normal.

It is important to determine whether a given laboratory reports total serum or ionized Ca^{++} levels on its lab reports; most only report ionized Ca^{++} levels. Serum Ca^{++} is largely bound to serum albumin; using the following formula will correct the serum Ca^{++} level using serum albumin levels:

$$\text{Corrected serum } Ca^{++} = \text{Serum } Ca^{++} \text{ mg/dL} + (0.8 \times [4.0 - \text{albumin grams/dL}])$$

PHARMACOTHERAPEUTIC OPTIONS

Calcium Salts

- calcium acetate (PhosLo)
- calcium carbonate (Rolaids, Os-Cal, Titralac, Tums, others); ♣ Apo-Cal, Caltrate 600, Maalox Quick Dissolve, Os-Cal
- calcium chloride
- calcium citrate (Citracal, Calcitrate); ♣ calcium citrate
- calcium gluconate; ♣ calcium gluconate

▥ Indications

Oral Ca^{++} is used in the treatment and management of mild hypocalcemia associated with hypoparathyroidism,

pseudohypoparathyroidism, achlorhydria, chronic diarrhea, pancreatitis, vitamin D deficiency, and hyperphosphatemia. Calcium carbonate has also been used as an antacid (see Chapter 45) and as an adjunct in the prevention of postmenopausal osteoporosis. Calcium acetate is used to control hyperphosphatemia in end-stage renal failure (see Chapter 44). Parenteral Ca^{++} salts include calcium chloride and gluconate. Intravenous (IV) calcium gluconate is the parenteral drug of choice. People needing supplemental calcium include children and adolescents, women who are pregnant or breast-feeding, older adults, and postmenopausal women.

▥ Pharmacodynamics

Ca^{++} is rapidly distributed to extracellular fluids to restore calcium levels and reestablish homeostasis. Its action is particularly important in the functioning of the nervous, cardiovascular, and skeletal systems. In the nervous system, Ca^{++} helps regulate neuron excitability and transmitter release. Decreasing excitability of the neuromuscular system produces a sedative effect on the body. In the cardiovascular system, Ca^{++} plays a crucial role in myocardial contraction and the coagulation of blood. Ca^{++} is also required for the structural integrity of the skeletal system.

▥ Pharmacokinetics

Orally administered Ca^{++} requires vitamin D for absorption in the duodenum and proximal jejunum. Under normal conditions, about one third of ingested Ca^{++} is absorbed. Absorption is facilitated by PTH and vitamin D. Absorption also depends on dietary factors, such as Ca^{++} binding to fiber and phytic, oxalic, and fatty acids. When Ca^{++} is taken with large amounts of foods containing these acids, Ca^{++} absorption is decreased. Ca^{++} readily enters extracellular fluid to be distributed to the bone.

Ca^{++} is primarily eliminated in the urine. The amount lost is determined by glomerular filtration rate and the extent of tubular reabsorption (see Table 54-2). Ca^{++} elimination is reduced by PTH and vitamin D. Likewise, elimination of Ca^{++} is increased with loop diuretics (e.g., furosemide) and by loading with Ca^{++}. Calcitonin also augments Ca^{++} elimination. Ca^{++} crosses the placenta, with significant amounts entering breast milk.

▥ Adverse Effects and Contraindications

The most common adverse effects of Ca^{++} salts include constipation, nausea, and vomiting. Ca^{++} causes GI distress from increased gas production. The most severe adverse effects include arrhythmias and cardiac arrest. Prolonged use of high doses of Ca^{++} produces other symptoms such as hypercalcemia with alkalosis, hypomagnesemia and hypophosphatemia, mood and mental changes, GI hemorrhage, and milk-alkali syndrome.

Ca^{++} formulations are contraindicated for use in patients with hypercalcemia, renal calculi, and ventricular fibrillation. Use them with caution in patients who are taking digoxin and in patients who have severe respiratory insufficiency or renal disease.

▥ Drug Interactions

All of the Ca^{++} salts enhance inotropic and toxic effects of cardiac glycosides. Ca^{++} competes with magnesium for GI absorption and decreases the absorption of tetracyclines and fluoroquinolone antibiotics. Ca^{++} is also an antagonist to the effects of verapamil and other Ca^{++} channel blockers. Cholestyramine, colestipol, and mineral oil decrease the absorption of vitamin D (see Table 54-3).

▥ Dosage Regimen

The National Institutes of Health recommend intake of 1000 to 1500 mg of Ca^{++} per day, depending on age, as part of a regimen to prevent bone loss associated with aging. Calcium carbonate products contain 40% absorbable Ca^{++}. Therefore, a 1500-mg tablet of calcium carbonate provides 600 mg of Ca^{++}. The various calcium salts differ in their percentage of elemental Ca^{++}. These differences must be accounted for when determining dosage (see Table 54-4).

▥ Lab Considerations

Intravenous Ca^{++} may falsely decrease serum and urine magnesium (Titan yellow method) levels and transiently elevate plasma II-hydroxycorticosteroids (OHCS) levels, although values usually normalize after 1 hour. Urinary steroid values (17-OHCS) may be decreased.

For more information, see the Evolve Resources Bonus Content "Influence of Selected Drugs on Laboratory Values," found at http://evolve.elsevier.com/Gutierrez/pharmacotherapeutics.

Vitamin D and Vitamin D Analogues

◆ calcitriol (cholecalciferol, Calcijex, vitamin D_3, Rocaltrol); ♣ Rocaltrol
◆ dihydrotachysterol (DHT, Hytakerol); ♣ Hytakerol
◆ ergocalciferol (Calciferol, Drisdol, D_2); ♣ Drisdol, Ostoforte

▥ Indications

The steroid hormone vitamin D is recognized as responsible for regulation of Ca^{++} and phosphorus levels in the body as well as bone mineralization. Calcitriol is used in the treatment of vitamin D deficiency, including rickets and osteomalacia.

Ergocalciferol is the form of vitamin D used in vitamin supplements. It is used for prophylaxis and treatment of vitamin D deficiency, hypophosphatemia, and hypocalcemia, as well as for the treatment of osteodystrophy, osteomalacia secondary to chronic antiepileptic drug use, and rickets, and to fortify foods. Dihydrotachysterol is used for the treatment of hypophosphatemia and hypocalcemia, as well as for the prevention and treatment of rickets, vitamin D deficiency, and postoperative and idiopathic tetany.

▥ Pharmacodynamics

The body's natural supply of vitamin D relies on exposure to the ultraviolet rays of the sun for the conversion of 7-dehydrocholesterol in the skin to vitamin D_3 (cholecalciferol). However, vitamin D must be activated by the liver and the kidneys before it can regulate Ca^{++} and phosphorus metabolism. It also regulates the homeostasis of Ca^{++} in conjunction with PTH and calcitonin (Fig. 54-2).

Activated vitamin D_3 is bound to receptors within the cell that act as transcription factors for gene expression. Vitamin D receptors can be found in most, if not all, bodily cells. The receptor for activated vitamin D_3 joins with a different intracellular receptor, the receptor for retinoid-X, to form a complex that in turn binds to DNA. This complex receptor unites

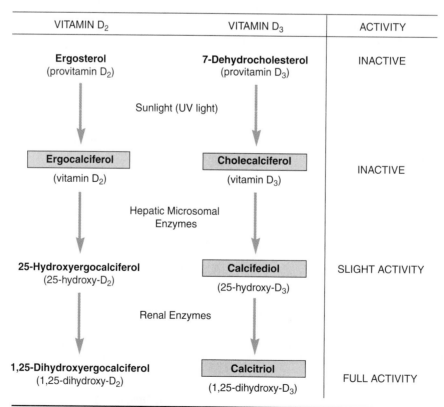

FIGURE 54-2 Activation of Vitamin D. (Adapted from Lehne, R. [2007]. *Pharmacology for nursing care* [6th ed., p. 852, Figure 73-2]. St. Louis: Saunders.)

several types of cholecalciferol, but primarily 1,25-dihydroxycholecalciferol.

Calcitriol enhances Ca^{++} absorption in the intestines, while also stimulating phosphate and magnesium ion absorption. The efficacy of dietary Ca^{++} absorption is greatly reduced when vitamin D is not available. Vitamin D stimulates a number of proteins responsible for moving Ca^{++} from the intestinal lumen, across epithelial cells, and into circulation.

Pharmacokinetics

Vitamin D analogues are readily absorbed from the GI tract. Calcitriol undergoes enterohepatic recycling and biliary excretion before being eliminated from the body. Its metabolites are eliminated primarily in feces.

Dihydrotachysterol and ergocalciferol are also well absorbed but in an inactive form. They are distributed to breast milk, lymph, liver, skin, brain, spleen, and bones and transformed to active metabolites by sunlight, the liver, and the kidneys. Fifty percent of vitamin D formulations is eliminated in feces or urine. The remainder is stored for months in body tissues, especially the liver and the bones (see Table 54-2).

Adverse Effects and Contraindications

The primary adverse effect of calcitriol is hypercalcemia. The symptoms of hypercalcemia include nausea, vomiting, constipation, anorexia, apathy, headache, thirst, sweating, and/or polyuria. Weakness, somnolence, photophobia, dry mouth, metallic taste, polydipsia, and weight loss have also been noted. Hypertension and arrhythmias, as well as muscle and bone pain, are possible. Calcitriol has a greater risk for inducing hypercalcemia compared to the other vitamin D compounds.

Vitamin D analogues are contraindicated for use in patients with hypersensitivity to the drugs and those with pre-existing hypercalcemia, and in the presence of vitamin D toxicity. The symptoms of progressive hypercalcemia can be severe enough as to require emergency attention. **Chronic hypercalcemia leads to generalized vascular calcification, nephrocalcinosis, and other soft-tissue calcification. The $Ca \times P$ value should not exceed 70.**

Use vitamin D and vitamin D analogues with caution in patients with hyperparathyroidism or sarcoidosis, and in patients taking digoxin. Excessive vitamin D intake in children may lead to mental and physical retardation and suppression of linear growth. Safe use during pregnancy has not been established.

Drug Interactions

Arrhythmias are more likely to appear in patients concurrently taking vitamin D analogues and digoxin. Thiazide diuretics can trigger hypercalcemia in patients with hypoparathyroidism who are taking vitamin D. A number of other drug interactions with vitamin D are identified in Table 54-3.

Dosage Regimen

The dosage of vitamin D analogues varies with the specific drug and is adjusted as needed to maintain serum Ca^{++} concentrations within a normal range (see Table 54-4).

Lab Considerations

Draw serum ionized Ca^{++} concentrations on a weekly basis during initial therapy. Measure the blood urea nitrogen

(BUN), serum creatinine, alkaline phosphatase, and PTH levels, the urinary calcium/creatinine ratio, and 24-hour urinary calcium levels periodically throughout therapy. A fall in alkaline phosphatase levels may signal the onset of hypercalcemia.

Overdosage of vitamin D compounds is associated with a $Ca \times P$ level over 70, and elevated BUN, alanine transaminase (ALT), and aspartate transaminase (AST) levels. Vitamin D analogues may cause a false increase in serum cholesterol values.

CLINICAL REASONING

Treatment Objectives

Regardless of the cause of hypoparathyroidism, the primary objectives are twofold: (1) Maintain serum Ca^{++} levels in an asymptomatic range. In keeping Ca^{++} levels on the low end of normal, (2) long-term complications such as renal stones and ectopic calcifications are avoided.

Treatment Options

Ca^{++} formulations are useful in patients who have low Ca^{++} levels, which are most often the result of a poor diet and avoidance of Ca^{++}. Replacement hormone therapy is indicated when Ca^{++} levels are below normal and the patient is symptomatic. Some literature suggests that once-daily doses of Ca^{++} supplements are better absorbed, and thus best taken, at bedtime.

Patient Variables

LIFE-SPAN CONSIDERATIONS

Pregnant and Nursing Women. PTH levels are not altered by pregnancy, and therefore diagnosis of hypoparathyroidism during pregnancy is similar to that of nonpregnant patients. More patients are diagnosed with symptomatic hypoparathyroidism during pregnancy than outside of pregnancy; however, this finding likely reflects a lack of routine screening of Ca^{++} levels rather than an increased severity of the disease. In fact, hypoparathyroidism in pregnancy is relatively uncommon.

The treatment of choice for hypoparathyroidism during pregnancy consists of calcium and vitamin D administration (Box 54-4). High maternal and fetal mortality ensues if hypoparathyroidism during pregnancy is not treated. Further, neonatal hyperparathyroidism may develop in response to the hypocalcemia. Breastfeeding can cause hypervitaminosis D in the infant because vitamin D is eliminated in the breast milk.

Neonates can have hypoparathyroidism, with 25% of the cases resulting in fetal death, 50% resulting in tetany, and 2% involving a congenital absence of parathyroid glands and thymus. The congenital absence of these structures frequently leads to an early death.

Children and Adolescents. Although the mechanisms involved in the accrual of bone are not well understood, the prepubertal years provide the greatest gains in bone mass and density when both Ca^{++} intake and physical activities are at or approach recommended levels. For the prevention of osteoporosis, the importance of bone gain early in life (i.e., during a period of relatively high plasticity of the skeleton to physical forces), has become an accepted truism. Because optimal amounts of Ca^{++} are not consumed by all children, the positive effect of

---

BOX 54-4

Dietary Calcium Intake Requirements by Age Group

AGE	CALCIUM PER DAY (MG)
Infants: 0–6 months	210
7–12 months	270
1–3 years	500
4–8 years	800
9–18 years	1300
19–50 years	1000
>50 years	1200
Pregnant and Lactating	
≤18	1300
19–50	1000

- Dairy products are the richest source of dietary calcium. If dairy products are not consumed as a regular part of the diet, it would be reasonable to seek nutritional counseling.
- For individuals who, for whatever reason, choose not to consume dairy products, other dietary sources of calcium should be used.
- Calcium taken together with vitamin D is more effective than calcium alone.
- Postmenopausal woman consuming high levels of calcium may reduce the risk of dying of heart disease, and this reduced risk may be achieved regardless of whether the higher intake of calcium is attributed to diet, supplements, or both.
- Milk and dairy products are more effective in the prevention and treatment of malnourishment in children than a grain-based diet.

Modified from the Food and Nutrition Board. Institute of Medicine. (1997). *Dietary reference intakes for calcium, phosphorus, magnesium, vitamin D, and fluoride.* Washington, DC: National Academy Press.

---

physical activity is important to offset low Ca^{++} intake in growing children and may dominate as an early determinant of bone mass and bone density.

As in the management of an adult, the management of hypoparathyroidism in a child is directed at maintenance of normal serum Ca^{++} levels. Some children may be treated with oral Ca^{++} salts alone, whereas others may also require supplemental vitamin D. Close follow-up is crucial to the well-being of the child. Serum Ca^{++} and phosphorus levels are checked twice weekly during initial therapy and then monthly thereafter.

The American Academy of Pediatrics (AAP) recently changed its recommendation for vitamin D supplementation in children, which may, in particular, affect those who do not drink much milk. The AAP now advises that to prevent rickets and vitamin D deficiency, children need a daily supplement of 200 units of vitamin D if they are exclusively breastfed or not drinking at least 500 mL (17 ounces) of vitamin D–fortified milk or infant formula. Older children and adolescents who do not have regular sunlight exposure and who do not drink at least 500 mL of vitamin D–fortified milk daily will also need a supplement.

Older Adults. Older adults may be susceptible to hypoparathyroidism because of dietary deficiencies of Ca^{++} and vitamin D, or because of decreased activity and lack of exposure to sunshine. Secondary causes of hypoparathyroidism that occur more often in older adults include cancer of the prostate, pancreatitis, and liver or renal disease. Older adults are more susceptible to osteoporosis and spontaneous fractures.

▓ *Drug Variables*

Calcium carbonate is the most efficient form of calcium available and is the drug of choice for the treatment of chronic hypocalcemia related to hypoparathyroidism. It is also less expensive than other formulations. Calcium carbonate is also a weak phosphate binder and is helpful in controlling the high serum phosphate levels associated with renal failure.

Start therapy with vitamin D as soon as oral calcium is begun. The drug of choice to supply vitamin D for chronic hypoparathyroidism is ergocalciferol (vitamin D_2). Ergocalciferol provides for more stable serum Ca^{++} levels than the shorter-acting vitamin D formulations. With proper dosages, serum Ca^{++} levels can be maintained within normal limits. Dihydrotachysterol has a shorter duration of action than ergocalciferol and is more effective in the mobilization of Ca^{++} from bone.

Patient Education

Orally administered Ca^{++} salts are taken with meals, although they should not be taken with foods containing large amounts of oxalic acid (e.g., spinach, Swiss chard, rhubarb, beets) or phytic acid (e.g., bran, whole-grain cereals). However, the concurrent administration of dairy products with Ca^{++} salts may produce milk-alkali syndrome, which is manifested as headache, confusion, nausea, and vomiting. This applies to anyone on vitamin D therapy (such as postmenopausal women taking Ca^{++} and vitamin D for prevention of osteoporosis).

Teach patients that Ca^{++} can cause constipation; thus, they should increase bulk and fluid in the diet and increase mobility. Severe constipation can indicate toxicity, necessitating contact with the health care provider.

Evaluation

The effectiveness of drug therapy for hypoparathyroidism is evidenced by resolution of hypoparathyroid symptoms and a return of serum Ca^{++} levels to a normal range. Monitoring serum Ca^{++} levels at regular intervals, at least every 3 months, is important. Urine Ca^{++} levels, with spot urine determinations, should also be monitored and kept below 30 mg/dL, if possible.

HYPERPARATHYROIDISM

EPIDEMIOLOGY AND ETIOLOGY

The saying that patients with hypercalcemia have difficulty with "bones, stones, abdominal groan, psychic moans, and fatigue overtones" is well known. *Hyperparathyroidism* (HPT), an increasingly recognized disorder, is defined as hypercalcemia secondary to excessive production of PTH. It is the third most common endocrine disorder following diabetes mellitus and thyroid disease. This disorder affects 1 in 500 to 1000 people and occurs 2 to 4 times more often in postmenopausal women than in men. It is rare before puberty, but the incidence increases dramatically after age 50.

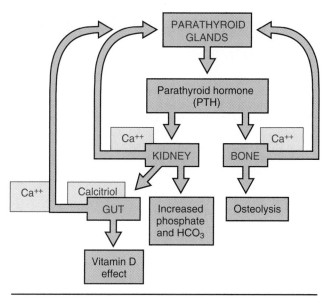

FIGURE 54-3 Parathyroid hormone secretion is regulated through a negative feedback loop involving the kidneys, the bones, and the intestine.

A single parathyroid adenoma accounts for 80% to 85% of cases of HPT. The etiology of the remaining cases is unknown. The adenoma is often clonal in nature, implying a defect in the gene that regulates PTH. Although in most cases HPT occurs sporadically, it also appears in assorted patterns as a familial disorder. Carcinoma of the parathyroid gland is rare, occurring in less than 2% of cases.

Secondary HPT is a response to vitamin D deficiency or the hypocalcemia of chronic renal disease. Hyperplasia of the parathyroid gland is found in 10% to 15% of cases. Eventually, the hyperplastic glands develop autonomous function and no longer respond to the normal feedback mechanisms (Fig. 54-3). Risk factors in the development of primary HPT include a history of radiation therapy to the neck or use of the drug lithium.

PATHOPHYSIOLOGY

Regardless of cause, the pathogenesis of primary HPT is related to the development of hypercalcemia. Increased quantities of PTH act directly on the kidneys, which in turn leads to Ca^{++} resorption (not *reabsorption*), and phosphate elimination increases in the renal tubules. Under ordinary circumstances, serum Ca^{++} levels are maintained within a narrow range despite large swings in calcium absorption during the day. These variations contribute to elevated serum Ca^{++} levels and low phosphorus levels.

The hallmarks of primary hypercalcemia are elevated ionized or total serum Ca^{++} levels and elevated PTH and PTH-C (C-terminal fragments). The C assays tend to have higher values and are more widely accepted as indicators of hyperparathyroidism. Increased levels of PTH lead to increased absorption of Ca^{++} by the intestines (in the presence of increased vitamin D production by the kidneys). Sodium phosphorus levels tend to be low; however, the results must be correlated with the patient's clinical picture.

Most patients with primary hypercalcemia show no evidence of bone disease. Extensive bone erosion results from

untreated, long-standing hyperparathyroidism. Bone resorption is readily demonstrated in the cortex of the phalanges. In the small number of patients who have significant bone erosion, serum alkaline phosphatase levels are also elevated. The elevation in alkaline phosphatase level reflects osteoblastic activity.

Increased osteoclastic activity and decreased osteoblastic activity results in the release of Ca^{++} and phosphorus to the circulation and decalcification of bone (e.g., osteopenia and osteoporosis). Only one third of patients with HPT show minor degrees of decalcification; 33% display obvious skeletal abnormalities, and the remaining 33% display advanced bone changes.

When the normal solubility of serum Ca^{++} is exceeded, Ca^{++} deposits in soft tissue such as the cornea, the conjunctiva, the myocardium, and the kidneys. The deposits are most likely to occur with long-standing hypercalcemia.

Hypertension may be noted in some cases of acute hypercalcemia, most likely as a result of vasoconstriction. In contrast, with a chronic hypercalcemic state, the development of hypertension is due to renal damage.

Increased bicarbonate elimination and decreased acid elimination produce metabolic acidosis, urinary alkalosis, and hypokalemia. Stones containing calcium oxalate or calcium phosphate may develop as a consequence of hypercalciuria. In addition, the glomerular filtration rate increases, and renal tubular acidosis (RTA) occurs.

CLINICAL REASONING

Treatment Objectives
The primary treatment objective for patients with hyperparathyroidism is to reduce the serum hypercalcemia caused by the excessive production of PTH.

Treatment Options
There is no totally acceptable treatment regimen for hypercalcemia associated with hyperparathyroidism. Surgical removal of the abnormal parathyroid gland has been the treatment of choice in patients who are symptomatic. However, a potentially dangerous trend has emerged over the last several years. Some health care providers have started using bisphosphonates to increase bone Ca^{++} rather than referring a patient for surgery. Bisphosphonate administration is not a substitute for removal of the overactive parathyroid gland.

Symptomatic patients are usually dehydrated; therefore hydration with isotonic saline is the first step in treatment. In addition, Ca^{++} intake is restricted and electrolyte deficits (i.e., potassium and magnesium) corrected. When expansion of plasma volume has been accomplished, a loop diuretic such as furosemide is given to promote urinary elimination of Ca^{++} (see Chapter 42). **If a loop diuretic (e.g., furosemide) ⚠ is used too early in the treatment of HPT, the diuretic may further dehydrate the patient and worsen the hypercalcemia. Use loop diuretics only after circulatory volume has been restored. Do not use thiazide diuretics, because they decrease the elimination of calcium and worsen the hypercalcemia.**

Glucocorticoids have been effective for hypercalcemia associated with sarcoidosis and hypervitaminosis D, because

ENDOCRINE

they decrease intestinal absorption of calcium (see Chapter 56). They are not useful for hypercalcemia that occurs with hyperparathyroidism or with production of a PTH-related hormone. At present, no PTH-inhibiting drug is available. Serum calcium levels can also be lowered by administering drugs that bind with calcium (i.e., edetate disodium [EDTA]) for elimination.

OSTEOPOROSIS

EPIDEMIOLOGY AND ETIOLOGY

Bone mass increases in males and females well into adulthood, with peak bone mass (i.e., the amount of bone present at the end of maturation) occurring during the second to fourth decades of life. Osteopenia and osteoporosis are major threats to the health of almost 44 million men and women over the age of 50 years. If measures aren't taken to stem this disease, which may be largely prevented with lifestyle changes and halted with treatment when appropriate, it is estimated that by the year 2010 over 52 million women and men in this age group will be affected; if current trends continue, the figure is expected to climb to over 61 million by 2020.

The rates of osteoporosis worldwide vary, but in every country, age is but one of the significant risk factors (Box 54-5). Given that people are living longer, the number of persons likely to develop osteoporosis is on the rise. In some countries, the hip fracture rate is increasing faster than the population. The reason for this trend is unknown, but it appears that decreasing levels of physical activity across populations may be one of the possible explanations.

There are also considerable ethnic differences in bone mineral density (BMD) and the prevalence of fractures. The lifetime risk of a fracture of the hip, the spine, or the forearm is 40% in white women and 13% in white men. Hispanic women have about half as many fractures as white women, but this is not explained by differences in BMD. Women of Asian descent have lower BMD compared with white women, but the hip fracture rate is not proportionally higher. There are several theories that may explain the discrepancy. Asian women have a shorter hip-axis length, their previous activity levels were higher, and they care for their older adults, confining them to their beds and thereby reducing the risk for falls and fractures. Higher BMDs and lower fracture rates are seen in persons of African descent.

Perhaps because many patients are unaware of vertebral fractures, calculating their incidence and prevalence is more difficult than doing so for hip and wrist fractures. To complicate matters, at present there are no standardized means for measuring the degree of compression necessary to define a vertebral fracture. The presence of a vertebral fracture increases the risk of a new fracture 4 times, even when adjusting for BMD. A fall to the side increases the risk of hip fracture 6 times compared to falls in other directions.

Osteopenia is defined as low BMD. Osteoporosis is the thinning of bone and loss of BMD over time. When analyzing BMD, a score is compared against two norms: "young normal" and "age-matched." The T-score compares a patient's BMD to the peak BMD of a 30-year-old healthy adult (i.e., young normal), and the risk for fracture is determined accordingly. The T-score for young normal adults increases as the

---

BOX 54-5

Risk Factors for Osteoporosis

- Advancing age
- Autoimmune deficiency syndrome or human immunodeficiency virus (HIV) infection
- Aluminum, antiepileptic drugs, cytotoxic drugs, immunosuppressants, lithium, heparin (long-term use), supraphysiologic dosages of thyroid hormones, tamoxifen (premenopausal)
- Amyloidosis
- Ankylosing spondylitis, rheumatoid arthritis
- Antineoplastic therapy, radiation therapy
- Caucasian or Asian descent
- Chronic obstructive pulmonary disease (COPD)
- Congenital porphyria
- Diet low in calcium, eating disorders, inadequate diet, vitamin D deficiency
- Early estrogen deficiency or menopause, hypogonadism (primary or secondary), progesterone administration (parenteral, long-acting)
- Female athlete triad (disordered eating patterns, amenorrhea, excessive exercise)
- Gastrectomy, colectomy, bariatric surgery; celiac disease; Crohn's disease
- Gaucher's disease
- Hemochromatosis, hemophilia, thalassemia
- Hyperparathyroidism (primary or secondary), thyrotoxicosis, Grave's disease, hypothyroidism, Cushing's syndrome
- Hypophosphatemia
- Idiopathic scoliosis
- Inflammatory bowel disease, malabsorption syndromes
- Insulin-dependent diabetes mellitus
- Low-trauma fracture as an adult
- Lymphoma, leukemias, multiple myeloma, resection of parathyroid gland
- Mastocytosis
- Low bone mineral density (e.g., >1 SD below the mean in healthy young adult women)
- Multiple sclerosis
- Oral or inhaled steroid therapy lasting longer than 3 months
- Osteoporosis in first-degree relative, hip fracture in a parent before age 80
- Prolonged use of thyroid hormones
- Prolonged or recurrent use of antiepileptic drugs, glucocorticoids, or sedatives
- Pernicious anemia
- Severe liver disease, especially primary biliary cirrhosis
- Smoker
- Spinal cord transection; cerebrovascular accident (CVA)
- Tall, thin, small bones, weight under 126 pounds
- Total parenteral nutrition
- Weight loss

SD, Standard deviation.

BMD drops below young-normal levels: an inverse relationship. The Z-score reports the patient's BMD in relation to that expected in a person of similar age and body size (i.e., age-matched). A low BMD is common in older adults, and therefore comparison with age-matched norms can be misleading.

The calculated difference between a patient's BMD and the BMD of a young, normal adult is referred to as a standard deviation (SD). Based on the diagnostic categories of the World Health Organization (WHO), patients whose T-score is within one SD of the "norm" have a "normal" BMD (WHO, 2003). Scores falling below the norm are noted with a minus sign (−). For example, a patient who has a score between −1 and −2.5 SD below the norm has a low BMD, or osteopenia, whereas a score of −2.5 SD below the norm is osteoporosis. Women in this group may have already sustained one or more fractures. For most BMD measurements, −1 SD equates to a 10% to 12% decrease in BMD.

PATHOPHYSIOLOGY

Normal bone undergoes remodeling, a process whereby bone is resorbed and reformed over a period of months. Bone is digested or dissolved by proteolytic enzymes and acids secreted by osteoclasts. Bone deposition by osteoblasts follows. The remodeling process allows bone to adapt to changes in physical stress, which stimulates osteoblast activity and bone formation. The rate of bone resorption exceeds that of bone formation after age 40 in both sexes, because of age-related decreases in osteoblast activity, dietary Ca^{++} intake, GI absorption of Ca^{++} and vitamin D, sex hormone production, exposure to ultraviolet light, physical activity and stress on bones, and liver and kidney function.

About one fourth of trabecular bone (i.e., the honeycomb-like material in the center of bones) is replaced every year. Trabecular bone is a major component of the vertebrae and the distal forearms. In contrast, only 3% of cortical bone (i.e., the major component of long bones) is replaced annually.

The balance between bone resorption and formation is maintained by the interactions and feedback between various hormones (e.g., PTH, 1,25-dihydroxyvitamin D, calcitonin, growth hormone, estrogens, androgens) and local regulators (e.g., cytokine interleukin-1, insulin-like growth factors, prostaglandins). Synthesized by bone cells or adjacent hematopoietic cells, these factors interact with each other and with systemic hormones. Excessive elevations in serum Ca^{++} levels are unlikely because the negative feedback system decreases the production of PTH. Calcitonin, a hormone from the thyroid gland, inhibits bone resorption. These actions help maintain Ca^{++} concentrations in the extracellular fluid within the narrow range necessary for the proper function of certain cells (e.g., cardiac muscle).

There are several biochemical markers of bone formation and bone resorption. Bone formation and resorption may not always be equivalent, as is the case in steroid-induced osteoporosis, where bone resorption is much higher than formation, so it is important to know which process is being assessed. Serum or urinary cross-linked N-telopeptides of type I collagen (NTx) provides a specific biochemical marker of human bone resorption. Generation of the NTx molecule is mediated by osteoclasts on bone, and it is found in the urine as a stable end product of degradation. Serum alkaline phosphatase (ALP) and urine Ca^{++} excretion, though less specific, may also give a useful measure of bone turnover and the effectiveness of therapy. Biochemical markers may be used to further knowledge of the physiology of osteoporosis, but they cannot be used to diagnose the disease. Although they are used to gain information in particularly complex cases, the markers do not have much use on the individual level. Consequently, using markers for screening or follow-up is discouraged.

PHARMACOTHERAPEUTIC OPTIONS

Bisphosphonates

- alendronate (alendronate, Fosamax, Fosamax-D); ◆ Fosalan, Fosamax, Fosavance
- etidronate (Didronel); ◆ Didronel
- ibandronate (Boniva); ◆ Boniva
- pamidronic acid (Aredia); ◆ Aredia
- risedronate (Actonel, Actonel with Calcium); ◆ Actonel
- zoledronic acid (Zometa); ◆ Zometa

Indications

Bisphosphonates are used in the treatment and prevention of osteoporosis. Bisphosphonates are also used for the treatment of glucocorticoid-induced osteoporosis in both genders receiving glucocorticoids in a daily dosage equivalent of 7.5 mg or greater. In addition, treatment reduces bone turnover and the number of bone remodeling sites.

Zoledronic acid, the newest drug on the market, is the most potent bisphosphonate. It is approved for the prevention of osteoporosis and skeletal fractures, particularly in patients with cancers such as multiple myeloma and prostate cancer. Zoledronic acid can also be used to treat hypercalcemia, particularly the hypercalcemia of malignancy, and is helpful in treating pain from osteolytic bony metastases and Paget's disease. Whether the drug offers clinically significant advantages over other bisphosphonates remains to be determined.

Pharmacodynamics

Bisphosphonates are structural analogues of pyrophosphate, a normal bone constituent. Bisphosphonates bind to bone crystals to specifically inhibit the activity of osteoclasts, which in turn reduces bone resorption without affecting bone formation. However, since bone formation and resorption come together in the bone turnover process, bone formation does ultimately decrease.

In studies of alendronate, an increase in BMD was shown in the spine and hip, with a 48% decrease in the rate of vertebral compression fractures (Black, Thompson, and Bauer, 2000). If the drug is taken for 6 years, no decrease in bone mass is noted for 2 years after therapy stops. One-year studies of ibandronate show that the once-monthly drug provides a significantly greater increase in lumbar spine BMD than placebo. Risedronate similarly reduced incidence of vertebral fractures by 41% over 3 years and reduced hip fractures by 40% in older adult women who had low BMD, but not in women who had risk factors for fracture alone (Iwamoto, Takeda, and Sato, 2006).

Pharmacokinetics

The extent of absorption of bisphosphonates in the upper GI tract is impaired by the presence of food or beverages (other than plain water). For example, when alendronate is taken concurrently with coffee or orange juice, bioavailability is decreased by about 60% (see Table 54-2). After absorption, bisphosphonates rapidly bind to bone. There is no evidence that bisphosphonates are biotransformed. The terminal half-life of bisphosphonates varies considerably, probably reflecting the release of the drug from the skeleton. Bisphosphonates are eliminated in the urine and the feces.

ENDOCRINE

⚏ *Adverse Effects and Contraindications*

⚠ **Bisphosphonates are contraindicated for use in patients with a history of esophageal disorders, gastritis, or peptic ulcer disease since they are more likely to cause esophagitis.** Esophagitis usually occurs within the first few months of therapy if the drugs are taken incorrectly. Other adverse effects include GI disturbance, diarrhea, and abdominal pain. Use caution when prescribing bisphosphonates for patients with serum creatinine levels over 3 mg/dL and for those who are taking nonsteroidal antiinflammatory drugs (NSAIDs) (because of the risk of GI disturbance). Alendronate should not be used in patients with a creatinine clearance less than 35 mL/min; risedronate should not be used if the creatinine clearance is less than 30 mL/min.

A rare complication of zoledronic acid and pamidronate is osteonecrosis of the jaw. This has primarily been seen in patients with multiple myeloma who were treated with zoledronate. Patients with cancer are generally at a higher risk for osteonecrosis because of other therapies (i.e., radiation, antineoplastic therapy, and drugs such as steroids) they may

⚠ undergo. **A causal relationship has not been established between use of bisphosphonates and osteonecrosis of the jaw, but patients with cancer should be advised to maintain good oral hygiene and have periodic dental checkups.** Any major dental work should be finished before starting therapy with bisphosphonates. In the case of a dental emergency, corrective strategies should be the least invasive possible.

⚏ *Drug Interactions*

Antacids, Ca^{++} salts, and multivitamins with minerals decrease absorption of the bisphosphonate, thereby reducing efficacy (see Table 54-3).

⚏ *Dosage Regimen*

Bisphosphonates must be taken regularly to suppress osteoclast activity on newly formed resorptive surfaces (see Table 54-4). The rate of bone formation is greater than the rate of bone resorption at these remodeling sites, resulting in accumulations in bone mass; in some cases, this may occur for as long as 10 years. Patients should also be taking supplemental Ca^{++} and vitamin D, particularly if dietary intake is inadequate.

Selective Estrogen Receptor Modulators
◆ raloxifene (Evista); ✦ Evista

⚏ *Indications*

Selective estrogen receptor modulators (SERMs) such as raloxifene are indicated for the prevention of osteoporosis in postmenopausal women.

⚏ *Pharmacodynamics*

Similar to those of estrogen, raloxifene's actions are mediated by binding to estrogen receptors, producing differential expression of multiple estrogen-regulated genes in different tissues. Raloxifene is an estrogen antagonist in uterine and breast tissues. This characteristic distinguishes SERMs from receptor agonists and antagonists.

Raloxifene also reduces overall bone turnover by decreasing bone resorption, which is manifested by a reduction in bone turnover markers in the serum and the urine and an increase in BMD. It also has estrogen-like activity on cholesterol and low-density lipoprotein (LDL) metabolism.

⚏ *Pharmacokinetics*

There is increased absorption of raloxifene following a high-fat meal, but the change in systemic exposure is not clinically relevant. Raloxifene has a significant first-pass effect, and the drug and its metabolites are highly bound to plasma proteins (see Table 54-2). Raloxifene is primarily eliminated in feces.

⚏ *Adverse Effects and Contraindications*

Common adverse events of raloxifene include hot flashes (25% of patients), which are ordinarily reported during the first 6 months of treatment, leg cramps, arthralgia, and sinusitis. Occasionally, weight gain, nausea, myalgias, pharyngitis, cough, dyspepsia, rash, and depression have occurred. Although rare, pneumonia, gastroenteritis, chest pain, vaginal bleeding, and breast pain have also been reported.

Raloxifene is contraindicated for use in women of child- ⚠ **bearing age and those who are lactating, in women with active or past history of deep vein thrombosis, pulmonary embolism, and retinal vein thrombosis, and in those hypersensitive to the drug or its ingredients.**

⚏ *Drug Interactions*

Cholestyramine reduces the absorption and enterohepatic cycling of raloxifene by 60% and thus should not be administered concomitantly (see Table 54-3). The international normalized ratio (INR) is decreased 10% in patients taking warfarin, so the risk of thromboembolism is higher. Be sure to monitor the INR more closely.

⚏ *Dosage Regimen*

The effect of raloxifene on BMD beyond 2 years of treatment is not known at this time. See Table 54-4 for the dosage recommendation.

⚏ *Lab Considerations*

Raloxifene raises apolipoprotein A_1 levels while reducing total cholesterol, LDL, apolipoprotein B, lipoprotein (a), and fibrinogen levels. Raloxifene produces a moderate increase in hormone-binding globulin concentrations, including sex steroid–binding globulin, thyroxine-binding globulin, and corticosteroid-binding globulin. Serum levels of total Ca^{++} and protein, albumin, inorganic phosphate, and platelets are slightly reduced, but the decreases are no more notable than those seen with estrogen or hormone replacement therapies.

Hormone Modifier Drugs
◆ teriparatide (Forteo)

⚏ *Indications*

Teriparatide is used for the treatment of osteoporosis in postmenopausal women who are at high risk for fracture. These include, most often, women who have had a previous osteoporosis-related fracture or who have multiple risk factors for a fracture, and those who have failed or are intolerant of other osteoporosis therapies. Teriparatide is also used to increase BMD in men with primary or hypogonadal osteoporosis who are at high risk for a fracture, although the effect of the drug on fracture risk in men has not been studied.

▓ Pharmacodynamics

Teriparatide is the only Food and Drug Administration (FDA)–approved drug for osteoporosis that increases bone formation (all others decrease bone resorption). Teriparatide is a form of PTH produced by recombinant DNA technology. Teriparatide increases serum Ca^{++} while decreasing serum phosphorus levels.

Once-daily administration of teriparatide stimulates new bone formation on trabecular and cortical bone surfaces by preferentially stimulating osteoblastic activity over osteoclastic activity. The outcome is an increase in BMD and improvement in bone turnover markers (e.g., Z-scores, NTX levels). In contrast, continuous overload of endogenous PTH, which occurs in hyperparathyroidism, may be harmful because bone resorption is stimulated more than bone formation.

▓ Pharmacokinetics

Teriparatide is well absorbed following subcutaneous (subQ) injection with an absolute bioavailability of about 95% (see Table 54-2). Biotransformation of teriparatide is thought to occur through nonspecific enzyme actions in the liver followed by elimination via the urine.

▓ Adverse Effects and Contraindications

The adverse effects of teriparatide treatment include leg cramps, nausea, dizziness, headache, orthostatic hypotension, tachycardia, and occasionally hypercalcemia. There may be injection site pain, swelling, erythema, localized bruising, and minor itching. Injection site reactions are usually mild and transient. Hypersensitivity reactions may appear shortly after injection and are manifested by acute dyspnea, orofacial edema, generalized urticaria, and chest pain.

Teriparatide is contraindicated for use in patients with a history of bony metastasis or metabolic diseases (other than osteoporosis), in those with an increased baseline risk for osteosarcoma, in patients with Paget's disease (elevations in alkaline phosphatase may warn of the disease), in children, and for patients who will be receiving external beam radiation.

▓ Dosage Regimen

Because of the risk for first-dose orthostatic hypotension, the first injection of teriparatide should be administered with the patient lying or sitting down (see Table 54-4). Minimize the time the pen is out of the refrigerator to reduce degradation of the drug. The prescribed dose may be administered immediately following removal from the refrigerator. The safety and efficacy of teriparatide treatment beyond 2 years is unknown, and consequently not advised.

▓ Drug Interactions

There are no known drug interactions with teriparatide, although in theory the drug may cause an elevation in INR levels for patients taking warfarin.

Miscellaneous Hypocalcemic Drugs

- ◆ calcitonin salmon (Calcimar, Miacalcin, Fortical, Osteocalcin); ◆ Calcimar, Caltine
- ◆ gallium nitrate (Ganite)
- ◆ plicamycin (Mithracin)

Calcitonin

Calcitonin salmon is useful for most forms of acute, severe hypercalcemia associated with increased bone resorption. It is safely used to decrease the rate of bone turnover, to lower serum calcium levels, and to more effectively relieve the pain of an osteoporotic fracture than other drugs. Any loss of efficacy may be due to calcitonin-induced reduction of serum phosphate levels. However, unidentified factors may also be involved.

Intranasal calcitonin increases spinal bone mass in women 5 years postmenopause who have established osteoporosis. It is also approved by the FDA for treatment of symptomatic Paget's disease. Injectable calcitonin is also indicated for hypercalcemic emergencies. Calcitonin has also been used in the treatment of osteogenesis imperfecta but is not approved by the FDA for that purpose at this time.

Much like the other hypocalcemic drugs, calcitonin salmon decreases serum Ca^{++} levels by directly inhibiting bone resorption, and by attaching to bone minerals for absorption into newly formed bone matrix. Single injections of calcitonin cause a marked, but transient, inhibition of bone resorption. There is a persistent, smaller reduction in the rate of bone resorption with continued use. It also promotes the renal excretion of Ca^{++}, but its effectiveness varies.

There are two sources of calcitonin, salmon and human. The salmon source of calcitonin is more potent than human sources on a milligram-to-milligram basis and has a longer duration of action. Because orally administered calcitonin is destroyed in the GI tract, calcitonin salmon requires parenteral administration. It is completely absorbed using subQ or intramuscular (IM) routes. Calcitonin does not appear to cross the placental membranes. It is rapidly biotransformed in the kidneys, blood, and tissues (see Table 54-2).

Calcitonin is generally devoid of serious adverse effects. However, anaphylaxis is more common with the salmon formulation of the drug. Nausea, vomiting, a strange taste in the mouth, and facial flushing have been reported. The common adverse effects of calcitonin include fatigue, anorexia, nausea, vomiting, constipation, and abdominal pain. Bone pain and generalized discomfort are relatively common. Supplemental use of vitamin D and calcium antagonize the calcium-lowering effect of hypocalcemic drugs (see Table 54-3). Nonetheless, a daily intake of 400 units of vitamin D and 1500 mg of calcium are recommended for patients receiving calcitonin for osteoporosis.

Although calcitonin salmon is most often administered as a nasal spray, the drug is available in parenteral form. Perform an intradermal skin test before beginning therapy with calcitonin salmon, regardless of the route. With the initial injection, watch the patient closely for anaphylaxis.

Plicamycin

Plicamycin (Mithracin), on the basis of limited clinical experience to date, may be considered in the treatment of certain symptomatic patients with hypercalcemia and hypercalciuria associated with a variety of advanced neoplasms (see Chapter 33). Plicamycin antagonizes the action of vitamin D and inhibits the action of PTH on osteoclasts.

The most common adverse effects include hypocalcemia and thrombocytopenia. CNS irritability or depression and GI upset have been noted, as well as fluid and electrolyte imbalances. Use the drug with caution in patients with hypersensitivity, bleeding disorders, depressed bone marrow reserve,

ENDOCRINE

hypocalcemia, or severe renal or liver disease. Plicamycin is contraindicated for use in patients with thrombocytopenia, thrombocytopathy, coagulation disorders, or an increased susceptibility to bleeding due to other causes. Plicamycin should not be administered to any patient with impairment of bone marrow function. Do not use plicamycin in women of childbearing years or during pregnancy since it may cause fetal harm. Safe use in children has not been established.

Do not give a patient vaccines that contain live strains of a virus (e.g., live oral polio vaccine) during treatment with plicamycin. In addition, prevent contact with persons who have recently received a live vaccine; there is a chance that the virus can be passed on.

Monitor the CBC and differential, platelet count, prothrombin time, bleeding times, and electrolyte levels before and periodically throughout therapy. Plicamycin may cause thrombocytopenia, leukemia, anemia, hypocalcemia, hypokalemia, and hypophosphatemia. Further evaluation by the health care provider is indicated if the platelet count drops below 150,000/mm^3, the INR is elevated, or the leukocyte count is less than 4000/mm^3.

Gallium Nitrate

Gallium nitrate (Ganite) inhibits Ca^{++} resorption from bone and is indicated for treatment of clearly symptomatic, cancer-related hypercalcemia that has not responded to adequate hydration.

Gallium nitrate is administered intravenously and eliminated unchanged by the kidneys. The half-life increases from 72 to 115 hours with prolonged infusions. Serum creatinine and BUN and serum Ca^{++} levels must be closely monitored during gallium nitrate therapy. In addition to baseline assessment, the suggested frequency of calcium and phosphorus determinations is daily and twice weekly, respectively. The most common adverse effects of gallium nitrate include renal toxicity and hypophosphatemia. Blood in urine, bone pain, greatly increased or decreased frequency of urination or amount of urine, increased thirst, loss of appetite, muscle weakness, and nausea or vomiting are also common. It is rare for the patient to have unusual levels of fatigue or weakness, abdominal cramping, or confusion, and muscle spasms are possible but rare. Hearing loss, optic neuritis, visual impairment, and hypocalcemia have been noted. Use of the drug is contraindicated in patients with severe renal impairment (serum creatinine exceeding 2.5 mg/dL), and it should be used with caution in patients with renal impairment. Safe use during pregnancy and lactation has not been established.

CLINICAL REASONING

Treatment Objectives

The goal of drug therapy for the patient with osteoporosis is to minimize bone loss and prevent fractures and fracture-related morbidity and mortality. To do this, bone strength must be increased and bone resorption reduced.

Treatment Options

Various non–drug and drug therapies may be used to prevent or treat osteoporosis (see Box 54-6). The approach used depends on the results of BMD testing, etiology, patient age, menopausal status (if female), sex, fracture risk, general health, and personal preference (see Case Study: Drugs for Calcium Disorders).

▓ Patient Variables

Osteoporosis is not a part of normal aging. Lifestyle modification, in the form of adequate calcium and vitamin D intake, weight-bearing exercise, and avoidance of smoking and excess alcohol intake, is an essential component in the prevention and treatment of osteoporosis. Include plans for hip protection (i.e., hip padding) for the frail older adults in the event of a fall.

Stopping corticosteroid therapy is the intervention of first choice for patients with, or at risk for, corticosteroid-induced osteoporosis. Unfortunately, in many cases this is not possible because of a chronic health condition. In these situations, using the lowest effective dosage (preferably of a topical or inhaled formulation) is recommended. However, using high-dose corticosteroids by inhalation also may adversely affect bone structure. Because bone loss is most rapid during the first 6 months of corticosteroid therapy, begin preventive intervention as soon as treatment begins.

At this time, the complexity of treatment of osteoporosis in men is compounded by a paucity of research. If testosterone deficiency underlies the patient's osteoporosis, testosterone replacement therapy is warranted, unless of course there are contraindications to such therapy. Only two drugs, alendronate and teriparatide, are approved for osteoporosis in men. Like alendronate, teriparatide increases BMD and reduces fracture risk. Calcitonin has been used for men, but proof of efficacy is lacking.

▓ Drug Variables

Currently, five types of drugs are approved for the prevention and/or treatment of osteoporosis: hormone therapy, bisphosphonates, SERMs, calcitonin, and PTH. The antiresorptive drugs, estrogen, raloxifene, bisphosphonates, and calcitonin are used most often. These drugs are effective at preventing bone loss, but not at restoring bone density once it is gone. Accordingly, antiresorptive drugs are most beneficial when used early on, before substantial bone loss has occurred. At this time, teriparatide is the only drug available that effectively promotes bone formation.

ESTROGEN. Estrogen therapy, with or without a progestin, is an established approached for osteoporosis prevention. Estrogen acts indirectly to suppress osteoclast proliferation and thereby puts a brake on bone resorption. As a result, when estrogen levels decline, either because of menopause or surgical removal of the ovaries, osteoclasts increase in number, causing bone resorption to dramatically increase (see Chapter 58). Estrogen replacement then helps restore the braking action on osteoclast proliferation and thereby suppress bone resorption.

In the Women's Health Initiative (WHI) study of more than 16,000 women, estrogen plus progestin increased BMD and reduced the risk of hip and vertebral fractures by about 34%, and fractures at other sites by about 23% (Lee, et al., 2006). The research study ended early because there were more breast cancers than expected, the interpretation being that the risk increased. It was established that women receiving the estrogen and progestin had a greater risk of breast cancer, myocardial infarction, stroke, and thromboembolic events than those taking the placebo. Nonetheless, because

BOX 54-6

Osteoporosis Studies

STUDY	PURPOSE AND OUTCOMES OF STUDY
Study of Osteoporotic Fractures (SOF) (Black, 1995)	*Primary Purpose:* To use previously collected data to develop osteoporosis guidelines, to estimate the cost-effectiveness of screening for osteoporosis, and to plan trials of osteoporosis therapies *Outcome:* Older age, previous nonspinal fracture, low BMD at all sites, a low body mass index (BMI), current smoking, low milk consumption during pregnancy, low levels of daily physical activity, having a fall, and regular use of aluminum-containing antacids independently increased the risk of a first vertebral fracture. Women using estrogen and those who engaged in recreational physical activity had a decreased risk.
Postmenopausal Evaluation and Risk Reduction with Lasofoxifene (PEARL) Study (Gennari, 2006)	*Primary Purpose:* To assess safety and efficacy on lasofoxifene treatment on reducing risk of osteoporotic fractures (especially vertebral fractures). *Outcome:* If found safe and effective, postmenopausal women will have another treatment option available for use.
Multiple Outcomes of Raloxifene Evaluation (MORE) Study (Cummings, 1999)	*Primary Purpose:* To evaluate raloxifene for the treatment of osteoporosis, rather than prevention for which it was previously FDA-approved *Outcome:* No significant difference in risk of nonspinal fractures between raloxifene and placebo groups was found.
Fracture Intervention Trial (FIT) (Chapurlat, 2005)	*Primary Purpose:* To evaluate the effects on bone density and fracture risk when treatment is discontinued vs. when it is continued over several years *Outcome:* As a result of the FIT study, the FDA approved alendronate for the treatment of osteoporosis in postmenopausal women.
Fracture Intervention trial Long-term Extension (FLEX) (Black, 2000).	*Primary Purpose:* To examine long-term efficacy, safety, and tolerability of oral alendronate in postmenopausal women previously treated with alendronate for 3 to 6 years in conjunction with the FIT study. *Outcome:* Compared with women who stopped alendronate after an average of 5 years, those continuing alendronate maintained a higher BMD and greater reduction of bone turnover, showing benefit of continued alendronate treatment on BMD and bone turnover. On discontinuation of alendronate therapy, rates of change in BMD at the hip and spine resumed at the background rate, but discontinuation did not result in either accelerated bone loss or a marked increase in bone turnover, showing persistence of alendronate's effects on bone.
Ibandronate and Bone Loss in Postmenopausal Women (McClung, 2004)	*Primary Purpose:* To assess the efficacy, dose response, and safety of oral ibandronate in the prevention of postmenopausal bone loss in women *Outcome:* If shown safe and effective, ibandronate will provide another treatment option to prevent osteoporosis in postmenopausal women.
PTH and alendronate in combination for the treatment of osteoporosis (PaTH) (Black, 2005)	*Primary Purpose:* To determine whether use of parathyroid hormone (PTH) and alendronate together is safe and effective for treating osteoporosis, possibly increasing BMD *Secondary Purpose:* To analyze the differences in treatment groups with regard to fractures and biochemical markers of bone metabolism *Outcome:* If combination safe and more effective compared with either drug alone, women with osteoporosis will have another treatment option.
Ultra Low Transdermal Estrogen Replacement Assessment (ULTRA) (Garcia-Perez, 2006)	*Primary Purpose:* To evaluate the efficacy of treatment using an ultralow dose of unopposed transdermal (TD) estradiol compared to placebo in the prevention of bone loss and osteoporosis of the lumbar spine in postmenopausal women without hysterectomy *Secondary Purpose:* To assess bone loss at the hip, quantifying biochemical parameters of bone metabolism, assess endometrial histology and bleeding patterns, measure metabolic effects, and consider treatment effects on postmenopausal quality of life and cognitive function *Outcome:* If low doses of unopposed TD estradiol are found to be safe and effective, another treatment option will become available to prevent osteoporosis in postmenopausal women.
Osteoporotic Fractures in Men (Mr. OS) (Cauley, 2006)	*Primary Purpose:* To examine the extent to which fracture risk is related to bone mass, bone geometry, lifestyle factors, biochemical measures, fall risk, and other variables *Secondary Purpose:* To determine the extent to which osteoporosis in men is associated with other age-related medical conditions such as prostate disease *Outcome:* The study is likely to have a significant impact on health care of older men, especially in formulating clinical algorithms for identifying those at risk for fractures and in the development of public health and research policies for osteoporosis detection and prevention.
Behavioral Strategies to Prevent Osteoporosis in Girls (Ievers-Landis, 2005)	*Primary Purpose:* To assess the feasibility and effectiveness of a 2-year behavioral program to increase calcium intake and physical activity among a cohort of fifth-grade girls (ages 9-11 years) enrolled in Girl Scout troops *Outcome:* If shown to be effective, this program could serve as a national model program for osteoporosis prevention among girls.

BMD, Bone mineral density; *FDA,* Food and Drug Administration; *TD,* transdermal.

ENDOCRINE

CASE STUDY | Drugs for Calcium Disorders

ASSESSMENT

History of Present Illness	SM is a 62-year-old newly divorced female who was involved in an MVA at age 43 that left her a paraplegic. The friend and neighbor who accompanies her at this visit reports SM had a syncopal episode that lasted 30 seconds. There was no known precipitating event or vertigo before the fall. She did not fall from her wheelchair. The neighbor also reports that SM never complains about anything, even when she sustained a non–trauma-related vertebral fracture 2 years ago that was slow to heal. She is worried that SM may have something wrong in her head.
Past Health History	SM had a total hysterectomy for large fibroids at age 48. She has little intake of daily products because of lactose intolerance; prefers not to use over-the-counter Lactaid products; stopped calcium supplements because of problems with constipation; and admits she does not follow a balanced diet or drink enough water, consuming primarily caffeinated diet sodas. She has no allergies and takes no other prescription or OTC drugs. Mother and father, both deceased, had osteoporosis, heart disease, and diabetes. Current meds: levothyroxine 200 mcg/daily for hypothyroidism: "It helps me keep my weight down so that I can fit in this damn chair."
Life-Span Considerations	SM lives alone and works as a radiation oncologist. She has been exposed to low level radiation since her career started, 22 years ago. A cat is her companion. She drives a van specially equipped for her wheelchair. She tries to swim once or twice a week at the local Easter Seal pool because the water is warm and there is a lift and an attendant who helps her into the pool.

SM has a 10-year history of alcohol abuse, consuming 1 to 2 fifths of bourbon a week: "It is how I used to cope with being in this wheelchair all the time." She has had no alcohol since joining Alcoholic's Anonymous in the last 8 months. Nonsmoker. SM has health insurance and a pharmacy plan. |
| **Physical Exam Findings** | *Height:* 5′6″. *Present weight:* 122 lb. *VS:* BP, 146/88, 98.6° F-88 (apical pulse)-24. Skin is warm and dry. ENT negative. EOMI, PERRLA. Fundoscopic exam unremarkable. No lymphadenopathy or thyromegaly. HRRR. BSCTA. Abdomen soft, flat, nontender. No vertebral tenderness. Left wrist painful to palpation with mild edema over lateral aspect. Radial and ulna pulses 2+. Patella and Achilles reflexes 0. Muscle wasting of lower extremities noted. No decubiti noted. |
| **Diagnostic Testing** | TSH 0.35 mg/dL. Total serum calcium level on last 3 visits high at 10.6 mg/dL, 13.9 mg/dL, and 12.0 mg/dL, respectively. Serum phosphorus level, 2.3 mg/dL. Serum magnesium, 1.1 mEq/L. BUN, creatinine, and other electrolytes WNL. BMD down from −1.5 to −2.1 in last 2 years. CXR negative. |

DIAGNOSIS: Postmenopausal osteoporosis

MANAGEMENT

Treatment Objectives	1. Maintain serum calcium and all lab values within the normal range. 2. Reduce risk of pathologic fractures secondary to osteoporosis. 3. Prevent long-term complications of fractures and their sequelae.
Treatment Plan	**Pharmacotherapy** • alendronate with vitamin D 70 mg PO weekly on an empty stomach • Increase calcium carbonate to 1500 mg/day and additional vitamin D 400 units/day • OTC magnesium gluconate 500 mg (i.e., 27 mg elemental magnesium) 3 times daily **Patient Teaching** 1. Correct way to take bisphosphonate (i.e., empty stomach first thing in the morning with 8 oz of water only; remain upright for at least 30 minutes) 2. Take calcium carbonate, vitamin D, and magnesium in divided doses with meals 3 times daily 3. Avoid intake of phosphoric acid–containing drinks and excessive meat intake. 4. Encourage swimming activities. 5. Teach about resources and patient education materials that are available from the National Osteoporosis Foundation. 6. Follow-up in office bimonthly initially, then every 6 months; BMD testing every 2 years

Evaluation

Six weeks later, serum calcium levels and other lab values were within normal limits. There have been no pathologic fractures to date. Long-term complications of fractures and their sequelae have not been evaluated at this time.

CLINICAL REASONING

Q1. Why did you choose alendronate rather than another bisphosphonate? How do you know which drug is the best one to use?

A. Information comes primarily from evidence-based research studies, but the bottom line is which drug has the better track record for fracture reduction. A study by Schousboe found it was cost-effective to treat women between the ages of 55 and 75 years with a clinical fracture or a T-score less than −2.5.with alendronate.

Q2. What other type of patients can take the alendronate? Can a man take bisphosphonates?

A. Male patients with osteoporosis and persons with glucocorticoid-induced osteoporosis or Paget's disease of the bone, as well as women with postmenopausal osteoporosis, may take alendronate. The only bisphosphonate that has been approved for men with osteoporosis is alendronate. Teriparatide has also been approved for men who are high risk for fracture; it actually deposits calcium in the bone rather than preventing resorption.

Q3. Why must SM also take vitamin D when she takes her calcium carbonate? Isn't one drug enough?

A. Orally administered calcium requires vitamin D for absorption to take place in the duodenum and the proximal jejunum. Absorption also depends on dietary factors, such as calcium binding to fiber and phytic, oxalic, and fatty acids. When calcium is taken with large amounts of foods containing these acids, calcium absorption is impaired. We will need to teach her what foods to avoid.

Q4. Let's say SM decides to stop taking the drug, or gets esophagitis and has to stop the alendronate. How long will the alendronate remain beneficial for her osteoporosis treatment?

A. Alendronate taken for up to 5 years has been shown to maintain bone for up to 5 years after the drug is stopped. We don't have enough research as to the length of time a bisphosphonate is beneficial.

EVIDENCE-BASED PHARMACOTHERAPEUTICS

Cost Effectiveness of Alendronate Therapy

■ Background

In the absence of fractures, the indications for bisphosphonates are controversial. Treatment guidelines recommend drug therapy to prevent fractures for some postmenopausal women who have low bone mass (osteopenia) but who do not have osteoporosis or a clinical history of fractures. The question is whether or not it is cost-effective to do so.

Many providers agree that patients who meet the World Health Organization (WHO) criteria (BMD T-score below −2.5) should be treated. Guidelines published by the National Osteoporosis Foundation (NOF) and the American College of Obstetrics and Gynecology (ACOG) recommend drug therapy for women who lack additional risk factors at a T-score of −2.0 or less, and for women with one or more additional risk factors at a T-score of −1.5. Nevertheless, many fractures occur in postmenopausal women whose T-scores are above the guidelines. Information about the cost-effectiveness of treating such women with bisphosphonate should guide clinical recommendations.

■ Research Article

Schousboe, J., Nyman, J., Kane, R. (2005). Cost-effectiveness of alendronate therapy for osteopenic postmenopausal women. *Annals of Internal Medicine, 142*(9), 734-741.

Purpose

The purpose of this study was to estimate the quality-adjusted life-years (QALYs) and cost of alendronate therapy to prevent fractures in postmenopausal women with osteopenia. The study used the societal perspective of pharmacoeconomics.

Design

The study was based on population-based studies of age-specific fracture rates and costs, prospectively measured estimates of disutility after fractures, and the Fracture Intervention Trial (FIT) of alendronate versus placebo to prevent fractures. Subjects included postmenopausal women ages 55 to 74 years with femoral neck T-scores between −1.5 and −2.4 on dual-energy X-ray absorptiometry (DEXA) scan.

Methods

A Markov cost-utility model containing eight health states (no fracture, post–distal forearm fracture, post–clinical vertebral fracture [clinically evident at onset], post–radiographic vertebral fracture [but clinically asymptomatic at onset], post–hip fracture, post–hip and vertebral fractures, and post–other fracture [e.g., proximal forearm fracture, distal femur], and death) was used to compare 5 years of treatment with alendronate with no drug therapy for women ages 55, 65, and 75 with varying levels of BMD T-scores (−1.5, −2.0, and −2.4). Many assumptions were identified during development of the model that included the probability of fracture, relative risk for fracture during drug therapy, mortality, yearly cost of alendronate, QALYs associated with each health state, and sensitivity analysis (including possible effects of nonadherence to therapy or inappropriate use of the drug).

Findings

For women with no additional fracture risk factors, the cost per QALY gained ranged from $70,000 to $332,000, depending on age and femoral

Continued

neck BMD. Results of the sensitivity analysis demonstrated that the results were sensitive to changes in fracture risk reduction attributable to alendronate and alendronate cost.

Conclusions

The results indicate that alendronate is not cost-effective, assuming a societal willingness to pay $50,000 per QALY gained, current U.S. drug costs, and available estimates of the efficacy of alendronate in postmenopausal women with femoral neck T-score better than −2.5 and no history of clinical fractures or other bone mineral density–independent risk factors. This conclusion should be reconsidered, however, if the cost of drug therapy is significantly lowered, if drug therapy is shown to reduce the risk for nonvertebral fractures in this population, or if the fracture reduction benefit persists longer than 10 years after a 5-year treatment course.

■ Implications for Practice

Recent publications and various guidelines recommend extending the accepted indications for drug therapy to postmenopausal women with osteopenia. These women are likely to be a growing segment of candidates for therapy even though they are less likely to experience fractures. If the T-score threshold for treatment was changed from −2.5 to −2.0 or −1.5, the percentages of women 65 years of age who are eligible for drug therapy would increase from 16% to 31% or 50%, respectively. The cost to society of treating osteopenic women must be considered before initiating public health campaigns targeted at this group. Results of this study are applicable only to white women living in the United States. Head-to-head studies should be conducted comparing other bisphosphonates with other therapies using the same outcome parameters.

---

this is as much a political issue as a medical one, neither a purely medical nor a purely political path is clear. In any case, in order for breast cancer to become detectable, most experts agree that it takes approximately 5 to 10 years. This means that any woman who developed breast cancer in the WHI study almost certainly had the cancer at the time of enrollment. A history of estrogen receptor–positive breast cancer contraindicates use of this therapy option.

BISPHOSPHONATES. Bisphosphonates are efficacious and generally well tolerated when taken properly. Calcium and vitamin D must also be taken for maximal benefits. However, recent post-marketing data has shown an association between the use of IV bisphosphonates and osteonecrosis of the jaw. Based on these data, precautions have been added to product labeling. Research is underway to assess whether this adverse effect represents a class effect. Preliminary data suggest it is associated mainly with IV bisphosphonate, but it has been reported in patients taking oral bisphosphonates (Delmas, et al., 2006).

SERMs. In the MORE trial, treatment with raloxifene for 36 months increased BMD and reduced fracture risk. The increase in BMD was 2.3% at the femoral neck and 2.7% in vertebrae. After 36 months, at least one new vertebral fracture was seen in 10.1% of women using the placebo, compared with 6.6% of those taking raloxifene. This represents a 52% decrease in risk of fracture. Although raloxifene reduced the risk of vertebral fractures, it failed to reduce the risk of nonspinal fractures (e.g., hip, wrist). The efficacy of raloxifene in preventing and treating corticosteroid-induced osteoporosis remains to be established.

CALCITONIN. Calcitonin has been used for over 20 years with no long-term adverse effects. Calcitonin is used to treat established osteoporosis, not prevent it. One 2-year study of women ages 68-72 treated with calcitonin nasal spray showed an increase in BMD in the spine by 3% compared with a 1% increase in BMD by women who were treated with placebo (Overgaard, Lindsay, and Christiansen, 1995). In younger postmenopausal women, calcitonin increased the average BMD by 2%, whereas the average BMD decreased by 7% in women taking the placebo. Not only is calcitonin moderately efficacious, but it is also safe and helps to relieve the discomfort of vertebral fractures associated with osteoporosis.

PTH. Teriparatide is the first and only drug for osteoporosis that works by increasing bone formation rather then decreasing bone resorption. Teriparatide increases BMD of the lumbar spine, the femoral neck, and the total body while significantly reducing the risk of vertebral fractures (Chen et al., 2007). As a general rule, however, reserve teriparatide for patients at high risk for fractures for three primary reasons: the drug is expensive; it is inconvenient in that it requires daily subQ injection; and it may contribute to development of potentially dangerous bone cancer.

Patient Education

Educate the patient about osteoporosis, its prevalence, and the importance of treating the condition to prevent fractures and other complications. Also educate patients about the various options for drug therapy to prevent and treat osteoporosis and work with the patient to develop a mutually agreeable treatment plan.

Most postmenopausal women, and some men, need Ca^{++} supplements. Advise the patient to take Ca^{++} supplements at a different time of day than the bisphosphonate or SERM, because Ca^{++} interferes with absorption of the drug. Drugs containing Ca^{++}, aluminum, and magnesium also interfere with the absorption of these drugs and should not be taken at the same time as the bisphosphonate or the SERM.

Instruct patients to take their bisphosphonate drug specifically as directed. To facilitate the delivery of a bisphosphonate to the stomach and reduce the risk for esophageal irritation, the patient takes the drug while in an upright position (sitting or standing), with 6 to 8 oz plain water. Advise the patient to not lie down for at least 30 minutes after taking the bisphosphonate. The tablet should not be chewed or sucked because of the risk of oropharyngeal irritation.

If using a subQ formulation of drug, include the correct technique for injection in patient teaching. Reassure the patient that the flushing and warm sensation following injection is transient and usually lasts about 1 hour.

Evaluation

The goal of drug therapy for the patient with osteoporosis is to minimize bone loss and prevent fractures and fracture-related morbidity and mortality. The effectiveness of drug therapy is evidenced by fewer fractures and reduced morbidity and mortality.

KEY POINTS

THYROID DISORDERS

- Hypothyroidism is the result of inadequate peripheral thyroid hormone levels. More than 90% of patients with hypothyroidism have primary thyroid atrophy. Hashimoto's thyroiditis is the most common cause.
- Insufficient thyroid hormones result in an overall decrease in the basal metabolic rate, producing multisystem manifestations.
- The primary aim of treatment is to restore a euthyroid state and alleviate symptoms.
- There are few adverse effects associated with thyroid hormone use except those that indicate overdosage. Development of chest pain and tachyarrhythmias signals overdosage.
- Teach the patient that therapy for hypothyroidism is lifelong. Notify the prescriber if brand changes are made.
- Therapeutic effectiveness of thyroid hormone therapy is determined by the presence of weight loss, greater energy levels, and an increased sense of well-being. Serum TSH and T_4 levels return to normal range.
- Hyperthyroidism occurs as a result of excessive secretion of thyroid hormones and is 4 times more common in females under the age of 40 than in males.
- Management of hyperthyroidism is aimed at reducing the levels of circulating thyroid hormones and alleviating symptoms.
- PTU is the drug of choice for pregnant hyperthyroid women because of its limited placental transfer and low potency. Methimazole, with its once-daily schedule, has decided advantages over PTU, including better adherence and more rapid improvement in serum concentrations of T_4 and T_3.
- Therapeutic effectiveness of antithyroid drugs is demonstrated by a decreased pulse rate and by weight gain. Thyroid hormone levels should return to normal, and the patient should reflect a clinically euthyroid state.

PARATHYROID DISORDERS

- Primary hyperparathyroidism is defined as hypercalcemia secondary to the excessive production of parathyroid hormone (PTH). Secondary hyperparathyroidism is a response to the hypocalcemia of chronic renal disease or vitamin D deficiency.
- Hyperparathyroidism is a relatively common disorder affecting postmenopausal women 2 to 4 times more often than men. It is the third most common endocrine disorder.
- The hallmarks of primary hyperparathyroidism are elevated total serum and ionized calcium levels with an elevated PTH level.
- The objective of treatment for hyperparathyroidism is to control the underlying disease and to restore calcium levels to a normal range.
- Therapeutic effectiveness of hypercalcemic drugs is demonstrated by lowered serum calcium levels and fewer complaints of bone pain and the absence of fractures.
- Hypoparathyroidism is related to insufficient amounts of PTH (true hypoparathyroidism), which is most often caused by surgical removal of the gland. Deficiency of PTH secretion leads to hypocalcemia and hyperphosphatemia.
- The primary objective of treatment for hypoparathyroidism is to maintain serum calcium levels in a slightly low, but asymptomatic range. In so doing, long-term complications are avoided.
- Calcium salts such as calcium carbonate and vitamin D preparations are the drugs of choice in the treatment of hypocalcemia.
- Therapeutic effectiveness of hypocalcemic therapy is noted, with resolution of hypocalcemic symptoms and an increase in serum calcium levels to normal range.

OSTEOPOROSIS

- Osteoporosis is characterized by low bone mineral density.
- The goal of drug therapy for the patient with osteoporosis is to minimize bone loss and prevent fractures and fracture-related morbidity and mortality.
- Five types of drugs are approved for the prevention and/or treatment of osteoporosis: bisphosphonates, selective estrogen receptor modulators, hormone therapy, calcitonin, and teriparatide (PTH).
- In treating osteopenia or osteoporosis, drug therapy will not work as well (if at all) in patients who have poor nutrition, vitamin D deficiency, or lack of exercise.

Bibliography

American Academy of Pediatrics. (2006). Update of newborn screening and therapy for congenital hypothyroidism. *Pediatrics, 117*(6), 2290–2303.

American College of Rheumatology Ad Hoc Committee on Glucocorticoid-induced Osteoporosis. (2001). 2001 update. *Arthritis and Rheumatism, 44*(7), 1496–1503.

Azizi, F. (2006). The safety and efficacy of antithyroid drugs. *Expert Opinions in Drug Safety, 5*(1), 107–116.

Bach-Huynh, T., and Jonklass, J. (2006). Thyroid medications during pregnancy. *Therapeutic Drug Monitoring, 28*(3), 431–441.

Baddoura, R., Awada, H., Okais, J., et al. (2006). An audit of bone densitometry practice with reference to ISCD, IOF and NOF guidelines. *Osteoporosis International, 17*(7), 1111–1115.

Bindra, A., and Braunstein, G. (2006). Thyroiditis. *American Family Physician, 73*(10), 1769–1776.

Black, D., Bilezikian, J., Ensrud, K., et al. (2005). One year of alendronate after one year of parathyroid hormone (1-84) for osteoporosis. *New England Journal of Medicine, 353*(6), 555–565.

Black, D., Palermo, M., Nevitt, M., et al. (1995). Comparison of methods for defining prevalent vertebral deformities: the Study of Osteoporotic Fractures. *Journal of Bone and Mineral Research, 10*(6), 890–902.

Black, D., Thompson, D., and Bauer, D. (2000). Fracture risk reduction with alendronate in women with osteoporosis: The Fracture Intervention Trial. *Journal of Clinical Endocrinology and Metabolism, 85*(11), 4118–4124.

Bryant, R., Cadogan, J., and Weaver, C. (1999). The new dietary reference intakes for calcium: Implications for osteoporosis. *Journal of the American College of Nutrition, 18*(90005), 406S–412S.

Cauley, J., Fullman, R., Stone, K., et al. (2005). Factors associated with the lumbar spine and proximal femur bone mineral density in older men. *Osteoporosis International, 16*(12), 1525–1537.

Chapurlat, R., Palermo, L., Ramsay, P., et al. (2005). Risk of fracture among women who lose bone density during treatment with alendronate: The Fracture Intervention Trial. *Osteoporosis International, 16*(7), 842–848.

ENDOCRINE

Chen, P., Miller, P., Recker, R., et al. Increases in bone mineral density correlate with improvements in bone microarchitecture with teriparatide treatment in postmenopausal women with osteoporosis. *Journal of Bone and Mineral Research* (In press).

Cooper, D. (2005). Antithyroid drugs. *New England Journal of Medicine, 352*(9), 905–917.

Crandall, C. (2003). Laboratory workup for osteoporosis. Which tests are most cost-effective? *Postgraduate Medicine, 114*(3), 35–38, 41–44.

Cummings, S., Eckert, S., Krueger, K., et al. (1999). The effect of raloxifene on risk of breast cancer in postmenopausal women: Results from the MORE randomized trial. Multiple Outcomes of Raloxifene Evaluation. *Journal of the American Medical Association, 281*(23), 2189–2197.

Davis, J., Ashe, M., Guy, P., et al. (2006). Undertreatment after hip fracture: A retrospective study of osteoporosis overlooked. *Journal of American Geriatric Society, 54*(6), 1019–1020.

Delmas, P., Adami, S., Strugula, C., et al. (2006). Intravenous ibandronate injections in postmenopausal women with osteoporosis: One-year results from the dosing intravenous administration study. *Arthritis and Rheumatology, 54*(6), 1838–1846.

Ensrud, K., Barrett-Connor, E., and Schwartz, A. (2004). Randomized trial of effect of alendronate continuation versus discontinuation in women with low BMD: Results from the Fracture Intervention Trial Long-Term Extension. *Journal of Bone and Mineral Research, 19*(8), 1259–1269.

Garber, J., Hennessey, J., and Liebermann, J. (2006). Managing the challenges of hypothyroidism. *Journal of Family Practice, 55*(6), S1–S8.

Garcia-Perez, M., Moreno-Mercer, J., Tarin, J., et al. (2006). Similar efficacy of low and standard doses of transdermal estradiol in controlling bone turnover in postmenopausal women. *Gynecological Endocrinology, 22*(4), 179–184.

Garwood, C., VanSchepen, K., McDonough, R., et al. (2006). Increased thyroid-stimulating hormone levels associated with concomitant administration of levothyroxine and raloxifene. *Pharmacotherapy, 26*(6), 881–885.

Gennari, L., Merlotti, D., Martini, G., et al. (2006). Lasofoxifene: A third-generation selective estrogen receptor modulator for the prevention and treatment of osteoporosis. *Expert Opinion on Investigational Drugs, 15*(9), 1091–1103.

Gold, D., Alexander, I., and Ettinger, P. (2006). How can osteoporosis patients benefit more from their therapy? Adherence issues with bisphosphonate therapy. *Annals of Pharmacotherapy, 40*(6), 1143–1150.

Ievers-Landis, C., Burant, C., Drotar, D., et al. (2005). A randomized controlled trial for the primary prevention of osteoporosis among preadolescent girl scouts: 1-year outcomes of a behavioral program. *Journal of Pediatric Psychology, 30*(2), 155–165.

Iwamoto, J., Takeda, T., and Sato, Y. (2006). Efficacy and safety of alendronate and risedronate for postmenopausal osteoporosis. *Current Medical Research Opinion, 22*(5), 919–928.

Kafilmout, I., Morris, L., Mayer, J., et al. (2006). What causes a low TSH level with a normal free T4 level? *Journal of Family Practice, 55*(6), 543–544.

Khamaisi, M., Regev, E., Yarom, N., et al. (2007). Possible association between diabetes and bisphosphonate-related jaw osteonecrosis. *Journal of Clinical Endocrinology and Metabolism, 92*(3), 1172–1175.

Lanhan-New, S. (2006). Fruit and vegetables: The unexpected natural answer to the question of osteoporosis prevention? *American Journal of Clinical Nutrition, 83*(6), 1254–1255.

Lee, E., Wutoh, A., Xue, Z., et al. (2006). Osteoporosis management in a Medicaid population after the Women's Health Initiative study. *Journal of Women's Health, 15*(2), 155–161.

Lieberman, U. (2006). Long-term safety of bisphosphonate therapy for osteoporosis: A review of the evidence. *Drugs and Aging, 23*(4), 289–298.

Marx, R., Sawatari, Y., Fortin, M., et al. (2005). Bisphosphonate-induced exposed bone (osteonecrosis/osteopetrosis) of the jaws: Risk factors, recognition, prevention, and treatment. *Journal of Oral and Maxillofacial Surgery, 63*(11), 1567–1575.

McClung, M., Wasnich, R., Recker, R., et al. (2004). Oral daily ibandronate prevents bone loss in early postmenopausal women without osteoporosis. *Journal of Bone and Mineral Research, 19*(1), 11–18.

Morganti, S., Ceda, G., Saccani, M., et al. (2006). Thyroid disease in the elderly: Sex-related differences in clinical expression. *Journal of Endocrinological Investigation, 28*(11 Suppl 2), 101–104.

Nevit, M., Cummings, S., Stone, K., et al. (2005). Risk factors for a first-incident radiographic vertebral fracture in women >65 years of age: The study of osteoporotic fractures. *Journal of Bone and Mineral Research, 20*(1), 131–140.

Overgaard, K., Lindsay, R., and Christiansen, C. (1995). Patient responsiveness to calcitonin salmon nasal spray: A subanalysis of a 2-year study. *Clinical Therapeutics, 17*(4), 680–685.

Pearce, E. (2006). Diagnosis and management of thyrotoxicosis. *British Medical Journal, 332*(7554), 1369–1373.

Pyon, E. (2006). Once-monthly ibandronate for postmenopausal osteoporosis: Review of a new dosing regimen. *Clinical Therapeutics, 28*(4), 475–490.

Recommendations for the prevention and treatment of glucocorticoid-induced osteoporosis: 2001 update. American College of Rheumatology Ad Hoc Committee on Glucocorticoid-Induced Osteoporosis. *Arthritis and Rheumatism, 44*(7), 1496–1503 update.

Riggs, B., and Hartmann, L. (2003). Selective estrogen-receptor modulators: Mechanisms of action and application to clinical practice. *New England Journal of Medicine, 348*(7), 618–629.

Sapountzi, P., Emanuele, N., Loutrianakis, E., et al. (2006). Diagnosis: Hypocalcemia due to primary hypoparathyroidism. *Endocrinology Practice, 12*(2), 233.

Siris, E., Harris, S., Eastell, R., et al. (2005). Skeletal effects of raloxifene after 8 years: Results from the continuing outcomes relevant to Evista (CORE) study. *Journal of Bone Mineral Research, 20*(9), 1514–1524.

Tran, H. (2006). Difficulties in diagnosing and managing coexisting primary hypothyroidism and resistance to thyroid hormone. *Endocrinology Practice, 12*(3), 288–293.

Tsai, W., Haghighi, K., and Placa, J. (2006). Bisphosphonate-induced osteonecrosis of the jaws: A case report and literature review. *General Dentistry, 54*(3), 215–219.

Unal, E., Abaci, A., Bober, E., et al. (2006). Efficacy and safety of oral alendronate treatment in children and adolescents with osteoporosis. *Journal of Pediatric Endocrinology and Metabolism, 19*(4), 523–528.

United States Department of Health and Human Services. Food and Drug Administration. Center for Drug Evaluation and Research. Office of Pharmaceutical Science. Office of Generic Drugs. (2006). *Approved drug products with therapeutic equivalency evaluations* (26th ed.). Available online: www.fda.gov/cder/orange/obannual.pdf. Accessed May 26, 2007.

Weitzman, R., Sauter, N., Eriksen, E., et al. (2006). Critical review: Updated recommendations for the prevention, diagnosis, and treatment of osteonecrosis of the jaw in cancer patients. *Critical Reviews in Oncology/Hematology, 62*(2), 148–152.

World Health Organization. (2003). Prevention and management of osteoporosis. Report of a WHO Scientific Group. *Technical Report Series, 921*, 1–164.

Woo, S., Hellstein, J., and Kalmar, J. (2006). Systematic review: Bisphosphonates and osteonecrosis of the jaws. *Annals of Internal Medicine, 144*(10), 753–761.

Wright, V. (2006). Osteoporosis in men. *Journal of the American Academy of Orthopedic Surgeons, 14*(6), 347–353.

55

Pituitary Drugs

Pituitary disorders are characterized by an excess or deficit of pituitary-secreted hormones. Hormonal excess or deficit may be caused by malfunctioning of the pituitary gland or by extrapituitary factors. Pituitary tumors are the major cause of hormone excess. Other causes of hormone excess can be related to ectopic hormone–secreting sites or the presence of substances, such as drugs, that enhance hormone secretion. In contrast, hormone deficits are usually related to defects in the pituitary gland itself.

PITUITARY PHYSIOLOGY

The pituitary gland is only about as big as the tip of the little finger, but it is one of the most important glands in the body. It produces a greater variety of hormones than any other gland. It sits directly under the brain in a pocket called the sella turcica of the sphenoid bone. It has three main parts: the anterior (adenohypophysis), posterior (neurohypophysis), and intermediate (or pars intermedium) lobes. In an adult the distinct pars intermedium disappears and the individual cells are distributed diffusely throughout the anterior and posterior lobes.

The lobes of the pituitary, like all endocrine glands, do not operate in isolation. They are part of classic feedback systems in which their responses to signals from body tissues are regulated to maintain a stable level of activity (Fig. 55-1).

Anterior Pituitary
The anterior pituitary serves multiple functions, and because of its ability to regulate other endocrine gland function, it is known as the "master gland." The anterior lobe (adenohypophysis) contains five cell types that synthesize six different polypeptide and glycoprotein hormones. The polypeptide hormones are *growth hormone (GH), prolactin (PRL),* and *adrenocorticotropin (ACTH, corticotropin).* The glycoprotein hormones are *thyroid-stimulating hormone [TSH, thyrotropin]), luteinizing hormone (LH),* and *follicle-stimulating hormone (FSH).* For each anterior pituitary hormone there is an appropriate, corresponding hypothalamic-releasing hormone (Table 55-1).

GH is the principal regulator of somatic growth. It has no specific target organ but rather influences carbohydrate, protein, and fat metabolism throughout the body, resulting in growth of skin, muscle, visceral tissues, bone, and cartilage. GH also induces insulin resistance and lipolysis. For GH to be released, the person must have at least 2 hours of sleep daily.

The primary action of PRL is to stimulate lactation and growth of mammary tissue. Dopamine is the predominant PRL inhibitory factor. PRL levels gradually increase throughout pregnancy with a tenfold elevation at term. Four to 12 weeks postpartum, PRL levels return to normal unless breastfeeding occurs.

The thyroid produces hormones that control the rates of metabolic processes throughout the body. TSH causes an immediate increase in the release of stored thyroid hormones, an increase in iodine uptake and oxidation, an increase in the synthesis and secretion of prostaglandins by the thyroid, and an increase in thyroid hormone synthesis (see Chapter 54).

FSH stimulates estrogen production, oogenesis, and follicular growth in females. LH stimulates ovulation and progesterone production, and estrogen release by the ovaries. LH also stimulates interstitial cells in males to promote spermatogenesis at the Leydig cells and testosterone secretion (see Chapter 58).

Posterior Pituitary
The posterior pituitary occupies an outpocketing of the ventral brain called the infundibulum, an extension of the central nervous system (CNS). Hormones secreted by the posterior pituitary gland are produced by nerve cells in the hypothalamus. The hormones produced include antidiuretic hormone (ADH, vasopressin) and oxytocin, which are stored in the pituitary.

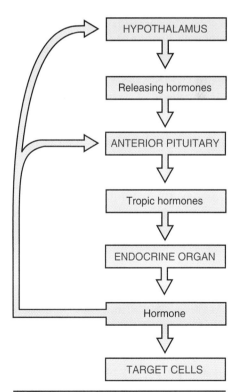

FIGURE 55-1 The Hypothalamic-Pituitary Control of Hormone Levels.

TABLE 55-1 Overview of Pituitary Hormones*

Hormone	Hypothalamic-Releasing Hormone	Desired Effects(s)	Effects of Hypersecretion	Effects of Hyposecretion
ANTERIOR PITUITARY HORMONES				
Growth hormone (GH)	GHRH (somatotropin)	Enhances systemic body growth	Gigantism in children; acromegaly in adults	Dwarfism
Prolactin (PRL)	Prolactin-inhibiting factor (dopamine)†	Stimulates the production of breast milk in mammary glands	Hyperprolactinemia, galactorrhea, hypogonadism	Reduced ability to lactate
Thyroid-stimulating hormone (TSH, thyrotropin)	Thyrotropin-releasing hormone	Stimulates the growth of the thyroid gland and secretion of thyroid hormones	Goiter, hyperthyroidism (thyrotoxicosis)	Hypothyroidism
Adrenocorticotropic hormone (ACTH, corticotropin)	Corticotropin-releasing hormone (CRH)	Stimulates secretion of glucocorticoids	Cushing's disease osteoporosis	Primary adrenal insufficiency, Addison's disease
Follicle-stimulating hormone (FSH)	Gonadotropin-releasing hormone (GnRH)	Stimulates ovarian follicles in females, estrogen secretion, and spermatogenesis in males	Infertility	Anovulation, aspermatogenesis
Luteinizing hormone (LH)	Gonadotropin-releasing hormone (GnRH)	Stimulates maturation of corpus luteum and production of progesterone after ovulation; stimulates production of testosterone	Primary gonadal failure, infertility	Fertility
POSTERIOR PITUITARY HORMONES				
Antidiuretic hormone (ADH)	—	Conserves water by concentrating urine and reducing urine volume; induces vasoconstriction of glomerulus	SIADH	Central diabetes insipidus
Oxytocin	—	Initiates uterine contraction	Uterine contraction; let-down reflex	Uterine atony

*There are many other mechanisms in play to reach the end points of hyper- and hyposecretion disorders.
†PRL is under inhibitory hypothalamic control with dopamine as the predominant inhibitory factor.
GHRH, Growth hormone–releasing hormone; *SIADH,* syndrome of inappropriate antidiuretic hormone secretion.

ADH increases water resorption in the distal tubules and collecting ducts of the nephron, concentrates urine, and causes vasoconstriction. ADH controls water balance in the body by increasing the permeability of cells of the distal tubules to water, thus decreasing the formation of urine. An increase in osmotic pressure or a decrease in volume increases ADH secretion. Osmolality, thirst, and blood volume regulate the secretion of ADH.

The uterus of a nonpregnant woman does not respond to normal concentrations of oxytocin, whereas the pregnant uterus is more sensitive. Oxytocin is secreted in response to sucking and mechanical distention of the female reproductive tract. Stimulated by sucking, oxytocin binds to its receptors on myoepithelial cells in the mammary tissues and causes contraction of those cells. During the third stage of labor, oxytocin functions to enhance the effectiveness of contractions, to promote delivery of the placenta, and to stimulate postpartum contractions to reduce excessive bleeding (see Chapter 59). Oxytocin is similar to ADH with respect to water homeostasis, response to secretory stimuli, and renal action.

PITUITARY DYSFUNCTION

EPIDEMIOLOGY AND ETIOLOGY

In general, pituitary disorders are rare, affecting only a few per 100,000 persons per year. A microadenoma (i.e., a benign tumor <10 mm in diameter) usually leads to hypersecretion of pituitary hormones (see Table 55-1). A few microadenomas secrete multiple hormones; GH and PRL is the most frequent

combination. Further, because the pituitary gland is enclosed in a small fossa, macroadenomas (i.e., a tumor >10 mm in diameter) lead to compression or destruction of the pituitary tissue, which in turn decreases secretion of all other pituitary hormones. Other disorders leading to pituitary hyposecretion include vascular thrombosis leading to pituitary necrosis, infiltrative granulomatous diseases, and idiopathic or perhaps autoimmune destruction of the pituitary gland.

Occasionally, a patient exhibits isolated pituitary hormone failure. Under these circumstances, the cause of the deficiency is likely to be in the hypothalamus and involve the corresponding releasing hormone.

PHARMACOTHERAPEUTIC OPTIONS

Pituitary hormone drugs have limited uses but primarily include replacement and suppressive therapies. All pituitary hormones are proteins (with the exception of dopamine). This makes them expensive and difficult to obtain in amounts sufficient to use therapeutically. In addition, protein increases the risk of allergic reactions. These problems make replacement therapy with target organ hormones safer and more economical. The therapeutic and adverse effects of these hormones are the same as those found with naturally existing hormones.

Anterior Pituitary Hormone Replacement Drugs

◆ corticotropin (ACTH, Acthar, HP Acthar Gel)
◆ cosyntropin (Cortrosyn); ♣ Synacthen Depot
◆ Recombinant somatrem (Protropin)
◆ Recombinant somatropin (Humatrope, Nutropin, Tev-Tropin); ♣ Nutropin AQ

Indications

Corticotropin is given diagnostically to stimulate synthesis of hormones by the adrenal cortex (i.e., glucocorticoids, mineralocorticoids, androgens) (see Chapter 56). It is not effective unless the adrenal cortex can respond. A corticotropin stimulation test is used to differentiate primary from secondary adrenocortical insufficiency. After injection of corticotropin, plasma cortisol levels rise in patients with secondary insufficiency. Corticotropin can also be used as an antiinflammatory or immunosuppressant drug when conventional glucocorticoid therapy fails, and is sometimes used to help manage adrenal crisis.

Cosyntropin is used to screen patients thought to have adrenocortical insufficiency. It may be used in an office or administered as an outpatient procedure because of its ability to stimulate a plasma cortisol response. Subnormal plasma cortisol levels may indicate hypofunction of the pituitary-adrenal axis; however, a low basal level is not as much diagnostic of adrenal insufficiency. Many patients with known adrenal insufficiency will develop signs of insufficiency only when stressed even though basal levels are normal. Further studies are needed to determine if an insufficiency is primary or secondary when found in a cosyntropin test.

Recombinant somatrem and recombinant somatropin are GH used to increase growth in children with growth failure, or those who have delayed physiologic development due to insufficient endogenous GH secretion, kidney disease, Prader-Willi syndrome (PWS), and Turner's syndrome. The drugs are ineffective when impaired growth results from other causes, or if they are used after puberty when the epiphyses of long bones have closed. These drugs are also used in adults to treat weight loss associated with acquired immunodeficiency syndrome (AIDS).

Pituitary extract was obtained from human cadavers when GH was first introduced, and therefore supplies were restricted. The extracts of GH were used to treat children with GH deficiency until 1985, when they were linked to Creutzfeldt-Jakob disease (CJD). CJD is a form of spongiform encephalopathy that is slow-developing but causes dementia and loss of muscle control. A transmissible protein particle, a prion, is the suspected cause. Since 1985, all GH in clinical use worldwide is derived from recombinant DNA technologies (rGH). The availability of rGH has ensured that all formulations currently available are free of the Creutzfeldt-Jakob prions.

Pharmacodynamics

Corticotropin is a polypeptide hormone that stimulates the adrenal cortex to the same extent as natural ACTH (maximal secretion of 17-OH corticosteroids, 17-ketosteroids, and/or 17-ketogenic steroids). It primarily boosts the synthesis of corticosteroids (primarily glucocorticoids) but also mineralocorticoids and androgens (see Chapter 57). Together with corticotropin the hormones lipotropin (whose major importance is as the precursor to beta-endorphin), melanocyte-stimulating hormone (known to control melanin pigmentation in the skin), and beta-endorphin and met-enkephalin (opioid peptides with pain-alleviating and euphoric effects) are also released. Corticotropin is also involved in the circadian rhythm in many organisms.

Recombinant somatrem and somatropin are therapeutically equivalent to endogenous GH. Specifically, somatrem and somatropin act by increasing cellular size and stimulating growth. They facilitate the transport of amino acids across cell membranes. Recombinant somatrem and somatropin also reduce the transport of glucose into cells and decrease its utilization, causing what is known as a diabetogenic effect. In addition, they facilitate the release of free fatty acids from adipose tissues, leading to increased fat storage in the liver and increased availability of fatty acids for energy. This effect is referred to as the ketogenic or lipolytic effect because it results from fat lipolysis.

Pharmacokinetics

Individual absorption rates of the anterior pituitary hormone drugs vary widely. In circulation, the drugs are extensively bound to plasma proteins, thus extending their half-lives (Table 55-2). Although the precise distribution of these drugs is unknown, it is thought that the hormones do not cross the placenta.

Adverse Effects and Contraindications

Corticotropin's adverse effects predominantly appear with chronic use of dosages exceeding 40 units/day. The most common adverse effects include depression, nausea, petechiae, hypokalemia, sodium retention, and adrenal suppression. Effects on the CNS include seizures, vertigo, headache, personality changes, and mental disturbances such as euphoria, mood swings, and psychosis. Impaired wound healing, thinning of the skin, petechiae, ecchymosis, facial erythema, increased diaphoresis, and hyperpigmentation may occur. Hypertension, heart failure, necrotizing angiitis, fluid volume overload, hypocalcemia, hypokalemia, alkalosis, and negative nitrogen balance have also occurred. Long-term use suppresses pituitary release of corticotropin, which in turn can cause adrenocortical hyperplasia, decreased glucose tolerance, suppression of growth in children, steroid myopathy, and muscle weakness. Patients who are sensitive to pork-based products may experience an allergic response from corticotropin. Corticotropin is contraindicated for use in patients with Cushing's syndrome. Because it exacerbates symptoms, it is also contraindicated for use in patients with diabetes mellitus and psychotic or psychopathic disorders. Avoid using corticotropin in patients with active tuberculosis or AIDS because it is immunosuppressive and increases the risk of gastrointestinal (GI) perforation and hemorrhage. Use it cautiously in patients with hypertension or heart failure because of sodium (Na^+) and water retention, and in patients who have myasthenia gravis because it causes muscle weakness.

The major adverse effects of corticotropin are related to its metabolic effects on GH and to the dosage amount. The most common adverse effect is fluid retention, which occurs in 5% to 18% of patients. Elevations in blood pressure are present with the fluid retention; this problem can be avoided with appropriate dosing. Other adverse effects include paresthesias, joint stiffness, peripheral edema, arthralgia, and myalgia. Carpal tunnel syndrome appears in less than 2% of adult patients treated with GH. Patients who are female, heavier, or older are more prone to these complications compared with other persons.

Somatrem and somatropin given to adults with adult-onset pituitary insufficiency are likely to cause a marked increase in high-density lipoproteins (HDL) levels, but low-density lipoprotein (LDL) values are unchanged.

Even though it has slight immunologic activity, cosyntropin is safer to use than ACTH because it does not contain

PHARMACOKINETICS
TABLE 55-2 Pituitary Drugs

Drugs	Route	Onset	Peak	Duration	PB (%)	t₁/₂	BioA (%)
ANTERIOR PITUITARY REPLACEMENT DRUGS							
cosyntropin	IM	UA	45–60 min	UA	UA	15 min	UA
	IV	Immed	UA	UA	UA	100	100
corticotropin	IM	5 min	3–12 hr	10–25 hr	UA	20 min	UA
	IV	Immed	1 hr	UA	UA	UA	100
Recombinant somatrem	SubQ, IM	3 mo	2–6 hr	12–48 hr	20–30 min	3–5 hr	UA
	IV	3 mo	2–6 hr	12–48 hr	20–30 min	20–30 min	100
Recombinant somatropin	SubQ, IM	3 mo	2–4 hr	36 hr	UA	20–25 min	UA
POSTERIOR PITUITARY REPLACEMENT DRUGS							
conivaptan	PO, IV	Rapid	1.1; 2.4 hr*	8–12 hr	98.5	3.1–7.8 hr	44
desmopressin	NS	60 min	0.9–1.5 hr	8–20 hr	UA	7.8 min; 75.5 min†	UA
vasopressin	IM, SubQ	60 min	2–4 hr	2–8 hr	UA	10–20 min	UA
vasopressin tannate in oil	IM	60 min	2–4 hr	48 hr‡	UA	UA	UA
HORMONE-SUPPRESSANT DRUGS							
bromocriptine	PO	2 hr; 1–2 hr§	8 hr; 4–8 wk§	24 hr; 4–8 hr§	93–96	4–4.5 hr; 45–50 hr‖	3–6
octreotide	SubQ	Rapid	30 min; 1 hr¶	12 hr; 3–5 days¶	41–65	1.5 hr	100

*Peak plasma concentrations of conivaptan are reached 1.11 hr following oral administration, and peak diuretic effect has been observed 2–4 hr following oral or intravenous administration.
†The half-life of desmopressin is biphasic. The initial phase is 7.8 min in duration and the terminal phase, 75.5 min.
‡The duration of action of vasopressin tannate in oil (PTO) for any given dose depends on how well the PTO is resuspended and may vary substantially.
§Effect of bromocriptine on serum prolactin levels and growth hormone levels, respectively.
‖The half-life of bromocriptine is biphasic. The initial phase is 4–4.5 hr in duration and the terminal phase, 45–50 hr.
¶Figures given are for the long-acting formulation of octreotide.
BioA, Bioavailability; *IM*, intramuscular; *IV*, intravenous; *LA*, long-acting; *NS*, nasal spray; *PB*, protein binding; *PO*, by mouth; *subQ*, subcutaneous; *t₁/₂*, half-life; *UA*, unavailable.

---

animal proteins. Most patients with a preexisting allergic disorder or a history of previous hypersensitivity to natural ACTH usually tolerate cosyntropin without incident.

Whether cosyntropin will cause fetal harm when administered during pregnancy or can affect reproduction capacity is unknown. It is also unknown whether this drug is excreted in human milk. The only contraindication to use of cosyntropin is a documented previous reaction to the drug.

Because of differences in age, body composition, and genetic predisposition, there is considerable variability in insulin sensitivity in patients taking anterior pituitary replacement hormone drugs. There is a slight risk for glucose intolerance and diabetes mellitus in patients using these drugs that may require changes in the antidiabetic drugs. Other adverse affects include hypothyroidism and slipped femoral epiphyses.

GH increases cellular protein synthesis, nitrogen retention, impaired glucose tolerance, lipid mobilization from fat stores, and increased plasma levels of fatty acids. GH also causes retention of Na⁺, K⁺, and phosphorus. **There have been concerns that GH therapy may lead to the development of malignancies or to their reoccurrence. However, no such increase has been demonstrated to date.**

GH replacement may lower serum free thyroxine (fT₄) levels as a result of increased deiodination of T₄. By reducing serum cortisol levels, GH uncovers central hypoadrenalism that was hidden by the enhanced conversion of cortisone to cortisol during the GH-deficient state. There has also been some concern about GH enhancing replication of human immunodeficiency virus (HIV).

Locally, somatrem and somatropin cause pain and swelling at the injection site. Furthermore, approximately 30% to 40% of all somatrem-treated patients and 7% to 20% of children develop antibodies to the drug. Treatment resistance is rare

and frequently can be overcome by increasing the dosage of the hormone.

Untreated hypothyroidism interferes with the growth response to GH. It is not known if the drug is eliminated in breast milk, and animal reproduction studies have not been conducted with GH drugs (pregnancy category C).

Drug Interactions

Table 55-3 lists the drug interactions of selected pituitary drugs. Enzyme-inducing drugs (e.g., barbiturates, phenytoin, and rifampin) increase the biotransformation of glucocorticoids when taken concurrently with corticotropin or cosyntropin.

Taking somatrem and somatropin concurrently with either glucocorticoids or corticotropin decreases the growth response. Anabolic steroids increase the growth response.

Dosage Regimens

In general, dosages of pituitary hormone replacement drugs are highly individualized and adjusted frequently according to patient response (Table 55-4). Although dose-response curves for recombinant somatrem and somatropin have been proposed, an optimal treatment schedule has not been established. Subcutaneous (subQ) and intramuscular (IM) routes are equally effective, although subQ injections are preferred because they are less painful. Even so, subQ administration of GH may lead to local lipoatrophy.

Lab Considerations

Corticotropin and cosyntropin have significant impact on blood glucose and plasma cortisol levels. When used to diagnose adrenal insufficiency, plasma cortisol concentrations and urine 17-ketosteroids and 17-hydroxycorticosteroids are measured

DRUG INTERACTIONS
TABLE **55-3** Selected Pituitary Drugs

Drug	Interactive Drugs	Interaction(s)
ANTERIOR PITUITARY HORMONE REPLACEMENT DRUGS		
cosyntropin	Blood or whole plasma	May inactivate cosyntropin
corticotropin	Barbiturates, phenytoin, rifampin	Increases glucocorticoid biotransformation
	Insulin, Oral hypoglycemic drugs	Increases requirements for interactive drug
	Estrogens, Oral contraceptives	Blocks biotransformation of corticotropin
	Salicylates	Increases risk for GI bleeding
	amphotericin B, furosemide, mezlocillin, piperacillin, ticarcillin	Additive hypokalemia
Recombinant somatrem and recombinant somatropin	Glucocorticoids	Inhibits growth response
POSTERIOR PITUITARY HORMONE REPLACEMENT DRUGS		
desmopressin, vasopressin	carbamazepine, chlorpropamide, clofibrate, fludrocortisone	Increases antidiuretic effects
	Alcohol, demeclocycline, heparin, lithium, norepinephrine	Decreases antidiuretic effects
	Ganglionic-blocking drugs	Increases vasopressor effects
	Barbiturates, cyclopropane	Synergistic effects
HORMONE SUPPRESSANTS		
bromocriptine	Alcohol, Antihistamines, Opioids, Sedative-hypnotics	Increases CNS depression
	levodopa	Additive neurologic effects of bromocriptine
	haloperidol, imipramine, methyldopa, reserpine, Phenothiazines, TCAs	Increases prolactin levels and decreases effectiveness of bromocriptine
	Antihypertensive drugs	Increases hypotensive effects
octreotide	cyclosporine	Reduces levels of interactive drug
	chlorpropamide, carbamazepine, Insulins, Oral hypoglycemics, glucagon, growth hormone	Alters glucose concentrations with interactive drug

CNS, Central nervous system; *GI*, gastrointestinal; *TCAs*, tricyclic antidepressants.

before and after drug administration. Therapeutic response is equated with a rise in the plasma and urine steroid concentrations. Corticotropin decreases white blood cell counts and serum potassium and calcium levels and suppresses reactions to allergy skin tests. It causes an increase in blood sugar levels, especially in patients with diabetes, and increases serum sodium, cholesterol, and lipid values. Serum protein-bound iodine and T_4 concentrations decrease.

Somatrem reduces glucose tolerance, total protein, and thyroid function test results (T_4-binding capacity and radioactive iodine uptake).

Posterior Pituitary Hormone Replacement Drugs
◆ conivaptan (Vaprisol)
◆ desmopressin acetate (DDAVP, Stimate); ◆ DDAVP
◆ vasopressin (Pitressin); ◆ Pressyn

▥ Indications
Vasopressin is used primarily to control neurogenic (i.e., central or hypothalamic) diabetes insipidus. It is not effective in treating nephrogenic diabetes insipidus, a condition in which the kidneys are unable to respond appropriately to this hormone. Vasopressin is also used in the emergency management of massive GI bleeding, to relieve postoperative flatus, and to dispel flatus before abdominal radiography. Vasopressin infusion is used for second-line management of patients in septic shock who are not responding to high dosages of inotropes (e.g., dopamine or epinephrine).

Therapeutic uses of desmopressin are the same as those of vasopressin. In addition, because of its dose-dependent increase in plasma factor VIII (antihemophilic factor), desmopressin is used to treat hemophilia A and B and von Willebrand's disease. Desmopressin is also used in the management

of unresponsive neurogenic diabetes insipidus, primary nocturnal enuresis, and the temporary polyuria and polydipsia following head trauma or surgery in the pituitary region.

Conivaptan is used to treat euvolemic hyponatremia caused by syndrome of inappropriate antidiuretic hormone secretion (SIADH), hypothyroidism, adrenal insufficiency, and pulmonary disorders in hospital patients. The safety of this drug in patients with underlying heart failure has not been determined.

▥ Pharmacodynamics
Vasopressin (V) acts at three receptors. V_{1a} causes vasoconstriction, promotes gluconeogenesis in the liver, and fosters platelet aggregation and the release of factor VIII and von Willebrand factor. V_{1b} causes corticotropin secretion from the pituitary gland. V_2 controls free water reabsorption in collecting ducts (especially the cortical and outer medullary collecting ducts). Activation of adenylate cyclase increases cyclic adenosine monophosphate (cAMP), which in turn leads to the insertion of water channels into the apical membrane of the cells lining the collecting duct. This allows water to be reabsorbed down an osmotic gradient, making the urine more concentrated. As much as 90% of the water that might otherwise be eliminated in the urine is conserved.

Direct administration of vasopressin into the superior mesenteric artery constricts the gastroduodenal, superior mesenteric, and splenic arteries, thus decreasing portal blood pressure and reducing blood loss. However, it is important to note that the dosage of vasopressin necessary to promote water conservation is seldom high enough to produce widespread pressor activity.

In large doses, desmopressin stimulates arteriolar smooth muscle contraction. The vasoconstriction, in turn, decreases blood flow to the spleen, the coronary arteries, the GI tract,

ENDOCRINE

DOSAGE
TABLE 55-4 Pituitary Drugs

Drug	Uses	Dosage	Implications
ANTERIOR PITUITARY HORMONE REPLACEMENT DRUGS			
corticotropin	ACTH replacement; treatment purposes	*Adult:* 20 units subQ or IM 4 times daily –or– 40–80 units of gel formulation every 25–72 hr	Refrigerate repository form and administer with 22-gauge needle.
	Diagnosis of ACTH deficiency	*Adult:* 10–25 units zinc formulation in 500 mL D5W by IV infusion over 8 hr –or– 20 units subQ or IM	Direct IV infusion should be given over 2 min.
cosyntropin	Diagnosis of ACTH deficiency	*Adult:* 0.25–0.75 mg subQ or IM for a single dose –or– 0.25 mg in D5W or NSS IV at 0.04 mg/hr *Child <2 yr:* 0.125 mg IM as single dose	Normal response in most patients is an approximate doubling of the basal level, provided that the basal level does not exceed the normal range. Check package insert for administration instructions.
Recombinant somatrem and somatropin	Long-term treatment GH deficiency in children	*Adult and Child:* Titrate dosages based on patient response.	**Dosages of somatrem and somatropin differ for each brand name product.**
POSTERIOR PITUITARY HORMONE REPLACEMENT DRUGS			
conivaptan	Hyponatremia secondary to SIADH or heart failure	*Adults:* 20-mg loading dose IV administered over 30 min, followed by 20 mg IV infusion over 24 hr for 1–3 days; not to exceed 4 days	If serum sodium is not rising at the desired rate, dosage may be titrated upward to 40 mg daily by continuous IV infusion.
desmopressin	Central diabetes insipidus	*Adult:* 10 mcg NS at HS –or– 2–4 mcg subQ or IV in 2 divided doses –or– 0.05 mg PO twice daily based on response. Increase by 2.5 mcg until satisfactory response. Maintenance: 10–40 mcg subQ in single or divided doses 1–3 times daily *Child:* 5 mcg NS at HS. Increase by 2.5 mcg increments. Maintenance: 2–4 mcg/kg/day (5–30 mcg) as single dose or in 2 divided doses	An oral LD$_{50}$ has not been established. Dosages are primarily based on patient response.
	GI bleeding	*Adult and Child >3 mo:* 0.3 mcg/kg repeated as needed *Adult and Child >50 kg:* 1 spray (150 mcg) in each nostril *Adult and Child >50 kg:* 1 spray (150 mcg) in one nostril	
	Primary nocturnal enuresis	*Child >6 yr:* 0.2 mg PO daily HS. Titrate dose based on patient response up to 0.6 mg/day	
vasopressin (oil formulation)	Neurogenic diabetes insipidus	*Adult:* 5–10 units subQ or IM 2–3 times daily –or– 2.5–5 units subQ or IM every 2–3 days *Child:* 2.5–10 units subQ or IM 3–4 times daily –or– 1.25–2.5 units subQ or IM every 2–3 days	**Watch for water intoxication.** In the case of toxicity, the drug should be withdrawn and the patient's fluid intake restricted until the urine specific gravity is at least 1.015.
HORMONE-SUPPRESSANT DRUGS			
bromocriptine	Hyperprolactinemia	*Adult:* 1.25–2.5 mg PO daily. Increase every 3–7 days up to 2.5 mg 2–3 times daily	Dosages for children are not yet established. Other uses may require different dosages.
	Acromegaly	*Adult:* 1.25–2.5 mg PO daily for 3 days. Increase by 1.25–2.5 mg PO every 3–7 days until optimal response obtained. Range: 10–30 mg PO daily up to 100 mg/day	
	Pituitary prolactinoma	*Adult:* 5–7.5 mg PO daily. Range 1.25–20 mg PO daily	
octreotide	Acromegaly associated with pituitary tumor	*Adult:* 100–200 mcg subQ 3 times daily –or– 20 mg of LA formulation IM every 4 wk for 3 mo. Max: 40 mg every 4 wk	LA formulation may be given only IM; preferred sites are the hip, the thigh, and the abdomen.
	VIPomas	*Adults:* 200–300 mcg IV/subQ in 2–4 divided doses	

ACTH, Adrenocorticotropic hormone; *GH,* growth hormone; *GI,* gastrointestinal; *HS,* hour of sleep (at bedtime); *IM,* intramuscular (route); *IN,* intranasal; *IV,* intravenous (route); *NSS,* normal saline solution; *PO,* by mouth; *SIADH,* syndrome of inappropriate antidiuretic hormone secretion; *subQ,* subcutaneous (route); *VIPomas,* vasoactive intestinal peptide tumors.

the pancreas, the skin, and the musculature. Also in large doses, desmopressin increases peristalsis of the large bowel and contraction of the smooth muscle of the gallbladder and the urinary bladder. Some oxytocic activity may also occur, causing uterine contractions.

Conivaptan is a non–peptide dual antagonist of arginine vasopressin (AVP) with an affinity for V_{1A} and V_2 receptors in vitro. V_2 receptors are thought to modify AVP-mediated vasoconstriction. The distribution of the V_{1a} and V_2 receptors within the renal cortex and medullary microcirculation has not been determined. The presence of AVP is critical for the regulation of water and electrolyte balance and is usually elevated in both euvolemic and hypervolemic hyponatremia.

V_2 receptors help maintain plasma osmolality within the normal range. The predominant effect of conivaptan in the treatment of hyponatremia is through its V_2 antagonism of AVP in the renal collecting ducts. The antagonism results in increased elimination of free water, which is generally accompanied by increased urine output and decreased urine osmolality.

▥ *Pharmacokinetics*
Pituitary replacement drugs are proteins that would be destroyed by enzyme activity if taken orally; therefore they are administered parenterally or by inhalation (see Table 55-2). The durations of action and half-lives vary a great deal.

ⅲ *Adverse Effects and Contraindications*

The adverse effects of vasopressin are usually mild in small dosages and most commonly include circumoral pallor, abdominal cramps, nausea, sweating, tremors, and a pounding headache. Uterine cramping and diarrhea may occur because of the oxytocic and smooth muscle–stimulant effects of vasopressin. Shifts in fluid volumes occur with initial therapy. Use caution in treating patients who may have difficulty tolerating the fluid shifts (e.g., those with heart failure).

⚠ **Vasopressin in large dosages results in blood pressure elevations, anginal pain, and arrhythmias, and possible myocardial infarction. The pressor effects are not usually evident with the amounts used to manage polyuria. However, in patients with coronary artery disease, even small doses have been found to precipitate angina, especially in the older adult.**

The adverse effects of desmopressin are usually mild and infrequent. The most common are rhinitis, local irritation of nasal passages, and heartburn. Headache, conjunctivitis, rhinorrhea, and nasal congestion have also occurred. Large doses of the intranasal and injectable formulations of desmopressin cause slight blood pressure elevations, transient headache, nausea, flushing, and mild abdominal cramps, although these are rare. Symptoms recede as the dosage is lowered.

⚠ **Use desmopressin cautiously in patients with fluid and electrolyte imbalances because of the risk of hyponatremia. The intravenous (IV) and intranasal formulations of desmopressin have been associated with anaphylaxis, but not the tablet formulation.**

Conivaptan is well tolerated with no serious adverse effects. Common adverse effects include hypotension, light-headedness, thirst, and constipation, although clinically significant changes in blood pressure and pulse have not been observed.

⚠ **Excessively rapid increase in serum sodium concentration (>12 mEq/L/24 hours) after administration of conivaptan can produce serious sequelae.** Conivaptan is contraindicated for use in patients with hypovolemic hyponatremia and in those hypersensitive to the drug or its ingredients.

ⅲ *Drug Interactions*

Several drug interactions are possible with pituitary hormone replacement drugs and their analogues. In general, antidiuretic effects may be increased or decreased by the concurrent use of alcohol, heparin, carbamazepine, or lithium (see Table 55-3). Conivaptan should not be used concurrently with potent CYP 3A4 inhibitors, such as clarithromycin, antivirals (e.g., ritonavir, indinavir), and azole antifungal drugs (e.g., ketoconazole, itraconazole).

ⅲ *Dosage Regimen*

As with many other endocrine system drugs, the dosages of vasopressin and its analogues are determined by patient response (see Table 55-4). Give vasopressin depot formulation with two large glasses of water to minimize adverse GI affects of the drug.

Desmopressin therapy is initiated in a stepwise fashion. After a nightly dose to control nocturia is established, a larger morning dose or two divided doses are used during the day. Desmopressin is administered intranasally using an insufflator, vaginally, or parenterally. Chronic intranasal use may cause tolerance, and tachyphylaxis may develop if IV

desmopressin is given more frequently than every 24 to 48 hours. IV desmopressin has 10 times the antidiuretic effect of intranasal desmopressin.

Conivaptan is only administered by continuous IV infusion. Raising the dosage titration upward to 40 mg daily may be done if the patient's serum sodium level is not increasing adequately.

ⅲ *Lab Considerations*

Throughout therapy with vasopressin, monitor patients for urine specific gravity, urine volume, and serum electrolytes. Measure plasma factor VIII concentrations and bleeding times when using vasopressin in patients with hemophilia A and B or von Willebrand's disease.

Hormone Inhibitor Drugs
◆ bromocriptine (Parlodel); ◆ Parlodel
◆ octreotide (Sandostatin); ♣ Sandostatin, Sandostatin LAR

ⅲ *Indications*

Bromocriptine is used to treat the signs and symptoms of hyperprolactinemia, including amenorrhea with or without galactorrhea, infertility, hypogonadism, and acromegaly. PRL-secreting macroadenomas may be the basic underlying endocrinopathy contributing to hyperprolactinemia. Bromocriptine reduces tumor size in both male and female patients with macroadenomas. When used alone or as an adjuvant to pituitary irradiation or surgery, bromocriptine lowers serum GH by 50% or more in approximately one half of patients treated. However, bromocriptine therapy will not typically reduce GH to normal levels.

Octreotide is the most prescribed and most studied drug for the treatment of the acromegaly associated with an excess production of GH in adults, and helps control symptoms in patients with carcinoid tumors and vasoactive intestinal peptide tumors (VIPomas), reducing the volume of secretions produced by the stomach and intestine. Carcinoid tumors are classified as benign or malignant, and can be found primarily in the appendix, the small intestine, the rectum, and the bronchus. Less frequently, the tumors can appear in the stomach, the pancreas, the colon, the liver, the ovary, the testis, and the cervix. Octreotide has also been used in the treatment of AIDS-related diarrhea, although it has not been approved by the Food and Drug Administration (FDA) for such use.

ⅲ *Pharmacodynamics*

Bromocriptine decreases PRL secretion through direct action on the pituitary gland. It is a nonhormonal, nonestrogenic, ergot derivative with potent postsynaptic dopamine receptor agonist activity. Bromocriptine significantly lowers plasma levels of PRL in patients with physiologically elevated PRL levels, as well as in patients with hyperprolactinemia. Secretion of other tropic hormones from the anterior pituitary is not disturbed by the dosages needed for the inhibition of physiologic lactation as well as galactorrhea in pathologic hyperprolactinemic states. Depending on mammary tissue stimulation before therapy, management of galactorrhea may take longer. Secretion reductions of at least 75% are usually noted after 8 to 12 weeks, but 12 months of therapy may still

ENDOCRINE

be insufficient to produce a response in some patients. Bromocriptine therapy results in a prompt and continued reduction in circulating levels of serum GH in many acromegalic patients.

Octreotide is a synthetic polypeptide that is structurally and pharmacologically related to somatostatin (growth hormone–releasing factor GHRF). Octreotide has 45 times the potency of somatostatin in inhibiting the effects of GH, glucagons, and insulin. Like somatostatin, octreotide suppresses LH response to gonadotropin-releasing hormone (GnRH), decreases splanchnic blood flow, and inhibits release of serotonin, gastrin, vasoactive intestinal peptide (VIP), secretin, motilin, and pancreatic polypeptide. Somatostatin is not used clinically owing to its short half-life (1 to 3 minutes). In the majority of patients, octreotide controls GH and insulin-like growth factor I (IGF-I) and reduces the size of tumors to help control symptoms of acromegaly.

Pharmacokinetics

Bromocriptine is partially absorbed from the GI tract, with the onset time varying depending on whether the drug is used for its effects on serum PRL levels or on GH (see Table 55-2). Over 90% of bromocriptine is bound to albumin. It is completely biotransformed in the liver by first-pass kinetics. The majority of the drug is eliminated via bile, with less than 5% eliminated in the urine. The half-life of bromocriptine is biphasic. The initial phase takes 4 to 4.5 hours, with a terminal phase of 45 to 50 hours.

Octreotide is rapidly absorbed after subQ administration, reaching peak plasma levels in 30 minutes. The half-life of octreotide is about 1.5 hours, with a duration of action of up to 12 hours. About one third of the dose is eliminated unchanged in the urine.

Adverse Effects and Contraindications

The adverse effects of bromocriptine are generally related to its activity as a dopamine agonist and are classified into two groups, those related to initial therapy and those associated with long-term use. Initial effects include nausea, vomiting, and postural hypotension. **Bromocriptine use carries a risk of first-dose phenomenon as evidenced by sudden cardiovascular collapse.** Long-term effects may include constipation, confusion, vivid dreams, delusions, hallucinations, dyskinesia, alcohol intolerance, and digital vasospasm. All adverse effects can be reduced by decreasing the dose or discontinuing the drug. When the dose of bromocriptine is increased gradually, the incidence of nausea decreases. Other adverse effects include nasal congestion, tinnitus, rash, and depression. Although rare, pleural effusions may occur with long-term therapy.

Bromocriptine use is contraindicated in patients with hepatic and renal dysfunction and in patients with hypersensitivity to the drug, to ergot alkaloids, or to bisulfites (capsules only). Do not use bromocriptine in breastfeeding mothers because it results in reduced quantities of breast milk. Use the drug cautiously in pregnancy and in patients with cardiac disease and mental disturbances. **Bromocriptine may restore fertility; thus additional contraception may be required if pregnancy is undesirable.**

There are many adverse effects with octreotide, but they are usually of short duration. GI adverse effects of octreotide are

milder than those seen with bromocriptine. Circumoral pallor, sweating, tremors, and a pounding headache may be noted.

Octreotide inhibits contraction of the gallbladder and bile secretion. Dosage reduction may be required in patients with renal failure. Hyperglycemia or hypoglycemia can occur, and the malabsorption of fats may be aggravated. The impact of bromocriptine and octreotide on pregnancy is not yet clear (category B).

Drug Interactions

Table 55-3 lists drug interactions of bromocriptine and octreotide. Drugs increasing PRL secretion (e.g., haloperidol, imipramine) reduce the effectiveness of bromocriptine. Octreotide alters the requirements for insulin or oral hypoglycemic drugs and reduces the blood levels of cyclosporine.

Dosage Regimens

The dosage of bromocriptine is adjusted every 3 to 7 days based on patient needs and response (see Table 55-4). Dosages of bromocriptine for children have not yet been established.

Octreotide depot formulation is administered by IM route immediately after mixing, usually every 4 weeks. Administration of the depot formulation at intervals longer than 4 weeks is not recommended because of a lack of information on patient tolerance and disease control. Deltoid injections are to be avoided because of significant discomfort at the injection site. **Never administer the depot octreotide by IV or subQ routes.**

Lab Considerations

Because of their impact on GH, bromocriptine and octreotide have a significant impact on plasma glucose levels. When using either drug, closely monitor the patient's plasma glucose levels.

Bromocriptine elevates the blood urea nitrogen (BUN), alanine transaminase (ALT), aspartate transaminase (AST), creatine kinase, alkaline phosphatase, and uric acid levels. The elevations are usually transient and usually clinically insignificant. Octreotide can aggravate fat malabsorption, so monitor the patients B₁₂ levels along with 72-hour fecal fat collections and serum carotene determinations.

CLINICAL REASONING

Treatment Objectives

Owing to the rarity of pituitary disorders and the rapidly advancing concepts of their management, consultation with an endocrinologist is usually indicated. However, the treatment objective overall is to bring the plasma levels of the affected hormone or hormones to within a normal range. With hormone excess, the relevant objective is to suppress the production of that hormone. With hormone deficits, the objective is to replace the deficient hormone and maintain or improve existing system functioning.

Treatment Options

In terms of hormone replacement, it is not important to differentiate whether the difficulty is coming from the hypothalamus, the pituitary, or the target organ. **It is critical to**

address any underlying neoplastic process if either neuro-surgical intervention or special drug therapy is required. Most drug therapy is used to replace or supplement naturally occurring hormones in situations involving inadequate function of the pituitary gland. Conditions resulting from excessive amounts of pituitary hormones are more often treated with surgery or radiation therapy.

▥ Patient Variables

Dosages of any pituitary hormone must be individualized because responsiveness of affected tissues varies. The benefits of treating GH deficiency manifest in the patients' body composition, bone health, cardiovascular risk factors, and quality of life. Extra caution is needed when pituitary drugs are used in children and older adults, because they may lack the ability to regulate drug activity. If drugs are used during pregnancy, monitor the mother and the fetus very closely.

Further, GH has great potential for misuse, primarily because of its real and perceived effects on body size and composition. Enhanced athletic performance is the most commonly desired result. GH is useless for stimulating linear growth in adults in light of the closure of epiphyseal plates. Yet adult athletes often seek GH to increase muscle mass and decrease body fat in a manner that is undetectable by current drug testing programs.

LIFE-SPAN CONSIDERATIONS

Pregnant and Nursing Women. Because of the lack of controlled human studies, the risks associated with pituitary hormone replacement or suppression during pregnancy and lactation is not well established. However, the risks and benefits for the use of a particular drug should be evaluated on individual basis.

A threefold increase in circulating levels of endogenous vasopressin has been reported during the last trimester of pregnancy and in labor compared with the nonpregnant state. Uterine contractions have been reported after administration of vasopressin, although tonic uterine contractions that may be harmful to the fetus or threaten a pregnancy are infrequent. Vasopressin is classified as a category C drug; use it during pregnancy only when the need is clearly indicated.

Bromocriptine use is usually stopped as soon as a pregnancy is diagnosed in patients who are receiving treatment for infertility because of the risk of hyperprolactinemia or pituitary tumors.

Children and Adolescents. Vasopressin deficiency may occur at any age including during infancy and childhood. Nephrogenic diabetes insipidus usually manifests in infancy. The use of pituitary drugs in children over 6 months of age has been fairly safe; however, because of the immaturity of the negative feedback mechanisms in children, plasma levels of exogenous pituitary hormones may be difficult to regulate. Caution is needed in evaluating the effectiveness of any of the pituitary drugs, because children are more susceptible to fluid volume disturbances than adults.

Older Adults. Owing to the age-related decline of hepatic and renal functioning, older adults are at higher risk for drug overdose and therefore should have routine monitoring of liver and kidney functioning.

Older adults are at increased risk for GH-related adverse effects. GH secretion normally decreases with age, as do GH

dosage requirements. Conversely, higher dosages may better suit young adults. In general, women undergoing oral estrogen replacement therapy require considerably higher doses of GH; women taking transdermal estrogen preparations may not need higher dosing.

▥ Drug Variables

Because of the limited choice of drugs available for treating pituitary disorders, it is difficult to establish criteria for selecting one drug over another. Even when more than one drug is available to treat the same disorder, they are likely to have comparable pharmacokinetics and pharmacodynamics.

DWARFISM. The dosing recommendations for GH have shifted to personalized dose-titration strategies from dosing based on weight. Adverse effects of GH are less than half as frequent when a dosage titration method is used (rather than using weight-based methods). Start with low doses and titrate upward based on the patient's response, adverse effects, and IGF-I (insulin-like growth factor) levels while considering age, sex, and estrogen status. During titration, monitor patients at 1- to 2-month intervals, and semiannually thereafter. It may take 6 months before clinical benefits become evident.

DIABETES INSIPIDUS. Neurogenic diabetes insipidus (i.e., vasopressin deficit) is treated most often with intranasal desmopressin given twice daily in dosages necessary to control polyuria or polydipsia. Drugs used in the treatment of central diabetes insipidus include chlorpropamide, an antidiabetic drug that reduces polyuria and polydipsia (see Chapter 53), and hydrochlorothiazide, a thiazide diuretic (see Chapter 42), although these drugs are not as predictable as desmopressin.

Nephrogenic diabetes insipidus (insensitivity to vasopressin) is treated with thiazide diuretics combined with amiloride, a K^+-sparing diuretic (see Chapter 42). Nephrogenic diabetes insipidus usually has an inherited (sex-linked recessive) origin. It is expressed primarily in males and is rare in females. Two gene defects involving response elements to arginine vasopressin have been identified.

The dosage of desmopressin is adjusted according to the patient's diurnal pattern of response. Response is measured by the parameters of adequate duration of sleep and adequate, not excessive, water turnover. For patients previously on intranasal desmopressin, begin tablet therapy 12 hours after the last intranasal dose. To ensure an adequate response, measure safety parameters and watch patients carefully during the initial dose titration period. Monitor patients at regular intervals throughout the course of desmopressin therapy to confirm adequate antidiuretic response. Adjust individual doses separately for adequate diurnal rhythm of water turnover. Increase or decrease total daily dosage as needed to obtain adequate antidiuresis.

PRIMARY NOCTURNAL ENURESIS. Patients previously using intranasal desmopressin therapy may start using tablet formulations; begin tablet therapy 24 hours after the last intranasal dose. The recommended initial dosage for patients 6 years of age and older is 0.2 mg at bedtime. The dosage is titrated to achieve the desired response.

SIADH. Hyponatremia characterizes SIADH. The disparity between water and Na^+ is the result of one of three conditions: (1) hypovolemic hyponatremia, in which water and Na^+ both leave the body, but more Na^+ is lost than water; (2) hypervolemic hyponatremia, in which the levels of both Na⁺ and water in the body rise, but the water gain is greater; or (3) euvolemic hyponatremia, in which the body's water content increases while Na⁺ levels remain stable.

Patient Education

Proper planning is important for the patient receiving hormonal therapy, and the amount of teaching varies according to the patient's diagnoses and the treatment plan. For example, for a child, make sure the family has a responsible caregiver who will ensure adherence with the treatment plan. Teach the caregiver and the patient how to administer injections. In addition, advise the patient and caregivers how and where to obtain the drugs and the supplies needed for injections. It is important to teach what to realistically expect from the treatment and what changes should be reported. Stress the necessity of routine monitoring of drug and hormone levels. Advise the patient to wear or carry medical alert identification, and to avoid use of over-the-counter (OTC) drugs without first consulting with the health care provider.

Evaluation

Evaluation of treatment outcomes is important and can be accomplished a number of different ways. If the goal is to bring the hormone level to the normal range, then routine monitoring of the plasma drug level of the hormone is sufficient. However, if the objective of treatment is to produce a change in organ function, then specific organ monitoring is needed. For example, if desmopressin is used for the treatment of diabetes insipidus, close monitoring of urine osmolarity and volume are vital (see Case Study). Finally, because of how the endocrine system is integrated, it is important to evaluate the functioning of the other endocrine glands, for example, by monitoring blood glucose levels.

A patient's clinical response to GH can be evaluated by the child's attainment of adult height. Monitor the patient for development of neutralizing antibodies if the growth rate does not exceed 2.5 cm in 6 months. A therapeutic response to GH is determined by the patient receiving an adequate amount of sleep, and adequate, but not excessive, intake and output of body water.

With vasopressin and its analogues, the effectiveness of treatment is evaluated by observing for decreased urinary output, increased urine specific gravity, decreased signs of dehydration, and decreased thirst. Do, however, monitor for evidence of water intoxication (e.g., drowsiness, listlessness, and headache).

To judge the effectiveness of treatment for hyperprolactinemia, measure serum PRL concentrations on a monthly basis during initial therapy and twice yearly thereafter. Periodically monitor serum GH levels and IGF-I concentrations. The effectiveness of therapy is demonstrated by a decrease in galactorrhea within 6 to 8 weeks, and decreased serum levels of GH in patients with acromegaly.

The effectiveness of treatment with octreotide is demonstrated by the relief of symptoms and suppressed tumor growth in patients with pituitary tumors associated with acromegaly.

CASE STUDY   Pituitary Drugs

ASSESSMENT

History of Present Illness	JS is a 53-year-old white male who came to be seen at the outpatient clinic today with complaints of increased thirst (particularly for ice-cold water) for the past 2 to 3 weeks, and increased urination that keeps him up at night. He adds that epigastric fullness and anorexia is a problem. States he has had an unintentional weight loss of 15 pounds over the last 2 to 3 weeks.
Past Health History	Positive for broken nose with obstructed right nares. He denies a history of brain tumor, head trauma, TIA, stroke, or granulomatous disease. He has no known drug or food allergies and denies use of prescription or over-the-counter drugs. JS states he has frequent, severe episodes of allergic rhinitis secondary to hay fever.
Life-Span Considerations	JS is a high-school teacher. He is married and has three grown children. He is planning to retire within the next 10 years and is concerned that his diagnosis will prevent the couple from traveling in Europe. JS has no significant age-related changes in hepatic, renal, or cardiac functioning. JS is covered by a private health insurance that includes pharmacy coverage with a $10 copay.
Physical Exam Findings	JS appears mildly dehydrated and restless. Skin warm and dry with poor skin turgor. *BP:* 104/62, 98.8° F-76-20.
Diagnostic Testing	Urine specific gravity, 1.001 with an osmolality of 175 mOsm/kg. Total 24-hour urinary output is, 10.4 L. Serum sodium is 129 mEq/L. Serum osmolality is 350 mOsm/kg. BUN: 20 mg/dL. Creatinine: 1.5 mg/dL. MRI of brain is unremarkable.

DIAGNOSIS: Diabetes Insipidus

MANAGEMENT

Treatment Objective	1. Restore renal function. 2. Prevent dehydration and hyponatremia.
Treatment Plan	**Pharmacotherapy** • desmopressin 0.05 mg PO twice daily. Increase by 2.5 mcg based on response. **Patient Education** 1. Meaning of the disease, sign and symptoms, drug therapy 2. Take fluids as directed by thirst with no water restriction (in most cases, but not all). 3. Avoid situations where a marked increase in water loss is possible (e.g., sports). 4. Stress importance of having access to fluids as thirst dictates. 5. Wear a medical identification neck tag or bracelet. 6. Follow-up in office every 2 to 3 weeks initially; every 3 to 4 months thereafter. 7. Treatment adjustments will be needed based on the urine and electrolyte concentrations and patient symptoms. **Evaluation** JS's renal function was restored, dehydration prevented, and a normal serum sodium level achieved.

CLINICAL REASONING ANALYSIS

Q1. We learned that drug therapy is the only treatment for diabetes insipidus. How do you know which of the drugs to use?

A. Vasopressin and desmopressin both mimic the action of ADH. Desmopressin is preferred over vasopressin because it requires fewer doses per day; however, this benefit may be offset by the cost of the drug. Vasopressin tannate in oil is dosed even less frequently than vasopressin, but it necessitates an injection every 2 to 3 days. The tablets will be the simplest to use.

Q2. Wouldn't the intranasal form of desmopressin be a better choice for him than the tablets?

A. JS has frequent, severe episodes of rhinitis; therefore intranasal routes of drug administration should be avoided. The desmopressin tablets have been found to be efficacious in treating his diabetes insipidus.

Q3. What do we look for to know if the desmopressin is working?

A. We would look for his renal function to be restored, dehydration prevented, and a normal serum sodium level achieved over the next couple of months. He will need to keep regular appointments so that we can watch for these positive outcomes.

KEY POINTS

- The anterior pituitary secretes polypeptide hormones (i.e., GH, ACTH, PRL) and glycoprotein hormones (i.e., LH, FSH, TSH).
- The posterior pituitary is responsible for storing and releasing vasopressin (ADH) and oxytocin, which are produced by the hypothalamus.
- Pituitary disorders are characterized as those with hypersecretion of hormones and those with deficient hormone production.
- Excessive pituitary hormones exert their effects on the target organs, causing hyperactivity of those organs. Hormone excess is associated with manifestations such as acromegaly, and galactorrhea or amenorrhea.
- Hormone deficits are associated with disorders such as diabetes insipidus and dwarfism.
- For patients with hormone excess, the goal is to suppress the production of the hormone and keep plasma levels within normal limits.
- For patients with hormone deficiency, the goal is to replace the hormone using an exogenous synthetic form of the hormone.

- Pituitary hormone replacement drugs include corticotropin and cosyntropin (ACTH preparations), somatrem and somatropin (GH preparations), and desmopressin and vasopressin (ADH preparations).
- Conivaptan is indicated for the treatment of euvolemic hyponatremia in hospitalized patients.
- Recombinant somatrem and recombinant somatropin increase growth and metabolic activity in children who lack sufficient GH.
- Vasopressin and its analogue desmopressin reduce urine formation, thus conserving water. Vasopressin is also a potent vasoconstrictor that is used in the management of GI bleeding.
- Pituitary hormone–suppressant drugs include bromocriptine and octreotide and are used to manage hypersecretion of anterior pituitary hormones.
- Drug effectiveness is evaluated by monitoring patient response and plasma levels of hormones.

ENDOCRINE

Bibliography

Adrogue, H., and Madias, N. (2000). Hyponatremia. *New England Journal of Medicine*, *342*(21), 1581–1589.

Ali, F., Guglin, M., Vaitkevicius, P., et al. (2007). Therapeutic potential of vasopressin receptor antagonists. *Drugs*, *67*(6), 847–858.

Arnaldi, G., Polenta, B., Cardinaletti, M., et al. (2005). Potential indications for somatostatin analogs in Cushing 's syndrome. *Journal of Endocrinological Investigation*, *28*(11 Suppl), 106–110.

Barton, J., Gardineri, H., and Cullen, S. (1995). The growth and cardiovascular effects of high dose growth hormone therapy in idiopathic short stature. *Clinical Endocrinology*, *42*(6), 619–626.

Caldwell, H., and Young, W. (2006). Oxytocin and vasopressin: Genetics and behavioral implications in Lim, R. (Ed.). *Handbook of neurochemistry and molecular neurobiology* (3rd ed.). New York: Springer.

Freda, P., Katznelson, L., vander Lely, A., et al. (2005). Long-acting somatostatin analog therapy of acromegaly: A meta-analysis. *Journal of Clinical Endocrinology and Metabolism*, *90*(8), 4465–4473.

Greenberg, A., and Verbalis, J. (2006). Vasopressin receptor antagonists. *Kidney International*, *69*(12), 2124–2130.

Hoffman, A., Strasburger, C., Zagar, A., et al. (2004). T002 Study Group. Efficacy and tolerability of an individualized dosing regimen for adult growth hormone replacement therapy in comparison with fixed body weight-based dosing. *Journal of Clinical Endocrinology and Metabolism*, *89*(7), 3224–3233.

Johannsson, G., Rosen, T., and Bengtsson, B. (2007). Individualized dose titration of growth hormone (GH) during GH replacement in hypopituitary adults. *Clinical Endocrinology*, *47*(5), 571–581.

Kanaka-Gantenbein, C. (2006). Hormone replacement treatment in Turner syndrome. *Pediatric Endocrinology*, *3*(Suppl 1), 214–218.

Kano, K., and Arisaka, O. (2006). Efficacy and safety of nasal desmopressin in the long-term treatment of primary nocturnal enuresis. *Pediatric Nephrology*, *21*(8), 1211.

Lindholm, J. (2006). Growth hormone: Historical notes. *Pituitary*, *9*(1), 5–10.

Motlich, M., Clemmons, D., Malozowski, S., et al. (2006). Evaluation and treatment of adult growth hormone deficiency: An Endocrine Society Clinical Practice Guideline. *Journal of Clinical Endocrinology and Metabolism*, *91*(5), 1621–1634.

Newell-Price, J., Bertagna, X., Grossman, A., et al. (2006). Cushing's syndrome. *Lancet*, *367*(9522), 1605–1607.

Oshino, S., Saitoh, Y., Kasayama, S., et al. (2006). Short-term preoperative octreotide treatment of GH-secreting pituitary adenoma: Predictors of tumor shrinkage. *Endocrine Journal*, *53*(1), 125–132.

Petersenn, S. (2005). Efficacy and limits of somatostatin analogs. *Journal of Endocrinological Investigation*, *28*(11 Suppl), 53–57.

Steiner, I., Kaehler, S., Sauermann, R., et al. (2006). Plasma pharmacokinetics of desmopressin following sublingual administration: An exploratory dose-escalation study in healthy male volunteers. *International Journal of Clinical Pharmacology and Therapeutics*, *44*(4), 172–179.

Van Dam, D. (2006). Somatropin therapy and cognitive function in adults with growth hormone deficiency: A critical review. *Treatments in Endocrinology*, *5*(3), 159–170.

Wyatt, D. (2004). Lessons from the national cooperative growth study. *European Journal of Endocrinology*, *151*(Suppl 1), S55–S59.

56

Adrenal Cortex Agonists and Inhibitors

The adrenal cortex generates the body's steroid hormones. In the adrenal cortex, which constitutes 80% of the total weight of the gland, three zones are responsible for *corticosteroid* synthesis. The outmost layer synthesizes *aldosterone*, which is the predominant *mineralcorticoid* responsible for sodium (Na^+) retention and potassium (K^+) excretion. The middle and inner layers produce *glucocorticoids* (primarily cortisol) and the androgenic steroids and their precursor, dehydroepiandrosterone (DHEA). Androgenic steroids are discussed in Chapter 57. *Cortisol* functions to promote protein and lipid catabolism and gluconeogenesis. Catecholamines such as norepinephrine are synthesized in the adrenal medulla, and are regulated via the autonomic nervous system.

All corticosteroids, which are found in large quantities in the adrenal cortex, are derived from cholesterol through a series of transformations mediated by enzymes. Cortisol is subject to the negative feedback regulation via *adrenocorticotropic hormone (ACTH, corticotropin)* and the *hypothalamic-pituitary-adrenal (HPA) axis* (Fig. 56-1). The majority of cortisol (i.e., 15 to 25 mg) is produced between 5 AM and 9 AM. Metabolic stressors such as myocardial infarction or sepsis can raise production levels to 250 mg/day.

Aldosterone is regulated by the renin-angiotensin feedback loop, through which low renal perfusion pressure stimulates increased production of aldosterone. Aldosterone secretion and the HPA axis affect extracellular K^+ levels, regulating about 15% of aldosterone production via ACTH stimulation.

Hyposecretion of adrenal hormones occurs either because of direct damage to the adrenal cortex (primary adrenal insufficiency) or because a pathologic process has impinged on the production or the secretion of adrenal cortex hormones (secondary adrenal insufficiency). In either case, secretion of adrenal hormones is insufficient (chronically or acutely) to support normal body functions.

ADRENAL INSUFFICIENCY

EPIDEMIOLOGY AND ETIOLOGY

Adrenocortical hypofunction is a rare condition affecting only 4 in 100,000 people. It can develop at any age, usually during the third to the fifth decade and to women slightly more often than men, and may be a temporary or permanent problem. The body's own immune system is most often responsible for the gradual destruction of the adrenal cortex. Autoimmune adrenal insufficiency shows some hereditary disposition. Familial glucocorticoid insufficiency may have a recessive pattern; adrenomyeloneuropathy is X-linked.

PATHOPHYSIOLOGY

Cortisol is needed for the maintenance of vascular tone and cardiovascular output based on its inotropic effects; thus hypotension may be present in either the primary or the secondary form. Hypoglycemia occurs because of the loss of the permissive effects of cortisol on glycogenolysis and gluconeogenesis. Elevated serum calcium (Ca^{++}) levels, hypercalcemia, occurs because of the loss of cortisol inhibition of intestinal absorption and renal reabsorption of Ca^{++} Hyponatremia can occur as a result of the Na^+-retentive properties of aldosterone. In both primary and secondary adrenal insufficiency the clinical manifestations are related to loss of cortisol, a hormone essential for survival. Adrenal insufficiency comes about when at least 90% of the adrenal cortex is destroyed. Cortisol levels less than 5 mcg/dL at 8 AM are diagnostic of adrenal insufficiency.

Primary Adrenal Insufficiency
In the United States, most cases of primary adrenal insufficiency (i.e., Addison's disease) are due to an autoimmune destruction of the adrenal cortex, with consequent loss of all corticosteroid hormone production. Although rare, there are other causes of adrenal gland destruction including tuberculosis (about 20% of cases), chronic infections, and invasion of the adrenal glands by cancer cells, amyloidosis (protein deposits), adrenoleukodystrophy, anticoagulants, and surgical removal of both adrenal glands.

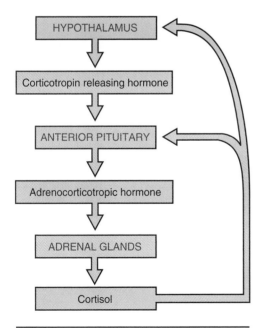

FIGURE 56-1 The hypothalamic-pituitary-adrenal axis shows that cortisol production is dependent on an intact hypothalamus, pituitary gland, and adrenal gland. It operates as a negative feedback system.

Acute adrenal crisis precipitated by infection, trauma, surgery, emotional turmoil, or other stress factors may be the initial presentation of adrenocortical hypofunction in as many as 25% of cases.

Hyperpigmentation is only seen in primary adrenal insufficiency and is due to increased secretion of β-lipotropin, a component of the precursor peptide that also contains ACTH.

Secondary Adrenal Insufficiency

Adrenal insufficiency may also be secondary to the result of diminished ACTH production by the pituitary gland. In the secondary form, only glucocorticoid and androgen production are affected, with mineralocorticoid production remaining largely intact. This is because ACTH plays only a small role in aldosterone regulation. Angiotensin II and potassium are the primary factors affecting aldosterone production, and the renin-angiotensin II–aldosterone system (RAAS) is independent of regulation by the pituitary gland.

Hyponatremia occurs despite normal aldosterone levels as a result of decreased cortisol-mediated renal free water clearance and compensatory elevations in antidiuretic hormone (ADH).

⚠ **The loss of aldosterone can result in potentially life-threatening hyperkalemia. Increased sodium elimination in the absence of aldosterone results in an overwhelming volume depletion.**

Secondary adrenal insufficiency can be related to panhypopituitarism, isolated ACTH loss, or exogenous glucocorticoid suppression of the HPA axis. Hypothalamic or pituitary tumors, postpartum necrosis of the pituitary gland (Sheehan's syndrome), high-dose radiation therapy of the pituitary or other intracranial lesions, and hypophysectomy are all contributing causes.

In addition to pathologic hyposecretion of hypothalamic or pituitary hormones, glucocorticoids, when administered in supraphysiologic levels, cause a suppression of the HPA axis via the negative feedback system.

hormones is insufficient to sustain life. In these cases, glucocorticoids are administered systemically at dosages calibrated to mimic normal physiologic activity (Box 56-1). This approach is called *replacement therapy*. Topical corticosteroid drugs used for ophthalmic, otic, and dermatologic disorders are discussed in Chapters 61, 62 and 63, respectively.

▌▌ *Pharmacodynamics*

Cortisone, the precursor to cortisol, is secreted in minute quantities and by itself has little physiologic activity. Cortisone is converted to its active form by hydroxylation of the 11-keto-group by the enzyme 11-beta-steroid dehydrogenase. Cortisol is thus sometimes referred to as hydrocortisone. Cortisol accounts for 95% of glucocorticoid activity as a group, with about 15 to 25 mg secreted daily.

Endogenous glucocorticoids are cyclically secreted, with the largest amount produced in the morning and lesser amounts during the evening hours (i.e., in people on a normal day-night schedule). Whether of endogenous or exogenous origin, glucocorticoids affect carbohydrate, protein, and fat metabolism. They also exert effects on inflammatory and immune responses; on the nervous, musculoskeletal, respiratory, and gastrointestinal systems; and on fluid and electrolyte balance.

It is important to distinguish between the physiologic effects of glucocorticoids and their pharmacologic effects. Physiologic effects occur at low levels (i.e., the levels produced by the release of glucocorticoids from healthy adrenals, or by the administration of low-dose exogenous glucocorticoids). Pharmacologic effects occur at supraphysiologic doses. These effects are achieved when glucocorticoids are required to treat disorders unrelated to adrenocortical function (e.g., allergic reactions, asthma, inflammation).

PHARMACOTHERAPEUTIC OPTIONS

Glucocorticoids

Short-Acting Glucocorticoids
- cortisone (Cortone); ◆ hydrocortisone, Cortate
- hydrocortisone (Cortef, Hydrocortone); ◆ hydrocortisone, Cortef, Emo-Cort, Hycort

Intermediate-Acting Glucocorticoids
- methylprednisolone (Depo-Medrol, Medrol, Solu-Medrol); ◆ methylprednisolone, Depo-Medrol, Medrol
- prednisolone (Delta-Cortef, Duepred, Hydeltra)
- prednisone (Deltasone, Meticorten); ◆ prednisone
- triamcinolone (Aristocort, Kenacort, Kenalog); ◆ Kenalog

Long-Acting Glucocorticoids
- dexamethasone (Decadron, Dexamethasone, Dexasone); ◆ dexamethasone, Dexasone
- betamethasone (Alphatrex, Betatrex, Beta-Val Celestone); ◆ Betnesol, Celestone SoluSpan

▌▌ *Indications*

Glucocorticoids are indicated in the treatment of adrenal insufficiency when the amount of naturally occurring adrenal

---

BOX 56-1

Indications for Adrenal Glucocorticoids

- Acute spinal cord injury
- Acute gouty arthritis
- Adrenal insufficiency, primary and secondary
- Allergic conjunctivitis
- Allergic reactions to foods, drugs, contact dermatitis
- Allergic rhinitis
- Ankylosing spondylitis
- Arthritis—degenerative
- Asthma
- Aspiration pneumonia
- Bursitis
- Carcinoma
- Cerebral edema
- Giant cell arteritis
- Hemolytic anemia
- Idiopathic thrombocytopenic purpura
- Inflammatory bowel disease
- Leukemia

- Multiple myeloma
- Myasthenia gravis
- Neoplastic conditions
- Nephrotic syndrome
- Optic neuritis
- Organ transplant
- Polymyalgia rheumatica
- Regional enteritis
- Rheumatoid arthritis
- Sarcoidosis
- Septic shock
- Systemic lupus erythematosus
- Severe erythema multiforme
- Severe seborrheic, contact, and atopic dermatitis
- Severe psoriasis
- Synovitis
- Tendinitis
- Thyroiditis
- Ulcerative colitis
- Uveitis

EFFECTS ON NUTRIENT METABOLISM. Glucocorticoids stimulate the formation of glucose (*gluconeogenesis*) by causing the breakdown of protein to amino acids. The amino acids are transported to the liver and converted to glucose through enzymatic action. The glucose is returned to the circulation for use by body tissues, or is stored in the liver as glycogen. There is a moderate decrease in the cell's use of glucose by an unknown mechanism (antiinsulin effects). In addition, there is increased production but decreased use of glucose. Higher glucose levels thus promote a diabetic-like state. These actions also increase the amount of glucose stored as glycogen in the liver, the skeletal muscles, and other tissues.

The effects of glucocorticoids on protein metabolism include an increased breakdown of protein to amino acids. The rate at which amino acids are transported to the liver and converted to glucose is increased. There is also a decrease in the rate at which new proteins are formed (antianabolic effects) from dietary and other amino acids. The combination of increased breakdown of cell protein and decreased protein synthesis produces protein depletion in almost all body cells except those of the liver. Thus glycogen stores are increased, whereas protein stores are decreased.

Fatty acids are mobilized from adipose tissue, resulting in increased fatty acid concentration in the plasma. The oxidation of fatty acids within body cells is also stimulated.

ANTIINFLAMMATORY AND IMMUNE EFFECTS. Glucocorticoids act to interrupt inflammatory and immune responses. Glucocorticoids inhibit the synthesis of prostaglandins, leukotrienes, and histamine, thereby reducing swelling, warmth, redness, and pain. In addition, glucocorticoids suppress the infiltration of phagocytes and avert damage from the release of lysosomal enzymes. Lastly, glucocorticoids suppress proliferation of lymphocytes, reducing the immune component of inflammation. A decrease in the number of eosinophils and lymphocytes as well as a decreased production of antibodies results in immunosuppressive effects.

Note, however, that the mechanisms by which glucocorticoids suppress inflammation are broader in scope than those of nonsteroidal antiinflammatory drugs (NSAIDs; see Chapter 17). The antiinflammatory effects of glucocorticoids are also related to the synthesis of specific regulatory proteins. Glucocorticoids penetrate cell membranes to bind to intracellular receptors. The receptor-steroid complex binds to chromatin in the DNA of the cell's nucleus. The interaction with chromatin triggers the transcription of messenger RNA molecules that, in turn, code for regulatory proteins, thereby increasing the synthesis of such proteins.

Normally, physiologic doses of glucocorticoids probably do not significantly affect inflammation and healing; however, large amounts inhibit all stages of the inflammatory and immune responses.

⚠ **Caution is necessary when using glucocorticoids for long-term therapy because of the risk of adrenal suppression. Glucocorticoids are used with caution in patients who have diabetes mellitus or peptic ulcers, and for those with immunosuppression from cancer, kidney disease, or human immunodeficiency virus (HIV).**

CENTRAL NERVOUS SYSTEM EFFECTS. Physiologic levels of glucocorticoids help maintain normal nerve excitability. Pharmacologic amounts decrease nerve excitability, slow activity in the cerebral cortex, and alter brain wave patterns. Secretion of corticotropin-releasing hormone (CRH) by the hypothalamus and of corticotropin by the anterior pituitary gland is decreased. There is further suppression of glucocorticoid secretion by the adrenal cortex.

MUSCULOSKELETAL EFFECTS. Muscle strength is maintained when glucocorticoids are present in physiologic amounts. Muscle atrophy (from protein breakdown) occurs when glucocorticoids are used in supraphysiologic doses. In addition, they inhibit bone formation and growth, increase bone breakdown, decrease intestinal absorption of calcium, and increase the renal excretion of calcium. These actions contribute to bone demineralization (osteopenia and osteoporosis) in adults and to a decrease in linear growth in children.

RESPIRATORY SYSTEM EFFECTS. Although glucocorticoids have no bronchodilating action, it is thought that they play a role in maintaining the bronchodilating responsiveness to endogenous catecholamines (e.g., epinephrine). Glucocorticoids stabilize mast cells as well as other cells to inhibit the release of bronchoconstrictive and inflammatory chemicals (e.g., histamine).

GASTROINTESTINAL SYSTEM EFFECTS. Glucocorticoids decrease the viscosity of gastric mucus. The decreased protective properties of the mucus are thought by some to contribute to the development of peptic ulcer disease.

FLUID AND ELECTROLYTE EFFECTS. Glucocorticoids cause the retention of Na^+ and therefore water, and increase the excretion of Ca^{++} and K^+.

STRESS PROTECTION. Glucocorticoids have a permissive effect on the action of catecholamines, thereby supporting blood pressure during times of stress. Working together, the catecholamines and glucocorticoids maintain blood pressure and plasma glucose content. If corticosteroid levels are insufficient, as they are in adrenal insufficiency, circulatory collapse and death can follow.

▦ Pharmacokinetics

The absorption of glucocorticoids depends on the route of administration and the specific drug. Glucocorticoid formulations are classified as short-acting, intermediate-acting, and long-acting according to their therapeutic effects (Table 56-1). The duration of action of glucocorticoids is a function of dosage, route of administration, and solubility. Approximately 75% of the cortisol in circulation is bound to plasma proteins and transcortin. Transcortin, a corticosteroid binding protein, is an α-globulin with high affinity for binding cortisol. Cortisol is biologically active only when it is not bound to transcortin.

For glucocorticoids administered orally or intravenously, the duration of action is determined largely by the biologic half-life. With intramuscular (IM) administration, the duration of action is a function of water-solubility. Highly soluble formulations have a shorter duration of action than that of less soluble formulations. For locally administered glucocorticoids, the duration of action is a function of solubility as well as of the specific site of administration.

Glucocorticoids are biotransformed by CYP450 enzymes in the liver. Prednisone and cortisone require hepatic conversion to prednisolone or cortisol, respectively, to achieve glucocorticoid effects. The durations of action of the various methylprednisolone drugs vary considerably from one drug to the other.

PHARMACOKINETICS

TABLE 56-1 Adrenal Cortex Agonists and Inhibitors

Drug	Route	Onset	Peak	Duration	PB (%)	$t_{1/2}$	BioA (%)
SHORT-ACTING CORTICOSTEROIDS							
cortisone	PO	Rapid	2 hr	30–36 hr	High	30 min	UA
	IM	Slow	20–48 hr	30–36 hr	High	30 min	100
hydrocortisone	PO	UA	1 hr	30–36 hr	High	1.5–2 hr	UA
	IM	Rapid	4–8 hr	1.2–1.5 days	High	1.5–2 hr	100
	IV	Rapid	1 hr	1.2–1.5 days	High	30 min	100
INTERMEDIATE-ACTING CORTICOSTEROIDS							
methylprednisolone	PO	UA	1–2 hr	1.2–1.5 days	High	>3.5 hr	UA
	IM	Rapid	4–8 days	1–4 wk	High	UA	100
prednisolone	PO	1 hr	1–2 hr	UA	UA	1 hr	70
	IV	Rapid	1 hr	UA	UA	2.1–3.8 hr	100
prednisone	PO	UA	1–2 hr	UA	Very high	18–36 hr	UA
triamcinolone	PO	UA	1–2 hr	2.25 days	High	2–5 hr	UA
LONG-ACTING CORTICOSTEROIDS							
dexamethasone	PO	UA	1–2 hr	66 hr	High	36–54 hr	UA
	IM	UA	8 hr	6 days	High	3–4.5 hr	100
betamethasone	PO	UA	1–2 hr	3.25 days	High	3–5 hr	UA
	IM	1–3 hr	UA	7 days	High	3–5 hr	100
MINERALOCORTICOID							
fludrocortisone	PO	10–20 min	1.7 hr	1–2 days	High	3.5 hr*	42
ADRENAL HORMONE INHIBITORS†							
aminoglutethimide	PO	3–5 days	1.5 hr	1.5–3 days	20–25	11–16 hr; 5–9 days‡	>95
metyrapone	PO	24 hr	1 hr	4 hr	UA	1–2.5 hr	UA
mitotane	PO	2–3 days	3–5 hr	UA	UA	0.14 hr	40

*Fludrocortisone remains therapeutically active for 24 to 48 hours.
†Time of onset of adrenal suppression with adrenal hormone inhibitors (e.g., corticosteroid excretion in urine).
‡During aminoglutethimide therapy, the half-life increases with prolonged therapy (1 yr of therapy). Initial $t_{1/2}$ of aminoglutethimide is biphasic: the first phase lasts 11–16 hr; the second phase lasts 5 to 9 days.
BioA, Bioavailability; IM, intramuscular; IV, intravenous; PB, protein binding; PO, by mouth; $t_{1/2}$, half-life; UA, unavailable.

Further biotransformation by the liver conjugates the glucocorticoids with glucuronic acid to permit excretion by the kidneys.

Adverse Effects and Contraindications

Glucocorticoids are naturally occurring substances, and at normal physiologic levels, they have no adverse effects or contraindications. Adverse effects occur when the dosage is greater than the body's requirements for the hormones (Box 56-2).

No contraindications exist when glucocorticoids are given for replacement therapy in adrenal insufficiency. However, their use is contraindicated in patients with systemic fungal infections and in those who are hypersensitive to the drug formulations. In patients with existing infections, or those who are at risk for infections because of immunosuppression, glucocorticoids may mask the signs and symptoms so that infections become more severe before being recognized and treated. Also exercise caution in patients with diabetes mellitus, peptic ulcer disease, inflammatory bowel disorders, hypertension, heart failure, and renal insufficiency. **Do not abruptly discontinue glucocorticoid therapy in any patient because of the possibility of causing HPA axis suppression. Do not give glucocorticoids to patients with Cushing's syndrome.**

Glucocorticoids cross into breast milk. Exogenous formulations ingested by the infant from breast milk suppress the HPA axis. Therefore, mothers whose corticosteroid levels exceed the normal are advised not to breastfeed their infants.

Drug Interactions

Various drug interactions are possible between glucocorticoids and other drugs (Table 56-2), especially when the dosage exceeds the physiologic norm. Drugs that induce CYP450 enzymes (e.g., barbiturates, phenytoin, rifampin, and other glucocorticoids) increase adrenal hormone biotransformation and may necessitate increased dosages of glucocorticoids. Conversely, drugs inhibiting CYP450 enzymes (e.g., erythromycin and oral contraceptives) decrease biotransformation, and may necessitate reduced dosage of the corticosteroid to achieve desired effects. NSAIDs and glucocorticoids taken concurrently increase the risk of gastrointestinal (GI) ulceration. **Do not give vaccines to patients on glucocorticoid therapy because the immune response will be suppressed.**

Glucocorticoids have weak mineralcorticoid activity and at high dosages cause Na^+ and fluid retention and K^+ excretion. Hence diuretic therapy may be compromised. In addition, thiazide diuretics, furosemide, and amphotericin B potentiate the K^+-depleting effects of glucocorticoids, leading to severe hypokalemia.

High doses of glucocorticoids increase serum glucose levels. Therefore, insulin and oral hypoglycemic drugs used for diabetes mellitus may appear ineffective. Increased dosages of the antidiabetic drugs may be required.

Higher than normal doses of glucocorticoids may also increase the biotransformation and renal clearance of salicylates. Therefore, therapeutic dosages of salicylates are more difficult to achieve, and rapid cessation of glucocorticoid therapy may result in salicylate toxicity.

Dosage Regimens

Glucocorticoid dosages are highly individualized (Tables 56-3 and 56-4). For any given patient, the dosage is determined

BOX 56-2

Effects of Supraphysiologic Doses of Corticosteroids

Cushingoid Features and Musculoskeletal Changes
- Facial rounding (moon face)
- Dorsal hump (buffalo hump)
- Supraclavicular fossa fullness
- Central obesity
- Osteoporosis
- Muscle wasting, myopathy
- Weakness

Nervous System Changes
- Headache, vertigo
- Insomnia
- Restlessness
- Seizures
- Pseudotumor cerebri

Mood Changes
- Depression, suicidal ideations and/or gestures
- Euphoria, psychoses

Fluid and Electrolyte Imbalances
- Heart failure, hypertension
- Hypernatremia, hypokalemia, hypocalcemia
- Metabolic alkalosis
- Fluid retention, peripheral edema

Skin Changes
- Violaceous striae
- Fragile skin
- Impaired wound healing, ecchymosis
- Hirsutism
- Acne

Ophthalmologic Complications
- Cataracts, glaucoma

Miscellaneous
- Increased susceptibility to infection
- Gastrointestinal irritation
- Glucose intolerance and diabetes mellitus
- Decreased growth in children

empirically. For patients whose disease is not an immediate threat to life, initiate drug therapy at a low dosage, and then increase gradually until symptoms are under control. **All patients taking glucocorticoids, either for adrenal insufficiency or therapeutically at supraphysiologic dosages, must be given stress doses because of the loss of regulation by the HPA axis.** Clinical practice guidelines may recommend doubling the dosage of glucocorticoids in patients who have anxiety or fever. Occasionally the dosages are tripled for patients having surgery, those who have an infection, or those who have undergone trauma. Dosages would then be tapered downward with resolution of the condition.

When glucocorticoids are used for prolonged periods, reduce the dosage (after the patient is stabilized) to the smallest effective dose possible. Maintain prolonged treatment with supraphysiologic doses only if the disorder is life-threatening or if it has the potential to cause permanent disability.

Lab Considerations

Testing of serum cortisol levels is possible but not practical for monitoring therapy. Normally, cortisol levels vary greatly throughout the day in a circadian rhythm, with peak levels occurring from 6 AM to 8 AM, to lower levels at 4 PM to 5 PM, and with the lowest levels at midnight. Serum cortisol levels can be drawn at different times but will be interpreted according to these expected variations. The normal range at 8 AM is 7 to 25 mcg/dL; and at 4 PM to 6 PM, the cortisol level should be less than 10 mcg/dL. However, the clinical presentation of the patient is a more reliable indicator of drug effectiveness.

Mineralocorticoids

◆ fludrocortisone (Florinef); ◆ Florinef

Indications

Fludrocortisone is the drug of choice for chronic mineralocorticoid replacement where normal aldosterone synthesis is absent or impaired. In most cases, however, concomitant therapy with a glucocorticoid such as cortisone or hydrocortisone is required.

Pharmacodynamics

Fludrocortisone is a synthetic analogue of aldosterone with very weak glucocorticoid but very potent mineralocorticoid activity. It binds to renal mineralcorticoid to promote the reabsorption of Na^+ and water and the elimination of K^+.

Pharmacokinetics

Fludrocortisone is readily absorbed when given orally. Once absorbed, mineralocorticoids are highly bound to plasma proteins. Biotransformation occurs primarily in the liver, with metabolites eliminated by the kidneys.

Adverse Effects and Contraindications

Fludrocortisone has no adverse effects or contraindications at normal physiologic levels. The drug may cause typical signs of mineralocorticoid excess including edema and low K^+. These effects on water and Na^+ result in expansion of blood volume, hypertension, edema, cardiac enlargement, and hypokalemia. Exercise caution when using fludrocortisone in patients with heart failure or hypertension. Although rare, fludrocortisone may cause anaphylaxis.

Drug Interactions

Drug interactions with fludrocortisone are often related to electrolyte changes caused by the drug. For example, hypokalemia caused by fludrocortisone increases the toxicity of digoxin and increases the risk with other drugs that cause hypokalemia, including many diuretics and beta agonists used as bronchodilators. Drugs or food containing large amounts of Na^+ may cause hypernatremia because the kidneys, under the influence of fludrocortisone, may be unable to clear the excess Na^+.

Drugs that induce CYP450 enzymes increase the biotransformation of fludrocortisone (see Table 56-2). Mineralocorticoids increase K^+ excretion. When they are taken concurrently, non–K^+-sparing diuretics may cause severe hypokalemia. Patients who need supplemental K^+ require greater than normal dosages.

Dosage Regimen

The adult dose of fludrocortisone varies widely, and adjustments are made to meet patient needs. If hypertension or fluid retention occurs, the dosage is reduced. The dosage is also

ENDOCRINE

DRUG INTERACTIONS
TABLE **56-2** Adrenal Cortex Agonists and Inhibitors

Drug	Interactive Drug	Interaction
CORTICOSTEROIDS		
cortisone, dexamethasone, hydrocortisone, methylprednisolone	aminoglutethimide, carbamazepine, phenobarbital, phenytoin, rifampicin	Induces microsomal enzymes, decreases effects of corticosteroid
prednisolone	erythromycin	Decreases biotransformation of corticosteroid
prednisone	Antacids	Decreases absorption of corticosteroid
	Anticoagulants	Effects increases or decreases in clotting
	Antihypertensives	Loss of antihypertensive effectiveness because of mineralocorticoid effects
	Oral contraceptives, Estrogens	Decreases renal clearance of corticosteroids; decreases metabolism of corticosteroids
	salicylic acid	Increases biotransformation of salicylic acid
	NSAIDs	Additive GI irritation
	Thiazide diuretics, furosemide, amphotericin B	Potentiates potassium depleting effects of glucocorticoid—possible severe hypokalemia
	Skin-testing agents	Decreases reactivity of the skin test—false-negative reactions
	isoniazid, ketoconazole	Decreases renal clearance of corticosteroid
	Insulins, Oral hypoglycemics	Decreases effectiveness of interactive drug
MINERALOCORTICOIDS		
fludrocortisone	aminoglutethimide, carbamazepine, phenobarbital, phenytoin, rifampicin	Induces microsomal enzymes
	Diuretics, potassium supplements	Decreases effectiveness of diuretics; significant potassium depletion with non–potassium-sparing diuretics
	digoxin	Increases risk of digoxin toxicity
ADRENAL HORMONE INHIBITORS		
aminoglutethimide	dexamethasone, hydrocortisone	Increases biotransformation of aminoglutethimide
	Oral anticoagulants	Increases biotransformation and decreases effectiveness of interacting drug
	digoxin, medroxyprogesterone, theophylline	Decreases steady state concentration of interacting drug
	Alcohol	Potentiates action of adrenal hormone–inhibiting drug
	Estrogens	Antagonizes effects of aminoglutethimide
metyrapone	phenytoin	Increases biotransformation of metyrapone—inaccurate test results
	Estrogens	Subtherapeutic response to metyrapone—inaccurate test results
mitotane	Antigout drugs	Decreases effect of antigout drugs
	Bone marrow depressants	Increases bone marrow depression
	Live virus vaccines	Potentiates virus replication, increasing adverse effects and decreasing patient antibody response to vaccine
	CNS depressants	Additive CNS depression

CNS, Central nervous system; *GI*, gastrointestinal; *NSAIDs*, nonsteroidal antiinflammatory drugs.

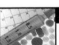

DOSAGE
TABLE **56-3** Adrenal Cortex Agonists and Inhibitors

Drug	Use(s)	Dosage*	Implications
SHORT-ACTING GLUCOCORTICOIDS			
cortisone	Adrenal insufficiency; congenital adrenal hyperplasia; inflammation and immunosuppression; local antiinflammatory effects	*Replacement:* *Adult:* 25–35 mg PO daily *Child:* 0.5–0.75 mg/kg PO daily in divided doses every 8 hr *Treatment:* *Adult:* 25–300 mg PO daily in divided doses every 12–24 hr *Child:* 2.5–10 mg/kg PO daily in divided doses every 8 hr	**Suppresses HPA axis at doses >20 mg/day.** Short-acting glucocorticoid. Carefully monitor growth and development in infants and children receiving prolonged therapy. Taper doses when discontinuing high-dose or long-term therapy. Dosage depends on degree of inflammation and location and size of area.
hydrocortisone	Adrenal insufficiency; congenital adrenal hyperplasia	*Replacement:* *Adult:* 15–25 mg PO daily in divided doses *Child:* 0.5–0.75 mg/kg PO daily	For adults, give two thirds of dose in morning and one third of dose in evening. May increase doses during periods of physical or emotional stress. Drug is also formulated for IV use.
INTERMEDIATE-ACTING CORTICOSTEROIDS			
methylprednisolone	Inflammation and immunosuppression	*Adult:* 8–240 mg PO daily –or– 10–1000 mg/day –or– 10–240 mg every 4 hr IM or IV *Child:* 0.117–1.66 mg/kg/day PO –or– 0.2–2 mg/kg/day IM or IV	**Suppresses adrenal function at chronic doses of 4 mg/day.** Practically devoid of mineralocorticoid activity

Drug	Use	Dosage	Notes	
prednisolone	Adrenal insufficiency; inflammation and immunosuppression	*Adult:* 5–60 mg PO daily in divided doses *Child:* 0.1–2 mg/kg PO day in 1–4 divided doses	**Do not confuse with prednisone.**	▲
prednisone	Adrenal insufficiency; congenital adrenal hyperplasia; inflammation and immunosuppression; local antiinflammatory effects	*Adult:* 5–60 mg PO in divided doses –or– 4–60 mg/day IM or IV –or– 2–30 mg every 3 days to every 3 wk by local injection. Individualize dosage. *Child:* 0.05–2 mg/kg PO daily in 1–4 divided doses	**Do not confuse with prednisolone.** Dosage depends on degree of inflammation and location and size of area. Use dosage that maintains satisfactory clinical response. **Suppresses adrenal function at chronic doses of 5 mg/day.** Minimal mineralocorticoid activity.	▲ ▲
triamcinolone	Inflammation and immunosuppression; local antiinflammatory effects on lungs	*Adult:* 4–60 mg PO daily –or– 40 mg IM weekly of acetonide formulation *Child 6–12 yr:* 100–200 mcg PO 3–4 times daily	**Suppresses adrenal function at chronic doses of 4 mg/day.** Suppression lasts 2.25 days.	▲

LONG-ACTING CORTICOSTEROIDS

Drug	Use	Dosage	Notes	
dexamethasone	Inflammation and immunosuppression	*Adult:* 0.75–9 mg PO daily in 3–4 divided doses every 6–8 hr –or– 8–16 mg IM every 1–3 wk of LA formula *Child:* 0.08–0.34 mg/kg/day PO in divided doses every 6–12 hr	**Suppresses HPA axis at chronic doses of 0.75 mg/day.** Suppression lasts 2.75 days. Dosage depends on degree of inflammation and location and size of area.	▲
betamethasone	Inflammation and immunosuppression	*Adult:* 0.6–7.2 mg/day *Child:* 0.063–0.25 mg/kg/day in 3–4 divided doses	Give single doses before 9 AM; multiple doses should be given at evenly spaced intervals.	

MINERALOCORTICOID

Drug	Use	Dosage	Notes
fludrocortisone	Adrenal insufficiency	*Adult:* 0.05–0.1 mg PO 3 times weekly to 0.2 mg PO daily *Child:* 0.1–0.2 mg PO daily	Administration with cortisone or hydrocortisone is preferred.

CORTICOSTEROID INHIBITORS

Drug	Use	Dosage	Notes
aminoglutethimide	Cushing's syndrome; ectopic ACTH-producing tumors; adrenal enzyme inhibition	*Adult:* 250 mg PO every 6 hr for 14 days. Increase until desired effects achieved or max of 2 grams/day is reached.	Dosages are decreased or discontinued if signs and symptoms of adrenal insufficiency appear.
mitotane	Cushing's syndrome	*Adult:* 500–1000 mg PO daily in divided doses. Increase every 2–4 wk based on patient response. Max: 4 grams/day. Maintenance: 500–2000 mg PO daily in divided doses	Larger dose given in the evening to lessen discomfort associated with therapy. Dosages are decreased or discontinued if signs and symptoms of adrenal insufficiency appear.
metyrapone	Testing of HPA axis function; adrenal enzyme inhibition	*Adult:* 750 mg PO every 4 hr for 6 doses, 4 days after administration of ACTH *Child:* 15 mg/kg every 4 hr for 6 doses	Used in conjunction with ACTH suppression test. Corticosteroids are discontinued before testing.

*All antiinflammatory and immunosuppressive doses are given as a typical range. Doses much higher than those indicated are used during emergency situations. Initial therapy may include multiple divided doses. With long-term therapy, early-morning administration and alternate-day therapy is recommended.
ACTH, Adrenocorticotropic hormone; *HPA,* hypothalamic-pituitary-adrenal axis; *IM,* intramuscular (route); *IV,* intravenous (route); *LA,* long-acting; *PO,* by mouth.

TABLE 56-4 Glucocorticoid Equivalencies

Drug	Dosage* (mg)	Relative GC Potency (Antiinflammatory)	Relative MC Potency (Sodium-Retaining)
SHORT-ACTING			
cortisol	20	1	2
cortisone	25	0.8	2
INTERMEDIATE-ACTING			
methylprednisolone	4	5	0
prednisone	5	4	1
prednisolone	5	4	1
triamcinolone	4	5	0
LONG-ACTING			
betamethasone	0.6	25–50	0
dexamethasone	0.5	25–50	0
MINERALOCORTICOIDS			
aldosterone	0.3	0	300
fludrocortisone	2	15	150

*Approximate oral or IV dose needed to produce equivalent antiinflammatory effects. These values refer to doses given systemically. This information does not apply to locally administered therapy.
GC, Glucocorticoid; *MC,* mineralocorticoid.

reduced in the presence of hypoalbuminemia. Normally, mineralocorticoids are highly bound to plasma proteins, especially albumin. With hypoalbuminemia, more drug is free in the circulation and pharmacologically active; the inverse is true when plasma proteins are elevated. This increases the incidence and severity of adverse effects if the dosage is not reduced.

For patients receiving chronic fludrocortisone therapy, the dosage must be increased during periods of stress. Although what is stressful to one patient may not be to another, some common stressors exist. Surgery and anesthesia, infections, anxiety, and temperature extremes may require an increased dosage of mineralocorticoid drug.

▌ Lab Considerations

Lab testing of serum drug levels is not considered practical. Drug efficacy is best determined by clinical presentation.

CLINICAL REASONING

Treatment Objectives

The objective of treatment for adrenal insufficiency is to reduce patient symptoms to a tolerable level. Set reasonable goals for drug therapy in collaboration with the patient.

ENDOCRINE

Antiinflammatory and immunosuppressive therapy is aimed at maintaining the lowest glucocorticoid dosage possible without the recurrence of symptoms of the original disorder. Special care is taken to determine the risks and benefits of initiating glucocorticoid therapy in supraphysiologic dosages.

Treatment Options

It is important that although basal cortisol and ACTH levels may be helpful, definitive cortisol stimulation testing is required to confirm a diagnosis of adrenal insufficiency (Box 56-3). Plasma ACTH levels are higher than normal in patients with primary adrenal insufficiency. Free cortisol and the metabolites of adrenal hormones (17-hydroxycorticosteroids and 17-ketosteroids) are eliminated in the urine. Levels are reduced with adrenal insufficiency. On initiation of drug therapy, metabolite excretion returns to normal levels.

▥ Patient Variables

The clinical manifestations of adrenal insufficiency vary from patient to patient, with the severity of signs and symptoms related to the degree of deficiency (see Case Study). When needed, plasma cortisol levels are drawn at specific times throughout the day and evening to determine whether the normal diurnal pattern is evident of a rise in the early morning (peaking around 8 AM to 7 to 25 mcg/dL) and a fall in the evening (less than 10 mcg/dL) to almost undetectable levels near midnight. Levels lower than expected suggest some form of adrenal insufficiency. Care providers should be familiar with the sleep patterns of the patient, because the expected diurnal pattern changes when the person habitually works throughout the night and sleeps in the daytime.

Life-Span Considerations

Pregnant and Nursing Women. Couples with a history of adrenal hormone disorders who are thinking about conception must consider the potential consequences to both the mother and fetus. Glucocorticoids taken for physiologic replacement therapy should not affect the pregnant woman or the fetus. However, maintaining exact physiologic drug requirements during pregnancy is difficult given the physical changes of pregnancy (see Chapter 6). Relative overdosage with glucocorticoids causes Na^+ and water retention, resulting in elevated blood pressure and edema. Further, glucocorticoids are teratogenic in lab animals, however, no clinical studies on humans exist that demonstrate an association between congenital malformations and the therapeutic use of adrenal hormones. Theoretically, use of glucocorticoids increases the risk of gestational diabetes.

Children and Adolescents. Infants born to mothers receiving large doses of glucocorticoids are monitored closely immediately after birth for signs and symptoms of adrenal insufficiency. Supplemental doses of steroids may be required temporarily by the newborn. The health care provider determines whether the infant's adrenal glands can be stimulated naturally by the gradual withdrawal of exogenous steroids.

The most significant concern with glucocorticoid replacement therapy in children is the suppression of growth hormone (GH), resulting in the child's failure to grow to normal adult stature. When given as replacement therapy for adrenal insufficiency, the dosage is adjusted to approximate minimal levels necessary for body functioning. Closely monitor the child,

---

BOX 56-3

Cortisol Stimulation Testing

Cosyntropin (Cortrosyn)

Cosyntropin is used diagnostically to distinguish between primary and secondary adrenal insufficiency (see also Chapter 55). Cosyntropin is a synthetic version of adrenocorticotropic hormone (ACTH) that contains the first 24 of the 39 amino acids found in natural ACTH. Like natural ACTH, cosyntropin directly simulates the adrenal cortex to synthesize adrenal steroids. Normal adrenal glands respond to ACTH by synthesizing and releasing cortisol into the blood stream, where it may be measured. In adrenal insufficiency, the adrenal gland cannot respond to ACTH and no excess cortisol is produced. In patients with low pituitary function, the adrenal gland may be suppressed and may respond less rapidly to ACTH than would a normal gland.

Corticorelin (ACTHREL)

Corticorelin is used to identify the source of high ACTH levels. The drug induces release of ACTH from the pituitary, but tumors or other ectopic sites of ACTH production usually do not respond. Thus persons with normal pituitary function or with oversecretion from the pituitary show a rise in ACTH and cortisol after administration of the drug. Production of ACTH or cortisol is not changed in response to the drug when the primary source of ACTH is a tumor. Assess patient for hypersensitivity to the drug or class, or a component. Use caution in administering the drug if the patient has an allergy to corticotropin.

Pharmacokinetics

Because they are peptides, cosyntropin and corticorelin are not effective orally and must be given by injection. Both are rapidly cleared from the circulation and produce peak increases in plasma cortisol levels 30 to 60 minutes after administration.

Adverse Effects

Principle adverse effects of either drug are a consequence of increased secretion of adrenal corticosteroids. Corticorelin may cause flushing after intravenous (IV) injection; dyspnea, hypotension, and tachycardia have been reported. Usually these effects are transient, lasting from 5 to 30 minutes. Cosyntropin is less antigenic than native ACTH, but it still may produce allergic reactions and anaphylaxis in susceptible persons.

Drug Interactions

Corticorelin may produce severe hypotension in the presence of heparin. It can accentuate electrolyte loss with diuretic therapy.

Cosyntropin Testing

- Hold cortisone, hydrocortisone, and spironolactone on test day.
- Draw preinjection baseline cortisol level or collect 24-hour urine specimen for 17-KS or 17-OCHS.
- *Dosage: Adults and children >2 years of age:* Give 0.25 mg by IM or 0.25 mg by IV route.
- *Dosage: Children <2 years of age:* Give 0.125 mg by IM or 0.125 mg by IV route.
- Draw baseline cortisol level, and then draw a second level 30 to 60 minutes after cosyntropin injection or after infusion complete.
- *Results:* Patients with adrenal insufficiency have values that do not rise above 10 mcg/dL.

IM, Intramuscular; *IV,* intravenous; *17-KS,* 17-ketosteroids; *17-OCHS,* 17-hydroxyglucocorticoids.

CASE STUDY | Adrenal Cortex Agonists

ASSESSMENT

History of Present Illness	PK is a 4-year-old boy accompanied to the clinic by his parents. He is complaining of tummy aches, muscle weakness, diarrhea, irritability, and a lack of ability to keep up with his 5-year-old brother in play. He has not been eating well for several weeks, and his mother believes that he has lost weight. For the last week, PK frequently asks to lie down and refuses to play outside with his brother. He complains of headache, and his mother states that he is frequently sweaty. The parents have seen no evidence of seizure activity.
Past Health History	PK has been well and developing normally until approximately 1 week ago. There have been discussions with a previous health care provider that he may have adrenal insufficiency, but the diagnosis was never confirmed. Other than for insignificant acute illnesses, PK has been seen only for regularly scheduled well-child examinations. He has no known allergies to drugs, foods, or environmental elements. Family history is noncontributory.
Life-Span Considerations	PK is more susceptible to suppression of the HPA axis and decreased secretion of growth hormone with treatment. **Psychosocial Considerations** Because PK is not yet in school and stays at home with his mother during the day, adapting his schedule to allow for his increased appetite, nutritional needs, needs for rest, and drug administration is not problematic. PK and his brother live with both parents in a middle-class neighborhood. The father works full time, and the mother is able to stay home with the boys. All family members are covered by an HMO through the father's employment. All prescription drugs are $5 per prescription, regardless of the drug cost.
Physical Exam Findings	PK is irritable but cooperates with exam. Vital signs are all well within normal limits for age except blood pressure, which is slightly lower than expected for age. Weight is down 2 lb since last visit 2 months ago. Skin is smooth, warm, pale, and moist with elastic turgor, with no evidence of infection or purpura. Normal male-pattern hair distribution with no flaking noted. Lungs are clear to auscultation. Normal sinus rhythm with no murmur. Abdomen is slightly distended and tender to deep palpation in all four quadrants. Pupils are equal, round, and reactive to light and accommodation. No nuchal rigidity elicited with Kernig's or Brudzinski's signs. Gait is symmetric and equal with no ataxia.
Diagnostic Testing	Serum Na^+, 134 mEq/L; serum K^+, 5.0 mEq/L; serum Ca^{++}, 12 mg/dL; BUN, 19 mg/dL; FBS, 62 mg/dL. CBC shows moderate neutropenia, lymphocytosis, and hemoconcentration.

DIAGNOSIS: Adrenal insufficiency

MANAGEMENT

Treatment Objectives	• Replace adrenal hormones to prevent life-threatening consequences associated with lack of naturally occurring corticosteroids.
Treatment Options	**Pharmacotherapy** • prednisone 4 to 5 mg/kg PO daily in divided doses at 8 AM and 5 PM • fludrocortisone 0.1 mg PO daily at 8 AM **Patient Education** 1. Hormone replacement is a lifelong need. 2. Take prednisone with food to protect the stomach from irritation. 3. Identify potential emotional and environmental stressors early and plan possible interventions. 4. Encourage a normal exercise regimen to prevent excessive muscle wasting. 5. Avoid crowds and people with known infections. Treatment for even minor infections is initiated quickly. 6. High-carbohydrate, high-protein diet. Generally, potassium and sodium are not restricted. Dietary sodium intake should remain constant after the requirements for fludrocortisone replacement have been determined. 7. Abrupt decreases in sodium intake can precipitate an adrenal crisis. Contact the health care provider right away.

Continued

ENDOCRINE

CASE STUDY   Adrenal Cortex Agonists—Cont'd

8. Keep appointments with health care provider and pediatric endocrinologist as scheduled.
9. Wear a medical alert identification bracelet or necklace.

Evaluation

Treatment effectiveness is apparent when blood pressure and other vital signs stabilize; fluid, electrolyte, and blood sugar levels return to normal; appetite and physical strength improve; and weight is regained. Likewise, the patient has minimal to no signs and symptoms of overtreatment. Maintenance of the child's growth in the 50th percentile for similar age groups is also indication of successful therapy.

CLINICAL REASONING

Q1. Why do you need to calculate the dosage of prednisone? Can't we simply use the drug reference here on the floor?

A. It's necessary for several reasons, but primarily it is because children are not small adults. All drug dosages for children should be calculated based on mg/kg of body weight. Further, the lowest possible dosage of glucocorticosteroid is used in an attempt to maintain PK's growth within the 50th percentile of children his own age.

Q2. But if he has a cortisol deficiency, why are you also giving him fludrocortisone.?

A. The adrenal gland produces both glucocorticoids, but also the mineralocorticoid aldosterone. We need to replace both. We will use prednisone for glucocorticoid hormone replacement and fludrocortisone for the mineralocorticoid component. Without fludrocortisone, he will have no end of problems with his fluid and electrolyte balance.

Q3. If PK has to take the prednisone twice a day, can't we tell his mom to give it to him at noon with his lunch so it won't upset his stomach after he has had his bath, and the other dose just before bedtime?

A. Endogenous glucocorticoids are cyclically secreted, with the largest amount produced in the morning and the smallest amount during the evening hours. The majority of cortisol is produced between 5 AM and 9 AM. It would be best to give him two thirds of his total daily dose in the morning and the other third in the evening, about 4 PM, when he eats his dinner. We want to mimic the body's normal rhythm of cortisol production.

Q4. PK is just a growing kid. What happens with his prednisone dosage during periods of emotional upset or infection—kids get a lot of colds—or if, heaven forbid, surgery is necessary?

A. His dosage will be adjusted upward, if needed, as he grows or if he becomes ill. Dosages are decreased with signs of relative overtreatment. However, when dosage adjustments are needed, he will be referred back to his pediatric endocrinologist, who specializes in adrenal insufficiency. He may also need human growth hormone.

---

attempting to maintain the child's growth in the 50th percentile for similar age groups. Supplemental doses of GH are controversial but may be used during predicted high-growth periods to stimulate normal development.

Older Adults. Administration of glucocorticoids to older patients poses many challenges. Although the pharmacodynamics of glucocorticoids are similar for both young and old adults, normal physiologic changes and pathophysiologic changes common with aging make monitoring for overdosing or underdosing difficult. Normal changes of aging such as weakness, fatigue, anorexia, and sparse hair are also seen in adrenal insufficiency. Slight to moderate immunosuppression, development of cataracts, redistribution of body mass, changes in vessel compliance, decreased glucose tolerance, alterations in GI functioning, and thinning of the skin are also associated with normal changes of aging and may be difficult to distinguish from the signs and symptoms of adrenal insufficiency. In addition, many older patients have preexisting fluid and Na^+ retention associated with hypertension and heart failure. The added burden of glucocorticoids further increases fluid and Na^+ retention, leading to further pathology. When used in older adults, the corticosteroid dose is usually reduced because of the decreased muscle mass, plasma volume, hepatic biotransformation, and renal elimination.

▌ Drug Variables

The adverse effects of glucocorticoids have been widely reported. Available data are scant, but suggest that low-dose glucocorticoids (<10 mg of prednisolone or prednisone equivalent) do not increase the risk for osteoporotic fractures, blood pressure elevation, or cardiovascular diseases, or the incidence of peptic ulcers. Weight gain is common, as are skin changes. However, adrenal insufficiency, regardless of the cause, necessitates replacement of both glucocorticoids and mineralocorticoids.

Hydrocortisone and cortisone are usually the drugs of choice because they have greater mineralocorticoid activity compared with other glucocorticoids (see Table 56-4). If additional mineralocorticoid activity is required, fludrocortisone can be given by mouth. Androgens normally produced in the adrenal cortex are also limited with adrenal insufficiency, but generally are not replaced unless clinically indicated (see Chapter 57).

Adults with adrenal insufficiency are maintained on consistent daily drug dosages once clinical signs and symptoms of adrenal insufficiency are stabilized. Medical or psychosocial stressors require increased dosages of the glucocorticoid to sustain the metabolic functions of adrenal hormones. Patients with preexisting medical conditions such as diabetes and hypertension may find regulation of both their adrenal insufficiency and other chronic conditions more difficult.

Use supraphysiologic dosages of glucocorticoids for antiinflammatory effects only after carefully weighing the potential benefits against the known adverse effects. Patients with severe pathologic signs and symptoms associated with a disease process causing inflammation or overactivation of the immune response may require corticosteroid therapy to preserve life or functional ability.

The classic corticosteroid used for its antiinflammatory effects is hydrocortisone (cortisol). A variety of other preparations are available with differing durations of action and potency. All have equal antiinflammatory effects when given in equivalent dosages. Selection of a specific drug to use is based on the relative antiinflammatory and mineralocorticoid (Na^+-retaining) potency, as well as the plasma and half-life of the drug. When drug therapy is aimed at antiinflammatory and immunosuppressive effects, drugs with relatively lower mineralocorticoid potency are desirable.

Recommended regimens for long-term glucocorticoids therapy vary from a regular, low daily dose of the drug of choice to intermittent dosing using moderate to high dosages. Many of the primary disorders treated with glucocorticoids lend themselves to intermittent therapy during periods of symptom exacerbation.

Some patients may only need drug therapy for a limited time. Short-term treatment regimens are often referred to as a "burst" or "pulse" of steroids. The patient is given a large dose initially and then slowly weaned off the drug. A burst can last from 7 to 10 days, although longer regimens are often used in clinical practice. An example of a 10-day burst schedule is shown in Box 56-4.

For patients with upper respiratory infections (e.g., viral), any febrile illness, strenuous exercise, gastroenteritis with vomiting and diarrhea, or minor surgery, doubling the daily maintenance dose is usually sufficient. Once the stressful period is over, the dosage may be reduced. If infection occurs during long-term glucocorticoid therapy, administration of appropriate antibiotics is indicated. In addition, prescribe increased doses of glucocorticoids to cope with the added stress of the infection.

If the patient must undergo anesthesia and surgery, even greater doses of glucocorticoids may be given for several days in advance of the procedure. For example, a patient undergoing abdominal surgery may require 300 to 400 mg of hydrocortisone on the day of surgery. The dose can be gradually reduced to the usual maintenance dose within about 5 days if postoperative recovery is uncomplicated. As a general rule, it is wise to administer high doses temporarily rather than to risk inadequate doses and an adrenal insufficiency crisis. However, specific regimens will vary according to the type of anesthesia, surgical procedure, health care provider preference, and patient condition.

Treatment of secondary adrenal insufficiency includes the administration of either the hypothalamic-releasing factor (i.e., CRH) or pituitary-stimulating hormone (i.e., ACTH) that signals the release of adrenal cortex hormones. However, hypothalamic and pituitary hormones drugs are expensive and must be administered parenterally.

WITHDRAWING GLUCOCORTICOID THERAPY. Sudden cessation of therapy following 3 weeks or more of supraphysiologic doses of glucocorticoids can precipitate acute adrenal insufficiency. Guidelines to prevent adrenal crisis during withdrawal from therapy are identified in Box 56-5. Changing therapy to shorter-acting drugs and using alternate-day therapy (ADT) are features that allow for HPA axis recovery. The rate of taper depends primarily on the underlying nonendocrine disorder for which the drug was used. As previously noted, there may be significant adrenal suppression for up to 1 year after discontinuing glucocorticoid therapy. If patients have symptoms of adrenal insufficiency on withdrawal of steroids, it may be reasonable to perform a cosyntropin stimulation test to assess adrenal responsiveness (see Box 56-3).

Patient Education

A diagnosis of adrenal insufficiency necessitates significant participation by the patient in the treatment plan. The patient must be made aware that hormone replacement is a lifelong need. In addition, by identifying potential emotional and environmental stressors and discussing possible interventions, the health care provider can help minimize crises. Careful attention by the health care provider to patient and family education may alleviate the anxiety that often surrounds chronic illness.

BOX 56-5

Principles of Glucocorticoid Use and Withdrawal

- Use the smallest dosage of glucocorticoid possible for the shortest time possible.
- Use shorter-acting drugs (e.g., prednisone, cortisol) given as early in the day as possible, and avoid twice-daily administration.
- Use alternate-day-therapy (ADT) when possible (if underlying condition is responsive to this regimen). A dosage equivalent to 2.5 to 3 times the minimal daily dosage is used for ADT. Surprisingly, administration of higher dosages of glucocorticoids on alternate days leads to fewer adverse effects than lower dosages given daily.
- Weaning a patient to ADT is accomplished in a variety of ways. One weaning method suggests a once-a-day schedule. When the patient demonstrates a tolerance for the ADT regimen, the dosage is gradually decreased while the patient is monitored for signs and symptoms of recurrence of the original disease.
- Give all patients supplemental calcium and vitamin D; consider pharmacologic prophylaxis for osteoporosis.
- Educate the patient as to the appropriate response to major medical and psychosocial stressors for 1 year following glucocorticoid replacement.
- To begin a taper after long-term therapy, change to the shortest-acting drug administered once daily, early in the day.
- Taper dosage further and switch to ADT as tolerated, based on the underlying disease.

BOX 56-4

Example of Prednisone Taper Instructions*

Using 10-mg tablets of prednisone:

Take 5 tablets today (_____[Insert date]); and then take
4 tablets tomorrow (_____[Insert date]); then take
3 tablets/day for 2 days, (_____[Insert dates]); then take
2 tablets/day for 3 days, (_____[Insert dates]); then take
1 tablet/day for 4 days (_____[Insert dates]).

*Be sure to take all of the tablets at once with food to reduce stomach upset.

ADT, Alternate day therapy.

Glucocorticoids, when used for adrenal insufficiency, are administered orally in the early morning and late afternoon to simulate natural glucocorticoid diurnal rhythms. Ideally, the drug is taken between 6 AM and 9 AM, with the second dose given between 4 PM and 6 PM. Patients who routinely work during the night may need to make scheduling adjustments.

Instruct patients and families about the possibility of overtreatment and undertreatment and the signs and symptoms to monitor, as well as the occasional need to temporarily increase drug dosages during times of stress. Also teach patients about the need to avoid stressful situations (where possible) and to practice stress-reducing techniques.

Patients should avoid becoming fatigued, even if steroid therapy has resulted in increased energy levels. A normal exercise regimen is needed to prevent excessive muscle wasting and to help maintain bone mass; however, it should be interspersed with adequate rest periods.

Patients with adrenal insufficiency are more prone to infections and are taught to avoid crowds and people with known infections. Treatment for even minor infections is initiated quickly.

Teach patients that when drug levels are maintained at near-normal physiologic levels, no dietary alterations are necessary. However, should drug dosages exceed physiologic levels, patients may need to limit foods high in Na^+ to prevent fluid retention, edema, and hypertension. In contrast, patients with adrenal insufficiency who do not have adequate hormone levels may require additional Na^+ to maintain homeostatic fluid balance.

Dietary adjustments are made based on the clinical presentation of the patient. Discuss nutritional needs, including the need for a high-carbohydrate, high-protein diet. Generally, potassium and Na^+ are not restricted. Dietary Na^+ intake should remain constant after the requirements for mineralocorticoid replacement have been determined. A shift of Na^+ intake in either direction necessitates a concomitant change in the dosage of fludrocortisone. Abrupt decreases in Na^+ intake can precipitate an adrenal crisis. In climates where there is great variation in temperatures, mineralocorticoid dosage may be adjusted. Patients should receive daily Ca^{++} supplementation to maintain bone mass.

Often patients regulate their own corticosteroid dosage based on personal responses and daily activities or stress levels. Advise patients to maintain dosages at the lowest possible levels to achieve therapeutic effects. Discuss the palliative nature of glucocorticoid therapy. Other treatment modalities used in the cure or direct treatment of the primary disease must not be discontinued because of improvement in physical abilities due to steroid therapy. Teach patients the importance of wearing a medical alert identification bracelet or necklace.

Evaluation

For the patient with adrenal insufficiency, adequate treatment is apparent when blood pressure and other vital signs stabilize; fluid, electrolyte, and blood sugar levels return to normal; appetite and physical strength improve; and weight is regained. Likewise, the patient has minimal to no signs and symptoms of overtreatment. With adequate replacement therapy, most people with adrenal insufficiency lead normal lives.

The best way to determine the effectiveness of glucocorticoid therapy for suppression of the immune and inflammatory responses is by evaluation of clinical presentation of the patient. When treatment is effective, pathologic signs and symptoms of the primary disease are resolved to an acceptable level.

Given the multitude of adverse effects possible with high-dose glucocorticoid therapy, an evaluation of the effectiveness of treatment is not complete until the patient has been assessed for the presence and extent of the less desirable effects of treatment. Keep dosages at the lowest level possible, administering oral drugs early in the morning, and using ADT when possible. Close monitoring for potentially dangerous adverse effects includes examination of skin integrity, bone-density studies to monitor for osteoporosis, laboratory analysis for early signs of infection (i.e., complete blood count), eye and vision checks for early detection of glaucoma and cataracts, and assessment of vital signs and fluid balance status.

ADRENAL HYPERSECRETION

EPIDEMIOLOGY AND ETIOLOGY

Adrenal hypersecretion, otherwise known as Cushing's syndrome or hypercortisolism, is a constellation of symptoms, signs, and biochemical abnormalities that result from prolonged exposure to excess levels of glucocorticoids. The disorder, although relatively rare, affects adults aged 20 to 50 years. An estimated 10 to 15 out of every 1 million people are affected each year. The disease predominantly affects women in an 8:1 ratio compared with men. Left untreated, it is linked to high morbidity and mortality.

PATHOPHYSIOLOGY

Excessive endogenous secretion of cortisol may be caused by increased production of ACTH by pituitary adenomas (Cushing's disease); ectopic production of ACTH by a tumor in the GI tract, the pancreas, or the lung; or production by an autonomously functioning adrenal tumor. Adrenal tumors are usually unilateral and are responsible for approximately 25% of all cases of Cushing's syndrome. In adults, approximately 50% of these tumors are malignant. The remainders of the cases are due to bilateral adrenal hyperplasia that is caused by pituitary or nonendocrine tumors that produce excessive ACTH.

Adrenocortical hyperplasia results in the loss of normal diurnal rhythms; a decreased responsiveness to prolactin, thyrotropin, and gonadotropin to their respective releasing hormones; and abnormal sleeping patterns. Although some of the changes are due to excessive amounts of glucocorticoids, others are linked to a yet unidentified hypothalamic abnormality.

Patients with Cushing's syndrome have a *cushingoid* appearance (i.e., moon face, buffalo hump, truncal obesity) as a result of alterations in nitrogen, carbohydrate, and mineral metabolism. An increase in total body fat results from a decreased turnover of plasma fatty acids, and a redistribution of bulk to a more truncal pattern. Moderate to marked increases in the breakdown of tissue protein and a marked increase in urinary nitrogen levels occur. These changes result in decreased muscle mass with a proximal myopathy, atrophic skin, decreased bone matrix, and a loss of total skeletal Ca^{++}. High levels of glucocorticoids kill lymphocytes within organs that contain these cells, such as the liver, the spleen, and the lymph nodes. Thus the immune response is reduced.

Hypersecretion by the adrenal cortex also leads to hyperaldosteronism and excessive amounts of androgens. In most cases, there is evidence of increased androgen production with acne, hirsutism, and in rare instances, clitoral hypertrophy. Increased androgen production also interrupts the normal pituitary-ovarian axis, thereby decreasing production of estrogens, and of progesterone from the ovary, causing oligomenorrhea.

Hypersecretion by the adrenal medulla results in excessive secretion of catecholamines, of which 80% is epinephrine and the remainder norepinephrine.

PHARMACOTHERAPEUTIC OPTIONS

Adrenal Corticosteroid Inhibitors
◆ aminoglutethimide (Cytadren)
◆ metyrapone (Metopirone)
◆ mitotane (Lysodren); ✦ Lysodren

▥ Indications
Although adrenal corticosteroid inhibitors relieve hypercortisolism in some patients, drugs are often not the preferred treatment modality. Bilateral adrenalectomy is now the first-line treatment for many patients with known Cushing's disease. Bilateral adrenalectomy is most often reserved for patients in whom radiotherapy and mitotane therapy do not alleviate Cushing's, or when the patient does not tolerate mitotane therapy. Several drugs are available to block the synthesis of cortisol and are used for testing the function of the HPA axis.

Aminoglutethimide is used as a temporary means of decreasing excessive corticosteroid production in patients awaiting more definitive therapy (e.g., surgery). In patients with adrenal adenomas and carcinomas, or ectopic ACTH-secreting tumors, morning plasma cortisol levels are reduced by about 50%. The drugs do not influence the underlying disease process; therefore, if the drug is discontinued, excessive production of glucocorticoids will resume.

Aminoglutethimide originated as an anticonvulsant, but its use resulted in adrenal insufficiency. Aminoglutethimide has also been used to produce a so-called medical adrenalectomy in patients with advanced breast cancer and in patients with metastatic cancer of the prostate.

Metyrapone is primarily used to test for and diagnose adrenal insufficiency, but it is sometimes used in the treatment of Cushing's syndrome.

Mitotane is an antineoplastic drug that selectively inhibits cortisol from the adrenal cortex. Mitotane is indicated to control the production of cortisol in patients with inoperable adrenal carcinoma, or in patients in which the carcinoma cannot be completely removed. Mitotane therapy does not offer a cure for adrenal carcinoma, but it may increase survival.

▥ Pharmacodynamics
Corticosteroid inhibitors act primarily by inhibiting enzyme activity in the adrenal cortex and to prevent conversion of cholesterol to pregnenolone. In turn, the synthesis of all adrenal

steroids is inhibited. Aminoglutethimide is a simple derivative of the sedative glutethimide.

As an aromatase inhibitor, aminoglutethimide is used in the treatment of Cushing's syndrome and breast cancer because it blocks estrogen synthesis. Aromatase inhibitors deplete estrogen by inhibiting aromatase, the enzyme that synthesizes estrogen from androgens. Aminoglutethimide is a mixture of D- and L-isomers which have different pharmacologic potencies.

Metyrapone inhibits 11-β hydroxylase in the adrenal cortex, thus blocking cortisol production. The blockade of this enzyme stimulates ACTH secretion, in turn leading to increased secretion of 11-deoxycortisol, which mildly suppresses the release of ACTH. The metyrapone test can help gauge pituitary responsiveness and therefore whether the source of hypercortisolism, when caused by excess ACTH, is pituitary or ectopic (nonpituitary). Adrenal insufficiency must be ruled out before administration of metyrapone.

Mitotane is a derivative of the insecticide dichlorodiphenyltrichloroethane (DDT) which causes direct necrosis and atrophy of the adrenal cortex. Mitotane also increases extra-adrenal metabolism of cortisol, so less is excreted in urine.

▥ Pharmacokinetics
Because there is limited use of corticosteroid inhibitors, little is known of their pharmacokinetic properties. They are absorbed when taken orally and generally have a half-life that ranges from minutes to several hours. Mitotane is the exception, with a half-life of 18 to 159 days (see Table 56-1). Biotransformation occurs in the liver, with metabolites eliminated by the kidneys.

▥ Adverse Effects and Contraindications
Adverse effects of corticosteroid inhibitors are common. Patients complain of nausea with abdominal distress, headaches, drowsiness, dizziness, and a morbilliform (measles-like) skin rash. Additional adverse effects include hematologic abnormalities, hypothyroidism, muscle pain, and fever. Masculinization may occur in females, and precocious sexual development may occur in males.

▥ Drug Interactions
Adrenal corticosteroid inhibitors inhibit or promote the biotransformation of synthetic adrenal hormones (see Table 56-2).

▥ Dosage Regimens
The dosage varies depending on the drug used (see Table 56-3). Patients are generally started on smaller doses and the dosage gradually increased as signs and symptoms of adverse effects, such as abdominal pain, lessen. Dosages are increased until clinical evidence of the hypersecretion syndrome is lessened. The drugs are administered in divided doses throughout the day, usually every 4 to 6 hours.

▥ Lab Considerations
No lab tests for drug effectiveness are available. Urine sampling helps validate the effects of therapy. Analyses of 24-hour urine samples for 17-hydroxyglucocorticoids and 17-ketogenic steroids reveals increased urinary elimination of corticosteroid by products.

ENDOCRINE

CLINICAL REASONING

Treatment Objectives

The primary treatment objective for the patient with hypercortisolism is to control excessive amounts of cortisol and the pathologic consequences.

Treatment Options

▌▎ Patient Variables

Various diagnostic tests are used to identify the etiology of Cushing's syndrome, including radiographic studies, magnetic resonance imaging, and dexamethasone suppression test. In addition, hypercortisolism has many metabolic consequences that may be identified through blood and urine testing. Plasma ACTH levels vary depending on the etiology of hypercortisolism. In Cushing's syndrome, ACTH levels are low to unmeasurable. In ectopic syndromes, the ACTH level is elevated. In hypercortisolism, basal levels of urinary free cortisol, 17-ketosteroids, and 17-hydroxyglucocorticoids are all elevated. Urinary calcium, potassium, and glucose levels are also elevated.

Plasma cortisol levels are measured the morning following a midnight oral dose of dexamethasone. Normally, plasma cortisol levels are less than 5 mg/dL. Further definitive testing for Cushing's syndrome is required if plasma levels are higher than 5 mg/dL. A 24-hour urine collection for cortisol is the preferred screening test for Cushing's.

The metyrapone test is used to assess HPA axis feedback responses. Metyrapone lowers serum cortisol levels and, therefore, stimulates ACTH secretion. A normal response is an increase in ACTH and 11-deoxycortisol levels.

LIFE-SPAN CONSIDERATIONS

Pregnant and Nursing Women. Little information exists about the safety of adrenal hormone–inhibitor use during pregnancy. Women with Cushing's syndrome are less likely to conceive. If the disorder occurs during pregnancy, the fetus also receives higher than normal cortisol levels, potentially resulting in negative consequences on fetal growth and development. Interestingly, treatment with metyrapone during the second and third trimesters may block enzyme activity, leading to adrenal insufficiency for the fetus.

Children and Adolescents. Cushing's syndrome has an effect on the growth and development of children. The physical changes associated with high levels of cortisol are particularly devastating for children and adolescents concerned with appearance. Little is known about treatment of children with adrenal hormone inhibitors, and the safety of pharmaceutical agents is not well established. Treatment is difficult given that the Food and Drug Administration (FDA) has no established dosage guidelines for corticosteroid inhibitor use in children.

Older Adults. Skin changes associated with Cushing's syndrome are exaggerated in older patients. Excessive skin thinning, blood vessel fragility, and fat redistribution occur as a natural part of aging and worsen with high levels of cortisol. Older patients are also more likely to have other chronic conditions complicating disease progression and treatment.

▌▎ Drug Variables

Drug therapy is used primarily for identification of the etiology and palliative treatment. Although all corticosteroid inhibitors have similar pharmacodynamic properties, the effectiveness of drug therapy can be erratic and less than satisfactory. Corticosteroid inhibitors potentially produce signs and symptoms associated with adrenal insufficiency. It is wise to refer these patients to an endocrinologist who specializes in adrenal disorders.

Adrenal hormone–inhibitor therapy requires multiple daily dosings. Patients are started on smaller doses, and increases are made to achieve desired effects. All preparations are administered orally, and dosages are decreased with the appearance of signs and symptoms of adrenal insufficiency.

Patient Education

Patients are usually aware of their symptoms; however, when taking corticosteroid inhibitors they should be taught the signs and symptoms of adrenal insufficiency. Unfortunately, many of the clinical indicators of adrenal insufficiency are not specific, nor are they very different from those of Cushing's syndrome. Warn patients of the sometimes erratic nature of drug therapy effectiveness and the possibility of recurrence in physical problems of Cushing's syndrome.

Evaluation

Effectiveness of therapy is noted when the signs and symptoms of Cushing's syndrome are lessened without complications of adrenal insufficiency. Vital signs stabilize, serum electrolytes including glucose levels return to normal, and emotional changes are less disruptive. Often, surgical removal of the adrenal glands is necessary, but this approach, in turn, results in acute adrenal insufficiency. Adequate treatment of the adrenal insufficiency is required thereafter.

KEY POINTS

- Adrenal insufficiency results in decreased levels of adrenal cortex hormones: glucocorticoids (cortisol and cortisone), mineralocorticoids (aldosterone), and androgens (testosterone).
- Dysfunction of the adrenal glands results in primary adrenal insufficiency.
- Pathologic conditions of the HPA axis lead to secondary adrenal insufficiency.
- The sodium and water depletion in adrenal insufficiency leads to hypovolemia and dehydration; shock may become evident.

- Physiologic symptoms of adrenal insufficiency include weakness, fluid and electrolyte imbalances, hypoglycemia, hypotension, weight loss, nausea, vomiting, anorexia, abdominal pain, and mental status changes.
- Glucocorticoid replacement is required to prevent life-threatening consequences associated with the lack of naturally occurring adrenal hormones.
- Treatment of primary adrenal insufficiency requires replacement of glucocorticoids and mineralocorticoids in some instances.

■ Extensive teaching about the drugs and the importance of taking the drug daily at the prescribed times is required.

■ Patients should be taught about their disease, appropriate treatment regimens, and the potential for complications.

■ Allow for changes in dosage to meet special physical and emotional needs such as stress, surgical procedures, trauma, and physical growth.

■ Treatment objectives for patients with an immune system response are to suppress the detrimental effects of inflammation and the immune response, and to lessen but not cure the primary pathologic process. Supraphysiologic doses of glucocorticoids are often needed.

■ Local rather than systemic administration of glucocorticoids is preferred when possible.

■ When long-term therapy is required, attempts are made to maintain the dosage at the smallest level possible, give the dose early in the morning, and administer on an ADT schedule.

■ Glucocorticoid therapy should be tapered downward when it is time for it to be discontinued. Sudden discontinuance of glucocorticoids can result of an inability of the HPA axis to effectively recover.

■ Adrenal hypersecretion, also known as Cushing's syndrome or hypercortisolism, is characterized by overproduction of the adrenal hormone cortisol.

■ The most common form is iatrogenic Cushing's syndrome caused by excessive amounts of exogenous adrenal hormones.

■ Adrenal corticosteroid inhibitors are administered in increasing dosages until signs and symptoms of hypercortisolism are diminished.

■ Therapy is effective when signs and symptoms of Cushing's syndrome are lessened without complications of adrenal insufficiency. Vital signs, electrolytes, and glucose levels return to normal, and emotional changes are less disruptive.

■ Surgery is the definitive treatment for Cushing's syndrome.

Bibliography

Arlt, W. (2005). Androgen replacement therapy in women. *Current Opinion in Investigational Drugs*, 6(10), 1028–1036.

Arlt, W., and Allolio, B. (2003). Adrenal insufficiency. *Lancet, 361* (9372), 1881–1893.

Bhattacharyya, A., Kaushal, K., Tymms, D., et al. (2005). Steroid withdrawal syndrome after successful treatment of Cushing's syndrome: A reminder. *European Journal of Endocrinology, 153*(2), 207–210.

Chrousos, G., and Lafferty, A. (2002). Glucocorticoid therapy and Cushing syndrome. *eMedicine*, December 6. Available online: www.emedicine.com/ped/topic1068.htm. Accessed May 28, 2007.

DaSilva, J., Jacobs, J., Kirwin, J., et al. (2006). Safety of low dose glucocorticoid treatment in rheumatoid arthritis: Published evidence and prospective trial data. *Annals of Rheumatic Diseases, 65*(3), 285–293.

DiPiro, J., Talbert, R., and Yee, G. (2005). *Pharmacotherapy: A pathophysiologic approach* (6th ed.). New York: McGraw-Hill.

Hardman, J., Limbird, L., and Gilman, A. (Eds.). (2001). *Goodman and Gilman's the pharmacologic basis of therapeutics* (10th ed.). New York: McGraw-Hill.

Lovas, K., and Husebye, E. (2005). Addison's disease. *The Lancet, 365* (9476), 2058–2061.

McCance, K., and Huether, S. (2002). *Pathophysiology: The biologic basis for disease in adults and children* (4th ed.). St. Louis: Mosby.

Nieman, L., and Ilias, I. (2005). Evaluation and treatment of Cushing's syndrome. *American Journal of Medicine, 118*(12), 1340–1346.

Nobel, J. (Ed.). (2001). *Textbook of Primary Care Medicine*, St. Louis: Mosby.

Schuff, K. (2003). Issues in the diagnosis of Cushing's syndrome for the primary care physician. *Primary Care, 30*(4), 791–799.

Sosino, N., Boscaro, M., and Fallo, F. (2005). Pharmacologic management of Cushing syndrome: New targets for therapy. *Treating Endocrinologist, 4*(2), 7–94.

Thomsen, A., Kvist, K., Anderson, P., et al. (2006). The risk of affective disorders in patients with adrenocortical insufficiency. *Psychoneuroendocrinology, 31*(5), 614–622.

ENDOCRINE

57

Androgens and Anabolic Steroids

Knowledge of androgens and their use for male reproductive disorders increased significantly during the 1930s. Androgenic substances were extracted from urine; also, testosterone was isolated from the testes, and its synthesis was accomplished. Additional study of the androgens noted two distinct actions: virilizing activity and protein anabolic activity. Current knowledge indicates an overlap in the actions of androgens and anabolic steroids; each drug group possesses some properties of the other group.

HYPOGONADISM

EPIDEMIOLOGY AND ETIOLOGY

Hypogonadism is commonly seen in primary care in both males and females (see also Chapter 58). Hypogonadism is caused by deficient secretion of testosterone by the testes. Both primary and secondary hypogonadism occur in the pre-pubertal or postpubertal male. It generally has significant effects on the psychosocial as well as the physical well-being of the male patient. Hypogonadism, whether from a chromosomal, pituitary, or testicular disorder, involves the non–development or regression of secondary male characteristics along with a fragile libido and waning potency. It is classified as a disease of the testes themselves (primary hypogonadism), or as insufficient gonadotropin secretion by the pituitary (secondary hypogonadism). The distinction and the differential diagnosis between the two disorders are essential to the choice of drug therapy.

PATHOPHYSIOLOGY

Testicular function is primarily controlled by the gonadotropin hormones, *luteinizing hormone (LH)* and *follicle-stimulating hormone (FSH)*, which are secreted by the anterior pituitary gland (Fig. 57-1). LH binds to receptors on Leydig's cells to stimulate testosterone production. FSH binds to receptors on Sertoli's cells and is important in the initiation and quantitative maintenance of spermatogenesis.

Gonadotropin secretion by the pituitary relies on stimulation by *gonadotropin-releasing hormone (GnRH),* a protein produced by the hypothalamus that stimulates secretion of LH and FSH. Pulsatile secretion of GnRH and stimulation of the pituitary are necessary for normal gonadotropin secretion. The hypothalamic secretion of GnRH relies on activation and ongoing stimulation by the central nervous system (CNS).

Delayed Puberty

In delayed puberty, there is deficient or absent androgenic stimulation of undifferentiated embryonic tissues. It can be caused by deficient production of testicular steroids (congenital and acquired), insensitivity syndrome of target organs (e.g., receptor defects, 5α-reductase deficiency), deficient secretion of pituitary gonadotropin, deficient hypothalamic secretion of GnRH, hyperprolactinemia, or other unknown factors. Male secondary sexual characteristics and behavior, accelerated growth, and the initiation of spermatogenesis do not occur.

Postpubertal Hypogonadism

Postpubertal hypogonadism is classified as primary or secondary. In primary hypogonadism, defects in testicular response to gonadotropin release lead to decreased secretion of testosterone and, as a result of normal feedback mechanisms, high levels of circulating gonadotropins (Case Study: Androgens). In the absence of adequate testosterone levels, spermatogenesis is impaired.

Secondary postpubertal hypogonadism in an adult is the result of pituitary failure and is usually associated with complete destruction or removal of the pituitary gland. In this situation, gonadotropin levels are low because the feedback mechanism is inhibited. In the absence of adequate gonadotropin secretion, Leydig's cells are not stimulated to secrete

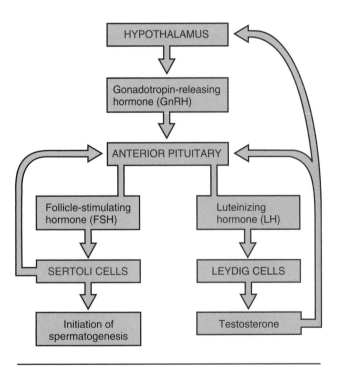

FIGURE 57-1 Feedback Mechanism for Testosterone. Testosterone production is dependent on an intact hypothalamus, pituitary gland, and Leydig's cells in the testis. Spermatogenesis requires both an intact pituitary gland and Sertoli's cell function. The two feedback loops influence continuous hormone production.

CASE STUDY   Androgens

ASSESSMENT

Patient History	AB is a 62-year-old male with vague complaints of decreased motivation and an inability to perform sexually for the last several months. He believes that his scrotum and penis have gotten smaller because of his age but wants verification.
Past Health History	AB denies history of cardiac, renal, hepatic, or prostate disease or carcinoma. No recent weight loss or gain. He exercises sporadically and takes no prescription or over-the-counter drugs. States he does not like taking drugs in general.
Life-Span Considerations	AB is married and given his age may be at risk for benign prostatic hypertrophy. Adult children live in the same community.
Psychosocial Considerations	Concerned about what he describes as symptoms of "aging." Reluctant to verbalize specific concerns about sexual performance, but states he feels like "less of a man." AB belongs to an HMO with pharmacy privileges. Income is derived from job in construction.
Physical Exam Findings	VSS. Decreased muscle mass relative to visit of 5 years ago. Relative atrophy of genitalia with loss of pubic and axillary hair. Prostate exam reveals 20- to 25-gram bilobular organ. Other systems exam unremarkable.
Diagnostic Testing	Electrolytes, liver function values, blood urea nitrogen, creatinine, lipid panel, hemoglobin WNL. Serum Ca^{++} levels, 8.5 mg/dL; testosterone, 220 mcg/mL; 24-hour urine LH, 25 international units/24 hr. FSH, 30 international units/24 hr.

DIAGNOSIS: Primary Hypogonadism

MANAGEMENT

Treatment Objectives	Restore sexual function, normalize behavior, and promote masculine and sexual characteristics.
Treatment Options	**Pharmacotherapy** • testosterone cypionate 100 mg IM every 2 to 4 weeks. Titrate to 400 mg IM monthly. **Patient Education** 1. Teach proper administration technique for IM testosterone cypionate into deep gluteal muscle. 2. Routine follow-up appointments, weight checks, and blood work for liver function tests because of the potential for hepatic damage and other adverse effects **Evaluation** Most men experience improvement in symptoms in 1 to 2 months after therapy is started. The efficacy of androgen replacement therapy is assessed primarily by monitoring the patient's clinical response.

CLINICAL REASONING ANALYSIS

Q1. How do you know that AB has a testicular hormone deficiency?
A. Along with his symptoms, AB's lab values reflect low testosterone levels and elevated LH and FSH levels.

Q2. Why would you choose testosterone cypionate in treating this patient over an oral testosterone such as fluoxymesterone?
A. Oral androgens generally have weaker therapeutic effect than injectable esters and are often more expensive. Testosterone cypionate has a greater efficacy, lower cost, and a longer duration. In addition, the patient dislikes taking drugs in general, and testosterone cypionate requires a less frequent dosing regimen than an oral testosterone.

Q3. What if AB dislikes IM injections? Is there another possible treatment for him?
A. We could offer AB a testosterone patch or gel, which he would apply once daily to upper arms, abdomen, or shoulders. We would need to caution him to properly dispose of either drug when changing his formulation so as not to expose others to the harmful effects of testosterone. In addition, oral testosterone formulations have a greater tendency for adverse effects compared with topical formulations.

Continued

ENDOCRINE

CASE STUDY   Androgens—Cont'd

Q4. What adverse effects are you talking about?
A. Female patients exposed to androgens should be monitored closely owing to the possibility of irreversible virilization. Clitoral enlargement may be noted, and there are alterations in metabolic and endocrine functioning including the development of hypercalcemia and facial hair growth, libido changes, a deepening of the voice, and menstrual irregularities.

Q5. Isn't AB at risk for benign prostatic hypertrophy? Would this alter your treatment choice?
A. Yes he is, given his age. However, because androgen use does increase the risk of BPH, we will proceed as planned but do so with caution and perform digital rectal exams and PSA levels more often.

testosterone, and sperm maturation is not promoted in Sertoli's cells.

Hypergonadotropic hypogonadism occurs as a result of testicular destruction (i.e., castration, radiation, mumps-related orchitis).

PHARMACOTHERAPEUTIC OPTIONS

Androgens
- fluoxymesterone (Halotestin, Android-F)
- methyltestosterone (Android, Oreton Methyl, Testred, Virilon)
- testosterone base (Andro, Histerone, Testamone, Testaqua, Testoject)
- testosterone cypionate (Andro-Cyp, Andronate, Depotest, Depo-Testosterone); ✦ Depotest, Everone
- testosterone enanthate (Delatest, Delatestryl, Testone LA, Andro L.A.)
- testosterone propionate (Testex)
- Transdermal testosterone (Androderm, Androgel, Testim, Testoderm)

▥ Indications

The primary use of the androgen testosterone, the prototype androgen, is in replacement therapy. In both delayed puberty and postpubertal primary and secondary hypogonadism, where the treatment goal is initiation and maintenance of spermatogenesis, other drugs are given along with the androgen therapy.

Another therapeutic use of testosterone is in secondary or tertiary hormonal treatment of advanced inoperable breast cancer in women who are 1 to 5 years postmenopause. Less common uses for testosterone and the 17 α-alkylated androgens (fluoxymesterone and methyltestosterone) are based on their ability to stimulate erythropoiesis by enhancing renal and extrarenal production of erythropoietin.

▥ Pharmacodynamics

Testosterone produces both androgenic and anabolic effects by binding to receptors in skeletal muscle, the prostate gland, and bone marrow. The binding of testosterone to receptors promotes the synthesis of specific messenger RNA molecules. In some tissues, testosterone is initially converted to dihydrotestosterone to permit binding with the androgen receptors. The hormone-receptor pairs also serve as models for production of specific proteins. The effects of testosterone are evidenced through these proteins.

▥ Pharmacokinetics

The pharmacokinetics of androgenic hormones vary with the individual drug. However, the onset of action of most

intramuscular (IM) formulations is slow, and their durations of action range from 1 to 3 days to 2 to 4 weeks (Table 57-1). The formulations are biotransformed in the liver and eliminated through the urine and the feces.

▥ Adverse Effects and Contraindications

Testosterone use can produce many adverse effects. The CNS effects include headache, anxiety, depression, sleeplessness, and excitement. Adverse cardiovascular effects include edema (with fluoxymesterone and methyltestosterone), polycythemia, and suppression of clotting factors II, V, VII, and X (with testosterone and fluoxymesterone). Bladder irritability, vaginitis, nausea, vomiting, gastric irritation, diarrhea, jaundice, hepatotoxicity, peliosis hepatitis, hepatic neoplasm, and cholestatic hepatitis (with methyltestosterone) have been documented. In prepubertal males, priapism (abnormal, continued, painful erection) and phallic enlargement have been seen. Premature epiphyseal closure, paresthesias, and acne may be noted in prepubertal males as well. Genitourinary adverse effects in postpubertal males include testicular atrophy, oligospermia, decreased ejaculatory volume, urinary hesitancy, epididymitis, impotence, and gynecomastia.

The adverse effects of androgens are often related to dosage and duration of administration. Male patients receiving androgens as replacement therapy are usually minimally affected. **Female patients taking androgens need to be monitored** ⓐ **closely owing to the possibility of irreversible virilization. Clitoral enlargement may be noted. Alterations in metabolic and endocrine functioning include the development of hypercalcemia and facial hair growth, libido changes, a deepening of the voice, and menstrual irregularities.**

Androgens are contraindicated for use in females during pregnancy (category X), in patients with serious cardiac, hepatic, or renal diseases, and in those with hypersensitivity to the drugs. Avoid using androgenic therapy in men with cancer of the breast or the prostate, and in patients who are hypersensitive to mercury compounds. It is not known whether androgens are excreted in breast milk.

▥ Drug Interactions

The effects of anticoagulants are increased when given in combination with androgens. The synthetic oral androgens exert stronger effects than testosterone (Table 57-2). Administration of imipramine with methyltestosterone may cause paranoia.

▥ Dosage Regimen

Testosterone is available as oral tablets, transdermal patches, gel formulations, and injectables. **The propionate,** ⓐ

PHARMACOKINETICS

TABLE 57-1 Androgens and Anabolic Steroids

Drug	Route	Onset	Peak	Duration	PB (%)	t½	BioA (%)
ANDROGENS							
fluoxymesterone	PO	Rapid	2 hr	UA	98	9–10 hr	UA
methyltestosterone	PO	Rapid	2 hr	UA	98	2.5–3.5 hr	UA
	Buccal	Rapid	1 hr	UA	98	UA	UA
testosterone	PO	Slow	UA	1–3 days	98	10–100 min	UA
	Patch	Rapid	2–4 hr	22–24 hr	98	10–100 min	UA
	Gel	Rapid	2 hr	1–5 days	98	10–100 min	UA
testosterone cypionate (LA)	IM	Slow	UA	2–4 wk	98	8 days	100
testosterone enanthate (LA)	IM	Slow	UA	2–4 wk	98	10–100 min	100
testosterone propionate (SA)	IM	Slow	UA	1–3 days	98	10–100 min	100
ANABOLIC STEROIDS							
danazol	PO	Rapid	2–8 hr	3–6 mo	98	24 hr	UA
nandrolone decanoate	IM	Slow	3–6 days	UA	98	6 days	100
oxandrolone	PO	Slow	UA	UA	98	0.5 hr; 9 hr*	97
oxymetholone	PO	Rapid	UA	UA	98	9 hr	95
ANTIANDROGENS							
bicalutamide	PO	UA	31.3 hr	UA	96	5.8 days	UA
flutamide	PO	UA	2 hr	UA	92–96	6 hr	UA
nilutamide	PO	Rapid	UA	UA	UA	40–60 hr	UA

*First-phase and second-phase half-lives, respectively.
BioA, Bioavailability; *IM,* intramuscular; *LA,* long-acting formulation; *PB,* protein binding; *PO,* by mouth; *SA,* short-acting formulation; *t½,* half-life; *UA,* unavailable.

cypionate, and enanthate esters of testosterone should not be confused; the drug formulations are not interchangeable. Because of the long durations of action of these drugs, their adverse effects cannot be quickly reversed by simply discontinuing the drug (Table 57-3).

▥ Lab Considerations

Androgen replacement therapy should provide normal physiologic serum testosterone levels as well as correction of the clinical manifestations of hypogonadism (Box 57-1). Testosterone levels should be in the midnormal range 1 week after the first testosterone injection and should exceed the lower limit of the normal range immediately before the next injection.

Because of androgens' potential for severe hepatic damage, periodic liver function tests are recommended. In patients receiving high dosages of androgens, regularly check hemoglobin and hematocrit levels to monitor for polycythemia. Serum cholesterol levels may increase during androgen therapy, particularly in patients with a history of coronary artery disease or myocardial infarction. Blood glucose and total serum thyroxine levels may decline. Increased creatinine and

DRUG INTERACTIONS

TABLE 57-2 Androgens and Anabolic Steroids

Drug	Interactive Drugs	Interaction(s)
ANDROGENS		
testosterone	Anticoagulants	Increases action of anticoagulants
methyltestosterone	imipramine	Paranoid response
Androgens	oxyphenbutazone	Increases serum levels of interactive agent
	Oral hypoglycemic agents, Insulins	Increases hypoglycemic response
ANABOLIC STEROIDS		
Anabolic steroids	Anticoagulants	Increases action of anticoagulants
	Sulfonylureas	Increases hypoglycemic effects
	Adrenal corticosteroid, ACTH	Increases edema formation
danazol	CYP 3A4 substrates	Potential for toxicity to danazol
ANTIANDROGENS		
flutamide	leuprolide	Synergism
	warfarin	Increases effects of warfarin
bicalutamide	warfarin	Possible increased effectiveness of interactive drug
	CYP 3A4 inducers	Decreases bicalutamide levels
	CYP 3A4 inhibitors	Increases bicalutamide levels
nilutamide	warfarin, theophylline, phenytoin	Possibly increases effectiveness of interactive drug
	Alcohol	Possible ethanol intolerance

ACTH, Adrenocorticotropic hormone.

ENDOCRINE

DOSAGE
TABLE 57-3 Androgens and Anabolic Steroids

Drug	Use(s)	Dosage	Implications	
ANDROGENS				
testosterone propionate	Androgen replacement	*Adult:* 10–25 mg IM 2–3 times weekly	**Do not confuse testosterone propionate, cypionate, and enanthate; each is a different formulation and has a different duration of action.**	⚠
	Delayed puberty	*Child:* 100 mg IM monthly for limited duration		
	Palliation of breast cancer in females	*Adult:* 50–100 mg IM 3 times weekly		
testosterone cypionate	Androgen replacement	*Adult:* 50–400 mg IM every 2–4 wk	**Adverse effects cannot be quickly reversed by stopping the drug because of its long duration of action.** For limited duration in delayed puberty	⚠
	Delayed puberty	*Child:* 50–200 mg IM every 2–4 wk		
	Palliation of breast cancer in females	*Adult:* 200–400 mg IM every 2–4 wk		
testosterone enanthate	Androgen replacement	*Adult:* 50–400 mg IM every 2–4 wk	**Adverse effects cannot be quickly reversed by stopping the drug because of its long duration of action.** Limit treatment duration to 4–6 mo.	⚠
	Delayed puberty	*Child:* 50–200 mg IM every 2–4 wk		
	Palliation of breast cancer in females	*Adult:* 200–400 mg IM every 2–4 wk		
testosterone patch	Androgen replacement	*Adult:* 1 patch daily (2.5–10 mg every day HS)	Discontinue after 6–8 wk if no results. For proper dosing, a morning serum testosterone level should be used.	
testosterone 1% gel	Androgen replacement	*Adult:* 5–10 grams gel every morning and titrate to response	Apply to dry intact skin of shoulders and/or abdomen and not directly to genitals.	
methyltestosterone	Hypogonadism; male climacteric and impotence	*Adult:* 10–50 mg PO daily	**Increases risk for hepatocellular carcinoma.**	⚠
	Delayed puberty (Testred)	*Child:* 10–25 mg PO daily	**Increases risk for hepatocellular carcinoma.** Give for maximum of 4–6 mo.	
	Postpubertal cryptorchidism	*Adult:* 30 mg PO daily in 3 divided doses	**Increases risk for hepatocellular carcinoma.**	
	Palliation of breast cancer in females	*Adult:* 50–200 mg PO daily –or– 25–100 mg buccal daily	**Increases risk for hepatocellular carcinoma.**	
fluoxymesterone	Replacement of endogenous testosterone	*Adult:* 5–20 mg PO daily in 3–4 divided doses	Monitor older adult male for evidence of prostatic hypertrophy and carcinoma.	
	Inoperable breast cancer in females	*Adult:* 10–40 mg PO daily in divided doses	Continue for 1 mo for subjective response; 2–3 mo for objective response.	
ANABOLIC STEROIDS				
danazol	Hereditary angioedema	*Adult:* 400–600 mg PO daily initially; then half dose every 1–3 mo	Titrate to lowest dose possible to prevent long-term adverse effects. For maintenance, use ADT or regimen of several days with drug followed by several days without drug.	
	Endometriosis	*Adult:* 100–200 mg PO twice daily for mild cases; 400 mg PO twice daily for moderate to severe cases	Treatment duration: 3–6 mo	
	Fibrocystic breast disease	*Adult:* 50–200 mg PO twice daily	Treatment duration: 2–6 mo	
oxymetholone	Anemias caused by deficient RBC production; acquired or congenital anemias; myelofibrosis; hypoplastic anemias due to myelotoxic drugs	*Adult:* 1–5 mg/kg PO daily	Treatment trial period: 3–6 mo; response not often immediate; continuous maintenance usually necessary with congenital aplastic anemia	
oxandrolone	Promote weight gain in medically related weight loss	*Adult:* 2.5 mg PO 2–4 times daily. Increase to 20 mg PO daily	A course of 2–4 wk is usually adequate, but it may be repeated.	
		Child: <0.1 mg/kg/day PO in divided doses 2–4 times daily		
nandrolone decanoate	Management of anemia in renal insufficiency	*Adult:* 50–100 mg IM weekly at 1- to 4-wk intervals for females; 50–200 mg IM weekly at 1- to 4-wk intervals for males	If possible, therapy should be intermittent.	
		Child 2–13 yr: 25–50 mg IM every 3–4 wk		
ANTIANDROGENS				
flutamide	Prostate cancer	*Adult:* 250 mg PO every 8 hr	Given in combination with luteinizing hormone	
bicalutamide	Prostate cancer	*Adult:* 50 mg PO daily		
nilutamide	Prostate cancer	*Adult:* Begin 300 mg PO daily on day of surgery; then decrease to 150 PO daily after 1 mo	Use in combination with surgical castration, with treatment beginning on day of or day after surgery.	

ADT, Alternate day therapy; *HS,* at bedtime; *IM,* intramuscular (route); *PO,* by mouth; *RBC,* red blood cell.

creatinine clearance values may last for 2 weeks after therapy is initiated.

In females with breast cancer receiving androgen therapy, frequently check urine and serum Ca^{++} levels, because androgens may induce hypercalcemia. Take care, however, to note whether a serum and/or urine Ca^{++} elevation is due to androgen therapy or to bony metastases.

Newer Androgens

Subcutaneously implanted testosterone pellets are available in the United States but have not been used extensively. The pellets are more commonly used in other countries. Two to six pellets containing 150 to 450 mg of testosterone are implanted, with the intent that testosterone levels will be within a normal range in 4 to 6 months. The need for a minor surgical procedure

---

BOX 57-1

Normal Hormone Levels

HORMONE	MALE	FEMALE
Follicle-stimulating hormone	2–18 million international units /mL	Follicular phase: 5–20 million international units /mL Peak midcycle: 30–50 million international units /mL Luteal phase: 5–15 million international units /mL Postmenopausal: >50 million international units /mL
Luteinizing hormone	2–18 million international units /mL	Basal: 5–22 million international units /mL Ovulation: 30–250 million international units /mL Postmenopausal: >30 million international units /mL
Testosterone (total plasma)	Adolescent (bound): <100 mcg/dL Adult (bound): 300–1100 mcg/dL Adult (unbound): 3–24 mcg/dL	(Bound): 215–90 mcg/dL (Unbound): 0.09–1.3 mcg/dL

---

to implant the pellets and the large number of pellets to be implanted have contributed to the unpopularity of this formulation. The rare possibility of pellet extrusion and the risk of local hematoma formation, inflammation, infection, and fibrosis have also contributed to its lack of use.

A longer-acting 17-β-hydroxyl testosterone ester, testosterone buciclate (20-Aet-1), has been developed and is in clinical trials. Another potent synthetic androgen, 7 α-methyl 19-nor-testosterone is under development in a depot formulation for androgen replacement and male contraception.

CLINICAL REASONING

Treatment Objectives

The treatment objectives for the adult male with primary hypogonadism is to restore sexual function, normalize behavior, and promote virilization. In males with delayed puberty, treatment interventions are directed at reestablishing and maintaining masculine characteristics and functions.

TREATMENT OPTIONS

▮ Patient Variables

The adult male with primary hypogonadism may first come to the health care provider with a history of infertility, reduced libido and potency, and alterations in behavior. Conditions that require androgen therapy require a sexual history for an accurate diagnosis. The patient may be reluctant to verbalize such intimate concerns. A teenage male with diminished secondary sex characteristics may be embarrassed to share such information. Further, at a time when an adolescent is striving for his or her own identity separate from that of the parents, in general, hypogonadism may increase parental involvement in the adolescent's life. Similarly, an adult male with decreased libido and impotence may have trouble expressing concerns, because the changes hypogonadism produces may be thought of as "normal" with increasing age.

Diagnostic studies are used to determine whether the suspected hypogonadal state exists because of a testicular, pituitary, or hypothalamic dysfunction. Evaluation and monitoring of hypogonadism consists of serum testosterone measurements. Testosterone levels fluctuate, generally being higher in the morning, so more than one assay may be necessary for evaluation. A low serum testosterone level is further evaluated in light of serum levels of LH and FSH. LH and FSH levels tend to be high in patients with primary hypogonadism but low or inappropriately normal in men with hypogonadotropic hypogonadism. Patients with low gonadotropin levels may undergo further evaluation for other pituitary abnormalities, such as hyperprolactinemia. The hemoglobin and hematocrit values may be slightly below the normal male range owing to hypogonadism. Obtain both urine and blood tests.

LIFE-SPAN CONSIDERATIONS

Pregnant and Nursing Women. Androgens and anabolic steroids are not used during pregnancy because of the teratogenic risk.

Children and Adolescents. Hypogonadism in the adolescent male is usually not diagnosed until the patient reaches 16 or 17 years of age, when delayed puberty can be ascertained. At that time, diagnostic testing consists of an endocrine evaluation to determine the specific cause of the dysfunction.

The adolescent male can benefit from androgen therapy; however, exercise caution since androgens accelerate epiphyseal closure and may affect linear growth. Perform x-ray studies of the epiphyseal area of the hand and wrist area on a regular basis, usually every 6 months, during androgen therapy.

Generally, in the male with delayed puberty, androgen therapy with testosterone is likely to be only one part of the drug regimen. Other drugs that may be used are luteinizing hormone–releasing hormone, human chorionic gonadotropin, and GnRH.

Older Adults. Administration of androgens increases the risk of prostatic hypertrophy and prostate cancer in elderly males. Furthermore, chronic disease is more common in older adults. Use caution when prescribing androgen therapy in the older adult with a history of liver, cardiac, or renal disease.

▮ Drug Variables

Injectable testosterone is available in short-acting aqueous solutions (e.g., Delatestryl) or long-acting solutions in oil (e.g., Depo-Testosterone). The short-acting solutions require more frequent administration, 2 to 3 times a week, and generally are not as readily available for use. The formulation of choice is usually a long-acting solution administered once or twice a month. The drug of choice for the hypogonadal adult male is either testosterone enanthate or testosterone cypionate because of the greater efficacy of these drugs, their lower cost, and their longer duration of action.

In general, the oral androgens (methyltestosterone and fluoxymesterone) have weaker therapeutic effects than injectable testosterone esters. Part of the reason for their lower efficacy is their biotransformation in the liver. In addition, oral, sublingual, and buccal formulations cost more than IM forms and carry a higher risk for adverse effects; the buccal and sublingual preparations have a bitter taste, as well.

Patient Education

Topical formulations vary in their instructions for use. Be sure to instruct the patient as to the appropriate application of these drugs to maximize efficacy and minimize adverse effects.

Testoderm is applied to clean, intact, dry-shaved scrotal skin for optimal skin contact; avoid chemical hair removers. Testoderm TTS is applied to the arm, the back, or the upper buttock. Each patch is worn for 22 to 24 hours, and then a new patch is applied.

Androderm is applied to an area on the back, the abdomen, the upper arms, or the thighs that is intact, clean, and dry. Avoid bony prominences or oily, damaged, or irritated skin areas. Do not apply Androderm patches to the scrotum, or another area likely to sustain prolonged pressure while sitting or during sleep. Rotate the site with each application of Androderm, returning to the same site every 7 days. The patch need not be removed when showering or bathing, or during intercourse.

AndroGel and Testim, the transdermal gel formulations of testosterone, are applied to clean, dry, intact skin of the shoulder, the upper arms, or the buttocks. Do not apply AndroGel to the scrotum, or Testim to the abdomen. Wait 2 hours after application of Testim, or 5 to 6 hours after application of AndroGel, before showering or swimming, although such activities have minimal effect on the absorption of testosterone, if done infrequently. The application site should be covered with clothing after it has dried to avoid transferring testosterone to others.

If skin-to-skin contact with another is likely, wash the application site thoroughly with soap and water before the encounter. If accidental transfer to another person does occur, wash the contacted area with soap and water as soon as possible. Fire, flame, and smoking should be avoided during AndroGel use; the gel is flammable.

Owing to the virilizing and masculinizing effects of androgens, patients need a full understanding of the potential changes in secondary sex characteristics that may accompany therapy. Remain sensitive to the emotional responses of both male and female patients to therapy and encourage the patient to discuss the emotional responses to a changing body image with the health care provider. Monitor the changes that do occur, because some changes may necessitate a reduction in dosage or discontinuation of the drug.

Advise patients of the importance of follow-up supervision. Laboratory tests must be performed periodically to monitor response to therapy.

Patient education includes information about the possibility of fluid retention with both oral and IM testosterone formulations. Fluid retention makes it necessary for the patient to monitor body weight on a regular basis. Advise the patient to report a weight gain of more than 2 pounds/week. The patient may need instruction regarding dietary sodium restriction and/or the use of diuretics. Patients also must be taught that if a dose of an orally administered androgen is missed, the next dose should not be doubled to correct the omission.

Evaluation

The efficacy of androgen replacement therapy is assessed by monitoring the patient's clinical response. Although there is variability in response, most men experience an awakening of libido, resumption of sexual activity, and improved sense of well-being 1 to 2 months after androgen therapy is started. Whether therapy continues depends on the patient's symptoms.

HEREDITARY ANGIOEDEMA

In 1882, Sir William Osler described the features of hereditary angioedema (HAE) that occurred in five generations of a family. Osler observed abdominal pain and both cutaneous and laryngeal edema in one family. Concluding that the symptoms were all one disorder, he commented on its hereditary nature. It was determined in 1917 that HAE is an autosomal dominant trait. Not until 1962 was more definitive work performed on this disorder. It was determined at that time that HAE results from a deficiency in the inhibition of complement. The causative factor, a low level of C1 esterase inhibitor (C1 INH), was discovered in 1963.

EPIDEMIOLOGY AND ETIOLOGY

HAE accounts for only 2% of clinical angioedema. HAE occurs in 1 of 50,000 to 150,000 individuals, with men and women equally affected. All races are affected; bias is not reported in different ethnic groups. Half of those affected have had significant symptoms by 7 years of age, and two thirds by adolescence. Laryngeal edema results in a 15% to 33% mortality rate.

C1-INH deficiency first appears during childhood, although there have been a few patients reported with perinatal angioedema. Patients typically experience minor swelling that goes unnoticed; the severity increases at puberty. While HAE is a lifelong malady, some report that symptoms decline with age. Adults carrying the C1-INH gene mutation (5%) are ordinarily asymptomatic. Ordinarily, these adults are identified only after their children become symptomatic.

Trauma (especially dental trauma), anxiety, menstruation, use of certain drugs such as estrogen or angiotensin-converting enzyme (ACE) inhibitors, infection, exercise, alcohol consumption, and stress are precipitating factors for HAE attacks. Other less common disorders precipitating HAE attacks include systemic lupus erythematosus, glomerulonephritis, rheumatoid arthritis, thyroiditis, Sjögren's syndrome, and pernicious anemia. Patients with HAE who develop a *Helicobacter pylori* infection are more likely to exhibit more symptoms than those who remain uninfected.

PATHOPHYSIOLOGY

As an immune response is initiated, reactions are triggered that enhance or expand the patient's original response to an antigen (Ag). The complement system consists of a group of sequentially acting proteins, C1 through C9, in the globulin portion of serum. Two activating systems, called the classic and alternative pathways, lead to a final common pathway that operates in cell lysis and stimulates the release of inflammatory mediators. The classic pathway is usually activated by antigen-antibody (Ag-Ab) complexes, but C1, its first component, can also be activated by a variety of serum proteins.

C1 INH is one of a group of serum protease enzyme inhibitors. C1 INH is the initial mediator in the classic complement pathway and is a major inhibitor of several steps of the formation of bradykinin as well. The primary function of C1 INH is to act as a regulatory brake on the complement activation process. Other examples of serum protease enzyme inhibitors in this group are antithrombin III, alpha$_1$-antitrypsin, and angiotensinogen. The proteins react with and inactivate their target proteases. Activated C1 esterase is the target for which C1 INH is named.

HAE results from a genetic deficiency of functional C1 INH. A deficiency of this enzyme inhibitor allows unopposed activation of the first component of complement, with the subsequent breakdown of its two substrates, C2 and C4. With this deficiency, there is a local release of vasoactive peptides and greater vascular permeability.

There are two types of HAE; both have essentially the same phenotype. In type I HAE, which accounts for about 80% of all cases, there is a lack of production of C1 INH synthesis because of the faulty gene. Twenty percent of individuals with HAE have type 2, which involves normal production of nonfunctional C1 INH. Gene mapping found that the gene for C1 INH is on chromosome 11.

Lab findings associated with HAE include a low level of C4 in the presence of normal C1 and C3 levels, and a low level of C1 INH in about 80% to 85% of patients with HAE. A C4 evaluation is usually recommended as a simple screening test for HAE, and the diagnosis is confirmed by measurement of C1 INH levels. In 20% of patients, this inhibitor protein may be present in normal or even increased amounts, but its function is abnormal (type 2 HAE). A functional or qualitative C1 INH assay is imperative before type 2 HAE can be ruled out. The C4 level is decreased in both types of HAE.

PHARMACOTHERAPEUTIC OPTIONS

Anabolic Steroids

◆ danazol (Danocrine); ✢ danazol, Cyclomen, Ladogal
◆ nandrolone decanoate (Deca Durab, Durabolin, Kabolin)
◆ oxandrolone (Oxandrin)
◆ oxymetholone (Anadrol-50)

▥ Indications

There are several uses for anabolic steroids (attenuated androgens), including HAE, endometriosis, and fibrocystic breast disease. Less commonly, these drugs are used in palliation of metastatic breast cancer (without hypercalcemia) and for treatment of anemias caused by deficiencies in red blood cell production.

▥ Pharmacodynamics

Anabolic steroids, which resemble testosterone, promote anabolic (rather than catabolic) activity by blocking cortisol uptake in muscle and liver cells. Cortisol normally acts as a catabolic agent, but by blocking cortisol uptake in muscle cells, anabolic steroids reduce muscle breakdown and increase muscle mass. When cortisol uptake is blocked in liver cells, the action of cortisol on the body's stress response is affected. In addition, these drugs decrease plasma protein synthesis in the liver and enhance their effects by increasing the amount of free drug in the plasma. The mechanism of action of the anabolic steroids in HAE is still unclear, but they appear to raise C1 inhibitor activity and C4 serum concentrations by increasing the synthesis of C1 INH in the liver.

▥ Pharmacokinetics

Anabolic steroids vary in onset from slow to rapid (see Table 57-1). These drugs are widely distributed, biotransformed in the liver, and eliminated in the urine.

▥ Adverse Effects and Contraindications

Like the androgens, anabolic steroids have a number of adverse effects. Excitement, insomnia, habituation, and depression are manifestations of CNS involvement. Gastrointestinal (GI) and genitourinary adverse effects include nausea, vomiting, diarrhea, cholestatic jaundice, hepatic necrosis, hepatocellular neoplasms, peliosis hepatitis (with long-term therapy), and death.

Endocrine effects in prepubertal males include phallic enlargement and greater frequency of erections; in the postpubertal male, acne, inhibition of testicular function with oligospermia, gynecomastia, testicular atrophy, chronic priapism, epididymitis, bladder irritability, change in libido, and impotence may occur.

In females, hirsutism, acne, hoarseness or a deepening of the voice, clitoral enlargement, changes in libido, menstrual irregularities, and male-pattern baldness have been noted. Other adverse effects of anabolic steroids are fluid retention and edema. Patients with seizure disorders may note increased activity.

Anabolic steroids are contraindicated for use during pregnancy (category X) and in lactating females and in male patients with hormone-dependent cancers (breast or prostatic). Other contraindications to use include any use intended to enhance physical appearance or athletic performance (see Controversy box), as well as the presence of nephrosis or the nephrotic phase of nephritis; use is also contraindicated in females with breast cancer who have accompanying hypercalcemia. **Anabolic steroids are unacceptable for use in patients with osteoporosis or alcoholic hepatitis and are contraindicated for use in patients with severe cardiac or hepatic disease.**

▥ Drug Interactions

The concurrent use of anticoagulants and anabolic steroids may potentiate anticoagulant activity (see Table 57-2). The hypoglycemic action of sulfonylureas increases when taken in conjunction with anabolic steroids. Administration of the anabolic steroids with an adrenal steroid adrenocorticotropic hormone may exacerbate edema.

▥ Dosage Regimen

Dosage regimens for patients taking anabolic steroids for therapeutic reasons vary with the specific use (see Table 57-3). In most cases, intermittent therapy is desirable. Use the minimal effective dose of anabolic steroids because of potential adverse effects. To calculate the minimal effective dose, consider the patient's clinical response, and not strictly the levels of C4 and C1 INH. At times a patient's C4 and C1 INH levels are below normal, but the patient remains asymptomatic. Response to treatment is slow, often taking weeks to months before therapeutic efficacy is noted.

Controversy

Androgens and Anabolic Steroids: Not Just in Pro Sports

Jonathan J. Wolfe

The emergence of abuse patterns has led many states to classify steroids as controlled substances. This is a reasonable response to a class of drugs whose role in therapy is limited, but whose potential for abuse is high. It is a sad fact that those who divert androgens and anabolic steroids reap monstrous profits from willing users desirous of enhancing athletic prowess. Even more appalling is the choice by some coaches, who have been entrusted to develop athletic skill among adolescents and young adults, to suggest using these products as adjuncts to strength training. The scandal attached to such practices in former Soviet Block countries, related to their development of Olympic athletes, seems to have lost its ability to chasten current athletes and trainers worldwide.

Body builders and sculptors of both sexes are also susceptible to the temptation to use androgens and steroids. Human growth hormone has also sparked the interest of those seeking larger and more impressive stature. It seems an unproductive quest to challenge such trends in a society that reveres physique and an advertising industry that links physical attributes to the promotion of every sort of consumable product.

However, health care practitioners increasingly see the regrettable effects of these bad choices. The human skeleton was not designed to carry the mass of a 340-pound (155-kg) lineman. Knees and hips racked by arthritis are poor thirtieth-birthday presents. The cardiac damage brought on by bulk-up diets and the fluid retention attributable to steroid use shortens life and diminishes its quality. Concentration on physical development toward unattainable and artificial standards curses those who abuse this class of drugs as well as others who fast and purge to attain an unrealistically slender body. The abuse of physical conditioning with or without steroids is a public health issue.

CLINICAL REASONING

- Your local high school football team regularly fields junior and senior defensive linemen weighing over 240 pounds. You have known these boys as normal-sized junior high school students. What techniques may they be using under proper supervision to achieve such mass? Are these players likely to resist using anabolic steroids if a trainer or older student role model offers them?
- Androgenic steroids produce gynecomastia and testicular atrophy in a significant number of abusers. What further history should you elicit when examining a 17-year-old athlete before fall football camp, when you note that this 220-pound young man was normomastic a year ago but now presents with obvious gynecomastia? He denies using marijuana.
- You have been asked to make a presentation about the hazards of steroid abuse to a seventh-grade class at your local junior high school. Your information includes coverage of the drugs banned by the International Olympic Committee. One young man challenges you, asserting that he intends to become a professional ball player, adding: "You can't make it for college scholarships or in the pros if you aren't man enough to do whatever it takes to be the strongest and the fastest!"

Anabolic steroids are controlled substances, listed under Schedule III of the Controlled Substances Act. Although non–prescription sale of the drugs is illegal, they are readily available.

▥ Lab Considerations

Anabolic steroids may influence the results of lab tests. Lab values for bromosulphalein test and aspartate transaminase (AST), alanine transaminase (ALT), serum bilirubin, and alkaline phosphatase measurements may rise in the presence of anabolic steroids. Cholesterol levels and prothrombin times may increase because of suppression of clotting factors II, V, VII, and X. Low-density lipoprotein levels and uptake of triiodothyronine and thyroxine also increase. Creatinine and creatine excretion may also increase.

Lab values that may decrease in the presence of anabolic steroids are serum high-density lipoprotein and protein-bound iodine levels, thyroxine-binding capacity, and radioactive iodine uptake. Free thyroxine levels remain normal. Other laboratory tests whose results are altered by anabolic steroid therapy are the metyrapone test (serum, plasma, or urine cortisol) and glucose tolerance tests.

For more information, see the Evolve Resources Bonus Content "Influence of Selected Drugs on Laboratory Values," found at http://evolve.elsevier.com/Gutierrez/pharmacotherapeutics.

CLINICAL REASONING

Treatment Objectives

The primary treatment objective in HAE is to decrease the frequency and severity of attacks.

Treatment Options

▥ Patient Variables

The clinical history of the patient with HAE varies greatly, making a diagnosis difficult. Diagnosis of HAE is suspected if there is a positive family history of the disease (Case Study: Hereditary Angioedema). Other support for the diagnosis includes a history of attacks of swelling and unexplained abdominal colic. A patient's age at the time of the initial attack is of little help in making the diagnosis. In most patients, the initial episode occurred in early childhood; however, a few patients with HAE have their first attack between the ages of 50 and 70 years. Some patients have weekly attacks, whereas others have occasional attacks spread over several decades.

During an acute attack, the patient exhibits facial and/or extremity swelling. Occasionally, abdominal palpation reveals a tender abdomen with crampy pain, accompanied by watery diarrhea. In extreme cases, partial to complete airway obstruction can occur.

The most important patient variables involve the past and present health history of the patient. A past medical history of cardiac, renal, or hepatic disease demands much caution in prescribing anabolic steroids. Give serious consideration to the risk-benefit ratio. Patients with diabetes who are receiving anabolic steroids may find that their blood glucose levels are decreased, thereby necessitating a reduction in their insulin or oral hypoglycemic dose, or a change in diet.

Life-Span Considerations

Pregnant and Nursing Women. Anabolic steroids are not used during pregnancy because of the teratogenic risk. Clitoral hypertrophy and fused labia have been noted in fetuses exposed to danazol.

CASE STUDY Anabolic Steroids

ASSESSMENT

History of Present Illness	JK, a 30-year-old female, reports swelling of her extremities, lips, and periorbital area. This attack of swelling has lasted 2 days. Several months ago, she had a similar episode that lasted for "several" days and included abdominal cramping and diarrhea.
Past Health History	Unremarkable. JK reports that she remembers her maternal aunts having occasional swelling of the face. She takes no drugs at present time but has documented history of compliance with drug therapy.
Life-Span Considerations	JK never married but is raising her sister's children.
Psychosocial Considerations	Patient expresses normal concerns about the unknown. JK's income is "satisfactory for my needs," although she does not have pharmacy insurance.
Physical Exam Findings	VSS. Physical exam unremarkable except for obvious edema of periorbital region and arms, with mild swelling in lower extremities.
Diagnostic Testing	Routine blood work WNL. hCG negative. C4 complement level, 8 mg/dL (normal: 10–30 mg/dL). C1 INH level, 4 mg/dL (normal: 8–24 mg/dL).

DIAGNOSIS: Hereditary angioedema

MANAGEMENT

Treatment Objectives	Decrease the frequency and severity of attacks.
Treatment Options	**Pharmacotherapy** • danazol 400 to 600 mg PO daily **Patient Education** 1. Explain to JK that treatment with danazol is prophylactic and that, although she may still experience attacks, the goal is to limit their frequency and severity and to reduce virilization symptoms as much as possible. 2. Inform JK of the potential adverse effects associated with danazol and that regular medical follow-up is essential to check lab work and monitor weight. **Evaluation** The effectiveness of danazol for the JK's treatment of HAE is evidenced by a reduction in the frequency and severity of attacks.

CLINICAL REASONING ANALYSIS

Q1. When a patient is taking danazol, why is it important to halve the dose after response is achieved?

A. It is imperative to titrate to the lowest effective dose possible to prevent long-term adverse effects. For maintenance, the patient can use an alternate-day dosing regimen to lower risks.

Q2. Don't we have to counsel JK on the importance of contraception while taking danazol?

A. Yes, absolutely. Anabolic steroids are not used during pregnancy because of the teratogenic risk. Danazol is a pregnancy category X drug, and JK must be cautious if sexually active while taking it. We need to do a pregnancy test before starting her on the drug.

Q3. Though JK has a history of adherence with medication regimes, why is it important to thoroughly discuss the potential adverse effects of danazol?

A. Adherence to a drug regimen is important in the prevention of hereditary angioedema. However, the masculinizing and virilizing effects of anabolic steroid therapy can lead to nonadherence. It is important for the health care provider to explain to JK the potential for changes in secondary sex characteristics, and to encourage her to report such changes since a reduction in drug dosage or discontinuation might be required.

ENDOCRINE

Danazol was originally developed as a drug for the treatment of endometriosis. Pregnancy has a suppressive effect on endometriosis, however, so it is unlikely that a pregnant woman would be taking danazol for this indication. Furthermore, when the drug is administered, ovulation is usually suppressed. Because danazol may be effective in the treatment of immune thrombocytopenic purpura, classic hemophilia, and alpha$_1$-antitrypsin deficiency, it is conceivable that health care providers will encounter more patients who began taking this drug while unknowingly pregnant.

Children and Adolescents. The adverse effects of giving anabolic steroids to young children are not fully understood. The risk-benefit ratio needs to be evaluated carefully before anabolic steroids are prescribed. In children, anabolic steroids may accelerate epiphyseal maturation out of proportion to the rate of linear growth, thus compromising adult height. The potential therapeutic benefit of anabolic steroids should offset the risk of premature epiphyseal closure. The drug effects may continue for up to 6 months after the drug has been discontinued.

Older Adults. Older adults often have hypertension and other cardiovascular disorders that may be aggravated by the sodium and water retention associated with anabolic steroids. In men, the drugs may increase prostate size and interfere with urination, raise the risk of prostate cancer, and cause excessive sexual stimulation and priapism.

Adherence to a drug regimen is important in prevention or control of any disease process. In anabolic steroid therapy, the presence of masculinizing and virilizing adverse effects could lead to nonadherence. Although these adverse effects would be more tolerable for males, females might discontinue the drug if such effects occur. Patients may also have concerns with taking anabolic steroids because of an awareness of their reputation for abuse. The health care provider must be sensitive to the patient's concerns and explain the different uses of the drugs.

▥ Drug Variables

Prophylaxis is warranted for patients who have frequent and/or severe episodes of HAE. It is unnecessary to normalize the levels of C1 INH; danazol is given in dosages that prevent attacks. Anabolic steroids such as danazol are highly effective and have been reported to control symptoms of HAE in more than 90% of cases. The drugs have similar pharmacodynamics, pharmacokinetics, and adverse effects. The major complication of long-term use of androgenic steroids is hypertension. Hepatotoxicity and liver tumors are rare with the 17 α-alkylated androgens, but use them at the lowest effective dosage.

Aminocaproic acid or tranexamic acid, which are antifibrinolytic drugs, can also be used for prophylaxis, although they are not as effective as the androgenic drugs. Surgical procedures, especially dental work, require short-term prophylaxis, and C1 INH infusions can be administered by intravenous (IV) route 24 hours or less before the procedure. Alternatives such as antifibrinolytics or androgens can be used; however, they should be started 5 days before the procedure and continue for 2 days afterwards.

Treating the underlying cause of the HAE attack, such as *H. pylori* or another infectious agent, may lead to resolution of symptoms. Pay careful attention to drugs taken by the patient, such as contraceptives, hormone replacement therapy, or ACE inhibitors that may have contributed to an attack.

Patient Education

Regular medical supervision is essential for patients taking anabolic steroids. Periodic lab tests to monitor liver function, lipids, hemoglobin, and hematocrit are needed. Because anabolic steroids cause sodium, chloride, water, potassium, phosphate, and calcium imbalances, monitor electrolytes closely. Advise patients to report ankle swelling or a weight gain of more than 2 lb/wk. Restriction of dietary sodium and/or the use of diuretics may be indicated.

Patients must be fully informed of the potential for changes in secondary sex characteristics when taking androgen or anabolic steroids. Monitor the changes that do occur, because certain changes necessitate a reduction in dosage or discontinuation of the drug. Remain sensitive to the emotional responses of both male and female patients to changes in body image. Patients must also be taught that if they miss a dose, they should not double up on the next dose, but should continue with the original dosage.

Evaluation

The effectiveness of anabolic steroids in the management of HAE is evidenced by reductions in frequency and severity of attacks. Comparing the frequency of attacks before and after a trial period of anabolic steroids is necessary.

Antiandrogens

◆ flutamide (Eulexin); ♣ Euflex
◆ bicalutamide (Casodex)
◆ nilutamide (Nilandron); ♣ Anandron

Antiandrogen drugs interfere with androgens at target tissues of the prostate gland, bone marrow, and skeletal muscle. These drugs are also discussed in Chapter 33.

Flutamide

Flutamide is a nonsteroidal antiandrogen used in combination with leuprolide, a synthetic luteinizing hormone–releasing hormone, for the treatment of prostate carcinoma. It acts by interfering with testosterone uptake in the nucleus or with testosterone activity in target tissues. It arrests tumor growth in androgen-sensitive tissues (i.e., prostate).

Table 57-1 identifies the pharmacokinetics; flutamide is rapidly and completely absorbed when taken by mouth, and its metabolites eliminated in the urine and the feces. ALT, AST, and alkaline phosphatase levels may be elevated in the presence of flutamide.

The most common adverse effects of flutamide are hot flashes, decreased libido, impotence, gynecomastia, diarrhea, nausea, and vomiting. The most serious adverse effect is drug-induced hepatitis. Flutamide is contraindicated for use in patients with hypersensitivity to the drug or hepatic disease, and during pregnancy.

Bicalutamide

Like flutamide, bicalutamide is a nonsteroidal antiandrogen agent. It is also used in the treatment of prostate cancer but in combination with leuprolide. It acts by binding to cytosol androgen in target tissues to competitively inhibit androgen actions.

Table 57-1 identifies the pharmacokinetics; briefly, bicalutamide is well absorbed taken by mouth, biotransformed in the liver, and eliminated in the urine and the feces. Use it with caution in patients also receiving anticoagulant therapy, because bicalutamide displaces the anticoagulant from its binding sites.

Blood urea nitrogen, creatinine, bilirubin, ALT, and AST levels may be elevated in the presence of bicalutamide.

The most common adverse effects of bicalutamide are similar to those of flutamide. Bicalutamide is contraindicated for use in patients with hypersensitivity and during pregnancy. Exercise caution when using it in patients with a history of renal or hepatic disease, in the older adult, and during lactation.

Nilutamide

Nilutamide is also a nonsteroidal antiandrogen used in combination with surgical castration for the treatment of metastatic prostate cancer. Nilutamide interacts with androgen receptors, blocking the effects of testosterone and preventing the normal androgenic response.

Table 57-1 identifies the pharmacokinetics; nilutamide is rapidly absorbed orally, extensively biotransformed in the liver, and eliminated in the urine and the feces. Nilutamide is contraindicated for use in patients with hypersensitivity and in patients with severe respiratory or hepatic impairment. Nilutamide has no indication for women, and its safety has not been determined for the pediatric population.

Common adverse effects of nilutamide include hot flashes, impotence, impaired adaptation to darkness, nausea, and hypertension. Severe reactions include hepatitis and interstitial pneumonia.

Nilutamide inhibits hepatic CYP450 enzymes responsible for biotransformation of many other drugs. Use it cautiously with drugs such as warfarin or theophylline.

KEY POINTS

- Hypogonadism is caused by a deficiency of testosterone secretion by the testes, whether a result of chromosomal, pituitary, or testicular disorders. It involves non–development or regression of the secondary male characteristics along with a fragile libido and waning potency.

- Hypogonadism is classified as primary (due to a disease in the testes) or secondary (due to insufficient gonadotropin secretion by the pituitary gland).

- The treatment objectives for the adult male with primary hypogonadism are to restore sexual function, normal behavior, and virilization.

- In males with delayed puberty, treatment interventions are directed at reestablishing and maintaining masculine characteristics and functions.

- Treatment options for the hypogonadal male include using oral androgens (fluoxymesterone or methyltestosterone) and IM solutions of testosterone enanthate and testosterone cypionate; topical and transdermal options are also available.

- Evaluation of the efficacy of androgen replacement is primarily based on the patient's clinical response and not strictly on serum testosterone levels.

- HAE is an autosomal dominant disorder that results from a genetic deficiency of functional C1 esterase inhibitor.

- C1 INH deficiency or dysfunction allows unopposed activation of the first component of the complement cascade, with the consequent breakdown of C2 and C4, allowing for local release of vasoactive peptides and greater vascular permeability.

- The objective of treatment for HAE is to decrease the frequency and severity of attacks.

- Anabolic steroids (i.e., danazol) are widely accepted in the long-term prevention of HAE attacks.

- Patients may require long-term therapy with anabolic steroids to decrease the symptoms of HAE.

- The effectiveness of anabolic steroids is evidenced by fewer and less severe attacks of HAE.

- Antiandrogen drugs interfere with androgens at target tissues of the prostate gland, bone marrow, and skeletal muscle.

- Flutamide is a nonsteroidal antiandrogen used in combination with leuprolide, a synthetic luteinizing hormone–releasing hormone, for the treatment of prostate carcinoma.

- Bicalutamide is a nonsteroidal antiandrogen used in the treatment of prostate cancer. It acts by binding to cytosol androgen in target tissues, thereby competitively inhibiting the action of androgens.

- Nilutamide is a nonsteroidal antiandrogen used in combination with surgical castration for the treatment of metastatic prostate cancer. Nilutamide interacts with androgen receptors, blocking the effects of testosterone and preventing the normal androgenic response.

Bibliography

Daskivich, T., and Oh, W. (2006). Recent progress in hormonal therapy for advanced prostate cancer. *Current Opinion in Urology, 16*(3), 173–178.

Fourcroy, J. (2006). Designer steroids: Past, present, and future. *Current Opinion in Endocrinology and Diabetes, 13*(3), 306–309.

Frank, M. (2005). Hereditary angioedema. *Current Opinion in Pediatrics, 17*(6), 686–689.

Khorram, O. (2001). Potential therapeutic effects of prescribed and over-the-counter androgens in women. *Clinical Obstetrics and Gynecology, 44*(4), 880–892.

T'Sjoen, G., and Kaufman, J. (2006). Androgen deficiency in aging men. *Current Opinion in Urology, 13*(3), 254–261.

Vermeulen, A. (2001). Androgen replacement therapy in the aging male: A critical evaluation. *The Journal of Clinical Endocrinology and Metabolism, 86*(6), 2380–2390.

ENDOCRINE

58

Hormonal Contraceptives and Related Drugs

Only in the last half of the twentieth century did it become acceptable to discuss issues related to the female reproductive cycle, such as conception and contraception, menstruation, and menopause. As knowledge of physiologic and pathophysiologic conditions has grown, so have the availability of treatment and management options. The management choices can become confusing, making an understanding necessary of the normal reproductive cycle as well as of the variations from normal.

Female hormones are administered in the clinical setting for both contraceptive and noncontraceptive purposes. Noncontraceptive uses of estrogens are the management of menopausal symptoms, prevention of osteoporosis, and palliative treatment of breast or prostatic cancer. Noncontraceptive uses of progestins include the treatment of amenorrhea, dysfunctional uterine bleeding, endometrial carcinoma, and endometriosis. Combinations of estrogens and progestins are used for contraception and for relief of menopausal symptoms.

MENSTRUAL CYCLE

The primary female reproductive organs, the ovaries, have two main functions. They secrete female sex hormones, and they develop and release ova. At birth, a female infant has 1 to 2 million egg cells. By puberty, approximately 300,000 to 400,000 inactive eggs remain. The process of ovulation begins after puberty, when the hypothalamic-pituitary-ovarian axis (HPO) is fully developed. During a woman's reproductive years, approximately 300 to 400 mature ova are released. The remainders fail to ovulate, and degenerate. The menstrual cycle occurs in two locations, the ovary and the endometrium.

OVULATORY RESPONSE

The ovulatory cycle is divided into three phases: the menstrual phase, the follicular phase, and the luteal phase (Fig. 58-1). The first day of menstrual bleeding is day 1 of the cycle. During the first 4 to 5 days, a large group of ovarian follicles begin to grow. The hypothalamus responds to low levels of estrogen and progesterone from the end of the previous cycle by producing *gonadotropin-releasing hormone (GnRH)*. GnRH is released in a pulsatile manner every 1 to 3 hours. Regular pulses of GnRH are important for regular cycling. Many menstrual disorders are related to abnormal GnRH pulsatility. GnRH travels to the anterior pituitary to stimulate the release of *follicle-stimulating hormone (FSH)*. As a result, the group of follicles continues to develop. One follicle becomes dominant as it matures over the next 8 to 12 days.

Granulosa cells in the dominant *graafian follicle* produce more estrogen and have more FSH and *luteinizing hormone (LH)* receptors than other follicles in the group. Through a negative feedback mechanism, estrogen reduces secretion of FSH from the anterior pituitary (Fig. 58-2).

The granulosa cells also produce *inhibin*, which suppresses FSH stimulation of other follicles. As a result, follicles with fewer FSH receptors fail to develop, and die. The dominant follicle also has theca cells that produce androgens in response to LH secretion from the pituitary.

By days 13 to 15 of the cycle, 1 to 2 days before ovulation, higher levels of estrogen stimulate LH release from the anterior pituitary, causing a sudden rise in LH. There are smaller increases in progesterone and inhibin at this time. The LH surge triggers the remaining events necessary for ovulation. Completion of the first meiotic division, along with production of prostaglandins and proteolytic enzymes, allows for rupture of the follicle and release of the ovum. The LH surge occurs approximately 34 to 36 hours before ovulation and lasts about 48 hours. As LH production peaks, estrogen levels drop.

Following ovulation, the ruptured ovarian follicle acquires additional LH receptors and becomes the *corpus luteum*. If fertilization occurs, the corpus luteum continues to produce large amounts of progesterone and lesser amounts of estrogen and androgens. If the ovum is not fertilized, the corpus luteum degenerates after approximately 14 days, and menstrual bleeding occurs. FSH levels again start to rise about 2 days before the menses begin, in response to decreased levels of progesterone and inhibin. Follicular development for the next cycle begins.

Estrogen is produced primarily in the ovaries and in lesser amounts by the adrenal cortex.

The most potent form of estrogen is 17β-estradiol. *Estradiol* is converted to the weaker estrogens estrone and estriol. Estradiol is synthesized from cholesterol or acetyl coenzyme A in the ovaries. During pregnancy, the placenta produces large quantities of estrogen.

Estrogen plays a key role in the development and maintenance of the female reproductive tract and the development of secondary sex characteristics. Estrogen increases the number and size of endometrial cells. Estrogens affect the release of pituitary hormones; cause capillary dilation, fluid retention, and protein anabolism; and inhibit ovulation. Estrogen stimulates increased secretion of angiotensin and thyroid-binding globulin. Estrogen inhibits the formation of comedones (blackheads) and acne. Endogenous estrogen lowers plasma cholesterol and inhibits atherosclerosis.

In the male, small amounts of testosterone are converted to estradiol and estrone by the testes. Additional estrogen is produced through enzymatic conversion of testosterone in peripheral tissues such as the liver, fat, and skeletal muscle.

Progesterone prepares the endometrium for implantation of a fertilized ovum. The target organs of progesterone are the uterus, the breast, and the brain. Progesterone is produced

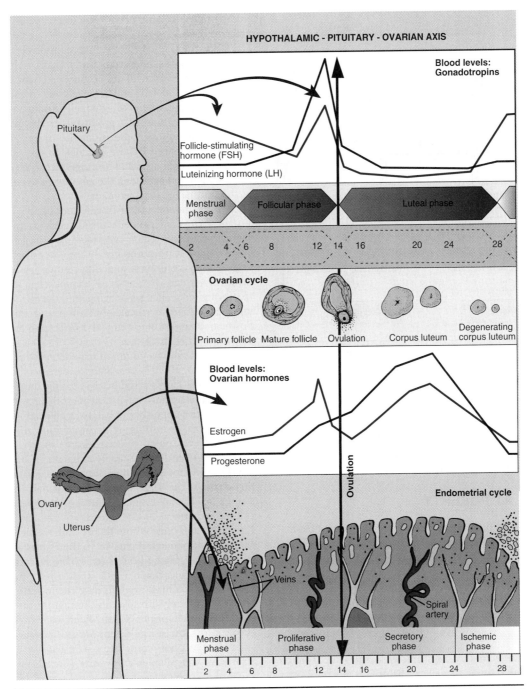

FIGURE 58-1 Hormonal Events During Menstrual Cycle. The female menstrual cycle is composed of an ovulatory response and an endometrial response, which is composed of a menstrual phase, a follicular phase, and a luteal phase. (Adapted from Nichols, F. H., and Zwelling, E. [1997]. Maternal-newborn nursing: Theory and practice, p. 193. Philadelphia: Saunders; data from Speroff, L., Glass, R., and Kase, N. [1994]. Clinical gynecologic endocrinology and infertility, 5th ed. Baltimore: Williams & Wilkins.)

largely by the corpus luteum (and in smaller amounts by the adrenal cortex) and is regulated by LH secretion from the anterior pituitary. If implantation takes place, the developing trophoblast produces its own luteotropic hormone *(human chorionic gonadotropin)*, which acts on the corpus luteum to promote continued progesterone secretion. Secretion of progesterone by the placenta during pregnancy is necessary for maintenance of the pregnancy.

ENDOMETRIAL RESPONSE

During the follicular phase of the menstrual cycle, estrogen produced by the developing follicle has a proliferative effect on the endometrium, increasing the number and size of endometrial cells. Following ovulation, progesterone produced by the corpus luteum suppresses follicular growth and initiates secretory changes in the endometrium. If implantation does

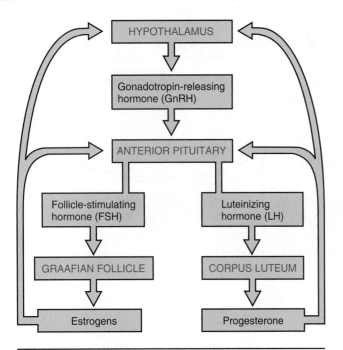

FIGURE 58-2 The hypothalamic-pituitary-ovarian (HPO) axis illustrates the pathways to the production of estrogen and progesterone with the feedback pathways identified.

not occur, the corpus luteum degenerates, and there is spasm of vessels in the endometrium. The endometrium becomes necrotic and starts to shed approximately 14 days after ovulation. The menstrual cycle thus begins anew.

CHANGES AT PUBERTY

Beginning in fetal life, the ovaries secrete low levels of estrogen. Estrogen secretion increases between the ages of 9 and 12 years, triggering sexual maturation. Puberty is complete with the first menstrual cycle, when the female is capable of sexual reproduction. As puberty begins, hypothalamic production of GnRH increases, as does secretion of LH and FSH from the anterior pituitary. As a result, the ovaries produce higher levels of the sex hormones, estrogen, progesterone, and androgen.

Genitalia and secondary sex characteristics develop, such as the breasts and pubic and axillary hair. The sex hormones stimulate ovulation, leading to menstruation. Estrogens are responsible for the brisk growth of long bones during puberty. They also guide epiphyseal closure, thereby bringing linear growth to a halt.

CHANGES AT MENOPAUSE

Menopause is defined as the permanent cessation of menstruation caused by the gradual decrease and cessation of ovarian function due to aging. The ovaries no longer respond to pituitary gonadotropin hormone stimulation. Estrogen levels drop and FSH and LH levels rise. Women are post-menopausal when a year has elapsed since their last menstrual period. Menopause is reached by most women between the ages of 40 and 58 years, with an average age of 51 years. Changes

leading to menopause occur over several years before menses actually cease.

During the period before menses completely cease, the menstrual cycle may become erratic and irregular. Although fertility is reduced, a woman may still become pregnant during this *perimenopausal* period. FSH and LH levels both rise until a few years after menopause, when they gradually decline.

Some estrogen is still produced in the postmenopausal woman from sources other than the ovary. *Androstenedione,* produced primarily by the adrenal cortex, is converted to estrone. The conversion of androgens to estrogen is variable. Body weight and age affect the amount of circulating estrogen in the postmenopausal woman.

In early menopause, estrogen production is adequate to sustain estrogen-dependent tissues such as breasts, urethra, vagina, and vulva. Later, symptoms of estrogen loss develop. They include vasomotor instability ("hot flashes"), atrophic vaginal mucosa, dryness and dyspareunia, and stress incontinence or urinary frequency. Atrophic changes, in addition to other normal changes of aging, and the effects of childbearing may lead to cystocele formation and uterine prolapse. Postmenopausal women are at higher risk for osteoporosis and cardiovascular disease.

The hot flash is a common experience of postmenopausal women. Forty to 70% of women experience hot flashes, and 25% to 49% have episodes of sweating during menopause. Many women report intense heat, with or without perspiration, over the upper body. It lasts a relatively short time but can be most disturbing at night, waking the patient from sleep. However, not all hot flashes are caused by estrogen deficiency; measure FSH to verify. The origin of hot flashes is poorly understood, but they seem to originate in the hypothalamus. At the same time that a hot flash begins, there is a surge in LH and an increase in GnRH secretion.

Loss of bone density affects approximately 25 million Americans and causes more than 1 million fractures each year. The rate of bone loss is greatest in the 5 years after a woman's last menses. Lifetime bone loss is 35% of cortical bone and 50% of trabecular bone. White women have the highest rates of osteoporosis. Black women have the lowest rates. Vertebral bone is commonly affected, accounting for the dorsal kyphosis (Dowager's hump) seen in older women. In addition to estrogen loss, the risk of osteoporosis increases with smoking, the use of alcohol, corticosteroids, excessive exercise, eating disorders, and slender body size. Weight-bearing exercise and Ca^{++} supplementation plus the use of bisphosphonates (see Chapter 54) reduce this risk. Recent evidence has suggested that intake of calcium and vitamin D supplements do not help reduce the risk for osteoporosis. The minimum daily requirement for Ca^{++} according to the National Institutes of Health (NIH) is 1200 mg/day; however, the NIH consensus statement lists 1000 mg if the patient is taking estrogen, or 1500 mg if not taking estrogen.

Cardiovascular disease is the principal cause of death in the United States. During reproductive years, women have 3.5 times lower risk of developing coronary artery disease than men. The risk of cardiovascular disease doubles after menopause, and postmenopausal women are more likely to die after a heart attack. High low-density lipoprotein (LDL) and low high-density lipoprotein (HDL) cholesterol levels are correlated with a greater incidence of atherosclerosis.

MENSTRUAL CYCLE DISRUPTIONS

AMENORRHEA

Amenorrhea is the absence of menses. It is further classified as primary or secondary amenorrhea. Primary amenorrhea is the lack of menarche or secondary sex characteristics by age 14 years; the absence of menses by age 16.5 years; or no menses within 2 years after breast and pubic hair development. Underdevelopment or malformation of the reproductive organ caused by endocrine disturbances, genetic disorders (e.g., Turner's syndrome, ovarian dysgenesis with dwarfism), or central nervous system (CNS) dysfunction may cause primary amenorrhea.

Secondary amenorrhea is defined as the absence of menses for at least three consecutive cycles in a woman with previously regular cycles, or for 6 to 12 months in a woman who normally has irregular menses. Causes of secondary amenorrhea include pregnancy, lactation, menopause, stress, endocrine imbalances, tumors, weight abnormalities, excessive exercise, certain drugs, anatomic abnormalities, genetic factors, and previous surgery.

Polycystic ovarian syndrome (PCOS) is a common cause of *oligomenorrhea* (interval between menses exceeds 35 days, but is less than 3 months). It is characterized by chronic anovulation, hyperandrogenism, and high serum levels of LH. Patients with PCOS do not ovulate regularly, and their menses are irregular, heavy, and prolonged. Many, but not all patients, are obese, hirsute, subfertile, and have acne. Because of their anovulatory cycles and the prolonged endometrial stimulation, they are at long-term risk for endometrial cancer. They have lipid and insulin abnormalities that place them at higher risk for coronary artery disease and diabetes mellitus.

DYSMENORRHEA

Dysmenorrhea is painful menstruation, and it affects a large number of women of childbearing age. The pain may radiate to the back, the sacrum, and/or the inner thighs. Nausea, vomiting, diarrhea, headache, weakness, and fainting can accompany it. Dysmenorrhea is classified as primary or secondary. Primary dysmenorrhea usually begins shortly after menarche. It is associated with ovulatory cycles, and occurs in the absence of pelvic disease. Excessive prostaglandin is produced in the endometrium, causing forceful uterine contractions. Secondary dysmenorrhea usually has a physical cause. It can be accompanied by dyspareunia and pelvic pain not associated with menses. Endometriosis, adenomyosis, fibroids, and adhesions are common causes. Diagnostic laparoscopy is often necessary to establish the cause.

PREMENSTRUAL SYNDROME

Premenstrual syndrome (PMS) is the cyclic presence of signs and symptoms before onset of menses followed by a symptom-free interval. Symptoms can include depression, irritability, anxiety, breast tenderness, abdominal bloating, appetite changes, and fluid retention. It is common: approximately 20% to 30% of women complain of moderate to severe PMS. The definition and diagnosis of premenstrual syndrome

depend on the timing and the cyclic nature of symptoms rather than on specific clinical manifestations. Symptoms appear during the late luteal phase and subside with the onset of menses. The cause is unknown but is suspected to be multifactorial.

ABNORMAL UTERINE BLEEDING

Abnormal uterine bleeding (AUB) is defined as menstrual cycles that are excessive in frequency, duration, or amount of flow. Normal cycles occur at 21- to 35-day intervals, are of 4 to 6 days' duration, and consist of approximately 20 to 80 mL of flow. Excessive bleeding with a normal cycle interval is termed *hypermenorrhea* or *menorrhagia*. Hypermenorrhea is blood loss in excess of 80 mL. *Menorrhagia* is bleeding that lasts for more than 7 days. *Polymenorrhea* is bleeding at intervals of less than 21 days. Excessive bleeding with an irregular cycle is termed *metrorrhagia* or *menometrorrhagia*. Metrorrhagia is irregular, frequent bleeding. Menometrorrhagia is irregular, prolonged bleeding. Intermenstrual bleeding is bleeding between the regular cycles. Bleeding after intercourse is referred to as postcoital bleeding.

Causes of AUB include complications of pregnancy, cervical or pelvic infection, polyps, endometriosis, fibroids, adenomyosis, endometrial hyperplasia, and cancer. Systemic disease such as thyroid dysfunction, blood dyscrasias, liver disease, and adrenal disorders can cause AUB. The use of hormonal contraceptives or intrauterine devices can also cause abnormal menstrual bleeding, as can trauma and foreign bodies.

Dysfunctional uterine bleeding (DUB) is a diagnosis of exclusion. It is abnormal uterine bleeding without a known or pathologic cause. It is further classified into anovulatory, the most common form, and ovulatory, which is less common. Anovulatory DUB is more common at the beginning and the end of the reproductive life span. For the first year after menarche, when the HPO axis is maturing, almost 55% of menstrual cycles are anovulatory. Irregular, sometimes excessive bleeding is caused by unopposed estrogen stimulation, inadequate production of progesterone, and excessive prostaglandin levels. During the perimenopausal period, as ovarian function declines, menstruation may become irregular.

Approximately 10% to 15% of cases of DUB are ovulatory. It occurs during the peak reproductive years and is due to prostaglandin imbalance.

PHARMACOTHERAPEUTIC OPTIONS

Estrogens

- ◆ conjugated estrogens (Premarin, Premphase, Prempro); ♣ C.E.S., Premarin
- ◆ conjugated estrogen A (Cenestin)
- ◆ ethinyl estradiol (Estinyl)
- ◆ esterified estrogens (Estratest, Menest); ♣ Neo-Estrone
- ◆ estradiol (Activella, Alora, Climara, Eselim, Estrace, Estraderm, Estrasorb, Estring, Estrogel, Femring, Femtrace, Menostar, Prefest, Vagifem, Vivelle); ♣ Climara, Estrace, Estraderm, Estradot, Estring, Vivelle
- ◆ estradiol cypionate (DepGynogen, Depo-Estradiol, DepoGen)

◆ estradiol valerate (Delestrogen, Dioval, Duragen, Estradiol la, Estra-L 40, Gynogen LA, Valergen); ◆ Delestrogenestrone (Kestrone 5)
◆ estropipate (Ogen, Ortho-Est); ◆ Ogen

Indications

Estrogens are most commonly found in combined oral contraceptives (COCs) and in formulations used for hormone replacement therapy in postmenopausal women. Estrogen replacement therapy (ERT) is also used for primary ovarian failure and female hypogonadism. Estrogen is effective in the prevention of osteoporosis. Estrogen can be useful for treating acute, severe DUB. Estrogens may also be used in palliative therapy for advanced inoperable breast or prostate cancer.

MENOPAUSAL SYMPTOMS. Most menopausal women have hot flashes, but responses to estrogen deficiency and estrogen therapy may vary. For example, many menstruating but perimenopausal women have estrogen-responsive hot flashes. However, hot flashes that do not respond to estrogen therapy occur in 20% of naturally menopausal women and 10% of surgically menopausal women. In addition, the intensity, frequency, and duration of the hot flashes vary. Twenty percent of women have persistent hot flashes, lasting for up to 15 years post after menopause.

Hormone therapy has been used for 50 years for the relief of menopausal symptoms. It is very effective in reducing the frequency of hot flushes and night sweats, reducing the frequency of hot flushes by 75%. Vaginal estrogen cream effectively relieves the symptoms of vaginal atrophy. In the last 25 years, hormone therapy was thought to be beneficial in the prevention and management of chronic disease—cardiovascular disease, osteoporosis, dementia. However, recent research suggests that risks of estrogen therapy outweigh benefits. Estrogen increases the risk for venous thromboembolism, stroke, dementia, and gallbladder disease. Although once thought to protect against cardiovascular disease, estrogen did not reduce incidence of coronary heart disease (CHD) in the Women's Health Initiative study (Department of Health and Human Services, 2002). Estrogen alone used for less than 5 years appears to have little impact on breast cancer risk.

Currently, estrogen replacement is reserved for treatment of moderate to severe vasomotor symptoms, or for treatment of moderate to severe vulvar and/or vaginal atrophy with urinary symptoms, vaginal dryness, and dyspareunia in women without a uterus. Short-term use at the lowest dose possible is recommended.

OVARIAN FAILURE. Low estradiol levels characterize ovarian failure. Gonadotropin levels are high in women with primary ovarian failure. Secondary ovarian failure is due to hypothalamic dysfunction, and gonadotropin levels are normal or low. Premature ovarian failure occurs when a woman younger than 35 years is depleted of estrogen-producing follicles. The cause is unknown. There may be an accelerated loss of follicles because of genetics, autoimmune disease, severe infection, exposure to ionizing radiation, or exposure to chemotherapy drugs.

When estrogens are used to manage primary ovarian failure, cyclic estrogen replacement begun at the time of puberty stimulates normal female reproductive tract maturation. Genital structures grow to normal size, breasts develop, axillary and pubic hair grows, and the body assumes a feminine contour.

Bone growth and maturation are stimulated. After puberty, ovarian failure is treated by ovulation induction for patients desiring pregnancy or by combination estrogen-progestin hormone therapy to maintain bone density and to prevent genital atrophy.

OSTEOPOROSIS. Estrogen receptors exist in osteoblasts and osteoclasts, and estrogen has a direct effect on osteoblasts. Estrogen is a very effective treatment for the prevention of osteoporosis in women. It increases bone density, promotes Ca^{++} retention, reduces bone resorption and slows postmenopausal bone loss. Estrogen reduces the risk of hip fractures by 25% to 50%, vertebral fractures by 50% and reduces risk for other fractures as well when started within a few years of menopause. Estrogen therapy may be considered in women at high risk of fracture in the next 5 to 10 years if other treatments are contraindicated and cardiovascular risk is low. Weight-bearing exercise, dietary Ca^{++} intake of 1000 to 1500 mg per day, and vitamin D 400 to 800 units per day are also useful. (See Chapter 54 for further discussion.)

Pharmacodynamics

Fifty percent to 80% of endogenous estrogens bind with the sex hormone–binding globulin and albumin in the blood stream for distribution to target cells, where they combine with receptor proteins in the cell nucleus. The estrogen-receptor complex then interacts with DNA to produce RNA, which codes for proteins that influence cell function. The estrogen receptors are located in the hypothalamus, the pituitary gland, the female reproductive tract, and the breast.

Pharmacokinetics

Oral estrogen is completely and rapidly absorbed. Exogenously administered estrogen is added to the existing supply of estrogens produced by the body. The additive estrogen influences the synthesis of sex hormone–binding globulin, altering the availability of endogenous estrogen. The availability of endogenous estrogen is also influenced by the type of estrogen prescribed, the dosage, and the route of administration. Some estrogen is excreted in the bile and undergoes enterohepatic circulation.

Estrogen is also readily absorbed from skin and mucous membranes. Transdermal estrogen produces therapeutic serum levels of estradiol with lower levels of estrone; therefore smaller dosages are needed. Injectable depot formulations are absorbed over a period of weeks. Vaginal estrogen creams do not significantly increase serum levels of estrogens.

Adverse Effects and Contraindications

Common minor adverse effects of estrogen pharmacotherapy include nausea, headache, midcycle bleeding, breast tenderness and enlargement, abdominal bloating, and increased vaginal discharge. These adverse effects may be alleviated by reducing the dosage, changing to another formulation, or discontinuing the drug.

A serious potential complication of estrogen therapy is the development of endometrial carcinoma. In postmenopausal women with an intact uterus, estrogen therapy without the concurrent use of progestins causes endometrial hyperplasia, atypia, and a fourfold to fourteenfold increase in the risk of endometrial cancer. As dosage and duration of use increases, the risk rises. Approximately 10% of women with endometrial hyperplasia and a larger percentage with atypia develop cancer. The addition of a progestin for 10 to 14 days of the cycle decreases hyperplasia and lowers the incidence of endometrial cancer.

Estrogens are not thought to be carcinogenic, nor do they cause breast cancer. However, they do promote the growth of estrogen-receptive tumors. Rule out breast cancer before beginning estrogen therapy.

Estrogen enhances blood coagulability and is associated with increased risk for thromboembolic disease. The risk is dose related. Hypertension can develop or be aggravated by the estrogen content of oral contraceptives.

Estrogen causes increased amounts of cholesterol to collect in bile and contributes to stone formation. The incidence of gallbladder disease is 2 to 4 times higher in postmenopausal women taking estrogen. Estrogens can cause jaundice in patients with preexisting liver disease (cholestatic jaundice).

Estrogen is contraindicated for use during pregnancy; it increases the risk for congenital birth defects. Females exposed in utero to diethylstilbestrol (DES) have a higher risk for a rare form of cervical or vaginal cancer later in life. DES was used in the 1960s and 1970s to prevent miscarriage. The cancer appears most commonly around the age of 19 years. It may also have caused congenital heart defects and limb reductions. Testicular hypoplasia has developed in males exposed in utero to DES.

Other contraindications to the use of estrogen include undiagnosed vaginal bleeding, acute liver disease, thromboembolic disease, and endometrial or breast carcinoma. Exercise caution when using estrogens in women with migraine headaches or hypertension.

Drug Interactions

A number of drugs interact with estrogens; they are listed in Table 58-1. Anticonvulsants such as phenobarbital, phenytoin, topiramate, carbamazepine, and primidone induce liver enzymes that accelerate the hepatic biotransformation of estrogen, thus reducing its therapeutic effects. Rifampin and St. John's wort also have this effect. The effects of estrogen are enhanced in the presence of ascorbic acid. Estrogen reduces the effects of oral anticoagulants. In addition, glucose tolerance is reduced, and estrogens may decrease the effectiveness of antidiabetic drugs.

The hepatic biotransformation of other drugs can be decreased by estrogen, thus increasing therapeutic effects or causing toxicity. These substances include corticosteroids and tricyclic antidepressants. Concurrent administration of estrogen with macrolides, itraconazole, or ketoconazole increases estrogen serum levels and can result in adverse effects.

Dosage Regimens

When using estrogen for replacement therapy, prescribe the lowest effective dose for the shortest possible time. Determine the dosage and the route of estrogen administration on an individual basis according to the indication and the patient's circumstances. The risks and benefits of therapy should be thoroughly discussed. Lower-than-standard dosages may be equally effective and better tolerated, and generally have a better risk-benefit profile.

Exogenous estrogen can be administered orally, parenterally, transdermally, or intravaginally (Table 58-2). Lower-than-standard dosages include 0.3 mg oral conjugated estrogens, 0.25 to 0.5 mg oral micronized 17β-estradiol, and the 0.025-mg β-estradiol patch. The transdermal patch may have a lower risk for deep venous thrombosis than oral forms of estrogen. For women with an intact uterus, add a progestin (see following discussion on progestins).

For acute, severe DUB, 2.5 mg of conjugated estrogens once daily or 50 mcg of COCs 2 to 4 times a day for 1 or 2 days can stop the bleeding.

Lab Considerations

Estrogens have favorable effects on cholesterol levels: LDL is reduced, and HDL and triglycerides increase. Estrogen alters coagulation factors VII, VIII, IX, and X and impairs glucose tolerance. Estrogens can also decrease serum folate and pyridoxine. Estrogen increases thyroid-binding globulin, thus altering the results of some thyroid function tests. Estradiol blood levels lower than 20 pg/mL can be helpful in establishing the diagnosis of menopause. In menstruating women, estradiol levels fluctuate throughout the menstrual cycle.

Progestins

- levonorgestrel (Mirena, Plan B); ◆ Mirena, Plan B
- medroxyprogesterone acetate (Provera, Amen, Curretab, Cycrin, Depo-Provera, MPA); ◆ medroxyprogesterone, Provera

DRUG INTERACTIONS
TABLE 58-1 Hormonal Contraceptives

Drug	Interactive Drug(s)	Interaction
Estrogens	Acetaminophen, aspirin, Benzodiazepines, clofibrate, Oral anticoagulants, phenytoin, Sulfonylureas	Decreases effects of interactive drugs
	ampicillin, Barbiturates, carbamazepine, griseofulvin, phenytoin, rifampin, tetracycline	Accelerates elimination of hormone, thus reducing its effectiveness
	dantrolene	Increases risk of hepatic toxicity to dantrolene
	Nicotine	Increases risk of thromboembolic phenomena
	Ascorbic acid	Increases effects of estrogen
	Glucocorticoids (systemic)	Enhances antiinflammatory effects and possible toxicity
	Benzodiazepines, Beta blockers, caffeine, theophylline, Tricyclic antidepressants	Increases effectiveness of interactive drug and possible toxicity
PROGESTINS		
norethindrone	rifampin	Reduces plasma levels of progestin
medroxyprogesterone	aminoglutethimide	Decreases effects of interactive drug

ENDOCRINE

DOSAGE
TABLE **58-2** Hormonal Therapies

Drug	Use(s)	Dosage
ESTROGEN AND ESTROGEN DERIVATIVES		
conjugated estrogen	Menopausal symptoms	0.3–0.625 mg PO daily; cyclically 3 wk on, 1 wk off.
	DUB	2.5 mg PO every 4–6 hr for 14–21 days until bleeding stops –or– 25 mg PO or IV every 4 hr until bleeding stops
	Primary ovarian failure	1.25 mg PO daily
	Primary hypogonadism	0.3–0.625 mg PO daily; cyclically
	Atrophic vaginitis	0.5–2 grams vaginal cream daily; cyclically, 3 wk on, 1 wk off
	Osteoporosis prophylaxis	0.3 mg PO daily; cyclically
Synthetic conjugated estrogens, A	Menopause	0.625, 0.9, or 1.25 mg PO taken daily
	Vulvar and vaginal atrophy	0.3 mg PO daily
Synthetic conjugated estrogens, B	Menopause	0.625 mg PO daily
estrone	Female hypogonadism, primary ovarian failure, vasomotor symptoms	0.1–1 mg IM weekly in single or divided doses; cyclically
	Atrophic vaginitis	0.1–0.5 mg IM 2–3 times per wk; cyclically
estropipate	Vasomotor symptoms	0.625–6 mg PO daily; cyclically 3 wk on, 1 wk off
	Female hypogonadism, primary ovarian failure	1.5–9 mg PO daily for 3 wk; 7–10 days off; repeat cycle
	Osteoporosis prophylaxis	0.625 mg PO daily (days 1–25 of a 31-day cycle)
	Atrophic vaginitis	2–4 grams/day per vagina; cyclically
esterified estrogens	Female hypogonadism	2.5–7.5 mg PO daily in divided doses for 3 wk; 7–10 days off
	Vasomotor symptoms, atrophic vaginitis	0.3–1.25 mg PO daily for 3 wk; 7–10 days off, repeat
	Inoperable breast cancer	10 mg PO 3 times daily for 3 mo
	Primary ovarian failure	1.25 mg PO daily; cycle 3 wk on, 1 wk off
estradiol	Menopausal symptoms, female hypogonadism, primary ovarian failure	1–2 mg PO daily for 3 wk; 7–10 days off; repeat sequence
	Osteoporosis prophylaxis	0.5 mg PO daily 23 days on, 5 days off.
	Advanced breast cancer	10 mg PO 3 times daily
estradiol TD patch	Osteoporosis prevention	0.025–0.1 mg/day; change patch once-twice weekly; frequency varies by manufacturer
estradiol valerate	Atrophic vaginitis, female hypogonadism, primary ovarian failure, vasomotor symptoms	10–20 mg IM every 4 wk
estradiol cypionate	Vasomotor symptoms	1–5 mg IM every 3–4 wk
	Female hypogonadism	1.5–2 mg IM every mo
ethinyl estradiol	Vasomotor symptoms	0.02–0.05 mg PO daily for 3 wk; 7–10 days off; repeat
	Female hypogonadism	0.05 mg PO 3 times daily during first 2 wk of menstrual cycle, followed by 2 wk of progestin; continue for 3–6 months; then 2 mo off
	Breast cancer	1 mg PO 3 times daily
conjugated estrogen and medroxyprogesterone acetate	Menopausal symptoms	0.625 mg CEG/2.5 mg MPA PO daily –or– 0.625 mg CEG/5 mg MPA PO daily; 0.625 mg CEG daily for 14 days; then 0.625 mg CEG/5 mg MPA days 15–28.
ethinyl estradiol and norethindrone	Vasomotor symptoms, osteoporosis prophylaxis	1 mg estradiol/0.5 mg NE daily; 2.5 mcg EE/0.5 mg NE daily; 5 mcg EE/1.0 mg NE daily; 0.05 mg EE/0.14 mg NE; 0.05 mg EE/0.25 mg NE. Replace patch formulation twice weekly.
esterified estrogen and methyltestosterone	Menopausal symptoms not relieved by estrogen alone	0.625 mg estrogen/1.25 mg MTT PO daily –or– 1.25 mg estrogen/ 2.5 mg MTT PO daily; cyclically 3 wk on, 1 wk off
ethinyl estradiol and levonorgestrel patch	Osteoporosis prevention, vasomotor symptoms	0.045 mg EE/0.015 mg LNG patch. Apply weekly.
ethinyl estradiol and levonorgestrel	Postcoital contraception	Two tablets PO every 12 hr for 2 doses
estradiol and norgestimate	Vasomotor symptoms, osteoporosis prevention	1 mg EE/0.09 mg NGE. One pink tab daily for 3 days, one white tab daily for 3 days, repeat

PROGESTERONE FORMULATIONS		
hydroxyprogesterone caproate	Amenorrhea, DUB	375 mg IM every 4 wk; may be followed by cyclic estrogen therapy
levonorgestrel	Emergency contraception	One tablet PO every 12 hr for 2 doses
medroxyprogesterone acetate	Secondary amenorrhea	5–10 mg PO daily for 5–10 days; start at any time in cycle
	DUB	As above, start day 16 or 21 of cycle
megestrol acetate	Breast cancer	40 mg PO 4 times daily
	Endometrial cancer	40–320 mg PO in divided doses
norethindrone	Secondary amenorrhea, DUB	5–20 mg PO on days for 5–10 days second half of menstrual cycle
	Endometriosis	10 mg PO daily initially, then 30 mg PO daily for maintenance
norethindrone acetate	Secondary amenorrhea, DUB	2.5–10 mg PO daily for 5–10 days second half of menstrual cycle
	Endometriosis	5 mg PO daily for 2 wk. Increase by 2.5 mg/day every 2 wk until 15 mg/day is reached.
progesterone	Amenorrhea	5–10 mg IM daily for 6–8 days, 8–10 days before menstrual period
	DUB	5–10 mg IM daily for 6 days; start progesterone therapy after 2 wk of estrogen therapy
	ART	8% gel vaginally daily until 10–12 wk of gestation

ART, Assisted reproductive technology; *CEG,* conjugated estrogens; *DUB,* dysfunctional uterine bleeding; *EE,* ethinyl estradiol; *IM,* intramuscular (route); *IV,* intravenous (route); *MPA,* medroxyprogesterone acetate; *MTT,* methyltestosterone; *NE,* norethindrone; *PO,* by mouth; *TD,* transdermal.

- megestrol acetate (Megace); ◆ megestrol, Megace, Megace OS
- norethindrone (Micronor, Nor QD, Errin, Camila); ◆ Micronor
- progesterone (Crinone, Femotrone, Gesterol, Progestaject, Prometrium); ◆ Crinone
- norgestrel (Ovrette)

▌▌▌ *Indications*

Progestins as a class of hormones are used for treatment of DUB, amenorrhea, and endometriosis, and for habitual abortion and infertility. Progestins are also used as adjunct therapy in postmenopausal hormone replacement. Progestins have been used for acquired immunodeficiency syndrome (AIDS) wasting syndrome and as a palliative measure in recurrent or metastatic endometrial cancer. The primary use of progestins in contraception is discussed later in this chapter.

MENOPAUSAL SYMPTOMS. Progestin is added to estrogen regimens in the postmenopausal patient with an intact uterus to decrease risk for endometrial cancer. Continuous therapy is more protective than cyclic therapy. Combined estrogen-progestin therapy decreases risk for osteoporosis and fractures as well as for colorectal cancer after 4 to 5 years of use. However, when colorectal cancer is diagnosed in hormone therapy users, it is more advanced. The beneficial effects of estrogen in the prevention of osteoporosis are not reduced by the addition of a progestin.

However, the harmful effects of long-term estrogen-progestin therapy for menopausal symptoms are likely to exceed the chronic disease–prevention benefits. Combined estrogen-progestin therapy increases risk for breast cancer, venous thromboembolism, stroke, cardiovascular disease, cholecystitis, and dementia. Breast cancer risk is increased in women who use combined therapy for more than 5 years. When breast cancer is diagnosed in hormone users, it is more advanced. Estrogen-progestin therapy confers no benefit regarding CHD and may actually increase the risk.

ANOVULATORY DUB. Irregular cycles and episodes of prolonged bleeding without pathologic cause characterize anovulatory DUB. It is a diagnosis of exclusion. The bleeding is caused by unopposed estrogen stimulation of the endometrium, by progesterone priming of prostaglandins, and by excessive amounts of vasodilating prostaglandins. Progesterone can be used daily to suppress the endometrium, or given the last half of each cycle to regulate it.

SECONDARY AMENORRHEA. Progesterone is used in the assessment of the amenorrheic patient after exclusion of pregnancy and the measurement of thyroid-stimulating hormone (TSH) and prolactin. The progestational challenge evaluates the presence of endogenous estrogen, the patency of the uterus and the vagina, and responsiveness of the endometrium to hormone stimulation. If endogenous estrogen levels are adequate, treatment with a progestin for 7 to 10 days is followed by withdrawal bleeding when the progestin is discontinued. If no withdrawal bleeding occurs, it may be necessary to induce endometrial proliferation with an estrogen in addition to a progestin. Obtain FSH and LH levels to assess ovarian function. Cyclic progesterone therapy can be used to promote regular monthly flow for women with anovulatory cycles.

ENDOMETRIOSIS. Endometriosis is a disorder in which endometrial tissue is transplanted to location other than the uterus, usually in the peritoneum. It is a common cause of pelvic pain and infertility. It can be asymptomatic or can cause debilitating pelvic pain and infertility. The cause is unknown, but retrograde menstruation with reflux of endometrial tissue through the fallopian tubes is thought to be a contributing factor.

Continuous oral or parenteral progestin therapy is given to thin the endometrium and cause regression of tissue. Treatment is effective for pain, but not as effective at restoring fertility. Continuous use of monophasic oral contraceptives with no hormone-free intervals is also effective. Danazol, an androgenic hormone (see Chapter 57) has been used in the past, but high cost and significant adverse effects limit its use.

INFERTILITY AND HABITUAL ABORTION. Progesterone deficiency, or a luteal-phase defect, may account for some cases of habitual abortion. Progesterone vaginal gel can be given

ENDOCRINE

to support the pregnancy. Progestins have also been used after assisted reproductive technology (ART) to promote a successful pregnancy, particularly if a woman is known to have low levels of endogenous progesterone. Keep progestin doses low, and discontinue the drug when placental production of progestins becomes sufficient to support the pregnancy (approximately 12 weeks of gestation). Since progestin therapy poses a risk to the fetus for congenital anomalies, the risk-benefit ratio of therapy must be considered.

PREMENSTRUAL SYNDROME. Progesterone suppositories have been used in the past to relieve symptoms of premenstrual syndrome with mixed results. Selective serotonin reuptake inhibitors (SSRIs) are more effective and now are considered the mainstay of treatment.

ENDOMETRIAL AND BREAST CANCER. Progestins can be used as palliative therapy for advanced endometrial or breast cancer when other treatment options such as surgery, radiation, or chemotherapy are not indicated. Medroxyprogesterone acetate (MPA), megestrol acetate, or depot medroxyprogesterone (DMPA) may be used for recurrent endometrial cancer. They help with tumor regression and remission of the cancer. The average duration of response is 20 months. Several months of therapy may be needed before a clinical response is seen. Megestrol acetate is used for palliative therapy for women with advanced breast or endometrial cancer.

Pharmacodynamics

Progesterone is secreted by the corpus luteum during the last half of the menstrual cycle, after ovulation. It converts the endometrium from a proliferative state to a secretory one. Progesterone causes the endocervical gland secretions to become scant and viscous, whereas estrogen causes the secretions to become profuse and watery. Progesterone has antiestrogenic effects. It reduces the number of estrogen receptors in the endometrium and decreases uterine contractility. Progesterone increases the biotransformation of estradiol to weaker estrogens.

Pharmacokinetics

Oral progestins are rapidly absorbed from the GI tract. They are biotransformed in the liver, the endometrium, and the myometrium. The half-life of progesterone in the circulation is a few minutes. It is converted in the liver to pregnanediol, which is then eliminated through the kidneys. Small amounts of progestins are stored in adipose tissue, and the remainder is highly protein bound. Long-acting parenteral formulations can maintain effective serum concentrations for 3 to 6 months.

Adverse Effects and Contraindications

Progestins can cause headaches, bloating, and breast tenderness and have an adverse effect on lipid levels. The most common adverse effect of progestin therapy is breakthrough bleeding. Nausea, vomiting, fatigue, depression, and uterine cramps can also accompany therapy.

Progestins given during the first 4 months of pregnancy have been associated with genital abnormalities of both male and female fetuses. Congenital heart defects and limb reduction defects have also been observed. Advise women who become pregnant while taking progestins of the potential risks to the fetus.

Contraindications to the use of progestins are similar to those for estrogen and include thromboembolic disorders, liver disease, breast or genital tract cancer, undiagnosed vaginal bleeding, and cerebrovascular bleeding.

Drug Interactions

Rifampin induces hepatic microsomal enzymes that speed biotransformation and may reduce serum norethindrone levels.

Dosage Regimens

Progestins are available in oral, parenteral, and vaginal gel forms (see Table 58-2). Different progestins are not equipotent, and dosages cannot be compared; they also have varying degrees of estrogenic or androgenic activity.

Cyclic progestin therapy can be used in DUB to establish regular monthly menstrual cycles. Ten mg of medroxyprogesterone is given once daily for 10 days beginning on day 16 of the cycle. Withdrawal bleeding usually occurs 3 to 7 days after discontinuation of therapy. This cycle promotes a repeating pattern of endometrial proliferation following endometrial breakdown and menstruation. If DUB is acute and heavy, estrogen is the drug of choice. For women desiring contraception, oral contraceptives are useful.

Norethindrone acetate may be used in the management of endometriosis. Oral doses of 5 mg daily are used for 2 weeks, after which the dosage is increased in increments of 2.5 mg per day every 2 weeks until 15 mg per day is reached. Therapy may be continued for 6 to 9 months. Pelvic pain is relieved in most patients, but fertility returns in only about 20% to 40% of patients. Daily oral MPA or COCs can also be used.

Lab Considerations

Progesterone generally has opposite effects on the metabolism of lipids from those of estrogen. Progesterone decreases HDL and increases LDL levels, thereby potentially raising the risk of cardiovascular disease. The effect of progestins on lipoproteins appears to be dose related. A physiologic dose of progestins appears not to alter the favorable effects of estrogen on lipoproteins. Either a decrease or no significant change in HDL cholesterol can be seen with low doses of progesterone. Progestins also have been shown to increase insulin resistance.

Hormonal Contraceptives

Oral contraceptives are one of the most popular methods of reversible birth control in the United States; as a class of drugs, they are among the most common. Current estimates suggest that over 10 million women in the United States, and 60 million worldwide, take oral contraceptives. These safe, effective, oral COCs have been on the market for more than 45 years. COCs have an efficacy rate of 99% when used correctly.

Progestin-only contraceptive pills (POPs) or "minipills" are also available and are useful for women in whom use of estrogen is contraindicated, or who are lactating. They are slightly less effective than COCs, and adverse effects such as breakthrough bleeding can be troublesome.

Short-Acting Contraceptives
Indications

Noncontraceptive uses for COCs include treatment of DUB, endometriosis, and functional ovarian cysts. They have beneficial effects on dysmenorrhea, hirsutism, acne, and PMS. COC use prevents anemia, ovarian cysts, benign breast disease, and ovarian cancer. COC users have a lower risk for endometrial cancer, ovarian cancer, ectopic pregnancy, and uterine leiomyofibromas. Noncontraceptive benefits of progestin-only methods include relief of dysmenorrhea, prevention of anemia, and lower risk of ovarian and endometrial cancer.

COCs suppress endogenous androgen production and are useful in the treatment of polycystic ovarian syndrome for women desiring contraception. A pill with low androgenic progestin activity such as drospirenone or norgestimate is the best choice.

For patients with endometriosis, COCs are used continuously with no hormone-free interval to suppress the endometrium.

Pharmacodynamics

Hormonal contraceptives prevent pregnancy by inhibiting ovulation, altering the endometrium, and changing cervical mucus. Ovulation is inhibited by the suppression of FSH and LH. Both estrogen and progestin alter the endometrium, making implantation less likely. Progestins thicken cervical mucus, which hampers sperm transport.

Newer forms of progestins now available for use in COCs include desogestrel, norgestimate, and drospirenone. Desogestrel and norgestimate are biologically similar. Drospirenone is chemically similar to spironalactone. It has antiandrogenic and antimineralocorticoid activity. The newer progestins have fewer androgenic adverse effects (e.g., acne), and do not adversely affect the LDL profile.

Pharmacokinetics

Hormonal contraceptives are well absorbed following oral administration. The hormones are slowly released when the drug is used transdermally, parenterally, as a vaginal ring, or in an intrauterine device (IUD). The duration of action varies according to formulation.

Adverse Effects and Contraindications

Although COCs are generally safe, the risk for thromboembolic disease, stroke, or myocardial infarction is somewhat higher in some women. **Risk factors for serious complications from COC use include smoking, age greater than 50 years, obesity, history of hypertension or heart disease, hyperlipidemia, and severe diabetes mellitus.** Employ great caution and close medical follow-up when giving COCs to patients with hypertension, gallbladder disease, migraine headaches without focal neurologic signs, or hyperlipidemia, or those using drugs affecting liver enzymes (anticonvulsants, rifampin, and griseofulvin). Absolute and relative contraindications to use of COCs are listed in Box 58-1.

Oral contraceptive users are at higher risk for chlamydia cervicitis because the pill can cause cervical ectopy, a condition where the columnar cells that normally line the cervical canal are present at the cervical os, or opening of the cervix.

Breakthrough bleeding is common the first few cycles of COC use. It usually improves with continued use, typically within 3 months. If it persists, changing to another formulation is useful. Women taking COCs normally have shorter and lighter periods.

The estrogenic adverse effects from COCs include nausea, vomiting, breast tenderness and enlargement, hypertension, and migraine headaches. Progestins can cause appetite increase, weight gain, fatigue, and depression, and decreased libido can occur in connection with the progestin.

The progestins used in oral contraceptives vary in androgenic activity, depending on the type and the dose. Androgenic adverse effects include acne, hirsutism, oily skin, sebaceous cysts, and increased libido.

Drug Interactions

Certain drugs alter the biotransformation of oral contraceptives, making them less effective. Anticonvulsants, rifampin, griseofulvin, and some anti–human immunodeficiency virus (HIV) protease inhibitors induce CYP450 enzymes that cause breakdown of estrogen or progestins. Phenobarbital, phenytoin, topiramate, carbamazepine, and primidone are the anticonvulsants most likely to do this (see Table 58-1).

There have been anecdotal reports that some antibiotics may decrease contraceptive hormone absorption and decrease effectiveness, but there is no firm pharmacokinetic evidence to support this. Nevertheless, COC users may wish to use a back-up method when taking antibiotics. Serum levels of fluoroquinolones are decreased in oral contraceptive users.

COCs affect the pharmacokinetics of other drugs. They decrease clearance of corticosteroids, cyclosporine, selegiline, beta blockers, tricyclic antidepressants, and theophylline, leading to possible toxicity. COCs can either increase or decrease the clearance of benzodiazepines, depending on the specific drug. Atorvastatin increases estrogen and progestin levels when taken with COCs. Drospirenone interacts with potassium-sparing drugs such as angiotensin-converting enzyme inhibitors (ACEIs), angiotensin II–receptor blockers (ARBs II), and NSAIDs.

Dosage Regimens

Contraceptive pills are taken daily for 21 or 28 days. The extended hormonal contraceptive Seasonale is taken daily for 84 days, with 1 week reserved every 3 months for menses to occur. Transdermal patches are replaced weekly. NuvaRing is removed and replaced every 3 weeks. Intramuscular (IM) depot medroxyprogesterone is given every 3 months. The hormonal IUD Mirena is removed and replaced after 5 years; Progestasert is removed and replaced after 1 year.

COCs are available in monophasic, biphasic, and triphasic regimens. Table 58-3 lists various formulations. With *monophasic* regimens, the daily estrogen and progestin dosage remains constant throughout the cycle. In *biphasic* or *triphasic* regimens, estrogen and progestin dosages are variable. **There are no clinical advantages to using biphasic or triphasic COC regimens**. Progestin-only pills come in a single dose and are taken continuously with no hormone-free interval.

COCs therapy is usually started with a low-dosage pill containing 20 to 35 mcg of estrogen. Older preparations containing 50 mcg are not a first choice for contraception. The pills are taken sequentially for 21 days, followed by 7 days in which either no pill is taken or an inert or iron-containing pill is taken. Before pills are started, ensure that the patient is not pregnant. Perform a urine pregnancy test for women who do not have regular periods or are unreliable historians.

Hormonal contraceptives are also available as progestin-only minipills. Unlike COCs, they are started on day 1 of

BOX 58-1

Contraindications to Use of Contraceptives

Absolute Contraindications to Use of COCs

- Active thrombophlebitis or thromboembolic disorder
- Breast cancer history
- Cerebrovascular disease or stroke
- Diabetes mellitus over 20 years or with complications or cardiovascular risk factors
- Known thrombogenic disorders (factor V Leiden, protein S, protein C, antithrombin deficiency)
- Liver cancer; active liver disease
- Major surgery with prolonged immobilization
- Migraine headaches with focal neurologic signs, or in women older than 35 years
- Moderate or severe hypertension ($\geq$160/100)
- Myocardial infarction or coronary artery disease
- Personal or family history of thrombophlebitis or thromboembolic disorder
- Pregnancy, postpartum less than 21 days, lactation less than 6 weeks postpartum
- Severe hyperlipidemia
- Smoking in a patient older than 35 years
- Undiagnosed vaginal bleeding
- Valvular heart disease with thrombogenic complications

Relative Contraindications to Use of COCs

- Elective surgery
- Gallbladder disease
- Gestational diabetes
- Hypertension

- Hyperlipidemia
- Migraine headaches without focal neurologic signs or aura
- Mitral valve prolapse
- Seizure disorder
- Sickle cell disease
- Systemic lupus erythematosus
- Use of drugs affecting liver enzymes (anticonvulsants, rifampin, griseofulvin)

Absolute Contraindications to Use of Progestin-Only Contraceptives

- Active deep vein thrombosis or pulmonary embolism
- Benign or malignant liver tumors or active liver disease
- Current coronary heart disease
- Diabetes mellitus with complications
- Known or suspected breast cancer
- Pregnancy
- Stroke
- Undiagnosed genital bleeding

Relative Contraindications to Use of Progestin-Only Contraceptives

- Concomitant use of phenytoin, phenobarbital, carbamazepine, rifampin, primidone, griseofulvin
- History of cardiovascular disease
- Hypercholesterolemia
- Hypertension (BP $\geq$160/100)

BP, Blood pressure; *COCs,* combined oral contraceptives.

the menstrual cycle and are taken continuously thereafter. There is no hormone-free break between cycles.

▥ Lab Considerations

COCs may increase levels of clotting factors VII, VIII, IX, and X, prothrombin, fibrinogen, thyroid-binding globulin, protein-bound iodine, thyroxine, and phospholipids. The estrogen component in OCs increases HDL levels and decreases LDL levels. Triglycerides and platelet aggregation are increased. Total cholesterol and LDL levels are increased by progestins, whereas levels of triglycerides and HDL are decreased. The newer generation of progestins (desogestrel and norgestimate) raises levels of HDL while leaving LDL essentially unchanged. High-dose contraceptives can cause decreased glucose tolerance and increased insulin resistance.

Longer-Acting Contraceptives

- ◆ depot medroxyprogesterone acetate (Depo-Provera, DMPA); ◆ medroxyprogesterone, Depo-Provera
- ◆ estradiol cypionate–medroxyprogesterone (Lunelle)
- ◆ ethinyl estradiol–norelgestromin transdermal patch (Ortho Evra); ◆ Ortho-Evra
- ◆ estradiol–etonogestrel (NuvaRing)
- ◆ etonorgestrel (Implanon)
- ◆ Intrauterine devices (Mirena, Paragard Copper-T, Progestasert)

Longer-acting contraceptives come in a variety of formulations. The Ortho Evra transdermal patch and the NuvaRing (a

silastic vaginal ring) combine estrogen and progestin. In rare cases, NuvaRing can be expelled from the body without the woman's knowledge, often as a result of constipation. Occasionally the transdermal patch formulation will come off. Depo-Provera and the Mirena and Progestasert IUDs are progestin-only formulations. The ParaGard IUD contains copper as the active ingredient. Longer-acting contraceptives are convenient to use, especially for women who have difficulty remembering to take a pill daily. The progestin-only formulations are useful for women with contraindications to estrogen use.

Transdermal Formulations

The transdermal patch, Ortho Evra, contains estradiol and norelgestromin in a patch that releases hormone slowly over a week. The patch releases 60% more estrogen than a 35-mcg OC and may increase the risk for thromboemboli. The patch is changed weekly for 3 weeks, and then 1 week is left patch-free. The patch can be applied to the abdomen, the buttock, the upper outer arm, or the upper torso (but not the breasts). The adverse effects profile is similar to other COCs. **A black box warning was added in 2006 to Ortho Evra's package insert noting that cigarette smoking increases the risk of serious cardiovascular adverse effects (i.e., the risk increases with over 15 cigarettes per day, particularly in women over the age of 35 years).** A disadvantage is that the patch is visible. It is less effective in women weighing more than 198 lb. It takes 2 days after applying the patch to achieve therapeutic hormone levels. Local skin irritation can occur.

TABLE 58-3 Comparison of Contraceptive Formulations

Brand Name	Estrogen Component	Progestin Component	EE Activity	PG Activity	Androgen Activity	Endometrial Activity	BTB (%)*
COMBINATION HIGH-DOSE MONOPHASIC COCS							
Ogestrel, Ovral 0.5/50	50 mcg EE	0.5 mg NG	Hi	Hi	Hi	Int	4.5
Genora 1/50, Norinyl 1/50, Necon 1/50, Ortho-Novum 1/50, Nelova 1/50M, Norethin 1/50M	50 mcg MS	1 mg NE	Lo-Int	Int	Lo	Int-Hi	10.6
Norethin 1/50M, Ovcon-50	50 mcg EE	1 mg NE	Hi	Int	Int	Int	11.9
Demulen 1/50, Zovia 1/50	50 mcg EE	1 mg EA	Lo	Hi	Lo	Int	13.9
Norlestrin 2.5/50	50 mcg EE	2.5 mg NEA	Lo	Int	Hi	Int-Hi	8.7
COMBINATION LOW-DOSE MONOPHASIC COCS							
Alesse, Aviane, Lessina, Levlite	20 mcg EE	0.1 mg LNG	Int	Lo	Int	Int	UA
Loestrin-21 1/20, Loestrin 28 1/20, Microgestin Fe 1/20	20 mcg EE	1 mg NE	Lo	Int-Hi	Int-Hi	Int	29.7
Apri, Desogen, Ortho-Cept	30 mcg EE	0.15 mg DG	Int	Int-Hi	Lo	Lo-Int	9.9
Junel Fe 1.5/30, Loestrin Fe 1.5/30 Loestrin 21–1.5/30, Microgestin Fe 1.5/30	30 mcg EE	1.5 mg NE	Lo	Hi	Hi	Int	25.2
Loestrin Fe 1/20	30 mcg EE	1.5 mg NEA	Lo	Hi	Hi	Int	25.2
Levlen, Levora, Nordette, Portia	30 mcg EE	0.15 mg LNG	Lo-Int	Lo-Int	Int	Int	14.0
Cryselle, Lo-Ovral, Low-Ogestrel	30 mcg EE	0.3 mg NG	Lo-Int	Lo-Int	Int	Lo-Int	9.6
Brevicon, Genora 0.5/35, NEE 0.5/35, Nelova 0.5/35E, Necon 0.5/35	35 mcg EE	0.5 mg NE	Int-Hi	Lo	Lo	Int	14.6
Demulen 1/35, NEE 1/35, Nelova 1/35E, Norethin 1/35E, Zovia 1/35	35 mcg EE	1 mg EA	Int	Hi	Int	Hi	37.4
Genora 1/35, Norinyl 1 + 35, Ortho-Novum 1/35	35 mcg EE	1 mg NE	Int-Hi	Int	Int	Int	14.7
Mononessa, Ortho-Cyclen, Sprintec	35 mcg EE	0.25 mg NRG	Int-Hi	Lo	Lo	Lo-Int	14.3
Ovcon-35	35 mcg EE	0.4 mg NE	Int-Hi	Lo	Lo	Int	11.0
Yasmin 28	30 mcg EE	3 mg DRSP	Int	Int-Hi	Lo	Lo-Int	UA
Yaz	20 mcg EE	0.3 mg DRSP	Lo-Int	Int-Hi	Lo	Lo-Int	UA
COMBINATION BIPHASIC COCS							
Kariva, Mircette	20 mg EE	21 days 0.15 mg DG	Int-Hi	Low-Int	Lo	Lo	3.5
	10 mg EE	—					
NEE 10/11, Nelova 10/11, Ortho-Novum 10/11	35 mcg EE	10 days 0.5 mg NE	Int-Hi	Lo-Int	Int	Int	19.6
	35 mcg EE	11 days 1 mg NE					
Jenest-28	35 mcg EE	7 days 0.5 mg NE	Int-Hi	Lo	Int	Int	14.1
	35 mcg EE	14 days 1.0 mg NE					
COMBINATION TRIPHASIC COCS							
Ortho Tri-Cyclen Lo	25 mcg EE	1.8 mg NRG	Lo-Int	Lo	Lo	Int	17.5
	25 mcg EE	0.125 mg NRG					
	25 mcg EE	0.25 mg NRG					
Necon 777, Nortrel	35 mcg EE	7 days 0.5 mg NE	Hi	Lo-Int	Int	Int	12.2
	35 mcg EE	7 days 0.75 mg NE					
	35 mcg EE	7 days 1 mg NE					
Tri-Levlen, Triphasil, Trivora-28, Enpresse	30 mcg EE	6 days 0.05 mg LNG	Int	Lo	Int	Int	15.1
	40 mcg EE	5 days 0.075 mg LNG					
	30 mcg EE	10 days 0.125 mg LNG					
Ortho Tri-Cyclen Trinessa, Tri-Sprintec	35 mcg EE	7 days 0.18 mg NRG	Int-Hi	Lo	Lo	Int	17.5
	35 mcg EE	7 days 0.215 NRG					
	35 mcg EE	7 days 0.25 NR					
Tri-Norinyl	35 mcg EE	7 days 0.5 mg NE	Int-Hi	Int	Int	Int	14.7
	35 mcg EE	9 days 1 mg NE					
	35 mcg EE	5 days 0.5 mg NE					
Estrostep 21, Estrostep Fe	20 mcg EE	5 days 1 mg NE	Lo-Int	Int-Hi	Int	Int	UA
	30 mcg EE	7 days 1 mg NE					
	35 mcg EE	9 days 1 mg NE					
PROGESTIN-ONLY MINIPILLS							
Ovrette	None	0.075 mg NG	None	Lo	Hi	Lo	34.9
Camila, Errin, Jolivette, Micronor, Ortho Micronor, Nora-BE, Nor-QD	None	0.35 mg NE	Very lo	Lo	Hi	Lo	42.3

Continued

ENDOCRINE

TABLE 58-3 Comparison of Contraceptive Formulations—Cont'd

Brand Name	Estrogen Component	Progestin Component	EE Activity	PG Activity	Androgen Activity	Endometrial Activity	BTB (%)*
OTHER CONTRACEPTIVE FORMULATIONS							
Depo-Provera (IM)	—	150 mg/mL DMPA	NA	Lo-Int	Hi	Lo	UA
Mirena (IUD)	—	52 mg LNG (20 mcg/day)	NA	Lo	Hi	Lo	UA
NuvaRing (vaginal ring)	2.7 mg EE (15 mcg/24 hr)	11.7 mg NRGT (0.12 mg/24 hr)	Lo-Int	Lo	Lo	Int	UA
Ortho Evra (transdermal patch)†	0.75 mg EE (20 mcg/24 hr)	6 mg NRGT (1.5 mg/24 hr)	Int	Lo	Int	Int	UA
Plan B‡	—	0.75 mg LNG	NA	Hi	NA	NA	NA
Seasonale (extended oral regimen)	30 mcg EE	0.15 mg LNG	Lo-Int	Lo-Int	Int	Int	12

*Reported prevalence of spotting and breakthrough bleeding during third cycle of use. Information should not be precisely compared.
†In 2005, the FDA approved updated labeling for the Ortho Evra contraceptive patch to warn health care providers and patients that this product exposes women to higher levels of estrogen than most birth control pills.
‡Plan B is an emergency contraception pill—the "morning-after pill"—two tablets taken as soon as possible but within 72 hr; repeat in 12 hr.
BTB, Break through bleeding; COCs, combined oral contraceptives; DG, desogestrel; DMPA, depot medroxyprogesterone acetate; DRSP, drospirenone; EA, ethynodiol diacetate; EE, ethinyl estradiol; ET, etonogestrel; FDA, Food and Drug Administration; IM, intramuscular; IUD, intrauterine device; LNG, levonorgestrel; MPA, medroxyprogesterone acetate; MS, megestrol; MTT, methyltestosterone; NA, not applicable; NE, norethindrone; NEA, norethindrone acetate; NG, norgestrel; NRG, norgestimate; NRGT, norelgestromin; PG, progestin; UA, unavailable.
Data extracted from Dickey, R. (2004). *Managing contraceptive pill patients* (12th ed.). Durant, OK: Essential Medical Information Systems; and *Mosby's Drug Consult*. (2006). St. Louis: Mosby.

The vaginal contraceptive ring, NuvaRing, is a flexible, silastic (non–latex) ring that slowly releases estradiol and etonorgestrel. The ring is inserted into the vagina and left in place for 3 weeks. One week after removal, a new ring is inserted. NuvaRing can be used in a "tri-cycle" plan—"in" for three cycles, "out" for one—resulting in the user only having three to four periods per year. The ring is not removed for intercourse. Withdrawal bleeding can continue beyond the ring-free period.

Implantable Progestin

The only implantable progestin available in the United States is Implanon. Implanon is a single, small, flexible rod that is inserted subdermally, usually in the upper arm. It contains the progestin and etonorgestrel, which is slowly released and provides effective contraception for up to 3 years. Eight hours after insertion, progestin levels are high enough to inhibit ovulation.

Implanon is a safe, highly effective, continuous method of long-term contraception. It is useful for women unable to use estrogen-containing preparations, or who have difficulty remembering to take a pill every day. Implanon can be used during breastfeeding and can be inserted immediately postpartum. Its effectiveness is not affected by body weight. Implanon is an excellent choice of contraception for obese women.

Compared to its predecessor, Norplant, Implanon is more effective and has fewer adverse effects. Hormone levels are less variable, and there is less irregular bleeding. Ovarian cysts are less common than with Norplant. Implanon is easier to insert and to remove. Fertility returns promptly after the rod is removed. Ovulation usually occurs within a month.

Implanon does not have any important clinical effects on lipoprotein profile or carbohydrate metabolism. It does not affect thyroid, adrenal, or liver function, nor does it affect clotting mechanisms. It does not have an adverse effect on bone density.

The most common adverse effects are irregular bleeding and amenorrhea due to constant low level progestin levels. Bleeding is less frequent and lighter compared with Norplant. Amenorrhea occurs in approximately 20% of users in the first year, and in about 30% to 40% of users after 1 year.

Injectable Contraceptives

Two injectable contraceptives have been formulated. Lunelle is a combination of estradiol cypionate and medroxyprogesterone that is given intramuscularly every 28 days. It is not yet available in the United States. The dosage of Lunelle is 0.5 mg given intramuscularly. The adverse effects profile is similar to that of the COCs. The initial dose should be within the first 5 days of onset of normal menses. The first period usually comes 2 to 3 weeks after the first injection, and there may be increased breakthrough bleeding the first month of use. Monthly injections may be inconvenient. Weight gain is the most common reason for discontinuation. The average weight gain is 2 to 6 lb.

DMPA is a progestin-only drug and is given intramuscularly every 3 months. Serum levels adequate to achieve contraception are obtained within 24 hours of injection and are maintained for at least 14 weeks. DMPA has no estrogenic or androgenic effects.

DMPA is convenient and reliable as long as the patient is conscientious about getting it every 3 months. It is useful for patients with contraindications to estrogen use, and for patients who have difficulty taking a pill every day. It can be used with anticonvulsants and has few significant drug interactions. In fact, DMPA is advantageous for women with seizures since it raises the seizure threshold. DMPA decreases menstrual flow significantly; 50% of women become amenorrheic after the first year of use. DMPA can be given postpartum and increases the quantity of breast milk in lactating mothers. Other advantages include lower risk for endometrial cancer and ectopic pregnancy and decreased endometriosis and uterine fibroids.

The most common problems with DMPA are irregular bleeding, weight gain, and depression. Seventy percent of women experience heavier or more frequent bleeding the first year of use. This lessens with continued use, and many women become amenorrheic after a year. Approximately 37% of women gain weight: 5 lb the first year, 8 lb after 2 years, and 16 lb after 5 years of DMPA use. **DMPA effects ▲ are not immediately reversible, and adverse effects may persist for 6 to 12 months after discontinuation. Fertility can**

take 6 to 12 months to return after discontinuing the drug. Long-term use of DMPA is associated with significant loss of bone density. Do not use DMPA for longer than 2 years unless other methods of contraception are inadequate. Women using DMPA should ensure adequate daily calcium intake. DMPA may have adverse effects on lipids, and obtaining an annual lipid profile is good clinical practice.

The dosage of DMPA is 150 mg administered intramuscularly every 3 months. The initial dose is given within the first 5 days of the menstrual cycle. Advise the use of a back-up contraceptive method for the first 7 days after initial administration.

A newer depot formulation of DMPA contains 104 mg of medroxyprogesterone acetate. It is also given subQ every 3 months. Blood levels are approximately 30% lower than with the 150-mg dose but are efficacious, and weight gain is less of a problem.

Intrauterine Devices

An IUD is a small, plastic contraceptive device inserted into the uterus. IUDs are cost-effective, easy to use, long-acting, reversible, and a highly effective method of contraception. Two IUDs are currently available in the United States; the Paragard Copper-T380A, and the levonorgestrel-containing Mirena. The Paragard IUD can remain in place for 5 years. The Mirena IUD is effective for at least 5 years.

IUDs are thought to work by preventing sperm from fertilizing ova and producing a spermicidal uterine environment. The copper IUD (Paragard) alters tubal and uterine transport of sperm. It can be used as an emergency contraceptive if inserted within 5 days of unprotected intercourse. The progestin IUD, Mirena, slowly releases levonorgestrel and works by local hormonal effect. Because fertilization does not occur, IUDs are not abortifacients.

The most common adverse effects of IUDs are increased menstrual bleeding and pain. The copper IUD can increase the number of days of bleeding and dysmenorrhea. Bleeding and cramping are more common the first few months after insertion. The levonorgestrel IUD reduces menstrual blood loss by 40% to 50%. After 1 year, almost 50% of women with the IUD are amenorrheic. The levonorgestrel IUD has also been used for menorrhagia, and to treat endometriosis.

▲   **Women who have an IUD may be at higher risk of pelvic inflammatory disease (PID), but serious complications resulting from IUDs rarely occur. The risk for PID is generally at its highest the first 20 days after insertion; the risk does not increase with duration of use.** Other complications are uterine perforation and abnormal bleeding; these complications are most often experienced during and immediately following insertion of the IUD. Although IUDs are highly effective, there is a risk of complications if pregnancy occurs. The risk for ectopic pregnancy is 50% lower in IUD users than in noncontraceptive users, but if pregnancy occurs with IUD use (rare), it has an increased likelihood of being ectopic.

Do not use IUDs in women with a history of frequent sexually transmitted diseases (STDs), those with multiple sexual partners, or those who have a history of PID. Thus it is preferred that the woman be in a mutually monogamous relationship. IUDs are not a first-choice method for nulliparous women. IUDs are not advised for women with uterine anatomic abnormalities such as cervical stenosis, uterine fibroids, or small or bicornuate uterus.

New and Future Contraceptives

Two new single-rod progestin implants are being developed. They contain newer progestins with fewer adverse effects compared to levonorgestrel. Uniplant contains nomegestrol and is effective for 1 year. Nestorone contains nestorone and is effective for 2 years.

Norethindrone enanthate is an injectable progestin similar to Depo-Provera and is effective for 2 months. A combination estrogen-progestin injectable, Mesigyna, contains norethindrone enanthate and estradiol valerate. It is administered monthly and causes less bleeding than Lunelle. Dihydroxyprogesterone acetophenide in combination with estradiol enanthate is an injectable contraceptive that is used widely in Latin America. It is administered monthly.

IUDs under development include Ombrelle, a more flexible IUD. Flexi-Gard is a frameless IUD suitable for women who have never been pregnant. FibroPlant is a very low–dose levonorgestrel IUD for use in perimenopausal and postmenopausal women.

CLINICAL REASONING

Treatment Objectives

Treatment objectives for the patient presenting with complaints of menstrual cycle disorders consist of accurate diagnosis followed by amelioration or elimination, when possible, of the symptoms. A primary management goal is to choose the method that is the most effective and carries the fewest risks and adverse effects, is the least invasive, and is appropriate for the patient's age and circumstances.

For the patient seeking contraception, the goals are similar to those just noted. Provide the patient with effective and reversible contraception that carries a minimum risk for adverse effects and that is consistent with the patient's preferences.

For the menopausal woman, the goals are relief of menopausal symptoms and reduction of the risks for osteoporosis.

Treatment Options

▥ Patient Variables

Human sexuality is a complex phenomenon encompassing biologic, psychologic, and sociocultural aspects. The biologic aspects include the anatomy and physiology of sexual development and sexual function. The psychologic aspects include gender identity, sexual self-concept, and developing intimate relationships. Sociocultural aspects include values systems of the family, peers, and community. All of these aspects are interrelated and interdependent.

Changing social norms have made discussion of sexual concerns more acceptable. However, some patients continue to feel extremely uncomfortable discussing these issues. Be tactful and nonjudgmental. The health care provider should be knowledgeable about sexuality and sexual norms, and use this knowledge to understand the patient's behavior and reactions to sexuality in health and illness. Maintain respect for differences in cultural and individual attitudes and perspectives regarding sexuality and the menstrual cycle. Pay attention to patient attitudes and the words used to describe the symptoms. In some cases, it may be well to begin the interview with discussion of other subjects, such as physical or family questions, and then move to questions about menarche, age of onset of sexual development, and the sexual history. Focus the discussion on the patient's general knowledge and expectations of the visit before moving to specific concerns.

▲ **Personal preference, adherence, cost, convenience, and medical contraindications are major factors to consider in the treatment plan. Even the best form of hormonal therapy is ineffective if improperly used or not used at all.** Discuss the available options with the patient. The choice of method is then made on the basis of a thorough discussion and informed consent.

In determining the patient's need or desire for hormonal therapy, many other factors must also be taken into account. They are the patient's specific complaints, age (developmental and physical), lifestyle, physical exam findings, and laboratory data. Therapy may require continuous use of hormones for a long time, and compliance may be an issue, especially if adverse effects are experienced. Ask about use of over-the-counter (OTC) drugs, nutritional supplements, and herbal formulations, and whether or not the patient smokes, uses alcohol, or engages in illicit drug use.

The first step in assessing the patient who seeks care because of disorders of the menstrual cycle or for contraception is to obtain the reason for the visit. Obtain the patient's age, information on concurrent drugs or contraceptives used, and a complete history of the current problem. A complete menstrual history, including age at menarche, and the usual interval and duration of menses, amount of flow, and presence of dysmenorrhea, should be noted.

Explore the signs and symptoms, such as the amount and duration of abnormal bleeding, and pain associated with bleeding or intercourse. If the patient reports heavy menses, estimate the amount by number of pads or tampons per day, or hour, and absorbency. Establish the degree to which the menstrual disorder is interfering with her normal activities.

Questions about the presence or absence of premenstrual symptoms such as breast tenderness or bloating, or abdominal pain that occur midway between menstrual periods (i.e., mittelschmerz), can be included. History of headaches, presence or absence of abdominal pain, hirsutism, vasomotor symptoms, vaginal dryness, vaginal discharge, mastalgia, and breast lumps or discharge are important.

In addition to a menstrual history, obtain a past health history: past illnesses, hospitalizations, and surgeries. Note any chronic diseases, particularly cardiac, thyroid, hepatic, renal, neurologic, or endocrine disorders. Ask about a history of coagulopathies, excessive bruising, varicose veins, or thrombophlebitis. Previous gynecologic surgery or treatment for gynecologic disorders, such as abnormal Papanicolaou smear, endometriosis, leiomyoma, or breast disease, is important to note. Previous history of sexually transmitted diseases should be investigated.

LIFE-SPAN CONSIDERATIONS

Pregnant and Nursing Women. Obtain a pregnancy test for women of childbearing age who seek care because of menstrual disorders. Urine tests for pregnancy are usually sufficient. Thyroid function tests (thyroxine and TSH) and prolactin levels are useful in evaluating amenorrhea. If the patient's history or exam findings so suggest, liver function tests, coagulation tests, and progesterone, FSH, and LH measurements may be helpful.

Contraception. The choice of contraceptive is individualized, determined by the patient's age, preferences, lifestyle, and overall health. Table 58-4 contains a quick overview of current contraceptive methods, their estimated effectiveness, and their availability. Many methods of contraception are currently available. Nonhormonal barrier methods include the diaphragm, the cervical cap, spermicides, and condoms. For women who wish to avoid hormonal contraceptives, the copper IUD is available. Hormonal options for contraception include COCs in various doses and combinations, transdermal patches, vaginal ring, progestin-only pills, progesterone-releasing IUDs, injectable progesterone, and a progesterone subdermal implant. Patients respond differently to COC drugs, dosages, and formulations. Low-dose (i.e., less than 50 mcg) pills carry fewer hormone-related risks than the previously available high-dose formulations. Nevertheless, COCs are contraindicated for use in some patients (see Box 58-1). A progestin-only or nonhormonal method of contraception is safer for some women. Multiphasic pills have no real advantages compared with monophasic pills.

TABLE 58-4 Estimated Effectiveness of Contraceptive Methods

Contraceptive Method	Percent of Women with Pregnancy		Availability
	Lowest Expected (%)	Typical Use (%)	
No method	85	85	NA
Withdrawal	4	23.6	NA
Periodic abstinence (calendar method)	1–9*	20	NA
Spermicide alone	3	21	OTC
Male condom	2	12	OTC
Female condom	5	21	OTC
Sponge (nulliparous women)	6	18	OTC
Sponge (multiparous women)	9	28	OTC
Diaphragm with spermicide	6	18	Rx
Cervical cap with spermicide†	9–20	20–40	Rx
Progestin-only oral contraceptive	0.5	3	Rx
Combination oral contraceptive	0.1	3	Rx
DMPA Injection	0.3	0.3	Rx
Implant (Implanon)	0.2	0.2	Rx
IUD with levonorgestrel (Mirena)	0.3	0.3	Rx
IUD with CuT ("Copper-T," Para-Guard, Mini-7)	0–1	0.8	Rx
IUD with progesterone (Progestasert)	1	UA	Rx
Surgical sterilization			
Female	0.2	0.4	Surgery
Male	0.1	0.15	Surgery

*Efficacy varies based on specific method used.
†Less effective in parous women, more difficult to achieve proper fit.
DMPA, Depot medroxyprogesterone acetate; *IUD,* intrauterine device; *NA,* not applicable; *OTC,* over-the-counter; *Rx,* prescription; *UA,* unavailable.

One of the ongoing controversies is whether hormonal therapy increases the risk for breast cancer in past and present users. **Research findings suggest than a woman's risk of breast cancer 10 years after discontinuing birth control pills is no higher than that of women who never have used them, and her risk for metastatic breast cancer is less** (Lund et al., 2007). There is no increased risk in women with a family history of breast cancer, or a personal history of breast disease. In fact, oral contraceptives decrease the incidence of benign breast disease by 40%.

Transdermal patches and the vaginal ring combine estrogen and progestin. They have essentially the same advantages, contraindications, and adverse effect profiles as COC pills. The advantage to these formulations is that they do not require daily pill-taking.

Progestin-only pills reduce cramps and bleeding associated with menses, as well as reducing the risk for PID and endometrial and ovarian cancers. Minipills do not carry the risk for thromboembolic events that are otherwise associated with the estrogen in COCs. They are a good option for women who have contraindications to estrogen use. They are commonly used by women who are breastfeeding.

Of the currently available contraceptive methods, IUDs have the lowest failure rates, and are a safe and effective method. Patients likely to consider an IUD are those who are in a stable, mutually monogamous relationship and who are not at risk for acquiring a sexually transmitted disease. (See Controversy box.)

Children and Adolescents. It takes approximately 2 years for the HPO axis to fully mature. As a result, menstrual cycles are frequently anovulatory immediately after menarche. Irregular menstrual bleeding and dysmenorrhea are common problems in the adolescent female. Inquire about the age of onset of secondary sexual characteristics and menses. Obtaining a history of sexual activity, including the number of partners and use of contraception and STD prevention, is important and offers an opportunity for teaching. Unless bleeding is heavy, a bimanual exam and/or ultrasound are usually sufficient for diagnosis in girls who have not had sexual intercourse. A vaginal examination can usually be performed, if necessary, by using a pediatric speculum. A full pelvic exam should be performed if the patient is sexually active.

The health care provider can offer support to adolescents when they are undergoing a number of physical and emotional changes that can be confusing. Being nonjudgmental and offering complete confidentiality is extremely important.

Older Adults

Menopausal Symptoms. Treatment of perimenopausal or postmenopausal problems depends on the diagnosis and individual needs. For perimenopausal or menopausal patients, an FSH level higher than 40 international units/mL indicates ovarian failure (5 to 20 international units/mL is normal). If abnormal vaginal bleeding is present, an endometrial biopsy is performed to assess for endometrial proliferation or hyperplasia. Office hysteroscopy can be used to visualize the endometrium and obtain directed sampling for the patient who is not actively bleeding.

Short term hormone replacement therapy (HRT) can be used in women with moderate to severe menopausal symptoms. **HRT is not indicated for the prevention of CHD.** The decision to start HRT is made only after a careful and thorough discussion of the risks and benefits (see Evidence-based Pharmacotherapeutics box).

Alternatives to HRT are available. Life-style changes, such as diet, exercise, weight loss, stress reduction, and smoking cessation are beneficial. Alternative and complementary therapies may be useful and appropriate (see Chapter 11). For women who are having few symptoms, life-style changes may be the only treatment needed. The patient should understand that although a decision to use a specific modality has been made, the choice is not life-long. The decision can always be re-evaluated as the woman's thinking and circumstances change. Table 58-5 provides an overview of HRT regimens.

Drug Variables

The choice of drug is largely determined by the cost and convenience to the patient. Oral therapy may be preferred: the action begins promptly and the treatment can be terminated at will. Parenteral, transdermal, and implant formulations are longer acting and can be more convenient.

AMENORRHEA. COC regimens preserve bone density and prevent genital atrophy. COCs are preferred in the patient who is sexually active, a non-smoker, and younger than 35 years of age who desires contraception. Another regimen is to use 0.625 mg conjugated estrogens days 1 to 25 of the cycle and 5 to 10 mg of medroxyprogesterone on days 16 to 25 of the cycle. A third regimen is to use medroxyprogesterone 10 mg daily for 10 to 13 days a month.

DUB. Treatment depends on the age of the woman. COCs are the drugs of choice for women under the age of menopause. If the patient does not need contraception, or pregnancy is not desired, oral MPA can be used. If the patient is experiencing heavy bleeding, estrogen may need to be added to the progestin regimen. Postmenopausal bleeding is more likely to be due to pathological factors.

DYSMENORRHEA. For patients with dysmenorrhea, NSAIDs are effective in relieving pain in 70% to 90% of cases. NSAIDs inhibit prostaglandin synthesis without affecting endometrial development. Begin NSAIDs just prior to or concurrent with the onset of menstrual flow. Examples include ibuprofen, naproxen, mefenamic acid, diflunisal, and ketoprofen and others.

If the patient also desires contraception, low-dose COC is indicated. They are effective in preventing dysmenorrhea in 60% to 80% of patients. Patients can use concomitant NSAIDs if needed. COCs induce endometrial hypoplasia and suppresses both menstrual fluid volume and prostaglandin release (but not synthesis).

PREMENSTRUAL SYNDROME. The first-line management options are not hormonal. Selective serotonin release inhibitors (SSRIs) are now considered the mainstay of treatment for PMS.

CONTRACEPTION. Factors that should be considered when choosing a contraceptive method include patient preference, age, frequency of intercourse, and motivation and ability to use the method correctly. For women who engage in intercourse frequently, COCs or a progestin implant may be appropriate. For women who have infrequent sexual activity, the use of condoms and spermicide may be adequate and offers protection against sexually transmitted diseases. If ease of use is an issue, an IUD, DMPA, or a progestin implant may be a reasonable choice. For couples whose family planning goals have already been met, sterilization of either partner may be a desirable alternative.

ENDOCRINE

Controversy

Hormonal Contraceptives

Jonathan J. Wolfe

No pharmaceutical has had as profound an impact on society during the past 40 years as hormonal contraceptives. The abilities to treat most infections, alter lipid metabolism, regulate cardiac function, and influence the course of mental illness, which are provided by other, concurrently developed agents, are remarkable in themselves. They pale, however, in comparison with the almost flawless control over reproductive function that hormonal contraceptives confer. Worldwide population trends clearly show the effect of access to these sophisticated drugs. In some cases, abortion rates testify to a willingness to substitute far riskier means of birth control in nations where contraceptives are either not available or unacceptable.

Oral contraceptives are often viewed by patients as benign products. Certainly, the risks of pregnancy and delivery are far greater than the risk of using hormonal contraceptives, especially the newer low-dose drug combinations. However, many patients stand at substantial risk; and indeed, the acceptance of any drug therapy is a matter for sober reflection. Patients who have either a personal history of clotting disorders, or a family history of certain malignancies, and patients who smoke have higher risk profiles. Many of them require careful counseling before hormonal contraceptives are chosen over other methods.

CLINICAL REASONING ANALYSIS

- What counseling should you offer a minor, 15 years of age, who requests an examination and prescription for oral contraceptives without the knowledge of her parents?
- Why are oral contraceptives more acceptable to American patients than contraceptive implants or rings?
- The privacy associated with oral contraceptives makes them highly desirable. What aspects of these products are least desirable for individual patients?
- Name the three most important interactions between hormonal contraceptives and other drugs. What is the best source for information about these potentially grave drug interactions? Is it fair for public health authorities to have access to hormonal contraceptives at prices far below those that community pharmacies must pay for the same drugs? Is it good public policy to subsidize access to these drugs for some citizens?

In choosing a COC, a 35 mcg estrogen formulation or lower is optimal. For patients with acne, hirsutism, or lipid abnormalities, a pill containing one of the new progestins (norgestimate, desogestrel or drospirenone) would be a good choice.

Progestin-only methods such as minipills, DMPA, the levonorgestrel IUD, and the progestin implant are appropriate choices for women with contraindications to estrogen. Although minipills are slightly less effective than COCs, they are useful for women who are breastfeeding. Contraceptive

EVIDENCE-BASED PHARMACOTHERAPEUTICS

Long-Term Hormone Therapy

■ **Background**

Hormone replacement therapy (HRT) and estrogen replacement therapy (ERT) are widely used for the relief of menopausal symptoms as well as for management and prevention of cardiovascular disease, osteoporosis, and dementia. However, evidence supporting the use for these purposes is primarily from observational studies.

■ **Research Article**

Farquhar, C., Marjoribanks, J., Lethaby, A., et al. (2005). Cochrane HT Study Group. Long-term hormone therapy for perimenopausal and postmenopausal women. *The Cochrane Database of Systematic Reviews. 2005,* Issue 3. Art. No. CD004143. DOI: 10.1002/14651858. CD004143.pub2.

Purpose

The purpose of this metaanalytical review was to evaluate the effects of long-term HRT on the following variables: fractures; heart disease; thromboembolic events; transient ischemic attacks; cancer of the breast, ovary, and endometrium and colorectal cancer; gallbladder disease; dementia; quality of life; and mortality.

Design

Two reviewers independently extracted data from 15 double-blind, randomized, controlled trials of ERT (estrogen alone) or HRT (estrogen with progestin) taken for at least 1 year by perimenopausal or postmenopausal women. A metaanalysis was not possible because of the heterogeneity of the trials.

Methods

All statistically significant results were extracted from the two biggest trials—Heart and Estrogen-Progestin Replacement Study (Barrett-Connor, et al., 1997) and the Women's Health Initiative (The Women's Health Initiative Study Group, 1998) trials. Women (*N* = 2763) were eligible for the HERS trial if they were postmenopausal, ages 50 to 88 years, and still had their uterus. Women (*N* = 161,808) were eligible for the WHI trials if they were ages 50 to 70 years, with or without a uterus. These trials compared 0.625 mg oral conjugated estrogens, with and without continuous 2.5 mg medroxyprogesterone. Smaller trials used different hormone therapies or had different populations and could not be used in the analysis.

Findings

Hormonal therapy used in healthy women caused significant increases in the risk for thromboembolic and cardiac events after 1 year of use. Hormonal therapy increased the risk for stroke after 3 years of use. Additionally, in this review, hormonal therapy increased the risk for breast cancer after 5 years of use. There is also an increased risk for gallbladder disease and dementia. The estrogen-only arm of the study noted significant increases in the risk for stroke and gallbladder disease. The only statistically significant findings were a reduced incidence of fractures and colorectal cancer.

Conclusion

Hormonal therapy is not indicated for the routine management of menopausal symptoms. Short-term HRT for menopausal symptoms in healthy younger women appears safe at this time.

■ **Implications for Practice**

Additional clinical trials are needed about the safety of short-term use of hormone therapy for control of menopausal symptoms. Randomized, placebo-controlled clinical trials would be appropriate.

TABLE 58-5 Hormonal Replacement Therapy*

Drug	Brand Name	Dosages Available
ESTROGEN, ORAL		
conjugated estrogens A	Cenestin	0.3, 0.45, 0.625, 0.9, 1.25 mg
conjugated estrogens B	Enjuvia	0.625, 1.25 mg
conjugated estrogens	Premarin	0.3, 0.45, 0.625, 0.9, 1.25, 2.5 mg
esterified estrogen	Menest, Estratab	0.3, 0.625. 1.25, 2.5 mg
estradiol	Femtrace	0.45, 0.9, 1.8 mg
estradiol micronized	Estrace	0.5, 1.0, 2.0 mg
estropipate	Ogen, Ortho-Est	0.625, 1.25 mg
ESTROGEN, TRANSDERMAL		
estradiol patch	Alora	0.025, 0.05, 0.075, 0.1 mg/day
	Climara	0.025, 0.0375, 0.05, 0.06, 0.075, 0.1 mg/day
	Esclim	0.025, 0.0375, 0.05, 0.075, 0.1 mg/day
	Estraderm	0.05, 0.1 mg/day
	Menostar	0.014 mg/day
	Vivelle	0.05, 0.1 mg/day
	Vivelle-dot	0.025, 0.0375, 0.05, 0.075, 0.1 mg/day
estradiol gel or emulsion	Estrogel	1.25 grams/pump
	Estrasorb	1.74 grams/pouch
ESTROGEN, VAGINAL		
conjugated estrogen cream	Premarin	0.625 mg/g/day
estradiol vaginal cream	Estrace	0.1 mg/g /day
estradiol vaginal tab	Vagifem	25 mcg daily
estradiol vaginal ring	Estring	7.5 mcg/day
	Femring	0.05, 0.1 mg/day
PROGESTIN, ORAL		
medroxyprogesterone	Provera	2.5, 5, 10 mg tabs daily
norethindrone acetate	Aygestin	5 mg daily
progesterone	Prometrium	100, 200 mg daily
COMBINATION ESTROGEN AND PROGESTIN, ORAL†		
conjugated estrogens and medroxyprogesterone	Premphase	0.625 mg/0.625 + 5 mg daily sequentially
	Prempro	0.3 mg +1.5 mg daily continuously –or– 0.45 mg + 1.5 mg; –or– 0.625 mg + 2.5 mg; –or– 0.625 mg + 5 mg
estradiol and norethindrone	Activella	1 mg + 0.5 mg daily
estradiol and norgestimate	Prefest	1 mg/ 1 mg + 0.9 mg daily sequentially
ethinyl estradiol and norethindrone	FemHRT	2.5 mcg + 0.5 mg daily continuously –or– 5 mcg + 1 mg
ESTROGEN AND PROGESTIN, TRANSDERMAL†		
estradiol and levonorgestrel	Climara Pro	0.045 + 0.015 mg/day
estradiol and norethindrone	Combipatch	0.05 + 0.14 mg/day; 0.05 + 0.25 mg/day

*Estrogen-only preparations only for women without an intact uterus.
†Estrogen dose listed first, progestin dose second.

implants are effective contraceptives. The adverse effects are similar to those of other progestin-only formulations. A disadvantage is that surgery is required for their insertion and removal.

MENOPAUSAL SYMPTOMS. Use of unopposed estrogen for menopausal symptoms in women with an intact uterus is associated with increased risk for endometrial cancer. Give progestins in addition to estrogen if hormone replacement therapy is elected.

Estrogen and estrogen-progestin therapy may be useful for moderate to severe menopausal symptoms (see Case Study). However, their use is associated with increased risk for venous thrombosis, stroke, dementia, breast cancer, and heart disease. In many instances, the risks outweigh the benefits, and the risks must be carefully considered before initiating therapy. Since vasomotor symptoms decline spontaneously over time, long-term use of hormones is not always necessary. The duration of treatment should not be limited to an arbitrary period (e.g., 5 years) but should be dictated by clinical needs and safety monitoring. Nonhormonal approaches to symptom relief are helpful.

Patient Education

For many women, a gynecologic exam is the time she is likely to seek medical care. Therefore it is a valuable time to provide education. Regular gynecologic exams, Pap smears, breast exams, mammograms, and bone density measurements, depending on age and medical history, are a part of good health care. The time of the exam is an opportunity to teach breast self-exam, and to answer health-related questions.

Stress the importance of a healthy diet and regular exercise in the prevention of osteoporosis and cardiovascular disease. Smoking cessation, STD prevention, and contraceptive

ENDOCRINE

CASE STUDY | Hormonal Therapy

ASSESSMENT

History of Present Illness	AD is a 59-year-old white female with a history of amenorrhea for 8 years. She also complains of hot flashes that awaken her at night, diaphoresis, dyspareunia, and stress incontinence. She believes that she is a little shorter than she used to be.
Past Health History	AD is allergic to sulfa. She denies tobacco or alcohol use. She takes no drugs other than acetaminophen or ibuprofen for occasional aches and pains, a multivitamin, and a daily calcium supplement. She has no history of cardiovascular disease or bone fractures. She has never taken hormonal replacement therapy. She has had three vaginal deliveries, but no gynecologic surgery. Her last Papanicolaou smear 2 years ago was normal. The lipid profile done at that time was normal. Her last mammogram 3 years ago was normal.
Life-Span Considerations	AD is within the normal menopausal age range and is experiencing menopausal symptoms. She is married and sexually active.
Physical Exam Findings	*Ht:* 5'4"; *Wt:* 150 lb. *BP:* 106/60. Small degree of kyphosis. Pelvic exam: labia atrophic, vagina pale pink, no rugae, first-degree cystocele, uterus small, nontender, normal size and shape, no adnexal mass or tenderness. No thyromegaly. Breasts without palpable masses or nipple discharge.
Diagnostic Testing	Papanicolaou smear normal. Endometrial biopsy reveals atrophic endometrium. TSH and fT_4 are within normal limits. Total cholesterol, 239 mg/dL; triglycerides, 135 mg/dL; HDL, 59 mg/dL; LDL, 96 mg/dL. BMD: −1 at lumbar vertebrae; −1.8 at head of femur. Mammogram is normal.

DIAGNOSIS: Postmenopausal symptoms

MANAGEMENT

Treatment Objectives	1. Relieve patient's symptoms (hot flushes, diaphoresis, dyspareunia, stress incontinence). 2. Initiate treatment plan using a drug that has the fewest risks and the greatest benefit for the patient.
Treatment Plan	**Pharmacotherapy** • estradiol 0.01% vaginal cream nightly for 2 weeks; then 1 gram per vagina nightly 1 to 3 times/week • medroxyprogesterone 2.5 mg PO daily **Patient Education** 1. Discussion of risks and benefits of short-term estrogen-progestin hormone replacement 2. Regular weight-bearing exercise 3. Diet rich in fruits, vegetables, and whole grains, avoidance of unhealthy fats (saturated fat and trans fats) 4. Continue daily intake of 1200 to 1500 mg calcium supplement along with 400 to 800 units of vitamin D **Evaluation** Follow-up office visit in 2 to 3 months to evaluate menopausal symptoms; response to estrogen cream; lipid levels; and to discuss hormone replacement therapy

CLINICAL REASONING ANALYSIS

Q1. What factors did you consider when deciding to use the estradiol vaginal cream?

A. There are many considerations before prescribing HRT, most of which are exclusionary criteria. Some are relative contraindications; others are absolute. If you will look again at the table I gave you earlier (see Table 58-5) and at AD's history, you will find that AD has none of the conditions that absolutely contraindicate hormone therapy. Her slightly abnormal total cholesterol level warrants attention but does not hinder hormonal therapy.

Q2. If she will be using the estradiol vaginal cream for her atrophic vaginitis, why does AD also need to take medroxyprogesterone? Isn't the estrogen enough?

A. The estrogen is not enough. AD still has her uterus. In a patient with a uterus, both hormones are required to prevent overgrowth of the endometrium and avert the subsequent risk of endometrial cancer later on.

Q3. Why did you tell AD to continue taking her daily calcium? Isn't the estrogen enough to prevent osteoporosis?
A. Additional calcium in the diet also reduces the rate of vertebral fractures by as much as 80%. Because only 35% of postmenopausal women develop significant osteoporosis, and because weight-bearing exercise and increased calcium intake are also effective, the routine prophylactic use of estrogen may be hard to justify in some instances. However, a great deal of evidence is available to show that estrogen replacement lowers the frequency of arm and hip fractures secondary to osteoporosis. The prophylactic effect of estrogens appears to be greatest when they are taken before significant osteoporosis occurs.

methods are topics that can be discussed, as appropriate. Discuss the benefits of breastfeeding in reducing the risk for breast cancer. And finally, ensure that the patient education is appropriate for the age and educational level of the patient.

Contraception

When starting a patient on oral contraceptives, explain how OC pills work. Clearly review the risks and benefits. The risks in most women are very low, and there are many benefits. Even so, many health care providers have the patient sign a consent when prescribing an OC. Advise all patients who smoke to quit.

Show a pill package to the patient using OCs for the first time, and explain how to use it. OCs can be started one of three ways: (1) Same-day start (use backup contraceptive method for 7 days for the first cycle). **A backup method of birth control (e.g., condoms, spermicides, diaphragm, and abstinence) is recommended during the first week of initial COC use.** (2) First-day start: start on first day of menses. (3) Sunday start: start on first Sunday after the period begins. OCs should be taken daily at approximately the same time of day (including weekends). The cycle is repeated every 28 days, regardless of whether breakthrough bleeding or spotting occurs.

Advise patients that they can start a COC or progestin-only pill 4 to 6 weeks postpartum. This period allows coagulation factors to return to normal levels and permits lactation to become well-established.

Provide instruction on what to do in the event of missed pills, if diarrhea or vomiting occurs, or there is concomitant use of drugs that may interfere with the pill's effectiveness. In each case, having a backup method and using it until the next menstrual period is indicated.

If one dose of a COC is missed, it should be taken as soon as it is remembered, and the pack finished. If two to four doses are missed in the first 2 weeks of the pill package, the patient should take pills as soon as remembered and then finish the pack. If two to four doses are missed in the third or fourth week of the package, she should discard the pack and start a new one. A backup birth control method should be used for 7 days. Some experts recommend using emergency contraception pills (ECPs) if any pills are missed in the first week of the package.

Breakthrough bleeding is the most common adverse effect with both COCs and progestin-only pills. With COCs, it is most common the first few months of use and improves with each cycle. Emphasize to the patient the importance of taking the pill at the same time daily, and to not forget pills. If bleeding persists despite correct use, perform an exam to rule out

infection or other problems. Scanty periods or amenorrhea is common with low-dose COCs. Irregular bleeding is to be expected with minipills.

Further, breakthrough bleeding is very common when first starting DMPA. It diminishes with time and length of use until at 1 year when most women are amenorrheic. Irregular bleeding and pain is more common with the copper IUD. Bleeding is common at first with the levonorgestrel IUD, but decreases dramatically with continued use.

Teach the woman using an IUD to check for the presence of the IUD strings in the vagina after each menses. The check is important because an IUD could be expelled during menses without the patient's being aware. Advise the patient to seek medical care if signs of infection appear, such as fever, pelvic pain, severe cramping, or increased bleeding. If she misses a period, she should contact the health care provider immediately to evaluate for the possibility of pregnancy.

Inform patients using a contraceptive implant that the implant becomes effective 24 hours after insertion and is most often effective for up to 3 years. Teach the patient to watch for signs of infection after insertion and to return to the health care provider if they occur. Irregular bleeding is common for the first few months to 1 year after insertion of the implants. Follow-up care is important if bleeding becomes heavy.

Teach healthy nonsmoking women they may continue to use OCs without increased risk until the age of 50 years. Do not use COCs in women over 35 years who smoke, because of the increased risk for thromboembolic disease. When pregnancy is desired, contraceptive pills should be stopped approximately 2 months ahead of conception to allow for accurate dating of the pregnancy. There does not appear to be a higher risk of birth defects if conception occurs within the first month after the contraceptive drug is discontinued.

For convenience, such as for a honeymoon, holidays, or athletics, it is possible to skip withdrawal bleeding for a month. Instead of taking the 7-day placebo pills, a new pill package is started. Also, Seasonale, an extended-regimen COC, is available. It consists of 12 weeks of active hormone pills followed by a week of hormone-free pills; women have withdrawal bleeding only 4 times a year.

For emergency contraception, the progestin-only formulation Plan B is now available upon the patient's request to the pharmacist. However, it may be prudent for some patients to have the drug available in advance of need. Emergency contraception is most effective when taken within 72 hours of unprotected intercourse, but can be taken up to 5 days afterwards, although effectiveness diminishes with length of time following unprotected intercourse. Two doses are taken 12 hours apart. Nausea is less of a problem with the

ENDOCRINE

progestin-only ECP (Plan B). Taking the pills with food or using an OTC antihistamine can help with nausea if it occurs. The patient should return for a pregnancy test if her menses does not occur within 3 weeks. Providing a prescription for ECPs is an opportunity to discuss other more effective methods of contraception with the patient and answer any questions she may have (see Box 58-2).

Advise the patient that non–barrier methods such as OCs, IUDs, subdermal implants, and contraceptive injections do not provide protection from STDs, including HIV. Advise the patient of the signs and symptoms of serious adverse effects of contraceptives. A useful acronym to remember is *ACHES: A* stands for severe abdominal pain, which could be a symptom of serious liver or gallbladder disease; *C* stands for chest pain, which could be a pulmonary embolus, myocardial infarction, angina, or a breast lump; *H* stands for headache, which could be a symptom of a stroke, or a migraine; *E* stands for eye problems, which could be a symptom of a stroke, migraine headache, thromboemboli, or corneal changes; *S* stands for severe leg pain, which could be the symptom of a thromboembolus.

▓▓ *Hormonal Replacement Therapy*

Reassure the perimenopausal or menopausal patient that her symptoms are a natural occurrence and that loss of ovarian function may result in physical changes such as hot flushes, diaphoresis, urinary symptoms, and vaginal dryness. Counsel her about the actions to take to reduce the risk for osteoporosis and cardiovascular disease. In addition, give the patient information appropriate to her age regarding recognition of disorders such as cardiovascular disease and diabetes.

A careful and thorough discussion about the risks and benefits of short-term HRT allows the woman to make an informed choice among her treatment options. Encourage the patient to incorporate exercise and dietary changes into her life, and to stop smoking. Teach her how to perform monthly breast self-examinations (BSEs) and the importance of a yearly pelvic exam, Pap smear, and mammogram. Perform a bone density test when indicated by age and medical history. Monitor the health of the vaginal epithelium by regularly testing the vaginal pH. For treatment of atrophic vaginitis, use low-dose vaginal estrogen, which can also supplement systemic estrogen therapy when indicated.

Evaluation

Schedule a return visit within 3 months of starting hormonal therapy, or sooner if problems develop. For women starting contraception, the follow-up visit is an opportunity to see if she is having any problems, and is an opportunity to answer questions. The method of choice is the one that is most effective and carries the fewest risks and adverse effects, is the least invasive, and is appropriate for the patient's age and circumstances.

BOX 58-2

Emergency Contraception

Scope of the Problem
Approximately 3 million unintended pregnancies occur in the United States each year. More than half of these end in abortion. The causes of unintended pregnancy include contraceptive failure (e.g., broken condom, missed oral contraceptives), failure to use contraception, and rape. Emergency contraception offers a safe, effective way to prevent many unintended pregnancies.

Emergency contraception used within 72 hours decreases pregnancy risk by 75% to 90%. ECPs can be taken up to 5 days after unprotected intercourse, but the efficacy diminishes rapidly. ECPs prevent fertilization and are not abortifacients. Contraindications to ECP use include known or suspected pregnancy (the method would have no effect), undiagnosed abnormal vaginal bleeding, and a history of thromboembolic disease.

Barriers to Emergency Contraception
Despite decades of availability, the rate of use of ECPs remains low. The reasons for low utilization rates include a lack of patient awareness, health care provider attitudes and practices, and the lack of timely availability. A 2004 California Kaiser Family Foundation study found that only 57% of teens and adults were aware of the availability of ECPs (Foster et al., 2007). The survey also identified confusion in the distinction between ECPs and medical abortion using mifepristone.

In most states, ECP requires a visit to the health care provider. A 2001 study found that 80% of gynecologists and 33% of general practitioners reported prescribing ECP within the past year, the majority doing so 6 or fewer times.

In a study by Trussell et al. (2000), 76% of attempts to obtain an appointment with the health care provider within 72 hours of intercourse were successful; but even if a prescription was obtained, it may not have been filled. Further, a study by Espey et al. (2003) found that only 11% of Albuquerque, New Mexico pharmacies had a stock of ECPs. However, a national movement now permits pharmacists to dispense ECPs without a prescription. Check with your state pharmacy board for further information.

Nonhormonal Methods for Emergency Contraception
Insertion of a copper-containing IUD (Paragard Copper-T380A) within 5 days of unprotected intercourse provides effective emergency contraception and reduces pregnancy by up to 95%.

Hormonal Methods for Emergency Contraception*

ECP	Formulation Per Pill	Pills per dose
Alesse	20 mcg EE + 0.1 mg LNG (pink pills)	5
Levlen	30 mcg EE + 0.15 mg LNG (light orange pills)	4
Levlite	20 mcg EE + 0.1 mg LNG (pink pills)	5
Levora	30 mcg EE + 0.15 mg LNG (white pills)	4
Ovral	50 mcg EE + 0.5 mg NG (white pills)	2
Plan B	0.75 mg LNG	2
Triphasil	30 mcg EE + 0.125 mg LNG (yellow pills)	4
Tri-Levlen	30 mcg EE + 0.125 mg LNG (yellow pills)	4
Nordette	30 mcg EE + 0.15 mg LNG (light orange pills)	4
Trivora	30 mcg EE + 0.125 mg LNG (pink pills)	4

*Levonorgestrel (Plan B), a progestin-only formulation, was FDA-approved specifically for ECP in 1999. However, other OCs may also be used for emergency contraception. *EE,* Ethinyl estradiol; *FDA,* Food and Drug Administration; *LNG,* levonorgestrel; *OCs,* oral contraceptives.

For the menopausal woman, the goals are relief of menopausal symptoms and reduction of the risks for osteoporosis. For the postmenopausal patient who was started on HRT, document response to therapy, noting improvement in menopausal symptoms as well as avoidance of adverse drug effects.

Evaluate the patient on HRT for endometrial cancer if ⚠ she develops persistent or recurrent vaginal bleeding. Additional follow-up depends on the particular condition and treatment regimen chosen.

KEY POINTS

■ There are three phases to the ovarian cycle: follicular phase, ovulatory phase, and luteal phase. The endometrial cycle prepares the endometrium for implantation by an ovum.

■ Estrogen secretion increases between ages 9 and 12 years, triggering sexual maturation, and begins to decline as the woman enters the perimenopausal period at about 40 years.

■ Disruptions of the normal menstrual cycle may occur; they include amenorrhea, dysmenorrhea, premenstrual syndrome, abnormal uterine bleeding, and polycystic ovarian syndrome.

■ A complete history and physical exam is performed to establish the diagnosis and to prescribe or recommend appropriate therapy for contraception or menopausal symptoms.

■ The best strategy when prescribing a hormonal drug is to use a drug at the lowest possible dosage and one that has the fewest adverse effects but which provides the desired therapeutic effects.

■ Many forms of hormonal preparations are available as contraceptives, including oral estrogen-progestin combination pills, patches, and vaginal rings; oral progestin-only pills; IM and subcutaneous long-acting progesterone; IM estrogen-progestin; subdermal implants; copper and progesterone-releasing IUDs.

■ The patient should be advised that non–barrier contraceptives do not provide protection against HIV or STDs.

■ For emergency contraception, the earlier the drug is taken, the more effective it is. It is most effective if taken within 3 days of unprotected intercourse. It can be taken up to 5 days after the event but is less effective. One dose is taken immediately; the second dose is taken 12 hours later.

■ Estrogen and progestin preparations are available for the treatment of menopausal symptoms. If the patient still has her uterus, progestin should be given concomitantly to avoid endometrial hyperplasia.

■ Initiation of menopausal hormonal therapy necessitates a follow-up visit in 3 months to evaluate its efficacy and adverse effects. This length of time is sufficient for the occurrence of improvement in menopausal symptoms to be noted, as well as the drug's adverse effects.

Bibliography

Barrett-Connor, E, Slone, S, Greendale, G, et al. (1997). The Postmenopausal Estrogen/Progestin Interventions Study: Primary outcomes in adherent women. *Maturatis, 27*(3), 261–274.

Bennett, W., Petraitis, C., D'Anella, A., et al. (2003). Pharmacists' knowledge and the difficulty obtaining emergency contraception. *Contraception, 68*(4), 261–267.

Davis, R. (2004). Alternative to hormone therapy: A clinical guide to menopausal transition. *Advance for Nurse Practitioners, 12*(10), 37–82.

DeCherney, A., and Nathan, L. (2003). *Current obstetrics and gynecologic diagnosis and treatment* (9th ed.). New York: Lange Medical Books.

Defective drugs. (2004). Norplant. Available online: http://adrugrecall.com/norplant/html. Accessed May 29, 2007.

Department of Health and Human Services. National Institutes of Health. (2002). *Women's Health Initiative Update.* Available online: www.whi.org. Accessed May 29, 2007.

Drug facts and comparisons 2007. (2007). St. Louis: Wolters Kluwer Health.

Espey, E., Ogburn, T., Howard, D., et al. (2003). Emergency contraception: Pharmacy access in Albuquerque, New Mexico. *Obstetrics and Gynecology, 102*(5 Part 1), 918–921.

Ethinyl estradiol/levonorgestrel (Seasonale). (2003). Package insert. Pomona, NY: Duramed Pharmaceuticals. Available online: www.seasonale.com/Seasonale_prescribing_info.pdf. Accessed May 29, 2007.

Farquhar, C., Marjoribanks, J., Lethaby, A., et al.Cochrane HT Study Group. (2005). Long term hormone therapy for perimenopausal and postmenopausal women. *The Cochrane Database of Systematic Reviews. 2005,* (Issue 3), Art. No. CD004143: 10.1002/14651858. CD004143. pub2.

Food and Drug Administration. (2005). Ortho-Evra. Available online: www.fda.gov/cder/foi/label/2005/021180s019lbl.pdf. Accessed May 29, 2007.

Foster, D., Landau, S., Monastersky, N., et al. (2006). Pharmacy access to emergency contraception in California. *Perspectives on Sexual and Reproductive Health, 38*(1), 46–52.

Foster, D., Ralph, L., Arons, A., et al. (2007). Trends in knowledge of emergency contraception among women in California, 1999–2004. *Women's Health Issues, 17*(1), 22–28.

Hatcher, R., Trussell, J., Stewart, F., et al. (2004). *Contraceptive technology* (18th rev. ed.). New York: Ardent Media.

Herrington, D. (1999). Clinical implications of HERS trial results. *Menopausal Medicine, 7*(20), 1–4.

Lund, E., Bakken, K., Dumeaux, V., et al. (2007). Hormone replacement therapy and breast cancer in former users of oral contraceptives—The Norwegian Women and Cancer study. *International Journal of Cancer, 121*(3), 645–648.

National Institutes of Health. (2006). WHI study finds no heart disease benefit, increased stroke risk with estrogen alone. Available online: www.nih.gov.news/pr. Accessed May 29, 2007.

National Institutes of Health Osteoporosis and Related Bone Diseases National Resource Center. (2006). *Osteoporosis overview.* Available online: www.osteo.org. Accessed May 29, 2007.

North American Menopause Society. (2004). 2004 Position Statement. *Menopause, 11*(6), 589–600.

Notelvitz, M. (2006). Clinical opinion: The biologic and pharmacologic principles of estrogen therapy for symptomatic menopause. *Medscape General Medicine, 8*(1), 85. Available online: www.medscape.com/viewarticle/523196_1. Accessed May 29, 2007.

Ogburn, T. (2006). Emergency contraception: Telling the secret. *The Female Patient, 31*(1), 14–19.

Organon USA. (2005). Product insert: NuvaRing. Roseland, NJ: Author.

Ortho-McNeil Pharmaceutical. (2001). Product insert: Ortho-Evra. Raritan, NJ: Author.

ENDOCRINE

Peterson, H., and Curtis, K. (2005). Long-acting contraceptives. *New England Journal of Medicine, 353*(20), 2169–2180.

Speroff, L., and Darney, P. (2005). *A clinical guide for contraception* (4th ed.). Philadelphia: Lippincott, Williams & Wilkins.

Stockwell, J. (2006). Endometriosis: Clinical assessment and medical management. *Advance for Nurse Practitioners, 14*(1), 43–45.

The Women's Health Initiative Study Group. (1998). Design of the Women's Health Initiative clinical trial and observational study. *Controlled Clinical Trials, 19*(1), 61–109.

Trussell, J., Duran, V., Shocket, T., et al. (2000). Access to emergency contraception. *Obstetrics and Gynecology, 95*(2), 267–270.

U.S. Preventive Services Task Force. (2005). Hormone therapy for the prevention of chronic conditions in postmenopausal women: Recommendation statement. AHRQ Publication No. 05–0576, May. Agency for Healthcare Research and Quality: Rockville, MD. Available online: www.ahrq.gov/uspst05/ht/htpostmenrs.htm. Accessed May 29, 2007.

59

Uterine Motility Drugs

The drug-induced induction and augmentation of labor has been practiced for hundreds of years in Europe and North America. The midwives of the Middle Ages knew of the labor-inducing qualities of ergot. Interestingly, though, ergot did not gain acceptance in medicine until the early nineteenth century. Around the same time, however, ergot's potential dangers to the fetus were recognized, leading to the recommendation that the drug only be used to control postpartum hemorrhage. Today, ergot is the source of only some of the collection of drugs relied on by modern obstetrics to suppress or stimulate uterine contractions.

To understand the actions of drugs that induce or suppress uterine contractions during pregnancy, one must consider the nature of a uterine contraction and its various quieting and stimulating factors.

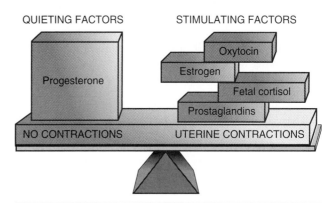

FIGURE 59-1 Balance of Factors Influencing Labor. A delicate balance exists between the biochemical factors related to gestation. Those factors identified on the right side of the fulcrum provide stimulus for uterine contractions and the initiation of labor. Progesterone on the left exerts a quieting effect on uterine contractions. Labor begins when the balance of these factors changes.

PHYSIOLOGY OF LABOR

INITIATION OF LABOR

Initiation of myometrial cell contraction occurs when an enzyme called myosin light-chain kinase (MLCK) attaches a phosphorus atom (phosphorylation) to myosin at a rate faster than another enzyme, myosin light-chain phosphatase (MLCP), removes the phosphorus atom (dephosphorylation). The phosphorylation by MCLK results in a linkage of the myosin head with a specific site on the actin filament, bringing about a subsequent change in arrangement such that the myosin head (now attached to the actin) tilts to about a 45-degree angle. The tilting of the myosin head pulls the attached actin fiber in the direction of the tilt, resulting in a sliding or "ratcheting" of the actin over the myosin. Uterine contraction results when millions of myosin and actin filaments slide over on one another. Adenosine triphosphate (ATP) binds to the tilted myosin head. Through its hydrolysis to adenosine diphosphate (ADP) and phosphorus, ATP provides energy to reestablish the myosin head in its original, upright position. Uterine relaxation occurs when phosphorylation of the myosin light-chain by MLCK ceases and dephosphorylation by MLCP occurs. Therefore, the rate at which MLCK phosphorylates myosin is crucial in controlling uterine contractility (see Fig. 59-1).

At the onset of labor, there is a heightened uterine sensitivity to oxytocin, which can be attributed to upregulation of oxytocin receptor mRNA levels as well as an increased density of myometrial oxytocin receptors. Receptor levels rise to 200 times that in the nonpregnant state. Hence levels of oxytocin that would not normally produce an effect can instead cause uterine contractions during labor. The density of the receptors sharply decreases after parturition. The decline downregulates uterine sensitivity and serves to prevent contractions during lactation.

Most births occur without the need for obstetric intervention. In some cases, however, drug therapy is necessary to maintain the safety of the woman and the fetus. Induction of labor is the attempt to initiate uterine contractions before their spontaneous onset. Uterine-stimulating drugs are used most frequently to induce or augment labor in selected pregnant women.

Indications for the induction of labor include situations in which the risk of continued pregnancy to the mother or fetus is considered to be greater than the risks of delivery or of pharmacologic induction. Maternal circumstances may include pregnancy-induced hypertension (PIH), isoimmunization, or maternal conditions such as renal disease or diabetes. Fetal indications that may require induction of labor include postmaturity syndrome, oligohydramnios, macrosomia (large baby), intrauterine growth restriction, or fetal death. Labor induction is accomplished through the use of cervical ripening drugs and drugs that cause contractions.

Augmentation of labor is any attempt to stimulate uterine contractions when labor has already begun but the contractions are found inadequate. Augmentation may be started when the cervix is not dilating, the fetus is not descending, or the contractions have proven to be weak via measurement by an intrauterine pressure monitor.

STAGES OF LABOR

The *first stage* of labor begins with uterine contractions causing progressive cervical change and is complete when the cervix is dilated to 10 cm. Contractions become progressively stronger and more rhythmic during the *latent phase,* and there is minimal discomfort. The cervix thins and dilates to about 4 cm. This phase lasts about 12 hours if this is the woman's first pregnancy, or 5 hours if she is a multipara.

During the active phase, the cervix opens from about 4 cm to the full 10 cm. The infant's head begins to descend into the woman's pelvis, and she begins to feel an urge to push. If this is the woman's first pregnancy, the phase lasts about 3 hours; it lasts 2 hours in subsequent pregnancies.

The *second stage* of labor begins with complete dilation of the cervix and ends with delivery of the infant. With a first pregnancy, the stage lasts 45 to 60 minutes; in later pregnancies 15 to 30 minutes. If monitoring indicates that the fetus is continuing its descent through the pelvis and is healthy, many times the woman will be allowed to continue past the 2-hour time frame.

The third stage of labor lasts a few minutes (but can be longer) and begins with delivery of the infant and the placenta.

PHARMACOTHERAPEUTIC OPTIONS

Uterine Stimulant

◆ oxytocin (Oxytocin Injection, Pitocin, Syntocinon, Syntocinon Nasal Spray)

▥ Indications

The principal use of uterine stimulants, such as oxytocin, is for the induction of labor. Oxytocin is used to initiate or improve uterine contractions, providing use of the uterine stimulant is appropriate. Acceptable reasons to initiate labor

with oxytocin include preeclampsia at or near term, when delivery is in the best interest of the mother and the fetus, when there is premature rupture of membranes (PROM) and delivery is warranted, in the presence of maternal diabetes or Rh problems, in women with uterine inertia, and as an adjunct in the management of abortion.

▥ Pharmacodynamics

Oxytocin stimulates uterine contractions by increasing the intracellular calcium (Ca^{++}). Patient response to oxytocin is very individualized, varying with the sensitivity of oxytocin receptors. However, health care providers should be aware of the fact that oxytocin, even in its pure form, has inherent hypotensive effects due to dilation of vasculature; administration can potentially result in rebound hypertension when oxytocin is stopped or reflex tachycardia sets in. Its antidiuretic properties manifest with large dosages.

In the breast, the myoepithelium, a type of smooth muscle, will contract in response to oxytocin. Milk is forced by these contractions into large sinuses within the breast, where it is readily available to the suckling infant.

▥ Pharmacokinetics

Oxytocin is readily absorbed from the oral mucosa and when given parenterally (Table 59-1). The nasal passages are a less efficient route of delivery for oxytocin, and it is not administered orally because it will be destroyed by chymotrypsin in the gastrointestinal (GI) tract.

Oxytocin is distributed throughout the extracellular fluid, with small amounts reaching fetal circulation. Oxytocinase,

PHARMACOKINETICS
TABLE 59-1 Uterine Motility Drugs

Drug	Route	Onset	Peak	Duration	PB (%)	t½	BioA (%)
OXYTOCIN							
oxytocin	IV	Immed	UA	1 hour	UA	1–6 min	100
	IM	3–5 min	UA	2–3 hr	UA	3–5 min	UA
	NS	Few min	UA	20 min	UA	<10 min	UA
PROSTAGLANDINS							
carboprost	IM	15 min	2 hr	2 hr	NA	UA	NA
dinoprostone*	IC	10 min	30–45 min	2–3 hr	NA	UA	NA
mifepristone	PO	Rapid	90 min	72 hr	98	18 hr	69
misoprostol	PO	30 min	60–90 min	3–6 hr	80–90	20–40 min	UA
ERGOT ALKALOIDS							
ergonovine maleate	IV	1 min	UA	45 min	UA	UA	100
	IM	2–5 min	UA	3 hr	UA	UA	UA
	PO	5–15 min	UA	3 hr	UA	UA	UA
methylergonovine	IV	Immed	UA	45 min–3 hr	UA	30–120 min	100
	IM	2–5 min	0.5 hr	3 hr	UA	30–120 min	78
	PO	5–10 min	UA	3 hr	UA	UA	60
BETA₂ AGONISTS							
ritodrine	IV	Immed	30–60 min	UA	32	6 min; 1.5–2.5 hr†	100
	PO	Rapid	30–60 min	UA	32	UA	30
terbutaline sulfate	IV, SubQ	6–15 min	15–30 min	1.5–4 hr	UA	3–4 hr	100
	PO	30 min	1–2 hr	4–8 hr	UA	UA	30–50
MISCELLANEOUS							
Magnesium sulfate	IV	Immed	UA	30 min	UA	UA	100
	IM	1 hr	UA	3–4 hr	UA	UA	UA

*Dinoprostone: time to onset of cervical ripening. Time to abortion via suppository is 10 min, with a peak of 12–24 hr and a 2- to 3-hour duration of action.
†Ritodrine: distribution half-life is 6 min; second phase is 1.5–2.5 hr, with an elimination half-life of over 10 hr.
BioA, Bioavailability; *IC*, intracervical; *IM*, intramuscular; *Immed*, immediate; *IV*, intravenous; *NA*, not applicable; *NS*, nasal spray; *PB*, protein binding; *PO*, by mouth; *PV*, per vagina; *t½*, half-life; *UA*, unavailable.

a circulating enzyme produced in early pregnancy, is also capable of inactivating the drug. Oxytocin is eliminated through the kidneys and the liver.

▒ Adverse Effects and Contraindications

Maternal adverse effects include both those caused by the drug and those caused by contractions. Excessive contractions, or increased strength of the contractions, may cause increased blood loss, uterine rupture, and pelvic hematoma. When excessive contractions are present, stopping the drug is usually sufficient to reverse the process. Rapid intravenous (IV) administration of a large dose of oxytocin may cause hypertonic uterine contractions and fetal distress. Potential fetal reactions to oxytocin include abruptio placentae, bradycardia, arrhythmias, fetal trauma, brain damage, and fetal death secondary to asphyxia. Tocolytic drugs may be used to reverse the hypertonic uterus and resuscitate the fetus.

Rare, but severe, reactions to oxytocin include fatal afibrinogenemia, anaphylaxis, arrhythmias (e.g., premature ventricular contractions), subarachnoid hemorrhage, coma, and death. Less severe reactions may include hypertension or hypotension, nausea, and vomiting. **Oxytocin is known to cause dose-related water intoxication and death with prolonged use.** Oxytocin use is contraindicated in the following circumstances:

* When there is considerable cephalopelvic disproportion
* When the fetus is in an unfavorable position for delivery (e.g., transverse position), and cannot be delivered without changing its position
* In an emergency where the benefit-risk ratio for mother and/or fetus warrants intervention
* When the fetus is in distress and delivery is delayed
* When uterine contractions do not bring about delivery
* In the presence of an hypertonic or hyperactive uterus
* In situations where vaginal delivery is also contraindicated (e.g., active genital herpes, total placenta previa,

cord prolapse); or in patients who have had two or more caesarian deliveries or cervical or uterine surgeries

▒ Drug Interactions

A number of drug interactions are associated with oxytocin. Vasoconstrictors (e.g., norepinephrine) given concurrently with oxytocin have been linked to severe hypertension (Table 59-2). Cyclopropane can cause tachycardia and hypotension or bradycardia with abnormal atrioventricular rhythms. Similarly, thiopental given with oxytocin has been associated with a delay in anesthesia induction. Prochlorperazine and warfarin sodium have also been cited as producing drug interactions with oxytocin.

▒ Dosage Regimen

The desired cervical dilation rate of 1 cm/hr is used as a **Ⓐ** **guide for increasing oxytocin infusion rates.** The initial dose of oxytocin is 0.5 to 1 milliunits/min (equal to 3 to 6 mL/hr). The dose may be gradually increased in 1 to 2 milliunits/min after the first half hour. Once the desirable contraction pattern is established and labor has progressed to 5- to 6-cm dilation, the dose may be reduced by 1 to 2 milliunits/min. Infusion rates up to 6 milliunits/min deliver the same levels of oxytocin as those found in spontaneous labor. Infusion rates higher than this are rarely needed (Table 59-3).

▒ Lab Considerations

Owing to its short-term use, therapeutic serum levels of oxytocin are not determined. Oxytocin is not known to interfere with other laboratory tests.

Prostaglandins

* dinoprostone (Cervidil, Prostin E$_2$); ◆ Cervidil, Prepidil, Prostin E2 Gel
* carboprost tromethamine (Hemabate); ◆ Prostin/15M
* mifepristone (Mifeprex)
* misoprostol (Cytotec); ◆ Cytotec

DRUG INTERACTIONS
TABLE 59-2 Uterine Motility Drugs

Drug	Interaction Drug	Interaction
UTERINE STIMULANTS		
oxytocin	Vasopressors	Severe hypertension
	cyclopropane	Excessive hypotension
PROSTAGLANDINS		
dinoprostone, carboprost	oxytocin	Augments effects of interacting drug
mifepristone	ketoconazole, itraconazole, erythromycin	Inhibits biotransformation of mifepristone
	carbamazepine, rifampin, phenytoin, phenobarbital	Increases biotransformation of mifepristone
misoprostol	Magnesium-containing antacids	Increases risk of diarrhea
ERGOT ALKALOIDS		
ergonovine, methylergonovine	Diuretics, nicotine, Vasopressors	Additive vasoconstriction
	CYP 3A4 inhibitors	Increases risk for ergot toxicity
BETA₂ AGONISTS		
ritodrine, terbutaline	Decongestants, Sympathomimetics, Vasopressors	Increases adrenergic effects of beta$_2$ agonist
	Beta blockers	Blocks effects of beta$_2$ agonist
	Corticosteroids	Fatal pulmonary edema
	Anticholinergics, MAO inhibitors, TCAs	Increases risk for hypertensive crisis
	Potent anesthetics, meperidine, diazoxide, IV magnesium sulfate	Significant risk of pulmonary edema, hypotension, arrhythmias

MAO, Monoamine oxidase; *TCA*, tricyclic antidepressants.

DOSAGE
TABLE 59-3 Uterine Motility Drugs

Drug	Uses	Dosage	Implications
OXYTOCIN			
oxytocin	Induction or augmentation of labor	*Adult:* 0.5–1 milliunits/min IV via infusion pump. Increase by 1 milliunit/min every 30–60 min. Titrate to minimum of 3 contractions in 10 min.	**Uterine response should start within 3–5 min and persist for 2–3 hr.** ▲
	Control of postpartum bleeding	*Adult:* 10 milliunits/min IV after delivery of placenta; IV drip: 10–40 milliunits/L titrated to control uterine atony	Not recommended for IV push administration
	Promote milk letdown	*Adult:* 1–2 sprays to each nostril, 2–3 min before breastfeeding or pumping	Hold bottle upright and squeeze into nostrils while sitting up.
PROSTAGLANDINS			
dinoprostone	Cervical ripening	*Adult:* 20-mg vaginal suppository every 3–5 hr. Max: 240 mg (0.3 mg/hr) –or– 10-mg vaginal insert over 12 hr –or– 0.5–5-mg vaginal gel every 4–6 hr for 1–2 doses. Max: 1.5 mg/24 hr.	Start oxytocin 60 min after last dose of PG if delivery has not occurred after 24–36 hr.
carboprost	Postpartum hemorrhage	*Adult:* 250 mcg IM; may repeat in 15–90 min for 2 doses. Max: 2 mg	Not for IV use. Must be refrigerated
	Pregnancy termination	*Adult:* 250 mcg IM every 1.5–3.5 hr based on patient response. Max: 12 mg in 48 hr	
mifepristone (RU486)	Pregnancy termination	*Adult:* 600 mg PO as single dose; then 400 mg PO 2 days later if abortion has not occurred	**Do not confuse with misoprostol.** Expect bleeding or spotting for an average of 9–16 days. Used with misoprostol ▲
misoprostol	Cervical ripening Pregnancy termination	*Adult:* 25- to 50-mcg tablets placed in posterior fornix every 3–6 hr *Adult:* 100–200 mcg every 12 hr intravaginally	**Do not confuse with mifepristone.** Oxytocin may be started 1–2 hr after the last dose of misoprostol. ▲
ERGOT ALKALOIDS			
ergonovine	Postpartum hemorrhage	*Adult:* 0.2–0.4 mg IM every 6–12 hr. Max: 1 mg	Usual course of treatment is 48 hr. Total dosage should not exceed five doses.
methylergonovine	Postpartum hemorrhage	*Adult:* 0.2–0.4 mg IM every 6–12 hr. Not to exceed 1 mg	
BETA₂ AGONISTS			
ritodrine	Tocolysis	*Adult:* 0.1 mg IV with 10 mg PO 30 min before stopping IV therapy. Follow with 10 mg PO every 2 hr for 24 hr. Increase by 0.05 mg every 10–15 min based on patient response. Maintenance: 0.15–0.35 mg/min for 12 hr; 10–20 mg PO every 4–6 hr. Total dose not to exceed 120 mg/day	Use of an IV infusion pump is recommended.
terbutaline sulfate	Tocolysis (unlabeled use)	*Adult:* 2.5 mg PO every 4–6 hr until term. Adjust dose based on maternal and fetal response. Not to exceed 15 mg/24hr. IV: 2.5–10 mcg/hr Max: 100 mcg/hr	**Limit use to less than 72 hr. Should not be used for continuous tocolysis.** Use infusion pump. ▲
MISCELLANEOUS			
magnesium sulfate	Tocolysis	*Adult:* 4–6 grams IV bolus then 1–4 grams/hr	Continued for 24–48 hr until patient is ready for subQ terbutaline.
nifedipine	Tocolysis	*Adult:* 10–20 mg PO every 4–8 hr to max of 4 doses	Limit use of drug to less than 48 hr.

IM, Intramuscular (route); *IV*, intravenous (route); *PG*, prostaglandin; *PO*, by mouth; *subQ*, subcutaneous (route).

▥ Indications

Dinoprostone and misoprostol are used to ripen an unfavorable cervix (Bishop's score <5) at or near term when induction of labor is warranted (Table 59-4).

Dinoprostone vaginal suppositories can be used (1) to terminate a pregnancy during the twelfth through twentieth weeks of gestation; (2) to evacuate uterine contents in situations of missed abortion or intrauterine fetal death up to 20 weeks of gestation; and (3) to manage trophoblastic disease (benign hydatidiform mole). It is vital that patients with trophoblastic disease be closely followed to ensure that they do not develop choriocarcinoma at a later date.

Carboprost is also used to abort pregnancy between the thirteenth and twentieth weeks of gestation, and in the following circumstances surrounding second trimester abortion: (1) failure to expulse the fetus using another method; (2) premature rupture of membranes with insufficient or absent uterine activity; (3) necessity of repeating intrauterine instillation of a drug to expel the fetus; (4) inadvertent or spontaneous rupture

of membranes in the presence of a fetus before it is viable; and (5) absence of sufficient uterine activity for expulsion.

Carboprost is also indicated for the treatment of postpartum hemorrhage due to uterine atony that has not responded to conventional methods of management such as uterine

TABLE 59-4 Bishop's Score

Criteria	Points			
	0	1	2	3
Cervical dilation (cm)	0	1–2	3–4	>5
Cervical effacement (%)	0–30	40–50	60–70	>80
Cervical consistency	Firm	Moderate	Soft	—
Cervical position	Posterior	Central	Anterior	—
Fetal station	−3	−2	−1	+1, +2

Adapted from Bishop, E. (1964). Pelvic scoring for elective induction. *Obstetrics and Gynecology, 24,* 266–288. Reprinted with permission from the American College of Obstetricians and Gynecologists.

massage and IV oxytocin. Carboprost is not recommended in patients with asthma or heart disease.

Mifepristone is also used to terminate an intrauterine pregnancy up to the forty-ninth gestational day. Prostaglandins are also used to maintain the patency of the ductus arteriosus in neonates with certain types of heart disease.

▥ Pharmacodynamics

Prostaglandin E_2 (PGE_2) and $PGF_{2\alpha}$ are active metabolites of arachidonic acid, derivatives of fatty acids. The amnion and chorion are responsible for the majority of PGE_2 production, whereas $PGF_{2\alpha}$ is preferentially produced in the decidua and myometrium. Unlike true hormones, however, prostaglandins do not travel to distant sites to produce effects. They act on the very tissues in which they are made. Exogenous prostaglandins induce uterine contractions that are comparable in frequency and duration to those occurring naturally. Further, the prostaglandin content of amniotic fluid, umbilical cord blood, and maternal blood increases at term and during labor. The ability of the uterus to synthesize prostaglandins increases at term. Lastly, labor is delayed and prolonged by drugs that inhibit prostaglandin synthesis.

However, the exact mechanism of action of prostaglandins is unknown. It is theorized that intracellular concentrations of cyclic 3′,5′-adenosine monophosphate (cAMP) or the regulation of cellular membrane calcium transport may be involved. Degradation of prostaglandins is so rapid that these substances rarely escape their tissue of origin intact. Unlike other abortifacients, however, prostaglandins are not feticidal. Hence, a fetus aborted by means of prostaglandins may show transient signs of life.

▥ Pharmacokinetics

Intravaginal dinoprostone is well absorbed through vaginal mucosa, with the onset of contractions noted in as little as 10 minutes after insertion. The effects last for 2 to 3 hours (see Table 59-1). Dinoprostone is biotransformed in the kidneys, the lungs, the spleen, and other body tissues. Elimination of the drug and its metabolites occurs through the kidneys, with small amounts in the feces.

Carboprost is absorbed slowly when given intramuscularly, with a drug onset of action of 15 minutes and peak action reached in 2 hours. Biotransformation takes place by the action of tissue enzymes. The pharmacokinetics of vaginal use of misoprostol are not available.

Misoprostol is rapidly absorbed from the GI tract and rapidly converted to an active metabolite. The metabolite is primarily eliminated through the urine.

Following oral administration, mifepristone is absorbed from the GI tract and rapidly converted to an active metabolite. Peak plasma concentrations are reached 90 minutes after ingestion. Biotransformation takes place in the liver. Fifty percent of mifepristone is eliminated between 12 and 72 hours after administration, with the remaining percentage having an elimination half-life of 18 hours.

▥ Adverse Effects and Contraindications

The adverse effects of prostaglandins depend in part on their formulation as well as their dosage. Nausea, vomiting, and diarrhea occur in up to 60% of patients as a result of prostaglandin stimulation of GI smooth muscle. These responses can be minimized by pretreatment with antiemetic and antidiarrheal drugs.

The endocervical prostaglandin gels most often cause back pain, fever, and uterine contraction abnormalities. **Intense ▲ uterine contractions can result in uterine rupture, cervical trauma, cervical lacerations, painful chemical cervicitis, and retained placenta.**

Patients receiving the suppository formulation of dinoprostone most often complain of headache and chills. Seventy percent of patients receiving dinoprostone in 20-mg doses have fevers as high as 101° F. The fevers may continue for approximately 6 hours after dosing and are resistant to aspirin. Vascular symptoms including hot flashes, flushing, headaches, lightheadedness, fainting sensations, a diastolic blood pressure drop of 20 mm Hg, arrhythmias, and death have been reported. Respiratory symptoms including wheezing, dyspnea, bronchospasm, coughing, and tightness of chest and chest pain have accompanied the administration of these drugs. Anaphylaxis is possible. Underlying cardiac disease and asthma are relative contraindications for prostaglandin administration.

Prolonged heavy bleeding (i.e., soaking through more ▲ than two thick full-size sanitary pads per hour for 2 consecutive hours) can be indicative of incomplete abortion or other complications. Patients experiencing prolonged heavy vaginal bleeding may need immediate medical intervention to prevent hypovolemic shock.

Serious bacterial infections, with some extremely rare cases leading to fatal septic shock, have resulted following the use of mifepristone for abortion. Mifepristone and misoprostol should not be used for pregnancy termination in patients who have a confirmed or suspected ectopic pregnancy (treatment will not terminate an ectopic pregnancy), or undiagnosed adnexal mass, and in women with an intrauterine device (IUD) in place.

▥ Drug Interactions

Drug interactions of prostaglandins are identified in Table 59-2.

▥ Dosage Regimens

Historically, *Laminaria digitata*, a species of kelp or seaweed, was used for induction of labor. Now, it may be used concurrently with prostaglandin administration for second-trimester terminations. When dried, *Laminaria* has the ability to absorb water and expand with substantial force. It has been used to dilate the cervical canal in induced abortion. Oxytocin may be started 1 to 2 hours after the last dose of misoprostol.

Induction of cervical ripening has been achieved with dinoprostone gel. The gel is placed in close proximity to the cervix at 4- to 6-hour intervals, followed by IV oxytocin administration 4 to 6 hours after the last gel administration. A diaphragm may be used to hold the gel next to the cervix. One or two doses are usually administered, although up to four doses have been used for some patients. The patient should remain in a supine position for at least 30 minutes after drug administration. The intraamniotic and extraamniotic routes are not recommended because of unacceptably high incidence of adverse affects.

Dinoprostone suppositories are used to terminate pregnancies in which the uterine size is equivalent to 20 weeks or less. If appropriate, IV oxytocin at doses of 10 to 100 milliunits/hour can be used if delivery has not occurred 24 to 36 hours after induction (see Table 59-3).

ENDOCRINE

Use carboprost for no longer than 48 hours. Dosages over 12 mg are contraindicated because of risk of bronchospasm, vomiting, hypertension, and anaphylaxis.

Termination of pregnancy using mifepristone and misoprostol requires three separate office visits. On the first visit, the patient is administered 600 mg of mifepristone. Two days later, a dose of 400 mcg of misoprostol should be given if complete abortion has not already been confirmed. The third visit is used as follow-up to verify that complete abortion of the fetus has occurred. Surgical termination of the pregnancy is recommended if the drugs fail.

Ergot Alkaloids

* ergonovine maleate (Ergotrate Maleate)
* methylergonovine (Methergine)

▓ *Indications*

Ergonovine and methylergonovine are used to increase the strength, the duration, and the frequency of uterine contractions in patients with uterine atony, and to decrease postpartum and postabortion bleeding. Their ability to induce sustained uterine contraction makes them particularly suited for these purposes.

▓ *Pharmacodynamics*

Ergot is a naturally occurring fungus found on rye plants. Spores of this fungus are spread by the wind or flying insects and carried to the ovaries of young grains. A growth of tissue forms and hardens. These hard purple growths are a major source of commercial ergot. Ergonovine has proved to be the most effective uterine stimulant. Methylergonovine is a derivative of ergonovine and produces effects similar to those of the natural alkaloid.

The uterine-stimulating effects of ergot alkaloids appear to be the result of interactions with receptors for biogenic amines. The prolactin-inhibiting effects are accomplished by direct action on the pituitary and hypothalamus, causing the release of prolactin-inhibiting factor via the dopamine receptors.

▓ *Pharmacokinetics*

Both orally and parenterally administered ergonovine maleate and methylergonovine maleate are rapidly absorbed. IV usage is limited to life-threatening situations only. The GI tract absorbs approximately 60% of methylergonovine (see Table 59-1). It is believed that ergonovine maleate undergoes extensive hepatic biotransformation followed by renal elimination of its metabolites. Methylergonovine is eliminated through nonrenal mechanisms in the feces.

▓ *Adverse Effects and Contraindications*

Nausea, vomiting, dizziness, and a headache are the most common adverse effects of ergot alkaloids. Other adverse effects include tinnitus, *ergotism* (a constellation of signs and symptoms that include blood pressure changes, weak pulse, dyspnea, chest pain, and numbness and coldness of the extremities), confusion, excitement, delirium, hallucinations, convulsions, and coma.

Hypertension has been recorded, especially in women with preeclampsia or underlying hypertension. **Ergot alkaloids are contraindicated for use in these patients due to instances of cerebrovascular accidents, seizures, and serious arrhythmias.** Use them cautiously in patients with hepatic or renal impairment.

▓ *Drug Interactions*

Ergot alkaloids can produce excessive vasoconstriction when they are used with other vasopressors, such as dopamine or nicotine (see Table 59-2).

▓ *Dosage Regimen*

Dosages for methylergonovine and ergonovine are exactly the same. Oral doses are given until heavy bleeding slows or up to 7 days of continued administration. The usual course, however, is 48 hours. Change to an oral formulation after administering five intramuscular (IM) doses. Administration is usually held until after passage of the placenta (see Table 59-3).

PRETERM LABOR

The largest cause of infant morbidity and mortality is preterm birth. Preterm labor (PTL) is defined as the onset of labor with cervical changes before completion of the thirty-seventh week of pregnancy. In the majority of patients with PTL, the exact cause of the condition is unknown.

Certain conditions are known to predispose women to PTL. Up to one third of preterm deliveries are due to infection. Chorioamnionitis, an infection of the membranes that cover the fetus, is implicated in the majority of these cases. Closely associated with infection and PTL is premature rupture of membranes. In the patient with PROM, onset of labor often occurs shortly after the rupture, especially when infection is the cause. The time between membrane rupture and delivery is known as the latency period. If infection is not the cause of PROM, this latency period may last from a few days to weeks.

An overdistended uterus, due to either multiple gestation or polyhydramnios, is known to increase the chance of PTL. Fetal anomalies, especially chromosomal abnormalities, and death of the fetus can precipitate early labor. Cervical incompetence and certain uterine anomalies predispose women to preterm deliveries. Placenta disorders such as placenta previa or abruptio placentae may cause PTL in a percentage of patients. The true cause of PTL is found in only a small percentage of patients. The majority of cases are classified as cause unknown.

PHARMACOTHERAPEUTIC OPTIONS

Alcohol was the first drug used to stop labor. It is rarely if ever used for that purpose today, particularly with the discovery of tocolytic drugs (see Controversy box). All drugs currently used for tocolysis were originally developed for the treatment of other diseases. The drugs covered in this chapter are discussed only for their therapeutic use as tocolytics.

Beta Agonists

* ritodrine (Yutopar)
* terbutaline (Bricanyl, Brethine)

▓ *Indications*

Beta$_2$ agonists are commonly used for the treatment of PTL. Ritodrine is the only drug approved by the Food and Drug Administration (FDA) for tocolytic use; however, terbutaline is more commonly used because it is less expensive. In general, ritodrine is reserved for pregnancies in which the

Controversy

Uterine Motility Drugs

Jonathan J. Wolfe

Therapy in response to inappropriately early labor has advanced radically in the past 3 decades. Formerly, obstetric care in the face of premature labor largely involved use of bed rest. In acute settings, the principal therapeutic intervention involved use of intravenous ethanol. Neither treatment offered great expectations of good outcomes. Complete bed rest in advanced pregnancy predictably enhanced the chance of clotting disorders, pneumonia, and the other sequelae one expects with inactivity. Alcohol infusion (in combination with dextrose) was not appropriate for long-term use.

In the 1970s, a new product for management of preterm labor was introduced. Ritodrine, a beta agonist, offered important improvement in responding to the condition. The good this drug may accomplish is clear, because prematurely delivered children suffer disproportionately from a variety of severe disorders. The premature neonate also is far more likely to die than the full-term child. Within the limits of maternal tolerance, ritodrine allows continuous and effective ablation of inappropriate labor.

Controversy involving the use of this drug is twofold. The first relates to the mother's exposure to potential harm. A trade-off is required in the case of a pregnant patient with diabetes mellitus, steroid-treated asthma, and a variety of cardiac ailments. Severe pulmonary complications, sometimes manifested postpartum, are also associated with the drug. The second dilemma stems from commercial use of ritodrine. Home care using labor monitoring devices is available in many markets. These devices can provide data over telephone links to prompt administration of tocolytics, such as ritodrine. However, in a managed care setting, it is difficult to establish the cost-benefit ratio of outpatient tocolysis.

CLINICAL REASONING

- In choosing to use monitoring and tocolytic interventions, what level of hazard to the neonate is acceptable in the case of a mother who is otherwise healthy and has had an uneventful pregnancy?
- What alternative use could be made of the money spent on monitoring for premature labor and providing home intravenous therapy?
- Imagine that a marketing representative from a home care company has met with you in your office to explain the labor monitoring and intravenous drug therapy available from his company. What ethical concerns would you, as a practitioner, have about recommending this provider to one of your patients?
- What harm might come to a patient as the result of choosing either to use or not to use tocolytic therapy?
- In an acute care setting, what additional monitoring would be appropriate for meeting the outcomes of tocolytic therapy?

---

gestational age is greater than 20 weeks but less than 34 to 36 weeks. Balance the use of a tocolytic drug (i.e., to prolong intrauterine development) against the risks of early delivery to both the mother and fetus.

Pharmacodynamics

Beta$_2$ agonists stimulate the production of cyclic cAMP by activating the enzyme adenyl cyclase. An increase in cAMP increases the uptake and sequestration of intracellular Ca^{++}. The lack of available Ca^{++} prevents activation of the contractile proteins of smooth muscle cell, creating uterine smooth muscle relaxation. The result is a decrease in the intensity and duration of contractions.

The optically pure R-isomer of the beta$_2$ agonist albuterol, substantially free of its corresponding S-isomer, is a potent inhibitor of premature uterine contractions and at the same time avoids the adverse effects associated with the corresponding S-isomer. A new method is in development which will use the optically pure R-isomer of albuterol to treat premature uterine contractions while minimizing the adverse effects of racemic albuterol.

Pharmacokinetics

The bioavailability of oral ritodrine is approximately 30%, with peak plasma levels attained in 30 to 60 minutes. IV ritodrine has an immediate onset. Elimination of both terbutaline and ritodrine is partially achieved through biotransformation in the liver to inactive metabolites. The majority of the drugs and the inactive conjugates are eliminated in urine (see Table 59-1).

Adverse Effects and Contraindications

As might be expected, beta$_2$ agonists produce a number of cardiovascular and metabolic adverse effects in the mother. Although there are few changes in the mean arterial pressure, a dose-related tachycardia as well as an increase in cardiac output occur. The response is probably the result of a reflex response to the lowered diastolic pressure and direct action on β_1 receptors in the heart. Other cardiac-related adverse effects include tachycardia, widening pulse pressure, chest pain or tightening, heart murmur, palpitations, and cardiac arrest. ST-T depression and T-wave inversion have been reported with terbutaline. Other adverse effects commonly seen include tremors, restlessness, jitteriness, nervousness, emotional upset, and anxiety. Headache, nausea, vomiting, erythema, malaise, and lethargy have also been reported.

There is decreased renal elimination of sodium, potassium, and water. This is presumably due to the enhanced secretion of renin. If hydration during beta$_2$ agonist therapy is overly vigorous, pulmonary edema may result, with or without evidence of myocardial failure. The patient is especially at high risk if she has concurrent preeclampsia. Evidence of cardiac disease is a contraindication to use of beta$_2$ agonists. Patients complaining or showing signs of severe cardiac symptoms should be worked up for occult cardiac disease.

Ritodrine can cause marked hyperglycemia. Although treatment is not usually required, persistent hyperglycemia may result in fetal tachycardia, hyperinsulinemia, and reactive hypoglycemia in the fetus should parturition proceed. The use of beta agonists in patients with diabetes is hazardous and is usually contraindicated.

Hypokalemia is another consequence of ritodrine administration. This state reflects a movement of potassium into the intracellular compartment, although total body stores are not reduced and treatment is not usually indicated. Ritodrine administration in patients with hyperthyroidism may result in arrhythmias.

Drug Interactions

Beta blockers antagonize the effects of ritodrine and terbutaline; therefore, avoid concurrent use. Simultaneous use with other sympathomimetic drugs is not recommended because of the possible additive effects (see Table 59-2).

Intravenous use of a beta₂ agonist increases the woman's risk for pulmonary edema. Additional use of corticosteroid to promote fetal lung maturity further increases the risk for pulmonary edema. Concomitant use of IV magnesium sulfate and a subcutaneous (subQ) beta₂ agonist is contraindicated except during emergency transport because of a significant risk of pulmonary edema, hypotension, and arrhythmias.

Dosage Regimen

The dosages of ritodrine and terbutaline are individualized by balancing uterine response and unwanted effects (see Table 59-3). Maternal and fetal heart rates are monitored, and the infusion is decreased if the heart rates exceed 130 and 170, respectively. The lowest effective dose is continued for at least 12 hours before discontinuing IV administration and starting the patient on subQ formulations.

Laboratory Considerations

Monitor serum glucose levels in patients with diabetes. In patients concurrently receiving potassium-depleting drugs, monitor serum electrolytes including sodium and potassium levels. Therapeutic serum levels of beta₂ agonists are not usually performed because the drug is titrated to uterine activity.

For more information, see the Evolve Resources Bonus Content "Influence of Selected Drugs on Laboratory Values," found at http://evolve.elsevier.com/Gutierrez/pharmacotherapeutics.

Miscellaneous Drugs
Magnesium Sulfate

The primary indication for use of magnesium sulfate is the treatment of seizures associated with preeclampsia. It was subsequently found to have tocolytic effects. Magnesium sulfate relaxes both the frequency and the force of contractions. Labor is arrested at magnesium levels ranging from 6 to 8 mEq/L. Because magnesium does not sensitize the heart to catecholamines or promote hyperglycemia, it may be preferred to beta₂ agonists in women with hyperthyroidism or diabetes. Prolonging the pregnancy for at least 48 hours allows time for drug-induced stimulation of surfactant production in the fetus.

Serum magnesium levels of 4 mEq/L and above may cause hot flashes, flushing, sweating, nausea, vomiting, headache, and depression of reflexes. At levels of 8 to 10 mEq/L, patients complain of blurry vision, double vision, and lethargy. The deep tendon reflexes are depressed or absent. Respiratory arrest, flaccid paralysis, and severe central nervous system (CNS) depression can occur at serum levels above 13 to 15 mEq/L. Levels equal to or greater than 25 mEq/L will cause circulatory collapse and cardiac arrest. Neonatal CNS depression may occur in infants born to mothers who are taking magnesium. An attendant who is familiar with neonatal resuscitation, preferably a neonatal nurse practitioner or neonatologist, should be attending the delivery. Calcium gluconate reverses magnesium sulfate toxicity.

Nifedipine

Nifedipine, a calcium channel blocker (see Chapter 37), rather than a tocolytic, is often considered the drug of choice for preterm labor, although it is not FDA-approved for such use. Nifedipine works to inhibit the transmembranous influx of calcium ions. This action inhibits the contractile process of uterine smooth muscle.

Nonsteroidal Antiinflammatory Drugs

Nonsteroidal antiinflammatory drugs (i.e., prostaglandin inhibitors; NSAIDs) such as indomethacin and sulindac have been used to prolong gestation in both term and preterm pregnancies. The overall experience with indomethacin is limited; however, it may be the drug of choice in the management of PTL if IV access is not possible (such as during transfer to high-risk care centers), or if polyhydramnios is present.

Indomethacin use in the management of PTL has the potential for fetal adverse effects. Do not use NSAIDs in gestations over 34 weeks and, when used, limit use to 48 hours. NSAIDs are ordinarily only used if PTL is thought to be caused by polyhydramnios. Of particular importance is the possibility of premature closure of the ductus arteriosus and the production of pulmonary hypertension. However, fetal echocardiography can detect early signs of constriction of the ductus, and its use may allow for continued administration of indomethacin or related drugs in those instances in which evidence of ductal constriction is absent. Indomethacin also causes a dose-dependent oligohydramnios owing to decreased fetal urinary output. Oligohydramnios is reversible by stopping the drug.

Drugs To Improve Neonatal Outcomes

It is believed that fetal lungs produce surfactant in response to a cascade of hormonal signals. Fetal corticosteroids are postulated to be involved in this process, although the exact mechanism of action is unknown. There is evidence that use of corticosteroids reduces the risk of fetal respiratory distress syndrome (RDS), necrotizing enterocolitis, electrolyte imbalances, and patent ductus arteriosus in premature infants who are treated prenatally.

CLINICAL REASONING

Treatment Objectives

The goal of treatment with a uterine stimulant is to establish regular contractions that occur every 3 to 5 minutes and last for 60 to 90 seconds. To effect cervical effacement and dilation, a rate that mimics normal spontaneous labor (approximately 1 cm/hr) is desired to deliver a fetus vaginally without increasing the risk to the mother or the fetus. The goal in abortifacient treatment is to cause expulsion of uterine contents without increasing maternal risk for complications.

The treatment goal in tocolysis is to stop uterine contractions and prevent progression of cervical effacement and dilation. In addition, corticosteroids are ordinarily used to delay delivery of the fetus for 24 to 48 hours in order to permit acceleration of fetal lung maturity if the gestation is of less than 32 weeks.

Treatment Options

▥ *Patient Variables*

Society as a whole tends to view labor as a natural process. "Women have been dropping babies in the fields for years" is a persuasive attitude that has been cited many times. Therefore, women who require induction of labor or who experience PTL may believe that they have failed or their body has failed them. Added to this problem is the anxiety and fear the patient and family have about the survival of the infant. Parents often experience tremendous apprehension about the survival and quality of life of their unborn child. Compounding this issue is the pervasive feeling of powerlessness the patient and partner often experience. In America's multicultural society, understanding the patient's cultural views of pregnancy and the labor experience influences how the health care provider perceives the patient's attitudes and influences the plan of care.

LIFE-SPAN CONSIDERATIONS. Obtain information about the outcome of all previous pregnancies. This includes information about any abortions (spontaneous or elective), and previous term or preterm deliveries. The length of labor, the type of delivery, the gestational age at delivery, the weight of the infant, and any complications are important to ascertain. Note the past use of drugs to prevent or to induce delivery.

A complete assessment of the current pregnancy includes reviewing the first, second, and third trimesters of pregnancy for any problems or complications. It is important to determine whether the mother has had previous contractions or bleeding episodes. If the answer is yes, query her as to what treatment was initiated and if it was effective. The fetus is also a patient; therefore ask questions about fetal movement.

It is exceedingly important to determine the gestational age of the fetus, because drug therapy may differ considerably based on the course of the pregnancy. If the patient is experiencing contractions, the assessment includes time of onset, duration, frequency, and the perceived strength of the contraction. Has the patient noted leakage of vaginal fluid? If yes, it is important to determine the quantity, the color, and the odor of the fluid. Recent sexual intercourse, owing to the release of prostaglandins from the cervix and prostaglandins in the semen, may cause the onset of contractions. Therefore, ask the patient in PTL about recent sexual intercourse.

Before the thirty-seventh week, or if it must be determined whether the patient is leaking amniotic fluid, perform a sterile speculum exam in place of the sterile vaginal exam. The speculum exam eliminates cervical stimulation, which can cause the release of prostaglandins, thus initiating contractions. The speculum exam also decreases the chance of vertical transmission of bacteria that can occur with a vaginal exam. Also check deep tendon reflexes to evaluate hyperreflexia associated with preeclampsia.

▥ *Drug Variables*

UTERINE STIMULANTS. Augmentation of labor may be indicated when non–drug measures such as amniotomy (artificial rupture of membranes) and nipple stimulation are unsuccessful. It may also be appropriate in cases in which prolongation of pregnancy is dangerous to the mother (e.g., hypertension, diabetes) or the fetus. Oxytocin is considered the initial treatment if Bishop's score is 5 or more in patients who are gravida one or two (see Table 59-4). **Do not use oxytocin to induce ⚠ labor for any reason other than medical necessity.** The convenience of the health care provider or patient is an unacceptable reason for induction.

Before administering oxytocin, assess fetal maturity and presentation, and pelvic adequacy. Monitor the character, the frequency, and the duration of uterine contractions, resting uterine tone, and fetal heart rate during treatment with oxytocin. Use a Y-connection when preparing the IV infusion so that the oxytocin solution can be discontinued if necessary while access to a vein is maintained. **Do not administer oxy- ⚠ tocin by more than one route simultaneously. Should any of the following conditions develop, discontinue oxytocin, turn the patient onto her left side (to prevent fetal anoxia), and give oxygen:**

- Contractions are less than 2 minutes apart
- Contractions are stronger than 50 to 65 mm Hg on the internal uterine pressure monitor
- Resting uterine pressure is greater than 15 to 20 mm Hg
- Contractions are lasting longer than 60 to 90 seconds
- A significant change in fetal heart rate occurs

Terbutaline 0.125 to 0.25 mg by IV push can be used for fetal distress. Magnesium sulfate should be available if excessive stimulation of the myometrium occurs and the patient has a known cardiac defect. In addition, monitor the patient for signs and symptoms of water intoxication (drowsiness, listlessness, confusion, headache, and anuria).

Selection of a uterine stimulant to be used as an abortifacient depends on gestational age. During weeks 1 through 12, suction dilation and curettage is the procedure of choice. Mifepristone may also be used in some instances. Other drugs are generally ineffective during this time. During weeks 13 to 20, dilation and evacuation is generally preferred. Oxytocin is less effective during this time but may be used as an adjunct, if necessary. Hypertonic solutions (e.g., saline, urea) behave as poisons to the placenta and fetus, thus acting as an abortifacient.

PROSTAGLANDINS. Induction of labor without cervical softening has a high failure rate. Prostaglandins stimulate effective preinduction cervical ripening. When prostaglandins are administered locally, they decrease the duration of labor, shorten the induction-to-delivery period, decrease the dosage of oxytocin required, and reduce the overall risk for failure of induction. Further, uterine response to oxytocin is enhanced in the presence of PGE$_2$. The time to induction and the duration of labor are longer with prostaglandin gel, although patient acceptance is greater.

Determine the degree of effacement before inserting the prostaglandin for cervical ripening. To avoid skin contact with prostaglandin, handle the drug carefully. For effective and proper administration, the patient should be in a dorsal recumbent position, with view of the cervix provided by the speculum. Use sterile technique when inserting the prostaglandin gel or suppository. After administration, instruct the patient to assume a supine position for 15 to 30 minutes to prevent leakage from the cervical canal. During low-dose prostaglandin use, monitor the fetus for 2 hours after the drug is administered.

During prostaglandin therapy, monitor the frequency, the duration, and the force of contractions, and uterine resting tone. Dinoprostone-induced adverse effects can be minimized by pretreatment with an antidiarrheal, antiemetic, and antipyretic (e.g., acetaminophen) drug before the use of high-dose prostaglandin.

Mifepristone is used in combination with prostaglandins (i.e., misoprostol) for termination of early pregnancy; it is given first, and the prostaglandin administered 48 hours later. The combination of the two drugs stimulates uterine contractions and the expulsion of uterine contents. The oral formulations of both drugs make the procedure more convenient and less expensive than using IM prostaglandins.

TOCOLYTICS. Tocolytics stop contractions for 24 to 48 hours, but there is debate about whether they improve perinatal outcomes or reduce the overall rate of preterm birth. There is a suggestion that tocolytics only decrease infant mortality in gestations of 24 to 27 weeks. Because perinatal morbidity and mortality are not altered, the purpose of tocolysis is to delay delivery long enough to administer corticosteroids to the mother. The corticosteroids hasten fetal lung maturity and reduce the incidence of respiratory distress in the premature newborn.

In general, tocolysis is indicated for preterm labor between 24 and 32 weeks' gestation, with documented cervical dilation and uterine contractions occurring every 7 to 10 minutes and lasting 30 seconds. Therapy is used only if there are no contraindications to stopping PTL; when major maternal illness cannot be controlled; in the presence of preeclampsia, abruptio placentae, chorioamnionitis, or severe fetal anomalies that are incompatible with life; or in the case of fetal demise.

When the decision to use a tocolytic drug is made, treatment is likely to be successful if cervical dilation is less than 4 cm and cervical effacement less than 80%. Tocolysis is usually not attempted if the membranes have ruptured, because there is a risk of infection. SubQ terbutaline is the drug of choice if the cervix is less than 3 cm dilated. IV magnesium sulfate or a beta$_2$ agonist is used for women with cervical dilation over 3 cm. After 48 hours, indomethacin or an NSAID may be added if IV tocolysis is not slowing uterine contractions.

Always administer magnesium sulfate infusions via IV pumps because of the serious consequences of extremely high magnesium levels. Monitor the patient's respiratory rate and patellar reflex before and throughout therapy. If the patient reports symptoms that reflect excessive dosages, decrease or discontinue the IV infusion and close observe the patient until lab results are available. Calcium gluconate, the reversal agent for magnesium sulfate, should be on hand. Monitor serum magnesium levels and renal function periodically throughout administration of parenteral magnesium sulfate.

Patient Education

ⅲ *Uterine Stimulants*

Advise patients receiving uterine stimulants to expect contractions, after administration is started, similar to those of menses. Inform them of the goal of therapy and that the infusion rate will be adjusted based on their response. Women receiving prostaglandins at high doses should be forewarned of the adverse effects of nausea, vomiting, diarrhea, and high temperatures that often occur and that they will be premedicated to lessen these effects.

When a prostaglandin is used as an abortifacient, instruct the patient to report any fever, chills, foul-smelling vaginal discharge, lower abdominal pain, or increased bleeding. Once expulsion of uterine contents and the placenta has occurred, thoroughly examine the patient for trauma (cervical or uterine lacerations).

ⅲ *Tocolytics*

Advise the patient receiving oral tocolytic therapy that contractions may resume even with therapy; in such cases advise the patient to contact the health care provider for reinstitution of IV therapy. Women taking beta$_2$ agonists should be aware of the drugs' common adverse effects.

Inform patients on magnesium sulfate that this drug may cause nausea and vomiting, especially with the loading dose. Other important information to include in patient education includes a flushed feeling, burning at the IV site, lethargy, blurred vision, and dry mouth.

Educate patients at risk for preterm delivery about the drugs that may be used to promote fetal lung maturity and the reasons for their use. Emotional support is vital during therapy.

Evaluation

The effectiveness of uterine stimulants such as oxytocin is demonstrated by the onset of effective contractions and an increase in uterine tone without the appearance of fluid volume excess. The effectiveness of prostaglandins is noted by cervical ripening and the induction of labor. If therapy is not successful in 10 or 12 hours, discontinue oxytocin and allow the patient to rest. The infusion may be restarted the following day.

The effectiveness of tocolysis is demonstrated by the discontinuation of uterine contractions and no further progression of cervical effacement and dilation. Additionally, tocolysis is considered a success if delivery of the fetus has been delayed long enough (24 to 48 hours) to permit acceleration of fetal lung maturity.

KEY POINTS

- The etiology for the initiation of labor is unknown, but several theories have been proposed.
- Labor is separated into three distinct stages: progressive cervical change, dilation of cervix and delivery of infant, and delivery of placenta.
- Induction or augmentation of labor, if needed, is accomplished through the use of cervical ripening drugs and drugs that cause uterine contractions.
- The goal of treatment with a uterine stimulant is to establish regular contractions that occur every 3 to 5 minutes and last 60 to 90 seconds.
- Oxytocins are used for the initial induction of labor in patients with a favorable cervix or in patients who are gravida three or greater.

- PTL is defined as the onset of labor with cervical change before completion of the thirty-seventh week of gestation. The etiology of PTL is often unknown.
- The treatment goal for tocolysis is to stop uterine contractions and to prevent the progression of cervical effacement and dilation.
- Prostaglandins are used to ripen an unfavorable cervix. The primary use of prostaglandins is for termination of pregnancy.
- Ergot alkaloids have been used to decrease postpartum bleeding secondary to uterine atony.
- Beta$_2$ agonists, magnesium sulfate, nifedipine, and NSAIDs are used in the treatment of PTL.

- Fetal maturity and presentation, pelvic adequacy, maternal vital signs, and fetal heart rate should be assessed before the start of therapy and periodically thereafter.
- The effectiveness of uterine stimulants is demonstrated by the onset of effective contractions and an increase in uterine tone without indications of fluid volume excess.
- The effectiveness of tocolysis is demonstrated by the discontinuation of uterine contractions, and progression of cervical effacement and dilation.
- The effectiveness of an abortifacient drug is demonstrated by expulsion of uterine contents.

Bibliography

Arias, F. (2000). Pharmacology of oxytocin and prostaglandins. *Clinical Obstetrics and Gynecology, 43*(3), 455–468.

Berkman, N., Thorp, J., Lohr, K., et al. (2003). Tocolytic treatment for the management of preterm labor: A review of the evidence. *American Journal of Obstetrics and Gynecology, 188*(6), 1648–1659.

Hofmeyr, G., and Gülmezoglu, A. (2003). Vaginal misoprostol for cervical ripening and induction of labour. *Cochrane Database of Systematic Reviews. 2003,* Issue 1. Art. No. CD000941. DOI: 10.1002/14651858.CD000941.

Iams, J. (2003). Prediction and early detection of preterm labor. *Obstetrics and Gynecology, 101*(2), 402–412.

Kelly, A., Kavanagh, J., and Thomas, J. (2003). Vaginal prostaglandin (PGE2 and PGF2a) for induction of labour at term. *Cochrane Database of Systematic Reviews. 2003,* Issue 4. Art. No. CD003101. DOI: 10.1002/14651858.CD003101.

Lopez, B. (2003). Mechanisms of labor: Biochemical aspects. *BJOG: An International Journal of Obstetrics and Gynecology, 110*(Suppl 20), 39–45.

Sanchez-Ramos, L., and Kaunitz, A. (2000). Misoprostol for cervical ripening and labor induction: A systematic review of the literature. *Clinical Obstetrics and Gynecology, 43*(3), 475–488.

Tenore, J. (2003). Methods for cervical ripening and induction of labor. *American Family Physician, 67*(10), 2213–2218.

ENDOCRINE

60

Fertility Drugs

The last decade brought a tremendous increase in the knowledge of the human reproductive system and a simultaneous expansion in medical interventions for the treatment of infertility. Fertility centers have come a long way from the first hush-hush consultations with specialists in obstetrics and gynecology, genetics, and urology; today's fertility centers are well-staffed with a range of health care professionals, and offer much more than testing, diagnosis, and treatment. Most fertility centers offer counseling as couples ride the roller coaster that will hopefully lead to conception, and many offer alternative family-building methods such as surrogacy opportunities. Still, only 50% to 60% of couples with diagnosed infertility expect to achieve pregnancy and carry the fetus to term even with the expert diagnosis and interventions available today.

INFERTILITY

EPIDEMIOLOGY AND ETIOLOGY

Infertility is defined as an inability to conceive after 1 year of unprotected coitus or an inability to carry a fetus to term. Primary infertility occurs in couples with no history of pregnancy with either partner. Secondary infertility occurs when there has been a previous pregnancy, regardless of the outcome.

In the United States, it is estimated that 1 to 2 million couples of child-bearing age (15 to 44 years old) are unsuccessful in their attempts to achieve pregnancy. In general, infertility rates increase with age and are more prevalent in certain populations. Blacks have a 1.5% greater incidence of infertility than whites. It is estimated that 40% of infertility is due to male factors, 40% due to female factors, and 20% due to both.

The physiologic events of normal fertility are discussed in Chapter 58. It is important to review the information on the menstrual cycle and the physiologic and pharmacologic effects of estrogens and progestins. Information on testosterone from Chapter 57 should also be reviewed. In particular, note the roles of luteinizing hormone (LH) and follicle-stimulating hormone (FSH) in male and female reproduction. Finally, consider the pulsatile nature of gonadotropin-releasing hormone (GnRH), the hormone that controls the release of LH and FSH and that is essential to normal reproductive function.

PATHOPHYSIOLOGY

Female Fertility Disorders

Female fertility disorders include problems related to follicular maturation, ovulation, pituitary disorders, or luteal-phase defects. Fertilization, implantation, and growth and development of the ovum may be a problem in patients with uterine,

tubal, and pelvic disorders that contribute to infertility (see Table 60-1).

▌▌ Ovulation Disorders

Disorders of ovulation are due to hypothalamic, pituitary, or ovarian dysfunction. Ovulatory dysfunction accounts for approximately 2% of female infertility. The hormonal system that sends feedback from the hypothalamus to the pituitary to the ovaries and then back can malfunction at any point.

Hypothalamic dysfunction produces a hypogonadotropic state. The inactivity of GnRH results in decreased secretion of gonadotropins, primarily LH, which in turn causes amenorrhea. Amenorrhea may be caused by disruption of estrogen production, which in turn has an impact on hypothalamic function. It has been shown that GnRH is inhibited by the feedback effects of ovarian steroids on the endogenous opiate system of the hypothalamus. Chronic stimulation of brain opioid activity is implicated as a cause of amenorrhea.

Prolactin levels are increased when gonadotropin levels are decreased. Opiate antagonists have been found to be effective in these women for increasing the LH pulse frequency suppressed by the excess opiates they produce.

Amenorrhea following the discontinuation of oral contraceptives is rare. It is possible that the woman had a history of undiagnosed abnormalities of the hypothalamic-pituitary-ovarian (HPO) axis before pill use or developed it during therapy. Because most women resume menstruation within 6 months, delay a definitive diagnosis until that time.

If the exact cause of amenorrhea is unknown, it is termed idiopathic hypothalamic dysfunction. Clinically, these patients have normal gonadotropin levels and exhibit withdrawal bleeding following progesterone challenge. When GnRH levels are low or GnRH is released improperly, however, most patients ovulate with pharmacotherapy.

Kallman's syndrome, a type of hypogonadotropic hypogonadism, is a rare congenital defect caused by a deficiency of GnRH. However, this syndrome predominates in males owing to the recessive nature of the X-chromosome. This syndrome appears to be genetically heterogeneous. Karyotyping reveals a normal female. Agenesis or hypoplasia of the olfactory lobes is associated with decreased luteinizing hormone–releasing factor (LRF). Patients manifest primary amenorrhea, decreased gonadotropin levels, and a lack of sexual development, as well as an inability to perceive odors. Although the ovaries are responsive to administered gonadotropins, ovulation cannot be induced.

▌▌ Pituitary Disorders

Examples of pituitary disorders affecting fertility include hyperprolactinemia and prolactin-secreting adenomas. Prolactin acts at the level of the gonads, the pituitary, or the hypothalamus to inhibit gonadotropin secretion. When prolactin

TABLE **60-1** Disorders of Fertility

Female Disorders of Fertility	Male Disorders of Fertility
OVULATION DISORDERS	**PRETESTICULAR DISORDERS**
Hypothalamic amenorrhea	Hypogonadotropic hypogonadism
Kallman's syndrome	Isolated gonadotropin deficiency
Birth control pills	Pituitary failure, hyperprolactinemia
Idiopathic hypothalamic dysfunction	Chronic disease
Stress, weight loss, anorexia	Kallman's syndrome
PITUITARY DISORDERS	**TESTICULAR DISORDERS**
Hyperprolactinemia	Dysfunctional spermatogenesis, varicocele
Sheehan's syndrome	Infection, toxins
Hypogonadotropic hypogonadism	Klinefelter's syndrome
OVARIAN DISORDERS	**POSTTESTICULAR DISORDERS**
Gonadotropin-resistant ovary syndrome	Absence of vas deferens, vasectomy, hypospadias
Polycystic ovary syndrome	Obstructions, retrograde ejaculation
Premature ovarian failure	Sperm autoimmunity
Luteinized, unruptured follicle syndrome	Physiologic or psychogenic dysfunction
Disorders of sexual development	Spinal cord injury
UTERINE, TUBAL, AND PELVIC DISORDERS	
Structural anomalies, tubal damage	
Endometriosis or endometritis	
Leiomyomas, unfavorable cervical mucus	
Asherman's syndrome (intrauterine adhesions)	
OTHER DISORDERS	
Heat, radiation, chemicals	
Endocrine disorders	
Complications of pregnancy	
LUTEAL-PHASE DEFECTS	

secretion is low, LH and estrogen levels may also be low. Hyperprolactinemia in women is associated with amenorrhea.

Many of the psychoactive drugs cause excess production of prolactin, as can stress and pituitary adenomas. In the postpartum period, the ovary is resistant to exogenous gonadotropin stimulation because of the hyperprolactinemic state induced by nipple stimulation. This often results in anovulation and is the basis for the belief that breastfeeding is a form of contraception. However, breastfeeding alone as a postpartum contraceptive has proved to be unreliable.

Postpartum hypopituitarism (i.e., Sheehan's syndrome) occurs as a result of acute necrosis of the anterior pituitary. During pregnancy, the anterior pituitary enlarges, increasing the oxygen demand and the blood flow to the gland. In cases of postpartum hemorrhage and shock, the pituitary is particularly vulnerable to damage from ischemia. Prompt diagnosis and volume replacement is essential for survival. The degree of hypopituitarism is highly variable, and the pituitary response to GnRH may be normal, diminished, or absent. Subsequent pregnancy has been reported after spontaneous complete or partial recovery.

Hypogonadotropic hypogonadism is associated with insufficient secretion of GnRH and subsequent deficiency of gonadotropins. The appearance of secondary sex characteristics is dependent on sex steroids, which are lacking in these patients. The syndrome often goes undetected until puberty, at which point patients display persistent sexual infantilism. A genetic or developmental defect, it is found in both males and females. Females have primary amenorrhea and immature ovaries that readily respond to gonadotropin.

Ovarian Dysfunction

Gonadotropin-resistant ovary syndrome is found in patients with both primary and secondary amenorrhea. In the presence of elevated gonadotropins, particularly FSH, the follicles fail to respond. Estrogen levels are low or low-normal, whereas FSH and LH levels are found to be normal or high. The etiology, then, is thought to be the presence of ovarian antigonadotropin-receptor antibodies, which may suggest an autoimmune disease. Ovarian biopsy is necessary to make a definitive diagnosis. These patients do not respond to gonadotropin administration, and therefore pregnancy is virtually impossible.

In polycystic ovary syndrome (PCOS), virtually all androgenic hormones are found to be elevated. Patients with PCOS frequently present with anovulation, hirsutism, hyperprolactinemia, and obesity. However, the combination of these symptoms and infertility is not unique to PCOS. It is important to assess the patient for other endocrinopathies. Elevated LH and low or normal FSH levels are secondary to decreased levels of GnRH. The follicular cysts in the ovaries do not mature fully. Chronic anovulation causes a lack in the negative feedback system that keeps estrogen levels in balance, further suppressing FSH. The administration of FSH to the patient with PCOS elevates estrogen levels and decreases androstenedione and testosterone. The result is ovulation.

Premature ovarian failure affects a group of patients with a history of menstrual infrequency or irregularity who have ceased menstruating before the age of 40, and who have no apparent genetic abnormalities. Their symptoms usually include amenorrhea, elevated gonadotropins, and decreased estrogens. Varying profiles of gonadotropins and steroid hormones are found, many of which are typical of postmenopausal women. It is thought that oocytes are prematurely depleted, a deficient number were developed prenatally, or excessive gonadotropic stimulation has occurred. Autoimmune response to gonadotropins or their receptors is also suspected. Hormone replacement therapy is often prescribed, and in some cases, ovulation induction has been successful.

The condition of regular menses without the normal release of an ovum has been described as luteinized, unruptured follicle syndrome. This syndrome has been found in women with normal cycles. It is considered to be a sporadic and infrequent cause of infertility, probably the result of occasional desynchronized mechanisms of ovulation.

There are many instances of developmental aberrations that inhibit or preclude fertility. Many go undetected until the etiology of infertility or recurrent abortion is investigated. Structural anomalies of the uterus, the vagina, and the cervix may be detected by manual exam, during delivery or surgery, or by sonogram or radiographic imaging. Examples include uterine didelphia (so-called double uterus); bicornuate uterus, and septate uterus. Uterine and cervical defects may be the result of developmental defects of unknown etiology or the effects of exposure to teratogenic substances during pregnancy.

Gonadal dysgenesis occurs as a result of an embryonic developmental defect. Examples of chromosomal anomalies adversely affecting fertility are Turner's syndrome, Klinefelter's syndrome, and pseudohermaphroditism or true hermaphroditism. Fertility is rarely possible in patients with disorders of sexual development.

▥ Luteal-Phase Defects

Approximately 3% to 4% of infertile women are diagnosed with luteal-phase defects. In women with a history of habitual abortion the incidence may be higher. An inadequate luteal phase is the result of a deficient secretion of progesterone by the corpus luteum after normal, spontaneous ovulation. This results in an inadequate stimulation of the endometrium and inability to conceive or maintain the pregnancy. Inadequate luteal function is often only a natural consequence of similarly inadequate folliculogenesis. Luteal-phase deficiency consistently accompanies follicular phase FSH deficiency.

▥ Uterine, Tubal, and Pelvic Disorders

A history of pelvic inflammatory disease, septic abortion, intrauterine device use, ruptured appendix, or ectopic pregnancy suggests the possibility of tubal damage. Fallopian tubes consist of three muscular layers and are lined with ciliated cells that wave in the direction of the uterus. Their secretory and contractile functions are vital to the transport of both the sperm and the ovum and, ultimately, the delivery of the embryo to the uterus after fertilization.

The secretory activity of the fallopian tubes, which is primarily under the influence of estrogen, varies in response to hormonal fluctuations of the menstrual cycle. As ovulation approaches and estrogen production increases, secretions accumulate in the tubal lumen to assist in sperm transport. After fertilization, owing to the effects of progesterone, the secretions decrease and the fluid becomes clear. This allows the cilia to move the embryo through the tubes to the uterus.

If the cilia are destroyed or the tubes are twisted, scarred, or blocked, this transport process is impaired.

Endometriosis is one of the most common gynecologic disorders resulting in infertility. It is defined as the presence of hormonally responsive endometrial tissue found implanted outside the endometrial cavity. Although the etiology and pathogenesis are not clear, it is postulated that during menstruation, endometrial cells reflux through the tubes and attach to the pelvic structures. Endometrial fragments are most commonly found in dependent pelvic structures but may also be carried by the lymphatic system and vasculature to distant sites.

Ectopic endometrial tissue contains receptors for estrogen, progesterone, and androgens. They respond to the fluctuating serum levels of these hormones in much the same way as normal endometrium, with monthly bleeding that results in inflammation and peritoneal scarring. When the ovaries and tubes are involved, ovum transport is often obstructed by adhesions and the distortion of the anatomic structures in relation to each other.

Endometriosis is suspected when there are complaints of dysmenorrhea, dyspareunia, and infertility. Symptoms, however, vary greatly and, by themselves, cannot be used to measure the severity of the disease. Use laparoscopy to confirm the diagnosis. Treatment options include surgery, medical therapy, or a combination of medical and surgical treatment.

Acquired uterine defects are commonly seen in cases of infertility. Uterine leiomyomas, or fibroids, are benign pelvic tumors affecting approximately 20% of American women. Interference with the proliferation of the endometrium prevents normal expansion of the uterus as pregnancy progresses. Fibroids may cause habitual abortion or abnormalities of implantation, predisposing the pregnancy to placenta previa and premature labor. They occur more often in later reproductive years and are 3 to 9 times more prevalent in blacks than in whites.

Between 1938 and 1971, an estimated 5 to 10 million persons in the United States were exposed to diethylstilbestrol (DES). DES, a nonsteroidal estrogen, was first used to prevent miscarriages and premature deliveries; it did not help. Women exposed to DES demonstrate a wide range of aberrations in fertility that range from cervical incompetencies to uterine cavity anomalies. Women exposed to DES in utero are also at a higher risk for clear cell adenocarcinoma of the vagina and cervix. Many of these problems are surgically repairable, and a nearly normal pregnancy may result. Others, however, require assisted reproductive techniques (ART) that have a marginal success rate.

Intrauterine adhesions (i.e., Asherman's syndrome) cause the destruction of a large area of the endometrium, usually as a result of postpartum curettage, curettage after missed abortion, or infection. Amenorrhea or recurrent abortions may ensue, owing to an insufficient amount of tissue left to provide for proper implantation. Hysteroscopy allows direct visualization of adhesions and a means by which lysis can be performed. High-dose estrogen-progestin treatment may be used for 2 to 3 months to promote reepithelialization of the endometrium.

Cervical factors also contribute to infertility. Inspection of the cervical mucus allows the health care provider to directly observe the effects and timing of hormonal activity. Further study of the chemical properties as well as the contents of the mucus provides detailed information that can be helpful in the diagnosis and treatment of infertility. In some cases, there is a lack of cervical mucus or cervical stenosis. These conditions can be seen in women who were exposed to DES in utero and women whose cervical glands have been destroyed by cervical cautery or conization.

Male Fertility Disorders

Infertility in men accounts for 40% to 60% of problems of conception. Disorders can be classified as pretesticular, testicular, and posttesticular.

Pretesticular Disorders

Pretesticular disorders include hypothalamic and pituitary disorders such as hypogonadotropic hypogonadism (Kallman's syndrome and isolated gonadotropin deficiency), pituitary failure, delayed or premature sexual development, and congenital adrenal hyperplasia. This category of patients has underlying defects of the hypothalamic-pituitary axis that are either acquired or hereditary.

In most of these patients, hypothalamic dysfunction results in decreased or absent release of GnRH. Testicular biopsy reveals immature testes with underdeveloped Leydig's cells that are unable to produce testosterone. Both sexual development and spermatogenesis are dependent on the quantity of gonadotropins secreted. Treatment with various hormones usually promotes sexual maturation and, hence, the restoration of fertility.

Prolactin plays a role in male fertility, as it does in females. Many studies suggest that prolactin synergizes LH and testosterone to increase reproductive function in the male. Almost all males with prolactin-producing pituitary tumors are impotent, regardless of their testosterone level. Suppression of prolactin with bromocriptine or removal of the tumor restores sexual function.

Chronic disease can be another source of pretesticular infertility. Diabetes mellitus can cause a lack of emission or retrograde ejaculation. Cystic fibrosis or recurrent upper respiratory infections may cause abnormalities of the seminal vesicles, vas deferens, and epididymis, or cause immotile cilia syndrome that interferes with the transport of sperm through the ductal system.

Testicular Disorders

Testicular disorders include dysfunctional spermatogenesis as a result of genetic or abnormal development or causes such as varicocele; exposure to toxins, drugs, and radiation; or infections. Semen studies are used to examine the cellular development of germ cells during various stages of spermatogenesis to classify disorders of sperm maturation. Drugs affecting spermatogenesis include alcohol, amebicides, anabolic steroids, cimetidine, homogenated hydrocarbons, nicotine, nitrofurantoin, sulfonamide drugs, and sulfasalazine.

Infertility may occur as a result of a recurrent or chronic infection that causes mechanical obstruction from scarring. Infection can cause epididymitis, orchitis, or epididymoorchitis (a combination of the two). Common causative organisms include *Escherichia coli*, streptococci, staphylococci, *Neisseria gonorrhoeae*, and *Chlamydia*. The mumps virus can cause acute orchitis and, in pubertal or adult males, can result in damage to seminiferous tubules and Leydig's cells, creating testosterone deficiency, hypogonadism, and infertility.

In some cases, infertility is reversible with surgical intervention. Varicocele is an abnormal dilatation or varicosity of the veins that drain the testicle. Varicoceles are found in up to 15% of males. Of those, approximately 50% have poor semen quality. Some studies have shown improved pregnancy rates in partners of men who have undergone surgery.

Posttesticular Disorders

Posttesticular causes of infertility include a congenital absence of the vas deferens, obstructive problems, retrograde ejaculation, and sexual dysfunction related to physiologic and psychogenic problems, or spinal cord injuries. New technologies are aimed at improving vasectomy resections. Electroejaculation implants may be used for voluntary nerve innervation in patients with spinal cord injuries. Improvement of semen processing for ART also promotes male fertility.

Sperm autoimmunity can occur if the man's immune system at puberty identifies the spermatozoa as foreign. When autoimmunity occurs, there is a decrease in sperm motility and viability due to agglutination or clumping and immobilization.

ASSISTIVE REPRODUCTION

In most cases, there are five options available to the couple who is attempting to conceive: (1) prepare for a biologic child using assistive reproductive technologies (ART); (2) accept donated eggs and/or sperm using a surrogate, and thus the child is biologically related to one of the parents; (3) accept a donated embryo, and thus the child is unrelated to either parent; (4) adopt a child; or (5) choose to remain childless.

The success rates of ART are variable, with many factors that must be overcome. ART is time-consuming and costly; however, ART have helped many couples to conceive who otherwise would have been unable to do so. For women with impaired ovaries or genetic diseases that could be passed on to the infant, donor eggs or frozen embryos may be used in ART procedures.

Intrauterine implants (IUI) use sperm that has been cleaned and concentrated. It is then inserted directly into the uterus, whence it travels to the fallopian tubes for fertilization. This is in contrast to sperm delivered through natural intercourse, in which only a percentage of the sperm make their way to the fallopian tubes.

In vitro fertilization (IVF) may be particularly useful with infertility due to (1) inflammation, blockage, absent tube, and so forth; (2) a low sperm count, poor morphology, or motility; (3) endometriosis; (4) immunology-based antibody issues; and (5) unexplained infertility. In IVF, specialized drugs excite the ovaries to turn out multiple eggs. The mature eggs are removed and combined with sperm for fertilization. The eggs are inspected after 40 hours to see if fertilization has taken place and if the cells are dividing. If so, the embryos are placed inside the uterus. *IVF with blastocyst transfer* is similar to the standard IVF procedure.

Intracytoplasmic sperm injection (ICSI) is an increasingly popular procedure whereby a single sperm is injected directly into an ovum. Then, as in IVF, the embryo is inserted into the uterus. Fifteen percent to 20% of these procedures result in pregnancy.

Frozen-embryo transfer involves the transfer into the uterus of extra IVF-produced embryos that have been frozen. Embryos may be frozen on days 1, 2, 3, 5, or 6 *(blastocyst transfer)* after fertilization.

Assisted hatching (AH) may help some women conceive. Embryos have an outer coating, the zona pellucida, which holds the cells of the embryo together. Once an embryo arrives in the uterus, the zona pellucida dissolves, allowing the embryo to "hatch" and grow. The embryo must hatch before implantation can take place.

Gamete intrafallopian transfer (GIFT) is much like IVF. Three to five ova are inserted into the fallopian tube along with the sperm. GIFT has a success rate of approximately 30% but requires that the woman have at least one functional fallopian tube.

Zygote intrafallopian transfer (ZIFT) combines the techniques of IVF and GIFT, achieving a success rate of about 28%. Also called tubal embryo transfer, the ova are fertilized in the lab and inserted into the fallopian tubes rather than the uterus.

PHARMACOTHERAPEUTIC OPTIONS

Many advances in the treatment of infertility have been made in the last few decades. Ovulatory dysfunction, once the root of a hopeless situation for achieving pregnancy, now constitutes one of the most successful areas of new technology. If the infertility problems are due solely to problems of ovulation, current drug preparations can increase the couple's chances of conceiving to near those of the general population. Treatment with the appropriate drugs can give patients about a 90% chance that the ovaries can be made to function correctly, unless the patient exhibits a raised baseline FSH level that may indicate ovarian failure. Before beginning treatment for ovulation induction, other endocrinopathies must first be eliminated.

Nonsteroidal Antiestrogen Drug
◆ clomiphene citrate (Clomid, Milophene, Serophene); ◆ Clomid, Serophene

▥ Indications
Clomiphene citrate is most often used for the patient who has PCOS, infrequent or rare ovulation, or a luteal-phase deficiency, and to increase the numbers of eggs available. Clomiphene has been used in a limited number of patients for menstrual disorders, endometrial anaplasia or hyperplasia, persistent lactation, and fibrocystic breast disease; however, it is not approved for these purposes. It is also used for the treatment of oligospermia and male infertility.

▥ Pharmacodynamics
Clomiphene is a nonsteroidal antiestrogen drug whose precise mechanism of action is unknown. It appears to compete with estradiol for estrogen binding sites in the hypothalamus, where it increases the release of GnRH to stimulate the pituitary to increase FSH and LH secretion. In other words, it "tricks" the pituitary gland into believing there is less estrogen around. Clomiphene has no progestational, androgenic, corticotropic, or antiandrogenic effects.

Patients with PCOS may benefit from treatment with clomiphene because the drug competes for the estrone-binding sites and inhibits negative feedback. If the high levels of estrogen are not inhibited, gonadotropin secretion continues to be inhibited, suppressing ovulation.

▥ Pharmacokinetics
Clomiphene citrate is taken orally and is readily absorbed in the gastrointestinal (GI) tract. Its half-life is about 5 days, but traces have been found in feces for up to 6 weeks. Biotransformation takes place in the liver, with elimination in the feces. There is evidence that some of the drug may be stored in body fat or undergo enterohepatic circulation to be slowly released from the body.

▥ Adverse Effects and Contraindications
The most common adverse effects of clomiphene citrate are menopause-like hot flashes. The hot flashes are related to the antiestrogenic properties of the drug. Abdominal bloating, distention, and discomfort have also been reported, as well as breast tenderness, nausea and vomiting, headache, and visual disturbances. Other adverse effects include hair loss or dryness, urinary frequency, increased appetite, weight gain, skin rash, tension, fatigue, insomnia, dizziness, and mood swings.

Clomiphene is contraindicated for use in women with pre-existing ovarian cysts and those with persistent ovarian enlargement after treatment has begun. The ovary may increase in size for several days after the drug is discontinued. Normally, the enlargement spontaneously subsides without any intervention or sequela. If ovarian enlargement does occur, stop treatment and decrease the dosage of the next cycle.

Some patients with PCOS are unusually sensitive to the gonadotropin levels induced by normal doses of clomiphene and may have an exaggerated response. Again, discontinuation of the drug is recommended, and the condition is expected to resolve spontaneously.

Clomiphene citrate is also contraindicated for use in patients who are hypersensitive to gonadotropins, in patients with liver disease or with a history of liver dysfunction, and in women with abnormal uterine bleeding of unknown etiology. Do not use it in women with pituitary tumors and thyroid and adrenal dysfunction. Warn the patient and her partner about the risk of multiple gestations, especially with higher doses, and about the risks inherent in a multiple-gestation pregnancy.

▥ Dosage Regimen
Following a negative pregnancy test, clomiphene therapy is started on the third to the fifth day of the cycle. In the absence of adverse effects, dosages above 150 mg/day are likely to be effective.

Treatment begins on day 5 of the menstrual cycle, which correlates with the day when the dominant follicle is being selected (see Pharmacodynamics section under Gonadotropins). Starting clomiphene earlier than day 5 more often results in multiple gestations. Earlier administration may be used in the recruitment of oocytes for ART such as in IVF, in which the goal is to mature a number of ova for retrieval in one cycle.

The gonadotropin surge is expected from 5 to 10 days after the last dose of clomiphene. The patient is instructed that for optimal results to be achieved, coitus should occur every day for 1 week, beginning 5 days after the last dose of drug. The majority of patients ovulate after the first course of treatment. Those with prolonged amenorrhea may be less responsive, but up to 80% can be expected to ovulate, and approximately 40% will become pregnant. The pregnancy rate in those without other causes of infertility approaches that of the general population, approximately 80% to 90%. The greater the number of cycles in which the drug is administered, regardless of the number of ovulations induced, the lower the pregnancy rate. Treatment should be discontinued if not successful after six cycles of clomiphene.

When the patient is unresponsive and the basal body temperature chart findings (used to detect progesterone levels from the corpus luteum) are inconclusive, human chorionic gonadotropin (hCG) may be added to the regimen (Fig. 60-1). This method improves the midcycle LH surge, but requires more accurate timing. If this supplemental treatment also fails to produce pregnancy, progesterone may be added, or treatment with human menopausal gonadotropin (hMG) started. In some practices, clomiphene is also used to regulate ovulation in patients receiving artificial insemination. Do not give gonadotropins if the ovaries are abnormally enlarged; over three follicles of 15 mm or larger are present; an ovarian cyst is present, or estradiol levels exceed 2000 pg/mL.

▥ Lab Considerations

No clinically important hematologic or renal abnormalities have been reported with clomiphene citrate. Alterations in liver function tests and cholesterol synthesis may occur, although rarely. It may cause increases in serum thyroxine and thyroid-binding globulin levels.

Close monitoring of follicle development and the determination of ovulation are accomplished by evaluating urine or serum estrogen levels. During cycles in which ovulation was assisted by hCG, endometrial growth is inhibited by the antiestrogenic activity of clomiphene. Endometrial thickness can be monitored by ultrasound and optimally should be 6 mm or more for successful implantation.

Gonadotropins

- follicle-stimulating hormone (FSH, human urofollitropin, Fertinex, Gonal-F, Metrodin)
- human chorionic gonadotropin (hCG, Profasi, Pregnyl, Novarel, choriogonadotropin alpha [r-hCG]); ◆ chorionic gonadotropin
- human menopausal gonadotropin (hMG, menotropin, Humegon, Pergonal); ◆ Repronex
- gonadorelin (Factrel, Lutrepulse); ◆ Suprefact

▥ Indications

Clinical indications for FSH include anovulation, luteal-phase defects, endometriosis, unexplained infertility, male infertility, and ART. Women in whom pregnancy is desired as soon as possible owing to advanced maternal age are also considered candidates. In women who have elevated LH levels, as in PCOS, the additional LH found in hMG may stimulate premature ovulation. Some studies have indicated that purified forms of FSH may decrease this complication and consequently produce a higher pregnancy rate. Other studies indicate that FSH, when used in addition to hMG, enhances the pregnancy rate, especially for hyporesponders.

In women whose cause of infertility is not primary ovarian failure, hCG is used in conjunction with hMG and FSH to stimulate ovulation. It is also used in combination with hMG to stimulate spermatogenesis in males who have primary or secondary hypogonadotropic hypogonadism.

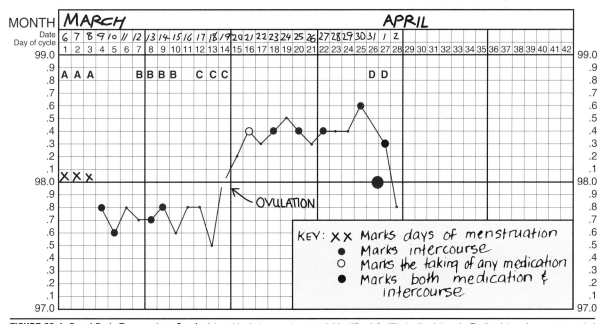

FIGURE 60-1 Basal Body Temperature Graph. A basal body temperature graph identifies infertility testing intervals. Testing intervals are represented by *A*, semen analysis; *B*, hysterosalpingography; *C*, postcoital test; and *D*, endometrial biopsy. (Reprinted with permission from Garner, C. [1991]. An overview of infertility. In Garner C. [Ed.]. *Principles of infertility nursing* [p. 4]. Boca Raton, FL: CRC Press, copyright CRC Press, Boca Raton, FL.)

Similar to FSH, the clinical indications for hMG include unexplained infertility, endometriosis, ovulatory dysfunction, and luteal-phase defects. Male infertility is also treated with hMG. In women for whom ART is indicated, hMG is also used to induce a large number of eggs to mature in one cycle, which are then retrieved for IVF, ZIFT, or GIFT.

Human menopausal gonadotropin is used for patients with hypothalamic pituitary failure, but who have ovarian function with normal gonadotropin levels, or who respond to the progesterone challenge with bleeding. Candidates for hMG therapy include women for whom clomiphene citrate and hCG have been ineffective and those taking clomiphene citrate who continue to have abnormal cervical mucus.

There are two formulations of gonadorelin (GnRH). Gonadorelin hydrochloride (Factrel) is the salt form of gonadorelin indicated for the diagnosis of hypogonadism, whereas gonadorelin acetate (Lutrepulse) is indicated for amenorrhea and infertility. Women with hypothalamic amenorrhea who have a deficiency of endogenous GnRH or a hypothalamic dysfunction are the best candidates for gonadorelin therapy. Multiple pregnancies are possible.

Some women with PCOS respond favorably to this treatment, but owing to their hypersensitivity to the drug, lower dosages must be used and the advantages are not as great. Hyperprolactinemic patients who cannot tolerate bromocriptine (see following discussion) have also been treated successfully with gonadorelin.

▥ Pharmacodynamics

FSH is a pituitary peptide hormone derived from urine or through recombinant DNA technology. FSH stimulates maturation of follicles by causing an elevation in endogenous FSH levels. During a normal menstrual cycle, as the follicular phase progresses, one follicle matures more rapidly and becomes the dominant follicle. When FSH levels begin to fall off during the mid- to late follicular phase, the less mature follicles begin to atrophy, whereas the dominant follicle continues to mature despite decreasing levels of FSH. Administration of exogenous FSH provides nondominant follicles the additional stimulation needed to mature; thus a larger number of mature follicles are recruited per ovulation cycle, increasing the potential for fertilization.

hCG is a polypeptide produced by the placenta and obtained from the urine of pregnant women. The action of human or recombinant hCG is identical to that of LH in that it stimulates the production of gonadal steroid hormones by inducing the production of androgen by Leydig's cells of the testes and progesterone by the corpus luteum of the ovary. In this way, male androgens cause the development of secondary sex characteristics and cause testicular descent. When given with hMG, hCG stimulates spermatogenesis. In the female, FSH stimulation in the ovary causes maturation of the follicle, whereas the LH surge promotes ovulation. hCG can substitute for LH in this capacity.

A pituitary peptide hormone, hMG is usually made from the urine of menopausal women. The FSH and LH contained in hMG bypass the hypothalamus and pituitary gland to bind to ovarian granulosa and thecal cells, respectively. This process leads to follicular proliferation and maturation, followed by development of the corpus luteum. To induce ovulation of the mature ovum, a single large dose of hCG, having LH

activity, is administered. In males, LH stimulates spermatogenesis. Men who have had adequate virilization with hCG treatment require 3 months of concomitant hMG treatment to promote spermatogenesis.

Gonadorelin replaces missing hormone and allows the pituitary gland to function. Pulsatile administration of exogenous gonadorelin acetate simulates the natural secretion pattern, stimulating FSH and LH secretion. In turn, the natural sequence of maturation of one follicle and ovulation occurs.

Endogenous GnRH is normally released in a pulsatile fashion from the hypothalamus to stimulate the release of gonadotropins from the pituitary. The frequency and amplitude of the pulses are critical to the stimulatory effects of GnRH. Before this knowledge was achieved, single-dose injections of gonadorelin were used; they were effective for the first 2 to 4 weeks of therapy, elevating the plasma level of gonadotropins. At that point, however, gonadorelin began to desensitize the receptor sites on the pituitary and suppressed the secretions of gonadotropins.

▥ Pharmacokinetics

Like other gonadotropins, FSH is given parenterally. Biotransformation takes place in the proximal tubules of the kidneys and in the liver.

Human chorionic gonadotropin is destroyed in the GI tract and, therefore, is administered parenterally. Distribution is primarily to the testes in males and the ovaries in females. Elimination is through the kidneys, with approximately 10% eliminated within the first 24 hours; the remainder may be detected for up to 3 to 4 days.

hMG is destroyed in the GI tract and, therefore, must be administered intramuscularly or subcutaneously. Its biotransformation is unclear. Like other gonadotropins, glomerular filtration with further breakdown in the proximal tubule is followed by completed clearance in the reticuloendothelial system of the liver. Blood levels decrease in a biphasic manner (see Table 60-2). Following a single intramuscular (IM) dose of hMG, approximately 8% of unchanged drug is eliminated in the urine.

Gonadorelin is poorly absorbed by the GI tract and therefore must be given by subcutaneous (subQ) or IV route. It is widely distributed in extracellular spaces and is primarily biotransformed and eliminated by the kidneys. Prolonged hypogonadism may be resistant to initial treatment and require priming with gonadorelin for several days before a response is elicited and gonadorelin levels increase.

▥ Adverse Effects and Contraindications

Adverse reactions to FSH are similar to those of hMG, the most prominent being ovarian hyperstimulation syndrome (OHSS). Other adverse reactions occur infrequently but include ovarian cysts, ovarian enlargement, pelvic or abdominal discomfort, headache, pain or swelling at the injection site, and breast tenderness. As with all gonadotropins, there is a risk for multiple births with the use of FSH.

FSH is contraindicated for use in women with primary ovarian failure, ovarian cysts, or enlargement unrelated to PCOS; abnormal uterine bleeding; uncontrolled thyroid or adrenal dysfunction; or pituitary tumor. FSH use is also contraindicated in men with oligospermia.

The likelihood of ovulation with hMG is dose related, as are the complications. Hot flashes are a common adverse

PHARMACOKINETICS

TABLE 60-2 Selected Fertility Drugs

Drug	Rte	Onset	Peak	Duration	PB (%)	t½	BioA (%)
bromocriptine	PO	30–90 min	1–2 hr	8–12 hr*	90–96	3–4.5; 45–50 hr†	UA
clomiphene citrate	PO	5–14 days	UA	UA	UA	5 days	UA
FSH	SubQ, IM	UA	6–18 hr	UA	UA	2.9 hr	UA
gonadorelin acetate	IV	Rapid	Min	3–5 hr	UA	2–8 min	100
gonadorelin hydrochloride	IV, subQ	Rapid to slow	2–6 hr	3–5 hr	UA	2–8 min	100
hMG	SubQ, IM	UA	Fe: 18 hr; M: 4 mo	UA	UA	LH: 4 hr; FSH: 70 hr	UA
hCG	SubQ, IM	2 hr	6 hr	36–72 hr	UA	23 hr	UA
leuprolide acetate	SubQ, IM	1–2 wk‡	2–4 hr	3–4 wk	7–15	3 hr	94

*The most therapeutic effects of bromocriptine when used in hyperprolactinemia are seen after 4 weeks of therapy.
†First-phase half-life of bromocriptine is 3–4.5 hr, whereas terminal phase is 45–50 hr.
‡Onset of leuprolide action follows a transient increase during the first week of therapy; depot formulation.
BioA, Bioavailability; *Fe*, female; *FSH*, follicle-stimulating hormone; *hCG*, human chorionic gonadotropin; *hMG*, human menopausal gonadotropin; *IM*, intramuscular; *IV*, intravenous; *LH*, luteinizing hormone; *M*, male; *PB*, protein binding; *PO*, by mouth; *SubQ*, subcutaneously; *t½*, half-life; *UA*, unavailable.

effect. Ovarian enlargement may be mild to moderate with the same symptoms as that of clomiphene, but the incidence of severe OHSS is greater.

OHSS develops in approximately 1% of patients and can be life-threatening. As ovaries are hyperstimulated, mild enlargement can progress to ascites, pleural effusion, hypovolemia, hypotension, oliguria, and electrolyte imbalance. **OHSS is a potentially life-threatening complication of ovarian stimulation. Any patient undergoing ovulation induction is at risk, although some more so than others. OHSS may be classified as mild, moderate, or severe based on its signs and symptoms** (Table 60-3). **To prevent OHSS, do not give hCG if estradiol levels are too high or follicle growth excessive, particularly if there are more than five large follicles.**

The ovaries are at risk for rupture from the development of multiple follicular cysts, corpora lutea, and stromal edema. Increased coagulability and decreased renal perfusion are the major complications. Hemoconcentration occurs, and renal hypoperfusion leads to hyperkalemia, and azotemia.

hMG is contraindicated for use in women with primary ovarian failure, thyroid or adrenal dysfunction, intracranial lesions, pituitary insufficiency, or genital bleeding of unknown etiology. In men, the contraindications include normal pituitary function, primary testicular failure, or infertility due to causes other than hypogonadotropic hypogonadism.

Cramping and occasional headaches are reported with gonadorelin as well as fatigue, irritability, depression, pain at the injection site, and edema. Owing to its profound effect on the ovaries, there is a higher incidence of OHSS in cycles during which hCG is used as the ovulation stimulant.

The contraindications to gonadorelin use are similar to those for hCG. Androgen secretion induced by hCG can cause fluid retention. Use it with caution in patients who have asthma, seizure disorders, migraines, and cardiac or renal problems. Persons with hamster allergies should not receive the recombinant formulation of hCG.

One of the advantages to gonadorelin treatment is a decreased incidence of OHSS. Although the drug must still

TABLE 60-3 Ovarian Hyperstimulation Syndrome (OHSS)

Signs and Symptoms	Possible Cause of Symptoms	Recommended Treatment
Mild: • Abdominal distention	• Ovaries larger than normal, tender and fragile • High level of estrogen and progesterone and fluid imbalance causing bloating	• Avoid sexual intercourse; do not have a pelvic exam • Reduce activities, no heavy lifting, straining or exercise
• Nausea • Diarrhea • Slight weight gain		• Clear fluids, ginger ale, cranberry juice, Gatorade
Moderate: As noted above, plus the following:	• High level of estrogen and progesterone and fluid imbalance causing bloating	*As noted above, plus the following:*
• Weight gain over 2 lb per day	• Fluid imbalance causes dehydration because body fluids collect in the abdomen and other tissues. • Increased abdominal girth	• Ultrasound if ordered • Twice-daily weights; record number of voidings per day
• Thirst, vomiting, and diarrhea • Urine concentrated; amount reduced • Dry skin and hair	• Abdominal distention	• Contact HCP if 5 lb weight gain over previous 24 hr; a 50% drop in voidings; increased pelvic pain
Severe: As noted above, plus the following:	• Extremely large ovaries	*As noted above, plus the following:*
• Marked abdominal distention	• Pleural effusion and/or ascites	• Notify health care provider
• Urine concentrated; amount reduced	• Peripheral edema	• Assessment at hospital or clinic
• Calf pains, chest pain, SOB • Lower abdominal pain	• Abnormal blood clotting	• Paracentesis may be needed

HCP, Health care provider; *SOB*, shortness of breath.

ENDOCRINE

be used cautiously and monitoring of ovarian stimulation is necessary, there have been fewer reported cases of OHSS than in women treated with hMG. Local infection at the injection site is also a problem; the subQ route may eliminate this problem.

Drug Interactions

There are no documented drug interactions with use of FSH or hMG. There are also no known drug interactions with gonadorelin; however, do not administer gonadorelin in conjunction with ovulation stimulators.

Dosage Regimen

The dosage of FSH is individualized. Instruct the couple to have daily coitus beginning the day before the dosage of hCG is administered. Treatment may continue for two to three more cycles if ultrasound measurement and estrogen levels indicate that adequate follicular growth has not been achieved. If treatment is still unsuccessful, some health care providers may increase the dosage in subsequent cycles.

Dosages of hCG are dependent on the particular use and the individual patient. When used concomitantly with hMG and FSH, a single injection is administered 24 hours after the last dose of hMG or FSH is given. The dosage of hCG recommended for ovulation induction is 5000 to 10,000 international units. Ovulation is expected 24 to 40 hours later. To avoid OHSS, do not give hCG if estradiol levels are too high or there are more than five large follicles.

hMG is a purified preparation of the gonadotropins LH and FSH extracted from the urine of postmenopausal women. The commercial formulation contains a 1:1 ratio of FSH (75 international units) and LH (75 international units) (see Table 60-4). It is an expensive drug, and because of its greater complication rate, it should be used only with careful evaluation and by a qualified reproductive technology specialist.

The dosage of hMG is individually determined to produce follicular maturation. Use the lowest possible dosage of hMG and hCG to minimize the risk for OHSS. The recommended dosage of hMG varies based on the product and patient situation but typically begins with the use of FH and/or LH for 9 to 12 days until follicular maturation has occurred. Then, a single dose of hCG is given 1 day after the last dose of hMG. This dose of hCG stimulates the midcycle LH surge and is necessary because the dosage of LH in hMG is not high enough to do so. The couple is then advised to have coitus the day of the hCG injection and the 2 days after. If there is evidence of ovarian hyperstimulation, owing to the fragility of the stimulated ovary, further coitus and strenuous exercise should be avoided.

If pregnancy does not occur but there is evidence of ovulation, this regimen may be repeated twice more. If ovulation did not occur, the dose of hMG can be increased to 150 international units each for both LH and FSH and the regimen repeated twice more.

In order to prevent OHSS, estrogen measurements and ultrasound determination of follicular size are necessary to determine the best time to administer the ovulatory dose of hCG. By day 7 of hMG therapy, urine or blood estrogen levels are measured and drug dosage adjusted for the rest of the cycle. Observation of cervical mucus changes is also noted.

To stimulate spermatogenesis with hMG, full masculinization, as evidenced by the presence of secondary sex characteristics, must first be achieved. Pretreatment with hCG is necessary in the case of primary or secondary hypogonadotropic hypogonadism. Once pretreatment is complete, concomitant use of hCG and hMG can begin. Spermatozoa should then be evident in the ejaculate. If they are not, the dosages of hMG can be increased and the regimen repeated.

Gonadorelin hydrochloride formulation (Factrel) is given subcutaneously or intravenously. The acetate formulation (Lutrepulse) is administered via the Lutrepulse pump. A 5-mcg dose is given every 90 minutes in doses of 1 to 20 mg. Observation of the ovaries by ultrasound and estradiol levels is initiated after 4 days and repeated every 3 to 4 days. The patient requires between 10 and 20 days of therapy for ovulation to occur. Some health care providers continue treatment for 2 more weeks to maintain the corpus luteum. Others add hCG or progesterone for luteal-phase support. For gonadorelin-resistant patients, priming with repeated doses for several days may be required.

Lab Considerations

hCG may interfere with the results of radioimmunoassays for gonadotropins, especially LH. When requesting assay levels, inform the laboratory of the therapy. **Because hCG is** ⒜ **the same hormone used to diagnose pregnancy, advise patients that false-positive test results may occur for up to 14 days after administration.**

Serum estradiol levels are measured beginning day 7 of hMG administration and repeated every 1 to 3 days. Depending on the estradiol level, a subsequent dose of hMG is individualized for the rest of the cycle. For best results, midcycle estradiol levels, which are taken early in the morning after an evening dose of hMG is given, should be between 1000 and 1500 pg/mL. The risk of hyperstimulation is increased when estradiol levels reach 1500 to 2000 pg/mL; above 2000 pg/mL, hMG is generally withheld.

In addition, ultrasound monitoring of follicular size is done. In a normal cycle, when the follicle reaches 20 to 24 mm, it is mature. In cycles induced by hMG, clomiphene citrate, and FSH, follicles may be ready for the dose of hCG when slightly smaller (16 to 18 mm). Measurement of endometrial thickness by ultrasound is also used to determine the optimal time for administration of hCG. Pregnancy success rates are greatest when endometrial thickness is greater than 6 mm.

As with all ovulation inducers, it is necessary to monitor the development of the follicle with gonadotropin therapy. Ultrasound and regular assessment of estradiol levels, as well as cervical mucus evaluation, are commonly done. Although it is less common, close observation for OHSS is advised.

Gonadotropin-Releasing Hormone Analogue

◆ leuprolide acetate (Lupron, Synarel, Zoladex); ◆ leuprolide acetate, Lupron Depot, Lupron Injection

Indications

Although not approved for such use, leuprolide acetate is often used to prevent premature release of eggs for ART, or to help induce a menopause-like state (by suppressing endogenous LH and FSH) to suppress endometriosis or fibroids. Leuprolide acetate is indicated in those patients with elevated baseline levels of these gonadotropins. The FDA-approved use of leuprolide is in advanced prostate cancer.

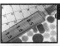

DOSAGE

TABLE 60-4 Fertility Drugs

Drug	Use(s)	Dosage	Comments	
bromocriptine	Hyperprolactinemia	*Female:* 1.25 mg PO daily; increase by 2.5 mg/day every 2–7 days. Max: 30 mg/daily.	Appears safe; should be stopped once pregnancy occurs. Approx cost: $65 for 30 2.5-mg tablets	
clomiphene citrate	Oligospermia, anovulation, PCOS	*Female:* 50 mg PO for 5 days; repeat in 30 days; 100 mg PO for 5 days. Increase to 150 mg daily if still unresponsive. *Male:* 25 mg daily with 5-day rest period and repeat −or− 100 mg on MWF	**First-line drug for primary infertility. Use for longer than 1 yr may increase risk for ovarian cancer.** Chance for multiple pregnancies: 8%. Approx cost: $1.50/50-mg tablet	▲
FSH (human urofollitropin)	Failed clomiphene therapy	*Female:* 150 international units subQ daily for 5–7 days beginning on cycle day 2 or 3. Ordinarily followed by 5,000–10,000 units hCG day 1 after last dose of FSH −or− 75–600 units subQ or IM daily of recombinant FSH for 6–10 days, beginning on cycle day 2 or 3. PCOS with elevated LH and FSH *Female:* 75 mg subQ daily for 1 wk or more	**If ovaries enlarged, hold hCG.** Chance for multiple pregnancies 25%–50%. Dosage must be carefully monitored and may be changed during treatment cycle. Approx cost: $28–$520/dose depending on specific drug used	▲
gonadorelin acetate or gonadorelin hydrochloride	Amenorrhea due to hypothalamus dysfunction	*Female:* HCl formulation: 100 mcg subQ or IV. Acetate formulation: 5 mcg IV initially every 90 min based on patient response. Range: 1–20 mcg every 90 min	No increase in risk for multiple pregnancies. Less risk for OHSS. Obtain U/S and estradiol levels every 3–4 days.	
hCG	Anovulatory women pretreated with menotropins; hypogonadotropic hypogonadism secondary to pituitary deficiency in males	*Female:* 5000–10,000 USP units IM or subQ day 1 after last dose of hMG *Male:* 500–1000 USP units IM or subQ 3 times/wk for 3 wk and then twice weekly for 3 wk −or− 4000 units 3 times/wk for 6–9 mo and then decrease to 2000 units 3 times/wk for 3 mo	**Do not give if ovaries abnormally enlarged to avoid OHSS. Chance for multiple births variable.** Approx cost: $22/10,000 units.	▲
hMG	Follicle stimulation for ART. Ovulation dysfunction, luteal-phase deficiency, idiopathic and male infertility	*Female:* 150 international units (FSH and LH) IM or subQ daily for 6–12 days, starting on day 2–3 of cycle. Repeat twice more before doubling dosage. *Male:* 150 international units IM or subQ 3 times/wk with 2000 units hCG 2 times/wk for 4 months to detect sperm in ejaculate. May increase to 300 mg international units	**Potential for ovarian cancer is unclear.** Chance for multiple pregnancies 25%–50%. Approx cost: $12–$38/dose	▲
leuprolide acetate	Controlled ovulation induction for ART	*Female:* Begin midluteal phase of previous cycle. Give 1 mg subQ daily for 2 wk; decrease to 0.5 mg subQ daily when hMG or FSH is started.	Not FDA-approved for this use. Also available as nasal spray and implant. Approx cost: $170–$270 for 14 days' course	
progesterone	Secondary amenorrhea caused by luteal-phase defect and ART	*Female:* 400 mg PO every evening for 10 days −or− 1 application 8% vaginal gel daily. If pregnancy occurs, continue for 10–12 wk.	Appears safe; other progestins associated with birth defects. No increase in risk for multiple pregnancies. One vaginal application = 90 mg progesterone. Approx cost: $90 for 15 days' treatment.	
testosterone cyprionate	Male hypogonadism	*Males:* 50–400 mg IM every 2–4 wk	Schedule III drug; often abused by athletes and body builders	

ART, Assisted reproductive techniques; *FDA,* Food and Drug Administration; *FSH,* follicle-stimulating hormone; *hCG,* human chorionic gonadotropin; *hMG,* human menopausal gonadotropin; *IM,* intramuscular (route); *IV,* intravenous (route); *LH,* luteinizing hormone; *MWF,* Monday, Wednesday, and Friday; *OHSS,* ovarian hyperstimulation syndrome; *PCOS,* polycystic ovary syndrome; *PO,* by mouth; *PRN,* as needed; *SubQ,* subcutaneous (route); *U/S,* ultrasound.

DRUG INTERACTIONS

TABLE 60-5 Fertility Drugs

Drug(s)	Interactive Drug(s)	Interaction
bromocriptine	amitriptyline, Butyrophenones, erythromycin, Estrogens, imipramine, methyldopa, Oral contraceptives, Phenothiazines, progesterone, reserpine, TCAs	Reduces effectiveness of bromocriptine
	levodopa	Additive neurologic effects
	Antihypertensives	Additive hypotensive effects
	Ergot alkaloids	Severe hypertension
	Alcohol	Decreased tolerance to alcohol
leuprolide	Antiandrogens, megestrol, flutamide	Additive antineoplastic effects
	Chasteberry or chaste tree fruit *(Vitex agnus-castus)*	Decreases effectiveness of leuprolide

TCAs, Tricyclic antidepressants.

ENDOCRINE

Pharmacodynamics

Leuprolide is an analogue of GnRH with an affinity for pituitary GnRH receptor sites. Initially, it has a stimulating effect, causing the LH and FSH levels to rise. In other words, it prevents premature release of eggs (daily form), and turns off the pituitary gland (monthly form). With 2 to 4 weeks of use it has the opposite effect, causing a suppression of the secretion of gonadotropin-releasing hormone and, hence, decreased LH and FSH ("chemical castration").

During ART, endogenous hormones may interfere with stimulation and maturation of the ovum. Excess FSH influences follicular response, resulting in suboptimal follicular development and inadequate estrogen production. When LH levels are abnormally elevated, the exact moment of the LH surge and subsequent rupture of mature follicles becomes more difficult to predict. Because timing of ovum retrieval is crucial to the success of ART procedures, a premature LH surge can result in cancelled cycles. Approximately 15% to 30% of ART cycles must be cancelled owing to unsatisfactory response to hormonal stimulation. This contributes to the loss of precious time and financial resources. It is generally believed that the addition of GnRH agonist to the ART cycle assists with scheduling and decreases cancellation rates.

Pharmacokinetics

Leuprolide is administered intramuscularly or subcutaneously. The biotransformation, distribution, and elimination of leuprolide are unknown.

Adverse Effects and Contraindications

Hot flashes and mild headache may be caused by leuprolide. Irritation, pain, or reaction at the injection site may also occur. It is safe for less than 6 to 9 months of use, and longer if estrogen is supplemented to minimize bone loss.

Drug Interactions

There are no known drug interactions with leuprolide.

Dosage Regimen

Depending on the desired effect, leuprolide can be used in short- and long-term regimens. Short cycles are beginning to gain popularity as ovulation inducers, being used much the same way as hCG. Compared with ovulation induction with hMG and hCG, it is believed to cause fewer cases of OHSS.

Long-term regimens started on day 3, early in the follicular phase of the preceding cycle, or on day 21, in the midluteal phase, are instituted when there is concern about controlling the maturation process of the follicles in ART. As mentioned, premature luteinization can occur when the endogenous LH level interferes with the rate of follicle maturation. The use of leuprolide to suppress the endogenous hormone may help control the stimulation process.

Lab Considerations

When leuprolide is used in place of hCG to induce ovulation, LH, and estradiol levels are monitored. Ultrasound is used to determine follicular growth, and leuprolide is administered after two or more follicles have reached adequate size.

Gonadal function test results may be abnormal for up to 12 weeks following treatment. Elevated aspartate transaminase (AST), lactate dehydrogenase (LDH), alkaline phosphatase, triglycerides, low-density lipoprotein (LDL), high-density lipoprotein (HDL), total cholesterol, and decreased levels of white blood cells (WBCs) may also be found.

Dopamine Agonist

◆ bromocriptine (Parlodel, Dostinex); ◆ Parlodel

Indications

Bromocriptine is indicated for patients with infertility associated with hyperprolactinemia and pituitary adenomas. It is also used for the restoration of menstrual function in patients who so desire it or for those in whom restoration of ovarian function is necessary for the prevention of bone loss. Oligospermia, if caused by elevated prolactin levels, may also be treated with bromocriptine. Sperm count increases when elevated prolactin levels are corrected.

Pharmacodynamics

Bromocriptine resembles the neurotransmitter dopamine in structure and binds to dopamine receptors in the pituitary gland. By substantially reducing elevated prolactin levels, bromocriptine restores ovulation and ovarian function in women with amenorrhea. This is accomplished by direct suppression of pituitary secretion or by stimulating dopamine receptors in the hypothalamus to release prolactin-inhibiting factor (PIF). Bromocriptine may also act on dopaminergic receptors in the ovary to restore ovulation. It may stimulate ovulation in women whose prolactin level is not elevated and does not decrease with use of the drug, indicating it may have an effect on hypothalamic release of LH-releasing hormone.

Pharmacokinetics

Bromocriptine is rapidly and completely absorbed in the GI tract (see Table 60-2). The most therapeutic effects in hyperprolactinemic patients are seen after 4 weeks of therapy. Bromocriptine is biotransformed in the liver and eliminated in the feces through biliary elimination. A small percentage is eliminated in the urine.

Adverse Effects and Contraindications

The most frequently experienced adverse effects of bromocriptine are weakness upon standing, nasal congestion, and nausea and vomiting. These symptoms usually resolve spontaneously within a few days but may be avoided by a slow increase of the dosage to achieve the desired effects. Some patients experience severe postural hypotension and syncope on initiation of therapy. Hypertension, although rare, occurs usually after about 2 weeks of therapy. Discontinue treatment if the following are present: hypertension; severe, progressive, or unremitting headache; or signs of central nervous system toxicity.

Patients wishing to breastfeed should not take bromocriptine owing to its suppressive effects on lactation. Prolactin levels in the fetus of pregnant women treated with bromocriptine are decreased in utero but returned to normal after birth. Bromocriptine is routinely discontinued when conception is verified. The drug should be used cautiously in women prone to pregnancy-induced hypertension (PIH).

Drug Interactions

Note that bromocriptine is a CYP 3A4 substrate; blood levels can be altered when bromocriptine is given along with

CYP 3A4 inhibitors or inducers. The effectiveness of bromocriptine in decreasing prolactin levels is antagonized by drugs known to elevate prolactin (e.g., amitriptyline, imipramine, Phenothiazines, methyldopa) (Table 60-5). Additive neurologic effects may occur with levodopa, as well as additive hypotension when the drug is used with antihypertensives. Severe hypertension may occur when bromocriptine is given concomitantly with certain ergot alkaloids, which may lead to severe cardiovascular and central nervous system (CNS) complications.

Sulfites contained in commercial food products may cause allergic reactions in susceptible patients taking bromocriptine. Alcohol use is contraindicated.

Dosage Regimen

For the treatment of hyperprolactinemic causes of amenorrhea, hypogonadism, and infertility, the usual dose of bromocriptine is 1.25 to 2.5 mg/day (see Table 60-4). If the initial 2.5-mg daily dose is well tolerated during the first week of treatment, a second 2.5-mg dose can be added. Prolactin levels should be rechecked, and if adequate suppression has not occurred, the dosage may be increased to 7.5 mg/day. Dosages up to 30 mg/day have been used in patients with amenorrhea or galactorrhea.

If oral administration is not possible, some have found perivaginal administration to be equally effective while reducing symptoms. There are also a delayed-release oral preparation, a nasal formulation, and an injectable form of bromocriptine available.

Lab Considerations

Assess prolactin levels to obtain the desired effect at the lowest possible dosage. Bromocriptine has been associated with transient elevations in plasma concentrations of alanine transaminase (ALT), AST, alkaline phosphatase, uric acid, and blood urea nitrogen (BUN). Transient increases in g-glutamyl transferase (GGT) and creatine kinase (CK) values may also be noted.

For more information, see the Evolve Resources Bonus Content "Influence of Selected Drugs on Laboratory Values," found at http://evolve.elsevier.com/Gutierrez/pharmacotherapeutics.

Adjunctive Therapies
Progesterone

Progesterone is used for secondary amenorrhea caused by luteal-phase deficiency (progesterone deficiency) and ART (see also Chapter 58). The drug supplements the naturally produced hormone found during the last half of the menstrual cycle and in pregnancy (see Table 60-4). Headache, breast tenderness, tiredness, fluid retention and weight changes, and nausea are the common adverse effects. Serious adverse effects include thromboembolism, cerebrovascular accident (CVA), myocardial infarction (MI), gallbladder disease, cholestatic jaundice, and hypertension.

Progesterone is contraindicated for use in patients with undiagnosed vaginal bleeding, liver dysfunction or disease, and thrombocytopenia. Caution is used in patients with heart failure or hypertension, and in those with impaired renal function.

Testosterone

Testosterone cyprionate (Depo-Testosterone) is used primarily for replacement of endogenous hormone when there is deficient endocrine function of the testes (see Chapter 57). Because the therapeutic efficacy of testosterone in the infertile male has not been established, the risks associated with synthetic androgens may outweigh the benefits. High dosages of testosterone can result in permanent azoospermia when the drug is used to induce rebound increases in sperm count. Because of the anabolic and androgenic effects of testosterone, nonmedical use by athletes and body builders is believed to be common.

Adverse reactions to testosterone include acne, flushing, gynecomastia, habituation, changes in libido, and edema. IM testosterone may cause local irritation, and the rate of absorption may vary. With prolonged therapy, or in excessive doses, oligospermia and decreased ejaculatory volume may occur. Adverse effects also include increased aggression, antisocial behavior, and psychotic manifestations. There is a long list of potential physical damage on the heart, the liver, and bone formation, as well as other associated adverse effects, making testosterone a potentially dangerous drug.

Tamoxifen

Tamoxifen citrate is an oral antiestrogen that has been used in conjunction with clomiphene citrate in the treatment of idiopathic male infertility. It is structurally similar to clomiphene citrate and has also been used to stimulate ovulation. The precise mechanism of action is not known. Antiestrogens are thought to block estrogen receptors in the hypothalamus, resulting in a decrease in the inhibition of GnRH. This allows an increase in the GnRH with a subsequent increase in the secretion of LH and FSH. Elevated gonadotropins stimulate the production of testosterone in the testes, leading to enhanced spermatogenesis. The course of treatment should be at least 3 months, which is the length of one spermatogenic cycle.

Testolactone

Testolactone is an antineoplastic drug with antiestrogenic effects. It prevents the conversion of androgens to estrogens. When testolactone is used with GnRH in men with hypothalamic GnRH deficiency, it enhances the release of LH and FSH and stimulates testicular maturation and spermatogenesis.

Dexamethasone

Men with high sperm antibody titers may benefit from treatment with immunosuppressive therapy with dexamethasone. Treatment for men with antisperm antibodies may be more successful if intrauterine insemination procedures are employed.

Dexamethasone is also being used as an adjunct for treatment in women with high circulating androgen levels. These women are hyporesponders to ovulation-inducing drugs, whereas dexamethasone inhibits corticotropin release and decreases adrenal androgen levels in ovarian follicles. Excess androgens cause elevated LH and FSH levels, which interfere with normal gonadotropin feedback mechanisms. Dexamethasone may be used in conjunction with clomiphene, hMG, or FSH during induction of ovulation.

CLINICAL REASONING

Treatment Objectives

The general objective in the treatment of infertility is to determine the cause of the infertility and to correct, if possible, endocrinopathies, infections, anatomic aberrations, and hormonal imbalances or deficiencies. The use of ART is very common in the field of infertility.

The goal of achieving pregnancy with minimal adverse reactions takes skill and timing to achieve. Ninety percent of patients taking hMG ovulate, whereas 50% to 70% will achieve pregnancy after an average of three treatment cycles. Some have noted improved cervical mucus with hMG that may be therapeutic in itself, making coitus more natural and efficient. Multiple pregnancy rates range from 10% to 30% and mostly result in twins, with 5% of the pregnancies resulting in three or more fetuses. The spontaneous abortion rate is 20% to 25%, which is slightly higher than the general norm (see Controversy box).

Treatment Options

ⅲ *Patient Variables*

Compliance with the complex regimen of fertility treatment requires a firm understanding of the plan of care, with attention to timing of drug administration and coital activities. An understanding of the couple's relationship and commitment to a treatment regimen is vital to treatment success.

For many couples, treatment for infertility represents a final chance to have biologic children before resorting to adoption. A waiting period of up to 7 years is not uncommon for couples attempting to adopt a child. Couples who choose to remain childless need as much support for their decision as does the couple who chooses to accept fertility treatment. Answers to questions that address the couple's self-image, guilt and blame, and sexuality are important data to obtain.

Before beginning the treatments, the couple must be made fully aware of the expense, the amounts they can expect to be reimbursed by their insurance if they are covered, and the expense that can be incurred if complications ensue. In other words they need to understand the economic implications of multiple births. Hospitalization costs for the antepartum woman and the potential cost of multiple premature infants can be devastating. (see Case Study).

ⅲ *Drug Variables*

Although clomiphene is a first-line drug, in the case of an anatomic abnormality such as fallopian tubes that are not patent, ovulation induction followed by coitus and normal fertilization, conception, and implantation is not an option. In this case, treatment ordinarily involves ART with drugs such as hMG, FSH, and hCG. The particular regimen chosen is largely based on the preference of the health care provider. Different providers routinely use drugs they are most familiar with and with which they have the most confidence of bringing about the best results.

Patient Education

Encourage the patient to maintain a healthy weight because even mild obesity may result in ovulation failure. For the obese patient, weight loss may produce spontaneous ovulation and may also improve responsiveness to treatment. Underweight patients may experience similar ovulation problems, and weight gain may cause resumption and spontaneous ovulation.

Although fertility centers offer a wide range of treatment and support services, they are expensive. Advise patients to ask questions before agreeing to participate in ARTs. The questions to be asked are found in Box 60-1.

When infertility treatment is initiated, the regimen should be clearly explained to the couple and also provided to them in writing. Teach the couple to self-administer injections.

Controversy

The Ethics of Using Fertility Drugs

Jonathan J. Wolfe

The use of assistive reproductive technologies (ARTs) presents the thorniest moral questions faced by health care providers. The topic of promoting fertility by drug administration may produce less ardent political arguments than abortion, but it contains clear conflicts and poses difficult choices.

Couples who want children but cannot conceive experience a unique type of emotional suffering. They live in a world where abortion is easily available, the adoption process is difficult and lengthy, and child abuse is the fodder of daily news. Every instance of child abuse appears an affront to justice, particularly to couples who find a bitter sting to their continued infertility. Surely one can argue that they deserve relief.

Other participants in the area of fertility promotion may hold complementary, if differing, viewpoints. The issue of justice is easy to assert. However, how many pregnancies come to disaster because prenatal care is lacking? How much prenatal care could be purchased for the price of a single in vitro fertilization or artificial insemination? Do numbers win out, or does the claim of the individual person?

The hazard of fertility treatments also demands a hearing. Preparation for harvesting ova requires painful and lengthy hormonal treatment. Aside from cost and short-term adverse effects, are long-term adverse health effects also possible? The use of ovulation-stimulating drugs can produce showers of ova, contributing to multiple births that may be complicated by prematurity. Do parents have the right to demand neonatal intensive care for quadruplets in order to overcome infertility? Is it ethical to advocate abortion for fetuses in a multiple pregnancy in order to improve the odds for one or two others? Furthermore, the entire issue of fertility treatment remains morally unacceptable when one's beliefs forbid any intervention in conception.

CLINICAL REASONING

- What increases in insurance premiums in your own plan are acceptable to ensure that all infertile participants have access to fertility treatment?
- Does a single woman who desires to bear children have the same right to treatment of infertility as a married couple?
- Is surrogacy a proper resource for an infertile couple when the woman cannot carry a pregnancy to successful termination?
- An insurance company denied a couple's request to use in vitro fertilization (IVF) because the couple specifically wanted to create a daughter. Should they have been allowed to pursue IVF?
- ART is not used exclusively by infertile couples. Should single straight adults, gay men, and lesbians also have access to the resources used by "regular" heterosexual folks who have a hard time conceiving?
- Is there an ethical difference between creating human embryos specifically for stem cell extraction versus extraction from embryos left over from fertility treatments?
- What about religious issues affecting infertility and ART?

CASE STUDY   Fertility Drugs

ASSESSMENT

History of Present Illness	DJ is a 25-year-old nullipara who visits her primary care provider with complaints of failure to become pregnant after 5 years of unprotected intercourse. She is accompanied by her husband.
Past Health History	DJ's history is benign for contributing factors to infertility. Her menses started at age 12 with 28–29 day cycles, lasting 4 to 5 days. She reports no unusual discomfort, bleeding, or symptoms of PMS. She has been told she has PCOS but it is not being treated. History is negative for STDs and PID. No family history of infertility. Mother had four spontaneous term pregnancies without complications.
Life-Span Considerations	DJ and her partner have experienced a wide range of emotions, from denial to anger and grief. They have experienced low self-esteem and marital discord for a time. Counseling provided the needed support while waiting for diagnosis. Relationship now stable and supportive. Couple willing and capable of doing whatever is necessary for DJ to conceive, including IVF. In light of diagnosis (obstructive pathology), she is an immediate candidate for ART. Possibility of multiple embryo development would satisfy the couple's desire for family in one pregnancy. DJ and husband are gainfully employed, have financial stability, and a large savings account from which they can draw funds if required to pay for one cycle of ovulation induction (approximately $10,000) and IVF procedure. Cost of laboratory and ultrasound monitoring covered by health insurance.
Physical Exam Findings	*Height:* 5′9″; *Weight:* 130 lb. VSS. Manual exam reveals slightly retroverted uterus with ovaries of normal size and location. Speculum exam reveals nulliparous cervix with no unusual findings. Remainder of physical unremarkable.
Diagnostic Testing	LH, FSH, and estradiol levels, thyroid function studies, prolactin levels, cervical mucus, Pap smear, genital cultures, hysterosalpingogram, and laparoscopy are WNL.

DIAGNOSIS: Infertility

MANAGEMENT

Treatment Objectives	1. Foster follicle stimulation in preparation for IVF. 2. Achieve and maintain pregnancy.

Treatment Options	**Pharmacotherapy**
	Refer to our fertility specialist, who will prescribe the following regimen after patient counseling:
	   • Step 1: leuprolide acetate 0.5 mg subQ twice initially; to start in midluteal phase of previous cycle until FSH started, and then single 0.5 mg doses subQ daily
	   • Step 2: FSH 150 international units IM daily for 7 to 12 days to start on day 3 of cycle
	   • Step 3: hCG 10,000 units IM 24 hours after last dose of leuprolide acetate and FSH
	
	Patient Education
	1. Hot flashes tend to decrease with continued therapy.
	2. Inform health care provider if regular menstruation persists or if pregnancy occurs.
	3. Avoid tasks that require alertness until response to drugs are established.
	4. Record daily basal temperature; initiate intercourse daily beginning the day preceding hCG treatment.
	5. Possibility of multiple births
	
	Evaluation
	Follicle stimulation has been successful. Pregnancy has been achieved.

CLINICAL REASONING ANALYSIS

Q1. Didn't DJ come to you because you are her primary care provider? Why are you sending her to a specialist?

A. Fertility treatment regimens are complicated. Regimens require close attention by the fertility specialist and the couple if they are to maximize their chances for pregnancy.

Q2. Okay. But don't you have to answer questions about her other health care issues while she is taking this treatment regimen?

A. Yes. Because we will still care for DJ's other health care issues, we need to understand the treatment regimen the specialist is providing; which also means we need to have knowledge of the drugs that she is taking.

Continued

ENDOCRINE

CASE STUDY | Fertility Drugs—Cont'd

Q3. DJ is always having an ultrasound. What is the purpose of the continual ultrasounds?

A. Ultrasounds are needed to monitor the ovaries for ovarian hyperstimulation syndrome. Despite careful monitoring, a small number of women may still develop OHSS. The cause of OHSS is unknown, but women at risk of developing OHSS include younger women with PCOS, those with high estrogen hormone levels and a large number of follicles or eggs; those receiving a GnRH agonist, (DJ is on leuprolide); and those receiving hCG for luteal-phase support (DJ will be taking hCG).

Q4. I thought hCG was a blood or urine test for pregnancy. Why is she taking it to produce pregnancy?

A. In the female, FSH stimulation in the ovary causes maturation of the follicle, whereas the LH surge promotes ovulation; therefore hCG can substitute for LH in this capacity.

BOX 60-1

Questions to Ask About ART

- What is the cause of our infertility?
- What are the chances for pregnancy and a live birth without treatment, and how much will the proposed treatment improve our chances of success?
- What are the alternatives?
- What, if any, aspects of treatment will be covered by our health insurance? Can we get itemized bills to submit to our insurance company?
- Should we expect to pay for the drugs out of pocket, or are they included in the cost of the fertility treatments? How much are the drugs?

- If it is needed, do the treatment fees include intracytoplasmic sperm injection, assisted hatching, or other procedures if needed? Do the costs include fees for cryopreservation and a thaw cycle?
- If needed, does the cost include the use of donor sperm (or eggs)?
- How long will we have to undergo treatment to give it a reasonable chance to work?
- What are the risks and complications?
- If we decide not to continue with infertility treatments after one cycle, is there a refund?

Include information on aseptic technique and what to watch for infection at the injection site. Warnings about the importance of adherence should be provided. Instruct the couple to report signs and symptoms of ovarian hyperstimulation as soon as possible. In addition, include the correct procedure for monitoring basal body temperature in the teaching. And finally, emphasize the importance of follow-up meetings.

Evaluation

The effectiveness of bromocriptine therapy can be demonstrated by the resumption of normal ovulatory menstrual cycles and the restoration of fertility. The effectiveness of clomiphene citrate is demonstrated by the occurrence of ovulation, as measured by estrogen elimination, biphasic body temperature elevations, and endometrial histologic changes.

If conception is not achieved after three to four treatment cycles, reevaluate the original diagnosis.

hMG effectiveness is evaluated by the maturation of follicles. hMG therapy is followed by hCG administration, which in turn should lead to ovulation. If ovulation does not occur after three to six menstrual cycles, therapy may be discontinued. For the male, effectiveness is evident by increased spermatogenesis after 4 months of therapy. Treatment effectiveness of hCG can be noted by an increase in spermatogenesis in males.

Although the couple may believe that the only successful outcome of treatment is a pregnancy, that outcome cannot, and should not, be guaranteed. However, when pregnancy has been detected and the embryonic sac and heart rate can be detected by ultrasound, treatment with fertility drugs is considered successful.

KEY POINTS

- Infertility is defined as an inability to conceive after 1 year of unprotected coitus or an inability to carry a fetus to term.
- Alterations in the HPO axis are responsible for a large proportion of female infertility.
- Female fertility disorders include problems related to follicular maturation, ovulation, pituitary disorders, luteal-phase defects, and uterine, tubal, and pelvic disorders.
- Male fertility problems include a variety of dysfunctions that can be classified as pretesticular, testicular, and posttesticular disorders.

- The primary objectives in the treatment of infertility are induction of ovulation, the control of interference with hormonal response, and the restoration of spermatogenesis.
- Drug therapy modifies the HPO axis that controls GnRH, FSH, and LH secretion.
- Drug options include clomiphene citrate, bromocriptine, FSH, GnRH, hCG, and leuprolide acetate.
- Treatment regimens often use a combination of drugs, and therefore therapy should be carried out by a specialist in infertility and the family referred to support groups as needed.

■ Treatment regimens require that the couple be highly educated about the drug therapy, appropriate timing of drug therapy in relation to coitus, and the importance of follow-up monitoring.

■ Treatment with fertility drugs is considered successful when pregnancy is detected and the embryonic sac and heart rate can be identified on ultrasound.

Bibliography

Balen, A., Mulders, A., Fauser, B., et al. (2004). Pharmacodynamics of a single low dose of long-acting recombinant follicle-stimulating hormone (FSH-carboxy terminal peptide, corifollitropin alfa) in women with World Health Organization group II anovulatory infertility. *Journal of Clinical Endocrinology and Metabolism, 89* (12), 6297–6304.

Bibbo, M., Haenszel, W., Wied, G., et al. (1978). A twenty-five year follow-up study of women exposed to diethylstilbestrol during pregnancy. *New England Journal of Medicine, 298*(14), 763–777.

Bibbo, M., Gill, W., Azizi, F., et al. (1977). Follow-up study of male and female offspring of DES-exposed mothers. *Obstetrics and Gynecology, 49*(1), 1–7.

Elder, K., Baker, D., and Ribes, J. (2005). *Infections, infertility, and assisted reproduction.* Cambridge, England: The Press Syndicate of the University of Cambridge.

Gill, W., Schumacher, G., and Bibbo, M. (1976). Structural and functional abnormalities in the sex organs of male offspring of mothers treated with diethylstilbestrol (DES). *Journal of Reproductive Medicine, 16*(4), 147–153.

Infertility. (2005). *Infertility Central.* Available online: Infertilitycentral.com. Accessed May 31, 2007.

Infertility. (2005). *IVF infertility.* Available online: www.ivf-infertility.com. Accessed May 31, 2007.

Meara, J., Vessey, M., and Fairweather, D. (1989). A randomized double-blind controlled trial of the value of diethylstilbestrol therapy in pregnancy: 35 year follow-up of mothers and their offspring. *British Journal of Obstetrics and Gynecology, 96*(5), 620–622.

Perloe, M. (1999). A cost efficient approach to the diagnosis and treatment of infertility for the OBGYN generalist. Available online: www.obgyn.net/infertility. Accessed May 31, 2007.

Rutstein, S., and Shag, I. (2004). *Infecundity, infertility, and childlessness in developing countries. DHS Comparative Reports No. 9.* Calverton, Maryland: ORC Macro and the World Health Organization.

Vayena, E., Rose, P., and Griffin, D. (Ed.). (2002). Current practices and controversies in assisted reproduction. Report of a meeting on medical, ethical and social aspects of assisted reproduction at WHO Headquarters, Geneva, Switzerland, 17–21 September, 2001.

Vessey, M., Fairweather, D., Norman-Smith, B., et al. (1983). A randomized double blind controlled trial of the value of stilbestrol therapy in pregnancy: Long-term follow-up of mothers and their offspring. *British Journal of Obstetrics and Gynecology, 90*(11), 1007–1017.

World Health Organization. (2000). *WHO manual for the standardized investigation, diagnosis and management of the infertile male.* Cambridge, England: Cambridge University Press.

Wurn, B., Wurn, L., and King, R. (2004). Treating female infertility and improving IVF pregnancy rates with a manual of physical therapy technique. *Medscape General Medicine, 6*(2), 51.

Yen, S., and Jaffe, R. (1986). *Reproductive endocrinology, physiology, pathophysiology, and clinical management* (2nd ed.). Philadelphia: WB Saunders.

ENDOCRINE

61

Ophthalmic Drugs

V isual disorders occur at any age and are a peril to patients, largely because vision is one of the most cherished of senses. Although many eye disorders are correctable with eyeglasses or contact lenses, others require drugs to control or treat the problem. This chapter focuses primarily on the pharmacokinetics, the pharmacodynamics, drug delivery issues, and specific uses for ocular drugs in patients with eye infections, inflammation, or glaucoma.

However, it is also important to briefly review the bewildering array of persons who care for the patient. Eye-care professionals include the ophthalmologist, the optician, the optometrist, and the ophthalmic technician. A distinction is also made between the terms ophthalmic and ocular for the purposes of this chapter. Ophthalmic refers to the drug or treatment modality, whereas ocular refers to the eye itself (e.g., ocular tear film). The terminology often confuses the uninformed (Box 61-1).

PHARMACOKINETICS OF OPHTHALMIC DRUGS

As would be expected, the classical pharmacokinetics based on systemically administered drugs do not fully apply to ophthalmic drugs. Although similar principles of absorption, distribution, biotransformation, and elimination determine the fate of drug disposition in the eye, alternative routes of drug administration, in addition to oral and intravenous (IV) routes, introduce other variables into the analysis.

ABSORPTION

The rate and extent of absorption of an ocular drug is determined by the time the drug remains in the cul-de-sac and precorneal tear film and the binding of the drug to tear proteins. The time that the drug remains in the cul-de-sac and precorneal tear film can be prolonged by changing its formulation from a suspension to an ointment. Most ocular drugs are delivered in aqueous solutions. When there is minimal solubility, a suspension form is used to assist in delivery.

The drug concentration between the tear film and the corneal and the conjunctival epithelium provides the driving force for passive diffusion across these tissues. Drug penetration into the eye is related to its concentration in the tear film.

Factors affecting the bioavailability of ocular drugs include pH, the salt form of the drug, structural forms of a given drug, vehicle composition, and osmolality, tonicity, and viscosity. Some formulations prolong the time a drug remains on the surface of the eye. These include gels, ointments, solid inserts, soft contact lenses, and collagen shields. For example, ocular gels (e.g., 4% pilocarpine gel) release drugs by diffusion following erosion of soluble polymers. Ointments usually contain mineral oil or a petroleum base and are helpful in delivering antibiotics, cycloplegic drugs, or miotics. Solid inserts, such as

---

BOX 61-1

Eye-Care Professionals

Ophthalmologist	A licensed physician and surgeon (MD) with extensive education and formal training: 4 years of college, 4 years of medical school, 1 year of internship, 3 to 4 years of residency training, and sometimes, 1 to 2 years of subspecialty fellowship training (12 to 15 years total). Diagnoses and treats all diseases and disorders of the eye, medically and surgically. Evaluates the effect of systemic disorders on the eye and assesses the risk of eye treatment on the patient's general health. Does eye exams; provides prescriptions for glasses and drugs.
Optometrist	A licensed primary eye care provider who has 4 years of college and 4 years of optometry school (OD, or Doctor of Optometry). Performs eye exams and some diagnostic work (i.e., screening for cataracts and glaucoma); prescribes and dispenses glasses and contact lenses. In many states, optometrists are allowed to prescribe selected ophthalmic drugs. Patient is referred to ophthalmologist if the optometrist discovers significant ocular disease or if surgery is needed.
Optician	A technician who completes a 2-year program in optometry at a community college or a technical school. Apprentice work may be optional or required, based on program objectives. Makes, fits, and dispenses eyeglasses and contact lens when provided with a prescription from an optometrist or an ophthalmologist. May be employed by an optical laboratory or in retail sales. Opticians do not perform eye exams or write prescriptions.
Ophthalmic technician	Usually works with an ophthalmologist; a technician who may complete a 2-year technical program. Performs selected tests (e.g., ultrasound and electrophysiology) and at times refractions for glasses and contact lens fitting.

---

the Ocuserts Pilo-20 and Pilo-40, provide a steady-state diffusion rate over time rather than as a bolus. The pharmacokinetics of ophthalmic drugs are identified in Table 61-1.

Absorption from the nasal mucosa avoids first-pass effect by the liver, and as a consequence, significant systemic adverse effects may be noted with topical ophthalmic drugs, particularly when used chronically.

DISTRIBUTION

Topically administered ophthalmic drugs are systemically distributed primarily by nasal mucosal absorption and by local distribution by the cornea and the conjunctiva. Drugs accumulate in the aqueous humor, which is then distributed to intraocular structures as well as the systemic circulation via the trabecular

PHARMACOKINETICS

TABLE 61-1 Glaucoma Drugs

Drug	Onset of Miosis	Peak Miosis; IOP Reduction	Duration of Miosis; IOP Reduction	Onset of Mydriasis, Cycloplegia	Maximal Mydriasis; Cycloplegia	Duration Mydriasis Cycloplegia	Effect on Aqueous Outflow
BETA BLOCKERS							
betaxolol	30–60 min	2 hr	12 hr	NA	NA	NA	*
carteolol	UA	12 hr	UA	NA	NA	NA	*
levobunolol	<60 min	2–6 hr	UA; 24 hr	NA	NA	NA	*
metipranolol	<30 min	UA	12–24 hr	NA	NA	NA	*
timolol	30 min	1–2 hr	6 hr	NA	NA	NA	*
PROSTAGLANDIN ANALOGUES							
latanoprost	UA	2 hr	UA	NA	NA	NA	Inc
bimatoprost	UA	7 days	45 min	NA	NA	NA	Inc
travoprost	30 min	1–7 days	45–60 min	NA	NA	NA	Inc
unoprostone	UA	14 min		NA	NA	NA	Inc
CARBONIC ANHYDRASE INHIBITORS							
acetazolamide	30 min–2 hr	NA; 18–24 hr	2–4 hr; 8–12 hr	NA	NA	NA	*
brinzolamide	UA	NA; 20–28 wk	111 days	NA	NA	NA	*
dichlorphenamide	NA	NA; 2–4 hr	6–12 hr	NA	NA	NA	*
dorzolamide	NA	NA; UA	4 mo	NA	NA	NA	*
methazolamide	NA	NA; 10–18 hr	NA; 10–18 hr	NA	NA	NA	*
ADRENERGICS							
apraclonidine	NA	NA	NA; UA	60 min; NA	3–5 hr; NA	12 hr; NA	Inc
brimonidine	NA	NA	NA; UA	UA	2 hr	4–6 hr; NA	Inc
dipivefrin	NA	NA	NA; 12 hr	Minutes	60 min	UA	Inc
phenylephrine	NA	NA	NA	<60 min; NA	15–60 min	3–7 hr; NA	Inc
CHOLINERGIC MIOTICS							
carbachol	2–5 min	UA; 6 hr	4–8 hr; 4 hr	NA	NA	NA	Inc
pilocarpine	10–30 min	30 min; 1–1.5 hr	4–8 hr; 4–14 hr†	NA	NA	NA	Inc
ANTICHOLINESTERASE MIOTICS							
echothiophate	10–30 min	2 hr; 24 hr	1–4 wk; days-wk‡	NA	NA	NA	Inc
ANTICHOLINERGIC MYDRIATICS AND CYCLOPLEGICS							
atropine	NA	NA	NA	30–40 min; 1–3 hr	30–40 min; 1–3 hr	7–12 days; 6–14 days	Dec
cyclopentolate	NA	NA	NA	30–60 min; 15–60 min	30–60 min; 25–75 min	24 hr; 0.25–1 day§	Dec
homatropine	NA	NA	NA	10–30 min; 30–90 min	10–30 min; 30–90 min	6 hr–3 days; 10–48 hr	Dec
scopolamine	NA	NA	NA	20–30 min; 30–60 min	20–30 min; 30–60 min	3–7 days; 3–7 days	Dec
tropicamide	NA	NA	NA	20–40 min; 20–35 min	20–40 min; 20–40 min	6–7 hr; 1–6 hr	Dec

*Ophthalmic beta blockers and carbonic anhydrase inhibitors reduce the production of aqueous humor rather than increasing its outflow.
†Pilocarpine's duration of IOP action depends on concentration.
‡Duration of decrease in IOP for demecarium, echothiophate, and isoflurophate may last up to 1 month.
§Cyclopentolate's recovery of accommodation; recovery from mydriasis may take several days.
Dec, Decrease; *Inc,* increase; *IOP,* intraocular pressure; *NA,* not applicable; *UA,* unavailable.

meshwork. Distribution is also affected by melanin binding of certain drugs. Black and brown irises contain more melanin than blue, green, or gray irises. The more pigment in the iris, the more the drug can bind to it, resulting in a slower onset but longer duration of action. For example, the onset of the mydriatic effects of alpha agonists is slower in a patient with a brown iris compared to someone with a blue iris.

BIOTRANSFORMATION AND ELIMINATION

Biotransformation of ophthalmic drugs is significant because local tissues in the eye express a variety of enzymes including esterases, lysosomal enzymes, peptidases, glucuronide and sulfate transferases, monoamine oxidase (MAO), and catechol-0-methyl-transferase (COMT). The esterases are of particular interest because of the development of prodrugs for enhanced corneal permeability. For example, dipivefrin is a prodrug of epinephrine, and latanoprost is a prodrug of prostaglandin $F_{2\alpha}$; both drugs are used in the management of glaucoma. Topically applied ophthalmic drugs are eliminated by the liver and the kidney after systemic absorption.

OCULAR INFECTIONS

ETIOLOGY

Ocular infections can involve the lid, the conjunctiva, the cornea, the socket, and the inside of the globe itself. Severity can range from mild annoyances to sight-destroying infections.

PATHOPHYSIOLOGY

The body's immune response to infection, whether from bacteria, viruses, fungi, or parasites, is to clear organisms, repair damage, and form a scar, has the potential to directly and permanently damage the eye. The immune response can, in fact, result in a greater loss of eye function than direct damage from the infecting organism. For example, one cannot see through a scar on the cornea; hence both the immune response and the infecting organism must be taken into account when planning treatment for an infection. The infection's type and location determine the significance of the potential damage caused by the immune response and the infecting organism.

Hordeolum and blepharitis are common. A hordeolum, or stye, is an infection of the glands at the lid margins. Blepharitis is a common bilateral inflammatory process of the eyelids characterized by irritation and burning. The common offending organism in both cases is usually *Staphylococcus aureus*. Ophthalmic antibiotics are used, usually in ointment form, particularly when the disease is accompanied by conjunctivitis and keratitis.

Orbital cellulitis is an infection in the bony socket of the eye, often the result of a recent hordeolum or blepharitis. Symptoms of cellulitis usually include pain, proptosis, or protuberance of the eye, decreased eye movement, redness, swelling, a fever of 102°F to 103°F, and in some cases, damage to the optic nerve. Meningitis may develop without timely treatment. Patients require immediate hospitalization, intensive IV antibiotics, and occasionally, surgical drainage of the abscess.

Dacryocystitis is an infection of the lacrimal gland. The infection is usually unilateral and secondary to an obstruction of the nasolacrimal duct in infants and children. In the past, the common organism was *Haemophilus influenzae*, but with the introduction in 1985 of the *H. influenzae* vaccine, the incidence has declined. In adults, dacryocystitis and canalicular infections may be caused by *S. aureus*, *Streptococcus*, *Candida*, or *Actinomyces israelii*.

Acute conjunctivitis is an inflammation of the bulbar or the scleral conjunctiva that lines the inside surface of the lid and covers the surface of the globe up to the junction of the sclera and the cornea. The more common causes of conjunctivitis include bacteria, viruses, allergies, environmental irritants, contact lenses, and chemicals. The less common causes include pathogens such as immune-mediated reactions, systemic diseases, and tumors of the conjunctiva or eyelid. The more commonly reported infectious agents include the adenovirus and the herpes simplex virus, followed by other viruses (e.g., enterovirus, coxsackievirus, measles virus, varicella zoster virus, vaccinia-variola virus) and bacteria such as *S. aureus* (common in adults), *Streptococcus pneumoniae*, *H. influenzae*, *Moraxella lacunata*, and the *Chlamydia* and *Neisseria* species. *Neisseria gonorrhoeae* and *Pseudomonas aeruginosa* bacteria are particularly dangerous. Instillation of an antibiotic at birth is a legally mandated prophylaxis for gonorrhea. *Rickettsiae*, fungi, and parasites, in both cyst and trophozoite form, are rare causes of conjunctivitis.

The most common symptom of conjunctivitis is red eye, but not all red eyes signify conjunctivitis (Table 61-2). The distinguishing feature of bacterial conjunctivitis is that the purulent discharge continues throughout the day, in contrast with the mostly watery discharge during the day occurring with viral or allergic conjunctivitis. The purulent discharge will be noticeable at the lid margins and in the corners of the eyes, and eyes may be stuck closed in the morning.

Experiences of health care providers suggest that the most infectious conjunctivitis is viral. Adenovirus typically causes the highly contagious viral conjunctivitis that is spread by direct contact with the patient and their secretions, or with contaminated objects. The clinical course of viral conjunctivitis coincides with the common cold.

Keratitis, or corneal ulcer, may occur at any level of the cornea. The mildest form of keratitis is usually caused by a virus. Keratitis caused by bacteria is the most serious form, carrying the risk of vision loss. Numerous organisms have been isolated including bacteria, viruses, fungi, spirochetes, and trophozoites. **Aggressive forms of bacterial keratitis must be treated A**

TABLE 61-2 Selected Differential Diagnoses for Red Eye

Disorder	Burn, Sting	Pain	Discharge	Vision	PP	PERRLA	Cornea	Redness	IOP	Itch	Lid
Viral Conjunctivitis	Yes	–	Watery	NL	None	Intact	Clear	Yes	NL	–	–
Bacterial conjunctivitis	Yes	–	Purulent	NL	–	Intact	Clear	Yes	NL	–	–
Allergic conjunctivitis	Yes	–	Ropy	NL	Yes	Intact	Clear	Yes	NL	Yes	Swell
Acute iritis	Yes	–	Clear	Blurry	Yes	*	Clear	–	NL	–	–
Acute glaucoma	–	FBS	None	Changed	Maybe	†	Clear	–	Up	–	–
Vernal keratoconjunctivitis	Yes	FBS	Thick, ropy	–	Yes	–	Central or diffuse; limbus	Yes	NL	Intense	Yes‡
Atopic keratoconjunctivitis	Yes	FBS	Tearing	–	Yes	–	–	Yes	NL	–	Yes‡; Swell
Giant papillary conjunctivitis	Yes	FBS	Mucus sheets; tearing	–	–	–	–	Yes	NL	Yes	Yes‡§; Swell
Drug-induced conjunctivitis	Yes	FBS	Thin, mucoid; tearing	–	Yes	–	Limbus	Yes	NL	–	Yes‡§; Swell

*Acute iritis: Small irregular pupil, ciliary flush, central redness, poor response to light, conjunctival and circumcorneal injection with acute iritis.
†Acute glaucoma: May also have nausea and vomiting, middilated and oval pupil with poor response to light; moderate to severe conjunctival and circumcorneal injection.
‡Cobblestone papillae on tarsal surface of lid; chemosis; limbus and/or central diffuse corneal involvement.
§Periorbital dermatitis; lid margin dysfunction with blockage; limbus and central and diffuse corneal involvement.
FBS, Foreign body sensation; *IOP*, intraocular pressure; *NL*, normal; *PERRLA*, pupils equal, round, reactive to light and accommodation; *PP*, photophobia.

SENSORY

empirically and intensively with the appropriate antibiotic to prevent blindness from corneal perforation and secondary scarring. The mainstay of treatment is steroids and specific antibiotics. Many patients require hospitalization. The outcome of treatment is determined by the degree of scarring.

Endophthalmitis is a potentially severe and devastating inflammatory, and usually infectious, process of the intraocular tissues. Endophthalmitis is usually caused by bacteria, fungi or, rarely, by spirochetes. The typical patient is one who has had cataract, glaucoma, corneal, or retinal surgery; but infection may also result from trauma, or endogenous seeding in an immunocompromised patient or IV-drug user. Recent literature estimates that as many as 50% of all laser-assisted in situ keratomileusis (Lasik) infections develop from atypical mycobacteria.

Interventions for endophthalmitis include vitrectomy (i.e., surgical removal of the vitreous) and empiric intravitreal antibiotics. Steroids are often used to reduce the immune response and the risk for subsequent scarring. In cases of endogenous seeding, parenteral antibiotics are used; however, in trauma, or in the postoperative patient, the efficacy of systemic antibiotics has not been established.

PHARMACOTHERAPEUTIC OPTIONS

Antibiotics

Topical antimicrobials used to treat ocular infections include a wide variety of antibacterial, antiviral, antifungal, and antiprotozoal drugs. Many of these drugs were discussed in detail in preceding chapters (Chapters 27, 28, and 30) (Box 61-2). The antibiotic chosen is based on exam findings and the results of culture and sensitivity testing. Although rarely done, a culture and sensitivity of exudate, or if needed, ocular fluid, can be obtained; but even when it is done, empiric treatment is often provided while awaiting culture results. Empiric antibiotic treatment covers most common pathogens responsible for bacterial eye infections. Patients who do not respond within 1 to 2 days with a decrease in discharge, redness, and irritation should be referred to an ophthalmologist.

Ophthalmic antibiotics work one of three ways to disrupt invading organisms. They may inhibit cell wall synthesis, inhibit protein synthesis, or alter permeability of the cell membrane. Drugs that destroy the causative organism are *bactericidal*, whereas *bacteriostatic* drugs simply inhibit the organism's growth, allowing the body's immune system to fight the infection. Whatever the mechanism, the desired outcome is elimination of the infecting organism.

The bioavailability of an ocular antibiotic depends on the specific pathogen, the site of infection, and the integrity of the hematoaqueous barrier. For example, quinolones penetrate the cornea, reaching therapeutic concentrations in the anterior chamber of the eye, whereas polymixin B–bacitracin has no penetrating powers and remains at the eye's surface.

Gatifloxacin, moxifloxacin, and levofloxacin have greater solubility than older-generation quinolones because of their increased corneal solubility and penetration, greater concentrations, more neutral pH levels, and greater bacterial susceptibility. Their neutral pH and greater solubility will decrease the precipitation of the drug and reduce burning symptoms. Their lower levels of preservatives reduce the risk for toxicity and burning even further.

The most common adverse effects of ophthalmic antibiotics are local and transient inflammation, burning, stinging,

---

BOX 61-2

Ophthalmic Antimicrobials

Antibiotics

Aminoglycosides
- gentamicin ophthalmic (Garamycin, Genoptic, Gentacidin, Gentak); ✦ Garamycin
- tobramycin ophthalmic (Tobrex); ✦ tobramycin, Tobrex

Sulfonamide Antibiotics
- sulfacetamide ophthalmic (AK-Sulf, Bleph-10, Cetamide, Sodium Sulamyd, Storz Sulf); ✦ sulfacetamide with prednisone (Blephamide Ophthalmic)
- sulfisoxazole (Gantrisin Ophthalmic)

Macrolides
- erythromycin (Ilotycin Ophthalmic and generics)

Quinolones
- ciprofloxacin HCL (Ciloxan); ✦ Ciloxan
- gatifloxacin (Zymar Ophthalmic); ✦ Zymar Eye Drops
- levofloxacin ophthalmic (Quixin)
- moxifloxacin ophthalmic (Vigamox); ✦ Vigamox
- ofloxacin ophthalmic (Ocuflox); ✦ Ocuflox Ophthalmic Solution

Polypeptides
- bacitracin ointment
- polymixin B sulfate with bacitracin zinc, and neomycin sulfate (Neosporin)

- polymixin B with bacitracin (Polysporin)
- polymixin B with trimethoprim (Polytrim); ✦ Polytrim

Miscellaneous
- chloramphenicol (AK-chlor, Chloroptic); ✦ chloramphenicol
- neomycin, polymixin B, hydrocortisone (Cortisporin Ophthalmic); ✦ Cortisporin suspension
- neomycin, polymixin B with gramicidin (solution) or bacitracin (ointment) (Neosporin Ophthalmic)

Antivirals
- fomivirsen (Vitravene)
- ganciclovir (Cytovene, Vitrasert); ✦ Cytovene
- idoxuridine (Herplex); ✦ Herplex-D
- trifluridine (Viroptic)
- vidarabine (Vira-A Ophthalmic)

Antifungals
- amphotericin B
- fluconazole
- ketoconazole
- miconazole
- natamycin (Natacyn)*

*Only natamycin is commercially available for ophthalmic use. It is structurally related to the sulfonamides, amphotericin B, and nystatin. Other antifungal drugs must be formulated for a given mode of administration.

and drug hypersensitivity. Other adverse effects and toxicities, and drug interactions are specific for individual drugs and were discussed in preceding chapters. Erythromycin and polymyxin B are ordinarily safe for use as topical applications in pregnant women and nursing mothers.

Organisms commonly associated with bacterial conjunctivitis, particularly gram-positive pathogens, are showing significant resistance to earlier quinolones. Ordinarily, administration 4 times daily of any quinolone for a period of 7 to 10 days is more than sufficient to eradicate the infection. When ophthalmic antibiotics are combined with corticosteroids, the immunosuppression that results may make it more difficult to rid the eye of infection.

Antivirals

Ophthalmic antiviral drugs are identified in Box 61-2. The primary targets for ophthalmic antiviral drugs are herpes simplex, viral keratitis, herpes zoster ophthalmicus, cytomegalovirus (CMV), and retinitis.

There are no specific antiviral treatments for *viral conjunctivitis*. Viral conjunctivitis is often caused by adenoviruses and usually has a self-limited course. Symptoms can persist for 2 to 3 weeks and will not be "cured" by topically administered drugs. Symptomatic relief can be gained from topical antihistamine and/or decongestants and warm or cool compresses. Encourage the use of non–antibiotic lubricating agents such as Hypotears, Refresh, Tears II, Lacri-Lube, and Refresh PM (see discussion that follows). Teach patients that these topical drugs treat the symptoms but not the disease. The irritation and discharge may get worse for 3 to 5 days before getting better.

Herpes simplex infection of the cornea is usually treated with idoxuridine, the first ophthalmic antiviral drug developed. It is invaluable because it prevents the virus from feeding off the cells of the corneal epithelium. Idoxuridine is poorly absorbed intraocularly. Vidarabine and trifluridine are found in trace amounts in the aqueous humor after application to a cornea with an epithelial defect or inflammation. Neither drug displays significant systemic absorption. To prevent recurrence of herpes, continue antiviral drugs for 5 to 7 days after healing has occurred. Improvement usually occurs in 7 to 8 days and may continue for as long as 21 days.

Herpes zoster ophthalmicus is a latent reactivation of a varicella zoster infection in the first division of the trigeminal cranial nerve. Systemic acyclovir is effective in reducing the severity and the complications of zoster. There are no ophthalmic formulations of acyclovir approved by the Food and Drug Administration (FDA), although there is an ointment available for investigational use.

Viral keratitis, an infection of the cornea, is most commonly caused by the herpes simplex I and varicella zoster viruses, and less commonly the Epstein-Barr virus, herpes zoster, and CMV. Topical antivirals are used for the treatment of epithelial disease due to herpes simplex. Because there is a very narrow margin between therapeutic topical antiviral activity and toxicity on the cornea, patients are followed very closely. Use of topical corticosteroids is avoided in patients with herpetic keratitis because of uncontrolled virus proliferation. In contrast, corticosteroids accelerate recovery for the patient with herpetic disciform keratitis, a cell-mediated immune reaction.

Viral retinitis may be caused by herpes simplex virus, CMV, adenovirus, or varicella zoster virus. CMV retinitis does not appear to progress when anti-CMV therapy is discontinued, provided highly active antiretroviral therapy has been used. Treatment of CMV requires long-term parenteral administration of an antiviral drug. An effective alternative to the systemic route of administration for ganciclovir is intravitreal administration.

Antifungal Drugs

The frequency of fungal corneal ulcers has increased in recent years, most likely because of the increased use of corticosteroids and the related depression of the immune system. In addition, use of broad-spectrum antibiotics has contributed to the incidence of ocular fungal infections. Antifungal drugs are discussed in more depth in Chapter 28.

Natamycin, as one of the few ophthalmic antifungal drugs available in the United States, is considered the drug of choice for initial treatment of fungal keratitis because of its broad spectrum. It is also effective in treatment of blepharitis, conjunctivitis, and in some cases, endophthalmitis, which occur frequently after an eye injury or eye surgery. Other antifungal drugs must be formulated for a given mode of administration.

Ocular fungal infections are a challenge to treat since the eyes absorb ophthalmic antifungal drugs only poorly. Natamycin does not reach measurable levels in the deeper corneal layers (unless a defect in the epithelium is present), and thus it may not reach deep corneal mycoses. The 5% suspension increases the permeability of the fungal cell membrane to the drug (see Table 61-1).

Antiprotozoal Drugs

Parasitic infections involving the eye usually become manifest as a form of uveitis, an inflammatory process of either the anterior or posterior eye segments, or at times as conjunctivitis, keratitis, or retinitis. Antiprotozoal drugs were discussed previously in Chapter 30.

In the United States, the most common protozoal infections are caused by *Acanthamoeba* and *Toxoplasma gondii*. Be highly suspicious of the presence of these organisms when contact lens wearers develop keratitis. Treatment of *Acanthamoeba*-caused keratitis usually consists of a combination of a topical antibiotic (e.g., polymyxin B, bacitracin zinc, neomycin sulfate [Neomycin]), and sometimes an imidazole such as clotrimazole, miconazole, or ketoconazole.

Toxoplasmosis may manifest as a posterior or occasionally as an anterior uveitis. Treatment is warranted when inflammatory lesions encroach upon the macula and threaten central vision. Several regimens have been recommended along with a systemic steroid (e.g., pyrimethamine, sulfadiazine, and folinic acid; pyrimethamine, sulfadiazine, clindamycin, and folinic acid; sulfadiazine and clindamycin; clindamycin; and trimethoprim-sulfamethoxazole, with or without clindamycin).

OCULAR INFLAMMATION AND ALLERGIES

The eye is constructed of several different layers of tissue, and all can become inflamed owing to infection, allergy, chemical burns, or other factors. Inflammation of the conjunctiva is termed conjunctivitis. Similarly, keratitis, uveitis, scleritis, and

SENSORY

neuritis describe inflammation of the cornea, the uveal tract, the sclera, and the nerves, respectively. It is of course possible that more than one tissue becomes inflamed at any given time. Systemic disease can manifest or become complicated by inflammatory symptoms in the eye. Although inflammation is generally associated with pain, this is not always the case.

PHARMACOTHERAPEUTIC OPTIONS

Nonsteroidal Antiinflammatory Drugs

Ophthalmic nonsteroidal antiinflammatory drugs (NSAIDs) inhibit prostaglandin synthesis and reduce prostaglandin-mediated effects (i.e., miosis, increased vascular permeability, conjunctival hyperemia, and changes in intraocular pressure) (Box 61-3). They are generally well tolerated but do produce transient burning and stinging when administered. Dendritic keratitis is also possible. Assess for abnormal bleeding, because

---

BOX 61-3

Ophthalmic Antiinflammatory Drugs

Nonsteroidal Antiinflammatory Drugs
- diclofenac (Voltaren Eye Drops); ♣ Voltaren
- flurbiprofen (Ocufen)
- ketorolac tromethamine (Acular); ♣ ketorolac tromethamine
- rimexolone (Vexol); ♣ Vexol
- suprofen (Profenal)

Glucocorticosteroids
- betamethasone
- clobetasone
- dexamethasone (Maxidex); ♣ Maxidex
- fluorometholone (Flarex, FML Liquifilm, FML Forte Liquifilm); ♣ Flarex, FML
- Forte Eye Drops, FML Liquifilm
- fluorometholone with sulfacetamide (FML-S Liquifilm)*
- hydrocortisone acetate
- prednisolone (Pred Mild, Pred Forte); ♣ Pred Forte
- prednisolone with sulfacetamide; ♣ Blephamide

Histamine₁ (H₁) Antagonists
- antazoline (Naphazoline)
- azelastine (Optivar)
- emedastine (Emadine)
- ketotifen fumarate (Zaditor); ♣ Zaditor†
- levocabastine (Livostin); ♣ Livostin
- olopatadine (Patanol); ♣ Patanol

Mast Cell Stabilizers
- cromolyn (Crolom, Opticrom); ♣ Cromolyn
- lodoxamide tromethamine (Alomide); ♣ Alomide
- nedocromil sodium (Alocril); ♣ Alocril
- pemirolast potassium (Alamast)

Alpha Adrenergic Agonists
- naphazoline (AK-Con, Albalon, Allerest Eye Drops, Naphcon, Naphcon Forte, others); ♣ Albalon eye drops, Naphcon Forte
- naphazoline hydrochloride–pheniramine (Naphcon-A, OcuHist, Opcon-A, Vascon-A); ♣ Visine Advance Allergy

*Used for patients with inflammation but who are also at risk of bacterial infection.
†Ketotifen ophthalmic has a dual action: it selectively inhibits H₁ but also stabilizes mast cells.

---

excessive systemic absorption may interfere with platelet aggregation. Chapter 17 discusses the NSAIDs in more depth.

Corticosteroids

Ophthalmic corticosteroids also reduce inflammation. The corticosteroids' mechanism of action was described in Chapter 56. However, these drugs are for short-term use only. With prolonged use they may cause a "steroid glaucoma" or cataracts. They should be used under the direction of an ophthalmologist. Systemic corticosteroids may be appropriate for severe eye disease such as scleritis, episcleritis, and blinding uveitis. A correct diagnosis is essential before using corticosteroids since these drugs will worsen an inflamed eye caused by a dendritic ulcer resulting from a herpes simplex viral infection, which may lead to blindness or even loss of the eye.

Ophthalmic corticosteroids may also be used for severe allergy. Ocular allergies such as seasonal allergic conjunctivitis may be managed with histamine₁ antagonists such as the ophthalmic formulation olopatadine. Mast cell stabilizers such as cromolyn sodium or nedocromil can be used for allergic conjunctivitis as well as vernal keratoconjunctivitis.

Antihistamines

Approximately 20% of the population is affected by ocular allergies on an annual basis. There is a history of personal or family history of allergies in half of the patients with ocular allergy. Patients with ocular allergies describe symptoms of itching, tearing, redness, burning, photophobia, and mucous discharge. The average age of onset for allergic conjunctivitis is 20 years of age; primarily it is a disease of young adults.

Ocular allergies primarily affect the conjunctiva and result from a combination of the following factors: amplified specific response to allergen recognition, increased immunoglobulin E (IgE) and IgG production, and hyperresponsiveness of ocular tissue.

The common pathway for all three of these ocular allergies is that an allergen binds to an IgE antibody in the tears and the conjunctiva. The IgE antibodies are bound to Fc receptors on mast cells; the mast cells then degranulate and release allergic mediators. This allergic response presents as itching, tearing, conjunctival edema, hyperemia, eyelid edema, watery discharge, and photophobia.

Acute allergic conjunctivitis is an acute hypersensitivity reaction caused by exposure to allergens. This hypersensitivity reaction is characterized by intense episodes of itching, hyperemia, tearing, and eyelid edema. Typically this acute allergic conjunctivitis resolves in less than 24 hours.

The primary treatment focus is to educate the patient about the importance of avoiding the allergen. Topical antihistamines or vasoconstrictors are usually the choice for treating these short exacerbations of symptoms. Mast cell stabilizers or a combination of antihistamine and mast cell stabilizers (e.g., olopatadine) can be used for patients with frequent attacks (episodes occurring more than 2 days per month). Prophylaxis may include oral antihistamines with the addition of artificial tears for the drying effect that oral antihistamines have on mucosal surfaces.

Seasonal allergic conjunctivitis is a mild form of ocular allergy and is frequently associated with rhinitis. As the term "seasonal" implies, eye symptoms appear in spring and late summer when the patient is exposed to pollen, grasses, and ragweed. *Perennial allergic conjunctivitis* is a year-round allergy caused by environmental exposure to allergens such as dust mites and molds.

The primary treatment for ocular allergies is the avoidance of the allergen. Instruct patients not to rub their eyes, since this can cause mechanical mast cell degranulation and worsening of symptoms. In addition, teach them to use topical antihistamines, to brush their hair before bedtime to remove pollens and dust that have settled during the day, to frequently use artificial tears, and to use cool compresses.

Since the onset of symptoms of seasonal and perennial allergic conjunctivitis is fairly predictable based on the patient's history, the goal is to start treatment in anticipation of the onset of symptoms. Olopatadine has become the first-line drug of choice. Start mast cell stabilizers 2 weeks before the onset of symptoms is anticipated. These drugs are not useful for acute conjunctivitis since the onset of action is 5 to 14 days after the start of therapy. Patient adherence is less likely given the slow onset, the multiple dosing regimen, and the sensation of burning and stinging upon instillation. If the patient continues with allergic conjunctivitis for 2 to 3 weeks, a short course (2 weeks) of ophthalmic corticosteroids may slow the immune response. Since these patients frequently use oral antihistamines for systemic symptoms, patients need to be instructed to use artificial tears at least 4 times a day.

GLAUCOMA

EPIDEMIOLOGY AND ETIOLOGY

Affecting approximately 2.5 million people, glaucoma is the primary cause of irreparable blindness worldwide. It is the second most common cause of legal blindness in the United States and the leading cause of blindness among blacks. Fifty percent of persons with glaucoma are unaware they have the disorder because there are no symptoms until damage to the optic nerve becomes severe.

Intraocular pressure (IOP), that is pressure over 21 mm Hg, and insults to the eye (trauma and steroid therapy) are the only known causes for open-angle glaucoma. Associated risk factors include increasing age, black heritage, and a first-degree family history of glaucoma. Commonly, persons aged 80 to 84 years of age are more likely to have primary open-angle glaucoma compared to 0.6% of people aged 60 to 64 years. Blacks develop glaucoma at an earlier age than whites. They are also 14 to 17 times more likely than whites to development blindness as a result. Also, persons with diabetes mellitus, migraines, myopia, and sleep apnea are at higher risk for glaucoma. Systemic drugs associated with vision difficulties are identified in Table 61-3.

Historically, glaucoma is characterized as an elevated IOP. A more accurate description is that of optic neuropathy, where the nerve cells in front of the optic nerve die. Damage to the optic nerve results in progressive loss of retinal axons. Many patients with glaucoma have a normal IOP and do not develop damage to the optic nerve or the characteristic pressure increases. Two thirds of patients with elevated IOP do not lose visual fields or develop cupping of the optic nerve. They do not have glaucoma but rather are considered "glaucoma suspects." The opposite is true for about 15% of patients who have characteristic glaucomatous nerve damage. These patients have "normal pressure" glaucoma.

There are two classifications of glaucoma based on the location of compromised aqueous humor circulation and reabsorption, open-angle and closed-angle glaucoma. *Open-angle glaucoma* is usually found during an adult eye exam

TABLE 61-3 Systemic Drugs Producing Ocular Adverse Effects

Drug Category	Drug	Effect(s) on Eye
Adrenergics	Nasal decongestants, reserpine	Reduced visual acuity, mydriasis, miosis, ocular palsies
Analgesics	ibuprofen	Reduced visual acuity (rare), miosis
	Opioids (including pentazocine)	Miosis. With opioid withdrawal, irregular pupils, diplopia, paresis of accommodation, tearing
Antiarrhythmics	amiodarone, quinidine	Cataracts, keratopathy, optic neuritis, reduced visual acuity
Anticholinergics	atropine, dicyclomine, glycopyrrolate, propantheline, scopolamine, trihexyphenidyl	Cycloplegia, decreased accommodation, mydriasis, photophobia
Anticoagulants	heparin, warfarin	Retinal hemorrhage
Anticonvulsants	carbamazepine, phenytoin, trimethadione	Blurred vision, diplopia, cataracts, nystagmus, visual glare
Anesthetics	propofol	Inability to open eyes
Antidepressants	Tricyclic antidepressants	Cycloplegia, mydriasis (most common)
	fluoxetine	Eye tics (paroxysmal contractions of lateral eye muscles)
Antidiabetic drugs	chlorpropamide	Mydriasis, optic neuritis, diplopia, conjunctivitis
Antihistamines	chlorpheniramine	Blurred vision, decreased lacrimal secretions, mydriasis
Antihypertensives	clonidine	Dry, itchy eyes, miosis
	diazoxide	Lacrimation
	guanethidine	Blurred vision, miosis, conjunctivitis, ptosis
	reserpine	Conjunctivitis, miosis
Antiinflammatory drugs	Gold salts	Corneal deposits, conjunctivitis, conjunctival deposits, nystagmus
	indomethacin	Reduced visual acuity, oculogyric crisis, color vision disturbances, change in tear quality
	phenylbutazone	Conjunctivitis, reduced visual acuity, retinal hemorrhage, optic neuritis, corneal erosions
	Salicylates	Retinal hemorrhages, mydriasis, conjunctivitis, optic neuritis, nystagmus
	chloroquine	Ptosis, pigment changes, optic atrophy
Antilipemic drugs	lovastatin	Cataracts

Continued

SENSORY

TABLE 61-3 Systemic Drugs Producing Ocular Adverse Effects—Cont'd

Drug Category	Drug	Effect(s) on Eye
Antimicrobial drugs	amantadine	Corneal lesions
	chloramphenicol	Optic neuritis, changes in visual acuity
	chloroquine	Corneal deposits, macular degeneration
	ethambutol	Retrobulbar neuritis
	gentamicin	Pseudotumor cerebri (rare)
	isoniazid	Optic neuritis
	nalidixic acid	Brightly colored appearance of objects
	Sulfonamides	Conjunctivitis, myopia, optic neuritis, nystagmus, photosensitivity
	streptomycin	Optic neuritis
	quinine	Diplopia
	piperazine	Reduced visual acuity
	ethionamide	Optic neuritis
	Tetracyclines	Myopia (rare, transient), papilledema
Antineoplastic drugs	busulfan	Cataracts
	carmustine	Arterial narrowing, intraretinal hemorrhages, nerve fiber layer infarcts
	cytarabine	Blurred vision, keratoconjunctivitis, ocular burning, photophobia
	doxorubicin	Conjunctivitis, excessive tearing
	fluorouracil	Lacrimation, ocular irritation
	tamoxifen	Corneal opacities, reduced visual acuity, retinopathy
	Vinca alkaloids	Extraocular muscle paresis, ptosis
Antiparkinsonian drugs	levodopa	Mydriasis
Barbiturates	All barbiturates	Ptosis, mydriasis, nystagmus, diplopia, conjunctivitis
Biologic response modifiers	interleukin-2	Diplopia, palinopsia, scotomas
Benzodiazepines	diazepam	Reduced visual acuity, nystagmus, diplopia
Calcium channel blockers	All calcium channel blockers	Blurred vision, transient blindness
Cardiac glycosides	digoxin	Altered color vision, acuity
Cholinergics	neostigmine	Ptosis, nystagmus
CNS depressants	Cannabis	Vision changes, diplopia
CNS stimulants	Amphetamines	Vision changes, mydriasis, oculogyric crises
Diuretics	CAIs, Thiazides	Myopia
Hormones	ACTH	Papilledema
	clomiphene	Blurred vision, mydriasis, visual field changes, visual sensations
	Oral contraceptives	Optic neuritis, pseudotumor cerebri, retrobulbar neuritis
Phenothiazines	chlorpromazine	Lens deposits, retinal pigment deposits
	prochlorperazine	Vision changes, oculogyric crises
	thioridazine	Pigmentary retinopathy
Sedative Hypnotics	chloral hydrate	Diplopia, conjunctivitis
	ethchlorvynol	Optic neuritis, nystagmus
	haloperidol	Vision changes, mydriasis, oculogyric crises
	trilafon	Oculogyric crisis, optic neuritis
	thioridazine, mellaril	Vision changes, mydriasis
Uricosurics	allopurinol	Cataracts; macular lesions (rare)
Others	Vitamin A	Nystagmus, diplopia, ocular palsies, papilledema, exophthalmia
	Vitamin D	Calcium deposits
	nicotinic acid	Optic neuritis
	chlorambucil	Papilledema
	Antihistamines	Miosis, vision changes, photophobia, reduced lacrimation

ACTH, Adrenocorticotropic hormone; *CAIs,* carbonic anhydrase inhibitors; *CNS,* central nervous system.

performed for other reasons and is the most common type; the drainage angle for aqueous humor remains patent. In contrast, 5% to 15% of all glaucoma is of the closed-angle type. Because of its higher prevalence in Asians, closed-angle glaucoma makes up about half of the cases of glaucoma worldwide. In closed-angle glaucoma, the iris is pushed against the lens, closing off the drainage angle.

The term "primary" refers to glaucoma occurring with evidence of preexisting ocular or systemic disease directly affecting IOP pressure on the optic nerve. When other conditions or diseases cause elevated IOP, it is known as "secondary" glaucoma. Diabetes mellitus, hypertension, hypothyroidism, sleep apnea, myopia, previous eye surgery, and physical injury

to the eye can contribute to the development of IOP. In patients with acute closed-angle glaucoma, there is a sudden, dramatic rise in IOP with the patient displaying significant symptoms. Acute-angle glaucoma is a medical emergency requiring care and treatment within hours to avoid loss of visual fields.

PATHOPHYSIOLOGY

Glaucoma results from interference with the drainage of aqueous humor from the anterior chamber of the eye. Aqueous humor, secreted by ciliary epithelium and transported to the posterior chamber, passes through the pupil to the anterior

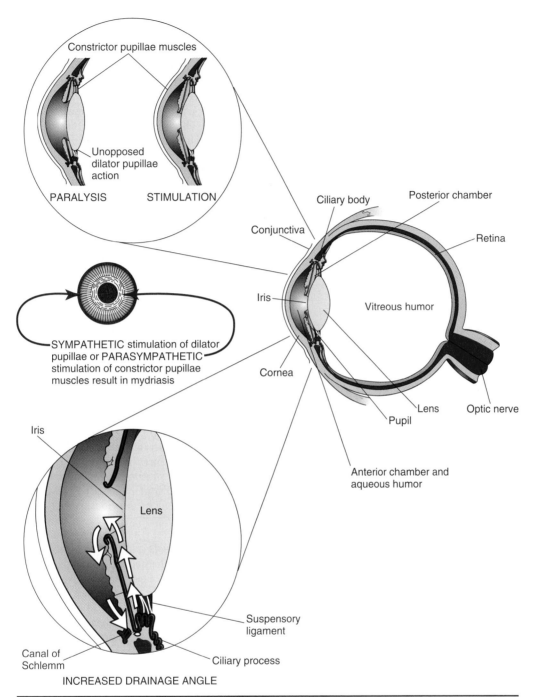

FIGURE 61-1 Ophthalmic Drug Action. Cholinergic miotics cause miosis by contracting the iridic and ciliary sphincters, leading to a deeper anterior chamber, a wider angle, and increased outflow of aqueous humor. Anticholinesterase miotics increase the amount of acetylcholine (ACh) available near ciliary muscles and the iridic sphincters, causing them to contract and the pupil to dilate. Adrenergics stimulate β_2 receptors to increase the outflow of aqueous humor. Anticholinergic drugs paralyze ciliary muscles and relax the iris, causing pupillary dilation and cycloplegia.

chamber (Fig. 61-1). Eighty percent of the total outflow of aqueous humor passes through the trabecular meshwork at the angle of the anterior chamber, enters the canal of Schlemm, and then appears in the ocular venous circulation. The remaining 20% flows through the uveoscleral pathway to the ciliary body and into the suprachoroidal space. From here it drains into venous circulation in the ciliary body, the choroid, and the sclera. IOP is the balance between the rate

of humor produced by the ciliary body, the resistance to outflow, and the level of episcleral venous pressure.

Visual impairment, either temporary or permanent, results from the degenerative changes in the retina and the optic nerve caused by increasing IOP. The elevated IOP causes progressive atrophy of axons with resulting pallor of the optic disk, increased size and depth of the optic cup, and permanently decreased visual fields.

With open-angle glaucoma there is no obstruction at the iridocorneal angle. The increase in IOP usually occurs because of an abnormality of the trabecular meshwork that controls the flow of aqueous humor into the canal of Schlemm. In contrast, **closed-angle glaucoma has a narrow anterior chamber and impaired outflow of aqueous humor due to the iris thickening as a result of papillary dilation. This disorder is a medical emergency.** The thickening of the iris leads to a reduction in or elimination of the access to the angle where aqueous humor reabsorption occurs.

PHARMACOTHERAPEUTIC OPTIONS

Drugs used for the management of glaucoma are aimed at reducing IOP and its fluctuations and essentially work by increasing the outflow of aqueous humor or decreasing its production (Table 61-4). The treatment of choice for open-angle glaucoma is topical ophthalmic drugs.

Ophthalmic Beta Blockers

* betaxolol (Betoptic); ✦ betaxol, Betoptic S
* carteolol (Ocupress); ✦ Ocupress
* levobetaxolol (Betaxan)
* levobunolol (AK-Beta, Betagan); ✦ Betagan
* metipranolol (OptiPranolol)
* timolol (timolol, Timoptic, Timoptic XE); ✦ Betimol

▥ Indications

Ophthalmic beta blockers are typically chosen as initial drug therapy for open-angle glaucoma. They are used for patients who also have cataracts because they cause much less eye irritation than some other ophthalmic drugs.

As the prototype ophthalmic beta blocker, timolol appears to be as effective as pilocarpine or epinephrine in lowering IOP in open-angle glaucoma; in addition, it may be more efficacious for nocturnal control of IOP, and it is often better tolerated. An abrupt rise in IOP may occur when timolol replaces other antiglaucoma drugs. Ocular hypotensive effects and the incidence of adverse effects are similar for both timolol and levobunolol. However, levobunolol is more expensive than timolol, whether it is administered once or twice daily.

The efficacy of betaxolol in decreasing IOP has been demonstrated, but the magnitude of the decrease may not be as great as with timolol. One percent betaxolol has been shown to cause fewer cardiovascular adverse effects than 0.5% timolol. It is also better tolerated than timolol in patients with chronic obstructive pulmonary disease (COPD)

and should be considered when use of topical beta blockers is contraindicated.

Topical metipranolol offers no advantage over timolol or levobunolol in the treatment of glaucoma, but like timolol, metipranolol reportedly produces corneal anesthesia. Metipranolol has been cited as the most cost-effective drug in treating primary open-angle glaucoma; however, the increased frequency of burning and stinging, as well as granulomatous anterior uveitis, may limit its use.

▥ Pharmacodynamics

Although the exact mechanism of action is unknown, all ophthalmic beta blockers antagonize the effect of circulating catecholamines on β_2 receptors in ciliary epithelium, thus causing a fall in the production of aqueous humor and a reduction in IOP.

The ophthalmic beta blockers differ in their affinity for cardiac (β_1) and noncardiac (β_2) receptors. Betaxolol and levobetaxolol are selective for the β_1 receptor. In concentrations of 0.125% to 0.5%, they are shown to effectively reduce IOP by as much as 35% from baseline. Levobunolol, metipranolol, and carteolol are nonselective beta blockers (i.e., they affect both β_1 and β_2 receptors) and are comparable to timolol in reducing IOP.

▥ Pharmacokinetics

The ability of metipranolol to reduce IOP is comparable to that of 0.5% timolol and 0.5% to 1% levobunolol. In combination therapy, metipranolol 0.1% and 2% pilocarpine produces a greater reduction in IOP in patients with open-angle glaucoma than either drug alone. In one study, the combination of pilocarpine and metipranolol stabilized IOP in up to 95% of patients whose glaucoma was inadequately controlled by previously used antiglaucoma drugs (see Table 61-1).

▥ Adverse Effects and Contraindications

Although ophthalmic beta blockers are effective and customarily well tolerated, some adverse effects have been reported. Most of the drug enters the circulation and can therefore cause systemic adverse effects. The adverse effects may include worsening of heart failure, bradycardia, heart block, increased airway resistance, and bronchospasms. The adverse effects of beta blockers are most noticeable in the first 2 weeks of therapy.

Betaxolol may cause more local eye irritation than timolol. Although it is safer than a nonselective beta blocker, β_1 selectivity is not absolute, and bronchospasm has occasionally occurred in patients with COPD (i.e., asthma, emphysema, chronic bronchitis). Bradycardia, syncope, and sinus arrest are rare. Other adverse effects are similar to timolol. Further, significantly fewer patients report stinging and burning with carteolol than with timolol.

Metipranolol has been associated with a greater incidence of stinging or burning on administration than other ophthalmic beta blockers, and it has also been associated with the development of granulomatous anterior uveitis.

Exercise extreme caution when using ophthalmic beta blockers in patients who have COPD because of the risk of airway obstruction, which has occurred even in patients without a history of airway disease. Other common systemic

---

TABLE 61-4 Antiglaucoma Drugs

DRUGS DECREASING PRODUCTION OF AQUEOUS HUMOR
* Beta blockers
* Adrenergics (alpha agonists)
* Carbonic anhydrase inhibitors

DRUGS INCREASING OUTFLOW OF AQUEOUS HUMOR
* Prostaglandin analogues
* Adrenergics
* Cholinergic miotics
* Anticholinesterase miotics

adverse effects include fatigue, anxiety, depression, nausea, vomiting, and a reduced libido.

Using selective beta blockers offers a lower risk of systemic adverse effects, especially pulmonary adverse effects, than nonselective ophthalmic beta blockers. Gentle eyelid closure or light pressure over the inner canthus of the eye following drug application reduces the likelihood of systemic reactions and increases ocular contact time.

▥ Drug Interactions

A fall in blood pressure and pulse can occur as a result of concomitant blockade of β receptors in the heart and vascular system. Therefore, discontinue all other beta-blocking drugs before using an ophthalmic beta blocker such as timolol. Perform frequent checks of blood pressure and pulse during the initial phase of therapy and later during maintenance. Further, a tendency toward tolerance has been noted with long-term ophthalmic beta blocker therapy; therefore, periodic measurements of IOP are warranted.

Systemically absorbed ophthalmic beta blockers also interact with orally administered calcium channel blockers and with the antiarrhythmic drug quinindine. Patients with diabetes mellitus who are taking insulin or oral antidiabetic drugs may note a masking of the symptoms of hypoglycemia (Table 61-5).

Although indomethacin, an NSAID, may potentiate the antihypertensive effect of oral beta blockers, it does not affect the ocular hypotensive action of ophthalmic beta blockers. Close observation is needed when administering a beta blocker concurrently with catecholamine-depleting drugs such as reserpine.

Prostaglandin Analogues
- latanoprost (Xalatan); ♣ Xalantan
- bimatoprost (Lumigan); ♣ Lumigan
- travoprost (Travaton); ♣ Amo-Timop, Gen-Timolol, Timoptic, Travatan,
- unoprostone (Rescula)

▥ Indications

Topical prostaglandin analogues are increasingly chosen as initial therapy in primary open-angle glaucoma because of their once-daily dosing, or as the second-line drug if a topical beta blocker alone does not sufficiently lower IOP.

Although latanoprost is now the most frequently prescribed glaucoma drug in the world, there are some who feel that the newer ophthalmic prostaglandin analogues, travoprost and bimatoprost, may be superior in treating glaucoma in black patients.

▥ Pharmacodynamics

Prostaglandins reduce IOP by increasing the outflow of aqueous humor through the uveoscleral pathway rather than the trabecular meshwork. These hormonelike substances also cause dilation of ocular vessels.

▥ Pharmacokinetics

Prostaglandin analogues are absorbed through the cornea and can be found in intraocular fluids within 4 hours (see Table 61-1). They reduce IOP by 45% to 71% with once-daily dosing.

▥ Adverse Effects and Contraindications

Ophthalmic prostaglandin analogues are effective and well tolerated, with few systemic adverse effects. These drugs do not cause bradycardia or the more severe respiratory adverse effects that ophthalmic beta blockers cause. The localized adverse effects include itching, redness, and burning upon administration. All ophthalmic prostaglandin analogues may permanently change eye color from blue or green to brown,

DRUG INTERACTIONS
TABLE 61-5 Ophthalmic Drugs

Drug	Interactive Drugs	Interaction
BETA BLOCKERS		
timolol	Calcium channel blockers, Carbonic anhydrase inhibitors, Cholinergic miotics, dipivefrin echothiophate, epinephrine	Additive mydriasis
	pilocarpine	Synergistic
	Oral beta blockers, quinidine	Additive bradycardia
	verapamil (oral formulation)	Bradycardia and asystole
	reserpine	Decreases "flight or fight" response
CARBONIC ANHYDRASE INHIBITORS		
acetazolamide	nethenamine, procainamide, quinidine	Decreases excretion of interactive drug
	diflunisol	Increases therapeutic and toxic levels of CAI
ADRENERGICS		
phenylephrine	atropine, guanethidine, MAO inhibitors, methyldopa, reserpine, TCAs	Enhances pressor effects of phenylephrine
CHOLINERGIC MIOTICS		
carbachol	flurbiprofen	Decreases effects of carbachol
ANTICHOLINESTERASE MIOTICS		
demecarium	Carbamates	Cardiovascular and respiratory arrest if used concurrently
echothiophate, isoflurophate	Organophosphate insecticides	
isoflurophate	chymotrypsin	Inhibits isoflurophate activity

CAI, Carbonic anhydrase inhibitor; *MAO,* monoamine oxidase; *TCAs,* tricyclic antidepressants.

with a more pronounced cosmetic problem in patients who treat only one eye. Some patients may experience thicker, longer eyelashes because of the increase in blood flow in the eye.

Carbonic Anhydrase Inhibitors
◆ acetazolamide (Diamox); ◆ Diamox
◆ brinzolamide (Azopt); ◆ Azopt
◆ dichlorphenamide (Daramide)
◆ dorzolamide (Cosopt, Trusopt); ◆ Cosopt, Trusopt
◆ methazolamide (Neptazane)

ⅢⅡ *Indications*
Carbonic anhydrase inhibitors (CAIs) are most often used as adjunctive therapy, rarely as initial therapy. They are used when other drugs have been ineffective as monotherapy in the long-term treatment of open-angle glaucoma and other chronic conditions refractory to beta blockers, cholinergic miotics, and epinephrine. Dorzolamide is more active in lowering IOP in primary open-angle glaucoma and ocular hypertension and may be somewhat better tolerated than other CAIs. Oral acetazolamide may have a more consistent pressure-lowering effect than methazolamide.

The CAIs are used also to decrease IOP for preoperative and postoperative eye surgery patients. In addition, they are used along with miotics, ophthalmic beta blockers, and osmotics for the emergency treatment of acute closed-angle glaucoma. Patients younger than 40 years of age tolerate these drugs better than older adults. Ophthalmic CAIs are useful in combination. For example, dorzolamide and timolol maleate (Cosopt) together decrease aqueous production by two different mechanisms.

The oral forms of CAI, acetazolamide, dichlorphenamide, and methazolamide, are rarely used in the long-term treatment of glaucoma because they carry significantly more adverse effects than the ophthalmic formulations.

ⅢⅡ *Pharmacodynamics*
Ophthalmic CAIs block the enzyme carbonic anhydrase in the ciliary epithelium, reducing the flow of aqueous humor by as much as 40% and usually resulting in miosis and opening of the angle of the anterior chamber. These drugs catalyze the reversible action involved in the hydration of carbon dioxide and carbonic acid. The systemic acidosis that results enhances the ocular hypotensive effects.

ⅢⅡ *Pharmacokinetics*
Most body tissues contain carbonic anhydrase in amounts greater than those needed for physiologic functioning. Almost 99% of carbonic anhydrase must be inhibited to significantly reduce aqueous humor formation.

Dorlazemide is the most potent CAI developed thus far. It is specific for CAI II, the isoenzyme present in ciliary processes. Because of the short duration of action of CAIs, topical application 3 times daily is recommended (Table 61-6).

ⅢⅡ *Adverse Effects and Contraindications*
CAIs are for short-term use only before iridectomy because the lowered IOP may mask the fact that the angle is still partly closed. Permanent closure of the angle can result.

Ten percent of patients using dorzolamide report fatigue, stinging in the eye, anorexia, and a change in taste. The newer

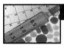

DOSAGE
TABLE **61-6 Ophthalmic Drugs**

Drug	Use(s)	Dosage	Implications
CHOLINERGIC MIOTICS			
carbachol	Primary open-angle glaucoma, chronic glaucoma, secondary glaucoma	*Adult:* 1–2 drops each eye initially every 6–8 hr	Drug concentration and dosage frequency adjusted to maintain IOP in desired range. Available in 0.75%–3% concentrations. Check label carefully.
pilocarpine		*Adult:* 1–2 drops each eye up to 6 times daily −*or*− 0.5 inch ribbon to lower conjunctival sac	Drug concentration and dosage frequency adjusted to maintain IOP in desired range. 1%–6% concentration solutions available in combination with 1% epinephrine bitartrate or 2% concentration with physostigmine. Check labels carefully.
pilocarpine ophthalmic system		*Adult:* One 20 mcg −*or*− 40 mcg ophthalmic system placed into lower conjunctival sac once weekly	Ophthalmic system gently moved to upper conjunctival sac by pressure through closed eyelids. Each system releases 20 or 40 mcg of drug per hr for 1 wk.
ANTICHOLINESTERASE MIOTICS			
echothiophate	Primary open-angle glaucoma, chronic glaucoma, refractory glaucoma, strabismus	*Adult:* 1 drop each eye every 12–48 hr	Available in 0.03%, 0.06%, 0.125%, and 0.25% solutions. Check labels carefully.
BETA BLOCKERS			
betaxolol, carteolol	Chronic open-angle glaucoma, aphakic glaucoma, some secondary glaucoma	*Adult:* 1 drop solution twice daily	Available in variety of concentrations. Check label carefully. May produce fewer local adverse effects than miotics and are better tolerated by patients with active accommodation or cataracts
levobunolol, metipranolol	Chronic open-angle glaucoma, aphakic glaucoma, some secondary glaucoma	*Adult:* 1 drop solution once to twice daily	Available in variety of concentrations. Check label carefully. May produce fewer local adverse effects than miotics and are better tolerated by patients with active accommodation or cataracts

timolol	Chronic open-angle glaucoma, aphakic glaucoma, some secondary glaucoma	*Adult:* 1 drop of 0.25% solution twice daily. Increase to 1 drop of 0.5% solution twice daily if response unsatisfactory. Gel formulation: 0.5% once daily	Available in variety of concentrations. Check label carefully. May produce fewer local adverse effects than miotics and are better tolerated by patients with active accommodation or cataracts
ADRENERGICS			
apraclonidine	Primary open-angle glaucoma, secondary glaucoma, ocular exams, uveitis, eye irritation	*Adult:* 1 drop in affected eye 1 hr before procedure	Use cautiously in patients with history of cardiovascular disease.
dipivefrine	Primary open-angle glaucoma, secondary glaucoma, ocular exams, uveitis, eye irritation	*Adult:* 1 drop of 0.1% solution twice daily. If miotic drug is also ordered, give miotic first.	To switch from another drug, continue other drug first day of dipivefrin therapy. To switch from epinephrine, administer dipivefrin when next epinephrine dose is due.
epinephrine	Primary open-angle glaucoma, secondary glaucoma, ocular exams, uveitis, eye irritation	*Adult: Glaucoma:* 1–2 drops of 0.1% solution to affected eye once-twice daily up to every 3 days *Mydriasis:* 1–2 drops into the eye; may repeat once	When used with miotics, instill miotic first.
phenylephrine	Primary open-angle glaucoma, secondary glaucoma, ocular exams, uveitis, eye irritation	*Adult: Mydriasis:* 1 drop of 2.5% –or– 10% solution on upper limbus. May be repeated in 1 hr. *Uveitis:* 1 drop of 2.5% *or* 10% solution on surface of cornea with atropine. *Glaucoma:* 1 drop of 10% solution repeated as often as necessary. May use in conjunction with miotics. *Intraocular surgery:* 2.5% –or– 10% solution 30–60 min before procedure. *Refraction:* 1 drop of cycloplegic followed in 5 min by 1 drop of 2.5% solution and in 10 min by another drop of cycloplegic drug. *Fundoscopic exam:* 1 drop of 2.5% solution each eye. *Eye irritation:* 1–2 drops of 0.12% solution to affected eye	Precede instillation with local anesthetic to prevent tearing and dilution of solution. Available as 0.8%–0.12% and 10% solutions. Check labels carefully.
ANTICHOLINERGICS			
atropine	Refraction; diagnosis of uveitis; keratitis, secondary glaucoma, intraoperative and postoperative mydriasis, and cycloplegia	*Adult:* 1–2 drops 1–4 times daily *Child:* 1–2 drops of 0.5% solution 1–3 times daily	Adult formulation available as 0.5%–3% solution or 0.5%–1% ointment. Check labels carefully.
cyclopentolate	Refraction; diagnosis of uveitis; keratitis, secondary glaucoma, intraoperative and postoperative mydriasis, and cycloplegia	*Adult: Refraction:* Single dose of 1–3 drops. *Fundoscopic exam:* 1 drop	Available as 0.55%, 1%, and 2% solutions. Check label carefully.
homatropine	Refraction; diagnosis of uveitis; keratitis, secondary glaucoma, intraoperative and postoperative mydriasis, and cycloplegia	*Adult: Refraction:* 1–2 drops 5% solution every 5 min for 2–3 doses –or– 1–2 drops of 2% solution every 10–15 min for 5 doses. *Uveitis:* 1 drop of 2%-5% solution 2–3 times daily	Available as 2%–5% solutions. Check label carefully.
scopolamine	Refraction; diagnosis of uveitis; keratitis, secondary glaucoma, intraoperative and postoperative mydriasis, and cycloplegia	*Adult: Refraction:* 1–2 drops 1 hr before exam	Available as 0.25% solution
tropicamide	Refraction; diagnosis of uveitis; keratitis, secondary glaucoma, intraoperative and postoperative mydriasis, and cycloplegia	*Adult:* 1–2 drops repeated in 5 min; then every 20–30 min PRN to maintain mydriasis.	Available as 0.5%–1% solutions. Check label carefully.
CARBONIC ANHYDRASE INHIBITORS			
acetazolamide	Glaucoma; preoperative and postoperative eye surgery	*Adult:* 62.5–250 mg tabs PO 2–4 times daily –or– 500 mg cap once-twice daily –or– 500 mg IV or IM and repeated PRN in 2–4 hours *Child:* 8–30 mg/kg PO daily in divided doses –or– 5–10 mg/kg IV or IM every 6 hr	The prolonged-release formulation given once daily is better tolerated by some patients.
dichlorphenamide	Glaucoma; preoperative and postoperative eye surgery	*Adult:* 100–200 mg PO every 12 hr initially; then maintenance dose of 25–50 mg 1–3 times daily	Take with food to minimize GI irritation. Long-acting capsules may be opened and sprinkled on soft food, but do not crush, chew, or swallow contents dry.
dorzolamide	Glaucoma; preoperative and postoperative eye surgery	*Adult:* 1 drop 3 times daily	
methazolamide	Glaucoma; preoperative and postoperative eye surgery	*Adult:* 25–50 mg PO 2–3 times daily	
OSMOTICS			
glycerine	Short-term reduction of IOP and vitreous volume, acute closed-angle glaucoma, preoperative and postoperative chronic glaucoma, retinal detachment, cataract extraction, keratoplasty, secondary glaucoma	*Adult:* 1–1.8 grams/kg PO of a 50%–75% solution. May be given more than once daily if necessary	Usually given 1–1.5 hr preoperatively. Ocular penetration is poor.

Continued

SENSORY

DOSAGE
TABLE 61-6 Ophthalmic Drugs—Cont'd

Drug	Use(s)	Dosage	Implications
isosorbide	Short-term reduction of IOP and vitreous volume, acute closed-angle glaucoma, preoperative and postoperative chronic glaucoma, retinal detachment, cataract extraction, keratoplasty, secondary glaucoma	*Adult:* 1.5 grams/kg PO initially; then 4 times daily if needed	Dosage range 1–3 grams/kg. Ocular penetration is good.
mannitol	Short-term reduction of IOP and vitreous volume, acute closed-angle glaucoma, preoperative and postoperative chronic glaucoma, retinal detachment, cataract extraction, keratoplasty, secondary glaucoma	*Adult and Child:* 0.5–2 grams/kg of a 20% solution infused IV over 30–60 min.	Ocular penetration is very poor.
urea	Short-term reduction of IOP and vitreous volume, acute closed-angle glaucoma, preoperative and postoperative chronic glaucoma, retinal detachment, cataract extraction, keratoplasty, secondary glaucoma	*Adult:* 0.5–2 grams/kg of a 30% solution IV at 60 drops/min. Usual dose is 1 gram/kg *Child:* 0.5–1.5 gram/kg of a 30% solution IV over 30 min	Ocular penetration is good.

GI, Gastrointestinal; *IOP*, intraocular pressure; *IM*, intramuscular (route); *IV*, intravenous (route); *PO*, by mouth; *PRN*, as needed.

drug of the class, brinzolamide, is chemically designed to be closer in pH to human tears, thereby causing less stinging than dorzolamide.

The adverse effects of the oral formulations of CAIs include frequent urination, fatigue, weight loss, sexual dysfunction, and failure to thrive in infants. Long-term use can cause serious anemia and kidney problems, thus requiring discontinuation of the drug.

Drug Interactions

Orally administered acetazolamide decreases the elimination of methenamine, procainamide, and quinidine. It also increases the elimination of lithium. The NSAID diflunisol competes with acetazolamide for plasma protein–binding sites, thereby increasing both the therapeutic and the adverse effects of acetazolamide.

Ophthalmic Adrenergics
◆ apraclonidine (Lopidine); ♣ lopidine
◆ brimonidine tartrate (Allergan, Alphagan); ♣ brimonidine, Alphagan P
◆ dipivefrin (Propine); ♣ Propine
◆ phenylephrine (AK-Dilate, AK-Nefrin, Neosynephrine, Phenoptic)

Indications

Adrenergics are used in the management of primary open-angle glaucoma and other chronic glaucomas. In addition, they are used to dilate the pupil for fundoscopic exams, to prevent hemorrhage of small ocular vessels, and as an ophthalmic decongestant during allergic reactions.

Adrenergic agonists may be administered alone, especially when beta blockers are ineffective or not tolerated. Phenylephrine is generally reserved for the short-term pupillary dilation needed for eye exams.

Apraclonidine and brimonidine are alpha$_2$ agonists generally used before glaucoma surgery. These drugs are also used in combination with ophthalmic beta blockers or other standard ophthalmic drugs as primary therapy in the treatment of glaucoma. Brimonidine may be effective for long-term glaucoma therapy, whereas apraclonidine is used for shorter-term therapy. Brimonidine is thought to be safer when used during pregnancy and for patients who have asthma. Further, brimonidine use results in a better quality of life than betaxolol, a beta blocker.

Pharmacodynamics

Data are conflicting regarding the mechanisms involved in adrenergic control of aqueous humor dynamics. Current evidence suggests that aqueous humor production and outflow is primarily mediated by beta mechanisms. Although the sphincter and ciliary muscles are largely under parasympathetic control, adrenergic receptors have also been found in these tissues. Both α and β receptors are found in the sphincter muscle of the iris. β receptors are primarily found in the ciliary muscles. Activation of β_2 receptors in the canal of Schlemm increases outflow, an action that may involve stimulation of prostaglandin synthesis and, hence, uveoscleral drainage. Activation of β receptors in the ciliary bodies produces a slight, transient, clinically unimportant increase in aqueous production, whereas blockade of β receptors decreases production. Concurrent use of adrenergics with CAIs may produce a 65% to 70% decrease in aqueous humor production.

As a prodrug, dipivefrin is converted to an active form, epinephrine, by ocular enzymes in the eye. Dipivefrin penetrates the cornea more readily than epinephrine because of its high lipid-solubility. Dipivefrin's effect on IOP is slightly less than that of epinephrine, but its mydriatic effect is comparable. In contrast to timolol, the outflow effects of adrenergic drugs appear to be preserved when used in combination with betaxolol.

Pharmacokinetics

The prodrug formulations are more efficiently delivered than the parent drug owing to their enhanced absorption; consequently less drug is needed to produce the desired therapeutic response. The onset of action of adrenergic ophthalmic drugs ranges from 5 minutes for epinephrine to 30 minutes for dipivefrin. Peak decrease in IOP occurs in 1 to 5 hours, with a duration of drug action of 12 to 24 hours (see Table 61-1).

Adverse Effects and Contraindications

The most common adverse effects of apraclonidine and brimonidine are dry nose and mouth and altered taste, occurring most often when 1% solutions are used. An allergic response to ophthalmic adrenergic drugs manifests as red, itching eyes, and eye lids. Brimonidine can cause lethargy and a mild drop in blood pressure but is less likely to cause an allergic response.

The ophthalmic and systemic adverse effects of dipivefrin are the same as for epinephrine but are generally less common and less severe. Adrenergics are contraindicated for use before iridectomy in closed-angle glaucoma because they can precipitate an acute rise in IOP.

The most important and common adverse effect of chronic phenylephrine use is rebound congestion of the conjunctiva, in which the vessels become progressively more dilated. Refer patients with rebound effects to an ophthalmologist for further management. Because phenylephrine is contained in a variety of over-the-counter (OTC) drugs; it may be used indiscriminately to quiet irritated eyes. The problem is that the drug causes pupillary dilation and may precipitate closed-angle glaucoma in susceptible patients. This adverse effect is more likely to occur if the cornea has been damaged or is diseased, allowing increased corneal drug penetration.

Use caution when prescribing phenylephrine for patients with a history of cardiovascular disease, diabetes mellitus, and in patients taking interactive drugs. Do not use phenylephrine as an ocular irrigant because of its potential adverse effects.

▥ Drug Interactions

Concurrent use of ophthalmic adrenergics is discouraged in patients taking atropine because of the risk of hypertension and tachycardia (see Table 61-5).

Cholinergic Miotics

◆ carbachol (Carboptic, Isopto Carbachol); ✦ Isopto Carbachol
◆ pilocarpine (Pilocar, Adsorbocarpine, Almocarpine, Isoptocarpine, Ocusert, others); ✦ Miocarpine, Pilocar, Pilopine

▥ Indications

A cholinergic miotic was historically the principal and initial drug used for chronic open-angle glaucoma; however, beta blockers are now preferred for initial therapy. Although miotics are beneficial in many forms of noninflammatory secondary glaucoma, they are not as effective when obstruction of the outflow channels is due to particulate matter (e.g., red blood cells, tumor cells, inflammatory cells).

▥ Pharmacodynamics

Cholinergic miotics produce effects similar to those produced by the parasympathetic nervous system neurohormone, acetylcholine (ACh). ACh action is stopped by hydrolysis of cholinesterase, resulting in contraction of the iridic sphincter and miosis. Contraction of the iritic sphincter and miosis pulls the iris away from the trabecular meshwork reducing the pressure inside the anterior chamber, thereby increasing the outflow of aqueous humor through the canal of Schlemm.

Vasodilation of blood vessels and collection channels peripheral to the canal of Schlemm help to increase the outflow of aqueous humor. Ciliary muscle action leaves the eye in accommodation for near vision. Although hydrolysis occurs at various rates, once it is complete, the pupil returns to the pretreated state. Pilocarpine does not appear to have a clinically significant effect on aqueous humor production.

▥ Pharmacokinetics

Miotic drug effects and the reduction in IOP persist for about 4 hours (see Table 61-1). Maximal reduction of IOP occurs in 1 to 1.5 hours, which correlates with the maximal decrease in outflow resistance. The duration of pilocarpine's miotic action is 4 to 8 hours, with IOP reduction lasting 4 to 14 hours.

Stronger concentrations of pilocarpine may be required in patients with dark irises. Melanin in the iris is a binding site for pilocarpine; thus reduction in IOP may be decreased in heavily pigmented eyes.

▥ Adverse Effects and Contraindications

In patients over age 50 years who do not have cataracts, pilocarpine is better tolerated than other available miotics. Carbachol is sometimes substituted when resistance or tolerance develops to pilocarpine or when a slightly longer acting drug is needed.

Although pilocarpine is ordinarily better tolerated than other miotics, adverse effects commonly associated with cholinergic miotics include irritation, conjunctivitis, and blepharitis. Allergic reactions and systemic effects are uncommon, although retinal detachment, obstruction of the lacrimal apparatus, synechiae (adhesion of the iris to the lens and cornea), iridic cysts, and cataracts have been noted with prolonged use. **Avoid using miotics when iritis is present ▲ because they can aggravate the inflammatory process.** Tolerance and resistance are possible.

Unusual hypersensitivity to or overdose of cholinergic miotics causes headache, salivation, diaphoresis, abdominal discomfort, diarrhea, respiratory distress, bradycardia, arrhythmias, and a drop in the blood pressure. Exercise caution when using cholinergic miotics in patients with a history of asthma, heart failure, peptic ulcer disease, Parkinson's disease, epilepsy, or hyperthyroidism.

▥ Drug Interactions

Carbachol and pilocarpine may be ineffective in reducing IOP when used concurrently with flurbiprofen, a NSAID (see Table 61-5).

Anticholinesterase Miotics

◆ demecarium (Humorsol)
◆ echothiophate (Phospholine Iodide)

▥ Indications

Anticholinesterase miotics (i.e., cholinesterase inhibitors) are used in the treatment of glaucoma in patients who have *aphakia* (an absence of a lens). These are long-acting, potent drugs and have been associated with cataract formation and therefore are reserved for patients refractory to short-acting miotics, beta blockers, dipervine, and CAIs.

If control of IOP is not achieved with optimal use of a cholinergic miotic such as pilocarpine, anticholinesterase drugs are usually prescribed as second-line therapy. However, these drugs have been associated with the formation of iris cysts. These may be prevented by the use of phenylephrine in combination with the anticholinesterase miotic.

Laser trabeculoplasty or filtering surgery (i.e., trephination, thermal sclerostomy, or sclerectomy) may be preferred over the long-acting miotics, especially if the lens is present. In the absence of a lens, or when there is no sign of an imminent retinal detachment, strong miotics can be used to treat chronic glaucoma. In addition to their use in glaucoma, anticholinesterase miotics have been used to diagnose and treat strabismus. By inducing accommodation peripherally, these drugs decrease accommodation and reduce convergence.

SENSORY

Pharmacodynamics

Anticholinesterase miotics are subclassified into two groups, those producing reversible activity and those with irreversible activity. Both groups reduce enzymatic destruction of ACh by inactivating cholinesterase, whereby ACh accumulates. The additional ACh acts on ciliary muscles and iridic sphincters to cause pupillary constriction and ciliary muscle contraction.

The reversible drugs demecarium and physostigmine act on plasma cholinesterase to halt its activity. In contrast, echothiophate and isoflurophate irreversibly impair the destructive function of cholinesterase. Destruction of ACh then depends on the synthesis of new enzyme. The effects of irreversible drugs may last several days or weeks, whereas reversible drug effects last 12 to 36 hours.

Pharmacokinetics

The onset of miosis from anticholinesterase miotics varies from 10 to 30 minutes (see Table 61-1). Pressure reduction can last as little as 12 hours or as much as several weeks, depending on the specific drug.

Adverse Effects and Contraindications

Anticholinesterase miotics produce a variety of adverse effects as a result of their local effects on ocular structures. Accommodative myopia can be problematic in young patients, and pupillary constriction may interfere with vision, especially in patients with cataracts.

Other common local effects include brow ache, headache, eye pain, ciliary and conjunctival congestion, and tearing. Anticholinesterase drugs may cause spasm of the blink reflex (eyelid twitching), which is annoying to the patient. Conjunctivitis and contact dermatitis may develop with localized allergy. Long-term use of potent miotics can cause conjunctival thickening and obstruction of the nasolacrimal canals.

Cataract development is hastened by anticholinesterase miotics, particularly in patients over age 60 years, with the drug echothiophate being a particular problem. In addition, pupillary blockade, local vascular congestion, and occasional forward movement of the lens may cause a sudden or, more often, an insidious angle closure and an increase in IOP (even in eyes with only moderately narrow angles). Patients with advanced cataracts may be particularly at risk.

Drug Interactions

Concurrent use of anticholinesterase miotics with organophosphate insecticides or pesticides can result in cardiovascular and respiratory arrest. Carbamates, succinylcholine, and systemic anticholinesterase inhibitors also increase the risk of cardiovascular and respiratory arrest if used concurrently with the anticholinesterase miotics (see Table 61-5). Chymotrypsin inhibits isoflurophate activity.

Ophthalmic Anticholinergics

◆ atropine (Isopto Atropine); ✦ Isopto Atropine
◆ cyclopentolate (Cyclogyl); ✦ Cyclogyl, Diopentolate
◆ homatropine (Isopto Homatropine); ✦ Isopto Homatropine, Minims Homatropine
◆ scopolamine (Isopto Hyoscine)
◆ tropicamide (Mydriacyl); ✦ Minims Tropicamide, Mydriacyl

Indications

Ophthalmic anticholinergic drugs (also commonly known as mydriatics and cycloplegics) are used to produce mydriasis for refraction and other diagnostic purposes. They also facilitate mydriasis during ocular surgery and decrease postoperative complications. Ophthalmic anticholinergic drugs can be used in the treatment of anterior uveitis and keratitis, as well as for some secondary forms of glaucoma. Atropine and scopolamine were discussed in Chapter 15, along with other muscarinic antagonists; thus, only ocular considerations are discussed here.

Pharmacodynamics

Ophthalmic anticholinergics block the action of parasympathetic nervous system stimulation. There is paralysis of ciliary muscles and relaxation of the muscles of the iris, resulting in pupil dilation and loss of accommodation (cycloplegia). A cycloplegic drug dilates the pupil and paralyzes accommodation, whereas a mydriatic drug dilates the pupil without affecting accommodation.

Pharmacokinetics

The majority of ophthalmic anticholinergics reach maximal mydriasis and cycloplegia 15 to 60 minutes after administration, depending on the specific drug (see Table 61-1). Their duration of action varies. Mydriatic effects can last from 6 hours to 12 days, whereas cycloplegic effects can last from 6 hours to 7 days.

Adverse Effects and Contraindications

Adverse effects, including toxic reactions, can occur with systemic absorption of an ophthalmic anticholinergic through the nasolacrimal ducts and episcleral blood vessels. Ocular responses include blurred vision, photophobia, and precipitation of closed-angle glaucoma. Systemic effects may include dry mouth, constipation, fever, tachycardia, and central nervous system effects.

Ophthalmic Decongestant

◆ naphazoline (AK-Con, Allerest, Naphcon A, Naphcon Forte); ✦ Naphcon A, Naphcon Forte, Vasocon

Ophthalmic decongestants stimulate α receptors in vascular smooth muscle of the eye, resulting in local vasoconstriction. These drugs are typically used for the short-term treatment of superficial corneal vascularity (i.e., congestion, itching, minor irritation, and hyperemia).

The most common adverse effects of ophthalmic decongestants include headache, nervousness, dizziness, weakness, hypertension, and arrhythmias with systemic absorption. Other adverse effects are transient burning, stinging, dryness, blurred vision, mydriasis, and increased or decreased IOP. Rebound congestion and eye redness may occur if the drug is overused.

The onset of the drug's effects occurs in 10 minutes, with a duration of action of 2 to 6 hours. Some systemic absorption does occur. The usual dose is one drop placed in the conjunctival sac every 3 to 4 hours. Do not use naphazoline for more than 3 days without the oversight of a health care provider.

Diagnostic Aids

◆ rose bengal
◆ fluorescein (AK-Fluor, Fluorescite, Fluor-I-Strip, others); ✦ Diofluor, Fluorescite, Fluorets
◆ fluorexon

Several drugs are available for diagnostic purposes. Rose bengal is a dye used for ordinary ocular examinations or when superficial corneal or conjunctival tissue changes are suspected.

Fluorescein sodium is a nontoxic water-soluble dye that is applied to the cornea or conjunctiva of the eye to identify denuded areas of epithelium, or foreign bodies. Fluorescein is also used in fitting hard contact lens, to test the patency of the nasolacrimal system, and to identify defects in corneal pigment. The dye stains denuded areas of epithelium a bright green color, and a green ring will surround a foreign body. Conjunctival loss is stained a yellow color. Staining of the eye disappears in about 30 minutes; staining of the skin can be washed off with mild soap and water.

Fluorexon, a high–molecular weight fluorescein, is used to fit soft contact lenses because it has less than 5% water content and does not stain soft lenses. The lenses are then flushed with saline after exposure to fluorexon (0.35% solution). If the nasolacrimal system is patent, the dye will appear in nasal secretions.

Ocular Anesthetics
◆ fluorescein-proparacaine ophthalmic (Fluoracaine)
◆ proparacaine (Alcaine, Ophthetic); ◆ Diocaine
◆ tetracaine (Pontocaine); ◆ Minims Tetracaine

Surgery and some diagnostic procedures involving the eye would be impossible without anesthetics since the cornea and conjunctiva contain delicate sensory nerves. Ocular anesthetics are also used for foreign body and suture removal, for conjunctival or corneal scraping, and for lacrimal canal manipulation. Local anesthetics are particularly helpful when general anesthesia is considered unnecessary or unduly risky. They should never be prescribed for home use.

Proparacaine and tetracaine anesthetize the corneal surface so that tonometry measurements can be taken. Fluoracaine, a combination of fluorescein and proparacaine, is used to facilitate removal of foreign bodies from the eye. Fluoracaine can also be administered intravenously as an aid in retinal angiography to identify retinal defects.

Proparacaine and tetracaine act by stabilizing neurons so neurons are less permeable to ions, thus interfering with cell activity. Additional drops may be required to anesthetize an inflamed eye because the vasculature carries the ocular anesthetic away. Systemic adverse effects can occur if the ocular anesthetic is absorbed through the nasolacrimal system.

Ocular anesthetics can cause transient eye pain and redness. Prolonged use can cause loss of visual acuity, keratitis, scarring, corneal opacities, and delayed corneal healing. **Use ocular anesthetics with caution, and advise patients not to rub their eyes. Explain that corneal abrasion may occur because the usual signal for pain is absent. Apply a protective eye patch while the eye is anesthetized.**

The only significant drug interaction is with tetracaine. Because tetracaine interferes with the antibacterial action of sulfonamides, administer tetracaine 30 minutes apart from the antibiotics.

Lubricants
◆ sodium chloride (Adsorbonac, Muro 128)
◆ polyvinyl alcohol (Hypotears); ◆ Hypotears
◆ petrolatum and mineral oil (Lacri-Lube); ◆ Lacri-Lube
◆ petrolatum, mineral oil, and lanolin (Duratears Naturale)

The availability of synthetic chemicals appropriate for topical use has permitted the development of various solutions that help alleviate dry eyes. The use of water-soluble polymer solutions and bland, nonmedicated ointments remains the primary therapy. Because these drugs are available OTC, the

health care provider and the pharmacist often carry the primary responsibility to assist and counsel the patient regarding the selection and proper use of almost all of these products. Although the purpose of ocular lubricants is to increase the viscosity of existing tears, it must be noted that high viscosity alone does not necessarily provide relief for all dry eye conditions.

Perhaps the most important property of the cellulose ethers in artificial tear formulations is that they stabilize the tear film and prevent tear evaporation. Beneficial effects generally occur without irritation or toxicity to ocular tissues. Clinical results and patient acceptance remain the final criteria for determining efficacy of treatment of dry eyes. **It must be emphasized that no single formulation has yet been identified that universally improves dry eyes while maintaining patient comfort and acceptance.**

Ocular Irrigants

Irrigating solutions (e.g., physiologic saline) for the eye are used to clear away unwanted materials or debris from the ocular surface while maintaining moisture. Ocular irrigants are used on a short-term basis only. They are not to be used for open wounds in or near the eyes. All ophthalmic irrigating solutions are available without a prescription and can be used by patients and health care providers alike.

One of the most useful applications of ocular irrigants is in ocular lavage following chemical injuries to the eyes. Penetrating chemicals, such as alkalis, must be washed out immediately. Although the ideal irrigating solution for this purpose is physiologic saline, water may be the only available, practical solution, and it can be used when no commercial ocular irrigant is available. In emergency situations involving alkali or acid burns, prompt professional evaluation and treatment by an ophthalmologist is required.

Advise patients not to use ocular irrigants with a contact lens in place because the solutions tend to cause contact lens irritation by reducing the mucin component of the tear film or, in the case of rigid gas-permeable lenses, by reducing the hydrophilicity of the lens surface. Further, absorption of the preservatives contained in the irrigant by a soft contact lens can have an adverse effect on the corneal epithelium.

CLINICAL REASONING

Treatment Objectives

The primary goal in the treatment of ocular disorders depends on the specific disorder. For example, the goal in treating glaucoma is to facilitate the outflow of aqueous humor, thus preventing damage to the ganglion cells and the optic nerve fibers and loss of visual field. The primary treatment goals in the management of infection and inflammation are to reduce symptoms and to prevent recurrence of the disorder while minimizing adverse effects. Other treatment goals include relief from ocular allergies and dry eyes, improved diagnostic capabilities, and pain that is avoided or relieved, when appropriate.

Treatment Options

▓ Patient Variables
Always do a visual acuity exam when examining and treating a patient with an eye disorder. Give special

consideration to treatment of open-angle glaucoma in patients with cataracts. An ophthalmic beta blocker or the adrenergic dipivefrin is usually preferred because miotics may further impair vision. In addition, the long-acting miotics may exacerbate cataracts and increase the risk of complications during or after cataract surgery. Furthermore, the prolonged use of miotics may lead to permanent miosis and thus interfere with the evaluation of the optic disc and the macula.

Laser iridotomy or conventional iridotomy is the definitive treatment for primary closed-angle glaucoma (see Case Study). The IOP is usually lowered with drugs before these procedures. A combination of two or more drugs, including osmotics, CAIs, ocular beta blockers, and adrenergics, is often used preoperatively. After surgery, any residual glaucoma is managed in a stepwise fashion with drug therapy, laser trabeculoplasty, and filtering surgery, as indicated.

LIFE-SPAN CONSIDERATIONS

Pregnant and Nursing Women. Just as with nonpregnant individuals, pregnant women may have visual disorders that necessitate pharmacotherapy. The normal changes of pregnancy may alter visual acuity in some cases. Consider systemic absorption of ocular drugs when assessing the patient's signs and symptoms. Question the woman about visual blurring or changes, or scotomata. The results of the fundoscopic exam should be recorded on the patient's record.

The elevated blood sugar levels that accompany gestational diabetes may cause alterations in vision. Check the woman's blood sugar at the appropriate time during the three gestational periods. A hypertensive crisis can also alter vision; therefore monitor the woman's blood pressure regularly and maintain a record.

Children and Adolescents. Few studies of ophthalmic drug use in children have been reported. Further, the conditions for which adults need therapy (e.g., glaucoma) rarely occur in children. Congenital glaucoma is present at birth, even though 50% of affected infants have symptoms that may not be readily apparent. Symptoms usually develop during the first year of life. In about 40% of cases, the IOP is elevated in the fetus, and the infant is born with ocular enlargement. Both eyes are affected in 75% of the infants, but the severity of the disorder varies.

Bacterial conjunctivitis is more common in children than in adults. The higher prevalence of bacterial conjunctivitis seen in children may reflect the greater likelihood that these children with copious discharge will be seen for care by a health care provider.

For children, patients with poor adherence, or those in whom it is difficult to administer eye drops, ointment formulations are preferred. Ointments stay on the lids and can have a therapeutic effect even if it is not clear if any of the ointment was applied directly to the conjunctiva. Drops are

---

CASE STUDY   Ophthalmic Drugs

ASSESSMENT

History of Present Illness	LH is a 65 year-old black man who returns to the glaucoma clinic today at the request of his health care provider. For weeks, he has been complaining of eye pain; reduced visual acuity, particularly peripheral vision; and persistent headaches, but he denies inflammation, itching, or discharge. Vision changes started about 6 weeks ago and have become progressively worse. LH reports taking an over-the-counter nonsteroidal antiinflammatory drug for daily arthritis pain and uses dipivefrin eye drops.
Past Health History	LH history is unremarkable for cardiovascular, respiratory, or renal disease. A cataract was found on his last eye exam about 6 months ago, when he had his last eyeglass prescription filled. No known drug allergies.
Life-Span Considerations	Although a widower, LH is active in his church, driving the van for church activities. LH states he is "one of the luckies" who does not have a problem with systemic hypertension but participates in his community to increase awareness in his culture. "My vision just can't go now. I have too much to do." LH receives a small retirement check and is covered by both Medicare and FHP insurance. He wants his care to be cost-effective and yet therapeutic without "draining the insurance" or himself.
Physical Exam Findings	Physical exam reveals clear white sclera, visible opacity to left cornea, pink bulbar conjunctiva; no inflammation or discharge noted. Lacrimal glands patent. Visual acuity 20/80 (large Snellen). Fundoscopic exam unremarkable at this time—no AV nicking, papilledema, exudates, or macula changes.
Diagnostic Testing	Left eye Schiøtz tonometry: 21 mm Hg (normal: 15 ± 2.5). Right eye: 19 mm Hg

DIAGNOSIS: Glaucoma

MANAGEMENT

Treatment Objectives	1. Facilitate outflow of aqueous humor, thus preventing damage to optic nerve and loss of visual acuity and visual field 2. Reduce eye discomfort and headache

Treatment Options

Pharmacotherapy
• timolol maleate 0.5% gel. Apply one-quarter inch to lower conjunctival sac of left eye HS.

Patient Education
1. Correct administration technique. Provide large-print written instructions and illustrations.
2. Provide positive reinforcement for adherence to therapy.
3. Advise patient to remove contact lens at bedtime before using the drug.
4. Stress importance of regular follow-up with ophthalmologist.
5. Teach what adverse effects indicate a worsening of the condition as well as the signs to watch for that signal improvement.
6. Do not stop ophthalmic drug without first contacting the health care provider.

Evaluation
LH has no further complaints of eye discomfort or headache. The outflow of aqueous humor has improved, thus preventing damage to optic nerve and loss of visual acuity and visual field.

CLINICAL REASONING ANALYSIS

Q1. Why was timolol chosen for LH's glaucoma when there are other drug classes that could be used?
A. Cholinergic miotics, anticholinesterase miotics, anticholinergics, adrenergics, CAIs, and osmotics are all appropriate for use with primary open-angle glaucoma. Beta blockers are efficacious, most commonly used, and usually considered standard of care. Timolol is as effective as pilocarpine, for example, in lowering IOP in open-angle glaucoma; in addition, it may also be more efficacious for nocturnal control of IOP, and it is often better tolerated.

Q2. According to my PDA drug database, timolol comes in drops and gels. Why did you choose to use the gel rather than the drops?
A. Drops are more likely to cause burning and stinging than gel formulations. The once-daily gel helps promote adherence because he can use it at bedtime when it is least likely to interfere with his activities of daily living. The problems with ointments are that a film or haze tends to form over the eye and interfering with vision, the majority are not sterile formulations, and they are associated with a higher incidence of contact dermatitis than solutions.

Q3. So, you chose the gel because it lasts longer than the drops would, right?
A. Yes. The effects of timolol persist for at least 24 hours, hence the once-daily dosing. And again, a once-daily regimen is more likely to promote adherence to therapy, an important aspect of treatment if he is to reduce future risk for complications of glaucoma.

---

preferred for most adults who need clear vision immediately after the drug is administered.

Older Adults. The incidence of cataracts, dry eye, retinal detachment, glaucoma, entropion (i.e., the turning in of the edges of the eyelid [usually the lower eyelid] so that the lashes rub against the eye surface), and ectropion (the turning out of the eyelid [usually the lower eyelid] so that the inner surface is exposed) increases with age. *Ptosis* (drooping eyelid) may also occur with aging but also results from edema, disorders of the third cranial nerve, and neuromuscular disorders. Older adults are at risk for ocular disorders, especially glaucoma and cataracts. They are also more likely to have cardiovascular disorders that can be aggravated by systemic absorption of ocular drugs. The principles of drug therapy are the same as those for young adults, however.

Drug Variables

FORMULATIONS. Ocular formulations are sterile, easily administered, and ordinarily do not interfere with vision. The disadvantage is that the solutions are in contact with the eye for a short time. Ointments, on the other hand, are comfortable upon administration and stay in contact with the eye for longer periods. The problems with ointments are that a film or haze tends to form over the eye interfering with vision, the

majority are not sterile formulations, and they are associated with a higher incidence of contact dermatitis than solutions. Gels and Ocuserts, the newer delivery systems, were developed to overcome the problems associated with conventional eye drops and ointments. The advantage to using Ocuserts is their longer duration of action, which in turn increases patient adherence to treatment. Use of Ocuserts also avoids the peak-and-valley responses associated with solutions and ointments.

ANTIBIOTICS. Prudent use of ocular antibiotics, either for prophylaxis or treatment, of course encompasses the needs of the individual patient, but also an awareness of larger issues. The health care provider must consider the impact of his or her actions upon our broader ability to maintain strong defensive and offensive lines against ocular pathogens. The one thing we know with certainty is that bacteria are relentless in their pursuit of self-preservation. Through mutation and natural selection, they eventually become resistant to the agents we create to kill them.

There are many options for empiric therapy. Initial choices of broad-spectrum antibiotics include ciprofloxacin, gentamicin, levofloxacin, ofloxacin, polymixin B–trimethoprim, and tobramycin. The fourth-generation ocular quinolones, moxifloxacin and gatifloxacin, provide gram-negative coverage similar to that of other quinolones but with greater coverage of gram-positive organisms. The aminoglycosides gentamicin and tobramycin have weak activity against *Staphylococcal* species, and some strains of *Pseudomonas* are resistant to aminoglycosides. Polyantimicrobial therapy may be needed to cover all possible organisms initially.

ANTIINFLAMMATORIES. Although antibiotics treat the bacterial infection, they do nothing to suppress coexisting inflammation. If there is no disruption of the cornea, corticosteroids such as prednisolone, fluorometholone, or loteprednol used concurrently with the antibiotics help to resolve the inflammation. Steroid-antibiotic combinations (neomycin–polymixin B–dexamethasone, gentamicin-prednisolone, tobramycin-dexamethasone) may be used when the cornea is intact.

GLAUCOMA TREATMENT. Treatment of glaucoma varies with the type of glaucoma and the presence of comorbid conditions. Most patients are treated first with ocular beta blockers, then with dipivefrin, pilocarpine, and anticholinesterase miotics, and finally with CAIs. However, drug selection for the patient with primary open-angle glaucoma largely depends on how well the patient tolerates adverse effects. If the first topical drug fails to reduce pressure sufficiently and nonadherence has been ruled out as a cause of treatment failure, substitution of another drug is recommended before proceeding to combination therapy. Laser trabeculoplasty is usually reserved for patients whose IOP has not been sufficiently lowered despite maximally tolerated drug therapy.

ADVERSE EFFECTS. All ocular drugs are potentially absorbed into the circulation, so undesirable systemic adverse effects may occur. Most ocular drugs are delivered locally to the eye, and the potential local toxic effects are due to hypersensitivity reactions or to direct toxic effects on the cornea, the conjunctiva, the periocular skin, and the nasal mucosa. Eye drops and contact lens solutions commonly contain preservatives such as benzalkonium chloride, chlorobutanol, chelating agents, and thimerisol for their antimicrobial effectiveness. In particular, benzalkonium chloride may cause a punctate keratopathy or ulcerative keratopathy, noninflammatory disorders of the cornea.

Patient Education

Patients with eye conditions, particularly glaucoma, often have high levels of anxiety because of the risk of blindness. As a result, patients may not understand simple verbal administration instructions during the encounter with the health care provider. Written instructions to fall back on when the initial stress has passed (larger print may be of assistance) are helpful to ensure proper administration and adherence with therapy.

⚠ **Advise the patient to use caution when administering drugs because many otic, ophthalmic, and hemooccult-developer drug containers are similar in appearance. Instilling something other than an ophthalmic drug into the eye can lead to permanent eye damage and blindness.**

Since some eye diseases are silent, much like hypertension, there is little positive reinforcement to continue therapy. Encourage patients to continue use of their prescribed drugs for effective treatment of glaucoma nonetheless. **Nonadherence is the major cause of, and should be suspected in, treatment failure in patients with glaucoma.**

Teach the patient to assess for redness, swelling or other irritation, and systemic effects that were not present before treatment was started. Explain the purpose for the formulation prescribed. Advise the patient to use caution when administering these drugs because many otic and ophthalmic drug containers are similar in appearance. Eye drops that have changed color or become cloudy should be discarded. Further, the use of eyecups is discouraged because of the potential for contamination and risk of spreading disease.

The normal healthy eye holds about 10 mcL of fluid. The average eyedropper delivers 25 to 50 mcl per drop. Thus, administering more than a drop is not useful. When more than one drop is to be administered, it is best to wait 5 minutes between drops. The wait ensures that the original drop is not rinsed away by the second or that the second drop is not diluted by the first.

Systemic absorption of eye drops can cause adverse reactions. Nasolacrimal occlusion is effective in decreasing drug loss through the nasolacrimal system into the posterior nasopharynx. The occlusion is accomplished by placing a finger over the inner canthus for a period of 3 to 5 minutes. This permits maximal drug effects in combination with using lower concentrations and less frequent administrations, and reduces the risk for systemic absorption.

Advise patients taking cholinergic miotics or anticholinesterase miotics that they may have difficulty adjusting to changes in lighting. This problem can be particularly serious for older adult patients because their adaptive abilities and visual acuity are often reduced, nighttime being especially dangerous. Instruct the patient to use the drug at bedtime to minimize interference caused by blurring. Because blurring and difficulty in focusing may occur, also instruct the patients to avoid hazardous activities (e.g., driving, operating machinery).

More than 200 contact lens–care products are available without prescription. Selection depends on the products' compatibility with each other as well as compatibility with the specific lens (i.e., contact lenses, extended-wear contact lenses, or rigid gas-permeable lenses). As a general rule, advise patients not to use any ocular product or drug when contact lenses are in place. However, there are products specifically formulated for use with contact lenses.

The potential for bacterial contamination of contact lens solution is great because of the daily use of the solution. Depending on the specific lens care procedure, a single container of solution may last for a month or more. Therefore the solution must contain a bacteriocidal agent that is both effective over the long term and nonirritating with daily use. Commonly used antibacterial agents include benzalkonium chloride, thimerosal, and sorbic acid, all of which cause irritation, depending on the concentration and patient sensitivity.

Many adverse effects have been reported when a patient who wears contact lens ingests or topically applies certain drugs. The effects of certain ocular drugs may be enhanced when soft lenses are in place. Soft contact lenses absorb the drug and release it over time, thus creating a sustained-release dosage form, and decreased peak drug effects (Table 61-7). Further, contact time of the drug with the eye is increased regardless of the type of contact lens. Finally, increased drug absorption can occur secondary to compromise of corneal epithelium, which can arise during contact lens wear. Variables that alter the integrity of contact lenses include the preservatives contained in the agent, its vehicle, and the tonicity and the pH of the solution. For example, 10% sodium

EVIDENCE-BASED PHARMACOTHERAPEUTICS

Patient Preferences for Eye Drop Characteristics

■ Background
The use of eye drops to lower intraocular pressure (IOP) has been the bastion of treatment for glaucoma. The practice is profitable for the drug companies but a major expense for patients and insurance companies. The last decade has seen the development of new, but relatively costly drugs for lowering IOP.

There are numerous reports in the literature about inadequate adherence with glaucoma drug therapy. Adverse effects, comfort, and convenience may influence adherence with a particular eye drop. Therefore, an eye drop's characteristics (i.e., dosing frequency, blurry vision, stinging, tearing, bad taste, drowsiness, and sexual inhibition) may in part determine adherence with a treatment regimen and outcomes of therapy. The most common undesirable adverse effects of glaucoma drug use are fatigue, blurry vision, and tearing. Understanding which characteristics are important to the patient increases adherence and improves the outcomes of therapy.

■ Research Article
Jampel, H., Schwartz, G., Robin, A., et al. (2003). Patient preferences for eye drop characteristics: A willingness-to-pay analysis. Archives in *Ophthalmology, 121*(4), 540–546.

Purpose
The purpose of this study was to determine which characteristic(s) of eye drops are most important to patients. Primary outcome: willingness to pay extra (in dollars) for an eye drop with generally positive characteristics.

Design
Over a period of 16 months, this qualitative, correlational study was done using a convenience sample of subjects ($N = 230$) from four glaucoma subspecialty practices and two private practices on the East Coast of the United States. The demographic information collected on subjects included economic status, educational level, attitudes toward systemic drugs in general and **eye** drops in particular, and toward their adverse effects. Subject demographics were then correlated with their willingness-to-pay (WTP) using two-part models.

Methods
The same experienced individual interviewed subjects (mean age 66 years; 46% men; 33% black) face-to-face during a 30-minute session. Subjects were asked if they had comorbid diseases (i.e., hypertension, diabetes, cardiac or pulmonary disease, or arthritis); if there was a family history of glaucoma; their level of formal education; employment status; drugs used for general health; the number of eye drops used; how long they had been taking the drug(s); if the cost of the drops was prohibitive; how often the subject forgot to take the drops or systemic drugs; and how much they worried about adverse effects of their systemic or ophthalmic drugs. A visual analogue scale was used to assess the perception of their vision where 0 equaled blindness and 100 implied ideal vision.

Following this first-part interview, subjects were read a vignette and then asked how much they would be willing to pay for each eye drop that did not produce a particular symptom (e.g., blurry vision for 2 hours). The same question was asked a second time (with the assumption that the patient had a prescription drug plan that had a $10 copayment per bottle of eye drops) during which patients were asked to identify how much, above and beyond their copayment, they were willing to pay to avoid this particular symptom. Information about the validity of the WTP instrument for assessing patient preference was assessed using a rank-ordering method (i.e., 1, most important; 2, second-to-most important reason, etc.). Patients were offered the opportunity to repeat the ranking if a disparity existed between the WTP value and the rank assigned to that attribute by the subject.

Data were analyzed using descriptive statistics. (1) Chi^2 statistics were used to compare frequency of adverse effects between those using eye drops and those who did not use eye drops. (2) Logistic regression was used to determine whether the patient was willing to pay extra for an eye drop that did not possess undesirable characteristics. (3) A log-normal model was then used to analyze patients who stated they were willing to pay extra for the eye drop that did not possess undesirable characteristics and how much more they would pay. (4) Univariate statistics were used for analysis of the two-part model to determine if key demographic variables were associated with a response to questions about eye drop characteristics on the WTP questionnaire. (5) Multivariate statistics were used to determine if various factors were associated with the patient response on the WTP questions (e.g., frequency of forgetting to take eye drugs; frequency of thinking about adverse effects of the eye drug).

Findings
Of the 230 subjects, 169 (77%) were using eye drops to lower IOP (i.e., ophthalmic beta blockers, prostaglandins, topical carbonic anhydrase inhibitors [CAIs], alpha agonists, and miotics). Eighty-five percent of the patients reported never, or almost never, forgetting to take their eye drop. Fatigue, blurry vision, and tearing were the most commonly reported symptoms.

The characteristics deemed most valuable by subjects included eye drops that did not result in blurring, tearing, or stinging; did not cause a bad taste, drowsiness, or fatigue; or did not inhibit sexual performance. A high percentage of subjects (i.e., 85% to 90%) were WTP 40% more for a drug that did not cause blurring. Patients with higher educational levels and income were likely to pay more for desirable attribute.

Conclusions
The only statistically significant relationship was for patients taking ophthalmic prostaglandins or CAIs. Subjects using prostaglandin analogues were less likely to pay more for an eye drop bottle containing two different drugs rather than for two bottles, each containing a different drug. Patients using a CAI were less likely to pay extra for an eye drop used once daily or that did not cause stinging or tearing. There was a tendency for patients to attribute blurry vision and fatigue to the alpha agonists, and blurry vision, stinging, and bad taste to ophthalmic CAIs. Avoiding blurry vision was the only characteristic for which patients were willing to pay extra.

The more highly educated patients (i.e., 27% with college degrees and 51% with graduate degrees) may well place greater value on convenience and the absence of adverse effects, but it is also possible these same patients had a better understanding of the study's purpose.

Patients tend to have conflicting perspectives on eye drop characteristics. An improved understanding of patient preference could lead to better adherence with therapy. Patient preferences for eye drop characteristics can be determined through the use of a WTP instrument.

One limitation to the WTP analysis is that it is entirely hypothetical. Regardless of the subjects' response to the WTP questionnaire, at the conclusion of the interview, the subjects had yet to spend their money for the drug. What subjects say they will do and what they actually do may be quite different.

■ Implications for Practice
Future studies should focus on whether subject adherence can be improved with the use of eye drops having desirable characteristics. The search for eye drops that are convenient to use, and which have minimal adverse effects, is key to effective treatment. It is justified only if new drug development results in better patient adherence with therapy.

SENSORY

TABLE 61-7 Drug Effects on Contact Lens

Effect on Contact Lens or Eye	Drug or Drug Group
Tear volume decreased	Anticholinergics, Antihistamines, Diuretics, TCAs, timolol
Tear volume increased	Cholinergics, reserpine
Color changes in lens	Diagnostic dyes, Phenothiazines, epinephrine (topical), phenylephrine, fluorescein (ophthalmic), rifampin, nicotine, nitrofurantoin, sulfasalazine, phenazopyridine, tetracycline, tetrahydrozoline (topical)
Changes in tonicity of lens	pilocarpine, sulfacetamide
Lid or corneal edema	chlorthalidone, Oral contraceptives, clomiphene, primodone
Ocular inflammation and/or irritation	Gold salts, isotretinoin, NSAIDs
Induction of myopia	acetazolamide, sulfadiazine, sulfamethizole, sulfasoxazole
Miscellaneous	digoxin (increased glare), ribavarin (cloudy lens)

NSAIDs, Nonsteroidal antiinflammatory drugs; *TCAs*, tricyclic antidepressants.

sulfacetamide or 8% pilocarpine may cause the contact lens to dehydrate, leading to a softening and disfigurement of the lens.

Systemic drugs may interact with contact lenses because they are found in eye fluids. For example, the urinary antiseptic phenazopyridine (Pyridium) and the antibiotic drug rifampin stain tears and contact lenses orange. Gold salts found in tears can cause ocular irritation. Refractory properties of the eye, the shape of the cornea, tear production, or the actual lens of the eye may affect tear production.

Counsel the patient regarding which adverse effects suggest worsening of the condition and signs to watch for that signal improvement. Be specific when providing instructions about what to do and who to contact if adverse effects appear, and when to contact the health care provider for follow-up. Instruct patients to avoid sharing ocular drugs with others. Also, advise the patient not to stop a drug without first consulting with the health care provider who ordered the drug.

Evaluation

Although primary health care providers can and do treat many eye ailments, refer the following patients to an ophthalmologist for further evaluation: the patient who (1) has keratitis near the visual axis; (2) has more than one infiltrate with the infiltrate over 3 mm in size; (3) is immunocompromised; or (4) manifests the keratitis after a previous surgery and is coming from a nosocomial environment.

Note any reduction in inflammation, discharge, and discomfort. In some cases, the use of the drug (e.g., antivirals) may continue for 5 to 7 days to prevent recurrence of the infection.

When evaluating the effectiveness of IOP-lowering drugs, measure the IOP at different times during the day, because variations of as much as 10 mm Hg or more may occur over a 24-hour period. In addition, the condition of the optic nerve and visual field status must be determined at least twice yearly, or more frequently when indicated. The close monitoring is necessary to ensure that there is no further progressive damage from insufficient lowering of pressure, intermittent noncompliance, or other causes.

KEY POINTS

- Eye disorders can occur at any age. The disorders can be due to a wide variety of causes, but the majority are categorized as infections, inflammation, glaucoma, or refractive disorders.
- Always do a visual acuity exam when examining or treating a patient with an eye disorder.
- Acute conjunctivitis can be classified as infectious or noninfectious. Infectious bacterial conjunctivitis is more common in children than in adults.
- The experiences of health care providers suggest that the most infectious conjunctivitis in all ages is viral. Usually there is greater tearing rather than discharge with viral conjunctivitis.
- Therapy directed at viral and allergic conjunctivitis reduces symptoms, but does nothing to alter the clinical course. Treatment of bacterial conjunctivitis probably shortens the clinical course and reduces the person-to-person spread, but in most cases, bacterial conjunctivitis is self-limited.
- There are no specific antiviral treatments for viral conjunctivitis. Symptomatic relief can be gained from topical antihistamines and decongestants.
- NSAIDs have a variety of uses including inhibition of intraoperative miosis, postoperative cataract surgery, and prevention or treatment of cystoid macular edema, iritis, iridocyclitis, episcleritis, seasonal allergic conjunctivitis, contact lens-associated conjunctivitis, and vernal conjunctivitis.

- The primary therapy for treating ocular allergies is the avoidance of the allergen. Topical antihistamines and decongestants are usually the choice for treating these short exacerbations of symptoms.
- Local anesthetics are helpful when general anesthesia is considered unnecessary or unduly risky, for use in foreign body and suture removal, for conjunctival or corneal scraping, and for lacrimal canal manipulation. They should never be prescribed for home use.
- The availability of lubricants for topical ophthalmic use has made it possible to alleviate dry eyes. The use of water-soluble polymer solutions and bland, nonmedicated ointments remains the primary therapy.
- Ocular irrigating solutions are used to clear away unwanted materials or debris from the ocular surface while maintaining their moisture, and as extraocular irrigants following chemical injuries to the eyes.
- Mydriatics and cycloplegics (anticholinergic drugs) are used to produce mydriasis for refraction and other diagnostic purposes.
- Glaucoma is an optic neuropathy in which the nerve cells in front of the optic nerve die.
- The two classifications of glaucoma are open-angle and closed-angle glaucoma. Most people with glaucoma have open-angle glaucoma, with the drainage angle remaining open.
- Closed-angle glaucoma is less common in the United States but comprises half of the world's glaucoma cases. This disorder is a medical emergency.

- The visual impairment with glaucoma, whether temporary or permanent, results from the degenerative changes in the retina and the optic nerve caused by increasing IOP.
- Drugs used for the management of open-angle glaucoma are aimed at reducing ocular pressure and its fluctuations and work by increasing aqueous humor outflow or decreasing aqueous humor production.
- Ophthalmic beta blockers are most often chosen as initial drug therapy for open-angle glaucoma. However, ophthalmic beta blockers should be avoided or used with extreme caution in patients with COPD since airway obstruction has been reported with systemic absorption.
- Ophthalmic prostaglandin analogues are used as initial therapy in primary open-angle glaucoma or as the next drug added if a ophthalmic beta blocker alone does not sufficiently lower the IOP. Latanoprost is the most frequently prescribed glaucoma drug in the world.
- Teach the patient and family how to administer the prescribed ophthalmic drug. Written instructions (larger print may be helpful) are helpful to ensure adherence to the treatment regimen.

Bibliography

American Academy of Ophthalmology, Glaucoma Panel. (2000). *Primary open-angle glaucoma. Preferred practice pattern.* San Francisco: American Academy of Ophthalmology.

Bartlett, J., and Jaanus, S. (2001). *Clinical ocular pharmacology* (4th ed.). London: Butterworth Heinemann.

Distelhorst, J., and Hughes, G. (2003). Open-angle glaucoma. *American Family Physician, 67*(9), 1937–1944.

Doughty, M., Bennett, E., Naase, T., et al. (2005). Use of a high molecular weight fluorescein (fluorexon) ophthalmic strip in assessments of tear film break-up time in contact lens wearers and non-contact lens wearers. *Ophthalmic and Physiologic Optic, 25* (2), 119–127.

Fleming, C., Whitlock, E., Beil, T., et al. (2005). Screening for primary open-angle glaucoma in the primary care setting: An update for the U.S. preventive services task force. *Annuals of Family Medicine, 3*(2), 167–170.

Fraunfelder, F.T., and Fraunfelder, F.W. (2001). *Drug-induced ocular side effects,* (5th ed.). London: Butterworth Heinemann.

Hwang, D. (2004). Fluoroquinolone resistance in ophthalmology and the potential role for newer ophthalmic fluoroquinolones. *Survey of Ophthalmology, 49*(Suppl 2), S79–S83.

Jampel, H., Parekh, P., Johnson, E., et al. (2005). Preferences for eye drop characteristics among glaucoma specialists: a willingness-to-pay analysis. *Journal of Glaucoma, 14*(2), 151–156.

Mather, R, Karenchak, L., Romanowski, E., et al. (2002). Fourth generation fluoroquinolones: New weapons in the arsenal of ophthalmic antibiotics. *American Journal of Ophthalmology, 133*(4), 463–466.

McCulley, J., Caudle, D., and Aronowicz, J. (2006). Fourth-generation fluoroquinolone penetration into the aqueous humor in humans. *Ophthalmology, 113*(6), 955–959.

Rakel, R., and Bope, E. (Eds.). (2006). *Conn's current therapy 2006.* Philadelphia: WB Saunders.

Tierney, L., McPhee, S., Papadakis, M., et al. (2007). *Current medical diagnosis and treatment* (46th ed.). New York: McGraw-Hill.

Robert, P., and Adenis, J. (2001). Comparative review of topical ophthalmic antibacterial preparations. *Drugs, 61*(2), 175–185.

Thomas, R., Sekhar, G., and Parikh, R. (2007). Primary angle closure glaucoma: A developing world perspective. *Clinical and Experimental Ophthalmology, 35*(4), 374–378.

Tielsch, J., Sommer, A., and Katz, J. (1991). Racial variations in the prevalence of primary open-angle glaucoma: The Baltimore Eye Survey. *Journal of the American Medical Association, 266*(3), 369–374.

Weinreb, R., and Khaw, P. (2004). Primary open-angle glaucoma. *Lancet, 363*(9422), 1711.

62

Otic Drugs

Treatment of middle and inner ear disease often requires oral or parenteral medications. External ear pathologies, however, depend on topical otic drugs administered locally to prevent or treat disorders. Otic drugs instilled directly into the external meatus of the ear include antibiotics, antiinfective drugs, antiinflammatory drugs, anesthetics, drying drugs, and cerumen solvents. These drugs are used exclusively for their local actions, and direct administration allows distribution to all surface areas of the external canal. Many otic drugs are combinations of two or more drugs and are primarily used to treat external ear infections, inflammation, and pain, and to remove excessive or impacted cerumen.

INFECTION

EPIDEMIOLOGY AND ETIOLOGY

Infection of the external ear *(otitis externa)* is common when the integrity of the external canal is compromised, allowing invasion of pathogenic organisms into the tissue. Patients whose ears are frequently exposed to water as a result of swimming, bathing, or environmental factors are at greatest risk for alterations in the integrity of the skin tissue of the external ear. In addition, patients who traumatize the skin with cotton swabs or other foreign objects inserted into the canal are at risk for development of an external ear infection. Pathogens causing external otitis include *Pseudomonas aeruginosa, Staphylococcus aureus, Escherichia coli, Proteus species,* and anaerobes.

PATHOPHYSIOLOGY

Infection results in inflammation and pain. External canal structures become red, edematous, and painful even to slight touch. The dermis in the inner osseous portion of the canal is in direct contact with the underlying periosteum, thus minimal inflammation or touching with an instrument causes significant pain. A telltale finding is when the patient complains of pain when the tragus is compressed or the auricle is pulled superiorly during an exam. However, in mild cases of otitis externa, these signs may not be present. Extensive swelling leads to a conductive type of hearing loss due to obstruction of the canal. Fever, malaise, anorexia, and fatigue reflect signs of systemic involvement and require systemic therapy rather than topical preparations. Acute otitis media and infections of the inner ear require systemic antibiotic therapy to combat the organism effectively.

There are five basic steps in the treatment of external otitis. These are to thoroughly clean the ear canal, treat inflammation and infection, control the pain, culture severe cases, and avoid promoting factors for external otitis.

PHARMACOTHERAPEUTIC OPTIONS

Antibiotics
- chloramphenicol otic (Chloromycetin Otic); ◆ Sopamycetin
- ciprofloxacin and dexamethasone (Cipro HC Otic)
- ofloxacin (Floxin Otic Solution); ◆ Floxin Otic Solution; Ocuflox
- polymyxin and neomycin combinations (Cortisporin, Coly-Mycin, Pediotic)

Indications
Otic antibiotics and antifungal drugs are used in the treatment of external otitis, a superficial infection of the ear. There are many topical solutions available. There are a number of factors that must be considered when the health care provider selects an ototopical antibiotic. Consideration has to be given to the coverage of the expected pathogens, the possibility of drug resistance, the patient's allergy sensitization, and the possibility of ototoxicity. Otic antimicrobials are sometimes prescribed in the treatment of chronic suppurative otitis media and otorrhea following tympanotomy tube insertion. Systemic antibiotics are used when the infection is extensive or resistant to antimicrobial therapy. Relief of symptoms of external otitis occurs within a week of the initial application of topical agents. Pain associated with the infection is generally severe enough to ensure adherence with the therapeutic regimen. However, untreated infections can progress to necrotizing external otitis, resulting in an increase in both morbidity and mortality.

Pharmacodynamics
Otic antimicrobials work via direct contact with the microorganism on the lining of the external canal. They are not designed for systemic absorption.

Broad-spectrum antibiotics acts on both gram-negative and gram-positive organisms such as *S. aureus, E. coli, Haemophilus influenzae, P. aeruginosa, Aerobacter aerogenes, Klebsiella pneumoniae,* and *Proteus* species. Antibiotics produce primarily bacteriostatic effects by inhibiting protein synthesis. Antifungal drugs are effective for candidiasis, the most common fungal infection.

Pharmacokinetics
Typical pharmacokinetic properties do not apply to topical otic antimicrobials. These drugs are not designed to be absorbed, biotransformed, or eliminated systemically. Absorption of otic antimicrobials occurs through the otic tissues. The otic drug must remain in direct contact with the infected tissue long enough to be effective. If possible, use warm water irrigation to remove all exudate, cerumen, debris, and other secretions before administering the otic antimicrobial (Fig. 62-1). Elimination is via evaporation, normal physiologic ear cleaning, and warm water irrigation.

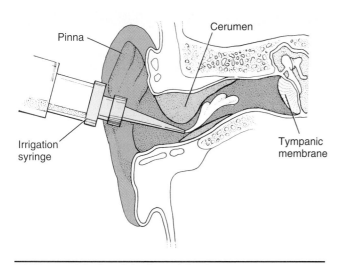

FIGURE 62-1 Irrigation of the External Canal. A stream of warm water is directed above or below the blockage. This allows back pressure to push out cerumen and other debris rather than further impact the external canal.

Pinna
Cerumen
Irrigation syringe
Tympanic membrane

▥ Adverse Effects and Contraindications

Health care providers need to be aware that some patients may be experiencing allergic contact dermatitis to their topical otic drug. These patients may be seen with persistent edema and erythema of the ear canal and auricle despite appropriate treatment. Itching, burning, angioedema (e.g., local wheals accompanied by swelling of subcutaneous tissue), urticaria, vesicular lesions, and maculopapular dermatitis are associated with allergic contact dermatitis. Prolonged use can lead to an overgrowth of nonsusceptible organisms including fungi. Certain otic antimicrobials (e.g., gentamicin and tobramycin) are contraindicated for use in patients with a perforated tympanic membrane. Chloramphenicol otic is ototoxic if it enters the inner ear and round window.

Cautious use of otic antimicrobials is warranted in pregnant or lactating women because these otics have not been studied in this patient group. They are probably safe, because systemic absorption is negligible. Patients with known adverse reactions to kanamycin, paromomycin, streptomycin, or gentamicin should use chloramphenicol with caution.

An allergy history for the patient must include preservatives such as benzethonium chloride, sulfites, and thiomersal. These possible allergies need to be considered because many otic preparations contain these products.

▥ Drug Interactions

Given the topical nature of otic preparations, the likelihood of drug interactions is rare. Topical otic antiinflammatory and otic analgesic drugs are often used concurrently to alleviate ear discomfort.

▥ Dosage Regimen

The usual dosage for topical antimicrobial solutions is four to six drops 3 to 4 times daily (Table 62-1).

▥ Lab Considerations

The effectiveness of ototopical antibiotics is well documented, rarely necessitating that exudate from the ear be cultured before administration. When otic therapy is ineffective and

signs and symptoms of external ear infection continue, cultures and sensitivities may be taken to determine the infecting organism and the best drug for treatment.

Audiology testing with tympanometry may be performed to assess hearing and to determine movement potential of the tympanic membrane. It is most often performed with persistent infection or when the infection is thought to have affected the patient's hearing.

Acidifying Solutions
◆ acetic acid
◆ acetic acid and Burow's solution (Otic Domeboro)
◆ boric acid and isopropyl alcohol (Dri/Ear, Ear-Dry, Swim-Ear)

▥ Indications

Acidifying solutions acidify the ear canal and inhibit bacterial growth. Drying drugs suppress the growth of organisms and help prevent recurrent ear canal infection. Swimmers who have repeated ear infections frequently use drying drugs.

▥ Pharmacodynamics

Acidifying solutions and drying otic drugs contain acetic or boric acid, antiseptics, weak antimicrobials (both antibacterial and antifungal), and isopropyl alcohol as a drying agent. The antimicrobial drugs eliminate and prevent susceptible organisms from accumulating in the external ear canal via weak antimicrobial action and drying of the external ear canal tissue. Otic drops that include a steroid with the acetic acid drops are more effective than the acetic acid drops alone.

▥ Pharmacokinetics

Acidifying solutions and drying drugs are designed to be effective through direct contact with external ear canal tissue. Normal pharmacokinetics do not apply to otic acidifying solutions and drying drugs because these are not designed for absorption, distribution, or biotransformation. Drug elimination is through evaporation, normal physiologic ear cleaning, or water irrigation.

▥ Adverse Effects and Contraindications

Adverse reactions include local irritation and contact dermatitis with burning, stinging, pruritus, tenderness, erythema, rash, urticaria, and edema. The external ear canal is observed closely for signs of local irritation or worsening of the pretreatment symptoms. Antibacterial solutions, acidifying solutions, and drying drugs are not used when the tympanic membrane has been perforated. Allergies to preservatives such as benzethonium chloride, sulfites, and thiomersal must be considered, because many otic preparations contain these products.

▥ Dosage Regimen

Four to six drops of the acidifying solution or drying solution are instilled into the external canal 1 to 4 times daily as needed (see Table 62-1).

INFLAMMATION AND PAIN

EPIDEMIOLOGY AND ETIOLOGY

Structures of the external ear become inflamed for a variety of reasons including allergic reactions, trauma, and infection.

SENSORY

DOSAGE
TABLE 62-1 Otic Drugs

Drug	Use(s)	Dosage	Implications	
ANTIBIOTICS				
chloramphenicol 0.5% otic solution	For superficial external ear canal infections	*Adult and Child:* 2–3 drops 3 times daily	**Do not use for more than 10 days.** Supplement with systemic antibiotics in all but superficial infections.	▲
ANTIBACTERIAL AND DRYING DRUGS				
acetic acid 2% + Burow's solution	For superficial infections of the external ear canal	*Adult and Child:* 4–6 drops every 2–3 hr PRN	Not to be used for extended periods	
boric acid + isopropyl alcohol; acetic acid	Infection prophylaxis for recurrent external otitis	*Adult and Child:* 5 drops 3–4 times daily	Not to be used for extended periods	
acetic acid + hydrocortisone	Infection prophylaxis for recurrent external otitis	*Adult and Child:* 5 drops 3–4 times daily	May replace with saturated cotton wick for first 24 hr	
STEROIDS				
desonide + acetic acid	Inflammation of external ear canal caused by infection or trauma	*Adult and Child:* 2–3 drops 3 times daily	**Treatment period not to exceed 4 days**	▲
dexamethasone sodium phosphate 0.1%	Steroid-responsive inflammation of external canal	*Adult and Child:* 3–4 drops 2–3 times daily	May replace with saturated cotton wick for first 24 hr	
STEROID-ANTIBIOTIC COMBINATIONS				
hydrocortisone + neomycin sulfate + polymixin B; hydrocortisone + polymixin B	Infections of external ear, fenestration cavities, mastoidectomy	*Adults:* 4 drops 3–4 times daily *Child:* 3 drops 3–4 times daily	**Ototoxicity possible with prolonged use.** Do not use longer than 10 days.	▲
hydrocortisone + neomycin sulfate	Infections of external ear, fenestration cavities, mastoidectomy	*Adults:* 4 drops 3–4 times daily *Child:* 3 drops 3–4 times daily	**Ototoxicity possible with prolonged use.** Do not use longer than 10 days.	▲
OTIC ANESTHETICS				
benzocaine	Analgesia in acute otitis media	*Adult and Child:* Fill ear canal	**Use with caution if allergic to local anesthetics.**	▲
benzocaine + antipyrine	Analgesia in acute otitis media; adjunct in cerumen removal	*Adult and Child:* Fill ear canal. May repeat every 1–2 hr PRN. Insert moistened cotton plug.	Treat infection with systemic antibiotics. Discard 6 months after initial use.	
benzocaine + antipyrine + phenylephrine	Analgesia in acute otitis media	*Adult and Child:* Fill ear canal.		
CERUMINOLYTICS				
triethanolamine + polypeptide oleate + condensate 10%	Cerumen removal	*Adult and Child:* Fill the ear canal and let remain for 15–30 min. May repeat 1 time as needed	Irrigate repeatedly with warm water after instilling drug.	
carbamide peroxide 6.5%	Cerumen removal	*Adult and Child:* 5–10 drops. May repeat twice daily for up to 4 days.	May irrigate with warm water	

PRN, As needed.

Patients living in areas of high humidity or who engage in water activities are more likely to have problems with external canal inflammation and infection.

PATHOPHYSIOLOGY

With inflammation, blood flow to the area increases, capillary permeability increases, and fluid flows into the affected tissues, producing edema and erythematous coloring. As a sensory organ, the ear contains many sensory nerve fibers that, when inflamed, produce significant pain. Thus drug therapy is designed to alleviate pain through either the reduction of inflammation or direct anesthetic effects.

PHARMACOTHERAPEUTIC OPTIONS

Steroids and Steroid-Antibiotic and Steroid-Antifungal Combinations
◆ desonide + acetic acid (Tridesilon)
◆ dexamethasone sodium phosphate (Decadron)

◆ dexamethasone phosphate + neomycin sulfate + polymyxin B (Cortisporin Otic, Drotic, Ear-Eze, Otomycin-HPN, Otosporin); ◆ Cortisporin
◆ hydrocortisone + neomycin sulfate; ◆ Coly-Mycin Otic
◆ hydrocortisone + pramoxine + chloroxylenol + propylene glycol diacetate + benzalkonium chloride (Cortic)
◆ hydrocortisone + acetic acid + propylene glycol diacetate + benzethonium chloride + sodium acetate (VoSol HC Otic)
◆ hydrocortisone + polymyxin B

▥ Indications

Inflammation of the external canal caused by infection or trauma leads to severe pain. Corticosteroids are given to reduce inflammation and control pain, either alone or in combination with an otic antibiotic and otic anesthetic. Hydrocortisone and dexamethasone are the most common corticosteroids used as otic drugs. The broad-spectrum antibiotic neomycin sulfate is used in combination with corticosteroids because of its bactericidal effect. Combinations of corticosteroids and antibiotics are used to treat superficial infections causing pain and inflammation. The corticosteroid helps alleviate discomfort, whereas the antibiotic treats the infection. The health care provider needs to be aware that inadequately treated cases of external otitis may be masked with analgesics.

Pharmacodynamics

Steroid and steroid-antibiotic combinations are given to reduce dermal reactions to inflammation, edema, pruritus, and pain. Similar to other topical steroids, the exact mechanism of action is not fully understood. Topical steroids most likely act to decrease formation, release, or activity of inflammatory mediators. They require direct contact with the skin and are given for their local topical effect.

Pharmacokinetics

Normal pharmacokinetics do not apply to steroids and steroid-antibiotic combinations because these are not designed for absorption, distribution, or biotransformation. Some drug may be absorbed unintentionally through the skin depending on the dosage, the integrity of the skin, the length of use, and whether an occlusive dressing was used. The drugs are eliminated via evaporation, normal physiologic ear cleaning, and water irrigation. Little fear of interactions among otic steroids and other drugs exists unless the otic steroid is systemically absorbed.

Adverse Effects and Contraindications

The most common adverse effects of steroid and steroid-antibiotic combinations are overgrowth of organisms, delayed healing, and contact dermatitis. Limiting the length of treatment to no more than 4 days helps prevent problems. Steroid and steroid-antibiotic combinations are contraindicated for use in patients with a perforated tympanic membrane, herpes simplex, vaccinia, and varicella. Cautious use of steroids and steroid-antibiotic combinations is warranted in pregnant or lactating women, because neither type has been studied in this group.

Once again, allergies to preservatives such as benzethonium chloride, sulfites, and thiomersal must be considered because many otic preparations contain these products.

Dosage Regimen

Two to three drops of solution are instilled into the external canal of the affected ear (see Table 62-1).

Lab Considerations

Rarely is the exudate from the ear cultured before administration of otic corticosteroids. When therapy is ineffective and signs and symptoms of external ear infection continue, cultures and sensitivities are taken to determine the infecting organism and the best drug for treatment.

Otic Anesthetics

- benzocaine (Americaine Otic, Otocain)
- benzocaine-antipyrine (Auralgan Otic, Otocalm Ear); ♣ Auralgan
- benzocaine + antipyrine + phenylephrine (Tympagesic)

Indications

Otic anesthetics contain benzocaine and are used for the relief of pain and pruritus associated with the acute congestion of serous otitis and external otitis.

Pharmacodynamics

Otic anesthetics temporarily stabilize the neuronal membranes to decrease membrane permeability to sodium ions. Depolarization of the neuronal membrane is inhibited, thereby blocking the initiation and conduction of nerve impulses and sensitivity to pain. Otic anesthetics have no effect on microorganisms or inflammation.

Pharmacokinetics

Much like the other otic drugs, to be effective, topical anesthetics must come in direct contact with ear tissue. Normal pharmacokinetics do not apply to topical anesthetics because these are not designed for absorption, distribution, or biotransformation.

Adverse Effects and Contraindications

Otic anesthetics tend not to blanch the tympanic membrane or mask the otoscopic landmarks; however, benzocaine may mask the symptoms of fulminating infection of the middle ear if it is used indiscriminately. Although rare, methemoglobinemia may result from the use of otic benzocaine. Methemoglobinemia causes respiratory distress and cyanosis, necessitating treatment with intravenous methylene blue.

Otic anesthetics are not to be used with patients who have ⚠ a perforated tympanic membrane. No teratogenic studies have been conducted with pregnant women; hence, safety in pregnancy has not been established. Allergies to preservatives such as benzethonium chloride, sulfites, and thiomersal must be considered because many otic drugs contain these products.

Drug Interactions

Benzocaine antagonizes the antibacterial activity of sulfonamides; do not administer these together. When both benzocaine and sulfonamides must be used concurrently, instill the benzocaine in the ear first to achieve anesthesia and thus avoid the potential for drug interaction. Then remove the pooled benzocaine before administering the sulfonamide.

Dosage Regimen

Four to five drops are instilled into the external canal. The dosage may be repeated every 1 to 2 hours while severe pain persists (see Table 62-1).

CERUMEN IMPACTION

EPIDEMIOLOGY AND ETIOLOGY

Cerumen, or earwax, is a normal sebaceous gland secretion with the function of protecting and lubricating the canal. The primary action of cerumen is to gather bacteria and debris for removal. Normally, when the external ear canal gets wet and drains, cerumen is eliminated. Various factors lead to decreased elimination of cerumen compared with production. When elimination is decreased, the cerumen may become impacted in the canal. The incidence of cerumen impaction is greater in the geriatric population.

PATHOPHYSIOLOGY

Patients with cerumen impaction may have no symptoms or may complain of a sensation of fullness in the ear, with or without associated conductive hearing loss. Complaints of pain, itching, or bleeding from the ear may also be noted. Treatment requires removal of the impacted cerumen via warm water irrigation. If the impaction is resistant to irrigation, commercially prepared ceruminolytics can be used to soften the cerumen for ease of removal.

PHARMACOTHERAPEUTIC OPTIONS

Ceruminolytics

* carbamide peroxide (Auro Ear Drops, Debrox ear drops, E-R-O Ear Drops, Murine Ear Drops); ♣ Murine Earwax Removal System, Murine Earwax Drops
* triethanolamine + polypeptide oleate + condensate (Cerumenex ear drops)

▓ *Indications*

Ceruminolytic drugs help soften cerumen for removal. They are used for removal of cerumen without painful instrumentation using a metal curette. Cerumen removal is necessary for otoscopic examination, audiometry, and tympanometry, and when the patient experiences discomfort or hearing loss from excessive or dry cerumen. Additionally, cerumen solvents provide antiseptic protection.

▓ *Pharmacodynamics*

Ceruminolytics contain glycerin to soften cerumen and carbamide peroxide to loosen debris by effervescence of oxygen. They act to emulsify and disperse excess or impacted cerumen. Carbamide peroxide slowly releases hydrogen peroxide and oxygen when exposed to moisture. The release of oxygen imparts a weak antibacterial action, and the effervescence resulting from the release of oxygen has the mechanical effect of removing cerumen from inaccessible spaces.

▓ *Pharmacokinetics*

Normal pharmacokinetics do not apply to cerumen solvents, because these are not designed for absorption, distribution, or biotransformation. The drug is placed directly on the affected tissue and is then mechanically eliminated using warm water irrigation.

▓ *Adverse Effects and Contraindications*

Ceruminolytics are irritating and may cause a severe eczematoid allergic reaction, especially with prolonged exposure. If the patient experiences excessive irritation, adequate softening of cerumen may often be achieved with plain anhydrous glycerin followed by flushing with plain warm water. The friability of older skin, especially of the external canal, may contribute to a greater incidence of contact dermatitis when ceruminolytics are used in the geriatric population.

⚠ **Ceruminolytics are not to be used in patients who have a perforated tympanic membrane.** Allergies to preservatives such as benzethonium chloride, sulfites, and thiomersal must be considered because many otic drugs contain these products.

▓ *Dosage Regimen*

Administration of the correct dosage requires filling of the ear canal with the drug while the patient's head is tilted at a 45-degree angle. Patients may use the ceruminolytic over a

2- to 3-day period and then once or twice weekly to prevent recurrence (see Table 62-1).

OTOTOXICITY

When inner ear structures or the auditory nerve (cranial nerve VIII) are damaged by drug therapies, the drugs are considered *ototoxic.* Two areas of the inner ear are commonly affected by toxic substances, the cochlea and the vestibular system. Damage occurs as different structures are affected. A variety of mechanisms, including toxic levels of drugs in the perilymphatic fluid, may damage the hair cells in the organ of Corti. In addition, drug therapy can change enzymatic activity in the inner ear, causing damage.

Topical and systemic drugs can be toxic, with ototoxicity resulting at therapeutic drug levels. The ototoxicity of topical otic drugs is primarily related to the drug's coming into direct contact with the inner ear structures. Therefore, consequences of ototoxicity are lessened if the tympanic membrane is intact, thus preventing direct contact with the inner ear. Some controversy exists regarding the use of otic drugs in the treatment of chronic otitis externa when the patient has a tympanic perforation.

The categories of drugs known to be ototoxic include the aminoglycosides and other antibiotics, loop diuretics, antimalarial, nonsteroidal antiinflammatory drugs (NSAIDs), and some antineoplastic drugs. Specific substances and the area most commonly affected are found in Table 62-2. Unfortunately, neomycin, a highly ototoxic drug, is commonly found in topical otic drugs. Assessment for an intact tympanic

TABLE 62-2 Impact of ototoxic Drugs on Auditory and Vestibular Function

Drug	Auditory Problems	Vestibular Problems
ANTIBIOTICS		
amikacin	++	+
chloramphenicol	+ to ++	+
erythromycin	+ to ++	+
gentamicin	++	+
kanamycin	++	+
neomycin	++	+
tobramycin	++	+
vancomycin	++	+
DIURETICS		
acetazolamide	+	+
ethacrynic acid	++	+
furosemide	++	+
NONSTEROIDAL ANTIINFLAMMATORY DRUGS		
ibuprofen	+	
indomethacin	+	+
naproxen	+	
Salicylates	++	
OTHER DRUGS		
Alcohol		++
cisplatin	+	+
nitrogen mustard	+	+
quinine	+	++
quinidine	+	++

+, Slight; ++, significant.

membrane is essential before the administration of any otic preparation containing neomycin. Neomycin may also cause a local allergic reaction.

Symptoms of ototoxicity depend on the inner ear structure most affected. Tinnitus and sensorineural hearing loss are present with damage to the cochlea. Damage to the vestibular apparatus produces vertigo, ataxia, lightheadedness, headache, giddiness, inability to focus or fixate on images, nausea, vomiting, and cold sweats. Factors such as dosage, renal function, concomitant use of other ototoxic chemicals, inherent susceptibility, age, and exposure to high-intensity noise have an impact on the ototoxic effects of different drugs.

Effects on hearing loss secondary to ototoxic drugs can be transient or permanent, unilateral or bilateral, and dose related or non–dose related. In addition to auditory function tests, monitoring of renal function is essential in patients who are being treated with ototoxic drugs. Renal function tests are indicators of drug and drug–by-product clearance. Ototoxicity is increased with decreased renal function. Older patients are especially prone to developing ototoxicity because of a normal age-related decline in renal function.

CLINICAL REASONING

Treatment Objectives

Treatment objectives for otic disorders are based on the purpose for the drug. The objectives may include relieving ear pain and reducing infection and inflammation. To prevent further episodes of external otitis, the use of otic drying drugs keep the external canal dry and less likely to support organism growth. When cerumen is the problem, the treatment objective is to soften and remove excessive cerumen from the external canal, decrease conductive hearing loss, and improve comfort.

Treatment Options

There are five basic components to the treatment of otic disorders. These are to thoroughly clean the ear canal, treat inflammation and infection, control the pain, culture severe cases, and avoid promoting factors for external otitis.

▥ Patient Variables

Patients known to have skin sensitivity to any topical preparation should use otic drugs with caution to avoid possible skin irritation.

LIFE-SPAN CONSIDERATIONS

Pregnant and Nursing Women. As a general rule, the incidence of otic disorders in the pregnant woman is no greater than that of the general population. However, use caution when giving systemic antibiotics because some of the drugs are teratogenic in nature. For example, chloramphenicol readily crosses the placental membranes and may produce gray baby syndrome (i.e., fetal abdominal distention, drowsiness, low body temperature, cyanosis, hypotension, and respiratory distress). Any otic drug absorbed systemically has teratogenic potential, although otic drugs are not appreciably absorbed.

Children and Adolescents. Children are more susceptible to disorders of the middle ear than to external otitis because of their relatively straight and short eustachian tube. The eustachian tube can easily be blocked by the adenoid tissue in the

nasopharynx, especially in conjunction with upper respiratory tract infections. The straight, short external canal of childhood makes children less susceptible to cerumen impaction than adults.

Generally, children who are diagnosed with otitis media are not treated with systemic antibiotics, given that the disorder is 70% to 80% virally mediated. Most otic preparations are not recommended for use in infants younger than 1 year of age because of the danger of potential systemic absorption. Systemic absorption may hinder the normal development of infants.

In addition, infants who feed from a bottle while lying down are more likely to have pooling of fluids in their nasopharynx and eustachian tubes, resulting in a greater risk of serous otitis and otitis media. The most common use of otic drops in infants and children with serous otitis and otitis media is for the treatment of ear pain. Systemic antibiotic drugs are necessary to treat the otitis media.

Older Adults. The friability of older skin, especially of the ear canal, contributes to a greater incidence of contact dermatitis and systemic absorption of otic drugs. A stiffening of the cilia of the ear, combined with a higher keratin content of cerumen, causes cerumen to impact easily, decreasing the ability to hear. In addition, physiologic changes of aging may alter the presentation of an otic disorder, causing the disorder to be overlooked. Monitor the older patient for adverse effects more frequently.

▥ Drug Variables

All otic antibacterial and drying drugs, and steroid and steroid-antibiotic combinations have similar pharmacokinetics and pharmacodynamics. Steroids and anesthetics are used primarily for pain control and relief of inflammation. Patients with minimal to no pain do not require steroids or anesthetic otic drugs. When they are used, treatment is provided for a limited time.

If patient is nonadherent to therapy, do not give otic anesthetics, or give them in a very limited quantity. Prolonged use of anesthetics may mask the signs and symptoms of fulminating infection.

Several commercial preparations are available to soften cerumen. Anhydrous glycerin is very inexpensive, and when used over several days can be as effective as other ceruminolytic products. The cost of different products varies, but all are relatively inexpensive.

Patient Education

Teach patients the general principles of otic drug storage and administration. Solutions are kept tightly closed and stored at 59°F to 86°F. Administration of cold otic drugs causes nausea, vomiting, and ataxia. Instruct the patient to warm the eardrop container passively to body temperature by holding it in the hands for 5 to 10 minutes. **Eardrops should never be warmed in a microwave oven.**

Otic drugs are more easily administered by someone other than the patient. Family members or friends can be instructed on the administration of otic drugs. Instruct the patient to lie on the unaffected side or tilt the head to the unaffected side. The person administering the eardrops should wash his or her hands thoroughly. In children, the pinna is displaced down and back to open the canal, whereas in adults, the pinna is displaced up and back. After administering the otic drug, hold this position for 2 to 5 minutes, allowing the drug to disperse into the canal. Repeat in the opposite ear if indicated. If the dropper accidentally touches the ear, the dropper is wiped clean with a tissue before placing it back in the bottle.

If the patient must administer the eardrops alone, have the patient sit in front of a mirror and tilt the head so the affected ear is up. The patient carefully drops the warmed solution into the ear without the dropper touching the ear or putting the dropper down. Caution the patient to avoid contact with the tip of the dropper to prevent contamination of the entire bottle of solution.

Otic discomfort often disrupts sleeping patterns. Appropriate use of otic drugs before retiring for the night may enhance sleeping patterns. Significant improvement is usually noted after a day or two of therapy. Teach patients to monitor symptoms and to contact the health care provider if symptoms persist or worsen.

Instruct patients to avoid activities that might dilute or wash out an otic drug from the ear. Such activities include showering without proper ear protection and swimming with the head exposed to water. Ideally, antibacterial, antifungal, and drying drugs are used upon rising, at bedtime, and after bathing, swimming, or any circumstance in which the ear has been exposed to added moisture. If an ear device (e.g., hearing aid, telephone ear piece, or ear plugs) is worn, it should be kept clean and free of debris. Ear devices should not be shared with others.

When administering otic antibiotics or antifungal drugs, a cotton pledget is inserted in the external canal to prevent the drug from leaking out and to permit the drug to reach the inner canal (Fig. 62-2). To prevent cross-contamination and infection, caution patients not to share otic drugs with other persons. Handwashing and proper disposal of contaminated ear drainage and soiled cotton pledgets prevents spread to others. Give special instructions, and caution the patient not to use otic drops in the eyes.

Special teaching needs with regard to steroid and steroid-antibiotic combinations and anesthetics include teaching the patient to limit the use of pain-controlling drugs so they are only administered when ear pain is present. Further, patients are also cautioned against keeping drugs from previous illnesses and self-medicating for recurrent ear problems. Patients are instructed that a change in the treatment regimen may be required if pain continues after 2 to 3 days of use.

Patients having cerumen problems are taught about the normal production, function, and elimination of cerumen (Case Study). They are also taught nonpharmacologic means for the removal of cerumen from the canal; note that cotton-tip applicators should not be used so as to avoid scratching

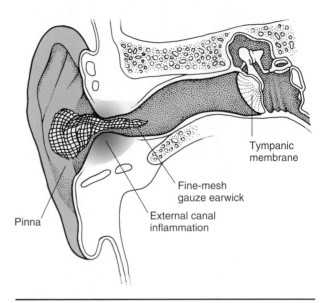

FIGURE 62-2 Earwick for Instillation of Antibiotics into the External Canal. Otic solutions are placed on the external portion of the earwick to be absorbed through the canal. This is particularly helpful when the canal is blocked by edema.

the external canal or accidentally perforating the tympanum. Allowing warm water from a shower to run in the ear and using a clean towel to wipe out the larger ear structures daily is effective. Finally, patients are told of the potential for hearing loss with impaction. If there has been a recent change in hearing associated with the impaction, the patient can expect hearing to markedly improve with removal of the impacted cerumen. If hearing does not return, the patient is instructed to contact a health care provider to have additional hearing testing and tympanometry conducted.

Evaluation

Evaluation involves determining the efficacy of the otic preparation. When the drugs are effective, the patient no longer complains of pain, edema, itching, or sensorial or perceptual alterations. Effectiveness of antibacterial and drying drugs is noted when external otitis does not recur.

When hearing loss persists after other signs and symptoms are resolved, audiology testing with tympanometry may be performed. Decreased movement of the tympanic membrane indicates conductive hearing loss, which necessitates additional diagnostic procedures as well as corrective measures to restore hearing.

CASE STUDY   Otic Drugs

ASSESSMENT

History of Present Illness	KZ is a 73-year-old Italian-American male. Complains of itching in the ears, feeling of fullness, and partial loss of hearing in both ears for the last month. No complaints of bleeding from the ear canals. Denies using any over-the-counter (OTC) otic preparations.
Past Health History	Throughout his life, KZ has had recurrent problems with excessive and dry cerumen. He has ear irrigations done by his health care provider but none for the last 2 years. He denies a history of otitis media and tympanic membrane perforation, history of skin irritation, or eczema. No known allergies to food preservatives. Current drugs include hydrochlorothiazide for hypertension.
Life-Span Considerations	KZ showers daily in the morning but avoids getting water in his ears. Denies swimming and resides in a very dry climate. KZ appears reliable and willing to comply with therapy recommendations. KZ is married, and his wife is willing to assist him as necessary. KZ is living on his retirement income and feels able to purchase OTC otic drugs. He owns and drives his own car for transportation. KZ may need assistance with administration of otic drugs.
Physical Exam Findings	Bilaterally pinna of equal size and appearance. Elongated lobes bilaterally. No tenderness with manipulation of the pinna nor compression of the tragus bilaterally. Unable to visualize either tympanic membrane due to excessive yellow-brown cerumen. No drainage noted in external canal opening. Decreased hearing demonstrated bilaterally by inability to hear whispered words from 1 to 2 feet away. Weber tuning fork test reveals lateralization to left ear.
Diagnostic Testing	None

DIAGNOSIS: Cerumen impaction

MANAGEMENT

Treatment Objective	Soften and remove excessive cerumen from the external canal, decrease conductive hearing loss, and improve comfort level.
Treatment Options	**Pharmacotherapy** • Cerumenex ear drops to affected ear daily per package instructions **Patient Education** 1. Do not use cotton applicators to remove cerumen. 2. Follow package instructions closely. 3. Administer ear drops at body temperature. 4. Lie on the side opposite the affected ear for 5 minutes after drug administration; a small cotton ball may be inserted into the ear canal to keep the drug in place. 5. May use 2 to 3 drops of olive oil to soften cerumen before warm water irrigations. 6. If no improvement in symptoms, make appointment with health care provider. **Evaluation** Cerumen has been removed without difficulty.

CLINICAL REASONING ANALYSIS

Q1. Why did you instruct the patient to avoid Q-tips? That's what I use to clean wax from my ears.
A. Because Q-tips and cotton applicators can scratch the external canal and even perforate the tympanum if the patient is too aggressive with the cleaning.

Q2. Aren't there adverse effects to Cerumenex ear drops?
A. There are adverse effects to every drug; some harmful, some of benefit. In the case of Cerumenex, patients have had severe eczematoid allergic reactions, especially with prolonged exposure. The drug should be stopped and the patient advised to return to the office for evaluation, if it occurs.

Q3. Couldn't KZ do a candling to remove the wax? It doesn't have to be a drug, does it?
A. No, KZ can do candling if he wishes. It is an alternative method for removing cerumen that many patients prefer, and it seems to work well in most cases.

KEY POINTS

- Treatment of otic disorders may necessitate the use of topical otic drugs as well as systemic drugs.
- Infection of the external ear *(otitis externa)* is common when the integrity of the external canal is compromised, allowing invasion of pathogenic organisms into the tissue.
- Patients whose ears are frequently exposed to water as a result of swimming, bathing, or environmental factors are at greatest risk for alterations in the integrity of the skin tissue of the external ear.
- Patients who traumatize the skin with cotton swabs or other foreign objects inserted into the canal are at risk for development of an external ear infection.
- There are a number of factors that must be considered when the health care provider selects an ototopical antibiotic. Consideration has to be given to the coverage of the expected pathogens, the possibility of drug resistance, the patient's allergy sensitization, tympanic membrane perforation, and the possibility of ototoxicity.
- Health care providers need to be aware that some patients may be experiencing allergic contact dermatitis to their ototopical medications.
- Otic drops that include a steroid with the acetic acid drops are more effective than the acetic acid drops alone.
- Corticosteroids are given to reduce inflammation and control pain, either alone or in combination with an otic antibiotic and otic anesthetic.
- Cerumen is a normal sebaceous gland secretion of the ear, functioning to protect and lubricate the external canal. Normally, cerumen is eliminated when the ear canals get wet; however, impaction is not uncommon.
- Categories of drugs known to be ototoxic include aminoglycosides and other antibiotics, loop diuretics, antimalarials, nonsteroidal antiinflammatory drugs, and some antineoplastic drugs.
- Tinnitus and sensorineural hearing loss are present with damage to the cochlea.
- Damage to the vestibular apparatus produces vertigo, lightheadedness, headache, giddiness, inability to focus or fixate on images, nausea, vomiting, and cold sweats.
- Factors such as dosage, renal function, concomitant use of other ototoxic drug, inherent susceptibility, age, and exposure to high-intensity noise affect ototoxicity.
- If conductive hearing loss is associated with the infection, hearing returns to normal with resolution of the infection.

Bibliography

Rosenfeld, R., Brown, L., Brow, C., et al. (2006). Clinical practice guideline: Acute otitis externa. *Otolaryngology Head and Neck Surgery, 134*(Suppl 4), S4–S23.

Rosenfeld, R., Singer, M., Wasserman, J., et al. (2006). Systematic review of topical antimicrobial therapy for acute otitis externa. *Otolaryngology Head and Neck Surgery, 134*(Suppl 4), S24–S28.

van Balen, F., Smit, W., Zuithoff, N., et al. (2003). Clinical efficacy of three common treatments in acute otitis externa in primary care:

Randomized controlled trial. *British Medical Journal, 321*(7425), 1201–1205.

Weber, P., Roland, P., Hannley, M., et al. (2004). The development of antibiotic resistant organisms with the use of ototopical medications. *Otolaryngology Head and Neck Surgery, 130*(Suppl 3), S89–S94.

Dermatologic Drugs

63

The skin has been described as the largest metabolically active organ in the body; it has vital functions such as protection, thermoregulation, immune responsiveness, biochemical synthesis, sensory detection, and social and sexual communications. It has a surface area of approximately 1.8 m² (for the average adult), makes up approximately 16% of our body weight, and acts as a shield from the environment. More importantly, the skin is a window through which the health care provider "sees" the entire body.

For most diseases, drugs are administered at a site that is distant from the target organ; however, in dermatology, drugs can be directly applied to the site. Topical therapy is a convenient method for treatment of skin disorders, but its efficacy depends on understanding the barrier function of the skin. Topical therapy can be used to restore skin hydration, alleviate symptoms, reduce inflammation, protect the skin, reduce scales and callus, cleanse and débride, and eradicate microorganisms. Some dermatologic problems, such as severe burns and decubitus ulcers, take extensive, aggressive, multifaceted interventions to resolve.

Since it is nearly impossible to discuss all skin disorders and their treatments within this chapter or even within this text, the more common disorders for which drug therapy is used are briefly discussed, after which follows a brief discussion of the major drug classifications used in treatment. Many of the drugs used to treat skin disorders have been discussed in previous chapters. The reader is referred to a comprehensive dermatologic text for further information.

STRUCTURE AND FUNCTIONS OF THE SKIN

In a strict sense, the skin is composed of two basic layers: the epidermis and dermis (Fig. 63-1). However, health care providers usually include the soft tissue underlying the dermis in a discussion of the skin because of its close apposition to and tendency to react as a unit with the overlying skin. A key question that must be posed when formulating differential diagnoses for skin disorders: Is there epidermal involvement?

EPIDERMIS

The *epidermis*, the top layer of the skin, is composed almost entirely of closely packed cells: keratinocytes, melanocytes (pigment cells), Langerhans' cells (antigen presentation), and Merkel cells (sensory). Most of the cells composing the epidermis are keratinocytes, the proliferative portion of the epidermis, which provide the internal structure of the skin. Each layer of epidermis expresses different keratins, which are often used as keratinocyte differentiation markers. Abnormal expression of keratin is a feature of many skin diseases including psoriasis and some ichthyotic disorders (i.e., skin disorders associated with dry, scaling, thick skin over widespread parts of the body).

Formation of the stratum corneum, or horny layer, is the most important function of the epidermis. It protects the skin against water loss and prevents the absorption of noxious agents. Corneocytes (the "bricks") and barrier lipids (the "mortar") form the scaffolding for the stratum corneum.

DERMIS

The *dermis* contains most of the structural components of the skin such as mast cells, fibroblasts, collagen, elastic fibers, sweat glands, sebaceous glands, and vasculature. The dermis is composed largely of collagen, and is approximately 40 times thicker than the epidermis. Within this 1- to 4-mm stratum is a rich supply of blood vessels, nerves, lymphatic tissues, glands, hair follicles, and structural matrix. Collagen fibers, the most abundant protein in the body, constitute about 70% of the dry weight of the dermis. This tough, but flexible layer of tissue provides for temperature regulation, sensation, and natural lubrication, and gives the skin many of the cosmetically important characteristics valued by all persons.

The hair and nails are considered appendages of the skin. Hair is made up of keratinized epithelial cells and grows in cycles at a rate of about 0.35 mm/day. The rate of hair growth is affected by various drugs and hormones. The nails are also made up of keratinized cells but with different anatomic components. The nail plate is highly adherent to the nail bed that grows beneath. Toenails tend to grow at a slower rate than fingernails. Factors affecting the growth of nails include genetics, age, and the weather.

Abnormalities of the dermis that provide clues to dermatologic dilemmas, and therefore their treatment, involves dilation and inflammation. Blanching is defined as redness of the skin, such as that seen with sunburn. The term implies that dilation and inflammation or both of these changes have occurred. Nonblanching redness of the skin usually results from extravasation of red blood cells (RBCs) into the dermis secondary to vascular damage, such as that seen with a bruise. A noninflammatory thickening or growth confined to the dermis (with normal overlying epidermis) usually develops from a benign or malignant tumor, or from an infiltrative disease of existing normal structures.

SOFT TISSUES

A layer of soft, subcutaneous tissue lies beneath the dermis. It is composed primarily of fat cells, which provide insulation, cushioning, and a reserve energy source.

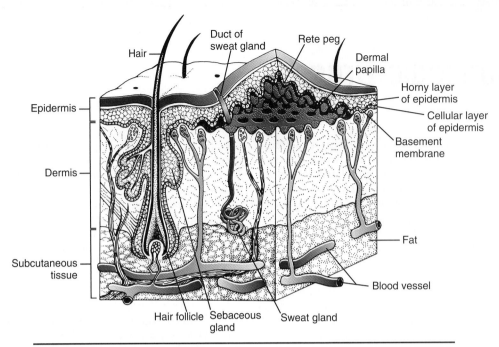

FIGURE 63-1 The Anatomy of the Skin. There are three growth layers of the epidermis and other structures.

SKIN DISORDERS

Skin disorders are classified in several ways. For the purpose of this chapter, they have been classified as noninfectious inflammatory diseases, infectious inflammatory diseases (caused by bacteria, fungi, or viruses), drug reactions, infestations and bites, and trauma.

Primary lesions develop without any preceding skin changes. In many cases, primary lesions are not seen and one must depend on the patient to describe how the lesion looked when it first appeared. Primary lesions include macules, papules, patches, plaques, nodules, wheals, vesicles, bullae, and pustules. Dermatologic diagnoses rely heavily on these primary lesions (Fig. 63-2). *Secondary lesions* result from changes in primary lesions and are influenced by scratching or infection. These changes may be brought about by the patient or the patient's environment and often occur in the epidermal layer of skin. Secondary lesions include scales, crusts, lichenification, keloids, scars, excoriations, atrophy, ulcers, and fissures.

NONINFECTIOUS INFLAMMATORY DERMATOSES

Dermatitis and eczema are noninfectious inflammatory dermatoses. *Dermatitis* is a general term that denotes an inflammation of the skin caused by exogenous irritants, allergens, or trauma. The term *eczema* is often used as a synonym for endogenous dermatitis. Regardless of the cause, dermatitis is usually characterized by erythema, vesicle formation, edema, oozing, excoriation, crusting, and scaling. With chronic scratching, the tissues become thickened *(lichenification).*

Atopic dermatitis (also known as atopic eczema) is a common pruritic dermatosis is responsible for 10% to 20% of

visits to dermatologists; it affects both sexes. Of patients with this disease, 40% to 65% have a family history of hay fever or asthma with a hereditary predisposition to a lowered cutaneous threshold for pruritus. Although the disorder may appear at any age, approximately 65% of patients develop symptoms during infancy and childhood. Infantile atopic dermatitis can start as early as 4 to 6 months of age, disappearing by about ages 3 to 5 years. Ninety percent of patients develop childhood atopic dermatitis, beginning at age 2 to 4 years and disappearing around age 10. In some cases, it continues into adulthood. Although it does so less frequently, atopic dermatitis can begin after age 30, usually as a result of skin exposure to either harsh or wet conditions. The debilitating effects of atopic dermatitis commonly lead to workplace disability.

Those more commonly affected live in cities and in dry climates. Most react to common foods and inhaled allergens by producing immunoglobulin E (IgE) antibodies. In adults, the dermatitis may be a response to harsh chemicals or scratching, with lesions most often noted on the forehead, wrists, feet, and sides of the neck. There may be lichenification on flexor surfaces from continued scratching and rubbing. Lesions in infants and young children are found primarily on the cheeks and the extensor surfaces of the antecubital or popliteal surfaces.

Contact dermatitis is a rash resulting from contact between an allergen or irritant and the skin. It is a form of allergic exogenous dermatitis and may be caused by chemicals or mechanical irritation. Contact dermatitis due to an irritant is not an allergic reaction but a result of direct tissue damage by the offending substance. The reaction can start within minutes to hours and does not require a previous exposure. The rash often stings at first, then becomes itchy. Solvents and fiberglass are common examples of substances that cause irritant contact dermatitis. In contrast, an allergic contact dermatitis (type IV hypersensitivity reaction) usually starts 2 to 10

SECONDARY LESIONS
(Modification of Original Appearance)

DAMAGED OR DIMINISHED SKIN SURFACE

 Erosion: Loss of epidermis that does not extend into dermis. **Example:** ruptured chicken pox vesicle.

PRIMARY LESIONS (Original Appearance)

NONPALPABLE

 Macule: A spot, circumscribed, up to 1 cm; not palpable; not elevated above or depressed below surrounding skin surface; hypopigmented, hyperpigmented, or erythematous. **Example:** freckles. Referred to as **patch** if greater than 1 cm. **Examples:** cafe´ au lait spots, mongolian spots.

 Ulcer: Loss of skin through the epidermis; healing results in scar formation. **Example:** stasis ulcer.

PALPABLE, SOLID

 Papule: A bump, palpable and circumscribed, elevated and less than 5 mm in diameter; may be pigmented, erythematous, or flesh-toned. **Example:** elevated nevus (mole).

 Fissure: A split in all epidermal layers of skin **Example:** athlete's foot.

 Nodule: A lesion similar to a papule, with a diameter of 5 mm to 2 cm; may have a significant palpable dermal component. **Examples:** fibroma, xanthoma, intradermal nevi.

 Atrophy : Diminution of epidermal surface; skin looks thinner and more translucent than normal; atrophy of the dermal layers may result in wasting or depression of the skin surface. **Example:** arterial insufficiency.

 Tumor: Any mass lesion; generally larger than a nodule; may be either malignant or benign. **Example:** lipoma.

 Excoriation: Loss of outer skin layers from scratching or rubbing. **Example:** scratched insect bite.

 Plaque: Usually well-circumscribed lesion with large surface area and slight elevation. **Examples:** psoriasis, lichen planus.

AUGMENTED OR INCREASED SKIN SURFACE

 Crust: A collection of serous exudate and debris on the surface of damaged or absent outer skin layers. **Example:** impetigo.

 Wheal: An elevation in the skin, with a smooth surface, sloping borders, and (usually) light pink color; caused by acute areas of edema in the skin; may appear, disappear, or change form abruptly within minutes or hours; size ranges from 3 mm to 20 cm. **Example:** mosquito bite.

PALPABLE, FLUID-FILLED

 Vesicle: A small blister (up to 5 mm in diameter); fluid collection may be subcorneal, intraepidermal, or subepidermal. **Example:** herpes simplex (early stages).

 Scale: A compact portion of desquamating stratum corneum; may vary in size, thickness, and consistency. **Examples:** psoriasis scale (compact and thick), pityriasis rosea scale (thin and small).

 Lichenification: Epidermal thickening and roughening of the skin with increased visibility of skin surface furrows. **Example:** chronic atopic dermatitis.

 Bulla: A blister larger than 5 mm; fluid may be located at various levels. **Examples:** pemphigus, pemphigoid.

 Scar : A collection of fibrous tissue that forms to replace lost epidermal and dermal tissue. **Examples:** surgical scar, acne scar.

 Pustule: An elevated, well-circumscribed lesion containing purulent exudate. **Example:** acne vulgaris.

 Keloid: Augmentation of scar tissue, creating a significant elevation on the skin surface after healing. **Examples:** postsurgical scar, post-acne scar.

FIGURE 63-2 Primary and Secondary Skin Lesions. Primary lesions are recognizable structural changes in the skin. Secondary lesions are primary lesions that have changed because of the natural progression of the lesion or because of scratching, irritation, or infection.

days after first exposure to the substance, but reactions can start in as early as 2 hours with repeated exposures. The most common causes of allergic contact dermatitis are urushiol from poison ivy, neomycin, nickel, fragrances, latex, lanolin, and benzocaine. Contact dermatitis has clinical features that include red, thick, crusty, fissured, suppurating areas in various stages.

Seborrheic dermatitis affects hairy areas, often appearing on the scalp, the eyebrows, the ears, or the sternum, as well as the beard area and the T-zone on the face with sebaceous glands. The lesions are red and greasy-looking with yellowish scale, and they often itch. Untreated patients may further excoriate the skin by scratching, thus allowing a secondary infection to develop. In babies, scalp seborrhea is called "cradle cap." In the adult, mild seborrhea may appear as dandruff. Patients with acquired immunodeficiency syndrome or parkinsonism may develop especially prominent seborrhea.

Urticaria (hives) is an IgE-mediated allergic response to external agents (e.g., insect bites) or to internal allergens (i.e., food allergies) that reach the skin through the blood stream. Urticaria occurs in about 15% to 20% of the population and is usually self-limiting, but may also become chronic. Chronic urticaria usually appears as a large hive without the sensation of itching, and is often accompanied by angioedema. The characteristic lesion of urticaria is itchy and edematous, and has an erythematous wheal with a pallid center. The lesions typically blanch with pressure and are transient in nature.

Psoriasis is a chronic, papulosquamous disorder that alters the appearance of the epidermis by increasing its thickness. The primary defect is an accelerated maturation of the epidermis. Instead of epidermal cells being replaced every 26 to 28 days, they complete their growth cycle in less than 7 days. Symmetric patches appear on extensor surfaces, knees, elbows, and/or buttocks, or on the scalp. Initial papules coalesce into red plaques. Both papules and plaques are covered with silvery scales that may be pruritic. Removal of the scales frequently leaves fine bleeding points called *Auspitz's sign.* The nails often become thick and irregular and exhibit pits of 1 mm or less. Psoriasis is sometimes associated with arthritic symptoms.

Pityriasis rosea, also a papulosquamous disease, is a self-limiting disorder of unknown cause. There is reason to believe that a virus or an autoimmune disorder is the underlying mechanism. It develops predominantly in patients of ages 10 to 35 years, with a typically seasonal onset during the fall and the spring. Pityriasis appears initially with a single oval salmon-colored patch (herald patch) 2 to 10 mm in diameter that is covered with scales. Within days to weeks, numerous similar but smaller patches appear. The major patches appear on the trunk, following the cleavage lines of the skin; smaller patches appear on peripheral areas. The rash usually resolves after about 6 to 8 weeks.

Lichen planus, another papulosquamous disease, produces 2- to 8-mm flat, purple lesions with polygonal borders. Its cause is unknown, but it is possibly a disease of keratinization or an autoimmune disorder. Emotional stress may be the antecedent event. The surfaces of the lesions are crisscrossed with white or silver lines called *Wickham's striae.* The lesions first appear on flexor surfaces of the wrists and forearm, the legs above the ankles, the sacral area, the penis, or mucous membranes. Onset of the disease usually occurs between the ages of 30 and 70 years.

INFECTIOUS INFLAMMATORY DERMATOSES

Bacterial Infections

Bacterial infections of the skin are most often caused by *Streptococcus* or *Staphylococcus* invasion of the skin where the barrier function has been compromised by damage or inflammation. Organisms may be introduced below the epidermis by trauma or by disturbances in normal anatomy (e.g., hair follicle or ingrown nail). Virulence of the organisms and host immune factors combine to determine whether an infection will occur and if so, the infection's extent.

Acne vulgaris is the most common skin disorder in the United States, affecting approximately 7% of the population each year, and is commonly found in 30% to 85% of adolescents and young adults. It is a disease of the pilosebaceous unit.

Acne is stimulated by the increased production of androgens during adolescence. Under androgen influence, acne typically originates from the blockage of skin pores with dead skin cells and oil. Acne vulgaris, or "common acne," appears as swollen red lesions primarily found on the face, the chest, the back, the shoulders, and the upper arms. In its more severe forms, acne can manifest as blackheads, whiteheads, pustules, papules, and cysts.

These symptoms are exacerbated by the activity of *Propionibacterium acnes,* a bacterial organism that converts sebum into irritating fatty acids. The bacterium releases chemotactic factors that promote inflammation. With the exception of open comedones, which are noninflammatory, lesions of acne can be thought of as either proinflammatory (closed comedones) or inflammatory (papules, pustules, nodules, and cysts). Open comedones are the most common lesions of mild acne. A comedo forms when sebum combines with keratin to form a plug within a skin pore. Oxidation causes the exposed surface of the sebum plug to turn black, hence the term blackhead. Closed comedones, known often as whiteheads, develop when pores fill below the skin surface with sebum and scales. Treatment regimens vary with the severity of the acneiform lesions.

Cellulitis, an infection and inflammation of the tissues beneath the skin, is typically caused by group A streptococci or *Staphylococcus aureus,* although other organisms such as non–group A beta hemolytic streptococci (i.e., group B, C, or G), *Enterobacteriaceae, Pseudomonas, Haemophilus influenzae,* and fungi may be present. Cellulitis is characterized by tenderness, edema, and erythema that spread to subcutaneous tissues; occasionally there are weeping lesions.

Erysipelas is a form of cellulitis caused by group A *Streptococcus pyogenes.* The visible signs include round or oval patches on the skin that promptly enlarge and spread, becoming swollen, tender, and red. The affected skin is hot to the touch, and occasionally the adjacent skin blisters. Systemic manifestations such as headache, malaise, fever, chills, vomiting, and prostration can occur.

Folliculitis is an infection of hair follicles. It most often occurs on the scalp or bearded areas of the face and can be caused by *S. aureus, Pseudomonas aeruginosa* as in hot-tub folliculitis, and gram-negative bacteria in patients on long-term antibiotics. *Candida albicans* is the culprit in patients who are taking immunosuppressants or who are on long-term antibiotics. Dermatophyte fungi are uncommon causes of folliculitis. Occasionally folliculitis is caused by herpes simplex I, herpes zoster, or molluscum contagiosum virus. Plastic occlusive dressings can also cause folliculitis in susceptible individuals.

Furuncles (boils) and *carbuncles* (a cluster of boils) are usually caused by coagulase-positive *S. aureus* (about 50% to 90% of cases). Beta hemolytic strep infections occur only about 10% of the time, but mixed infections are common. They are often a symptom of poor health. Furuncles tend to recur as a result of folliculitis. They usually appear on the neck, the face, the axillae, the buttocks, the thighs, and the perineum. Carbuncles involve multiple hair follicles with pustules. Like furuncles, carbuncles are caused by pus-forming bacteria. Systemic manifestations can develop and include malaise, fever, leukocytosis, and bacteremia. Scar tissue forms with healing.

Impetigo is a highly contagious, superficial skin infection usually found on exposed skin surfaces in children. It is caused by group A *S. pyogenes, S. aureus,* or both. It is not uncommon to find the infection in adolescents involved in wrestling activities because the organisms seem to thrive on the wrestling mats. The lesions are rapidly crusting, clear vesicles, 2 to 3 mm to 2 cm in diameter. The honey-colored crusts are moist and oozing. If the crusts are removed, the base is red and eroded.

Methicillin-resistant S. aureus (MRSA) is one of the most important pathogens in terms of increasing prevalence and impact. Historically, MRSA was a hospital-acquired organism (HA-MRSA) found most often in immunocompromised patients. Since MRSA first emerged as a pathogen in U.S. health care facilities in the late 1970s, infectious disease experts have noted an emergence of infections not associated with hospitalization. In the last decade, community-acquired MRSA (CA-MRSA) has developed in healthy people who would not normally be expected to develop this infection.

Despite the fact that MRSA is frequently cultured, the total number of patients colonized or infected and the impact of the MRSA infections on our U.S. health care facilities and patients is unclear. Current estimates of the incidence and prevalence of HA-MRSA are based on either (1) patients in intensive care units at a small number of hospitals, or (2) analyses of United States hospital discharge data. Both of these sources of information have major limitations. Furthermore, neither of these sources distinguishes between HA-MRSA and CA-MRSA.

According to the Centers for Disease Control and Prevention (CDC), MRSA infection is considered community acquired if (1) the diagnosis is made in an outpatient setting or a positive culture result is obtained within 48 hours of hospitalization; (2) there is no history of MRSA infection or colonization; (3) there is no history in the past year of hospitalization, admission to a nursing home or skilled nursing facility or hospice, dialysis, or surgery; and (4) the patient has no permanent indwelling catheters or medical devices that pass through the skin into the body. In general, CA-MRSA is more sensitive to antibiotic therapy and there is a wider choice of antibiotic treatment options available compared with HA-MRSA.

Perioral dermatitis affects up to 1% of the population, primarily young women ages 25 to 45. Since perioral dermatitis is far more common in developed countries, it is thought that the environment is somehow involved. The exact cause of perioral dermatitis is unclear, but there may be a linkage between the disorder and rapidly multiplying bacteria or yeast harbored in the hair follicles.

The rash of perioral dermatitis is likely caused by a number of factors. Topical steroids are the most frequent cause. Unknowingly, the patient's fingers may move the steroid cream from the site of application to other parts of the body. The speed and severity of the development of perioral dermatitis increase with the strength of the steroid cream. Other factors contributing to perioral dermatitis include (1) not washing the face with water; (2) using soap or a soap-free cleanser; (3) the application of face cream around the cheek folds and the chin, or around the eyes as occurs with periocular dermatitis; and (4) the use of moisturizers, cream cleansers, make-up foundation, and sunscreens.

The rash of perioral dermatitis looks like a cross between acne and eczema. The rash of some patients looks more like acne and that of others more like eczema, and some patients have equal attributes of both. Basically, acne-like blemishes form that are red, rough, scaling, and very sensitive, with itching and burning.

Rosacea is a common but little-known disorder of the facial skin that affects an estimated 14 million Americans. Redness on the forehead, cheeks, nose, and chin, acneiform lesions, small visible blood vessels on the face, and watery or irritated eyes characterize rosacea. The results of a 2005 survey conducted by the National Rosacea Society showed that 70% of patients with rosacea have declining self-confidence and self-esteem. Over 50% of patients reported stares, rude comments, and jokes. Further, 41% avoided going out in public or reported having canceled social engagements. Seventy percent of patients who had severe rosacea noted that their disorder affected professional relationships, with approximately 30% missing work because of their appearance.

Viral Infections

Viral skin lesions are caused by replication of the virus in the skin, by immune responses of the host, or both. Viral infections of the skin include herpes simplex, herpes zoster, varicella (chickenpox), verrucae, and other dermatoses.

Herpes simplex is caused by the *Herpes simplex* virus (HSV), a DNA virus of two major types, HSV_1 and HSV_2. Primary infections have an incubation period of up to 2 weeks. Type 1 herpes infections most often involve the skin and the oral cavity, although other body parts may be involved. Type 2 herpes infections most often appear on the genital mucosa. Neonates can be exposed to the virus as they exit the birth canal, developing severe infections that can lead to encephalitis, seizures, learning disorders, blindness, and death. Recurrent infection is due to either a reactivation of an older infection or acquisition of new infections. Lesions appear as vesicles on an inflamed base. In immunocompromised individuals, herpes infections can spread to the lungs and the brain.

Herpes zoster ("shingles") is caused by reactivation of the varicella virus, the virus causing chickenpox. Once contracted, the virus survives in a latent form in dorsal root ganglia. Certain stimuli (e.g., stress, immunocompromise) allow the virus to travel down the axon to the skin, where vesicles appear in a dermatomal distribution pattern. Pain, itching, or irritation precede the skin eruption by 48 to 72 hours. The lesions begin with a red base, on which appears a small but enlarging clear vesicle. The vesicle becomes white and then yellow before rupturing. Fluid oozes to form a crust that may require 7 to 10 days to heal. Systemic symptoms may be present. Postherpetic neuralgia, debilitating pain persisting months after the skin lesions have resolved, afflicts 1 in 5 patients with zoster.

Verrucae (warts) are of various types and often associated with hyperkeratosis. Verrucae are most often caused by the human papilloma virus (HPV). Verruca vulgaris ("common wart") is a papilloma infection of the hands and fingers. Verrucae plana are flat warts located on the dorsum of the hands and on the face. Verruca plantaris ("plantar wart") appear as an inward growth on the sole of the foot, often containing visible ends of capillaries, which appear as black specks. Unlike common and flat warts, plantar warts are often painful. They may be covered by a callus. *Condylomata acuminatum*, cauliflower-like growths in the anogenital area ("genital warts"), are caused by HPV (most commonly by types 6 and 11) and are spread through sexual contact. Cervical dysplasia and carcinoma in situ, other manifestations of sexually-transmitted HPV, are likely caused by HPV of types 16, 18, 31, 33, and 35. Often asymptomatic, HPV infection is exceedingly common; 80% of women age 50 years and older have been infected.

Fungal Infections

Fungal infections of the skin, the hair, and the nails are a major source of morbidity throughout the world. It is estimated that fungal infections account for 5% of new outpatient referrals to dermatologists in temperate climates, and as many as 20% in tropical climates. Most infections are caused by either dermatophytes or by yeasts, most commonly the *Candida* species.

Tinea ("ringworm") is a superficial infection in which the fungus lives on the dead horny layer of the skin. It causes the skin to scale and disintegrate, the nails to crumble, and hair to break off. Lesions appear as circular, scaly, and erythematous. *Tinea pedis* affects the feet ("athlete's foot"); *tinea capitis*, the scalp; *tinea barbae*, the beard; *tinea cruris*, the groin ("jock itch"); *tinea corporis*, the body; and *tinea manus*, the hand. *Tinea versicolor* is caused by the organism *Pityrosporum ovale* (formally known as *Mallassezia furfur*). Tinea versicolor is estimated to affect 2% to 8% of the population of the United States. This skin disease commonly affects adolescents and young adults, especially in warm and humid climates. It is thought that yeast feeds on skin oils as well as dead skin cells.

Tinea unguium (otherwise known as onychomycosis) is a fungal infection of toenails often seen in persons who have long-standing tinea pedis or who have traumatic nail damage. The affected nails appear dull and thick. The distal edge becomes separated from the nail bed (onycholysis), causing a misshapen appearance. Fingernails may also become infected. This infection is very difficult to treat and easily returns.

Candidiasis is a yeast infection caused by *C. albicans*. Predisposition to candidiasis occurs in people treated with antibiotics, oral contraceptives, corticosteroids, or antineoplastic therapies; babies and adults in diapers; and in people who are immunosuppressed (e.g., with diabetes mellitus or acquired immunodeficiency syndrome). *Candida* has a predilection for warm, moist sites; thus intertriginous sites (skin folds), the mouth, and the vagina are common sites for infection. With candidal growth, the skin may be denuded, leaving

a raw, glistening base. Red papules (satellite lesions) are scattered away from the margins of the raw areas. The presence of the scattered papules is useful in distinguishing candidiasis from *tinea*. The most prominent symptom of vaginal candidiasis is severe itching. A thick, "cottage cheese–like" discharge may also occur, but colored discharges or odors suggest that the patient may need referral for a sexually transmitted infection.

DRUG REACTIONS

Drug reactions take on many morbillous forms and are caused by a variety of mechanisms. A rather common form is a fine, reddish maculopapular rash over the trunk (or any part of the body). Five percent of patients have an extended hospital stay as the result of adverse drug reactions, with 10% of hospitalized patients experiencing at least one adverse drug reaction. **Allergic drug reactions may or may not result in specific antibody formation or sensitized lymphocytes. For this reason, the recognition of the signs and symptoms of a drug reaction is of utmost importance.** Adverse cutaneous reactions to drugs are noted in Table 63-1.

INFESTATIONS AND BITES

The bites of bees, wasps, hornets, and yellow jackets are potential causes of skin lesions, and are responsible for 50 to 100 reported deaths a year. Most victims are under 20 years of age. Males are affected twice as often as females, possibly because they are more likely to be involved in outdoor work. Reactions are more frequent when stings occur around the head and neck, but reactions can occur from bites in other areas as well. Reactions may range in severity from transient redness, edema, and pain or pruritus to acute anaphylactic shock (usually within 15 minutes). Reactions peak within 48 to 72 hours of exposure and last up to 7 days. Neurologic or vascular reactions or immune-complex disease may also be seen. Anaphylaxis is the major cause of death in sensitive individuals.

Pediculosis, an infestation of the ectoparasites known as lice (see Chapter 30), affects 6 to 12 million people annually in the United States. Pediculus humanus capitis (head louse), Pediculus humanus corporis (body louse), and Pthirus pubis (pubic louse) are the three types of lice that infest humans. P. capitis is common among school children. Head lice are very rare among blacks; possibly because of the twisted nature of the hair shaft and the use of hair pomades. Pediculosis is spread by close physical contact and through the sharing of combs, hats, clothes, and linens. Overcrowding encourages pediculosis spread. Infestation with P. pubis is a sexually transmitted disease (STD).

TRAUMA

Trauma contributes to infection when physical injury disrupts the integrity of the skin. Common wounds include lacerations (cuts or tears), abrasions (shearing or scraping of the skin), puncture wounds, surgical avulsions, traumatic amputations, incisions, and burns. In many cases, decubitus ulcers have been considered as trauma given the associated shearing forces and friction, and the pressure exerted on bony prominences.

DRUG INTERACTIONS

TABLE 63-1 Common Dermatologic Adverse Reactions Induced by Topical Dermatologic Preparations

Common Drug-Induced Dermatologic Reactions					
Acneiform Reactions		**Urticaria**		**Alopecia**	
ACTH	Iodides	ACTH	meprobamate	Alkylating drugs	levodopa
Androgenic hormones	isoniazid	amitriptyline	nitrofurantoin	allopurinol	norethindrone acetate
Bromides	lithium	Barbiturates	Opioids	Anticoagulants	Oral contraceptives
Corticosteroids	Oral contraceptives	Bromides	Penicillins	Antimetabolites	propranolol
cyanocobalamin	trimethadione	chloramphenicol	pentazocine	Antithyroid drugs	Retinoids
ethambutol	phenytoin	Dextran	Phenothiazines	colchicine	trimethadione
ethionamide	phenobarbital	Enzymes	Salicylates	Heavy metals	Vitamin A
Hydantoins		erythromycin	Serums	indomethacin	
		griseofulvin	streptomycin		
		Hydantoins	Sulfonamides		
		Insulins	Tetracyclines		
		Iodides	thiouracil		
		meperidin			
Photosensitive Reactions		**Purpura**		**Contact Dermatitis**	
acetohexamide	Oral contraceptives	ACTH	Gold salts	bacitracin	meprobamate
amitriptyline	phenytoin	allopurinol	griseofulvin	benzocaine	neomycin
Antimalarials	phenothiazines	amitriptyline	Iodides	benzoyl peroxide	nitrofurazone
Barbiturates	Salicylates	Anticoagulants	meprobamate	chloramphenicol	PABA
carbamazepine	Sulfonamides	Barbiturates	Penicillins	chlorpromazine	Penicillins
Citrus fruits	Sulfonylureas	chloral hydrate	quinidine	ephedrine	Phenol
doxycycline	Tetracyclines	chlorpropamide	rifampin	formaldehyde	streptomycin
Gold salts	Thiazides	chlorpromazine	Sulfonamides	Iodine	Sulfonamides
griseofulvin	Topical steroids	Corticosteroids	Thiazides	isoniazid	Thiamine
haloperidol	TCAs	digoxin	trifluoperazine	Lanolin	thimerosal
nortriptyline					
Life-Threatening Drug-Induced Skin Eruptions					
Stevens-Johnson Syndrome		**Exfoliative Dermatitis**		**Lupus Erythematosus**	
ampicillin	Penicillins	PAS	isoniazid	aminosalicylic acid	Oral contraceptives
Barbiturates	pentazocine	Barbiturates	isosorbide	chlorpromazine	penicillamine
carbamazepine	phenobarbital	carbamazepine	Measles vaccine	Steroid withdrawal	Penicillins
chloramphenicol	phenytoin	chlorpropamide	nitroglycerine	digoxin	phenobarbital
chlorpropamide	procaine penicillin	demeclocycline	Hypoglycemics	ethosuximide	Phenothiazines
clindamycin	Sulfonamides	Diphtheria vaccine	Penicillins	Gold compounds	primidone
codeine	Tetracyclines		Phenothiazines	griseofulvin	propylthiouracil
novobiocin		furosemide	phenytoin	Hydantoins	rifampin
		Gold	Sulfonamides	hydralazine	streptomycin
		griseofulvin	Tetracyclines	isoniazid	Sulfonamides
		Tetracyclines		methyldopa	Tetracyclines
				methysergide	Thiazides

ACTH, Adrenocorticotropic hormone; *PABA,* para-aminobenzoic acid; *PAS,* aminosalicylic acid; *TCAs,* tricyclic antidepressants.

BURNS

Burns are classified according to the depth of destruction. *Superficial burns* (formerly known as "first-degree burns") involve the epidermal layer only, are painful, and appear red or pink and dry. There are no blisters. An example of a superficial burn is mild sunburn, which is caused by the shorter ultraviolet (UV) wavelengths known as ultraviolet B (UVB). A longer wavelength, ultraviolet A (UVA), also penetrates skin and damages connective tissue at deeper levels, even if the skin's surface feels cool. UVA is implicated in skin cancer and aging but does not contribute to sunburn. Severe sunburn may blister, manifesting as a superficial partial-thickness burn (see below).

Partial-thickness ("second-degree") burns involve the epidermis and parts of the dermis. These burns are red, moist, blistered, and painful. Mottling, and pink or red to waxy, white areas with blisters and edema are often present. These are characterized as superficial or deep partial-thickness burns, depending on the degree to which the dermis is damaged. The entire epidermal and dermal layers are affected in deep partial-thickness burns. Sweat glands and hair follicles remain intact. If more than a tenth or so of the body surface area is compromised by weeping wounds or denuded skin, evaporation of body water can be severe enough to cause serious dehydration and necessitate fluid replacement.

Full-thickness ("third-degree") burn injuries involve the loss of the entire skin layer. They are generally painless because nerve fibers are destroyed. The burn lesions vary in color, often turning white over the first 24 hours after injury, with much edema noted. The eschar is hard, dry, and leathery, but the wound leaks fluid absorbed from the underlying tissues. A blackened, depressed, full-thickness burn that involves muscle, fascia, and bone (full-thickness plus some underlying tissue) is sometimes called a "fourth-degree burn." Exposure of bones and ligaments is common. When bone is involved, the wound appears dull and dry.

DECUBITUS ULCERS

Decubitus ulcers are an ulceration of the skin and the subcutaneous tissue over or near a bony prominence, sometimes known as a "bedsore." Decubitus ulcers are caused by sustained pressure or friction of a body part resting against an external object. The 10 most common reasons for hospitalizations during which the patients also had decubitus ulcers were (1) septicemia; (2) pneumonia; (3) urinary tract infections; (4) aspiration pneumonitis; (5) heart failure; (6) rehabilitation; (7) fluid and electrolyte disorders; (8) complications of a device, implant, or graft; (9) respiratory failure; and (10) diabetes mellitus with complications.

Obstruction of capillary blood flow by externally applied pressure causes tissue hypoxia. An early sign of pressure is blanching erythema, an area of redness that turns white when pressed. Nonblanching erythema is the first serious sign of impaired blood supply to the tissues. Deeper, irreversible tissue damage is likely if hyperemia persists; necrotic tissue may appear yellow or black. Muscle damage develops when ischemia persists for long periods and the wound extends through the entire skin layer and underlying structures. A cycle of cellular death and release of metabolic wastes into the surrounding tissues accompanies ischemia. Edema encroaches on interstitial spaces, slowing tissue perfusion and increasing the hypoxia. Decubitus ulcers are categorized by stages (Table 63-2).

PHARMACOTHERAPEUTIC OPTIONS

Pharmacokinetics

There are several factors that influence transdermal absorption of drugs. Drug penetration and absorption are increased as much as 10% with hydration of the stratum corneum. Hydration causes the cells to swell, decreasing their density and thereby decreasing their resistance to diffusion. High ambient humidity increases hydration of the skin, as do certain drug formulations. Occlusion under impermeable plastic film enhances drug absorption by preventing transepidermal water loss and increasing epidermal hydration. Further, the more occlusive the formulation (e.g., emulsions, ointments) the more hydrated the skin and the greater the permeability becomes. However, the low solubility of some formulations limits drug concentration and reduces the rate of absorption.

Because absorption of topical drugs occurs by passive diffusion, higher drug concentrations increase the amount of drug absorbed. Absorption from abraded or damaged skin surfaces is also much greater than that from intact skin. When drugs are left in place for prolonged periods or applied over large surface areas, more absorption will occur.

Mucous membranes and facial skin are sites of enhanced drug penetration, and often toxicity, because of the thinness of the stratum corneum. Intertriginous areas also show enhanced drug penetration because of their inherent occlusion. In addition, hair follicles and sweat ducts provide epidermal fenestrations that provide limited but low-resistance pathways for drug penetration.

Transdermal, systemic drug absorption from areas with thick skin (e.g., the palms of the hand and the soles of the feet) is relatively slow. Peak rates are not achieved for 12 to 24 hours. However, large fluctuations in plasma concentrations and increased first-pass effects commonly seen with some orally administered drugs can sometimes be avoided with transdermal administration. The use of topical rather than systemic drugs also may improve the therapeutic index of many compounds and enhance patient adherence to therapy.

TABLE 63-2 Staging and Treatment of Decubitus Ulcers

Stage	Signs and Symptoms	Treatment Options	Time to Healing
I	• Blanchable erythema, with warmth and induration that does not resolve within 30 minutes of pressure relief • Continued pressure causes erythema with no blanching—first outward sign of tissue destruction is skin that is white from ischemia	• No drug therapy • Relieve pressure	14 days
II	• Partial-thickness loss involving epidermis and possibly dermis. • Lesion may first appear as abrasion, blister, or superficial ulceration • Wound base is moist, pink, and painful	• Hydrocolloid occlusive dressing (e.g., DuoDerm) • Silicon sprays • Transparent dressings (e.g., Tegaderm, Opsite) • Sharp débridement in severely contaminated, necrotic wounds	45 days
III	• Full-thickness loss with extension into subcutaneous tissue but not through the underlying fascia • Ulcer is 2.075 mm or deeper* • Lesion presents as a crater with or without undermining of adjacent tissue • Eschar, necrotic tissue, tunneling, exudate, and infection appear • No pain in most cases	• Débridement with wet-to-dry dressings (e.g., saline, Dakin's solution) • Proteolytic enzyme débridement • Hydrocolloidal dressings	90 days
IV	• Full-thickness loss of skin and subcutaneous tissue and extension into muscle, bone, tendon, or joint capsule • Osteomyelitis with bone destruction, dislocations, or pathologic fractures possible • Sinus tracts and severe undermining commonly present	• Daily whirlpool • Wet-to-dry dressings (e.g., saline, Dakin's solution) • Enzymatic débridement • Surgical débridement • Vacuum-assisted closure (VAC) sponges	Over 120 days (may be much longer; ulcer may even be unable to heal)

*Examples of the thickness of a stage III decubitus ulcer are an ordinary house key, a U.S. nickel, and a plastic ruler.

Most topically administered dermatologic drugs have limited distribution. However, the skin functions as a reservoir for some drugs. For example, a topical corticosteroid under occlusion for 24 hours establishes a drug reservoir in the stratum corneum that can persist for as long as 2 weeks. Most drugs passing through the stratum corneum to the epidermis are biotransformed there. Drugs not biotransformed in the epidermis pass unchanged into systemic circulation. Drugs reaching the systemic circulation are eliminated through the kidneys, or by biotransformation in the liver.

Antibiotics

There is little definitive evidence on which to base empiric antibiotic selection for bacterial skin infections. Numerous topical antibiotics are available for the treatment of acne (Table 63-3) and minor bacterial skin problems. Patients can develop allergic contact dermatitis to topical application of neomycin and bacitracin. A newer topical agent, mupirocin (Bactroban ointment), is effective against infections with gram-positive cocci. This antibiotic is particularly useful in patients who are carriers of *S. aureus* in the nares. Topical clindamycin (Cleocin-T) and metronidazole (Metrogyl) have become standards of care in the treatment of acne and rosacea, respectively. Gram-positive and gram-negative infections can be effectively treated with silver sulfadiazine (Silvadene) but may cause neutropenia in children.

Systemic antibiotics are useful for most bacterial skin infections, including acne, rosacea, hidradenitis suppurativa, and folliculitis. Commonly used drugs include cephalexin (Keflex), dicloxacillin (Dynapen), doxycycline (Vibramycin), minocycline (Minocin), tetracycline (Sumycin), erythromycin (E-mycin), trimethoprim-sulfamethoxazole (Bactrim), and clindamycin (Cleocin) (see Chapter 27).

The antiinflammatory effects of the tetracycline and erythromycin drug classes are as important as their antibacterial effects in the treatment of inflammatory skin disorders. If after 24 to 48 hours the patient is still febrile or not improving, a penicillinase-resistant drug can be substituted. Continue antibiotic therapy for 10 to 14 days, depending on the rate of clinical resolution. In patients with a *Pseudomonas* or a mixed infection, the drug of choice may be a quinolone and treatment may be extended beyond the usual 10 to 14 days. Antibiotics change the nature of protein structure in the pathogen, causing coagulation of proteins, inhibition of cell wall synthesis, and disturbance of enzymatic processes.

Antiseptics

Antiseptics are organic or inorganic preparations that kill or inhibit the growth of bacteria, fungi, and viruses; however, antiseptics are used primarily to prevent infections rather than for treatment. According to the Food and Drug Administration (FDA), antiseptics in general are classified as unsafe or ineffective in the management of minor wounds, and are not considered necessary. Antiseptics are available in many formulations and differ in spectrum and effectiveness, and thus are not interchangeable. Vegetative forms of bacteria are most sensitive to antiseptics, followed by fungi, lipophilic viruses, tubercle bacilli, and hydrophilic viruses. Bacterial and fungal spores are resistant to most antiseptics. The therapeutic index of an antiseptic is a crucial consideration, because any useful agent must be considerably more toxic to surface pathogens than to adjacent living tissues.

The adverse effects of antiseptics vary with the specific drug; however, most are irritating to skin surfaces. **In some cases, ▲ antiseptics interfere with the body's natural healing; they should be applied around but not in a wound. Further, most antiseptics are drying to the skin.** Table 63-4 summarizes the uses and characteristics of various antiseptics.

Antiviral Drugs

Claims of unique efficacy are made for each new antiviral drug that appears. All have a cure rate of approximately 85% for acute infections but a much lower rate for chronic ones. Acyclovir (Zovirax) and penciclovir (Denavir) reduce healing time and viral shedding in patients who have herpes simplex or herpes zoster. The antiviral activity of acyclovir requires activation by the viral enzyme thymidine kinase. Because of this requirement, acyclovir has little toxicity to human cells and therefore has relatively few systemic adverse effects. Docosanol (Abreva) is an over-the-counter (OTC) topical agent for facial herpes outbreaks.

Valacyclovir (Valtrex) is used for the same purposes as acyclovir. It achieves higher blood levels than acyclovir with oral dosing. Once absorbed, valacyclovir is biotransformed to acyclovir.

Famciclovir (Famvir) is used in the treatment of acute herpes zoster and recurrent HSV. Its pharmacologic action is similar to that of acyclovir and valacyclovir.

Condylomata can be treated with podophyllin (25% solution) and podofilox (Condylox, 0.5% solution or gel). Imiquimod (Aldara), which induces interferon production, is also

TABLE **63-3 Treatment Options for Acne**				
Drug	**Reduces Sebum Production**	**Comedolytic-Keratolytic**	**Antimicrobial Action**	**Antiinflammatory Action**
Oral contraceptives	+++	+++	0	0
Oral isotretinoin	+++	+++	++	++
Oral antibiotics	0	+	++	++
Benzoyl peroxide	0	+	+++	++
Topical antibiotics	0	+	+++	+
Topical retinoids	0	+++	0	+
azelaic acid	0	++	++	+
adapalene	0	+++	+	++
spironolactone	++	++	0	++
Salicylic acid	0	+	0	0

0, no activity; +, low activity; ++, moderate activity; +++, high activity.

TABLE **63-4** Antiseptics		
Antiseptic	**Example**	**Uses and Characteristics**
Ethanols	Isopropyl alcohol	• Bacteriocidal; kills 90% of bacteria in 2 minutes if area remains moist; 75% of bacteria with a single swipe; less effective for viruses and fungi • Used to clean intact skin before injections or surgical incisions • Is drying to healthy skin • Is irritating to open wounds, causing burning type of pain
Oxidizing antiseptics	Hydrogen peroxide; benzoyl peroxide	• Alters surface tension, thus increasing the permeability of the organism's cell wall and leakage of cell contents • Used for wound cleansing, cleansing of tracheostomy tubes, cerumen removal; diluted as a mouthwash; used to treat acne vulgaris • Hydrogen peroxide more effective as a débriding and cleansing agent than an antiseptic; doubtful value on intact skin • Benzoyl peroxide is bactericidal for anaerobic bacteria (e.g., *Corynebacterium*)
Biguanides	chlorhexidine gluconate (Hibiclens)	• Effective against gram-positive and gram-negative organisms • Used primarily as a skin cleanser
Iodines	povidone-iodine, (Betadine)	• Bactericidal to most bacteria, fungi, and viruses, but effectiveness dependent on concentration • 1% solution kills 90% of bacteria in 90 seconds • Prevention and treatment of infections of the skin, scalp, and mucous membranes of the mouth and vagina
Chlorine preparations	Dakin's solutions	• Bactericidal; dissolves necrotic materials and blood clots. Used with infected wounds when other drugs or methods not effective or available • May interfere with wound healing by delaying blood clotting
Metallics	silver nitrate, silver sulfadiazine, zinc oxide	• Treatment of burn wounds; cauterizing warts or wounds • Effective against *Pseudomonas* and other organisms, eczema, impetigo, tinea, venous stasis ulcers, pruritus, psoriasis, and seborrhea • Ingredient in over-the-counter dandruff shampoos
Phenol derivatives	hexachlorophene (Phisohex)	• Bacteriostatic against gram-positive bacteria • Handwashing and preoperative skin cleansing • Ineffective against gram-negative bacteria and fungi • Systemically absorbed with repeated use
Other	Acetic acid Gentian violet Sulfur	• 5% concentration is bactericidal to many organisms including *Pseudomonas;* less than 5% concentration is bacteriostatic • Use for wound, bladder, vaginal, and otic irrigations; dressing surgical wounds • Effective against gram-positive bacteria and many fungi • Used therapeutically as a topical antimicrobial • Fungicidal and keratolytic properties • Widely used for the treatment of psoriasis, seborrhea, and dermatitis • May be used alone or in combination with other keratolytic drugs (e.g., coal tar, resorcinol, salicylic acid)

approved for the treatment of condylomata and is effective in treating verrucae, molluscum contagiosum, and superficial basal cell carcinomas.

Antifungal Drugs

In the past several years, a variety of oral and topical antifungal drugs have been developed (Table 63-5). Topical antifungal therapy is effective for tinea pedis (excluding onychomycosis), tinea cruris, tinea versicolor, and seborrheic dermatitis. Griseofulvin, the first systemic antifungal drug for use in dermatology, is now limited in use. Its primary use is in tinea capitis in children. Recent research suggests that terbinafine and itraconazole may be as effective and will likely replace griseofulvin.

Terbinafine (Lamisil, Lamisil AT) is an allylamine derivative that is effective against most superficial antifungal infections. The risks for hepatotoxicity and drug interactions is less than with the imidazole antifungals. It is approved for treatment of onychomycosis for a period of 3 months.

Itraconazole (Sporanox) is an imidazole antifungal; it is approved for treatment of onychomycosis using a pulse regimen twice daily for 1 week per month for a total of 3 months. Both terbinafine and itraconazole are quick to raise drug levels in the nail of the patient with onychomycosis that persists after therapy is stopped. **For the patient taking itraconazole, monthly monitoring of liver function tests for hepatotoxicity**

is required. Follow-up is also required because of the many drug interactions associated with itraconazole.

Fluconazole's (Diflucan's) high concentrations in skin and mucous membranes recommend it for use in the treatment of oral candidiasis (thrush) and vaginal candidiasis. It is also effective as single-dose therapy for tinea versicolor and as a weekly administered therapy for onychomycosis. Hepatotoxicity is rare, but drug interactions can be significant.

Ketoconazole (Nizoral, Nizoral Topical) is no longer used routinely because of the potential for liver toxicity and because newer, less toxic, and more effective antifungals are available.

Systemic antifungal drugs may be indicated for the treatment of severe tinea corporis, tinea capitis, onychomycosis, and all deep fungal infections that occur in the setting of human immunodeficiency virus (HIV) infection. The pharmacology, the indications, and the toxicities of antifungal drugs are discussed in Chapter 28.

Antiinflammatory Drugs

Many skin conditions respond to topical or intralesional corticosteroids (see also Chapter 56). Most often applied topically, they may also be taken systemically for severe disorders. The vehicle containing a corticosteroid is as important as the steroid itself. Creams and lotions are composed of a combination of

TABLE **63-5** Treatment Options for Topical Fungal Infections

Disorder	Topical Drugs	Oral Drugs
Candidiasis, localized	Azoles	N/A
Candidiasis, generalized	N/A	ketoconazole, itraconazole, fluconazole
Candidiasis, mucocutaneous	nystatin, clotrimazole*	ketoconazole, itraconazole, fluconazole
Tinea corporis, localized	Azoles, Allylamines	N/A
Onychomycosis†	N/A	terbinafine, itraconazole, fluconazole
Tinea corporis, generalized	N/A	griseofulvin, terbinafine ketoconazole, itraconazole, fluconazole
Tinea pedis	Azoles, Allylamines	griseofulvin, terbinafine, ketoconazole, itraconazole, fluconazole
Tinea versicolor, localized	Azoles, Allylamines	N/A
Tinea versicolor, generalized	N/A	ketoconazole, itraconazole, fluconazole

*Nystatin and clotrimazole may be combined with a topical steroid to help reduce inflammation.
†Systemic therapy is needed for onychomycosis. Terbinafine and itraconazole are quick to raise drug levels in the nail that persist after therapy is stopped. There are fewer drug interactions with terbinafine, and itraconazole is broad-spectrum. Treatment for toenail onychomycosis with terbinafine (250 mg daily) is 3 mo (76% effective); with itraconazole, 3 mo on pulsed dosing (200 mg twice daily for 1 wk/mo for 3 to 4 mo) (63% effective).
N/A, Not applicable.

oil and water. The higher the ratio of oil to water, the thicker the formulation. The presence of water in the vehicle may contribute to skin drying through evaporation. Vehicles containing water must also contain preservatives to prevent contamination with bacteria and fungi. Some of the preservatives (e.g., quaternium 15 and imidazolidinyl urea) can cause allergic contact dermatitis. In general, patients tolerate creams and lotions better than ointments, but ointments have adherent properties that enhance penetration. Creams and lotions are more effective in intertriginous or moist areas because of their drying properties. Use ointments on dry skin, because their occlusive properties retard drying. Solutions contain alcohol and are best used on the scalp.

In general, potency correlates with chlorination or fluorination of steroids. Fluorinated, high-potency topical steroids (i.e., class I) are used for the most recalcitrant dermatoses (e.g., ▲ psoriasis) as short term treatment only (Table 63-6). **Never use class I steroids on the face**. Fluorinated steroids are used in the treatment of these disorders because of their antimitotic, antiinflammatory, antipruritic, and vasoconstrictive actions. Switch the patient to less potent steroids before stopping treatment to minimize the risk of rebound flare of the disease.

Class I steroids are also the most likely to cause permanent atrophy, telangiectasia, purpura, striae, and acneiform eruptions. Thin-skinned areas are particularly susceptible to the development of atrophy. Purpura can be seen on the dorsal aspect of the forearms and hands with long-term use of potent corticosteroids. Allergic contact dermatitis, burning sensations, dryness, itching, hypopigmentation, facial hirsutism, folliculitis, moon facies, and alopecia (usually of the scalp) are also possible. Other adverse effects include overgrowth of bacteria, fungi, and viruses, and immunosuppression. When potent steroids are used topically for long periods over broken skin, or under occlusion, systemic absorption resulting in hypothalamic-pituitary-adrenal (HPA) axis suppression can occur.

Classes II through V steroids can be used on open skin areas for up to several months without concern but are to be avoided in intertriginous areas. The weakest classes, VI and VII, are generally safe on the face and in intertriginous areas.

Occasionally, when recalcitrant dermatoses are of limited size, the use of intralesional steroids (e.g., betamethasone valerate [Celestone] or triamcinolone acetonide [Kenalog]) can be helpful. Skin atrophy is a risk whenever intralesional steroids are used.

Emollients and Lubricants
Emollients and lubricants are oily or fatty substances used to keep the skin soft and to prevent water evaporation. They lubricate psoriatic plaques, for example, thereby easing the removal of scales and reducing formation of fissures in intertriginous areas. Mineral oil, lanolin, or petrolatum is used to relieve pruritus and skin dryness. Emollients are best applied after the skin has been exposed to water through a bath, shower, or soak. Even dry skin absorbs some moisture through gentle bathing, especially if soap is avoided.

The most common adverse effects of emollients and ▲ lubricants is excessive greasiness of the skin and an increased incidence of acne. Other adverse effects of emollients and lubricants are related specifically to the active ingredient in the formulation.

Keratolytics
Keratolytics, such as salicylic acid and urea, soften scales and loosen the horny layer of skin. They are used in the treatment of warts, corns, calluses, and other keratin-containing skin lesions. Some of the products are sold over the counter.

Patients may have hypersensitivity reactions to keratolytics, and the products may burn skin or cause excessive desquamation if the preparation is too concentrated and/or gets on neighboring intact skin. Renal damage has been reported in patients using cantharidin and podophyllin. **Do not use keratolytics ▲ on reddened, irritated skin or on any area that is infected, or if the patient has uncontrolled diabetes mellitus or poor peripheral circulation.**

Proteolytic Enzymes
Proteolytic enzymes (e.g., fibrinolysin [Elase]) are used to chemically débride burn wounds, decubitus ulcers, and venous stasis ulcers. Enzymatic débridement removes sloughing tissue and helps facilitate granulation of the wound. **To ▲ prevent delayed healing, discontinue the proteolytic enzyme when the wound is clean and healthy, pink, granulation tissue is present.** Surgical débridement may be required if a decubitus ulcer is very serious or if complications, such as osteomyelitis, are present. Surgical skin closure or grafting may be required after chemical débridement.

Adverse effects of proteolytic enzymes consist of mild, transient pain, paresthesias, bleeding, and transient dermatitis. Even with high concentrations, adverse effects are minimal,

TABLE **63-6** Potency of Selected Topical Corticosteroids

Vasoconstrictive Potency*	Formulation
GROUP I—HIGHEST-POTENCY STEROIDS (FOR MODERATE TO SEVERE ATOPIC DERMATITIS)	
Augmented betamethasone dipropionate 0.05% (Diprolene)	Ointment, lotion, gel, cream
clobetasol propionate 0.05% (Temovate)	Cream, ointment, solution
halobetasol propionate 0.05% (Ultravate)	Cream, ointment
GROUP II—HIGH-POTENCY STEROIDS	
amcinonide 0.1% (Cyclocort)	Ointment, lotion
betamethasone dipropionate 0.05% (Diprosone, Maxivate)	Ointment
desoximetasone 0.25% (Topicort)	Cream, ointment
fluocinonide 0.05% (Lidex)	Cream, gel, ointment
halcinonide 0.1% (Halog)	Cream
GROUP III—MEDIUM-HIGH–POTENCY STEROID	
amcinonide 0.1% (Cyclocort)	Cream
betamethasone dipropionate 0.05% (Diprosone, Maxivate)	Cream
diflorasone diacetate 0.05% (Florone, Maxiflor, Psorcon)	Cream
fluticasone propionate 0.05% ointment (Cutivate)	Ointment
GROUP IV—MEDIUM-POTENCY STEROIDS (for eczema or resistant rashes)	
flurandrenolide 0.05% (Cordran)	Ointment
hydrocortisone valerate 0.2% (Westcort)	Ointment
mometasone furoate 0.1% (Elocon)	Cream
triamcinolone acetonide 0.1% (Aristocort, Kenalog)	Ointment
GROUP V—LOW-POTENCY STEROIDS (for eczema or resistant rashes)	
alclometasone dipropionate 0.05% (Aclovate)	Ointment
betamethasone valerate 0.1% (Beta-Val)	Cream
flurandrenolide 0.05% (Cordran)	Cream
fluocinolone acetonide 0.025% (Synalar)	Cream
hydrocortisone butyrate 0.1% (Locoid)	Cream
hydrocortisone valerate 0.2% (Westcort)	Cream
triamcinolone acetonide 0.1% (Kenalog)	Lotion
GROUP VI—MILD-POTENCY STEROIDS (for facial dermatitis or rashes)	
desonide 0.05% (Desowen)	Cream, lotion, ointment
fluocinolone acetonide 0.01% (Synalar)	Cream, solution
GROUP VII—LOWEST-POTENCY STEROIDS (for facial dermatitis or rashes)	
dexamethasone 0.1% (Decadron)	Gel
hydrocortisone 0.5%, 1%, 2.5% (Hytone, Synacort)	Cream, ointment, lotion

*It is recommended that one become familiar with and use one drug from each category, making the selection on the basis of cost, cosmetic acceptability, and efficacy.
Adapted from Goroll, A., May, L., and Mulley, A. (1995). *Primary care medicine: Office evaluation and management of the adult patient* (p. 907). Philadelphia: JB Lippincott. Used with permission.

primarily consisting of local hyperemia. Adverse effects severe enough to warrant discontinuation of therapy are rare. No systemic toxicity has been observed as a result of topical application of proteolytic enzymes.

Astringents

Astringents (e.g., aluminum and zinc salts) are generally classified as ineffective; only aluminum acetate (Burow's solution) and witch hazel are recognized by the FDA. They promote drying through vasoconstriction and coagulating proteins on cell surfaces, which reduces weeping and helps exudates crust over. The adverse effects of astringents are related to the degree of vasoconstriction produced by the drug and the frequency of use.

Sunscreens

Sunlight causes skin damage with continued exposure. Sunburn does not have to occur for damage to the skin to take place. In addition to the risk of sunburn and skin cancers, signs of premature aging appear; these include wrinkling, and in time, an almost leathery appearance of the skin

develops. It is also thought that excessive UV exposure may disturb the body's immune system.

Sunscreens are an important component of a total program aimed at reducing the harmful effects of the sun. The first component is to limit sun exposure and wear protective clothing. The sun protection factor (SPF) numbers on sunscreens and cosmetics supply information on how long one can stay in the sun without burning.

The majority of sunscreens contain two basic active ingredients. "Reflectants" (i.e., inorganic agents such as talc, titanium dioxide, zinc oxide) physically block UVA and UVB rays. Unfortunately, products containing reflectants have been thick, opaque ointments usually reserved for skin areas at high risk of burn, such as the nose. However, more cosmetically acceptable formulations are now in the marketplace. Some moisturizers now contain the reflectant ingredients of sunscreens.

"Chemical absorbers" (i.e., organic compounds such as oxybenzone and dioxybenzone, aminobenzoates, camphor derivatives, cinnamates, and salicylates) block UVB rays. Chemical absorbers are weak absorbers of UV light rays, but are highly water-insoluble, and hypersensitivity to the product or its ingredients is rare. The salicylate ingredients, octylsalicylate and homosalate, provide modest protection against UVB light. Even when used in high concentrations, they are among the safest sunscreens. However, they adhere poorly to the skin and must be reapplied often.

Para-aminobenzoic acid (PABA), an ingredient in early sunscreens, was often associated with photosensitivity and contact reactions, had a poor consistency, and frequently discolored clothing. It is rarely found in sunscreens today. The acid esters (octyl dimethyl para-aminobenzoic acid) of PABA that are now used instead in many sunscreens seem to be devoid of the photosensitivity and contact reactions found with PABA.

CLINICAL REASONING

Treatment Objectives
Prevention is a key objective to controlling dermatologic disorders. That said, general treatment objectives for the patient with a skin disorder include identifying and removing the cause (when possible). Additional objectives may include restoring, protecting, and maintaining normal structure and function of the skin, reducing inflammation, reducing scales and calluses, cleansing and débriding, eradicating microorganisms, and providing symptom relief.

Treatment Options
There are many topical drugs and formulations used to prevent or manage the many dermatoses. The decision as to which drugs to use for dermatoses include the following variables: (1) whether the lesion is dry or moist, pruritic, or inflammatory; (2) any presence of an infectious agent; and (3) the location and spread of the lesions. **In general, it is better for the health care provider to be thoroughly familiar with a few dermatologic drugs and treatment methods than to attempt to use many forms.** Naturally, the course of some endogenous skin diseases cannot be altered. However, steps can be taken to prevent their occurrence and to minimize their effects.

Patient Variables
At every pharmacy, the cost to the patient for drugs is calculated using a specific formula. Usually, a pharmacy charge is added to the result. One large prescription is usually less costly (although not necessarily inexpensive) than the same amount of drug given using refills because the pharmacy charge is added to each refill. This may be particularly true with inexpensive drugs, when the pharmacy charge composes most of the patient cost.

The Norton scale or the Braden Scale for Predicting Pressure Sore Risk can help identify patients and the specific factors that place them at risk for decubitus ulcers. **All patients at risk for decubitus ulcers should undergo a thorough and systematic skin examination at least once daily, or at each office visit, particularly concentrating on any bony prominences.**

Life-Span Considerations
Pregnant and Nursing Women. Alterations in hormonal balance, mechanical stretching of tissues, and stress are responsible for melasma (chloasma), the mask of pregnancy. Dependent on sun exposure, it is caused by increased melanin and appears as a blotchy, brownish tone to the skin over the cheeks and the forehead of some women. *Striae gravidarum*

(stretch marks) may also appear. Vascular abnormalities can cause spider angiomas and palmar erythema. Oily skin, acne, hirsutism, and fingernail changes are other skin abnormalities sometimes seen during pregnancy.

Children and Adolescents. Children are at increased risk for systemic toxicity from topically applied drugs for two reasons. First, because of the child's greater surface–area to weight ratio, a given amount of applied drug represents a greater dose (mg/kg) compared with the same amount given to an adult. Secondly, at least in preterm neonates, the permeability of the skin is increased (see Chapter 7).

The most common skin disease of the adolescent is acne, which can be devastating. Acne and the associated hormonal changes in adolescents are accompanied by feelings of self-doubt and self-consciousness. When dealing with an adolescent with skin problems, body-image considerations become a basic part of the treatment care plan (see Controversy box).

Older Adults. Physiologic changes of aging affect the skin. Progressive impairment of the peripheral vascular circulation alters the cutaneous response to physical trauma, cold, and infection. In contrast to the skin of children and adolescents, the skin of older adults is less permeable to drugs, perhaps because of the altered lipid content and loss of subcutaneous tissue (see Chapter 8). Changes in the central nervous system (CNS) modify the perception of itching and pain, and atrophy of the reticuloendothelial system may impair the immune response. Also, emotional factors are certainly important and may prolong or exacerbate a skin disorder.

Drug Variables
The most effective results are obtained when the degree of moisturizing or drying associated with a specific drug is tailored to the patient's skin type. The most effective topical drug is the one that produces just enough moisture or dryness to meet the patient's needs. **A general principle to follow in regard to what formulation to use when treating dermatoses is this: "If the lesion is wet, dry it. If the lesion is dry, wet it!"**

Figure 63-3 provides an overview of the continuum of topical bases and demonstrates the range of OTC products on the market today. The formulation used for the base affects potency and cosmetic acceptability. A description of the various vehicles and formulations can be found in Table 63-7.

Because there are a vast number of preparations and formulations available, it would be impossible to discuss them all. Further, not all generic topical drugs are equivalent to their brand-name counterparts, either in potency (due to differences in vehicle), or in the presence of ingredients that may cause irritation or allergy. When in doubt about the proper method of treatment or the quantity to prescribe, it is generally considered prudent to undertreat rather than overtreat the disorder. **The following quantities provide a guideline for how much topical drug to prescribe:**

- **45 grams for the hands or feet**
- **60 to 90 grams for one arm or leg**
- **60 to 90 grams for the trunk**
- **360 to 450 grams or more for coverage of entire body**

Application frequency depends on the site, response to the drug, and the application technique. Use less potent formulations on thin-skinned and/or cosmetically important areas such as the face, the dorsum of the hands, the groin, the scrotum, and the axillae, because of the risk of atrophy and striae

SENSORY

CASE STUDY   Dermatologic Drugs

ASSESSMENT

History of Present Illness	MZ is a 62-year-old retired horticulturist who comes to be seen at the office this Friday afternoon with complaints of periorbital redness, itching, and weeping and a red, irritated rash on the inside of her forearms for the last 48 hours. She thinks it is poison ivy. She rubbed her face and eyes 2 days ago while she had her work gloves on. She was pulling weeds and putting in new plants in the neighborhood park that morning. She denies any visual changes. She had one other mild episode with similar characteristics about 2 months ago while she was on vacation, which she treated with Calamine lotion. Character of lesions and distribution has not changed. Current drugs: hydrochlorothiazide 25 mg PO daily for mild hypertension.
Past Health History	MZ denies history of drug or food allergies but has a family history of asthma. She has mild "seasonal hay fever."
Life-Span Considerations	MZ is a widow; her husband died in battle in the Afghanistan mountains within the last year. She volunteers as a landscaper occasionally during busy seasonal periods and fills in when other employees are on vacation. She enjoys sewing in her shop at home and refinishing furniture, and spends Sunday afternoons leading children's tours at the botanical garden.
Physical Exam Findings	Afebrile. Erythematous blotches over forehead, periorbital region, and cheeks. No vesicular lesions noted. Bilateral forearms from wrists to elbows covered with papules, vesicles, bullae with surrounding erythema. Crusting and oozing are present with evidence of scratching and secondary infection. No evidence of systemic involvement.
Diagnostic Testing	Facial lesions cultured *Staphylococcus aureus,* characteristic of cellulitis of the face.

DIAGNOSIS: Contact dermatitis

MANAGEMENT

Treatment Objectives	1. Identify, avoid, and/or remove allergen. 2. Reduce severity of pruritus. 3. Eradicate existing infection. 4. Reduce inflammatory process and risk for further infection. 5. Promote comfort.
Treatment Options	**Pharmacotherapy** • methylprednisolone acetate 60 mg IM as single dose now • prednisone taper per written instructions (i.e., 50 mg today, 40 mg tomorrow, 30 mg for 2 days, 20 mg for 3 days, and 10 mg for 4 days) • dicloxacillin 500 mg PO every 6 hours for 10 days • diphenhydramine OTC at bedtime per package instructions if needed for sleep **Patient Education** 1. Be sure patient has washed thoroughly to remove any residual plant oils 2. Regular, thorough handwashing; gently cleanse lesions as part of normal bathing using a mild, fragrance-free, dye-free cleanser and pat dry 3. Keep hands away from face. Avoid scratching and direct contact with others. 4. Avoid OTC cortisone creams. and do not cover lesions with plastic wrap. To prevent lesion contact with unclean surfaces in the environment, the patient may need to cover lesions on her arms with light, nonadherent, breathable, sterile dressings. 5. Acute nature of lesions and pruritus may lessen in 3 to 4 days, but it may take 2 to 3 weeks before the lesions have resolved. To keep the skin from becoming too dry, light, fragrance-free, dye-free moisturizer or OTC antibiotic cream (without neomycin) may have to be sparingly applied later in the lesions' progression as the vesicles crust over and dry out. 6. Cleanse all clothing, linens, and surfaces that have been in contact with patient; consider disposing of boots worn at time of exposure. 7. Take dicloxacillin on empty stomach; take prednisone with food as directed until drugs are gone. 8. Adverse effects of antibiotic and steroid 9. Importance of follow-up in office in 24 to 48 hours or sooner if lesions on face worsen

Evaluation

Pruritus is reduced, and secondary infection is improving. Inflammation of lesions on arms and face has lessened. Patient can now identify the plant commonly associated with poison ivy exposure and vows to avoid it in the future.

CLINICAL REASONING ANALYSIS

Q1. Why did you use dicloxacillin for MZ? I thought the best treatment for poison ivy was the steroid.

A. I ordered dicloxacillin for MZ because of the secondary infection she has developed from scratching the lesions. According to the *Sanford Guide,* it is one of the drugs of choice for *S. aureus* infection.

Q2. Why did you order a prednisone taper for her rather than a topical steroid? Wouldn't the topical drug have been a safer alternative?

A. Yes, a topical drug would have been a safe alternative. However, since secondary infection is already present, she could potentially spread the infection. And besides, the oral prednisone will be much more effective than a topical given the extent of her lesions.

Q3. I see, but then she shouldn't have needed the steroid shot, right?

A. Perhaps, but I happen to know she is leaving for her home town in Czechoslovakia early next week. It was appropriate to give her a drug that would be 100% bioavailable and would have a long half-life, given that she was leaving the country in 3 days. In this way if something happens and she is unable to complete the steroid taper, she will be covered for inflammation.

Q4. What do you think about her using an OTC like diphenhydramine for sleep? Wouldn't it be better to use a sleeping pill instead?

A. We certainly could consider a sedative-hypnotic for MZ but those drugs have no antipruritic action. We use the diphenhydramine to help her with the itching even though it's primarily to help her sleep.

Q5. Going back to my question on the prednisone. Couldn't she have used a topical steroid and covered the involved areas with plastic wrap to keep the drug from getting on clothing or linens and to keep the rash from spreading? Why does she need a prednisone taper?

A. There are a couple of reasons. The lesions cover a large surface area of her arms, about 9% to be exact. If she used a topical steroid on the lesions and then covered it with an occlusive dressing, she would risk suppression of the HPA axis. Remember, we gave her a methylprednisolone injection as well as an oral prednisone taper. As long as we taper the prednisone and avoid occlusive dressings, the risk of HPA axis suppression is not a major concern.

---

with more potent preparations. Restrict use of the highest-potency corticosteroids to no more than 45 grams/week for no longer than 2 weeks. Retention of the drug in the stratum corneum makes one to two applications per day sufficient. For children, preparations in the low-potent or mildly potent category of preparations are recommended.

Many patients use OTC skin care products such as moisturizers, cleansers, and sunscreens. Sometimes these products are optimal for the patient's skin type and are compatible with topical drugs. However, many times this is not the case. For example, oily moisturizers used by patients with acne are likely to undermine the beneficial effect that would be obtained from drying agents. Although the effectiveness of the drying agent could still be achieved without taking this factor into consideration, better outcomes can be achieved when the use of both products is coordinated with the patient's skin type.

Patient Education

It is vital for the patient to understand the importance of handwashing. Good hygiene of the unaffected areas of the body should be maintained and the affected area cleansed only in the prescribed fashion. Advise the patient to avoid touching the affected areas as much as possible and to dress in a manner that will minimize contact with the involved area.

Teach patients with dry or irritated skin that soaps, strong cleansers, and detergents should be used only in the axillae and the groin and on the feet. Unless the patient's occupation exposes him or her to excessive soiling, most patients need not use soap on all body surfaces. When informed, most patients often comply with this restriction rather than to a total ban on soap. Baths containing a small amount of bath oil may be used but are less effective than the application of oils to the skin after bathing.

Teach the patient how to apply the prescribed drug and to continue its use for the recommended time, even if results are not immediate or the symptoms are slow in subsiding. They should be told that acute skin disorders do not clear in 3 to 4 days. In some cases, it can take several weeks or months before significant improvement is noted. However, if the condition worsens, the patient should contact the health care provider. Prudent handwashing prevents self-inoculation of other body parts and minimizes the possibility of spreading the condition to others.

Advise the patient to follow manufacturers' instructions for application of a topical drug and to avoid applying one drug on top of another unless otherwise indicated. Before applying topical drugs, the patient must ensure that dirt, soil, organic matter, or other contaminants are removed from the skin surface. Such materials not only harbor organisms but provide a

SENSORY

Controversy

Dermatologic Drugs

Jonathan J. Wolfe

Drugs used in dermatology are usually unexceptionable. Local anesthetics in small doses make minor surgery tolerable. Doses of epinephrine too small for systemic actions enhance the effect of those anesthetics. Lastly, topical drugs, even those containing potent steroids, represent a low risk when used correctly. Not many systemic medications are regularly used for dermatologic effect. However, the decision to use this last group of drugs demands careful thought and monitoring.

The classic systemic drug taken for dermatologic effect is surely tetracycline. The antibiotic is used at a low dose over a long time for acne treatment. It seems innocuous but may not be so. The female patient taking this drug may also be sexually active and taking oral contraceptives. Controversy remains regarding the theoretical possibility of tetracycline reducing the efficacy of oral contraceptives, although the data do not support an increased risk of pregnancy in women taking tetracycline. Regardless, effective birth control is extremely important for women taking tetracycline or related antibiotics, because tetracycline exposure *in utero* can cause discolored teeth and possibly abnormal bone development to occur in the fetus.

Isotretinoin, an antiacne drug derived from vitamin A, poses a special risk. Again, it is women and neonates who bear most of the risk. Isotretinoin is a known teratogenic agent. Its use in pregnancy is associated with grave birth defects. The sexually active woman who takes this class of drug must not, under any circumstances, become pregnant. The prohibition extends after the drug is stopped until it is fully eliminated (which is a lengthy matter with a lipid-soluble vitamin). The iPLEDGE program for isotretinoin prescribing and dispensing requires women to use birth control for a month before therapy, during it, and for a month afterward.

Sunscreen, although invaluable in skin protection, may offer a false sense of security to the unsuspecting person. The average consumer uses the sun protection factor (SPF) to gauge the strength of the sunscreen. People are quick to understand that the higher the SPF number, the higher the protection. Yet people often associate the increase in SPF with an increase in the amount of the time they can spend in the sun. Sunscreen is not meant to extend time in the sun.

CLINICAL REASONING ANALYSIS

- An 18-year-old female patient suffers from disfiguring cystic acne. She has been taking isotretinoin since she was 17 years old. She now is planning her wedding, but needs to remain on the drug for another 6 months. Her liver tests have remained normal, and her progress is good. She tells you that her fiancé's religion does not permit contraception or abortion. What choices do you have as her caregiver?
- A 15-year-old boy takes 250 mg of tetracycline once daily for moderate to severe acne. He seeks care for a rash that disappears when the drug is discontinued. What alternatives can you suggest for oral antiacne therapy?
- A 22-year-old woman is planning her honeymoon in the Bahamas. She takes 250 mg of tetracycline daily for her moderate acne. She has been sexually active for the past 4 years. You have worked with her to meet her outcome of effective contraception. How can you help assure her that her stay in the tropics will be a happy memory under this regimen?
- An 18-month-old child and her parents just arrived from the north to vacation on Mexico's beaches. The parents have come by the medical clinic at the hotel to inquire about which sunscreen they should use for their child. How will you respond to their inquiry for information?

Moisturizing ◄───────────		Neutral ──────────►			Drying
Oleaginous Bases	Water-in-Oil Emulsions	Oil-in-Water Emulsions	Oil-Free Emulsions with Emollient Esters	Strictly Oil-Free Emulsions	Alcohol Solutions
–	–	–	–	–	–
–	–	–		–	–
–	–	–		Gels	–
–	–	–	–	–	–
–	–	–	–	–	–
Water-Free Products	Oil-Based Products	Water-Based Products	Glycerin/ P.Glycol Bases	Water Solutions	Other Volatile Solutions

FIGURE 63-3 Continuum of Topical Bases. Products to the left in this model become increasingly moisturizing. Products toward the right of the model are increasingly drying. The more moisturizing the product, the greasier it becomes and the less acceptable it is to patients. The ideal product is one that is neither too moisturizing nor too drying. (From Scheman, A., and Severson, D. [1997]. *Pocket guide to medications used in dermatology* [5th ed., p. 6]. Baltimore: Williams & Wilkins. Used with permission.)

physical barrier that restricts access of the drug to the skin and may chemically inactivate specific agents. Water and mild soap is usually sufficient with the lesions cleansed (except for burns) during ordinary bathing activity.

▌▌▌ Sunscreens

Sun damage can be minimized by avoiding long periods in the sun; wearing loose, tight-weave, light clothing covering as much of the body as possible; wearing a hat; and using a sunscreen (Box 63-1). The best way to choose a sunscreen is by skin type, the length of time to be spent in the sun, the usual intensity of the sun in the patient's geographic area, and the formulation preferred. Sunscreen products are labeled in terms of SPF. The higher the SPF value, the greater the protection; however, the SPF number applies to UVB rays only. Suncreens typically offer protection against UVA rays at approximately 10% of the UVB rating. Nevertheless, the patient should not depend on sunscreens to prevent against skin cancer—covering up is essential. Advise the patient not to use tanning beds at a tanning salon or at home.

▌▌▌ Prevention and Treatment of Decubitus Ulcers

The most effective way to treat a decubitus ulcer is to prevent it in the first place. Skin care should be individualized, but at a minimum, skin should be cleansed regularly and when soiled. Inform the patient of the environmental factors (i.e., low humidity and exposure to cold) that can result in dry skin. Patients should avoid massage over bony prominences as well as exposure to moisture due to incontinence, perspiration, or wound drainage. The use of proper positioning, transferring, and turning techniques minimizes skin injury due to friction and shearing forces. Adequate protein and calorie intake are necessary to promote tissue integrity and healing. Nutritional supplements or support should be available as required. Institute rehabilitation efforts as early as possible in the treatment regimen.

Evaluation

How fast skin lesions heal is dependent upon the patient's general health, which determines the amount of natural

TABLE 63-7 Vehicles and Formulations*

Vehicle	Physical Characteristics	Advantages and Disadvantages	Examples
Ointments	Active ingredients in a semisolid preparation built on a fatty base (such as petrolatum or lanolin), or a nongreasy base (such as a white petrolatum with aqueous propylene glycol emulsion)†	*Advantages:* Very moisturizing owing to thick barrier that prevents water loss. Best reserved for thick, scaling, or keratotic lesions. Prolonged, protective action when applied at night *Disadvantages:* Greasier than creams. Not suitable on hairy or intertriginous areas or on oozing surfaces. Clog pores. See lanolin warning below.	Augmented betamethasone dipropionate 0.05% ointment (Diprolene), acyclovir 5% ointment (Zovirax), antibiotic first-aid ointments (Neosporin, Bacitracin), Aquaphor, Whitfield's ointment
Emollients	Formulations based on fixed oils such as olive oil, cotton seed, or flaxseed (i.e., any cream or ointment that softens skin by trapping water)	*Advantages:* Keep skin soft. Prevent evaporation of water and development of dryness. *Disadvantages:* Avoid lanolin-based drugs if allergic to wool.	Lanolin, petrolatum, vitamin A and D creams and ointments, vitamin E oil, cream, liquid, ointment, Lubriderm, Nivea Moisturizing Creme
Creams (solid emulsions)	Active ingredients incorporated into water-in-oil or oil-in-water emulsions. "Vanishing creams" are generally oil-in-water emulsions; water evaporates and the cream "vanishes" when rubbed in	*Advantages:* Good for daytime use, particularly with potent active ingredients that are effective when rubbed into oozing, denuded surfaces	Hydrocortisone 1% cream, AmLactin 12% cream (ammonium lactate)
Lotions (liquid emulsions)	Powdered active ingredients suspended in oil or water. Require shaking to disperse ingredients	*Advantages:* Best suited for hairy areas or wet and oozing lesions. Protect and cool acutely inflamed areas on face and on hairy body surfaces *Disadvantages:* Are more drying than creams	Calamine lotion (Caladryl); benzoyl peroxide 5% lotion
Solutions (aqueous) or tinctures (alcohol solutions)	Active ingredients incorporated into liquid containing water or alcohol as solvent	*Advantages:* Mildly drying owing to a slow evaporation of water *Disadvantages:* Alcohol solutions are very drying; ethanol and other low–molecular weight alcohols are volatile and rapidly evaporate	Aluminum acetate (Burow's solution), Dakin's solution
Pastes	Ointments into which relatively larger amounts of powders are mixed (e.g., zinc oxide, starch, talc)	*Advantages:* Prolonged protective and occlusive action. Porous. Permit heat to escape from skin *Disadvantages:* Not suited for hairy surfaces or on oozing areas	Zinc oxide paste
Powders	Materials in fine particles for dusting on surfaces	*Advantages:* Absorb moisture and reduce friction from large areas. Exert cooling or protective effects *Disadvantages:* Irritation of respiratory tract in susceptible adults and small children	Pedi-Dri powder (nystatin), talcum powder, Zeasorb-AF powder (miconazole 2%)
Gels	Semisolid product of precipitated or coagulated colloid. Contain large amounts of water. Deposit film of active ingredients on skin	*Advantages:* Used on hairy areas and smooth skin *Disadvantages:* Somewhat drying when used on nonhairy areas	Augmented betamethasone dipropionate 0.05% gel (Diprolene Gel), Coppertone Aloe Vera gel
Rubs (semisolid) and liniments (liquid)	Preparations intended to be rubbed into the skin; liniments have higher proportions of oil (fixed or volatile) than ordinary lotions or solutions. Often contain counterirritants such as methyl salicylate, camphor, oil of cloves, capsaicin	*Advantages:* Pain relief on intact skin. May include antiseptic, analgesic, anesthetic additives. Formulated as gel, cream, lotions, or ointment *Disadvantages:* Ingredients irritating to abraded skin. Some preparations greasy	Vicks VapoRub, Myoflex Creme, Ben-Gay, Aspercreme Rub lotion, Heet liniment
Colloidal baths and emollient bath oils	Added to bath water to decrease the drying effect of water	*Advantages:* Soothing to irritated skin and helps relieve itching *Disadvantages:* Bathtub may become slippery, increasing the risk for falls	Alpha Keri bath oil, Aveeno Daily Moisturizing Bath, Aveeno Soothing Bath
Soaps	Sodium salts of palmitic, oleic, and stearic fatty acids. Made by mixing fats or oils with alkalis. Consistency depends on the acid and the alkali used	*Advantages:* Some contain antiseptics but only work to the degree to which they mechanically clean the skin *Disadvantages:* Dry and irritating if used excessively	Yardley Aloe-Vera soap, Boraxo powdered hand soap
Cleansers	Contain emollient substance with pH adjusted to neutral or slightly acidic	*Advantages:* For persons with sensitive, dry, or irritated skin, or those who have had a previous reaction to a soap product *Disadvantages:* May contain soaps	Aveeno Cleansing Bar, Phisoderm, Lowila Cake
Hydrocolloid dressings	Composed of hydrophilic granules embedded in polymer base. Absorb water from wound to form protective gel	*Advantages:* Stimulate tissue granulation. Breathable. Exclude bacteria. Waterproof. Easy application. Reduce pain; nonstick. Permits less frequent changes than ordinary dressings	DuoDerm, Restore, Ultec
Transparent dressings	Thin, polyurethane adhesive dressings. Permeable to vapor and gas. Support cellular regeneration	*Advantages:* Wound visible. Exclude bacteria. Breathable. Waterproof. Good adhesion. Cost-effective. Infrequent changes. *Disadvantages:* Nonabsorbent. Difficult to apply. Limited to superficial lesions	Tegaderm, Opsite

*It is recommended that one become familiar with and use one drug from each category, making the selection on the basis of cost, cosmetic acceptability, and efficacy. This table reflects vasoconstrictive potency rating, not USP potency rating (different scale: low, medium, high, very high).

†To make it easier to understand, one could say "built on a fatty or greasy base" because even the "nongreasy" preps might more accurately be called "less greasy."

Adapted from Goroll, A., and Mulley, A. (2005). *Primary care medicine: Office evaluation and management of the adult patient* (5th ed.). Philadelphia: Lippincott, Williams & Wilkins.

SENSORY

BOX 63-1

"Slip, Slop, and Slap"*

- **DO** cover skin with protective clothing and wear a wide-brimmed hat outdoors.
- **DO** wear 100% UV-protective sunglasses to protect against cataract development.
- **DO** apply sunscreen liberally to all exposed parts of the skin, including scalp (if hair is thin or very short), eyelids, ears, nose, and neck.
- **DO** use a sunscreen-containing lip balm—many patients good about using sunscreen lotions neglect their lips entirely.
- **DO** avoid sun exposure between the peak hours of 10 AM and 3 PM. Sunlight reflects off sand, snow, ice, and concrete, increasing direct sunlight exposure by 10% to 50%. Remember, the intensity of sunlight at 5000 feet elevation is 20% greater than at sea level.

- **DO** Apply sunscreens 30 minutes to 1 hour before sun exposure to allow absorption into the skin. Reapply after swimming, sweating, and every 2 hours while in the sun. Even sunscreens labeled as "waterproof" or "water resistant" are removed by toweling and perspiration.
- **DO** apply sunscreen on cloudy days. Though often forgotten, UV rays, and especially UVA rays, can cause skin damage even on cloudy days.
- **DO** use a sunscreen when photosensitizing drugs such as tetracyclines are used.
- **DO** take supplements, not megadoses, of vitamin D_3 and β-carotene as necessary. The absorption of vitamin D is impaired with the use of sunscreens.

*Adapted from the "Slip, Slop, Slap" slogan of an Australian skin cancer prevention campaign. The campaign recommends that anyone out in the sun *slip* on a shirt, *slop* on sunscreen, and *slap* on a hat.
UV, Ultraviolet; UVA, ultraviolet A.

---

resources that the body can provide for healing. The frail older adult or those under stress from other health conditions will require a longer healing time. Most importantly, however: ordinarily they will heal.

Acute skin lesions should decrease in severity and eventually disappear when treatment has been successful. However, it should be noted that acute skin lesions do not resolve in 3 to 4 days. They require time and frequent observation. Chronic skin conditions, some decubitus ulcers, and severe burns may take weeks to months or even years to heal. Recording changes helps determine progress toward achieving the desired outcome or resolution of the skin disorder. Furthermore, because the affected area is visible, drug therapy can be directly and continuously monitored, although not always quantitatively.

KEY POINTS

- The primary function of the epidermis is to retard the loss of fluids from the inner body to the outside environment and to shield the inner body from environmental pathogens and chemicals. The dermis contributes to the support and nourishment of the epidermis. Subcutaneous tissues insulate the body from cold, cushion deep tissues from trauma, and serve as a reserve source of calories.
- Noninfectious, inflammatory dermatoses include atopic dermatitis, contact dermatitis, seborrheic dermatitis, urticaria, psoriasis, pityriasis rosea, and lichen planus.
- Infectious, inflammatory dermatoses include bacterial, fungal, and viral infections.
- Drug reactions can manifest as a variety of skin disorders including local and diffuse lesions as well as life-threatening systemic reactions.
- Infestations and insect bites are potential causes of skin lesions with reactions that range from redness and itching to anaphylaxis.
- Decubitus ulcers have been considered as trauma given the associated shearing forces and friction, and the pressure exerted on bony prominences.
- Topical drug classifications include antimicrobials (antibiotics, antivirals, antifungals), antiseptics, antiinflammatory drugs, astringents, emollients and lubricants, proteolytic enzymes, keratolytics, and sunscreens.
- Adverse effects of topical drugs range from local drying, pruritus, urticaria, erythema, blistering, and peeling to systemic effects such as Stevens-Johnson syndrome and anaphylaxis.

- Factors influencing the absorption of topical dermatologic drugs include the degree of skin hydration and humidity, occlusion, drug concentration, and the site of administration.
- Management of the patient with a dermatologic disorder may require monitoring of systemic laboratory parameters as well as monitoring of the lesions.
- General treatment objectives for the patient with a skin disorder include prevention, identifying and removing the cause, restoring and maintaining normal structure and function of the skin, and providing symptom relief.
- Become thoroughly familiar with a few dermatologic drugs and treatment methods rather than attempting to use many.
- Educate patients and their families as to the cause of the skin disorder and how to minimize its recurrence and spread to other body surfaces or other persons.
- Clear instructions regarding application of the topical dermatologic drug should be provided. Adherence with the plan of care will improve with documented patient understanding of the regimen.
- Subacute skin lesions should decrease in size and severity and eventually disappear when treatment has been successful. Chronic skin conditions, some decubitus ulcers, and severe burns may take weeks to months or even years to heal.

Bibliography

Agency for Healthcare Research and Quality (AHRQ). (2006) Number of patients with pressure sores increasing. *Medscape Business of Medicine.* 7(1). Available online: http://hcup.ahrq.gov/HCUPnet.asp. Accessed June 2, 2007.

Berardi, R. (2004). *Handbook of nonprescription drugs* (14th ed.). Washington, DC: American Pharmaceutical Association.

Barankin, B., and Freiman, A. (2006). *Derm notes: Dermatology clinical pocket guide.* Philadelphia: FA Davis.

Centers for Disease Control and Prevention. (2005). Methicillin-resistant *Staphylococcus aureus* (MRSA) information for clinicians. Available online: www.cdc.gov/ncidod/dhqp/ar_mrsa_ca_clinicials.html. Accessed June 2, 2007.

DiPiro, J., Talbert, R., Yee, G., et al. (2005). *Pharmacotherapy: A pathophysiologic approach* (6th ed.). New York: McGraw-Hill.

Freedberg, I., Eisen, Z., Wolff, K., et al. (Eds.). (2003). *Fitzpatrick's dermatology in general medicine* (5th ed., *Vol. 1*). New York: McGraw-Hill.

Gilbert, D., Moellering, R., Eliopoulos, G., et al (2007). *The Sanford guide to antimicrobial therapy* (37th ed.). Hyde Park: VT: Antimicrobial Therapy.

Hardman, J., Limbird, L., and Gilman, A. (Eds.). (2001). *Goodman and Gilman's the pharmacologic basis of therapeutics* (10th ed.). New York: McGraw-Hill.

Lindow, K., Shelestak, D., and Lappin, J. (2005). Perceptions of self in persons with rosacea. *Dermatology Nursing, 17*(4), 249–254.

National Rosacea Society. (2005). Rosacea often affects patients' social lives, new survey finds. Rosacea Review, Summer 2005. Available online: www.rosacea.org/rr/2005/summer/article_3.php. Accessed June 2, 2007.

Panel on the Prediction and Prevention of Pressure Ulcers in Adults. (May 1992). *Pressure ulcers in adults: Prediction and prevention. Quick reference guide for clinicians.* AHCPR Publication No. 92-0050. Rockville, MD: Agency for Health Care Policy and Research. Public Health Service, U.S. Department of Health and Human Services.

Scheinfield, N. (2006). Schools of pharmacology: Retinoid update. *Journal of Drugs in Dermatology, 5*(9), 921–922.

Title 21 of the Code of Federal Regulations (CFR), Part 352, Sunscreen drug products for over-the-counter human use. Available online:http://www.access.gpo.gov/nara/cfr/waisidx_07/21cfr352_07.html. Accessed July 30, 2007.

van Zuuren, E., Gupta, A., Gover, M., et al. (2007). Systematic review of rosacea treatments. *Journal of the American Academy of Dermatology, 56*(1), 107–115.

Wolff, K., Johnson, R., and Suurmond, R. (2005). *Fitzpatrick's color atlas and synopsis of clinical dermatology* (5th ed.). New York: McGraw-Hill.

SENSORY

Index

Note: Page numbers followed by f, indicate
figures; t, tables; and b, boxes.

Pituitary hormone inhibitor drugs, 1039–1040
    clinical reasoning for, 1041, 1042
    dosages for, 1038t
    drug interactions with, 1037t
    pharmacokinetics of, 1036t
Pituitary hormones, 1033–1034, 1034t
Pityriasis rosea, 1158
pKa value, 40
Placebos
    in clinical trials, 3
    for pain management, 237, 240
    response to, 67
Placenta, properties of 73–75, 74f.
        See also Fetal-placental pharmacokinetics.
Plague, 599
Plan B (levonorgestrel), 1079–1080, 1079t,
    1084t, 1092
Planning vs. management, 17b
Plants. See also Herbal remedies.
    medicinal, 2, 137, 140
    poisonous, 182b, 187
Plaque
    atherosclerotic, 665–666, 666f, 737, 771
    neuritic, 203
    skin, 1157f
Plaquenil (hydroxychloroquine), 264t, 265t,
    266t, 268, 271, 566
Plasma volume in pregnancy, 70, 72
Plasmids, bacterial, 461, 604
Plasmodium species, 564, 567
Platelets
    antineoplastic drug effects on, 626–627, 643,
        644t
    in hemostasis, 753, 756f
    in inflammatory response, 246
Platinol, Platinol AQ (cisplatin), 627, 628t, 629,
    630t, 631–632, 631t, 644t
Plavix (clopidogrel), 679, 757t, 759t, 761t, 763–
    765, 768
Plenaxis (abarelix), 640
Plendil (felodipine), 668t, 669t, 670t, 672–673,
    716
Plicamycin, 636–637
    drug interactions with, 632t
    indications for, 629t
    for osteoporosis, 1005t, 1006t, 1008t, 1026–
        1027
    pharmacokinetics of, 630t
PMS-Benztropine (benztropine), 430t, 432t,
    434–435, 437t, 441
PMS-Chlorate Hydrate (chloral hydrate), 307t,
    308t, 309t, 310–311
PMS-Dicitra (sodium citrate), 846
PMS-Isoniazid. See Isoniazid.
PMS-Propranolol (propranolol), 685t, 686t,
    689t, 690t, 694–695
PMS-Pyrazinamide (pyrazinamide), 536–541,
    538t, 539t, 540t, 544–545
PMS Sulfasalazine (sulfasalazine), 264t, 265t,
    266t, 268–269, 271
Pneumococcal disease, 587
Pneumococcal vaccine, 581t, 587
Pneumococcal 7-valent, 581t
Pneumonia
    enfuvirtide and, 506
    lipid, mineral oil aspiration and, 882, 883
    pneumococcal, 581t, 587

Pneumonitis
    antineoplastic drugs and, 634, 636–637
    inhaled anesthetics and, 294
Pneumovax 23 (pneumococcal vaccine), 581t,
    587
Pnu-Imune 23 (pneumococcal vaccine), 581t
Podofilox, 1163
Podophyllin, 1163
Poison control centers, 183, 184b
Poisondex, 184
Poisoning or overdose, 182–188
    amphetamine, 165, 187
    antidotes for, 185, 186–187, 186t
    barbiturate, 170
    benzodiazepine, 172
    caffeine, 164
    cyanide, 106, 718b
    epidemiology and etiology of, 182
    evaluation of, 187
    nicotine, 163
    opioid, 169–170, 184, 187
    patient education for, 187
    toxidromes in, 183–184, 184b
    treatment objectives for, 182–183
    treatment options for, 183–187
Poison Prevention Packaging Act (PPPA), 183
Poisons, 182
    examples of, 182b
    identification of, 184–185
Polifeprosan 20 with carmustine implant, 627,
    628t, 629, 631–632
Poliomyelitis, 587–588
Poliovirus vaccines, 581t, 587–588, 594t
Polocaine (mepivacaine), 279, 282t, 284
Polycarbophil, 875–876, 877t, 878t
Polyclonal antibodies, 604
Polycystic ovary syndrome, 1075, 1107
Polydrug drug abuse, 159b
Polyene antifungals, 518–519, 518b
    action of, 519f
    dosages for, 523t
    drug interactions with, 522t
    pharmacokinetics of, 520t
Polyethylene glycol, 185–186
Polymenorrhea, 1075
Polymerases, viral, 490
Polymorphism, genetic, 66
Polymyxin + neomycin, otic, 1146–1147
Polymyxins, action of, 461f
Polypeptide antibiotics, ophthalmic, 1126b
Polypharmacy
    among older adults, 97–98
    drug response and, 67
    poisoning related to, 183
Polysaccharide-based vaccines, 580, 583
Polystyrene glycol electrolyte solution, 877t,
    878t, 880, 883
Polyvinyl alcohol, ophthalmic, 1139
Pontocaine (tetracaine), 279, 282t, 283, 1139
Porin, bacterial, 462
Pork insulin, 979
Pork tapeworm, 556t
Porphyria
    carisoprodol and, 376–377
    fosphenytoin and, 409
Posaconazole, 520t, 521–522, 523t
Positive symptoms of schizophrenia, 348, 349b

Postantibiotic effects, 474, 486
Posterior pituitary hormone replacement
        drugs, 1037–1039
    clinical reasoning for, 1041, 1042
    dosages for, 1038t
    drug interactions with, 1037t
    pharmacokinetics of, 1036t
Posterior pituitary hormones, 1033–1034,
    1034t
Postexposure prophylaxis for HIV, 511, 512t
Postganglionic neurons, 189, 191f, 192f
Postherpetic neuralgia, 1160
Postmarketing surveillance, 4
Postoperative nausea and vomiting, 904
Postoperative pain, analgesia for, 234,
    235b–236b
Postpartum depression, 332, 334
Postpartum hemorrhage
    ergot alkaloids for, 1100
    prostaglandins for, 1098–1099
Postpartum hypopituitarism, 1003, 1107
Postrenal failure, 834, 835f
Posttraumatic stress disorder (PTSD), 300t, 301
Postural instability in Parkinson's disease, 428,
    438
Potassium 132, 908, 909f.
        See also Hyperkalemia; Hypokalemia.
Potassium-sparing diuretics, 804–806
    combination drugs with, 728b, 812b
    dosages for, 805t
    drug interactions with, 804t
    for hypertension, 709, 726t
    pharmacokinetics of, 803t
    site of action of, 709f, 802f
    treatment options for, 811, 812
Potency vs. efficacy, 58
Potentiation vs. synergism, 64–65
Poultice, herbal, 140
Povidone-iodine, 1164t
Powders, 39t, 1171t
PPD. See Tuberculin skin test.
Practice-based knowledge, 13
Pramipexole, 430t, 431t, 432–434, 432t, 437t,
    440
Pramlintide, 984t, 985t, 986t, 989–990
Pramoxine, 282t
Prandase (acarbose), 984t, 985t, 986t, 988–989
Prandin (repaglinide), 984t, 985t, 986t, 988
Pravachol (pravastatin), 737–738, 738t, 739t, 740t
Pravastatin, 737–738, 738t, 739t, 740t
Praziquantel, 559t, 560, 561t, 562
Prazosin
    for benign prostatic hyperplasia, 817t, 818t,
        821
    for hypertension, 716
Preclinical drug development, 2–3, 3f
Precose (acarbose), 984t, 985t, 986t, 988–989
Prediabetes, 977
Prednisolone, 1046–1049, 1048t,
    1050t, 1051t
Prednisone
    for adrenal insufficiency, 1046–1049, 1048t,
        1050t, 1051t
    for gout, 276
    for myasthenia gravis, 446–448, 446t, 447t,
        448t, 452
    taper instructions for, 1055b

Pharmacotherapeutic Terms and Phrases in English and Spanish

English	Spanish
Basic Greetings and Questions	
Saludos y Preguntas Básicas	
Hello	Hola
Good morning, good afternoon, good evening.	Buenos días, buenas tardes, buenas noches.
What is your name? How old are you?	¿Cómo se llama usted? ¿Cuántos años tiene?
What is your phone number?	¿Cuál es su número de teléfono?
What is your address?	¿Cuál es su dirección?
How are you? How are you doing?	¿Cómo esta usted? ¿Cómo le va?
How many..., What..., Where..., Who..., Why..., How...	Cuántos(as)..., Qué..., Dónde..., Quién..., Por qué..., Cómo...
Are you ready?	¿Está listo(a)?
Terms for Health History	
Expresiones Para la Histórica Clínica	
How do you feel? Good, bad, tired, dizzy.	¿Cómo se siente? Bien, mal, cansado(a), mareado(a).
Are you constipated? Do you have diarrhea?	¿Está estreñido(a)? ¿Tiene diarrea?
Do you have nausea?	¿Tiene náuseas?
Do you have a fever?	¿Tiene usted fiebre?
Is this affecting your daily activities?	¿Le afecta esto sus actividades diarias?
Have you had these symptoms before? For how long? Minutes, hours, days, months, more than six months?	¿Ha tenido estos síntomas antes? ¿Por cuánto tiempo? ¿Minutos, horas, días, meses, más de seis meses?
Are you taking any medications now? Do you know what drugs you are taking? What color is the medicine? Green, yellow, clear, white, dark, brown, blue, pink?	¿Está tomando alguna medicina ahora? ¿Sabes que drogas está utilizada para tratar la enfermedad? ¿De qué color es la medicina? ¿Verde, amarilla, transparente, blanca, oscura, marrón/café, azule, rosa?
Do you have the medicine with you now?	¿Tiene la medicina en este momento?
Show me, please. How many pills do you take? One, two, three, four, five, six, seven, eight, nine, ten?	Enséñemela, por favor. ¿Cuántas pastillas? ¿Una, dos, tres, cuatro, cinco, seis, siete, ocho, nueve, diez?
Do you use street drugs?	¿Usted usa calle drogas?
Do you use home remedies?	¿Usted usa remedios caseros?
Do you take pills for your diabetes or insulin?	¿Aceptan píldoras para su diabetes o insulina?
Do you use prescriptions from another health care provider?	¿Usted utiliza recetas de otro proveedor de atención médica?
Did the medicine work?	¿Trabajó la medicina?
Have you had an allergic reaction to the medicine?	¿Tenido una reacción alérgica a la medicina?
Are you allergic to any medicines? Are you allergic to any foods?	¿Tiene alergias a algunas medicinas? ¿Tiene alergias de algunas comidas?
Do you have pain? Where is the pain?	¿Tiene algún dolor? ¿Dónde le duele?
Describe the pain. Annoying, bothering; brief; burning; cold; constant; doesn't let me rest; crushing; cramping; discomfort; dull; excruciating; heavy; hot; itching; periodic; comes and goes; strong/severe; throbbing	Descríbanse el dolor. Un dolor molesto; breve; que quema, que arde, "como que le quema;" frío; constante, "que no le deja descansar;" aplastastante, "como que lo están moliendo;" como calambre; incómodo; no agudo; agudísimo; pesado, "como que tiene un gran peso encima;" caliente; de picazón; no constante, "que va y viene;" fuerte; "como que le palpita"
What color is your urine?	¿De qué color es la orina?
Do you drink alcohol? Do you smoke?	¿Toma alcohol? ¿Fuma?
What types of food do you eat?	¿Qué tipo de alimentos te comes?
How many years of school did you complete?	¿Cómo muchos años de la escuela hizo usted completa?
Terms for Physical Exam	
Expresiones Para el Exámen Físico	
We need to draw some blood.	Necesitamos extraer un poco de sangre.
You need to have an x-ray.	Necesita sacar rayos-x.
I am going to listen to your heart/lungs/stomach.	Voy a escuchar tu corazón/los pulmones/tu estómago.
Can you feel this? Left, right. Let me feel your pulse;...blood pressure. Let me see your abdomen, chest, ears, eye, forehead, heart, lungs, mouth, nose, skin, stomach, throat, tongue...	¿Puede sentir esto? A la izquierda, a la derecha. Permítame tomarle el pulso;...la presión arterial. Permítame examinarle el vientre, el pecho, las orejas, el ojo, la frente, el corazón, los pulmones, la boca, la nariz, la piel, el estomago, la garganta, la lengua...
Cough. Take a deep breath. Cough again.	Tosa. Respire profundo. Tosa otra vez.